Focus on Nursing Pharmacology

SEVENTH EDITION

Focus on Nursing Pharmacology

SEVENTH EDITION

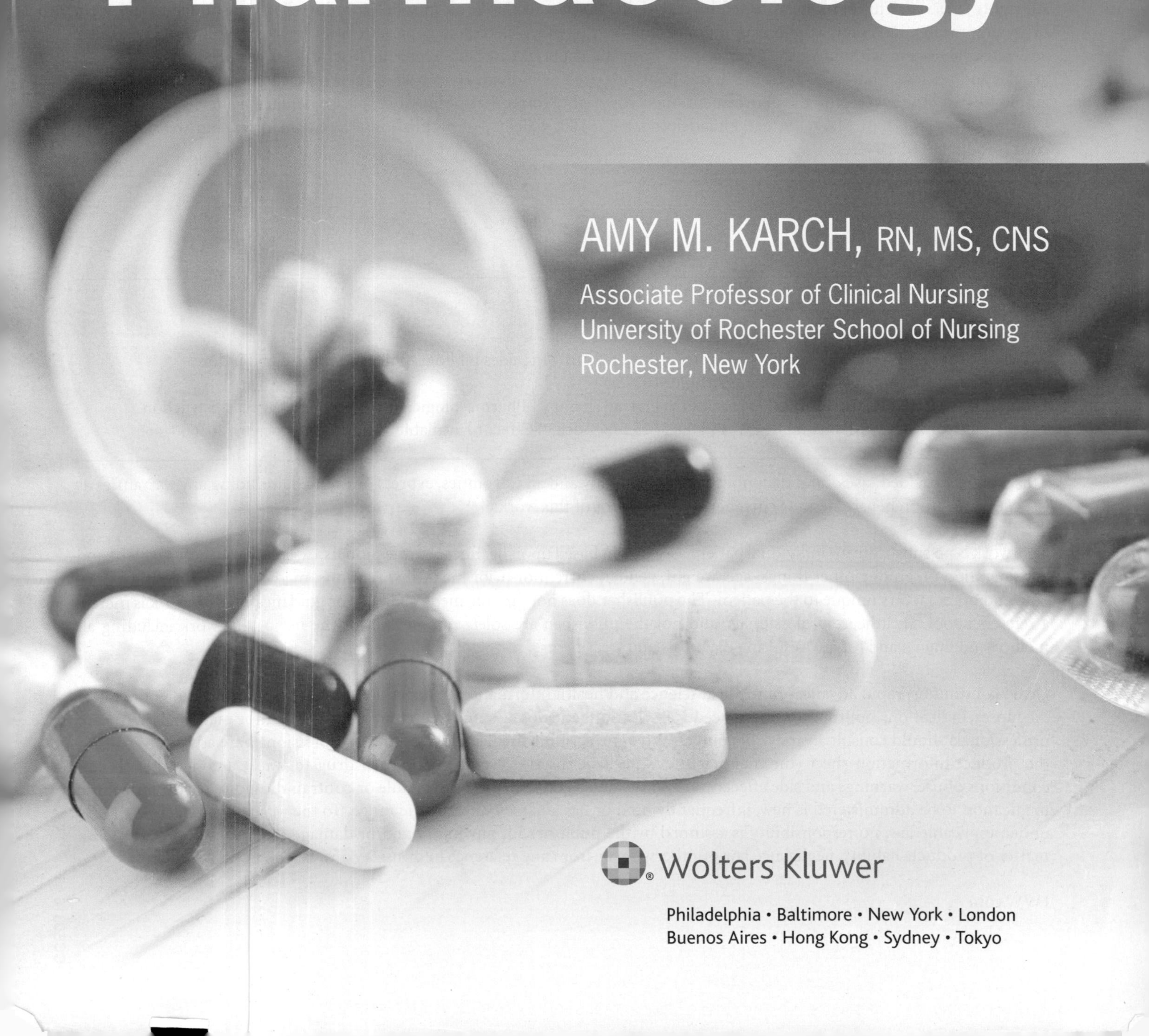

AMY M. KARCH, RN, MS, CNS

Associate Professor of Clinical Nursing
University of Rochester School of Nursing
Rochester, New York

Wolters Kluwer

Philadelphia • Baltimore • New York • London
Buenos Aires • Hong Kong • Sydney • Tokyo

Vice President and Publisher: Julie K. Stegman
Director of Product Development: Jennifer K. Forestieri
Executive Editor: Sherry Dickinson
Project Development Editor: Shana Murph
Production Project Manager: Priscilla Crater
Marketing Manager: Todd McQueston
Editorial Assistant: Dan Reilly
Designer: Stephen Druding
Art Director: Jennifer Clements
Manufacturing Coordinator: Karin Duffield
Production Service: SPi Global

Seventh edition

9 8 7 6 5 4 3 2 1

Printed in China

Library of Congress Cataloging-in-Publication Data
Names: Karch, Amy Morrison, 1949- , author.
Title: Focus on nursing pharmacology / Amy M. Karch.
Description: Edition 7. | Philadelphia : Wolters Kluwer, 2016. | Includes bibliographical references and index.
Identifiers: LCCN 2016004466 | ISBN 9781496318213
Subjects: | MESH: Pharmaceutical Preparations | Drug Therapy | Pharmacological Phenomena | Nurses' Instruction
Classification: LCC RM300 | NLM QV 4 | DDC 615.5/8—dc23 LC record available at http://lccn.loc.gov/2016004466

LWW.com

CCS0816

It is important to have a dream.... I have learned that it takes many people to make a dream come true. Those people become your heroes and your inspiration; teaching compassion, perseverance, and instilling the love of learning; helping you to always make good things come from bad things. To the inspirations in my life... Dr. Todd Wihlen, the MVA team, Amy Laukatitis, Jen Bidwell, Pam Holt, Dr. Patrick Hopkins, Dr. Rebecca Tucker.

Amy M. Karch

Reviewers

Carol Agana, MNSc, CNP, APRN
Faculty
Eleanor Mann School of Nursing
University of Arkansas
Fayetteville, Arkansas

Stephanie Bailey, RN, BA (Psychology), MHS
Registered Nurse, Nursing Instructor
British Columbia Institute of Technology
Vancouver, British Columbia, Canada

Nancy Barker, MSN, RN, EdD(c)
Instructor
Director, Nursing Arts and Clinical Simulation Lab
Division of Nursing
Immaculata University
Immaculata, Pennsylvania

Joy Borrero, MSN, RN, ANP
Associate Professor of Nursing
Suffolk County Community College
Brentwood, New York

Theresa Buchanan, DNP, APRN, FNP
Associate Professor of Nursing
Gordon State College
Barnesville, Georgia

Sandy Carroll, EdD, MSN, RN, CNE
Professor
College of the Canyons
Valencia, California

Elicia S. Collins, MSN, RN
Clinical Instructor
Clayton State University School of Nursing
Morrow, Georgia

Elizabeth Cooper, DNP, RN
Dean, School of Nursing
Director, MSN and BSN Programs
Aquinas College
Nashville, Tennessee

Carrie Davis, MS, RN
Nursing Faculty
Gwinnett Technical College
Lawrenceville, Georgia

Claire DeCristofaro, MD
Clinical Assistant Professor
College of Nursing
Medical University of South Carolina
Charleston, South Carolina

Leeann Denning, DNP, RN, CNE
Associate Professor of Nursing
Shawnee State University
Portsmouth, Ohio

Carol Diehl, MSN, MSEd, RN
Simulation Coordinator
Reading Hospital School of Health Sciences
Reading, Pennsylvania

Annette Ferguson, MSN
Assistant Professor
Ohio University
Athens, Ohio

Deborah Brooks Flaherty, MSN, APN-C, CNE
Associate Professor of Nursing
Cumberland County College
Vineland, New Jersey

Charlene Beach Gagliardi, MSN, BSN, RN
Assistant Professor
Mount St. Mary's University
Los Angeles, California

Edith Gerdes, MSN
Program Chair
Ivy Tech Community College
Indianapolis, Indiana

Betsy D. Gulledge, PhD, RN, CNE, NEA-BC
Associate Dean of Nursing/Assistant Professor
Jacksonville State University
Jacksonville, Alabama

Connie Houser, MSN, RNC-OB, CNE
ADN Instructor
Central Carolina Technical College
Sumter, South Carolina

Patrick LaRose, DNP, MSN, RN
Nursing Program Director
Keiser University–Sarasota
Sarasota, Florida

Melanie McClure, MSN, APRN, FNP-BC
Associate Professor of Nursing
University of Saint Mary
Leavenworth, Kansas

Maria Sheilla C. Membrebe, MSNEd, RN, RN, ONC, CMSRN
Assistant Professor
Community College of Baltimore County
Essex Campus, Maryland

Monica S. Messer, DNP, PhD, RN, CWS
Adjunct Faculty
University of South Florida College of Nursing
Tampa, Florida

Helen Mills, MSN, RN, RMA, AHI, LXMO
Clinical Education Consultant
Keiser University and Martin Health Systems
Stuart, Florida

Linda Mollino, MSN, RN
Director of Career and Technical Programs
Oregon Coast Community College
Newport, Oregon

Vicki Moran, PhD, RN, CNE
Assistant Professor
Saint Louis University
St. Louis, Missouri

Cynthia Parker, PhD, RN, MSPH, COI
Professor
Kettering College
Kettering, Ohio

Nancy Petges, EdD, MSN, RN
Associate Professor of Nursing
Aurora University, School of Nursing
Aurora, Illinois

Sarah E. Plunkett, PhD, RN, CNE
Assistant Dean of Health Sciences
Tulsa Community College
Tulsa, Oklahoma

Lisa Bridwell Robinson, DNP, CCRN, CNE, NP-C
Assistant Professor
Tanner Health System School of Nursing
University of West Georgia
Carrollton, Georgia

Dana L. Scott, MSN, RN, RVT, LMT
Assistant Professor of Nursing
College of Nursing
Ohio University
Ironton, Ohio

Martha Shemin, MSN, RN
Nursing Faculty
Holy Name Medical Center
Teaneck, New Jersey

Nadia Torresan-Doodnaught, MN, RNC
Professor of Nursing
Seneca College of Applied Arts and Technology
King City, Ontario, Canada

Kimberly Valich, MSN, RN
Assistant Professor
Advanced Medical Surgical Nursing Course Coordinator
University of Saint Francis
Crown Point, Indiana

Shannon van Wiltenburg, MSN, BScN, BA, RN
Nursing Faculty
Douglas College
Vancouver, British Columbia, Canada

Shannon Vorlick, MSN, RN
Nursing Faculty
Trident Technical College
Charleston, South Carolina

Cynthia Watson, MSN, APRN, FNP-BC, ADM-BC
Nursing Instructor
University of Louisiana at Lafayette
Lafayette, Louisiana

Preface

Pharmacology is a difficult course to teach in a standard nursing curriculum, whether it be a diploma, associate, baccalaureate, or graduate program. Teachers are difficult to find, and time and money often dictate that the invaluable content of such a course be incorporated into other courses. As a result, the content is often lost. At the same time, changes in medical care delivery—more outpatient and home care, shorter hospital stays, and more self-care—have resulted in additional legal and professional responsibilities for nurses, making them more responsible for the safe and effective delivery of drug therapy. Prevention of medication errors has become a national challenge.

Pharmacology should not be such a formidable obstacle in the nursing curriculum. The study of drug therapy incorporates physiology, pathophysiology, chemistry, and nursing fundamentals—subjects that are already taught in most schools. A textbook that approaches pharmacology as an understandable, teachable, and learnable subject would greatly facilitate the incorporation of this subject into nursing curricula. Yet many nursing pharmacology texts are large and burdensome, mainly because they need to cover not only the basic pharmacology but also the particulars included in each area considered.

The seventh edition of *Focus on Nursing Pharmacology* is based on the premise that students first need to have a solid and clearly focused concept of the principles of drug therapy before they can easily grasp the myriad details associated with individual drugs.

Armed with a fundamental knowledge of pharmacology, the student can appreciate and use the specific details that are so readily available in the many annually updated and published nursing drug guides, such as the *Lippincott Nursing Drug Guide*.

With this goal in mind, *Focus on Nursing Pharmacology* provides a concise, user-friendly, and uncluttered text for the modern student. This difficult subject is presented in a streamlined, understandable, teachable, and learnable manner. Because this book is designed to be used in conjunction with a handbook of current drug information, it remains streamlined. This seventh edition of *Focus on Nursing Pharmacology* continues to emphasize "need-to-know" concepts.

The text reviews and integrates previously learned knowledge of physiology, chemistry, and nursing fundamentals into chapters focused on helping students conceptualize what is important to know about each group of drugs. Illustrations, sidebars, and tables sum up concepts to enhance learning. Special features further focus student learning on clinical application, critical thinking, patient safety, life span issues related to drug therapy, evidence-based practice, patient teaching, and case study–based critical thinking exercises that incorporate nursing process principles. The text incorporates study materials that conclude each chapter. Check Your Understanding sections provide both new- and old-format National Council Licensure Examination (NCLEX)-style review questions, as well as study guide review questions to help the student master the material and prepare for the national licensing exam.

Focus on Teaching/Learning Activities

thePoint® (available at http://thepoint.lww.com/), a trademark of Wolters Kluwer Health, is a Web-based course and content management system that provides every resource instructors and students need in one easy-to-use site. thePoint® ... where teaching, learning, and technology click!

Student Resources

Students can visit thePoint® to access supplemental multimedia resources to enhance their learning experience, download content, upload assignments, and join an online study group. thePoint® offers a variety of free student resources, including NCLEX-Style Student Review Questions, Watch and Learn video clips, Practice and Learn activities, an Alternate-Format NCLEX Tutorial, and a Spanish-English Audioglossary. It also has free journal articles related to topics discussed in the Focus on Safe Medication Administration boxes from the book. Also included are videos on preventing medication errors and three-dimensional animated depictions of pharmacology concepts. In addition, an online course is available that includes interactive activities.

Instructor Resources

Advanced technology and superior content combine at thePoint® to allow instructors to design and deliver online and offline courses, maintain grades and class rosters, and communicate with students. thePoint® also provides additional resources, including Pre-lecture Quizzes,

PowerPoints with Guided Lecture Notes, Discussion Topics, Assignments, and over 1700 Test Generator questions—almost 1200 of which are brand new to this edition!

Organization

Focus on Nursing Pharmacology is organized following a "simple-to-complex" approach, much like the syllabus for a basic nursing pharmacology course. Because students learn best "from the bottom up," the text is divided into distinct parts.

Part I begins with an overview of basic nursing pharmacology, including such new challenges as bioterrorism, street drugs, herbal therapies, the importance of preventing medication errors and the information overload; each of the other parts begins with a review of the physiology of the system affected by the specific drugs being discussed. This review refreshes the information for the student and provides a quick and easy reference when he or she is reading about drug actions.

Part II of the text introduces the drug classes, starting with the chemotherapeutic agents—both antimicrobial and antineoplastic drugs. Because the effectiveness of these drugs depends on their interference with the most basic element of body physiology—the cell—students can easily understand the pharmacology of this class. Mastering the pharmacotherapeutic effects of this drug class helps the student to establish a firm grasp of the basic principles taught in Part I. Once the easiest pharmacological concepts are understood, the student is prepared to move on to the more challenging physiological and pharmacological concepts.

Part III focuses on drugs affecting the immune system because recent knowledge about the immune system has made it the cornerstone of modern therapy. All of the immune system drugs act in ways in which the immune system would act if it were able. Recent immunological research has contributed to a much greater understanding of this system, making it important to position information about drugs affecting this system close to the beginning of the text instead of at the end as has been the custom.

Parts IV and **V** of the text address drugs that affect the nervous system, the basic functioning system of the body. Following the discussion of the nervous system, and closely linked with it in **Part VI**, is the endocrine system. The sequence of these parts introduces students to the concept of control, teaches them about the interrelatedness of these two systems, and prepares them for understanding many aspects of shared physiological function and the inevitable linking of the two systems into one: the neuroendocrine system.

Parts VII, **VIII**, and **IX** discuss drugs affecting the reproductive, cardiovascular, and renal systems, respectively. The sequencing of cardiovascular and renal drugs is logical because most of the augmenting cardiovascular drugs (such as diuretics) affect the renal system.

Part X covers drugs that act on the respiratory system, which provides the link between the left and right ventricles of the heart.

Part XI addresses drugs acting on the gastrointestinal system. The gastrointestinal system stands on its own; it does not share any actions with any other system.

Text Features

The features in this text are skillfully designed to support the text discussion, encouraging the student to look at the whole patient and to focus on the essential information that is important to learn about each drug class. Important features in the seventh edition focus on incorporating basic nursing skills, patient safety, critical thinking, and application of the material learned to the clinical scenario, helping the student to understand the pharmacology material.

Special Elements and Learning Aids

Each chapter opens with a list of learning objectives for that chapter, helping the student to understand what the key learning points will be. A list of featured drugs and a glossary of key terms are also found on the opening chapter page. Key points appear periodically throughout each chapter to summarize important concepts. The text of each chapter ends with a summary of important concepts. This is followed by a series of review exercises, Check Your Understanding, which includes NCLEX-style questions in the new format to focus student learning on the seminal information presented in the chapter. New to this edition, the nursing process sections related to each drug class include the planning step in the nursing process, to help direct the interventions that will be needed for patients taking those drugs; the Drugs affecting blood glucose chapter has been expanded and revised to include all of the new drugs being used and the need for patient education; the Cardiotonic agents chapter includes the new approaches to heart failure in an revised presentation; other chapters include newly released drugs and effects on the patient and need for patient teaching.

- In the *Nursing Considerations* section of each chapter, *italics* highlight the *rationale* for each nursing intervention, helping the student to apply the information in a clinical situation. Elsewhere in the text, the rationale is consistently provided for therapeutic drug actions, contraindications, and adverse effects.
- In the *Drug List* at the beginning of each chapter, a special icon appears next to the drug that is considered the prototype drug of each class. In each chapter, *prototype summary* boxes spotlight need to know information for each prototype drug.
- *Drugs in Focus* tables clearly summarize and identify the drugs within a class, highlighting them by generic and trade names, usual dosage, and indications. The icon

appears in these tables next to each drug that is considered to be the prototype for its specific class.

- *Focus on Safe Medication Administration* boxes present important safety information to help keep the patient safe, prevent medication errors, and increase the therapeutic effectiveness of the drugs.
- *Focus on the Evidence* boxes compile information based on research to identify the best nursing practices associated with specific drug therapy.
- *Focus on Herbal and Alternative Therapies* displays highlight known interactions with specific herbs or alternative therapies that could affect the actions of the drugs being discussed.
- *Focus on Calculations* reviews are designed to help the student hone calculation and measurement skills while learning about the drugs for which doses might need to be calculated.
- *Focus on Drug Therapy Across the Lifespan* boxes concisely summarize points to consider when using the drugs of each class with children, adults, and the elderly.
- *Focus on Gender Considerations* and *Focus on Cultural Considerations* discussions encourage the student to think about cultural awareness and to consider the patient as a unique individual with a special set of characteristics that not only influences variations in drug effectiveness but also could influence a patient's perspective on drug therapy.
- *Critical Thinking Scenarios* tie each chapter's content together by presenting clinical scenarios about a patient using a particular drug from the class being discussed. Included in the case study are hints to guide critical thinking about the case and a discussion of *drug- and nondrug-related nursing considerations* for that particular patient and situation. Most important, the case study provides a *plan of nursing care* specifically developed for that patient and specifically based on the nursing process. The care plan is followed by a checklist of *patient teaching points* designed for the patient presented in the case study. This approach helps the student to see how assessment and the collected data are applied in the clinical situation.
- *Check Your Understanding* sections present NCLEX-style questions, including alternate format questions, to help the student prepare for that exam. Other questions and activities in this section are designed to help students test their knowledge of the information that has been learned in the chapter.

To the Student Using This Text

As you begin your study of pharmacology, don't be overwhelmed or confused by all of the details. The study of drugs fits perfectly into your study of the human body—anatomy, physiology, chemistry, nutrition, psychology, and sociology. Approach the study of pharmacology from the perspective of putting all of the pieces together; this can be not only fun but also challenging! Work to understand the concepts, and all of the details will fall into place and it will be easy to remember and apply to the clinical situation. This understanding will help you in creating the picture of the whole patient as you are learning to provide comprehensive nursing care. This text is designed to help you accomplish all of this in a simple and concise manner. Good luck!

Amy M. Karch, RN, MS, CNS

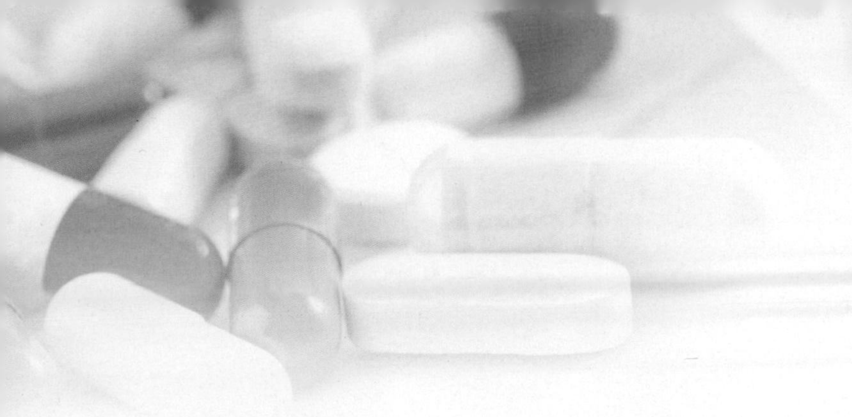

Acknowledgments

I would like to thank the various people who have worked so hard to make this book a reality, especially the many students and colleagues who have for so long pushed for a pharmacology book that was straightforward and user-friendly and who have taken the time to make suggestions to improve each edition. Thanks to Sherry Dinckinson, the executive editor at Wolters Kluwer; to Shana Murph, my amazing development editor, who had the vision and helped to make it reality and always responded; to Stephen Druding and Jennifer Clements, who saw it all come together; to Todd Chennell, Walter Peppers, Daniel Hovey, and Jennifer Netkin for support, laughs, and providing hope for the future; to Tim, Jyoti, Mark, Tracey, Cortney, Kathryn, and Jason, who continue to thrive and grow and have become the wonderful, supportive people in my life and usually my harshest critics; to the new generation—Vikas, Nisha, Zara, Logan, Connor, Jack, Madelyn, and Eli—who have returned the sunshine and joy of learning to our lives; and lastly to Dixie and Brodie, whose happily wagging tails never fail to bring smiles and peace and who help to keep everything in perspective.

Contents

PART 1

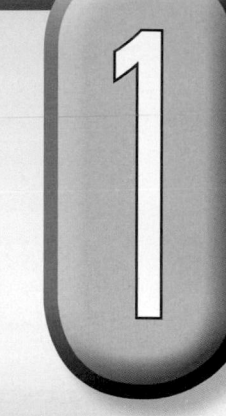

INTRODUCTION TO NURSING PHARMACOLOGY

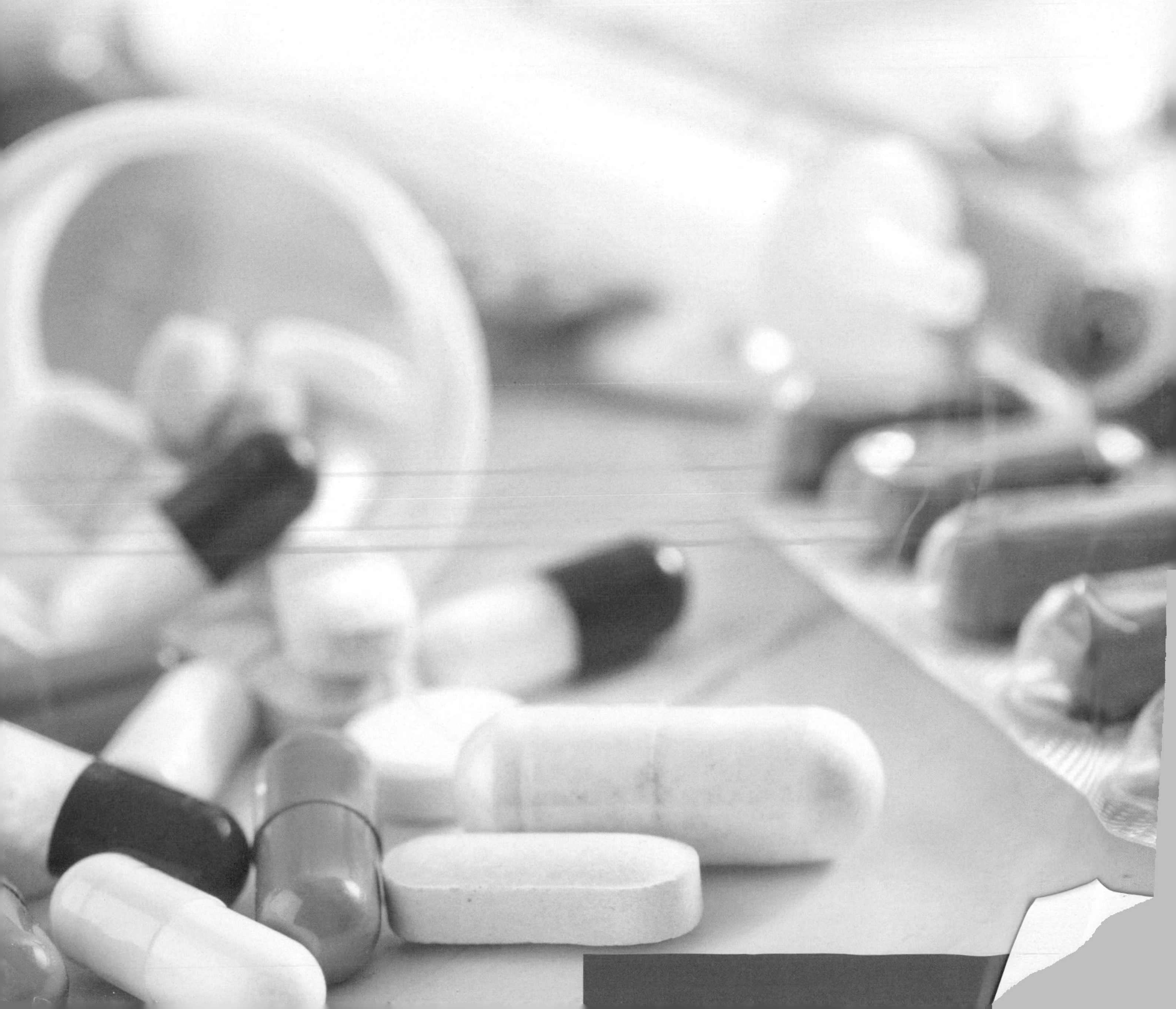

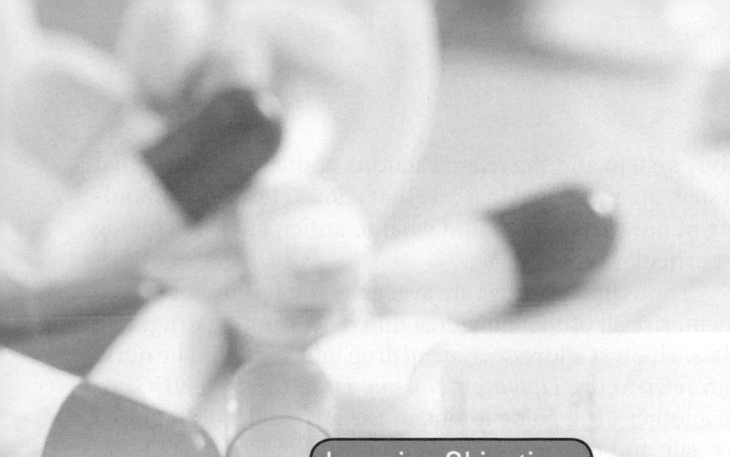

Introduction to Drugs 1

Learning Objectives

Upon completion of this chapter, you will be able to:

1. Define the word pharmacology.
2. Outline the steps involved in developing and approving a new drug in the United States.
3. Describe the federal controls on drugs that have abuse potential.
4. Differentiate between generic and brand-name drugs and over-the-counter and prescription drugs.
5. Explain the benefits and risks associated with the use of over-the-counter drugs.

Glossary of Key Terms

adverse effects: Drug effects, sometimes called side effects, that are not the desired therapeutic effects; may be unpleasant or even dangerous

brand name: name given to a drug by the pharmaceutical company that developed it; also called a trade name or proprietary name

chemical name: name that reflects the chemical structure of a drug

drugs: chemicals that are introduced into the body to bring about some sort of change

Food and Drug Administration (FDA): federal agency responsible for the regulation and enforcement of drug evaluation and distribution policies

generic drugs: drugs sold by their generic name; not brand name or trade name product

generic name: the original designation that a drug is given when the drug company that developed it applies for the approval process

genetic engineering: process of altering DNA, usually of bacteria, to produce a chemical to be used as a drug

orphan drugs: drugs that have been discovered but would not be profitable for a drug company to develop; usually drugs that would treat only a small number of people; these orphans can be adopted by drug companies to develop

over-the-counter (OTC) drugs: drugs that are available without a prescription for self-treatment of a variety of complaints; deemed to be safe when used as directed

pharmacology: the study of the biological effects of chemicals

pharmacotherapeutics: clinical pharmacology—the branch of pharmacology that deals with drugs; chemicals that are used in medicine for the treatment, prevention, and diagnosis of disease in humans

phase I study: a pilot study of a potential drug using a small number of selected, usually healthy human volunteers

phase II study: a clinical study of a proposed drug by selected physicians using actual patients who have the disorder the drug is designed to treat; patients must provide informed consent

phase III study: use of a proposed drug on a wide scale in the clinical setting with patients who have the disease the drug is thought to treat

phase IV study: continuous evaluation of a drug after it has been released for marketing

preclinical trials: initial trial of a chemical thought to have therapeutic potential; uses laboratory animals, not human subjects

teratogenic: having adverse effects on the fetus

The human body works through a complicated series of chemical reactions and processes. **Pharmacology** is the study of the biological effects of chemicals. **Drugs** are chemicals that are introduced into the body to cause some sort of change. When drugs are administered the body begins a sequence of processes designed to handle the new chemicals. These processes, which involve breaking down and eliminating the drugs, affect the body's complex series of chemical reactions. In clinical practice, health care providers focus on how chemicals act on people.

Nurses deal with **pharmacotherapeutics**, or clinical pharmacology, the branch of pharmacology that uses drugs to treat, prevent, and diagnose disease. Clinical pharmacology addresses two key concerns: the drug's effects on the body and the body's response to the drug.

For many reasons, understanding how drugs act on the body to cause changes and applying that knowledge in the clinical setting are important aspects of nursing practice. For instance, patients today often follow complicated drug regimens and receive potentially toxic drugs and/or drug combinations. Also, many patients need to manage their care at home. A drug can have many effects, and the nurse must know which ones may occur when a particular drug is administered. Some drug effects are therapeutic, or helpful, but others are undesirable or potentially dangerous. These negative effects are called **adverse effects**, or side effects, of the drug. (See Chapter 3 for a detailed discussion of adverse effects.)

The nurse is in a unique position regarding drug therapy because nursing responsibilities include the following:

- Administering drugs
- Assessing drug effects
- Intervening to make the drug regimen more tolerable
- Providing patient teaching about drugs and drug regimens
- Monitoring the overall patient care plan to prevent medication errors

Knowing how drugs work makes these tasks easier to handle, thus enhancing the effectiveness of drug therapy.

This text is designed to provide the pharmacological basis for understanding drug therapy. The physiology of a body system and the related actions of many drugs on that system are presented in a way that allows clear understanding of how drugs work and what to anticipate when giving a particular type of drug.

Thousands of drugs are available, and it is impossible to memorize all of the individual differences among drugs in a class. This text addresses *general* drug information. The nurse can refer to the *Lippincott Nursing Drug Guide* (*LNDG*) or to another drug guide to obtain the *specific* details required for safe and effective drug administration. Drug details are changing constantly. The practicing nurse must be knowledgeable about these changes and rely on an up-to-date and comprehensive drug guide in the clinical setting.

A section related to nursing considerations for patients receiving particular drugs will be found in each chapter of this book. This includes assessment points, nursing diagnoses to consider, planning for patient-centered care, implementation of particular interventions that should be considered, and evaluation points that will provide a guide for using the nursing process to effectively incorporate drug therapy into patient care. This information can be used to develop an individual nursing care plan for your patient. The monographs in *LNDG* (Table 1.1) or

Table 1.1 Sample Nursing Care Plan from *Lippincott's Nursing Drug Guide* for a Patient Receiving Oral Linezolid

Assessment	Nursing Diagnosis	Implementation	Evaluation
History (contraindications/cautions) Hypertension Hyperthyroidism Blood dyscrasias Hepatic dysfunction Pheochromocytoma Phenylketonuria Carcinoid syndrome Pregnancy Lactation Known allergy to: linezolid **Medication History** (possible drug–drug interactions) Pseudoephedrine Selective serotonin reuptake inhibitors MAOIs Antiplatelet drugs **Diet History** (possible drug–food interactions) Foods high in tyramine **Physical Assessment** (screen for contraindications and to establish a baseline for evaluating effects and adverse effects) Local: Culture site of infection CNS: Affect, reflexes, orientation CV: P, BP, peripheral perfusion GI: Bowel sounds, liver evaluation Skin: Color, lesions Hematologic: CBC with differential, liver function tests	Imbalanced nutrition, less than body requirements, related to GI effects Acute pain related to GI effects, headache Ineffective peripheral tissue perfusion related to bone marrow effects Deficient knowledge related to drug therapy	Safe and appropriate administration of drug: Culture infection site to ensure appropriate use of drug Provision of safety and comfort measures: • Monitor BP periodically • Monitor platelet counts before and periodically during therapy • Alleviation of GI upset • Ready access to bathroom facilities • Nutritional consult • Safety provisions if dizziness and CNS effects occur • Avoidance of tyramine-rich foods Patient teaching regarding: Drug Side effects to anticipate Warnings Reactions to report Support and encouragement to cope with disease, high cost of therapy, and side effects Provision of emergency and life support measures in cases of acute hypersensitivity	Monitor for therapeutic effects of drug: resolution of infection. If resolution does not occur, reculture site. Monitor for adverse effects of drug: • GI upset—nausea, vomiting, diarrhea • Liver function changes • Pseudomembranous colitis • Blood dyscrasias—changes in platelet counts • Fever • Rash • Sweating • Photosensitivity • Acute hypersensitivity reactions Evaluate effectiveness of patient-teaching program: patient can name drug, dose of drug, use of drug, adverse effects to expect, and reactions to report. Evaluate effectiveness of comfort and safety measures. Monitor for drug–drug and drug–food interactions as appropriate. Evaluate effectiveness of life support measures if needed.

MAOI, monoamine oxidase inhibitor; CNS, central nervous system; CV, cardiovascular; P, pulse; BP, blood pressure; GI, gastrointestinal; CBC, complete blood count.

any other nursing drug guide can be used to provide the specific information that you need to plan care for each particular drug you might be giving. The various sections of each drug monograph (Figure 1.1) can provide information to help in the development of patient teaching guides and drug cards for reference in the clinical setting. The Patient Drug Sheet: Oral Linezolid (Figure 1.2) is an example of how this information can be used to develop a patient teaching guide.

The patient teaching guides for all of the drugs found in *LNDG* can be found on thePoint®. The nurse can use this text as a resource for basic concepts of pharmacology and a nursing drug guide as an easy-to-use reference in the clinical setting.

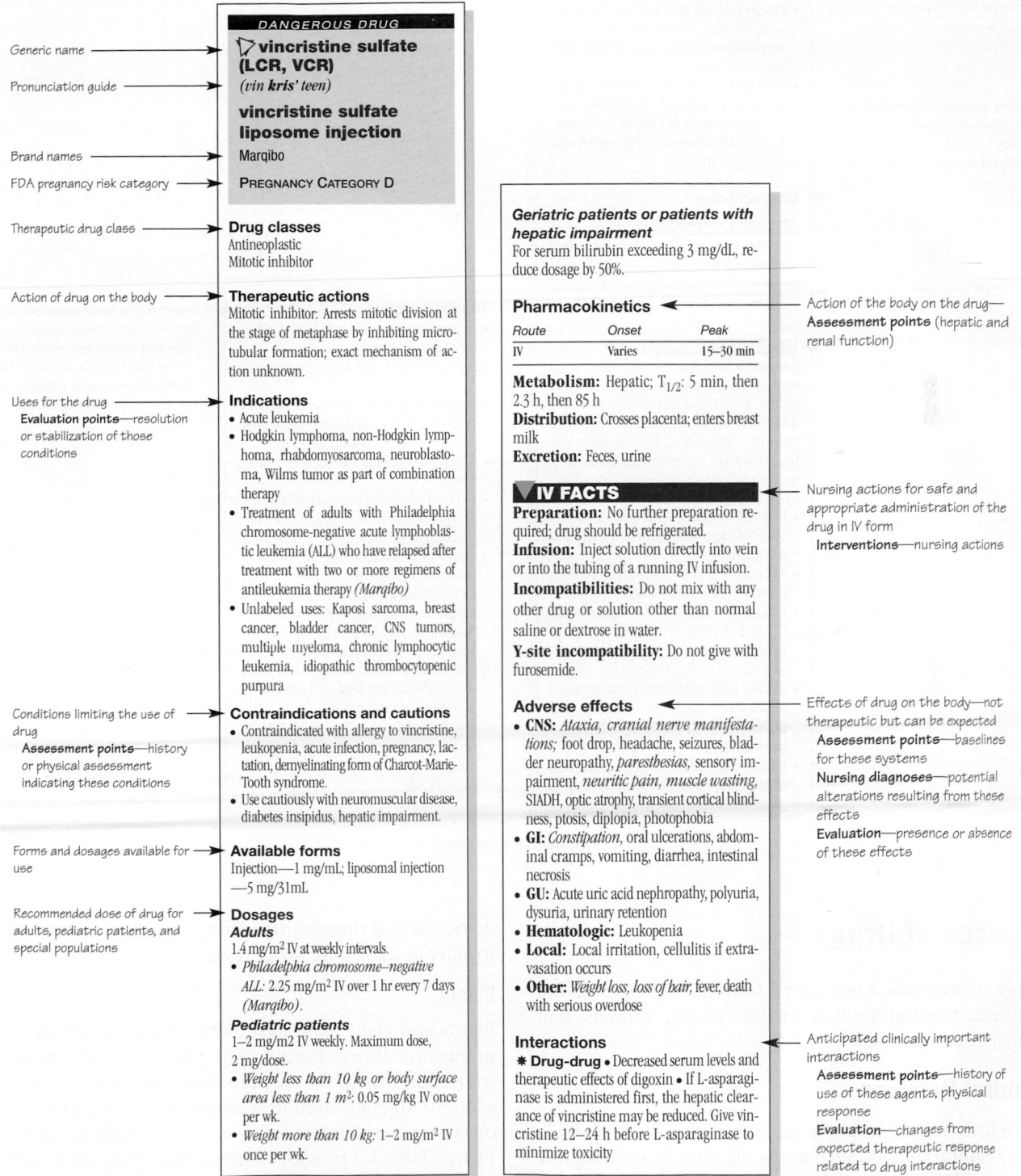

DANGEROUS DRUG

Generic name

vincristine sulfate (LCR, VCR)

Pronunciation guide

*(vin **kris'** teen)*

vincristine sulfate liposome injection

Brand names

Marqibo

FDA pregnancy risk category

PREGNANCY CATEGORY D

Therapeutic drug class

Drug classes

Antineoplastic
Mitotic inhibitor

Action of drug on the body

Therapeutic actions

Mitotic inhibitor: Arrests mitotic division at the stage of metaphase by inhibiting microtubular formation; exact mechanism of action unknown.

Uses for the drug
***Evaluation points**—resolution or stabilization of those conditions*

Indications

- Acute leukemia
- Hodgkin lymphoma, non-Hodgkin lymphoma, rhabdomyosarcoma, neuroblastoma, Wilms tumor as part of combination therapy
- Treatment of adults with Philadelphia chromosome-negative acute lymphoblastic leukemia (ALL) who have relapsed after treatment with two or more regimens of antileukemia therapy *(Marqibo)*
- Unlabeled uses: Kaposi sarcoma, breast cancer, bladder cancer, CNS tumors, multiple myeloma, chronic lymphocytic leukemia, idiopathic thrombocytopenic purpura

Conditions limiting the use of drug
***Assessment points**—history or physical assessment indicating these conditions*

Contraindications and cautions

- Contraindicated with allergy to vincristine, leukopenia, acute infection, pregnancy, lactation, demyelinating form of Charcot-Marie-Tooth syndrome.
- Use cautiously with neuromuscular disease, diabetes insipidus, hepatic impairment.

Forms and dosages available for use

Available forms

Injection—1 mg/mL; liposomal injection —5 mg/31mL

Recommended dose of drug for adults, pediatric patients, and special populations

Dosages

Adults

1.4 mg/m² IV at weekly intervals.

- *Philadelphia chromosome–negative ALL:* 2.25 mg/m² IV over 1 hr every 7 days *(Marqibo)*.

Pediatric patients

1–2 mg/m2 IV weekly. Maximum dose, 2 mg/dose.

- *Weight less than 10 kg or body surface area less than 1 m²:* 0.05 mg/kg IV once per wk.
- *Weight more than 10 kg:* 1–2 mg/m² IV once per wk.

Geriatric patients or patients with hepatic impairment

For serum bilirubin exceeding 3 mg/dL, reduce dosage by 50%.

*Action of the body on the drug—**Assessment points** (hepatic and renal function)*

Pharmacokinetics

Route	Onset	Peak
IV	Varies	15–30 min

Metabolism: Hepatic; $T_{1/2}$: 5 min, then 2.3 h, then 85 h
Distribution: Crosses placenta; enters breast milk
Excretion: Feces, urine

Nursing actions for safe and appropriate administration of the drug in IV form
***Interventions**—nursing actions*

IV FACTS

Preparation: No further preparation required; drug should be refrigerated.
Infusion: Inject solution directly into vein or into the tubing of a running IV infusion.
Incompatibilities: Do not mix with any other drug or solution other than normal saline or dextrose in water.
Y-site incompatibility: Do not give with furosemide.

Effects of drug on the body—not therapeutic but can be expected
***Assessment points**—baselines for these systems*
***Nursing diagnoses**—potential alterations resulting from these effects*
***Evaluation**—presence or absence of these effects*

Adverse effects

- **CNS:** *Ataxia, cranial nerve manifestations;* foot drop, headache, seizures, bladder neuropathy, *paresthesias,* sensory impairment, *neuritic pain, muscle wasting,* SIADH, optic atrophy, transient cortical blindness, ptosis, diplopia, photophobia
- **GI:** *Constipation,* oral ulcerations, abdominal cramps, vomiting, diarrhea, intestinal necrosis
- **GU:** Acute uric acid nephropathy, polyuria, dysuria, urinary retention
- **Hematologic:** Leukopenia
- **Local:** Local irritation, cellulitis if extravasation occurs
- **Other:** *Weight loss, loss of hair,* fever, death with serious overdose

Anticipated clinically important interactions
***Assessment points**—history of use of these agents, physical response*
***Evaluation**—changes from expected therapeutic response related to drug interactions*

Interactions

✱ **Drug-drug** • Decreased serum levels and therapeutic effects of digoxin • If L-asparaginase is administered first, the hepatic clearance of vincristine may be reduced. Give vincristine 12–24 h before L-asparaginase to minimize toxicity

FIGURE 1.1 Example of a drug monograph from *Lippincott Nursing Drug Guide.*

✱ Drug-food • Decreased metabolism and risk of toxic effects if combined with grapefruit juice; avoid this combination

■ **Nursing considerations**

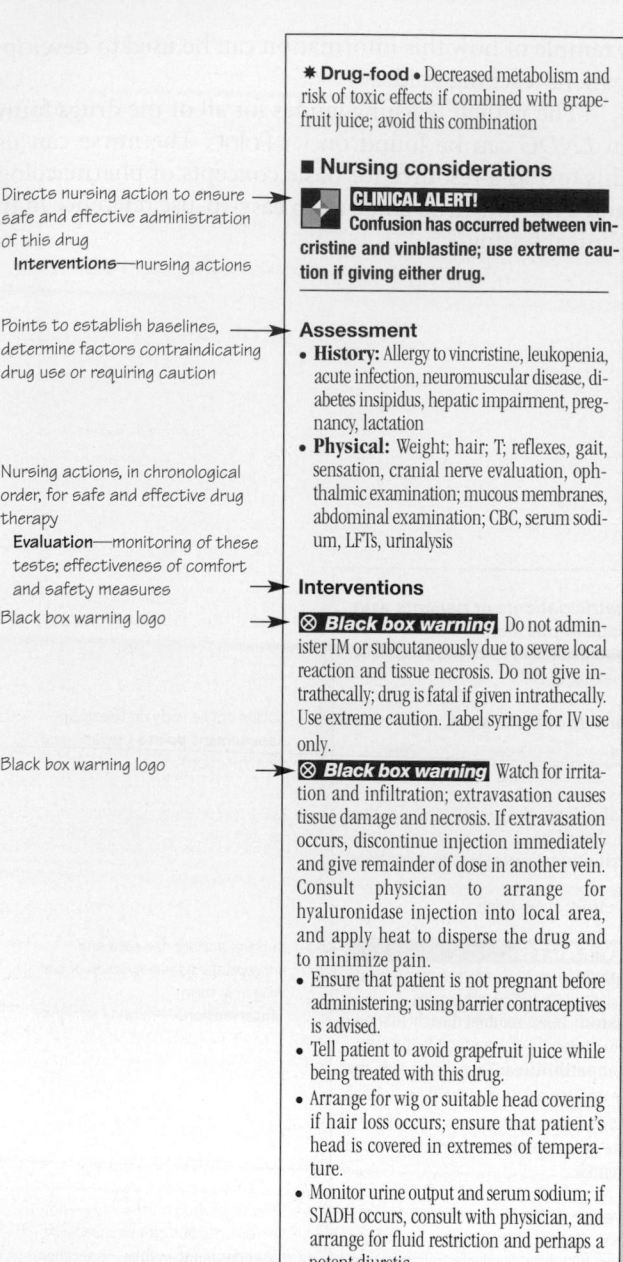

Directs nursing action to ensure safe and effective administration of this drug
Interventions—nursing actions

CLINICAL ALERT!
Confusion has occurred between vincristine and vinblastine; use extreme caution if giving either drug.

Points to establish baselines, determine factors contraindicating drug use or requiring caution

Assessment

- **History:** Allergy to vincristine, leukopenia, acute infection, neuromuscular disease, diabetes insipidus, hepatic impairment, pregnancy, lactation
- **Physical:** Weight; hair; T; reflexes, gait, sensation, cranial nerve evaluation, ophthalmic examination; mucous membranes, abdominal examination; CBC, serum sodium, LFTs, urinalysis

Nursing actions, in chronological order, for safe and effective drug therapy
Evaluation—monitoring of these tests; effectiveness of comfort and safety measures

Interventions

Black box warning logo

- ⊗ **Black box warning** Do not administer IM or subcutaneously due to severe local reaction and tissue necrosis. Do not give intrathecally; drug is fatal if given intrathecally. Use extreme caution. Label syringe for IV use only.

Black box warning logo

- ⊗ **Black box warning** Watch for irritation and infiltration; extravasation causes tissue damage and necrosis. If extravasation occurs, discontinue injection immediately and give remainder of dose in another vein. Consult physician to arrange for hyaluronidase injection into local area, and apply heat to disperse the drug and to minimize pain.
- Ensure that patient is not pregnant before administering; using barrier contraceptives is advised.
- Tell patient to avoid grapefruit juice while being treated with this drug.
- Arrange for wig or suitable head covering if hair loss occurs; ensure that patient's head is covered in extremes of temperature.
- Monitor urine output and serum sodium; if SIADH occurs, consult with physician, and arrange for fluid restriction and perhaps a potent diuretic.
- Consider stimulant laxative to prevent or treat constipation.

Teaching points

Drug-specific teaching points to include in patient-teaching program
Nursing diagnoses—deficient knowledge regarding drug therapy
Evaluation—points patient should be able to repeat

- Prepare a calendar of dates to return for treatment and additional therapy.
- Avoid grapefruit juice while you are using this drug.
- This drug cannot be taken during pregnancy; use birth control. If you become pregnant, consult your health care provider.
- Have regular blood tests to monitor the drug's effects.
- You may experience these side effects: Loss of appetite, nausea, vomiting, mouth sores (frequent mouth care, frequent small meals may help; maintain nutrition; request an antiemetic); constipation (bowel program may be ordered); sensitivity to light (wear sunglasses; avoid bright lights); numbness, tingling, change in style of walking (reversible; may persist for up to 6 weeks); hair loss (transient; obtain a wig or other suitable head covering; keep the head covered at extremes of temperature).
- Report change in frequency of voiding; swelling of ankles, fingers, and so forth; changes in vision; severe constipation, abdominal pain.

FIGURE 1.1 *(continued)*

Sources of Drugs

Drugs are available from varied sources, both natural and synthetic. Natural sources include plants, animals, and inorganic compounds.

Natural Sources

Chemicals that might prove useful as drugs can come from many natural sources, such as plants, animals, or inorganic compounds. To become a drug, a chemical must have a demonstrated therapeutic value or efficacy without severe toxicity or damaging properties.

Plants

Plants and plant parts have been used as medicines since prehistoric times. Even today, plants are an important source of chemicals that are developed into drugs. For example, digitalis used to treat cardiac disorders and various opiates used for sedation were originally derived from plants. Table 1.2 provides examples of drugs derived from plant sources.

Patient Drug Sheet: Oral Linezolid

Patient's Name: Mr. Kors
Prescriber's Name: J. Smith, ANP
Phone Number: 555-555-5555

Instructions:

1. The name of your drug is *linezolid*; the brand name is *Zyvox*. This drug is an antibiotic that is being used to treat your *pneumonia*. This drug is very specific in its action and is only indicated for your particular infection. Take the full course of your drug. Do not share this drug with other people or save tablets for future use.
2. The dose of the drug that has been prescribed for you is: *600 mg* (*1 tablet*).
3. The drug should be taken *once every 12 hours*. The best time for you to take this drug will be *8:00 in the morning and 8:00 in the evening*. Do not skip any doses. Do not take two doses at once if you forget a dose. If you miss a dose, take the dose as soon as you remember and then again in 12 hours.
4. The drug can be taken with food if GI upset is a problem. Avoid foods that are rich in tyramine (list is below) while you are taking this drug.
5. The following side effects may occur:
   Nausea, vomiting, abdominal pain (taking the drug with food and eating frequent small meals may help).
   Diarrhea (ensure ready access to bathroom facilities). Notify your health care provider if this becomes severe.
6. Do not take this drug with over-the-counter drugs or herbal remedies without first checking with your health care provider. Many of these agents can cause problems with your drug.
7. Tell any nurse, physician, or dentist who is taking care of you that you are on this drug.
8. Keep this and all medications out of the reach of children.

Notify your health care provider if any of the following occur:
Rash, severe GI problems, bloody or excessive diarrhea, weakness, tremors, increased bleeding or bruising, anxiety.

Foods high in tyramine to avoid: Aged cheeses, avocados, bananas, beer, bologna (polony), caffeinated beverages, chocolate, liver, over-ripe fruit, pepperoni, pickled fish, red wine, salami, smoked fish, yeast, yogurt.

FIGURE 1.2 Example of a patient teaching sheet from *Lippincott Nursing Drug Guide*.

Drugs also may be processed using a synthetic version of the active chemical found in a plant. An example of this type of drug is dronabinol (*Marinol*), which contains the active ingredient delta-9-tetrahydrocannabinol found in marijuana. This drug helps to prevent nausea and vomiting in cancer patients but does not have all the adverse effects that occur when the marijuana leaf is smoked. Marijuana leaf is a controlled substance with high abuse potential and is legal for medical use in some states, but not approved for recreational use in most states. The synthetic version of the active ingredient allows for an accepted form to achieve the desired therapeutic effect in cancer patients.

Ingestion of a plant-derived food can sometimes lead to a drug effect. For instance, the body converts natural licorice to a false aldosterone—a hormone found in the body—resulting in fluid retention and hypokalemia or low serum potassium levels if large amounts of licorice are eaten. However, people seldom think of licorice as a drug.

Finally, plants and plant byproducts have become the main component of the growing herbal and alternative therapy movement. Chapter 6 discusses the alternative therapy movement and its impact on today's drug regimens.

Table 1.2 Drugs Derived from Plants

Plant	Product
Ricinus communis	Seed Oil Castor oil (*Neolid*)
Digitalis purpurea (foxglove)	Leaves Dried leaves Digitalis leaf
Papaver somniferum (poppy)	Unripe capsule Juice Opium (paregoric) Morphine (*Roxanol*) Codeine Papaverine (*Pavabid*)

Animal Products

Animal products are used to replace human chemicals that fail to be produced because of disease or genetic problems. Until recently, insulin for treating diabetes was obtained exclusively from the pancreas of cows and pigs. Now **genetic engineering**—the process of altering DNA—permits scientists to produce human insulin by altering *Escherichia coli* bacteria, making insulin a better product without some of the impurities that come with animal products.

Thyroid drugs and growth hormone preparations also may be obtained from animal thyroid and hypothalamic tissues. Many of these preparations are now created synthetically, however, and the synthetic preparations are considered to be purer and safer than preparations derived from animals.

Inorganic Compounds

Salts of various chemical elements can have therapeutic effects in the human body. Aluminum, fluoride, iron, and even gold are used to treat various conditions. The effects of these elements usually were discovered accidentally when a cause–effect relationship was observed. Table 1.3 shows examples of some elements used for their therapeutic benefit.

Table 1.3 Elements Used for Their Therapeutic Effects

Element	Therapeutic Use
Aluminum	Antacid to decrease gastric acidity Management of hyperphosphatemia Prevention of the formation of phosphate urinary stones
Fluorine (as fluoride)	Prevention of dental cavities Prevention of osteoporosis
Gold	Treatment of rheumatoid arthritis
Iron	Treatment of iron deficiency anemia

Synthetic Sources

Today, many drugs are developed synthetically after chemicals in plants, animals, or the environment have been tested and found to have therapeutic activity. Scientists use genetic engineering to alter bacteria to produce chemicals that are therapeutic and effective. Other technical advances allow scientists to alter a chemical with proven therapeutic effectiveness to make it better. Sometimes, a small change in a chemical's structure can make that chemical more useful as a drug—more potent, more stable, and less toxic. These technological advances have led to the development of groups of similar drugs, all of which are derived from an original prototype, but each of which has slightly different properties, making a particular drug more desirable in a specific situation.

Throughout this book, the icon Ⓟ will be used to designate those drugs of a class that are considered the prototype of the class, the original drug in the class, or the drug that has emerged as the most effective. For example, the cephalosporins are a large group of antibiotics derived from the same chemical structure. Alterations in the chemical rings or attachments to that structure make it possible for some of these drugs to be absorbed orally, whereas others must be given parenterally. Some of these drugs cause severe toxic effects (e.g., renal toxicity), but others do not.

KEY POINTS

- Clinical pharmacology is the study of drugs used to treat, diagnose, or prevent a disease.
- Drugs are chemicals that are introduced into the body and affect the body's chemical processes.
- Drugs can come from natural sources including plants, foods, animals, salts of inorganic compounds, or synthetic sources.

Drug Evaluation

After a chemical that might have therapeutic value is identified, it must undergo a series of scientific tests to evaluate its actual therapeutic and toxic effects. This process is tightly controlled by the U.S. **Food and Drug Administration (FDA)**, an agency of the U.S. Department of Health and Human Services that regulates the development and sale of drugs. FDA-regulated tests are designed to ensure the safety and reliability of any drug approved in this country. For every 100,000 chemicals that are identified as being potential drugs, only about 5 end up being marketed. Before receiving final FDA approval to be marketed to the public, drugs must pass through several stages of development. These include preclinical trials and phase I, II, and III studies. The drugs listed in this book have been through rigorous testing and are approved for sale to the public, either with or without a prescription from a health care provider.

Preclinical Trials

In **preclinical trials**, chemicals that may have therapeutic value are tested on laboratory animals for two main purposes: (1) to determine whether they have the presumed effects in living tissue and (2) to evaluate any adverse effects. Animal testing is important because unique biological differences can cause very different reactions to the chemical.

These differences can be found only in living organisms, so computer-generated models alone are often inadequate.

At the end of the preclinical trials, some chemicals are discarded for the following reasons:

- The chemical lacks therapeutic activity when used with living animals.
- The chemical is too toxic to living animals to be worth the risk of developing into a drug.
- The chemical is highly **teratogenic** (causing adverse effects to the fetus).
- The safety margins are so small that the chemical would not be useful in the clinical setting.

Some chemicals, however, are found to have therapeutic effects and reasonable safety margins. This means that the chemicals are therapeutic at doses that are reasonably different from doses that cause toxic effects. Such chemicals will pass the preclinical trials and advance to phase I studies.

Phase I Studies

A **phase I study** uses human volunteers to test the drugs. These studies are more tightly controlled than preclinical trials and are performed by specially trained clinical investigators. The volunteers are fully informed of possible risks and may be paid for their participation. Usually, the volunteers are healthy, young men and often women. Women of childbearing potential are sometimes not good candidates for phase I studies because the chemicals may exert unknown and harmful effects on a woman's ova, and too much risk is involved in taking a drug that might destroy or alter the ova. Women do not make new ova after birth. Men produce sperm daily, so there is less potential for complete destruction or alteration of the sperm. Volunteers who elect to participate in phase I studies have to be informed of the potential risks and must sign a consent form outlining the possible effects.

Some chemicals are therapeutic in other animals but have no effects in humans. Investigators in phase I studies scrutinize the drugs being tested for effects in humans. They also look for adverse effects and toxicity. At the end of phase I studies, many chemicals are dropped from the process for the following reasons:

- They lack evidence of potential therapeutic effect in humans.
- They cause unacceptable adverse effects.
- They are highly teratogenic.
- They are too toxic.

Some chemicals move to the next stage of testing despite undesirable effects. For example, the antihypertensive drug minoxidil was found to effectively treat malignant hypertension, but it caused unusual hair growth on the palms and other body areas. However, because it was so much more effective for treating malignant hypertension at the time of its development than any other antihypertensive drug and because the undesired effects were not dangerous, it proceeded to phase II studies. (Now, its hair-growing effect has been channeled for therapeutic use into various topical hair-growth preparations such as *Rogaine.*)

Phase II Studies

A **phase II study** allows clinical investigators to try out the drug in patients who have the disease that the drug is designed to treat. Patients are told about the possible benefits of the drug and are invited to participate in the study. Those who consent to participate are fully informed about possible risks and are monitored very closely, often at no charge to them, to evaluate the drug's effects. Usually, phase II studies are performed at various sites across the country—in hospitals, clinics, and doctors' offices—and are monitored by representatives of the pharmaceutical company studying the drug. At the end of phase II studies a drug may be removed from further investigation for the following reasons:

- It is less effective than anticipated.
- It is too toxic when used with patients.
- It produces unacceptable adverse effects.
- It has a low benefit-to-risk ratio, meaning that the therapeutic benefit it provides does not outweigh the risk of potential adverse effects that it causes.
- It is no more effective than other drugs already on the market, making the cost of continued research and production less attractive to the drug company.

A drug that continues to show promise as a therapeutic agent receives additional scrutiny in phase III studies.

Phase III Studies

A **phase III study** involves use of the drug in a vast clinical market. Prescribers are informed of all the known reactions to the drug and precautions required for its safe use. Prescribers observe patients very closely, monitoring them for any adverse effects. Often, prescribers ask patients to keep journals and record any symptoms they experience. Prescribers then evaluate the reported effects to determine whether they are caused by the disease or by the drug. This information is collected by the drug company that is developing the drug and is shared with the FDA. When a drug is used widely and within uncontrolled environments, totally unexpected responses may occur. A drug that produces unacceptable adverse effects or unforeseen reactions is usually removed from further study by the drug company. In some cases the FDA may have to request that a drug be removed from the market.

Food and Drug Administration Approval

Drugs that finish phase III studies are evaluated by the FDA, which relies on committees of experts familiar with the specialty area in which the drugs will be used. Only those drugs that receive FDA committee approval may be marketed. Figure 1.3 recaps the various phases of drug development discussed.

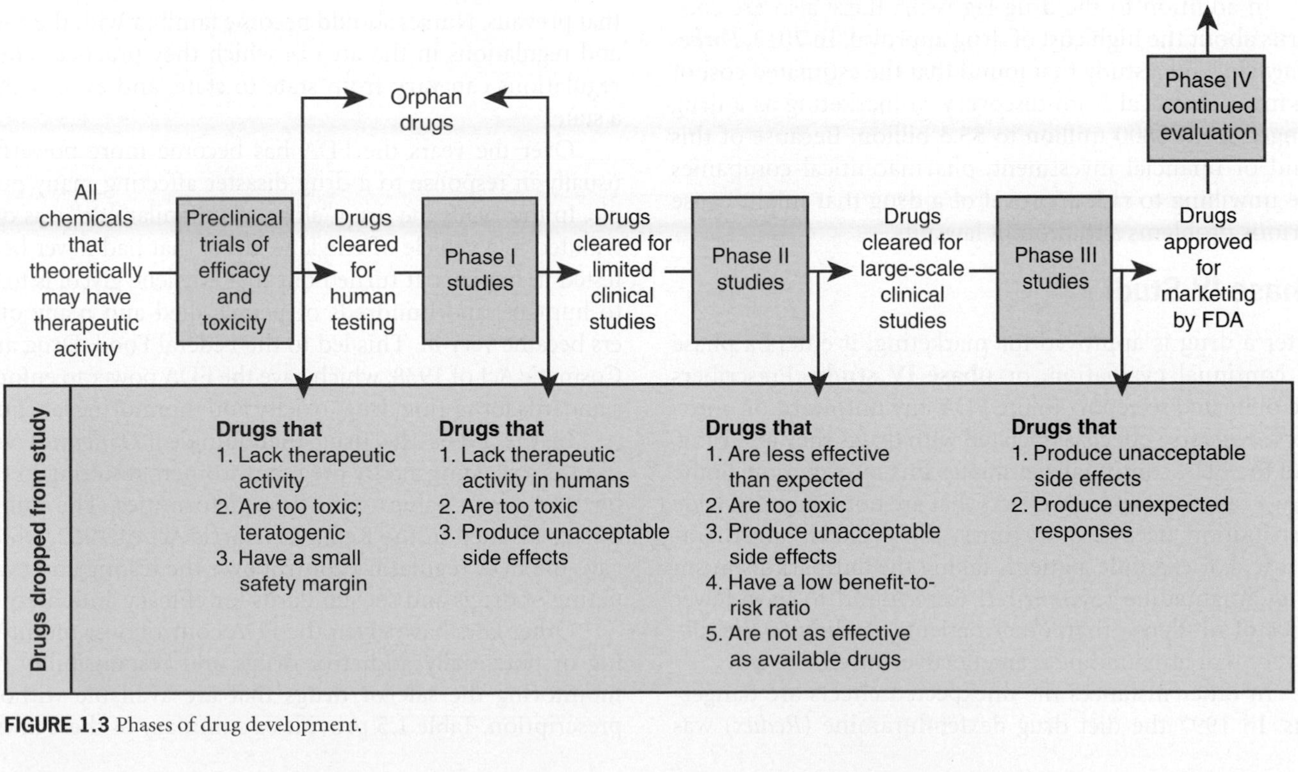

FIGURE 1.3 Phases of drug development.

Table 1.4 Comparison of Generic, Chemical, and Brand Names of Drugs

Levothyroxine sodium	←	Generic name	→	Dronabinol
L-thyroxine, T_4	←	Chemical name	→	Delta-9-tetrahydrocannabinol
Levothroid, Levoxyl, Synthroid	←	Brand names	→	*Marinol*

An approved drug is given a **brand name** (trade name) by the pharmaceutical company that developed it. The **generic name** of a drug is the original designation that the drug was given when the drug company applied for the approval process. **Chemical names** are names that reflect the chemical structure of a drug. Some drugs are known by all three names. It can be confusing to study drugs when so many different names are used for the same compound. In this text the generic and chemical names always appear in straight print, and the brand name is always italicized (e.g., minoxidil [*Rogaine*]). Table 1.4 compares examples of drug names.

The entire drug development and approval process can take 5 to 6 years, resulting in a so-called drug lag in the United States. In some instances, a drug that is available in another country may not become available here for years. The FDA regards public safety as primary in drug approval, so the process remains strict; however, it can be accelerated in certain instances involving the treatment of deadly diseases. For example, some drugs (e.g., delavirdine [*Rescriptor*] and efavirenz [*Sustiva*]) that were thought to offer a benefit to patients with acquired immune deficiency syndrome (AIDS), a potentially fatal immune disorder, were pushed through because of the progressive nature of AIDS and the lack of a cure. All literature associated with these drugs indicates that long-term effects and other information about the drug may not yet be known.

In addition to the drug lag issue, there also are concerns about the high cost of drug approval. In 2013, *Forbes Magazine* did a study that found that the estimated cost of taking a chemical from discovery to marketing as a drug ranged from $800 million to $5.3 billion. Because of this kind of financial investment, pharmaceutical companies are unwilling to risk approval of a drug that might cause serious problems and prompt lawsuits.

Phase IV Studies

After a drug is approved for marketing, it enters a phase of continual evaluation, or **phase IV study**. Prescribers are obligated to report to the FDA any untoward or unexpected adverse effects associated with drugs they are using, and the FDA continually evaluates this information. Some drugs cause unexpected effects that are not seen until wide distribution occurs. Sometimes, those effects are therapeutic. For example, patients taking the antiparkinsonism drug amantadine (*Symmetrel*) were found to have fewer cases of influenza than other patients, leading to the discovery that amantadine is an effective antiviral agent.

In other instances the unexpected effects are dangerous. In 1997 the diet drug dexfenfluramine (*Redux*) was removed from the market only months after its release because patients taking it developed serious heart problems. In 2004 the drug company Merck withdrew its cyclooxygenase-2 (Cox-2) specific nonsteroidal anti-inflammatory drug rofecoxib (*Vioxx*) from the market when postmarketing studies seemed to show a significant increase in cardiovascular mortality in patients who were taking the drug. These problems were not seen in any of the premarketing studies of the drug. The effects were only seen with a much wider use of the drug after it had been marketed.

KEY POINTS

- The FDA carefully regulates the testing and approval of all drugs in this country.
- To be approved for marketing a drug must pass through animal testing, testing on healthy humans, selected testing on people with the disease being treated, and then broad testing on people with the disease being treated.

Legal Regulation of Drugs

The FDA regulates the development and sale of drugs. Local laws further regulate the distribution and administration of drugs. In most cases, the strictest law is the one that prevails. Nurses should become familiar with the rules and regulations in the area in which they practice. These regulations can vary from state to state, and even within a state.

Over the years the FDA has become more powerful, usually in response to a drug disaster affecting many people. In the 1930s the drug "elixir of sulfanilamide" was distributed in a vehicle of ethylene glycol that had never been tested in humans. It turned out that ethylene glycol is toxic to humans, and hundreds of people died and many others became very ill. This led to the Federal Food, Drug and Cosmetic Act of 1938, which gave the FDA power to enforce standards for testing drug toxicity and monitoring labeling.

In the 1960s the drug thalidomide (*Thalomid*) was used as a sleeping aid by pregnant women, resulting in the birth of many babies with limb deformities. The public outcry resulted in the Kefauver-Harris Act of 1962, which gave the FDA regulatory control over the testing and evaluating of drugs and set standards for efficacy and safety.

Other laws have given the FDA control over monitoring of potentially addictive drugs and responsibility for monitoring the sale of drugs that are available without prescription. Table 1.5 provides a summary of these laws.

Table 1.5 Federal Legislation Affecting the Clinical Use of Drugs

Year Enacted	Law	Impact
1906	Pure Food and Drug Act	Prevented the marketing of adulterated drugs; required labeling to eliminate false or misleading claims
1938	Federal Food, Drug and Cosmetic Act	Mandated tests for drug toxicity and provided means for recall of drugs; established procedures for introducing new drugs; gave FDA the power of enforcement
1951	Durham-Humphrey Amendment	Tightened control of certain drugs; specified drugs to be labeled "may not be distributed without a prescription"
1962	Kefauver-Harris Act	Tightened control over the quality of drugs; gave FDA regulatory power over the procedure of drug investigations; stated that efficacy as well as safety of drugs had to be established
1970	Controlled Substances Act	Defined drug abuse and classified drugs as to their potential for abuse; provided strict controls over the distribution, storage, and use of these drugs
1983	Orphan Drug Act	Provided incentives for the development of orphan drugs for treatment of rare diseases

Safety during Pregnancy

As part of the standards for testing and safety the FDA requires that each new drug be assigned to a pregnancy category (Box 1.1). The categories indicate a drug's potential or actual teratogenic effects, thus offering guidelines for use of that particular drug in pregnancy. Research into the development of the human fetus, especially the nervous system, has led many health care providers to recommend that no drug should be used during pregnancy because of potential effects on the developing fetus. In cases in which a drug is needed, it is recommended that the drug of choice be one for which the benefit outweighs the potential risk. In 2014 the FDA established guidelines that will lead to categories related to the presence of the drug in breast milk, indicating the possibility of effects on a baby who is breastfed. This has been an ongoing issue, with increasing numbers of mothers electing to breastfeed and no clinical studies or accurate information available for many drugs. It will take time to see this information appear in prescribing information. In 2015 the FDA elected to do away with the pregnancy categories. The classes were confusing at times and not helpful to many people. Moving forward, drugs will not have a pregnancy category listed but will have a risk level for effects on fertility, pregnancy, and when used in breastfeeding. It will take time for drug companies to reevaluate all drugs and relabel them.

BOX 1.1

Food and Drug Administration Pregnancy Categories

The FDA has established five categories to indicate the potential for a systemically absorbed drug to cause birth defects. The key differentiation among the categories rests on the degree (reliability) of documentation and the risk–benefit ratio. These labels have often been confusing and in December 2014 the FDA passed a new rule which will phase out these categories. In their place the prescribing information will have more information under the section "Use in Specific Populations." This area will outline the risk of using the drug during pregnancy and lactation with data to support the clinical information and information to help health care providers make prescribing and counseling decisions about the use of these drugs in pregnancy and lactation. This change will occur over time and it is thought that it will provide safer use of drugs in these two groups. While the transition is occurring the following categories will still appear and will eventually be phased out.

Category A: Adequate studies in pregnant women have not demonstrated a risk to the fetus in the first trimester of pregnancy, and there is no evidence of risk in later trimesters.

Category B: Animal studies have not demonstrated a risk to the fetus but there are no adequate studies in pregnant women, *or* animal studies have shown an adverse effect, but adequate studies in pregnant women have not demonstrated a risk to the fetus during the first trimester of pregnancy, and there is no evidence of risk in later trimesters.

Category C: Animal studies have shown an adverse effect on the fetus but there are no adequate studies in humans; the benefits from the use of the drug in pregnant women may be acceptable despite its potential risks, *or* there are no animal reproduction studies and no adequate studies in humans.

Category D: There is evidence of human fetal risk, but the potential benefits from the use of the drug in pregnant women may be acceptable despite its potential risks.

Category X: Studies in animals or humans demonstrate fetal abnormalities or adverse reactions; reports indicate evidence of fetal risk. The risk of use in a pregnant woman clearly outweighs any possible benefit.

Regardless of the designated pregnancy category or presumed safety, *no* drug should be administered during pregnancy unless it is clearly needed.

Controlled Substances

The Controlled Substances Act of 1970 established categories for ranking of the abuse potential of various drugs. This same act gave control over the coding of drugs and the enforcement of these codes to the FDA and the Drug Enforcement Agency (DEA), a part of the U.S. Department

BOX 1.2

Drug Enforcement Agency Schedules of Controlled Substances

The Controlled Substances Act of 1970 regulates the manufacturing, distribution, and dispensing of drugs that are known to have abuse potential. The DEA is responsible for the enforcement of these regulations. The controlled drugs are divided into five DEA schedules based on their potential for abuse and physical and psychological dependence:

Schedule I ***(C-I):*** High abuse potential and no accepted medical use (heroin, marijuana, LSD)
Schedule II ***(C-II):*** High abuse potential with severe dependence liability (narcotics, amphetamines, and barbiturates)
Schedule III ***(C-III):*** Less abuse potential than schedule II drugs and moderate dependence liability (nonbarbiturate sedatives, nonamphetamine stimulants, limited amounts of certain narcotics)
Schedule IV ***(C-IV):*** Less abuse potential than schedule III and limited dependence liability (some sedatives, antianxiety agents, and nonnarcotic analgesics)
Schedule V ***(C-V):*** Limited abuse potential. Primarily small amounts of narcotics (codeine) used as antitussives or antidiarrheals. Under federal law, limited quantities of certain schedule V drugs may be purchased without a prescription directly from a pharmacist. The purchaser must be at least 18 years of age and must furnish suitable identification. All such transactions must be recorded by the dispensing pharmacist.

Prescribing physicians and dispensing pharmacists must be registered with the DEA, which also provides forms for the transfer of schedule I and II substances and establishes criteria for the inventory and prescribing of controlled substances. State and local laws are often more stringent than federal law. In any given situation, the more stringent law applies.

of Justice. The FDA studies the drugs and determines their abuse potential; the DEA enforces their control. Drugs with abuse potential are called *controlled substances.* Box 1.2 contains descriptions of each category, or schedule.

The prescription, distribution, storage, and use of controlled substances drugs are closely monitored by the DEA in an attempt to decrease substance abuse of prescribed medications. Each prescriber has a DEA number, which allows the DEA to monitor prescription patterns and possible abuse. A nurse should be familiar with not only the DEA guidelines for controlled substances but also the local policies and procedures, which might be even more rigorous.

Generic Drugs

When a drug receives approval for marketing from the FDA the drug formula is given a time-limited patent, in much the same way as an invention is patented. The length of time for which the patent is good depends on the type of chemical involved. When the patent runs out on a brand-name drug, the drug can be produced by other manufacturers. **Generic drugs** are chemicals that are produced by companies involved solely in the manufacturing of drugs. Because they do not have the research, the advertising, or, sometimes, the quality control departments that the pharmaceutical companies developing the drugs have, they can produce the generic drugs more cheaply. In the past, some quality-control problems were found with generic products. For example, the binders used in a generic drug might not be the same as those used in the brand name product. As a result, the way the body breaks down and uses the generic drug may differ from that of the brand name product. In that case the bioavailability of the drug is different from that of the brand name product.

Many states require that a drug be dispensed in the generic form if one is available. This requirement helps to keep down the cost of drugs and health care. Some prescribers, however, specify that a drug prescription be "dispensed as written" (DAW) (i.e., that the brand name product be used). By doing so the prescriber ensures the quality control and the action and effect expected with that drug. These elements may be most important in drugs that have narrow safety margins, such as digoxin (*Lanoxin*), a heart drug, and warfarin (*Coumadin*), an anticoagulant. The initial cost may be higher, because some insurance companies will not pay for these brand name drugs when the generic is available, but some prescribers believe that, in the long run, the cost to the patient will be less.

Orphan Drugs

Orphan drugs are drugs that have been discovered but are not financially viable and therefore have not been "adopted" by any drug company. Orphan drugs may be useful in treating a rare disease, or they may have potentially dangerous adverse effects. Orphan drugs are often abandoned after preclinical trials or phase I studies. The Orphan Drug Act of 1983 provided tremendous financial incentives to drug companies to adopt these drugs and develop them. These incentives help the drug company put the drug through the rest of the testing process, even though the market for the drug in the long run may be very small (as in the case of a drug to treat a rare neurological disease that affects only a small number of people). Some drugs in this book have orphan drug uses listed.

Over-the-Counter Drugs

Over-the-counter (OTC) **drugs** are products that are available without prescription for self-treatment of a variety of complaints. Some of these agents were approved as prescription drugs but later were found to be very safe and useful for patients without the need of a prescription. Some were not rigorously screened and tested by the current drug evaluation protocols because they were developed and marketed before the current laws were put into effect. Many of these drugs were "grandfathered" into use because they had been used for so long. The FDA is currently testing the effectiveness of many of these products and, in time, will evaluate all of them. Although OTC drugs have been found to be safe when taken as directed, nurses should consider several problems related to OTC drug use:

- Taking these drugs could mask the signs and symptoms of underlying disease, making diagnosis difficult.
- Taking these drugs with prescription medications could result in drug interactions and interfere with drug therapy.
- Not taking these drugs as directed could result in serious overdoses.

Many patients do not consider OTC drugs to be medications and therefore do not report their use. Nurses must always include specific questions about OTC drug use when taking a drug history and should provide information in all drug-teaching protocols about avoiding OTC use while taking prescription drugs or checking with the health care provider first if the patient feels a need for one of these drugs.

KEY POINTS

- Generic drugs are drugs no longer protected by patent and can be produced by companies other than the one that developed it.
- OTC drugs are available without a prescription and are deemed safe when used as directed.
- Orphan drugs are drugs that have been discovered but that are not financially viable because they have a limited market or a narrow margin of safety. These drugs may have then been adopted for development by a drug company in exchange for tax incentives.

Sources of Drug Information

The fields of pharmacology and drug therapy change so quickly that it is important to have access to sources of information about drug doses, therapeutic and adverse effects, and nursing-related implications. Textbooks provide valuable background and basic information to help in the understanding of pharmacology, but in clinical practice it is important to have access to up-to-the-minute information. Several sources of drug information are readily available. Nurses often need to consult more than one source.

Drug Labels

Drug labels have specific information that identifies a specific drug. For example, a drug label identifies the brand and generic names for the drug, the drug dosage, the expiration date, and special drug warnings. Some labels also indicate the route and dose for administration. Figure 1.4 illustrates an example of a drug label.

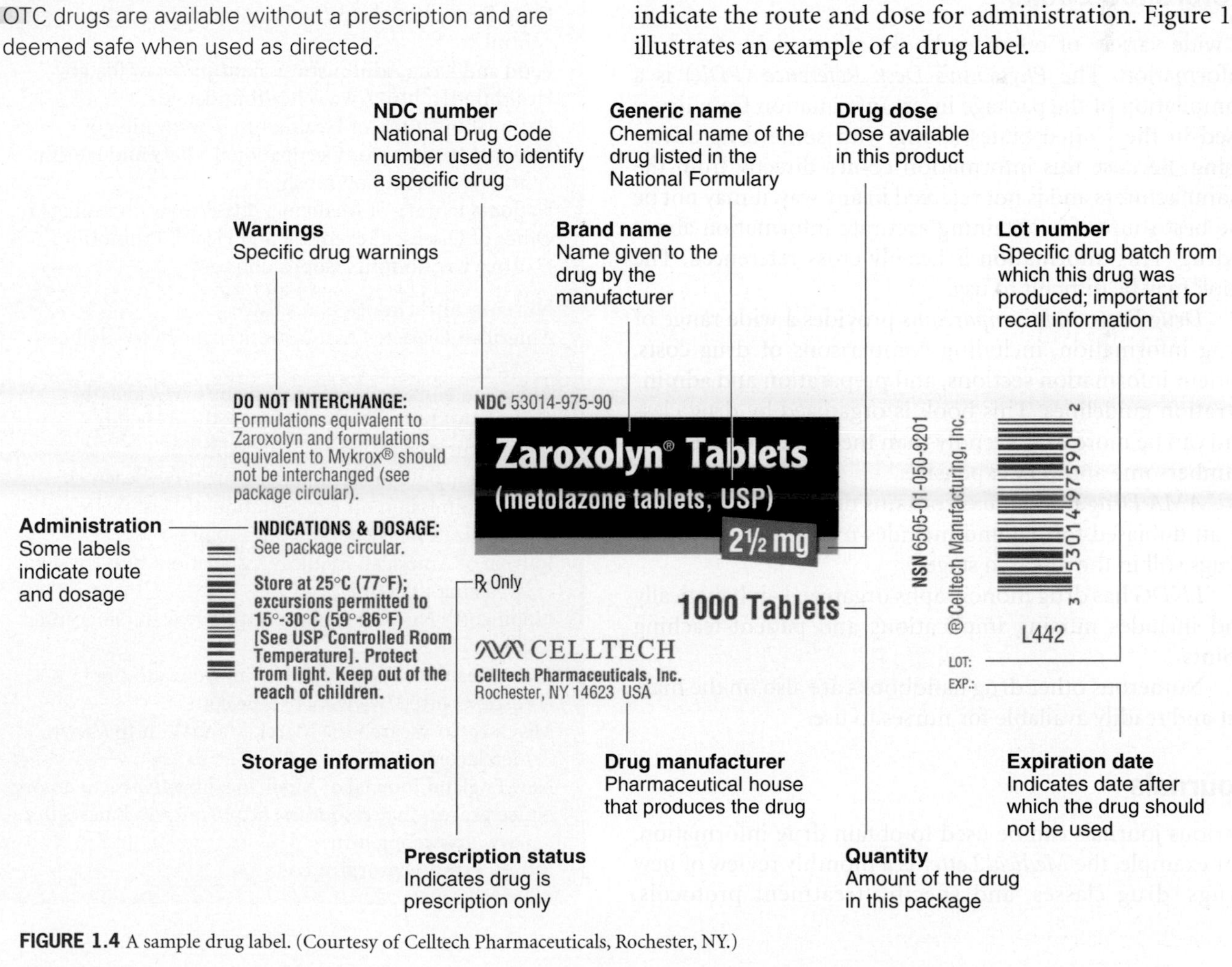

FIGURE 1.4 A sample drug label. (Courtesy of Celltech Pharmaceuticals, Rochester, NY.)

Understanding how to read a drug label is essential. Nurses need to become familiar with each aspect of the label.

Package Inserts

All drugs come with a package insert prepared by the manufacturer according to strict FDA regulations. The package insert, or full prescribing information, contains all of the chemical and study information that led to the drug's approval. Package inserts sometimes are difficult to understand and are almost always in very small print, making them difficult to read. The FDA is in the process of revising the format for all of the required package insert information to make it more readily useable. New and revised package inserts will contain a highlights section at the beginning of the insert that highlights the most essential information for the health care provider. The FDA Web site has also been revised to make it more user friendly, so information is much easier to access. The FDA Web site, www.fda.gov, is a good resource for finding the full prescribing information for most drugs.

Reference Books

A wide variety of reference books are available for drug information. The *Physician's Desk Reference* (*PDR*) is a compilation of the package insert information from drugs used in the United States, along with some drug advertising. Because this information comes directly from the manufacturers and is not refereed in any way, it may not be the best source for obtaining accurate information about a drug. This information is heavily cross-referenced. The book may be difficult to use.

Drug Facts and Comparisons provides a wide range of drug information, including comparisons of drug costs, patient information sections, and preparation and administration guidelines. This book is organized by drug class and can be more user friendly than the *PDR*. However, it is cumbersome and very expensive.

AMA Drug Evaluations contains detailed monographs in an unbiased format and includes many new drugs and drugs still in the research stage.

LNDG has drug monographs organized alphabetically and includes nursing implications and patient-teaching points.

Numerous other drug handbooks are also on the market and readily available for nurses to use.

Journals

Various journals can be used to obtain drug information. For example, the *Medical Letter* is a monthly review of new drugs, drug classes, and specific treatment protocols. The *American Journal of Nursing* offers information on new drugs, drug errors, and nursing implications.

Internet Information

Many patients now use the Internet as a source of medical information and advice. Box 1.3 lists some informative Internet sites for obtaining drug information, patient information, or therapeutic information related to specific disease states. Nurses need to become familiar with what is available on the Internet and what patients may be referencing.

BOX 1.3

Sources of Internet Information

Evaluate sites with drug information on the Internet

Government Sites

Agency for Health Care Research and Quality: http://www.ahcpr.gov
CancerNet (National Cancer Institute): http://www.cancer.gov
Centers for Disease Control: http://www.cdc.gov
Drug Formulary: http://www.intmed.mcw.edu/drug.html
Food and Drug Administration: http://www.fda.gov
Healthfinder: http://www.healthfinder.gov
National Institutes of Health: http://www.nih.gov
National Institute for Occupational Safety and Health: http://www.cdc.gov/niosh
National Library of Medicine: http://www.nlm.nih.gov
Office of Disease Prevention and Health Promotion: http://www.odphp.osophs.dhhs.gov

Nursing and Health Care Sites

American Diabetes Association: http://www.diabetes.org
American Nurses Association: http://www.ana.org
Cumulative Index to Nursing and Allied Health Literature: http://www.cinahl.com
International Council of Nurses: http://www.icn.ch
Joint Commission on Accreditation of Healthcare Organizations: http://www.jcaho.org
Journal of American Medical Association: http://www.jama.ama-assn.org
Lippincott's Nursing Center: http://www.nursingcenter.com
Mayo Health Oasis: http://www.mayohealth.org
Medscape: http://www.medscape.com
Merck & Co. (search the Merck Manual): http://www.merck.com
New England Journal of Medicine: http://www.nejm.org
Nurse practitioner resources: http://nurseweb.ucsf.edu/www/arwwebpg.htm
RxList: http://www.rxlist.com

SUMMARY

- Drugs are chemicals that are introduced into the body to bring about some sort of change.
- Drugs can come from many sources: plants, animals, inorganic elements, and synthetic preparations.
- The FDA regulates the development and marketing of drugs to ensure safety and efficacy.
- Preclinical trials involve testing of potential drugs on laboratory animals to determine their therapeutic and adverse effects.
- Phase I studies test potential drugs on healthy human subjects.
- Phase II studies test potential drugs on patients who have the disease the drugs are designed to treat.
- Phase III studies test drugs in the clinical setting to determine any unanticipated effects or lack of effectiveness.
- FDA pregnancy categories indicate the potential or actual teratogenic effects of a drug.
- DEA controlled substance categories indicate the abuse potential and associated regulation of a drug.
- Generic drugs are sold under their generic names, not brand names; they may be cheaper but in some situations are not necessarily as safe as brand name drugs.
- Orphan drugs are chemicals that have been discovered to have some therapeutic effect but that are not financially advantageous for development into drugs.
- OTC drugs are available without prescription for the self-treatment of various complaints.
- Information about drugs can be obtained from a variety of sources, including the drug label, reference books, journals, and Internet sites.

CHECK YOUR UNDERSTANDING

Answers to the questions in this chapter can be found in Answers to Check Your Understanding Questions on thePoint®.

MULTIPLE CHOICE

Select the best answer to the following.

1. Clinical pharmacology is the study of
  a. the biological effects of chemicals.
  b. drugs used to treat, prevent, or diagnose disease.
  c. plant components that can be used as medicines.
  d. binders and other vehicles for delivering medication.

2. Phase I drug studies involve
  a. the use of laboratory animals to test chemicals.
  b. patients with the disease the drug is designed to treat.
  c. mass marketing surveys of drug effects in large numbers of people.
  d. healthy human volunteers who are often paid for their participation.

3. The generic name of a drug is
  a. the name assigned to the drug by the pharmaceutical company developing it.
  b. the chemical name of the drug based on its chemical structure.
  c. the original name assigned to the drug at the beginning of the evaluation process.
  d. the name that is often used in advertising campaigns.

4. An orphan drug is a drug that
  a. has failed to go through the approval process.
  b. is available in a foreign country but not in this country.
  c. has been tested but is not considered to be financially viable.
  d. is available without a prescription.

5. The FDA pregnancy categories
  a. indicate a drug's potential or actual teratogenic effects.
  b. are used for research purposes only.
  c. list drugs that are more likely to have addicting properties.
  d. are tightly regulated by the DEA.

6. The storing, prescribing, and distributing of controlled substances—drugs that are more apt to be addictive—are monitored by
  a. the FDA.
  b. the Department of Commerce.
  c. the Federal Bureau of Investigation.
  d. the DEA.

(continues on page 16)

7. Healthy young women are sometimes not able to be involved in phase I studies of drugs because
- **a.** male bodies are more predictable and responsive to chemicals.
- **b.** females are more apt to suffer problems with ova, which are formed only before birth.
- **c.** males can tolerate the unknown adverse effects of many drugs better than females.
- **d.** there are no standards to use to evaluate the female response.

8. A patient has been taking fluoxetine (*Prozac*) for several years, but when picking up the prescription this month found that the tablets looked different and became concerned. The nurse, checking with the pharmacist, found that fluoxetine had just become available in the generic form and the prescription had been filled with the generic product. The nurse should tell the patient
- **a.** that the new tablet may have similar effects or may not so the patient should carefully monitor response.
- **b.** that generic drugs are available without a prescription and they are just as safe as the brand name medication.
- **c.** that the law requires that prescriptions be filled with the generic form if available to cut down the cost of medications.
- **d.** that the pharmacist filled the prescription with the wrong drug and it should be returned to the pharmacy for a refund.

MULTIPLE RESPONSE

Select all that apply.

1. When teaching a patient about OTC drugs, which points should the nurse include?
- **a.** These drugs are very safe and can be used freely to relieve your complaints.
- **b.** These compounds are called drugs, but they aren't really drugs.
- **c.** Some of these drugs were once prescription drugs, but are now thought to be safe when used as directed.
- **d.** Reading the label of these drugs is very important; the name of the active ingredient is prominent; you should always check the ingredient name.
- **e.** It is important to read the label and to see what the recommended dose of the drug is; some of these drugs can cause serious problems if too much of the drug is taken.
- **f.** It is important to report the use of any OTC drug to your health care provider because many of them can interact with drugs that might be prescribed for you.

2. A patient asks what generic drugs are and if he should be using them to treat his infection. Which of the following statements should be included in the nurse's explanation?
- **a.** A generic drug is a drug that is sold by the name of the ingredient, not the brand name.
- **b.** Generic drugs are always the best drugs to use because they are never any different from the familiar brand names.
- **c.** Generic drugs are not available until the patent expires on a specific drug.
- **d.** Generic drugs are usually cheaper than the well-known brand names, and some insurance companies require that you receive the generic drug if one is available.
- **e.** Generic drugs are forms of a drug that are available over the counter and do not require a prescription.
- **f.** Your physician may want you to have the brand name of a drug, not the generic form, and DAW will be on your prescription form.
- **g.** Generic drugs are less likely to cause adverse effects than brand name drugs.

BIBLIOGRAPHY

Anderson, P. O. (2007). *Handbook of critical drug data* (11th ed.). Hamilton, IL: Drug Intelligence.

Barton, J. H., & Emanuel, E. J. (2005). The patient-based pharmaceutical development process: Rationale, problems and potential reforms. *Journal of the American Medical Association, 294*, 2075–2082.

Brunton, L., Chabner, B., & Knollman, B. (2011). *Goodman & Gilman's the pharmacological basis of therapeutics* (12th ed.). New York: McGraw-Hill.

Cardinale, V. (1998). Consumers looking for more answers, clearer directions. *Drug Topics Supplement, 142*(11), 23a.

Creigle, V. (2007) MedWatch: The FDA safety information and adverse event reporting program. *Journal of the Medical Library Association, 95*(2), 224–225.

Drug Enforcement Agency. (2011). *Guidelines for pain prescriptions*. Washington, DC: U.S. Government Printing Office.

Ebadi, M. (2007). *Pharmacodynamic basis of herbal medications* (2nd ed.). Boca Raton, FL: CRC Press.

Federal Register. (2014, February 12). Content and format of labeling for human prescription drugs and biological products, requirements for pregnancy and lactation labeling. Available online at: https://www.federalregister.gov

Fitzgerald, M. (1994). Pharmacological highlights: Principles of pharmacokinetics. *Journal of the American Academy of Nursing Practice, 6*(12), 581.

Focus on Intellectual Property Rights. (2006). United States Department of State. Washington, DC. Available online at: http://www.america.gov/publications/books/ipr.html

Herper, M. (2013). The cost of creating a new drug now $5 billion, pushing pharma to change [*Forbes*]. Available online at: http://www.forbes.com/sites/matthewherper/2013/08/11/how-the-staggering-cost-of-inventing-new-drugs-is-shaping-the-future-of-medicine/

Karch, A. M. (2014). *Lippincott nursing drug guide.* Philadelphia, PA: Lippincott Williams & Wilkins.

Koo, M. M., Krass, I., & Aslani, P. (2003). Factors influencing consumer use of written drug information. *Annals of Pharmacotherapy, 37*(2), 259–267.

Medical Letter. (2015). *The medical letter on drugs and therapeutics* New Rochelle, NY: Author.

Sun, S. X., Lee, K. Y., Bertram, C. T., & Goldstein, J. L. (2007). Withdrawal of COX-2 selective inhibitors rofecoxib and valdecoxib: Impact on NSAID and gastroprotective drug prescribing and utilization. *Current Medical Research and Opinion, 23*(8), 1859–1866.

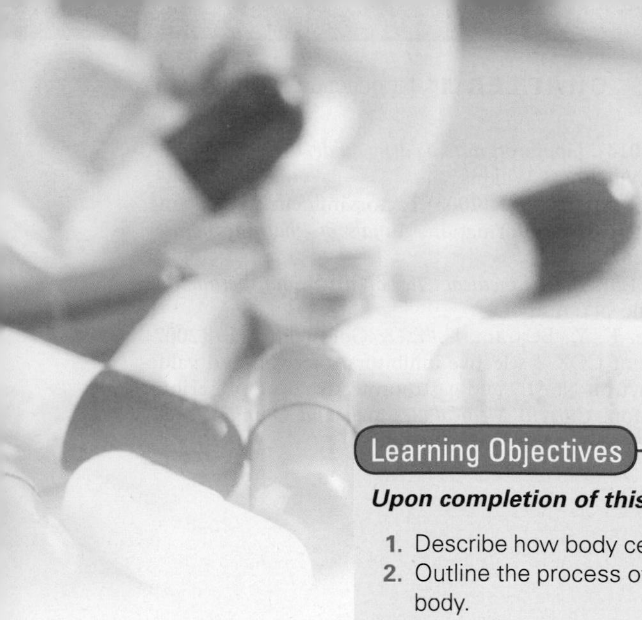

Drugs and the Body 2

Learning Objectives

Upon completion of this chapter, you will be able to:

1. Describe how body cells respond to the presence of drugs that are capable of altering their function.
2. Outline the process of dynamic equilibrium that determines the actual concentration of a drug in the body.
3. Explain the meaning of half-life of a drug and calculate the half-life of given drugs.
4. List at least six factors that can influence the actual effectiveness of drugs in the body.
5. Define drug–drug, drug–alternative therapy, drug–food, and drug–laboratory test interactions.

Glossary of Key Terms

absorption: what happens to a drug from the time it enters the body until it enters the circulating fluid; intravenous administration causes the drug to directly enter the circulating blood, bypassing the many complications of absorption from other routes

active transport: the movement of substances across a cell membrane against the concentration gradient; this process requires the use of energy

chemotherapeutic agents: synthetic chemicals used to interfere with the functioning of foreign cell populations, causing cell death; this term is frequently used to refer to the drug therapy of neoplasms, but it also refers to drug therapy affecting any foreign cell

critical concentration: the concentration a drug must reach in the tissues that respond to the particular drug to cause the desired therapeutic effect

distribution: movement of a drug to body tissues; the places where a drug may be distributed depend on the drug's solubility, perfusion of the area, cardiac output, and binding of the drug to plasma proteins

enzyme induction: process by which the presence of a chemical that is biotransformed by a particular enzyme system in the liver causes increased activity of that enzyme system

excretion: removal of a drug from the body; primarily occurs in the kidneys, but can also occur through the skin, lungs, bile, or feces

first-pass effect: a phenomenon in which drugs given orally are carried directly to the liver after absorption, where they may be largely inactivated by liver enzymes before they can enter the general circulation; oral drugs frequently are given in higher doses than drugs given by other routes because of this early breakdown

glomerular filtration: the passage of water and water-soluble components from the plasma into the renal tubule

half-life: the time it takes for the amount of drug in the body to decrease to one half of the peak level it previously achieved

hepatic microsomal system: liver enzymes tightly packed together in the hepatic intracellular structure, responsible for the biotransformation of chemicals, including drugs

loading dose: use of a higher dose than what is usually used for treatment to allow the drug to reach the critical concentration sooner

passive diffusion: movement of substances across a semipermeable membrane with the concentration gradient; this process does not require energy

pharmacodynamics: the study of the interactions between the chemical components of living systems and the foreign chemicals, including drugs, that enter living organisms; the way a drug affects a body

pharmacogenomics: the study of genetically determined variations in the response to drugs

pharmacokinetics: the way the body deals with a drug, including absorption, distribution, biotransformation, and excretion

placebo effect: documented effect of the mind on drug therapy; if a person perceives that a drug will be effective, the drug is much more likely to actually be effective

receptor sites: specific areas on cell membranes that react with certain chemicals to cause an effect within the cell

selective toxicity: property of a chemotherapeutic agent that affects only systems found in foreign cells without affecting healthy human cells (e.g., specific antibiotics can affect certain proteins or enzyme systems used by bacteria but not by human cells)

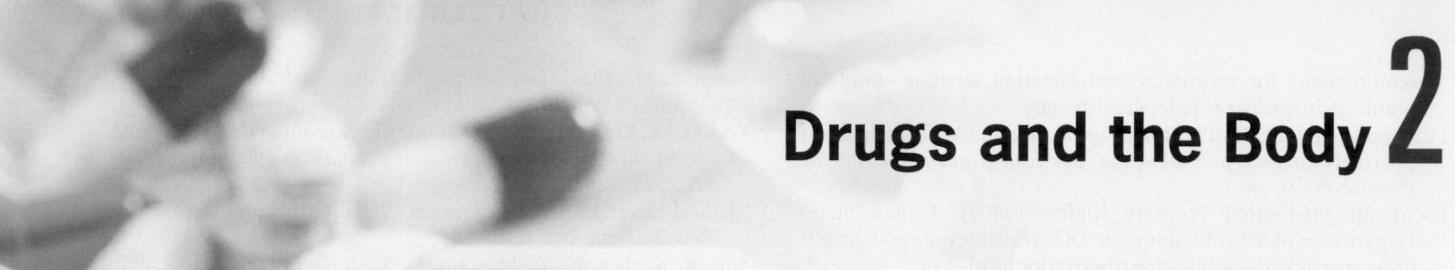

To understand what happens when a drug is administered, the nurse must understand **pharmacodynamics**—how the drug affects the body—and **pharmacokinetics**—how the body acts on the drug. These processes form the basis for the guidelines that have been established regarding drug administration—for example, why certain agents are given intramuscularly (IM) and not intravenously (IV), why some drugs are taken with food and others are not, and the standard dose that should be used to achieve the desired effect. Knowing the basic principles of pharmacodynamics and pharmacokinetics helps the nurse to anticipate therapeutic and adverse drug effects and to intervene in ways that ensure the most effective drug regimen for the patient.

Pharmacodynamics

Pharmacodynamics is the study of the interactions between the chemical components of living systems and the foreign chemicals, including drugs, that enter those systems. All living organisms function by a series of complicated, continuous chemical reactions.

When a new chemical enters the system, multiple changes in and interferences with cell functioning may occur. To avoid such problems, drug development works to provide the most effective and least toxic chemicals for therapeutic use.

Drugs usually work in one of four ways:

1. To replace or act as substitutes for missing chemicals
2. To increase or stimulate certain cellular activities
3. To depress or slow cellular activities
4. To interfere with the functioning of foreign cells, such as invading microorganisms or neoplasms leading to cell death (drugs that act in this way are called **chemotherapeutic agents**).

Drugs can act in several different ways to achieve these results.

Receptor Sites

Many drugs are thought to act at specific areas on cell membranes called **receptor sites**. The receptor sites react with certain chemicals to cause an effect within the cell. In many situations, nearby enzymes break down the reacting chemicals and open the receptor site for further stimulation.

To better understand this process, think of how a key works in a lock. The specific chemical (the key) approaches a cell membrane and finds a perfect fit (the lock) at a receptor site (Figure 2.1). The interaction between the chemical and the receptor site affects enzyme systems within the cell. The activated enzyme systems then produce certain effects, such as increased or decreased cellular activity, changes in cell membrane permeability, or alterations in cellular metabolism.

Some drugs interact directly with receptor sites to cause the same activity that natural chemicals would cause at that site. These drugs are called *agonists* (Figure 2.1A). For example, insulin reacts with specific insulin-receptor sites to change cell membrane permeability, thus promoting the movement of glucose into the cell.

Other drugs act to prevent the breakdown of natural chemicals that are stimulating the receptor site. For example, monoamine oxidase (MAO) inhibitors block the breakdown of norepinephrine by the enzyme MAO. (Normally, MAO breaks down norepinephrine, removes it from the receptor site, and recycles the components to form new norepinephrine.) The blocking action of MAO inhibitors allows norepinephrine to stay on the receptor site, stimulating the cell longer and leading to prolonged norepinephrine effects. Those effects can be therapeutic (e.g., relieving depression) or adverse (e.g., increasing heart rate and blood pressure). Selective serotonin reuptake inhibitors work similarly to MAO inhibitors in that they also exert a blocking action. Specifically, they block removal of serotonin from the nerve synapse, allowing it to remain in the synapse longer, leading to further stimulation of receptor sites. This action leads to prolonged stimulation of certain brain cells, which is thought to provide relief from depression.

Some drugs react with receptor sites to block normal stimulation, producing no effect. For example, curare (a drug used on the tips of spears by inhabitants of the Amazon basin to paralyze prey and cause death) occupies receptor sites for acetylcholine, which is necessary for muscle contraction and movement. By blocking the action of acetylcholine at this receptor site, curare prevents muscle stimulation, causing paralysis. Curare is said to be a *competitive antagonist* of acetylcholine (Figure 2.1B).

Still other drugs react with specific receptor sites on a cell and, by reacting there, prevent the reaction of another chemical with a different receptor site on that cell. Such drugs are called *noncompetitive antagonists* (Figure 2.1C). For some drugs the actual mechanisms of action are unknown. Speculation exists, however, that many drugs use receptor site mechanisms to bring about their effects.

Drug–Enzyme Interactions

Drugs also can cause their effects by interfering with the enzyme systems that act as catalysts for various chemical reactions. Enzyme systems work in a cascade fashion, with one enzyme activating another, and then that enzyme activating another, until a cellular reaction eventually occurs. If a single step in one of the many enzyme systems is blocked, normal cell function is disrupted. Acetazolamide (*Diamox*) is a diuretic that blocks the enzyme carbonic anhydrase, which subsequently causes alterations in the hydrogen ion and water exchange system in the kidney, as well as in the eye.

Selective Toxicity

Ideally, all chemotherapeutic agents would act only on enzyme systems that are essential for the life of a pathogen

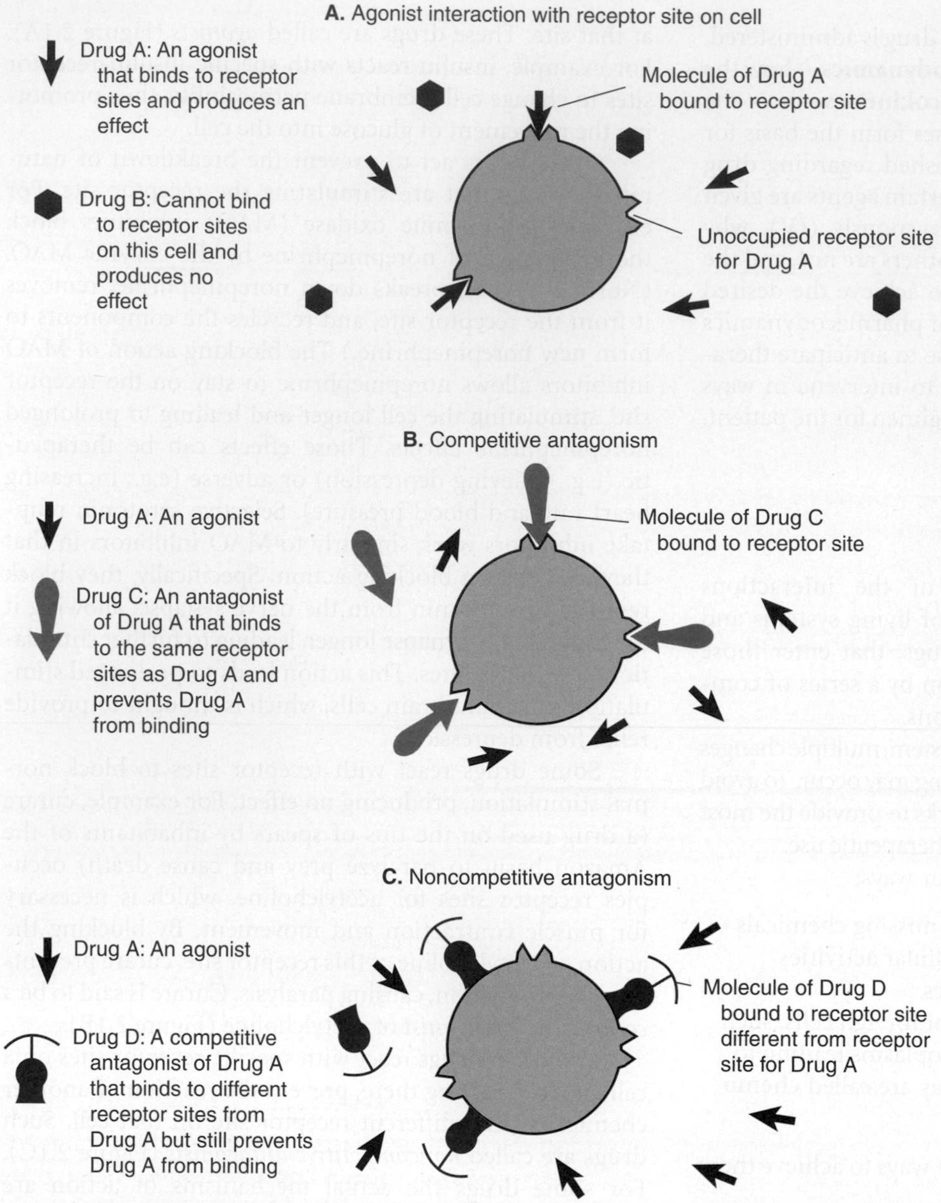
A. Agonist interaction with receptor site on cell
Drug A: An agonist that binds to receptor sites and produces an effect
Molecule of Drug A bound to receptor site
Drug B: Cannot bind to receptor sites on this cell and produces no effect
Unoccupied receptor site for Drug A
B. Competitive antagonism
Drug A: An agonist
Molecule of Drug C bound to receptor site
Drug C: An antagonist of Drug A that binds to the same receptor sites as Drug A and prevents Drug A from binding
C. Noncompetitive antagonism
Drug A: An agonist
Molecule of Drug D bound to receptor site different from receptor site for Drug A
Drug D: A competitive antagonist of Drug A that binds to different receptor sites from Drug A but still prevents Drug A from binding

FIGURE 2.1 Receptor theory of drug action. A. Agonist interaction with receptor site on cell. Molecules of drug A react with specific receptor sites on cells of effector organs and change the cells' activity. Competitive antagonism. **B.** Drug A and drug C have an affinity for the same receptor sites and compete for these sites; drug C has a greater affinity, occupies more of the sites, and antagonizes drug A. **C.** Noncompetitive antagonism. Drug D reacts with a receptor site that is different from the receptor site for drug A but still somehow prevents drug A from binding with its receptor sites. Drugs that act by inhibiting enzymes can be pictured as acting similarly to the receptor site antagonists illustrated in panels (B) and (C). Enzyme inhibitors block the binding of molecules of normal substrate to active sites on the enzyme.

or neoplastic cell and would not affect healthy cells. The ability of a drug to attack only those systems found in foreign cells is known as **selective toxicity**. Penicillin, an antibiotic used to treat bacterial infections, has selective toxicity. It affects an enzyme system unique to bacteria, causing bacterial cell death without disrupting normal human cell functioning.

Unfortunately, most other chemotherapeutic agents also destroy normal human cells, causing many of the adverse effects associated with antipathogen and antineoplastic chemotherapy. Cells that reproduce or are replaced rapidly (e.g., bone marrow cells, gastrointestinal [GI] cells, hair follicles) are more easily affected by these agents. Consequently, the goal of many chemotherapeutic regimens is to deliver a dose that will be toxic to the invading cells yet cause the least amount of toxicity to the host.

KEY POINTS

- Pharmacodynamics is the process by which a drug works or affects the body.
- Drugs may work by replacing a missing body chemical, by stimulating or depressing cellular activity, or by interfering with the functioning of foreign cells.
- Drugs are thought to work by reacting with specific receptor sites or by interfering with enzyme systems in the body.

Pharmacokinetics

Pharmacokinetics involves the study of absorption, distribution, metabolism (biotransformation), and excretion of drugs. In clinical practice, pharmacokinetic considerations include the onset of drug action (how long it will take to

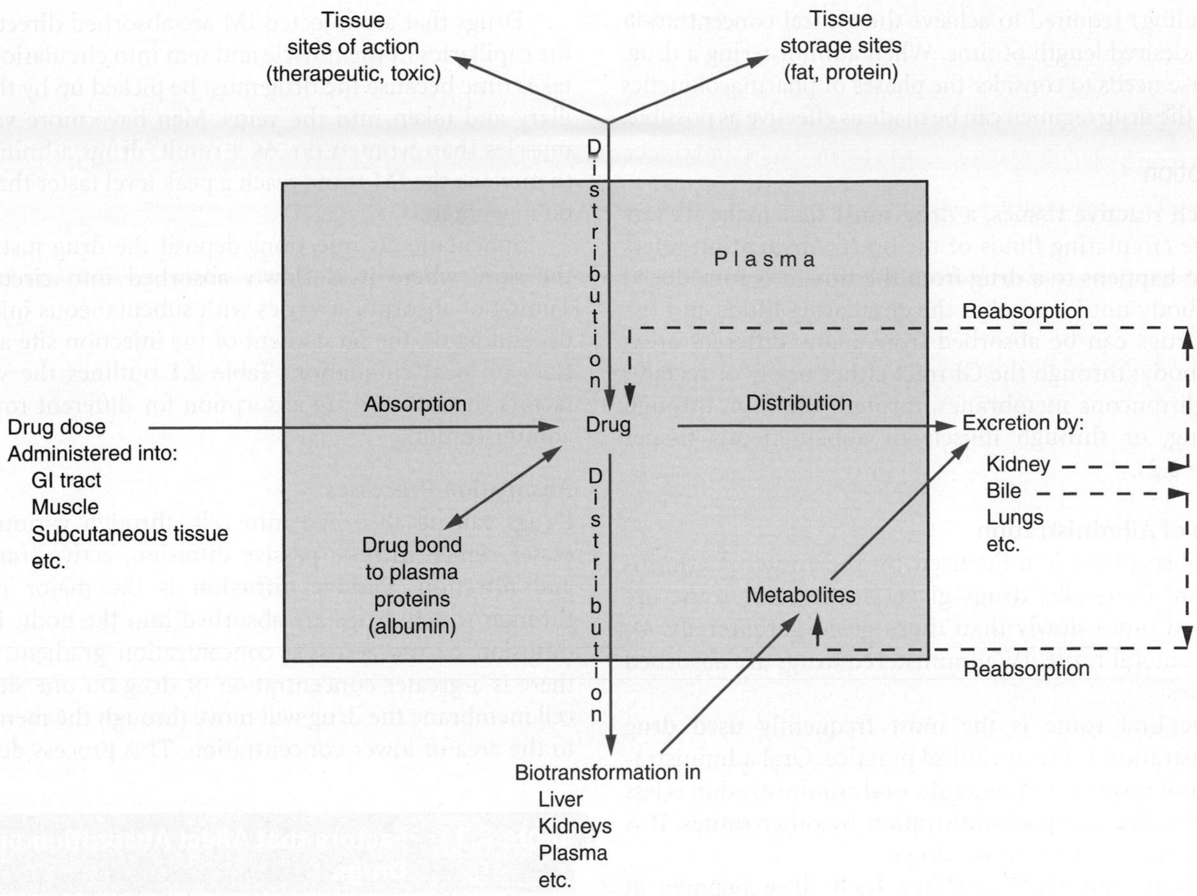

FIGURE 2.2 The processes by which a drug is handled by the body. *Dashed lines* indicate that some portion of a drug and its metabolites may be reabsorbed from the excretory organs. The dynamic equilibrium of pharmacokinetics is shown.

see the beginning of the therapeutic effect), drug half-life, timing of the peak effect (how long it will take to see the maximum effect of the drug), duration of drug effects (how long the patient will experience the drug effects), metabolism or biotransformation of the drug, and the site of excretion. Figure 2.2 outlines these processes, which are described in the following sections.

Critical Concentration

After a drug is administered, its molecules first must be absorbed into the body; then they make their way to the reactive tissues. If a drug is going to work properly on these reactive tissues, and thereby have a therapeutic effect, it must attain a sufficiently high concentration in the body. The amount of a drug that is needed to cause a therapeutic effect is called the **critical concentration.**

Drug evaluation studies determine the critical concentration required to cause a desired therapeutic effect. The recommended dose of a drug is based on the amount that must be given to eventually reach the critical concentration. Too much of a drug will produce toxic (poisonous) effects, and too little will not produce the desired therapeutic effects.

Loading Dose

Some drugs may take a prolonged period to reach a critical concentration. If their effects are needed quickly, a loading dose is recommended. Digoxin (*Lanoxin*)—a drug used to increase the strength of heart contractions—and many of the xanthine bronchodilators (e.g., aminophylline, theophylline) used to treat asthma attacks are often started with a **loading dose** (a higher dose than that usually used for treatment) to reach the critical concentration. The critical concentration then is maintained by using the recommended dosing schedule.

Dynamic Equilibrium

The actual concentration that a drug reaches in the body results from a dynamic equilibrium involving several processes:

- Absorption from the site of entry
- Distribution to the active site
- Biotransformation (metabolism) in the liver
- Excretion from the body

These processes are key elements in determining the amount of drug (dose) and the frequency of dose repetition (scheduling) required to achieve the critical concentration for the desired length of time. When administering a drug, the nurse needs to consider the phases of pharmacokinetics so that the drug regimen can be made as effective as possible.

Absorption

To reach reactive tissues, a drug must first make its way into the circulating fluids of the body. **Absorption** refers to what happens to a drug from the time it is introduced to the body until it reaches the circulating fluids and tissues. Drugs can be absorbed from many different areas in the body: through the GI tract either orally or rectally, through mucous membranes, through the skin, through the lung, or through muscle or subcutaneous tissues (Figure 2.2).

Routes of Administration

Drug absorption is influenced by the route of administration. Generally, drugs given by the oral route are absorbed more slowly than those given parenterally. Of the parenteral route, IV administered drugs are absorbed the fastest.

The oral route is the most frequently used drug administration route in clinical practice. Oral administration is not invasive and, as a rule, oral administration is less expensive than drug administration by other routes. It is also the safest way to deliver drugs.

Patients can easily continue their drug regimen at home when they are taking oral medications.

Oral administration subjects the drug to a number of barriers aimed at destroying ingested foreign chemicals. The acidic environment of the stomach is one of the first barriers to foreign chemicals. The acid breaks down many compounds and inactivates others. This fact is taken into account by pharmaceutical companies when preparing drugs in capsule or tablet form. The binders that are used often are designed to break down in a certain acidity and release the active drug to be absorbed.

When food is present, stomach acidity is higher and the stomach empties more slowly, thus exposing the drug to the acidic environment for a longer period. Certain foods that increase stomach acidity, such as milk products, alcohol, and protein, also speed the breakdown of many drugs. Other foods may chemically bind drugs or block their absorption. To decrease the effects of this acid barrier and the direct effects of certain foods, oral drugs ideally are to be given 1 hour before or 2 hours after a meal.

Some drugs that cannot survive in sufficient quantity when given orally are administered via injection directly into the body. Drugs that are injected IV reach their full strength at the time of injection, avoiding initial breakdown. Basically, these drugs have an immediate onset and are fully absorbed at administration because they directly enter the blood stream. These drugs are more likely to cause toxic effects because the margin for error in dose is much smaller.

Drugs that are injected IM are absorbed directly into the capillaries in the muscle and sent into circulation. This takes time because the drug must be picked up by the capillary and taken into the veins. Men have more vascular muscles than women do. As a result, drugs administered to men via the IM route reach a peak level faster than they do in women.

Subcutaneous injections deposit the drug just under the skin, where it is slowly absorbed into circulation. Timing of absorption varies with subcutaneous injection, depending on the fat content of the injection site and the state of local circulation. Table 2.1 outlines the various factors that affect drug absorption for different routes of administration.

Absorption Processes

Drugs can be absorbed into cells through various processes, which include passive diffusion, active transport, and filtration. **Passive diffusion** is the major process through which drugs are absorbed into the body. Passive diffusion occurs across a concentration gradient. When there is a greater concentration of drug on one side of a cell membrane the drug will move through the membrane to the area of lower concentration. This process does not

Table 2.1 Factors that Affect Absorption of Drugs

Route	Factors Affecting Absorption
Intravenous	None: direct entry into the venous system
Intramuscular	Perfusion or blood flow to the muscle Fat content of the muscle Temperature of the muscle: cold causes vasoconstriction and decreases absorption; heat causes vasodilation and increases absorption
Subcutaneous	Perfusion or blood flow to the tissue Fat content of the tissue Temperature of the tissue: cold causes vasoconstriction and decreases absorption; heat causes vasodilation and increases absorption
PO (oral)	Acidity of stomach Length of time in stomach Blood flow to gastrointestinal tract Presence of interacting foods or drugs
PR (rectal)	Perfusion or blood flow to the rectum Lesions in the rectum Length of time retained for absorption
Mucous membranes (sublingual, buccal)	Perfusion or blood flow to the area Integrity of the mucous membranes Presence of food or smoking Length of time retained in area
Topical (skin)	Perfusion or blood flow to the area Integrity of skin
Inhalation	Perfusion or blood flow to the area Integrity of lung lining Ability to administer drug properly

PO, oral perfusion; PR, rectal perfusion.

require any cellular energy. It occurs more quickly if the drug molecule is small, is soluble in water and in lipids (cell membranes are made of lipids and proteins—see Chapter 7), and has no electrical charge that could repel it from the cell membrane.

Unlike passive diffusion, **active transport** is a process that uses energy to actively move a molecule across a cell membrane. The molecule may be large, or it may be moving against a concentration gradient. This process is not very important in the absorption of most drugs, but it is often a very important process in drug excretion in the kidney.

Filtration involves movement through pores in the cell membrane, either down a concentration gradient or as a result of the pull of plasma proteins (when pushed by hydrostatic, blood, or osmotic pressure). Filtration is another process the body commonly uses in drug excretion.

Distribution

Distribution involves the movement of a drug to the body's tissues (Figure 2.2). As with absorption, factors that can affect distribution include the drug's lipid solubility and ionization and the perfusion of the reactive tissue.

For example, tissue perfusion is a factor in treating a patient with diabetes who has a lower-leg infection and needs antibiotics to destroy the bacteria in the area. In this case, systemic drugs may not be effective because part of the disease process involves changes in the vasculature and decreased blood flow to some areas, particularly the lower limbs. If there is not adequate blood flow to the area, little antibiotic can be delivered to the tissues, and little antibiotic effect will be seen.

In the same way, patients in a cold environment may have constricted blood vessels (vasoconstriction) in the extremities, which would prevent blood flow to those areas. The circulating blood would be unable to deliver drugs to those areas, and the patient would receive little therapeutic effect from drugs intended to react with those tissues.

Many drugs are bound to proteins and are not lipid soluble. These drugs cannot be distributed to the central nervous system (CNS) because of the effective blood–brain barrier (see later discussion), which is highly selective in allowing lipid-soluble substances to pass into the CNS.

Protein Binding

Most drugs are bound to some extent to proteins in the blood to be carried into circulation. The protein–drug complex is relatively large and cannot enter into capillaries and then into tissues to react. The drug must be freed from the protein's binding site at the tissues.

Some drugs are tightly bound and are released very slowly. These drugs have a very long duration of action because they are not free to be broken down or excreted. Therefore, they are released very slowly into the reactive tissue. Some drugs are loosely bound; they tend to act quickly and to be excreted quickly. Some drugs compete with each other for protein-binding sites, altering effectiveness or causing toxicity when the two drugs are given together.

Blood–Brain Barrier

The blood–brain barrier is a protective system of cellular activity that keeps many things (e.g., foreign invaders, poisons) away from the CNS. Drugs that are highly lipid soluble are more likely to pass through the blood–brain barrier and reach the CNS. Drugs that are not lipid soluble are not able to pass the blood–brain barrier. This is clinically significant in treating a brain infection with antibiotics. Almost all antibiotics are not lipid soluble and cannot cross the blood–brain barrier. Effective antibiotic treatment can occur only when the infection is severe enough to alter the blood–brain barrier and allow antibiotics to cross.

Although many drugs can cause adverse CNS effects, these are often the result of indirect drug effects and not the actual reaction of the drug with CNS tissue. For example, alterations in glucose levels and electrolyte changes can interfere with nerve functioning and produce CNS effects such as dizziness, confusion, or changes in thinking ability.

Placenta and Breast Milk

Many drugs readily pass through the placenta and affect the developing fetus in pregnant women. As stated earlier, it is best not to administer any drugs to pregnant women because of the possible risk to the fetus. Drugs should be given only when the benefit clearly outweighs any risk. Many other drugs are secreted into breast milk and therefore have the potential to affect the neonate. Because of this possibility the nurse must always check the ability of a drug to pass into breast milk when giving a drug to a breastfeeding mother. With the new regulations, prescribing information will eventually state the risk of drugs passing into breast milk.

Biotransformation (Metabolism)

The body is well prepared to deal with a myriad of foreign chemicals. Enzymes in the liver, in many cells, in the lining of the GI tract, and even circulating in the body detoxify foreign chemicals to protect the fragile homeostasis that keeps the body functioning (Figure 2.2). Almost all of the chemical reactions that the body uses to convert drugs and other chemicals into nontoxic substances are based on a few processes that work to make the chemical less active and more easily excreted from the body.

The liver is the most important site of drug metabolism, or biotransformation, the process by which drugs are changed into new, less active chemicals. Think of the liver as a sewage treatment plant. Everything that is absorbed from the GI tract first enters the liver to be "treated." The liver detoxifies many chemicals and uses others to produce needed enzymes and structures.

First-Pass Effect

Drugs that are taken orally are usually absorbed from the small intestine directly into the portal venous system (the blood vessels that flow through the liver on their way back to the heart). Aspirin and alcohol are two drugs that are known to be absorbed from the lower end of the stomach. The portal veins deliver these absorbed molecules into the liver, which immediately transforms most of the chemicals delivered to it by a series of liver enzymes. These enzymes break the drug into metabolites, some of which are active and cause effects in the body, and some of which are deactivated and can be readily excreted from the body. As a result, a large percentage of the oral dose is destroyed at this point and never reaches the tissues. This phenomenon is known as the **first-pass effect**. The portion of the drug that gets through the first-pass effect is delivered to the circulatory system for transport throughout the body.

Injected drugs and drugs absorbed from sites other than the GI tract undergo a similar biotransformation when they pass through the liver. Because some of the active drug already has had a chance to reach the reactive tissues before reaching the liver the injected drug is often more effective at a lower dose than the oral equivalent. Thus, the recommended dose for oral drugs can be considerably higher than the recommended dose for parenteral drugs, taking the first-pass effect into account.

Hepatic Enzyme System

The intracellular structures of the hepatic cells are lined with enzymes packed together in what is called the **hepatic microsomal system**. Because orally administered drugs enter the liver first, the enzyme systems immediately work on the absorbed drug to biotransform it. As explained earlier, this first-pass effect is responsible for neutralizing most of the drugs that are taken. Phase I biotransformation involves oxidation, reduction, or hydrolysis of the drug via the cytochrome P450 system of enzymes. These enzymes are found in most cells but are especially abundant in the liver. Table 2.2 gives some examples of drugs that induce or inhibit the cytochrome P450 system. Phase II biotransformation usually involves a conjugation reaction that makes the drug more polar and more readily excreted by the kidneys.

The presence of a chemical that is metabolized by a particular enzyme system often increases the activity of that enzyme system. This process is referred to as **enzyme induction**. Only a few basic enzyme systems are responsible for metabolizing most of the chemicals that pass through the liver. Increased activity in an enzyme system speeds the metabolism of the drug that caused the enzyme induction, as well as any other drug that is metabolized via that same enzyme system. This explains why some drugs cannot be taken together effectively. The presence of one drug speeds the metabolism of others, preventing them from reaching their therapeutic levels. Some drugs inhibit an enzyme system, making it less effective. As a consequence, any drug that is metabolized by that system will not be broken down for excretion, and the blood levels of that drug will increase, often to toxic levels. These actions also explain why liver disease is often a contraindication or a reason to use caution when administering certain drugs. If the liver is not functioning effectively the drug will not be metabolized as it should be, and toxic levels could develop rather quickly.

Table 2.2 Examples of Drugs that Alter the Effects of the Cytochrome P450 Hepatic Enzyme System

Drugs that Induce or Increase Activity	Drugs that Inhibit or Decrease Activity
Nicotine (cigarette smoking) Alcohol (drinking) Glucocorticoids (cortisone, others)	Ketoconazole (*Nizoral*) Mexiletine (generic) Quinidine (generic)

Excretion

Excretion is the removal of a drug from the body. The skin, saliva, lungs, bile, and feces are some of the routes used to excrete drugs. The kidneys, however, play the most important role in drug excretion (Figure 2.2).

Drugs that have been made water soluble in the liver are often readily excreted from the kidney by **glomerular filtration**—the passage of water and water-soluble components from the plasma into the renal tubule. Other drugs are secreted or reabsorbed through the renal tubule by active transport systems. The active transport systems that move the drug into the tubule often do so by exchanging it for acid or bicarbonate molecules. Therefore, the acidity of urine can play an important role in drug excretion. This concept is important to

FOCUS ON Safe Medication Administration

The liver is very important in metabolizing drugs in the body, and the kidneys are responsible for a large part of the excretion of drugs from the body. One should get into the habit of always checking a patient's liver and renal function before a patient starts a drug regimen. If the liver is not functioning properly the drug may not be metabolized correctly and may reach toxic levels in the body. If the kidneys are not functioning properly the drug may not be excreted properly and could accumulate in the body. Dose adjustment needs to be considered if a patient has problems with either the liver or the kidneys.

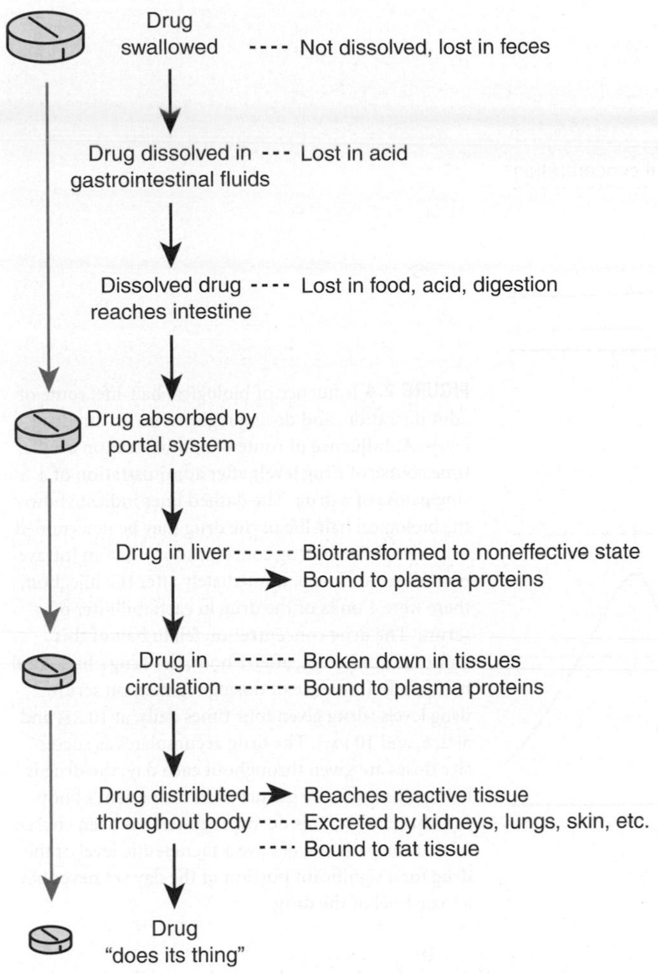

FIGURE 2.3 Pharmacokinetics affects the amount of a drug that reaches reactive tissues. Very little of an oral dose of a drug actually reaches reactive sites.

remember when trying to clear a drug rapidly from the system or trying to understand why a drug is being given at the usual dose but is reaching toxic levels in the system. One should always consider the patient's kidney function and urine acidity before administering a drug. Kidney dysfunction can lead to toxic levels of a drug in the body because the drug cannot be excreted. Figure 2.3 outlines the pharmacokinetic processes that occur when a drug is administered orally.

Half-Life

The **half-life** of a drug is the time it takes for the amount of drug in the body to decrease to one half of the peak level it previously achieved. For instance, if a patient takes 20 mg of a drug with a half-life of 2 hours, 10 mg of the drug will remain 2 hours after administration. Two hours later, 5 mg will be left (one half of the previous level); in 2 more hours, only 2.5 mg will remain. This information is important in determining the appropriate timing for a drug dose or determining the duration of a drug's effect on the body. (See Box 2.1.)

BOX 2.1 FOCUS ON Calculations

DETERMINING THE IMPACT OF HALF-LIFE ON DRUG LEVELS

A patient is taking a drug that has a half-life of 12 hours. You are trying to determine when a 50-mg dose of the drug will be gone from the body:

- In 12 hours, half of the 50 mg (25 mg) would be in the body.
- In another 12 hours (24 hours), half of 25 mg (12.5 mg) would remain in the body.
- After 36 hours, half of 12.5 mg (6.25 mg) would remain.
- After 48 hours, half of 6.25 mg (3.125 mg) would remain.
- After 60 hours, half of 3.125 (1.56 mg) would remain.
- After 72 hours, half of 1.56 (0.78 mg) would remain.
- After 84 hours, half of 0.78 (0.39 mg) would remain.
- Twelve more hours (for a total of 96 hours) would reduce the drug amount to 0.195 mg.
- Finally, 12 more hours (108 hours) would reduce the amount of the drug in the body to 0.097 mg, which would be quite negligible.
- Therefore, it would take 4½ to 5 days to clear the drug from the body.

The absorption rate, the distribution to the tissues, the speed of biotransformation, and how fast a drug is excreted are all taken into consideration when determining the half-life of the drug. The half-life that is indicated in any drug monograph is the half-life for a healthy person. Using this information, one can estimate the half-life of a drug for a patient with kidney or liver dysfunction (which could prolong the biotransformation and the time required for excretion of a drug), allowing the prescriber to make changes in the dosing schedule.

The timing of drug administration is important to achieve the most effective drug therapy. Nurses can use their knowledge of drug half-life to explain the importance of following a schedule of drug administration in the hospital or at home. Figure 2.4 shows the effects of drug administration on the critical concentration of a drug.

KEY POINTS

- Pharmacokinetics is the study of how the body deals with a drug.
- The concentration of a drug in the body is determined by the balance of absorption, distribution, metabolism, and excretion of the drug.
- In determining the amount, route, and appropriate timing of a drug dose, the pharmacokinetics of that drug has to be considered.

Factors Influencing Drug Effects

When administering a drug to a patient, the nurse must be aware that the human factor has a tremendous influence on what actually happens to a drug when it enters

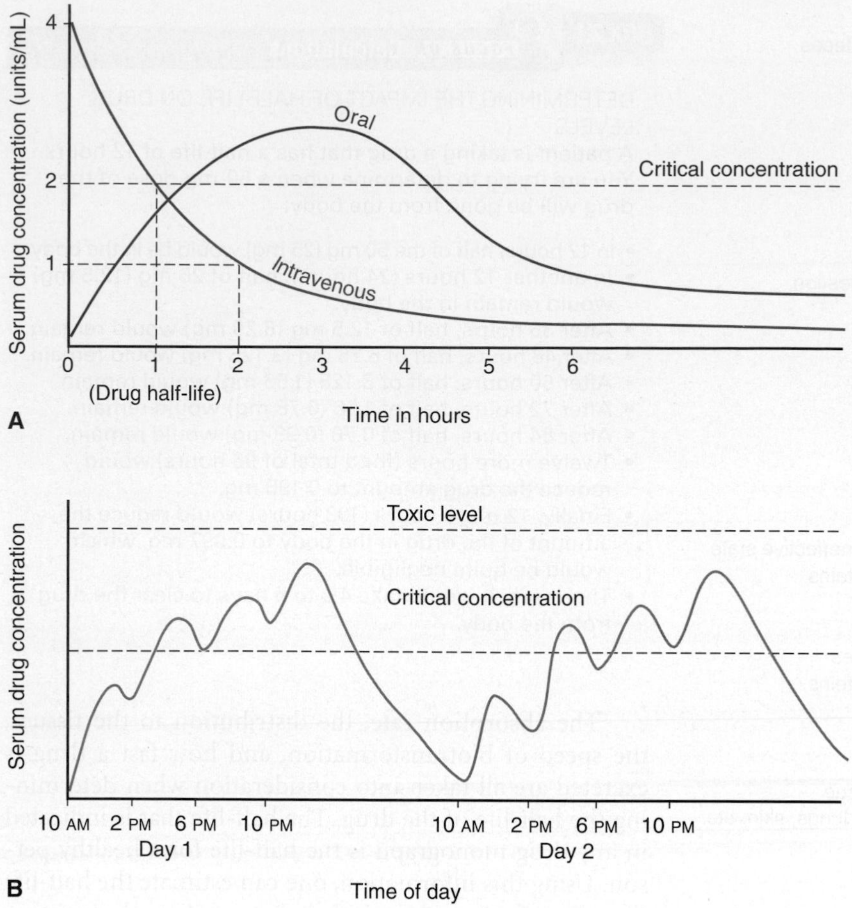

FIGURE 2.4 Influence of biological half-life, route of administration, and dosing regimen on serum drug levels. **A.** Influence of route of administration on the time course of drug levels after administration of a single dose of a drug. The dashed lines indicate how the biological half-life of the drug may be determined from the curve of drug concentration after an intravenous dose. At time 0, immediately after the injection, there were 4 units of the drug in each milliliter of serum. The drug concentration fell to half of this amount, 2 units/mL, after 1 hour, the drug's biological half-life. **B.** Influence of dosing regimen on serum drug levels (drug given four times daily, at 10 AM and at 2, 6, and 10 PM). The drug accumulates as successive doses are given throughout each day; the drug is being given at a rate greater than the patient's body can eliminate it. This dosing regimen has been chosen so that the patient will have a therapeutic level of the drug for a significant portion of the day yet never have a toxic level of the drug.

the body. No two people react in exactly the same way to any given drug. Even though textbooks and drug guides explain the pharmacodynamics and pharmacokinetics of a drug, it must be remembered that much of that information is based on controlled studies of both healthy adults and patients. Circumstances may be very different in the clinical setting. Consequently, before administering any drug, the nurse must consider a number of factors. These are discussed in detail in the following sections and summarized in Box 2.2.

Weight

The recommended dose of a drug is based on drug evaluation studies and is targeted at a 150-pound person. People who are much heavier may require larger doses to get a therapeutic effect from a drug because they have increased tissues to perfuse and increased receptor sites in some reactive tissue. People who weigh less than the norm may require smaller doses of a drug. Toxic effects may occur at the recommended dose if the person is very small.

Age

Age is a factor primarily in children and older adults. Children are not just little adults. Children metabolize many drugs differently than adults do, and they have immature systems for handling drugs. Many drugs come with recommended pediatric doses, and others can be converted to pediatric doses using one of several conversion formulas (Box 2.3).

BOX 2.2

Factors Affecting the Body's Response to a Drug

Weight
Age
Gender
Physiological factors—diurnal rhythm, electrolyte balance, acid–base balance, hydration
Pathological factors—disease, hepatic dysfunction, renal dysfunction, gastrointestinal dysfunction, vascular disorders, low blood pressure
Genetic factors
Immunological factors—allergy
Psychological factors—placebo effect, health beliefs, compliance
Environmental factors—temperature, light, noise
Drug tolerance
Cumulation effects
Interactions

BOX 2.3 FOCUS ON Calculations

PEDIATRIC DOSES

Children often require different doses of drugs than adults because children's bodies often handle drugs very differently from adults' bodies. The "standard" drug doses listed in package inserts and references such as the *Physician's Desk Reference* (*PDR*) refer to the adult dose. In some cases a pediatric dose is suggested, but in many cases it will need to be calculated based on the child's age, weight, or body surface. The following are some standard formulas for calculating the pediatric dose.

Fried's Rule

$$\text{infant's dose } (<1 \text{ year}) = \frac{\text{infant's age (in months)}}{150 \text{ months}} \times \text{average adult dose}$$

Young's Rule

$$\text{child's dose } (1\text{–}12 \text{ year}) = \frac{\text{child's age (in years)}}{\text{child's age (in years)} + 12} \times \text{average adult dose}$$

The surface area of a child is determined using a nomogram that determines surface area based on height and weight measurements.

Pediatric dose calculations should be checked by two persons. Many institutions have procedures for double-checking the dose calculation of those drugs (e.g., digoxin) used most frequently in the pediatric area.

Clark's Rule

$$\text{child's dose} = \frac{\text{weight of child (in pounds)}}{150} \times \text{average adult dose}$$

Surface Area Rule

$$\text{child's dose} = \frac{\text{surface area of child (in square meters)}}{1.73} \times \text{average adult dose}$$

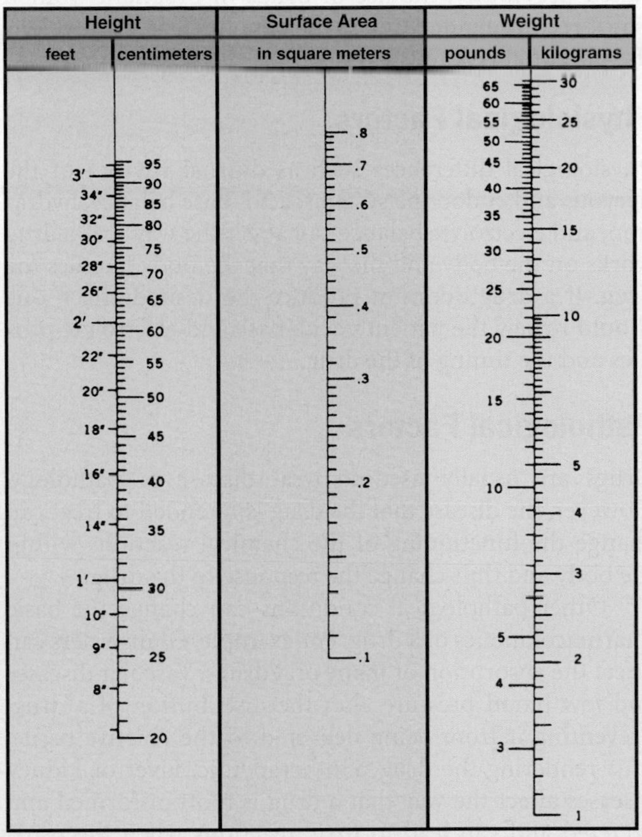

Nomogram for estimating surface area of infants and young children. To determine the surface area of the patient, draw a straight line between the point representing the height on the left vertical scale and the point representing the weight on the right vertical scale. The point at which this line intersects the middle vertical scale represents the patient's surface area in square meters.

Older adults undergo many physical changes that are a part of the aging process. They are more likely to be taking multiple drugs for various conditions. Their bodies may respond very differently in all aspects of pharmacokinetics—less effective absorption, less efficient distribution because of fewer plasma proteins and less efficient perfusion, altered biotransformation or metabolism of drugs because of age-related liver changes, and less effective excretion owing to less efficient kidneys. Many drugs now come with recommended doses for patients who are older. The doses of other drugs also may need to be decreased for the older adult.

When administering drugs to a patient at either end of the age spectrum, one should monitor the patient closely for the desired effects. If the effects are not what would normally be expected, one should consider the need for a dose adjustment.

Gender

Physiological differences between men and women can influence a drug's effect. When giving IM injections, for example, it is important to remember that men have more vascular muscles, so the effects of the drug will be seen sooner in men than in women.

Women have more fat cells than men do, so drugs that deposit in fat may be slowly released and cause effects for a prolonged period. For example, gas anesthetics have an affinity for depositing in fat and can cause drowsiness and sedation sometimes weeks after surgery.

Women who are given any drug should always be questioned about the possibility of pregnancy because, as stated previously, the use of drugs in pregnant women is not recommended unless the benefit clearly outweighs the potential risk to the fetus.

Physiological Factors

Physiological differences such as diurnal rhythm of the nervous and endocrine systems, acid–base balance, hydration, and electrolyte balance can affect the way that a drug works on the body and the way that the body handles the drug. If a drug does not produce the desired effect, one should review the patient's acid–base and electrolyte profiles and the timing of the drug.

Pathological Factors

Drugs are usually used to treat disease or pathology. However, the disease that the drug is intended to treat can change the functioning of the chemical reactions within the body and thus change the response to the drug.

Other pathological conditions can change the basic pharmacokinetics of a drug. For example, GI disorders can affect the absorption of many oral drugs. Vascular diseases and low blood pressure alter the distribution of a drug, preventing it from being delivered to the reactive tissue, thus rendering the drug nontherapeutic. Liver or kidney diseases affect the way that a drug is biotransformed and excreted and can lead to toxic reactions when the usual dose is given.

Genetic Factors

Genetic differences can sometimes explain patients' varied responses to a given drug. Some people lack certain enzyme systems necessary for metabolizing a drug, whereas others have overactive enzyme systems that cause drugs to be broken down more quickly. Still others have differing metabolisms or slightly different enzymatic makeups that alter their chemical reactions and the effects of a given drug.

Predictable differences in the pharmacokinetics and pharmacodynamic effects of drugs can be anticipated with people of particular cultural backgrounds because of their genetic makeup. **Pharmacogenomics** is a new area of study that explores the unique differences in response to drugs that each individual possesses based on genetic makeup. The mapping of the human genome has accelerated research in this area. It is thought that, in the future, medical care and drug regimens could be individually designed based on each person's unique genetic makeup. Trastuzumab (*Herceptin*) (see Chapter 17) is a drug that was developed to treat breast cancer when the tumor expresses human epidermal growth factor receptor 2—a genetic defect seen in some tumors. The drug has no effect on tumors that do not express that genetic defect. This drug was developed as a personalized or targeted medicine based on genetic factors. Such differences are highlighted throughout this book. In late 2007 the U.S. Food and Drug Administration approved a blood test to check for specific genetic markers that would indicate that a patient would metabolize warfarin (*Coumadin*), an oral anticoagulant, differently than the standard patient. The test will give the prescriber information that would change the dosing schedule for the drug and could save the patient many adverse effects while achieving the therapeutic dose for that patient.

Immunological Factors

People can develop an allergy to a drug. After exposure to its proteins, a person can develop antibodies to a drug. With future exposure to the same drug, that person may experience a full-blown allergic reaction. Sensitivity to a drug can range from mild (e.g., dermatological reactions such as a rash) to more severe (e.g., anaphylaxis, shock, and death). (Drug allergies are discussed in detail in Chapter 3.)

Psychological Factors

The patient's attitude about a drug has been shown to have an effect on how that drug works. A drug is more likely to be effective if the patient thinks it will work than if the patient believes it will not work. This is called the **placebo effect**.

The patient's personality also influences compliance with the drug regimen. Some people who believe that they can influence their health actively seek health care and willingly follow a prescribed regimen. These people usually trust the medical system and believe that their efforts will be positive. Other people do not trust the medical system. They may believe that they have no control over their health and may be unwilling to comply with any prescribed therapy. Knowing a patient's health-seeking history and feelings about health care is important in planning an educational program that will work for that patient. It is also important to know this information when arranging for necessary follow-up procedures and evaluations.

As the caregiver most often involved in drug administration the nurse is in a position to influence the patient's attitude about drug effectiveness. Frequently, the nurse's positive attitude, combined with additional comfort measures, can improve the patient's response to a medication.

Environmental Factors

The environment can affect the success of drug therapy. Some drug effects are enhanced by a quiet, cool, nonstimulating environment. For example, sedating drugs are given to help a patient relax or to decrease tension. Reducing external stimuli to decrease tension and stimulation help the drug be more effective. Other drug effects may be influenced by temperature. For example, antihypertensives that work well during cold, winter months may become too effective in warmer environments, when natural vasodilation may lead to a release of heat that tends to lower the blood pressure. If a patient's response to a medication is not as expected, look for possible changes in environmental conditions.

Tolerance

The body may develop a tolerance to some drugs over time. Tolerance may arise because of increased biotransformation of the drug, increased resistance to its effects, or other pharmacokinetic factors. When tolerance occurs the drug no longer causes the same reaction. Therefore, increasingly larger doses are needed to achieve a therapeutic effect. An example is morphine, an opiate used for pain relief. The longer morphine is taken, the more tolerant the body becomes to the drug, so that larger and larger doses are needed to relieve pain. Clinically, this situation can be avoided by giving the drug in smaller doses or in combination with other drugs that may also relieve pain. Cross-tolerance—or resistance to drugs within the same class or similar classes—may also occur in some situations.

Cumulation

If a drug is taken in successive doses at intervals that are shorter than recommended, or if the body is unable to eliminate a drug properly, the drug can accumulate in the body, leading to toxic levels and adverse effects. This can be avoided by following the drug regimen precisely. In reality, with many people managing their therapy at home, strict compliance with a drug regimen seldom occurs. Some people take all of their medications first thing in the morning, so that they won't forget to take the pills later in the day. Others realize that they forgot a dose and then take two to make up for it. Many interruptions of everyday life can interfere with strict adherence to a drug regimen. If a drug is causing serious adverse effects, review the drug regimen with the patient to find out how the drug is being taken, and then educate the patient appropriately.

Interactions

When two or more drugs or substances are taken together, there is a possibility that an interaction can occur, causing unanticipated effects in the body. Alternative therapies, such as herbal products, act as drugs in the body and can cause these same interactions. Certain foods can interact with drugs in much the same way. Usually, this is an increase or decrease in the desired therapeutic effect of one or all of the drugs or an increase in adverse effects.

Drug–Drug or Drug–Alternative Therapy Interactions

Clinically significant drug–drug interactions occur with drugs that have small margins of safety. If there is very little difference between a therapeutic dose and a toxic dose of the drug, interference with the drug's pharmacokinetics or pharmacodynamics can produce serious problems. For example, drug–drug interactions can occur in the following situations:

- *At the site of absorption:* One drug prevents or accelerates absorption of the other drug. For example, the antibiotic tetracycline is not absorbed from the GI tract if calcium or calcium products (milk) are present in the stomach.
- *During distribution:* One drug competes for the protein-binding site of another drug, so the second drug cannot be transported to the reactive tissue. For example, aspirin competes with the drug methotrexate (*Rheumatrex*) for protein-binding sites. Because aspirin is more competitive for the sites the methotrexate is bumped off, resulting in increased release of methotrexate and increased toxicity to the tissues.
- *During biotransformation:* One drug stimulates or blocks the metabolism of the other drug. For example, warfarin (*Coumadin*), an oral anticoagulant, is biotransformed more quickly if it is taken at the same time as barbiturates, rifampin, or many other drugs. Because the warfarin is biotransformed to an inactive state more quickly, higher doses will be needed to achieve the desired effect. Patients who use St. John's wort may experience altered effectiveness of several drugs that are affected by that herb's effects on the liver. Digoxin, theophylline, oral contraceptives, anticancer drugs, drugs used to treat HIV, and antidepressants are all reported to have serious interactions with St. John's wort.
- *During excretion:* One drug competes for excretion with the other drug, leading to accumulation and toxic effects of one of the drugs. For example, digoxin (*Lanoxin*) and quinidine are both excreted from the same sites in the kidney. If they are given together the quinidine is more competitive for these sites and is excreted, resulting in increased serum levels of digoxin, which cannot be excreted.
- *At the site of action:* One drug may be an antagonist of the other drug or may cause effects that oppose those of the other drug, leading to no therapeutic effect. This is seen, for example, when an antihypertensive drug is taken with an antiallergy drug that also increases blood pressure. The effects on blood pressure are negated, and there is a loss of the antihypertensive effectiveness of the drug. If a patient is taking antidiabetic medication and also takes the herb ginseng, which lowers blood glucose levels, he or she may experience episodes of hypoglycemia and loss of blood glucose control.

Whenever two or more drugs are being given together, first consult a drug guide for a listing of clinically significant drug–drug interactions. Sometimes problems can be avoided by staggering the administration of the drugs or adjusting their doses. (See the Critical Thinking Scenario.)

Drug–Food Interactions

For the most part a drug–food interaction occurs when the drug and the food are in direct contact in the stomach. Some foods increase acid production, speeding the breakdown of the drug molecule and preventing absorption and distribution of the drug. Some foods chemically react with

CRITICAL THINKING SCENARIO

Drug Interactions

THE SITUATION

R.D. is a 68-year-old male from Wisconsin, who has now lived in his Florida home for 6 months. He has a history of hyperlipidemia and was started on treatment with atorvastatin (*Lipitor*), combined with a diet and exercise regimen 6 weeks ago. He has lowered his lipid levels to the upper level of normal. He comes into the clinic complaining of low-grade fever and severe muscle pain.

Critical Thinking

What are the important nursing implications in this case?
What are the effects of this drug and what issues should be considered?
What specific issues should be discussed?
What teaching points need to be clarified?

Discussion

When a person presents with new signs and symptoms it is important to do a complete history and physical and to do a thorough drug history. Dealing with the chief complaint is the patient's highest priority and should be the initial focus when dealing with the patient. Ensure the patient's comfort and arrange for any additional tests that might be needed. In this situation, looking up atorvastatin shows that rhabdomyolysis is a potentially serious adverse effect associated with the use of atorvastatin, a lipid lowering drug known as a hydroxymethylglutaryl (HMG) coenzyme A inhibitor. Rhabdomyolysis is a disease of muscle breakdown and presents with low-grade fever and acute muscle pain. In severe cases it can lead to renal failure and even death. Could this have happened after 6 weeks, or could something else be involved? Further reading about this drug shows that it cannot be combined with many other prescription drugs (which he denies using) or with grapefruit juice, which will block the biotransformation of the drug and lead to potentially toxic atorvastatin levels. R.D.'s blood tests reveal high creatine kinase levels, consistent with the diagnosis of rhabdomyolysis.

Discussing the drug therapy with R.D. needs to include an explanation of what seems to have happened to him. Encourage him to present when he experiences these signs and symptoms. Reviewing the need to avoid grapefruit juice reveals that he did not understand his previous instructions. He has been drinking a lot of grapefruit juice because he has a grapefruit tree on his patio, but he never takes the drug with grapefruit juice. He always takes the pill with water and then has the grapefruit juice later. This is a common misunderstanding when telling patients not to take a drug with grapefruit juice. The nurse should explain that this is a common misunderstanding and that it takes 48 hours to clear the chemical in grapefruit juice that interferes with atorvastatin, so he really should not drink grapefruit juice at all. This leads to a discussion about other ways to treat his hyperlipidemia because he really enjoys his fresh grapefruit juice and does not want to give it up. By listening to the patient's needs and priorities, the health care team begins a plan to help him lower his lipids safely while still allowing him to enjoy his favorite Florida beverage.

NURSING CARE GUIDE FOR R.D.

Assessment: History and Examination

Allergies to any drugs
Use of any over-the-counter (OTC) drugs or herbal therapies
CNS: affect, reflexes
Musculoskeletal: ROM (range of motion)
CV: P, BP
Hematological: lipid levels, creatine kinase

Nursing Diagnoses

Acute pain related to muscle breakdown effects
Deficient knowledge related to drug therapy

Planning

When leaving the clinic, the patient will have a good understanding of his drug therapy and will have means of adjusting his lifestyle to keep his lipids lowered.

Interventions

Provide patient teaching regarding drug effects, safe use of the drug, ways to avoid adverse effects.

Provide referral for evaluation of other drugs available to help keep lipids lowered

Evaluation

Monitor for adverse effects related to drug therapy

Monitor effectiveness of referral for alternate therapy.

Patient Teaching

- Atorvastatin has been prescribed to help keep your lipid levels in a normal range. This drug must be combined with diet and exercise to be most effective. It should be taken with the evening meal to be most effective.

Drug Interactions (continued)

- Common adverse effects you might experience include headache, abdominal pain, constipation, nausea.
- Serious adverse effects that may occur include liver damage (report changes in color of urine or stool, extreme fatigue), rhabdomyolysis (report acute muscle pain with fever).
- This drug cannot be combined with many other drugs. Always report the addition of any other drug to your drug regimen, this includes OTC drugs and herbal therapies.
- This drug cannot be combined with grapefruit juice. The chemical in grapefruit juice that affects atorvastatin stays in the body for 48 hours so when on this drug you should not use any grapefruit juice.
- We will be arranging for a referral to discuss changing your lipid lowering plans so that you will be able to enjoy your grapefruit juice. Please continue your current therapy and avoid all grapefruit juice until that appointment.

FOCUS ON Safe Medication Administration

Always check the monograph of any drug that is being given to monitor for clinically important drug–drug, drug–alternative therapy, or drug–food interactions.

certain drugs and prevent their absorption into the body. The antibiotic tetracycline cannot be taken with iron products for this reason. Tetracycline also binds with calcium to some extent and should not be taken with foods or other drugs containing calcium. Grapefruit juice has been found to affect liver enzyme systems for up to 48 hours after it has been ingested. This can result in increased or decreased serum levels of certain drugs. Many drugs come with the warning that they should not be combined with grapefruit juice. This drug–food interaction does not take place in the stomach, so grapefruit juice needs to be avoided the entire time the drug is being used, not just while the drug is in the stomach.

In most cases, oral drugs are best taken on an empty stomach. If the patient cannot tolerate the drug on an empty stomach the food selected for ingestion with the drug should be something that is known not to interact with it. Drug monographs usually list important drug–food interactions and give guidelines for avoiding problems and optimizing the drug's therapeutic effects.

Drug–Laboratory Test Interactions

As explained previously, the body works through a series of chemical reactions. Because of this, administration of a particular drug may alter results of tests that are done on various chemical levels or reactions as part of a diagnostic study. This drug–laboratory test interaction is caused by the drug being given and not necessarily by a change in the body's responses or actions. Keep these interactions in mind when evaluating a patient's diagnostic tests. If one test result is altered and does not fit in with the clinical picture or other test results, consider the possibility of a drug–laboratory test interference. For example, dalteparin (*Fragmin*), a low-molecular-weight heparin used to prevent deep vein thrombosis after abdominal surgery, may cause increased levels of the liver enzymes aspartate aminotransferase and alanine aminotransferase with no injury to liver cells or hepatitis.

Optimal Therapeutic Effect

As overwhelming as all of this information may seem, most patients can follow a drug regimen to achieve optimal therapeutic effects without serious adverse effects. Avoiding problems is the best way to treat adverse or ineffective drug effects. One should incorporate basic history and physical assessment factors into any plan of care so that obvious problems can be spotted and handled promptly. In the patient-centered approach to care the nurse needs to also consider cultural, emotional, psychological, and environmental factors. If a drug just does not do what it is expected to do, further examine the factors that are known to influence drug effects (Box 2.2). Frequently, the drug regimen can be modified to deal with that influence. Rarely is it necessary to completely stop a needed drug regimen because of adverse or intolerable effects. In many cases the nurse is the caregiver in the best position to assess problems early.

SUMMARY

- Pharmacodynamics is the study of the way that drugs affect the body.
- Most drugs work by replacing natural chemicals, by stimulating normal cell activity, or by depressing normal cell activity.
- Chemotherapeutic agents work by interfering with normal cell functioning, causing cell death. The most desirable chemotherapeutic agents are those with selective toxicity to foreign cells and foreign cell activities.
- Drugs frequently act at specific receptor sites on cell membranes to stimulate enzyme systems within the cell and to alter the cell's activities.

- Pharmacokinetics—the study of the way the body deals with drugs—includes absorption, distribution, biotransformation, and excretion of drugs.
- The goal of established dosing schedules is to achieve a critical concentration of the drug in the body. This critical concentration is the amount of the drug necessary to achieve the drug's therapeutic effects.
- Arriving at a critical concentration involves a dynamic equilibrium among the processes of drug absorption, distribution, metabolism or biotransformation, and excretion.
- Absorption involves moving a drug into the body for circulation. Oral drugs are absorbed from the small intestine, undergo many changes, and are affected by many things in the process. IV drugs are injected directly into the circulation and do not need additional absorption.
- Drugs are distributed to various tissues throughout the body depending on their solubility and ionization. Most drugs are bound to plasma proteins for transport to reactive tissues.
- Drugs are metabolized or biotransformed into less toxic chemicals by various enzyme systems in the body. The liver is the primary site of drug metabolism or biotransformation. The liver uses the cytochrome P450 enzyme system to alter the drug and start its biotransformation.
- The first-pass effect is the breakdown of oral drugs in the liver immediately after absorption. Drugs given by other routes often reach reactive tissues before passing through the liver for biotransformation.
- Drug excretion is removal of the drug from the body. This occurs mainly through the kidneys.
- The half-life of a drug is the period of time it takes for an amount of drug in the body to decrease to one half of the peak level it previously achieved. The half-life is affected by all aspects of pharmacokinetics. Knowing the half-life of a drug helps in predicting dosing schedules and duration of effects.
- The actual effects of a drug are determined by its pharmacokinetics, its pharmacodynamics, and many human factors that can change the drug's effectiveness.
- To provide the safest and most effective drug therapy the nurse must consider all of the possible factors that influence drug concentration and effectiveness.

CHECK YOUR UNDERSTANDING

Answers to the questions in this chapter can be found in Answers to Check Your Understanding Questions on thePoint®.

MULTIPLE CHOICE

Select the best answer to the following.

1. Chemotherapeutic agents are drugs that
a. are used only to treat cancers.
b. replace normal body chemicals that are missing because of disease.
c. interfere with foreign cell functioning causing cell death, such as invading microorganisms or neoplasms.
d. stimulate the normal functioning of a cell.

2. Receptor sites
a. are a normal part of enzyme substrates.
b. are protein areas on cell membranes that react with specific chemicals.
c. can usually be stimulated by many different chemicals.
d. are responsible for all drug effects in the body.

3. Selective toxicity is
a. the ability of a drug to seek out a specific bacterial species or microorganism.
b. the ability of a drug to cause only specific adverse effects.
c. the ability of a drug to cause fetal damage.
d. the ability of a drug to attack only those systems found in foreign or abnormal cells.

4. When trying to determine why the desired therapeutic effect is not being seen with an oral drug the nurse should consider
a. the blood flow to muscle beds.
b. food altering the makeup of gastric juices.
c. the weight of the patient.
d. the temperature of the peripheral environment.

5. Much of the biotransformation that occurs when a drug is taken occurs as part of
a. the protein-binding effect of the drug.
b. the functioning of the renal system.
c. the first-pass effect through the liver.
d. the distribution of the drug to the reactive tissues.

6. The half-life of a drug
   a. is determined by a balance of all pharmacokinetic processes.
   b. is a constant factor for all drugs taken by a patient.
   c. is influenced by the fat distribution of the patient.
   d. can be calculated with the use of a body surface nomogram.

7. J.B. has Parkinson's disease that has been controlled for several years with levodopa. After he begins a health food regimen with lots of vitamin B6, his tremors return, and he develops a rapid heart rate, hypertension, and anxiety. The nurse investigating the problem discovers that vitamin B6 can speed the conversion of levodopa to dopamine in the periphery, leading to these problems. The nurse would consider this problem
   a. a drug–laboratory test interaction.
   b. a drug–drug interaction.
   c. a cumulation effect.
   d. a sensitivity reaction.

MULTIPLE RESPONSE

Select all that apply.

1. When reviewing a drug to be given the nurse notes that the drug is excreted in the urine. What points should be included in the nurse's assessment of the patient?
   a. The patient's liver function tests
   b. The patient's bladder tone
   c. The patient's renal function tests
   d. The patient's fluid intake
   e. Other drugs being taken that could affect the kidney
   f. The patient's intake and output for the day

2. When considering the pharmacokinetics of a drug, what points would the nurse need to consider?
   a. How the drug will be absorbed
   b. The way the drug affects the body
   c. Receptor site activation and suppression
   d. How the drug will be excreted
   e. How the drug will be metabolized
   f. The half-life of the drug

3. Drug–drug interactions are important considerations in clinical practice. When evaluating a patient for potential drug–drug interactions, what would the nurse expect to address?
   a. Bizarre drug effects on the body
   b. The need to adjust drug dose or timing of administration
   c. The need for more drugs to balance the effects of the drugs being given
   d. A new therapeutic effect not encountered with either drug alone
   e. Increased adverse effects
   f. The use of herbal or alternative therapies

BIBLIOGRAPHY AND REFERENCES

Agency for Health Care Research and Quality. (2014). Twenty tips to help prevent medical errors. [*Author*]. Available online at: http://www.ahrq.gov/patients-consumers/care-planning/errors/20tips/index.html

Barat, I., Anreassen, F., & Damsgaard, E. M. S. (2001). Drug therapy in the elderly: What doctors believe and what patients actually do. *British Journal of Clinical Pharmacology, 51*(6), 615–622.

Brunton, L., Chabner, B., & Knollman, B. (2011). *Goodman and Gilman's the pharmacological basis of therapeutics* (12th ed.). New York: McGraw-Hill.

Gray, C., & Gandher, C. (2009). Adverse drug events in the elderly: An ongoing problem. *Journal of Managed Care Pharmacy, 15*(7), 568–571.

Horne, R. (2004). Non-adherence with drugs more likely if patients' beliefs are ignored. *The Pharmaceutical Journal, 273*(7320), 525.

King, R. L. (2004). Nurses' perceptions of their pharmacology educational needs. *Journal of Advanced Nursing, 45*(4), 392–400.

Kudzma, E., & Carey, E. (2009). Pharmacogenomics: Personalizing drug therapy. *American Journal of Nursing, 109*(10), 50–57.

Mangoni, A. A., & Jackson, S. H. D. (2004). Age related changes in pharmacokinetics and pharmacodynamics: Basic principle and practical applications. *British Journal of Clinical Pharmacology, 57*(1), 6–14.

Medical Letter. (2015). *The medical letter on drugs and therapeutics*. New Rochelle, NY: Author.

Milos, P. M., & Seymour, A. B. (2004). Emerging strategies and applications of pharmacogenomics. *Human Genomics, 1*(6), 444–445.

Murphy, A. (2012). *Clinical pharmacokinetics*. Bethesda, MD: American Society of Health-System Pharmacists.

Ray, W. A. (2004). Population based studies of adverse effects. *New England Journal of Medicine, 349*, 1592–1594.

Schwab, M., & Ratain, M. J. (Eds.). (2015). *Pharmacogenetics and genomics*. Philadelphia, PA: Lippincott Williams & Wilkins.

Swonger, A. and Burbank, P. (2010). Drug therapy and the elderly. http://www.worldcat.org/title/drug-therapy-and-the-elderly/oclc/45732586.

Wessling, S. (2013). Ethnopharmacology: What nurses need to know. Available online at: http://minoritynurse.com

Zhou, S. F. (2008). Potential strategies for minimizing mechanism based inhibition or CP450-3A4. *Current Pharmaceutical Design, 14*(10), 990–1000.

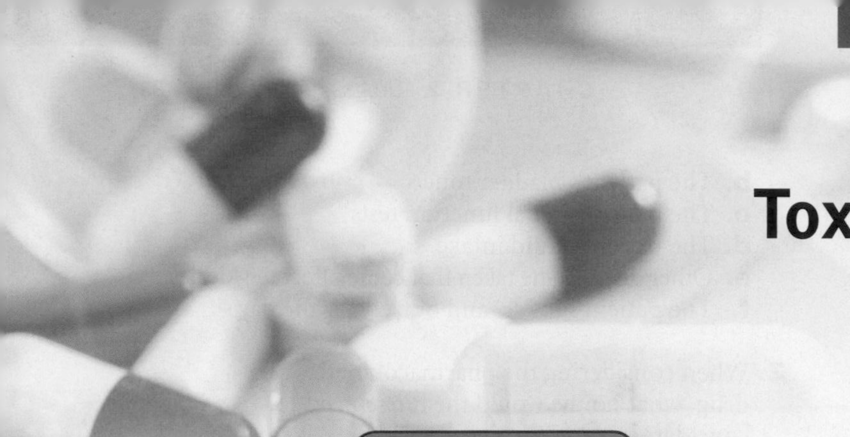

Toxic Effects of Drugs 3

Learning Objectives

Upon completion of this chapter, you will be able to:

1. Define the term adverse drug reaction and explain the clinical significance of this reaction.
2. List four types of allergic responses to drug therapy.
3. Discuss five common examples of drug-induced tissue damage.
4. Define the term poison.
5. Outline the important factors to consider when applying the nursing process to selected situations of drug toxicity.

Glossary of Key Terms

blood dyscrasia: bone marrow depression caused by drug effects on the rapidly multiplying cells of the bone marrow; lower-than-normal levels of blood components can be seen

dermatological reactions: skin reactions commonly seen as adverse effects of drugs; can range from simple rash to potentially fatal exfoliative dermatitis

drug allergy: formation of antibodies to a drug or drug protein; causes an immune response when the person is next exposed to that drug

hypersensitivity: excessive responsiveness to either the primary or the secondary effects of a drug; may be caused by a pathological condition or, in the absence of one, by a particular patient's individual response

poisoning: overdose of a drug that causes damage to multiple body systems and has the potential for fatal reactions

stomatitis: inflammation of the mucous membranes related to drug effects; can lead to alterations in nutrition and dental problems

superinfections: infections caused by the destruction of normal flora bacteria by certain drugs, which allow other bacteria to enter the body and cause infection; may occur during the course of antibiotic therapy

All drugs are potentially dangerous. Even though chemicals are carefully screened and tested in animals and in people before they are approved for sale, drug products often cause unexpected or unacceptable reactions when they are administered. Drugs are chemicals, and the human body operates by a vast series of chemical reactions. Consequently, many effects can be seen when just one chemical factor is altered. Today's potent and amazing drugs can cause a great variety of reactions, many of which are more extreme than those seen previously.

Adverse Effects

Adverse effects are undesired effects that may be unpleasant or even dangerous. They can occur for many reasons, including the following:

- The drug may have other effects on the body besides the therapeutic effect.
- The patient may be sensitive to the drug being given.
- The drug's action on the body may cause other responses that are undesirable or unpleasant.
- The patient may be taking too much or too little of the drug, leading to adverse effects.

The nurse, as the caregiver who most frequently administers medications, must be constantly alert for signs of drug reactions of various types. Patients and their families need to be taught what to look for when taking drugs at home. Some adverse effects can be countered with specific comfort measures or precautions. Knowing that these effects may occur and what actions can be taken to prevent or cope with them may be the most critical factor in helping the patient to comply with drug therapy. Adverse drug effects can be one of several

FOCUS ON Safe Medication Administration

Before administering any drug to a patient, it is important to review the contraindications and cautions associated with that drug, as well as the anticipated adverse effects of the drug. This information will direct your assessment of the patient, helping you to focus on particular signs and symptoms that would alert you to contraindications or to proceed cautiously, and helping you to establish a baseline for that patient so that you will be able to identify the adverse effects that occur. When teaching the patient about a drug, you should list the adverse effects that should be anticipated, along with the appropriate actions that the patient can take to alleviate any discomfort associated with these effects. Being alert to adverse effects—what to assess and how to intervene appropriately—can increase the effectiveness of a drug regimen, provide for patient safety, and improve patient compliance to the drug regimen.

types: primary actions, secondary actions, and hypersensitivity reactions.

Primary Actions

One of the most common occurrences in drug therapy is the development of adverse effects from simple overdose. In such cases the patient suffers from effects that are merely an extension of the desired effect. For example, an anticoagulant may act so effectively that the patient experiences excessive and spontaneous bleeding. This type of adverse effect can be avoided by monitoring the patient carefully and adjusting the prescribed dose to fit that particular patient's needs.

In the same way, a patient taking an antihypertensive drug may become dizzy, weak, or faint when taking the standard recommended dose but will be able to tolerate the drug therapy with a reduced dose. These effects can be caused by individual response to the drug, high or low body weight, age, or underlying pathology that alters the effects of the drug.

Secondary Actions

Drugs can produce a wide variety of effects in addition to the desired pharmacological effect. Sometimes the drug dose can be adjusted so that the desired effect is achieved without producing undesired secondary reactions. Sometimes this is not possible, however, and the adverse effects are almost inevitable. In such cases, the patient needs to be informed that these effects may occur and counseled about ways to cope with the undesired effects. For example, many antihistamines are very effective in drying up secretions and helping breathing, but they also cause drowsiness. The patient who is taking antihistamines needs to know that driving a car or operating power tools or machinery should be avoided because the drowsiness could be dangerous. A patient taking an oral antibiotic needs to know that frequently the effects of the antibiotic on the gastrointestinal (GI) tract result in diarrhea, nausea, and sometimes vomiting. The patient should be advised to eat small, frequent meals to help alleviate this problem.

Hypersensitivity

Some patients are excessively responsive to either the primary or the secondary effects of a drug. This is known as **hypersensitivity**, and it may result from a pathological or underlying condition. For example, many drugs are excreted through the kidneys; a patient who has kidney problems may not be able to excrete the drug and may accumulate the drug in the body, causing toxic effects. The patient will exhibit exaggerated adverse effects from a standard dose of the medication because of the accumulation of the drug. In some cases, individuals exhibit increased therapeutic and adverse effects with no definite pathological condition. Each person has slightly different receptors and cellular responses. Frequently, older people will react to narcotics with increased stimulation and hyperactivity, not with the sedation that is expected. It is thought that this response is related to a change in receptors with age leading to an increased sensitivity to a drug's effects.

Hypersensitivity also can occur if a patient has an underlying condition that makes the drug's effects especially unpleasant or dangerous. For example, a patient with an enlarged prostate who takes an anticholinergic drug may develop urinary retention or even bladder paralysis when the drug's effects block the urinary sphincters. This patient needs to be taught to empty the bladder before taking the drug. A reduced dose also may be required to avoid potentially serious effects on the urinary system.

Drug Allergy

A **drug allergy** occurs when the body forms antibodies to a particular drug, causing an immune response when the person is reexposed to the drug. A patient cannot be allergic to a drug that has never been taken, although patients can have cross-allergies to drugs within the same drug class as one formerly taken. Many people state that they have a drug allergy because of the effects of a drug. For example, one patient stated that she was allergic to the diuretic furosemide (*Lasix*). On further questioning the nurse discovered that the patient considered herself to be "allergic" to the drug because it made her urinate frequently—the desired drug effect, but one that the patient thought was a reaction to the drug. Ask additional questions of patients who state that they have a drug allergy to ascertain the exact nature of the response and whether or not it is a true drug allergy.

Many patients do not receive needed treatment because the response to the drug is not understood.

Drug allergies fall into four main classifications: anaphylactic reactions, cytotoxic reactions, serum sickness, and delayed reactions (Table 3.1). The nurse, as the primary caregiver involved in administering drugs, must constantly assess for potential drug allergies and must be prepared to intervene appropriately.

Table 3.1 Interventions for Types of Drug Allergies

Allergy Type	Assessment	Interventions
Anaphylactic reaction		
This allergy involves an antibody that reacts with specific sites in the body to cause the release of chemicals, including histamine, that produce immediate reactions (mucous membrane swelling and constricting bronchi) that can lead to respiratory distress and even respiratory arrest	Hives, rash, difficulty breathing, increased BP, dilated pupils, diaphoresis, "panic" feeling, increased heart rate, respiratory arrest	Administer epinephrine, 0.3 mL of a 1:1,000 solution, subcutaneously for adults or 0.01 mg/kg of 1:1,000 subcutaneously for pediatric patients. Massage the site to speed absorption rate. Repeat the dose every 15–20 min, as appropriate. Notify the prescriber and/or primary caregiver and discontinue the drug. Be aware that prevention is the best treatment. Counsel patients with known allergies to wear Medic-Alert identification and, if appropriate, to carry an emergency epinephrine kit
Cytotoxic reaction		
This allergy involves antibodies that circulate in the blood and attack antigens (the drug) on cell sites, causing death of that cell. This reaction is not immediate but may be seen over a few days	Complete blood count showing damage to blood-forming cells (decreased hematocrit, white blood cell count, and platelets); liver function tests show elevated liver enzymes; renal function test shows decreased renal function	Notify the prescriber and/or primary caregiver and discontinue the drug. Support the patient to prevent infection and conserve energy until the allergic response is over
Serum sickness reaction		
This allergy involves antibodies that circulate in the blood and cause damage to various tissues by depositing in blood vessels. This reaction may occur up to 1 wk or more after exposure to the drug	Itchy rash, high fever, swollen lymph nodes, swollen and painful joints, edema of the face and limbs	Notify the prescriber and/or primary caregiver and discontinue the drug. Provide comfort measures to help the patient cope with the signs and symptoms (cool environment, skin care, positioning, ice to joints, administer antipyretics or anti-inflammatory agents, as appropriate)
Delayed allergic reaction		
This reaction occurs several hours after exposure and involves antibodies that are bound to specific white blood cells	Rash, hives, swollen joints (similar to the reaction to poison ivy)	Notify the prescriber and/or primary caregiver and discontinue drug. Provide skin care and comfort measures that may include antihistamines or topical corticosteroids

KEY POINTS

- All drugs have effects other than the desired therapeutic effect.
- Primary actions of the drug can be extensions of the desired effect.
- Secondary actions of the drug are effects that the drug causes in the body that are not related to the therapeutic effect.
- Hypersensitivity reactions to a drug are individual reactions that may be caused by increased sensitivity to the drug's therapeutic or adverse effects.
- Drug allergies occur when a patient develops antibodies to a drug after exposure to the drug.

Drug-Induced Tissue and Organ Damage

Drugs can act directly or indirectly to cause many types of adverse effects in various tissues, structures, and organs (Figure 3.1). These drug effects account for many of the cautions that are noted before drug administration begins. The possibility that these effects can occur also accounts for the contraindications for the use of some drugs in patients with a particular history or underlying pathology. The specific contraindications and cautions for the administration of a given drug are noted with each drug type discussed in this book and in the individual monographs found in various

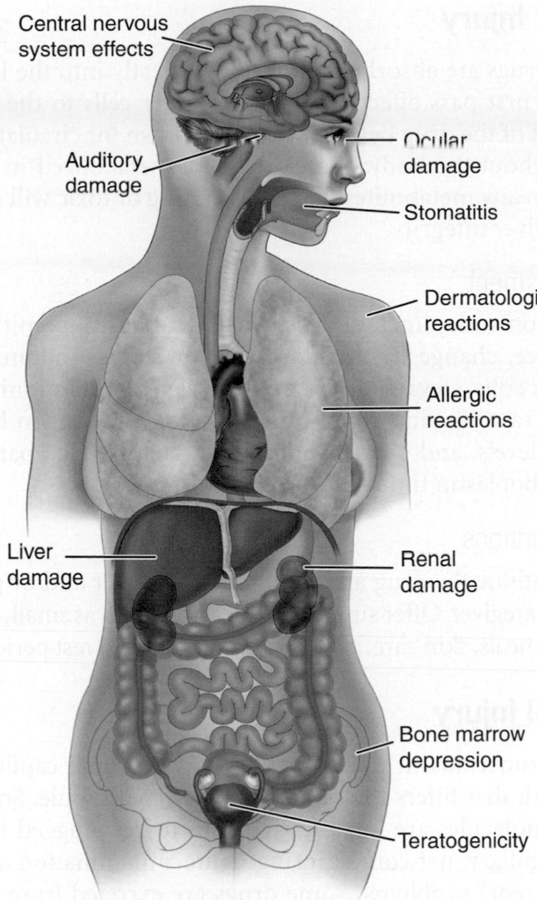

FIGURE 3.1 Variety of adverse effects and toxicities associated with drug use.

drug guides. These effects occur frequently enough that the nurse should be knowledgeable about the presentation of drug-induced damage and about appropriate interventions to be used should it occur.

Dermatological Reactions

Dermatological reactions are adverse reactions involving the skin. These can range from a simple rash to potentially fatal exfoliative dermatitis. Many adverse reactions involve the skin because many drugs can deposit there or cause direct irritation to the tissue.

Rashes, Hives

Many drugs are known to cause skin reactions. Meprobamate (generic), a drug used to treat anxiety, is associated with an itchy, red rash and in some patients has caused a serious and potentially fatal skin reaction, Stevens-Johnson syndrome. Although many patients will report that they are allergic to a drug because they develop a skin rash when taking the drug, it is important to determine whether a rash is a commonly associated adverse effect of the drug.

Assessment

Hives, rashes, and other dermatological lesions may be seen. Severe reactions may include exfoliative dermatitis, which is characterized by rash and scaling, fever, enlarged lymph nodes, enlarged liver, and the potentially fatal erythema multiforme exudativum (Stevens-Johnson syndrome), which is characterized by dark red papules appearing on the extremities with no pain or itching, often in rings or disk-shaped patches.

Interventions

In mild cases, or when the benefit of the drug outweighs the discomfort of the skin lesion, provide frequent skin care; instruct the patient to avoid rubbing, wearing tight or rough clothing, and using harsh soaps or perfumed lotions; and administer antihistamines, as appropriate. In severe cases, discontinue the drug and notify the prescriber and/or primary caregiver. Be aware that, in addition to these interventions, topical corticosteroids, antihistamines, and emollients are often used.

Stomatitis

Stomatitis, or inflammation of the mucous membranes, can occur because of a direct toxic reaction to the drug or because the drug deposits in the end capillaries in the mucous membranes, leading to inflammation. Many drugs are known to cause stomatitis. Antineoplastic drugs commonly cause these problems because they are toxic to rapidly turning-over cells such as those found in the GI tract. Patients receiving antineoplastic drugs are usually given instructions for proper mouth care when the drugs are started.

Assessment

Symptoms can include swollen gums, inflamed gums (gingivitis), and swollen and red tongue (glossitis). Other symptoms include difficulty swallowing, bad breath, and pain in the mouth and throat.

Interventions

Provide frequent mouth care with a nonirritating solution. Offer nutrition evaluation and development of a tolerated diet, which usually involves frequent, small meals. If necessary, arrange for a dental consultation. Note that antifungal agents and/or local anesthetics are sometimes used.

Superinfections

One of the body's protective mechanisms is provided by the wide variety of bacteria that live within or on the surface of the body and in the GI tract. This bacterial growth is called the *normal flora*. The normal flora protect the body from invasion by other bacteria, viruses, fungi, and so on. Several kinds of drugs (especially antibiotics) destroy the normal flora, leading to the development of **superinfections**, or infections caused by organisms that are usually controlled by the normal flora.

Assessment

Symptoms can include fever, diarrhea, black or hairy tongue, inflamed and swollen tongue (glossitis), mucous membrane lesions, and vaginal discharge with or without itching.

Interventions

Provide supportive measures (frequent mouth care, skin care, access to bathroom facilities, small and frequent meals). Administer antifungal therapy as appropriate. In severe cases, discontinue the drug responsible for the superinfection.

Blood Dyscrasia

Blood dyscrasia is bone marrow suppression caused by drug effects. This occurs when drugs that can cause cell death (e.g., antineoplastics, antibiotics) are used. Bone marrow cells multiply rapidly; they are said to be rapidly turning over. Because they go through cell division and multiply so often, they are highly susceptible to any agent that disrupts cell function.

Assessment

Symptoms include fever, chills, sore throat, weakness, back pain, dark urine, decreased hematocrit (anemia), low platelet count (thrombocytopenia), low white blood cell count (leukopenia), and a reduction of all cellular elements of the complete blood count (pancytopenia).

Interventions

Monitor blood counts. Provide supportive measures (rest, protection from exposure to infections, protection from injury, avoidance of activities that might result in injury or bleeding). In severe cases, discontinue the drug or stop administration until the bone marrow recovers to a safe level.

KEY POINTS

- Adverse drug effects can include skin irritation ranging from rashes and hives to potentially fatal Stevens-Johnson syndrome.
- Superinfections, or infections caused by destruction of protective normal flora bacteria; blood dyscrasias caused by bone marrow suppression of blood-forming cells; and stomatitis or mucous membrane eruptions are common adverse drug effects.

Toxicity

Introducing chemicals into the body can sometimes affect the body in a very noxious or toxic way. These effects are not acceptable adverse effects but are potentially serious reactions to a drug. When a drug is known to have toxic effects the benefit of the drug to the patient must be weighed against the possibility of toxic effects which may cause the patient harm.

Liver Injury

Oral drugs are absorbed and passed directly into the liver in the first-pass effect. This exposes liver cells to the full impact of the drug before it is broken down for circulation throughout the body. Most drugs are metabolized in the liver, so any metabolites that are irritating or toxic will also affect liver integrity.

Assessment

Symptoms may include fever, malaise, nausea, vomiting, jaundice, change in color of urine or stools, abdominal pain or colic, elevated liver enzymes (e.g., aspartate aminotransferase, alanine aminotransferase), alterations in bilirubin levels, and changes in clotting factors (e.g., partial thromboplastin time).

Interventions

Discontinue the drug and notify the prescriber and/or primary caregiver. Offer supportive measures such as small, frequent meals, skin care, a cool environment, and rest periods.

Renal Injury

The glomerulus in the kidney has a very small capillary network that filters the blood into the renal tubule. Some drug molecules are just the right size to get plugged into the capillary network, causing acute inflammation and severe renal problems. Some drugs are excreted from the kidney unchanged; they have the potential to directly irritate the renal tubule and alter normal absorption and secretion processes. Gentamicin (generic), a potent antibiotic, is frequently associated with renal toxicity.

Assessment

Elevated blood urea nitrogen, elevated creatinine concentration, decreased hematocrit, electrolyte imbalances, fatigue, malaise, edema, irritability, and skin rash may be seen.

Interventions

Notify the prescriber and/or primary caregiver and discontinue the drug as needed. Offer supportive measures—for example, positioning, diet and fluid restrictions, skin care, electrolyte therapy, rest periods, and a controlled environment. In severe cases, be aware that dialysis may be required for survival.

Poisoning

Poisoning occurs when an overdose of a drug damages multiple body systems, leading to the potential for fatal reactions. Assessment parameters vary with the particular drug. Treatment of drug poisoning also varies, depending on the drug. Throughout this book, specific antidotes or treatments for poisoning are identified, if known. Emergency and life support measures often are needed in severe cases.

Alterations in Glucose Metabolism

All cells need glucose for energy; the cells of the central nervous system (CNS) are especially dependent on constant glucose levels to function properly. The control of glucose in the body is an integrated process that involves a series of hormones and enzymes that use the liver as the place for glucose storage or release. Many drugs have an impact on glucose levels because of their effects on the liver or the endocrine system.

Hypoglycemia

Some drugs affect metabolism and the use of glucose, causing a low serum blood glucose concentration, or hypoglycemia. Glipizide (*Glucotrol*) and glyburide (*DiaBeta*) are antidiabetic agents that have the desired action of lowering the blood glucose level but can lower blood glucose too far, causing hypoglycemia.

Assessment

Symptoms may include fatigue; drowsiness; hunger; anxiety; headache; cold, clammy skin; shaking and lack of coordination (tremulousness); increased heart rate; increased blood pressure; numbness and tingling of the mouth, tongue, and/or lips; confusion; and rapid and shallow respirations. In severe cases, seizures and/or coma may occur.

Interventions

Restore glucose—orally, if possible, or intravenously. Provide supportive measures (e.g., skin care, environmental control of light and temperature, rest). Institute safety measures to prevent injury or falls. Monitor blood glucose levels to help stabilize the situation. Offer reassurance to help the patient cope with the experience.

Hyperglycemia

Some drugs stimulate the breakdown of glycogen or alter metabolism in such a way as to cause high serum glucose levels, or hyperglycemia. Ephedrine (generic), a drug used as a bronchodilator and antiasthma drug and to relieve nasal congestion, can break down stored glycogen and cause an elevation of blood glucose by its effects on the sympathetic nervous system.

Assessment

Fatigue, increased urination (polyuria), increased thirst (polydipsia), deep respirations (Kussmaul respirations), restlessness, increased hunger (polyphagia), nausea, hot or flushed skin, and fruity odor to breath may be observed.

Interventions

Administer insulin therapy to decrease blood glucose as appropriate, while carefully monitoring glucose levels. Provide support to help the patient deal with signs and symptoms (e.g., provide access to bathroom facilities, control the temperature of the room, decrease stimulation while the patient is in crisis, offer reassurance, provide mouth care—the patient will experience dry mouth and bad breath with the ensuing acidosis, and mouth care will help to make this more tolerable).

Electrolyte Imbalances

Because they are chemicals acting in a body that works by chemical reactions, drugs can have an effect on various electrolyte levels in the body. The electrolyte that can cause the most serious effects when it is altered, even a little, is potassium.

Hypokalemia

Some drugs affecting the kidney can cause low serum potassium levels (hypokalemia) by altering the renal exchange system. For example, loop diuretics function by causing the loss of potassium, as well as of sodium and water. Potassium is essential for the normal functioning of nerves and muscles.

Assessment

Symptoms include a serum potassium concentration ($[K^+]$) lower than 3.5 mEq/L, weakness, numbness and tingling in the extremities, muscle cramps, nausea, vomiting, diarrhea, decreased bowel sounds, irregular pulse, weak pulse, orthostatic hypotension, and disorientation. In severe cases, paralytic ileus (absent bowel sounds, abdominal distention, and acute abdomen) may occur.

Interventions

Replace serum potassium and carefully monitor serum levels and patient response; achieving the desired level can take time, and the patient may experience high potassium levels in the process. Provide supportive therapy (e.g., safety precautions to prevent injury or falls, reorientation of the patient, comfort measures for pain and discomfort). Cardiac monitoring may be needed to evaluate the effect of the fluctuating potassium levels on heart rhythm.

Hyperkalemia

Some drugs that affect the kidney, such as the potassium-sparing diuretics, can lead to potassium retention and a resultant increase in serum potassium levels (hyperkalemia). Other drugs that cause cell death or injury, such as many antineoplastic agents, also can cause the cells to release potassium, leading to hyperkalemia.

Assessment

Symptoms include a serum potassium level higher than 5.0 mEq/L, weakness, muscle cramps, diarrhea, numbness and tingling, slow heart rate, low blood pressure, decreased urine output, and difficulty breathing.

Interventions

Institute measures to decrease the serum potassium concentration, including use of sodium polystyrene sulfonate. When trying to stabilize the potassium level, it is possible that the patient may experience low potassium levels. Careful monitoring is important until the patient's potassium levels are stable. Offer supportive measures to cope with discomfort. Institute safety measures to prevent injury or falls. Monitor for cardiac irregularities because potassium is an important electrolyte in the action potential, which is needed for cell membrane stability. When potassium levels are too high the cells of the heart become very irritable and rhythm disturbances can occur. Be prepared for a possible cardiac emergency. In severe cases, be aware that dialysis may be needed.

Sensory Effects

Drugs can affect the special senses, including the eyes and ears. Alterations in seeing and hearing can pose safety problems for patients.

Ocular Damage

The blood vessels in the retina are very tiny and are called "end arteries," that is, they stop and do not interconnect with other arteries feeding the same cells. Some drugs are deposited into these tiny arteries, causing inflammation and tissue damage. Chloroquine (*Aralen*), a drug used to treat some rheumatoid diseases, can cause retinal damage and even blindness.

Assessment

Blurring of vision, color vision changes, corneal damage, and blindness may be noted.

Interventions

Monitor the patient's vision carefully when the patient is receiving known oculotoxic drugs. Consult with the prescriber and/or primary caregiver and discontinue the drug as appropriate. Provide supportive measures, especially if vision loss is not reversible. Monitor lighting and exposure to sunlight.

Auditory Damage

Tiny vessels and nerves in the eighth cranial nerve are easily irritated and damaged by certain drugs. The macrolide antibiotics, streptomycin in particular, can cause severe auditory nerve damage. Aspirin, one of the most commonly used drugs, is often linked to auditory ringing and eighth cranial nerve effects.

Assessment

Dizziness, ringing in the ears (tinnitus), loss of balance, and loss of hearing may be assessed.

Interventions

Monitor the patient's perceptual losses or changes. Provide protective measures to prevent falling or injury. Consult with the prescriber to decrease dose or discontinue the drug. Provide supportive measures to cope with drug effects.

Neurological Effects

Many drugs can affect the functioning of the nerves in the periphery and the CNS. Nerves function by using a constant source of energy to maintain the resting membrane potential and allow excitation. This requires glucose, oxygen, and a balance of electrolytes.

General Central Nervous System Effects

Although the brain is fairly well protected from many drug effects by the blood–brain barrier, some drugs do affect neurological functioning, either directly or by altering electrolyte or glucose levels. Beta-blockers, which are used to treat hypertension, angina, and many other conditions, can cause feelings of anxiety, insomnia, and nightmares.

Assessment

Symptoms may include confusion, delirium, insomnia, drowsiness, hyperreflexia or hyporeflexia, bizarre dreams, hallucinations, numbness, tingling, and paresthesias.

Interventions

Provide safety measures to prevent injury. Caution the patient to avoid dangerous situations such as driving a car or operating dangerous machinery. Orient the patient and provide support. Consult with the prescriber to decrease drug dose or discontinue the drug.

Atropine-like (Anticholinergic) Effects

Some drugs block the effects of the parasympathetic nervous system by directly or indirectly blocking cholinergic receptors. Atropine, a drug used preoperatively to dry up secretions and any other indications, is the prototype anticholinergic drug. Many cold remedies and antihistamines also cause anticholinergic effects.

Assessment

Dry mouth, altered taste perception, dysphagia, heartburn, constipation, bloating, paralytic ileus, urinary hesitancy and retention, impotence, blurred vision, cycloplegia, photophobia, headache, mental confusion, nasal congestion, palpitations, tachycardia, decreased sweating, and dry skin may be noted.

Interventions

Provide sugarless lozenges and mouth care to help mouth dryness. Arrange for bowel program as appropriate. Have the patient void before taking the drug, to aid voiding.

Provide safety measures if vision changes occur. Arrange for medication for headache and nasal congestion as appropriate. Advise the patient to avoid hot environments and to take protective measures to prevent falling and to prevent dehydration, which may be caused by exposure to heat owing to decreased sweating.

Parkinson-like Syndrome

Drugs that directly or indirectly affect dopamine levels in the brain can cause a syndrome that resembles Parkinson's disease. Many of the antipsychotic and neuroleptic drugs can cause this effect. In most cases the effects go away when the drug is withdrawn.

Assessment

Lack of activity, akinesia, muscular tremors, drooling, changes in gait, rigidity, extreme restlessness or "jitters" (akathisia), or spasms (dyskinesia) may be observed.

Interventions

Discontinue the drug, if necessary. Know that treatment with anticholinergics or antiparkinson drugs may be recommended if the benefit of the drug outweighs the discomfort of its adverse effects. Provide small, frequent meals if swallowing becomes difficult. Provide safety measures if ambulation becomes a problem.

Neuroleptic Malignant Syndrome

General anesthetics and other drugs that have direct CNS effects can cause neuroleptic malignant syndrome (NMS), a generalized syndrome that includes high fever.

Assessment

Neurological symptoms, including slowed reflexes, rigidity, involuntary movements; hyperthermia; and autonomic disturbances, such as hypertension, fast heart rate, and fever, may be noted.

Interventions

Discontinue the drug, if necessary. Know that treatment with anticholinergics or antiparkinson drugs may be required. Provide supportive care to lower the body temperature. Institute safety precautions as needed.

Teratogenicity

Many drugs that reach the developing fetus or embryo can cause death or congenital defects, which can include skeletal and limb abnormalities, CNS alterations, heart defects, and the like. The exact effects of a drug on the fetus may not be known. In some cases a predictable syndrome occurs when a drug is given to a pregnant woman. In any situation, inform any pregnant woman who requires drug therapy about the possible effects on the baby. Before a drug is administered to a pregnant patient the actual benefits should be weighed against the potential risks. All pregnant women should be advised not to self-medicate during pregnancy. Emotional and physical support is needed to assist the woman in dealing with the possibility of fetal death or birth defects.

Box 3.1 summarizes all of the adverse effects that have been described throughout this chapter.

BOX 3.1

Summary of Adverse Drug Effects

- Extension of primary action
- Occurrence of secondary action
- Allergic reactions
  - Anaphylactic reactions
  - Cytotoxic reactions
  - Serum sickness reactions
  - Delayed allergic reactions
- Tissue and organ damage
  - Dermatological reactions
  - Stomatitis
  - Superinfections
  - Blood dyscrasia
- Toxicity
  - Liver injury
  - Renal injury
  - Poisoning
- Alterations in glucose metabolism
  - Hypoglycemia
  - Hyperglycemia
- Electrolyte imbalances
  - Hypokalemia
  - Hyperkalemia
- Sensory effects
  - Ocular toxicity
  - Auditory damage
- Neurological effects
  - General CNS effects
  - Atropine-like (cholinergic) effects
  - Parkinson-like syndrome
  - Neuroleptic malignant syndrome
- Teratogenicity

SUMMARY

- No drug does only what is desired of it. All drugs have adverse effects associated with them.
- Adverse drug effects can range from allergic reactions to tissue and cellular damage. The nurse, as the health care provider most associated with drug administration, needs to assess each situation for potential adverse effects and intervene appropriately to minimize those effects.
- Adverse effects can be extensions of the primary action of a drug or secondary effects that are not necessarily desirable but are unavoidable.
- Allergic reactions can occur when a person's body makes antibodies to a drug or drug protein. If the person is exposed to that drug at another time an immune response may occur. Allergic reactions can be of various types. The exact response should be noted to avoid future confusion in patient care.
- Tissue damage can include skin problems, mucous membrane inflammation, blood dyscrasias, superinfections, liver or renal toxicity, poisoning, hypoglycemia or hyperglycemia, electrolyte disturbances, various CNS problems (ocular damage, auditory damage, atropine-like effects, Parkinson-like syndrome, NMS), and teratogenicity.

CHECK YOUR UNDERSTANDING

Answers to the questions in this chapter can be found in Answers to Check Your Understanding Questions on thePoint®.

MULTIPLE CHOICE

Select the best answer to the following.

1. An example of a drug allergy is
   a. dry mouth occurring with use of an antihistamine.
   b. increased urination occurring with use of a thiazide diuretic.
   c. breathing difficulty after an injection of penicillin.
   d. urinary retention associated with atropine use.

2. A patient taking glyburide (an antidiabetic drug) has his morning dose and then does not have a chance to eat for several hours. An adverse effect that might be expected from this would be
   a. a teratogenic effect.
   b. a skin rash.
   c. an anticholinergic effect.
   d. hypoglycemia.

3. A patient with a severe infection is given gentamicin, the only antibiotic shown to be effective in culture and sensitivity tests. A few hours after the drug is started intravenously the patient becomes very restless and develops edema. Blood tests reveal abnormal electrolytes and elevated blood urea nitrogen. This reaction was most likely caused by
   a. an anaphylactic reaction.
   b. renal toxicity associated with gentamicin.
   c. superinfection related to the antibiotic.
   d. hypoglycemia.

4. Patients receiving antineoplastic drugs that disrupt cell function often have adverse effects involving cells that turn over rapidly in the body. These cells include
   a. ovarian cells.
   b. liver cells.
   c. cardiac cells.
   d. bone marrow cells.

5. A woman has had repeated bouts of bronchitis throughout the fall and has been taking antibiotics. She calls the clinic with complaints of vaginal pain and itching. When she is seen, it is discovered that she has developed a yeast infection. You understand that
   a. her bronchitis has moved to the vaginal area.
   b. she has developed a superinfection, because the antibiotics kill bacteria that normally provide protection.
   c. she probably has developed a sexually transmitted disease related to her lifestyle.
   d. she will need to take even more antibiotics to treat this new infection.

6. Knowing that a patient is taking a loop diuretic and is at risk for developing hypokalemia the nurse would assess the patient for
   a. hypertension, headache, and cold and clammy skin.
   b. decreased urinary output and yellowing of the sclera.
   c. weak pulse, low blood pressure, and muscle cramping.
   d. diarrhea and flatulence.

MULTIPLE RESPONSE

Select the best answer to the following.

1. A patient is taking a drug that is known to be toxic to the liver. The patient is being discharged to home. What teaching points related to liver toxicity and the drug should the nurse teach the patient to report to the physician?
   a. Fever; changes in the color of urine
   b. Changes in the color of stool; malaise
   c. Rapid, deep respirations; increased sweating
   d. Dizziness; drowsiness; dry mouth
   e. Rash, black or hairy tongue; white spots in the mouth or throat
   f. Yellowing of the skin or the whites of the eyes

2. Pregnant women should be advised of the potential risk to the fetus any time they take a drug during pregnancy. What fetal problems can be related to drug exposure in utero?
   a. Fetal death
   b. Nervous system disruption
   c. Skeletal and limb abnormalities
   d. Cardiac defects
   e. Low-set ears
   f. Deafness

3. A client is experiencing a reaction to the penicillin injection that the nurse administered approximately ½ hour ago. The nurse is concerned that it might be an anaphylactic reaction. What signs and symptoms would validate her suspicion?
   a. Rapid heart rate
   b. Diaphoresis
   c. Constricted pupils
   d. Hypotension
   e. Rash
   f. Client report of a panicky feeling

4. A client is experiencing a serum sickness reaction to a recent rubella vaccination. Which of the following interventions would be appropriate when caring for this client?
   a. Administration of epinephrine
   b. Cool environment
   c. Positioning to provide comfort
   d. Ice to joints as needed
   e. Administration of anti-inflammatory agents
   f. Administration of topical corticosteroids

BIBLIOGRAPHY AND REFERENCES

Armitage, G., & Knapman, H. (2003). Adverse events in drug administration: A literature review. *Journal of Nursing Management, 11*(2), 130–140.

Benkirane, R. R., Abouqal, R., Haimeur, C. C., et al. (2009). Incidence of adverse drug events and medication errors in intensive care units. *Journal of Patient Safety, 5*(1), 16–22.

Bennett, C. L., Nebekar, J. R., Lyons, E. A., et al. (2005). The research on adverse drug events and report project. *Journal of the American Medical Association, 293*, 2131–2140.

Brunton, L., Chabner, B., & Knollman, B. (2011). *Goodman & Gilman's the pharmacological basis of therapeutics* (12th ed.). New York: McGraw-Hill.

Budnitz, D. A., Pollack, D. A., Weindenbach, K. N., et al. (2006). National surveillance of emergency department visits for outpatient adverse drug events. *Journal of the American Medical Association, 296*, 1858–1866.

Facts and Comparisons. (2015). *Drug facts and comparisons.* St. Louis, MO: Author.

FDA. (2015). FDA MEDWATCH program: Monitoring adverse drug reactions. [*Food and Drug Administration*]. Available online at: fda.gov.

Karch, A. M. (2014). *Lippincott nursing drug guide.* Philadelphia, PA: Lippincott Williams & Wilkins.

Lewis, J. L., Dorman, T., Taylor, D., et al. (2009). Prevalence, incidence and nature of prescribing errors in hospital inpatients. *Drug Safety, 32*(5), 379–389.

Medical Letter. (2015). *The medical letter on drugs and therapeutics.* New Rochelle, NY: Author.

Minneman, K. (2010). *Brody's human pharmacology: Molecular to clinical.* St. Louis, MO: Elsevier.

Stefanacci, R. G. (2006). Preventing medication errors in long term care. *Clinical Geriatrics, 14*(10), 9–11.

Thomsen, L. A., Winterstein, A. G., Sandergaard, B., et al. (2007). Systematic review of the incidence and characteristic of preventable adverse drug events in ambulatory care. *Annals of Pharmacotherapy, 41*(9), 1411–1426.

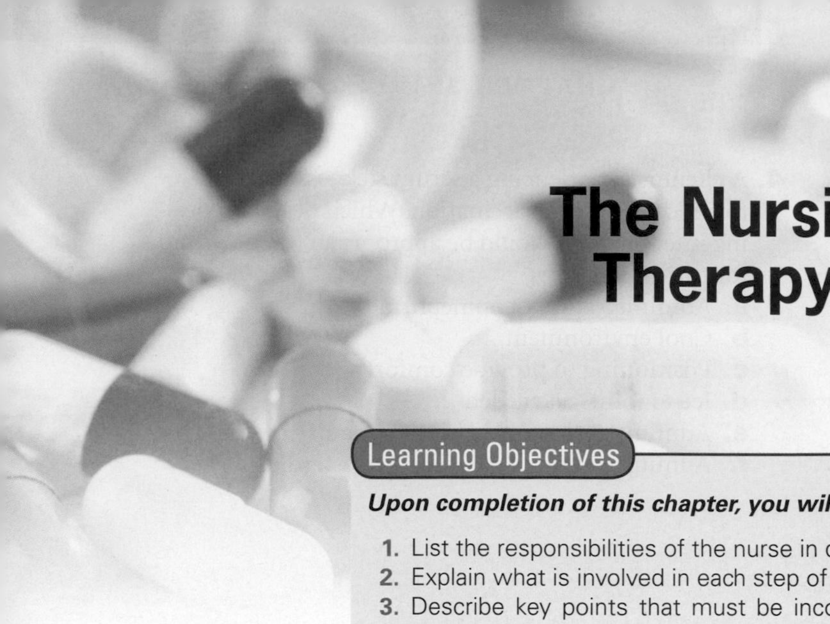

4 The Nursing Process in Drug Therapy and Patient Safety

Learning Objectives

Upon completion of this chapter, you will be able to:

1. List the responsibilities of the nurse in drug therapy.
2. Explain what is involved in each step of the nursing process as it relates to drug therapy.
3. Describe key points that must be incorporated into the assessment of a patient receiving drug therapy.
4. Describe the essential elements of a medication order.
5. Outline the important points that must be assessed and considered before administering a drug, combining knowledge about the drug with knowledge of the patient and the environment.
6. Describe the role of the nurse and the patient in preventing medication errors.

Glossary of Key Terms

assessment: information gathering regarding the current status of a particular patient, including evaluation of past history and physical examination; provides a baseline of information and clues to effectiveness of therapy

evaluation: part of the nursing process; determining the effects of the interventions that were instituted for the patient and leading to further assessment and intervention

implementation: actions undertaken to meet a patient's needs, such as administration of drugs, comfort measures, or patient teaching

nursing: the art of nurturing and administering to the sick, combined with the scientific application of chemistry, anatomy, physiology, biology, nutrition, psychology, and pharmacology to the particular clinical situation

nursing diagnosis: statement of an actual or potential problem, based on the assessment of a particular clinical situation, which directs needed nursing interventions

nursing process: the problem-solving process used to provide efficient nursing care; it involves gathering information, formulating a nursing diagnosis statement, prioritizing the diagnoses, developing goals and desired outcomes for the patient, carrying out interventions, and evaluating the process

planning: the process of prioritizing the information gathered in assessment and, using the established nursing diagnoses, to develop goals and desired outcomes for the patient

The delivery of medical care today is in a constant state of change, at times reaching crisis levels. The population is aging, resulting in an increased incidence and prevalence of chronic disease and more complex care issues. The population also is more transient, with individuals and families more mobile, often resulting in unstable support systems and fewer at-home care providers and helpers. At the same time, health care is undergoing a technological boom, including greater use of more sophisticated diagnostic methods and treatments, new, specialized drugs, including experimental drugs, and so on. Moreover, patients are being discharged earlier from acute care facilities or are not being admitted at all for procedures that used to be treated in-hospital with follow-up support and monitoring. Patients also are becoming more responsible for their care and for adhering to complicated medical regimens at home. The wide use of the Internet and an emphasis in the media on the need to question all aspects of health care has led to more knowledgeable and challenging patients. Patients may no longer accept a drug regimen or therapy without question and often feel confident in adjusting it on their own because of information that they have found on the Internet—information that might not be very accurate or even relevant to their particular situation.

Nursing: Art and Science

Nursing is a unique and complex science, as well as a nurturing and caring art. In the traditional sense, nursing has been viewed as ministering to and soothing the sick. In the current state of medical changes, nursing also has become increasingly technical and scientific. Nurses are assuming increasing responsibilities that involve not only nurturing and caring but also assessing, diagnosing, and intervening with patients to treat, to prevent, and to educate as they assist patients in coping with various health states.

The nurse deals with the whole person, including physical, emotional, intellectual, social, cultural, and spiritual aspects. Nurses must consider how a person responds to disease and its treatment, including the changes in lifestyle that may be required. Therefore, a nurse is a key health care provider who is in a position to assess the whole patient, to administer therapy as well as medications, to teach the patient how best to cope with the therapy so as to ensure the most favorable outcome, and to evaluate the effectiveness of the therapy.

The nurse is a key component in developing and implementing patient-centered care. Nurses accomplish these tasks by integrating knowledge of the basic sciences (anatomy, physiology, nutrition, chemistry, pharmacology), the social sciences (sociology, psychology), education, and many other disciplines and applying the nursing process.

The Nursing Process

Nurses use the **nursing process**—a decision-making, problem-solving process—to provide efficient and effective care. Although not all nursing theorists completely agree on this process that defines the practice of nursing, most do include certain key elements: assessment, nursing diagnosis, planning, implementation, and evaluation. Application of the nursing process with drug therapy ensures that the patient receives the best, safest, most efficient, scientifically based, holistic care. Box 4.1 outlines the steps of the nursing process, which are discussed in detail in the following paragraphs.

Assessment

Assessment (gathering information) is the first step of the nursing process. This involves systematic, organized collection of data about the patient. Because the nurse is responsible for holistic care, data must include information about physical, intellectual, emotional, social, cultural, and environmental factors. When viewed together, this information provides the nurse with the facts needed to plan educational and discharge programs, arrange for appropriate consultations, and monitor the physical response to treatment or to disease.

Each nurse develops a unique approach to the organization of the assessment, an approach that is functional and useful in the clinical setting and that makes sense to that nurse and in the particular clinical situation. Regardless of the approach the process of assessment never ends because the patient is in a dynamic state, continuously adjusting to physical, emotional, and environmental influences.

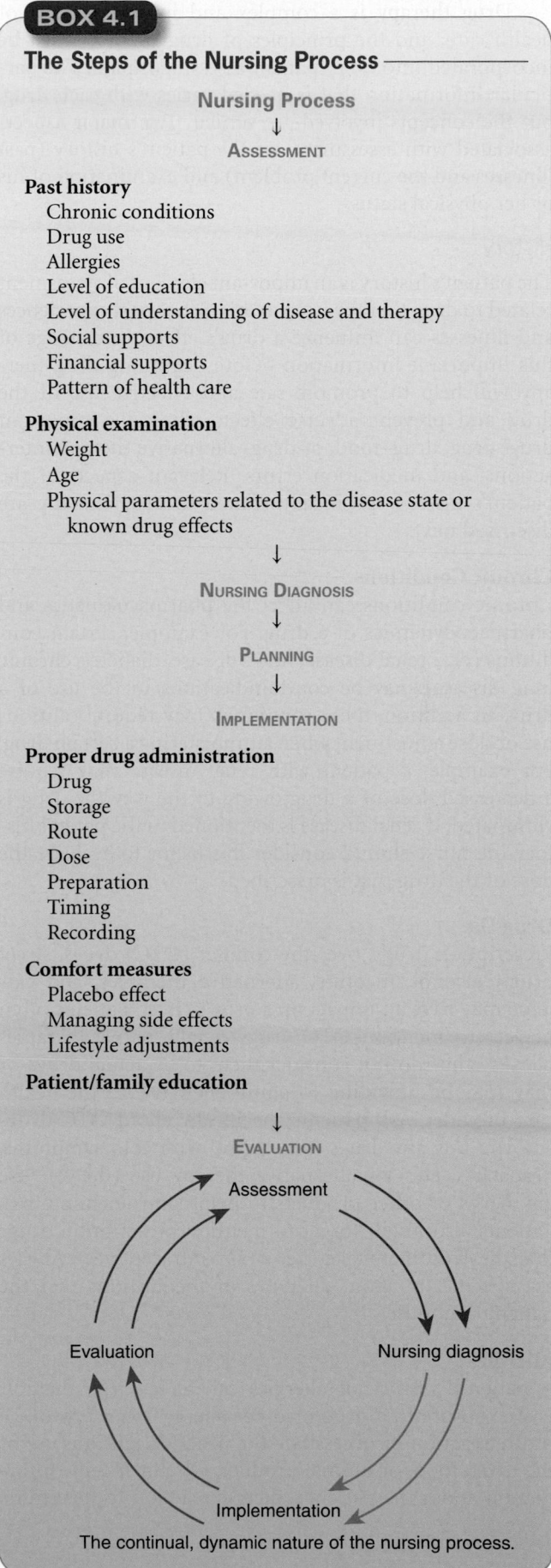

BOX 4.1

The Steps of the Nursing Process

Nursing Process

↓

ASSESSMENT

Past history
- Chronic conditions
- Drug use
- Allergies
- Level of education
- Level of understanding of disease and therapy
- Social supports
- Financial supports
- Pattern of health care

Physical examination
- Weight
- Age
- Physical parameters related to the disease state or known drug effects

↓

NURSING DIAGNOSIS

↓

PLANNING

↓

IMPLEMENTATION

Proper drug administration
- Drug
- Storage
- Route
- Dose
- Preparation
- Timing
- Recording

Comfort measures
- Placebo effect
- Managing side effects
- Lifestyle adjustments

Patient/family education

↓

EVALUATION

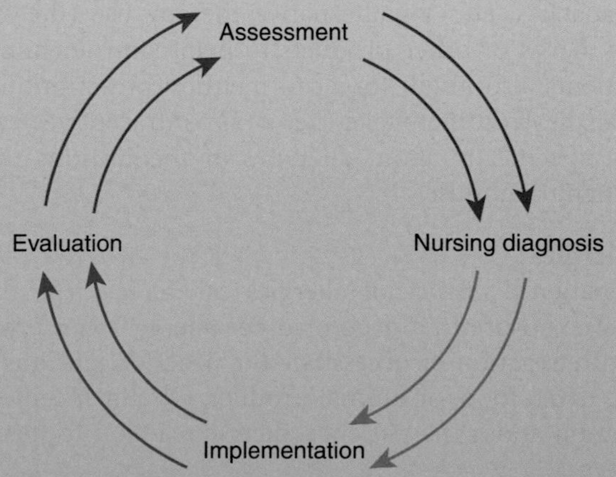

The continual, dynamic nature of the nursing process.

Drug therapy is a complex and important part of health care, and the principles of drug therapy must be incorporated into every patient assessment plan. The particular information that is needed varies with each drug, but the concepts involved are similar. Two major aspects associated with assessment are the patient's history (past illnesses and the current problem) and examination of his or her physical status.

History

The patient's history is an important element of assessment related to drug therapy because his or her past experiences and illnesses can influence a drug's effect. Knowledge of this important information before beginning drug therapy will help to promote safe and effective use of the drug and prevent adverse effects, clinically important drug–drug, drug–food, or drug–alternative therapy interactions, and medication errors. Relevant aspects of the patient's history specifically related to drug therapy are discussed next.

Chronic Conditions

Chronic conditions can affect the pharmacokinetics and pharmacodynamics of a drug. For example, certain conditions (e.g., renal disease, heart disease, diabetes, chronic lung disease) may be contraindications to the use of a drug. In addition, these conditions may require cautious use or dose adjustment when administering a certain drug. For example, a patient with renal disease may require a decreased dose of a drug owing to the way the drug is eliminated. If renal disease is mentioned in the patient history the nurse should consider this factor to evaluate the dose of the drug that is prescribed.

Drug Use

Prescription drugs, over-the-counter (OTC) drugs, street drugs, alcohol, nicotine, alternative therapies, and caffeine may have an impact on a drug's effect. Patients often neglect to mention OTC drugs or alternative therapies because they do not consider them to be actual drugs or they may be unwilling to admit their use to the health care provider. Ask patients specifically about OTC drugs (do you buy any drugs to help you with cold symptoms, headaches, etc.) or alternative therapy use (do you use any herbs or other products to help control symptoms). Patients also might forget to mention prescription drugs that they routinely take (i.e., oral contraceptives). Always ask specifically about all types of medications that the patient might use.

Allergies

A patient's history of allergies can affect drug therapy. Past exposure to a drug or other allergens can provoke a future reaction or necessitate the need for cautious use of the drug, food, or animal product. Obtain specific information about the patient's allergic reaction to determine whether the patient has experienced a true drug allergy or was experiencing an actual effect or adverse effect of the drug.

Level of Education and Understanding

Information about the patient's level of education provides a baseline from which the nurse can determine the appropriate types of teaching information to use with the patient. A patient with a fifth-grade education may require materials at a different level than a patient with a graduate degree. Gathering information about the patient's level of understanding about his or her condition, illness, or drug therapy helps the nurse to determine where the patient is in terms of his or her status and the level of explanation that will be required. It also provides additional baseline information for developing a patient education program. It is important not to assume anything about the patient's ability to understand based on his or her reported education level. Stress, disease, and environmental factors can all affect a patient's learning readiness and ability. Direct assessment of actual learning abilities is critical for good patient education.

Social Supports

Patients are being discharged from health care facilities earlier than ever before, often with continuing care needs. In addition, earlier discharges leave minimal time for teaching. Often patients need help at home with care and drug therapy. A key aspect of discharge planning involves determining what support, if any, is available to the patient at home. In many situations, it also involves referral to appropriate community resources.

Financial Supports

The high cost of health care, in general, and of medications, in particular, must be considered when initiating drug therapy and promoting patient compliance. Financial constraints may cause a patient not to follow through with a prescribed drug regimen. For example, the drug may be too expensive or the patient may lack the means to get to a pharmacy to obtain the drug. In some situations a less expensive drug might be appropriate in place of a very expensive drug. In addition, the nurse may need to refer the patient to appropriate resources that might offer financial assistance.

Pattern of Health Care

Knowing how a patient seeks health care provides the nurse with valuable information to include when preparing the patient's teaching plan. Does this patient routinely seek follow-up care, or does he or she wait for emergency situations? Does the patient tend to self-treat many complaints, or is every problem brought to a health care provider? Information about patterns of health care also provides insight into conditions that the patient may have but has not reported or medication use that has not been stated.

Physical Examination

It is important to assess the patient's physical status before beginning drug therapy to determine if any conditions exist that would be contraindications or cautions for using the drug and to develop a baseline for evaluating the effectiveness of the drug and the occurrence of any adverse effects. Relevant aspects of the patient's physical examination specifically related to drug therapy are discussed in the following text.

Weight

A patient's weight helps to determine whether the recommended drug dose is appropriate. Because the recommended dose typically is based on a 150-pound adult man, patients who are much lighter or much heavier often need a dose adjustment.

Age

Patients at the extremes of the age spectrum—children and older adults—often require dose adjustments based on the functional level of the liver and kidneys and the responsiveness of other organs. The child's age and developmental level will also alert the nurse to possible problems with drug delivery, such as the ability to swallow pills or follow directions related to other delivery methods. The child's developmental age will also influence pharmacokinetics and pharmacodynamics; the immature liver may not metabolize drugs in the same way as in the adult, or the kidneys may not be as efficient as those of an adult. As patients age the body undergoes many normal changes that can affect drug therapy, such as decreased blood volume, decreased gastrointestinal absorption, reduced blood flow to muscles or skin, and changes in receptor site responsiveness. Older adults may often have a variety of chronic medical conditions and could be receiving a number of medications that need to be evaluated for possible interactions. Older adults with various central nervous system disorders, like Alzheimer's disease or Parkinson's disease, may develop difficulty swallowing and might require liquid forms of medication. Throughout this book, Drug Therapy Across the Life Span features will present information related to the drug class being discussed as it pertains specifically to children, adults, and the older population. These boxes highlight points that the nurse should consider to assure safe and effective therapy in each age group.

Physical Parameters Related to Disease or Drug Effects

The specific parameters that need to be assessed depend on the disease process being treated and on the expected therapeutic and adverse effects of the drug therapy. Assessing these factors before drug therapy begins provides a baseline level with which future assessments can be compared to determine the effects of drug therapy. For example, if a patient is being treated for chronic pulmonary disease, his or her respiratory status and reserve need to be assessed, especially if a drug is being given that is known to affect the respiratory tract. In contrast, a thorough respiratory evaluation would not be warranted in a patient with no known pulmonary disease who is taking a drug with little or no known effects on the respiratory system. Because the nurse has the greatest direct and continued contact with the patient the nurse is in the best position to detect subtle changes that ultimately determine the course of drug therapy—therapeutic success or discontinuation because of adverse or unacceptable responses.

FOCUS ON Safe Medication Administration

Review the monographs in a drug guide or handbook for specific parameters to be assessed in relation to the particular drug being discussed. This assessment provides not only the baseline information needed before giving that drug but also the data required to evaluate the effects of that drug on the patient. This information should supplement the overall nursing assessment of the patient, which includes social, intellectual, financial, environmental, and other factors.

Nursing Diagnosis

A **nursing diagnosis** is simply a statement of the patient's status from a nursing perspective. The nurse analyzes the information gathered during assessment to arrive at some conclusions that lead to a particular goal and set of interventions. A nursing diagnosis shows actual or potential alterations in patient function based on assessment of the clinical situation. Because drug therapy is only a small part of the overall patient situation, nursing diagnoses that are related to drug therapy must be incorporated into a total picture of the patient.

In the nursing considerations sections of this book the nursing diagnoses listed are those that reflect potential alteration of function based only on the particular drug's actions (i.e., therapeutic and adverse effects). No consideration is given to environmental or disease-related problems. These diagnoses, culled from the North American Nursing Diagnosis Association (NANDA-I) list of accepted nursing diagnoses, are only a part of the overall nursing diagnoses related to the patient's situation. See Box 4.2 for a list of accepted NANDA-1 nursing diagnoses.

Planning

Planning involves taking and prioritizing the information gathered and synthesized in the nursing diagnoses to plan the patient care. This process includes setting goals and desired patient outcomes to assure safe and effective drug therapy. These outcomes usually involve ensuring effective response to drug therapy, minimizing adverse effects, and understanding the drug regimen.

BOX 4.2

NANDA-I Approved Nursing Diagnoses

The North American Nursing Diagnosis Association (NANDA-I) endorsed its first nursing diagnosis taxonomic structure, NANDA-I Taxonomy I, in 1986. This taxonomy has been revised and updated several times. The new Taxonomy II has a code structure that is compliant with recommendations from the National Library of Medicine concerning health care terminology codes. The taxonomy that appears here represents the currently accepted classification system for nursing diagnosis (2011).

Activity Intolerance
Activity Intolerance, Risk for
Ineffective Activity Planning
Airway Clearance, Ineffective
Allergy Response, Latex
Allergy Response, Risk for Latex
Anxiety
Anxiety, Death
Aspiration, Risk for
Attachment, Risk for Impaired Parent/Child
Autonomic Dysreflexia
Autonomic Dysreflexia, Risk for
Behavior, Risk-Prone Health
Risk for Bleeding
Body Image, Disturbed
Body Temperature, Risk for Imbalanced
Bowel Incontinence
Breast-feeding, Effective
Breast-feeding, Ineffective
Breast-feeding, Interrupted
Breathing Pattern, Ineffective
Cardiac Output, Decreased
Caregiver Role Strain
Caregiver Role Strain, Risk for
Readiness for Enhanced Childbearing Process
Comfort, Readiness for Enhanced
Impaired Comfort
Communication, Impaired Verbal
Communication, Readiness for Enhanced
Conflict, Decisional
Conflict, Parental Role
Confusion, Acute
Confusion, Chronic
Confusion, Risk for Acute
Constipation
Constipation, Perceived
Constipation, Risk for
Contamination
Contamination, Risk for
Coping, Compromised Family
Coping, Defensive
Coping, Disabled Family
Coping, Ineffective
Coping, Ineffective Community
Coping, Readiness for Enhanced
Coping, Readiness for Enhanced Community
Coping, Readiness for Enhanced Family
Death Syndrome, Risk for Sudden Infant
Decision Making, Readiness for Enhanced
Denial, Ineffective
Dentition, Impaired
Development, Risk for Delayed
Diarrhea
Dignity, Risk for Compromised Human
Distress, Moral
Disuse Syndrome, Risk for
Diversional Activity, Deficient
Risk for Disturbed Maternal/Fetal Dyad
Risk for Electrolyte Imbalance
Energy Field, Disturbed
Environmental Interpretation Syndrome, Impaired
Failure to Thrive, Adult
Falls, Risk for
Family Processes, Dysfunctional: Alcoholism
Family Processes, Interrupted
Family Processes, Readiness for Enhanced
Fatigue
Fear
Fluid Balance, Readiness for Enhanced
Fluid Volume, Deficient
Fluid Volume, Excess
Fluid Volume, Risk for Deficient
Fluid Volume, Risk for Imbalanced
Gas Exchange, Impaired
Dysfunctional Gastrointestinal (GI) Motility
Risk for Dysfunctional GI Motility
Glucose, Risk for Unstable Blood
Grieving, Anticipatory
Grieving, Complicated
Grieving, Risk for Complicated
Growth and Development, Delayed
Growth, Risk for Disproportionate
Health Maintenance, Ineffective
Ineffective Self Health Maintenance
Health-Seeking Behaviors (Specify)
Home Maintenance, Impaired
Hope, Readiness for Enhanced
Hopelessness
Hyperthermia
Hypothermia
Identity, Disturbed Personal
Immunization Status, Readiness for Enhanced
Incontinence, Functional Urinary
Incontinence, Overflow Urinary
Incontinence, Reflex Urinary
Incontinence, Stress Urinary
Incontinence, Urge Urinary
Incontinence, Risk for Urge Urinary
Infant Behavior, Disorganized
Infant Behavior, Risk for Disorganized
Infant Behavior, Readiness for Enhanced Organized
Infant Feeding Pattern, Ineffective

BOX 4.2

NANDA-I Approved Nursing Diagnoses (continued)

Infection, Risk for
Injury, Risk for
Injury, Risk for Perioperative-Positioning
Insomnia
Intracranial Adaptive Capacity, Decreased
Knowledge, Deficient (Specify)
Knowledge, Readiness for Enhanced
Lifestyle, Sedentary
Liver Function, Risk for Impaired
Loneliness, Risk for
Memory, Impaired
Mobility, Impaired Bed
Mobility, Impaired Physical
Mobility, Impaired Wheelchair
Nausea
Neglect, Unilateral
Neonatal Jaundice
Noncompliance
Nutrition, Imbalanced: Less than Body Requirements
Nutrition, Imbalanced: More than Body Requirements
Nutrition, Readiness for Enhanced
Nutrition, Risk for Imbalanced: More than Body Requirements
Oral Mucous Membrane, Impaired
Pain, Acute
Pain, Chronic
Parenting, Readiness for Enhanced
Parenting, Impaired
Parenting, Risk for Impaired
Peripheral Neurovascular Dysfunction, Risk for
Poisoning, Risk for
Post-Trauma Syndrome
Post-Trauma Syndrome, Risk for
Power, Readiness for Enhanced
Powerlessness
Powerlessness, Risk for
Protection, Ineffective
Rape Trauma Syndrome
Readiness for Enhanced Relationship
Religiosity, Impaired
Religiosity, Readiness for Enhanced
Religiosity, Risk for Impaired
Relocation Stress Syndrome
Relocation Stress Syndrome, Risk for
Risk for Compromised Resilience
Readiness for Enhanced Resilience
Impaired Individual Resilience
Role Performance, Ineffective
Self-Care, Readiness for Enhanced
Self-Care Deficit, Bathing/Hygiene
Self-Care Deficit, Dressing/Grooming
Self-Care Deficit, Feeding
Self-Care Deficit, Toileting
Self-Concept, Readiness for Enhanced
Self-Esteem, Chronic Low
Self-Esteem, Situational Low
Self-Esteem, Risk for Situational Low
Readiness for Enhanced Self Health Management
Self-Mutilation
Self-Mutilation, Risk for
Self Neglect
Sensory Perception, Disturbed (Specify: Visual, Auditory, Kinesthetic, Gustatory, Tactile, Olfactory)
Sexual Dysfunction
Sexuality Pattern, Ineffective
Risk for Shock
Skin Integrity, Impaired
Skin Integrity, Risk for Impaired
Sleep Deprivation
Sleep Pattern, Disturbed
Sleep, Readiness for Enhanced
Social Interaction, Impaired
Social Isolation
Sorrow, Chronic
Spiritual Distress
Spiritual Distress, Risk for
Spiritual Well-Being, Readiness for Enhanced
Stress Overload
Suffocation, Risk for
Suicide, Risk for
Surgical Recovery, Delayed
Swallowing, Impaired
Therapeutic Regimen Management, Ineffective
Therapeutic Regimen Management, Ineffective Family
Therapeutic Regimen Management, Readiness for Enhanced
Thermoregulation, Ineffective
Tissue Integrity, Impaired
Tissue Perfusion, Ineffective Peripheral (Specify Type: Renal, Cerebral, Cardiopulmonary, GI, Peripheral)
Tissue Perfusion, Ineffective Cardiac
Transfer Ability, Impaired
Trauma, Risk for
Risk for Vascular Trauma
Urinary Elimination, Impaired
Urinary Elimination, Readiness for Enhanced
Urinary Retention
Ventilation, Impaired Spontaneous
Ventilatory Weaning Response, Dysfunctional
Violence, Risk for Other-Directed
Violence, Risk for Self-Directed
Walking, Impaired
Wandering

Implementation

Implementation involves nursing interventions aimed at achieving the goals of outcomes determined in the planning phase. Three types of nursing interventions are frequently involved in drug therapy: drug administration, provision of comfort measures, and patient/family education.

Proper Drug Administration

The nurse must consider seven points, or "rights," to ensure safe and effective drug administration. These are right drug and patient, right storage of drug, right and most effective route, right dose, right preparation, right timing, and right recording of administration. See the later section on the prevention of medication errors for a detailed explanation of the nurse's role in implementing these rights. Remembering to review each point before administering a drug will help to prevent medication errors and improve patient outcomes.

Comfort Measures

Nurses are in a unique position to help the patient cope with the effects of drug therapy. A patient is more likely to be compliant with a drug regimen if the effects of the regimen are not too uncomfortable or overwhelming.

Placebo Effect

The anticipation that a drug will be helpful (placebo effect) has proven to have tremendous impact on the actual success of drug therapy. Therefore, the nurse's attitude and support can be a critical part of drug therapy. For example, a back rub, a kind word, and a positive approach may be as beneficial as the drug itself.

Managing Adverse Effects

Interventions can be directed at promoting patient safety and decreasing the impact of the anticipated adverse effects of a drug. Such interventions include environmental control (e.g., temperature, light), safety measures (e.g., avoiding driving, avoiding the sun, using side rails), and physical comfort measures (e.g., skin care, laxatives, frequent meals).

Lifestyle Adjustment

Some medications and their effects require that a patient make changes in his or her lifestyle. For example, patients taking diuretics may have to rearrange their day so as to be near toilet facilities when the drug action peaks. Patients taking bisphosphonates will need to plan their morning so they can take the drug on an empty stomach, stay upright for at least half an hour, and plan their first food of the day at least half an hour after taking the drug. Many drugs come with similar guidelines for assuring effectiveness and decreasing adverse effects. Patients taking monoamine oxidase inhibitors must adjust their diet to prevent serious adverse effects due to potential drug–food interactions. In some cases the change in lifestyle that is needed can have a tremendous impact on the patient and can affect his or her ability to cope and comply with any medical regimen. Lifestyle changes are quite difficult for patients to accomplish, and therefore compliance with drug therapy requires a great deal of support, education, and encouragement.

FOCUS ON Safe Medication Administration

Special points regarding drug administration and related comfort measures are noted with each drug class discussed in this book. Refer to the individual drug monographs in a drug guide or handbook for more detailed interventions regarding a specific drug.

Patient and Family Education

With patients becoming increasingly responsible for their own care, it is essential that they have all of the information necessary to ensure safe and effective drug therapy at home. In fact, many states now require that patients be given written information. Box 4.3 includes key elements for any drug education program. Also see the later section on prevention of medication errors for patient-teaching tips related to the patient's role in preventing medication errors.

Evaluation

Evaluation is part of the continuing process of patient care that leads to changes in assessment, diagnosis, planning, and intervention. The patient is continually evaluated for therapeutic response, the occurrence of adverse drug effects, and the occurrence of drug–drug, drug–food, drug–alternative therapy, or drug–laboratory test interactions. Some drug therapy requires evaluation of specific therapeutic drug levels. In addition, the efficacy of the nursing interventions and the education program also are evaluated. In some situations the nurse evaluates the patient simply by reapplying the beginning steps of the nursing process and then analyzing for changes, either positive or negative. The process of evaluation may lead to changes in the nursing interventions being used to provide better and safer patient care.

KEY POINTS

- Nurses use the nursing process to provide a framework for organizing the information that is needed to provide safe and effective patient care.
- The steps of the nursing process (assessment, nursing diagnosis, planning, implementation, and evaluation) are constantly being repeated to meet the ever-changing needs of the patient.
- The nursing process provides an effective method for handling all of the scientific and technical information, as well as the unique emotional, social, and physical factors that each patient brings to a given situation.

BOX 4.3 FOCUS ON Patient and Family Teaching

Include the following key elements in any drug education program:

1. *Name, dose, and action of drug:* Ensure that patients know this information. Many patients see more than one health care provider; this knowledge is crucial to ensuring safe and effective drug therapy and avoiding drug–drug interactions. Urge patients to keep a written list of the drugs that they are taking to show to any health care provider taking care of them and in case of an emergency when they are not able to report their drug history.
2. *Timing of administration:* Teach patients when to take the drug with respect to frequency, other drugs, and meals.
3. *Special storage and preparation instructions:* Inform patients about any special handling or storing required. Some drugs may require refrigeration; others may need to be mixed with a specific liquid such as water or fruit juice. Be sure that patients know how to carry out these requirements.
4. *Specific OTC drugs or alternative therapies to avoid:* Prevent possible interactions between prescribed drugs and other drugs or remedies the patient may be using or taking. Many patients do not consider OTC drugs or herbal or alternative therapies to be actual drugs and may inadvertently take them along with their prescribed medications, causing unwanted or even dangerous drug–drug interactions. Prevent these situations by explaining which drugs or therapies should be avoided. Encourage patients to always report all of the drugs or therapies that they are using to health care providers to reduce the risk of possible inadvertent adverse effects.
5. *Special comfort measures:* Teach patients how to cope with anticipated adverse effects to ease anxiety and avoid noncompliance with drug therapy. If a patient knows that a diuretic is going to lead to increased urination the day can be scheduled so that bathrooms are nearby when they might be needed. Also educate patients about the importance of follow-up tests or evaluation.
6. *Safety measures:* Instruct all patients to keep drugs out of the reach of children. Remind all patients to inform any health care provider they see about the drugs they are taking; this can prevent drug–drug interactions and misdiagnoses based on drug effects. Also alert patients to possible safety issues that could arise as a result of drug therapy. For example, teach patients to avoid driving or performing hazardous tasks if they are taking drugs that can make them dizzy or alter their thinking or response time.
7. *Specific points about drug toxicity:* Give patients a list of warning signs of drug toxicity. Advise patients to notify their health care provider if any of these effects occur.
8. *Specific warnings about drug discontinuation:* Remember that some drugs with a small margin of safety and drugs with particular systemic effects cannot be stopped abruptly without dangerous effects. Alert patients who are taking these types of drugs to this problem and encourage them to call their health care provider immediately if they cannot take their medication for any reason (e.g., illness, financial constraints).

NOTE: Refer to the CD-ROM accompanying this book for teaching guides that can be used for patients in the actual clinical setting.

Medication Errors

With the increase in the older adult patient population, the increase in the number of available drugs and OTC and alternative therapy preparations, and the reduced length of hospital stays for patients, the risk for medication errors is ever increasing. In 2000 the Institute of Medicine published a large-scale study of medication errors in the United States, entitled *To Err Is Human: Building a Safer Health System*. It reported that 44,000 reported deaths in hospitals each year occurred from medication errors, and that the number could probably be closer to 98,000. The study brought to light the many places in the system where a medication error could occur and suggested methods for improving the problem.

The drug regimen process, which includes prescribing, dispensing, and administering a drug to a patient, has a series of checks along the way to help to catch errors before they occur. These include the physician or nurse practitioner who prescribes a drug, the pharmacist who dispenses the drug, and the nurse who administers the drug. Each serves as a check within the system to catch errors—the wrong drug, the wrong patient, the wrong dose, the wrong route, the wrong time, the wrong storage, or the wrong documentation. Often the nurse is the final check in the process because the nurse is the one who administers the drug and is the one responsible for patient education before the patient is discharged to home.

Nurse's Role

The monumental task of ensuring medication safety with all of the potential problems that could confront the patient can best be managed by consistently using the "rights" of medication administration. These rights are as follows:

FOCUS ON Safe Medication Administration

1. *Right patient. It is always important to make sure that you are giving the drug to the correct patient. Checking the patient's wrist band and asking the patient to repeat his/her name and often birthdate are good policies to make sure it is the patient you think it is. Avoid the error of asking a patient, "Are you Mr. Jones?" The patient could respond yes without thinking or may not have heard you correctly. Rely on the patient telling you his/her name and read it from the identification band. It is also important to make sure this patient does not have allergies to the drug being given and that the patient is not taking interacting drugs, food, or alternative therapies.*
2. *Right drug. To prevent medication errors, always check to make sure the drug you are going to administer is the one that was prescribed. Many drugs may look alike and or have sound-alike names. Ask for the generic as well as the brand name if you are unsure. Never assume the computer is correct; always double-check. Avoid abbreviations, and if you are not sure about abbreviations that were used, ask. Make sure the drug makes sense for the patient for whom it is ordered.*
3. *Right storage. Be aware that some drugs require specific storage environments (e.g., refrigeration, protection from light). Check to make sure that general guidelines have been followed.*
4. *Right route. Determine the best route of administration; this is frequently established by the formulation of the drug. Nurses can often have an impact in modifying the route to arrive at the most efficient, comfortable method for the patient based on the patient's specific situation. For example, perhaps a patient is having trouble swallowing, and a large capsule would be very difficult for the patient to handle. The nurse could check and see if the drug is available in a liquid form and bring this information to the attention of the person prescribing the drug. When establishing the prescribed route, check the proper method of administering a drug by that route. Review drug administration methods periodically to make sure you have not forgotten important techniques. If you have instructed a patient in the proper administration of a drug, be sure to have the patient explain it back to you and demonstrate the proper technique. This should be done not only when the patient first learns this technique, but also periodically to make sure he or she has not forgotten any important points. Throughout this book, Focus on Safe Medication Administration boxes will provide review of proper medication administration technique.*
5. *Right dose. Always double-check calculations, and always do the calculations if the drug is not available in the dose ordered. Calculate the drug dose appropriately, based on the available drug form, the patient's body weight or surface area, or the patient's kidney function. Do not assume that the computer or the pharmacy is always right; you are one more check in the system. Do not cut tablets to get to a correct dose without checking to make sure the tablet can be cut, crushed, or chewed. Many tablets cannot be altered this way. Be very cautious if you see an order that starts with a decimal point; these orders are often the cause of medication errors. You should never see .5 mg as an order because it could be interpreted as 5 mg, 10 times the ordered dose. The proper dose would be 0.5 mg. If you see an order for 5.0 mg, be cautious; it could be interpreted as 50 mg. If a dose seems too big, question it. Throughout this book, Focus on Calculations boxes will provide review for calculating dose properly.*
6. *Right preparation. Know the specific preparation required before administering any drug. For example, oral drugs may need to be crushed or shaken; parenteral drugs may need to be reconstituted or diluted with specific solutions; and topical drugs may require specific handling, such as the use of gloves during administration or shaving of a body area before application. Many current oral drugs cannot be cut, crushed, or chewed. Checking that information can help to prevent serious adverse effects. If a drug needs to be diluted or reconstituted, check the manufacturer's instructions to make sure that this is done correctly.*
7. *Right time. When drugs are studied and evaluated, a suggested timing of administration is established. This timing takes into account all aspects of pharmacokinetics to determine a dosing schedule that will provide the needed therapeutic level of the drug. Recognize that the administration of one drug may require coordination with the administration of other drugs, foods, or physical parameters. In a busy hospital setting, getting the drug to the patient at the prescribed time can be a real challenge. As the caregiver most frequently involved in administering drugs the nurse must be aware of and manage all of these factors, as well as educate the patient to do this on his or her own. Organizing the day and the drug regimen to make it the least intrusive on a patient's lifestyle can help to prevent errors and improve compliance.*
8. *Right recording. Always document drug administration. If it isn't written, it didn't happen. Document the information in accordance with the local requirements for recording medication administration after assessing the patient, making the appropriate nursing diagnoses, and delivering the correct drug, by the correct route, in the correct dose, and at the correct time. Accurately record the drug given and the time given only once you have given the drug to avoid inadvertent overdoses or missing doses, which would lead to a lack of therapeutic effect. Encourage patients to keep track of their drugs at home, what they take, and when they take it, especially if they could be confused.*

The Patient's Role

With so many patients managing their drug regimens at home, one other very important check in the system also exists: the patient. Only the patient really knows what is being taken and when, and only the patient can report the actual as opposed to the prescribed drug regimen being followed. Patient and family education plays a vital role in the prevention of medication errors. Encourage patients to be their own advocates and to speak up and ask questions. Doing so helps to prevent medication errors. The following teaching points help to reduce the risk of medication errors in the home setting:

- *Keep a written list of all medications you are taking, including prescription, OTC, and herbal medications.* Keep this list with you at all times in case you are in an emergency situation and to keep your health care providers up to date. This list can be essential if you are traveling and need to refill a prescription while away from home.
- *Know what each of your drugs is being used to treat.* If you know why you are taking each drug, you will have a better understanding of what to report, what to watch for, and when to report to your health care provider if the drug is not working.
- *Read the labels, and follow the directions.* It is easy to make up your own schedule or to just take everything all at once in the morning. Always check the labels to see if there are specific times you should be taking your drugs. Make a calendar if you take drugs on alternating days. Using a weekly pillbox may also help to keep things straight.
- *Store drugs in a dry place, away from children and pets.* Humid and hot storage areas (like the bathroom) tend to cause drugs to break down faster. Storing drugs away from children and pets can prevent possible toxic effects if these drugs are inadvertently ingested by children or your family pet.
- *Speak up.* You are the most important member of the health care team, and you have information to share that no one else knows. Don't be shy about reporting the use of OTC or herbal therapies; these are your choices and are important to you. Sharing information about the use of these products will help your health care provider to incorporate them into your total drug regimen in a safe and effective way.

Children present unique challenges related to medication errors. Children often cannot speak for themselves and rely on a caregiver or caregivers to manage their drug regimen. Because their bodies are still developing and respond differently than those of adults to many drugs the risk of serious adverse reactions is greater with children. The margin of safety with many drugs is very small when dealing with a child. When teaching parents about their children's drug regimens, be sure to include the following instructions:

- *Keep a list of all medications you are giving your child, including prescription, OTC, and herbal medications.* Share this list with any health care provider who cares for your child. Never assume that a health care provider already knows what your child is taking.
- *Never use adult medications to treat a child.* The body organs and systems of children, primarily their livers and kidneys, are very different from those of an adult. As a result, children respond differently to drugs.
- *Read all labels before giving your child a drug.* Many OTC drugs contain the same ingredients, and you could accidentally overdose your child if you are not careful. In addition, some OTC drugs are not to be used with children younger than a certain age. Doses also may differ for children.
- *Measure liquid medications using appropriate measuring devices.* Never use your flatware teaspoon or tablespoon to measure your child's drugs. Always use a measured dosing device or the spoon from a measuring set.
- *Call your health care provider immediately if your child seems to get worse or seems to be having trouble with a drug.* Do not hesitate; many drugs can cause serious or life-threatening problems with children, and you should act immediately.
- *When in doubt, do not hesitate to ask questions.* You are your child's best advocate.

Reporting of Medication Errors

Medication errors must be reported on a national level as well as on an institutional level. National reporting programs are coordinated by the US Pharmacopeia, and they help to gather information about errors to prevent their recurrence at other health care sites and by other health care providers. These reports might prompt the issuing of health care provider warnings, which point out potential or actual medication errors and suggest ways to avoid these errors in the future. For example, in 2007 the name of the drug *Omacor* (omega-3 fatty acid) was changed to *Lovaza* after many reports of confusion between *Omacor* and *Amicar* (aminocaproic acid). Other reports have led to public warnings about look-alike or sound-alike drug names and common dosing errors and transcribing issues.

Institutions also have their own policies for reporting medication errors that protect patients and staff and identify particular areas in which education or system changes may be needed. Always be aware of the policies of your employing institution or agency. If you see or participate in a medication error, report it to your institution and then report it to the national reporting program. Box 4.4 provides information about reporting medication errors. Your report will be shared with all of the appropriate agencies—the U.S. Food and Drug Administration, the drug manufacturer, and the Institute for Safe Medication Practices. Health care providers working together and sharing information can make a big impact in decreasing the occurrence of medication errors.

BOX 4.4

Reporting Medication Errors

National center for reporting actual or potential medication errors (U.S. Pharmacopeia/Institute for Safe Medication Practices Medication Errors Reporting Program):

Call 1-800-23-ERROR.
Go online to http://www.usp.org

SUMMARY

- Nursing is a complex art and science that provides for nurturing and care of the sick, as well as prevention and education services.
- Components of the nursing assessment (history of past illnesses and the current complaint, as well as a physical examination) provide a database of baseline information to ensure safe administration of a drug and to evaluate the drug's effectiveness and adverse effects.
- Nursing assessment must include information on the history of past illnesses and the current complaint as well as a complete drug history and a physical examination; this provides a database of baseline information to ensure safe administration of a drug and to evaluate the drug's effectiveness and adverse effects.
- Nursing diagnoses are developed from the information gathered during the assessment phase of the nursing process. A nursing diagnosis states the actual or potential response of a patient to a clinical situation.
- Planning uses the information gathered and the resultant nursing diagnoses to determine the desired patient outcomes, setting goals for safe and effective drug administration. The plan will lead to the necessary nursing interventions.
- Implementation puts the nursing interventions into action. Interventions related to drug therapy include safely administering the drug, providing comfort measures to help the patient cope with the therapeutic or adverse effects of a drug, and providing patient and family education to ensure safe and effective drug therapy.
- Evaluation is part of the continuing process of patient care that leads to changes in assessment, diagnosis, and intervention. The patient is continually evaluated for therapeutic response, the occurrence of adverse drug effects, and the occurrence of drug–drug, drug–food, drug–alternative therapy, or drug–laboratory test interactions.
- A nursing care guide and patient education materials can be prepared for each drug being given, using information about a drug's therapeutic effects, adverse effects, and special considerations.
- Prevention of medication errors is a complicated task that involves the prescriber, the pharmacist, the nurse administering the drugs, and the patient. The nurse needs to be vigilant in administering drugs to check the seven "rights" of drug administration. The patient needs to be educated to be his or her own advocate and to take steps to avoid medication errors.

CHECK YOUR UNDERSTANDING

Answers to the questions in this chapter can be found in Answers to Check Your Understanding Questions on thePoint®.

MULTIPLE CHOICE

Select the best answer to the following.

1. A patient reports that she has a drug allergy. In exploring the allergic reaction with the patient, which of the following might indicate an allergic response?
   a. Increased urination
   b. Dry mouth
   c. Rash
   d. Drowsiness

2. The nurse obtains a medical history from a patient before beginning drug therapy based on an understanding of which of the following?
   a. Medical conditions can alter a drug's pharmacokinetics and pharmacodynamics.
   b. A medical history is a key component of any nursing protocol.
   c. A baseline of information is necessary to evaluate a drug's effects.
   d. The medical history is the first step in the nursing process.

3. The nurse writes a nursing diagnosis for which reason?
   a. Direct medical care
   b. Help to increase patient compliance
   c. Identify actual or potential alteration in patient function
   d. Determine insurance reimbursement in most cases

4. A patient receiving an antihistamine complains of dry mouth and nose. An appropriate comfort measure for this patient would be to
   a. suggest that the patient use a humidifier.
   b. encourage voiding before taking the drug.
   c. have the patient avoid sun exposure.
   d. give the patient a back rub.

5. When establishing the nursing interventions appropriate for a given patient
   a. the patient should not be actively involved.
   b. the patient support systems should be included only at discharge.

c. teaching should be done when the patient states he or she is ready to learn.
d. an evaluation of all of the data accumulated should be incorporated to achieve an effective care plan.

6. The evaluation step of the nursing process
a. is often used as a last resort.
b. is important primarily in the acute setting.
c. is a continuous process.
d. includes making nursing diagnoses.

7. After teaching a patient about digoxin (generic)—a drug used to increase the effectiveness of the heart's contractions—which statement indicates that the teaching was effective?
a. "I need to take my pulse every morning before I take my pill."
b. "If I forget my pills, I usually make up the missed dose once I remember."
c. "This pill might help my hay fever when it becomes a problem."
d. "I don't remember the name of it, but it is the white one."

MULTIPLE RESPONSE

Select all that apply.

1. A client is being started on a laxative regimen. Before beginning the regimen the nurse performs which of the following assessments?
a. Liver function test
b. Abdominal examination
c. Skin color and lesion evaluation
d. Lung auscultation
e. 24-hour urine analysis
f. Cardiac assessment

2. The nursing care of a patient receiving drug therapy should include measures to decrease the anticipated adverse effects of the drug. Which of the following measures would a nurse consider?
a. A positive approach
b. Environmental temperature control
c. Safety measures
d. Skin care
e. Refrigeration of the drug
f. Involvement of the family

3. A nurse is preparing to administer a drug to a client for the first time. What questions should the nurse consider before actually administering the drug?
a. Is this the right patient?
b. Is this the right drug?
c. Is there a generic drug available?
d. Is this the right route for this patient?
e. Is this the right dose, as ordered?
f. Did I record this properly?

BIBLIOGRAPHY AND REFERENCES

Bickley, L. (2012). *Bates' guide to physical examination and history taking* (11th ed.). Philadelphia, PA: Lippincott Williams & Wilkins.

Buchanan, L. M. (1994). Therapeutic nursing intervention knowledge development and outcome measures for advanced practice. *Nursing and Health Care, 15*(4), 190–195.

Carpenito, L. J. (2008). *Nursing care plans and documentation* (5th ed.). Philadelphia, PA: Lippincott Williams & Wilkins.

Carpenito, L. J. (2012). *Handbook of nursing diagnoses* (14th ed.). Philadelphia, PA: Lippincott Williams & Wilkins.

Carpenito, L. J. (2012). *Nursing diagnosis: Application in clinical practice* (12th ed.). Philadelphia, PA: Lippincott Williams & Wilkins.

Cohen, M. (1994). Medication errors… misprinted doses: FDA precautions. *Nursing, 94*(3), 14.

Jones, J. H., & Treiber, L. (2010). When the rights go wrong: Medication errors from a nursing perspective. *Journal of Nursing Care Quality, 25*(3), 240–247.

Karch, A. (2003). *Lippincott's guide to preventing medication errors.* Philadelphia, PA: Lippincott Williams & Wilkins.

Kohn, L., Corrigan, J., & Donaldson, M. (Eds.). (2000). *To err is human: Building a safer health system.* Washington, DC: National Academy Press.

McCloskey, J., & Bulechek, G. (Eds.). (2008). *Nursing interventions classification* (5th ed.). St. Louis, MO: Elsevier Mosby.

Redman, B. (2007). *The practice of patient education* (10th ed.). St. Louis, MO: Elsevier/Mosby-Year Book.

Spath, P. L. (2011). *Error reduction in health care: A systems approach to improving patient safety* (2nd ed.). San Francisco, CA: Jossey-Bass.

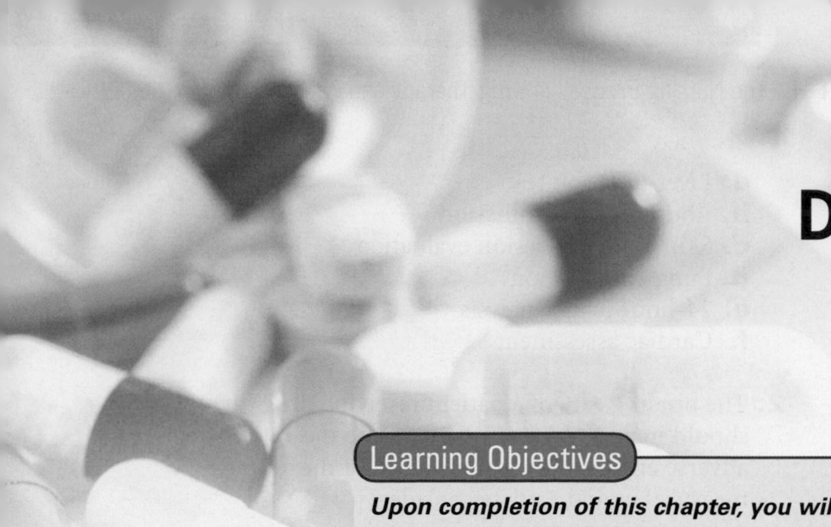

Dosage Calculations 5

Learning Objectives

Upon completion of this chapter, you will be able to:

1. Describe four measuring systems that can be used in drug therapy.
2. Convert between different measuring systems when given drug orders and available forms of the drugs.
3. Calculate the correct dose of a drug when given examples of drug orders and available forms of the drugs ordered.
4. Discuss why children require different dosages of drugs than adults.
5. Explain the calculations used to determine a safe pediatric dose of a drug.

Glossary of Key Terms

apothecary system: a very old system of measure that was specifically developed for use by apothecaries or pharmacists; it uses the minim as the basic unit of liquid measure and the grain as the basic unit of solid measure

Clark's rule: a method of determining the correct drug dose for a child based on the known adult dose (assumes that the adult dose is based on a 150-pound person); it states

$$\text{child's dose} = \frac{\text{weight of child (lb)}}{150\ \text{lb}} \times \text{average adult dose}$$

conversion: finding the equivalent values between two systems of measure

Fried's rule: a method of determining a pediatric drug dose for a child younger than 1 year of age, based on the child's age and the usual adult dose (assumes that an adult dose would be appropriate for a 12.5-year-old child); it states

$$\text{child's dose (age 1 y)} = \frac{\text{weight of child (lb)}}{150\ \text{lb}} \times \text{average adult dose}$$

metric system: the most widely used system of measure, based on the decimal system; all units in the system are determined as multiples of 10

ratio and proportion: an equation in which a ratio containing two known equivalent amounts is on one side and a ratio containing the amount desired to convert and its unknown equivalent is on the other side

Young's rule: a method for determining pediatric drug dose based on the child's age and the usual adult dose; it states

$$\text{child's dose (age 1 – 12 y)} = \frac{\text{child's age (y)}}{\text{child's age (y)} + 12} \times \text{average adult dose}$$

To determine the correct dose of a particular drug for a patient, we consider the patient's sex, weight, age, and physical condition, as well as the other drugs that the patient is taking. Frequently, the dose that is needed for a patient is not the dose that is available, and it is necessary to convert the dose form available into the prescribed dose. Doing the necessary mathematical calculations to determine what should be given is the responsibility of the prescriber who orders the drug, the pharmacist who dispenses the drug, and the nurse who administers the drug. This allows the necessary checks on the dose being given before the patient actually receives the drug. Another check to help prevent medication errors is that in many institutions, drugs arrive at the patient care area in unit-dose form, prepackaged for each individual patient. The nurse who will administer the drug may come to rely on this prepackaged system, forgoing any recalculation or rechecking of the dose to match the written order. Unfortunately, mistakes still happen, and the nurse, as the person who is administering the drug, is legally and professionally responsible for any error that might occur. Practicing nurses must know how to convert drug-dosing orders into appropriate doses of available forms of a drug to ensure that the right patient is getting the right dose of a drug.

Measuring Systems

At least four different systems are currently used in drug preparation and delivery: the metric system, the apothecary system, the household system, and the avoirdupois system. Table 5.1 compares the basic units of measure of three of the measuring systems. With the growing number of drugs available and increasing awareness of medication errors that occur in daily practice, efforts have been made to decrease the dependence on so many different systems. In 1995 the U.S. Pharmacopeia Convention established standards requiring that all prescriptions, regardless of the system that was used in the drug dosing, include the metric measure for the quantity and strength of drug. It was also established that drugs may be dispensed only in the metric form. Prescribers are not totally converted to this new standard, however, so the nurse must be able to convert the dose ordered into the available dose form to ensure patient safety. It is important to be able to perform **conversions**—finding the equivalent values between two types of measure, within each system of measure, and between systems of measure.

Metric System

The **metric system** is the most widely used system of measure. It is based on the decimal system, so all units are determined as multiples of 10. This system is used worldwide and makes the sharing of knowledge and research information easier. The metric system uses the gram as the basic unit of solid measure and the liter as the basic unit of liquid measure (see Table 5.1).

Apothecary System

The **apothecary system** is a very old system of measurement that was specifically developed for use by apothecaries or pharmacists. The apothecary system uses the minim as the basic unit of liquid measure and the grain as the basic unit of solid measure (see Table 5.1). This system is much harder to use than the metric system and is rarely seen in most clinical settings. Occasionally, a prescriber will write an order in this system, and the dose will have to be converted to an available form. An interesting feature of this system is that it uses Roman numerals placed after the unit of measure to denote amount. For example, 15 grains would be written "gr xv."

Household System

The household system is the measuring system that is found in recipe books. This system uses the teaspoon as the basic unit of fluid measure and the pound as the basic unit of solid measure (see Table 5.1). Although efforts have been made in recent years to standardize these measuring devices, wide variations have been noted in the capacity of some of them. Patients need to be advised that flatware teaspoons and drinking cups vary tremendously in the volume that they contain. A flatware teaspoon could hold up to two measuring teaspoons of quantity. When a patient is using a liquid medication at home, it is important to clarify that the measures indicated in the instructions refer to a standardized measuring device.

Avoirdupois System

The avoirdupois system is another older system that was very popular when pharmacists routinely had to compound medications. This system uses ounces and

Table 5.1 Comparing Basic Units of Measure by Measuring Systems

System	Solid Measure	Liquid Measure
Metric	gram (g) 1 milligram (mg) = 0.001 g 1 microgram (mcg) = 0.000001 g 1 kilogram (kg) = 1,000 g	liter (L) 1 milliliter (mL) = 0.001 L 1 mL = 1 cubic centimeter = 1 cc
Apothecary	grain (gr) 60 gr = 1 dram (dr) 8 dr = 1 ounce (oz)	minim (min) 60 min = 1 fluidram (fl dr) 8 fl dr = 1 fluid ounce (fl oz)
Household	pound (lb) 1 lb = 16 ounces (oz)	pint (pt) 2 pt = 1 quart (qt) 4 qt = 1 gallon (gal) 16 oz = 1 pt = 2 cups (c) 32 tablespoons (tbsp) = 1 pt 3 teaspoons (tsp) = 1 tbsp 60 drops (gtt) = 1 tsp

grains, but they measure differently than those of the apothecary and household systems. The avoirdupois system is seldom used by prescribers but may be used for bulk medications that come directly from the manufacturer.

Other Systems

Some drugs are measured in units other than those already discussed. These measures may reflect chemical activity or biological equivalence. One of these measures is the unit. A unit usually reflects the biological activity of the drug in 1 mL of solution. The unit is unique for the drug it measures; a unit of heparin is not comparable with a unit of insulin. Milliequivalents (mEq) are used to measure electrolytes (e.g., potassium, sodium, calcium, fluoride). The milliequivalent refers to the ionic activity of the drug in question; the order is usually written for a number of milliequivalents instead of a volume of drug. International units are sometimes used to measure certain vitamins or enzymes. These are also unique to each drug and cannot be converted to another measuring form.

KEY POINTS

- At least four different systems are currently used in drug preparation and delivery. These are the metric system, the apothecary system, the household system, and the avoirdupois system.
- The metric system is the most widely used system of measure. The U.S. Pharmacopeia Convention established standards requiring that all prescriptions, regardless of the system that was used in drug dosing, include the metric measure for the quantity and strength of drug. All drugs are dispensed in the metric system.

Conversion between Systems

The simplest way to convert measurements from one system to another is to set up a **ratio and proportion** equation. The ratio containing two known equivalent amounts is placed on one side of an equation, and the ratio containing the amount you wish to convert and its unknown equivalent is placed on the other side. To do this, it is necessary to first check a table of conversions to determine the equivalent measure in the two systems you are using. Table 5.2 presents some accepted conversions equivalents between systems of measurement. It is a good idea to post a conversion guide in the medication room or on the medication cart for easy access. When conversions are used frequently, it is easy to remember them. When conversions are not used frequently, it is best to look them up.

Try the following conversion using Table 5.2. Convert 6 fl oz (apothecary system) to the metric system of measure.

Table 5.2 Commonly Accepted Conversions between Systems of Measurement

Metric System	Apothecary System	Household System
Solid Measure		
1 kg		2.2 lb
454 g		1.0 lb
1 g = 1,000 mg	15 gr (gr xv)	
60 mg	1 gr (gr i)	
30 mg	½ gr (gr ss)	
Liquid Measure		
1 L = 1,000 mL		about 1 qt
240 mL	8 fl oz (fl oz viii)	1 c
30 mL	1 fl oz (fl oz i)	2 tbsp
15–16 mL	4 fl dr (fl dr iv)	1 tbsp = 3 tsp
8 mL	2 fl dr (fl dr ii)	2 tsp
4–5 mL	1 fl dr (fl dr i)	1 tsp = 60 gtt
1 mL	15–16 min (min xv or min xvi)	
0.06 mL	1 min (min i)	

According to Table 5.2, 1 fl oz is equivalent to 30 mL. Use this information to set up a ratio:

$$\frac{1 \text{ fl oz}}{30 \text{ mL}} = \frac{6 \text{ fl oz}}{X}$$

The known ratio—1 fl oz (apothecary system) is equivalent to 30 mL (metric system)—is on one side of the equation. The other side of the equation contains 6 fl oz, the amount (apothecary system) that you want to convert, and its unknown (metric system) equivalent, *X*. Because the fluid ounce measurement is in the numerator (top number) on the left side of the equation, it must also be in the numerator on the right side of the equation. This equation would read as follows: 1 fl oz is to 30 mL as 6 fl oz is to how many milliliters?

The first step in the conversion is to cross-multiply (multiply the numerator from one side of the equation by the denominator from the other side, and vice versa):

$$\frac{1 \text{ fl oz}}{30 \text{ mL}} = \frac{6 \text{ fl oz}}{X}$$

$$1 \text{ fl oz} \times X = 6 \text{ fl oz} \times 30 \text{ mL}$$

This could also be written as:

$$(1 \text{ fl oz})(X) = (6 \text{ fl oz})(30 \text{ mL})$$

After multiplying the numbers, you have:

$$1(\text{fl oz})X = 180(\text{fl oz})(\text{mL})$$

Next, rearrange the terms to let the unknown quantity stand alone on one side of the equation:

$$X = \frac{180(\text{mL})(\text{fl oz})}{1 \text{ fl oz}}$$

Whenever possible, cancel out numbers, as well as units of measure. In this example, canceling out leaves $X = 180$ mL.

By canceling out, you are left with the appropriate amount and unit of measure. The answer to the problem is that 6 fl oz is equivalent to 180 mL.

Try another conversion. Convert 32 gr (apothecary system) to its equivalent in the metric system, expressing the answer in milligrams. First, find the conversion in Table 5.2: 1 gr is equal to 60 mg. Set up the ratio

$$\frac{1\ \text{gr}}{60\ \text{mg}} = \frac{32\ \text{gr}}{X}$$

Cross-multiply:

$$(1\ \text{gr})(X) = (32\ \text{gr})(60\ \text{mg})$$

$$1(\text{gr})X = 1{,}920(\text{gr})(\text{mg})$$

Rearrange:

$$X = \frac{1{,}920\ (\text{gr})(\text{mg})}{1\ \text{gr}}$$

Finally, cancel out like units and numbers:

$$X = 1{,}920\ \text{mg}$$

Therefore, 32 gr is equivalent to 1,920 mg.

Calculating Dose

As mentioned earlier, because there are several systems of measurement available that might be used when a drug is ordered and because drugs are made available only in certain forms or doses, it may be necessary to calculate what the patient should be receiving.

Oral Drugs

Frequently, tablets or capsules for oral administration are not available in the exact dose that has been ordered. In these situations the nurse who is administering the drug must calculate the number of tablets or capsules to give for the ordered dose. The easiest way to determine this is to set up a ratio and proportion equation. The ratio containing the two known equivalent amounts is put on one side of the equation, and the ratio containing the unknown value is put on the other side. The known equivalent is the amount of drug available in one tablet or capsule; the unknown is the number of tablets or capsules that are needed for the prescribed dose:

$$\frac{\text{amount of drug available}}{\text{one tablet or capsule}} = \frac{\text{amount of drug prescribed}}{\text{number of tablets or capsules to give}}$$

The phrase "amount of drug" serves as the unit, so this information must be in the numerator of each ratio.

Try this example: An order is written for 10 grains of aspirin (gr x, aspirin). The tablets that are available each contain 5 grains. How many tablets should the nurse give? First, set up the equation:

$$\frac{5\ \text{gr}}{\text{one tablet}} = \frac{10\ \text{gr}}{X}$$

Cross-multiply the ratio:

$$5(\text{gr})X = 10(\text{gr})(\text{tablet})$$

Rearrange and cancel like units and numbers:

$$X = \frac{10(\text{gr})(\text{tablets})}{5(\text{gr})}$$

Therefore, the nurse would administer two tablets.

Try another example: An order is written for 0.05 g *Aldactone* (spironolactone) to be given orally (per os, PO). *Aldactone* is available in 25-mg tablets. How many tablets would you have to give? First, you will need to convert the grams to milligrams:

$$\frac{1\ \text{g}}{1{,}000\ \text{mg}} = \frac{0.05\ \text{g}}{X}$$

Cross-multiply:

$$1(\text{g})X = (0.05 \times 1{,}000)(\text{g})(\text{mg})$$

Simplify:

$$X = \frac{50(\text{g})(\text{mg})}{1(\text{g})}$$

So 0.05 g of *Aldactone* is equal to 50 mg of *Aldactone*.

The order has been converted to the same measurement as the available tablets. Now solve for the number of tablets that you will need, letting X be the number of tablets to equal the desired dose of 50 mg:

$$\frac{25\ \text{mg}}{1\ \text{tablet}} = \frac{50\ \text{mg}}{X}$$

$$25\ (\text{mg})X = (50 \times 1)\ (\text{mg})(\text{tablet})$$

$$X = 2\ \text{tablets}$$

Sometimes the desired dose will be a fraction of a tablet or capsule, 1/2 or 1/4. Some tablets come with scored markings that allow them to be cut. Pill cutters are readily available in most pharmacies to help patients cut tablets appropriately. However, one must use caution when advising a patient to cut a tablet. Many tablets come in a matrix system that allows for slow and steady release of the active drug. These drugs cannot be cut, crushed, or chewed. Always consult a drug reference before cutting a tablet. However, as a quick reference, any tablet that is designated as having delayed or sustained release may very well be one that cannot be cut. Capsules can be very difficult to divide precisely, and some of them also come with warnings that they cannot be cut, crushed, or chewed. If the only way to deliver the correct dose to a patient is by cutting one of these preparations a different formulation of the drug, a different drug, or a different approach to treating the patient should be tried.

Other oral drugs come in liquid preparations. Many of the drugs used in pediatrics and for adults who might have difficulty swallowing a pill or tablet are prepared in a liquid form. Some drugs that do not come in a standard liquid form can be prepared as a liquid by the pharmacist. If the patient is not able to swallow a tablet or capsule, check for other available forms and consult with the pharmacist about the possibility of preparing the drug in a liquid as a suspension or a solution. The same principle used to determine the number of tablets needed to arrive at a prescribed dose can be used to determine the volume of liquid that will be required to administer the prescribed dose. The ratio on the left of the equation shows the known equivalents, and the ratio on the right side contains the unknown. The phrase "amount of drug" must appear in the numerator of both ratios, and the volume to administer is the unknown (X).

Try this example: An order has been written for 250 mg of amoxicillin. The bottle states that the solution contains 125 mg/5 mL. How much of the liquid should you give?

Cross-multiply:

$$125(\text{mg})X = (250 \times 5)(\text{mg})(\text{mL})$$

Simplify:

$$X = \frac{1{,}250(\text{mg})(\text{mL})}{125(\text{mg})}$$

So the desired dose is $X = 10$ mL.

Even if you are working in an institution that provides unit-dose medications, practice your calculation skills occasionally to keep them sharp. Power can be lost, computers can go down, and the ability to determine conversions is a skill that anyone who administers drugs should have in reserve. Periodically throughout this text you will find a Focus on Calculations box to help you refresh your dose calculation skills as they apply to the drugs being discussed.

Parenteral Drugs

All drugs administered parenterally must be administered in liquid form. The person administering the drug needs to calculate the volume of the liquid that must be given to administer the prescribed dose. The same formula can be used for this determination that was used for determining the dose of an oral liquid drug:

$$\frac{\text{amount of drug available}}{\text{volume available}} = \frac{\text{amount of drug prescribed}}{\text{volume to administer}}$$

Try this example: An order has been written for 75 mg of meperidine to be given intramuscularly. The vial states that it contains meperidine, 1.0 mL=50.0 mg. Set up the equation just as before:

$$\frac{50 \text{ mg}}{1 \text{ mL}} = \frac{75 \text{ mg}}{X}$$

$$50 \text{ (mg)}X = (75 \times 1) \text{ (mg)(mL)}$$

$$X = \frac{75 \text{ (mg)(mL)}}{50 \text{ (mg)}}$$

Thus, $X = 1.5$ mL.

Intravenous Solutions

Intravenous (IV) solutions are used to deliver a prescribed amount of fluid, electrolytes, vitamins, nutrients, or drugs directly into the bloodstream. Although most institutions now use electronically monitored delivery systems, it is still important to be able to determine the amount of an IV solution that should be given, using standard calculations. Most IV delivery systems come with a standard control called a microdrip, by which each milliliter delivered contains 60 drops. Macrodrip systems, which usually deliver 15 drops/mL, are also available; they are usually used when a large volume must be delivered quickly. Always check the packaging of the IV tubing to see how many drops/mL are delivered by that particular device if you have any doubts or are unfamiliar with the system.

Use the following ratio to determine how many drops of fluid to administer per minute:

$$\frac{\text{drops}}{\text{minute}} = \frac{\text{(mL of solution prescribed per hour)}\,\text{(drops delivered per mL)}}{(60\text{min})/(1\text{h})}$$

That is, the number of drops per minute, or the rate that you will set by adjusting the valve on the IV tubing, is equal to the amount of solution that has been prescribed per hour times the number of drops delivered per milliliter (mL), divided by 60 minutes in an hour.

Try this example: An order has been written for a patient to receive 400 mL of 5% dextrose in water (D5W) over a period of 4 hours in a standard microdrip system (i.e., 60 drops/mL). Calculate the correct setting (drops per minute):

$$X = \frac{(400 \text{ mL/4 h})(60 \text{ drops/min})}{(60 \text{ min})/(1 \text{ h})}$$

Simplify:

$$X = \frac{(100 \text{ mL/h})(60 \text{ drops/min})}{(60 \text{ min})/(1 \text{ h})}$$

$$X = \frac{6{,}000 \text{ drops/h}}{(60 \text{ min})/(1 \text{ h})}$$

Therefore, $X = 100$ drops/min.

Now calculate the same order for an IV set that delivers 15 drops/mL:

$$X = \frac{(400\text{ mL}/4\text{ h})(15\text{ drops/min})}{(60\text{ min})/(1\text{ h})}$$

$$X = \frac{(100\text{ mL/h})(15\text{ drops/min})}{(60\text{ min})/(1\text{ h})}$$

$$X = \frac{1{,}500\text{ drops/h}}{(60\text{ min})/(1\text{ h})}$$

Therefore, $X = 25$ drops/min.

If a patient has an order for an IV drug, the same principle can be used to calculate the speed of the delivery. For example, an order is written for a patient to receive 50 mL of an antibiotic over 30 minutes. The IV set used dispenses 60 drops/mL, which allows greater control. Calculate how fast the delivery should be:

$$X = \frac{(50\text{ mL}/0.5\text{ h})(60\text{ drops/min})}{(60\text{ min})/(1\text{ h})}$$

$$X = \frac{(100\text{ mL/h})(60\text{ drops/min})}{(60\text{ min})/(1\text{ h})}$$

$$X = \frac{6{,}000\text{ drops/h}}{(60\text{ min})/(1\text{ h})}$$

Therefore, $X = 100$ drops/min.

Pediatric Considerations

For most drugs, children require doses different from those given to adults. The "standard" drug dose that is listed on package inserts and in many references refers to the dose that has been found to be most effective in the adult male. An adult's body handles drugs differently and may respond to drugs differently than a child's. For example, a child's body may handle a drug differently in all areas of pharmacokinetics—absorption, distribution, metabolism, and excretion. In addition, the responses of the child's organs to the effects of the drug also may vary because of the immaturity of the organs. Most of the time a child requires a smaller dose of a drug to achieve the comparable critical concentration as that for an adult. On rare occasions, a child may require a higher dose of a drug. For ethical reasons, drug research per se is not done on children. Over time, however, enough information can be accumulated from experience with the drug to have a recommended pediatric dose. The drug guide that you have selected to use in the clinical setting will have the pediatric dose listed if this information is available.

Unfortunately, there may be times when no recommended dose for a child is available but that particular drug is needed. In these situations, established formulas can be used to estimate the appropriate dose. These methods of determining a pediatric dose take into consideration the child's age, weight, or body surface. Box 5.1 highlights **Fried's rule**, which considers age for a child under the age of 1 year; **Young's rule**, which calculates doses for children 1 to 12 years of age; and **Clark's rule**, which accounts for weight in the dose formula. These rules are not usually used today; the nomogram that uses body surface area is more accurate for determining doses (see Figure 5.1). If such a nomogram is not available, however, it is good to know that other methods can be used.

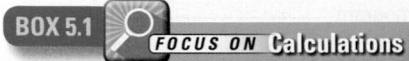

BOX 5.1 FOCUS ON Calculations

FORMULAS FOR CALCULATING PEDIATRIC DOSES

Fried's rule is a calculation method that applies to a child younger than 1 year of age. The rule assumes that an adult dose would be appropriate for a child who is 12.5 years (150 months) old. Fried's rule states:

$$\text{child's dose (age} < 1\text{ y)} = \frac{\text{child's age (mo)}}{150\text{ mo}} \times \text{average adult dose}$$

Young's rule is a calculation method that applies to children 1 to 12 years of age. It states:

$$\text{child's dose (age 1} - 12\text{ y)} = \frac{\text{child's age (y)}}{\text{child's age (y)} + 12} \times \text{average adult dose}$$

Clark's rule uses the child's weight to calculate the appropriate dose and assumes that the adult dose is based on a 150-pound person. It states:

$$\text{child's dose} = \frac{\text{weight of child (in lb)}}{150\text{ lb}} \times \text{average adult dose}$$

For example, a 3-year-old child weighing 30 lb is to receive a therapeutic dose of aspirin. The average adult dose is 5 gr, and the dose to be given is the unknown (X). The calculation may be made from the child's age by Young's rule:

$$X = \frac{3\text{ y}}{3 + 12\text{ y}} \times 5\text{ gr}$$

$$X = \frac{15\text{ (y)(gr)}}{15\text{ y}}$$

Therefore, $X = 1$ gr.

Alternatively, the calculation could be based on the child's weight, using Clark's rule:

$$X = \frac{30\text{ lb}}{150\text{ lb}} \times 5\text{ gr}$$

$$X = \frac{150\text{ (lb)(gr)}}{150\text{ lb}}$$

This again yields $X = 1$ gr.

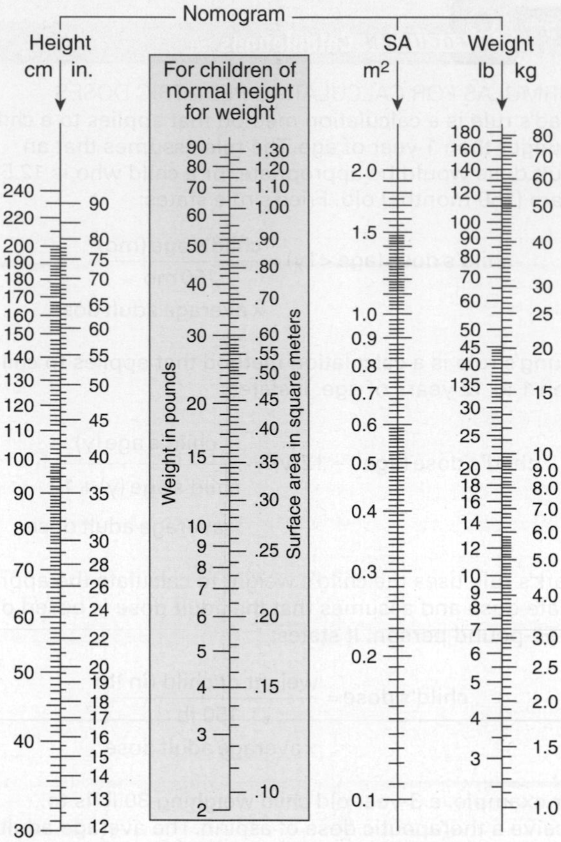

FIGURE 5.1 The West nomogram for calculating body surface area (BSA). Draw a straight line connecting the child's height (*left scale*) to the child's weight (*right scale*). The BSA value, which is calculated in square meters, is found at the point where the line intersects the SA column. The formula for estimating a child's dose is as follows: child's BSA (in m^2) × adult dose ÷ 1.73. Normal values are shown in the box.

Regardless of the calculation method used for children, even a tiny dose error can be critical. When working in pediatrics, one needs to be familiar with at least one of these methods of determining the drug dose. Many institutions require that two nurses check critical pediatric doses. This is a good practice when working with small children.

Body Surface Area

The surface area of a child's body may also be used to determine the approximate dose that should be used. To do this, the child's surface area is determined with the use of a nomogram (Figure 5.1). The height and weight of the child are taken into consideration in this chart. The following formula is then used:

$$\text{child's dose} = \frac{\text{surface area } (\text{m}^2)}{1.73} \times \text{average adult dose}$$

This method is more precise than the formula methods, but you have to have a nomogram available to determine the surface area.

Milligrams/Kilograms of Body Weight

When a safe and effective pediatric dose has been established the orders for the drug dose are often written in milligrams/kilograms. This method of prescribing takes into consideration the varying weights of children and the need for a higher dose of the drug when the weight increases. For example, if a child with postoperative nausea is to be treated with *Vistaril* (hydroxyzine) the recommended dose is 1.1 mg/kg by intramuscular injection. If the child weighs 22 kg, the dose for this child would be 1.1 mg/kg times 22 kg, or 24.2 mg, rounded down to24 mg. If a child weighed only 6 kg, the recommended dose would be 1.1 mg/kg times 6 kg, or 6.6 mg. The established guidelines allow the drug to be used safely within a large range of children. Some adult doses will also be written in this way. This is usually found in drugs with a small margin of safety or high potential for toxic effects, such as antineoplastic drugs.

SUMMARY

- At least four different systems are currently used in drug preparation and delivery. These are the metric system, the apothecary system, the household system, and the avoirdupois system.
- The metric system is the most widely used system of measure. The U.S. Pharmacopeia Convention established standards requiring that all prescriptions, regardless of the system that was used in drug dosing, include the metric measure for the quantity and strength of drug. All drugs are dispensed in the metric system.
- It is important to know how to convert doses from one system to another. The method of ratio and proportion, which uses basic principles of algebra to find an unknown, is the easiest method of converting doses within and between systems.
- Children require doses of most drugs different from those of adults due to the way their bodies handle drugs and the way that drugs affect their tissues and organs.
- Standard formulas, such as Fried's rule (for age <1 year), Clark's rule (which considers the child's weight), and Young's rule (which considers weight and age >1 year) can be used to determine the approximate dose that should be given to a child when the average adult dose is known. However, these rules are used less frequently today. Instead, most pediatric doses are based on body surface area, which requires the use of a nomogram, and milligrams per kilogram of body weight.

CHECK YOUR UNDERSTANDING

Answers to the questions in this chapter can be found in Answers to Check Your Understanding Questions on thePoint®.

MULTIPLE CHOICE

Select the best answer to the following.

1. Digoxin 0.125 mg is ordered for a patient who is having trouble swallowing. The bottle of digoxin elixir reads 0.05 mg/mL. How much would you give?
a. 5 mL
b. 0.5 mL
c. 2.5 mL
d. 2 mL

2. The usual adult dose of diphenhydramine (*Benadryl*) is 50 mg. What would be the safe dose for a child weighing 27 lb?
a. 0.9 mg
b. 1.8 mg
c. 9.0 mg
d. 18 mg

3. An order is written for 700 mg of ampicillin PO. The drug is supplied in liquid form as 1 g/3.5 mL. How much of the liquid should be given?
a. 5 mL
b. 2.5 mL
c. 6.2 mL
d. 2.45 mL

4. An order is written for 1,000 mL of normal saline to be administered IV over 10 hours. The drop factor on the IV tubing states 15 drops/mL. What is the IV flow rate?
a. 50 mL/h at 50 drops/min
b. 100 mL/h at 25 drops/min
c. 100 mL/h at 100 drops/min
d. 100 mL/h at 15 drops/min

5. The average adult dose of meperidine is 75 mg. What dose would be appropriate for a 10-month-old infant?
a. 50 mg
b. 5 mg
c. 25 mg
d. 0.5 mg

6. A patient needs to take 0.75 g of tetracycline PO. The drug comes in 250-mg tablets. How many tablets should the patient take?
a. 2 tablets
b. 3 tablets
c. 4 tablets
d. 30 tablets

7. Aminophylline is supplied in a 500 mg/2.5 mL solution. How much would be given if an order were written for 100 mg of aminophylline IV?
a. 5 mL
b. 1.5 mL
c. 2.5 mL
d. 0.5 mL

8. Heparin 800 units is ordered for a patient. The heparin is supplied in a multidose vial that is labeled 10,000 units/mL. How many milliliters of heparin would be needed to treat this patient?
a. 0.8 mL
b. 0.08 mL
c. 8.0 mL
d. 0.4 mL

COMPLETE THE FOLLOWING PROBLEMS

1. Change to equivalents within the system:
a. 100 mg =_____ g
b. 1,500 g =_____ kg
c. 0.1 L =_____ mL
d. 500 mL =_____ L

2. Convert to units in the metric system:
a. 150 gr =_____ g
b. gr =_____ mg
c. 45 min =_____ Ml
d. 2 qt =_____ L

3. Convert to units in the household system:
a. 5 mL =_____ tsp
b. 30 mL =_____ tbsp

(continues on page 64)

4. Convert the weights in the following problems:
   a. A patient weighs 170 lb. What is the patient's weight in kilograms?
   b. 170 lb =_____ kg
   c. A patient weighs 3,200 g. What is the patient's weight in pounds?
   d. 3,200 g =_____ lb

5. Robitussin cough syrup 225 mg PO is ordered. The bottle reads: 600 mg in 1 oz. How much cough syrup should be given? _____ mL

6. A postoperative order is written for 15 gr of codeine every 4 hours as needed (pro re nata, PRN) for pain. Each dose given will contain how many milligrams of codeine? _____ mg

7. Ordered: 6.5 mg. Available: 10 mg/mL. Proper dose: _____ mL.

8. Ordered: 0.35 mg. Available: 1.2 mg/2 mL. Proper dose: _____ mL.

9. Ordered: 80 mg. Available: 50 mg/mL. Proper dose: _____ mL.

10. Ordered: 150,000 units. Available: 400,000 units/5 mL. Proper dose: _____ mL.

BIBLIOGRAPHY AND REFERENCES

Broussard, M. C., & Pire, S. (1996). Medication problems in the elderly: A home healthcare nurse's perspective. *Home Healthcare Nurse, 14*, 441–443.

Brunton, L., Chabner, B., & Knollman, B. (2011). *Goodman and Gilman's the pharmacological basis of therapeutics* (12th ed.). New York: McGraw-Hill.

Craig, G. (2011). *Clinical calculations made easy*. Philadelphia, PA: Lippincott Williams & Wilkins.

DeCastillo, S., & Werner-McCullough, M. (2012). *Calculating drug dosages: An interactive approach* (3rd ed.). Philadelphia, PA: Davis.

Karch, A. (2003). *Lippincott's guide to preventing medication errors*. Philadelphia, PA: Lippincott Williams & Wilkins.

Morrison, G. (2007). Drug dosing in the intensive care unit: The patient with renal failure. In J. M. Rippe, R. S. Irwin, & M. P. Fink (Eds.), *Intensive care medicine* (3rd ed., pp. 951–986). Boston, MA: Little, Brown.

Ogden, S. (2015). *Calculation of drug dosages* (10th ed.). St. Louis, MO: Mosby.

Springhouse, Corp. (2009). *Dosage calculations made incredibly easy*. Ambler, PA: Author.

Tyreman, C. (2008). *How to master nursing calculations*. London, UK: Kogan Page Limited.

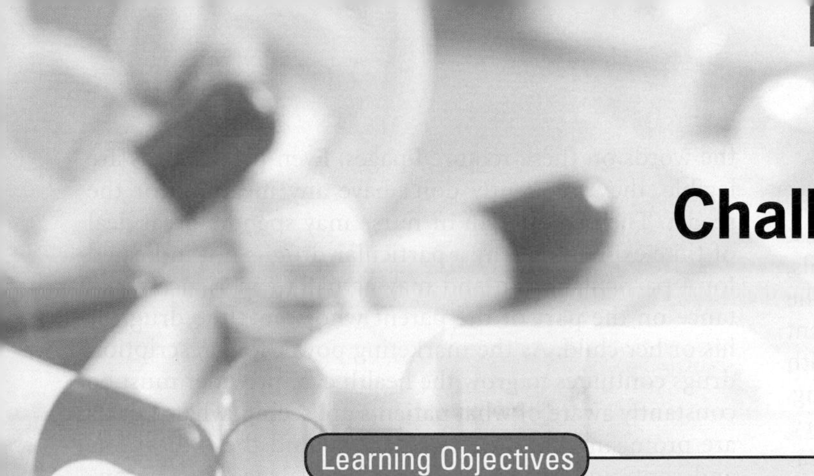

6 Challenges to Effective Drug Therapy

Learning Objectives

Upon completion of this chapter, you will be able to:

1. Discuss the impact of the media, the Internet, and direct-to-consumer advertising on consumers and health care professionals.
2. Explain the growing use of over-the-counter drugs and the impact it has on safe medical care.
3. Discuss the lack of controls on herbal or alternative therapies and the impact this has on safe drug therapy.
4. Define the off-label use of a drug.
5. Describe measures being taken to protect the public in cases of bioterrorism.

Glossary of Key Terms

alternative therapy: includes herbs and other "natural" products as often found in ancient records; these products are not controlled or tested by the U.S. Food and Drug Administration and are considered to be dietary supplements; however, they are often the basis for discovery of an active ingredient that is later developed into a regulated medication

biological weapons: so-called germ warfare; the use of bacteria, viruses, and parasites on a large scale to incapacitate or destroy a population

cost comparison: a comparison of the relative cost of the same drug provided by different manufacturers to determine the costs to the consumer

Internet: the worldwide digital information system accessed through computer systems

off-label uses: uses of a drug that are not part of the stated therapeutic indications for which the drug was approved by the FDA; off-label uses may lead to new indications for a drug

self-care: patients self-diagnosing and determining their own treatment needs

street drugs: nonprescription drugs with no known therapeutic use; used to enhance mood or increase pleasure

The dawn of the 21st century arrived with myriad new considerations and pressures in the health care industry. For the first time, consumers have access to medical and pharmacological information from many sources. Consumers are taking steps to demand specific treatments and considerations. Alternative therapies are being offered and advertised at a record pace, and this is causing people to rethink their approach to medical care and the medical system. At the same time, financial pressures have led to early discharge of patients from health care facilities and to provision of outpatient care for patients who, in the past, would have been hospitalized and monitored closely. Health care providers are being pushed to make decisions about patient care and prescriptions based on finances in addition to medical judgment. The events of 9/11 and the increased threat of terrorism have led to serious concerns about dealing with exposure to biological or chemical weapons. Illicit drug use is at an all-time high, bringing increased health risks and safety concerns. Concerns about the environment and the need to protect it from contamination are increasing. The nurse is caught in the middle of all of this change. Patients are demanding information but may not understand it when they have it. Patient teaching and home care provisions are vital to the success of any health regimen. The nurse is frequently in the best position to listen, teach, and explain some of this confusing information to the patient and to facilitate the care of the patient in the health system. In the push for patient-centered care, where each individual's unique concerns, culture, and needs are incorporated into the overall health regimen, the nurse is most often the one in the best position to provide that support, incentive, and advocacy to the patient and patient's family.

Consumer Awareness

Access to information has become so broad over the last decade that consumers are often overwhelmed with details, facts, and choices that affect their health care. Gone is the era when the health care provider was seen as omniscient and always right. The patient now comes into the health care system burdened with the influence of advertising, the Internet, and a growing alternative therapy industry. Many patients no longer calmly accept whatever medication is selected for them. They often come with requests and demands, and they partake of a complex array of over-the-counter (OTC) and alternative medicines that further complicate the safety and efficacy of standard drug therapy.

Media Influence

The last 25 years have seen an explosion of drug advertising in the mass media. It became legal to advertise prescription drugs directly to the public in the 1990s, and it is now impossible to watch television, listen to the radio, or flip through a magazine without encountering numerous drug advertisements. The goal behind the wide advertising of prescription drugs was to open a good discussion between the patient and the heath care provider to improve patient-centered care.

Federal guidelines determine what can be said in an advertisement, but in some cases this further confuses the issue for many consumers. If a drug advertisement states what the drug is used for, it must also state contraindications, adverse effects, and precautions. Because in many cases listing the possible adverse effects is not a good selling point, many advertisements are pure business ploys intended to interest consumers in the drug and to have them request it from their health care providers (even if it is unclear what the drug is used for). It is not unusual to see an ad featuring a smiling, healthy-looking person romping through a field of beautiful flowers on a sunny day with a cute baby or puppy in tow. The ad might simply state how wonderful it is to be outside on a day like today—contact your health care provider if you, too, would like to take drug X. Although most people now know what the erectile dysfunction drug *Viagra* (sildenafil) is used for, some of the ads for this drug simply show a happy older couple smiling and dancing the night away and then encourage viewers to ask their health care providers about *Viagra.* What older person wouldn't want a drug that makes him or her feel young, happy, and energetic?

Parenting magazines, which are often found in pediatricians' offices, are full of advertisements for antibiotics and asthma medications. These ads picture smiling, cute children and encourage readers to check with their pediatricians about the use of these drugs. If the drug's indication is mentioned the second page of the ad may well have the U.S. Food and Drug Administration (FDA)–approved drug insert printed in extremely tiny print and in full medical lingo. Most readers have trouble reading the words on these required pages. Even if the words are legible, they frequently don't have any meaning for the reader. The pediatrician or nurse may spend a great deal of time explaining why a particular drug is not indicated for a particular child and may actually experience resistance on the part of the parent who wants the drug for his or her child. As the marketing power for prescription drugs continues to grow the health care provider must be constantly aware of what patients are seeing, what the ads are promising, and the real data behind the indications and contraindications for these "hot" drugs. It is a continuing challenge to stay up to date and knowledgeable about drug therapy.

The media also look for headlines in current medical research or reports. It is not unusual for the media to take a headline or research title and make it into news. Sometimes the interpretation of the medical report is not accurate, and this can influence a patient's response to suggested therapy or provide a whole new set of demands or requests for the health care provider. Many of the usual television talk shows include a medical segment that presents just a tiny bit of information, frequently out of context, which opens a whole new area of interest for the viewer. Some health care providers have learned to deal with the "disease of the week" as seen on these shows; others can be unprepared to deal with what was presented and may lose credibility with the patient.

The Internet

The **Internet**, the worldwide digital information system accessed through computer systems, and World Wide Web are now readily accessible to most consumers. People who do not have Internet access at home can find it readily available at the local library, at work, or even in computer centers that allow community access. An increasingly large number of people have constant Internet access through the widespread use of smartphones, tablets, and other hand-held devices. The information available over the Internet is completely overwhelming to most people. A person can spend hours looking up information on a drug—including pharmaceutical company information sites, chat rooms with other people who are taking the drug, online pharmacies, lists of government regulations, and research reports about the drug and its effectiveness. Many people do not know how to evaluate the information that they access. Is it accurate or anecdotal? Patients often come into the health care system with pages of information downloaded from the Internet that they think pertains to their particular situation. The nurse or physician can spend a tremendous amount of time deciphering and interpreting the information and explaining it to the patient. Some tips that might be helpful in determining the usefulness or accuracy of information found on the Internet are given in Box 6.1.

BOX 6.1

Evaluating Internet Sites

Address Identification

- *.com:* commercial, advertising, selling, business site
- *.edu:* education site—school system, university, college
- *.gov:* government site
- *.net:* part of a linked network system, may include any of the above
- *.org:* sponsored by an organization, including professional, charitable, and educational groups

Site Evaluation

- *Navigation*—Is the site easy to access and navigate or confusing?
- *Contributors*—Who prepared the site? Is it reviewed? Is it purely commercial? What are the qualifications of the person(s) maintaining the site? Is there a mechanism for feedback or interaction with the site?
- *Dates*—Is the site updated frequently? When was the site last updated?
- *Accuracy/reliability*—Is the information supported by other sites? Is the information accurate and in agreement with other sources you have reviewed? Does the site list other links that are reasonable and reliable?

KEY POINTS

- An overwhelming amount of readily accessible information is available to consumers. This information has changed the way people approach the health care system.
- Consumer advertising of prescription drugs, mass media health reports and suggestions, and the Internet influence some patients to request specific treatments, to question therapy, and to challenge the health care provider, opening up dialogue for a discussion about treatments between the patient and the health care provider.

Over-the-Counter Drugs

OTC (over-the-counter) medications allow people to take care of simple medical problems without seeking advice from their health care providers. Although OTC drugs have been deemed to be safe when used as directed, many of these medications were "grandfathered in" as drugs when stringent testing and evaluation systems became law and have not been tested or evaluated to the extent that new drugs are today. Aspirin, one of the nonprescription standbys for many years, falls into this category. Slowly, the FDA is looking at all of these drugs to determine their effectiveness and safety. Ipecac, a former standard OTC drug, was used for many years by parents to induce vomiting in children in cases of suspected poisoning or suspected drug overdose. The drug was finally tested, and in 2003 the FDA announced that it was not found to be effective for its intended use. New guidelines have since been established for parents regarding possible poisoning, and parents were advised to dispose of any ipecac that they had at home. Some well-known approved OTC drugs are cimetidine (*Tagamet*) for decreasing gastric upset and heartburn; various vaginal antifungal medications for treating yeast infections (*Mycelex, Gyne-Lotrimin*); and omeprazole (*Prilosec*) and famotidine (*Pepcid*), two other drugs for dealing with heartburn.

Each year, several prescription drugs are reviewed for possible OTC status. One factor involved in the review process is the ability of the patient for **self-care**, which is the act of self-diagnosing and determining one's treatment needs. In 2009 and again in 2010, lovastatin, an antihyperlipidemic drug, was considered for OTC status. The FDA eventually decided that the public would have a hard time self-prescribing this drug because high lipid levels can be determined only with a blood test and present no signs and symptoms, so the drug's OTC status was not approved. OTC drugs can also mask the signs and symptoms of an underlying problem, making it difficult to arrive at an accurate diagnosis if the condition persists. These drugs are safe when used as directed, but many times the directions are not followed or even read. The idea that "If one makes me feel better, two will make me feel really good" is not always safe in the use of these drugs. Many people are not aware of which drugs are contained in these preparations and can inadvertently overdose when taking one preparation for each symptom they have. Table 6.1 gives an example of the ingredients that are found in some common cold and allergy preparations. Patients who take doses of different preparations to cover their various symptoms could easily wind up with an unintended overdose or toxic reaction.

Because many OTC drugs interact with prescription drugs, with possibly serious adverse or toxic effects for the patient, it is important that the health care provider specifically ask the patient when taking a drug history whether he or she is taking any OTC drugs or other medications. Many patients do not consider OTC drugs to be "real" drugs and do not mention their use when reporting a drug history to the health care provider. Specifically asking a patient about the use of any products for headache, colds, constipation, etc. can often prompt a patient to remember and report the use of these products. Every patient drug-teaching session should include information on which particular OTC drugs must be avoided or advice to check with the health care provider before taking any other medications or OTC products.

Table 6.1 Ingredients Found in Some Common Cold and Flu Over-the-Counter Preparations[a]

Drug Name	Ingredients	Use
Vicks Nyquil Severe Cold and Flu Nighttime	acetaminophen, dextromethorphan, phenylephrine, doxylamine	Runny nose, cough, headache, sore throat, aches and pains, sinus pressure, fever, sneezing
Vicks Dayquil Cold & Flu	acetaminophen, phenylephrine, dextromethorphan	Nasal congestion, fever, sore throat, aches, cough
Theraflu Nighttime Severe Cold & Cough	diphenhydramine, phenylephrine	Nasal congestion, sore throat, cough, sneezing
Theraflu Daytime Severe Cold & Cough	phenylephrine, dextromethorphan	Nasal congestion, sore throat, cough, headache
Theraflu Multisymptom Severe Cold	phenylephrine, dextromethorphan	Stuffy head, nasal congestion, sore throat, cough, headache, body aches, fever

[a]Safety precautions: A patient could take one preparation for cough, a second to cover sinus pressure, a third to cover the aches and pains, and a fourth to stay awake or fall asleep—when the total amounts of the drugs contained in these products are calculated a serious overdose of pseudoephedrine or dextromethorphan could easily occur.

Alternative Therapies and Herbal Medicine

Another aspect of the increasing self-care movement is the rapidly growing market of alternative therapies and herbal medicines. Herbal medicines and **alternative therapies** are found in ancient records and have often been the basis for the discovery of an active ingredient that is later developed into a regulated medication. Today, alternative therapies can also include nondrug measures, such as imaging and relaxation. There is an element of the placebo effect in using some of these therapies. The power of believing that something will work and that there is some control over the problem is often very beneficial in achieving relief from pain and suffering. The challenge for the health care provider is to balance the therapies that the patient wishes to use with the medical regimen that is prescribed. This may involve altering doses or timing of various drugs. See Appendix E for an extensive listing of alternative and complementary therapies.

Currently, these products are not controlled or tested by the FDA; they are considered to be dietary supplements, and therefore the advertising surrounding these products is not as restricted or as accurate as with classic drugs. Consumers are urged to use the "natural" approach to medical care and to self-treat with a wide variety of products. Numerous Internet sites point out natural treatments that can be used to cure various disorders. Television ads and magazine spreads push the use of these products in place of prescribed medications. Many people who want to gain control of their medical care or who do not want to take "drugs" for their diabetes, depression, or fatigue are drawn to these products. The Dietary Supplement Health and Education Act of 1994, updated in 2000, classifies herbal products, vitamins and minerals, and amino acids as "dietary supplements" that are not required to go through premarketing testing. The advertising that is permitted for these products does not allow direct claims to cure, treat, diagnose, or prevent a specific disease but does allow for nondisease claims such as "for muscle enhancement," "for hot flashes," or "for memory loss." Appendix E lists common alternative therapies and their suggested uses.

Several issues are of concern to the health care provider when a patient elects to self-treat with alternative therapies. The active ingredients in these products have not been tested by the FDA; when test results are available, often the tests were for only a very small number of people with no reproducible results. When a patient decides to take bilberry to control diabetes, for example, the reaction that will occur is not really known. In some patients the blood glucose level might decrease; in others, it might increase. Also, the incidental ingredients in many of these products are unknown. Many ingredients come directly from plants or from the conditions under which they grow, such as the fertilizer used for the plant, or depend on the time of the year when the plant was harvested. The other ingredients that are compounded with the product have a direct effect on its efficacy. Saw palmetto, an herb that has been used successfully to alleviate the symptoms of benign prostatic hypertrophy, is available in a wide variety of preparations from different manufacturers. A random sampling of these products performed in 2000 revealed that the contents of the identified active ingredient varied from 20% to 400% of the recommended dose. It is difficult to guide patients to the correct product with such a wide range of variability.

Patients often do not mention the use of alternative therapies to the health care provider. Some patients believe that the health care provider will disapprove of the use of these products and do not want to discuss it; others believe that these are just natural products and do not need to be mentioned. With the increasing use of these products, however, several drug interactions that can cause serious complications for patients taking prescription medication have been reported to the FDA. Diabetic patients who decide to use juniper berries, ginseng, garlic, fenugreek, coriander, dandelion root, or celery to "maintain their blood glucose level" may run into serious problems with hypoglycemia when they also use their prescription antidiabetic drugs. If the patient does not report the use of these alternative therapies to the health care provider, extensive medical tests and dose adjustments might be done to no avail.

St. John's wort, a highly advertised and popular alternative therapy, has been found to interact with oral contraceptives, digoxin (a heart medication), the selective serotonin reuptake inhibitors (used for depression), theophylline (a drug used to treat lung disease), various antineoplastic drugs used to treat cancer, and the antivirals used to treat acquired immune deficiency syndrome. Patients using St. John's wort for the symptoms of depression who are also taking *Prozac* (fluoxetine) for depression may experience serious side effects and toxic reactions. If the health care provider is not told about the use of St. John's wort, treatment of the toxicity can become very complicated.

Asking patients specifically about the use of any herbal or alternative therapies should become a routine part of any health history. If a patient presents with an unexpected reaction to a medication, ask the patient about any herbal or natural remedies he or she may be using. If a patient reports the use of an unusual or difficult-to-find remedy, try looking it up on the Internet at http://nccam.nih.gov, a site with general information about complementary and alternative medicines.

KEY POINTS

- OTC drugs have been deemed safe when used as directed and do not require a prescription or advice from a health care provider.
- OTC drugs can mask the signs and symptoms of disease, can interact with prescription drugs, and can be taken in greater than the recommended dose, leading to toxicity.
- Herbal or alternative therapies are considered to be dietary supplements and are not tightly regulated by the FDA.
- Herbal therapies can produce unexpected effects and toxic reactions, can interact with prescription drugs, and can contain various unknown ingredients that alter their effectiveness and toxicity.

Off-Label Uses

When a drug is approved by the FDA the therapeutic indications for which the drug is approved are stated. **Off-label use** refers to uses of a drug that are not part of the stated therapeutic indications for which the drug was approved by the FDA. Once a drug becomes available for use, it may be found to be effective in a situation not on the approved list. Using it for this indication may eventually lead to an approval of the drug for that new indication. Off-label use is commonly done for groups of patients for which there is little premarketing testing, particularly pediatric and geriatric groups. With the ethical issues involved in testing drugs on children the use of particular drugs in children often occurs by trial and error when the drug is released with adult indications. Dosing calculations and nomograms become very important in determining the approximate dose that should be used for a child. Drugs often used for off-label indications include the drugs used to treat various psychiatric problems. The fact that little is really known about the way the brain works and what happens when chemicals in the brain are altered has led to a polypharmacy approach in psychiatry—mixing and juggling drugs until the wanted effect is achieved. That same combination might not work in another patient with the same diagnosis because of brain and chemical differences in that patient.

Off-label use of drugs is widespread and often leads to discovery of a new use for a drug. The nurse needs to be cognizant of off-label uses, and know when to question the use of a drug before administering it. Liability issues surrounding many of these uses are very fuzzy, and the nurse should be clear about the intended use, why the drug is being tried, and its potential for problems.

Costs of Health Care and the Importance of Patient Teaching

The health care crisis in the United States has caused the cost of medical care and drugs to skyrocket in the last few years. This is partly due to the demand to have the best possible, most up-to-date, and safest care and drug therapies. The research and equipment requirements to meet these demands are huge. At the same time, the rising cost of health insurance to pay for all of this is a major complaint for employers and consumers. As a result, health maintenance organizations (HMOs) have surged in popularity. These groups treat the medical care system like a business, with financial aspects becoming the overriding concern. Decisions are often made by nonmedical personnel with a keen eye on the bottom line. To save costs, patients are being discharged from hospitals far earlier than ever before, and many are not even admitted to hospitals for surgical or invasive procedures that used to require several days of hospitalization and monitoring. As a result, there is less monitoring of the patient, and more responsibility for care falls on the patient or the patient's significant others. Teaching the patient about self-care, drug therapies, and what to expect is even more crucial now. The nurse is the one who most often is responsible for this teaching. The Affordable Care Act was designed to help relieve some of these costs and ensure access to care for more people, the full impact of this act on the health care system won't be known for many years.

Health Maintenance Organizations and Regulations

HMOs maintain a centralized control system to provide patient medical care within a budget. In many communities the HMO provides a centralized building with participating physicians and services housed in one area. Consumers are often provided with all of their health care at this facility and find the HMO insurance is less expensive than traditional medical insurance. The tradeoff is often a loss of choice.

The health care providers in the organization are the only ones who can be consulted. The HMO may regulate access to emergency facilities, types and timing of tests allowed, and procedures covered. Accessibility to prescription drugs is also controlled. The formulary for each HMO differs. Sometimes only generic products are covered, and newer drugs must be paid for by the patient; in other instances, a tier system exists, and the patient may urge the provider to choose a drug from a lower tier, at a lower cost. Many health care providers believe that their ability to make decisions is limited by such regulations and that decisions are often made by nonmedical personnel at the other end of a telephone, who have no contact with the patient.

Home Care

The home care industry is one of the most rapidly growing responses to the changes in costs and medical care delivery. Patients go home directly from surgery with the responsibility for changing dressings, assessing wounds, administering medications, and monitoring their recovery. Patients are being discharged from hospitals because the hospital days allowed for a particular diagnosis have run out. These patients may be responsible for their monitoring, rehabilitation, and drug regimens. At the same time, the population is aging and may be less accepting of all of this responsibility. The aging population brings additional issues that go with the changes in the aging body. *Beer's List* is a good resource of high risk medications to avoid in the elderly. Home health aides, visiting nurses, and home care programs are taking over some of the responsibilities that used to be handled in the hospital.

The responsibility of meeting the tremendous increase in teaching needs of patients frequently resides with the nurse. Patients need to know exactly what medications they are taking (generic and brand names), the dose of each medication, and what each is supposed to do. Patients also need to know what they can do to alleviate some of the adverse effects that are expected with each drug (e.g., small meals if gastrointestinal upset is common, use of a humidifier if secretions will be dried and make breathing difficult); which OTC drugs or alternative therapies they need to avoid while taking their prescribed drugs; and what to watch for that would indicate a need to call the health care provider; how to properly store drugs (humidity and heat in bathrooms is not good for drug storage, controlled substances need to be secured, particular drugs may need to refrigerated, etc.). With patients who are taking many drugs at the same time, this information should be provided in writing, in language that is clear and understandable. Many pharmacies provide written information with each drug that is dispensed, but trying to organize these sheets of information into a usable and understandable form is difficult for many patients. The nurse is often the one who needs to sort through the provided information to organize, simplify, and make sense of it for the patient. The cost of dealing with toxic or adverse effects is often much higher, in the long run, than the cost of the time spent teaching and explaining things to the patient.

The projections for trends in health care indicate even greater expansion of the home health care system, with hospitals being used for only the most critically ill patients. The role of the nurse in this home health system is crucial—as teacher, assessor, diagnostician, and patient advocate.

Cost Considerations

Despite the insurance coverage a patient may have for prescription medications, it is often necessary for the health care provider to choose a drug therapy based on the costs of the drugs available. With more and more of the population reaching retirement age and depending on a fixed income, costs are a real issue. Patients may be forced into a situation where they have to decide whether to "treat or eat." Sometimes patients do not tell the health care provider that they are not filling a prescription because of cost and lose the therapeutic benefit that the drug could offer. Sometimes this may mean not selecting a first-choice drug but settling for a drug that should be effective. Patients who take antibiotics must be reminded to take the full course and not to stop the drug when they feel better. Patients may be tempted to stop taking the antibiotic in order to save the remaining pills for the next time they feel sick and to save the costs of another health care visit and a new prescription. This practice has contributed to the problem of resistant bacteria, which is becoming more dangerous all the time.

Patients also need to be advised not to split tablets in half unless specifically advised to do so. Some drugs can be split, and it is cheaper to order the larger size and have the patient cut the tablet. Some patients think that by cutting the drug in half, they will have coverage for twice the time allowed by the prescription and will not be as dependent on the drug. With the new matrix delivery systems used for many medications, however, splitting the drug can cause it to become toxic or ineffective. Patients should be specifically alerted to avoid cutting drugs when it could be dangerous, especially if they are being advised to cut other tablets to be economical. The cost of treating the toxic reactions may far exceed the cost of the original drug.

Generic drug availability in many cases reduces the cost of a drug. Generic drugs are preparations that are off-patent and therefore can be sold by their generic name, without the cost associated with brand name products. Generic drugs are tested for bioequivalence with the brand name product, and resulting information is available to prescribers. When a drug has a small margin of safety (a small difference between the therapeutic and the toxic dose) a prescriber may feel more comfortable ordering the drug by brand name to ensure that the dose and binders are what the prescriber expects. When "DAW" (dispense as written) is on a prescription the prescription is filled with the brand name drug—such as *Lanoxin* instead of digoxin, or *Coumadin* instead of warfarin. In some situations, the generic drug is not less expensive than the brand name drug, so using only generic drugs does not guarantee that the patient is getting the least expensive preparation. Many pharmacies post the costs of commonly used drugs, and patients may do **cost comparisons** to compare the relative cost of the same drug among various pharmacies or the cost differences among manufacturers of drugs and request that a different drug be prescribed. The nurse is often the person who is in the middle of this issue and must be able to explain the reason for the drug choice or request that the prescriber consider an alternative treatment.

Table 6.2 presents an example of a cost comparison of some beta-blockers commonly used to treat hypertension. When deciding which drug to use the patient or nurse may need to consider the range of costs. *Drug Facts and Comparisons* provides a cost comparison of drugs in each class, and *The Medical Letter on Drugs and Therapeutics* provides cost comparisons of drugs that are reviewed in each issue.

In the last few years, with the cost of drugs becoming a political as well as a social issue, many people have begun ordering drugs on the Internet, often from other countries. These drugs may be cheaper, do not require the patient to see a health care provider (many of these sites simply have customers fill out a questionnaire that is reviewed by a doctor), and are delivered right to the patient's door. The FDA has begun checking these drugs as they arrive in this country and have found many discrepancies between what was ordered and what is in the product, as well as problems in the storage of these products. Some foreign brand names are the same as brand names in this country but are associated with different generic drugs. The FDA has issued many warnings to consumers about the risk of taking some of these drugs without medical supervision, reminding consumers that they are not protected by US laws or regulations when they purchase drugs from other countries. The FDA website, http://www.fda.gov, provides important information and guidelines for people who elect to use the Internet to get cheaper drugs.

Table 6.2 Generic or Trade Name Drugs? What Do They Cost?

Drug Name	Maximum Daily Dose (mg)	Cost of a 1-wk Supply
acetaminophen (generic)	4000	0.09
Tylenol		3.60
diclofenac potassium (generic)	200	9.80
Cataflam		74.80
diclofenac sodium (generic)	200	15.70
Voltaren-XR		65.80
duloxetine (generic)	120	44.00
Cymbalta		50.90
fenoprofen (generic)	3200	53.80
Nalfon		55.90
ibuprofen (generic)	2400	1.30
Advil		6.50
meloxicam (generic)	15	0.50
Mobic		40.30
naproxen (generic)	1250	1.30
Naprosyn		36.30
celecoxib (generic)	600	1.60
Celebrex		49.10

This table shows general prescription analgesic drug prices in September 2014. It is presented to illustrate the wide price range between generic and trade name drugs.

Emergency Preparedness

The events of 9/11 brought a change in the sense of security and safety that generally prevailed in the United States. Now there are terrorist alerts, long lines for security at airports, and increased inspection of bags and carryalls at sporting events and theme parks. One of the potential threats that is being addressed by the Centers for Disease Control and Prevention (CDC) and the Office of Homeland Security is the risk of exposure to biological and chemical weapons. Chemical weapons have been encountered in the wars in the Middle East, as well as in terrorist attacks in Japan. The threat of exposure to **biological weapons**, so-called germ warfare, is somewhat theoretical but very real, as seen in the anthrax mail scares in Washington, DC, Pennsylvania, and New York. The CDC has worked diligently to establish guidelines for treating possible exposure to biological weapons. For complete information on presenting signs and symptoms, diagnoses, and current research in this area, go to www.cdc.gov and click on Emergency Preparedness. Education of health care providers and the public is one of the central points in coping effectively with any biological assault. The CDC posts regularly updated information on signs and symptoms of infection by various biological agents, guidelines for management of patients who are exposed and those who are actually infected, and ongoing research into detection, diagnosis, prevention, and management of diseases associated with biological agents. The nurse is often called upon to answer questions, reassure the public, offer educational programs, and serve on emergency preparedness committees. Go to http://www.cdc.gov and click on Emergency Preparedness to keep up to date and informed about these issues.

Drug Abuse

Illicit drug use in the United States is a growing problem. Professional athletes are cited regularly for abusing anabolic steroids. Hollywood stars are often part of the drug scene, using **street drugs**—nonprescription drugs with no known therapeutic use—to enhance their moods and increase pleasure. Alcohol and nicotine are two commonly abused drugs that cause serious problems for the abuser or can interact with various drugs and alter a patient's response to a prescribed drug but that are often not seen as drug addiction issues. Parents are often very concerned that their children will use street drugs. The "everyone is doing it" argument is hard to counter when today's heroes are thought to be heavily involved. Some people abuse and become addicted to prescription drugs following an injury, when confronted with chronic pain, when their occupation puts them in contact with readily available drugs, or when someone else in the home is using a prescription drug. Many of the drugs used illicitly are addictive and can change a person's entire life, with drug-seeking behavior becoming a major factor. Researchers have identified actual changes in the brain and neurotransmitter patterns of people who abuse and become addicted to such drugs. Trying to reverse these changes and return the person to a nonaddicted state is a physiological, as well as a psychological, challenge. The use of these drugs can have severe consequences on health, can mask underlying signs and symptoms of medical problems, and can interact with other medications that the user may need (Table 6.3).

Being informed about drugs available in the community, current trends among teenagers or young adults, and community resources available to help patients can guide parents and health care professionals while dealing with this drug culture problem. Education provides a crucial defense against drug abuse and helps the public and health care professionals recognize the problem and deal with it when it occurs. The National Institutes of Health has a division called the National Institute

Table 6.3 Frequently Abused Street Drugs and Their Potential Health Consequences

Drug	Street Names	Class	Health Consequences
Amphetamines	Uppers, whites, dexies	Stimulant	Hypertension, tachycardia, insomnia, restlessness
Amyl nitrate	Boppers, pearls	Stimulant	Tachycardia, restlessness, hypotension, vertigo
Anabolic steroids	Roids, muscle	Steroid	Hypertension, hyperlipidemia, acne, cancer, cardiomyopathy
Barbiturates	Downers, reds	Depressant	Bradycardia, hypotension, laryngospasm, ataxia, impaired thinking
Benzodiazepines	M & Ms, Uncle Milty	Depressant	Confusion, fatigue, impaired memory, impaired coordination
Cannabis With formaldehyde With cocaine	Pot, grass, weed, THC; fry sticks; primo	Mixed CNS	Drowsiness, elation, dizziness, memory lapse, hallucinations
Cocaine	Snow, blow, crack	Stimulant	Tachycardia, hypertension, hallucinations, confused thinking
Fentanyl	Jackpot, China white	Opioid	Sedation, arrhythmias, shock, cardiac arrest, decreased respirations, constipation
Gamma-hydroxybutyrate	GHB, fantasy, liquid X, liquid E, date rape drug	Depressant	Memory loss, hypotension, somnolence
Heroin	Brown sugar, joy, crank, fairy dust	Opioid	Sedation, arrhythmias, shock, cardiac arrest, decreased respirations, constipation
Ketamine	Super acid, special K	Depressant	Paralysis, loss of sensation, disorientation, psychic changes
LSD	Acid, sunshine, blotter acid	Hallucinogen	Hallucinations, hypotension, changes in thinking, loss of social control
MDMA	Ecstasy, b-bombs, go, Scooby snacks	Hallucinogen	Hallucinations, psychic change, loss of memory, hypotension, cardiac arrest
Methamphetamine	Crystal, glass, speed, crystal meth, working mother's cocaine	Stimulant	Hypertension, tachycardia, restlessness, changes in thinking
Methylphenidate	Ritalin	Stimulant	Agitation, tachycardia, hypertension, hyperreflexia, fever
Morphine	Mort, Miss Emma	Opioid	Sedation, arrhythmias, shock, cardiac arrest, decreased respirations, constipation
OxyContin	Oxy, Oxycotton, Oxy 80s, hillbilly heroin, poor man's heroin, cotton	Opioid	Sedation, arrhythmias, shock, cardiac arrest, decreased respirations, constipation
PCP with steroids	Angel dust, zombie; juices	Hallucinogen	Acute psychosis, heart failure, death, seizures, memory loss
Peyote	Button, mesc	Hallucinogen	Acute psychosis, tremor, altered perception, death
Rohypnol	Rophies	Amnesiac	Date rape drug, loss of memory, immobility
Viagra/MDMA	Sextasy	Hallucinogen, ED drug	Severe hypotension, hallucinations, increased sexual function

CNS, central nervous system; ED, erectile dysfunction; LSD, lysergic acid diethylamide; MDMA, methylenedioxymethamphetamine; PCP, phencyclidine; THC, tetrahydrocannabinol.

on Drug Abuse. Go to http://www.nida.nih.gov to find educational programs for teens, parents, and health care professionals; the latest information on the hottest fads in illicit drugs; research on dealing with drug abuse problems; and links to sites for identifying unknown drugs, community resources, and laws.

Protecting the Environment

In March 2008, many news services across the United States reported studies showing that many prescription drugs had been found in the drinking water of various large cities. These studies showed ground and watershed contamination with many pharmaceutical products. The levels of these drugs were small, but the question was raised about what this would mean for the future and for the people, animals, and crops that were being affected by the presence of these drugs. The problem is quite real. Patients get a prescription and then get switched to a different drug. Some patients end up with extra pills at the end of a prescription because they did not follow the dosing guidelines exactly. Many people store these extra pills and end up with a medicine cabinet full of prescription drugs. In the past, people would often just flush these extras down the toilet, where they would enter the water system. Some people just threw them out, where they would eventually enter the ground of various landfills or would be diverted for illicit use by drug seekers going through garbage sites. With these issues in mind and the push to protect the environment, the Office of National Drug Control Policy has released specific guidelines for the proper disposal of prescription drugs. See Box 6.2 for the guidelines for drug disposal. It is important to teach patients how to dispose of drugs properly. Encourage patients to clean out their medicine cabinet at least yearly and to properly dispose of the drugs that they are no longer using. Most local governments now have drug take-back events to promote the safe disposal of drugs.

BOX 6.2 FOCUS ON **Patient and Family Teaching**

Proper Disposal of Unused, Unneeded, or Expired Medications

- Take unused, unneeded, or expired prescription drugs out of their original containers.
- Mix the prescription drugs with an undesirable substance, such as used coffee grounds or kitty litter, and put them in impermeable, nondescript containers, such as empty cans or sealable bags, further ensuring that the drugs are not diverted or accidentally ingested by children or pets.
- Throw these closed containers in the trash.
- Flush prescription drugs down the toilet **only** if the accompanying patient information **specifically instructs** that this is safe to do.
- Return unused, unneeded, or expired prescription drugs to pharmaceutical take-back locations that allow the public to bring unused drugs to a central location for safe disposal. Many hospitals have these locations. Many local governments have regular take-back days or drop-off sites. Check with your local hospital or Health Department.

SUMMARY

- In the 21st century, drugs pose new challenges for patients and health care providers, including information overload, demands for specific treatments, increased access to self-care systems, and financial pressures to provide cost-effective care.
- The mass media bombard consumers with medical reviews, research updates, and advertising for prescription drugs. If the use of a drug is stated the adverse effects and cautions also must be stated. If the use is not stated the drug advertisement is free to use any images and suggestions to sell the drug.
- Increasing access to the Internet and World Wide Web has increased consumer access to drug information, advertising, and even purchasing without a mediator of this information. Determining the reliability of an Internet site is a challenge for the consumer and the health care provider.
- OTC drugs and herbal and alternative therapies allow patients to make medical decisions and self-treat many common signs and symptoms. Problems arise when they are used inappropriately, when they interact with prescription drugs, or when they mask signs and symptoms, making diagnosis difficult.
- Off-label uses of drugs occur when a drug has been released and is available for use. The use of a drug for an indication that is not approved by the FDA occurs commonly in pediatric and in psychiatric medicine, in which testing is limited or made ineffective by individual differences.
- Increasing costs of drugs and health care has led to the emergence of HMOs and tight regulations on medical therapy and drug therapy alternatives. The choice of a drug to be used may be determined by the HMO formulary or insurance company database or by cost comparison with other drugs in the same or a similar class. Cost comparison is a major consideration in the use of many drugs.
- Home care is one of the most rapidly growing areas of medical care. Patients are increasingly more responsible for managing their medical regimens from home with dependence on home health providers and teaching and support from knowledgeable nurses.
- Emergency preparedness in the post-9/11 era includes awareness of risks associated with biological or chemical weapon exposure and medical management for the victims.

- Illicit drug use can lead to dependence on the drug and physiological changes, causing health problems and changing the body's response to traditional drugs.
- Proper disposal of unused or expired medications can help to protect the environment and may decrease drug-searching behaviors in some situations.

CHECK YOUR UNDERSTANDING

Answers to the questions in this chapter can be found in Answers to Check Your Understanding Questions on thePoint®.

MULTIPLE CHOICE

Select the best answer to the following.

1. Drugs can be advertised in the mass media only if
a. the FDA indication is clearly stated.
b. the actual use is never stated.
c. adverse effects and precautions are stated if the use is stated.
d. all adverse effects are clearly stated.

2. Herbal treatments and alternative therapies
a. are considered drugs and regulated by the FDA.
b. are considered dietary supplements and are not regulated by the FDA.
c. have no restrictions on claims and advertising.
d. contain no drugs, only natural substances.

3. OTC drugs are drugs that are
a. deemed to be safe when used as directed.
b. harmless to the public.
c. too old to be tested.
d. cheaper to use than prescription drugs.

4. The home health care industry is booming because
a. there is a shortage of hospital beds.
b. patients feel safer at home and prefer to be cared for at home.
c. patients are going home sooner and becoming responsible for their own care sooner than in the past.
d. the nursing shortage makes it difficult to care for patients in hospitals.

5. The cost of drug therapy is a major consideration in most areas because
a. generic drugs are always cheaper.
b. the high cost of drugs combined with more fixed income consumers puts constraints on drug use.
c. pharmacies usually carry only one drug from each class.
d. patients like to shop around and get the best drug for their money.

6. An off-label use of a drug means that the drug
a. was found without a label and its actual contents are not known.
b. has been found to be safe when used as directed and no restrictions are needed.
c. is being used for an indication not listed in the approved indications noted by the FDA.
d. has expired but is still found to be useful when used as directed.

MULTIPLE RESPONSE

Select all that apply.

1. When taking a health history the nurse should include specific questions about the use of OTC drugs and alternative therapies. This is an important aspect of the health history because
a. many insurance policies cover these drugs.
b. patients should be reprimanded about the use of these products.
c. patients often do not consider them to be drugs and do not report their use.
d. patients should never use these products when taking prescription drugs.
e. these products can mask or alter presenting signs and symptoms.
f. many of these products interact with traditional prescription drugs.

2. A nurse is caring for a patient who has been diagnosed with type 2 diabetes. The patient has reported that he frequently uses herbal remedies. Before administering any antidiabetic medications the nurse should caution the patient about the use of which of the following herbal therapies?
a. Glucosamine
b. Ginseng
c. St. John's wort
d. Juniper berries
e. Garlic
f. Kava

BIBLIOGRAPHY AND REFERENCES

Barton, J. H., & Emmanuel, E. J. (2005). The patient-based pharmaceutical development process: Rationale, problems and potential reforms. *Journal of the American Medical Association, 294,* 2075–2082.

Beers List of Medications. (2015). Available online at: http://www.web-wordline.rhcloud.com/get/beers-list-of-medications-2015

Brunton, L., Chabner, B., & Knollman, B. (2011). *Goodman and Gilman's the pharmacological basis of therapeutics* (12th ed.). New York: McGraw-Hill.

Cruipi, R. S., Asnis, D. S., Lee, C. C., et al. (2003). Meeting the challenge of bioterrorism: Lessons learned from the West Nile virus and anthrax. *American Journal of Emergency Medicine, 21*(1), 77–79.

DerMarderosian, A. (Ed.). (2010). *The review of natural products* (6th ed.). St. Louis, MO: Facts and Comparisons.

Ebadi, M. (2006). *Pharmacodynamic basis of herbal medicine* (2nd ed.). Abingdon, UK: Taylor & Francis.

Facts and Comparisons. (2015). *Drug facts and comparisons.* St. Louis, MO: Author.

Karch, A. M. (2014). *Lippincott nursing drug guide.* Philadelphia, PA: Lippincott Williams & Wilkins.

Koo, M. M., Krass, I., & Aslani, P. (2003). Factors influencing consumer use of written drug information. *Annals of Pharmacotherapy, 37*(2), 259–267.

Medical Letter. (2015). *The medical letter on drugs and therapeutics* New Rochelle, NY: Author.

Office of National Drug Control Policy. (2007). Proper disposal of prescription drugs. Available online at: http://www.whitehousedrugpolicy.gov/publications/pdf/prescrip_disposal.pdf

Pizzorno, J. E., & Murray, M. T. (2012). *Textbook of natural medicine* (4th ed.). St. Louis, MO: Elsevier.

Pizzorno, J. E., Murray, M. T., & Joiner-Bey, H. (2008). *The clinician's handbook of natural medicine.* London, UK: Churchill-Livingstone.

Smith, K., Richie, D., & Henyon, N. (2010). *Handbook of critical drug data* (11th ed.). Mississauga, ON: McGraw Hill Medical.

Stargrove, M. B., Treasure, J., & McKee, D. L. (2008). *Herb, nutrient and drug interactions: Clinical implications and therapeutic strategies.* St. Louis, MO: Mosby.

PART 2

CHEMOTHERAPEUTIC AGENTS

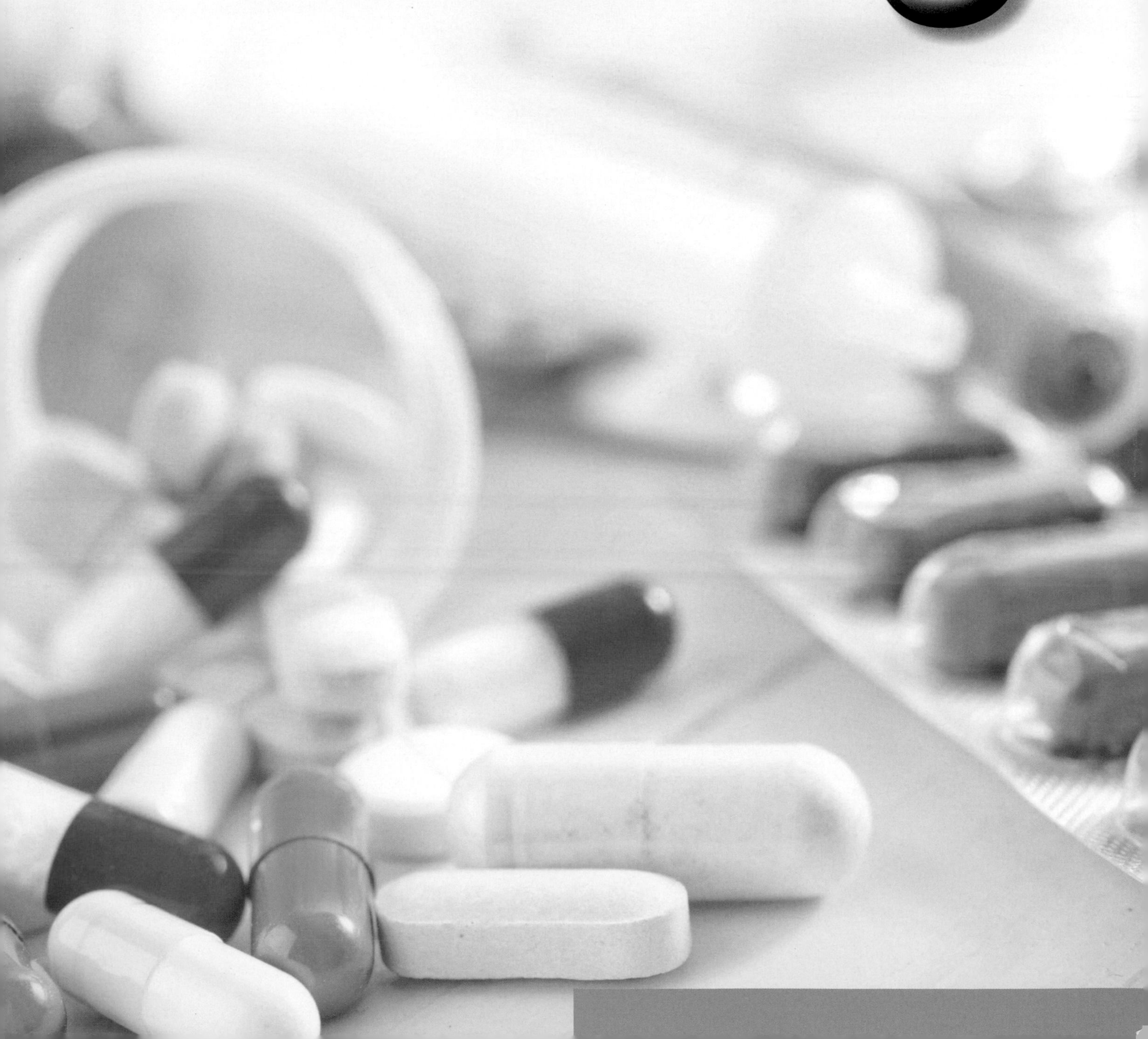

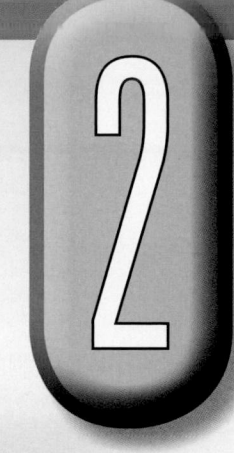

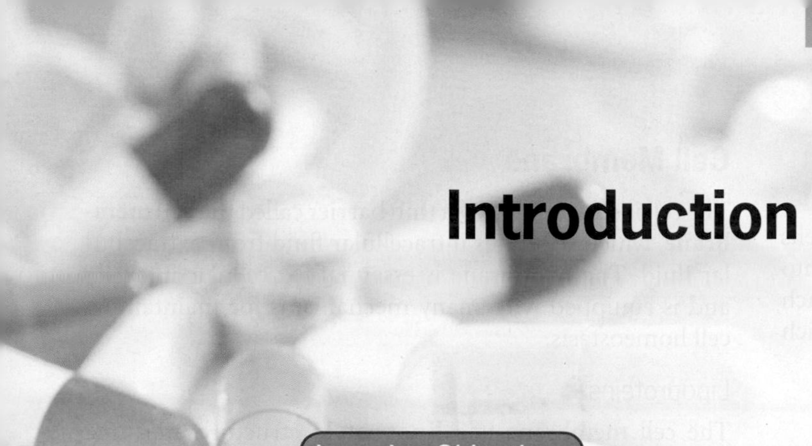

Introduction to Cell Physiology 7

Learning Objectives

Upon completion of this chapter, you will be able to:

1. Identify the parts of the human cell.
2. Describe the role of each organelle found within the cell cytoplasm.
3. Explain the unique properties of the cell membrane.
4. Describe three processes used by the cell to move things across the cell membrane.
5. Outline the cell cycle, including the activities going on within the cell in each phase.

Glossary of Key Terms

cell cycle: life cycle of a cell, which includes the phases G_0, G_1, S, G_2, and M; during the M phase the cell divides into two identical daughter cells

cell membrane: lipoprotein structure that separates the interior of a cell from the external environment; regulates what can enter and leave a cell

cytoplasm: lies within the cell membrane; contains organelles for producing proteins, energy, and so on

diffusion: movement of solutes from an area of high concentration to an area of low concentration across a concentration gradient

endocytosis: the process of engulfing substances and moving them into a cell by extending the cell membrane around the substance; pinocytosis and phagocytosis are two kinds of endocytosis

endoplasmic reticulum: fine network of interconnected channels known as cisternae found in the cytoplasm; site of chemical reactions within the cell

exocytosis: removal of substances from a cell by pushing them through the cell membrane

genes: sequences of DNA that control basic cell functions and allow for cell division

Golgi apparatus: a series of flattened sacs in the cytoplasm that prepare hormones or other substances for secretion and may produce lysosomes and store other synthesized proteins

histocompatibility antigens: proteins found on the surface of the cell membrane; they are determined by the genetic code and provide cellular identity as a self-cell (i.e., a cell belonging to that individual)

lipoprotein: structure composed of proteins and lipids; the bipolar arrangement of the lipids monitors substances passing in and out of the cell

lysosomes: encapsulated digestive enzymes found within a cell; they digest old or damaged areas of the cell and are responsible for destroying the cell when the membrane ruptures and the cell dies

mitochondria: rod-shaped organelles that produce energy within the cell in the form of adenosine triphosphate (ATP)

nucleus: the part of a cell that contains the DNA and genetic material; regulates cellular protein production and cellular properties

organelles: distinct structures found within the cell cytoplasm

osmosis: movement of water from an area of low solute concentration to an area of high solute concentration in an attempt to equalize the concentrations

ribosomes: membranous structures that are the sites of protein production within a cell

Chemotherapeutic drugs are used to destroy both organisms that invade the body (e.g., bacteria, viruses, parasites, protozoa, fungi) and abnormal cells within the body (e.g., neoplasms, cancers). These drugs affect cells by altering cellular function or disrupting cellular integrity, causing cell death, or by preventing cellular reproduction, eventually leading to cell death. Because most chemotherapeutic agents do not possess complete selective toxicity, they also to some extent affect the normal cells of patients. To understand the actions and adverse effects caused by chemotherapeutic agents and to determine interventions that increase therapeutic effectiveness, it is important to understand the various properties and the basic structure and function of the cell.

The Cell

The cell is the basic structural unit of the body. The cells that make up living organisms, which are arranged into tissues and organs, all have the same basic structure. Each cell has a nucleus, a cell membrane, and cytoplasm, which contains a variety of organelles (Figure 7.1).

Cell Nucleus

Each cell is "programmed" by the **genes**, or sequences of DNA, that allow for cell division, produce specific proteins that allow the cell to carry out its functions, and maintain cell homeostasis or stability. The **nucleus** is the part of a cell that contains all genetic material necessary for cell reproduction and for the regulation of cellular production of proteins. The nucleus is encapsulated in its own membrane and remains distinct from the rest of the cytoplasm. A small spherical mass, called the nucleolus, is located within the nucleus. Within this mass are dense fibers and proteins that will eventually become **ribosomes**, the sites of protein synthesis within the cell. Genes are responsible for the formation of messenger RNA and transcription RNA, which are involved in production of the proteins unique to the cell. The DNA necessary for cell division is found on long strains called chromatin. These structures line up and enlarge during the process of cell division.

Cell Membrane

The cell is surrounded by a thin barrier called the **cell membrane**, which separates intracellular fluid from extracellular fluid. The membrane is essential for cellular integrity and is equipped with many mechanisms for maintaining cell homeostasis.

Lipoproteins

The cell membrane is a **lipoprotein** structure, meaning that it is mainly composed of proteins and lipids—phospholipids, glycolipids, and cholesterol; the bipolar arrangement of the lipids monitors substances passing in and out of the cell. The phospholipids, which are bipolar in nature, line up with their polar regions pointing toward the interior or exterior of the cell and their nonpolar region lying within the cell membrane. The polar regions mix well with water, and the nonpolar region repels water. These properties allow the membrane to act as a barrier to regulate what can enter the cell (Figure 7.2). The freely moving nature of the membrane allows it to adjust to the changing shape of the cell so that areas of the membrane can move together to repair the membrane should it become torn or injured. Some of the outward-facing phospholipids have a sugar group attached to them; these are called glycolipids. Cholesterol is found in large quantities in the membrane, and it works to keep the phospholipids in place and the cell membrane stable.

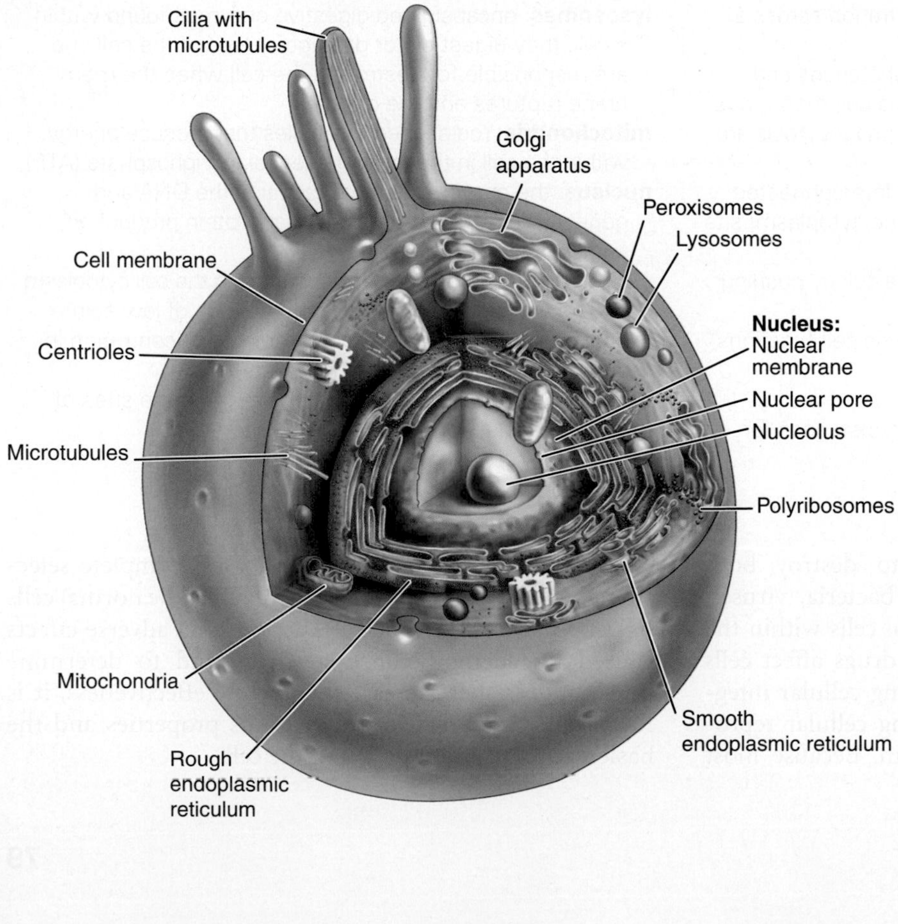

FIGURE 7.1 General structure of a cell and the location of its organelles.

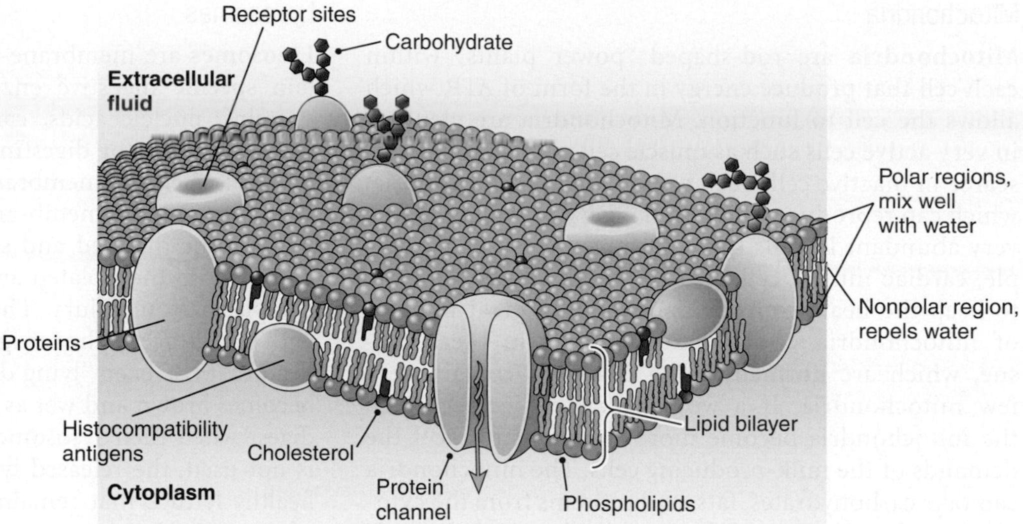

FIGURE 7.2 Structure of the lipid bilayer of the cell membrane.

Receptor Sites

Embedded in the cell membrane are a series of peripheral proteins with several functions. As discussed in Chapter 2, one type of protein located on the cell membrane is known as a receptor site. This protein reacts with specific chemicals outside the cell to stimulate a reaction within the cell. For example, the receptor site for insulin reacts with the hormone insulin to cause activation of ATP within the cell. This reaction alters the cell's permeability to glucose. Receptor sites are very important in the functioning of neurons, muscle cells, endocrine glands, and other cell types, and they play a very important role in clinical pharmacology.

Identifying Markers

Other surface proteins are surface antigens, or genetically determined identifying markers. These proteins are called **histocompatibility antigens** or human leukocyte antigens, which the body uses to identify a cell as a self-cell (i.e., a cell belonging to that individual). The body's immune system recognizes these proteins and acts to protect self-cells and to destroy non–self-cells. When an organ is transplanted from one person to another a great effort is made to match as many histocompatibility antigens as possible to reduce the chance that the "new" body will reject the transplanted organ.

Histocompatibility antigens can be changed in several ways: by cell injury, with viral invasion of a cell, with age, and so on. If the markers are altered the body's immune system reacts to the change and can ignore it, allowing neoplasms to grow and develop. The immune system may also attack the cell, leading to many of the problems associated with autoimmune disorders and chronic inflammatory conditions.

Channels

Channels or pores within the cell membrane are made by proteins in the cell wall that allow the passage of small substances in or out of the cell. Specific channels have been identified for sodium, potassium, calcium, chloride, bicarbonate, and water; other channels may also exist. Some drugs are designed to affect certain channels specifically. For example, calcium-channel blockers prevent the movement of calcium into a cell through calcium channels.

KEY POINTS

- The cell is the basic structure of all living organisms.
- The cell membrane features specific receptor sites that allow interaction with various chemicals, histocompatibility proteins that allow for self-identification, and channels or pores that allow for the passage of substances into and out of the cell.

Cytoplasm

The cell **cytoplasm** lies within the cell membrane and outside the nucleus and is the site of activities of cellular metabolism and special cellular functions. The cytoplasm contains many organelles, which are structures with specific functions such as producing proteins and energy. The **organelles** within the cytoplasm include the mitochondria, the endoplasmic reticulum, free ribosomes, the Golgi apparatus, and the lysosomes.

Mitochondria

Mitochondria are rod-shaped "power plants" within each cell that produce energy in the form of ATP, which allows the cell to function. Mitochondria are plentiful in very active cells such as muscle cells and are relatively scarce in inactive cells such as bone cells. Mitochondria, which can reproduce when a cell is very active, are always very abundant in cells that consume energy. For example, cardiac muscle cells, which must work continually to keep the heart contracting, contain a great number of mitochondria. Milk-producing cells in breast tissue, which are normally quite dormant, contain very few mitochondria. If a woman is lactating, however, the mitochondria become more abundant to meet the demands of the milk-producing cells. The mitochondria can take carbohydrates, fats, and proteins from the cytoplasm and make ATP via the Krebs cycle, which depends on oxygen. Cells use the ATP to maintain homeostasis, produce proteins, and carry out specific functions. If oxygen is not available, lactic acid builds up as a byproduct of cellular respiration. Lactic acid leaves the cell and is transported to the liver for conversion to glycogen and carbon dioxide.

Endoplasmic Reticulum

Much of the cytoplasm of a cell is made up of a fine network of interconnected channels known as cisternae, which form the **endoplasmic reticulum**. The undulating surface of the endoplasmic reticulum provides a large surface for chemical reactions within the cell. Many granules that contain enzymes and ribosomes, which produce protein, are scattered over the surface of the rough endoplasmic reticulum. Production of proteins, phospholipids, and cholesterol takes place in the rough endoplasmic reticulum. The smooth endoplasmic reticulum is the site of further lipid and cholesterol production and the production of cell products, such as hormones. The breakdown of many toxic substances may also occur here in particular cells.

Free Ribosomes

Other ribosomes that are not bound to the surface of the endoplasmic reticulum exist throughout the cytoplasm. These free-floating ribosomes produce proteins that are important to the structure of the cell and some of the enzymes that are necessary for cellular activity.

Golgi Apparatus

The **Golgi apparatus** is a series of flattened sacs that may be part of the endoplasmic reticulum. These structures prepare hormones or other substances for secretion by processing them and packaging them in vesicles to be moved to the cell membrane for excretion from the cell. In addition, the Golgi apparatus may produce lysosomes and store other synthesized proteins and enzymes until they are needed.

Lysosomes

Lysosomes are membrane-covered organelles that contain specific digestive enzymes that can break down proteins, nucleic acids, carbohydrates, and lipids and are responsible for digesting worn or damaged sections of a cell when the membrane ruptures and the cell dies. Lysosomes form a membrane around any substance that needs to be digested and secrete the digestive enzymes directly into the isolated area, protecting the rest of the cytoplasm from injury. This phenomenon can be seen with old lettuce in the refrigerator. The side of the lettuce head that has been "lying down" for a prolonged period becomes brown and wet as the lettuce cells die and self-digest when their lysosomes are released. If the lettuce is not used, the released lysosomes begin to digest any healthy lettuce that remains, with eventual destruction of the entire head. Lysosomes are important in ecology. Dead trees, animals, and other organisms self-digest. Lysosomes become very important clinically when cell death (from disease or a drug effect) leads to the death of neighboring cells when lysosomes are released from the dead cell and lyse or digest the proteins and membrane of neighboring cells, causing those cells to die and release their lysozymes. A decubitus ulcer is a good example of cell death leading to the death of neighboring cells and becoming a potentially out-of-control reaction.

KEY POINTS

- The cytoplasm of the cell contains various organelles that are important for cellular function.
- The mitochondria produce energy for the cell; the endoplasmic reticulum contains ribosomes that produce proteins; the Golgi apparatus packages proteins; and lysosomes contain protein-dissolving enzymes that are important for digestion and the recycling of organisms in nature.

Cell Properties

Cells have certain properties that allow them to survive. **Endocytosis** involves incorporation of material into the cell by extending the cell membrane around the substance. Pinocytosis, a form of endocytosis, refers to the engulfing of specific substances that have reacted with a receptor site on the cell membrane. This process allows cells to absorb nutrients, enzymes, and other materials. Phagocytosis is a similar process; it allows the cell, usually a neutrophil or macrophage, to engulf a bacterium or a foreign protein and destroy it within the cell by secreting digestive enzymes into the area. **Exocytosis** is the opposite of endocytosis and involves removing substances from a cell by pushing them through the cell membrane. Hormones, neurotransmitters, enzymes, and other substances produced within a cell are excreted into the body by this process (Figure 7.3).

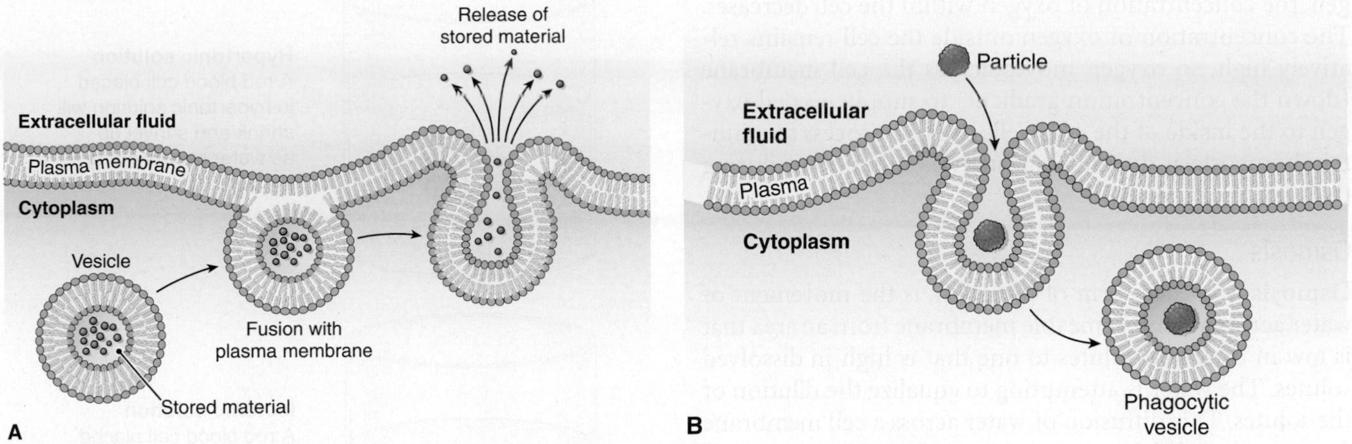

FIGURE 7.3 Schematic representation of endocytosis and exocytosis. **A:** Exocytosis is the movement of substances (waste products, hormones, neurotransmitters) out of the cell. **B:** Endocytosis involves the destruction of engulfed proteins or bacteria.

Homeostasis

The main goal of a cell is to maintain homeostasis, which means keeping the cytoplasm stable within the cell membrane. Each cell uses a series of active and passive transport systems to achieve homeostasis; the exact system used depends on the type of cell and its reactions with the immediate environment. For a cell to produce the energy needed to carry out cellular metabolism and other processes the cell must have a means to obtain necessary elements from the outside environment. In addition, it must have a way to dispose of waste products that could be toxic to its cytoplasm. To accomplish this, the cell moves substances across the cell membrane, either by passive transport or by active (energy-requiring) transport (Figure 7.4).

Passive Transport

Passive transport happens without the expenditure of energy and can occur across any semipermeable membrane. There are essentially three types of passive transport: diffusion, osmosis, and facilitated diffusion.

Diffusion

Diffusion is the movement of a substance from a region of higher concentration to a region of lower concentration. The difference between the concentrations of the substance in the two regions is called the *concentration gradient* of the substance; usually, the greater the concentration gradient the faster the substance moves. Movement into and out of a cell is regulated by the cell membrane. Some substances move through channels or pores in the cell membrane. Small substances and materials with no ionic charge move most freely through the channels. Substances with a negative charge move more freely than substances with a positive charge. Substances that move into and out of a cell by diffusion include sodium, potassium, calcium, carbonate, oxygen, bicarbonate, and water.

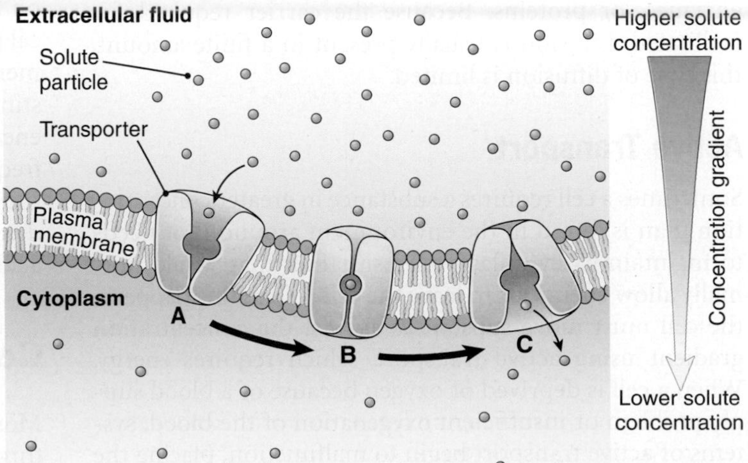

FIGURE 7.4 Schematic representation of transport across a cell membrane (**A**), which includes *diffusion* through the cell membrane (**B**) and *pore diffusion* through a protein channel (**C**).

When a cell is very active and is using energy and oxygen, the concentration of oxygen within the cell decreases. The concentration of oxygen outside the cell remains relatively high, so oxygen moves across the cell membrane (down the concentration gradient) to supply needed oxygen to the inside of the cell. Cells use this process to maintain homeostasis during many activities that occur during their life.

Osmosis

Osmosis, a special form of diffusion, is the movement of water across a semipermeable membrane from an area that is low in dissolved solutes to one that is high in dissolved solutes. The water is attempting to equalize the dilution of the solutes. This diffusion of water across a cell membrane from an area of high concentration (of water) to an area of low concentration creates pressure on the cell membrane called *osmotic pressure.* The greater the concentration of solutes in the solution to which the water is flowing the higher the osmotic pressure.

A fluid that contains the same concentration of solutes as human plasma is called an *isotonic* solution. A fluid that contains a higher concentration of solutes than human plasma is a *hypertonic* solution, and it draws water from cells. A fluid that contains a lower concentration of solutes than human plasma is hypotonic; it loses water to cells. If a human red blood cell, which has a cytoplasm that is isotonic with human plasma, is placed into a hypertonic solution, it shrinks and shrivels because the water inside the cell diffuses out of the cell into the solution. If the same cell is placed into a hypotonic solution the cell swells and bursts because water moves from the solution into the cell (Figure 7.5).

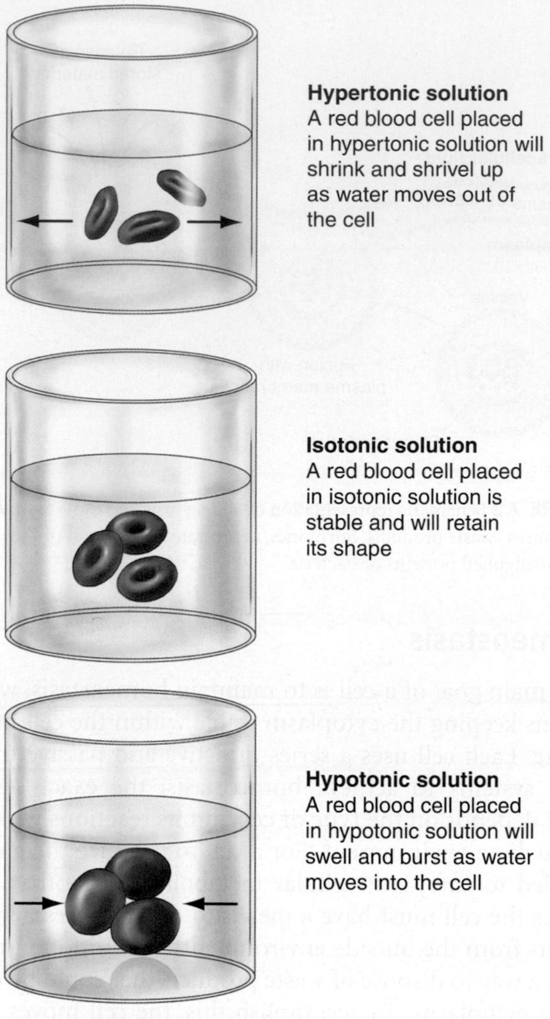
Hypertonic solution
A red blood cell placed in hypertonic solution will shrink and shrivel up as water moves out of the cell
Isotonic solution
A red blood cell placed in isotonic solution is stable and will retain its shape
Hypotonic solution
A red blood cell placed in hypotonic solution will swell and burst as water moves into the cell

FIGURE 7.5 Red blood cell, showing the cell's response to hypertonic, isotonic, and hypotonic solutions.

Facilitated Diffusion

Sometimes a substance cannot move freely on its own in or out of a cell. Such a substance may attach to another molecule, called a carrier, to be diffused. This form of diffusion, known as *facilitated diffusion*, does not require energy, just the presence of the carrier. Carriers may be hormones, enzymes, or proteins. Because the carrier required for facilitated diffusion is usually present in a finite amount, this type of diffusion is limited.

Active Transport

Sometimes a cell requires a substance in greater concentration than is found in the environment around it or needs to maintain its cytoplasm in a situation that would normally allow chemicals to leave the cell. When this happens, the cell must move substances against the concentration gradient using active transport, which requires energy. When a cell is deprived of oxygen because of a blood supply problem or insufficient oxygenation of the blood, systems of active transport begin to malfunction, placing the cell's integrity in jeopardy.

One of the best-known systems of active transport is the sodium–potassium pump. Cells use active transport to maintain a cytoplasm with a higher level of potassium and a lower level of sodium than the extracellular fluid contains. This allows the cell to maintain an electrical charge on the cell membrane, which gives many cells the electrical properties of excitation (the ability to generate a movement of electrons) and conduction (the ability to send this stimulus to other areas of the membrane). Some drugs use energy to move into cells by active transport. Drugs are frequently bonded with a carrier when they are moved into the cell. Cells in the kidney use active transport to excrete drugs from the body, as well as to maintain electrolyte and acid–base balances.

Cell Cycle

Most cells have the ability to reproduce themselves through the process of mitosis. The genetic makeup of a particular cell determines the rate at which that cell can

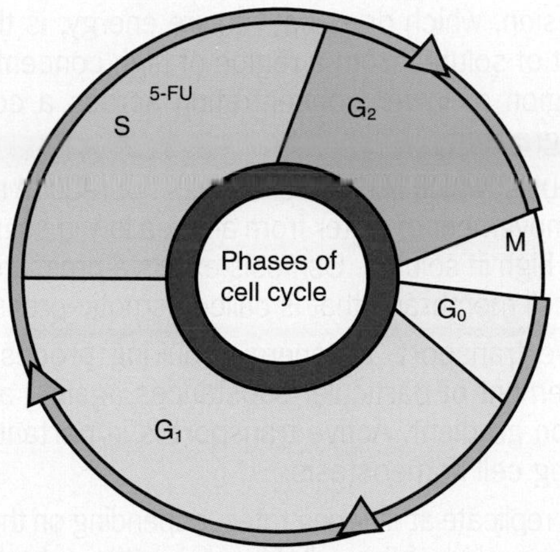

FIGURE 7.6 Diagram of the cell cycle, showing G_0, G_1, S, G_2, and M phases.

multiply. Some cells reproduce very quickly (e.g., the cells lining the gastrointestinal tract have a generation time of 72 hours), and some reproduce very slowly (e.g., the cells found in breast tissue have a generation time of a few months). In some cases, certain factors influence cell reproduction. Erythropoietin, a hormone produced by the kidney, can stimulate the production of new red blood cells. Active leukocytes release chemicals that stimulate the production of white blood cells when the body needs new ones. Regardless of the rate of reproduction, each cell has approximately the same life cycle. The life cycle of a cell, called the **cell cycle**, consists of four active phases and a resting phase (Figure 7.6).

G_0 Phase

During the G_0 phase, or resting phase, the cell is stable. It is not making any proteins associated with cell division and is basically dormant as far as reproduction goes. These cells are just functioning to do whatever they are supposed to do. Cells in the G_0 phase cause a problem in the treatment of some cancers. Cancer chemotherapy usually works on active, dividing cells, leaving resting cells fairly untouched. When the resting cells are stimulated to become active and regenerate the cancer can return, which is why cancer chemotherapeutic regimens are complicated and extended over time, and why a 5-year cancer-free period is usually the basic guide for considering a cancer to be cured.

G_1 Phase

When a cell is stimulated to emerge from its resting phase, it enters what is called the G_1 phase, which lasts from the time of stimulation from the resting phase until the formation of DNA. During this period the cell synthesizes substances needed for DNA formation. The cell is actively collecting materials to make these substances and producing the building blocks for DNA.

S Phase

The next phase, called the S phase, involves the actual synthesis of DNA, which is an energy-consuming activity. The cell remains in this phase until the amount of cellular DNA has doubled.

G_2 Phase

After the cellular DNA has doubled in preparation for replication the G_2 phase begins. During this phase the cell produces all of the substances required for the manufacture of the mitotic spindles.

M Phase

After the cell has produced all of the substances necessary for formation of a new cell, or daughter cell, it undergoes cell division. This occurs during the M phase of the cell cycle. During this phase the cell splits to form two identical daughter cells, a process called mitosis.

KEY POINTS

- All cells progress through a cell cycle, which allows them to reproduce.
- Each cell goes through a resting phase (G_0); a gathering phase (G_1), when the components needed for cell division are collected by the cell; a synthesizing phase (S), when DNA and other components are produced; a final gathering phase (G_2), when the last substances needed for division are collected and produced; and an M phase, when actual cell division occurs, producing two identical daughter cells.

SUMMARY

- The cell is composed of a nucleus, which contains genetic material and controls the production of proteins by the cell; a cell membrane, which separates the inside of the cell from the outside environment; and a cytoplasm, which contains various organelles important to cell function.
- The cell membrane functions as a fluid barrier made of lipids and proteins. The arrangement of the lipoprotein membrane controls what enters and leaves the cell.
- Proteins on the cell membrane surface can act either as receptor sites for specific substances or as histocompatibility markers that identify the cell as a self-cell (i.e., a cell belonging to that individual).
- Channels or pores in the cell membrane allow for easier movement of specific substances needed by the cell for normal functioning.
- Mitochondria are rod-shaped organelles that produce energy in the form of ATP for use by cells.

- Ribosomes are sites of protein production within the cell cytoplasm. The specific proteins produced by a cell are determined by the genetic material within the cell nucleus.
- The Golgi apparatus packages particular substances for removal from the cell (e.g., neurotransmitters, hormones).
- Lysosomes are packets of digestive enzymes located in the cell cytoplasm. These enzymes are responsible for destroying injured or nonfunctioning parts of the cell and for promoting cellular disintegration when the cell dies.
- Endocytosis is the process of moving substances into a cell by extending the cell membrane around the substance and engulfing it. Pinocytosis refers to the engulfing of necessary materials, and phagocytosis refers to the engulfing and destroying of bacteria or other proteins by white blood cells.
- Exocytosis is the process of removing substances from a cell by moving them toward the cell membrane and then changing the cell membrane to allow passage of the substance out of the cell.
- Cells maintain homeostasis by regulating the movement of solutes and water into and out of the cell.
- Diffusion, which does not require energy, is the movement of solutes from a region of high concentration to a region of lower concentration across a concentration gradient.
- Osmosis, which like diffusion does not require energy, is the movement of water from an area low in solutes to an area high in solutes. Osmosis exerts a pressure against the cell membrane that is called osmotic pressure.
- Active transport, an energy-requiring process, is the movement of particular substances against a concentration gradient. Active transport is important in maintaining cell homeostasis.
- Cells replicate at differing rates, depending on the genetic programming of the cell. All cells go through a life cycle consisting of the following phases: G_0, the resting phase; G_1, which involves the production of proteins for DNA synthesis; S, which involves the synthesis of DNA; G_2, which involves manufacture of the materials needed for mitotic spindle production; and M, the mitotic phase, in which the cell splits to form two identical daughter cells.
- Chemotherapeutic drugs act on cells to cause cell death or alteration. All properties of the drug that affect cells should be considered when administering a chemotherapeutic agent.

CHECK YOUR UNDERSTANDING

Answers to the questions in this chapter can be found in Answers to Check Your Understanding Questions on thePoint®.

MULTIPLE CHOICE

Select the best answer to the following.

1. The basic unit of human structure is
   a. the mitochondria.
   b. the nucleus.
   c. the nucleolus.
   d. the cell.

2. The cell membrane is composed of
   a. a phospholipid structure.
   b. channels of protein.
   c. a cholesterol-based membrane.
   d. Golgi apparatus.

3. The saying, "One rotten apple can spoil the whole barrel," can be used to refer to the cell-degrading properties of
   a. calcium channels.
   b. lysosomes.
   c. histocompatibility receptors.
   d. nuclear spindles.

4. The ribosomes are important sites for
   a. digestion of nutrients.
   b. excretion of waste products.
   c. production of proteins.
   d. hormone receptors.

5. A human cell placed in salty seawater will
   a. burst from water entering the cell.
   b. shrivel and die from water leaving the cell.
   c. not be affected in any way.
   d. break apart from the salt effect.

6. The sodium–potassium pump maintains a negative charge on the cell membrane by
   a. osmosis.
   b. diffusion.
   c. active transport.
   d. facilitated diffusion.

7. All cells progress through basically the same cell cycle, including
   a. two phases.
   b. four active phases and a resting phase.
   c. three periods of rest and a splitting phase.
   d. four active phases.

MULTIPLE RESPONSE

Select all that apply.

1. The amount of time that a cell takes to progress through the cell cycle is determined by which of the following?
   a. The acidity of the environment
   b. The genetic makeup of the cell
   c. The location of the cell in the body
   d. The number of ribosomes in the cell
   e. The cell response to contact inhibition
   f. The availability of nutrients and oxygen

2. Some substances will pass into the human cell by simple diffusion. Which of the following substances diffuse into the cell?
   a. Calcium
   b. Nitrogen
   c. Sodium
   d. Carbon dioxide
   e. Oxygen
   f. Potassium

3. Some substances require a channel or pore to enter a cell membrane. Which of the following substances use a channel to enter the cell?
   a. Calcium
   b. Urea
   c. Fat-soluble vitamins
   d. Sodium
   e. Oxygen
   f. Potassium

BIBLIOGRAPHY AND REFERENCES

Alberts, B., Johnson, A., Lewis, J., et al. (2012). *Molecular biology of the cell* (5th ed.). New York: Garland Science.

Barrett, K., Barman, S., Boitano, S., et al. (2012). *Ganong's review of medical physiology* (24th ed.). New York: McGraw-Hill.

Brunton, L., Chabner, B., & Knollman, B. (2011). *Goodman and Gilman's the pharmacological basis of therapeutics* (12th ed.). New York: McGraw-Hill.

Cooper, G., & Hausman, R. (2013). *The cell: A molecular approach* (6th ed.). London, UK: ASM Press/Sinauer Associates.

Guyton, A., & Hall, J. (2015). *Textbook of medical physiology* (13th ed.). Philadelphia, PA: W.B. Saunders.

Landowne, D. (2006). *Cell physiology*. New York: McGraw Hill.

Lodish, H., Berk, A., Kaiser, C. A., et al. (2012). *Molecular cell biology* (7th ed.). New York: W. H. Freeman.

Morgan, D. (2014). *The cell cycle: Principles of control* (2nd ed.). London, UK: New Science Press.

Porth, C. M. (2013). *Pathophysiology: Concepts of altered health states* (9th ed.). Philadelphia, PA: Lippincott Williams & Wilkins.

Sherwood, L. (2012). *Human physiology from cells to systems* (8th ed.). Florence, KY: Brooks Cole Thomson Learning.

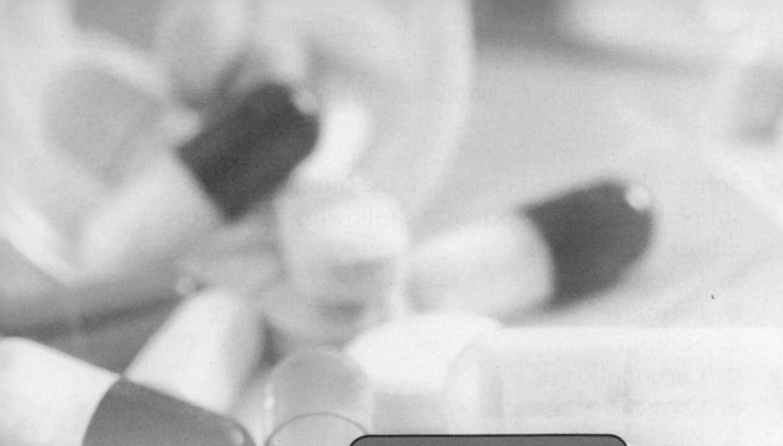

Anti-infective Agents 8

Learning Objectives

Upon completion of this chapter, you will be able to:

1. Explain what is meant by selective toxicity and discuss its importance in anti-infective therapies.
2. Differentiate between broad-spectrum and narrow-spectrum drugs.
3. Define resistance to anti-infectives and discuss the emergence of resistant strains.
4. Explain three ways to minimize resistance.
5. Describe three common adverse reactions associated with the use of anti-infectives.

Glossary of Key Terms

bactericidal: substance that causes the death of bacteria, usually by interfering with cell membrane stability or with proteins or enzymes necessary to maintain the cellular integrity of the bacteria

bacteriostatic: substance that prevents the replication of bacteria, usually by interfering with proteins or enzyme systems necessary for reproduction of the bacteria

culture: sample of the bacteria (e.g., from sputum, cell scrapings, urine) to be grown in a laboratory to determine the species of bacteria that is causing an infection

prophylaxis: treatment to prevent an infection before it occurs, as in the use of antibiotics to prevent bacterial endocarditis in high-risk patients or antiprotozoals to prevent malaria

resistance: ability of pathogens over time to adapt to an anti-infective to produce cells that are no longer affected by a particular drug

selective toxicity: the ability to affect certain proteins or enzyme systems that are used by the infecting organism but not by human cells

sensitivity testing: evaluation of pathogens obtained in a culture to determine the anti-infectives to which the organisms are sensitive and which agent would be appropriate for treatment of a particular infection

spectrum: range of bacteria against which an antibiotic is effective (e.g., broad-spectrum antibiotics are effective against a wide range of bacteria, narrow-spectrum antibiotics are effective only against very selective bacteria)

superinfection: infections that occur when opportunistic pathogens that were kept in check by the "normal" bacteria have the opportunity to invade tissues and cause infections because the normal flora bacteria have been destroyed by antibiotic therapy

Drug List

bacitracin
chloramphenicol
meropenem
polymyxin B
vancomycin

Anti-infective agents are drugs designed to target foreign organisms that have invaded and infected the body of a human host. For centuries, people have used various naturally occurring chemicals in an effort to treat disease. Often this was a random act that proved useful. For instance, the ancient Chinese found that applying moldy soybean curds to boils and infected wounds helped prevent infection or hastened cure. Their finding was, perhaps, a forerunner to the penicillins used today.

The use of drugs to treat systemic infections is a relatively new concept, beginning with Paul Ehrlich in the 1920s. Ehrlich's research to develop a synthetic chemical that would be effective only against infection-causing cells, not human cells, led the way for the scientific investigation of anti-infective agents. In the late 1920s scientists discovered penicillin in a mold sample; in 1935 the sulfonamides were introduced. Since then the number of anti-infectives available for use has grown tremendously. However, many of the organisms these drugs were designed to treat are rapidly adapting to repel the effects of anti-infectives, and, therefore, much work remains to deal with these emergent or resistant strains.

Although anti-infective agents target foreign organisms infecting the body of a human host, they do not possess total **selective toxicity**, which is the ability to affect certain proteins or enzyme systems used only by the infecting organism but not by human cells. Because all living cells are somewhat similar, no anti-infective drug has yet been developed that does not affect the host.

This chapter focuses on the principles involved in the use of anti-infective therapy and presents some anti-infectives as examples of these principles. The following chapters discuss specific agents used to treat particular infections: antibiotics for bacterial infections; antivirals; antifungals; antiprotozoals for infections caused by specific protozoa, including malaria; and anthelmintics for infections caused by worms. The final chapter in this section discusses antineoplastics—drugs used for treating diseases caused by abnormal human cells such as cancers. Antineoplastics specifically affect human cells to cause cell death or prevent cell growth and reproduction. The effects of anti-infectives on various age groups are discussed in Box 8.1.

Therapeutic Actions

Anti-infective agents may act on the cells of invading organisms in several different ways. The goal is interference with the normal function of the invading organism to prevent it from reproducing and to cause cell death without affecting host cells. Various mechanisms of action are briefly described here and shown in Figure 8.1. The specific mechanism of action for each drug class is discussed in the chapters that follow.

- Some anti-infectives interfere with biosynthesis of the pathogen cell wall. Because bacterial cells have a slightly different composition than human cells, this is an effective way to destroy the bacteria without interfering with the host (Box 8.2). The penicillins work in this way.
- Some anti-infectives prevent the cells of the invading organism from using substances essential to their growth and development, leading to an inability to divide and eventually to cell death. The sulfonamides, the antimycobacterial drugs, and trimethoprim-sulfamethoxazole (a combination drug frequently used to treat urinary tract infections) work in this way.
- Many anti-infectives interfere with the steps involved in protein synthesis, a function necessary to maintain the cell and allow for cell division. The aminoglycosides, the macrolides, and chloramphenicol (see the section on adverse effects for a box on chloramphenicol) work in this way.
- Some anti-infectives interfere with DNA synthesis in the cell, leading to inability to divide and cell death. The fluoroquinolones work in this way.
- Other anti-infectives alter the permeability of the cell membrane to allow essential cellular components to leak out, causing cell death. Some antibiotics, antifungals, and antiprotozoal drugs work in this manner.

BOX 8.1 FOCUS ON Drug Therapy Across the Lifespan

This box presents general principles of use of anti-infectives across the lifespan. Specifics for each type of anti-infective agent are discussed in their respective chapters within this unit.

Anti-infective Agents

CHILDREN

Use anti-infectives with caution; early exposure can lead to early sensitivity.

Controversy is widespread regarding the use of antibiotics to treat ear infections, a common pediatric problem. Some believe that the habitual use of antibiotics for what might well be a viral infection has contributed greatly to the development of resistant strains.

Because children can have increased susceptibility to the gastrointestinal (GI) and nervous system effects of anti-infectives, monitor hydration and nutritional status carefully.

ADULTS

Adults often demand anti-infectives for a "quick cure" of various signs and symptoms. Drug allergies and the emergence of resistant strains can be a big problem with this group.

Extreme caution must be exercised in the use of anti-infectives in pregnant and nursing women. Many anti-infectives can affect the fetus and also cross into breast milk, leading to toxic effects in the neonate.

OLDER ADULTS

Older patients often do not present with the same signs and symptoms of infection that are seen in younger people.

Culture and sensitivity tests are important to determine the type and extent of many infections.

The older patient is susceptible to severe adverse GI, renal, and neurological effects and must be monitored for nutritional status and hydration during drug therapy.

Anti-infectives that adversely affect the liver and kidneys must be used with caution in older patients, who may have decreased organ function.

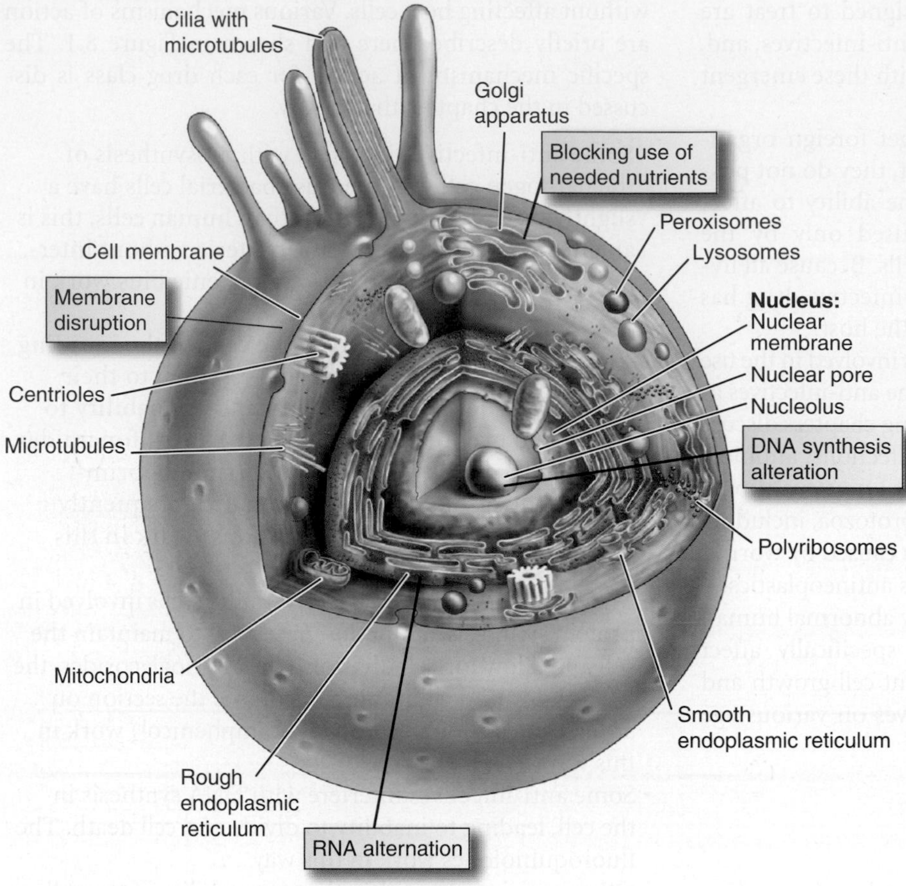

FIGURE 8.1 Anti-infectives can affect cells by disrupting the cell membrane, interfering with DNA synthesis, altering RNA, or blocking the use of essential nutrients.

BOX 8.2

Anti-infective Mechanism: Interference with Cell Wall Synthesis

Bacitracin (*Baci-IM, AK-Tracin, Baciguent*) is an antibiotic that interferes with the cell wall synthesis of susceptible staphylococcal bacteria. Adverse effects include nephrotoxicity and superinfection. Because of the development of resistant strains and more potent antibiotics, bacitracin is now indicated only for the treatment of respiratory infections in infants caused by susceptible staphylococci, treatment of eye infections, prevention of infections in minor skin wounds, and treatment of minor skin infections caused by susceptible strains of staphylococci. Bacitracin is available in intramuscular, ophthalmic, and topical preparations.

Usual Dosage

Infants <2.5 kg: 900 units/kg/d IM in three divided doses; *>2.5* kg: 1,000 units/kg/d IM in two to three divided doses.

Ophthalmic use: ½-in. ribbon to affected eye, b.i.d. to q3–4h.

Topical use: apply to affected area one to five times per day.

Anti-infective Activity

The anti-infectives used today vary in their **spectrum** of activity; that is, they vary in their effectiveness against invading organisms. Some anti-infectives are so selective in their action that they are effective against only a few microorganisms with a very specific metabolic pathway or enzyme. These drugs are said to have a narrow spectrum of activity. Other drugs interfere with biochemical reactions in many different kinds of microorganisms, making them useful in the treatment of a wide variety of infections. Such drugs are said to have a broad spectrum of activity.

Some anti-infectives are so active against the infective microorganisms that they actually cause the death of the cells they affect. These drugs are said to be **bactericidal** or fungicidal, etc. Some anti-infectives are not as aggressive against invading organisms; they interfere with the ability of the cells to reproduce or divide. These drugs are said to be **bacteriostatic** or fungastatic, etc. Several drugs are both "cidal" and "static," often depending on the concentration of the drug that is present. Many of the adverse effects noted with the use of anti-infectives are associated with the aggressive properties of the drugs and their effect on the cells of the host in addition to those of the pathogen.

Human Immune Response

The goal of anti-infective therapy is reduction of the population of the invading organism to a point at which the human immune response can take care of the infection. If a drug were aggressive enough to eliminate all traces of any invading pathogen, it also might be toxic to the host. The immune response (see Chapter 15) involves a complex interaction among chemical mediators, leukocytes, lymphocytes, antibodies, and locally released enzymes and chemicals. When this response is completely functional and all of the necessary proteins, cells, and chemicals are being produced by the body, it can isolate and eliminate foreign proteins, including bacteria, fungi, and viruses. However, if a person is immunocompromised for any reason (e.g., malnutrition, age, acquired immune deficiency syndrome, use of immunosuppressant drugs), the immune system may be incapable of dealing effectively with the invading organisms. It is difficult to treat any infections in such patients for two reasons: (1) Anti-infective drugs cannot totally eliminate the pathogen without causing severe toxicity in the host, and (2) these patients do not have the inflammatory or immune response in place to deal with even a few invading organisms. Immunocompromised patients present a significant challenge to health care providers. In helping these people cope with infections, prevention of infection and proper nutrition are often as important as drug therapy.

Resistance

Resistance can be natural or acquired, and refers to the ability over time to adapt to an anti-infective drug and produce cells that are no longer affected by a particular drug. Because anti-infectives act on specific enzyme systems or biological processes, many microorganisms that do not use that system or process are not affected by a particular anti-infective drug and are said to have a natural or intrinsic resistance. When prescribing a drug for treatment of an infection, this innate resistance should be anticipated. The selected drug should be one that is known to affect the specific microorganism causing the infection.

Since the advent of anti-infective drugs, microorganisms that were once very sensitive to the effects of particular drugs have begun to develop acquired resistance to the agents (Box 8.3). This can result in a serious clinical problem. The emergence of resistant strains of bacteria and other organisms poses a threat: Anti-infective drugs may no longer control potentially life-threatening diseases, and uncontrollable epidemics may occur.

Acquiring Resistance

Microorganisms develop resistance in a number of ways, including the following:

- Producing an enzyme that deactivates the antimicrobial drug. For example, some strains of bacteria that were once controlled by penicillin now produce an enzyme called penicillinase, which inactivates penicillin before it can affect the bacteria. This occurrence led to the development of new drugs that are resistant to penicillinase.
- Changing cellular permeability to prevent the drug from entering the cell or altering transport systems to exclude the drug from active transport into the cell.
- Altering binding sites on the membranes or ribosomes, which then no longer accept the drug.
- Producing a chemical that acts as an antagonist to the drug.

Most commonly, the development of resistance depends on the degree to which the drug acts to eliminate the invading microorganisms that are most sensitive to its effects. The cells that remain may be somewhat resistant to the effects of the drug, and with time these cells form the majority in the population. These cells differ from the general population of the species because of slight variations in their biochemical processes or biochemicals. The drug does not cause a mutation of these cells; it simply allows the somewhat different cells to become the majority or dominant group after elimination of the sensitive cells. Other microbes may develop resistance through actual genetic mutation. A mutant cell survives the effects of an anti-infective agent and divides, forming a new colony of resistant microbes with a genetic composition that provides resistance to the anti-infective agent.

BOX 8.3

Bacterial Resistance to an Anti-infective Drug

Vancomycin (*Vancocin*) is an antibiotic that interferes with cell wall synthesis in susceptible bacteria. It was developed as a result of a need for a drug that could be used both in patients who are intolerant to or allergic to penicillin and/or cephalosporins and in the treatment of patients with staphylococcal infections that no longer respond to penicillin or cephalosporins. This anti-infective drug can be used orally or intravenously to treat life-threatening infections when less toxic drugs cannot be used. It is used orally as prophylaxis against bacterial endocarditis in patients who cannot take penicillins or cephalosporins and to treat staphylococcal infections in people who cannot take these groups of drugs.

Because vancomycin may be highly toxic, its use is reserved for very special situations. It can cause renal failure, ototoxicity, superinfections, and a condition known as "red man syndrome," which is characterized by sudden and severe hypotension, fever, chills, paresthesias, and erythema or redness of the neck and back. When it is the only antibiotic that is effective against a specific bacterium, however, the benefits may outweigh the risks.

Usual Dosage

Adult: 500 mg to 1 g PO or IV q6h for 7–10 days.
Pediatric: 40 mg/kg/d PO or IV in four divided doses; do not exceed 2 g/d.

Preventing Resistance

Because the emergence of resistant strains of microbes is a serious public health problem that continues to grow, health care providers must work together to prevent the emergence of resistant pathogens. Exposure to an antimicrobial agent leads to the development of resistance, so it is important to limit the use of antimicrobial agents to the treatment of specific pathogens known to be sensitive to the drug being used.

Drug dosing is important in preventing the development of resistance. Doses should be high enough and the duration of drug therapy should be long enough to eradicate even slightly resistant microorganisms. The recommended dosage for a specific anti-infective agent takes this issue into account. Around-the-clock dosing eliminates the peaks and valleys in drug concentration and helps to maintain a constant therapeutic level to prevent the emergence of resistant microbes during times of low concentration. The duration of drug use is critical to ensure that the microbes are completely, not partially, eliminated and are not given the chance to grow and develop resistant strains. It has proved to be difficult to convince people who are taking anti-infective drugs that the timing of doses and the length of time they continue to take the drug are important. Many people stop taking a drug once they start to feel better and then keep the remaining pills to treat themselves at some time in the future when they do not feel well. This practice favors the emergence of resistant strains. Box 8.4 gives tips on patient teaching.

Health care providers should also be cautious about the indiscriminate use of anti-infectives. Antibiotics are not effective in the treatment of viral infections or illnesses such as the common cold. However, many patients demand prescriptions for these drugs when they visit practitioners because they are convinced that they need to take something to feel better. Health care providers who prescribe anti-infectives without knowing the causative organism and which drugs might be appropriate are promoting the emergence of resistant strains of microbes. With many serious illnesses, including pneumonias for which the causative organism is suspected, antibiotic therapy may be started as soon as a sample of the bacteria, or culture, is taken and before the results are known. Health care providers also tend to try newly introduced, more powerful drugs when a more established drug may be just as effective. Use of a powerful drug in this way leads to the rapid emergence of resistant strains to that drug, perhaps limiting its potential usefulness when it might be truly necessary.

BOX 8.4 FOCUS ON Patient and Family Teaching

Using Anti-infective Agents

When teaching patients who are prescribed an anti-infective agent, it is important to always include some general points:

- This drug is prescribed for treating the particular infection that you have now. Do not use this drug to treat other infections.
- This drug needs to be taken as prescribed—for the correct number of times each day and for the full number of days. Do not stop taking the drug if you start feeling better. You need to take the drug for the full number of treatment days to ensure that the infection has been destroyed.

KEY POINTS

- The goal of anti-infective therapy is the reduction of the invading organisms to a point at which the human immune response can take care of the infection.
- Anti-infectives can act to destroy an infective pathogen (bactericidal) or to prevent the pathogen from reproducing (bacteriostatic).
- Anti-infectives can have a small group of pathogens against which they are effective (narrow spectrum), or they can be effective against many pathogens (broad spectrum).

Using Anti-infective Agents

Anti-infective agents are used to treat systemic infections and sometimes as a means of prophylaxis (to prevent infections before they occur).

Treatment of Systemic Infections

Many infections that once led to lengthy, organ-damaging, or even fatal illnesses are now managed quickly and efficiently with the use of systemic anti-infective agents. Before the introduction of penicillin to treat streptococcal infections, many people developed rheumatic fever with serious cardiac complications. Today, rheumatic fever and the resultant cardiac valve defects are seldom seen. Several factors should be considered before beginning one of these chemotherapeutic regimens to ensure that the patient obtains the greatest benefit possible with the fewest adverse effects. These factors include identification of the correct pathogen and selection of a drug that is most likely to (1) cause the least complications for that patient and (2) be most effective against the pathogen involved.

Identification of the Pathogen

Identification of the infecting pathogen is done by culturing a tissue sample from the infected area. **Cultures** are performed in a laboratory, in which a swab of infected tissue is allowed to grow on an agar plate. Staining techniques and microscopic examination are used to identify the offending bacterium. When investigators search for parasitic sources of infection, they may examine stool for ova and parasites. Microscopic examination of other samples is also used to detect fungal and protozoal infections. The correct identification of the organism causing the infection is an important first step in determining which anti-infective drug should be used.

Sensitivity of the Pathogen

In many situations, health care providers use a broad-spectrum anti-infective agent that has been shown to be most effective in treating an infection with certain presenting signs and symptoms. In other cases of severe infection a broad-spectrum antibiotic is started after a culture is taken but before the exact causative organism has been identified. Again, experience influences selection of the drug, based on the presenting signs and symptoms. In many cases, it is necessary to perform **sensitivity testing** on the cultured microbes to evaluate bacteria and determine which drugs are capable of controlling the particular microorganism. This testing is especially important with microorganisms that have known resistant strains. In these cases, culture and sensitivity testing identify the causal pathogen and the most appropriate drug for treating the infection.

Combination Therapy

In some situations a combination of two or more types of drugs effectively treats the infection. When the offending pathogen is known, combination drugs may be effective in interfering with its cellular structure in different areas or developmental phases.

Combination therapy may be used for several reasons:

- The health care provider may be encouraged to use a smaller dose of each drug, leading to fewer adverse effects but still having a therapeutic impact on the pathogen.
- Some drugs are synergistic, which means that they are more powerful when given in combination.
- Many microbial infections are caused by more than one organism, and each pathogen may react to a different anti-infective agent.
- Sometimes, the combined effects of the different drugs delay the emergence of resistant strains. This is important in the treatment of tuberculosis (a mycobacterial infection), malaria (a protozoal infection), HIV infection (a viral infection), and some bacterial infections. Resistant strains may be more likely to emerge when fixed combinations are used over time; however, this may be prevented by individualizing the combination.

Prophylaxis

Sometimes it is clinically useful to use anti-infectives as a means of **prophylaxis** to prevent infections before they occur. For example, when patients anticipate traveling to an area where malaria is endemic, they may begin taking antimalarial drugs before the journey and continue taking them periodically during the trip. Patients who are undergoing gastrointestinal (GI) or genitourinary surgery, which might introduce bacteria from those areas into the system, often have antibiotics ordered immediately after the surgery and periodically thereafter, as appropriate, to prevent infection. Patients with known cardiac valve disease, valve replacements, and other conditions are especially prone to the development of subacute bacterial endocarditis because of the vulnerability of their heart valves. When these patients are at high risk for developing one of these infections, they may use prophylactic antibiotic therapy as a precaution when undergoing certain invasive procedures, including dental work. Refer to the American Heart Association's recommended schedule for this prophylaxis.

KEY POINTS

- Resistance of a pathogen to an anti-infective agent can be natural (the pathogen does not use the process on which the anti-infective works) or acquired (the pathogen develops a process to oppose the anti-infective agent).
- The emergence of resistant strains is a serious public health problem. Health care providers need to be alert to preventing the emergence of resistant strains by not using antibiotics inappropriately, assuring that the anti-infective is taken at a high enough dose for a long enough period of time, and avoiding the use of newer, powerful anti-infectives if other drugs would be just as effective.

Adverse Reactions to Anti-infective Therapy

Because anti-infective agents affect cells, it is always possible that the host cells will also be damaged (Box 8.5). No anti-infective agent has been developed that is completely free of adverse effects. The most commonly encountered adverse effects associated with the use of anti-infective agents are direct toxic effects on the kidney, GI tract, and nervous system. Hypersensitivity reactions and superinfections also can occur.

Kidney Damage

Kidney damage occurs most frequently with drugs that are metabolized by the kidney and then eliminated in the urine. Such drugs, which have a direct toxic effect on the fragile cells in the kidney, can cause conditions ranging from renal dysfunction to full-blown renal failure. When

BOX 8.5

Serious Adverse Effects of Antibiotic Treatment

Chloramphenicol (generic), an older antibiotic, prevents bacterial cell division in susceptible bacteria. Because of the potential toxic effects of this drug, its use is limited to serious infections for which no other antibiotic is effective. Chloramphenicol produces a "gray syndrome" in neonates and premature babies, which is characterized by abdominal distention, pallid cyanosis, vasomotor collapse, irregular respirations, and even death. In addition, the drug may cause bone marrow depression, including aplastic anemia that can result in death. These effects are seen even with the use of the ophthalmic and otic forms of the drug. Although the use of chloramphenicol is severely limited, it has stayed on the market because it is used to treat serious infections caused by bacteria that are not sensitive to any other antibiotic. It is now available in IV form only.

Usual Dosage

Adult or pediatric: 50 mg/kg/d IV in divided doses.

BOX 8.6

Severe Gastrointestinal Toxicity Resulting from Anti-infective Treatment

Meropenem (*Merrem IV*), an IV antibiotic, inhibits the synthesis of bacterial cell walls in susceptible bacteria. It is used to treat intra-abdominal infections and some cases of meningitis caused by susceptible bacteria. Meropenem almost always causes very uncomfortable GI effects; in fact, use of this drug has been associated with potentially fatal pseudomembranous colitis. It also results in headache, dizziness, rash, and superinfections. Because of its toxic effects on GI cells, it is used only in those infections with proven sensitivity to meropenem and reduced sensitivity to less toxic antibiotics.

Usual Dosage

Adult: 1 g IV q8h.

Pediatric: younger than 3 mo: not recommended; older than 3 mo: 20–40 mg/kg IV q8h; if >50 kg, 1–2 g IV q8h.

Geriatric: lower dose in accordance with creatinine clearance levels.

patients are taking these drugs (e.g., aminoglycosides), they should be monitored closely for any sign of renal dysfunction. To prevent any accumulation of the drug in the kidney, patients should be well hydrated throughout the course of the drug therapy.

Gastrointestinal Toxicity

GI toxicity is very common with many anti-infectives. Many of these agents have direct toxic effects on the cells lining the GI tract, causing nausea, vomiting, stomach upset, or diarrhea, and such effects are sometimes severe (Box 8.6). There is also some evidence that the death of the microorganisms releases chemicals and toxins into the body, which can stimulate the chemoreceptor trigger zone in the medulla and induce nausea and vomiting.

In addition, some anti-infectives are toxic to the liver. These drugs can cause hepatitis and even liver failure. When patients are taking drugs known to be toxic to the liver (e.g., many of the cephalosporins), they should be monitored closely, and the drug should be stopped at any sign of liver dysfunction.

Neurotoxicity

Some anti-infectives can damage or interfere with the function of nerve tissue, usually in areas where drugs tend to accumulate in high concentrations (Box 8.7). For example, the aminoglycoside antibiotics collect in the eighth cranial nerve and can cause dizziness, vertigo, and loss of hearing. Chloroquine, which is used to treat malaria and some other rheumatoid disorders, can accumulate in the retina and optic nerve and cause blindness. Other anti-infectives can cause dizziness, drowsiness, lethargy, changes in reflexes, and even hallucinations when they irritate specific nerve tissues.

BOX 8.7

Nerve Damage Caused by an Anti-infective Agent

Polymyxin B (generic), an older antibiotic, uses a surfactant-like reaction to enter the bacterial cell membrane and disrupt it, leading to cell death in susceptible gram-negative bacteria. This drug is available for IM, IV, or intrathecal use, as well as an ophthalmic agent for the treatment of infections caused by susceptible bacteria. Because of the actions of polymyxin B on cell membranes, however, it can be toxic to the human host, leading to nephrotoxicity, neurotoxicity (facial flushing, dizziness, ataxia, paresthesias, and drowsiness), and drug fever and rashes. Therefore, it is reserved for use in acute situations when the invading bacterium has been proven to be sensitive to polymyxin B and less sensitive to other, less toxic antibiotics.

Usual Dosage

Adult and pediatric: 15,000–25,000 units/kg/d IV may be divided into two doses *or*

25,000–30,000 units/kg/d IM divided into four to six doses *or*

50,000 units intrathecal daily for 3–4 days, then every other day for at least 2 weeks *or*

1–2 drops (gtt) ophthalmic preparation in affected eye b.i.d. q4h.

Hypersensitivity Reactions

Allergic or hypersensitivity reactions reportedly occur with many antimicrobial agents. Most of these agents, which are protein bound for transfer through the cardiovascular system, are able to induce antibody formation in susceptible people. With the next exposure to the drug, immediate or delayed allergic responses may occur. In severe cases, anaphylaxis can occur, which can be life threatening. Some of these drugs have demonstrated cross-sensitivity (e.g., penicillins, cephalosporins), and care must be taken to obtain a complete patient history before administering one of these drugs. It is important to determine what the allergic reaction was (what actually happened that made the patient think an allergy existed) and when the patient experienced it (e.g., after first use of the drug, or after years of use). Some patients report having a drug allergy, but closer investigation indicates that their reaction actually constituted an anticipated effect or a known adverse effect of the drug such as nausea or diarrhea. Proper interpretation of this information is important to allow treatment of a patient with a drug to which the patient reported a supposed allergic reaction but that would be very effective against a known pathogen.

Superinfections

One offshoot of the use of anti-infectives, especially broad-spectrum anti-infectives, is destruction of the normal flora. **Superinfections** are infections that occur when opportunistic pathogens that were kept in check by the "normal" flora bacteria have the opportunity to invade tissues. Common superinfections include vaginal or GI yeast infections, which are associated with antibiotic therapy, and infections caused by *Proteus* and *Pseudomonas* throughout the body, which are a result of broad-spectrum antibiotic use. In recent years the emergence of *Clostridium difficile* infections has been associated with the use of specific antibiotics. If patients receive drugs that are known to induce superinfections, they should be monitored closely for any signs of a new infection—sore patches in the mouth, vaginal itching, diarrhea—and the appropriate treatment for any superinfection should be started as soon as possible.

SUMMARY

- Anti-infectives are drugs designed to act with selective toxicity on foreign organisms that have invaded and infected the human host, which means that they affect biological systems or structures found in the invading organisms but not in the host.
- Anti-infectives include antibiotics, antivirals, antifungals, antiprotozoals, and anthelmintic agents.
- The goal of anti-infective therapy is interference with the normal function of invading organisms to prevent them from reproducing, and promotion of cell death without negative effects on the host cells. The infection should be eradicated with the least toxicity to the host and the least likelihood for development of resistance.
- Anti-infectives can work by altering the cell membrane of the pathogen, by interfering with protein synthesis, or by interfering with the ability of the pathogen to obtain needed nutrients.
- Anti-infectives also work to kill invading organisms or to prevent them from reproducing, thus depleting the size of the invasion to one that can be dealt with by the human immune system.
- Pathogens can develop resistance to the effects of anti-infectives over time when (1) mutant organisms that do not respond to the anti-infective become the majority of the pathogen population or (2) the pathogen develops enzymes to block the anti-infectives or alternative routes to obtain nutrients or maintain the cell membrane.
- An important aspect of clinical care involving anti-infective agents is preventing or delaying the development of resistance. This can be done by ensuring that the particular anti-infective agent is the drug of choice for the specific pathogen involved and that it is given in high enough doses for sufficiently long periods to rid the body of the pathogen.
- Culture and sensitivity testing of a suspected infection ensures that the correct drug is being used to treat the infection effectively. Culture and sensitivity testing should be performed before an anti-infective agent is prescribed.
- Anti-infectives can have several adverse effects on the human host, including renal toxicity, multiple GI effects, neurotoxicity, hypersensitivity reactions, and superinfections.
- Some anti-infectives are used as a means of prophylaxis when patients expect to be in situations that will expose them to a known pathogen, such as travel to an area where malaria is endemic, or oral or invasive GI surgery in a high-risk person who is susceptible to subacute bacterial endocarditis.

CHECK YOUR UNDERSTANDING

Answers to the questions in this chapter can be found in Answers to Check Your Understanding Questions on thePoint®.

MULTIPLE CHOICE

Select the best answer to the following.

1. The spectrum of activity of an anti-infective indicates
   a. the acidity of the environment in which they are most effective.
   b. the cell membrane type that the anti-infective affects.
   c. the anti-infective's effectiveness against different invading organisms.
   d. the resistance factor that bacteria have developed to this anti-infective.

2. The emergence of resistant strains of microbes is a serious public health problem. Health care providers can work to prevent the emergence of resistant strains by
   a. encouraging the patient to stop the antibiotic as soon as the symptoms are resolved to prevent overexposure to the drug.
   b. encouraging the use of antibiotics when patients feel they will help.
   c. limiting the use of antimicrobial agents to the treatment of specific pathogens known to be sensitive to the drug being used.
   d. using the most recent powerful drug available to treat an infection to ensure eradication of the microbe.

3. Sensitivity testing of a culture shows
   a. drugs that are capable of controlling that particular microorganism.
   b. the patient's potential for allergic reactions to a drug.
   c. the offending microorganism.
   d. an immune reaction to the infecting organism.

4. Combination therapy is often used in treating infections. An important consideration for using combination therapy would be that
   a. it is cheaper to use two drugs in one tablet than one drug alone.
   b. most infections are caused by multiple organisms.
   c. the combination of drugs can delay the emergence of resistant strains.
   d. combining anti-infectives will prevent adverse effects from occurring.

5. Superinfections can occur when anti-infective agents destroy the normal flora of the body. *Candida* infections are commonly associated with antibiotic use. A patient with this type of superinfection would exhibit
   a. difficulty breathing.
   b. vaginal discharge or white patches in the mouth.
   c. elevated blood urea nitrogen.
   d. dark lesions on the skin.

6. An example of an anti-infective used as a means of prophylaxis would be
   a. amoxicillin used for tonsillitis.
   b. penicillin used to treat an abscess.
   c. an antibiotic used before dental surgery.
   d. norfloxacin used for a bladder infection.

7. A broad-spectrum antibiotic would be the drug of choice when
   a. the patient has many known allergies.
   b. one is waiting for culture and sensitivity results.
   c. the infection is caused by one specific bacterium.
   d. treatment is being given for an upper respiratory infection of unknown cause.

MULTIPLE RESPONSE

Select all that apply.

1. Bacterial resistance to an anti-infective could be the result of which of the following?
   a. Natural or intrinsic properties of the bacteria
   b. Changes in cellular permeability or cellular transport systems
   c. The production of chemicals that antagonize the drug
   d. Initial exposure to the anti-infective
   e. Combination of too many antibiotics for one infection
   f. Narrow spectrum of activity

2. Anti-infective drugs destroy cells that have invaded the body. They do not specifically destroy only the cell of the invader, and because of this many adverse effects can be anticipated when an anti-infective is used. Which of the following adverse effects are often associated with anti-infective use?
   a. Superinfections
   b. Hypotension
   c. Renal toxicity
   d. Diarrhea
   e. Loss of hearing
   f. Constipation

BIBLIOGRAPHY AND REFERENCES

Bassler, B., & Winans, S. C. (2008). *Chemical communication among bacteria.* Hoboken, NJ: John Wiley & Sons.

Brunton, L., Chabner, B., & Knollman, B. (2011). *Goodman and Gilman's the pharmacological basis of therapeutics* (12th ed.). New York: McGraw-Hill.

CDC Vital Signs. (2013). Lethal drug-resistant bacteria spreading in US healthcare facilities. [*Centers for Disease Control*]. Available online at: http://www.cdc.gov/media/dpk/2013/dpk-vs-hai.html

Chopra, I., O'Neill, A. J., & Miller, K. (2003). The role of mutators in the emergence of antibiotic-resistant bacteria. *Drug Resistance Updates, 6*, 137–145.

Donadio, S., Maffioli, S., Monciardini, P., et al. (2010). Antibiotic discovery in the twenty-first century: Current trends and future perspectives. *Journal of Antibiotics, 63*, 423–430.

Facts and Comparisons. (2015). *Drug facts and comparisons.* St. Louis, MO: Author.

Karch, A. M. (2014). *Lippincott nursing drug guide.* Philadelphia, PA: Lippincott Williams & Wilkins.

Medical Letter. (2013). *The choice of antibacterial drugs* (Treatment Guidelines No. 131). New Rochelle, NY. Author.

Medical Letter. (2015). *The medical letter on drugs and therapeutics.* New Rochelle, NY: Author.

Porth, C. M. (2013). *Pathophysiology: Concepts of altered health states* (9th ed.). Philadelphia, PA: Lippincott Williams & Wilkins.

Shnayerson, M., & Plotkin, M. (2003). *The killers within: The deadly rise of drug-resistant bacteria.* New York: Little, Brown and Co.

Stephenson, J. (2008). Drug-resistant bacteria. *Journal of the American Medical Association, 299*(7), 755.

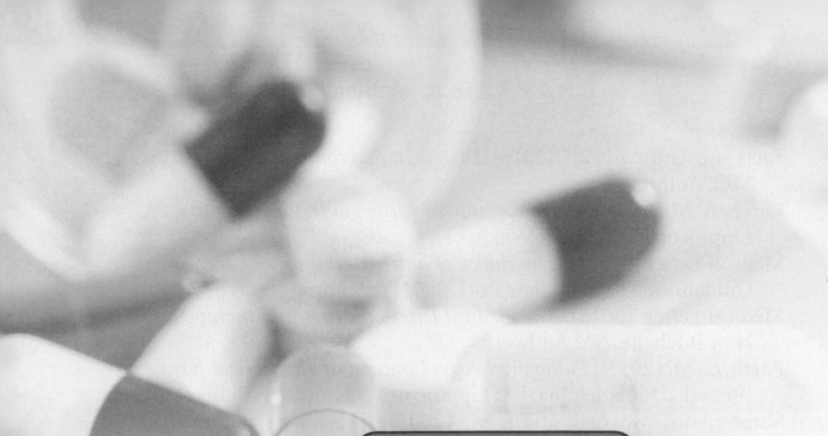

Antibiotics 9

Learning Objectives

Upon completion of this chapter, you will be able to:

1. Explain how an antibiotic is selected for use in a particular clinical situation.
2. Describe therapeutic actions, indications, pharmacokinetics, contraindications, most common adverse reactions, and important drug–drug interactions associated with each of the classes of antibiotics.
3. Discuss the use of antibiotics across the lifespan.
4. Compare and contrast prototype drugs for each class of antibiotics with other drugs in that class.
5. Outline nursing considerations for patients receiving each class of antibiotic.

Glossary of Key Terms

aerobic: bacteria that depend on oxygen for survival

anaerobic: bacteria that survive without oxygen, which are often seen when blood flow is cut off to an area of the body

antibiotic: chemical that is able to inhibit the growth of specific bacteria or cause the death of susceptible bacteria

gram-negative: bacteria that accept a negative stain and are frequently associated with infections of the genitourinary or gastrointestinal (GI) tract

gram-positive: bacteria that take a positive stain and are frequently associated with infections of the respiratory tract and soft tissues

synergistic: drugs that work together to increase drug effectiveness

Drug List

Aminoglycosides
amikacin
(P) gentamicin
neomycin
streptomycin
tobramycin

Carbapenems
doripenem
(P) ertapenem
imipenem–cilastatin
meropenem

Cephalosporins
First Generation
cefadroxil
cephalexin

Second Generation
(P) cefaclor
cefoxitin
cefprozil
cefuroxime

Third Generation
cefdinir
cefpodoxime
ceftazidime
ceftibuten
ceftizoxime
ceftriaxone

Fourth Generation
(P) cefditoren
cefepime
ceftaroline

Fluoroquinolones
(P) ciprofloxacin
finafloxacin
gemifloxacin
levofloxacin
moxifloxacin
ofloxacin

Penicillins and Penicillinase-Resistant Antibiotics
Penicillins
penicillin G benzathine
penicillin G potassium
penicillin G procaine
penicillin V

Extended-Spectrum Penicillins
(P) amoxicillin
ampicillin

Penicillinase-Resistant Antibiotics
nafcillin
oxacillin

Sulfonamides
(P) cotrimoxazole
sulfadiazine
sulfasalazine

Tetracyclines
demeclocycline
doxycycline
minocycline
(P) tetracycline

Antimycobacterials
Antituberculosis Drugs
capreomycin
cycloserine
ethambutol
ethionamide
(P) isoniazid
pyrazinamide
rifampin

rifapentine
streptomycin

Leprostatic Drugs
(P) dapsone

Other Antibiotics
Ketolides
(P) telithromycin

Lincosamides
(P) clindamycin
lincomycin

Lipoglycopeptide
dalbavanicin
oritavancin
televancin

Macrolides
azithromycin
clarithromycin
(P) erythromycin

Oxazolidinones
linezolid
tedizolid

Monobactams
(P) aztreonam

New Antibiotics and Adjuncts
New Antibiotics
daptomycin
fidaxomicin
quinupristin/dalfopristin
rifaximin
tigecycline

Adjuncts to Antibiotic Therapy
clavulanic acid
thalidomide
sulbactam

Many new bacteria appear each year, and researchers are challenged to develop new **antibiotics**—chemicals that inhibit specific bacteria—to deal with each new threat. Antibiotics are made in three ways: by living microorganisms, by synthetic manufacture, and in some cases through genetic engineering. Antibiotics may either be bacteriostatic (preventing the growth of bacteria) or bactericidal (killing bacteria directly), although several antibiotics are both bactericidal and bacteriostatic, depending on the concentration of the particular drug.

This chapter discusses the major classes of antibiotics: aminoglycosides, carbapenems, cephalosporins, fluoroquinolones, penicillins and penicillinase-resistant drugs, sulfonamides, tetracyclines, and the disease-specific antimycobacterials, including the antitubercular and leprostatic drugs. Antibiotics that do not fit into the large antibiotic classes include ketolides, lincosamides, lipoglycopeptides, macrolides, monobactams and oxazolidinones. Figures 9.1 and 9.2 show sites of cellular action of these classes of antibiotics.

FOCUS ON Safe Medication Administration

Many antibiotics used to treat childhood infections, such as otitis media and other upper respiratory infections, come in an oral suspension, suitable for children. The order for these solutions is usually written in teaspoons for the convenience of the parent who will be dispensing the medication. It is very important to make sure that the parent understands that the teaspoon in the prescription refers to a measuring teaspoon (5 mL). Inadvertent overdoses have been reported when parents used a flatware teaspoon to measure out the child's dose. Flatware teaspoons vary greatly in volume. If a parent calls to report that the medicine is all gone on day 4 and it was supposed to be given for 7 days, check to see how the medicine is being measured. Teaching the parent when the drug is first ordered can prevent problems during the course of treatment.

Bacteria and Antibiotics

Bacteria can invade the human body through many routes, for example, respiratory, gastrointestinal (GI), and skin. Once the bacteria invade the body the human inflammatory response is activated, and signs and symptoms of an infection occur as the body tries to rid itself of the foreign cells. Fever, lethargy, slow-wave sleep induction, and the classic signs of inflammation (e.g., redness, swelling, heat, and pain) all indicate that the body is responding to an invader. The body becomes the host for the bacteria and supplies proteins and enzymes the bacteria need for reproduction. Unchallenged, the invading bacteria can multiply and send out other bacteria to further invade tissue.

The goal of antibiotic therapy is to decrease the population of invading bacteria to a point at which the human immune system can effectively deal with the invader. To determine which antibiotic will effectively interfere with the specific proteins or enzyme systems for treatment of a specific infection the causative organism must be identified through a culture. Sensitivity testing is also done to determine the antibiotic to which that particular organism is most sensitive (e.g., which antibiotic best kills or controls the bacteria).

Gram-positive bacteria are those whose cell wall retains a stain known as Gram's stain or resists decolorization with alcohol during culture and sensitivity testing. Gram-positive bacteria are commonly associated with infections of the respiratory tract and soft tissues. An example of a gram-positive bacterium is *Streptococcus pneumoniae*, a common cause of pneumonia. In contrast, **gram-negative** bacteria are those whose cell walls lose a stain or are decolorized by alcohol. These bacteria are frequently associated with infections of the genitourinary (GU) or GI tract. An example of a gram-negative bacterium is *Escherichia coli*, a common cause of cystitis. **Aerobic** bacteria depend on oxygen for survival, whereas **anaerobic** bacteria (e.g., those bacteria associated with gangrene) do not use oxygen.

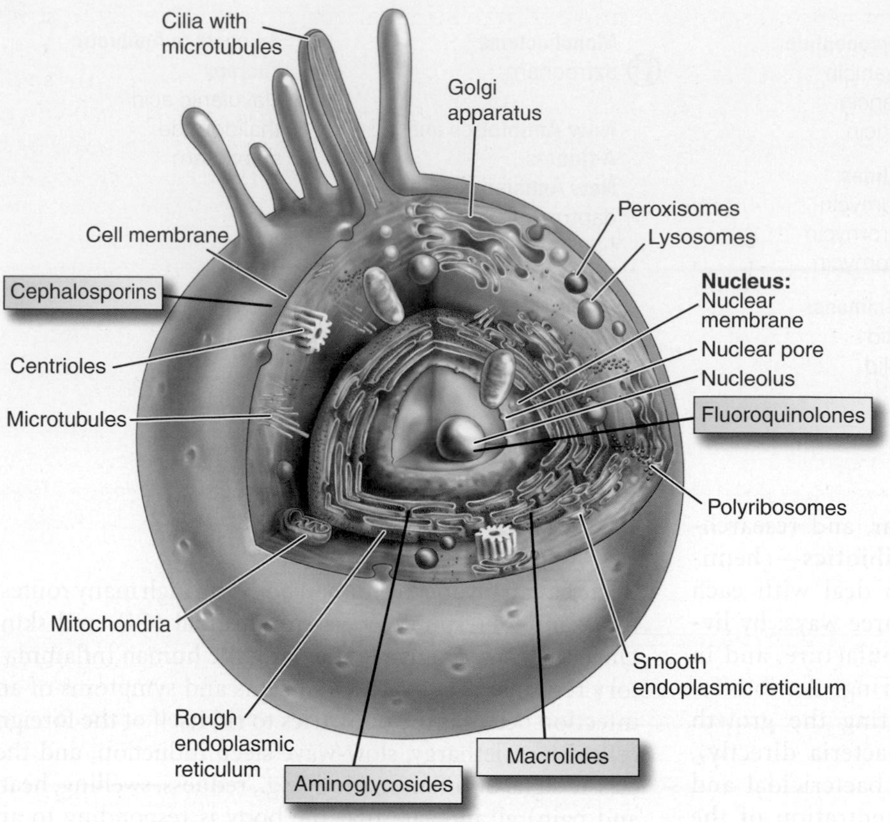

FIGURE 9.1 Sites of cellular action of aminoglycosides, cephalosporins, fluoroquinolones, oxazolidinones, and macrolides. Cephalosporins cause bacteria to build weak cell walls when dividing. Fluoroquinolones interfere with the DNA enzymes needed for growth and reproduction. Aminoglycosides, macrolides, and oxazolidinones change protein synthesis by binding to ribosome within the cell to cause cell death or prevent cell division.

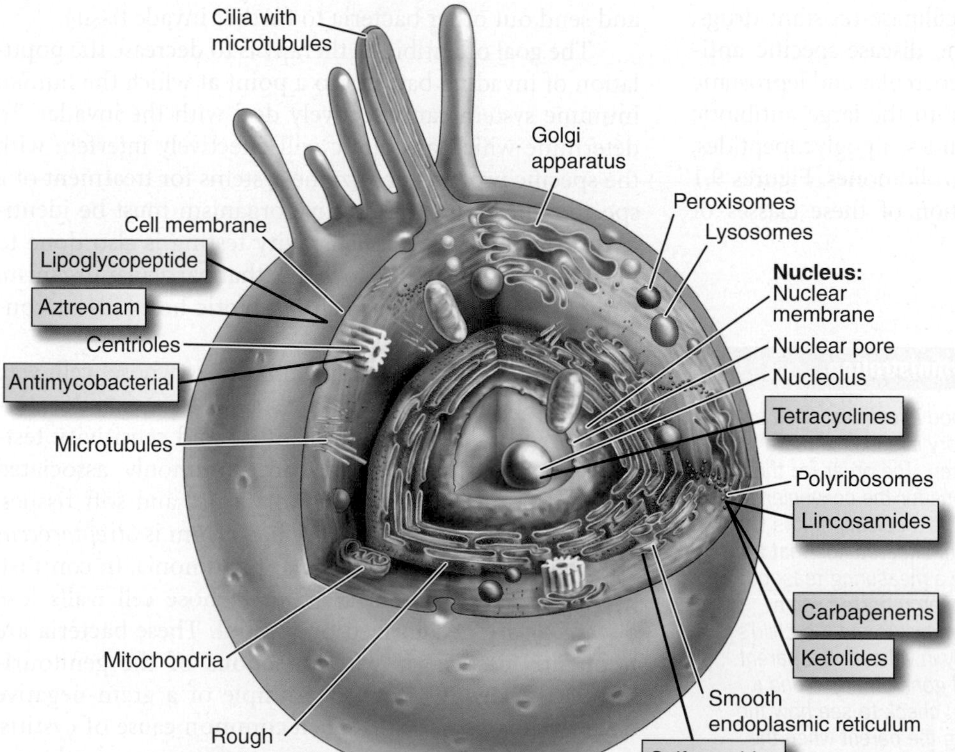

FIGURE 9.2 Sites of cellular action of carbapenems, ketolides, lincosamides, lipoglycopeptides, aztreonam, penicillins, sulfonamides, tetracyclines, and antimycobacterials. Carbapenems, ketolides, and lincosamides change protein function and prevent cell division or cause cell death. Aztreonam and lipoglycopeptides alter cell membranes to allow leakage of intracellular substances and cause cell death. Penicillins prevent bacteria from building their cells during division. Sulfonamides inhibit folic acid synthesis for RNA and DNA production. Tetracyclines inhibit protein synthesis, thereby preventing reproduction. Antimycobacterial drugs affect mycobacteria in three ways: They (1) affect the mycotic coat of the bacteria, (2) alter DNA and RNA, and (3) prevent cell division.

If culture and sensitivity testing is not possible, either because the source of the infection is not identifiable or because the patient is too sick to wait for test results to determine the best treatment, clinicians attempt to administer a drug with a broad spectrum of activity against gram-positive or gram-negative bacteria or against anaerobic bacteria. Antibiotics that interfere with a biochemical reaction common to many organisms are known as broad-spectrum antibiotics. These drugs are often given at the beginning of treatment until the exact organism and sensitivity can be established. Because these antibiotics have such a wide range of effects, they are frequently associated with adverse effects. Human cells have many of the same properties as bacterial cells and can be affected in much the same way, so damage may occur to the human cells, as well as to the bacterial cells.

Because there is no perfect antibiotic that is without effect on the human host, clinicians try to select an antibiotic with selective toxicity, or the ability to strike foreign cells with little or no effect on human cells. Certain antibiotics may be contraindicated in some patients because of known adverse effects; this includes those patients who are immunocompromised, who have severe GI disease, or who are debilitated (see Box 9.1 for effects of antibiotics across the lifespan). The antibiotic of choice is one that affects the causative organism and leads to the fewest adverse effects for the patient involved.

In some cases, antibiotics are given in combination because they are **synergistic**, meaning their combined effect is greater than their effect if they are given individually (Box 9.2). Use of synergistic antibiotics also allows the patient to take a lower dose of each antibiotic to achieve the desired effect, which helps to reduce the adverse effects that a particular drug may have.

read for exam

BOX 9.1 *FOCUS ON* **Drug Therapy Across the Lifespan**

Antibiotics

CHILDREN

Children are very sensitive to the GI and CNS effects of most antibiotics, and more severe reactions can be expected when these drugs are used in children. It is important to monitor the hydration and nutritional status of children who are adversely affected by drug-induced diarrhea, anorexia, nausea, and vomiting. Superinfections can be a problem for small children as well. For example, thrush (oral candidiasis) is a common superinfection that makes eating and drinking difficult.

Many antibiotics do not have proven safety and efficacy in pediatric use, and extreme caution should be used when giving them to children. The fluoroquinolones, for instance, are associated with damage to developing cartilage and are not recommended for growing children. Tetracyclines are not indicated for children because of effects on growing bones and teeth.

Pediatric dosages of antibiotics should be double-checked to make sure that the child is receiving the correct dose, thereby improving the chance of eradicating the infection and decreasing the risk of adverse effects.

Antibiotic treatment of ear infections, a common pediatric problem, is controversial. Ongoing research suggests that judicious use of decongestants and anti-inflammatories may be just as successful as the use of antibiotics without the risk of development of resistant bacterial strains.

Parents, not wanting to see their child sick, may demand antibiotics as a cure-all whenever their child is fussy or feverish. Parent education is very important in helping to cut down the unnecessary use of antibiotics in children.

ADULTS

Many adults believe that antibiotics are a cure-all for any discomfort and fever. It is very important to explain that antibiotics are useful against only specific bacteria and actually can cause problems when used unnecessarily for viral infections, such as the common cold.

Adults need to be cautioned to take the entire course of the medication as prescribed and not to store unused pills for future infections or share antibiotics with symptomatic friends.

Pregnant and breastfeeding women should not take antibiotics unless the benefit clearly outweighs the potential risk to the fetus or neonate. Tetracyclines, for example, are associated with pitting of enamel in developing teeth and with calcium deposits in growing bones. These drugs can cause serious problems for neonates. Women of childbearing age should be advised to use barrier contraceptives if any of these drugs are used.

Many antibiotics interfere with the effectiveness of hormonal contraceptives, and unplanned pregnancies can occur.

OLDER ADULTS

In many instances, older adults do not present with the same signs and symptoms of infections as other patients. Therefore, assessing the problem and obtaining appropriate specimens for culture is especially important with this population.

Older patients may be more susceptible to the adverse effects associated with antibiotic therapy. Their hydration and nutritional status should be monitored closely, as should the need for safety precautions if CNS effects occur. If hepatic or renal dysfunction is expected (particularly in very old patients, those who may depend on alcohol, and those who are taking other hepatotoxic or nephrotoxic drugs) the dose may need to be lowered and the patient should be monitored more frequently.

Elderly patients also need to be cautioned to complete the full course of drug therapy, even when they feel better, and not to save pills for self-medication at a future time.

BOX 9.2

Using Combination Drugs to Fight Resistant Bacteria

Clavulanic acid protects certain beta-lactam antibiotics from breakdown in the presence of penicillinase enzymes.

A combination of amoxicillin and clavulanic acid (*Augmentin*) is commonly used to allow the amoxicillin to remain effective against certain strains of resistant bacteria (usual dosage, 250–500 mg PO q8h for adults or 20–40 mg/kg/d PO in divided doses for children). The theory behind the combination of ticarcillin and clavulanic acid (*Timentin*) is similar (usual dosage 3.1 g IM q4–6h for adults; safety not established for children).

Sulbactam is another drug that increases the effectiveness of antibiotics against certain resistant bacteria. When combined with ampicillin in the drug *Unasyn*, sulbactam inhibits many bacterial penicillinase enzymes, broadening the spectrum of the ampicillin. In this combination, sulbactam is also slightly antibacterial (usual adult dosage, 0.5–1 g sulbactam, with 1–2 g ampicillin IM or IV q6–8h).

In some situations, antibiotics are used as a means of prophylaxis, or prevention of potential infection.

Patients who will soon be in a situation that commonly results in a specific infection (e.g., patients undergoing GI surgical procedures, which may introduce GI bacteria into the bloodstream or peritoneum; patients traveling to other countries with endemic bacteria that are not in their home area) may be given antibiotics before they are exposed to the bacteria. Usually a large, one-time dose of an antibiotic is given to destroy any bacteria that enter the host immediately and thereby prevent a serious infection.

Bacteria and Resistance to Antibiotics

Bacteria have survived for hundreds of years because they can adapt to their environment. They do this by altering their cell wall or enzyme systems to become resistant to (e.g., protect themselves from) unfavorable conditions or situations. Many species of bacteria have developed resistance to certain antibiotics. For example, bacteria that were once very sensitive to penicillin have developed an enzyme called penicillinase, which effectively inactivates many of the penicillin-type drugs. New drugs had to be developed to effectively treat infections involving these once-controlled bacteria. It is very important to use these drugs only when the identity and sensitivity of the offending bacterium have been established. Indiscriminate use of these new drugs can lead to the development of more resistant strains for which there is no effective antibiotic (see later discussion of new antibiotics for additional information on *Synercid* and linezolid).

The longer an antibiotic has been in use, the greater the chance that the bacteria will develop into a resistant strain. Efforts to control the emergence of resistant strains involve intensive educational programs that advocate the use of antibiotics only when necessary and effective and not for the treatment of viral infections such as the common cold (Box 9.3).

In addition, the use of antibiotics may result in the development of superinfections or overgrowth of resistant pathogens, such as bacteria, fungi, or yeasts, because antibiotics (particularly broad-spectrum agents) destroy bacteria in the flora that normally work to keep these opportunistic invaders in check (Figure 9.3). When "normal" bacteria are

BOX 9.3 FOCUS ON The Evidence

Using Antibiotics Properly

The Food and Drug Administration (FDA) and Centers for Disease Control and Prevention (CDC) have joined efforts to educate the public and health care providers about the dangers of inappropriate use of antibiotics. The evidence-based practice guidelines combine data from many studies to outline the most efficacious use of antibiotics. To review some of the studies, look at the references listed in the Bibliography and References section. Nurses should include some of the following points about the risks and dangers of antibiotic abuse in the patient education plan:

- Explain clearly that a particular antibiotic is effective against only certain bacteria and that a culture needs to be taken to identify the bacteria.
- Explain that bacteria can develop resistant strains that will not be affected by antibiotics in the future, so use of antibiotics now may make them less effective in situations in which they are really necessary.
- Ensure that patients understand the importance of taking the full course of medication as prescribed, even if they feel better. Stopping an antibiotic midway through a regimen often leads to the development of resistant bacteria. Using all of the medication will also prevent patients from saving unused medication to self-treat future infections or to share with other family members.
- Tell patients that allergies may develop with repeated exposures to certain antibiotics. In addition, explain to patients that saving antibiotics to take later, when they think they need them again, may lead to earlier development of an allergy, which will negate important tests that could identify the bacteria making them sick.
- Offer other medications, such as antihistamines, decongestants, or even chicken soup, to patients who request antibiotics; this may satisfy their need for something to take. Explaining that viral infections do not respond to antibiotics usually offers little consolation to patients who are suffering from a cold or the flu.

The publicity that many emergent, resistant strains of bacteria have received in recent years may help to get the message across to patients about the need to take the full course of an antibiotic and to use antibiotics only when they are appropriate. To view the educational program developed by the FDA and the CDC for use with patients and the data behind these efforts, go to http://www.cdc.gov/drugresistance/community/.

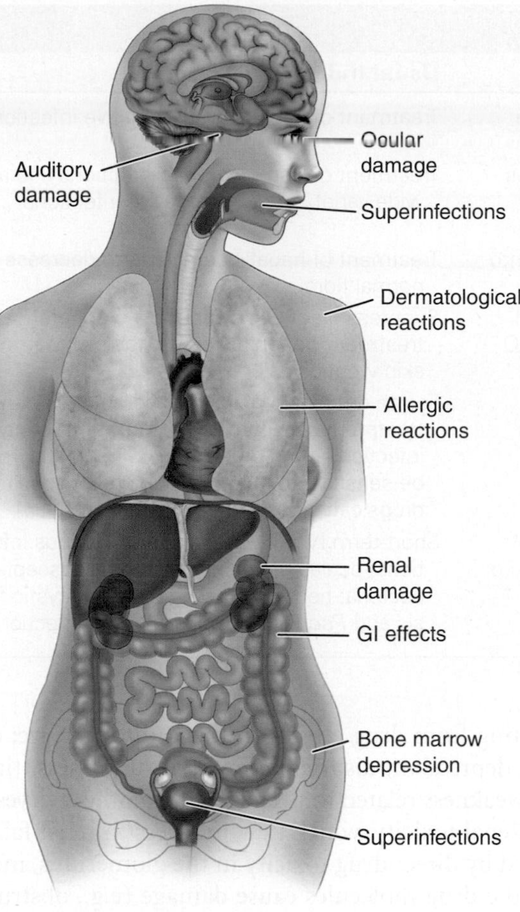

FIGURE 9.3 Common adverse effects associated with antibiotics.

destroyed or greatly reduced in number, there is nothing to prevent the invaders from occupying the host. In most cases the superinfection is an irritating adverse effect (e.g., vaginal yeast infection, candidiasis, diarrhea), but in some cases the superinfection can be more severe than the infection that was originally being treated. Treatment of the superinfection leads to new adverse effects and the potential for different superinfections. A vicious cycle of treatment and resistance is the result.

KEY POINTS

- The goal of antibiotic therapy is to reduce the population of invading bacteria to a size that the human immune response can deal with.
- Bacteria can be classified as gram-positive (frequently found in respiratory infections) or gram-negative (frequently found in GI and GU infections). They can also be classified as anaerobic (not needing oxygen) or aerobic (dependent on oxygen).
- Culture and sensitivity testing ensures that the correct antibiotic is chosen for each infection, a practice that may help to decrease the number of emerging resistant-strain bacteria.

Aminoglycosides

The aminoglycosides (Table 9.1) are a group of powerful antibiotics used to treat serious infections caused by gram-negative aerobic bacilli. Because most of these drugs have potentially serious adverse effects, newer, less-toxic drugs have replaced aminoglycosides in the treatment of less serious infections. Aminoglycosides include amikacin (*Amikin*), gentamicin (generic), neomycin (*Mycifradin*), streptomycin (generic), and tobramycin (*TOBI, TobrexOpthalmic*).

Therapeutic Actions and Indications

The aminoglycosides are bactericidal. They inhibit protein synthesis in susceptible strains of gram-negative bacteria. They irreversibly bind to a unit of the bacteria ribosomes, leading to misreading of the genetic code and cell death (Figure 9.1). These drugs are used to treat serious infections caused by susceptible strains of gram-negative bacteria, including *Pseudomonas aeruginosa, Escherichia coli, Proteus* spp., the *Klebsiella–Enterobacter–Serratia* group, *Citrobacter* spp., and *Staphylococcus* spp. such as *Staphylococcus aureus.* Aminoglycosides are indicated for the treatment of serious infections that are susceptible to penicillin when penicillin is contraindicated, and they can be used in severe infections before culture and sensitivity results have been obtained. See Table 9.1 for usual indications for each of these drugs.

Pharmacokinetics

The aminoglycosides are poorly absorbed from the GI tract but rapidly absorbed after intramuscular (IM) injection, reaching peak levels within 1 hour. These drugs have an average half-life of 2 to 3 hours. They are widely distributed throughout the body, cross the placenta and enter breast milk, and are excreted unchanged in the urine (see Contraindications and Cautions).

Amikacin is available for short-term IM or intravenous (IV) use.
Gentamicin is available in many forms: ophthalmic, topical, IV, IM, intrathecal
Neomycin is available in topical and oral forms.
Streptomycin is only available for IM use.
Tobramycin is used for short-term IM or IV treatment and is also available in an ophthalmic form and as a nebulizer solution.

Contraindications and Cautions

Aminoglycosides are contraindicated in the following conditions: known allergy to any of the aminoglycosides; renal or hepatic disease *that could be exacerbated by toxic aminoglycoside effects and that could interfere with drug metabolism and excretion, leading to higher toxicity*; preexisting

Table 9.1 *Drugs in Focus:* Aminoglycosides

Drug Name	Dosage/Route	Usual Indications
amikacin (*Amikin*)	15 mg/kg/d IM or IV divided into two or three equal doses; reduce dose in renal failure	Treatment of serious gram-negative infections
gentamicin (*Garamycin*)	*Adult:* 3 mg/kg/d IM or IV in three equal doses q8h; reduce dose in renal failure *Pediatric:* 2–2.5 mg/kg/d q8h IV or IM	Treatment of *Pseudomonas* infections and a wide variety of gram-negative infections
kanamycin (*generic*)	7.5 mg/kg q12h IM or 15 mg/kg/d IV divided into two to three equal doses given slowly	Treatment of hepatic coma and to decrease GI normal flora
neomycin (*Mycifradin*)	*Adult:* 4–12 g/d in divided doses PO for 5–6 d *Pediatric:* 50–100 mg/kg/d in divided doses PO for hepatic coma	Suppression of GI normal flora preoperatively; treatment of hepatic coma; topical treatment of skin wounds
streptomycin (generic)	*Adult:* 1–2 g/d IM in divided doses q6–12h *Pediatric:* 20–40 mg/kg/d IM in divided doses q6–12h	Fourth drug in combination therapy regimen for treatment of tuberculosis; treatment of severe infections if the organism has been shown to be sensitive to streptomycin and no less toxic drugs can be used
tobramycin (*TOBI, Tobrex*)	*Adult:* 3 mg/kg/d in three equal doses IM or IV q8h; reduce dose in renal failure; 300 mg b.i.d. by nebulizer *Pediatric:* 300 mg b.i.d. by nebulizer	Short-term IV or IM treatment of serious infections; ocular infections caused by susceptible bacteria; nebulizer management of cystic fibrosis and *Pseudomonas aeruginosa* infections

hearing loss, *which could be intensified by toxic drug effects on the auditory nerve*; active infection with herpes or mycobacterial infections *that could be worsened by the effects of an aminoglycoside on normal defense mechanisms*; myasthenia gravis or parkinsonism, *which often are exacerbated by the effects of a particular aminoglycoside on the nervous system*; and lactation, *because aminoglycosides are excreted in breast milk and potentially could cause serious effects in the infant.*

Caution is necessary when these agents are administered during pregnancy *because aminoglycosides are used to treat only severe infections, and the benefits of the drug must be carefully weighed against potential adverse effects on the fetus.* It is necessary to test urine function frequently when these drugs are used *because they depend on the kidney for excretion and are toxic to the kidney.*

The potential for nephrotoxicity and ototoxicity with amikacin is very high, so the drug is used only as long as absolutely necessary. Streptomycin, once a commonly used drug, is reserved for use in special situations *because it is very toxic to the eighth cranial nerve and kidney*. It can be used in severe infections if the organism has been shown to be sensitive to streptomycin and no less toxic drugs can be used.

Adverse Effects

The many serious adverse effects associated with aminoglycosides limit their usefulness. The drugs come with a black box warning alerting health care professionals to the serious risk of ototoxicity and nephrotoxicity. Central nervous system (CNS) effects include ototoxicity, possibly leading to irreversible deafness; vestibular paralysis resulting from drug effects on the auditory nerve; confusion; depression; disorientation; and numbness, tingling, and weakness related to drug effects on other nerves.

Renal toxicity, which may progress to renal failure, is caused by direct drug toxicity in the glomerulus, meaning that the drug molecules cause damage (e.g., obstruction) directly to the kidney. Bone marrow depression may result from direct drug effects on the rapidly dividing cells in the bone marrow, leading, for example, to immune suppression and resultant superinfections.

GI effects include nausea, vomiting, diarrhea, weight loss, stomatitis, and hepatic toxicity. These effects are a result of direct GI irritation, loss of bacteria of the normal flora with resultant superinfections, and toxic effects in the mucous membranes and liver as the drug is metabolized.

Cardiac effects can include palpitations, hypotension, and hypertension. Hypersensitivity reactions include purpura, rash, urticaria, and exfoliative dermatitis.

Clinically Important Drug–Drug Interactions

Most aminoglycosides have a synergistic bactericidal effect when given with penicillins or cephalosporins. In certain conditions, this synergism is used therapeutically to increase the effectiveness of treatment. Avoid combining aminoglycosides with potent diuretics; this increases the incidence of ototoxicity, nephrotoxicity, and neurotoxicity. If these antibiotics are given with anesthetics, nondepolarizing neuromuscular blockers, succinylcholine, or citrate anticoagulated blood, increased neuromuscular blockade with paralysis is possible. If a patient who has been receiving an aminoglycoside requires surgery and will be receiving any of these drugs, indicate prominently on the patient's chart the fact that the aminoglycoside has been given. Provide extended monitoring and support after surgery.

Ⓟ Prototype Summary: Gentamicin

Indications: Treatment of serious infections caused by susceptible bacteria.

Actions: Inhibits protein synthesis in susceptible strains of gram-negative bacteria, disrupting functional integrity of the cell membrane and causing cell death.

Pharmacokinetics:

Route	Onset	Peak
IM, IV	Rapid	30–90 min

$T_{1/2}$: 2 to 3 hours; metabolized in the liver and excreted in the urine.

Adverse Effects: Sinusitis, dizziness, rash, fever, risk of nephrotoxicity.

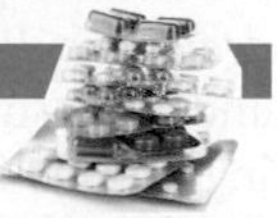

Nursing Considerations for Patients Receiving Aminoglycosides

Assessment: History and Examination

- Assess for *possible contraindications or cautions:* known allergy to any aminoglycoside (obtain specific information about the nature and occurrence of allergic reactions); history of renal or hepatic disease; preexisting hearing loss; active infection with herpes, vaccinia, varicella, or fungal or mycobacterial organisms; myasthenia gravis; parkinsonism; infant botulism; and current pregnancy or lactation status.
- Perform a physical assessment *to establish baseline data for assessing the effectiveness of the drug and the occurrence of any adverse effects associated with drug therapy.*
- Perform culture and sensitivity tests at the site of infection *to ensure appropriate use of the drug.*
- Conduct orientation and reflex assessment, as well as auditory testing, *to evaluate any CNS effects of the drug.*
- Assess vital signs: Respiratory rate and adventitious sounds *to monitor for signs of infection or hypersensitivity reactions;* temperature *to assess for signs and symptoms of infection;* and blood pressure *to monitor for cardiovascular effects of the drug.*
- Perform renal and hepatic function tests *to determine baseline function of these organs and, possibly, the need to adjust dose.*

Nursing Diagnoses

Nursing diagnoses related to drug therapy might include the following:

- Acute pain related to GI or CNS effects of drug
- Disturbed sensory perception (auditory) related to CNS effects of drug
- Risk for infection related to bone marrow suppression
- Excess fluid volume related to nephrotoxicity
- Deficient knowledge regarding drug therapy

Planning

- The patient will receive the best therapeutic effect from the drug therapy.
- The patient will have limited adverse effects to the drug therapy.
- The patient will have an understanding of the drug therapy, adverse effects to anticipate and measures to relieve discomfort and improve safety.

Implementation with Rationale

- Check culture and sensitivity reports *to ensure that this is the drug of choice for this patient.*
- Ensure that the patient receives a full course of aminoglycoside as prescribed, divided around the clock, *to increase effectiveness and decrease the risk for development of resistant strains of bacteria.*
- Monitor the infection site and presenting signs and symptoms (e.g., fever, lethargy) throughout the course of drug therapy. *Failure of these signs and symptoms to resolve may indicate the need to reculture the site.* Arrange to continue drug therapy for at least 2 days after all signs and symptoms resolve *to decrease the development of resistant strains of bacteria.*
- Monitor the patient regularly for signs of nephrotoxicity, neurotoxicity, and bone marrow suppression *to effectively arrange for discontinuation of drug or decreased dose, as appropriate, if any of these toxicities occurs.*
- Provide safety measures *to protect the patient if CNS effects, such as confusion, disorientation, or numbness and tingling, occur.*
- Provide small, frequent meals as tolerated; frequent mouth care; and ice chips or sugarless candy to suck if stomatitis and sore mouth are problems, *to relieve discomfort.*
- Provide *adequate fluids to replace fluid lost with diarrhea.*
- Ensure that patient is hydrated at all times during drug therapy *to minimize renal toxicity from drug exposure.*
- Instruct the patient about the appropriate dosage regimen and possible adverse effects to enhance patient knowledge about drug therapy and *to promote compliance.*

(continues on page 106)

- Provide the following patient teaching:
  - Take safety precautions, such as changing position slowly and avoiding driving and hazardous tasks, if CNS effects occur.
  - Try to drink a lot of fluids and to maintain nutrition (very important) even though nausea, vomiting, and diarrhea may occur.
  - Avoid exposure to other infections (e.g., avoid crowded areas and people with known infectious diseases).
  - Report difficulty breathing, severe headache, loss of hearing or ringing in the ears, or changes in urine output.

Evaluation

- Monitor patient response to the drug (resolution of bacterial infection).
- Monitor for adverse effects (orientation and affect, hearing changes, bone marrow suppression, renal toxicity, hepatic dysfunction, GI effects).
- Evaluate effectiveness of the teaching plan (patient can name drug, dosage, possible adverse effects to watch for, and specific measures to help avoid adverse effects).
- Monitor effectiveness of comfort and safety measures and compliance with the therapeutic regimen.

KEY POINTS

- Aminoglycosides inhibit protein synthesis in susceptible strains of gram-negative bacteria.
- These drugs are reserved for use in serious infections because of potentially serious adverse effects. Monitor for ototoxicity, renal toxicity, GI disturbances, bone marrow depression, and superinfections.

Carbapenems

The carbapenems (Table 9.2) are a relatively new class of broad-spectrum antibiotics effective against gram-positive and gram-negative bacteria. Meropenem, the first drug of the class, was discussed in Chapter 8 and has limited use because of the severe risk for potentially fatal GI toxicities. Newer carbapenems are not as toxic. Carbapenems discussed here include doripenem (*Doribax*), ertapenem (*Invanz*), imipenem–cilastatin (*Primaxin*), and meropenem (*Merrem IV*).

Therapeutic Actions and Indications

The carbapenems are bactericidal. They inhibit cell membrane synthesis in susceptible bacteria, leading to cell death (Figure 9.2). These drugs are used to treat serious infections caused by susceptible strains of *Streptococcus pneumoniae, Haemophilus influenzae, Moraxella catarrhalis, Streptococcus aureus, Streptococcus pyogenes, Escherichia coli, Peptostreptococcus* spp., *Klebsiella pneumoniae, Clostridium clostridioforme, Eubacterium lentum, Bacteroides fragilis, Bacteroides distasonis, Bacteroides ovatus, Bacteroides thetaiotamicron, Bacteroides uniformis, Proteus mirabilis, Proteus aeruginosa, Acinetobacter baumannii, Streptococcus agalactiae, Porphyromonas asaccharolytica, Prevotella bivia,* and other susceptible bacteria. They are indicated for treating serious intra-abdominal, urinary tract, skin and skin structure, bone and joint, and gynecological infections. See Table 9.2 for usual indications for each of these drugs.

Pharmacokinetics

These drugs are rapidly absorbed if given IM and reach peak levels at the end of the infusion if given IV. They are widely distributed throughout the body, although it is not known whether they cross the placenta or enter breast milk (see Contraindications and Cautions). Carbapenems

Table 9.2 ***Drugs in Focus:* Carbapenems**

Drug Name	Dosage/Route	Usual Indications
doripenem (*Doribax*)	500 mg IV, over 1 h every 8 h for 5–14 d	Treatment of complicated intra-abdominal infections or complicated UTIs, including pyelonephritis, caused by susceptible bacteria
ertapenem (*Invanz*)	1 g/d IV or IM for 5–14 d	Treatment of community-acquired pneumonia, complicated GU infections, acute pelvic infections, complicated intra-abdominal infections, skin and skin structure infections
imipenem–cilastatin (*Primaxin*)	250–500 mg IV q6–8h *or* 500–750 mg IM q12h *Pediatric <1 wk:* 25 mg 25 mg/kg q12h IV; *1–4 wk:* 25 mg/kg q8h IV; *4 wk–3 mo:* 25 mg/kg q6h IV; *≥3 mo:* 15–25 mg/kg q6h IV	Treatment of serious respiratory, intra-abdominal, urinary tract, gynecological, bone and joint, skin and skin structure infections; septicemia, endocarditis, bone and joint infections, and polymicrobic infections
meropenem (*Merrem IV*)	*Adult:* 500–1,000 mg IV q8h *Pediatric:* 500 mg–2 g IV q8h, depending on infection being treated	Treatment of bacterial meningitis, complicated skin and skin structure infections, intra-abdominal infections

are excreted unchanged in the urine and have an average half-life of 1 to 4 hours.

Doripenem is one of the newer drugs of the class. It is given IV every 8 hours by a 1-hour IV infusion for 5 to 14 days.

Ertapenem can be given IV or IM. It is given once a day for 5 to 14 days, depending on the infection.

Imipenem–cilastatin is a combination of imipenem, which interferes with cell wall synthesis and causes bacterial cell death, and cilastatin, which inactivates the imipenem and leads to increased urinary excretion of the drug and decreased renal toxicity. It can be given IM or IV and is approved for use in children.

Meropenem, the first drug of this class, is given IV over 1 hour, every 8 hours for 5 to 14 days.

Contraindications and Cautions

Carbapenems are contraindicated in the following conditions: known allergy to any of the carbanems or beta-lactams; seizure disorders, *which could be exacerbated by the drug*; meningitis, *because safety in patients with meningitis has not been established*; and lactation, *because it is not known whether these drugs enter breast milk, but potentially, they could cause serious effects in the infant.*

Use caution during pregnancy *because carbapenems are used to treat only severe infections, and the benefits of the drug must be carefully weighed against potential adverse effects on the fetus.* Test urine function regularly when these drugs are used *because they depend on the kidney for excretion and are toxic to the kidney.*

Ertapenem is not recommended for use in patients younger than 18 years of age.

Meropenem is associated with the development of pseudomembranous colitis and should be used with caution in patients with inflammatory bowel disorders.

FOCUS ON Safe Medication Administration

Name confusion has occurred between Invanz (ertapenem) and Avinza (extended-release morphine). Use extreme caution if your patient is prescribed either of these drugs to avoid possible confusion.

Adverse Effects

Toxic effects on the GI tract can limit the use of carbapenems in some patients. Pseudomembranous colitis, *Clostridium difficile* diarrhea, and nausea and vomiting can lead to serious dehydration and electrolyte imbalances, as well as to new serious infections.

Superinfections can occur with any of the carbapenems. Closely monitor patients to deal with the new infection before it becomes overwhelming.

CNS effects can include headache, dizziness, and altered mental state. Seizures have been reported when carbapenems are combined with other drugs. Monitor patients to provide safety measures if any of these occur.

Clinically Important Drug–Drug Interactions

Consider an alternative antibiotic treatment if a patient is on valproic acid. Combination of these drugs can cause serum valproic acid levels to fall and increase the risk of seizures. Avoid concurrent use of imipenem with ganciclovir because this combination may also cause seizures. Meropenem should not be combined with probenecid because this combination can lead to toxic levels of meropenem.

Prototype Summary: Ertapenem

Indications: Treatment of community-acquired pneumonia, complicated GU infections, complicated intra-abdominal infections, skin and skin structure infections, and acute pelvic infections caused by susceptible bacteria.

Actions: Inhibits protein synthesis in susceptible strains of gram-negative bacteria, disrupting functional integrity of the cell membrane and causing cell death.

Pharmacokinetics:

Route	Onset	Peak
IM, IV	Rapid	30–120 min

$T_{1/2}$: 4 hours; excreted unchanged in the urine.

Adverse Effects: Headache, dizziness, nausea, vomiting, pseudomembranous colitis, rash, pain at injection site.

Nursing Considerations for Patients Receiving Carbapenems

Assessment: History and Examination

- Assess for *possible contraindications or cautions*: Known allergy to any carbapenem or beta-lactam (obtain specific information about the nature and occurrence of allergic reactions), history of renal disease, history of seizures and current pregnancy or lactation status, and inflammatory bowel disorders.
- Perform physical assessment *to establish baseline data for assessing the effectiveness of the drug and the occurrence of any adverse effects associated with drug therapy.*
- Perform culture and sensitivity tests at the site of infection *to ensure appropriate use of the drug.*
- Conduct orientation and reflex assessment *to evaluate any CNS effects of the drug.*

(continues on page 108)

- Assess vital signs: Respiratory rate and adventitious sounds *to monitor for signs of infection or hypersensitivity reactions; temperature to assess for signs and symptoms of infection.*
- Perform renal function tests *to determine baseline function of the kidneys and, possibly, the need to adjust dose.*

Nursing Diagnoses

Nursing diagnoses related to drug therapy might include the following:

- Acute pain related to GI or CNS effects of the drug
- Risk for infection related to loss of normal flora
- Deficient knowledge regarding drug therapy

Planning

- The patient will receive the best therapeutic effect from the drug therapy
- The patient will have limited adverse effects to the drug therapy
- The patient will have an understanding of the drug therapy, adverse effects to anticipate, and measures to relieve discomfort and improve safety

Implementation with Rationale

- Check culture and sensitivity reports *to ensure that this is the drug of choice for this patient.*
- Ensure that the patient receives the full course of the carbapenem as prescribed *to increase effectiveness and decrease the risk for the development of resistant strains of bacteria.*
- Monitor the site of infection and presenting signs and symptoms (e.g., fever, lethargy) throughout the course of drug therapy. Failure of these signs and symptoms to resolve may indicate the need to reculture the site. Arrange to continue drug therapy for at least 2 days after all signs and symptoms resolve *to decrease the development of resistant strains of bacteria.*
- Monitor the patient regularly for signs of pseudomembranous colitis, severe diarrhea, or superinfections *to effectively arrange for discontinuation of drug or decreased dose, as appropriate, if any of these toxicities occur.*
- Provide safety measures *to protect the patient if CNS effects, such as confusion, dizziness, or seizures, occur.*
- Provide small, frequent meals as tolerated *to relieve GI discomfort. Also provide adequate fluids to replace fluid lost with diarrhea, if appropriate.*
- Ensure that the patient is hydrated at all times during drug therapy *to minimize renal toxicity from drug exposure.*
- Instruct the patient about the appropriate dosage regimen and possible adverse effects *to enhance patient knowledge about drug therapy and to promote compliance.*
- Provide the following patient teaching:
  - Take safety precautions, such as changing position slowly and avoiding driving and hazardous tasks, if CNS effects occur.
  - Try to drink a lot of fluids and to maintain nutrition (very important) even though nausea, vomiting, and diarrhea may occur.
  - Report difficulty breathing, severe headache, severe diarrhea, fever, and signs of infection.

Evaluation

- Monitor patient response to the drug (resolution of bacterial infection).
- Monitor for adverse effects (orientation and affect, superinfections, GI toxicity, severe diarrhea effects).
- Evaluate effectiveness of the teaching plan (patient can name drug, dosage, possible adverse effects to watch for, and specific measures to help avoid adverse effects).
- Monitor effectiveness of comfort and safety measures and compliance with the therapeutic regimen.

KEY POINTS

- Carbapenems are used to treat serious infections caused by a wide range of bacteria.
- Monitor for GI effects, serious diarrhea, dizziness, and superinfections.

Cephalosporins

The cephalosporins (Table 9.3) were first introduced in the 1960s. These drugs are similar to the penicillins in structure and in activity. Over time, four generations of cephalosporins have been introduced, each group with its own spectrum of activity.

First-generation cephalosporins are largely effective against the same gram-positive bacteria that are affected by penicillin G, as well as the gram-negative bacteria *Proteus mirabilis*, *Escherichia coli*, and *Klebsiella pneumoniae* (use the letters *PEcK* as a mnemonic device to remember which bacteria are susceptible to the first-generation cephalosporins). First-generation drugs include cefadroxil (generic) and cephalexin (*Keflex*).

Second-generation cephalosporins are effective against the previously mentioned strains, as well as *Haemophilus influenzae*, *Enterobacter aerogenes*, and *Neisseria* spp. (remember *HENPeCK*). Second-generation drugs are less effective against gram-positive bacteria. These include cefaclor (*Ceclor*), cefoxitin (generic), cefprozil (generic), and cefuroxime (*Zinacef*).

Third-generation cephalosporins, which are effective against all of the previously mentioned strains, are relatively weak against gram-positive bacteria but are more potent against the gram-negative bacilli, as well as against

Table 9.3 ***Drugs in Focus:*** **Cephalosporins**

Drug Name	Dosage/Route	Usual Indications
First-Generation Cephalosporins		
cefadroxil (generic)	*Adult:* 1–2 g PO in a single or two divided doses; reduce dose in renal impairment *Pediatric:* 30 mg/kg/d PO in divided doses q12h	Treatment of UTIs, pharyngitis, and tonsillitis caused by group A beta-hemolytic streptococci, as well as skin infections
cephalexin (*Keflex*)	*Adult:* 250 mg PO q6h *Pediatric:* 25–50 mg/kg/d PO in divided doses	Treatment of respiratory, skin, bone, and GU infections; used for otitis media in children
Second-Generation Cephalosporins		
cefaclor (*Ceclor*)	*Adult:* 250 mg PO q8h—do not exceed 4 g/d; must be taken every 8–12 h around the clock *Pediatric:* 20 mg/kg/d PO in divided doses q8h; do not exceed 1 g/d	Treatment of respiratory tract infections, skin infections, UTIs, otitis media, typhoid fever, anthrax exposure
cefoxitin (generic)	*Adult:* 1–2 g IM or IV q6–8h; reduce dose with renal impairment *Pediatric:* 80–160 mg/kg/d IM or IV in divided doses q4–6h	Treatment of severe infections; preoperative prophylaxis for cesarean section and abdominal, vaginal, biliary, or colorectal surgery; more effective in gynecological and intra-abdominal infections than some other agents
cefprozil (generic)	*Adult:* 250–500 mg PO q12h for 10 d; reduce dose with renal impairment *Pediatric:* 7.5–20 mg/kg PO q12h for 10 d; for child 6 mo–2 y of age, 7.5–15 mg/kg PO q12h for 10 d	Treatment of pharyngitis, tonsillitis, otitis media, sinusitis, secondary bronchial infections, and skin infections
cefuroxime (*Zinacef*)	*Adult:* 250 mg PO b.i.d.; 750 mg–1.5 g IM q8h; reduce dose with renal impairment *Pediatric:* 125–250 mg PO b.i.d.; 50–100 mg/kg/d IM or IV in divided doses q6–8h	Treatment of a wide range of infections, as listed for other second-generation drugs; Lyme disease; preferred treatment in situations involving an anticipated switch from parenteral to oral drug use
Third-Generation Cephalosporins		
cefdinir (generic; a suspension form is available for children)	*Adult:* 300 mg PO q12h for 10 d; reduce dose with renal impairment *Pediatric:* 7 mg/kg PO q12h	Treatment of respiratory infections, otitis media, sinusitis, laryngitis, bronchitis, skin infections
cefotaxime (*Claforan*)	*Adult:* 2–8 g/d IM or IV in divided doses q6–8h; reduce dose with renal impairment *Pediatric:* 50–180 mg/kg/d IM or IV in divided doses q4–6h	Treatment of moderate to severe skin, urinary tract, and respiratory tract infections; pelvic inflammatory disease; intra-abdominal infections; peritonitis; septicemia; bone infections; CNS infections; preoperative prophylaxis
cefpodoxime (*Vantin*)	*Adult:* 100–400 mg PO q12h; reduce dose with renal impairment *Pediatric:* 5–10 mg/kg PO q12h for 7–14 d	Treatment of respiratory infections, UTIs, gonorrhea, skin infections, and otitis media
ceftazidime (*Ceptaz, Tazicef*)	*Adult:* 1 g q8–12h IM or IV; reduce dose with renal impairment *Pediatric:* 30–50 mg/kg q8–12h IM or IV	Treatment of moderate to severe skin, urinary tract, and respiratory tract infections; intra-abdominal infections; septicemia; bone infections; CNS infections
ceftibuten (*Cedax*; available in a suspension form for children)	*Adult:* 400 mg PO every day for 10 d; reduce dose with renal impairment *Pediatric:* 9 mg/kg/d PO for 10 d *Note:* Once-a-day dosing increases compliance	Treatment of pharyngitis, tonsillitis, exacerbations of bronchitis, otitis media
ceftriaxone (*Rocephin*)	*Adult:* 1–2 g/d IM or IV in divided doses b.i.d.–q.i.d. *Pediatric:* 50–75 mg/kg/d IV or IM in divided doses q12h	Treatment of moderate to severe skin, urinary tract, and respiratory tract infections; pelvic inflammatory disease; intra-abdominal infections; peritonitis; septicemia; bone infections; CNS infections; preoperative prophylaxis; off-label use for treatment of Lyme disease

(table continues on page 110)

Table 9.3 *Drugs in Focus:* Cephalosporins (*continued*)

Drug Name	Dosage/Route	Usual Indications
Fourth-Generation Cephalosporins		
cefditoren (*Spectracef*)	*Adult and pediatric (>12 y):* 200–400 mg PO b.i.d.; reduce dose with renal impairment	Treatment of acute exacerbations of chronic bronchitis; pharyngitis and tonsillitis; skin and skin structure infections
cefepime (*Maxipime*)	*Adult:* 0.5–2 g IM or IV q12h; must be injected for greatest effectiveness q12h for 7–10 d; reduce dose with renal impairment *Pediatric:* 50 mg/kg per dose q12h IV or IM for 7–10 d	Treatment of moderate to severe skin, urinary tract, and respiratory tract infections
ceftaroline (*Teflaro*)	600 mg IV over 1 h for 5–7 d community-acquired pneumonia or 5–14 d skin infections	Treatment of skin and skin structure infections; community-acquired pneumonia

Serratia marcescens (remember *HENPeCKS*). Third-generation drugs include cefdinir (*Omnicef*), cefotaxime (*Claforan*), cefpodoxime (generic), ceftazidime (*Ceptaz, Tazicef*), ceftibuten (*Cedax*), and ceftriaxone (*Rocephin*).

Fourth-generation cephalosporins are in development. The first drug of this group, cefepime (generic), is active against gram-negative and gram-positive organisms, including cephalosporin-resistant staphylococci and *Pseudomonas aeruginosa.* Fourth-generation drugs also include cefditoren (*Spectracef*) and ceftaroline (*Teflaro*) which is effective with some methicillin-resistant organisms

Therapeutic Actions and Indications

The cephalosporins are both bactericidal and bacteriostatic, depending on the dose used and the specific drug involved. In susceptible species, these agents basically interfere with the cell wall–building ability of bacteria when they divide; that is, they prevent the bacteria from biosynthesizing the framework of their cell walls. The bacteria with weakened cell walls swell and burst as a result of the osmotic pressure within the cell (see Figure 9.1).

Cephalosporins are indicated for the treatment of infections caused by susceptible bacteria. See Table 9.3 for usual indications for each of these agents. Selection of an antibiotic from this class depends on the sensitivity of the involved organism, the route of choice, and sometimes the cost involved. It is important to reserve cephalosporins for appropriate situations because cephalosporin-resistant bacteria are appearing in increasing numbers. Before therapy begins, a culture and sensitivity test should be performed to evaluate the causative organism and appropriate sensitivity to the antibiotic being used.

Pharmacokinetics

The following cephalosporins are well absorbed from the GI tract: The first-generation drugs cefadroxil and cephalexin; the second-generation drugs cefaclor and cefprozil; the third-generation drugs cefdinir, cefpodoxime, and ceftibuten; and the fourth-generation drugs cefditoren and cefepime. The others are absorbed well after IM injection or IV administration. (Box 9.4 provides calculation practice using cefdinir.)

The cephalosporins are primarily metabolized in the liver and excreted in the urine. These drugs cross the placenta and enter breast milk (see Contraindications and Cautions).

Contraindications and Cautions

Avoid the use of cephalosporins in patients with known allergies to cephalosporins or penicillins *because cross-sensitivity is common.* Use with caution in patients with hepatic or renal impairment *because these drugs are toxic to the kidneys and could interfere with the metabolism and excretion of the drug.* In addition, use with caution in pregnant or lactating patients *because potential effects on the fetus and infant are not known; use only if the benefits clearly outweigh the potential risk of toxicity to the fetus or infant.*

Reserve cephalosporins for appropriate situations because cephalosporin-resistant bacteria are appearing in increasing numbers. Before therapy begins, perform a culture and sensitivity test to evaluate the causative organism and appropriate sensitivity to the antibiotic being used.

BOX 9.4 FOCUS ON Calculations

Your patient is a 20-kg child with a severe case of tonsillitis. An order is written for cefdinir (14 mg/kg/d PO for 10 days). The drug comes in an oral suspension 125 mg/mL. What should you administer at each dose?

The order is for 14 mg/kg, so 14 mg/kg × 20 kg = 280 mg. The available form is 125 mg/mL. Use the following formula:

$$\frac{\text{amount of drug available}}{\text{volume available}} = \frac{\text{amount of drug prescribed}}{\text{volume to administer}}$$

$$\frac{125\text{ mg}}{1\text{ mL}} = \frac{280\text{ mg}}{X}$$

$$125\text{ mg}/(X) = 280\text{ mg/mL}$$

$$X = \frac{280\text{ mg/mL}}{125\text{ mg}}$$

$$X = 2.24\text{ mL}$$

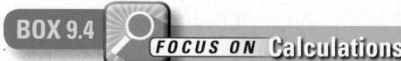

Adverse Effects

The most common adverse effects of the cephalosporins involve the GI tract and include nausea, vomiting, diarrhea, anorexia, abdominal pain, and flatulence. Pseudomembranous colitis—a potentially dangerous disorder—has also been reported with some cephalosporins. A particular drug should be discontinued immediately at any sign of violent, bloody diarrhea or abdominal pain.

CNS symptoms include headache, dizziness, lethargy, and paresthesias. Nephrotoxicity is also associated with the use of cephalosporins, most particularly in patients who have a predisposing renal insufficiency. Other adverse effects include superinfections, which occur frequently because of the death of protective bacteria of the normal flora. Monitor patients receiving parenteral cephalosporins for the possibility of phlebitis with IV administration or local abscess at the site of an IM injection.

Clinically Important Drug–Drug Interactions

Concurrent administration of cephalosporins with aminoglycosides increases the risk for nephrotoxicity. Frequently monitor patients receiving this combination, and evaluate serum blood urea nitrogen (BUN) and creatinine levels.

Patients who receive oral anticoagulants in addition to cephalosporins may experience increased bleeding. Teach these patients how to monitor for blood loss (e.g., bleeding gums, easy bruising) and to be aware that the dose of the oral anticoagulant may need to be reduced.

Instruct the patient receiving cephalosporins to avoid alcohol for up to 72 hours after discontinuation of the drug to prevent a disulfiram-like reaction, which results in unpleasant symptoms such as flushing, throbbing headache, nausea and vomiting, chest pain, palpitations, dyspnea, syncope, vertigo, blurred vision, and, in extreme reactions, cardiovascular collapse, convulsions, or even death.

Prototype Summary: Cefaclor

Indications: Treatment of respiratory, dermatological, urinary tract, and middle ear infections caused by susceptible strains of bacteria.

Actions: Inhibits the synthesis of bacterial cell walls, causing cell death in susceptible bacteria.

Pharmacokinetics:

Route	Peak	Duration
Oral	30–60 min	8–10 h

$T_{1/2}$: 30 to 60 minutes; excreted unchanged in the urine.

Adverse Effects: Nausea, vomiting, diarrhea, rash, superinfection, bone marrow depression, risk for pseudomembranous colitis.

Nursing Considerations for Patients Receiving Cephalosporins

Assessment: History and Examination

- Assess for *possible contraindications or cautions*: known allergy to any cephalosporin, penicillin, or any other allergens *because cross-sensitivity often occurs* (obtain specific information about the nature and occurrence of the allergic reactions); history of renal disease, *which could exacerbate nephrotoxicity related to the cephalosporin*; and current pregnancy or lactation status.
- Perform physical assessment to *establish baseline data for assessing the effectiveness of the drug and the occurrence of any adverse effects associated with drug therapy.*
- Examine the skin for any rash or lesions, examine injection sites for abscess formation, and note respiratory status—including rate, depth, and adventitious sounds—*to provide a baseline for determining adverse reactions.*
- Perform culture and sensitivity tests at the site of infection *to ensure appropriate use of the drug.*
- Check renal function test results, including BUN and creatinine clearance, *to assess the status of renal functioning and to detect the possible need to alter dose.*

Nursing Diagnoses

Nursing diagnoses related to drug therapy might include the following:

- Acute pain related to GI or CNS effects of drug
- Risk for infection related to repeated injections
- Deficient fluid volume and imbalanced nutrition: Less than body requirements, related to diarrhea
- Deficient knowledge regarding drug therapy

Planning

- The patient will receive the best therapeutic effect from the drug therapy
- The patient will have limited adverse effects to the drug therapy
- The patient will have an understanding of the drug therapy, adverse effects to anticipate, and measures to relieve discomfort and improve safety

Implementation with Rationale

- Check culture and sensitivity reports *to ensure that this is the drug of choice for this patient.*
- Monitor renal function test values before and periodically during therapy *to arrange for appropriate dose reduction as needed.*
- Ensure that patient receives the full course of the cephalosporin as prescribed, divided around the clock *to*

(continues on page 112)

increase effectiveness and to decrease the risk of development of resistant strains.

- Monitor the infection site and presenting signs and symptoms (e.g., fever, lethargy) throughout the course of drug therapy. *Failure of these signs and symptoms to resolve may indicate the need to reculture the site.* Arrange to continue drug therapy for at least 2 days after the resolution of all signs and symptoms *to help prevent the development of resistant strains of bacteria.*
- Provide small, frequent meals as tolerated, frequent mouth care, and ice chips or sugarless candy to suck if stomatitis and sore mouth are problems *to relieve discomfort and provide nutrition.*
- Provide *adequate fluids to replace fluid lost with diarrhea.*
- Monitor the patient for any signs of superinfection *to arrange for treatment if superinfection occurs.*
- Monitor injection sites regularly *and provide warm compresses and gentle massage to injection sites if they are painful or swollen.* If signs of phlebitis occur, remove the IV line and reinsert in a different vein.
- Initiate safety measures, including adequate lighting, side rails on the bed, and assistance with ambulation *to protect the patient from injury if CNS effects occur.*
- Instruct the patient about the appropriate dosage schedule and about possible side effects *to enhance patient knowledge about drug therapy and to promote compliance.*
- Provide the following patient teaching:
  - Take safety precautions, including changing position slowly and avoiding driving and hazardous tasks, if CNS effects occur.
  - Try to drink a lot of fluids and to maintain nutrition (very important) even though nausea, vomiting, and diarrhea may occur.
  - Report difficulty breathing, severe headache, severe diarrhea, dizziness, or weakness.
  - Avoid consuming alcoholic beverages while receiving cephalosporins and for at least 72 hours after completing the drug course because serious side effects could occur.

Evaluation

- Monitor patient response to the drug (resolution of bacterial infection).
- Monitor for adverse effects (orientation and affect; renal toxicity; hepatic dysfunction; GI effects; and local irritation, including phlebitis at injection and IV sites).
- Evaluate effectiveness of the teaching plan (patient can name drug, dosage, possible adverse effects to expect, and specific measures to help avoid adverse effects).
- Monitor effectiveness of comfort and safety measures and the patient's compliance with the regimen.

KEY POINTS

- Cephalosporins are a large group of antibiotics, similar to penicillin, that are effective against a wide range of bacteria.
- Monitor for GI upsets and diarrhea, pseudomembranous colitis, headache, dizziness, and superinfections.

Fluoroquinolones

The fluoroquinolones (Table 9.4) are a relatively new synthetic class of antibiotics with a broad spectrum of activity. Fluoroquinolones include ciprofloxacin (*Cipro*), which is the most widely used fluoroquinolone, gemifloxacin (*Factive*), levofloxacin (*Levaquin*), moxifloxacin (*Avelox*), ofloxacin (*Floxin, Ocuflox*), and finafloxacin (*Xtoro*).

Therapeutic Actions and Indications

The fluoroquinolones enter the bacterial cell by passive diffusion through channels in the cell membrane. Once inside, they interfere with the action of DNA enzymes necessary for the growth and reproduction of the bacteria (see Figure 9.1). This leads to cell death because the bacterial DNA is damaged and the cell cannot be maintained. The fluoroquinolones have the advantage of a unique way of disrupting bacterial activity. There is little cross-resistance with other forms of antibiotics. However, misuse of these drugs in the short time the class has been available has led to the existence of resistant strains of bacteria (see Contraindications and Cautions).

The fluoroquinolones are indicated for treating infections caused by susceptible strains of gram-negative bacteria, including *Escherichia coli*, *Proteus mirabilis*, *Klebsiella pneumoniae*, *Enterobacter cloacae*, *Proteus vulgaris*, *Proteus rettgeri*, *Morganella morganii*, *Moraxella catarrhalis*, *Haemophilus influenzae*, *Haemophilus parainfluenzae*, *Pseudomonas aeruginosa*, *Citrobacter freundii*, *Staphylococcus aureus*, *Staphylococcus epidermidis*, some *Neisseria gonorrhoeae*, and group D streptococci. These infections frequently include urinary tract, respiratory tract, and skin infections. Ciprofloxacin is effective against a wide spectrum of gram-negative bacteria. It has been approved for prevention of anthrax infection in areas that might be exposed to germ warfare. It is also effective against typhoid fever. See Table 9.4 for usual indications for each of these agents.

Pharmacokinetics

The fluoroquinolones are absorbed from the GI tract, metabolized in the liver, and excreted in the urine and feces. These drugs are widely distributed in the body and cross the placenta and enter breast milk (see Contraindications and Cautions).

Table 9.4 *Drugs in Focus:* Fluoroquinolones

Drug Name	Dosage/Route	Usual Indications
ciprofloxacin (*Cipro*)	*Adult:* 100–500 mg b.i.d. PO for up to 6 wk; reduce dose in renal failure *Pediatric:* Not recommended because of potential effects on developing cartilage	Treatment of infections caused by a wide spectrum of gram-negative bacteria
finafloxacin (*Xtoro*)	*Adult and pediatric:* 4 drops in affected ear(s) b.i.d. for 7 days	Treatment of acute otitis externa (swimmer's ear) caused by *Staphylococcus aureus, Pseudomonas aeruginosa*
gemifloxacin (*Factive*)	*Adult:* 320 mg/d PO for 5–7 d	Treatment of acute exacerbations of chronic bronchitis, community-acquired pneumonia
levofloxacin (*Levaquin*)	*Adult:* 250–750 mg/d PO or IV; reduce dose in renal impairment *After exposure to anthrax:* 500 mg/d PO or IV for 60 d	Treatment of respiratory, urinary tract, skin, and sinus infections caused by susceptible gram-negative bacteria in adults; treatment after exposure to anthrax
moxifloxacin (*Avelox*)	*Adult:* 400 mg/d PO or IV for 5–10 d; reduce dose in renal impairment	Treatment of adults with sinusitis, bronchitis, or community-acquired pneumonia
ofloxacin (*Floxin, Ocuflox*)	*Adult:* 200–400 mg q12h PO for up to 10 d; reduce dose in renal impairment	Treatment of respiratory, skin, and urinary tract infections; pelvic inflammatory disease; ocular infections; otic form available for otitis media

Ciprofloxacin is available in injectable, oral, and topical forms. Gemifloxacin, lomefloxacin, and moxifloxacin are oral agents. Levofloxacin is available in oral and IV forms. Because of its parenteral availability, it may be preferred for severe infections or for use when the patient cannot take oral drugs. Ofloxacin can be given IV or orally and is also available as an ophthalmic agent for the treatment of ocular infections caused by susceptible bacteria. The newest drug in this class, finafloxacin, is available in otic drops for topical treatment of swimmer's ear.

Contraindications and Cautions

Fluoroquinolones are contraindicated in patients with known allergy to any fluoroquinolone and in pregnant or lactating patients *because potential effects on the fetus and infant are not known.* Use with caution in the presence of renal dysfunction, *which could interfere with the metabolism and excretion of the drug,* and seizures, *which could be exacerbated by the drugs' effects on cell membrane channels.*

Because so many resistant strains are emerging, always perform culture and sensitivity tests of infected tissue *to determine the exact bacterial cause and sensitivity.* These drugs have been associated with lesions in developing cartilage and therefore are not recommended for use in patients younger than 18 years of age.

Adverse Effects

These drugs are generally associated with relatively mild adverse reactions. The most common are headache, dizziness, insomnia, and depression related to possible effects on the CNS membranes. GI effects include nausea, vomiting, diarrhea, and dry mouth, related to direct drug effect on the GI tract and possibly to stimulation of the chemoreceptor trigger zone in the CNS. A black box warning was added to all drugs in this class in 2009 reporting the risk of tendinitis and tendon rupture when using these antibiotics. The risk is increased in patients over the age of 60, those on concurrent steroids, and those with renal, heart, or lung transplants.

Immunological effects include bone marrow depression, which may be related to drug effects on the cells of the bone marrow that rapidly turn over. Other adverse effects include fever, rash, and photosensitivity, a potentially serious adverse effect that can cause severe skin reactions. Advise patients to avoid sun and ultraviolet light exposure and to use protective clothing and sunscreens.

Clinically Important Drug–Drug Interactions

When fluoroquinolones are taken concurrently with iron salts, sucralfate, mineral supplements, or antacids the therapeutic effect of the fluoroquinolone is decreased. If this drug combination is necessary, administration of the two agents should be separated by at least 4 hours.

If fluoroquinolones are taken with drugs that increase the QTc interval or cause torsades de pointes (quinidine, procainamide, amiodarone, sotalol, erythromycin, terfenadine, pentamidine, tricyclics, phenothiazines), severe-to-fatal cardiac reactions are possible. These combinations should be avoided, but if they must be used patients should be hospitalized with continual cardiac monitoring.

Combining fluoroquinolones with theophylline leads to increased theophylline levels because the two drugs use similar metabolic pathways. The theophylline dose should be decreased by one-half, and serum theophylline levels monitored carefully. In addition, when fluoroquinolones are combined with nonsteroidal anti-inflammatory drugs, an increased risk of CNS stimulation is possible. If this combination is used, closely monitor patients, especially those who have a history of seizures or CNS problems. Combining a fluoroquinolone with corticosteroids can lead to an increased risk of tendonitis and tendon rupture. If this combination must be used, instruct the patient to report any tendon pain or weakness.

Prototype Summary: Ciprofloxacin

Indications: Treatment of respiratory, dermatological, urinary tract, ear, eye, bone, and joint infections; treatment after anthrax exposure, typhoid fever.

Actions: Interferes with DNA replication in susceptible gram-negative bacteria, preventing cell reproduction.

Pharmacokinetics:

Route	Onset	Peak	Duration
Oral	Varies	60–90 min	4–5 h
IV	10 min	30 min	4–5 h

$T_{1/2}$: 3.5 to 4 hours; metabolized in the liver, excreted in bile and urine.

Adverse Effects: Headache, dizziness, hypotension, nausea, vomiting, diarrhea, fever, rash.

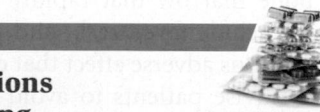

Nursing Considerations for Patients Receiving Fluoroquinolones

Assessment: History and Examination

- Assess for *possible contraindications or cautions*: Known allergy to any fluoroquinolone (obtain specific information about the nature and occurrence of allergic reactions); history of renal disease, *which could interfere with excretion of the drug*; and current pregnancy or lactation status *because of potential adverse effects on the fetus or infant.*
- Perform physical assessment to *establish baseline data for assessing the effectiveness of the drug and the occurrence of any adverse effects associated with drug therapy.*
- Examine the skin for any rash or lesions to *provide a baseline for possible adverse effects.*
- Perform culture and sensitivity tests at the site of infection *to ensure appropriate use of the drug.*
- Conduct assessment of orientation, affect, and reflexes *to establish a baseline for any CNS effects of the drug.*
- Perform renal function tests, including BUN and creatinine clearance, to *evaluate the status of renal functioning and to assess necessary changes in dose.*

Nursing Diagnoses

Nursing diagnoses related to drug therapy might include the following:

- Acute pain related to GI, CNS, or skin effects of the drug
- Deficient fluid volume and imbalanced nutrition: Less than body requirements, related to GI effects of the drug
- Deficient knowledge regarding drug therapy

Planning

- The patient will receive the best therapeutic effect from the drug therapy
- The patient will have limited adverse effects to the drug therapy
- The patient will have an understanding of the drug therapy, adverse effects to anticipate, and measures to relieve discomfort and improve safety

Implementation with Rationale

- Check culture and sensitivity reports to *ensure that this is the drug of choice for this patient.*
- Monitor renal function tests before initiating therapy *to appropriately arrange for dose reduction if necessary.*
- Ensure that the patient receives the full course of the fluoroquinolone as prescribed *to eradicate the infection and to help prevent the emergence of resistant strains.*
- Monitor the site of infection and presenting signs and symptoms (e.g., fever, lethargy, urinary tract signs and symptoms) throughout the course of drug therapy. *Failure of these signs and symptoms to resolve may indicate the need to reculture the site.* Arrange to continue drug therapy for at least 2 days after resolution of all signs and symptoms *to help decrease the development of resistant strains.*
- Provide small, frequent meals as tolerated, frequent mouth care, and ice chips or sugarless candy to suck if dry mouth is a problem *to relieve discomfort and provide nutrition*, and provide *adequate fluids to replace those lost with diarrhea.*
- Implement safety measures, including adequate lighting, use of side rails, and assistance with ambulation *to protect the patient from injury if CNS effects occur.*
- Instruct the patient about the appropriate dosage schedule and possible adverse effects *to enhance patient knowledge about drug therapy and to promote compliance.*

- Provide the following patient teaching:
  - Take safety precautions, including changing position slowly and avoiding driving and hazardous tasks, if CNS effects occur.
  - Try to drink a lot of fluids and to maintain nutrition (very important), although nausea, vomiting, and diarrhea may occur.
  - Avoid ultraviolet light and sun exposure, using protective clothing and sunscreens.
  - Report difficulty breathing, severe headache, severe diarrhea, severe skin rash, fainting spells, and heart palpitations, tendon pain, or weakness.

Evaluation

- Monitor patient response to the drug (resolution of bacterial infection).
- Monitor for adverse effects (orientation and affect, GI effects, photosensitivity).
- Evaluate effectiveness of the teaching plan (patient can name drug, dosage, possible adverse effects to expect, and specific measures to help avoid adverse effects).
- Monitor effectiveness of comfort and safety measures and compliance with the therapeutic regimen.

KEY POINTS

- Fluoroquinolones inhibit the action of DNA enzymes in susceptible gram-negative bacteria. They are used to treat a wide range of infections.
- Monitor the patient for headache, dizziness, GI upsets, and bone marrow depression, and caution the patient about the risk of photosensitivity reactions. Be aware that the patient may be at increased risk for tendonitis and tendon rupture.

Penicillins and Penicillinase-Resistant Antibiotics

Penicillin (Table 9.5) was the first antibiotic introduced for clinical use. Sir Alexander Fleming used *Penicillium* molds to produce the original penicillin in the 1920s. Subsequent versions of penicillin were developed to decrease the adverse effects of the drug and to modify it to act on resistant bacteria. Penicillins include penicillin G benzathine (*Bicillin, Permapen*), penicillin G potassium (*Pfizerpen*), penicillin G procaine (*Wycillin*), penicillin V (generic), amoxicillin (*Amoxil, Trimox*), and ampicillin (*Principen*).

Table 9.5 ***Drugs in Focus:*** **Penicillins and Penicillinase-Resistant Antibiotics**

Drug Name	Dosage/Route	Usual Indications
Penicillins		
penicillin G benzathine (*Bicillin, Permapen*)	*Adult:* 1.2–2.4 million units IM *Pediatric:* 900,000–1.2 million units IM as a single injection	Severe infections caused by sensitive organisms; treatment of syphilis and erysipeloid infections
penicillin G potassium (*Pfizerpen*)	*Adult:* 1–20 million units/d IM or IV, depending on condition *Pediatric:* 100,000–1 million units/d IM or IV	Treatment of severe infections; used for several days in some cases
penicillin G procaine (*Wycillin*)	*Adult:* 600,000–1.2 million units/d IM *Pediatric:* 50,000 units/kg/d IM	Treatment of moderately severe infections daily for 8–12 d
penicillin V (generic)	*Adult:* 250–500 mg q6–8h PO *Pediatric:* 15–62.5 mg/kg/d PO in divided doses q6–8h	Used for prophylaxis for bacterial endocarditis, Lyme disease, UTIs
Extended-Spectrum Penicillins		
amoxicillin (*Amoxil, Trimox*)	*Adult:* 250–500 mg PO q8h *Pediatric:* 20 mg/kg/d PO in divided doses q8h	Broad spectrum of uses for adults and children
ampicillin (*Principen*)	*Adult:* 250–500 mg IM or IV q6h, then 500 mg PO q6h when oral use is feasible *Pediatric:* 60 mg/kg/d IM or IV in four to six divided doses, then 250 mg PO q6h	Broad spectrum of activity; useful form if switch from parenteral to oral is anticipated; monitor for nephritis
Penicillinase-Resistant Antibiotics		
nafcillin	*Adult:* 500–1,000 mg IV q4h, 500 mg IM q6h *or* 250–500 mg PO q4–6h *Pediatric:* 25 mg/kg IM b.i.d. *or* 25–50 mg/kg/d PO in four divided doses	Infections by penicillinase-producing staphylococci as well as group A hemolytic streptococci, plus *Streptococcus viridans*; drug of choice if switch to oral form is anticipated
oxacillin	*Adult:* 500 mg PO q4–6h *or* 250–500 mg IM or IV q4–6h *Pediatric:* 50 mg/kg/d IM, IV, or PO in equally divided doses q4–6h	Infections by penicillinase-producing staphylococci; streptococci; drug of choice if switch to oral form is anticipated

With the prolonged use of penicillin, more and more bacterial species have synthesized the enzyme penicillinase to counteract the effects of penicillin. Researchers have developed a group of drugs with a resistance to penicillinase, which allows them to remain effective against bacteria that are now resistant to the penicillins. Penicillinase-resistant antibiotics include nafcillin and oxacillin. The actual drug chosen depends on the sensitivity of the bacteria causing the infection, the desired and available routes, and the personal experience of the clinician with the particular agent.

Therapeutic Actions and Indications

The penicillins and penicillinase-resistant antibiotics produce bactericidal effects by interfering with the ability of susceptible bacteria to build their cell walls when they are dividing (see Figure 9.2). These drugs prevent the bacteria from biosynthesizing the framework of the cell wall, and the bacteria with weakened cell walls swell and then burst from osmotic pressure within the cell. Because human cells do not use the biochemical process that the bacteria use to form the cell wall, this effect is a selective toxicity.

The penicillins are indicated for the treatment of streptococcal infections, including pharyngitis, tonsillitis, scarlet fever, and endocarditis; pneumococcal infections; staphylococcal infections; fusospirochetal infections; rat-bite fever; diphtheria; anthrax; syphilis; and uncomplicated gonococcal infections. At high doses, these drugs are also used to treat meningococcal meningitis. See Table 9.5 for usual indications for each agent. (See the Critical Thinking Scenario.)

CRITICAL THINKING SCENARIO

Antibiotics and Adverse Effects

THE SITUATION

N.S., an 18-month-old girl, was diagnosed with acute otitis media when her mother brought her to the clinic following a sleepless night of inconsolable crying, low-grade fever, and inability to take her bottle. A prescription was given for amoxicillin and the mother was told to return in 10 days for a follow-up appointment.

In talking with the mother, you discover that this is her first child and this is the first time the child has been sick.

Critical Thinking

What does amoxicillin affect a child with an ear infection?

What adverse effects and safety issues need to be considered?

What nursing interventions are appropriate for N.S. and her mother?

What teaching points should be stressed with the mother?

What potential medication errors should you consider?

What points do you need to include to help the mother safely administer the drug and evaluate its effectiveness?

DISCUSSION

Amoxicillin is a broad-spectrum antibiotic that interferes with the bacterial cell wall to cause bacterial cell death. It needs to be taken for 7–10 days. The adverse effects most frequently seen with this antibiotic are nausea, diarrhea, rash, and superinfections. The pain and discomfort of the ear infection may persist for a day or two after starting the drug and the toddler may require additional comfort measures.

The mother in this case will need clear, concise written information. This is her first child and the first time the child has been sick so the mother may also need support and encouragement to get through the experience. The medication will be prepared in a suspension form so the child can swallow it safely. Measuring out the dosage should be a top discussion. Many times a pharmacy will supply a measuring device, often a dosing syringe, to ensure that the correct dose is given. If the mother elects to use a teaspoon from home, it is key to explain that this needs to be a measuring teaspoon, not a tableware teaspoon. Proper storage of the drug may require refrigeration. The bottle will need to be shaken before each use. It will be important to explain that the toddler needs to receive the full prescribed dose, giving the drug for 7–10 days as prescribed. The mother needs to understand that the toddler may seem to feel just fine, but the bacteria may still be present and the full dose needs to be given.

N.S.'s mother will need to understand that some adverse effects are possible. Diarrhea is very common when this drug is used in this age group. The mother will need to be encouraged to watch for any signs of dehydration, to encourage lots of fluid intake, and to take special care in frequently changing the diaper and cleansing with each diaper change because diarrhea can be very irritating to the skin. She may also notice white patches in the mouth if a superinfection should occur. This may first present with the toddler unable to suck a

Antibiotics and Adverse Effects (continued)

bottle and unable to eat without crying. A mild rash may also occur; the mother might want to have this evaluated if she is concerned. The child may need further comfort measures until the infection resolves; N.S. could have a standby order for ibuprofen or acetaminophen in proper dosage for this age group. Warm compresses on the affected ear(s) and holding the child against the mother's body to provide warmth to the ear are appropriate comfort measures. The mother should be taught that over-the-counter (OTC) cold medicines are not approved for this age group and should be discouraged from using them. She should offer the child yogurt with live cultures to help balance any diarrhea that might occur. Encourage the mother to call if she cannot control the discomfort her child is experiencing.

The mother should be encouraged to monitor the toddler's reactions. Is she still feverish, is she now playing and eating, can she sleep soundly again? If there is any indication that things might be getting worse (continued high fever, persistent crying, drainage from the ears), the mother should be encouraged to call or bring the toddler back into the clinic. She should be praised for bringing the child to the clinic and encouraged to call with reports of the child's progress.

This first encounter with the health care system with a sick child is a unique opportunity for the nurse to do preventative and safety teaching around the experience, drug administration, use of OTC products, and safety measures when giving drugs.

NURSING CARE GUIDE FOR N.S.: AMOXICILLIN

Assessment: History and Examination

Allergy to any amoxicillin
Concurrent use of any other drugs
General: Site of infection, culture, and sensitivity
Skin: Color, lesions
Respiratory: Respiration, adventitious sounds
GI: Bowel sounds, usual output
Laboratory data: Liver and renal function tests if warranted.

Nursing Diagnoses

Imbalanced nutrition: Less Than Body Requirements related to GI effects
Potential for injury related to possible dehydration
Deficient knowledge regarding drug therapy

Planning

- The patient will receive the best therapeutic effect from the drug therapy
- The patient will have limited adverse effects to the drug therapy
- The patient's family will have an understanding of the drug therapy, adverse effects to anticipate, and measures to relieve discomfort and improve safety

Implementation

Perform culture and sensitivity tests before beginning therapy.
Store suspension in refrigerator; shake before each use; use appropriate measuring device.
Monitor for and provide hygiene measures and treatment if superinfections occur.
Monitor nutritional status and fluid intake if diarrhea occurs.
Provide appropriate perianal cleansing and care if diarrhea is a problem.
Provide comfort measures to deal with ear pain; warm compresses, analgesic as appropriate.
Provide patient's family with teaching regarding drug name, dosage, storage, measuring, adverse effects, possible adverse effects, warnings to report

Evaluation

Evaluate drug effects: Resolution of bacterial infections.
Monitor for adverse effects: Diarrhea, superinfections
Evaluate effectiveness of patient-teaching program.
Evaluate effectiveness of comfort and safety measures.

Patient Teaching the Mother of N.S.

- Amoxicillin is an antibiotic that is specific for your child's ear infection. You need to store the drug in the refrigerator, shake the bottle before each use. Use the measuring device provided, or use a measuring teaspoon, not a flatware teaspoon to administer the drug.
- Make sure you give your child the full course of this antibiotic. Do not stop giving it if the child seems better. It is very important to give the full course of the drug to prevent another infection or the development of resistant bacteria.
- Your child may experience stomach upset or diarrhea. If diarrhea occurs, make sure you change the diaper often and cleanse the diaper area well. Monitor your child for any signs of dehydration and try to encourage fluid intake.
- Your child may develop other infections in the mouth or vagina. You may notice that it is difficult for your child to suck a nipple or to swallow, you may notice white patches in the mouth or vaginal area. If this occurs, consult your provider for appropriate treatment; do not stop taking the drug.
- Your child may still experience pain for the first few days; a prescription for an analgesic may be given to you; warm compresses on the ear may help; holding the child close to your body will also provide warmth and may help ease the ear pain.
- Report any of the following to your health care provider if your child experiences: Worsening pain, higher fever, inability to swallow, lethargy, dry skin, severe diaper rash.

Pharmacokinetics

Most of the penicillins are rapidly absorbed from the GI tract, reaching peak levels in 1 hour. They are sensitive to gastric acid levels in the stomach and should be taken on an empty stomach to ensure adequate absorption. Penicillins are excreted unchanged in the urine, making renal function an important factor in safe use of the drug. Penicillins enter breast milk and can cause adverse reactions (see Contraindications and Cautions).

Contraindications and Cautions

These drugs are contraindicated in patients with allergies to penicillin or cephalosporins or other allergens. Penicillin sensitivity tests are available if the patient's history of allergy is unclear and a penicillin is the drug of choice. Use with caution in patients with renal disease (lowered doses are necessary *because excretion is reduced*). Although there are no adequate studies of use during pregnancy, use in patients who are pregnant or lactating should be limited to situations in which the mother clearly would benefit from the drug, *because diarrhea and superinfections may occur in the infant*.

Perform culture and sensitivity tests *to ensure that the causative organism is sensitive to the penicillin selected for use*. With the emergence of many resistant strains of bacteria, this has become increasingly important.

Adverse Effects

The major adverse effects of penicillin therapy involve the GI tract. Common adverse effects include nausea, vomiting, diarrhea, abdominal pain, glossitis, stomatitis, gastritis, sore mouth, and furry tongue. These effects are primarily related to the loss of bacteria from the normal flora and the subsequent opportunistic infections that occur. Superinfections, including yeast infections, are also very common and are again associated with the loss of bacteria from the normal flora. Pain and inflammation at the injection site can occur with injectable forms of the drugs. Hypersensitivity reactions may include rash, fever, wheezing, and with repeated exposure anaphylaxis that can progress to anaphylactic shock and death.

Clinically Important Drug–Drug Interactions

If penicillins and penicillinase-resistant antibiotics are taken concurrently with tetracyclines a decrease in the effectiveness of the penicillins results. This combination should be avoided if at all possible, or the penicillin doses should be raised, which could increase the occurrence of adverse effects.

In addition, when the parenteral forms of penicillins and penicillinase-resistant drugs are administered in combination with any of the parenteral aminoglycosides, inactivation of the aminoglycosides occurs. These combinations should also be avoided.

Ⓟ Prototype Summary: Amoxicillin

Indications: Treatment of infections caused by susceptible strains of bacteria, postexposure prophylaxis for anthrax, treatment of Helicobacter infections as part of combination therapy.

Actions: Inhibits synthesis of the cell wall in susceptible bacteria, causing cell death.

Pharmacokinetics:

Route	Onset	Peak	Duration
Oral	Varies	1 h	6–8 h

$T_{1/2}$: 1 to 1.4 hours; excreted unchanged in the urine.

Adverse Effects: Nausea, vomiting, diarrhea, glossitis, stomatitis, bone marrow suppression, rash, fever, superinfections, lethargy.

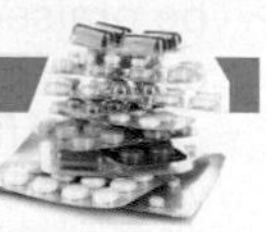

Nursing Considerations for Patients Receiving Penicillins and Penicillinase-Resistant Antibiotics

Assessment: History and Examination

- Assess for *possible contraindications or cautions*: Known allergy to any cephalosporins, penicillins, or other allergens *because cross-sensitivity often occurs* (obtain specific information about the nature and occurrence of allergic reactions); history of renal disease *that could interfere with excretion of the drug*; and current pregnancy or lactation status.
- Perform a physical assessment *to establish baseline data for evaluating the effectiveness of the drug and the occurrence of any adverse effects associated with drug therapy.*
- Examine skin and mucous membranes for any rashes or lesions and injection sites for abscess formation *to provide a baseline for possible adverse effects.*
- Perform culture and sensitivity tests at the site of infection *to ensure that this is the drug of choice for this patient.*
- Note respiratory status *to provide a baseline for the occurrence of hypersensitivity reactions.*
- Examine the abdomen *to monitor for adverse effects.* Evaluate renal function test findings, including BUN and creatinine clearance, *to assess the status of renal functioning and to determine any needed alteration in dose.*

Nursing Diagnoses

Nursing diagnoses related to drug therapy might include the following:

- Acute pain related to GI effects of drug
- Imbalanced nutrition: Less than body requirements related to multiple GI effects of the drug or to superinfections
- Deficient knowledge regarding drug therapy

Planning

- The patient will receive the best therapeutic effect from the drug therapy
- The patient will have limited adverse effects to the drug therapy
- The patient will have an understanding of the drug therapy, adverse effects to anticipate, and measures to relieve discomfort and improve safety

Implementation with Rationale

- Check culture and sensitivity reports *to ensure that this is the drug of choice for this patient.*
- Monitor renal function tests before and periodically during therapy *to arrange for dose reduction as needed.*
- Ensure that the patient receives the full course of the penicillin as prescribed, in doses around the clock, *to increase effectiveness.*
- Explain storage requirements for suspensions and the importance of completing the prescribed therapeutic course even if signs and symptoms have disappeared *to increase the effectiveness of the drug and decrease the risk of developing resistant strains.*
- Monitor the site of infection and presenting signs and symptoms (e.g., fever, lethargy) throughout the course of drug therapy. *Failure of these signs and symptoms to resolve may indicate the need to reculture the site.* Arrange to continue drug therapy for at least 2 days after the resolution of all signs and symptoms *to reduce the risk of development of resistant strains.*
- Provide small, frequent meals as tolerated, ensure frequent mouth care, and offer ice chips or sugarless candy to suck if stomatitis and sore mouth are problems *to relieve discomfort and ensure nutrition.*
- Provide adequate fluids *to replace fluid lost with diarrhea.*
- Monitor the patient for any signs of superinfection *to arrange for treatment if superinfections occur.*
- Monitor injection sites regularly, and *provide warm compresses and gentle massage to injection sites if they are painful or swollen.* If signs of phlebitis occur, remove the IV line and reinsert it in a different vein to continue the drug regimen.
- Instruct the patient regarding the appropriate dosage regimen and possible adverse effects *to enhance the patient's knowledge about drug therapy and promote compliance.*
- Provide the following patient teaching:
  - Try to drink a lot of fluids and to maintain nutrition (very important) even though nausea, vomiting, and diarrhea may occur.
  - Report difficulty breathing, severe headache, severe diarrhea, dizziness, weakness, mouth sores, and vaginal itching or sores to a health care provider. Box 9.5 contains a teaching checklist for penicillins.

Evaluation

- Monitor patient response to the drug (resolution of bacterial infection).
- Monitor for adverse effects (GI effects; local irritation, phlebitis at injection and IV sites; superinfections).
- Evaluate the effectiveness of the teaching plan (patient can name the drug, dosage, possible adverse effects to expect, and specific measures to help avoid adverse effects).
- Monitor the effectiveness of comfort and safety measures and compliance with the regimen.

BOX 9.5 FOCUS ON Patient and Family Teaching

Penicillins

- The penicillins are used to help destroy specific bacteria that are causing infections in the body. They are effective against only certain bacteria; they are not effective against viruses (such as cold germs) or other bacteria. To clear up a bacterial infection the penicillins must act on the bacteria over a period of time, so it is very important to complete the full course of this penicillin to avoid recurrence of the infection.
- The drug should be taken on an empty stomach with a full 8-oz glass of water—1 hour before meals or 2 to 3 hours after meals is best. Do not use fruit juice, soft drinks, or milk to take your drug, because these foods may interfere with its effectiveness. (This does not apply to amoxicillin, or penicillin V.)
- Common effects of these drugs include stomach upset, diarrhea, changes in taste, and change in the color of the tongue. Small, frequent meals may help. It is important to try to maintain good nutrition. These effects should go away when the drug is stopped.
- Report any of the following to your health care provider: hives, rash, fever, difficulty breathing, and severe diarrhea.
- Tell any doctor, nurse, or other health care provider that you are taking this drug.
- Keep this drug and all medications out of the reach of children and pets.
- Do not share this drug with other people, and do not use this medication to self-treat other infections.
- It is very important that you complete the full course of your prescription, even if you feel better before you finish it.

KEY POINTS

- The penicillins are one of the oldest classes of antibiotics, and many resistant strains have developed. The penicillinase-resistant antibiotics were created to combat bacteria that produce an enzyme to destroy the penicillin. Penicillins are used to treat a broad spectrum of infections, including respiratory tract infections and urinary tract infections (UTIs).
- Monitor the patient on penicillin for nausea, vomiting, diarrhea, superinfections, and the possibility of hypersensitivity reactions.

Sulfonamides

The sulfonamides, or sulfa drugs (Table 9.6), are drugs that inhibit folic acid synthesis. Sulfonamides include sulfadiazine (generic), sulfasalazine (*Azulfidine*), and cotrimoxazole (*Septra, Bactrim*).

Therapeutic Actions and Indications

Folic acid is necessary for the synthesis of purines and pyrimidines, which are precursors of RNA and DNA. For cells to grow and reproduce, they require folic acid. Humans cannot synthesize folic acid and depend on the folate in their diet to obtain this essential substance. Bacteria are impermeable to folic acid and must synthesize it inside the cell. The sulfonamides competitively block *para*-aminobenzoic acid to prevent the synthesis of folic acid in susceptible bacteria that synthesize their own folates for the production of RNA and DNA (see Figure 9.2). This includes gram-negative and gram-positive bacteria such as *Chlamydia trachomatis* and *Nocardia* and some strains of *Haemophilus influenzae*, *Escherichia coli*, and *Proteus mirabilis*.

Because of the emergence of resistant bacterial strains and the development of newer antibiotics the sulfa drugs are no longer used much. However, they remain an inexpensive and effective treatment for UTIs and trachoma, especially in developing countries and when cost is an issue. These drugs are used to treat trachoma (a leading cause of blindness), nocardiosis (which causes pneumonias, as well as brain abscesses and inflammation), UTIs, and sexually transmitted diseases. See Table 9.6 for usual indications for each of these agents. Sulfasalazine is used in the treatment of ulcerative colitis and rheumatoid arthritis.

Pharmacokinetics

The sulfonamides are teratogenic; they are distributed into breast milk (see Contraindications and Cautions). These drugs, given orally, are absorbed from the GI tract, metabolized in the liver, and excreted in the urine. The time to peak level and the half-life of the individual drug vary.

Sulfadiazine is an oral agent slowly absorbed from the GI tract, reaching peak levels in 3 to 6 hours.

Sulfasalazine is a sulfapyridine that is carried by aminosalicylic acids (aspirin), which release the aminosalicylic acid in the colon where it provides direct anti-inflammatory effects. In a delayed release form, this sulfa drug is also used to treat rheumatoid arthritis that does not respond to other treatments. It is rapidly absorbed from the GI tract, reaching peak levels in 2 to 6 hours. After being metabolized in the liver, it is excreted in the urine with a half-life of 5 to 10 hours.

Cotrimoxazole is a combination drug that contains sulfamethoxazole and trimethoprim, another antibacterial drug. It is rapidly absorbed from the GI tract, reaching peak levels in 2 hours. After being metabolized in the liver, it is excreted in the urine with a half-life of 7 to 12 hours.

Contraindications and Cautions

The sulfonamides are contraindicated with any known allergy to any sulfonamide, to sulfonylureas, or to thiazide diuretics *because cross-sensitivities occur*; during pregnancy *because the drugs can cause birth defects, as well as kernicterus*; and during lactation *because of a risk of*

Table 9.6 ***Drugs in Focus:* Sulfonamides**

Drug Name	Dosage/Route	Usual Indications
sulfadiazine (generic)	*Adult:* 2–4 g PO loading dose, then 2–4 g/d PO in four to six divided doses *Pediatric:* 75 mg/kg PO, then 120–150 mg/kg/d PO in four to six divided doses	Treatment of a broad spectrum of infections
sulfasalazine (*Azulfidine*)	*Adult:* 3–4 g/d PO in evenly divided doses, then 500 mg PO q.i.d.; 500 mg PO q.i.d. (arthritis) *Pediatric:* 40–60 mg/kg/d PO in divided doses, then 20–30 mg/kg/d PO in four equally divided doses	Treatment of ulcerative colitis and Crohn's disease; rheumatoid arthritis
cotrimoxazole (*Septra, Bactrim*)	*Adult:* 2 tablets PO q12h; reduce dose with renal impairment *Pediatric:* 8 mg/kg/d trimethoprim plus 40 mg sulfamethoxazole PO q12h	Treatment of otitis media, bronchitis, urinary tract infections, and pneumonitis caused by *Pneumocystis jiroveci*

kernicterus, diarrhea, and rash in the infant. They should be used with caution in patients with renal disease or a history of kidney stones *because of the possibility of increased toxic effects of the drugs.* They should be used with caution in the elderly *because of the increased incidence of CNS effects and safety issues with the elderly.*

Adverse Effects

Adverse effects associated with sulfonamides include GI effects such as nausea, vomiting, diarrhea, abdominal pain, anorexia, stomatitis, and hepatic injury, which are all related to direct irritation of the GI tract and the death of normal bacteria. Renal effects are related to the filtration of the drug in the glomerulus and include crystalluria, hematuria, and proteinuria, which can progress to a nephrotic syndrome and possible toxic nephrosis. CNS effects include headache, dizziness, vertigo, ataxia, convulsions, and depression (possibly related to drug effects on the nerves and more pronounced in the elderly). Bone marrow depression may occur and is related to drug effects on the cells that turn over rapidly in the bone marrow.

Dermatological effects include photosensitivity and rash related to direct effects on dermal cells. A wide range of hypersensitivity reactions may also occur.

Clinically Important Drug–Drug Interactions

If sulfonamides are taken with tolbutamide, tolazamide, glyburide, glipizide, or chlorpropamide the risk of hypoglycemia increases. If this combination is needed the patient should be monitored and a dose adjustment of the antidiabetic agent should be made. An increase in dose will then be needed when sulfonamide therapy stops.

When sulfonamides are taken with cyclosporine the risk of nephrotoxicity rises. If this combination is essential the patient should be monitored closely and the sulfonamide stopped at any sign of renal dysfunction.

Ⓟ Prototype Summary: Cotrimoxazole

Indications: Treatment of urinary tract infection, acute otitis media in children, exacerbations of chronic bronchitis in adults, traveler's diarrhea in adults, and Pneumocystis jiroveci pneumonia when caused by susceptible strains of bacteria.

Actions: Blocks two consecutive steps in protein and nucleic acid production, leading to inability for cells to multiply.

Pharmacokinetics:

Route	Onset	Peak
Oral	Rapid	1–4 h

$T_{1/2}$: 8 to 10 hours; excreted in the urine.

Adverse Effects: Nausea, vomiting, diarrhea, hepatocellular necrosis, hematuria, bone marrow suppression, Stevens-Johnson syndrome, rash, urticaria, photophobia, fever, chills.

Nursing Considerations for Patients Receiving Sulfonamides

Assessment: History and Examination

- Assess for *possible contraindications or cautions*: Known allergy to any sulfonamide, sulfonylureas, or thiazide diuretic *because cross-sensitivity often results* (obtain specific information about the nature and occurrence of allergic reactions); history of renal disease *that could interfere with excretion of the drug and lead to increased toxicity*; and current pregnancy or lactation status *because of potential adverse effects on the fetus or baby.*
- Perform a physical assessment *to establish baseline data for assessing the effectiveness of the drug and the occurrence of any adverse effects associated with drug therapy.*
- Examine skin and mucous membranes for any rash or lesions *to provide a baseline for possible adverse effects.*
- Obtain specimens for culture and sensitivity tests at the site of infection *to ensure that this is the appropriate drug for this patient.*
- Note respiratory status *to provide a baseline for the occurrence of hypersensitivity reactions.*
- Conduct assessment of orientation, affect, and reflexes *to monitor for adverse drug effects* and examination of the abdomen *to monitor for adverse effects.*
- Monitor renal function test findings, including BUN and creatinine clearance, *to evaluate the status of renal functioning and to determine any needed alteration in dosage.* Also perform a complete blood count (CBC) *to establish a baseline to monitor for adverse effects.*

Nursing Diagnoses

Nursing diagnoses related to drug therapy might include the following:

- Acute pain related to GI, CNS, or skin effects of the drug
- Disturbed sensory perception related to CNS effects
- Imbalanced nutrition: Less than body requirements related to multiple GI effects of the drug
- Deficient knowledge regarding drug therapy

Planning

- The patient will receive the best therapeutic effect from the drug therapy
- The patient will have limited adverse effects to the drug therapy
- The patient will have an understanding of the drug therapy, adverse effects to anticipate, and measures to relieve discomfort and improve safety

Implementation with Rationale

- Check culture and sensitivity reports *to ensure that this is the drug of choice for this patient and repeat cultures if response is not as anticipated.*

(continues on page 122)

- Monitor renal function tests before and periodically during therapy *to arrange for a dose reduction as necessary.*
- Ensure that the patient receives the full course of the sulfonamide as prescribed *to increase therapeutic effects and decrease the risk for development of resistant strains.*
- Administer oral drug on an empty stomach 1 hour before or 2 hours after meals with a full glass of water *to promote adequate absorption of the drug.*
- Discontinue immediately if hypersensitivity reactions occur *to prevent potentially fatal reactions.*
- Provide small, frequent meals and adequate fluids as tolerated, encourage frequent mouth care, and offer ice chips or sugarless candy to suck if stomatitis and sore mouth are problems *to relieve discomfort, ensure nutrition, and replace fluid lost with diarrhea.*
- Monitor CBC and urinalysis test results before and periodically during therapy *to check for adverse effects.*
- Instruct the patient about the appropriate dosage regimen, the proper way to take the drug (on an empty stomach with a full glass of water), and possible adverse effects, *to enhance patient knowledge about drug therapy and to promote compliance.*
- Provide the following patient teaching:
  - Avoid driving or operating dangerous machinery because dizziness, lethargy, and ataxia may occur.
  - Try to drink a lot of fluids and maintain nutrition (very important), even though nausea, vomiting, and diarrhea may occur.
  - Report difficulty in breathing, rash, ringing in the ears, fever, sore throat, or blood in the urine.

Evaluation

- Monitor patient response to the drug (resolution of bacterial infection).
- Monitor for adverse effects (GI effects, CNS effects, rash, and crystalluria).
- Evaluate the effectiveness of the teaching plan (patient can name the drug, dosage, possible adverse effects to expect, and specific measures to help avoid adverse effects).
- Monitor the effectiveness of comfort and safety measures and compliance with the regimen.

KEY POINTS

- Sulfonamides are older drugs; many strains have developed resistance to the sulfonamides, so they are no longer widely used.
- Monitor the patient for CNS toxicity, nausea, vomiting, diarrhea, liver injury, renal toxicity, and bone marrow depression.

Tetracyclines

The tetracyclines (Table 9.7) were developed as semisynthetic antibiotics based on the structure of a common soil mold. They are composed of four rings, which is how they got their name. Researchers have developed newer tetracyclines to increase absorption and tissue penetration. Widespread resistance to the tetracyclines has limited their use in recent years. Tetracyclines include tetracycline (generic), demeclocycline (generic), doxycycline (*Doryx, Vibromycin*), and minocycline (*Arestin, Minocin*).

Therapeutic Actions and Indications

The tetracyclines work by inhibiting protein synthesis in a wide range of bacteria, leading to the inability of the bacteria to multiply (see Figure 9.2). Because the affected protein is similar to a protein found in human cells, these drugs can be toxic to humans at high concentrations.

Tetracyclines are indicated for treatment of infections caused by *Rickettsia* spp., *Mycoplasma pneumoniae, Borrelia recurrentis, Haemophilus influenzae, Haemophilus ducreyi, Pasteurella pestis, Pasteurella tularensis, Bartonella bacilliformis, Bacteroides* spp., *Vibrio comma, Vibrio fetus, Brucella* spp., *Escherichia coli, Enterobacter aerogenes, Shigella* spp., *Acinetobacter calcoaceticus, Klebsiella* spp., *Diplococcus pneumoniae*, and *Staphylococcus aureus*; against agents that cause psittacosis, ornithosis, lymphogranuloma venereum, and granuloma inguinale; when penicillin is contraindicated in susceptible infections; and for treatment of acne and uncomplicated GU infections caused by *Chlamydia trachomatis.* Some of the tetracyclines are also used as adjuncts in the treatment of certain protozoal infections. See Table 9.7 for usual indications for each agent.

Pharmacokinetics

Tetracyclines are absorbed adequately, but not completely, from the GI tract. Their absorption is affected by food, iron, calcium, and other drugs in the stomach. Tetracyclines are concentrated in the liver and excreted unchanged in the urine, with half-lives ranging from 12 to 25 hours. These drugs cross the placenta and pass into breast milk (see Contraindications and Cautions).

Tetracycline is available in oral and topical forms, in addition to being available as an ophthalmic agent. Demeclocycline is available in oral form. Doxycycline and minocycline are available in IV and oral forms.

Contraindications and Cautions

Tetracyclines are contraindicated in patients with known allergy to tetracyclines or to tartrazine (e.g., in specific oral preparations that contain tartrazine) and during pregnancy and lactation *because of effects on developing bones and teeth.* The ophthalmic preparation is contraindicated in patients who have fungal, mycobacterial, or viral ocular infections *because the drug kills not only the undesired bacteria but also bacteria of the normal flora, which increases the risk for exacerbation of the ocular infection that is being treated.*

Tetracyclines should be used with caution in children younger than 8 years of age *because they can potentially*

Table 9.7 Drugs in Focus: Tetracyclines

Drug Name	Dosage/Route	Usual Indications
demeclocycline (generic)	*Adult:* 150 mg PO q.i.d. *or* 300 mg PO b.i.d. *Pediatric (>8 y):* 6–12 mg/kg/d PO in two to four divided doses	Treatment of a wide variety of infections when penicillin cannot be used
doxycycline (*Doryx, Vibramycin*)	*Adult:* 200 mg/d IV in two infusions of 1–4 h each *or* 100–300 mg/d PO *Pediatric (>8 y):* 4.4 mg/kg/d PO	Treatment of a wide variety of infections, including traveler's diarrhea and sexually transmitted diseases; periodontal disease
minocycline (*Arestin, Minocin*)	*Adult:* 200 mg IV, followed by 100 mg IV q12h *or* 200 mg PO, then 100 mg PO q12h *Pediatric (>8 y):* 4 mg/kg IV followed by 2 mg/kg IV or PO q12h	Treatment of meningococcal carriers and of various uncomplicated genitourinary and gynecological infections
tetracycline (generic)	*Adult:* 1–2 g/d PO in divided doses; topical applied generously to affected area *Pediatric (>8 y):* 25–50 mg/kg/d PO in four divided doses	Treatment of a wide variety of infections when penicillin is contraindicated, including acne vulgaris and minor skin infections caused by susceptible organisms; as an ophthalmic agent to treat superficial ocular lesions caused by susceptible microorganisms; as a prophylactic agent for ophthalmia neonatorum caused by *Neisseria gonorrhoeae* and *Chlamydia trachomatis*

damage developing bones and teeth and in patients with hepatic or renal dysfunction *because they are concentrated in the bile and excreted in the urine.*

Adverse Effects

The major adverse effects of tetracycline therapy involve direct irritation of the GI tract and include nausea, vomiting, diarrhea, abdominal pain, glossitis, and dysphagia. Fatal hepatotoxicity related to the drug's irritating effect on the liver has also been reported. Skeletal effects involve damage to the teeth and bones. Because tetracyclines have an affinity for teeth and bones, they accumulate there, weakening the structure and causing staining and pitting of teeth and bones. Dermatological effects include photosensitivity and rash. Superinfections, including yeast infections, occur when bacteria of the normal flora are destroyed. Local effects, such as pain and stinging with topical or ocular application, are fairly common. Hematological effects are less frequent, such as hemolytic anemia and bone marrow depression secondary to the effects on bone marrow cells that turn over rapidly. Hypersensitivity reactions reportedly range from urticaria to anaphylaxis and also include intracranial hypertension.

Clinically Important Drug–Drug Interactions

When penicillin G and tetracyclines are taken concurrently the effectiveness of penicillin G decreases. If this combination is used, the dose of the penicillin should be increased.

When oral contraceptives are taken with tetracyclines the effectiveness of the contraceptives decreases, and patients who take oral contraceptives should be advised to use an additional form of birth control while receiving the tetracycline (see Critical Thinking Scenario).

Digoxin toxicity rises when tetracyclines are taken concurrently. Digoxin levels should be monitored and the dose adjusted appropriately during treatment and after

CRITICAL THINKING SCENARIO

Antibiotics and Oral Contraceptives

THE SITUATION

You first see G.S., a 27-year-old married female graduate student, in the student health clinic a few weeks into the fall semester. She has developed a severe sinusitis and complains of head pressure, difficulty sleeping, fever, and muscle aches and pains. A culture is done, and the next day the culture and sensitivity report identifies the infecting organism as a strain of *Klebsiella* that is sensitive to tetracycline. G.S. returns to the clinic to get the prescription for tetracycline.

G.S. tells you that she began graduate school with plans to start a family in 2 years, after completing her program. She is a very organized person and has carefully planned her rigorous course work and her nonacademic activities so that almost every hour is scheduled. She states that she has successfully used low-dose oral contraceptives for 4 years and plans to continue this method of birth control.

(continues on page 124)

Antibiotics and Oral Contraceptives (continued)

Critical Thinking

How do tetracyclines and some other antibiotics and oral contraceptives interact?

What are the possible ramifications of continuing to take oral contraceptives during a pregnancy?

What nursing interventions are appropriate for G.S.?

What teaching points should be stressed with G.S.? Think about the nature of her personality and the problems that an unplanned pregnancy might cause.

How can you help G.S. to cope with her infection, her drug regimen, and her rigorous schedule?

DISCUSSION

Several antibiotics, including tetracycline, are known to lead to the failure of oral contraceptives as evidenced by breakthrough bleeding and unplanned pregnancy. Although the exact way in which these drugs interact is incompletely understood, it is thought that the antibiotics destroy certain bacteria in the normal flora of the gastrointestinal tract. These bacteria are necessary for the breakdown and eventual absorption of the female hormones contained in the contraceptives. The 5 days of antibiotic treatment together with the time necessary for rebuilding the normal flora can be long enough for the hypothalamus to lose the negative feedback signal provided by the contraceptives that prevents ovulation and preparation of the uterus. Sensing the low hormone levels, the hypothalamus releases gonadotropin-releasing hormone, which leads to the release of follicle-stimulating hormone and luteinizing hormone, with subsequent ovulation.

G.S. will need a clear explanation and follow-up in written form about the risks of oral contraceptive failure while she is receiving tetracycline therapy. She should be encouraged to use an additional form of birth control during the course of her antibiotic use and to read all of the literature that comes with oral contraceptives, as well as patient-teaching information that should be provided with the antibiotic.

G.S. also may need a great deal of support and encouragement at this time. The sinus infection may increase her stress by interfering with her ability to stick to her rigid schedule. Discussing the possibility of an unplanned pregnancy may cause even more stress. The health clinic visit could be used as an opportunity to allow G.S. to talk, to vent any frustrations and stress, and then to encourage her to make time for herself. The nurse should stress the importance of a good diet, which will ensure that her body has the components she will need to fight this infection and to heal and to ward off other infections, as well as the importance of adequate rest and exercise. The nurse should also make sure that G.S. is receiving annual gynecological exams and has been advised not to smoke.

All health care professionals who are involved with G.S. should consider the impact that an unplanned pregnancy could have on this very organized woman and use this as an example of the importance of clear, concise patient teaching in the administration of drug therapy.

NURSING CARE GUIDE FOR G.S.: TETRACYCLINE

Assessment: History and Examination

Allergy to any tetracycline

Hepatic or renal dysfunction

Pregnancy or lactation

Concurrent use of oral contraceptives, antacids, iron products, digoxin, or penicillins

General: Site of infection, culture, and sensitivity

Skin: Color, lesions

Respiratory: Respiration, adventitious sounds

GI: Liver evaluation, bowel sounds, usual output

Laboratory data: Liver and renal function tests, urinalysis

Nursing Diagnoses

Acute pain related to GI effects, superinfections

Imbalanced nutrition: Less than body requirements related to GI effects

Potential for injury related to CNS effects

Deficient knowledge regarding drug therapy

Planning

- The patient will receive the best therapeutic effect from the drug therapy
- The patient will have limited adverse effects to the drug therapy
- The patient will have an understanding of the drug therapy, adverse effects to anticipate, and measures to relieve discomfort and improve safety

Implementation

Perform culture and sensitivity tests before beginning therapy.

Administer drug on an empty stomach, 1 hour before or 2 to 3 hours after meals. Do not give with antacids, milk, or iron products.

Do not use outdated drug because of the risk of nephrotoxicity.

Monitor for and provide hygiene measures and treatment if superinfections occur.

Monitor nutritional status and fluid intake.

Provide ready access to bathroom facilities if diarrhea is a problem.

Provide support and reassurance for dealing with the drug effects and infection.

Provide patient teaching regarding drug name, dosage, adverse effects, precautions, warnings to report, and drugs that might cause a drug–drug interaction, including the need to use a second form of contraception if using oral contraceptives.

Antibiotics and Oral Contraceptives (continued)

Evaluation

Evaluate drug effects: Resolution of bacterial infections.
Monitor for adverse effects: GI effects, superinfections, CNS effects.
Monitor for drug–drug interactions: Lack of effectiveness of oral contraceptives, lack of antibacterial effect with antacids or iron.
Evaluate effectiveness of patient-teaching program.
Evaluate effectiveness of comfort and safety measures.

Patient Teaching for G.S.

- Tetracycline is an antibiotic that is specific for your infection. You should take it throughout the day for best results.
- Take this drug on an empty stomach, 1 hour before or 2 to 3 hours after meals, with a full glass of water.
- Do not take this drug with food, dairy products, iron preparations, or antacids.
- Take the full course of this antibiotic. Do not stop taking it if you feel better.
- Do not save tetracycline; outdated products can be very toxic to your kidneys.
- Hormonal contraceptives may become ineffective while you are taking this drug. If you rely on hormonal contraceptives for birth control, use a second form of contraceptive while on this drug.
- You may experience stomach upset or diarrhea.
- You may develop other infections in your mouth or vagina. (If this occurs, consult with your health care provider for appropriate treatment.)
- Tell any health care provider who is caring for you that you are taking this drug.
- Keep this, and all medications, out of the reach of children and pets.
- Report any of the following to your health care provider: Changes in color of urine or stool, severe cramps, difficulty breathing, rash or itching, yellowing of the skin or eyes.

tetracycline therapy is discontinued. Finally, decreased absorption of tetracyclines results from oral combinations with calcium salts, magnesium salts, zinc salts, aluminum salts, bismuth salts, iron, urinary alkalinizers, and charcoal.

Clinically Important Drug–Food Interactions

Because oral tetracyclines are not absorbed effectively if taken with food or dairy products, they should be administered on an empty stomach 1 hour before or 2 to 3 hours after any meal or other medication.

Ⓟ Prototype Summary: Tetracycline

Indications: Treatment of various infections caused by susceptible strains of bacteria; acne; when penicillin is contraindicated for eradication of susceptible organisms.

Actions: Inhibits protein synthesis in susceptible bacteria, preventing cell replication.

Pharmacokinetics:

Route	Onset	Peak
Oral	Varies	2–4 h
Topical	Minimal absorption occurs	

$T_{1/2}$: 6 to 12 hours; excreted unchanged in the urine.

Adverse Effects: Nausea, vomiting, diarrhea, glossitis, discoloring and inadequate calcification of primary teeth of fetus when used in pregnant women or of secondary teeth when used in children, bone marrow suppression, photosensitivity, superinfections, rash, local irritation with topical forms.

Nursing Considerations for Patients Receiving Tetracyclines

Assessment: History and Examination

- Assess for *possible contraindications or cautions*: Known allergy to any tetracycline or to tartrazine in certain oral preparations *because cross-sensitivity often occurs* (obtain specific information about the nature and occurrence of allergic reactions), any history of renal or hepatic disease *that could interfere with metabolism and excretion of the drug and lead to increased toxicity*, current pregnancy or lactation status *because of the potential for adverse effects to the fetus or infant*, and age *because of the risk of damage to bones and teeth.*
- Perform a physical examination *to establish baseline data for assessing the effectiveness of the drug and the occurrence of any adverse effects associated with drug therapy.*
- Examine the skin for any rash or lesions *to provide a baseline for possible adverse effects.*
- Perform culture and sensitivity tests at the site of infection *to ensure that this is the appropriate drug for this patient.*
- Note respiratory status *to provide a baseline for the occurrence of hypersensitivity reactions.*
- Evaluate renal and liver function test reports, including BUN and creatinine clearance, *to assess the status of renal and liver functioning, which helps to determine any needed changes in dose.*

(continues on page 126)

Nursing Diagnoses

Nursing diagnoses related to drug therapy might include the following:

- Diarrhea related to drug effects
- Imbalanced nutrition: Less than body requirements related to GI effects, alteration in taste, and superinfections
- Impaired skin integrity related to rash and photosensitivity
- Deficient knowledge regarding drug therapy

Planning

- The patient will receive the best therapeutic effect from the drug therapy
- The patient will have limited adverse effects to the drug therapy
- The patient will have an understanding of the drug therapy, adverse effects to anticipate, and measures to relieve discomfort and improve safety

Implementation with Rationale

- Check culture and sensitivity reports *to ensure that this is the drug of choice for this patient.* Arrange for repeated cultures if response is not as anticipated.
- Monitor renal and liver function test results before and periodically during therapy *to arrange for a dose reduction as needed.*
- Ensure that the patient receives the full course of the tetracycline as prescribed. The oral drug should be taken on an empty stomach 1 hour before or 2 hours after meals with a full 8-oz glass of water. Concomitant use of antacids or salts should be avoided because they interfere with drug absorption. *These precautions will increase drug effectiveness and decrease the development of resistant strains of bacteria.*
- Discontinue the drug immediately if hypersensitivity reactions occur *to avoid the possibility of severe reactions.*
- Provide small, frequent meals as tolerated, frequent mouth care, and ice chips or sugarless candy to suck if stomatitis and sore mouth are problems *to relieve discomfort and ensure nutrition.* Also provide adequate fluids *to replace fluid lost with diarrhea.*
- Monitor for signs of superinfections *to arrange for treatment as appropriate.*
- Encourage the patient to apply sunscreen and wear clothing *to protect exposed skin from skin rashes and sunburn associated with photosensitivity reactions.*
- Instruct the patient about the appropriate dosage regimen, how to take the oral drug, and possible side effects *to enhance patient knowledge about drug therapy and to promote compliance.*
- Provide the following patient teaching:
  - Try to drink a lot of fluids and maintain nutrition (very important) even though nausea, vomiting, and diarrhea may occur.
  - Use a barrier contraceptive method because hormonal contraceptives may not be effective while a tetracycline is being used.
  - Know that superinfections may occur. Appropriate treatment can be arranged through the health care provider.
  - Use sunscreens and protective clothing if sensitivity to the sun occurs.
  - Know when to report dangerous adverse effects, such as difficulty breathing, rash, itching, watery diarrhea, cramps, or changes in color of urine or stool.

Evaluation

- Monitor the patient's response to the drug (resolution of bacterial infection).
- Monitor for adverse effects (GI effects, rash, and superinfections).
- Evaluate the effectiveness of the teaching plan (patient can name the drug, dosage, possible adverse effects to expect, and specific measures to help avoid adverse effects).
- Monitor the effectiveness of comfort and safety measures and compliance with the regimen.

KEY POINTS

- Tetracyclines inhibit protein synthesis and prevent bacteria from multiplying.
- Tetracyclines can cause damage to developing teeth and bones and should not be used with pregnant women or children.
- Monitor the patient for GI effects, bone marrow depression, rash, and superinfections. Caution women that tetracyclines may make oral contraceptives ineffective.

Antimycobacterials

Mycobacteria—the group of bacteria that contain the pathogens that cause tuberculosis and leprosy—are classified on the basis of their ability to hold a stain even in the presence of a "destaining" agent such as acid. Because of this property, they are called "acid-fast" bacteria. The mycobacteria have an outer coat of mycolic acid that protects them from many disinfectants and allows them to survive for long periods in the environment. It may be necessary to treat these slow-growing bacteria for several years before they can be eradicated.

Mycobacteria cause serious infectious diseases. The bacterium *Mycobacterium tuberculosis* causes tuberculosis, the leading cause of death from infectious disease in the world. For several years the disease was thought to be under control, but with the increasing number of people with compromised immune systems and the emergence of resistant bacterial strains, tuberculosis is once again on the rise.

Mycobacterium leprae causes leprosy, also known as Hansen's disease, which is characterized by disfiguring skin lesions and destructive effects on the respiratory tract. Leprosy is also a worldwide health problem; it is infectious when the mycobacteria invade the skin or respiratory tract of susceptible individuals. *Mycobacterium avium-intracellulare,* which causes mycobacterium avium complex, is seen in patients with AIDS or in other patients who are severely immunocompromised. Rifabutin (*Mycobutin*), which was developed as an antituberculosis drug, is most effective against *M. avium-intracellulare.*

Antituberculosis Drugs

Tuberculosis can lead to serious damage in the lungs, the GU tract, bones, and the meninges. Because *Mycobacterium tuberculosis* is so slow growing the treatment must be continued for 6 months to 2 years. Using the drugs in combination helps to decrease the emergence of resistant strains and to affect the bacteria at various phases during their long and slow life cycle (Table 9.8).

First-line drugs for treating tuberculosis are used in combinations of two or more agents until bacterial conversion occurs or maximum improvement is seen. The first-line drugs for treating tuberculosis are isoniazid (generic), rifampin (*Rifadin*), pyrazinamide (generic), ethambutol (*Myambutol*), streptomycin (generic), and rifapentine (*Priftin*).

If the patient cannot take one or more of the first-line drugs, or if the disease continues to progress because of the emergence of a resistant strain, second-line drugs can be used. The second-line drugs include ethionamide (*Trecator-SC*), capreomycin (*Capastat*), cycloserine (*Seromycin*), rifabutin (*Mycobutin*), and bedaquiline (*Sirturo*).

Table 9.8 ***Drugs in Focus:*** **Antimycobacterials**

Drug Name	Dosage/Route	Usual Indications
Antituberculosis Drugs ***First-Line Drugs***		
ethambutol (*Myambutol*)	*Adult:* 15 mg/kg/d PO as a single dose *Pediatric:* Not recommended for children <13 y	Treatment of *Mycobacterium tuberculosis*
INH (*Nydrazid*)	*Adult:* 5 mg/kg/d PO *Pediatric:* 10–12 mg/kg/d PO	Treatment of *M. tuberculosis*
pyrazinamide (generic)	*Adult and pediatric:* 15–30 mg/kg/d PO	Treatment of *M. tuberculosis*
rifampin (*Rifadin, Rimactane*)	*Adult:* 600 mg PO or IV as a single daily dose *Pediatric:* 10–20 mg/kg/d PO or IV	Treatment of *M. tuberculosis*
rifapentine (*Priftin*)	*Adult:* 600 mg PO 2 times a week for 2 mo *Pediatric:* Safety not established	Treatment of *M. tuberculosis*
streptomycin (generic)	*Adult:* 15 mg/kg/d IM *or* 25/30 mg/kg IM given 2–3 times a week *Pediatric:* 20–40 mg/kg/d IM or 25–30 mg/kg IM given 2–3 times a week	Treatment of *M. tuberculosis*, tularemia, plague, subacute bacterial endocarditis
Second-Line Drugs		
bedaquiline (*Sirturo*)	*Adult:* 400 mg/d PO for 2 wk, then 200 mg PO 3 times a week for 22 wk	Second-line treatment of resistant *M. tuberculosis*; not for use in extrapulmonary, latent, or drug-sensitive TB
capreomycin (*Capastat*)	*Adult:* 1 g/d IM for 60–120 d, followed by 1 g IM 2–3 times a week for 18–24 mo; reduce dose with renal impairment *Pediatric:* 15 mg/kg/d IM	Second-line drug for treatment of *M. tuberculosis*
cycloserine (*Seromycin*)	*Adult:* 250 mg PO b.i.d. for 2 wk, then 500 mg–1 g/d PO in divided doses *Pediatric:* Safety not established	Second-line treatment of *M. tuberculosis*
ethionamide (*Trecator-SC*)	*Adult:* 15–20 mg/kg/d PO in divided doses with pyridoxine *Pediatric:* 10–20 mg/kg/d PO in divided doses with pyridoxine	Second-line treatment of *M. tuberculosis*
rifabutin (*Mycobutin*)	*Adult:* 300 mg PO daily *Pediatric:* 10–20 mg/kg/d PO or IV	Second-line treatment of *M. tuberculosis*
Leprostatic Drug		
dapsone (generic)	*Adult:* 50–100 mg/d PO *Pediatric:* 1 × 2 mg/kg/d PO for 3 y; do not exceed 100 mg/d	Treatment of leprosy, *Pneumocystic jiroveci* pneumonia in AIDS patients, and a variety of infections caused by susceptible bacteria and brown recluse spider bites

In addition, drugs from other antibiotic classes have been found to be effective in second-line treatment, such as ciprofloxacin (*Cipro*), ofloxacin (*Floxin*), and levofloxacin (*Levaquin*), which are fluoroquinolones.

Leprostatic Drugs

The antibiotic used to treat leprosy is dapsone (generic), which has been the mainstay of leprosy treatment for many years, although resistant strains are emerging (Table 9.8). Similar to the sulfonamides, dapsone inhibits folate synthesis in susceptible bacteria. In addition to its use in leprosy, dapsone is used to treat *Pneumocystic jiroveci* pneumonia in AIDS patients and for a variety of infections caused by susceptible bacteria, as well as for brown recluse spider bites.

Recently, the hypnotic drug thalidomide (*Thalomid*) was approved for use in a condition that occurs after treatment for leprosy (Box 9.6).

Therapeutic Actions and Indications

Most of the antimycobacterial agents act on the DNA and/or RNA of the bacteria, leading to a lack of growth and eventually to bacterial death (see Figure 9.2). Isoniazid (INH) specifically affects the mycolic acid coat around the bacterium. Although many of the antimycobacterial agents are effective against other species of susceptible bacteria, their primary indications are in the treatment of tuberculosis or leprosy (as previously indicated). The antituberculosis drugs are always used in combination to affect the bacteria at various stages and to help to decrease the emergence of resistant strains (see Table 9.8).

BOX 9.6

New Indication for Thalidomide

In the 1950s the drug thalidomide became internationally known because it caused serious abnormalities (e.g., lack of limbs, defective limbs) in the fetuses of many women who received the drug during pregnancy to help them sleep and to decrease stress. This tragedy led to the recall of thalidomide in the United States and the establishment of more stringent standards for drug testing and labeling. In 1998 the FDA approved the use of this controversial drug for the treatment of erythema nodosum leprosum, which is a painful inflammatory condition related to an immune reaction to dead bacteria that occurs after treatment for leprosy. It is also approved for use in the treatment of multiple myeloma, brain tumors, Crohn's disease, human immunodeficiency virus–wasting syndrome, and graft–host reaction in bone marrow transplant.

To take thalidomide a woman must have a monthly negative pregnancy test with results posted in her medical record, receive instruction in using birth control, and sign a release stating that she understands the risks associated with the drug. These limits on the use of a drug were the first such restrictions ever ordered by the FDA.

Thalidomide (*Thalomid*) is given in doses of 100–300 mg/d PO at bedtime for at least 2 weeks, followed by tapered doses in 50-mg increments over the next 2 to 4 weeks.

Pharmacokinetics

The antimycobacterial agents are generally well absorbed from the GI tract. These drugs, given orally, are metabolized in the liver and excreted in the urine; they cross the placenta and enter breast milk, placing the fetus or child at risk for adverse reactions (see Contraindications and Cautions).

Contraindications and Cautions

Antimycobacterials are contraindicated for patients with any known allergy to these agents; in those with severe renal or hepatic failure, *which could interfere with the metabolism or excretion of the drug*; in those with severe CNS dysfunction, *which could be exacerbated by the actions of the drug*; and in pregnancy *because of possible adverse effects on the fetus.* If an antituberculosis regimen is necessary during pregnancy, the combination of isoniazid, ethambutol, and rifampin is considered the safest.

Adverse Effects

CNS effects, such as neuritis, dizziness, headache, malaise, drowsiness, and hallucinations, are often reported and are related to direct effects of the drugs on neurons. These drugs also are irritating to the GI tract, causing nausea, vomiting, anorexia, stomach upset, and abdominal pain. Rifampin, rifabutin, and rifapentine cause discoloration of body fluids from urine to sweat and tears. Alert patients that in many instances orange-tinged urine, sweat, and tears may stain clothing and permanently stain contact lenses. This can be frightening if the patient is not alerted to the possibility that it will happen. As with other antibiotics, there is always a possibility of hypersensitivity reactions. Monitor the patient on a regular basis. The newest drug in this group, bedaquiline, has a black box warning that an increased risk of death has been reported when this drug is used so the drug should be reserved for use when no other drug is effective. This same drug also has a black box warning that QTc intervals may be increased when using the drugs; a baseline ECG should be done as well as periodic checks of the QTc interval during treatment.

Clinically Important Drug–Drug Interactions

When rifampin and INH are used in combination the possibility of toxic liver reactions increases. Patients should be monitored closely.

Increased metabolism and decreased drug effectiveness occur as a result of administration of quinidine, metoprolol, propranolol, corticosteroids, oral contraceptives, oral anticoagulants, oral antidiabetic agents, digoxin, theophylline, methadone, phenytoin, verapamil, cyclosporine, or ketoconazole in combination with rifampin or rifabutin. Patients taking bedaquiline should avoid any other drugs that prolong the QTc interval. Patients who are taking these drug combinations should be monitored closely and dose adjustments made as needed.

Prototype Summary: Isoniazid

Indications: Treatment of tuberculosis as part of combination therapy; prophylactic treatment of household members of recently diagnosed tuberculars.

Actions: Interferes with lipid and nucleic acid synthesis in actively growing tubercle bacilli.

Pharmacokinetics:

Route	Onset	Peak	Duration
Oral	Varies	1–2 h	24 h

$T_{1/2}$: 1 to 4 hours; metabolized in the liver, excreted in the urine.

Adverse Effects: Peripheral neuropathies, nausea, vomiting, hepatitis, bone marrow suppression, fever, local irritation at injection sites, gynecomastia, lupus syndrome.

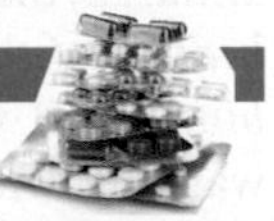

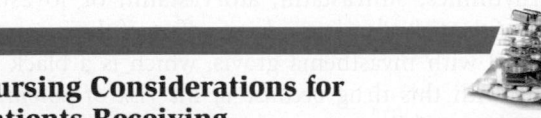

Nursing Considerations for Patients Receiving Antimycobacterials

Assessment: History and Examination

- Assess for *possible contraindications or cautions*: Known allergy to any antimycobacterial drug (obtain specific information about the nature and occurrence of allergic reactions); history of renal or hepatic disease, *which could interfere with metabolism and excretion of the drug and lead to toxicity*; history of CNS dysfunction, including seizure disorders and neuritis, *which could be exacerbated by adverse drug effects*; and current pregnancy status *to ensure appropriate drug selection to prevent adverse effects on the fetus.*
- Perform a physical examination *to establish baseline data for assessing the effectiveness of the drug and the occurrence of any adverse effects associated with drug therapy.*
- Examine the skin for any rash or lesions *to provide a baseline for possible adverse effects.*
- Obtain specimens for culture and sensitivity testing *to establish the sensitivity of the organism being treated.*
- Evaluate CNS for orientation, affect, and reflexes *to establish a baseline and to monitor for adverse effects.*
- Note respiratory status *to provide a baseline for the occurrence of hypersensitivity reactions.*
- Evaluate renal and liver function tests, including BUN and creatinine clearance, *to assess the status of renal and liver functioning so as to determine any needed alteration in dose.*

Nursing Diagnoses

Nursing diagnoses related to drug therapy might include the following:

- Imbalanced nutrition: Less than body requirements related to GI effects
- Disturbed sensory perception (kinesthetic) related to CNS effects of the drug
- Acute pain related to GI effects of the drug
- Deficient knowledge regarding drug therapy

Planning

- The patient will receive the best therapeutic effect from the drug therapy
- The patient will have limited adverse effects to the drug therapy
- The patient will have an understanding of the drug therapy, adverse effects to anticipate, and measures to relieve discomfort and improve safety

Implementation with Rationale

- Check culture and sensitivity reports *to ensure that this is the drug of choice for this patient, and arrange repeated cultures if response is not as anticipated.*
- Monitor renal and liver function test results before and periodically during therapy *to arrange for dose reduction as needed.*
- Ensure that the patient receives the full course of the drugs *to improve effectiveness and decrease the risk of development of resistant bacterial strains.* These drugs are taken for years and often in combination. Periodic medical evaluation and reteaching are often essential to ensure compliance.
- Discontinue drug immediately if hypersensitivity reactions occur *to avert potentially serious reactions.*
- Encourage the patient to eat small, frequent meals as tolerated, perform frequent mouth care, and drink adequate fluids *to ensure adequate nutrition and hydration.* Monitor nutrition if GI effects become a problem.
- Instruct the patient about the appropriate dosage regimen, use of drug combinations, and possible adverse effects *to enhance patient knowledge about drug therapy and to promote compliance.*
- Provide the following patient teaching:
  - Try to drink a lot of fluids to maintain nutrition (very important) even though nausea, vomiting, and diarrhea may occur.

(continues on page 130)

- Use barrier contraceptives, and understand that hormonal contraceptives may not be effective if antimycobacterials are being used.
- Understand that normally some of these drugs impart an orange stain to body fluids. If this occurs the fluids may stain clothing and tears may stain contact lenses.
- Report difficulty breathing, hallucinations, numbness and tingling, worsening of condition, fever and chills, or changes in color of urine or stool.

Evaluation

- Monitor patient response to the drug (resolution of mycobacterial infection).
- Monitor for adverse effects (GI effects, CNS changes, and hypersensitivity reactions).
- Evaluate the effectiveness of the teaching plan (patient can name the drug, dosage, possible adverse effects to expect, and specific measures to help avoid adverse effects).
- Monitor the effectiveness of comfort and safety measures and compliance with the regimen.

KEY POINTS

- The mycobacteria have an outer coat of mycolic acid that protects them from many disinfectants and allows them to survive for long periods in the environment. These slow-growing bacteria may need to be treated for several years before they can be eradicated. They cause tuberculosis and leprosy.
- Antituberculosis drugs are used in combination to increase effectiveness and decrease the emergence of resistant strains. These drugs are divided into first-line and second-line drugs. Adverse effects include rashes, an orange tint to body fluids, and GI reactions.
- Dapsone is the only antibiotic now used to treat leprosy. Thalidomide recently was reintroduced to treat an unusual reaction many patients develop after being on dapsone.

Other Antibiotics

There are other antibiotics that do not fit into the large antibiotic classes These drugs—the ketolides, lincosamides, lipoglycopeptides, macrolides, oxazolidinones, and monobactams—work in unique ways and are effective against specific bacteria (Table 9.9).

Ketolides

The ketolide class of antibiotics was first introduced in 2004. Now (2016), telithromycin (*Ketek*) is the only approved drug in the class.

Therapeutic Actions and Indications

The ketolides block protein synthesis within susceptible bacteria, leading to cell death, which makes them structurally related to the macrolide antibiotics (see later discussion of macrolides). Telithromycin binds to specific ribosome subunits, leading to cell death in susceptible bacteria, which includes several strains resistant to other antibiotics. Telithromycin is effective against *Streptococcus pneumoniae*, including certain multidrug-resistant strains, *Haemophilus influenzae, Moraxella catarrhalis, Chlamydophila pneumoniae*, and *Mycoplasma pneumoniae*.

It is only approved for use in treating mild to moderate community-acquired pneumonia (see Table 9.9).

Pharmacokinetics

Telithromycin is available as an oral drug only. It is rapidly absorbed through the GI tract, reaching peak levels in 1 hour. The drug is widely distributed, may cross the placenta, and does pass into breast milk. It is metabolized in the liver with a half-life of 10 hours. It is excreted in the urine and feces.

Contraindications and Cautions

Telithromycin is contraindicated with known allergy to any component of the drug or to macrolide antibiotics *to avoid hypersensitivity reactions*; with known congenital prolonged QT interval, bradycardia, or any proarrhythmic condition such as hypokalemia *to avoid potentially serious cardiac effects*; with concurrent use of pimozide, cardiac antiarrhythmics, simvastatin, atorvastatin, or lovastatin *because of the risk of serious adverse effects if these are combined*; and with myasthenia gravis, which is a black box warning with this drug *because of the risk of potentially fatal respiratory failure.*

Use with caution in cases of renal or hepatic impairment *because this could alter the metabolism and excretion of the drug, leading to serious adverse effects.* Use with caution with pregnant and lactating patients *because of the potential for toxic effects on the fetus or infant.*

Perform culture and sensitivity testing *to ensure that the drug is used appropriately.*

Adverse Effects

The adverse effects associated with telithromycin are largely secondary to toxic effects on the GI tract: nausea, vomiting, taste alterations, and the potential for pseudomembranous colitis. Superinfections are common, related to the loss of normal flora bacteria. Serious hypersensitivity reactions, including anaphylaxis, have occurred.

Clinically Important Drug–Drug Interactions

There is a risk of increased serum levels of telithromycin and potentially serious adverse effects if it is combined with

Table 9.9 *Drugs in Focus:* Other Antibiotics

Drug Name	Dosage/Route	Usual Indications
Ketolide		
telithromycin (*Ketek*)	800 mg/d PO for 7–10 d; reduce dose with renal impairment	Treatment of mild to moderate community-acquired pneumonia caused by susceptible bacteria
Lincosamides		
clindamycin (*Cleocin*)	*Adult:* 150–300 mg PO q6h *or* 600–2,700 mg/d in two to four equal doses; reduce dose with renal impairment *Pediatric:* 8–25 mg/kg/d PO *or* 15–40 mg/kg/d IM or IV in three to four divided doses	Treatment of severe infections when penicillin or other, less toxic antibiotics cannot be used
lincomycin (*Lincocin*)	*Adult:* 500 mg PO q6–8h, 600 mg IM q12–24h *or* 600 mg–1 g q8–12h; reduce dose with renal impairment *Pediatric:* 30–60 mg/kg/d PO in three to four divided doses, 10 mg/kg IM q12–24h *or* 10–20 mg/kg/d IV in divided doses	Treatment of severe infections when penicillin or other less toxic antibiotics cannot be used
Lipoglycopeptides		
dalbavancin (*Dalvance*)	*Adult:* 1,000 mg IV as a single dose followed by 500 mg IV one week later	Treatment of complicated skin and skin structure infections caused by susceptible strains of gram-positive bacteria
oritavancin (*Orbitiv*)	*Adult:* Single dose of 1,200 mg IV over 3 hours	Treatment of complicated skin and skin structure infections caused by susceptible strains of gram-positive organisms
televancin (*Vibativ*)	*Adult:* 10 mg/kg IV over 60 min once a day for 7–14 d	Treatment of complicated skin and skin structure infections caused by susceptible strains of gram-positive organisms including methicillin-resistant strains
Oxazolidinones		
linezolid (*Zyvox*)	*Adult:* 400–600 mg PO or IV q12h for 10–28 days *Pediatric:* 10 mg/kg PO or IV q12h for 10–14 days	Treatment of pneumonia, skin, and skin structure infections caused by susceptible strains, including resistant strains; diabetic foot ulcers
tedizolid (*Sivextro*)	*Adult:* 200 mg/day PO for 6 days	Treatment of acute skin and skin structure infections by susceptible strains
Macrolides		
azithromycin (*Zithromax*)	*Adult:* 500 mg PO as a single dose on day 1, then 250 mg/d PO to a total dose of 1.5 g or 1–2 g as a single dose *Pediatric:* 10 mg/kg PO as a single dose on day 1, then 5 mg/kg PO on day 2–5 or 30 mg/k PO as a single dose	Treatment of mild to moderate respiratory infections and urethritis in adults and otitis media and pharyngitis/tonsillitis in children
clarithromycin (*Biaxin*)	*Adult:* 250–500 mg q12h PO for 7–14 d; reduce dose with renal impairment *Pediatric:* 15 mg/kg/d PO given q12h for 10 d	Treatment of various respiratory, skin, sinus, and maxillary infections; effective against mycobacteria
erythromycin (*Ery-Tab, Eryc*)	*Adult:* 15–20 mg/kg/d IV or PO *Pediatric:* 30–50 mg/kg/d PO in divided doses	Treatment of infections in patients allergic to penicillin; drug of choice for treatment of Legionnaire's disease, infections caused by *Corynebacterium diphtheriae, Ureaplasma* spp., syphilis, mycoplasma pneumonia, and chlamydial infections
Monobactam		
aztreonam (*Azactam*)	*Adult:* 500 mg–1 g q8–12h IM or IV; reduce dose in renal and hepatic impairment *Pediatric:* 30 mg/kg IM or IV q6–8h	Treatment of gram-negative enterobacterial infections; safe alternative for treating infections caused by susceptible bacteria in patients who may be allergic to penicillins or cephalosporins

pimozide, simvastatin, lovastatin, or atorvastatin. These combinations should be avoided. There is risk of increased serum levels of digoxin and metoprolol if they are combined with telithromycin; if this combination is used, the patient should be monitored closely and dose adjustments made.

There is a risk of decreased serum levels of telithromycin and loss of therapeutic effects if it is taken with rifampin, phenytoin, carbamazepine, or phenobarbital; if these drugs are needed a different antibiotic should be used. Increased GI toxicity associated with theophylline can occur if the two drugs are used together. Separate the doses by at least 1 hour if both drugs are needed.

Ⓟ Prototype Summary: Telithromycin

Indications: Treatment of community-acquired pneumonia caused by susceptible bacteria.

Actions: Binds to bacterial ribosomes, altering protein function and leading to bacterial cell death.

Pharmacokinetics:

Route	Onset	Peak
Oral	Rapid	0.5–4 h

$T_{1/2}$: 10 hours; metabolized in the liver and excreted in the feces and urine.

Adverse Effects: Headache, dizziness, nausea, vomiting, pseudomembranous colitis, superinfections.

Lincosamides

The lincosamides (Table 9.9) are similar to the macrolides but are more toxic. These drugs include clindamycin (*Cleocin*) and lincomycin (*Lincocin*).

Therapeutic Actions and Indications

The lincosamides react at almost the same site in bacterial protein synthesis and are effective against the same strains of bacteria (Figure 9.2). These drugs are used in the treatment of severe infections when a less toxic antibiotic cannot be used.

Pharmacokinetics

The lincosamides are rapidly absorbed from the GI tract or from IM injections and are metabolized in the liver and excreted in the urine and feces. These drugs cross the placenta and enter breast milk (see Contraindications and Cautions).

Clindamycin has a half-life of 2 to 3 hours. It is available in parenteral and oral forms, as well as in topical and vaginal forms for the treatment of local infections.

Lincomycin has a half-life of 5 hours. It can be given orally, IM, or IV.

Contraindications and Cautions

Use lincosamides with caution in patients with hepatic or renal impairment, which could interfere with the metabolism and excretion of the drug. Use during pregnancy and lactation only if the benefit clearly outweighs the risk to the fetus or neonate.

Adverse Effects

Severe GI reactions, including fatal pseudomembranous colitis, have occurred, limiting the usefulness of lincosamides. However, for a serious infection caused by a susceptible bacterium a lincosamide may be the drug of choice. Some other toxic effects that limit usefulness are pain, skin infections, and bone marrow depression.

Ⓟ Prototype Summary: Clindamycin

Indications: Treatment of serious infections caused by susceptible strains of bacteria, including some anaerobes; useful in septicemia and chronic bone and joint infections.

Actions: Inhibits protein synthesis in susceptible bacteria, causing cell death.

Pharmacokinetics:

Route	Onset	Peak	Duration
Oral	Varies	1–2 h	8–12 h
IM	20–30 min	1–3 h	8–12 h
IV	Immediate	Minutes	8–12 h
Topical	Minimal absorption		

$T_{1/2}$: 2 to 3 hours; metabolized in the liver, excreted in the urine and feces.

Adverse Effects: Nausea, vomiting, diarrhea, pseudomembranous colitis, bone marrow suppression.

Lipoglycopeptides

The lipoglycopeptides class of antibiotics was first introduced in 2010. Drugs in this class include televancin (*Vibativ*), dalbavancin (*Dalvance*), and oritavancin (*Orbactiv*).

Therapeutic Actions and Indications

Lipoglycopeptides are semisynthetic derivatives of vancomycin (see Chapter 8). They inhibit bacterial cell wall synthesis by interfering with the polymerization and cross-linking of peptidoglycans. They bind to the bacterial membrane and disrupt the membrane barrier function causing bacterial cell death. The lipoglycopeptides are effective against susceptible strains of the gram-positive organisms: *Staphylococcus aureus* (including methicillin-susceptible and methicillin-resistant isolates), *Streptococcus pyogenes*, *Streptococcus agalactiae*, *Streptococcus anginosus*, *Enterococcus faecalis* (vancomycin-susceptible isolates only), *Streptococcus intermedius*, and *Streptococcus constellatus*.

The only approved use for these drugs is treating complicated skin and skin structure infections in adults (see Table 9.9). Oritavancin is approved as a single IV dose, making it a good choice if follow-up or compliance is an issue.

Pharmacokinetics

Lipoglycopeptides are available as IV drugs only. They are rapidly absorbed with peak levels occurring at the end of the infusion. These drugs are widely distributed, may cross the placenta, and may pass into breast milk. The site of metabolism is not known; half-life ranges from 4 to 8 or 9 hours. It is excreted in the urine.

Contraindications and Cautions

These drugs are contraindicated with known allergy to any component of the drug *to avoid hypersensitivity reactions*; with pregnant and lactating patients *because of the potential for toxic effects on the fetus or infant.* Televancin has a black box warning regarding serious fetal risk and is not recommended for women who are pregnant or who might become pregnant.

Perform culture and sensitivity testing *to ensure that the drug is used appropriately.*

Adverse Effects

The adverse effects associated with the lipoglycopeptides are largely secondary to toxic effects on the GI tract: Nausea, vomiting, taste alterations, diarrhea, loss of appetite, and risk of *Clostridium difficile* diarrhea. Nephrotoxicity has been reported, and many patients experience foamy urine, something they should be alerted to when the drug is started. There is a risk of prolonged QTc interval. A transfusion reaction called red man syndrome with flushing, sweating, and hypotension can occur with rapid infusion. Infusion site reactions with pain and redness have also been reported.

Clinically Important Drug–Drug Interactions

There is an increased risk of prolonged QT interval and resultant arrhythmias if lipoglycopeptides are combined with other drugs known to prolong the QT interval; if this combination is used the patient's ECG should be monitored. There is increased risk of nephrotoxicity if combined with other nephrotoxic drugs; if this combination must be used the patient's renal function should be monitored.

Ⓟ Prototype Summary: Televancin

Indications: Treatment of complicated skin and skin structure infections caused by susceptible bacteria.

Actions: Affects bacterial cell wall synthesis leading to disruption of cell membrane function and bacterial cell death

Pharmacokinetics:

Route	Onset	Peak
IV	Rapid	End of infusion

$T_{1/2}$: 8 to 9.5 hours; site of metabolism unknown; excreted in the urine.

Adverse Effects: Nausea, vomiting, diarrhea, taste alterations, QT prolongation, nephrotoxicity, foamy urine.

Macrolides

The macrolides (Table 9.9) are antibiotics that bind to the subunit of the ribosome within the bacterial cell and interfere with protein synthesis in susceptible bacteria. Macrolides include erythromycin (*Ery-Tab, Eryc*, and others), azithromycin (*Zithromax*), clarithromycin (*Biaxin*).

Therapeutic Actions and Indications

The macrolides, which may be bactericidal or bacteriostatic, exert their effect by binding to the ribosomes within the cell and changing protein synthesis (see Figure 9.1). This action can prevent the cell from dividing or cause cell death, depending on the sensitivity of the bacteria and the concentration of the drug.

Macrolides are indicated for treatment of the following conditions: Acute infections caused by susceptible strains of *Streptococcus pneumoniae*, *Mycoplasma pneumoniae*, *Listeria monocytogenes*, and *Legionella pneumophila*; infections caused by group A beta-hemolytic streptococci; pelvic inflammatory disease caused by *Neisseria gonorrhoeae*; upper respiratory tract infections caused by *Haemophilus influenzae* (with sulfonamides); infections caused by *Corynebacterium diphtheriae* and *Corynebacterium minutissimum* (with antitoxin); intestinal amebiasis; and infections caused by *Chlamydia trachomatis*. See Table 9.9 for usual indications for each of these agents.

In addition, macrolides may be used as prophylaxis for endocarditis before dental procedures in high-risk patients with valvular heart disease who are allergic to penicillin. Topical macrolides are indicated for the treatment of ocular infections caused by susceptible organisms and for acne vulgaris, and they may also be used prophylactically against infection in minor skin abrasions and for the treatment of skin infections caused by sensitive organisms.

Pharmacokinetics

The macrolides are widely distributed throughout the body; they cross the placenta and enter the breast milk (see Contraindications and Cautions). These drugs are absorbed in the GI tract.

Erythromycin is metabolized in the liver, with excretion mainly in the bile to feces. The half-life of erythromycin is 1.6 hours.

Azithromycin and clarithromycin are mainly excreted unchanged in the urine, making it necessary to monitor renal function when patients are taking these drugs. The half-life of azithromycin is 68 hours, making it useful for patients who have trouble remembering to take pills because it can be given once a day. The half-life of clarithromycin is 3 to 7 hours.

Contraindications and Cautions

Macrolides are contraindicated in patients with a known allergy to any macrolide *because cross-sensitivity occurs.* Ocular preparations are contraindicated for viral, fungal, or mycobacterial infections of the eye, *which could be exacerbated by loss of bacteria of the normal flora.* Use with caution in patients with hepatic dysfunction, *which could alter the metabolism of the drug,* and in those with renal disease, *which could interfere with the excretion of some of the drug.* Also use with caution in lactating women *because macrolides secreted in breast milk can cause diarrhea and superinfections in the infant,* and in pregnant women *because of potential adverse effects on the developing fetus;* use only if the benefit clearly outweighs the risk to the fetus or the infant.

Adverse Effects

Relatively few adverse effects are associated with the macrolides. The most frequent ones, which involve the direct effects of the drug on the GI tract, are often uncomfortable enough to limit the use of the drug. These include abdominal cramping, anorexia, diarrhea, vomiting, and pseudomembranous colitis. Other effects include neurological symptoms such as confusion, abnormal thinking, and uncontrollable emotions, which could be related to drug effects on the CNS membranes; hypersensitivity reactions ranging from rash to anaphylaxis; and superinfections related to the loss of normal flora.

Clinically Important Drug–Drug Interactions

Increased serum levels of digoxin occur when digoxin is taken concurrently with macrolides. Patients who receive both drugs should have their digoxin levels monitored and dose adjusted during and after treatment with the macrolide.

In addition, when oral anticoagulants, theophyllines, carbamazepine, or corticosteroids are administered concurrently with macrolides the effects of these drugs reportedly increase as a result of metabolic changes in the liver. Patients who take any of these combinations may require reduced dose of the particular drug and careful monitoring.

When cycloserine is taken with macrolides, increased serum levels of cycloserine have occurred, with a resultant risk of renal toxicity. This combination should be avoided if at all possible.

Clinically Important Drug–Food Interactions

Food in the stomach decreases absorption of oral macrolides. Therefore, the antibiotic should be taken on an empty stomach with a full, 8-oz glass of water 1 hour before or at least 2 to 3 hours after meals.

Ⓟ Prototype Summary: Erythromycin

Indications: Treatment of respiratory, dermatological, urinary tract, and gastrointestinal infections caused by susceptible strains of bacteria.

Actions: Binds to ribosomes within the bacterial cell, causing a change in protein synthesis and cell death; can be bacteriostatic or bactericidal.

Pharmacokinetics:

Route	Onset	Peak
Oral	1–2 h	1–4 h
IV	Rapid	1 h

$T_{1/2}$: 3 to 5 hours; metabolized in the liver, excreted in bile and urine.

Adverse Effects: Abdominal cramping, vomiting, diarrhea, rash, superinfection, liver toxicity, risk for pseudomembranous colitis, potential for hearing loss.

Oxazolidinones

There are currently two antibiotics available in this class: Tedizolid (*Sivextra*) and linezolid (*Zyvox*).

Therapeutic Actions and Indications

The oxazolidinones interfere with protein synthesis on the bacterial ribosome, within the bacterial cell. They also act as MAO (monoamine oxidase) inhibitors. They are effective against vancomycin-resistant strains of enterococci (VRE), *Staphylococcus* and methicillin-resistant *Staphylococcus aureus* (MRSA), and penicillin-resistant pneumococci and *S. aureus.*

Tedizolid is specific for skin and skin structure infections caused by susceptible organisms. Linezolid is used in pneumonia, skin, and skin structure infections caused by susceptible strains as well as diabetic foot infections without osteomyelitis.

Pharmacokinetics

Tedizolid is available for oral or IV use. It is rapidly absorbed, has a half-life of 12 hours, is metabolized in the liver, and excreted in urine and feces. Linezolid is also available for IV or oral use. It is rapidly absorbed, has a half-life of 5 hours, is metabolized in the liver, and excreted in the urine.

Contraindications and Cautions

These drugs are contraindicated with any known allergy to the drug or drug components; with phenylketonuria (with the oral suspension of linezolid) *because crisis could occur*; patients taking MAO inhibitors *because these drugs can act as reversible MAO inhibitors* and in breastfeeding women *because the drug enters breast milk and can be toxic to the baby.* They should be used with caution with hepatic impairment, pheochromocytoma, hypertension, hyperthyroidism, and bone marrow suppression *because the effects of the drugs could exacerbate these conditions.* Caution should also be used during pregnancy *because the effects on the fetus are not known.*

Adverse Effects

Adverse effects of the oxazolidinones include CNS effects of headache, insomnia, dizziness; GI effects of dry mouth, nausea, vomiting, and diarrhea with the potential for pseudomembranous colitis; and thrombocytopenia and hypertension.

Drug–Drug Interactions

Oxazolidinones have a risk of hypertension and related adverse effects if combined with other drugs that increase blood pressure. An increased risk of bleeding and further thrombocytopenia occurs if oxazolidinones are combined with drugs that affect bleeding including nonsteroidal anti-inflammatory drugs (NSAIDs) and platelet inhibitors. Potentially serious serotonin syndrome can occur if used with other serotogenic drugs; this combination should be avoided unless these drugs are needed for treatment of resistant strains. The serotogenic drugs should be stopped 2 weeks before therapy begins.

Drug–Food Interactions

Potential for serious to life-threatening hypertension is combined with large amounts of tyramine-containing foods. These should be avoided.

Prototype Summary: Linezolid

Indications: Treatment of infections caused by resistant strains, pneumonias, skin and skin structure infections, diabetic foot infections

Actions: Binds to ribosomes within the bacterial cell, causing a change in protein function and cell death in susceptible strains of bacteria

Pharmacokinetics:

Route	Onset	Peak
Oral	Rapid	1–2 h
IV	Rapid	90 min

$T_{1/2}$: 5 hours; metabolized in the liver, excreted in urine.

Adverse Effects: Headache, dizziness, vomiting, diarrhea, thrombocytopenia, risk for pseudomembranous colitis

Monobactam Antibiotic

The only monobactam antibiotic currently available for use is aztreonam (*Azactam*) (Table 9.9).

Therapeutic Actions and Indications

Among the antibiotics, aztreonam's structure is unique, and little cross-resistance occurs. It is effective against gram-negative enterobacteria and has no effect on gram-positive or anaerobic bacteria. Aztreonam disrupts bacterial cell wall synthesis, which promotes leakage of cellular contents and cell death in susceptible bacteria (see Figure 9.2). The drug is indicated for the treatment of urinary tract, skin, intra-abdominal, and gynecological infections, as well as septicemia caused by susceptible bacteria, including *Escherichia coli*, *Enterobacter* spp., *Serratia* spp., *Proteus* spp., *Salmonella* spp., *Providencia* spp., *Pseudomonas* spp., *Citrobacter* spp., *Haemophilus* spp., *Neisseria* spp., and *Klebsiella* spp.

Pharmacokinetics

Aztreonam is available for IV and IM use only and reaches peak effect levels in 1 to 1.5 hours. Its half-life is 1.5 to 2 hours. The drug is excreted unchanged in the urine. It crosses the placenta and enters breast milk (see Contraindications and Cautions).

Contraindications and Cautions

Aztreonam is contraindicated with any known allergy to aztreonam. Use with caution in patients with a history of acute allergic reaction to penicillins or cephalosporins *because of the possibility of cross-reactivity*, in those with renal or hepatic dysfunction *that could interfere with the clearance and excretion of the drug*, and in pregnant and lactating women *because of potential adverse effects on the fetus or neonate.*

Adverse Effects

The adverse effects associated with the use of aztreonam are relatively mild. Local GI effects include nausea, GI upset, vomiting, and diarrhea. Hepatic enzyme elevations related to direct drug effects on the liver may also occur. Other effects include inflammation, phlebitis, and discomfort at injection sites, as well as the potential for allergic response, including anaphylaxis.

Clinically Important Drug–Drug Interactions

Aztreonam is incompatible in solution with nafcillin, cephradine, and metronidazole.

Ⓟ Prototype Summary: Aztreonam

Indications: Treatment of lower respiratory, dermatological, urinary tract, intra-abdominal, and gynecological infections caused by susceptible strains of gram-negative bacteria.

Actions: Interferes with bacterial cell wall synthesis, causing cell death in susceptible gram-negative bacteria; is not effective against gram-positive or anaerobic bacteria.

Pharmacokinetics:

Route	Onset	Peak	Duration
IM	Varies	60–90 min	6–8 h
IV	Immediate	30 min	6–8 h

$T_{1/2}$: 1.5 to 2 hours; excreted unchanged in the urine.

Adverse Effects: Nausea, vomiting, diarrhea, rash, superinfection, anaphylaxis, local discomfort at injection sites.

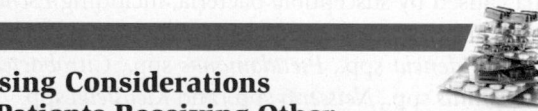

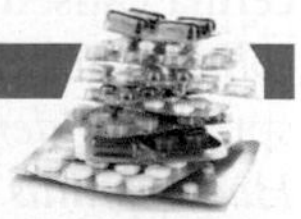

Nursing Considerations for Patients Receiving Other Antibiotics

Assessment: History and Examination

- Assess for *possible contraindications or precautions*: known allergy to ketolides, lincosamides, lipoglycopeptides, macrolides, oxazolidinones, and monobactams (obtain specific information about the nature and occurrence of allergic reactions); history of liver disease *that could interfere with metabolism of the drug*; history of renal disease, *which could be aggravated by the drug*; and current pregnancy or lactation status *because of potential adverse effects on the fetus or infant.*
- Perform a physical assessment *to establish baseline data for assessing the effectiveness of the drug and the occurrence of any adverse effects associated with drug therapy.*
- Examine the skin for any rash or lesions *to provide a baseline for possible adverse effects.*
- Obtain specimens for culture and sensitivity testing from the site of infection *to ensure appropriate use of the drug.*
- Monitor temperature *to detect infection.*
- Conduct assessment of orientation, affect, and reflexes *to establish a baseline for any CNS effects of the drug.*
- Assess liver and renal function test values *to determine the status of renal and liver functioning and to determine any needed alteration in dosage.*
- Obtain baseline electrocardiogram *to rule out conditions that could put the patient at risk for serious arrhythmias.*

Nursing Diagnoses

Nursing diagnoses related to drug therapy might include the following:

- Acute pain related to GI or CNS effects of the drug
- Risk for infection related to potential for superinfections
- Deficient knowledge regarding drug therapy

Planning

- The patient will receive the best therapeutic effect from the drug therapy
- The patient will have limited adverse effects to the drug therapy
- The patient will have an understanding of the drug therapy, adverse effects to anticipate, and measures to relieve discomfort and improve safety

Implementation with Rationale

- Check culture and sensitivity reports *to ensure that this is the drug of choice for this patient.*
- Monitor hepatic and renal function test values before therapy begins *to arrange to reduce dose as needed.*
- Ensure that the patient receives the full course of the medication as prescribed *to eradicate the infection and to help prevent the emergence of resistant strains.*
- Ensure that the patient swallows the tablet whole; it should not be cut, crushed, or chewed, *to ensure therapeutic dose of the drug.*
- Monitor the site of infection and presenting signs and symptoms (e.g., fever, lethargy, urinary tract signs and symptoms) throughout the course of drug therapy. *Failure of these signs and symptoms to resolve may indicate the need to reculture the site.* Arrange to continue drug therapy for at least 2 days after all signs and symptoms resolve, *to help prevent the development of resistant strains.*
- Provide small, frequent meals as tolerated *to ensure adequate nutrition with GI upset*; frequent mouth care and ice chips or sugarless candy to suck *to provide relief of discomfort if dry mouth is a problem*; and adequate fluids *to replace fluid lost with diarrhea.*
- Ensure ready access to bathroom facilities *to assist patients with problems associated with diarrhea.*

- Institute safety measures *to protect patient from injury if CNS effects occur.*
- Arrange for appropriate treatment of superinfections as needed *to decrease the severity of infection and complications.*
- Instruct the patient about the appropriate dosage regimen and possible adverse effects *to enhance patient knowledge about drug therapy and to promote compliance.* The monobactam agent aztreonam and televancin can be given only IV or IM, so the patient will not be responsible for administering the drug.
- For lincosamides, take additional precautions that include careful monitoring of GI activity and fluid balance and stopping the drug at the first sign of severe or bloody diarrhea.
- For lipoglycopeptides, take additional precautions to obtain a baseline QT interval on the ECG, alert the patient to the possibility of foamy urine, and ensure that the patient is not pregnant or planning to become pregnant when on the drug.
- Provide the following patient teaching:
  - Take safety precautions, including changing position slowly and avoiding driving and hazardous tasks, if CNS effects occur.
  - Try to drink a lot of fluids and to maintain nutrition (very important) even though nausea, vomiting, and diarrhea may occur.
  - Report difficulty breathing, severe headache, severe diarrhea, severe skin rash, and mouth or vaginal sores.

Evaluation

- Monitor patient response to the drug (resolution of bacterial infection).
- Monitor for adverse effects (orientation and affect, GI effects, superinfections).
- Evaluate the effectiveness of the teaching plan (patient can name the drug, dosage, possible adverse effects to expect, and specific measures to help avoid adverse effects).
- Monitor the effectiveness of comfort and safety measures and compliance with the regimen.

KEY POINTS

- Ketolides block protein synthesis in susceptible bacteria, leading to cell death. Telithromycin is the only ketolide currently available. It is used to treat community-acquired pneumonia. Monitor the patient for nausea, vomiting, diarrhea, and CNS effects, including dizziness and headache.
- Lincosamides are similar to macrolides but are more toxic. They are used to treat severe infections. Monitor the patient for pseudomembranous colitis, bone marrow depression, pain, and CNS effects.
- Lipoglycopeptides are a very new class of antibiotic and are similar to vancomycin. They prevent the synthesis of the bacterial cell wall, which leads to cell death. They are associated with high risk to the fetus. Monitor patients for prolonged QT interval, changes in renal function, GI effects, and foamy urine.
- Macrolides are in a class of older antibiotics that can be bactericidal or bacteriostatic. They are used to treat upper respiratory infections (URIs) and UTIs, and are often used when patients are allergic to penicillin. Monitor the patient for nausea, vomiting, diarrhea, dizziness, and other CNS effects.
- Oxazolidinones are newer drugs that are especially effective against various resistant strains. They are used for skin and skin structure infections, pneumonias, or any infection caused by a resistant bacteria that is sensitive to the drug. These drugs are also MAO inhibitors and caution must be used to prevent serotonin syndrome and hypertension-related effects.
- The monobactam antibiotic aztreonam is effective against only gram-negative enterobacteria; it is safely used when patients are allergic to penicillin or cephalosporins. Monitor the patient taking aztreonam for GI problems, liver toxicity, and pain at the injection site.

New Antibiotics and Adjuncts

Research is constantly being done to develop new antibiotics to affect the emerging resistant strains of bacteria. New antibiotics are daptomycin (*Cubicin*), tigecycline (*Tygacil*), quinupristin and dalfopristin (available only in a combination form called *Synercid*), fidaxomicin (*Dificid*), and rifixamin (*Xifaxan*). See the following for additional information about each of these agents.

Adjuncts to antibiotic therapy include clavulanic acid and sulbactam (see Box 9.2) and thalidomide (see Box 9.6).

- Daptomycin was introduced in the fall of 2003 as the first in a class of drugs called cyclic lipopeptide antibiotics. This class of drugs binds to bacterial cell membranes, causing a rapid depolarization of membrane potential. The loss of membrane potential leads to the inhibition of protein and DNA and RNA synthesis, which results in bacterial cell death. Daptomycin is approved for treating complicated skin and skin structure infections caused by susceptible gram-positive bacteria, including methicillin-resistant strains of *Staphylococcus aureus.* It must be given IV over 30 minutes, once each day for 7 to 14 days, which makes its use inconvenient. Patients should be monitored for pseudomembranous colitis and myopathies.
- Fidaxomicin (*Dificid*) was approved in 2011 as an orphan drug to treat *Clostridium difficile* infections. It belongs to a new class of narrow spectrum antibiotics called macrocycles. These drugs inhibit bacterial RNA polymerase and cause rapid death of *C. difficile* bacteria, which is very sensitive to its effects. It undergoes little systemic absorption and causes its effects directly in the GI tract. It is approved to treat *C. difficile* diarrhea and to prevent recurrence. It is given orally twice a day.

- Tigecycline (*Tygacil*) is the first drug of a new class of antibiotics called glycylcyclines. This antibiotic inhibits protein translation on ribosomes of certain bacteria, leading to their inability to maintain their integrity and culminating in the death of the bacterium. It is approved for use in the treatment of complicated skin and skin structure infections and intra-abdominal infections caused by susceptible bacteria. Caution should be used with a known allergy to tetracycline antibiotics because cross-sensitivity may occur. Women should be advised to use a barrier form of contraceptive when on this drug. Patients should be monitored for pseudomembranous colitis, rash, and superinfections. *Tygacil* is given as 100 mg IV followed by 50 mg IV every 12 hours, infused over 30 to 60 minutes for 5 to 14 days.
- Streptogramins became available in 1999 and include quinupristin and dalfopristin, which are available only in a combination form called *Synercid.* Together, they work synergistically and have been effective in treating VRE, resistant *Staphylococcus aureus*, and resistant *Staphylococcus epidermidis.* The drug is approved for VRE and methicillin-sensitive *S. aureus* infections. The drug also seems to be active against penicillin-resistant pneumococcus. The usual dosage of this drug for patients 16 years old and older is 7.5 mg/kg IV every 12 hours for 7 days. The drug should not be used unless the bacterium is clearly identified as being resistant to other antibiotics and sensitive to this one. Indiscriminate use of this new drug can lead to the development of even more invasive and resistant bacteria.
- Rifaximin (*Xifaxan)* was approved specifically for the treatment of traveler's diarrhea. It is similar to rifampin and blocks bacterial RNA synthesis, which leads to bacterial death; 97% of the drug passes through the GI tract unchanged, and it directly affects *Escherichia coli* bacteria, which cause traveler's diarrhea. It is also approved for treating hepatic encephalopathy. The usual dose is 200 mg, orally, three times a day. It should not be used if diarrhea is bloody and accompanied by fever, which might indicate that another pathogen is involved.

SUMMARY

- Antibiotics work by disrupting protein or enzyme systems within a bacterium, causing cell death (bactericidal) or preventing multiplication (bacteriostatic).
- The proteins or enzyme systems affected by antibiotics are more likely to be found or used in bacteria than in human cells.
- The primary therapeutic use of each antibiotic is determined by the bacterial species that are sensitive to that drug, the clinical condition of the patient receiving the drug, and the benefit-to-risk ratio for the patient.
- The longer an antibiotic has been available the more likely that mutant bacterial strains resistant to the mechanisms of antibiotic activity will have developed.
- The most common adverse effects of antibiotic therapy involve the GI tract (nausea, vomiting, diarrhea, anorexia, abdominal pain) and superinfections (invasion of the body by normally occurring microorganisms that are usually kept in check by the normal flora).
- To prevent or contain the growing threat of drug-resistant strains of bacteria, it is very important to use antibiotics cautiously, to complete the full course of an antibiotic prescription, and to avoid saving antibiotics for self-medication in the future. A patient and family–teaching program should address these issues, as well as the proper dosing procedure for the drug (even if the patient feels better) and the importance of keeping a record of any reactions to antibiotics.

CHECK YOUR UNDERSTANDING

Answers to the questions in this chapter can be found in Answers to Check Your Understanding Questions on thePoint®.

MULTIPLE CHOICE

Select the best answer to the following.

1. A bacteriostatic substance is one that

a. directly kills any bacteria it comes in contact with.

b. directly kills any bacteria that are sensitive to the substance.

c. prevents the growth of any bacteria.

d. prevents the growth of specific bacteria that are sensitive to the substance.

2. Gram-negative bacteria

a. are mostly found in the respiratory tract.

b. are mostly associated with soft tissue infections.

c. are mostly found in the GI and GU tracts.

d. accept a positive stain when tested.

3. Antibiotics that are used together to increase their effectiveness and limit the associated adverse effects are said to be

a. broad spectrum.

b. synergistic.

c. bactericidal.

d. anaerobic.

4. An aminoglycoside antibiotic might be the drug of choice in treating
   a. serious infections caused by susceptible strains of gram-negative bacteria.
   b. otitis media in an infant.
   c. cystitis in a woman who is 4 months pregnant.
   d. suspected pneumonia before the culture results are available.

5. Which of the following is not a caution for the use of cephalosporins?
   a. Allergy to penicillin
   b. Renal failure
   c. Allergy to aspirin
   d. Concurrent treatment with aminoglycosides

6. The fluoroquinolones
   a. are found freely in nature.
   b. are associated with severe adverse reactions.
   c. are widely used to treat gram-positive infections.
   d. are broad-spectrum antibiotics with few associated adverse effects.

7. Cipro, a widely used antibiotic, is an example of
   a. a penicillin.
   b. a fluoroquinolone.
   c. an aminoglycoside.
   d. a macrolide antibiotic.

8. A patient receiving a fluoroquinolone should be cautioned to anticipate
   a. increased salivation.
   b. constipation.
   c. photosensitivity.
   d. cough.

9. The goal of antibiotic therapy is
   a. to eradicate all bacteria from the system.
   b. to suppress resistant strains of bacteria.
   c. to reduce the number of invading bacteria so that the immune system can deal with the infection.
   d. to stop the drug as soon as the patient feels better.

10. The penicillins
   a. are bacteriostatic.
   b. are bactericidal, interfering with bacteria cell walls.
   c. are effective only if given intravenously.
   d. do not produce cross-sensitivity within their class.

MULTIPLE RESPONSE

Select all that apply.

1. A young woman is found to have a soft-tissue infection that is most responsive to tetracycline. Your teaching plan for this woman should include which of the following points?
   a. Tetracycline can cause gray baby syndrome.
   b. Do not use this drug if you are pregnant because it can cause tooth and bone defects in the fetus.
   c. Tetracycline can cause severe acne.
   d. You should use a second form of contraception if you are using oral contraceptives because tetracycline can make them ineffective.
   e. This drug should be taken in the middle of a meal to decrease GI upset.
   f. You may experience a vaginal yeast infection as a result of this drug therapy.

2. In general, all patients receiving antibiotics should receive teaching that includes which of the following points?
   a. The need to complete the full course of drug therapy
   b. The possibility of oral contraceptive failure
   c. When to take the drug related to food and other drugs
   d. The need for assessment of blood tests
   e. Advisability of saving any leftover medication for future use
   f. How to detect superinfections and what to do if they occur

BIBLIOGRAPHY AND REFERENCES

Anon. (2009). Tuberculosis. *Annals of Internal Medicine, 150,* ITC6-1.

Bancroft, E. (2007). Antimicrobial resistance. *Journal of the American Medical Association, 298,* 1803–1804.

Brunton, L., Chabner, B., & Knollman, B. (2011). *Goodman and Gilman's the pharmacological basis of therapeutics* (12th ed.). New York: McGraw-Hill.

Facts and Comparisons. (2015a). *Drug facts and comparisons.* St. Louis, MO: Author.

Facts and Comparisons. (2015b). *Professional's guide to patient drug facts.* St. Louis, MO: Author.

Gonzales, R., Bartlett, J. G., Besser, R. E., et al. (2001). Principles of appropriate antibiotic use for the treatment of acute respiratory tract infections in adults: Background, specific aims, and methods. *Annals of Internal Medicine, 134,* 479–486.

Karch, A. M. (2014). *Lippincott nursing drug guide*. Philadelphia, PA: Lippincott Williams & Wilkins.

Klevens, R. M., Morrison, M. A., Nadle, J., et al. (2007). Invasive methicillin-resistant. *Staphylococcus aureus* infections in the United States. *Journal of the American Medical Association, 298*, 1763–1771.

Medical Letter. (2013). *The choice of antibacterial drugs*. (Treatment Guidelines No. 123). New Rochelle, NY: Author.

Porth, C. M. (2013). *Pathophysiology: Concepts of altered health states* (9th ed.). Philadelphia, PA: Lippincott Williams & Wilkins.

Rosenstein, N., Phillips, W. R., Gerber, M. A., et al. (1998). The common cold—Principles of judicious use of antimicrobial agents. *Pediatrics, 100*, 181–184.

Workowski, K., Berman, S., & Douglas, J. (2008). Emerging antimicrobial resistance in *Neisseria gonorrhoeae*: Urgent need to strengthen prevention strategies. *Annals of Internal Medicine, 148*, 606–613.

Antiviral Agents 10

Learning Objectives

Upon completion of this chapter, you will be able to:

1. Discuss problems with treating viral infections in humans and the use of antivirals across the lifespan.
2. Describe characteristics of common viruses and the resultant clinical presentations of common viral infections.
3. Describe the therapeutic actions, indications, pharmacokinetics, contraindications, most common adverse reactions, and important drug–drug interactions associated with each of the types of antivirals discussed in the chapter.
4. Compare and contrast the prototype drugs for each type of antiviral with the other drugs within that group.
5. Outline the nursing considerations for patients receiving each class of antiviral agent.

Glossary of Key Terms

acquired immunodeficiency syndrome (AIDS): collection of opportunistic infections and cancers that occurs when the immune system is severely depressed by a decrease in the number of functioning helper T cells; caused by infection with human immunodeficiency virus (HIV)

AIDS-related complex (ARC): collection of less serious opportunistic infections with HIV infection; the decrease in the number of helper T cells is less severe than in fully developed AIDS

CCR5 coreceptor antagonist: a drug that blocks the receptor site on the T cell membrane that the HIV virus needs to interact with in order to enter the cell.

cytomegalovirus (CMV): DNA virus that accounts for many respiratory, ophthalmic, and liver infections

fusion inhibitor: a drug that prevents the fusion of the HIV-1 virus with the human cellular membrane, preventing it from entering the cell

helper T cell: human lymphocyte that helps to initiate immune reactions in response to tissue invasion

hepatitis B: a serious to potentially fatal viral infection of the liver, transmitted by body fluids

hepatitis C: a usually mild viral infection of the liver that can progress to chronic inflammation; most often seen hepatitis after blood transfusions

herpes: DNA virus that accounts for many diseases, including shingles, cold sores, genital herpes, and encephalitis

human immunodeficiency virus (HIV): retrovirus that attacks helper T cells, leading to a decrease in immune function and AIDS or ARC

influenza A: RNA virus that invades tissues of the respiratory tract, causing the signs and symptoms of the common cold or "flu"

integrase inhibitor: a drug that inhibits the activity of the virus-specific enzyme integrase, an encoded enzyme needed for viral replication; blocking this enzyme prevents the formation of the HIV-1 provirus

interferon: tissue hormone that is released in response to viral invasion; blocks viral replication

nonnucleoside reverse transcriptase inhibitors: drugs that bind to sites on the reverse transcriptase within the cell cytoplasm, preventing RNA- and DNA-dependent DNA polymerase activities needed to carry out viral DNA synthesis; prevents the transfer of information that allows the virus to replicate and survive

nucleoside reverse transcriptase inhibitors: drugs that prevent the growth of the viral DNA chain, preventing it from inserting into the host DNA, so viral replication cannot occur

protease inhibitors: drugs that block the activity of the enzyme protease in HIV; protease is essential for the maturation of infectious virus, and its absence leads to the formation of an immature and noninfective HIV particle

virus: particle of DNA or RNA surrounded by a protein coat that survives by invading a cell to alter its functioning

Agent List

Agents for Influenza A and Respiratory Viruses
- amantadine
- oseltamivir
- peramivir
- ribavirin
- (P) rimantadine
- zanamivir

Agents for Herpes Virus and Cytomegalovirus
- (P) acyclovir
- cidofovir
- famciclovir
- foscarnet
- ganciclovir
- valacyclovir
- valganciclovir

Agents for HIV and AIDS

Nonnucleoside Reverse Transcriptase Inhibitors
- delavirdine
- efavirenz
- etravirine
- (P) nevirapine
- rilpivirine

Nucleoside Reverse Transcriptase Inhibitors
- abacavir
- didanosine
- emtricitabine
- lamivudine
- stavudine
- tenofovir
- (P) zidovudine

Protease Inhibitors
- atazanavir
- darunavir
- (P) fosamprenavir
- indinavir
- lopinavir
- nelfinavir
- ritonavir
- saquinavir
- tipranavir

Fusion Inhibitor
- (P) enfuvirtide

CCR5 Coreceptor Antagonist
- (P) maraviroc

Integrase Inhibitor
- (P) dolutegravir
- raltegravir

Anti–Hepatitis B Agents
- (P) adefovir
- entecavir
- telbivudine

Anti–Hepatitis C Agents
- boceprevir
- simeprevir
- sofosbuvir

Locally Active Antiviral Agents
- docosanol
- ganciclovir
- imiquimod
- penciclovir
- trifluridine

Viruses cause a variety of conditions, ranging from warts, to the common cold and "flu," to diseases such as chickenpox and measles. A single virus particle is composed of a piece of either DNA or RNA inside a protein coat. To carry on any metabolic processes, including replication, a virus must enter a host cell. Once a virus has fused with a cell wall and injected its DNA or RNA into the host cell, that cell is altered (i.e., it is "programmed" to control the metabolic processes that the virus needs to survive). The virus, including the protein coat, replicates in the host cell (Figure 10.1). When the host cell can no longer carry out its own metabolic functions because of the viral invader,

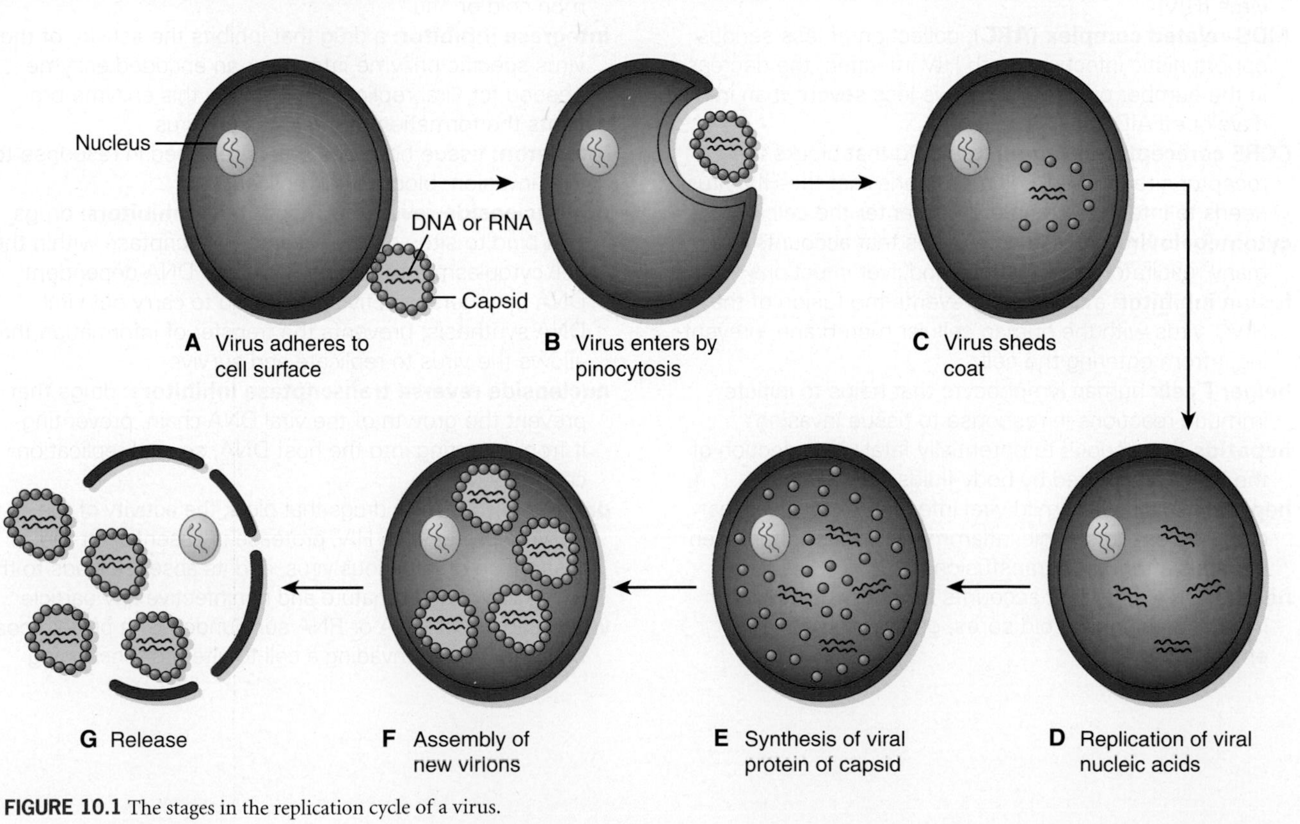

FIGURE 10.1 The stages in the replication cycle of a virus.

the host cell dies and releases the new viruses into the body to invade other cells.

Because viruses are contained inside human cells while they are in the body, researchers have difficulty developing effective drugs that destroy a virus without harming the human host. **Interferons** (see Chapter 15) are released by the host in response to viral invasion of a cell and act to prevent the replication of that particular virus. Some interferons that affect particular viruses can now be genetically engineered to treat particular viral infections. Other drugs that are used in treating viral infections are not natural substances and have been effective against only a limited number of viruses.

Viruses that respond to some antiviral therapy include influenza A and some respiratory viruses, herpes viruses, cytomegalovirus (CMV), HIV which causes AIDS, hepatitis B, hepatitis C, and some viruses that cause warts and certain eye infections. Patients need to be cautioned against using certain alternative therapies while on antiviral medication (Box 10.1). Box 10.2 discusses the use of antivirals across the lifespan. Figures 10.2 and 10.3 show sites of action for these agents.

BOX 10.1 FOCUS ON **Herbal and Alternative Therapies**

Alternative Therapies and Antiviral Drugs

An increasing number of people are using alternative therapies as part of their daily regimen. St. John's wort is one of the more popular alternative therapies sold today. This herb has been used as an anti-inflammatory agent, as an antidepressant, as a diuretic, and as a treatment for gastritis and insomnia. Multimedia advertisements urge the use of St. John's wort to increase one's sense of well-being and to decrease depression "without the use of drugs." Many people with viral infections just do not feel well. They are tired, have muscle aches and pains, and feel feverish and low on energy. This herbal remedy seems to be aimed at these people. Unfortunately, St. John's wort has been shown to interact with many prescription drugs. When taken with St. John's wort the protease inhibitors used in treating HIV were found to have decreased serum levels, leading to possible treatment failure. Because St. John's wort may induce the cytochrome P450 system in the liver, there is a possibility that it could increase the metabolism of many other antiviral drugs that are metabolized by that system and cause treatment failures with those drugs.

Patients may be reluctant to discuss their use of alternative therapies with the health care provider because they want to maintain control over that aspect of their medical regimen or because they believe that the health care provider would not approve of the use of these therapies. When a patient is prescribed an antiviral agent, it is important to ask specifically about the use of herbal or alternative medicines. Explain to the patient that antiviral drugs may interact with some herbal medicines and that it is important to try to avoid any adverse effects or drug failures.

Agents for Influenza A and Respiratory Viruses

Influenza A and other respiratory viruses, including influenza B and respiratory syncytial virus (RSV), invade the respiratory tract and cause the signs and symptoms of respiratory "flu." Vaccines have been developed (see Chapter 18) to stimulate immunity against influenza A and RSV. Preventing the viral infection is the best option, but if patients do develop a viral infection, some drug therapies are available. Agents for Influenza A and respiratory viruses include amantadine (*Symmetrel*), oseltamivir (*Tamiflu*), peramivir (*Rapivab*), ribavirin (*Virazole*), rimantadine (*Flumadine*), and zanamivir (*Relenza*) These drugs are described in detail in Table 10.1.

Therapeutic Actions and Indications

The exact mechanism of action of drugs that combat influenza A and respiratory viruses is not known. The belief is that these agents prevent shedding of the viral protein coat and entry of the virus into the cell (Figure 10.2). This action prevents viral replication, causing viral death. These agents for influenza A and respiratory viruses are especially important for health care workers and other high-risk individuals and for reducing the severity of infection if it occurs. See Table 10.1 for usual indications specific to each antiviral drug. Oseltamivir is the only antiviral agent that has been shown to be effective in treating H1N1 and avian flu.

Pharmacokinetics

Amantadine is slowly absorbed from the gastrointestinal (GI) tract, reaching peak levels in 4 hours. Excretion occurs unchanged through the urine, with a half-life of 15 hours. Oseltamivir is readily absorbed from the GI tract, extensively metabolized in the urine, and excreted in the urine with a half-life of 6 to 10 hours.

Peramivir is given intravenously (IV) as a single dose, reaches peak levels at the end of the infusion, and has a half-life of 20 hours.

Ribavirin, an inhaled drug, is slowly absorbed through the respiratory tract. It is metabolized at the cellular level and is excreted in the feces and urine with a half-life of 9.5 hours. It is teratogenic and is rated pregnancy category X.

Rimantadine is absorbed from the GI tract with peak levels achieved in 6 hours. This drug is extensively metabolized in the liver and excreted in the urine.

Zanamivir must be delivered by a Diskhaler device, which comes with every prescription of zanamivir. It is absorbed through the respiratory tract and excreted unchanged in the urine with a half-life of 2.5 to 5.1 hours.

read for exam

BOX 10.2 FOCUS ON **Drug Therapy Across the Lifespan**

Antivirals

CHILDREN

Children are very sensitive to the effects of most antiviral drugs, and more severe reactions can be expected when these drugs are used in children.

Many of these drugs do not have proven safety and efficacy in children, and extreme caution should be used.

Most of the drugs for prevention and treatment of influenza virus infections can be used, in smaller doses, for children.

Acyclovir is the drug of choice for children with herpes virus or CMV infections.

The drugs used in the treatment of AIDS are frequently used in children, many now have recommended pediatric dosing but others may be used without the evidence of safety because of the seriousness of the disease. Dose should be lowered according to body weight, and children must be monitored very closely for adverse effects on kidneys, bone marrow, and liver.

ADULTS

Adults need to know that these drugs are specific for the treatment of viral infections. The use of antibiotics to treat such infections can lead to the development of resistant strains and superinfections that can cause more problems.

Patients with HIV infection who are taking antiviral medications need to be taught that these drugs do not cure the disease, that opportunistic infections can still occur, and that precautions to prevent transmission of the disease need to be taken.

Pregnant women, for the most part, should not use these drugs unless the benefit clearly outweighs the potential risk to the fetus or neonate. Women of childbearing age should be advised to use barrier contraceptives if they take any of these drugs. Zidovudine has been safely used in pregnant women.

The Centers for Disease Control and Prevention advises that women with HIV infection should not breast-feed to protect the neonate from the virus.

OLDER ADULTS

Older patients may be more susceptible to the adverse effects associated with these drugs; they should be monitored closely.

Patients with hepatic dysfunction are at increased risk for worsening hepatic problems and toxic effects of those drugs that are metabolized in the liver. Drugs that are excreted unchanged in the urine can be especially toxic to patients who have renal dysfunction. If hepatic or renal dysfunction is expected (extreme age, alcohol abuse, use of other hepatotoxic or nephrotoxic drugs), the dose may need to be lowered and the patient should be monitored more frequently.

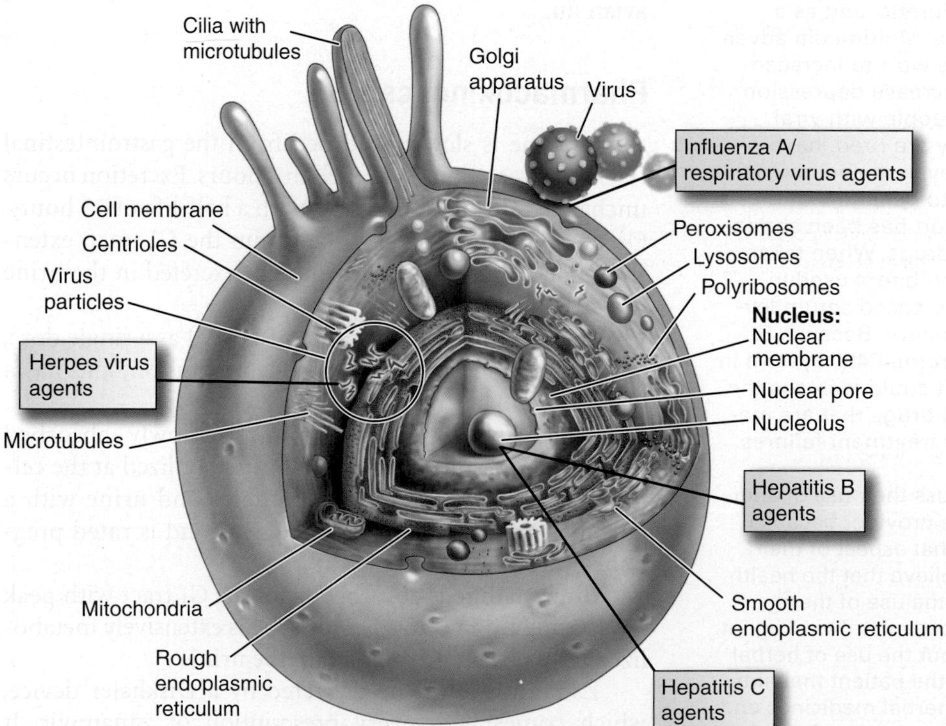

FIGURE 10.2 Agents for treating influenza A and respiratory viruses prevent shedding of the protein coat and entry of virus into the cell. Herpes virus agents alter viral DNA production. Anti–hepatitis B and C agents block DNA formation, preventing the formation of new viruses.

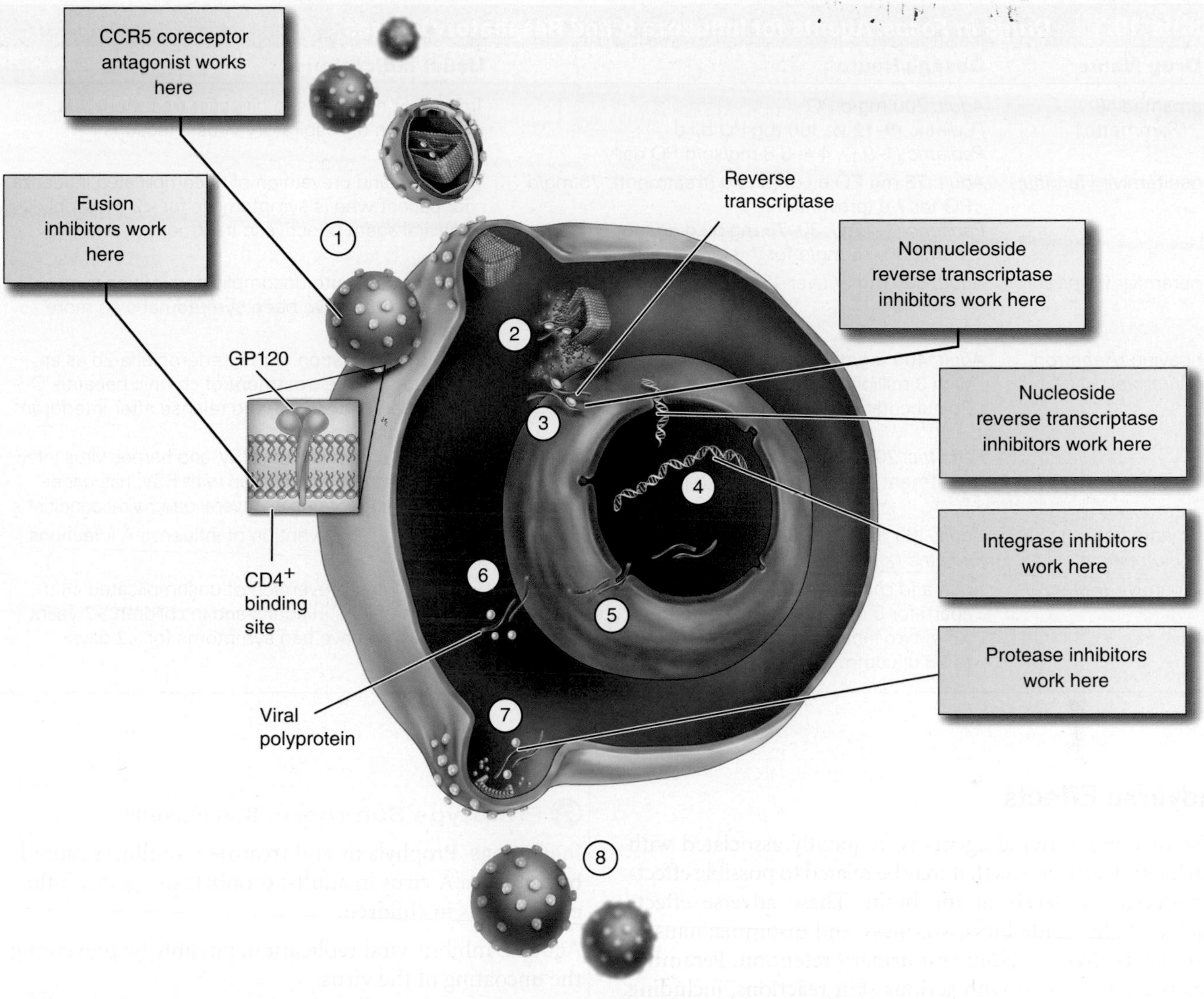

FIGURE 10.3 Agents that attempt to control HIV and AIDS work in the following ways: Interference with HIV replication by blocking synthesis of viral DNA (nonnucleoside and nucleoside reverse transcriptase inhibitors); blockage of protease within the virus, leading to immature, noninfective virus particles (protease inhibitors); prevention of virus from fusing with the cellular membrane, thereby preventing the HIV-1 virus from entering the cell (fusion inhibitors); blockage of HIV virus reaction with the receptor site that would allow it to enter the cell (CCR5 coreceptor antagonists); and prevention of necessary encoded enzyme action for viral reproduction (integrase inhibitors).

Contraindications and Cautions

Because of its renal clearance, amantadine must be used at reduced doses and with caution in patients who have any renal impairment *to avoid altered metabolism and excretion of the drug. Because it is embryotoxic in animals and crosses into breast milk*, amantadine should be used during pregnancy and lactation only if the benefits clearly outweigh the risks to the fetus or neonate.

Patients with renal dysfunction who are taking oseltamivir require reduced doses and close monitoring *to avoid altered metabolism and excretion of the drug*. Oseltamivir should be used during pregnancy and lactation only if the benefits clearly outweigh the risks to the fetus or neonate *because there are no adequate studies in pregnancy and lactation*.

Women of childbearing age should be advised to use barrier contraceptives if they are taking ribavirin. *The drug has been associated with serious fetal effects.*

Rimantadine and peramivir are *embryotoxic in animals* and should be used during pregnancy only if the benefits clearly outweigh the risks. These drugs should not be used by nursing mothers *because they cross into breast milk and can cause toxic reactions in the neonate.* Use in children should be limited to prevention of influenza A infections.

Because of the renal excretion, zanamivir must be used cautiously in patients with any renal impairment. It should be used during pregnancy and lactation only if the benefits clearly outweigh the risks to the fetus or neonate.

Table 10.1 *Drugs in Focus:* Agents for Influenza A and Respiratory Viruses

Drug Name	Dosage/Route	Usual Indications
amantadine (*Symmetrel*)	*Adult:* 200 mg/d PO *Pediatric (9–12 y):* 100 mg PO b.i.d. *Pediatric (1–9 y):* 4.4–8.8 mg/kg/d PO daily	Treatment of Parkinson disease; treatment and prevention of respiratory virus infections
oseltamivir (*Tamiflu*)	*Adult:* 75 mg PO b.i.d. for 5 d (treatment); 75 mg/d PO for 7 d (prevention) *Pediatric (1–12 y):* 30–75 mg b.i.d. PO for 5 d (treatment); 30–75 mg/d for 7 d (prevention)	Treatment and prevention of uncomplicated influenza for patient who is symptomatic for <2 days; only antiviral agent effective in treatment of avian flu
peramivir (*Rapivab*)	*Adult:* 600 mg IV over 15 min	Treatment of acute uncomplicated influenza in patients who have been symptomatic no more than 2 days
ribavirin (*Rebetron, Virazole*)	*Adult:* 400 mg/d PO in AM and 600 mg/d PO in PM with 3 million international units of interferon alfa-2b subcutaneous three times per week	Used in combination with interferon alfa-2b as an oral drug for the treatment of chronic hepatitis C in children and adults who relapse after interferon alpha therapy
	Pediatric: 20 mg/mL in the reservoir for aerosol treatment over 12–18 h each day for 3–7 d	Treatment of influenza A, RSV, and herpes virus infections; treatment of children with RSV; has undergone testing for use in several other viral conditions
rimantadine (*Flumadine*)	*Adult:* 100 mg PO b.i.d. *Pediatric (≥10 y):* 5 mg/kg PO daily	Treatment and prevention of influenza A infections
zanamivir (*Relenza*)	*Adult and children ≥7 y:* Two inhalations b.i.d. (12 h apart) for 5 d; prevention of influenza in patients >5 y; two inhalations per day for 10 d (houschold) to 28 d (community)	Treatment and prevention of uncomplicated influenza infections in adults and in children >7 years of age who have had symptoms for <2 days

RSV, respiratory syncytial virus.

Adverse Effects

Use of these antiviral agents is frequently associated with various adverse effects that may be related to possible effects on dopamine levels in the brain. These adverse effects include light-headedness, dizziness, and insomnia; nausea; orthostatic hypotension; and urinary retention. Peramivir has been associated with serious skin reactions, including Stevens-Johnson syndrome and erythema multiforme.

Clinically Important Drug–Drug Interactions

Patients who receive amantadine or rimantadine may experience increased atropine-like effects if either of these drugs is given with an anticholinergic drug. Patients taking rimantadine may also experience a loss of effectiveness of aspirin and acetaminophen if these are also being used. Ribavirin levels may be reduced if it is given with antacids. The use of ribavirin should be avoided if the patient is also receiving a nucleoside reverse transcriptase inhibitor (NRTI). Rifampin is known to decrease the effectiveness of many drugs, including antiarrhythmics, digoxin, hormonal contraceptives, corticosteroids, antifungals, and central nervous system (CNS) depressants. Patients should be monitored closely for loss of effectiveness of these drugs if this combination is used. There is an increased incidence of rifampin-related hepatitis if it is used concurrently with isoniazid. This combination should be avoided. Live attenuated nasal influenza vaccine should not be used within 2 weeks before or 48 hours after peramavir to avoid adverse reactions.

Prototype Summary: Rimantadine

Indications: Prophylaxis and treatment of illness caused by influenza A virus in adults; prophylaxis against influenza A virus in children.

Actions: Inhibits viral replication, possibly by preventing the uncoating of the virus.

Pharmacokinetics:

Route	Onset	Peak
Oral	Slow	6 h

$T_{1/2}$: 25.4 hours; excreted unchanged in the urine.

Adverse Effects: Light-headedness, dizziness, insomnia, nausea, dyspnea, orthostatic hypotension, depression.

Nursing Considerations for Patients Receiving Agents for Influenza A and Respiratory Viruses

Assessment: History and Examination

- Assess for *contraindications or cautions*: Known history of allergy to antivirals *to avoid hypersensitivity reactions*; history of liver or renal dysfunction *that might interfere with drug metabolism and excretion*; and current status

related to pregnancy or lactation *to prevent adverse effects on the fetus or nursing baby.*
- Perform a physical assessment to *establish baseline data for evaluating the effectiveness of the drug and the occurrence of any adverse effects associated with drug therapy.*
- Assess for orientation and reflexes *to evaluate any CNS effects of the drug*; vital signs (temperature, respiratory rate, breath sounds for adventitious sounds) *to assess for signs and symptoms of the viral infection;* blood pressure *to monitor for orthostatic hypotension;* urinary output *to monitor genitourinary (GU) effects of the drug*; and renal and hepatic function tests *to determine baseline function of these organs and to assess adverse effects on the kidney or liver and need to adjust the dose of the drug*; skin *to evaluate for potentially serious dermatological reactions.*

Nursing Diagnoses

Nursing diagnoses related to drug therapy might include the following:

- Acute pain related to GI, CNS, or GU effects of the drug
- Disturbed sensory perception (kinesthetic) related to CNS effects of the drug
- Deficient knowledge regarding drug therapy

Planning

- The patient will receive the best therapeutic effect from the drug therapy.
- The patient will have limited adverse effects to the drug therapy.
- The patient will have an understanding of the drug therapy, adverse effects to anticipate, and measures to relieve discomfort and improve safety.

Implementation with Rationale

- Start the drug regimen as soon after exposure to the virus as possible, usually within 2 days of the start of symptoms *to enhance effectiveness and decrease the risk of complications due to viral infection.*
- Administer influenza A vaccine before the flu season begins, if at all possible, *to decrease the risk of contracting the flu and decrease the risk of complications.*
- Administer the full course of the drug *to obtain the full beneficial effects.*
- Provide safety provisions if CNS effects occur *to protect the patient from injury.*
- Instruct the patient about the appropriate dosage-scheduling regimen; safety precautions, including changing position slowly and avoiding driving and hazardous tasks that should be taken if CNS effects occur; and the need to report any adverse effects such as difficulty walking or talking *to enhance patient knowledge about drug therapy and to promote compliance.*

Evaluation

- Monitor patient response to the drug (prevention of respiratory flu-like symptoms; alleviation of flu-like symptoms).
- Monitor for adverse effects (changes in orientation and affect, blood pressure, urinary output, skin changes, liver or renal function test changes).
- Determine the effectiveness of the teaching plan (patient can name the drug, dosage, possible adverse effects to watch for, and specific measures to help to avoid or minimize adverse effects).
- Monitor the effectiveness of comfort and safety measures and compliance with the regimen.

KEY POINTS

- Viruses are segments of RNA or DNA enclosed in a protein coat.
- A virus must enter a human cell to survive, making it difficult to treat without serious toxic effects for the host.
- Antiviral drugs that prevent the viral replication of respiratory viruses can be used to prevent or treat influenza A or other respiratory viruses.

Agents for Herpes and Cytomegalovirus

Herpes viruses account for a broad range of conditions, including cold sores, encephalitis, shingles, and genital infections. **Cytomegalovirus** (CMV), although slightly different from the herpes virus, can affect the eye, respiratory tract, and liver and reacts to many of the same drugs. Antiviral drugs used to combat these infections include acyclovir (*Zovirax*), cidofovir (*Vistide*), famciclovir (*Famvir*), foscarnet (*Foscavir*), ganciclovir (*Cytovene*), valacyclovir (*Valtrex*), and valganciclovir (*Valcyte*)—see Table 10.2.

Therapeutic Actions and Indications

Drugs that combat herpes and CMV inhibit viral DNA replication by competing with viral substrates to form shorter, noneffective DNA chains (see Figure 10.2). This action prevents replication of the virus, but it has little effect on the host cells of humans because human cell DNA uses different substrates. These antiviral agents are indicated for treatment of the DNA viruses herpes simplex, herpes zoster, and CMV. Research has shown that they are very effective in immunocompromised individuals, such as patients with AIDS, those taking immunosuppressants,elderly patients, and those with multiple infections. See Table 10.2 for usual indications for each of these agents.

Table 10.2 ***Drugs in Focus:* Agents for Herpes Virus and Cytomegalovirus**

Drug Name	Dosage/Route	Usual Indications
✱acyclovir (*Zovirax*)	*Adult:* 5–10 mg/kg q8h IV, IM, or subcutaneous *or* 200 mg q4h per day for 10 d and then 400 mg PO b.i.d. for 12 mo *Pediatric:* 250–500 mg/m² q8h IV, IM, or subcutaneous for 7–10 d *or* 20 mg/kg q.i.d. PO for 5 d	Treatment of herpes virus infections
cidofovir (*Vistide*)	5 mg/kg IV (over 1 h) once weekly for 2 wk, then every other week, with probenecid 2 g PO at 3 h before and 1 g PO at 2 and 8 h after cidofovir infusion	Treatment of CMV retinitis in AIDS patients
famciclovir (*Famvir*)	*Herpes zoster:* 500 mg PO q8h for 7 d *Genital herpes:* 125 mg b.i.d. PO for 5 d	Treatment of herpes virus infections such as herpes zoster or shingles and for recurrent episodes of genital herpes
foscarnet (*Foscavir*)	*Adult:* 40–60 mg/kg q8–12h IV given as a 2-h infusion *Pediatric:* Safety and efficacy not established	Treatment of CMV and acyclovir-resistant mucocutaneous herpes simplex infections in immunocompromised patients
ganciclovir (*Cytovene*)	*Adult:* 5 m/kg q12h IV given over 1 h for 14–21 d, then over 1 h daily 7 d/wk or 6 mg/kg/d for 5 d/wk for prophylaxis	Long-term treatment and prevention of CMV infection
valacyclovir (*Valtrex*)	*Herpes zoster:* 1 g PO t.i.d. for 7 d *Genital herpes:* 500 mg b.i.d. PO for 5 d	Treatment of herpes zoster and recurrent genital herpes; cold sores (herpes labialis)
valganciclovir (*Valcyte*)	900 mg PO b.i.d. for 21 d, then 900 mg PO once a day for maintenance; reduce dose with renal impairment	Treatment of CMV retinitis in AIDS patients

CMV, cytomegalovirus.

Pharmacokinetics

Most of the agents for herpes and CMV are readily absorbed and excreted through the kidney. Although cidofovir has been proven to be embryotoxic in animals, no adequate studies have been completed for the other agents.

Acyclovir, which can be given orally and parenterally or applied topically, reaches peak levels within 1 hour and has a half-life of 2.5 to 5 hours. It is excreted unchanged in the urine. It crosses into breast milk, which exposes the neonate to high levels of the drug.

Cidofovir, which is given by IV infusion, reaches peak levels at the end of the infusion and in studies was cleared from the system within 15 minutes after the infusion. It is excreted unchanged in the urine and must be given with probenecid to increase renal clearance of the drug. The dose must be decreased according to renal function and creatinine clearance; renal function tests must be done before each dose and the dose planned accordingly.

Famciclovir, an oral drug, is well absorbed from the GI tract, reaching peak levels in 2 to 3 hours. Famciclovir is metabolized in the liver and excreted in the urine and feces. It has a half-life of 2 hours and is known to cross the placenta.

Foscarnet is available in IV form only. It reaches peak levels at the end of the infusion and has a half-life of 4 hours. About 90% of foscarnet is excreted unchanged in the urine, making it highly toxic to the kidneys. Use caution and at reduced dose in patients with renal impairment.

Ganciclovir is available in IV and oral forms. It has a slow onset and reaches peak levels at 1 hour if given IV and 2 to 4 hours if given orally. This drug is primarily excreted unchanged in the feces with some urinary excretion, with a half-life of 2 to 4 hours.

Valacyclovir is an oral agent and is rapidly absorbed from the GI tract and metabolized in the liver to acyclovir. Excretion occurs through the urine, so caution should be used in patients with renal impairment.

Valganciclovir is an oral prodrug (i.e., it is immediately converted to ganciclovir once it is in the body). It is rapidly absorbed and reaches peak levels in 3 hours. It is primarily excreted unchanged in the feces with some urinary excretion, with a half-life of 2.5 to 3 hours.

Contraindications and Cautions

Drugs indicated for the treatment of herpes and CMV are highly toxic and should not be used during pregnancy or lactation *to prevent adverse effects on the fetus or infant*; use only if the benefits clearly outweigh the potential risks to the fetus or infant. Avoid use in patients with known allergies to antiviral agents *to prevent serious hypersensitivity reactions*; in patients with renal disease, *which could interfere with excretion of the drug*; or in patients with severe CNS disorders *because the drug can affect the CNS, causing headache, neuropathy, paresthesias, confusion, and hallucinations.*

Cidofovir has been proven to be embryotoxic in animals. Use cidofovir with caution in children with AIDS *because of the potential carcinogenic effects and effects on fertility*. If no other treatment option is available, monitor the child very closely.

For famciclovir, safety of use in children younger than 18 years of age has not been established.

Foscarnet *has been shown to affect bone development and growth.* Foscarnet, as well as ganciclovir and valganciclovir, should not be used in children unless the benefit clearly outweighs the risk and the child is monitored very closely.

Adverse Effects

The adverse effects most commonly associated with these antivirals include nausea and vomiting, headache, depression, paresthesias, neuropathy, rash, and hair loss (Figure 10.4). Rash, inflammation, and burning often occur at sites of IV injection and topical application. Renal dysfunction and renal failure also have been reported. Cidofovir is associated with severe renal toxicity and granulocytopenia. Ganciclovir and valganciclovir have been associated with bone marrow suppression. Foscarnet has been associated with seizures, especially in patients with electrolyte imbalance.

Clinically Important Drug–Drug Interactions

The risk of nephrotoxicity increases when agents indicated for the treatment of herpes and CMV are used in combination with other nephrotoxic drugs, such as the aminoglycoside antibiotics.

The risk of drowsiness also rises when these antiviral agents are taken with zidovudine, an antiretroviral agent.

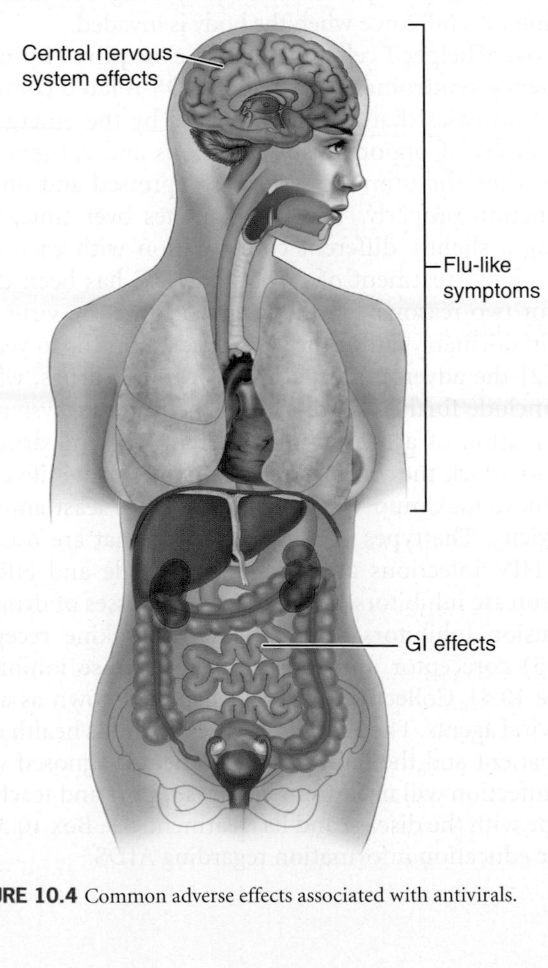

FIGURE 10.4 Common adverse effects associated with antivirals.

Ⓟ Prototype Summary: Acyclovir

Indications: Treatment of herpes simplex virus (HSV) 1 and 2 infections; treatment of severe genital HSV infections, treatment of HSV encephalitis; acute treatment of shingles and chickenpox; ointment for the treatment of genital herpes infections; cream for the treatment of cold sores (herpes labialis).

Actions: Inhibits viral DNA replication.

Pharmacokinetics:

Route	Onset	Peak	Duration
Oral	Varies	1.5–2 h	Not known
IV	Immediate	1 h	8 h
Topical	Not generally absorbed systemically		

$T_{1/2}$: 2.5 to 5 hours; excreted unchanged in the urine.

Adverse Effects: Headache, vertigo, tremors, nausea, vomiting, rash.

Nursing Considerations for Patients Receiving Agents for Herpes Virus and Cytomegalovirus

Assessment: History and Examination

- Assess patients receiving DNA-active antiviral agents for *contraindications or cautions*: any history of allergy to antivirals *to avoid hypersensitivity reactions*; renal dysfunction *that might interfere with the metabolism and excretion of the drug and increase the risk of renal toxicity*; severe CNS disorders *that could be aggravated*; and pregnancy or lactation *to prevent adverse effects on the fetus or nursing baby.*
- Perform a physical assessment *to establish baseline data for assessing the effectiveness of the DNA-active antiviral drug and the occurrence of any adverse effects associated with drug therapy.*
- Assess orientation and reflexes *to monitor CNS baseline and adverse effects of the drug.*
- Examine skin (color, temperature, and lesions) *to monitor adverse effects such as rashes.*
- Evaluate renal function tests *to determine baseline function of the kidneys and to assess adverse effects on the kidney and need to adjust the dose of the drug.*

Nursing Diagnoses

Nursing diagnoses related to drug therapy might include the following:

- Acute pain related to GI, CNS, or local effects of the drug
- Disturbed sensory perception (kinesthetic) related to CNS effects of the drug
- Deficient knowledge regarding drug therapy

(continues on page 150)

Planning

- The patient will receive the best therapeutic effect from the drug therapy.
- The patient will have limited adverse effects to the drug therapy.
- The patient will have an understanding of the drug therapy, adverse effects to anticipate, and measures to relieve discomfort and improve safety.

Implementation with Rationale

- Administer the drug as soon as possible after the diagnosis has been made *to improve effectiveness of the antiviral activity.*
- Ensure good hydration *to decrease the toxic effects on the kidneys.*
- Ensure that the patient takes the complete course of the drug regimen *to improve effectiveness and decrease the risk of the emergence of resistant viruses.*
- Wear protective gloves when applying the drug topically *to decrease the risk of exposure to the drug and inadvertent absorption.*
- Provide safety precautions (e.g., use of side rails, appropriate lighting, orientation, assistance) if CNS effects occur *to protect the patient from injury.*
- Warn the patient that GI upset, nausea, and vomiting can occur *to prevent undue anxiety and increase awareness of the importance of nutrition.*
- Monitor renal function tests periodically during treatment *to ensure prompt detection and early intervention, should renal toxicity develop.*
- Instruct the patient about the drug *to enhance patient knowledge about drug therapy and to promote compliance.*
- Provide the following patient teaching:
  - Avoid sexual intercourse if genital herpes is being treated because these drugs do not cure the disease.
  - Wear protective gloves when applying topical agents.
  - Avoid driving and hazardous tasks if dizziness or drowsiness occurs.

Evaluation

- Monitor patient response to the drug (alleviation of signs and symptoms of herpes or CMV infection).
- Monitor for adverse effects (orientation and affect, GI upset, and renal function).
- Evaluate the effectiveness of the teaching plan (patient can name the drug, dosage, possible adverse effects to watch for, and specific measures to help avoid adverse effects).
- Monitor the effectiveness of comfort and safety measures and compliance with the regimen.

KEY POINTS

- Drugs that interfere with viral DNA replication are used to treat herpes infections and CMV infections.
- These antiviral drugs are associated with GI upset and nausea, confusion, insomnia, and dizziness.

Agents for HIV and AIDS

Human immunodeficiency virus (HIV) attacks the **helper T cells** [CD4 (cluster of differentiation 4) cells] within the immune system. This virus (an RNA strand) reacts with a receptor site on the CD cell, fuses with the membrane, and then enters the helper T cell, where it uses reverse transcriptase to copy the RNA and produce a double-stranded viral DNA. The virus uses various nucleosides found in the cell to synthesize this DNA strand. The DNA enters the host cell nucleus and slides into the chromosomal DNA to change the cell's processes to ones that produce new viruses. This changes the cell into a virus-producing cell. As a result, the cell loses its ability to perform normal immune functions. The newly produced viruses mature through the action of various proteases and then are released from the cell. Upon release, they find a new cell to invade, and the process begins again. Eventually, as more and more viruses are released and invade more CD4 cells the immune system loses an important mechanism responsible for propelling the immune reaction into full force when the body is invaded.

Loss of helper T cell function causes **acquired immune deficiency syndrome (AIDS)** and **AIDS-related complex (ARC)**, diseases that are characterized by the emergence of a variety of opportunistic infections and cancers that occur when the immune system is depressed and unable to function properly. The HIV mutates over time, presenting a slightly different configuration with each new generation. Treatment of AIDS and ARC has been difficult for two reasons: (1) the length of time the virus can remain dormant within the T cells (i.e., months to years), and (2) the adverse effects of many potent drugs, which may include further depression of the immune system. A combination of at least three different antiviral drugs is used to attack the virus at various points in its life cycle to achieve maximum effectiveness with the least amount of toxicity. The types of antiviral agents that are used to treat HIV infections are the nonnucleoside and NRTIs, the protease inhibitors, and three newer classes of drugs—the fusion inhibitors, CCR5 (C–C chemokine receptor type 5) coreceptor antagonists, and integrase inhibitors (Table 10.3). Collectively, these drugs are known as antiretroviral agents. The HIV virus poses a serious health risk. The patient and the family of the patient diagnosed with HIV infection will need tremendous support and teaching to cope with the disease and its treatment. See Box 10.3 for public education information regarding AIDS.

Table 10.3 ***Drugs in Focus:*** **Agents for HIV and AIDS**

Drug Name	Dosage/Route	Usual Indications
Nonnucleoside Reverse Transcriptase Inhibitors		
delavirdine (*Rescriptor*)	*Adult:* 400 mg PO t.i.d.	Part of combination therapy regimens for treatment of HIV in adults
efavirenz (*Sustiva*)	*Adult:* 600 mg/d PO *Pediatric:* Dose determined by age and weight	Treatment of adults and children with HIV in combination with other antiretroviral agents
etravirine (*Intelance*)	*Adult:* 200 mg PO b.i.d after a meal *Pediatric:* Based on weight, 100–200 mg PO b.i.d	Treatment of HIV in adults with treatment experience who have evidence of viral replication and HIV strains resistant to standard therapy
nevirapine (*Viramune*)	*Adult:* 200 mg/d PO for 14 d, then 200 mg PO b.i.d. *Pediatric:* 4 mg/kg PO for 14 d, then 4–7 mg/kg PO b.i.d.	Treatment of adults or children with HIV in combination with other antiretroviral agents
Rilpivirine (*Edurant*)	*Adult:* 25 mg/d PO with food	Combination treatment of adults with HIV-1 infection
Nucleoside Reverse Transcriptase Inhibitors		
abacavir (*Ziagen*)	*Adult:* 300 mg PO b.i.d. *Pediatric:* 8 mg/kg PO b.i.d.	Combination therapy for the treatment of adults and children with HIV
didanosine (*Videx*)	*Adult:* 250–400 mg/d PO *or* 125–200 mg PO b.i.d. *Pediatric:* 120 mg/m^2 PO b.i.d.	Treatment of advanced infections in adults and children with HIV as part of combination therapy
emtricitabine (*Emtriva*)	*Adult:* 200 mg/d PO *or* 240 mg oral solution/d *Pediatric (3 mo–17 y):* 6 mg/kg/d PO to a maximum 240 mg	Part of combination therapy for treatment of HIV-1 infection
lamivudine (*Epivir*)	*Adult:* 150 mg PO b.i.d.; for chronic hepatitis B, 100 mg PO q.d. *Pediatric (3 mo–16 y):* 4 mg/kg PO b.i.d.	With other antiretroviral agents for the treatment of adults and children with HIV; as an oral solution for the treatment of chronic hepatitis B
stavudine (*Zerit XR*)	*Adult (≥60 kg):* 100 mg/d PO *Adult (30–60 kg):* 75 mg/d PO *Pediatric:* based on weight	Treatment of patients with HIV in combination with other antiretroviral agents
tenofovir (*Viread*)	*Adult:* 300 mg/d PO *Pediatric:* 8 mg/kg/day PO (for HIV, not recommended for hepatitis B)	Treatment of adults with HIV infection in combination with other antiretroviral drugs; treatment of chronic hepatitis B
AZT (*Retrovir, Aztec*)	*Adult:* 100 mg PO q4h *Pediatric (6 wk–12 y):* 90–180 mg/m^2 PO q6h *Maternal:* 100 mg PO five times per day from 14-wk gestation until start of labor	Treatment of symptomatic HIV in adults and children as part of combination therapy; prevention of maternal transmission of HIV
Protease Inhibitors		
atazanavir (*Reyataz*)	*Adult:* 400 mg PO, q8h	Treatment of adults with HIV as part of combination therapy
darunavir (*Prezista*)	*Adult:* 600 mg PO b.i.d with ritonavir 100 mg PO b.i.d	Treatment of adults with advanced HIV disease with progression following standard treatment, used as part of combination therapy that must contain ritonavir
fosamprenavir (*Lexiva*)	*Adult:* 1,400 mg/d PO with 100 mg/d ritonavir PO *or* 700 mg PO b.i.d. with ritonavir 100 mg PO b.i.d. *Pediatric:* 18–30 mg/kg b.i.d oral suspension, based on weight with ritonavir 3 mg/kg PO b.i.d	Part of combination therapy for the treatment of HIV
indinavir (*Crixivan*)	*Adult:* 800 mg PO q8h	Treatment of adults with HIV as part of combination therapy
lopinavir (*Kaletra*)	*Adult:* 3 capsules *or* 5 mL PO b.i.d. *Pediatric (6 mo–12 y):* 10–12 mg/kg PO b.i.d.	Treatment of adults and children with HIV in combination with other antiretroviral agents
nelfinavir (*Viracept*)	*Adult:* 750 mg PO t.i.d. *Pediatric (2–13 y):* 20–30 mg/kg per dose PO t.i.d.	Combination therapy for the treatment of adults and children with HIV
ritonavir (*Norvir*)	*Adult and pediatric (>2 y):* 600 mg PO b.i.d.	Part of combination therapy for the treatment of adults and children with HIV
saquinavir (*Invirase*)	*Adult:* 1,000 mg PO b.i.d with ritonavir 100 mg PO b.i.d	Treatment of adults with HIV as part of combination therapy
tipranavir (*Aptivus*)	*Adult:* 500 mg/d PO with 200 mg ritonavir	Treatment of adults with HIV in combination with ritonavir

(table continues on page 152)

Table 10.3 *Drugs in Focus:* Agents for HIV and AIDS (continued)

Drug Name	Dosage/Route	Usual Indications
Fusion Inhibitor		
enfuvirtide (*Fuzeon*)	*Adult:* 90 mg PO b.i.d. by subcutaneous injection *Pediatric 6–16 y:* 2 mg/kg b.i.d. by subcutaneous injection	Part of combination therapy in treatment of HIV patients with evidence of HIV replication despite antiretroviral therapy
CCR5 Coreceptor Antagonist		
maraviroc (*Selzentry*)	*Adult:* 150 mg PO b.i.d.	Part of combination therapy for treatment of HIV-1 infections
Integrase Inhibitor		
dolutegravir (*Tivicay*)	*Adult and children 12 and older:* 50 mg/day PO in combination with other antiretrovirals	Part of combination therapy for treatment of HIV-1 infections
raltegravir (*Isentress*)	*Adult:* 400 mg PO b.i.d.	Part of combination therapy for treatment of HIV-1 infections

AZT, zidovudine.

Nonnucleoside Reverse Transcriptase Inhibitors

The nonnucleoside reverse transcriptase inhibitors have direct effects on the HIV virus activities within the cell. The **nonnucleoside reverse transcriptase inhibitors** available include delavirdine (*Rescriptor*), efavirenz (*Sustiva*), etravirine (*Intelence*), nevirapine (*Viramune*), and rilpivirine (*Edurant*).

Therapeutic Actions and Indications

The nonnucleoside reverse transcriptase inhibitors bind directly to HIV reverse transcriptase, blocking both RNA- and DNA-dependent DNA polymerase activities. They prevent the transfer of information that would allow the virus to carry on the formation of viral DNA. As a result, the virus is unable to take over the cell and reproduce. These antiviral agents are indicated for the treatment of patients with documented AIDS or ARC who have decreased numbers of helper T cells and evidence of increased opportunistic infections in combination with other antiviral drugs (see Table 10.3).

Pharmacokinetics

Delavirdine is rapidly absorbed from the GI tract, with peak levels occurring within 1 hour. Delavirdine is extensively metabolized by the cytochrome P450 system in the liver and is excreted through the urine.

BOX 10.3 FOCUS ON The Evidence

Public Education about AIDS

When acquired immune deficiency syndrome (AIDS) was first diagnosed in the early 1980s, it was found in a certain population in New York City. The people in this group tended to be homosexuals, IV drug users, and debilitated persons with poor hygiene and nutrition habits. Originally, a number of health care practitioners thought that the disease was a syndrome of opportunistic infections that occurred in a population with repeated exposures to infections that naturally deplete the immune system. It was not until several years later that the human immunodeficiency virus (HIV) was identified. Since then, it has been discovered that HIV infection is rampant in many African countries. The infection also has spread throughout the United States in populations that are neither homosexual nor IV drug users, who have good nutrition and hygiene habits. As health care practitioners have learned, HIV is not particular about the body it invades. Once introduced into a body, it infects T cells and causes HIV infection.

The evidence shows that when a patient is diagnosed with HIV infection the nurse faces a tremendous challenge for patient education and support. The patient and any significant others should be counseled about the risks of transmission and reassured about ways in which the virus is not transmitted. They will need to learn about drug protocols, T cell levels, adverse drug effects, and anticipated progress of the disease. They also will need consistent support and a telephone number to call with questions at any time. Many communities have AIDS support groups and other resources that can be very helpful; the nurse can direct the patient to these resources as appropriate.

The combinations of drugs that are being used today and the constant development of more drugs make the disease less of a death sentence than it was in the past. The result, however, is that many people must take a large number of pills each day, at tremendous cost and inconvenience. Many people today do live for many years with HIV infection. An AIDS vaccine is currently being studied and offers hope for preventing this disease in the future.

Public education is key for promoting the acceptance and support of patients with HIV infection or AIDS, who need a great deal of support and assistance. Nurses can be role models for dealing with HIV patients and can provide informal public education whenever the opportunity presents.

Efavirenz is absorbed rapidly from the GI tract, reaching peak levels in 3 to 5 hours. Efavirenz is metabolized in the liver by the cytochrome P450 system and is excreted in the urine and feces with a half-life of 52 to 76 hours.

Etravirine is rapidly absorbed from the GI tract, reaching peak levels in 2.5 to 4 hours. Etravirine is metabolized in the liver by the cytochrome P450 system and is excreted in feces and urine with a half-life of 21 to 61 hours.

Nevirapine is recommended for use in adults and children older than 2 months. After rapid GI absorption with a peak effect occurring at 4 hours, nevirapine is metabolized by the cytochrome P450 system in the liver. Excretion is through the urine with a half-life of 45 hours. Box 10.4 provides information about the emergence of resistance to certain reverse transcriptase inhibitor combinations.

Rilpivirine (*Edurant*) is the newest drug in this class. It is rapidly absorbed from the GI tract, reaching peak levels in 4 to 5 hours. It is metabolized in the liver and excreted in feces and urine with a half-life of 50 hours.

Contraindications and Cautions

There are no adequate studies of nonnucleoside reverse transcriptase inhibitors in pregnancy, so use should be limited to situations in which the benefits clearly outweigh any risks. It is suggested that women not breastfeed if they are infected with HIV. Safety for the use of delavirdine in children has not been established.

Adverse Effects

The adverse effects most commonly experienced with these drugs are GI related—dry mouth, constipation or diarrhea, nausea, abdominal pain, and dyspepsia. Dizziness, blurred vision, and headache have also been reported. A flu-like syndrome of fever, muscle aches and pains, fatigue, and loss of appetite often occurs with the anti-HIV drugs, but these signs and symptoms may also be related to the underlying disease.

Clinically Important Drug–Drug Interactions

Life-threatening effects can occur if delavirdine is combined with antiarrhythmics, clarithromycin, dapsone, antituberculosis drugs, calcium-channel blockers, warfarin, quinidine, indinavir, saquinavir, or dapsone. These combinations should be avoided if at all possible. There is a risk of serious adverse effects if efavirenz is combined with midazolam, rifabutin, triazolam, or ergot derivatives; these combinations should be avoided. There may be a lack of effectiveness if nevirapine is combined with hormonal contraceptives or protease inhibitors. St. John's wort should not be used with these drugs; a decrease in antiviral effects can occur.

Prototype Summary: Nevirapine

Indications: Treatment of HIV-1–infected patients who have experienced clinical or immunological deterioration, in combination with other antiretrovirals.

Actions: Binds to HIV-1 reverse transcriptase and blocks replication of the HIV by changing the structure of the HIV enzyme.

Pharmacokinetics:

Route	Onset	Peak
Oral	Rapid	4 h

$T_{1/2}$: 45 hours, then 25 to 30 hours; metabolized in the liver and excreted in the urine.

Adverse Effects: Headache, nausea, vomiting, diarrhea, rash, liver dysfunction, chills, fever.

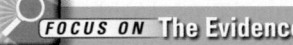

BOX 10.4 FOCUS ON The Evidence

HIV Resistance

In late 2003 Gilead Sciences, Inc. notified health care professionals of a high rate of early virological failure and the emergence of nucleoside reverse transcriptase inhibitor (NRTI) resistance–associated mutations. This was observed in a clinical study of HIV-infected, treatment-naive patients receiving a once-daily triple NRTI regimen containing didanosine enteric-coated beadlets (*Videx EC*), lamivudine (*Epivir*), and tenofovir disoproxil fumarate (*Viread*).

Based on these studies, tenofovir in combination with didanosine and lamivudine is not recommended when considering a new treatment regimen for therapy-naive or experienced patients with HIV infection. Patients currently on this regimen should be considered for treatment modification.

In a similar study, patients receiving unboosted *Reyataz* (atazanavir sulfate) and *Viread* (tenofovir) showed less decrease in viral concentrations and loss of virological response, which could show a possible resistance to *Reyataz*. For patients taking atazanavir and tenofovir, the Food and Drug Administration advises that a boosted dose of atazanavir should be used to overcome a decrease in concentration of the drug that seems to occur when it is used with tenofovir.

Nucleoside Reverse Transcriptase Inhibitors

The **nucleoside reverse transcriptase inhibitors (NRTIs)** (Table 10.3) were the first class of drugs developed to treat HIV infections. These are drugs that compete with the naturally occurring nucleosides within a human cell that the virus would need to develop. The NRTIs include the following agents: abacavir (*Ziagen*), didanosine (*Videx*), emtricitabine (*Emtriva*), lamivudine (*Epivir*), stavudine (*Zerit XR*), tenofovir (*Viread*), and zidovudine (*Retrovir*).

Therapeutic Actions and Indications

NRTIs compete with the naturally occurring nucleosides within the cell that the virus would use to build the DNA chain. These nucleosides, however, lack a substance needed to extend the DNA chain. As a result, the DNA chain cannot lengthen and cannot insert itself into the host DNA. Thus the virus cannot reproduce. They are used as part of combination therapy for the treatment of HIV infection. See Table 10.3 for usual indications for each of these agents.

Pharmacokinetics

Abacavir is an oral drug that is rapidly absorbed from the GI tract. It is metabolized in the liver and excreted in feces and urine with a half-life of 1 to 2 hours.

Didanosine is rapidly destroyed in an acid environment and therefore must be taken in a buffered form. It reaches peak levels in 15 to 75 minutes. Didanosine undergoes intracellular metabolism with a half-life of 8 to 24 hours. It is excreted in the urine.

Emtricitabine has the advantage of being a one-capsule-a-day therapy. Emtricitabine has a rapid onset and peaks in 1 to 2 hours. It has a half-life of 10 hours, and after being metabolized in the liver is excreted in the urine and feces. Dose needs to be reduced in patients with renal impairment. It has been associated with severe and even fatal hepatomegaly with steatosis, a fatty degeneration of the liver.

Lamivudine is rapidly absorbed from the GI tract and is excreted primarily unchanged in the urine. It peaks within 4 hours and has a half-life of 5 to 7 hours. Because excretion depends on renal function, dose reduction is recommended in the presence of renal impairment. The drug is available as an oral solution, *Epivir-HBV*; it is also recommended for the treatment of chronic hepatitis B.

Stavudine is rapidly absorbed from the GI tract, reaching peak levels in 1 hour. Most of the drug is excreted unchanged in the urine, making it important to reduce dose and monitor patients carefully in the presence of renal dysfunction. It can be used for adults and children and is only available in an extended release form, allowing for once-a-day dosing.

Tenofovir is a newer drug that affects the virus at a slightly different point in replication—a nucleotide that becomes a nucleoside. It is used only in combination with other antiretroviral agents. It is rapidly absorbed from the GI tract, reaching peak levels in 45 to 75 minutes. Its metabolism is not known, but it is excreted in the urine.

Zidovudine was one of the first drugs found to be effective in the treatment of AIDS. It is rapidly absorbed from the GI tract, with peak levels occurring within 30 to 75 minutes. Zidovudine is metabolized in the liver and excreted in the urine, with a half-life of 1 hour.

Contraindications and Cautions

Of the nucleosides, zidovudine is the only agent that has been proven to be safe when used during pregnancy. Of the other agents, *there have been no adequate studies in pregnancy*, so use should be limited to situations in which the benefits clearly outweigh any risks. Women infected with HIV are urged not to breastfeed. Tenofovir, zidovudine, and emtricitabine should be used with caution in the presence of hepatic dysfunction or severe renal impairment *because of their effects on the liver and kidneys.* Zidovudine should also be used with caution with any bone marrow suppression *because it could aggravate the suppression.*

Adverse Effects

Serious-to-fatal hypersensitivity reactions have occurred with abacavir, and it must be stopped immediately at any sign of a hypersensitivity reaction (fever, chills, rash, fatigue, GI upset, flu-like symptoms). Patients exhibiting any signs of hypersensitivity should be listed with the Abacavir Hypersensitivity Registry, a drug follow-up registry that is maintained by the drug company and reported to the U.S. Food and Drug Administration.

Serious pancreatitis, hepatomegaly, and neurological problems have been reported with didanosine, which is why its use is limited to the treatment of advanced infections.

Emtricitabine has been associated with severe and even fatal hepatomegaly with steatosis.

Severe hepatomegaly with steatosis has been reported with tenofovir, so it must be used with extreme caution in any patient with hepatic impairment or lactic acidosis. Patients also need to be alerted that the drug may cause changes in body fat distribution, with loss of fat from arms, legs, and face and deposition of fat on the trunk, neck, and breasts.

Severe bone marrow suppression has occurred with zidovudine.

Clinically Significant Drug–Drug Interactions

Tenofovir can cause large increases in the serum level of didanosine. If both of these drugs are given, tenofovir should be given 2 hours before or 1 hour after didanosine. Lamivudine and zalcitabine inhibit the effects of each other and should not be used together. Severe toxicity can occur if abacavir is combined with alcohol; this combination should be avoided. Didanosine can cause decreased effects of several antibiotics and antifungals; any antibiotic or antifungal started with didanosine should be evaluated carefully. There is an increased risk of potentially fatal pancreatitis if stavudine is combined with didanosine and increased risk of severe hepatomegaly if it is combined with other nonnucleoside antivirals; these combinations are often used, and the patient needs to be monitored very closely. There have been reports of severe drowsiness and lethargy if zidovudine is combined with cyclosporine; warn the patient to take appropriate safety precautions.

Ⓟ Prototype Summary: Zidovudine

Indications: Management of adults with symptomatic HIV infection in combination with other antiretrovirals; prevention of maternal–fetal HIV transmission.

Actions: A thymidine analogue that is activated to a triphosphate form, which inhibits the replication of various retroviruses, including HIV.

Pharmacokinetics:

Route	Onset	Peak
Oral	Varies	30–90 min
IV	Rapid	End of infusion

$T_{1/2}$: 30 to 60 minutes; metabolized in the liver and excreted in the urine.

Adverse Effects: Headache, insomnia, dizziness, nausea, diarrhea, fever, rash, bone marrow suppression.

Protease Inhibitors

The **protease inhibitors** block protease activity within the HIV virus. The protease inhibitors that are available for use include atazanavir (*Reyataz*), darunavir (Prezista), fosamprenavir (*Lexiva*), indinavir (*Crixivan*), lopinavir (*Kaletra*), nelfinavir (*Viracept*), ritonavir (*Norvir*), saquinavir (*Fortovase*), and tipranavir (*Aptivus*).

Therapeutic Actions and Indications

Protease is essential for the maturation of an infectious virus; without it an HIV particle is immature and noninfective, unable to fuse with and inject itself into a cell. All of these drugs are used as part of combination therapy for the treatment of HIV infection (see Table 10.3).

Pharmacokinetics

Atazanavir is rapidly absorbed from the GI tract and can be taken with food. After metabolism in the liver, it is excreted in the urine and feces with a half-life of 6.5 to 7.9 hours. It is not recommended for patients with severe hepatic impairment; for those with moderate hepatic impairment the dose should be reduced.

Darunavir is well absorbed from the GI tract, reaching peak levels in 2.5 to 4 hours. It is metabolized in the liver and excreted in the urine and feces with a half life of 15 hours. It is not recommended for patients with severe hepatic impairment.

Fosamprenavir is rapidly absorbed after oral administration, reaching peak levels in 1.5 to 4 hours. It is metabolized in the liver and excreted in the urine and feces.

Indinavir is rapidly absorbed from the GI tract, reaching peak levels in 0.8 hour. Indinavir is metabolized in the liver by the cytochrome P450 system. It is excreted in the urine with a half-life of 1.8 hours. Patients with hepatic or renal impairment are at risk for increased toxic effects, necessitating a reduction in dose.

Lopinavir is used as a fixed combination drug that combines lopinavir and ritonavir. The ritonavir inhibits the metabolism of lopinavir, leading to increased lopinavir serum levels and effectiveness. (Box 10.5 reviews the dose calculation with lopinavir.). It is readily absorbed from the GI tract, reaching peak levels in 3 to 4 hours, and undergoes extensive hepatic metabolism by the cytochrome P450 system. Lopinavir is excreted in urine and feces.

Tipranavir is used for the treatment of HIV infection in adults in combination with 200 mg of ritonavir. It is taken orally with food, two 250-mg capsules each day with the ritonavir. It is slowly absorbed, reaching peak levels in 2.9 hours. It is metabolized in the liver with a half-life of 4.8 to 6 hours; excretion is through urine and feces.

BOX 10.5 FOCUS ON Calculations

The health care provider prescribes lopinavir (*Kaletra*), 10 mg/kg, PO b.i.d. for a 14-year-old child weighing 50 kg. The drug comes in 200-mg tablets. How many tablets should the child receive at each dose?

To figure out the ordered dose, perform the following calculation:

$$10\ \text{mg/kg} \times 50\ \text{kg} = 500\ \text{mg/dose}$$

Then use

$$200\ \text{mg}\ (X) = 500\ \text{mg (tablets)}$$
$$X = \frac{500\ \text{mg (tablets)}}{200\ \text{mg}}$$
$$X = 2.5\ \text{mg (tablets)}$$

You would give 2.5 of the 200-mg tablets.

You notice that it is also available in an 80-mg/mL solution. How much solution would you give?

$$\frac{500\ \text{mg}}{\text{dose}} = \frac{80\ \text{mg}}{\text{mL}}$$
$$80\ \text{mg(dose)} = 500\ \text{mg(mL)}$$
$$\text{Dose} = \frac{500\ \text{mg/(mL)}}{80\ \text{mg}}$$
$$\text{Dose} = 6.25\ \text{mL.}$$

You would give 6.25 mL of the 80-mg/mL solution.

Nelfinavir is well absorbed from the GI tract, reaching peak levels in 2 to 4 hours. Nelfinavir is metabolized in the liver using the cytochrome P450 CY3A system, and caution must be used in patients with any hepatic dysfunction. It is primarily excreted in the feces, with a half-life of 3.5 to 5 hours. Because there is little renal excretion, this is considered a good drug for patients with renal impairment.

Ritonavir is rapidly absorbed from the GI tract, reaching peak levels in 2 to 4 hours. Ritonavir undergoes extensive metabolism in the liver and is excreted in the feces and urine.

Saquinavir is slowly absorbed from the GI tract and is metabolized in the liver by the cytochrome P450 mediator, so it must be used cautiously in the presence of hepatic dysfunction. It is primarily excreted in the feces with a short half-life.

Because therapy for HIV infection involves the use of several different antiviral drugs, many are now available as combination drugs, which reduces the number of tablets a patient has to take each day. Box 10.6 discusses combination drugs.

BOX 10.6

Fixed Combination Drugs for Treatment of HIV Infection

Patients who are taking combination drug therapy for HIV infection may have to take a very large number of pills each day. Keeping track of these pills and swallowing such a large number each day can be an overwhelming task. In an effort to improve patient compliance and make it easier for some of these patients, some anti-HIV agents are now available in combination products.

Combivir is a combination of 150-mg lamivudine and 300-mg zidovudine. The patient takes one tablet twice a day. Because this is a fixed combination drug, it is not the drug of choice for patients who require a dose reduction owing to renal impairment or adverse effects that limit dose tolerance.

Trizivir combines 300-mg abacavir, 150-mg lamivudine, and 300-mg zidovudine. The patient takes one tablet twice a day. Because this is a fixed combination drug, it is not the drug of choice for patients who require a dose reduction owing to renal impairment or adverse effects that limit dose tolerance. Patients taking *Trizivir* should be warned at the time the prescription is filled about the potentially serious hypersensitivity reactions associated with abacavir and should be given a written list of warning signs to watch for.

Epzicom (600-mg abacavir with 300-mg lamivudine) is taken as one tablet once a day. *Truvada* (200-mg emtricitabine with 300-mg tenofovir) is also a once-a-day tablet. The patient should be stabilized on each antiviral individually before being switched to the combination form *Atripla*—600-mg efavirenz, 200-mg emtricitabine, and 300-mg tenofovir. *Atripla* is recommended for patients 18 years old and older who have already been stabilized on each antiviral individually. *Complera* combines 200-mg emtricitabine, 25-mg rilpivirine, and 300-mg tenofovir. It is also approved for patients who have taken the individual drugs before. *Triumeq* combines 50-mg dolutegravir, 600-mg abacavir, and 300-mg lamivudine and is recommended for adults who experience success with each of the drugs alone.

Contraindications and Cautions

Of the protease inhibitors listed, saquinavir is the only agent that has not been shown to be teratogenic; however, its use during pregnancy should be limited. Saquinavir crosses into breast milk, and women are advised not to breastfeed while taking this drug. For the other agents, there are no adequate studies in pregnancy, so use should be limited to situations in which the benefits clearly outweigh any risks. It is suggested that women not breastfeed if they are infected with HIV.

Patients with mild to moderate hepatic dysfunction should receive a lower dose of fosamprenavir, and patients with severe hepatic dysfunction should not receive this drug or darunavir because of their toxic effects on the liver. Patients receiving tipranavir must have liver function monitored regularly because of the possibility of potentially fatal liver dysfunction. Saquinavir must also be used cautiously in the presence of hepatic dysfunction.

Patients receiving darunavir may also be at risk for developing diabetes mellitus or hyperglycemia and may require dosage adjustments if being treated with antidiabetic drugs. Darunavir is also associated with mild to severe dermatologic reactions including Stevens-Johnson syndrome and the drug should be stopped if a severe reaction develops.

The safety of indinavir for use in children younger than 12 years has not been established.

Darunavir should not be used in children younger than 3 years of age because of the potential for toxic effects.

Adverse Effects

As with the other antivirals, patients taking these drugs often experience GI effects, including nausea, vomiting, diarrhea, anorexia, and changes in liver function. Elevated cholesterol and triglyceride levels may occur. There is often a redistribution of fat to a buffalo hump with thinning of arms and legs. Rashes, pruritus, and the potentially fatal Stevens-Johnson syndrome have also occurred.

Clinically Significant Drug–Drug Interactions

Fosamprenavir should not be used in patients who are receiving ritonavir if they have used protease inhibitors to treat their disease because of a risk of serious adverse effects. If nelfinavir is combined with pimozide, rifampin, triazolam, or midazolam, severe toxic effects and life-threatening arrhythmias may occur. Such combinations should be avoided.

Indinavir and nevirapine interact to cause severe toxicity. If these two drugs are given in combination the doses should be adjusted and the patient should be monitored closely

Tipranavir, darunavir, and fosamprenavir have been shown to interact with many other drugs. Before administering these drugs, it is important to check a drug guide to assess for potential interactions with other drugs being given.

Many potentially serious toxic effects can occur when ritonavir is taken with nonsedating antihistamines, sedatives/hypnotics, or antiarrhythmics because of the activity of ritonavir in the liver. Patients with hepatic dysfunction are at increased risk for serious effects when taking ritonavir and require a reduced dose and close monitoring.

Prototype Summary: Fosamprenavir

Indications: Management of adults with symptomatic HIV infection in combination with other antiretrovirals.

Actions: Inhibits protease activity, leading to the formation of immature, noninfectious virus particles.

Pharmacokinetics:

Route	Onset	Peak
Oral	Varies	1.5–4 min

$T_{1/2}$: 7.7 hours; metabolized in the liver and excreted in the feces and urine.

Adverse Effects: Headache, mood changes, nausea, diarrhea, fatigue, rash, Stevens-Johnson syndrome, redistribution of body fat (buffalo hump, thin arms and legs).

Fusion Inhibitor

A newer class of drug is the **fusion inhibitor** (Table 10.3). This agent acts at a different site than do other HIV antivirals. The fusion inhibitor prevents the fusion of the virus with the human cellular membrane, which prevents the HIV-1 virus from entering the cell. Enfuvirtide (*Fuzeon*) is used in combination with other antiretroviral agents to treat adults and children older than 6 years who have evidence of HIV-1 replication despite ongoing antiretroviral therapy.

Enfuvirtide is given by subcutaneous injection and peaks in effect in 4 to 8 hours. After metabolism in the liver, it is recycled in the tissues and not excreted. The half-life of enfuvirtide is 3.2 to 4.4 hours. Enfuvirtide is contraindicated with hypersensitivity to any component of the drug and in nursing mothers. It should be used with caution in the presence of lung disease or pregnancy. The drug has been associated with insomnia, depression, peripheral neuropathy, nausea, diarrhea, pneumonia, and injection site reactions. There are no reported drug interactions, but caution should be used when it is combined with any other drug.

Prototype Summary: Enfuvirtide

Indications: Treatment of HIV-1–infected patients who have experienced clinical or immunological deterioration after treatment with other agents, in combination with other antiretrovirals.

Actions: Prevents the entry of the HIV-1 virus into cells by inhibiting the fusion of the virus membrane with the cellular membrane.

Pharmacokinetics:

Route	Onset	Peak
Subcutaneous	Slow	4–8 h

$T_{1/2}$: 3.2 to 4.4 hours; metabolized in the liver, tissues recycle the amino acids, not excreted.

Adverse Effects: Headache, nausea, vomiting, diarrhea, rash, anorexia, pneumonia, chills, injection site reactions.

CCR5 Coreceptor Antagonist

In 2007 another new class of drugs was introduced for the treatment of HIV. Maraviroc (*Selzentry*) is a **CCR5 coreceptor antagonist**. It blocks the receptor site on the cell membrane to which the HIV virus needs to interact to enter the cell. It is indicated for the treatment of HIV in adults as part of combination therapy with other antivirals. Maraviroc is rapidly absorbed from the GI tract, metabolized in the liver, and excreted primarily through the feces. It has a half-life of 14 to 18 hours. Maraviroc should not be used with known hypersensitivity to any component of the drug or by nursing mothers. The safety and efficacy of maraviroc in children has not been established. Caution should be used in the presence of liver disease or coinfection with hepatitis B, because of the risk of serious hepatic toxicity. Patients at increased risk for cardiovascular events or with hypotension should be monitored very closely if this is the drug of choice for them. As with other antivirals, it should be used in pregnancy only if the benefit outweighs the potential risk to the fetus.

Severe hepatotoxicity has been reported with this drug, often preceded by a systemic allergic reaction with eosinophilia and rash. Maraviroc has a black box warning regarding the risk for serious hepatotoxicity. Regular monitoring of liver function should be routine when using this drug. CNS effects including dizziness, and changes in consciousness have been reported; patients experiencing these should be cautioned to take measures to assure safety. Patients may also be at increased risk of infections because of the way the drug affects the cell membrane of the CD4 cells. Appropriate precautions are necessary.

There is a risk of increased serum levels and toxicity when combined with cytochrome P450 CYP3A inhibitors (ketoconazole, lopinavir/ritonavir, ritonavir, saquinavir, atazanavir, delavirdine), and the maraviroc dose should be adjusted accordingly. Decreased serum levels and loss of effectiveness may occur if maraviroc is combined with CYP3A inducers (nevirapine, rifampin, efavirenz), and the maraviroc dose should be adjusted accordingly. Patients should not use St. John's wort while on this drug because there is a loss of antiviral effects when the two are combined.

Prototype Summary: Maraviroc

Indications: Combination antiretroviral treatment of adults infected with CCR5-tropic HIV-1 who have evidence of viral replication and HIV-1 strains resistant to multiple antiretroviral agents.

Actions: Selectively binds to the human chemokine receptor CCR5 on the cell membrane, preventing interaction of HIV-1 and CCR5, which is necessary for the HIV to enter the cell; HIV cannot enter the cell and cannot multiply.

Pharmacokinetics:

Route	Onset	Peak
Oral	Slow	0.5–4 h

$T_{1/2}$: 14 to 28 hours; metabolized in the liver, excreted in the feces and urine.

Adverse Effects: Dizziness, paresthesias, nausea, vomiting, diarrhea, cough, upper respiratory infection (URI), fever, musculoskeletal symptoms, hepatotoxicity.

Integrase Inhibitors

In late 2007, another class of drugs—**integrase inhibitors**—was introduced to treat HIV infection. There are now two drugs in this class, dolutegravir (*Tivicay*) and raltegravir (*Isentress*). These drugs inhibit the activity of the virus-specific enzyme integrase, an encoded enzyme needed for viral replication. Blocking this enzyme prevents the formation of the HIV-1 provirus and leads to a decrease in viral load and increase in active CD4 cells. It is reserved for use in patients who have been treated with other antivirals and have evidence of a return to viral replication. Raltegravir is rapidly absorbed from the GI tract and metabolized in the liver. It has a half-life of 9 hours and is excreted primarily in the feces. Dolutegravir is rapidly absorbed, reaching peak levels in 2 to 3 hours. It is metabolized in the liver and excreted in the feces with a half-life of 14 hours.

Integrase inhibitors are contraindicated with known hypersensitivity to any component of the drug, as initial treatment in adults, for use in children, and for nursing mothers. Caution should be used if the patient is at risk for rhabdomyolysis or myopathy and during pregnancy. Patients taking either drug must be very careful to continue the drug regimen to help decrease the development of resistant strains of the virus.

Common adverse effects include headache, dizziness, and an increased risk for the development of rhabdomyolysis and myopathy. There is a risk of decreased serum levels of either drug if combined with rifampin; the patient should be monitored and the dose adjusted if this combination must be used. Patients should avoid the use of St. Johns wort, which can interfere with the drugs' effectiveness.

Prototype Summary: Raltegravir

Indications: In combination with other antiviral agents for the treatment of HIV-1 infection in treatment-experienced adult patients who have evidence of viral replication and HIV-1 strains resistant to multiple antiretroviral agents.

Actions: Inhibits the activity of the virus-specific enzyme integrase, an encoded enzyme needed for viral replication. Blocking this enzyme prevents the formation of the HIV-1 provirus and leads to a decrease in viral load and an increase in active CD4 cells.

Pharmacokinetics:

Route	Onset	Peak
Oral	Rapid	3 h

$T_{1/2}$: 9 hours; metabolized in the liver, excreted in the feces and urine.

Adverse Effects: Headache, dizziness, nausea, vomiting, diarrhea, fever, rhabdomyolysis.

Nursing Considerations for Patients Receiving Agents for HIV and AIDS

Assessment: History and Examination

- Assess for *contraindications and cautions to the use of these drugs*: any history of allergy to antivirals *to avoid hypersensitivity reactions*; renal or hepatic dysfunction *that might interfere with the metabolism and excretion of the drug*; and pregnancy or lactation *because of possible adverse effects on the fetus or infant.*

- Perform a physical assessment *to establish baseline data for assessing the effectiveness of the drug and the occurrence of any adverse effects associated with drug therapy.*
- Assess level of orientation and reflexes *to evaluate any CNS effects of the drug.*
- Examine the skin (color, temperature, and lesions) *to monitor for adverse effects of the drug.*
- Check temperature *to monitor for infections.*
- Evaluate hepatic and renal function tests *to determine baseline function of the kidneys and liver.* Check results of a complete blood count with differential *to monitor bone marrow activity* and helper T cell number *to determine the severity of the disease and indicate the effectiveness of the drugs.*

Nursing Diagnoses

Nursing diagnoses related to drug therapy might include the following:

- Acute pain related to GI, CNS, or dermatological effects of the drugs
- Disturbed sensory perception (kinesthetic) related to CNS effects of the drugs
- Imbalanced nutrition: Less than body requirements related to GI effects of the drugs
- Risk for injury related to CNS effects of the drugs.
- Deficient knowledge regarding drug therapy

Planning

- The patient will receive the best therapeutic effect from the drug therapy.
- The patient will have limited adverse effects to the drug therapy.
- The patient will have an understanding of the drug therapy, adverse effects to anticipate, and measures to relieve discomfort and improve safety.

Implementation with Rationale

- Monitor renal and hepatic function before and periodically during therapy *to detect changes requiring dose adjustments or additional treatment as needed.*
- Ensure that the patient takes the complete course of the drug regimen and takes all drugs included in a particular combination *to improve the effectiveness of the drug and decrease the risk of emergence of resistant viral strains.*
- Administer the drug around the clock, if indicated, *to provide the critical concentration needed for the drug to be effective.*
- Monitor nutritional status if GI effects are severe, and take appropriate action *to maintain nutrition, including small, frequent meals and balanced nutrition to provide protein and other nutrients.*
- Stop drug if severe rash occurs, especially if accompanied by blisters, fever, and other signs, *to avert potentially serious reactions.*
- Provide safety precautions (e.g., the use of side rails, appropriate lighting, orientation, assistance) if CNS effects occur, *to protect patient from injury.*
- Teach the patient about the drugs prescribed *to enhance patient knowledge about drug therapy and to promote compliance.* Include as a teaching point the fact that these drugs do not cure the disease, so appropriate precautions should still be taken *to prevent transmission.*
- Provide the following patient teaching:
  - Have regular medical care.
  - Set up a regular schedule for taking all of your drugs at the correct time during the day.
  - Have periodic blood tests for renal and hepatic function and a complete blood count (CBC), which are necessary to monitor the effectiveness and toxicity of the drug.
  - Realize that GI upset, nausea, and vomiting may occur but that efforts must be taken to maintain adequate nutrition.
  - Avoid driving and hazardous tasks if dizziness or drowsiness occurs.

Report extreme fatigue, severe headache, difficulty breathing, or severe rash to a health care provider.

See the Critical Thinking Scenario for a case study and focused follow-up for the antiviral agents used for HIV and AIDS. See Box 10.7 for information on new antidiarrheal drugs available to help patients with diarrhea caused by antiretroviral drugs.

BOX 10.7

Antidiarrheal Drug for Patients on Antiretroviral Agents

One of the potentially serious adverse effects of antiretroviral drugs is diarrhea which can lead to dehydration, skin breakdown, and infection. Crofelemer (*Fulyzaq*) is an antidiarrheal agent that works in the GI tract to stimulate chloride ion channels and calcium channels which blocks chloride secretion and high-volume water loss in diarrhea and helps to normalize the flow of chloride and water in the GI tract. It is approved for symptomatic diarrhea in adults on antiretroviral therapy. It is very important to make sure that the diarrhea is not being caused by an infectious process. The oral tablets (125-mg extended release) must be swallowed whole and are taken b.i.d. The drug is not recommended for use in pregnancy, so women of childbearing age should be encouraged to use contraceptive measures. Women who are breastfeeding need to be advised to find another method of feeding the baby.

CRITICAL THINKING SCENARIO

Antiviral Agents for HIV and AIDS

THE SITUATION

H.P. is a 34-year-old attorney who was diagnosed with AIDS, having had a positive HIV test 3 years ago. Although his helper T cell count had been stabilized with treatment with zidovudine and efavirenz, it recently dropped remarkably. He presents with numerous opportunistic infections and Kaposi sarcoma. H.P. admits that he has been under tremendous stress at work and at home in the last few weeks. He begins a combination regimen of lamivudine, zidovudine, ritonavir, and zalcitabine.

Critical Thinking

What are the important nursing implications in this case?
What role would stress play in the progress of this disease?
What specific issues should be discussed?
What other clinical implications should be considered?

DISCUSSION

Combination therapy with antivirals has been found to be effective in decreasing some of the morbidity and mortality associated with HIV and AIDS. However, this treatment does not cure the disease. H.P. needs to understand that opportunistic infections can still occur and that regular medical help should be sought. He also needs to understand that these drugs do not decrease the risk of transmitting HIV by sexual contact or through blood contamination and he should be encouraged to take appropriate precautions.

It is important to make a dosing schedule for H.P., or even to prepare a weekly drug box, to ensure that all medications are taken as indicated. H.P. should also receive interventions to help him decrease his stress because activation of the sympathetic nervous system during periods of stress depresses the immune system. Further depression of his immune system could accelerate the development of opportunistic infections and decrease the effectiveness of his antiviral drugs. Measures that could be used to decrease stress should be discussed and tried with H.P.

Discussing the adverse effects that H.P. may experience is important because GI upset, diarrhea, and discomfort may occur while he is taking all of these anti-HIV/AIDS medications. Small, frequent meals may help alleviate the discomfort. It is important that every effort be made to maintain H.P.'s nutritional state, and a nutritional consultation may be necessary if GI effects are severe. H.P. also may experience dizziness, fatigue, and confusion, which could cause more problems for him at work and may necessitate changes in his workload. Because some of the prescribed drugs must be taken around the clock, provisions may be needed to allow H.P. to take his drugs on time throughout the day. For example, he may need to wear an alarm wristwatch, establish planned breaks in his schedule at dosing times, or devise other ways to follow his drug regimen without interfering with his work schedule. The adverse effects and inconvenience of taking this many drugs may add to his stress. It is important that a health care provider work consistently with him to help him to manage his disease and treatment as effectively as possible.

NURSING CARE GUIDE FOR H.P.: ANTIVIRAL AGENTS FOR HIV AND AIDS

Assessment: History and Examination

Allergies to any of these drugs
Bone marrow depression
Renal or liver dysfunction
Skin: color, lesions, texture
CNS: affect, reflexes, orientation
GI: abdominal and liver evaluation
Hematological: complete blood count (CBC) and differential; viral load; T-cell levels; renal and hepatic function tests

Nursing Diagnoses

Acute pain related to GI, skin, CNS effects
Disturbed sensory perception (kinesthetic) related to CNS effects
Imbalanced nutrition: Less than body requirements related to GI effects
Deficient knowledge regarding drug therapy

Planning

The patient will receive the best therapeutic effect from the drug therapy
The patient will have limited adverse effects to the drug therapy
The patient will have an understanding of the drug therapy, adverse effects to anticipate, and measures to relieve discomfort and improve safety

Implementation

Monitor CBC and differential before and every 2 weeks during therapy.
Provide comfort and implement safety measures: assistance, temperature control, lighting control, mouth care, back rubs.
Provide small, frequent meals and monitor nutritional status.
Monitor for opportunistic infections and arrange treatment as indicated.
Provide support and reassurance for dealing with drug effects and discomfort.

Antiviral Agents for HIV and AIDS (continued)

Provide patient teaching regarding drug name, dosage, adverse effects, warnings, precautions, use of OTC or herbal remedies, and signs to report.

Evaluation

Evaluate drug effects: relief of signs and symptoms of AIDS and ARC stabilization of helper T cell levels.
Monitor for adverse effects: GI alterations, dizziness, confusion, headache, fever.
Monitor for drug–drug interactions as indicated for each drug.
Evaluate effectiveness of patient-teaching plan.
Evaluate effectiveness of comfort and safety measures.

PATIENT TEACHING FOR H.P.

A combination of antiviral drugs has been prescribed to treat your HIV infection. These drugs work in combination to stop the replication of HIV, to control AIDS, and to maintain the functioning of your immune system. A schedule will be plotted out to show exactly when to take each of the drugs. It is very important that you take all of the drugs and that you stick to this schedule to ensure that the drugs can be effective and won't encourage the development of resistant strains of the virus.

These drugs are not a cure for HIV, AIDS, or ARC. Opportunistic infections may occur, and regular medical follow-up should be sought to deal with the disease.

These drugs do not reduce the risk of transmission of HIV to others by sexual contact or by blood contamination; use appropriate precautions.

Common effects of these drugs include the following:

- Dizziness, weakness, and loss of feeling: Change positions slowly. If you feel drowsy, avoid driving and dangerous activities.
- Headache, fever, muscle aches: Analgesics may be ordered to alleviate this discomfort. Consult with your health care provider.
- Nausea, loss of appetite, change in taste: Small, frequent meals may help. It is important to try to maintain good nutrition. Consult your health care provider if this becomes a severe problem.
- Report any of the following to your health care provider: Excessive fatigue, lethargy, severe headache, difficulty breathing, or skin rash.
- Avoid OTC medications and herbal therapies; many of them interact with your drugs and may make them ineffective. If you feel that you need one of these, check with your health care provider first.
- Schedule regular medical evaluations, including blood tests, which are needed to monitor the effects of these drugs on your body and to adjust doses as needed.
- Tell any doctor, nurse, or other health care provider that you are taking these drugs.
- Keep these drugs and all medications out of the reach of children. Do not share these drugs with other people.

EVALUATION

- Monitor patient response to the drug (alleviation or reduction of signs and symptoms of AIDS or ARC and maintenance of helper T cell levels).
- Monitor for adverse effects (level of orientation and affect, GI upset, renal and hepatic function, skin, levels of blood components).
- Evaluate the effectiveness of the teaching plan (patient can name the drug, dosage, possible adverse effects to watch for, and specific measures to help avoid adverse effects).
- Monitor the effectiveness of comfort and safety measures and compliance with the regimen.

KEY POINTS

- The HIV virus infects helper T cells, leading to a loss of immune function and the development of opportunistic infections.
- Drugs used to treat HIV usually are given in combination to affect the virus at various points in the body: nonnucleoside and NRTIs block RNA and DNA activity in the cell; protease inhibitors prevent maturation of the virus; fusion inhibitors prevent the entry of the virus into the cell; CCR5 coreceptor antagonists prevent the virus from reacting with the receptor on the cell membrane, preventing its entry into the cell; and integrase inhibitors block an enzyme essential for formation of the provirus within the cell, leading to decrease in the number of viruses.
- Patients taking drugs to treat HIV need to take all of the medications continuously as prescribed and take precautions to prevent the spread of the disease to others.

Anti–Hepatitis B Agents

Hepatitis B is a serious to potentially fatal viral infection of the liver. The hepatitis B virus can be spread by blood or blood products, sexual contact, or contaminated needles or instruments. Health care workers are at especially high risk for contracting hepatitis B due to needle sticks. Hepatitis B has a higher mortality than other types of hepatitis. Individuals infected may also develop a chronic

Table 10.4 *Drugs in Focus:* Anti–Hepatitis B Agents

Drug Name	Dosage/Route	Usual Indications
Anti–Hepatitis B		
adefovir (*Hepsera*)	*Adult:* 10 mg/d PO *Renal impairment:* CrCl 20–40 mL/min: 10 mg PO q48h CrCl 10–19 mL/min: 10 mg PO q72h	Treatment of hepatitis B with evidence of active viral replication and persistent elevations in liver enzymes
entecavir (*Baraclude*)	*Adults and children (≥16 y):* 0.5 mg/d; also receiving lamivudine: 1 mg/d Reduce dose with renal impairment	Treatment of chronic hepatitis B in adults with evidence of active viral replication and persistent liver enzyme elevations
telbivudine (*Tyzeka*)	*Adults and children >16 y:* 600 mg/d PO; reduce dose with renal impairment	Treatment of chronic hepatitis B in patients >16 y with evidence of viral replication and persistent liver enzyme elevations
Anti–Hepatitis C		
boceprevir (*Victrelis*)	*Adult:* 800 mg PO t.i.d at intervals of 7–9 h	Treatment of hepatitis C in adults with compensated liver disease; must be given with peginterferon and ribavirin
simeprevir (*Olysio*)	*Adult:* 150 mg/day PO for 12–36 wk	Treatment of hepatitis C in adults with compensated liver disease, must be given with peginterferon and ribavirin
sofosbuvir (*Sovaldi*)	*Adult:* 400 mg/day PO for 12–24 wk	Treatment of hepatitis C in adults with compensated liver disease, must be given with peginterferon and ribavirin

condition or become a carrier. In the past, hepatitis B was treated with interferons (see Chapter 17). In 2004 and 2005, adefovir (*Hepsera*) and entecavir (*Baraclude*) were approved specifically for treating chronic hepatitis B. In 2006 another NRTI, telbivudine (*Tyzeka*) was found to be very effective in preventing viral replication in active hepatitis B patients (see Table 10.4).

Therapeutic Actions and Indications

All three of these antiviral drugs are indicated for the treatment of adults with chronic hepatitis B who have evidence of active viral replication and either evidence of persistent elevations in serum aminotransferases or histologically active disease. The drugs inhibit reverse transcriptase in the hepatitis B virus and cause DNA chain termination, leading to blocked viral replication and decreased viral load (see Table 10.4).

Pharmacokinetics

These drugs are rapidly absorbed from the GI tract, with peak effects occurring in 0.5 to 1.5 hours (entecavir), 0.5 to 4 hours (adefovir), and 1 to 4 hours (telbivudine). Entecavir and adefovir are metabolized in the liver and excreted in the urine. Telbivudine is excreted unchanged in the urine. Adefovir has a half-life of 7.5 hours; entecavir has a half-life of 128 to 149 hours; and telbivudine has a half-life of 40 to 49 hours. It is not known whether any of these drugs crosses the placenta or enters breast milk.

Contraindications and Cautions

These drugs are contraindicated with any known allergy to the drugs *to prevent hypersensitivity reactions* and with lactation *because of potential toxicity to the infant.* Use caution when administering these drugs to patients with renal impairment and severe liver disease *because of increased toxicity with these drugs* and those who are pregnant *because the effects on the fetus are not known.*

Adverse Effects

The adverse effects most frequently seen with these drugs are headache, dizziness, nausea, diarrhea, and elevated liver enzymes. Severe hepatomegaly with steatosis, sometimes fatal, has been reported with adefovir and telbivudine use. Lactic acidosis and renal impairment have been reported with entecavir and adefovir. A potential risk for hepatitis B exacerbation could occur when the drugs are stopped. Therefore, teach patients the importance of not running out of their drugs and use extreme caution when discontinuing these drugs.

Clinically Important Drug–Drug Interactions

There is an increased risk of renal toxicity if these drugs are taken with other nephrotoxic drugs. If such a combination is used, monitor the patient closely. An evaluation of risks versus benefits may be necessary if renal function begins to deteriorate.

Prototype Summary: Adefovir

Indications: Treatment of chronic hepatitis B in adults with evidence of active viral replication and either evidence of persistent elevations in alanine aminotransferase and aspartate aminotransferase or histologically active disease.

Actions: Inhibits hepatitis B virus reverse transcriptase, causes DNA chain termination, and blocks viral replication.

Pharmacokinetics:

Route	Onset	Peak	Duration
Oral	Rapid	0.6–4 h	Unknown

$T_{1/2}$: 7.5 hours; excreted in the urine.

Adverse Effects: Headache, asthenia, nausea, severe to fatal hepatomegaly with steatosis, nephrotoxicity, lactic acidosis, exacerbation of hepatitis B when discontinued.

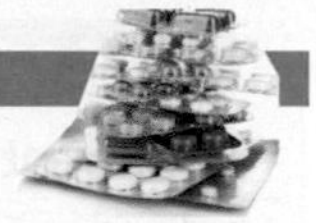

Nursing Considerations for Patients Receiving Anti–Hepatitis B Agents

Assessment: History and Examination

- Assess for *contraindications or cautions*: any history of allergy to adefovir, entecavir, or telbivudine *to avoid hypersensitivity reactions*; renal dysfunction, *which could be exacerbated by the nephrotoxic effects of these drugs*; severe liver impairment, *which could affect the metabolism and exacerbate the liver toxicity of these drugs*; and pregnancy and lactation *because the potential effects of these drugs on the fetus or baby are not known.*
- Perform a physical assessment *to establish baseline data for assessing the effectiveness of these drugs and the occurrence of any adverse effects associated with drug toxicity.*
- Assess body temperature *to monitor underlying disease.*
- Assess level of orientation and reflexes *to assess for CNS changes.*
- Evaluate renal and liver function tests *to monitor for developing toxicity and to determine drug effectiveness.*

Nursing Diagnoses

Nursing diagnoses related to the drug therapy might include the following:

- Acute pain related to the CNS and GI effects of the drug
- Imbalanced nutrition: Less than body requirements related to the GI effects of the drug
- Deficient knowledge regarding drug therapy

Planning

- The patient will receive the best therapeutic effect from the drug therapy.
- The patient will have limited adverse effects to the drug therapy.
- The patient will have an understanding of the drug therapy, adverse effects to anticipate, and measures to relieve discomfort and improve safety.

Implementation with Rationale

- Monitor renal and hepatic function prior to and periodically during therapy *to detect renal or hepatic function changes and determine the need for possible dose reduction or institute treatment as needed.*
- Withdraw the drug and monitor the patient if he or she develops signs of lactic acidosis or hepatotoxicity *because these adverse effects can be life threatening.*
- Caution patient to not run out of this drug but to take it continually *because acute exacerbation of hepatitis B can occur when the drug is stopped.*
- Advise women of childbearing age to use barrier contraceptives *because the potential adverse effects of this drug on the fetus are not known.*
- Advise women who are breastfeeding to find another method of feeding the baby while using the drug *because the potential toxic effects on the baby are not known.*
- Advise patients that these drugs do not cure the disease and there is still a risk of transferring the disease, *so the patient should continue to take appropriate steps to prevent transmission of hepatitis B.*
- Instruct the patient about the drug prescribed *to enhance patient knowledge about drug therapy and to promote compliance.*
- Provide the following patient teaching:
  - Have regular blood tests and medical follow-up.
  - Take precautions to avoid running out of the drug because it must be taken continually.
  - Realize that GI upset, with nausea and diarrhea, is common with this drug.
  - Report severe weakness, muscle pain, palpitations, yellowing of the eyes or skin, and trouble breathing.

Evaluation

- Monitor patient response to the drug (decreased viral load of hepatitis B).
- Monitor for adverse effects (liver or renal dysfunction, headache, nausea, diarrhea).
- Evaluate the effectiveness of the teaching plan (patient can name the drug, dosage, possible adverse effects to watch for, and specific measures to avoid adverse effects).
- Monitor the effectiveness of comfort and safety measures and compliance with the drug regimen.

KEY POINTS

- Hepatitis B is a serious to potentially fatal viral infection of the liver spread by blood or blood products, sexual contact, or contaminated needles or instruments. Hepatitis B has a higher mortality than other types of hepatitis.
- Prevention of infection through use of hepatitis B vaccines and avoiding exposure is essential in stopping the spread of this disease.
- Hepatitis B used to be treated only with interferons and rest. Entecavir, adefovir, and telbivudine are antivirals now available for the treatment of hepatitis B.

Anti–Hepatitis C Agents

In 2011 two new drugs were approved for the treatment of hepatitis C, boceprevir (*Victrelis*) and telaprevir (*Incivek*). In 2014 simeprevir (*Olysio*) and sofosbuvir (*Sovaldi*) as well as a number of drugs only available in a combination product were also approved. The introduction of these drugs led to the removal of telaprevir from the market. Most liver transplants performed in the United States are due to progressive liver disease caused by **hepatitis C** virus (HCV) infection. After initial infection with HCV, most people develop chronic hepatitis C. Some will develop cirrhosis of the liver over many years. People can get HCV in a number of ways including exposure to blood that is infected with the virus, being born to a mother with HCV, sharing a needle, having sex with an infected person, sharing personal items such as a razor or toothbrush with someone who is infected with the virus, or from unsterilized tattoo or piercing tools. Box 10.8 discusses new drugs for hepatitis C.

Therapeutic Effects and Indications

The new drugs approved for treating this disease are protease inhibitors. They can be used in combination with ribavirin or ribavirin and peginterferon to treat chronic hepatitis C in patients with compromised liver function.

BOX 10.8

More New Drugs for Hepatitis C

In 2015 two more drugs were introduced for the treatment of hepatitis C. *Technivie*—a combination of ombitasvir (a hepatitis C virus protease inhibitor), paritaprevir (a heptatitis C virus protease inhibitor), and ritonavir (a CYP3A inhibitor)—is indicated for use with ribavirin for the treatment of patients with genotype 4 chronic hepatitis C without cirrhosis. It is an oral agent taken twice a day for 12 weeks with ribavirin. *Daklinza* (daclatasvir) is a hepatitis C protease inhibitor that is indicated with sofosbuvir for the treatment of chronic hepatitis C genotype 3 without cirrhosis. It is taken once a day for 12 weeks.

Pharmacokinetics

These are oral drugs that are readily absorbed from the GI tract, metabolized in the liver, and excreted in the urine. Half-lives range from 4 to 10 hours. These drugs must also be taken with peginterferon and ribavirin.

Contraindications and Cautions

These drugs are contraindicated with any known allergy to the drugs *to prevent hypersensitivity reactions* and with lactation and pregnancy because these drugs must be given with ribavirin *which has known toxicity to the infant.* Use caution when administering these drugs to patients with severe liver disease *because of increased toxicity with these drugs.* Safety has not been established for use in patients who also have hepatitis B and/or HIV infections *because exacerbations of these diseases might occur.* The financial burden of these drugs caused a lot of problems when they were introduced. See Box 10.9 for a discussion of the impact of very costly new drugs on the health care system and Box 10.10 for fixed combination hepatitis C drugs.

BOX 10.9

High Cost of Hepatitis C drugs

The introduction of drugs to treat hepatitis C opened a new therapeutic option for patients with the disease. It is estimated that most of the people awaiting liver transplant are in need of a transplant because of hepatitis C. Most people with the disease, however, do not experience serious liver problems and would do fine without treatment. However, treatment is now available at a very high cost. Simeprevir (*Olysio*) comes with a $66,320/ course price tag. Sofosbuvir (*Sovaldi*) costs about $1,000 a pill or $84,000 for a bottle for one full course of therapy. The newest combination drug *Harvoni* is $1,125 per pill or approximately $94,500 for a 12-week supply. Drug companies argue that in the long run the cost of a liver transplant would be higher. Some experts have suggested, based on studies, that the drugs should be reserved for use in only those with more advanced liver scarring and risk. However, multimedia advertisements have marketed the drug to all people who have known chronic hepatitis C, which has raised demand considerably. Insurance companies are very concerned about the ability to cover the cost of these drugs. Medicaid, the Veterans Affairs (VA) system, and other insurance providers will have to make significant decisions regarding the possibilities of cutting off health care to others to cover these enormous costs. Fears of hospitals closing have arisen and the US government is getting involved. This raises concerns of US governmental influence over one drug at a time and the equity this would have for all patients and all drugs. The ability to treat this disease that once had no pharmacological options has caused a heated debate and raised much needed discussion about the cost of developing drugs and the price of this development on the whole health care system in the United States.

BOX 10.10

Fixed Combination Drugs for Treatment of Hepatitis C

Fixed combination drugs for the treatment of hepatitis C include drugs that are not available as standalone products.

Viekira Pak is a combination of 12.5-mg ombitasvir, 75-mg paritaprevir, and 50-mg ritonavir packaged with 250-mg dasabuvir as a separate tablet. It is not recommended for patients with decompensated liver disease.

Harvoni is a combination of 90-mg ledipasvir and 400-mg sofosbuvir. This combination is taken once a day for 12–24 weeks.

Adverse Effects

The most common adverse effects are fatigue, nausea, diarrhea, rash. Severe skin reactions can occur.

Clinically Important Drug Interactions

Toxic effects or loss of therapeutic effect could occur if combined with other protease inhibitors or other antivirals. If combining any of these, check a drug reference to make sure dosage is adjusted as needed. St. John's wort should be avoided as it leads to loss of effectiveness.

P Prototype Summary: Simeprevir

Indications: Treatment of chronic hepatitis C in adults with compensated liver dysfunction in combination with peginterferon and ribavirin.

Actions: Inhibits hepatitis C protease formation preventing viral replication.

Pharmacokinetics:

Route	Onset	Peak	Duration
Oral	Rapid	4–6 h	Unknown

$T_{1/2}$: 10–12 hours; excreted in the feces.

Adverse Effects: Fatigue, nausea, diarrhea, rash.

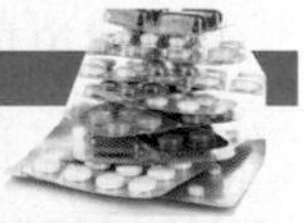

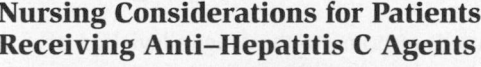

Nursing Considerations for Patients Receiving Anti–Hepatitis C Agents

Assessment: History and Examination

- Assess for *contraindications or cautions*: any history of allergy to drug or drug components *to avoid hypersensitivity reactions*; severe liver impairment, *which could affect the metabolism and exacerbate the liver toxicity of these drugs*; and pregnancy and lactation *because the potential effects of these drugs on the fetus or baby are not known.*
- Perform a physical assessment *to establish baseline data for assessing the effectiveness of these drugs and the occurrence of any adverse effects associated with drug toxicity.*
- Assess body temperature *to monitor underlying disease.*
- Assess level of orientation and reflexes *to assess for CNS changes.*
- Evaluate liver function tests *to monitor for developing toxicity and to determine drug effectiveness.*

Nursing Diagnoses

Nursing diagnoses related the drug therapy might include the following:

- Acute pain related to the CNS and GI effects of the drug
- Imbalanced nutrition: Less than body requirements related to the GI effects of the drug
- Deficient knowledge regarding drug therapy

Planning

- The patient will receive the best therapeutic effect from the drug therapy.
- The patient will have limited adverse effects to the drug therapy.
- The patient will have an understanding of the drug therapy, adverse effects to anticipate, and measures to relieve discomfort and improve safety.

Implementation with Rationale

- Ensure that this patient is also receiving peginterferon and ribavirin *to ensure therapeutic effectiveness.*
- Monitor hepatic function prior to and periodically during therapy *to detect hepatic function changes and determine the need for possible dose reduction or institute treatment as needed.*
- Advise women of childbearing age to use barrier contraceptives *because the potential adverse effects of this drug on the fetus are not known.*
- Advise women who are breastfeeding to find another method of feeding the baby while using the drug *because the potential toxic effects on the baby are not known.*
- Advise patients that these drugs do not cure the disease and there is still a risk of transferring the disease, *so the patient should continue to take appropriate steps to prevent transmission of hepatitis C.*
- Instruct the patient about the drug prescribed *to enhance patient knowledge about drug therapy and to promote compliance.*
- Provide the following patient teaching:
  - Have regular blood tests of hepatic function and viral load and medical follow-up.
  - Always take this drug with peginterferon and ribavirin.

(continues on page 166)

- Realize that GI upset, with nausea and diarrhea, is common with this drug.
- Report severe changes in color of urine or stool, rash, lethargy.

Evaluation

- Monitor patient response to the drug (decreased viral load of hepatitis C).
- Monitor for adverse effects (liver dysfunction, headache, nausea, diarrhea, rash).
- Evaluate the effectiveness of the teaching plan (patient can name the drug, dosage, possible adverse effects to watch for, and specific measures to avoid adverse effects).
- Monitor the effectiveness of comfort and safety measures and compliance with the drug regimen.

Locally Active Antiviral Agents

Some antiviral agents are given locally to treat local viral infections. These agents include docosanol (*Abreva*), ganciclovir (*Vitrasert*), imiquimod (*Aldara*), penciclovir (*Denavir*), and trifluridine (*Viroptic*).

Therapeutic Actions and Indications

These antiviral agents act on viruses by interfering with normal viral replication and metabolic processes. They are indicated for specific, local viral infections (see Table 10.5).

Contraindications and Cautions

Locally active antiviral drugs are not absorbed systemically, but caution must be used in patients with known allergic reactions to any topical drugs.

Adverse Effects

Because these drugs are not absorbed systemically the adverse effects most commonly reported are local burning, stinging, and discomfort. These effects usually occur at the time of administration and pass with time.

Table 10.5 *Drugs in Focus:* Locally Active Antiviral Agents

Drug Name	Usual Indications
docosanol (*Abreva*)	Local treatment of oral and facial herpes simplex cold sores and fever blisters
ganciclovir (*Vitrasert*)	Implanted for treatment of CMV in patients with AIDS
imiquimod (*Aldara*)	Local treatment of genital and perianal warts
penciclovir (*Denavir*)	Local treatment of herpes labialis (cold sores) on the face and lips
trifluridine (Viroptic)	Ophthalmic ointment to treat herpes simplex infections in the eye

CMV, cytomegalovirus.

Nursing Considerations for Patients Receiving Locally Active Antiviral Agents

Assessment: History and Examination

- Assess for history of allergy to antivirals *to avoid allergic response to these drugs.*
- Perform a physical assessment *to establish baseline data for evaluating the effectiveness of the drug and the occurrence of any adverse effects associated with drug therapy.*
- Assess the infected area, including location, size, and character of lesions *to provide baseline information and evaluation of drug effects.*
- Evaluate for signs of inflammation at the site of infection *to ensure safe use of the drug.*

Nursing Diagnoses

Nursing diagnoses related to drug therapy might include the following:

- Acute pain related to local effects of the drug
- Deficient knowledge regarding drug therapy

Planning

- The patient will receive the best therapeutic effect from the drug therapy.
- The patient will have limited adverse effects to the drug therapy.
- The patient will have an understanding of the drug therapy, adverse effects to anticipate and measures to relieve discomfort and improve safety.

Implementation with Rationale

- Ensure proper administration of the drug *to improve effectiveness and decrease risk of adverse effects.*
- Stop the drug if severe local reaction occurs or if open lesions occur near the site of administration *to prevent systemic absorption and adverse effects.*
- Instruct the patient about the drug being used *to enhance patient knowledge about drug therapy and to promote compliance.* Include as a teaching point the fact that these drugs do not cure the disease but should alleviate discomfort and prevent damage to healthy tissues. Encourage the patient to report severe local reaction or discomfort.

Evaluation

- Monitor patient response to the drug (alleviation of signs and symptoms of viral infection).
- Monitor for adverse effects (local irritation and discomfort).
- Evaluate the effectiveness of the teaching plan (patient can name the drug, the dosage, proper administration technique, and adverse effects to watch for and report to a health care provider).
- Monitor the effectiveness of comfort and safety measures and compliance with the regimen.

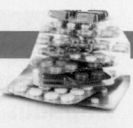

KEY POINTS

- Antihepatitis C drugs are relatively new. They are protease inhibitors specific to the hepatitis C virus. They must be combined with ribavirin and peginterferon.
- Some antivirals are available only for the local treatment of viral infections, including warts and eye infections.
- Topical antivirals should not be applied to open wounds; local reactions can occur with administration.

SUMMARY

- Viruses are particles of DNA or RNA surrounded by a protein coat that survive by injecting their own DNA or RNA into a healthy cell and taking over its functioning.
- Because viruses are contained within human cells, it has been difficult to develop drugs that are effective antivirals and yet do not destroy human cells. Antiviral agents are available that are effective against only a few types of viruses.
- Influenza A and respiratory viruses cause the signs and symptoms of the common cold or "flu." The drugs that are available to prevent the replication of these viruses are used for prophylaxis against these diseases during peak seasons and to treat disease when it occurs.
- Herpes viruses and CMV are DNA viruses that cause a multitude of problems, including cold sores, encephalitis, infections of the eye and liver, and genital herpes.
- Helper T cells are essential for maintaining a vigilant, effective immune system. When these cells are decreased in number or effectiveness, opportunistic infections occur. AIDS and ARC are syndromes of opportunistic infections that occur when the immune system is depressed.
- HIV, which specifically attacks helper T cells, may remain dormant in these cells for long periods and has been known to mutate easily.
- Antiviral agents that are effective against HIV and AIDS include nonnucleoside and NRTIs, protease inhibitors, fusion inhibitors, CCR5 coreceptor antagonists, and integrase inhibitors, all of which affect the way the virus communicates, replicates, or matures within the cell. These drugs are known as antiretroviral agents. They are given in combination to most effectively destroy the HIV virus and prevent mutation.
- Three drugs have been approved to treat hepatitis B infection: Adefovir, entecavir, and telbivudine.
- Three standalone drugs and several combination drugs are now available to treat hepatitis C. They must be combined with peginterferon and ribavirin.
- Some antivirals are available only for the local treatment of viral infections, including warts and eye infections. These drugs are not absorbed systemically.

CHECK YOUR UNDERSTANDING

Answers to the questions in this chapter can be found in Answers to Check Your Understanding Questions on thePoint®.

MULTIPLE CHOICE

Select the best answer to the following.

1. In assessing a patient a viral cause might be suspected if the patient was diagnosed with
- **a.** tuberculosis.
- **b.** leprosy.
- **c.** the common cold.
- **d.** gonorrhea.

2. Virus infections have proved difficult to treat because they
- **a.** have a protein coat.
- **b.** inject themselves into human cells to survive and to reproduce.
- **c.** are bits of RNA or DNA.
- **d.** easily resist drug therapy.

3. Naturally occurring substances that are released in the body in response to viral invasion are called
- **a.** antibodies.
- **b.** immunoglobulins.
- **c.** interferons.
- **d.** interleukins.

4. Herpes viruses cause a broad range of conditions but have not been identified as the causative agent in
- **a.** cold sores.
- **b.** shingles.
- **c.** genital infections.
- **d.** leprosy.

(continues on page 168)

5. Which of the following would be an important teaching point for the patient receiving an agent to treat herpes virus or CMV?

a. Stop taking the drug as soon as the lesions have disappeared.
b. Sexual intercourse is fine—as long as you are taking the drug, you are not contagious.
c. Drink plenty of fluids to decrease the drug's toxic effects on the kidneys.
d. There are few if any associated GI adverse effects.

6. HIV selectively enters which of the following cells?

a. B clones
b. Helper T cells
c. Suppressor T cells
d. Cytotoxic T cells

7. Nursing interventions for the patient receiving antiviral drugs for the treatment of HIV probably would include

a. monitoring renal and hepatic function periodically during therapy.
b. administering the drugs just once a day to increase drug effectiveness.
c. encouraging the patient to avoid eating if GI upset is severe.
d. stopping the drugs and notifying the prescriber if severe rash occurs.

8. Locally active antiviral agents can be used to treat

a. HIV infection.
b. warts.
c. RSV.
d. CMV systemic infections.

MULTIPLE RESPONSE

Select all that apply.

1. When explaining to a client the reasoning behind using combination therapy in the treatment of HIV the nurse would include which of the following points?

a. The virus can remain dormant within the T cell for a very long time; it can mutate while in the T cell.
b. Adverse effects of many of the drugs used to treat this virus include immunosuppression, so the disease could become worse.
c. The drugs are cheaper if used in combination.
d. The virus slowly mutates with each generation.
e. Attacking the virus at many points in its life cycle has been shown to be most effective.
f. Research has shown that using only one type of drug that targeted only one point in the virus life cycle led to more mutations and more difficulty in controlling the disease.

2. Appropriate nursing diagnoses related to the drug therapy for a patient receiving combination antiviral therapy for the treatment of HIV infection would include the following:

a. Disturbed sensory perception (kinesthetic) related to the CNS effects of the drugs.
b. Imbalanced nutrition: More than body requirements related to appetite stimulation.
c. Heart failure related to cardiac effects of the drugs.
d. Adrenal insufficiency related to endocrine effects of the drugs.
e. Acute pain related to GI, CNS, or dermatological effects of the drugs.
f. Deficient knowledge regarding drug therapy.

BIBLIOGRAPHY AND REFERENCES

AASLD/IDSA/IAS–USA. (2016). HCV testing and linkage to care. Recommendations for testing, managing, and treating hepatitis C [*International Antiviral Society–USA*]. Available online at: http://www.hcvguidelines.org/full-report/hcv-testing-and-linkage-care

Brunton, L., Chabner, B., & Knollman, B. (2011). *Goodman and Gilman's the pharmacological basis of therapeutics* (12th ed.). New York: McGraw-Hill.

CDC. (2015). Guidelines for management of AIDS [*Centers for Disease Control and Prevention*]. Available online at: http://www.cdc.gov/hiv/guidelines/index.html

Facts and Comparisons. (2015). *Drug facts and comparisons.* St. Louis, MO: Author.

Facts and Comparisons. (2015). *Professional's guide to patient drug facts.* St. Louis, MO: Author.

Kaiser, L., Wat, C., Mills, T., et al. (2003). Impact of oseltamivir treatment on influenza-related lower respiratory tract complications and hospitalizations. *Archives of Internal Medicine, 163,* 1667–1672.

Karch, A. M. (2014). *Lippincott's nursing drug guide.* Philadelphia, PA: Lippincott Williams & Wilkins.

Mandell, G., Bennett, J., & Dolin, R. (Eds.). (2014). *Mandell, Douglas and Bennett's principles and practice of infectious diseases* (8th ed.). St. Louis, MO: Elsevier.

Pasternak, B., & Hvid, A. (2010) Use of acyclovir, valacyclovir and famiciclovir in the first trimester of pregnancy and the risk of birth defects. *Journal of the American Medical Association, 304*(8), 859–866.

Porth, C. M. (2013). *Pathophysiology: Concepts of altered health states* (9th ed.). Philadelphia, PA: Lippincott Williams & Wilkins.

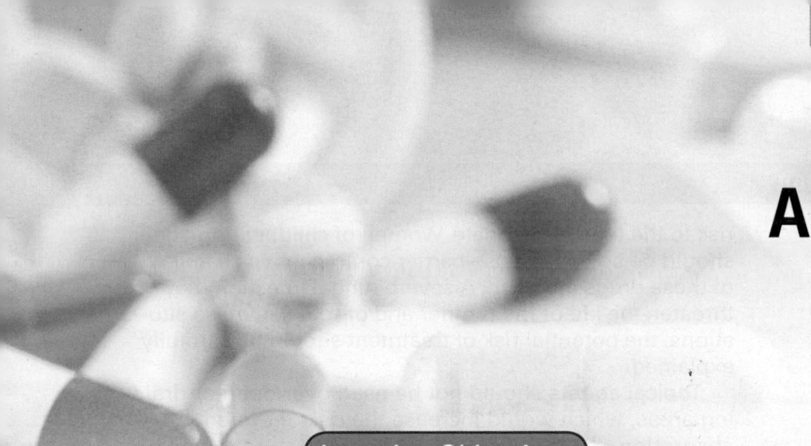

Antifungal Agents 11

Learning Objectives

Upon completion of this chapter, you will be able to:

1. Describe the characteristics of a fungus and a fungal infection.
2. Discuss the therapeutic actions, indications, pharmacokinetics, contraindications, proper administration, most common adverse reactions, and important drug–drug interactions associated with systemic and topical antifungals.
3. Compare and contrast the prototype drugs for systemic and topical antifungals with the other drugs in each class.
4. Discuss the impact of using antifungals across the lifespan.
5. Outline the nursing considerations for patients receiving a systemic or topical antifungal.

Glossary of Key Terms

azoles: a group of drugs used to treat fungal infections

***Candida*:** fungus that is normally found on mucous membranes; can cause yeast infections or thrush of the gastrointestinal (GI) tract and vagina in immunosuppressed patients

ergosterol: steroid-type protein found in the cell membrane of fungi; similar in configuration to adrenal hormones and testosterone

fungus: a cellular organism with a hard cell wall that contains chitin and many polysaccharides, as well as a cell membrane that contains ergosterols

mycosis: disease caused by a fungus

tinea: fungus called ringworm that causes such infections as athlete's foot, jock itch, and others

Drug List

Systemic Antifungals

Azole Topical Antifungals

butoconazole

(P) clotrimazole

econazole

efinaconazole

ketoconazole

miconazole

oxiconazole

sertaconazole

sulconazole

terbinafine

terconazole

tioconazole

Topical Antifungals

Azole Antifungals

(P) fluconazole

itraconazole

ketoconazole

posaconazole

terbinafine

voriconazole

Echinocandin Antifungals

anidulafungin

caspofungin

micafungin

Other Antifungals

amphotericin B

flucytosine

griseofulvin

nystatin

Other Topical Antifungals

butenafine

ciclopirox

gentian violet

naftifine

tolnaftate

undecylenic acid

Fungal infections in humans range from conditions such as the annoying "athlete's foot" to potentially fatal systemic infections. An infection caused by a **fungus** is called a **mycosis**. Fungi differ from bacteria in that the fungus has a rigid cell wall that is made up of chitin and various polysaccharides and a cell membrane that contains **ergosterol**. The composition of the protective layers of the fungal cell makes the organism resistant to antibiotics.

BOX 11.1 FOCUS ON Drug Therapy Across the Lifespan

Antifungal Agents

CHILDREN

Children are very sensitive to the effects of most antifungal drugs, and more severe reactions can be expected when these drugs are used in children.

Many of these drugs do not have proven safety and efficacy in children, and extreme caution should be exercised when using them. Fluconazole, ketoconazole, terbinafine, and griseofulvin have established pediatric doses and would be drugs of choice if appropriate for a particular infection.

Topical agents should not be used over open or draining areas that would increase the risk of systemic absorption and toxicity. Occlusive dressings, including tight diapers, should be avoided over the affected areas.

ADULTS

These drugs can be very toxic to the body, and their use should be reserved for situations in which the causative organism has been identified. Over-the-counter topical preparations are widely used, and patients should be cautioned to follow the instructions and to report continued problems to their health care provider.

Pregnant and nursing women should not use these drugs unless the benefit clearly outweighs the potential risk to the fetus or neonate. Women of childbearing age should be advised to use barrier contraceptives if any of these drugs are used. A severe fungal infection may threaten the life of the mother and/or fetus; in these situations, the potential risk of treatment should be carefully explained.

Topical agents should not be used over open or draining areas, which would increase the risk of systemic absorption.

OLDER ADULTS

Older patients may be more susceptible to the adverse effects associated with these drugs and should be monitored closely.

Patients with hepatic dysfunction are at increased risk for worsening hepatic problems and toxic effects of many of these drugs (ketoconazole, itraconazole, griseofulvin). If hepatic dysfunction is expected (extreme age, alcohol abuse, use of other hepatotoxic drugs), the dose may need to be lowered and the patient monitored more frequently.

Other agents are associated with renal toxicity (flucytosine, fluconazole, griseofulvin) and should be used cautiously in the presence of renal impairment. Patients at risk for renal toxicity should be monitored carefully.

Conversely, because of their cellular makeup, bacteria are resistant to antifungal drugs.

The incidence of fungal infections has increased with the rising number of immunocompromised individuals—patients with AIDS and AIDS-related complex, those taking immunosuppressant drugs, those who have undergone transplantation surgery or cancer treatment, and members of the increasingly large elderly population, whose body is no longer able to protect itself from the many fungi that are found throughout the environment (Box 11.1). For example, ***Candida***, a fungus that is normally found on mucous membranes, can cause yeast infections or "thrush" in the gastrointestinal (GI) tract and yeast infections or "vaginitis" in the vagina.

Systemic Antifungals

The drugs used to treat systemic fungal infections (Table 11.1) can be toxic to the host and are not to be used indiscriminately. It is important to get a culture of the fungus causing the infection to ensure that the right drug is being used so that the patient is not put at additional risk from the toxic adverse effects associated with these drugs.

Azole Antifungals

The **azoles** are a large group of antifungals used to treat systemic and topical fungal infections (Table 11.1). The azoles include fluconazole (*Diflucan*), itraconazole (*Sporanox*), ketoconazole (*Nizoral*), posaconazole (*Noxafil*), terbinafine (*Lamisil*), and voriconazole (*Vfend*). Although azoles are considered less toxic than some other antifungals, such as amphotericin B, they may also be less effective in very severe and progressive infections.

Therapeutic Actions and Indications

These drugs bind to sterols and can cause cell death (a fungicidal effect) or interfere with cell replication (a fungistatic effect), depending on the type of fungus being affected and the concentration of the drug (see Figure 11.1).

Ketoconazole, fluconazole, and itraconazole work by blocking the activity of a sterol in the fungal wall. In addition, they may block the activity of human steroids, including testosterone and cortisol (see Usual Indications in Table 11.1).

Posaconazole is one of the newest antifungals (see Table 11.1 for uses). This drug and voriconazole inhibit the synthesis of ergosterol, which leads to the inability of the fungus to form a cell wall, which results in cell death. Terbinafine is a similar drug that blocks the formation of ergosterol. It inhibits the cytochrome P450 2D6 (CYP2D6) enzyme system; therefore, it may be a better choice for patients who need to take drugs metabolized by the cytochrome P450 (CYP450) system. It is available in a sprinkle formulation for children.

Pharmacokinetics

Ketoconazole, itraconazole, posaconazole, and terbinafine are administered orally. Ketoconazole is also available as a

Table 11.1 ***Drugs in Focus:* Systemic Antifungals**

Drug Name	Dosage/Route	Usual Indications
Azole Antifungals		
fluconazole (*Diflucan*)	*Adult:* 200–400 mg PO on day 1, followed by 100 mg/d PO; IV route can be used, but do not exceed 200 mg/h *Pediatric:* 3–6 mg/kg PO; do not exceed 12 mg/kg	Treatment of candidiasis, cryptococcal meningitis, other systemic fungal infections; prophylaxis for reducing the incidence of candidiasis in bone marrow transplant recipients
itraconazole (*Sporanox*)	*Adult:* 100–400 mg/d PO *Pediatric:* Safety and efficacy not established	Treatment of blastomycosis, histoplasmosis, and aspergillosis
ketoconazole (*Nizoral, Xolegel*)	*Adult:* 200 mg/d PO, up to 400 mg/d PO in severe cases *Pediatric (□2 y):* 3.3–6.6 mg/kg/d PO *Pediatric (<2 y):* safety not established *Topical:* As a shampoo and topical	Treatment of aspergillosis, leishmaniasis, cryptococcosis, blastomycosis, moniliasis, coccidioidomycosis, histoplasmosis, and mucormycosis; topical treatment of mycoses (cream), and to reduce the scaling of dandruff (shampoo)
posaconazole (*Noxafil*)	*Adult and pediatric (□13 y):* 200 mg PO t.i.d. with food	Prophylaxis of invasive *Aspergillus* and *Candida* infections in adults and children >13 y who are immunosuppressed secondary to antineoplastic, chemotherapy, graft-vs.-host disease following transplants, or hematological malignancies
terbinafine (*Lamisil*)	*Adult:* 250 mg/d PO for 6 wk (fingernail) or 12 wk (toenail) *Pediatric:* 125–250 mg/d PO for 6 wk (sprinkle capsules)	Treatment of onychomycosis of the fingernail or toenail caused by dermatophytes; the drug was approved in late 2007 for treatment of tinea capitis (ringworm of the scalp) in children ≥4 y
voriconazole (*Vfend*)	*Adult and pediatric (>12 y):* 6 mg/kg IV q12h for two doses, then 4 mg/kg IV q12h; switch to oral dose as soon as possible *>40 kg:* 200 mg PO q12h *<40 kg:* 100 mg PO q12h	Treatment of invasive aspergillosis; treatment of serious fungal infections caused by *Scedosporium apiospermum* or *Fusarium* spp. when the patient is intolerant to or not responding to other therapy
Echinocandin Antifungals		
anidulafungin (*Eraxis*)	100–200 mg IV on day 1, then 50–100 mg/d IV for 14 d; dose varies with infection being treated	Treatment of candidemia (infection of the blood stream) and other forms of *Candida* infection, intra-abdominal infections, and esophageal candidiasis
caspofungin acetate (*Cancidas*)	*Adult:* 70 mg/d IV loading dose, then 50 mg/d IV infusion; dose should be reduced to 35 mg/d IV infusion with hepatic impairment	Treatment of invasive aspergillosis in patients who do not respond or are intolerant to other therapies
micafungin (*Mycamine*)	***Esophageal candidiasis:*** *Adult:* 150 mg/d IV over 1 h for 6–30 d *Prophylaxis:* 50 mg/d IV over 1 h for about 19 d	Treatment of patients with esophageal candidiasis; prophylaxis of *Candida* infections in patients with hematopoietic stem cell transplant
Other Antifungals		
amphotericin B (*Abelcet, Amphotec, AmBisome*)	0.25–1.5 mg/kg/d IV based on the infection being treated; each brand name has different dosages	Treatment of aspergillosis, leishmaniasis, cryptococcosis, blastomycosis, moniliasis, coccidioidomycosis, histoplasmosis and mucormycosis; use is reserved for progressive, potential fatal infections due to many associated adverse effects
flucytosine (*Ancobon*)	50–150 mg/kg/d PO in divided doses at 6-h intervals	Treatment of systemic infections caused by *Candida* or *Cryptococcus*
griseofulvin (generic)	***Tinea corporis, tinea cruris, and tinea capitis:*** *Adult:* 500 mg (microsize) or 330–375 mg/d (ultramicrosize) PO *Tinea pedis and tinea unguium:* *Adult:* 0.75–1 g (microsize) or 660–750 mg (ultramicrosize) PO daily *Pediatric (>2 y):* 11 mg/kg/d (microsize) or 7.3 mg (ultramicrosize) PO daily (not recommended for children ≤2 y)	Treatment of variety of ringworm or tinea infections caused by susceptible *Trichophyton* spp., including tinea corporis, tinea pedis, tinea cruris, tinea barbae, tinea capitis, and tinea unguium
nystatin (*Mycostatin, Nilstat*)	*Adult and pediatric:* 500,000–1,000,000 units t.i.d. PO; continue for 48 h after resolution to prevent relapse; also used topically	Treatment of candidiasis (oral form); treatment of local candidiasis, vaginal candidiasis, and cutaneous and mucocutaneous infections caused by *Candida* spp.

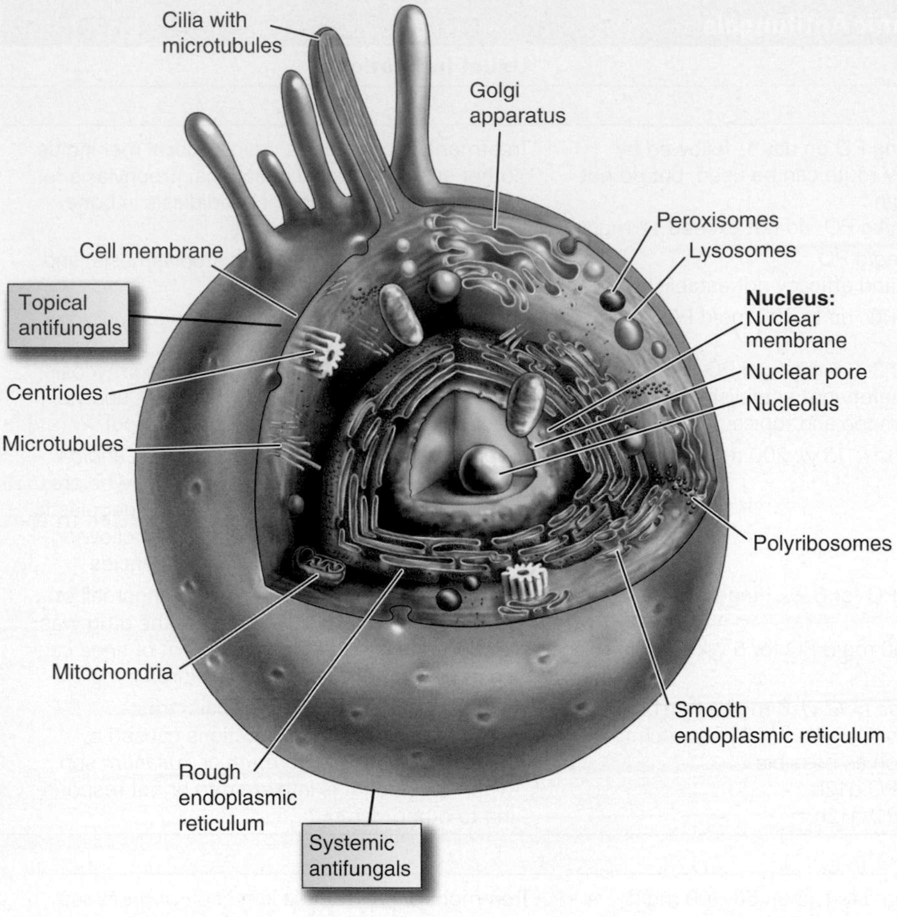

FIGURE 11.1 Sites of action of antifungal agents. Both systemic and topical antifungals alter fungal cell permeability, leading to prevention of replication and cell death.

shampoo and a cream, and terbinafine is also available in a sprinkle formulation for children.

Fluconazole and voriconazole are available in oral and IV preparations, making it possible to start the drug intravenously for a serious infection and then switch to an oral form when the patient's condition improves and he or she is able to take oral medications.

Ketoconazole is absorbed rapidly from the GI tract, with peak levels occurring within 1 to 3 hours. It is extensively metabolized in the liver and excreted through the feces. Fluconazole reaches peak levels within 1 to 2 hours after administration. Most of the drug is excreted unchanged in the urine, so extreme caution should be used in the presence of renal dysfunction. Itraconazole is slowly absorbed from the GI tract and is metabolized in the liver by the CYP450 system. It is excreted in the urine and feces. Posaconazole is given orally, has a rapid onset of action, and peaks within 3 to 5 hours. It is metabolized in the liver and excreted in the feces. Terbinafine is rapidly absorbed from the GI tract, extensively metabolized in the liver, and excreted in the urine with a half-life of 36 hours. Voriconazole reaches peak levels in 1 to 2 hours if given orally, and at the onset of the infusion if given IV. It is metabolized in the liver with a half-life of 24 hours and is excreted in the urine.

Contraindications and Cautions

Ketoconazole has been associated with severe hepatic toxicity and should be avoided in patients with hepatic dysfunction *to prevent serious hepatic toxicity.* In addition, ketoconazole is not the drug of choice for patients with endocrine or fertility problems *because of its effects on these processes.* Although fluconazole should be used with caution in the presence of liver or renal impairment, *because it could cause liver or renal toxicity*, fluconazole is not associated with the endocrine problems seen with ketoconazole.

Because itraconazole has been associated with hepatic failure, it should not be used in patients with hepatic failure, and should be used with caution in those with hepatic impairment. It is not known whether posaconazole crosses the placenta or enters breast milk, so it should not be used during pregnancy or lactation unless the benefits clearly outweigh the potential risks. Caution should be used if posaconazole is used in the presence of liver impairment *because it can cause liver toxicity.* Carefully monitor patients for bone marrow suppression and GI and liver toxicity if using this drug. *Terbinafine has been associated with severe liver toxicity* and is contraindicated with liver failure. *It may cross the placenta and may enter breast milk*, and so it should not be used in pregnant or nursing women because of the potential toxic effects on the fetus or baby.

Voriconazole should not be used with any other drugs that prolong the QTc interval (corrected QT Interval) *because that could be worsened* and *can cause ergotism if taken with ergot alkaloid*; so it should not be combined with ergots.

FOCUS ON Safe Medication Administration

*Name confusion has occurred between **Lamisil** (terbinafine) and **Lamictal** (lamotrigine, an antiepileptic agent). Use extreme caution if your patient is receiving either of these drugs to make sure that the correct drug is being used.*

Adverse Effects

Many of the azoles are associated with liver toxicity and can cause severe effects on a fetus or a nursing baby.

Clinically Important Drug–Drug Interactions

Ketoconazole and fluconazole strongly inhibit the CYP450 enzyme system in the liver and are associated with many drug–drug interactions, such as increased serum levels of the following agents: cyclosporine, digoxin, oral hypoglycemics, warfarin, oral anticoagulants, and phenytoin. If these combinations cannot be avoided, closely monitor patients and anticipate the need for dose adjustments. A drug guide should be consulted any time one of these drugs is added to or removed from a drug regimen. Itraconazole has a black box warning regarding the potential for serious cardiovascular effects if it is given with lovastatin, simvastatin, triazolam, midazolam, pimozide, or dofetilide. These combinations should be avoided. Voriconazole and posaconazole should not be used with any other drugs that prolong the QTc interval and can cause ergotism if taken with ergot alkaloids. Box 11.2 highlights important information about hazardous interactions between voriconazole and posaconazole and the herb ergot.

BOX 11.2 FOCUS ON Herbal and Alternative Therapies

Patients being treated with voriconazole or posaconazole should be cautioned about the risk of ergotism if they combine this drug with ergot, an herb frequently used to treat migraine headache and menstrual problems. If the patient is using either of these drugs, it should be suggested that ergot not be used until the antifungal therapy is finished.

Prototype Summary: Fluconazole

Indications: Treatment of oropharyngeal, esophageal, and vaginal candidiasis; cryptococcal meningitis; systemic fungal infections; prophylaxis to decrease the incidence of candidiasis in bone marrow transplants.

Actions: Binds to sterols in the fungal cell membrane, changing membrane permeability; fungicidal or fungistatic, depending on the concentration of drug and the organism.

Pharmacokinetics:

Route	Onset	Peak	Duration
Oral	Slow	1–2 h	2–4 d
IV	Rapid	1 h	2–4 d

$T_{1/2}$: 30 hours; metabolized in the liver and excreted in the urine.

Adverse Effects: Headache, nausea, vomiting, diarrhea, abdominal pain, rash.

Echinocandin Antifungals

The echinocandin antifungals are another group of antifungals. Drugs in this class include anidulafungin, caspofungin, and micafungin.

Therapeutic Actions and Indications

The echinocandins work by inhibiting glucan synthesis. Glucan is an enzyme that is present in the fungal cell wall but not in human cell walls. If this enzyme is inhibited the fungal cell wall cannot form, leading to death of the cell wall. See Table 11.1 for Usual Indications for each of these agents.

Pharmacokinetics

Anidulafungin is given as a daily IV infusion for at least 14 days. It has a rapid onset of action, is metabolized by degradation, and has a half-life of 40 to 50 hours. This drug is excreted in the feces.

Caspofungin is available for IV use. This drug is slowly metabolized in the liver, with half-lives of 9 to 11 hours, then 6 to 48 hours, and then 40 to 50 hours. It is bound to protein and widely distributed throughout the body. It is excreted through the urine.

Micafungin is an IV drug. It has a rapid onset, a half-life of 14 to 17 hours, and is excreted in the urine.

Contraindications and Cautions

Anidulafungin may cross the placenta and enter breast milk and should not be used by pregnant or lactating women. Caution must be used in the presence of hepatic impairment *because it can be toxic to the liver. Caspofungin can be toxic to the liver*; therefore, reduced doses must be used if a patient has known hepatic impairment. *Caspofungin is embryotoxic in animal studies and is known to enter breast milk*; therefore, it should be used with great caution during pregnancy and lactation. *Because of the potential for adverse reactions in the fetus or the neonate*, micafungin should be used during pregnancy and lactation only if the benefits clearly outweigh the risks.

Adverse Effects

Anidulafungin and caspofungin are associated with hepatic toxicity, and liver function should be monitored closely when using these drugs. Potentially serious hypersensitivity reactions have occurred with micafungin. In addition, bone marrow suppression can occur; monitor patients closely.

Clinically Important Drug–Drug Interactions

Concurrent use of cyclosporine with caspofungin is contraindicated unless the benefit clearly outweighs the risk of hepatic injury.

Other Antifungal Agents

Other antifungal drugs that are available do not fit into either of these classes. These include amphotericin B (*Abelcet, AmBisome, Amphotec*), flucytosine (*Ancobon*), griseofulvin (generic), and nystatin (*Mycostatin, Nilstat*).

Therapeutic Actions and Indications

Other antifungal agents work to cause fungal cell death or to prevent fungal cell reproduction. Amphotericin B is a very potent drug with many unpleasant adverse effects (see Adverse Effects). The drug binds to the sterols in the fungus cell wall, changing cell wall permeability. This change can lead to cell death (fungicidal effect) or prevent the fungal cells from reproducing (fungistatic effect). (See Table 11.1 for Usual Indications.) Because of the many adverse effects associated with this agent, its use is reserved for progressive, potentially fatal infections.

Flucytosine is a less toxic drug that alters the cell membrane of susceptible fungi, causing cell death (see Table 11.1 for Usual Indications).

Griseofulvin is an older antifungal that acts in much the same way, changing cell membrane permeability and causing cell death.

Nystatin binds to sterols in the cell wall, changing membrane permeability and allowing leaking of the cellular components, which will result in cell death.

Pharmacokinetics

Amphotericin B and flucytosine are available in IV form. They are excreted in the urine, with an initial half-life of 24 hours and then a 15-day half-life. Their metabolism is not fully understood. Flucytosine is well absorbed from the GI tract, with peak levels occurring in 2 hours. Most of the drug is excreted unchanged in the urine and a small amount in the feces, with a half-life of 2.4 to 4.8 hours. Griseofulvin is administered orally and reaches peak levels in around 4 hours. It is metabolized in the liver and excreted in the urine with a half-life of 24 hours. Nystatin is not absorbed from the GI tract and passes unchanged in the stool.

Contraindications and Cautions

Amphotericin B is available in several brand names; caution must be used to differentiate the brand used as the dosages vary. Amphotericin B has been used successfully during pregnancy, but it should be used cautiously. It crosses into breast milk and should not be used during lactation *because of the potential risk to the neonate. Because flucytosine is excreted primarily in the urine*, extreme caution is needed in the presence of renal impairment because drug accumulation and toxicity can occur. Toxicity is associated with serum levels higher than 100 mcg/mL. *Because of the potential for adverse reactions in the fetus or neonate*, flucytosine should be used during pregnancy and lactation only if the benefits clearly outweigh the risks. *It is not known whether nystatin crosses the placenta or enters breast milk*, so it should not be used during pregnancy or lactation unless the benefits clearly outweigh the potential risks.

Adverse Effects

The adverse effects of these drugs are related to their toxic effects on the liver and kidneys. Patients should be monitored closely for any changes in liver or kidney functions. Bone marrow suppression has also been reported with the use of these drugs. Rash and dermatological changes have been reported with these antifungals. Amphotericin B is associated with severe renal impairment, bone marrow suppression, GI irritation with nausea, vomiting, and potentially severe diarrhea, anorexia and weight loss, and pain at the injection site with the possibility of phlebitis or thrombophlebitis. The adverse effects of griseofulvin are relatively mild, with headache and central nervous system (CNS) changes occurring most frequently (Figure 11.2).

Clinically Important Drug–Drug Interactions

Patients who receive amphotericin B should not take other nephrotoxic drugs such as nephrotoxic antibiotics or antineoplastics, cyclosporine, or corticosteroids unless absolutely necessary *because of the increased risk of severe renal toxicity.*

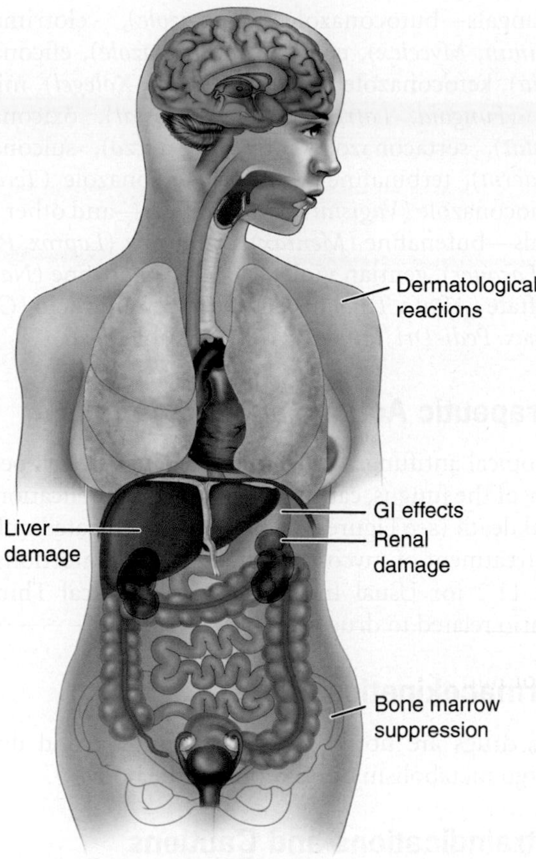

FIGURE 11.2 Common adverse effects associated with antifungals.

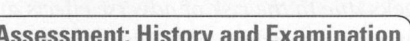

Nursing Considerations for Patients Receiving Systemic Antifungals

Assessment: History and Examination

- Assess the patient for *contraindications or cautions:* History of allergy to antifungals *to prevent potential hypersensitivity reactions*; history of liver or renal dysfunction *that might interfere with metabolism and excretion of the drug*; and pregnancy or lactation *because of potential adverse effects to the fetus or infant.*
- Perform a physical assessment *to establish baseline data for assessing the effectiveness of the drug and the occurrence of any adverse effects associated with drug therapy*; test orientation and reflexes *to evaluate any CNS effects*; and examine skin for color and lesions *to monitor for any dermatological effects.*
- Obtain a culture of the infected area *to make an accurate determination of the type and responsiveness of the fungus.*
- Evaluate renal and hepatic function tests and complete blood count *to determine baseline function of these organs and to assess possible toxicity during drug therapy.*

Nursing Diagnoses

Nursing diagnoses related to drug therapy might include the following:

- Acute pain related to GI, CNS, and local effects of the drug
- Disturbed sensory perception (kinesthetic) related to CNS effects
- Deficient knowledge regarding drug therapy

Planning

- The patient will receive the best therapeutic effect from the drug therapy.
- The patient will have limited adverse effects to the drug therapy.
- The patient will have an understanding of the drug therapy, adverse effects to anticipate, and measures to relieve discomfort and improve safety.

Implementation with Rationale

- Arrange for appropriate culture and sensitivity tests before beginning therapy *to ensure that the appropriate drug is being used.* However, in some cases, treatment can begin before test results are known because of the seriousness of the systemic infections.
- Administer the entire course of the drug *to get the full beneficial effects*; this may take as long as 6 months for some chronic infections.
- Monitor IV sites *to ensure that phlebitis or infiltration does not occur.* Treat appropriately and restart IV at another site if phlebitis occurs.
- Monitor renal and hepatic function before and periodically during treatment to assess for possible dysfunction *and arrange to stop the drug if signs of renal or hepatic failure occur.*
- Provide comfort and safety provisions if CNS effects occur (e.g., side rails and assistance with ambulation for dizziness and weakness, analgesics for headache, antipyretics for fever and chills, temperature regulation for fever) *to protect the patient from injury.*
- Provide small, frequent, nutritious meals if GI upset is severe. Monitor nutritional status and arrange a dietary consultation as needed *to ensure nutritional status.* GI upset may be decreased by taking an oral drug with food.
- Instruct the patient *to enhance patient knowledge about drug therapy and to promote compliance.*
- Provide the following patient teaching:
  - Follow the appropriate dosage regimen.
  - Take safety precautions, including changing position slowly and avoiding driving and hazardous tasks, if CNS effects occur.
  - Take an oral drug with meals and try small, frequent meals if GI upset is a problem.

(continues on page 176)

- Report to a health care provider any of the following: Sore throat, unusual bruising and bleeding, or yellowing of the eyes or skin, all of which could indicate hepatic toxicity; or severe nausea and vomiting, which could interfere with nutritional state and slow recovery.

Evaluation

- Monitor patient response to the drug (resolution of fungal infection).
- Monitor for adverse effects (orientation and affect, nutritional state, skin color and lesions, renal and hepatic function).
- Evaluate the effectiveness of the teaching plan (patient can name the drug, dosage, possible adverse effects to watch for, and specific measures to help avoid adverse effects).
- Monitor the effectiveness of comfort and safety measures and compliance with the regimen.

KEY POINTS

- Fungi can cause many different infections in humans.
- Fungi differ from bacteria in that a fungus has a rigid cell wall that is made up of chitin and various polysaccharides and a cell membrane that contains ergosterol.
- Systemic antifungal drugs can be very toxic; extreme care should be taken to ensure that the right drug is used to treat an infection and that the patient is monitored closely to prevent severe toxicity.
- Systemic antifungals are associated with many drug–drug interactions because of their effects on the liver. Monitor a patient closely when adding or removing a drug from a drug regimen if the patient is receiving a systemic antifungal.

Topical Antifungals

Some antifungal drugs are available only in topical forms for treating a variety of mycoses of the skin and mucous membranes. Some of the systemic antifungals are also available in topical forms. Fungi that cause these mycoses are called *dermatophytes.* These diseases include a variety of tinea infections, which are often referred to as ringworm, although the causal organism is a fungus, not a worm. These mycoses include **tinea** infections such as athlete's foot (tinea pedis), jock itch (tinea cruris), and yeast infections of the mouth and vagina often caused by *Candida.* Because the antifungal drugs reserved for use as topical agents are often too toxic for systemic administration, care is necessary when using them near open or draining wounds that might permit systemic absorption. Topical antifungals include the azole-type antifungals—butoconazole (*Gynazole*), clotrimazole (*Lotrimin, Mycelex*), econazole (*Spectazole*), eficonazole (*Jublia*), ketoconazole (*Extina, Nizoral, Xolegel*), miconazole (*Fungoid, Lotrimin AF, Monistat*), oxiconazole (*Oxistat*), sertaconazole nitrate (*Ertaczo*), sulconazole (*Exelderm*), terbinafine (*Lamisil*), terconazole (*Terazol*), and tioconazole (*Vagistat-1, Monistat-1*)—and other antifungals—butenafine (*Mentax*), ciclopirox (*Loprox, Penlac Nail Lacquer*), gentian violet (generic), naftifine (*Naftin*), tolnaftate (*Aftate, Tinactin*), and undecylenic acid (*Cruex, Desenex, Pedi-Dri, Fungoid AF*) (see Table 11.2).

Therapeutic Actions and Indications

The topical antifungal drugs work to alter the cell permeability of the fungus, causing prevention of replication and fungal death (see Figure 11.1). They are indicated only for local treatment of mycoses, including tinea infections. See Table 11.2 for Usual Indications (see Critical Thinking Scenario related to drug therapy).

Pharmacokinetics

These drugs are not absorbed systemically and do not undergo metabolism or excretion in the body.

Contraindications and Cautions

Because these drugs are not absorbed systemically, contraindications are limited to a known allergy to any of these drugs and open lesions. Econazole can cause intense, local burning and irritation and should be discontinued if these conditions become severe. Gentian violet stains skin and clothing bright purple; in addition, *it is very toxic when absorbed*, so it cannot be used near active lesions. Naftifine, oxiconazole, and sertaconazole nitrate should not be used for longer than 4 weeks *due to the risk of adverse effects and possible emergence of resistant strains of fungi.* Sulconazole should not be used for longer than 6 weeks *due to the risk of adverse effects and possible emergence of resistant strains of fungi.* Terbinafine should not be used for longer than 4 weeks. This drug should be stopped when the fungal condition appears to be improved or if local irritation and pain become too great to avoid toxic effects. Eficonazole must be applied with the supplied flow-through brush applicator.

Adverse Effects

When these drugs are applied locally as a cream, lotion, or spray, local effects include irritation, burning, rash, and swelling. When they are taken as a suppository or troche, adverse effects include nausea, vomiting, and hepatic dysfunction (related to absorption of some of the drug by the GI tract) or urinary frequency, burning, and change in sexual activity (related to local absorption in the vagina).

Table 11.2 *Drugs in Focus:* Topical Antifungals

Drug Name	Application/Available Form	Usual Indications
Azole Topical Antifungals		
butoconazole (*Gynazole I*)	Vaginal cream; applied only once a day for 4 wk	Available OTC for treatment of vaginal *Candida* infections
clotrimazole (*Lotrimin, Mycelex*)	Available OTC as a cream, lotion, or solution; applied as a thin layer twice a day for 2–4 wk	Available OTC for treatment of oral and vaginal *Candida* infections; tinea infections
econazole (*Spectazole*)	Available OTC as a cream; applied as a thin layer once or twice daily for 2 wk	Treatment of tinea
efinaconazole (*Jublia*)	Topical solution, applied with flow-through brush to affected toenails daily for 48 wk, completely cover all aspects of the involved toe(s)	Treatment of onychomycosis of the toenails due to *Trichophyton rubrum, Trichophyton mentagrophytes*
ketoconazole (*Extina, Xolegel*)	Available in cream, gel, foam, and shampoo form; applied once to twice daily for 2–4 wk	Treatment of seborrheic dermatitis, tinea corporis, tinea cruris, tinea pedis
miconazole (*Monistat, Fungoid, Lotrimin AF, Monistat*)	Available as an OTC product in several topical forms (vaginal suppository, cream, powder, solution, ointment, gel, and spray); applied twice daily for 2–4 wk	Treatment of local, topical mycoses, including bladder and vaginal infections and athlete's foot
oxiconazole (*Oxistat*)	Available as a cream or lotion; applied once daily or twice daily as needed	Short-term (up to 4 wk) treatment of topical mycosis
sertaconazole nitrate (*Ertaczo*)	Available as a topical cream; applied between toes affected by tinea pedis and to the surrounding healthy tissue two times a day for 4 wk	Treatment of tinea pedis infections (up to 4 wk)
sulconazole (*Exelderm*)	Available as a cream for athlete's foot and a solution for other tinea injections; applied once or twice a day for 4–6 wk	Treatment of tinea infections
terbinafine (*Lamisil*)	Available as a cream or gel; used for 1–4 wk; applied twice daily	Short-term (1–4 wk) treatment of topical mycosis; treatment of tinea infections
terconazole (*Terazol*)	Available as a suppository or a vaginal cream; applied for 3–7 consecutive days; used for 1–4 wk; applied twice daily	Local treatment of *Candida* infections
tioconazole (*Monistat-1, Vagistat-1*)	Vaginal ointment, meant for one-dose treatment only; one applicator full of ointment is inserted vaginally at bedtime	Treatment of recurrent vaginal *Candida* infections
Other Topical Antifungals		
butenafine (*Mentax*)	Topical cream; applied in a thin layer once to twice daily for up to 4 wk	Treatment of tinea infections
ciclopirox (*Loprox, Penlac Nail Lacquer*)	Available as a gel, cream, lotion, suspension, solution, and shampoo; applied twice daily for up to 4 wk	Treatment of topical tinea infections; solution for treatment of toenail and fingernail tinea infections caused by *Trichophyton rubrum*
gentian violet	Available as a topical solution; applied twice a day to affected area	Treatment of topical mycosis
naftifine (*Naftin*)	Available as a cream or gel; applied twice a day for up to 4 wk	Short-term treatment of severe topical mycosis (up to 4 wk)
tolnaftate (*Aftate, Tinactin*)	Available as a cream, solution, gel, powder, and spray; applied twice a day for 2–4 wk	Available OTC for treatment of athlete's foot
undecylenic acid (*Cruex, Desenex, Fungoid AF, Pedi-Dri*)	Available as a powder, cream, or ointment; used as needed	Available OTC for treatment of athlete's foot, jock itch, diaper rash, burning, and chafing in the groin area

OTC, over the counter.

Prototype Summary: Clotrimazole

Indications: Treatment of oropharyngeal candidiasis (troche); prevention of oropharyngeal candidiasis in patients receiving radiation or chemotherapy; local treatment of vulvovaginal candidiasis (vaginal preparations); topical treatment of tinea pedia, tinea cruris, and tinea corporis.

Actions: Binds to sterols in the fungal cell membrane, changing membrane permeability and allowing leakage of intracellular components, causing cell death.

Pharmacokinetics: Not absorbed systemically; pharmacokinetics is unknown.

Adverse Effects: Troche: Nausea, vomiting, abnormal liver function tests. Topical: Stinging, redness, urticaria, edema. Vaginal: Lower abdominal pain, urinary frequency, burning or irritation in sexual partner.

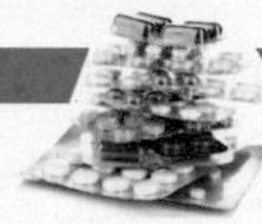

Nursing Considerations for Patients Receiving Topical Antifungals

Assessment: History and Examination

- Assess for known allergy to any topical antifungal agent *to prevent hypersensitivity reactions.*
- Perform a physical assessment *to establish baseline data for evaluation of the effectiveness of the drug and the occurrence of any adverse effects associated with drug therapy.*
- Perform culture and sensitivity testing of the affected area *to determine the causative fungus and appropriate medication.*
- Inspect the area of application for color, temperature, and evidence of lesions to establish a baseline *to monitor the effectiveness of the drug and to monitor for local adverse effects of the drug.*

Nursing Diagnoses

Nursing diagnoses related to drug therapy might include the following:

- Acute pain related to local effects of the drug
- Deficient knowledge regarding drug therapy
- Risk for impaired skin integrity

Planning

- The patient will receive the best therapeutic effect from the drug therapy.
- The patient will have limited adverse effects to the drug therapy.
- The patient will have an understanding of the drug therapy, adverse effects to anticipate, and measures to relieve discomfort and improve safety

Implementation with Rationale

- Culture the affected area before beginning therapy *to identify the causative fungus.*
- Ensure that the patient takes the complete course of the drug regimen *to achieve maximal results.*
- Instruct the patient in the correct method of administration, depending on the route, *to improve effectiveness and decrease the risk of adverse effects:*
  - Troches should be dissolved slowly in the mouth.
  - Vaginal suppositories, creams, and tablets should be inserted high into the vagina with the patient remaining recumbent for at least 10 to 15 minutes after insertion.
  - Topical creams and lotions should be gently rubbed into the affected area after it has been cleansed with soap and water and patted dry. Occlusive bandages should be avoided.
- Advise the patient to stop the drug if a severe rash occurs, especially if it is accompanied by blisters or if local irritation and pain are very severe. *This development may indicate a sensitivity to the drug or worsening of the condition being treated.*
- Provide patient instruction *to enhance patient knowledge about drug therapy and to promote compliance.*
- Provide the following patient teaching:
  - The correct method of drug administration; demonstrate proper application.
  - The length of time necessary to treat the infection adequately.
  - Use of clean, dry socks when treating athlete's foot, to help eradicate the infection.
  - The need to keep the infected area clean, washing with mild soap and water and patting dry; keep area dry.
  - The need to avoid scratching the infected area; use of cool compresses to decrease itching can be advised.
  - The need to avoid occlusive dressings because of the risk of increasing systemic absorption.
  - The importance of not placing drugs near open wounds or active lesions because these agents are not intended to be absorbed systemically.
  - The need to report severe local irritation, burning, or worsening of the infection to a health care provider.

Evaluation

- Monitor patient response to the drug (alleviation of signs and symptoms of the fungal infection).
- Monitor for adverse effects: Rash, local irritation, and burning.
- Evaluate the effectiveness of the teaching plan (patient can name the drug, dosage, possible adverse effects to watch for, and specific measures to help avoid adverse effects).
- Monitor the effectiveness of comfort and safety measures and compliance with the regimen.

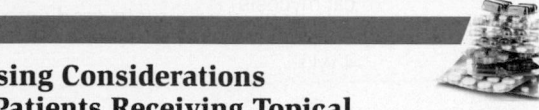

CRITICAL THINKING SCENARIO

Poor Nutrition and Opportunistic Infection

THE SITUATION

P.P., a 19-year-old woman and aspiring model, complains of abdominal pain, difficulty swallowing, and a very sore throat. The strict diets she has followed for long periods have sometimes amounted to a starvation regimen. In the last 18 months, she has received treatment for a variety of bacterial infections (e.g., pneumonia, cystitis) with a series of antibiotics.

P.P. appears to be a very thin, extremely pale young woman who looks older than her stated age. Her mouth is moist, and small, white colonies that extend down the pharynx cover the mucosa. A vaginal examination reveals similar colonies. Cultures are performed, and it is determined that she has mucocutaneous candidiasis. Ketoconazole (*Nizoral*) is prescribed, and P.P. is asked to return in 10 days for follow-up.

CRITICAL THINKING

What are the effects of taking a variety of antibiotics on the normal flora? *Think about the possible cause of the mycosis.*

What happens to the immune system and to the skin and mucous membranes when a person's nutritional status deteriorates?

How is P.P.'s chosen profession affecting her health?

What are the possible ramifications of suggesting that P.P. change her profession or her lifestyle?

What are the important nursing implications for P.P.?

Think about how the nurse can work with P.P. to ensure some compliance with therapy and a return to a healthy state.

DISCUSSION

Because of P.P.'s appearance a complete physical examination should be performed before drug therapy is initiated. It is necessary to know baseline functioning to evaluate any underlying problems that may exist. Poor nutrition and total starvation result in characteristic deficiencies that predispose individuals to opportunistic infections and prevent their bodies from protecting themselves adequately through inflammatory and immune responses. In this case, the fact that liver changes often occur with poor nutrition is particularly important; such hepatic dysfunction may cause deficient drug metabolism and lead to toxicity.

An intensive program of teaching and support should be started for P.P., who should have an opportunity to vent her feelings and fears. She needs help accepting her diagnosis and adapting to the drug therapy and nutritional changes that are necessary for the effective treatment of this infection. She should understand the possible causes of her infection (poor nutrition and the loss of normal flora secondary to antibiotic therapy); the specifics of her drug therapy, including timing and administration; and adverse effects and warning signs that should be reported. P.P. should be monitored closely for adverse effects and should return for follow-up regularly while taking the ketoconazole. Nutritional counseling or referral to a dietitian for thorough nutritional teaching may prove beneficial.

The actual resolution of the fungal infection may occur only after a combination of prolonged drug and nutritional therapy. Because the required therapy will affect P.P.'s lifestyle tremendously, she will need a great deal of support and encouragement to make the necessary changes and to maintain compliance. A health care provider, such as a nurse who P.P. trusts and with whom she can regularly discuss her concerns, may be an essential element in helping to eradicate the fungal infection.

NURSING CARE GUIDE FOR P.P.: ANTIFUNGAL AGENTS

Assessment: History and Examination

Assess history of allergy to any antifungal drug.

Also check history of renal or hepatic dysfunction and pregnancy or breastfeeding status.

Focus the physical examination on the following:

Local: Culture of infected site

Skin: Color, lesions, texture

GU: Urinary output

GI: Abdominal, liver evaluation

Hematological: Renal and hepatic function tests

Nursing Diagnoses

Acute pain related to GI, local, CNS effects

Disturbed sensory perception (kinesthetic) related to CNS effects

Imbalanced nutrition: Less than body requirements related to GI effects

Deficient knowledge regarding drug therapy

Planning

The patient will receive the best therapeutic effect from the drug therapy.

The patient will have limited adverse effects to the drug therapy.

The patient will have an understanding of the drug therapy, adverse effects to anticipate, and measures to relieve discomfort and improve safety.

Implementation

Culture infection before beginning therapy.

Provide comfort and implement safety measures (e.g., provide assistance and raise side rails).

(continues on page 180)

Poor Nutrition and Opportunistic Infection (continued)

Ensure temperature control, lighting control, mouth care, and skin care.
Provide small, frequent meals and monitor nutritional status.
Provide support and reassurance for dealing with drug effects and discomfort.
Provide patient teaching regarding drug name, dosage, adverse effects, precautions, and warning signs to report.

Evaluation

Evaluate drug effects: Relief of signs and symptoms of fungal infection.
Monitor for adverse effects: GI alterations, dizziness, confusion, headache, fever, renal or hepatic dysfunction, local pain, discomfort.
Monitor for drug–drug interactions as indicated for each drug.
Evaluate effectiveness of patient-teaching program and of comfort and safety measures.

PATIENT TEACHING FOR P.P.

- Ketoconazole is an antifungal drug that works to destroy the fungi that have invaded the body. Because of the way that antifungal drugs work, they may need to be taken over a long period of time.
- It is very important to take all of the prescribed medication.
- Common adverse effects of this drug include the following:
  - *Headache and weakness*—Change positions slowly. An analgesic may be ordered to help alleviate the headache. If you feel drowsy, avoid driving or dangerous activities.
  - *Stomach upset, nausea, and vomiting*—Small, frequent meals may help. Take the drug with food if appropriate because this may decrease the GI upset associated with these drugs. (Ketoconazole must be taken on an empty stomach at least 2 hours before taking a meal, antacids, milk products, or any other drugs.) Try to maintain adequate nutrition.
- Report any of the following to your health care provider: Severe vomiting, abdominal pain, fever or chills, yellowing of the skin or eyes, dark urine or pale stools, or skin rash.
- Avoid over-the-counter medications. If you feel that you need one of these, check with your health care provider first.
- Take the full course of your prescription. Never use this drug to self-treat any other infection, and never give this drug to any other person.
- Tell any doctor, nurse, or other health care provider involved in your care that you are taking this drug.
- Keep this drug and all medications out of the reach of children.

KEY POINTS

- Local fungal infections include vaginal and oral yeast infections (*Candida*) and a variety of tinea infections, including athlete's foot and jock itch.
- Topical antifungals are agents that are too toxic to be used systemically but are effective in the treatment of local fungal infections.
- Proper administration of topical antifungals improves their effectiveness. They should not be used near open wounds or lesions.
- Topical antifungals can cause serious local irritation, burning, and pain. The drug should be stopped if these conditions occur.

SUMMARY

- A fungus is a cellular organism with a hard cell wall that contains chitin and polysaccharides and a cell membrane that contains ergosterols.
- Any infection with a fungus is called a mycosis. Systemic fungal infections, which can be life threatening, are increasing with the rise in the number of immunocompromised patients.
- Systemic antifungals alter the cell permeability, leading to leakage of cellular components. This causes prevention of cell replication and cell death.
- Because systemic antifungals can be very toxic, patients should be monitored closely while receiving them. Adverse effects may include hepatic and renal failure.
- Local fungal infections include vaginal and oral yeast infections (*Candida*) and a variety of tinea infections, including athlete's foot and jock itch.
- Topical antifungals are agents that are too toxic to be used systemically but are effective in the treatment of local fungal infections.
- Proper administration of topical antifungals improves their effectiveness. They should not be used near open wounds or lesions.
- Topical antifungals can cause serious local irritation, burning, and pain. The drug should be stopped if these conditions occur.

CHECK YOUR UNDERSTANDING

Answers to the questions in this chapter can be found in Answers to Check Your Understanding Questions on thePoint®.

MULTIPLE CHOICE

Select the best answer to the following.

1. A patient with a fungal infection asks the nurse why she cannot take antibiotics. The nurse explains that the reason for this is that a fungus is resistant to antibiotics because
   a. a fungal cell wall has fewer but more selective protective layers.
   b. the composition of the fungal cell wall is highly rigid and protective.
   c. a fungus does not reproduce by the usual methods of cell division.
   d. antibiotics are developed to affect only bacterial cell walls.

2. When administering a systemic antifungal agent, the nurse incorporates understanding that all systemic antifungal drugs function to
   a. break apart the fungus nucleus.
   b. interfere with fungus DNA production.
   c. alter cell permeability of the fungus, leading to cell death.
   d. prevent the fungus from absorbing needed nutrients.

3. After assessing a patient the nurse would question an order for amphotericin B to prevent the possibility of serious nephrotoxicity if the patient was also receiving which of the following?
   a. digoxin
   b. oral anticoagulants
   c. phenytoin
   d. corticosteroids

4. The nurse is describing fungi that cause infections of the skin and mucous membranes, appropriately calling these which of the following?
   a. mycoses
   b. meningeal fungi
   c. dermatophytes
   d. worms

5. After teaching a group of students about topical fungal infections the instructor determines that the students need additional instruction when they identify which of the following as an example?
   a. athlete's foot
   b. Rocky Mountain spotted fever
   c. jock itch
   d. vaginal yeast infections

6. Which of the following would the nurse recommend that a woman with repeated vaginal yeast infections keep on hand?
   a. tolnaftate
   b. butenafine
   c. clotrimazole
   d. naftifine

7. The nurse instructs the patient to use care when applying topical antifungal agents to prevent systemic absorption because
   a. the fungus is only on the surface.
   b. these drugs are too toxic to be given systemically.
   c. absorption would prevent drug effectiveness.
   d. these drugs can cause serious local burning and pain.

8. A patient with a severe case of athlete's foot is seen with lesions between the toes, which are oozing blood and serum. After teaching the patient, the nurse determines that the instruction was effective if the patient states which of the following?
   a. "I have to wear black socks and must be careful not to change them very often because it could pull more skin off of my feet."
   b. "I need to apply a thick layer of the antifungal cream between my toes, making sure that all of the lesions are full of cream."
   c. "I should wear white socks and keep my feet clean and dry. I shouldn't use the antifungal cream in areas where I have open lesions."
   d. "After I apply the cream to my feet, I should cover my feet in plastic wrap for several hours to make sure the drug is absorbed."

(continues on page 182)

MULTIPLE RESPONSE

Select all that apply.

1. When administering a systemic antifungal, the nurse would include which of the following in the patient's plan of care?

a. Ensuring that a culture of the affected area had been done.
b. Having the patient swallow the troche used for oral *Candida* infections.
c. Ensuring that the patient stays flat for at least 1 hour if receiving a vaginal suppository.
d. Monitoring the IV site to prevent phlebitis.
e. Keeping the patient NPO (nothing by mouth) if GI upset occurs to prevent vomiting.
f. Providing antipyretics if fever occurs with IV antifungals.

2. The nurse would include which of the following in a teaching plan for a patient who is receiving an oral antifungal drug?

a. It is important that you complete the full course of your drug therapy.
b. You can share this drug with other family members if they develop the same symptoms.
c. If you feel drowsy or dizzy, you should avoid driving or operating dangerous machinery.
d. If GI upset occurs, avoid eating and drinking so you don't vomit and lose the drug.
e. Use over-the-counter drugs to counteract any adverse effects like headache, fever, or rash.
f. Notify your health care provider if you experience yellowing of the skin or eyes, dark urine or light-colored stools, or fever and chills.

BIBLIOGRAPHY AND REFERENCES

Brunton, L., Chabner, B., & Knollman, B. (2011). *Goodman and Gilman's the pharmacological basis of therapeutics* (12th ed.). New York: McGraw-Hill.

Eschenauer, G., Lam, S., & Carver, P. (2009) Antifungal prophylaxis in liver transplant recipients. *Liver Transplantation, 15*(8) 842–858.

Facts and Comparisons. (2015). *Drug facts and comparisons*. St. Louis, MO: Author.

Facts and Comparisons. (2015). *Professional's guide to patient drug facts*. St. Louis, MO: Author.

Gupta, A., & Cooper, E. (2008). Update in antifungal therapy of dermatophytosis. *Mycopathologia, 116*(5/6), 353–367.

Herbrecht, R., Maertens, J., Baila, L. (2010) Caspofungin first-line therapy for invasive aspergillosis in allogeneic hematopoietic stem cell transplant patients. *Bone Marrow Transplantation, 45*(7), 1227–1233.

Juang, P. (2007). Update on new antifungal therapy. *ACNN Advanced Critical Care, 18*(3), 253–260.

Karch, A. M. (2014). *Lippincott's nursing drug guide*. Philadelphia, PA: Lippincott Williams & Wilkins.

Kuse, E., Chetchotisakd, P., Arns da Cunha, C. (2007). Micafungin versus liposomal amphotericin B for candidemia and invasive candidosis. *The Lancet, 369*(9572), 1519–1527.

Masur, H., & Kaplan, J. (2009). New guidelines for the management of HIV-related opportunistic infections. *Journal of the American Medical Association, 301*(22), 2378–2380.

Porth, C. M. (2013). *Pathophysiology: Concepts of altered health states* (9th ed.). Philadelphia, PA: Lippincott Williams & Wilkins.

12 Antiprotozoal Agents

Learning Objectives

Upon completion of this chapter, you will be able to:

1. Outline the life cycle of the protozoan that causes malaria.
2. Describe the therapeutic actions, indications, pharmacokinetics, contraindications, proper administration, most common adverse reactions, and important drug–drug interactions associated with drugs used to treat malaria.
3. Describe other common protozoal infections, including cause and clinical presentation.
4. Compare and contrast the antimalarials with other drugs used to treat protozoal infections.
5. Outline the nursing considerations for patients receiving an antiprotozoal agent across the lifespan.

Glossary of Key Terms

amebiasis: amebic dysentery, which is caused by intestinal invasion of the trophozoite stage of the protozoan *Entamoeba histolytica*

***Anopheles* mosquito:** type of mosquito that is essential to the life cycle of *Plasmodium*; injects the protozoa into humans for further maturation

cinchonism: syndrome of quinine toxicity characterized by nausea, vomiting, tinnitus, and vertigo

giardiasis: protozoal intestinal infection that causes severe diarrhea and epigastric distress; may lead to serious malnutrition

leishmaniasis: skin, mucous membrane, or visceral infection caused by a protozoan passed to humans by the bites of sand flies

malaria: protozoal infection with *Plasmodium,* characterized by cyclic fever and chills as the parasite is released from ruptured red blood cells; causes serious liver, central nervous system (CNS), heart, and lung damage

Plasmodium: a protozoan that causes malaria in humans; its life cycle includes the *Anopheles* mosquito, which injects protozoa into humans

***Pneumocystis jiroveci* pneumonia:** opportunistic infection that occurs when the immune system is depressed; a frequent cause of pneumonia in patients with AIDS and in those who are receiving immunosuppressive therapy

protozoa: single-celled organisms that pass through several stages in their life cycle, including at least one phase as a human parasite; found in areas of poor sanitation and hygiene and crowded living conditions

trichomoniasis: infestation with a protozoan that causes vaginitis in women but no signs or symptoms in men

trophozoite: a developing stage of a parasite, which uses the host for essential nutrients needed for growth

trypanosomiasis: African sleeping sickness, which is caused by a protozoan that inflames the CNS and is spread to humans by the bite of the tsetse fly; also, Chagas' disease, which causes a serious cardiomyopathy after the bite of the housefly

Drug List

Antimalarials
- (P) chloroquine
- mefloquine
- primaquine
- pyrimethamine
- quinine

Other Antiprotozoals
- atovaquone
- (P) metronidazole
- nitazoxanide
- pentamidine
- tinidazole

Infections caused by **protozoa**—single-celled organisms that pass through several stages in their life cycles, including at least one phase as a human parasite—are very common in several parts of the world. In tropical areas, where protozoal infections are most prevalent, many people suffer multiple infestations at the same time. These illnesses are relatively rare in the United States, but with people traveling throughout the world in increasing numbers, it is not unusual to find an individual who returns home from a trip to Africa, Asia, or South America with fully developed protozoal infections. Protozoa thrive in tropical climates, but they may also survive and reproduce in any area where people live in very crowded and unsanitary conditions. This chapter focuses on agents used for protozoal infections that are caused by insect bites (malaria, trypanosomiasis, and leishmaniasis) and those that result from ingestion or contact with the causal organism (amebiasis, giardiasis, and trichomoniasis). Box 12.1 discusses the use of antiprotozoals across the lifespan. Figure 12.1 shows sites of action for these agents.

Malaria

Malaria is a parasitic disease that has killed hundreds of millions of people and even changed the course of history. The progress of several African battles and the building of the Panama Canal were altered by outbreaks of malaria. Even with the introduction of drugs for the treatment of this disease, it remains endemic in many parts of the world. The only known method of transmission of malaria is through the bite of a female *Anopheles* **mosquito**, an insect that harbors the protozoal parasite and carries it to humans.

Four protozoal parasites, all in the genus ***Plasmodium***, have been identified as causes of malaria:

- *Plasmodium falciparum* is considered to be the most dangerous type of protozoan. Infection with this protozoan results in an acute, rapidly fulminating disease with high fever, severe hypotension, swelling and reddening of the limbs, loss of red blood cells, and even death.
- *Plasmodium vivax* causes a milder form of the disease, which seldom results in death.
- *Plasmodium malariae* is endemic in many tropical countries and causes very mild signs and symptoms in the local population. It can cause more acute disease in travelers to endemic areas.
- *Plasmodium ovale,* which is rarely seen, seems to be in the process of being eradicated.

A major problem with controlling malaria involves the mosquito that is responsible for transmitting the disease; the mosquito has developed a resistance to the insecticides designed to eradicate it. Over the years, widespread efforts at mosquito control were successful, with fewer cases of malaria being seen each year. However, the rise of insecticide-resistant mosquitoes has allowed malaria to continue to flourish, increasing the incidence of the disease. In addition, the protozoa that cause malaria have developed strains resistant to the usual antimalarial drugs. This combination of factors has led to a worldwide public health challenge.

BOX 12.1 FOCUS ON **Drug Therapy Across the Lifespan**

Antiprotozoal Agents

CHILDREN

Children are very sensitive to the effects of most antiprotozoal drugs, and more severe reactions can be expected when these drugs are used in children.

Many of these drugs do not have proven safety and efficacy in children, and extreme caution should be used. The dangers of infection resulting from travel to areas endemic with many of these diseases are often much more severe than the potential risks associated with cautious use of these drugs.

If a child needs to travel to an area with endemic protozoal infections, the CDC or local health department should be consulted about the safest possible preventative measures.

ADULTS

Adults should be well advised about the need for prophylaxis against various protozoal infections and the need for immediate treatment if the disease is contracted. It is very helpful to mark calendars as reminders of the days before, during, and after exposure on which the drugs should be taken.

Pregnant and nursing women should not use these drugs unless the benefit clearly outweighs the potential risk to the fetus or neonate. Women of childbearing age should be advised to use barrier contraceptives if any of these drugs are used. A pregnant woman traveling to an area endemic with protozoal infections should be advised of the serious risks to the fetus associated with both preventive therapy and treatment of acute attacks, as well as the risks associated with contracting the disease.

OLDER ADULTS

Older patients may be more susceptible to the adverse effects associated with these drugs. They should be monitored closely.

Patients with hepatic dysfunction are at increased risk for worsening hepatic problems and toxic effects of many of these drugs. If hepatic dysfunction is expected (extreme age, alcohol abuse, use of other hepatotoxic drugs), the dose may need to be lowered and the patient monitored more frequently.

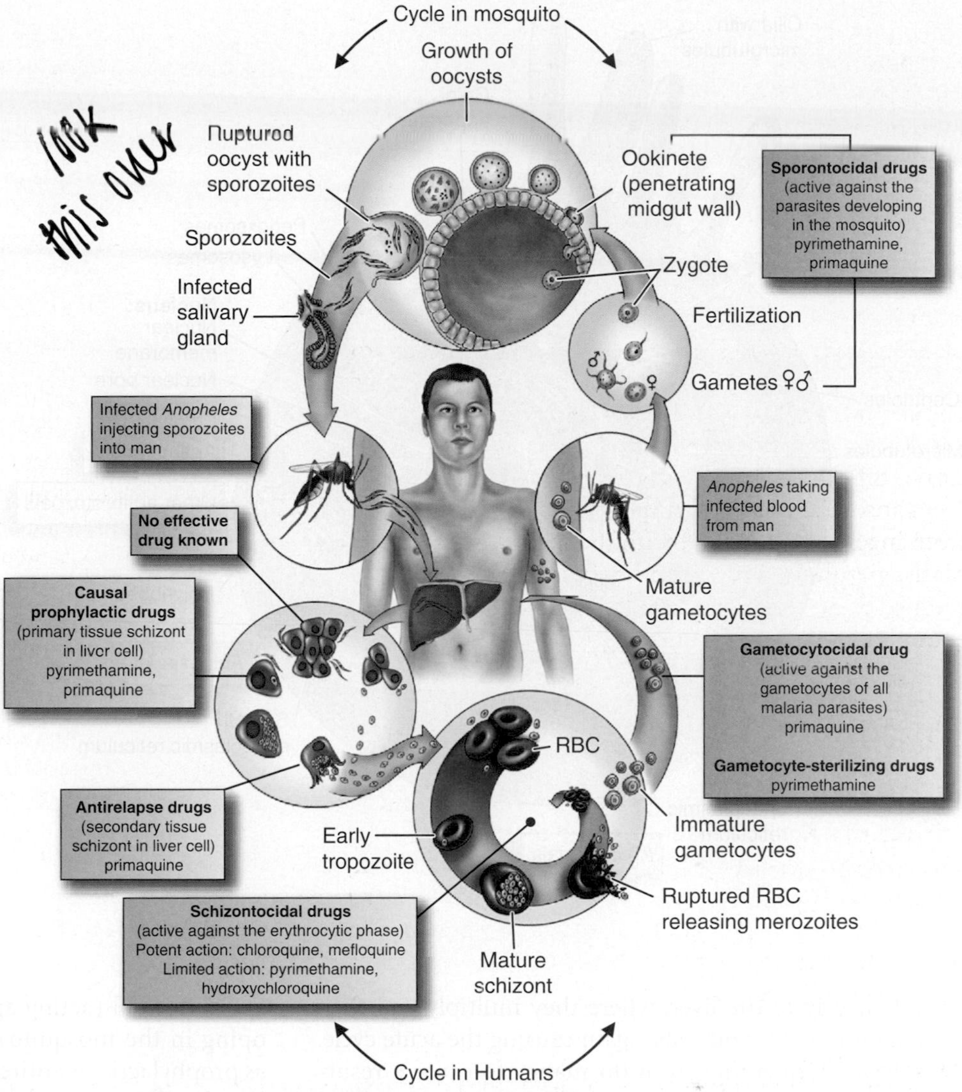

FIGURE 12.1 Sites of action of antimalarials and other antiprotozoals. Antimalarials block protein synthesis and cause cell death. Other antiprotozoals block DNA synthesis, prevent cell reproduction, and lead to cell death. RBC, red blood cell.

Life Cycle of *Plasmodium*

The parasites that cause human malaria spend part of their life in the *Anopheles* mosquito and part in the human host (Figure 12.2). When a mosquito bites a human who is infected with malaria, it sucks blood infested with gametocytes, which are male and female forms of the *Plasmodium*. These gametocytes mate in the stomach of the mosquito and produce a zygote that goes through several phases before forming sporozoites (spore animals) that make their way to the mosquito's salivary glands. The next person who is bitten by that mosquito is injected with thousands of sporozoites. These organisms travel through the bloodstream, where they quickly become lodged in the human liver and other tissues and invade the cells.

Inside human cells the organisms undergo asexual cell division and reproduction. Over the next 7 to 10 days, these primary tissue organisms called schizonts grow and multiply within their invaded cells, using the cell for needed nutrients (as **trophozoites**). Merozoites are then formed from the primary schizonts and burst from invaded cells when they rupture because of overexpansion. These merozoites enter the circulation and invade red blood cells. Here they continue to divide until the blood cells also burst, sending more merozoites into the circulation to invade yet more red blood cells.

Eventually, there are a large number of merozoites in the body, as well as many ruptured and invaded red blood cells. At this point the acute malarial attack occurs. The rupture of the red blood cells causes a massive inflammatory reaction with chills and fever related to the pyrogenic effects of the protozoa and the toxic effects of the red blood cell components on the system. This cycle of chills and fever usually occurs about every 72 hours.

With *Plasmodium vivax* and *Plasmodium malariae* malaria, this cycle may continue for a long period. Many of the tissue schizonts lay dormant until they eventually

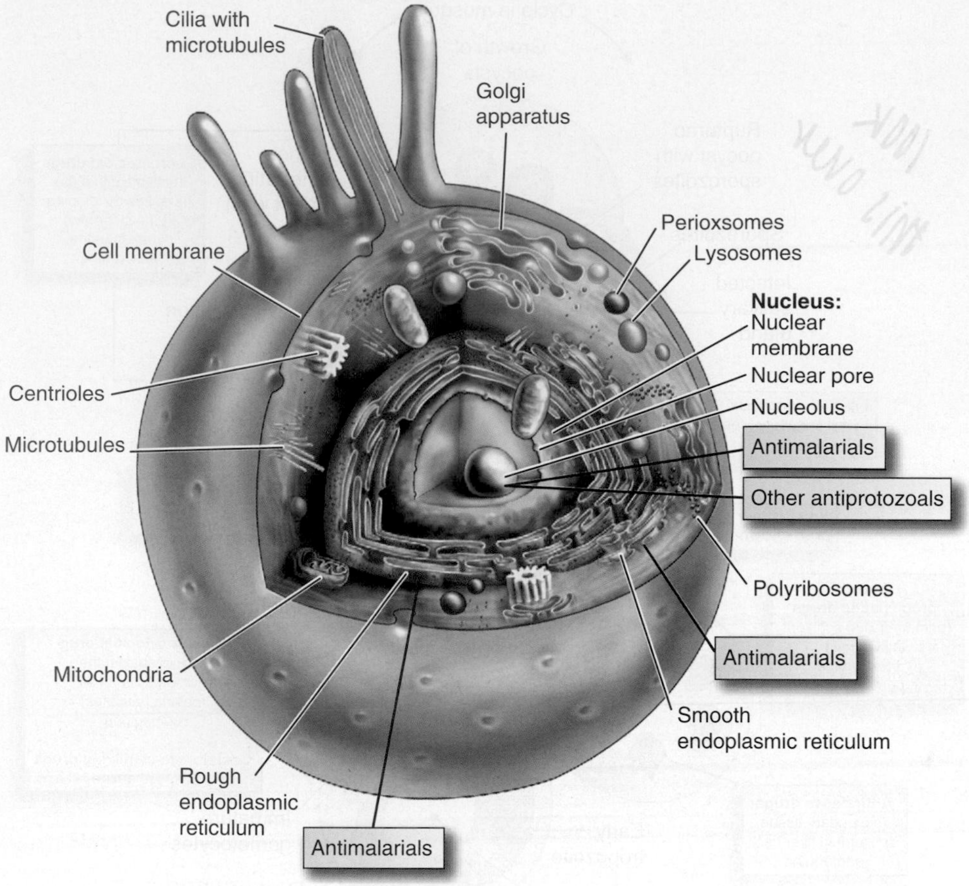

FIGURE 12.2 Types of antimalarial drugs in relation to the stages in the life cycle of *Plasmodium*.

find their way to the liver, where they multiply and then invade more red blood cells, again causing the acute cycle. This cycle of emerging from dormancy to cause a resurgence of the acute cycle may occur for years in an untreated patient.

With *Plasmodium falciparum* malaria, there are no extrahepatic sites for the schizonts. If the patient survives an acute attack, no prolonged periods of relapse occur. The first attack of this type of malaria can destroy so many red blood cells that the patient's capillaries become clogged and the circulation to vital organs is interrupted, leading to death.

Antimalarials

Antimalarial drugs (Table 12.1) are usually given in combination form to attack the *Plasmodium* at various stages of its life cycle. Using this approach, it is possible to prevent the acute malarial reaction in individuals who have been infected by the parasite. These drugs can be schizonticidal (acting against the red blood cell phase of the life cycle), gametocytocidal (acting against the gametocytes), sporontocidal (acting against the parasites that are developing in the mosquito), or work against tissue schizonts as prophylactic or antirelapse agents. Quinine (*Qualaquin)* was the first drug found to be effective in the treatment of malaria; it was absent from the market for a while but is now available for the treatment of uncomplicated malaria. Other antimalarials used today include chloroquine (*Aralen Phosphate*), mefloquine (generic), primaquine (generic), and pyrimethamine (*Daraprim*). Fixed dose combination drugs for malaria prevention and treatment are discussed in Box 12.2.

Therapeutic Actions and Indications

Chloroquine is currently the mainstay of antimalarial therapy. This drug enters human red blood cells and changes the metabolic pathways necessary for the reproduction of the *Plasmodium* (Figure 12.1). In addition, this agent is directly toxic to parasites that absorb it; it is acidic, and it decreases the ability of the parasite to synthesize DNA, leading to a blockage of reproduction. Because many strains of the parasite are developing resistance to chloroquine, the CDC (Centers for Disease Control and Prevention) often recommends the use of certain antibiotics as part

*

Table 12.1 ***Drugs in Focus:* Antimalarials**

Drug Name	Dosage/Route	Usual Indications
chloroquine (*Aralen*)	***Suppression:*** *Adult:* 300 mg PO every week beginning 1–2 wk before exposure and continuing for 4 wk after leaving endemic area *Pediatric:* 5 mg/kg/wk PO, using same schedule as for an adult ***Acute attacks:*** *Adult:* 600 mg PO, followed by 300 mg PO in 6 h; then 300 mg PO on days 2 and 3 *Pediatric:* 10 mg/kg PO, followed by 5 mg/kg PO in 6 h and on days 2 and 3	Prevention and treatment of *Plasmodium* malaria; treatment of extraintestinal amebiasis
mefloquine (*Lariam*)	***Treatment:*** *Adult:* 1,250 mg PO as a single dose ***Prevention:*** *Adult:* 250 mg PO once weekly, starting 1 wk before travel and continuing for 4 wk after leaving endemic area *Pediatric:* 15–19 kg, 1/4 tablet; 20–30 kg, 1/2 tablet; 31–45 kg, 3/4 tablet; >45 kg, 1 tablet; once a week, starting 1 wk before travel and continuing until 4 wk after leaving area	Prevention and treatment of *Plasmodium* malaria in combination with other drugs
primaquine (generic)	*Adult:* 26.3 mg/d PO for 14 d *Pediatric:* 0.5 mg/kg per day PO for 14 d; begin therapy during last 2 wk of (or after) therapy with chloroquine or other drugs	Prevention of relapses of *Plasmodium vivax* and *Plasmodium malariae* infections; radical cure of *P. vivax* malaria
pyrimethamine (*Daraprim*)	***Prevention:*** *Adult:* 25 mg PO every week *Pediatric (>10 y):* Same as adult *Pediatric (4–10 y):* 12.5 mg PO every week *Pediatric (<4 y):* 6.25 mg PO every week	Prevention of *Plasmodium* malaria, in combination with other agents to suppress transmission; treatment of toxoplasmosis
quinine (*Qualaquin*)	*Adult:* 648 mg every 8 h for 7 days	Treatment of uncomplicated malaria caused by *Plasmodium falciparum*

of combination therapy for treatment of malaria caused by these resistant strains. Box 12.3 lists the antibiotics used to treat malaria. See Table 12.1 for usual indications. Mechanisms of action are as follows:

Mefloquine increases the acidity of plasmodial food vacuoles, causing cell rupture and death. In combination therapy, mefloquine is used in malarial prevention, as well as treatment.

Primaquine, another very old drug for treating malaria, similar to quinine, disrupts the mitochondria of the *Plasmodium*. It also causes death of gametocytes and exoerythrocytic (outside of the red blood cell) forms and prevents other forms from reproducing.

Pyrimethamine is used in combination with agents that act more rapidly to suppress malaria; it acts by blocking the use of folic acid in protein synthesis by the *Plasmodium*, eventually leading to inability to reproduce and cell death.

Quinine inhibits nucleic acid synthesis, protein synthesis, and glycolysis in *Plasmodium falciparum*. It is used to treat uncomplicated malaria and is used effectively in regions where chloroquine resistance has been documented.

Pharmacokinetics

Chloroquine is readily absorbed from the gastrointestinal (GI) tract, with peak serum levels occurring in 1 to 6 hours. It is concentrated in the liver, spleen, kidney, and brain and is excreted very slowly in the urine, primarily as unchanged drug.

Mefloquine is a mixture of molecules that are absorbed, metabolized, and excreted at different rates. The terminal half-life is 13 to 24 days. Metabolism occurs in the liver; caution should be used in patients with hepatic dysfunction.

Primaquine is readily absorbed and metabolized in the liver. Excretion occurs primarily in the urine. Safety for use during pregnancy has not been established.

Pyrimethamine is readily absorbed from the GI tract, with peak levels occurring within 2 to 6 hours. It is

BOX 12.2

Combination Drugs Used for Malaria Prevention and Treatment

Two fixed combination drugs are available for use in the prevention and treatment of malaria. Combining two different preparations in one drug may increase compliance by reducing the number of pills a patient has to take, and it conforms to the treatment protocol of taking drugs that affect the protozoa at different stages on their life cycle.

Malarone and *Malarone Pediatric* combine atovaquone and proguanil. They are indicated for the prevention of *Plasmodium falciparum* malaria when chloroquine resistance has been reported. They are used for the treatment of uncomplicated *P. falciparum* malaria when chloroquine, halofantrine, and mefloquine have not proved successful, most likely because of resistance. This combination should be used in pregnancy and lactation only if the benefit clearly outweighs the potential risk to the fetus or neonate.

Usual dosage, acute attack:

Adult: Four tablets PO as a single daily dose for 3 consecutive days
Pediatric (11–20 kg): One adult tablet PO daily for 3 consecutive days
Pediatric (21–30 kg): Two adult tablets PO daily as a single daily dose for 3 consecutive days
Pediatric (31–40 kg): Three adult tablets PO daily as a single daily dose for 3 consecutive days
Pediatric (>40 kg): Four adult tablets PO daily as a single daily dose for 3 consecutive days

Prevention:

Adult: One tablet PO daily
Pediatric (11–20 kg): One pediatric tablet PO daily
Pediatric (21–30 kg): Two pediatric tablets PO daily
Pediatric (31–40 kg): Three pediatric tablets PO daily
Pediatric (>40 kg): One adult tablet PO daily

Prevention should start 1–2 days before exposure and continue throughout and 7 days after leaving the area.

The newest combination drug is *Coartem*, a combination of artemether and lumefantrine, antimalarials only available in this combination. This drug is approved for the treatment of acute, uncomplicated malaria caused by *Plasmodium falciparum* in patients weighing 5 kg or more. It should only be used with extreme caution in patients with severe hepatic impairment. It should be taken with food to improve absorption. This drug is known to prolong the QT interval and should be avoided in patients with known prolonged QT interval and should not be used in combination with other drugs known to prolong the QT interval.

Usual dosage:

Adults: Four tablets as one dose followed by four tablets 8 hours later, then four tablets twice a day for the following 2 days for a total of 24 tablets over 3 days.
Pediatric ≥35 kg: Use an adult dose.
Pediatric 25 to <35 kg: Three tablets as one dose, then three tablets in 8 hours followed by three tablets twice a day for the next 2 days for a total of 18 tablets over 3 days.
Pediatric 15 kg to <25 kg: Two tablets as one dose followed by two tablets in 8 hours, then two tablets twice a day for the next 2 days for a total of 12 tablets over 3 days.
Pediatric 5 kg to <15 kg: One tablet, followed by one tablet in 8 hours, then one tablet twice daily for the next 2 days for a total of six tablets over 3 days.

BOX 12.3

Antibiotics Used to Treat Malaria

With the emergence of chloroquine-resistant strains of *Plasmodium*, the CDC recommends the use of quinine and one of the following antibiotics as a combination therapy for the treatment of uncomplicated or severe malaria caused by chloroquine-resistant strains or uncomplicated malaria caused by strains with unknown resistance:

doxycycline: 100 mg/d PO for 7 days for adults; 2.2 mg/kg PO q12h for 7 days for children
tetracycline: 250 mg PO for 7 days for adults; 25 mg/kg/d PO in divided doses q.i.d. for 7 days for children
clindamycin: 20 mg base/kg/d PO in divided doses t.i.d. for 7 days for adults and children

In severe cases, the antibiotics can be started IV and then switched to oral forms as soon as the patient is able to take oral drugs

See Chapter 10 for a full discussion of these drugs.

metabolized in the liver and has a half-life of 4 days. It usually maintains suppressive concentrations in the body for about 2 weeks.

Quinine is rapidly absorbed from the GI tract, with peak serum levels occurring in 1 to 3 hours. It is metabolized in the liver with a half-life of 4 to 6 hours and is excreted in the urine.

Contraindications and Cautions

Antimalarials are contraindicated in the presence of known patient allergy to any of these drugs; liver disease or alcoholism, *both because of the parasitic invasion of the liver and because of the need for the hepatic metabolism to prevent toxicity*; and lactation *because the drugs can enter breast milk and could be toxic to the infant.* Another method of feeding the baby should be used if treatment is necessary. These drugs should be avoided during pregnancy *because they are associated with birth defects.* With mefloquine, which is teratogenic in preclinical studies, pregnancy should be avoided during and for 2 months

BOX 12.4 FOCUS ON **Cultural Considerations**

Potential for Hemolytic Crisis

Patients with glucose-6-phosphate dehydrogenase (G6PD) deficiency—which is more likely to occur in Greeks, Italians, and other people of Mediterranean descent—may experience a hemolytic crisis if they are taking the antimalarial agent chloroquine or primaquine. Patients of Greek, Italian, or other Mediterranean ancestry should be questioned about any history of potential G6PD deficiency. If no history is known the patient should be tested before any of these drugs are prescribed. If testing is not possible and the drugs are needed the patient should be monitored very closely and informed about the potential need for hospitalization and emergency services.

after completion of therapy. Use caution in patients with retinal disease or damage *because many of these drugs can affect vision and the retina, and the likelihood of problems increases if the retina is already damaged*; with psoriasis or porphyria *because of skin damage*; or with damage to mucous membranes, *which can occur as a result of the effects of the drug on proteins and protein synthesis.* There have been some genetic enzyme differences identified in various groups that predispose them to adverse effects associated with these drugs. See Box 12.4 for Cultural Considerations and the use of some antimalarials.

Adverse Effects

A number of adverse effects may be encountered with the use of these antimalarial agents (Figure 12.3). Central nervous system (CNS) effects include headache and dizziness. Immune reaction effects related to the release of merozoites include fever, shaking, chills, and malaise. Nausea, vomiting, dyspepsia, and anorexia are associated with direct effects of the drug on the GI tract and the effects on CNS control of vomiting caused by the products of cell death and protein changes. Hepatic dysfunction is associated with the toxic effects of the drug on the liver and the effects of the disease on the liver. Dermatological effects include rash, pruritus, and loss of hair associated with changes in protein synthesis of the hair follicles. Visual changes, including possible blindness related to retinal damage from the drug, and ototoxicity related to other nerve damage may occur. **Cinchonism** (nausea, vomiting, tinnitus, and vertigo) may occur with high levels of quinine or primaquine.

Clinically Important Drug–Drug Interactions

The patient who is receiving combinations of the quinine derivatives and quinine is at increased risk for cardiac toxicity and convulsions. Therefore, monitor the patient closely, checking drug levels and anticipating dose adjustments as needed.

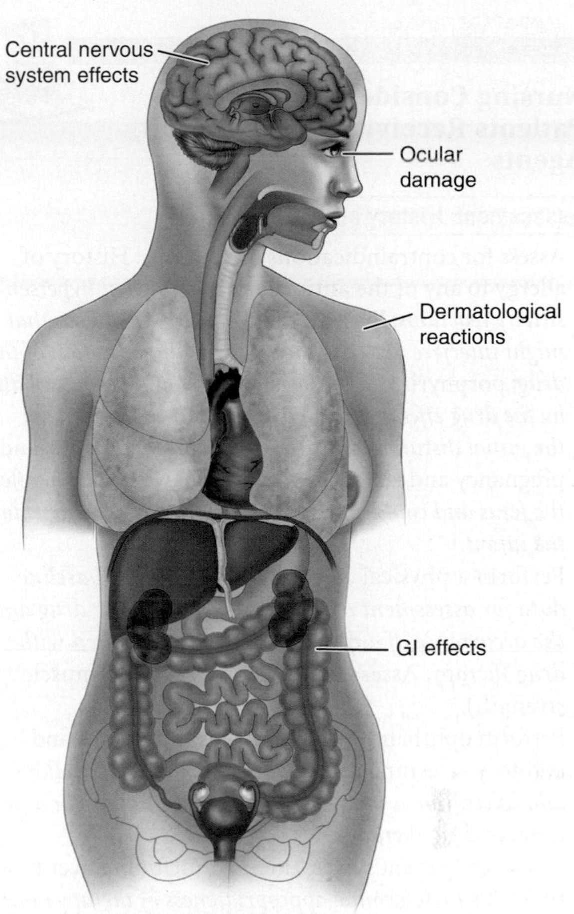

FIGURE 12.3 Common adverse effects associated with antiprotozoals.

Increased bone marrow suppression may occur if antifolate drugs (methotrexate, sulfonamides, etc.) are combined with pyrimethamine; discontinue pyrimethamine if signs of folate deficiency develop (diarrhea, fatigue, weight loss, anemia).

Prototype Summary: Chloroquine

Indications: Treatment and prophylaxis of acute attacks of malaria caused by susceptible strains of *Plasmodium*; treatment of extraintestinal amebiasis.

Actions: Inhibits protozoal reproduction and protein synthesis.

Pharmacokinetics:

Route	Onset	Peak	Duration
Oral	Varies	1–2 h	1 wk

$T_{1/2}$: 70 to 120 hours; metabolized in the liver and excreted in the urine.

Adverse Effects: Visual disturbances, retinal changes, hypotension, nausea, vomiting, diarrhea.

Nursing Considerations for Patients Receiving Antimalarial Agents

Assessment: History and Examination

- Assess for contraindications or cautions: History of allergy to any of the antimalarials *to prevent hypersensitivity reactions*; liver dysfunction or alcoholism *that might interfere with the metabolism and excretion of the drug*; porphyria or psoriasis, *which could be exacerbated by the drug effects*; retinal disease *that could increase the visual disturbances associated with these drugs*; and pregnancy and lactation *because these drugs could affect the fetus and could enter the breast milk and be toxic to the infant.*
- Perform a physical assessment *to establish baseline data for assessment of the effectiveness of the drug and the occurrence of any adverse effects associated with drug therapy.* Assess the CNS (reflexes and muscle strength).
- Perform ophthalmic and retinal examinations and auditory screening *to determine the need for cautious administration and to evaluate changes that occur as a result of drug therapy.*
- Assess the patient's liver function, including liver function tests *to determine appropriateness of therapy and to monitor for toxicity.*
- Obtain blood culture *to identify the causative Plasmodium spp. and ensure appropriate use of the drug.*
- Inspect the skin closely for color, temperature, texture, and evidence of lesions *to monitor for adverse effects.*

Nursing Diagnoses

Nursing diagnoses related to drug therapy might include the following:

- Acute pain related to GI, CNS, and skin effects of the drug
- Disturbed sensory perception (kinesthetic, visual) related to CNS effects
- Risk for injury related to CNS changes
- Deficient knowledge regarding drug therapy

Planning

- The patient will receive the best therapeutic effect from the drug therapy.
- The patient will have limited adverse effects to the drug therapy.
- The patient will have an understanding of the drug therapy, adverse effects to anticipate, and measures to relieve discomfort and improve safety.

Implementation with Rationale

- Arrange for appropriate culture and sensitivity tests before beginning therapy *to ensure proper drug for susceptible **Plasmodium** spp.* Treatment may begin before test results are known.
- Administer the complete course of the drug *to get the full beneficial effects.* Mark a calendar for prophylactic doses. Use combination therapy as indicated.
- Monitor hepatic function and perform ophthalmological examination before and periodically during treatment *to ensure early detection and prompt intervention with cessation of drug if signs of failure or deteriorating vision occur.*
- Provide comfort and safety measures if CNS effects occur (e.g., side rails and assistance with ambulation if dizziness and weakness are present) *to prevent patient injury.* Provide oral hygiene and ready access to bathroom facilities as needed *to cope with GI effects.*
- Provide small, frequent, nutritious meals if GI upset is severe *to ensure adequate nutrition.* Monitor nutritional status and arrange a dietary consultation as needed. Taking the drug with food may also decrease GI upset.
- Instruct the patient concerning the appropriate dosage regimen and the importance of adhering to the drug schedule *to enhance patient knowledge about drug therapy and to promote compliance.*
- Provide the following patient teaching:
  - Take safety precautions, including changing position slowly and avoiding driving and hazardous tasks, if CNS effects occur.
  - Take the drug with meals and try small, frequent meals if GI upset is a problem.
  - Report blurring of vision, which could indicate retinal damage; loss of hearing or ringing in the ears, which could indicate CNS toxicity; and fever or worsening of condition, which could indicate a resistant strain or noneffective therapy.

Evaluation

- Monitor patient response to the drug (resolution of malaria or prevention of malaria).
- Monitor for adverse effects (orientation and affect, nutritional state, skin color and lesions, hepatic function, and visual and auditory changes).
- Evaluate the effectiveness of the teaching plan (patient can name the drug, dosage, possible adverse effects to watch for, and specific measures to help avoid adverse effects).
- Monitor the effectiveness of comfort and safety measures and compliance with the regimen.

KEY POINTS

- A protozoan is a parasitic cellular organism. Its life cycle includes a parasitic phase inside human tissues or cells.
- Malaria is the most common protozoal infection and is spread to humans by the bite of an *Anopheles* mosquito. The signs and symptoms of malaria are related to the destruction of red blood cells and toxicity to the liver.
- Antimalarial agents attack the parasite at the various stages of its development inside and outside the human body.

Other Protozoal Infections

Other protozoal infections that are encountered in clinical practice include amebiasis, leishmaniasis, trypanosomiasis, trichomoniasis, and giardiasis. These infections, which are caused by single-celled protozoa, are usually associated with unsanitary, crowded conditions, and use of poor hygienic practices. Patients traveling to other countries may encounter these infections, which also appear increasingly in the United States. Box 12.5 discusses the impact of travel and tourism on the spread of pathogens.

Amebiasis

Amebiasis, an intestinal infection caused by *Entamoeba histolytica*, is often known as amebic dysentery. *E. histolytica* has a two-stage life cycle (Figure 12.4). The organism exists in two stages: (1) a cystic, dormant stage, in which the protozoan can live for long periods outside the body or in the human intestine, and (2) a trophozoite stage in the ideal environment—the human large intestine.

The disease is transmitted while the protozoan is in the cystic stage in fecal matter, from which it can enter water and the ground. It can be passed to other humans who drink this water or eat food that has been grown in this ground. The cysts are swallowed and pass, unaffected by gastric acid, into the intestine. Some of these cysts are passed in fecal matter, and some of them become trophozoites that grow and reproduce. The trophozoites migrate into the mucosa of the colon, where they penetrate into the intestinal wall, forming erosions. These forms of *Entamoeba* release a chemical that dissolves mucosal cells, and eventually they eat away tissue until they reach the vascular system, which carries them throughout the body. The trophozoites lodge in the liver, lungs, heart, brain, and so on.

Early signs of amebiasis include mild to fulminate diarrhea. In the worst cases, if the protozoan is able to invade extraintestinal tissue, it can dissolve the tissue and eventually cause the death of the host. Some individuals can become carriers of the disease without having any overt signs or symptoms. These people seem to be resistant to the intestinal invasion but pass the cysts in the stool.

Leishmaniasis

Leishmaniasis is a disease caused by a protozoan that is passed from sand flies to humans. The sand fly injects an asexual form of this flagellated protozoan, called a promastigote, into the body of a human, where it is rapidly attacked and digested by human macrophages. Inside the macrophages, the promastigote divides, developing many new forms called amastigotes, which keep dividing and eventually kill the macrophage, releasing the amastigotes into the system to be devoured by more macrophages. Thus, a cyclic pattern of infection is established. These amastigotes can cause serious lesions in the skin, the viscera, or the mucous membranes of the host.

BOX 12.5 FOCUS ON The Evidence

World Travel and the Spread of Pathogens

Nowadays, people are traveling to more exotic areas of the world than ever before. Because of this, people are being exposed to more pathogens than ever before, and they also are potentially spreading pathogens to different areas of the world. Pathogens that are endemic in one area of the world and cause mild disease to the local population can be quite devastating in a population that has not previously been exposed to that pathogen.

World health agencies and governments have established guidelines for prophylaxis and treatment of such diseases for travelers. People who are planning to travel out of the United States should contact their local health department or the CDC (http://www.cdc/gov/travel) for the latest information on what prophylactic measures are required in the area they plan to visit and to learn about potential health hazards in that area. The information is updated frequently; treatment and prophylaxis suggestions are based on current clinical experience in the area and should be consulted regularly. Nurses should access this information when working with patients who are traveling to provide pertinent teaching points and to ensure that appropriate prophylactic measures are taken. Nurses caring for patients with tropical diseases should access this information regularly for best treatment practices.

Patients who have been traveling to other areas of the world and who present with any illness should be questioned about where they traveled, what precautions (including prophylactic measures) they took, and when they first experienced any signs or symptoms of illness. The CDC can be consulted about diagnosis and treatment guidelines for any tropical disease that is unfamiliar to a health care provider, as well as about what precautions should be used in caring for such patients.

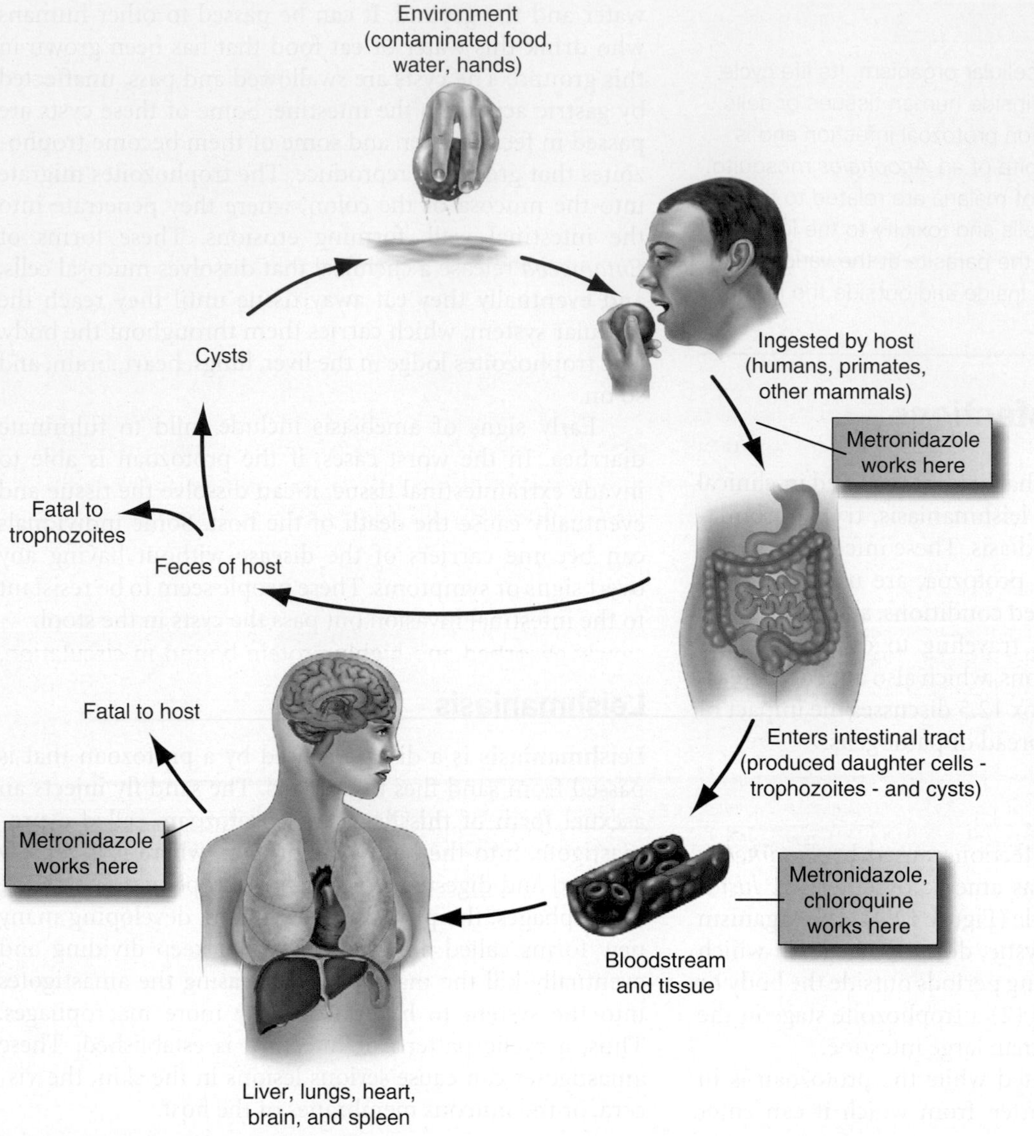

FIGURE 12.4 Life cycle of *Entamoeba histolytica* and the sites of action of metronidazole and chloroquine, which are used to treat amebiasis. Cysts ingested by the host enter the intestinal tract and produce trophozoites. Trophozoites enter the bloodstream to reach tissue. Trophozoites enter the liver, lungs, heart, brain, and spleen, which can be fatal to the host. Trophozoites are excreted in the stool and die. Cysts excreted in the stool contaminate water and can be ingested by the host.

Trypanosomiasis

Trypanosomiasis is caused by infection with *Trypanosoma.* Two parasitic protozoal species cause very serious and often fatal diseases in humans:

- African sleeping sickness, which is caused by *Trypanosoma brucei gambiense*, is transmitted by the tsetse fly. After the pathogenic organism has lived and grown in human blood, it eventually invades the CNS, leading to an acute inflammation that results in lethargy, prolonged sleep, and even death.
- Chagas' disease, which is caused by *Trypanosoma cruzi*, is almost endemic in many South American countries. It is passed to humans by the common housefly. This protozoan results in a severe cardiomyopathy that accounts for numerous deaths and disabilities in certain regions.

Trichomoniasis

Trichomoniasis, which is caused by another flagellated protozoan, *Trichomonas vaginalis*, is a common cause of vaginitis. This infection is usually spread during sexual intercourse by men who have no signs and symptoms of infection. In women, this protozoan causes reddened, inflamed vaginal mucosa, itching, burning, and a yellowish-green discharge.

Giardiasis

Giardiasis, which is caused by *Giardia lamblia*, is the most commonly diagnosed intestinal parasite in the United States. This protozoan forms cysts, which survive outside the body and allow transmission through contaminated water or food, and trophozoites, which break out of the cysts in the upper small intestine and eventually cause signs and symptoms of disease. Diarrhea, rotten egg–smelling stool, and pale and mucus-filled stool are commonly seen. Some patients experience epigastric distress, weight loss, and malnutrition as a result of the invasion of the mucosa.

Pneumocystis jiroveci Pneumonia

Pneumocystis jiroveci is an endemic protozoan that does not usually cause illness in humans. When an individual's immune system becomes suppressed because of AIDS or AIDS-related complex, the use of immunosuppressant drugs, or advanced age, this parasite is able to invade the lungs, leading to severe inflammation and the condition known as ***Pneumocystis jiroveci* pneumonia**. This disease is the most common opportunistic respiratory infection in patients with AIDS.

Other Antiprotozoal Agents

Drugs that are available specifically for the treatment of these various protozoan infections include many of the malarial drugs; chloroquine is effective against extraintestinal amebiasis, and pyrimethamine is also effective in treating toxoplasmosis. Other drugs, including some tetracyclines and aminoglycosides, are used for treating these conditions at various stages of the disease. Other antiprotozoals include atovaquone (*Mepron*), metronidazole (*Flagyl, MetroGel, Noritate*), nitazoxanide (*Alinia*), pentamidine (*Pentam 300, NebuPent*), and tinidazole (*Tindamax*) (see Table 12.2).

Therapeutic Actions and Indications

These antiprotozoal agents act to inhibit DNA synthesis in susceptible protozoa, interfering with the cell's ability to reproduce, subsequently leading to cell death (see Figure 12.1). These drugs are indicated for the treatment of infections caused by susceptible protozoa. See Table 12.2 for Usual Indications for each of these agents.

Pharmacokinetics

Atovaquone is available only as an oral suspension and is slowly absorbed and highly protein bound in circulation. It is excreted slowly through the feces, with a half-life of 67 to 76 hours.

Table 12.2 ***Drugs in Focus:* Other Antiprotozoals**

Drug Name	Dosage/Route	Usual Indications
atovaquone (*Mepron*)	***Prevention:*** *Adult and pediatric (>13 y):* 1,500 mg/d PO ***Treatment:*** *Adult and pediatric (>13 y):* 750 mg PO b.i.d. with meals for 12 d	Prevention and treatment of *Pneumocystis jiroveci* pneumonia; used in combination with proguanil for treatment of chloroquine-resistant malaria
metronidazole (*Flagyl, MetroGel, Noritate*)	***Amebiasis:*** *Adult:* 750 mg PO t.i.d. for 5–10 d *Pediatric:* 35–50 mg/kg/d PO in three divided doses for 10 d ***Trichomoniasis:*** *Adult:* 2 g PO as one dose, or divided into two doses given on the same day *or* 250 mg PO t.i.d. for 7 d *Pediatric:* 5 mg/kg per dose PO t.i.d. for 7 d	Treatment of amebiasis, trichomoniasis, giardiasis
nitazoxanide (*Alinia*)	***Giardia:*** *Pediatric (12–47 mo):* 100 mg PO q12h for 3 d *Pediatric (4–11 y):* 200 mg PO q12h for 3 d ***Cryptosporidium parvum:*** *Pediatric (1–11 y):* Same as for *Giardia* *Adult and pediatric (≥12 y):* 500 mg PO q12h for 3 d	Treatment of diarrhea associated with *Cryptosporidium parvum* or *Giardia lamblia*
pentamidine (*Pentam 300, NebuPent*)	*Inhalation:* 300 mg once every 4 wk *Injection:* 4 mg/kg/d IM or IV for 14 d	As inhalation treatment of *Pneumocystis jiroveci* pneumonia; as a systemic agent in the treatment of trypanosomiasis and leishmaniasis
tinidazole (*Tindamax*)	***Trichomoniasis, giardiasis:*** *Adult:* 2 g PO as a single dose with food *Pediatric (≥3 y):* 50 mg/kg PO as a single dose with food ***Amebiasis:*** *Adult:* 2 g/d PO with food for 3 d *Pediatric (≥3 y):* 50 mg/kg/d PO with food, do not exceed 2 g/d	Treatment of trichomoniasis, giardiasis, amebiasis

Metronidazole is well absorbed orally, reaching peak levels in 1 to 2 hours. It is metabolized in the liver with a half-life of 8 to 15 hours. Excretion occurs primarily through the urine.

Nitazoxanide is rapidly absorbed after oral administration, reaching peak levels in 1 to 4 hours. Nitazoxanide is metabolized in the liver and excreted in the urine and feces; it has a half-life of 8 to 12 hours.

Pentamidine is readily absorbed through the lungs. Excretion occurs in the urine, with traces found in the urine for up to 6 weeks.

Tinidazole is rapidly absorbed after oral administration, reaching peak levels within 60 to 90 minutes. It is excreted in the urine with a half-life of 12 to 14 hours.

Contraindications and Cautions

Contraindications include the presence of any known allergy or hypersensitivity to any of these drugs *to prevent hypersensitivity reactions* and pregnancy *because drug effects on developing fetal DNA and proteins can cause fetal abnormalities and even death.* Use caution when administering these drugs to patients with CNS disease *because of possible disease exacerbation due to drug effects on the CNS*; hepatic disease *because of possible exacerbation when hepatic drug effects occur*; candidiasis *because of the risk of superinfections*; and women who are lactating *because these drugs may pass into breast milk and could have severe adverse effects on the infant.* The safety and efficacy of pentamidine in children have not been established. Tinidazole should never be combined with alcohol and should be used with caution in patients with renal dysfunction, *which could interfere with excretion of the drug.*

Adverse Effects

Adverse effects that can be seen with these antiprotozoal agents include CNS effects such as headache, dizziness, ataxia, loss of coordination, and peripheral neuropathy related to drug effects on the neurons. GI effects include nausea, vomiting, diarrhea, unpleasant taste, cramps, and changes in liver function. Superinfections also can occur when the normal flora are disrupted.

Clinically Important Drug–Drug Interactions

Tinidazole and metronidazole should not be combined with alcohol, which could cause severe adverse effects; patients are advised to avoid alcohol for at least 3 days after treatment has ended. Metronidazole and tinidazole combined with oral anticoagulants can lead to increased bleeding; patients should be monitored closely and dose adjustments made to the anticoagulant during therapy and for up to 8 days after stopping therapy. Psychotic reactions have been reported when tinidazole or metronidazole is combined with disulfiram; this combination should be avoided, and 2 weeks should elapse between tinidazole therapy and the starting of disulfiram.

Ⓟ Prototype Summary: Metronidazole

Indications: Acute intestinal amebiasis, amebic liver abscess, trichomoniasis, acute infections caused by susceptible strains of anaerobic bacteria, and preoperative and postoperative prophylaxis for patients undergoing colorectal surgery.

Actions: Inhibits DNA synthesis of specific anaerobes, causing cell death; mechanism of action as an antiprotozoal and amebicidal is not known.

Pharmacokinetics:

Route	Onset	Peak
Oral	Varies	1–2 h
IV	Rapid	1–2 h

$T_{1/2}$: 6 to 8 hours; metabolized in the liver and excreted in the urine and feces.

Adverse Effects: Headache, dizziness, ataxia, nausea, vomiting, metallic taste, diarrhea, darkening of the urine.

Nursing Considerations for Patients Receiving Antiprotozoal Agents

Assessment: History and Examination

- Assess for contraindications and cautions: History of allergy to any of the antiprotozoals *to prevent hypersensitivity reactions*; liver dysfunction *that might interfere with metabolism and excretion of the drug or be exacerbated by the drug*; pregnancy, *which is a contraindication*, and lactation *because these drugs could enter the breast milk and be toxic to the infant*; CNS disease *that could be exacerbated by the drug*; and candidiasis *that could become severe as a result of the effects of these drugs on the normal flora.*
- Perform a physical assessment *to establish baseline data for determining the effectiveness of the drug and the occurrence of any adverse effects associated with drug therapy.*
- Evaluate the CNS *to check reflexes and muscle strength to identify the need for cautious drug use and to evaluate changes that occur as a result of drug therapy.*
- Examine the skin and mucous membranes to check for lesions, color, temperature, and texture *to monitor for adverse effects and superinfections.*
- Evaluate liver function, including liver function tests, *to determine the appropriateness of therapy and to monitor for toxicity.*
- Obtain cultures *to determine the exact protozoal species causing the disease.*

Nursing Diagnoses

Nursing diagnoses related to drug therapy might include the following:

- Acute pain related to GI and CNS effects of the drug
- Imbalanced nutrition: Less than body requirements related to severe GI effects of the drug
- Disturbed sensory perception (kinesthetic, visual) related to CNS effects
- Deficient knowledge regarding drug therapy

Planning

- The patient will receive the best therapeutic effect from the drug therapy.
- The patient will have limited adverse effects to the drug therapy.
- The patient will have an understanding of the drug therapy, adverse effects to anticipate, and measures to relieve discomfort and improve safety.

Implementation with Rationale

- Arrange for appropriate culture and sensitivity tests before beginning therapy *to ensure proper drug for susceptible organisms.* Treatment may begin before test results are known.
- Administer a complete course of the drug *to get the full beneficial effects.* Use combination therapy as indicated.
- Monitor hepatic function before and periodically during treatment *to arrange to effectively stop the drug if signs of failure or worsening liver function occur.*
- Provide comfort and safety measures if CNS effects occur, such as side rails and assistance with ambulation if dizziness and weakness are present, *to prevent injury to the patient.*
- Provide oral hygiene and ready access to bathroom facilities as needed *to cope with GI effects.*
- Arrange for the treatment of superinfections as appropriate *to prevent severe infections.*
- Provide small, frequent, nutritious meals if GI upset is severe *to ensure proper nutrition.* Monitor nutritional status and arrange a dietary consultation as needed. Taking the drug with food may also decrease GI upset.
- Instruct the patient about the appropriate dosage regimen *to enhance patient knowledge about drug therapy and to promote compliance.*
- Provide the following patient teaching:
- Take safety precautions, including changing position slowly and avoiding driving and hazardous tasks, if CNS effects occur.
- Take the drug with meals and try small, frequent meals if GI upset is a problem.
- Follow drug dosing guidelines carefully.
- Report severe GI problems and interference with nutrition; fever and chills, which may indicate the presence of a superinfection, and dizziness, unusual fatigue, or weakness, which may indicate CNS effects.

Evaluation

- Monitor patient response to the drug (resolution of infection and negative cultures for parasite).
- Monitor for adverse effects (orientation and affect, nutritional state, skin color and lesions, hepatic function, and occurrence of superinfections).
- Evaluate the effectiveness of the teaching plan (patient can name the drug, dosage, possible adverse effects to watch for, and specific measures to help avoid adverse effects).
- Monitor the effectiveness of comfort and safety measures and compliance with the regimen.

See Critical Thinking Scenario *for additional information related to coping with amebiasis and the use of metronidazole.*

CRITICAL THINKING SCENARIO

Coping with Amebiasis

THE SITUATION

J.C., a 20-year-old male college student, reported to the university health center complaining of severe diarrhea, abdominal pain, and, most recently, blood in his stool. He had a mild fever and appeared to be dehydrated and very tired. The young man, who denied travel outside the country, reported eating most of his meals at the local beer joint, where he worked in the kitchen each night making pizza.

A stool sample for ova and parasites (O&P) was obtained, and a diagnosis of amebiasis was made. Metronidazole was prescribed. A public health referral was sent to find the source of the infection, which was the kitchen of the beer joint where J.C. worked. The kitchen was shut down until all the food, utensils, and environment passed state health inspection. Although a potential epidemic was averted (only three other cases of amebiasis were reported) the action of the public health officials added new stress to this student's life because he was unemployed for several months.

(continues on page 196)

Coping with Amebiasis (continued)

CRITICAL THINKING

What are the important nursing implications for J.C.? *Think about the usual nutritional state of a college student who eats most of his meals in a pizza place.*

What are the implications for recovery when a patient is malnourished and then has a disease that causes severe diarrhea, dehydration, and potential malnourishment? *Consider how difficult it will be for J.C. to be a full-time student while trying to cope with the signs and symptoms of his disease, as well as the adverse effects associated with his drug therapy and the need to maintain adequate nutrition to allow some healing and recovery.*

What potential problems could the added stress of being out of work have for J.C.? *Consider the physiological impact of stress, as well as the psychological problems of trying to cope with one more stressor.*

DISCUSSION

J.C. needed a great deal of reassurance and an explanation of his disease. He learned that oral hygiene and small, frequent meals would help alleviate some of his discomfort until the metronidazole could control the amebiasis and that good hygiene and strict hand washing when the disease is active would help to prevent transmission. He was advised to watch for the occurrence of specific adverse drug effects, such as a possible severe reaction to alcohol (he was advised to avoid alcoholic beverages while taking this drug); GI upset and a strange metallic taste (the importance of good nutrition to promote healing of the GI tract was stressed); dizziness or light-headedness; and superinfections.

J.C. was scheduled for a follow-up examination for stool O&P and nutritional status. Metronidazole was continued until the stool sample came back negative. He needed and received a great deal of support and encouragement because he was far from home and the disease and the drug effects were sometimes difficult to cope with. The effects of stress—decreasing blood flow to the GI tract, for example—can make it more difficult for patients such as J.C. to recover from this disease. Support and encouragement can be major factors in their eventual recovery. J.C. was given a telephone number to call if he needed information or support and a complete set of written instructions regarding the disease and the drug therapy.

NURSING CARE GUIDE FOR J.C.: METRONIDAZOLE

Assessment: History and Examination

Allergies to metronidazole, renal or liver dysfunction

Concurrent use of barbiturates, oral anticoagulants, alcohol

Local: Culture of stool for accurate diagnosis of infection

CNS: Orientation, affect, vision, reflexes

Skin: Color, lesions, texture

GI: Abdominal, liver evaluation

Hematological: CBC, liver function tests

Nursing Diagnoses

Acute pain related to GI, superinfection effects

Disturbed sensory perception (kinesthetic, visual) related to CNS effects

Imbalanced nutrition: Less than body requirements related to GI effects

Deficient knowledge regarding drug therapy

Planning

The patient will receive the best therapeutic effect from the drug therapy.

The patient will have limited adverse effects to the drug therapy.

The patient will have an understanding of the drug therapy, adverse effects to anticipate, and measures to relieve discomfort and improve safety.

Implementation

Culture infection before beginning therapy.

Provide comfort and safety measures: Oral hygiene, safety precautions, treatment of superinfections, maintenance of nutrition.

Provide small, frequent meals and monitor nutritional status.

Provide support and reassurance for dealing with drug effects and discomfort.

Provide patient teaching regarding drug name, dosage, adverse effects, precautions, and warning signs to report and hygiene measures to observe.

Evaluation

Evaluate drug effects: Resolution of protozoal infection.

Monitor for adverse effects: GI alterations, dizziness, confusion, CNS changes, vision loss, hepatic function, superinfections.

Monitor for drug–drug interactions with oral anticoagulants, alcohol, or barbiturates.

Evaluate effectiveness of patient-teaching program.

Evaluate effectiveness of comfort and safety measures.

PATIENT TEACHING FOR J.C.

You have been prescribed metronidazole to treat your amebic infection. This antiprotozoal drug acts to destroy certain protozoa that have invaded your body. Because it affects specific phases of the protozoal life cycle, it must be taken over a period of time to be effective. It is very important to take all the drug that has been ordered for you.

Coping with Amebiasis (continued)

- This drug frequently causes stomach upset. If it causes you to have nausea, heartburn, or vomiting, take the drug with meals or a light snack.
- Common effects of this drug include the following:
  - *Nausea, vomiting, and loss of appetite:* Take the drug with food and have small, frequent meals.
  - *Superinfections of the mouth, skin:* These go away when the course of the drug has been completed. If they become uncomfortable, notify your health care provider for an appropriate solution.
  - *Dry mouth, strange metallic taste:* Frequent mouth care and sucking sugarless lozenges may help. This effect will also go away when the course of the drug is finished.
  - *Intolerance to alcohol (nausea, vomiting, flushing, headache, and stomach pain)*: Avoid alcoholic beverages or products containing alcohol while taking this drug.
- Report any of the following to your health care provider: sore throat, fever, or chills; skin rash or redness; severe GI upset; and unusual fatigue, clumsiness, or weakness.
- Take the full course of your prescription. Never use this drug to self-treat any other infection or give it to any other person.
- Tell any doctor, nurse, or other health care provider that you are taking this drug.
- Keep this drug and all medications out of the reach of children.

KEY POINTS

- Other protozoal infections include amebiasis, leishmaniasis, trypanosomiasis, trichomoniasis, giardiasis, and *Pneumocystis carinii.*
- Patients receiving antiprotozoal agents should be monitored regularly to detect any serious adverse effects, including loss of vision, liver toxicity, and so on.

SUMMARY

- A protozoan is a parasitic cellular organism. Its life cycle includes a parasitic phase inside human tissues or cells.
- Malaria is caused by *Plasmodium* protozoa, which must go through a cycle in the *Anopheles* mosquito before being passed to humans by the mosquito bite. Once inside a human the protozoa invade red blood cells.
- The characteristic cyclic chills and fever of malaria occur when red blood cells burst, releasing more protozoa into the bloodstream.
- Malaria is treated with a combination of drugs that attack the protozoan at various stages in its life cycle.
- Amebiasis is caused by the protozoan *Entamoeba histolytica*, which invades human intestinal tissue after being passed to humans through unsanitary food or water. It is best treated with metronidazole or tinidazole.
- Leishmaniasis, a protozoan-caused disease, can result in serious lesions in the mucosa, viscera, and skin. It is treated with systemic pentamidine.
- Trypanosomiasis, which is caused by infection with a *Trypanosoma* parasite, may assume two forms. African sleeping sickness leads to inflammation of the CNS, and Chagas' disease results in serious cardiomyopathy. These diseases can be treated with systemic pentamidine.
- Trichomoniasis is caused by *Trichomonas vaginalis*. This common cause of vaginitis results in no signs or symptoms in men but serious vaginal inflammation in women. It is treated with metronidazole and tinidazole.
- Giardiasis, which is caused by *Giardia lamblia*, is the most commonly diagnosed intestinal parasite in the United States. This disease may lead to serious malnutrition when the pathogen invades intestinal mucosa. It is treated with nitazoxanide, metronidazole, and tinidazole.
- *Pneumocystis jiroveci* is an endemic protozoan that does not usually cause illness in humans unless they become immunosuppressed. This is the most common opportunistic infection seen in AIDS patients. It is treated with inhaled pentamidine and oral atovaquone.
- Patients receiving antiprotozoal agents should be monitored regularly to detect any serious adverse effects, including loss of vision, liver toxicity, and so on.

CHECK YOUR UNDERSTANDING

Answers to the questions in this chapter can be found in the Answers to Check Your Understanding Questions on thePoint®.

MULTIPLE CHOICE

Select the best answer to the following.

1. After a group of students is taught about protozoal infections, which infection, if stated by the group as caused by an insect bite, would indicate the need for additional teaching?
   a. Malaria
   b. Trypanosomiasis
   c. Leishmaniasis
   d. Giardiasis

2. When describing the development of malaria caused by the *Plasmodium* protozoan the instructor would explain that the organism depends on
   a. a snail to act as intermediary in the life cycle of the protozoan.
   b. a mosquito and a red blood cell for maturation.
   c. a human liver cell for cell division and reproduction.
   d. stagnant water for maturation.

3. A patient who is receiving a combination drug to treat malaria asks the nurse why. The nurse responds to the patient based on the understanding that combination drugs are
   a. associated with a much lower degree of toxicity when used in combination.
   b. absorbed more completely when administered and taken together.
   c. more effective in preventing mosquitoes from biting the individual.
   d. effective at various stages in the life cycle of the protozoan.

4. A patient traveling to an area of the world where malaria is known to be endemic should be taught to
   a. avoid drinking the water.
   b. begin prophylactic antimalarial therapy before traveling and continue it through the visit and for 2 to 3 weeks after the visit.
   c. take a supply of antimalarial drugs in case he or she gets a mosquito bite.
   d. begin prophylactic antimalarial therapy 2 weeks before traveling and stop the drugs on arriving at the destination.

5. Amebiasis or amebic dysentery
   a. is seen only in Third World countries.
   b. is caused by a protozoan that enters the body through an insect bite.
   c. is caused by a protozoan that can enter the body in the cyst stage in water or food.
   d. usually has no signs and symptoms.

6. Giardiasis is the most common intestinal parasite seen in the United States, and it
   a. does not respond to drug therapy.
   b. can invade the liver and cause death.
   c. is seen only in areas with no sanitation.
   d. is associated with rotten egg–smelling stool, diarrhea, and mucus-filled stool.

7. *Pneumocystis jiroveci* pneumonia is
   a. an endemic protozoan found in the human respiratory system.
   b. responsive to inhaled pentamidine.
   c. an opportunistic bacterial infection.
   d. frequently associated with children in day care settings.

8. Trypanosomiasis may assume which of the following two different forms?
   a. African sleeping sickness and Chagas' disease
   b. Elephantiasis and malaria
   c. Dysentery and African sleeping sickness
   d. Malaria and Chagas' disease

9. A nurse would note that a patient had a good understanding of his antimalarial drug regimen if the patient reported,
   a. "I keep these pills with me at all times while I'm away and take them only when I have been bitten by a mosquito."
   b. "I will need to start these pills now and then continue to take them every day for the rest of my life."
   c. "I'll start the pills before my trip, keep taking them during the trip, and for a period of time after I'm home."
   d. "I start taking these pills as soon as I arrive at my vacation destination, but before I get off the plane."

MULTIPLE RESPONSE

Select all that apply.

1. A mother calls in concerned that her son, a college freshman, has been diagnosed with giardiasis. The nurse would respond to the mother's concerns by telling her which of the following?

a. You should have your son come home immediately so that he can be treated appropriately.

b. This is a very rare disorder; it is not usually seen in this country.

c. This is the most common protozoal infection seen in this country and is usually transmitted through food or water.

d. This infection can be treated with oral drugs, and he should be able to get the drugs where his infection was diagnosed.

e. This is an infection that has to be treated quickly with IV medications.

f. Encourage your son to get the medicine and to try very hard to eat nutritious food.

2. Your patient is a 32-year-old HIV-positive male being treated for *Pneumocystis jiroveci* pneumonia; he did well on a course of atovaquone and is now being discharged on pentamidine to prevent a recurrence of the infection. In preparing his teaching plan, you would need to include which of the following?

a. Pentamidine is an inhaled drug used once every 4 weeks.

b. Pentamidine is an oral drug that will need to be taken daily for a very long time.

c. Pentamidine requires very special handling to prevent toxicity.

d. Pentamidine must be inhaled using the Respigard inhaler.

e. The patient may also need to be put on an antihypertensive drug while using pentamidine.

f. Periodic renal, hepatic, and complete blood count (CBC) blood tests will be needed while using this drug.

BIBLIOGRAPHY AND REFERENCES

Ambachew, M., Yohannes, A., Bergqvist, Y., et al. (2011). Confirmed vivax resistance to chloroquine and effectiveness of artemether-lumefantrine for the treatment of vivax malaria in Ethiopia. *American Journal of Tropical Medicine and Hygiene, 84*(1), 137–140.

Andrews, M., & Boyle, J. (2011). *Transcultural concepts in nursing care* (6th ed.). Philadelphia, PA: Lippincott Williams & Wilkins.

Bailey, J. M., & Erramouspe, J. (2004). Nitazoxanide treatment for giardiasis and cryptosporidiosis in children. *Annals of Pharmacotherapy, 38*, 634–640.

Brunton, L., Chabner, B., & Knollman, B. (2011). *Goodman and Gilman's the pharmacological basis of therapeutics* (12th ed.). New York: McGraw-Hill.

CDC. (2012). *Malaria risk assessment for travelers [Centers for Disease Control and Prevention]*. Available online at: http://www.cdc.gov/malaria/travelers/risk_assessment.html

Facts and Comparisons. (2015). *Drug facts and comparisons*. St. Louis, MO: Author.

Facts and Comparisons. (2015). *Professional's guide to patient drug facts*. St. Louis, MO: Author.

Griffith, K. S., Lewis, L. S., Mali, S. (2007). Treatment of malaria in the United States. *Journal of the American Medical Association, 297*(20), 2264–2277.

Karch, A. M. (2014). *Lippincott's nursing drug guide*. Philadelphia, PA: Lippincott Williams & Wilkins.

Kovacs, J., & Masur, H. (2009) Evolving health effects of *Pneumocystis*: One hundred years of progress in diagnosis and treatment. *Journal of the American Medical Association, 301*(24), 2578–2585.

Porth, C. M. (2013). *Pathophysiology: Concepts of altered health states* (9th ed.). Philadelphia, PA: Lippincott Williams & Wilkins.

WHO. (2010). *Guidelines for the treatment of malaria* (2nd ed.). Geneva, Switzerland: WHO.

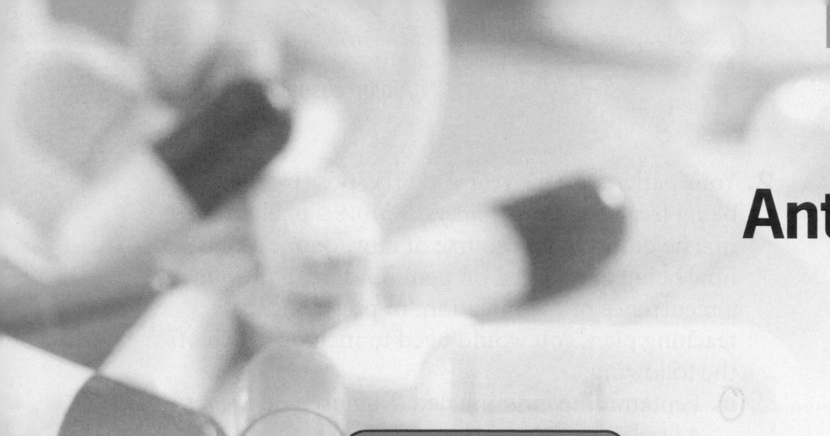

Anthelmintic Agents 13

Learning Objectives

Upon completion of this chapter, you will be able to:

1. List the common worms that cause disease in humans.
2. Describe the therapeutic actions, indications, pharmacokinetics, contraindications, most common adverse reactions, and important drug–drug interactions associated with the anthelmintics.
3. Discuss the use of anthelmintics across the lifespan.
4. Compare and contrast the prototype drug mebendazole with other anthelmintics.
5. Outline the nursing considerations, including important teaching points to stress for patients receiving an anthelmintic.

Glossary of Key Terms

Ascaris**:** the most prevalent helminthic infection; fertilized roundworm eggs are ingested, which hatch in the small intestine and then make their way to the lungs, where they may cause cough, fever, and other signs of a pulmonary infiltrate

cestode: tapeworm with a head and segmented body parts that is capable of growing to several yards in the human intestine

filariasis: infection of the blood and tissues of healthy individuals by worm embryos or filariae

helminth: worm that can cause disease by invading the human body

hookworms: worms that attach themselves to the small intestine of infected individuals, where they suck blood from the walls of the intestine, damaging the intestinal wall and leading to severe anemia with lethargy, weakness, and fatigue

nematode: roundworms such as the commonly encountered pinworm, whipworm, threadworm, *Ascaris*, or hookworm that cause a common helminthic infection in humans; can cause intestinal obstruction as the adult worms clog the intestinal lumen or severe pneumonia when the larvae migrate to the lungs and form a pulmonary infiltrate

pinworm: nematode that causes a common helminthic infection in humans; lives in the intestine and causes anal and possible vaginal irritation and itching

platyhelminth: flatworms, including the cestodes or tapeworms; a worm that can live in the human intestine or can invade other human tissues (flukes)

schistosomiasis: infection with a blood fluke that is carried by a snail; it poses a common problem in tropical countries, where the snail is the intermediary in the life cycle of the worm; larvae burrow into the skin in fresh water and migrate throughout the human body, causing a rash, diarrhea, and liver and brain inflammation

threadworm: pervasive nematode that can send larvae into the lungs, liver, and central nervous system (CNS); can cause severe pneumonia or liver abscess

trichinosis: disease that results from ingestion of encysted roundworm larvae in undercooked pork; larvae migrate throughout the body to invade muscles, nerves, and other tissues; can cause pneumonia, heart failure, and encephalitis

whipworm: worm that attaches itself to the intestinal mucosa and sucks blood; may cause severe anemia and disintegration of the intestinal mucosa

Drug List

Anthelmintics
albendazole
ivermectin
(P) mebendazole
praziquantel
pyrantel

BOX 13.1 FOCUS ON **Cultural Considerations**

Travelers and Helminths

People who come from or travel to areas of the world where schistosomiasis is endemic should always be assessed for the possibility of infection with such a disease when seen for health care. Areas of the world in which this disease is endemic are mainly tropical settings, such as Puerto Rico, islands of the West Indies, Africa, parts of South America, the Philippines, China, Japan, and Southeast Asia. People traveling to these areas should be warned about wading, swimming, or bathing in freshwater streams, ponds, or lakes. For example, swimming in the Nile River is a popular attraction on Egyptian vacation tours; however, this activity may result in a lasting (unhappy) memory when the traveler returns home and is diagnosed with schistosomiasis. The nurse can suggest to patients who are planning a visit to one of these areas that they contact the CDC for health and safety guidelines, as well as what signs and symptoms to watch for after returning home. The CDC can be found at http://www.cdc.gov/travel.

Helminthic infections, or infections in the gastrointestinal (GI) tract or other tissues due to worm infestation, affect about 1 billion people, making these types of infections among the most common of all diseases. These infestations are very common in tropical areas, but they are also often found in other regions, including countries such as the United States and Canada. With so many people traveling to many parts of the world, it is not uncommon for a traveler to contract a helminthic infection in one country and inadvertently bring it home, where the worms then can infect other individuals (Box 13.1). The **helminths** that most commonly infect humans are of two types: the nematodes (or roundworms) and the platyhelminths (or flatworms) that cause intestine-invading worm infections and tissue-invading worms.

Frequently, patients have a very difficult time dealing with a diagnosis of worm infestation. It is very important for the nurse to understand the disease process and to explain the disease and treatment carefully to help the patient to cope with both the diagnosis and the treatment.

Intestine-Invading Worm Infections

Many of the worms that infect humans live only in the intestinal tract. Proper diagnosis of a helminthic infection requires a stool examination for ova (eggs) and parasites. Treatment of a helminthic infection entails the use of an anthelmintic drug. Another important part of therapy for helminthic infections involves the prevention of reinfection or spread of an existing infection. Measures such as thorough hand washing after use of the toilet; frequent laundering of bed linens and underwear in very hot, chlorine-treated water; disinfection of toilets and bathroom areas after each use; and good personal hygiene to wash away ova are important to prevent the spread of the disease. See Table 13.1 for a summary of worms that cause intestinal infections.

Infections by Nematodes

Nematodes, or roundworms, include the commonly encountered pinworms, whipworms, threadworms, *Ascaris*, and hookworms. These worms cause diseases that range in severity from mild to potentially fatal.

Pinworm Infections

Pinworms are usually transmitted when the worm eggs are ingested, either by transfer by touching the eggs when they are shed to clothing, toys, or bedding; or by the inhalation of eggs that become airborne and are then swallowed. Pinworms, which remain in the intestine, cause little discomfort except for perianal itching or occasionally vaginal itching. Infection with pinworms is the most common helminthic infection among school-aged children. (See Critical Thinking Scenario for a case study of a child exposed to pinworm.)

Whipworm Infections

Whipworms are transmitted when eggs found in the soil are ingested. Whipworms attach to the wall of the colon. In large numbers, they cause colic and bloody diarrhea. In severe cases, whipworm infestation may result in prolapse of the intestinal wall and anemia related to blood loss.

Table 13.1 Helminthic Infections

Intestine-Invading Worm	Mechanism of Disease	Manifestations
Pinworms	Remain in intestine	Perianal itching; occasionally, vaginal itching
Whipworms	Attach to wall of colon	Bloody diarrhea (with large numbers of worms)
Threadworms	Burrow into intestine; can enter lungs, liver, and other tissue	Pneumonia, liver abscess
Ascaris	Burrow into intestine; enter the blood and infect lungs	Cough, fever, pulmonary infiltrates; abdominal distention and pain
Hookworms	Attach to the wall of the intestine	Anemia, fatigue, malabsorption
Cestodes	Live in the intestine, ingesting nutrients from the host	Weight loss, abdominal distention

CRITICAL THINKING SCENARIO

Treating Pinworm Infections

THE SITUATION

J.K. is a 4-year-old boy who attends pre-kindergarten classes 5 days a week at a local childhood development center. He brought a note home from the director of the school explaining that pinworm infections had been diagnosed in two of his classmates. The director outlined steps that the school was taking to prevent spread of the disease, but stated that since it is very contagious all families were being advised to contact their health care provider, mentioning that treatment with mebendazole had been suggested. J.K.'s mother became very upset and immediately called to make an appointment at the clinic. At the clinic, J.K. was diagnosed with a pinworm infection.

CRITICAL THINKING

What are the important nursing implications for J.K. and his family *Think about the impact a diagnosis of a worm infection in a child would have on a young mother. Think about how contagious this disease is and how the whole family needs to be involved in the treatment regimen.*

What drug therapy would most likely be suggested and who will need to take the drug?

What nondrug interventions are crucial in the treatment and prevention of further spread of this disease?

Is there any risk of spreading this disease in the clinic?

What steps should be taken to ensure the safety of other children who might come into the clinic? *Think about the way that pinworms spread and how the spread can be prevented.*

DISCUSSION

Pinworm infections are the most common helminth infection in young children. Hearing that your child has "worms" can be very upsetting to a parent. It will be important to explain what a pinworm infection is, how easy it is to spread, and how easy it is to treat. Assure the mother that it happens all the time and a pinworm infection in her young child is not a reflection on her or her family. It will be important to discuss the need for the whole family to be treated, just in case. It will be key to covering all of the hygiene measures that will be needed to eradicate any infection: Strict handwashing, showering the child every morning, cleaning bedding and undergarments in hot water, with chlorine if possible, cleaning the toilet area daily. Assure her that it will be a 3-day treatment course and few, if any, adverse effects would be expected from the drug. Keeping the child and family calm will be a major part of this visit. Many recommend that the whole family be treated if pinworms have been in his system. The 3-day drug treatment is easy and very few adverse effects are experienced. The mother might feel better knowing that since the possibility of cross infection exists something is being done to take care of the issue. Since pinworms are very contagious, it would be important to know if the child used the toilet facilities at the clinic, and have the area properly cleaned if needed. Toys or other objects the child might have played with might also need to be sanitized; if the child had long fingernails or had not washed his hands the worms could be spread. It would be a good exercise to help him wash his hands at the clinic—singing the *Happy Birthday* song is often a guideline for how long should be spent washing the hands and the child might relax and enjoy the activity while you are talking to his mother.

NURSING CARE GUIDE FOR J.K. PINWORM TREATMENT

Assessment: History and Examination

Allergies to this drug, any history of liver or renal issues

Local: Culture of infection, stool for ova and parasites

Skin: Color, lesions, texture; perianal inspection

GI: Abdominal evaluation

Nursing Diagnoses

Acute pain related to GI or central nervous system (CNS) effects

Disturbed personal identity related to diagnosis and treatment

Deficient knowledge regarding drug therapy

Planning

The patient will receive the best therapeutic effect from the drug therapy.

The patient will have limited adverse effects to the drug therapy.

The patient will have an understanding of the drug therapy, adverse effects to anticipate, and measures to relieve discomfort and improve safety

Implementation

Culture for ova and parasites before beginning therapy.

Provide support and reassurance to deal with drug effects, discomfort, and diagnosis.

Provide parent/patient teaching regarding drug name, dosage regimen, adverse effects, precautions to report, and hygiene measures to observe.

Stress the importance of hygiene measures in eradicating the infection.

Treating Pinworm Infections (continued)

Evaluation

Evaluate drug effects: Resolution of helminth infection.
Monitor for adverse effects: GI alterations
Evaluate effectiveness of parent/patient-teaching program.
Evaluate effectiveness of comfort and safety measures.

PARENT/PATIENT TEACHING FOR J.K.

- This drug is called an anthelmintic. It works by destroying certain helminths, or worms, that have invaded your body.
- It is important that you take/give the full course of the drug—chew the tablets thoroughly and take one tablet twice a day for 3 days.
- Other measures will be very important to eradicate the infection: Trim fingernails, encourage handwashing, shower in the morning, wash bedding and underwear everyday in hot water (with chlorine if possible), clean the toilet and toilet area daily.
- Common effects of this drug include
- *Nausea, loss of appetite*: Eat small, frequent meals.
- Report any of the following conditions to your health care provider: diarrhea, abdominal pain.
- Take/give all of the drug that has been prescribed, over 3 days. Never use this drug to self-treat any other infection or give it to any other person.
- Tell any doctor, nurse, or other health care provider that you/your child are/is taking this drug.
- Keep this drug and all medications out of the reach of children.

Threadworm Infestation

Threadworms can cause more damage to humans than most of the other helminths. Threadworms are transmitted as larvae found in the soil and inadvertently ingested. The larvae mature into worms, and after burrowing into the wall of the small intestine female worms lay eggs. These eggs hatch into larvae that invade many body tissues, including the lungs, liver, and heart. In very severe cases, death may occur from pneumonia or from lung or liver abscesses that result from larval invasion.

Ascaris

Worldwide, ***Ascaris*** infection is the most prevalent helminthic infection. It may occur wherever sanitation is poor. Eggs in the soil are ingested with vegetables or other improperly washed foods. Many individuals are unaware that they have this infestation unless they see a worm in their stool. However, others become quite ill.

Initially, the individual ingests fertilized roundworm eggs, which hatch in the small intestine and then make their way to the lungs, where they may cause cough, fever, and other signs of a pulmonary infiltrate. The larvae then migrate back to the intestine, where they grow to adult size (i.e., about as long and as big around as an earthworm), causing abdominal distention and pain. In the most severe cases, intestinal obstruction by masses of worms can occur.

Hookworm Infections

Hookworm eggs are found in the soil, where they hatch into a larva that molts and becomes infective to humans. The larvae penetrate the skin and then enter the blood and within about a week reach the intestine. Hookworms attach to the small intestine of infected individuals. The worms suck blood from the walls of the intestine, damaging the intestinal wall and leading to severe anemia with lethargy, weakness, and fatigue. Malabsorption problems may occur as the small intestinal mucosa is altered. Treatment for anemia and fluid and electrolyte disturbances is an important part of the therapy for this infection.

Infections Caused by Platyhelminths

The **platyhelminths** (flatworms) include the cestodes (tapeworms) that live in the human intestine and the flukes (schistosomes) that live in the intestine and also invade other tissues as part of their life cycle. Because schistosomes invade tissues, they are discussed in the following section on tissue-invading worm infections.

Cestodes

Cestodes are segmented flatworms with a head, or scolex, and a variable number of segments that grow from the head. Cestodes enter the body as larvae that are found in undercooked meat or fish; they sometimes form worms that are several yards long. Persons with a tapeworm may experience some abdominal discomfort and distention, as well as weight loss because the worm eats ingested nutrients. Many infected patients require a great deal of psychological support when they excrete parts of the tapeworm or when the worm occasionally exits through the mouth or nose.

Tissue-Invading Worm Infections

Some of the worms that invade the body exist outside of the intestinal tract and can seriously damage the tissues they invade. Because of their location within healthy tissue, they can also be more difficult to treat.

Trichinosis

Trichinosis is the disease caused by ingestion of the encysted larvae of the roundworm, *Trichinella spiralis*, in undercooked pork. Once ingested the larvae are deposited in the intestinal mucosa, pass into the bloodstream, and are carried throughout the body. They can penetrate skeletal muscle and can cause an inflammatory reaction in cardiac muscle and in the brain. Fatal pneumonia, heart failure, and encephalitis may occur.

The best treatment for trichinosis is prevention. Because the larvae are ingested by humans in undercooked pork, instructing individuals about freezing pork meat, monitoring the food eaten by pigs, and properly cooking pork can be most beneficial.

Filariasis

Filariasis refers to infection of the blood and tissues of healthy individuals by worm embryos, which enter the body via insect bites. These thread-like embryos, or filariae, can overwhelm the lymphatic system and cause massive inflammatory reactions. This may lead to severe swelling of the hands, feet, legs, arms, scrotum, or breast—a condition called elephantiasis.

Schistosomiasis

Schistosomiasis (Figure 13.1) is a platyhelminthic infection by a fluke that is carried by a snail. This disease is a common problem in parts of Africa, Asia, and certain South American and Caribbean countries that have climates and snails conducive to the life cycle of schistosomes.

Eggs that are excreted in the urine and feces of infected individuals hatch in fresh water into a form that infects a certain snail. In the snail, larvae known as cercariae develop. The snail sheds the cercariae back into the freshwater pond or lake. People become infected when they come in contact with the infested water. The larvae attach to the skin and quickly burrow into the bloodstream and lymphatics. Then they move into the lungs, and later to the liver, where they mature into adult worms that mate and migrate to the intestines and urinary bladder. The female worms then lay large numbers of eggs,

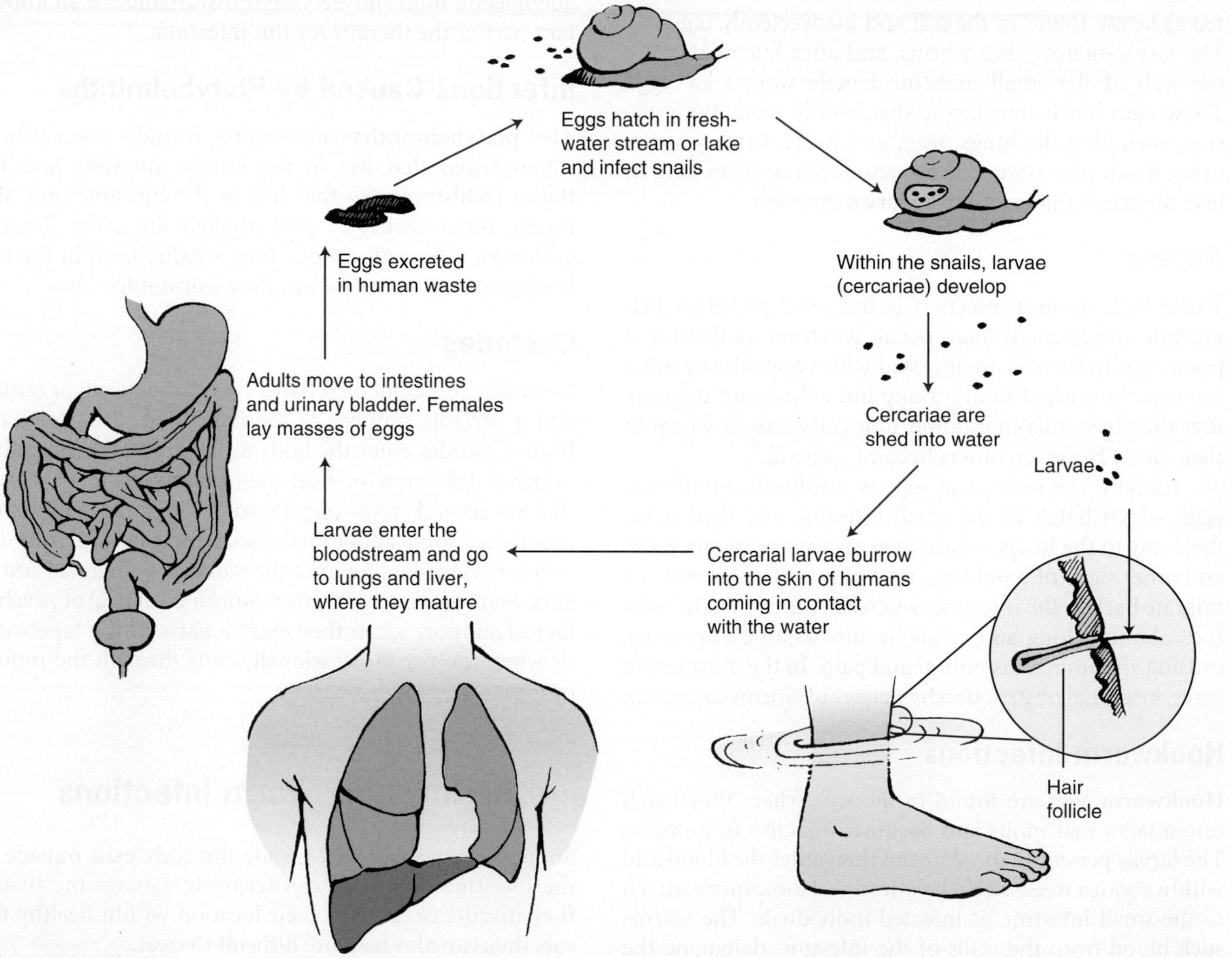
Eggs hatch in fresh-water stream or lake and infect snails
Within the snails, larvae (cercariae) develop
Cercariae are shed into water
Larvae
Cercarial larvae burrow into the skin of humans coming in contact with the water
Hair follicle
Larvae enter the bloodstream and go to lungs and liver, where they mature
Adults move to intestines and urinary bladder. Females lay masses of eggs
Eggs excreted in human waste

FIGURE 13.1 Life cycle of schistosomes.

which are expelled in the feces and urine, and the cycle begins again.

Signs and symptoms may include a pruritic rash, often called swimmer's itch, where the larva attaches to the skin. About 1 or 2 months later, affected individuals may experience several weeks of fever, chills, headache, and other symptoms. Chronic or severe infestation may lead to abdominal pain and diarrhea, as well as blockage of blood flow to areas of the liver, lungs, and CNS. These blockages can lead to liver and spleen enlargement, as well as signs of CNS and cardiac ischemia. (See Critical Thinking Scenario for a case study of a patient diagnosed with chronic schistosomiasis.)

KEY POINTS

- Helminths are worms that cause disease by invading the human body. Some helminths invade body tissues and can seriously damage lymphatic tissue, lungs, CNS, heart, or liver.
- Pinworms are the most frequent cause of helminth infection in the United States, and roundworms called *Ascaris* are the most frequent cause of helminth infections throughout the world.
- Patient teaching is important for decreasing the stress and anxiety that may occur when individuals are diagnosed with a worm infestation.

CRITICAL THINKING SCENARIO

Anthelmintics

THE SITUATION

V.Y., a 33-year-old man from Vietnam, underwent a complete physical examination in preparation for a training job in custodial work at a local hospital. He was a refugee who had come to the United States 6 months ago as part of a church-sponsored resettlement program. In the course of the examination, it was found that he had a history of chronic diarrhea, hepatomegaly, pulmonary rales, and splenomegaly. Further tests indicated that he had chronic schistosomiasis. Because of V.Y.'s limited use of the English language, he was hospitalized so that his disease, which was unfamiliar to most of the associated health care providers, could be monitored. He was treated with praziquantel.

CRITICAL THINKING

What are the important nursing implications for V.Y.?
Think about the serious limitations that are placed on medical care, particularly patient teaching, when the patient and the health care workers do not speak the same language.
What innovative techniques could be used to teach this patient about the disease, the drugs, and the hygiene measures that are important for him to follow?
Are the other patients or workers in the hospital exposed to any health risks?
What sort of educational program should be developed to teach them about this disease and to allay any fears or anxieties they may have?
What special interventions are needed to explain the drug therapy and any adverse effects or warning signs that V.Y. should be watching for?

DISCUSSION

A language barrier can be a real handicap in the health care system. In many cases, pictures can assist communication. For example, the need for nutritious food is conveyed by using appropriate pictures of foods that should be eaten. The patient is prepared for discharge through careful patient teaching that may involve pictures, calendars, and clocks so that he is given every opportunity to comply with his medical regimen.

In addition, the nursing staff should contact the local health department to determine whether the local sewer system can properly handle contaminated wastes. In this case the staff learned from the CDC (Centers for Disease Control and Prevention) that the snail's intermediate host does not live in this country, so the hazards posed by this waste are small, and normal disposal of the wastes should be appropriate.

V.Y. should also be observed for signs of adverse effects, although praziquantel is a relatively mild drug. Drug fever, abdominal pain, or dizziness may occur. If dizziness occurs, safety precautions, such as assistance with ambulation, use of side rails, and adequate lighting, need to be taken without alarming the patient.

NURSING CARE GUIDE FOR V.Y.: ANTHELMINTIC AGENTS

Assessment: History and Examination

Allergies to this drug, renal or liver dysfunction
Drug history: Use of albendazole
Local: Culture of infection
CNS: Orientation, affect
Skin: Color, lesions, texture
GI: Abdominal and liver evaluation, including hepatic function tests
GU: Renal function tests

Nursing Diagnoses

Acute pain related to GI or CNS effects
Disturbed personal identity related to diagnosis and treatment

(continues on page 206)

Anthelmintics (continued)

Fear related to communication problems, health issues

Deficient knowledge regarding drug therapy

PLANNING

The patient will receive the best therapeutic effect from the drug therapy.

The patient will have limited adverse effects to the drug therapy.

The patient will have an understanding of the drug therapy, adverse effects to anticipate, and measures to relieve discomfort and improve safety.

Implementation

Culture for ova and parasites before beginning therapy.

Provide comfort and safety measures: Small, frequent meals; safety precautions; hygiene measures; maintenance of nutrition.

Monitor nutritional status as needed.

Provide support and reassurance to deal with drug effects, discomfort, and diagnosis.

Provide patient teaching regarding drug name, dosage regimen, adverse effects, precautions to report, and hygiene measures to observe.

Evaluation

Evaluate drug effects: Resolution of helminth infection.

Monitor for adverse effects: GI alterations, CNS changes, dizziness and confusion, renal and hepatic function.

Monitor for drug–drug interactions: Concurrent use of albendazole.

Evaluate effectiveness of patient-teaching program.

Evaluate effectiveness of comfort and safety measures.

PATIENT TEACHING FOR V.Y.

- This drug is called an anthelmintic. It works by destroying certain helminths, or worms, that have invaded your body.
- It is important that you take the full course of the drug—three doses the first day, then retesting to repeat this course if needed to ensure that all of the worms, in all phases of their life cycle, have disappeared from your body.
- You may take this drug with meals or with a light snack to help decrease any stomach upset that you may experience. Swallow the tablets whole and avoid holding them in your mouth for any length of time because a very unpleasant taste may occur.
- Common effects of this drug include
- *Nausea, vomiting, and loss of appetite*: Take the drug with food, and eat small, frequent meals.
- *Dizziness and drowsiness*: If this occurs, avoid driving a car or operating dangerous machinery. Change positions slowly to avoid falling or injury.
- Report any of the following conditions to your health care provider: fever, chills, rash, headache, weakness, or tremors.
- Take all of the drug that has been prescribed. Never use this drug to self-treat any other infection or give it to any other person.
- Tell any doctor, nurse, or other health care provider that you are taking this drug.
- Keep this drug and all medications out of the reach of children.

Anthelmintics

The anthelmintic drugs (Table 13.2) act on metabolic pathways that are present in the invading worm but are absent or significantly different in the human host. Anthelmintic drugs include albendazole (*Albenza*), ivermectin (*Stromectol*), mebendazole (generic), praziquantel (*Biltricide*), and pyrantel (*Antiminth, Pin-Rid, Pin-X, Reese's Pinworm*). Box 13.2 includes information about use of these drugs across the lifespan. See the Critical Thinking Scenario for a case study of a patient receiving anthelmintics.

Therapeutic Actions and Indications

Anthelmintic agents are indicated for the treatment of infections by certain susceptible worms and are very specific in the worms that they affect; they are not interchangeable for treating various worm infections. See Table 13.2 for usual indications for each of these agents. Anthelmintics interfere with metabolic processes in particular worms, as described previously. Figure 13.2 shows sites of actions for these drugs.

Pharmacokinetics

Mebendazole is available in the form of a chewable tablet, and a typical 3-day course can be repeated in 3 weeks if needed. Very little of the mebendazole is absorbed systemically, so adverse effects are few. The drug is not metabolized in the body, and most of it is excreted unchanged in the feces. A small amount may be excreted in the urine.

Albendazole is poorly absorbed from the GI tract, reaching peak plasma levels in about 5 hours. It is metabolized in the liver and primarily excreted in urine.

Ivermectin is readily absorbed from the GI tract and reaches peak plasma levels in 4 hours. It is completely metabolized in the liver with a half-life of 16 hours; excretion is through the feces.

Table 13.2 Drugs in Focus: Anthelmintics

Drug Name	Dosage/Route	Usual Indications
albendazole (*Albenza*)	***Hydatid disease:*** *≥60 kg:* 400 mg b.i.d. *<60 kg:* 15 mg/kg/d PO in divided doses, b.i.d., on a 28-d cycle, followed by 14 d of rest, for a total of three cycles ***Neurocysticercosis:*** *≥60 kg:* 400 mg b.i.d. *<60 kg:* 15/mg/kg/d PO in divided doses, b.i.d., for 8–30 d of treatment	Treatment of active lesions caused by pork tapeworm and cystic disease of the liver, lungs, and peritoneum caused by dog tapeworm
ivermectin (*Stromectol*)	150–200 mg/kg PO as a single dose	Treatment of threadworm disease or strongyloidiasis; onchocerciasis or river blindness, which is found in tropical areas of Africa, Mexico, and South America
mebendazole (generic)	100 mg PO morning and evening on 3 consecutive days Enterobiasis: 100 mg PO as a single dose	Treatment of diseases caused by pinworms, roundworms, whipworms, and hookworms
praziquantel (*Biltricide*)	Three doses of 20–25 mg/kg PO as a 1-d treatment	Treatment of a wide number of schistosomes or flukes
pyrantel (*Antiminth, Pin-Rid, Pin-X, Reese's Pinworm*)	11 mg/kg PO as a single dose; maximum dose, 1 g	Treatment of diseases caused by pinworms and roundworms; because administered in single dose, may be preferred for patients who could have trouble remembering to take medication or following drug regimens

Praziquantel is taken in a series of three oral doses at 4- to 6-hour intervals. It is rapidly absorbed from the GI tract and reaches peak plasma levels within 1 to 3 hours. It is metabolized in the liver with a half-life of 0.8 to 1.5 hours. Excretion of praziquantel occurs primarily through the urine.

Pyrantel is poorly absorbed, and most of the drug is excreted unchanged in the feces, although a small amount may be found in the urine.

Contraindications and Cautions

Overall contraindications to the use of anthelmintic drugs include the presence of known allergy to any of these drugs *to prevent hypersensitivity reactions*; lactation, *because the drugs can enter breast milk and could be toxic to the infant*—women are advised to refrain from breastfeeding when using these drugs; and pregnancy (in most cases), *because of reported associated fetal abnormalities or death.* Women of childbearing age should be advised to use barrier contraceptives while taking these drugs. Pyrantel has not been established as safe for use in children younger than 2 years. Albendazole should be used only after the causative worm has been identified *because it can cause adverse effects on the liver, which could be problematic if the patient has liver involvement.*

Use caution in the presence of renal or hepatic disease *that interferes with the metabolism or excretion of drugs that are absorbed systemically* and in cases of severe diarrhea and malnourishment, *which could alter the effects of the drug on the intestine and any preexisting helminths.*

BOX 13.2 FOCUS ON Drug Therapy Across the Lifespan

Anthelmintic Agents

CHILDREN

A culture of the suspected worm is important before beginning any drug therapy.

The more toxic drugs—albendazole, ivermectin, and praziquantel—should be avoided in children.

The most commonly used anthelmintic, mebendazole, comes in a chewable tablet that is convenient for use in children.

Nutritional status and hydration are major concerns with children taking these drugs who develop serious GI effects.

ADULTS

Adults may be somewhat repulsed by the idea that they have a worm infestation, and they may be reluctant to discuss the needed lifestyle adjustments and treatment plans.

Pregnant and nursing women should not use these drugs unless the benefit clearly outweighs the potential risk to the fetus or neonate. If a severe helminth infestation threatens the mother, some of the drugs can be used as long as the mother is informed of the potential risk.

OLDER ADULTS

Older patients may be more susceptible to the CNS and GI effects of some of these drugs. Dose adjustment is needed for these agents.

Monitor hydration and nutritional status carefully.

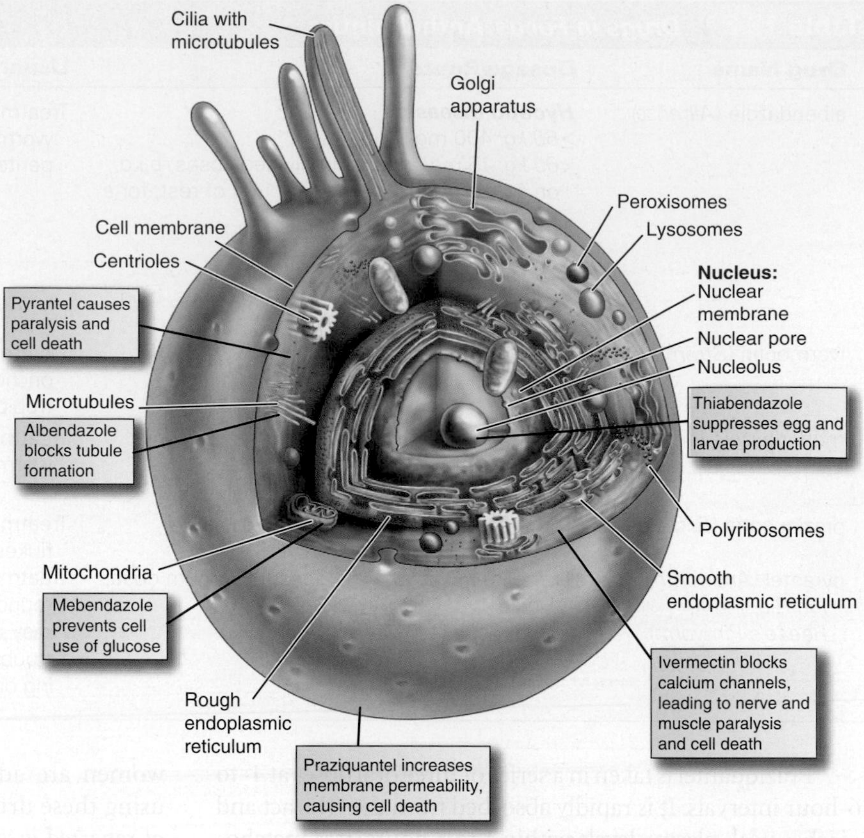

FIGURE 13.2 General structure of a cell, showing the sites of action of anthelmintic agents. Mebendazole interferes with the ability to use glucose, leading to an inability to reproduce and cell death. Albendazole blocks tubule formation, resulting in cell death. Ivermectin blocks calcium channels, leading to nerve and muscle paralysis and cell death. Pyrantel is a neuromuscular polarizing agent that causes paralysis and cell death. Praziquantel increases membrane permeability, leading to a loss of intracellular calcium and muscular paralysis; it may also result in disintegration of the integument.

Adverse Effects

Adverse effects frequently encountered with the use of these anthelmintic agents are related to their absorption or direct action in the intestine. Mebendazole and pyrantel, which are not absorbed systemically, may cause abdominal discomfort, diarrhea, or pain but have very few other effects and are well tolerated. Anthelmintics that are absorbed systemically may cause the following effects: Headache and dizziness; fever, shaking, chills, and malaise associated with an immune reaction to the death of the worms; rash; pruritus; and loss of hair.

Renal failure and severe bone marrow depression are associated with albendazole, which is toxic to some human tissues. Patients taking this drug require careful monitoring (Figure 13.3).

Clinically Important Drug–Drug Interactions

The effects of albendazole, which are already severe, may increase if the drug is combined with dexamethasone, praziquantel, or cimetidine. These combinations should be avoided if at all possible; if they are necessary, patients should be monitored closely for the occurrence of adverse effects.

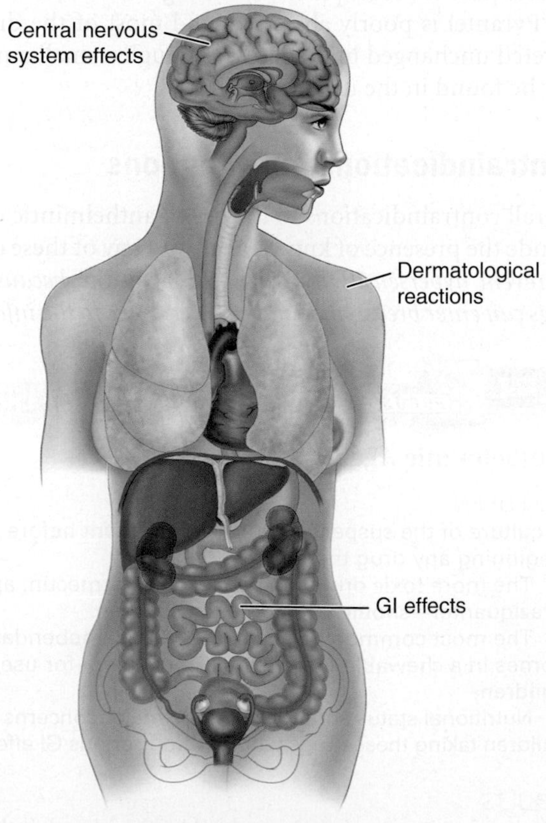

FIGURE 13.3 Common adverse effects associated with anthelmintics.

Ⓟ Prototype Summary: Mebendazole

Indications: Treatment of whipworm, pinworm, roundworm, and hookworm infections.

Actions: Irreversibly blocks glucose uptake by susceptible helminths, depleting glycogen stores needed for survival and reproduction, causing the death of the helminth.

Pharmacokinetics:

Route	Onset	Peak
Oral	Slow	2–4 h

$T_{1/2}$: 2.5 to 9 hours; metabolized in the liver and excreted in the feces.

Adverse Effects: Transient abdominal pain, diarrhea, fever.

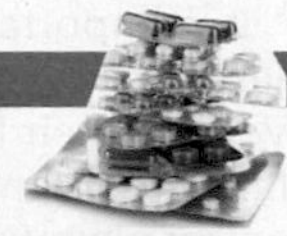

Nursing Considerations for Patients Receiving Anthelmintics

Assessment: History and Examination

- Assess for possible contraindications or cautions: History of allergy to any of the anthelmintics *to avoid hypersensitivity reactions*; history of hepatic or renal dysfunction *that might interfere with drug metabolism and excretion of the drug*; and current status related to pregnancy and lactation, *which are contraindications to the use of these drugs.*
- Perform a physical assessment to *establish baseline data for determining the effectiveness of the drug and the occurrence of any adverse effects associated with drug therapy.*
- Obtain a culture of stool for ova and parasites *to determine the infecting worm and establish appropriate treatment.*
- Examine reflexes and muscle strength *to evaluate changes that occur as a result of drug therapy.*
- Evaluate liver function and renal function tests *to determine appropriateness of therapy and to monitor for toxicity.*
- Examine skin, including color, temperature, and texture, and note any lesions *to assess for possible adverse effects.*
- Assess the abdomen *to evaluate for any changes from baseline related to the infection, identify possible adverse effects, and monitor for improvement.*

Nursing Diagnoses

Nursing diagnoses related to drug therapy might include:

- Acute pain related to GI, CNS, or skin effects of drug
- Disturbed personal identity related to diagnosis and treatment
- Deficient knowledge regarding drug therapy

Planning

- The patient will receive the best therapeutic effect from the drug therapy.
- The patient will have limited adverse effects to the drug therapy.
- The patient will have an understanding of the drug therapy, adverse effects to anticipate, and measures to relieve discomfort and improve safety.

Implementation with Rationale

- Arrange for appropriate culture and sensitivity tests before beginning therapy *to ensure identification of the correct cause and use of the appropriate drug.*
- Administer the complete course of the drug *to obtain the full beneficial effects*. Ensure that chewable tablets are chewed. Give the drug with food if necessary, but avoid giving the drug with high-fat meals, which might interfere with drug effectiveness.
- Monitor hepatic and renal function before and periodically during treatment *to allow for early identification and prompt intervention if signs of failure due to albendazole administration occur.*
- Provide comfort and safety measures if CNS effects occur (e.g., side rails and assistance with ambulation in the presence of dizziness and weakness) *to protect the patient from injury*. Provide oral hygiene and ready access to bathroom facilities as needed *to cope with GI effects.*
- Provide small, frequent, nutritious meals if GI upset is severe *to ensure adequate nutrition*. Monitor nutritional status and arrange a dietary consultation as needed. Taking the drug with food may also decrease GI upset.
- Instruct the patient about the appropriate dosage regimen and other measures *to enhance patient knowledge about drug therapy and to promote compliance.*
- Provide the following patient teaching:
  - Take safety precautions, including changing position slowly and avoiding driving and hazardous tasks, if CNS effects occur.
  - Take the drug with meals and try small, frequent meals if GI upset is a problem.
  - Identify the importance of strict hand washing and hygiene measures, including daily laundering of underwear and bed linens, daily disinfection of toilet facilities, and periodic disinfection of bathroom floors (Box 13.3).
  - Report fever, severe diarrhea, or aggravation of condition, which could indicate a resistant strain or noneffective therapy, to a health care provider.

Evaluation

- Monitor patient response to the drug (resolution of helminth infestation and improvement in signs and symptoms).
- Monitor for adverse effects (changes in orientation and affect, nutritional state, skin color and evidence of lesions, hepatic and renal function, and reports of abdominal discomfort and pain).
- Evaluate the effectiveness of the teaching plan (patient can name the drug, dosage, possible adverse effects to watch for, and specific measures to help avoid adverse effects).
- Monitor the effectiveness of comfort and safety measures and compliance with the regimen.

BOX 13.3 FOCUS ON Patient and Family Teaching

Managing Pinworm Infections

Infestation with worms can be a frightening and traumatic experience for most people. Seeing the worm can be an especially difficult experience. Some worm infestations are not that uncommon in the United States, especially infestation with pinworms.

Pinworms can spread very rapidly among children in schools, summer camps, and other institutions. Once the infestation starts, careful hygiene measures and drug therapy are required to eradicate the disease. After the diagnosis has been made and appropriate drug therapy started, proper hygiene measures are essential. Some suggested hygiene measures that might help to control the infection include the following:

- Keep the child's nails cut short and hands well scrubbed because reinfection results from the worm's eggs being carried back to the mouth after becoming lodged under the fingernails when the child scratches the pruritic perianal area.
- Give the child a shower in the morning to wash away any ova deposited in the anal area during the night.
- Change and launder undergarments, bed linens, and pajamas every day.
- Disinfect toilet seats daily and the floors of bathrooms and bedrooms periodically.
- Encourage the child to wash hands vigorously after using the toilet.

In some areas of the United States, parents are asked to check for worm ova by pressing sticky tape against the anal area in the morning before bathing. The sticky tape is then pressed against a slide that can be taken or sent to a clinical laboratory for evaluation. It may take 5–6 weeks to get a clear reading with this method of testing. Some health care providers believe that the psychological trauma involved in doing this type of follow-up, especially with a school age child, makes this task too onerous to ask parents to do. Instead, many believe that the ease of treating this relatively harmless disease makes it more prudent to continue to treat as prescribed and to forgo the follow-up testing.

It is important to reassure patients and families that these types of infections do not necessarily reflect negatively on their hygiene or lifestyle. It takes a coordinated effort among medical personnel, families, and patients to control a pinworm infestation.

KEY POINTS

- Anthelmintic drugs affect metabolic processes that are either different in worms than in human hosts or are not found in humans. These agents all cause death of the worm by interfering with normal functioning.
- Proper hygiene and sanitation processes are an important part in preventing the spread of helminths, including good hand hygiene and preparation and storage of food.

SUMMARY

- Helminths are worms that cause disease by invading the human body. Helminths that affect humans include nematodes (round-shaped worms) such as pinworms, hookworms, threadworms, whipworms, and roundworms; and platyhelminths (flatworms), which include tapeworms and flukes.
- Pinworms are the most frequent cause of helminth infection in the United States, and roundworms called *Ascaris* are the most frequent cause of helminth infections throughout the world.
- Some helminths invade body tissues and can seriously damage lymphatic tissue, lungs, CNS, heart, liver, and so on. These include trichinosis-causing tapeworms, which are found in undercooked pork; filariae, which occur when thread-like worm embryos clog up vascular spaces; and schistosomiasis-causing flukes. Schistosomiasis is a common problem in many tropical areas where the snail that is necessary in the life cycle of the fluke lives.
- Anthelmintic drugs affect metabolic processes that are either different in worms than in human hosts or are not found in humans. These agents all cause death of the worm by interfering with normal functioning.
- Prevention is a very important part of the treatment of helminths. Thorough handwashing; laundering of bed linens, pajamas, and underwear to destroy ova that are shed during the night; and disinfection of toilet facilities at least daily and of bathroom floors periodically help to stop the spread of these diseases. In addition, proper sanitation and hygiene in food preparation and storage is essential for reducing the incidence of these infestations.
- Patient teaching is important for decreasing the stress and anxiety that may occur when individuals are diagnosed with a worm infestation.

CHECK YOUR UNDERSTANDING

Answers to the questions in this chapter can be found in Answers to Check Your Understanding Questions on thePoint®.

MULTIPLE CHOICE

Select the best answer to the following.

1. To ensure effective treatment of pinworm infections, which instruction would be most important to emphasize to the patient and family?
   a. Keeping nails long so cutting will not introduce more infection
   b. Laundering undergarments, bed linens, and pajamas every day
   c. Boiling all drinking water
   d. Maintaining a clear liquid diet for at least 7 to 10 days

2. Which of the following would the nurse expect to assess in a patient who is suspected of having an *Ascaris* infection?
   a. Cough and signs of pulmonary infestation
   b. Cardiac arrhythmias and low blood pressure
   c. Seizures and disorientation
   d. Bloody diarrhea and excessive vomiting

3. The nurse describes schistosomiasis to a group of students as an infection caused by
   a. a protozoan carried by a mosquito.
   b. improperly cooked pork.
   c. a fluke carried by a snail.
   d. eating food contaminated by fecal material.

4. A patient has traveled to Egypt and come home with schistosomiasis. The family is very concerned about spreading the disease. Which of the following would be most helpful to teach the family?
   a. Strict hand washing will stop the spread of the disease.
   b. Isolating the patient will be necessary to stop the spread of the disease.
   c. Carefully cooking all of the patient's food will help to stop the spread of the disease.
   d. The snail needed for the life cycle of this worm does not live in this climate.

5. A patient is prescribed mebendazole. The nurse knows that this is the most commonly used anthelmintic, being the drug of choice for treating
   a. pinworms, roundworms, whipworms, and hookworms.
   b. trichinosis, flukes, cestodes, and hookworms.
   c. pork tapeworm, threadworms, cestodes, and whipworms.
   d. all stages of schistosomal infections.

6. Patient teaching regarding the use of anthelmintics should include counseling about
   a. the use of oral contraceptives.
   b. maintenance of nutrition during therapy.
   c. the use of oral anticoagulants.
   d. cardiac drug effects.

7. Patients may experience anxiety about the diagnosis and treatment of helminthic infections. Teaching may help to alleviate this anxiety and should include
   a. what they may experience if the worms are passed from the body.
   b. focus on the cleanliness of the home.
   c. measures to isolate the organism in the home.
   d. criticism of their personal hygiene practices.

MULTIPLE RESPONSE

Select all that apply.

1. An adult client is being treated with mebendazole for a pinworm infection. Appropriate nursing diagnoses that might apply to this patient would include
   a. Disturbed personal identity related to treatment.
   b. Abdominal distention related to worm infestation.
   c. Acute pain related to GI effects.
   d. Risk for social isolation related to quarantine conditions.
   e. Impaired physical mobility related to muscle infestation.
   f. Deficient knowledge related to drug therapy.

BIBLIOGRAPHY AND REFERENCES

Andrews, M., & Boyle, J. (2011). *Transcultural concepts in nursing care* (6th ed.). Philadelphia, PA: Lippincott Williams & Wilkins.

Brunton, L., Chabner, B., & Knollman, B. (2011). *Goodman and Gilman's the pharmacological basis of therapeutics* (12th ed.). New York: McGraw-Hill.

Facts and Comparisons. (2015). *Drug facts and comparisons*. St. Louis, MO: Author.

Facts and Comparisons. (2015). *Professional's guide to patient drug facts*. St. Louis, MO: Author.

Falcone, F., & Pritchard, D. (2005). Parasite reversal: Worms on trial. *Trends in Parasitology, 21*, 157–160.

Hotez, P. J., Brooker, S., Bethony, J., et al. (2004). Hookworm infection. *New England Journal of Medicine, 351*, 799–807.

James, D. T., Breman, J. G., Measham, A. (Eds). (2006). *Disease control priorities in developing countries* (2nd ed.). Washington, DC: World Bank Publications.

Karch, A. M. (2014). *Lippincott's nursing drug guide*. Philadelphia, PA: Lippincott Williams & Wilkins.

Keiser, J., & Utzinger, J. (2008). Efficacy of current drugs against soil transmitted helminth infections: Systematic review. *Journal of American Medical Association, 299*, 1937–1948.

Petri, W. (2008). *Diagnostic medical parasitology* (5th ed.). Washington, DC: ASM Press.

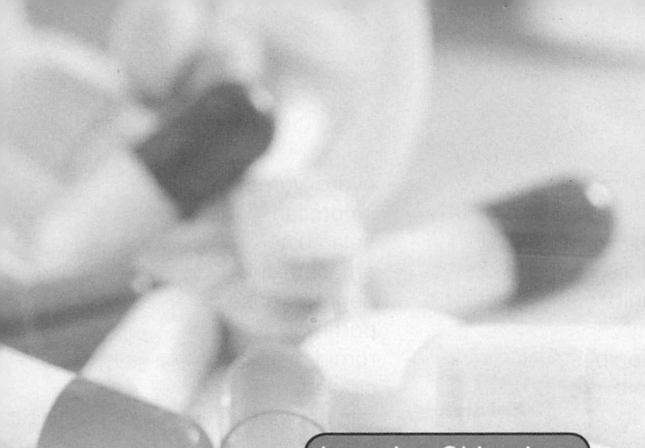

Antineoplastic Agents 14

Learning Objectives

Upon completion of this chapter, you will be able to:

1. Describe the nature of cancer and the changes the body undergoes when cancer occurs.
2. Describe the therapeutic actions, indications, pharmacokinetics, contraindications, most common adverse reactions, and important drug–drug interactions associated with each class of antineoplastic agents and with adjunctive therapy use with these drugs.
3. Discuss the use of antineoplastic drugs across the lifespan.
4. Compare and contrast the prototype drugs for each class of antineoplastic agents with the other drugs in that class.
5. Outline the nursing considerations and teaching needs for patients receiving each class of antineoplastic agents.

Glossary of Key Terms

alopecia: hair loss; a common adverse effect of many antineoplastic drugs, which are more effective against rapidly multiplying cells such as those of hair follicles

anaplasia: loss of organization and structure; property of cancer cells

angiogenesis: the generation of new blood vessels; cancer cells release an enzyme that will cause angiogenesis or the growth of new blood vessels to feed the cancer cells

antineoplastic agent: drug used to combat cancer or the growth of neoplasms

autonomy: loss of the normal controls and reactions that inhibit growth and spreading; property of cancer cells

bone marrow suppression: inhibition of the blood-forming components of the bone marrow; a common adverse effect of many antineoplastic drugs, which are more effective against rapidly multiplying cells, such as those in bone marrow; seen as anemia, thrombocytopenia, and leukopenia

carcinoma: tumor that originates in epithelial cells

metastasis: ability to enter the circulatory or lymphatic system and travel to other areas of the body that are conducive to growth and survival; property of cancer cells

neoplasm: new or cancerous growth; occurs when abnormal cells have the opportunity to multiply and grow

sarcoma: tumor that originates in the mesenchyme and is made up of embryonic connective tissue cells

Drug List

Alkylating Agents
altretamine
bendamustine
busulfan
carboplatin
carmustine
(P) chlorambucil
cisplatin
cyclophosphamide
dacarbazine
ifosfamide
lomustine
mechlorethamine
melphalan
oxaliplatin
procarbazine
streptozocin
temozolomide

Antimetabolites
capecitabine
cladribine
clofarabine
cytarabine
floxuridine
fludarabine
fluorouracil
gemcitabine
mercaptopurine
(P) methotrexate
pemetrexed
pentostatin
pralatrexate
thioguanine

Antineoplastic Antibiotics
bleomycin
dactinomycin
daunorubicin
(P) doxorubicin
epirubicin
idarubicin
mitomycin
mitoxantrone
valrubicin

(continues on page 214)

Mitotic Inhibitors
cabazitaxel
docetaxel
eribulin
etoposide
ixabepilone
paclitaxel
teniposide
vinblastine
(P) vincristine
vinorelbine

Hormones and Hormone Modulators
abiraterone
anastrazole
bicalutamide
degarelix
enzalutamide
estramustine
exemestane
flutamide
fulvestrant
goserelin
histrelin
letrozole
leuprolide
megestrol
mitotane
nilutamide
(P) tamoxifen
toremifene
triptorelin pamoate

Cancer Cell–Specific Agents
afatinib
axitinib
bortezomib
bosutinib
cabozantinib
ceretinib
crizotinib
dabrafenib
erlotinib
everolimus
ibrutinib
idelalisib
(P) imatinib
lapatinib
nilotinib
palbociclib
pazopanib
ponatinib
regorafenib
ruxolitinib
sorafenib
sunitinib
temsirolimus
trametinib
vemurafenib
ziv-aflibercept

Miscellaneous Antineoplastics
arsenic trioxide
asparaginase *Erwinia chrysanthemi*
azacitidine
belinostat
bexarotene
decitabine
hydroxyurea
irinotecan
nelarabine
omacetaxine
pegaspargase
porfimer
romidepsin
sipuleucel-T
talc powder
topotecan
tretinoin
vismodegib
vorinostat

Antineoplastic Adjunctive Therapy
allopurinol
amifostine
dexrazoxane
leucovorin
levoleucovorin
mesna
rasburicase

The use of the term chemotherapy implies cancer treatment to most people. However, only one branch of chemotherapy involves drugs developed to act on and kill or alter human cells—the **antineoplastic agents**, which are designed to fight **neoplasms**, or cancers.

Antineoplastic drugs alter human cells in a variety of ways. Their action is intended to target the abnormal cells that compose the neoplasm or cancer, having a greater impact on them than on normal cells. Unfortunately, normal cells also are affected by antineoplastic agents.

This area of pharmacology, which has grown tremendously in recent years, now includes many drugs that act on or are part of the immune system. These substances fight the cancerous cells using components of the immune system instead of destroying cells directly (see Chapter 15). This chapter discusses the classic antineoplastic agents, those drugs that are used in cancer chemotherapy.

Cancer

Cancer is a disease that can strike a person at any age. It remains second only to coronary disease as the leading cause of death in the United States. Treatment of cancer can be prolonged and often debilitating. The patient can experience numerous and wide-ranging complications and effects.

All cancers start with a single cell that is genetically different from the other cells in the surrounding tissue. This cell divides, passing along its abnormalities to daughter cells, eventually producing a tumor or neoplasm that has characteristics quite different from those of the original tissue (Figure 14.1). As the abnormal cells continue to divide, they lose more and more of their original cell characteristics. The cancerous cells exhibit **anaplasia**—a loss of cellular differentiation and organization, which leads to a loss of their ability to function normally. They also exhibit **autonomy**, growing without the usual homeostatic restrictions that regulate cell growth and control. This loss of control allows the cells to form a tumor.

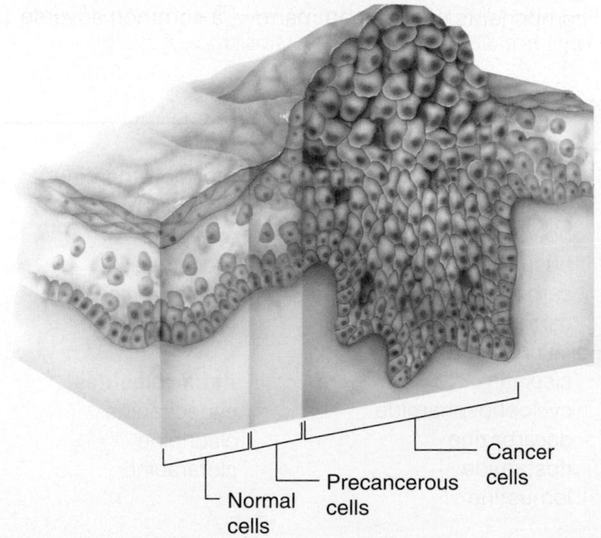

FIGURE 14.1 Malignant tumors develop from one cell, with somatic mutations occurring during cell division as the tumor grows.

Primary tumor
↓
Grows and invades surrounding tissue
↓
Moves into basement membrane of capillaries surrounding the tumor
↓
Enters the bloodstream
↓
Leaves the bloodstream through capillary walls
↓
Proliferates at this new site, grows, and invades surrounding tissue

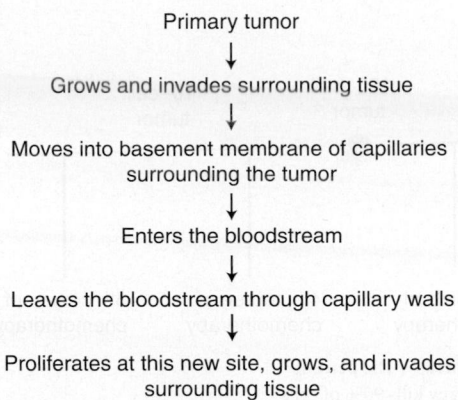

FIGURE 14.2 Metastasis of cancer cells.

Over time, these neoplastic cells grow uncontrollably, invading and damaging healthy tissue in the area and even undergoing **metastasis**, or traveling from the place of origin to develop new tumors in other areas of the body where conditions are favorable for cell growth (Figure 14.2). The abnormal cells release enzymes that generate blood vessels (**angiogenesis**) in the area to supply both oxygen and nutrients to the cells, thus contributing to their growth. Overall, the cancerous cells rob the host cells of energy and nutrients and block normal lymph and vascular vessels as the result of pressure and intrusion on normal cells, leading to a loss of normal cellular function.

The body's immune system can damage or destroy some neoplastic cells. T cells, which recognize the abnormal cells and destroy them; antibodies, which form in response to parts of the abnormal cell protein; interferons; and tissue necrosis factor all play a role in the body's attempt to eliminate the abnormal cells before they become uncontrollable and threaten the life of the host. Once the neoplasm has grown and enlarged, it may overwhelm the immune system, which is no longer able to manage the problem.

Causes of Cancer

What causes the cells to mutate and become genetically different is not clearly understood. In some cases a genetic predisposition to such a mutation can be found. Some breast cancers, for example, seem to have a definite genetic link. In other cases, viral infection, constant irritation and cell turnover, and even stress have been blamed for the ensuing cancer. Stress reactions suppress the activities of the immune system (see Chapter 29), so if a cell is mutating while a person is under prolonged stress, research suggests that the cell has a better chance of growing into a neoplasm than when the person's immune system is fully active. Pipe smokers are at increased risk for development of tongue and mouth cancers because the heat of the pipe and chemicals in the pipe tobaccos and smoke continuously destroy normal cells, which must be replaced rapidly, increasing the chances for development of a mutant cell. People living in areas with carcinogenic or cancer-causing chemicals in the air, water, or even the ground are at increased risk of developing mutant cells in response to exposure to these toxic chemicals.

Cancer clusters are often identified in such high-risk areas. Not everyone exposed to carcinogens or undergoing stress or having a genetic predisposition to develop cancer actually develops cancer. Researchers have not discovered what the actual trigger for cancer development is or what protective abilities some people have that other people lack. Most likely, a mosaic of factors coming together in one person leads to development of the neoplasm.

Types of Cancer

Cancers can be divided into two groups: (1) solid tumors and (2) hematological malignancies such as the leukemias and lymphomas, which occur in the blood-forming organs. Solid tumors may originate in any body organ and may be further divided into **carcinomas**, or tumors that originate in epithelial cells, and **sarcomas**, or tumors that originate in the mesenchyme and are made up of embryonic connective tissue cells. Examples of carcinomas include granular cell tumors of the breast, bronchogenic tumors arising in cells that line the bronchial tubes, and squamous and basal tumors of the skin. Sarcomas include osteogenic tumors, which form in the primitive cells of the bone, and rhabdomyosarcomas, which occur in striated muscles. Hematological malignancies involve the blood-forming organs of the body, the bone marrow, and the lymphatic system. These malignancies alter the body's ability to produce and regulate the cells found in the blood.

KEY POINTS

- Cancers arise from a single abnormal cell that multiplies and grows.
- Cancer cells lose their normal function (anaplasia), develop characteristics that allow them to grow in an uninhibited way (autonomy), and have the ability to travel to other sites in the body that are conducive to their growth (metastasis). They also have the ability to grow new blood vessels to feed the tumor (angiogenesis).
- The goal of cancer chemotherapy is to decrease the size of the neoplasm so that the human immune system can deal with it.

Antineoplastic Drugs

Antineoplastic drugs can work by affecting cell survival or by boosting the immune system in its efforts to combat the abnormal cells (Figure 14.3). Chapter 17 discusses the immune agents that are used to combat cancer. The present chapter focuses on those drugs that affect cell survival. The antineoplastic drugs that are commonly used today include alkylating agents, antimetabolites, antineoplastic antibiotics, mitotic inhibitors, hormones and hormone modulators, cancer cell–specific agents, protein tyrosine kinase inhibitors (which target enzymes specific to the cancer cells), and a group of antineoplastic agents that cannot be classified elsewhere. Other drugs are used to combat

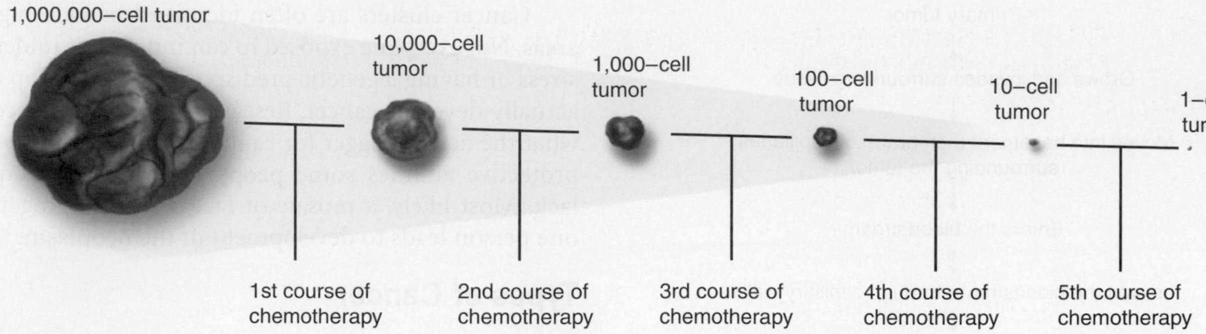

FIGURE 14.3 Cell kill theory. A set percentage of cells is killed after each dose of chemotherapy. The percentage killed is dependent upon the drug therapy. In this example, each course of chemotherapy kills 90% of cells in a cancerous tumor. After the fifth course of chemotherapy in this example a single-cell tumor remains; the patient's immune system would destroy this malignant cell.

the serious adverse effects that can be associated with the antineoplastic drugs. These drugs are used as adjunctive therapy. Figure 14.4 shows sites of action of these drugs. Box 14.1 discusses use of these drugs across the lifespan.

As discussed in Chapter 7, all cells progress through a cell cycle. Different types of cells progress at different rates (see Figure 7.6). Rapidly multiplying cells, or cells that replace themselves quickly, include those lining the

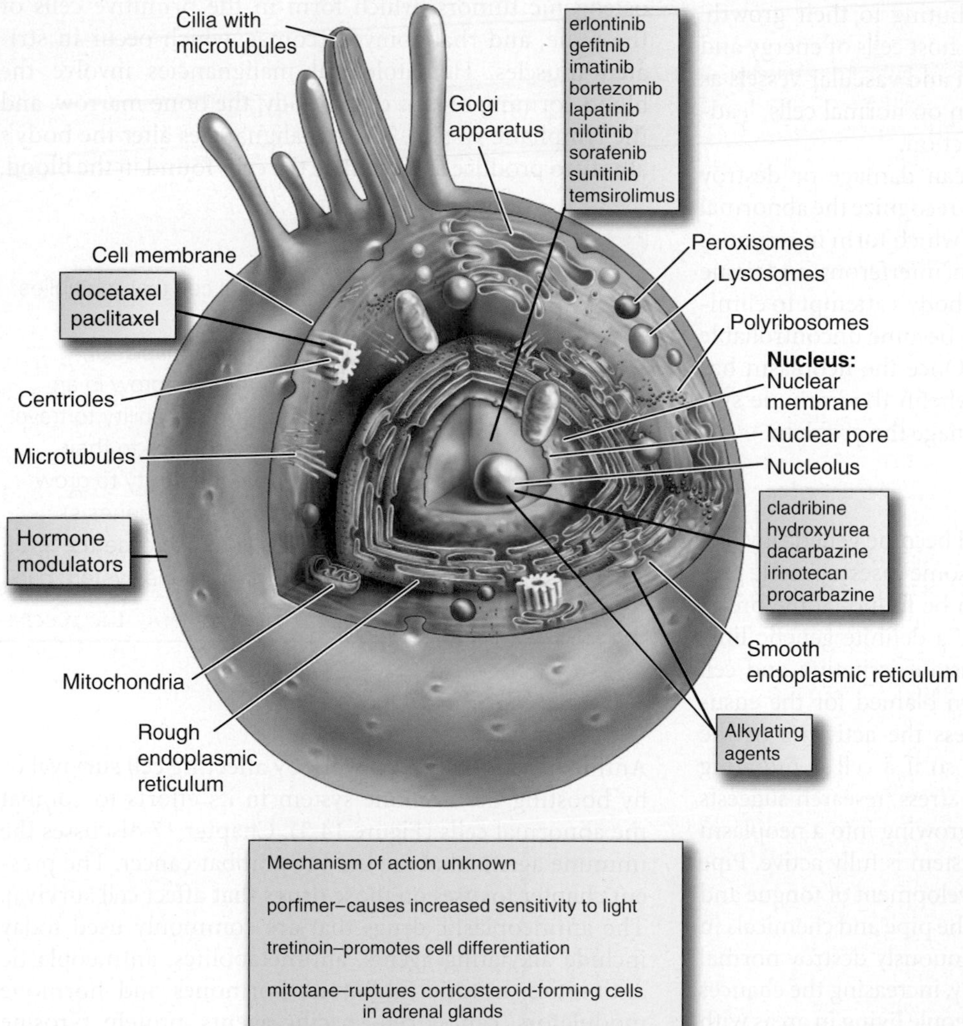

FIGURE 14.4 Sites of action of non–cell cycle specific antineoplastic agents. Alkylating agents interfere with RNA, DNA, or other cellular proteins. For example, dacarbazine blocks DNA and RNA synthesis, whereas procarbazine blocks DNA, RNA, and protein synthesis. Hormone modulators react with specific receptor sites to block cell growth and activity. Mitotic inhibitors such as docetaxel and paclitaxel inhibit microtubular reorganization. The antimetabolite cladribine and miscellaneous agent hydroxyurea block DNA synthesis. The miscellaneous agent irinotecan disrupts DNA strands. Cell-specific agents inhibit protein tyrosine kinases. Bortezomib is a proteasome inhibitor.

BOX 14.1 FOCUS ON Drug Therapy Across the Lifespan

Antineoplastic Agents

CHILDREN

Antineoplastic protocols have been developed for the treatment of most pediatric cancers. Combination therapy is stressed to eliminate as many of the mutant cells as possible. Dose and timing of these combinations are crucial.

Double-checking of dose, including recalculating desired dose and verifying the drug amount with another nurse, is good practice when giving these toxic drugs to children.

Children need to be monitored closely for hydration and nutritional status. The nutritional needs of a child are greater than those of an adult, and this needs to be considered when formulating a care plan.

These children need support and comfort and also need to be allowed to explore and learn like any other children. Body image problems, lack of energy, and the need to protect the child from exposure to infection can isolate a child receiving antineoplastic agents. The total care plan of the child needs to include social, emotional, and intellectual stimulation.

Monitor bone marrow activity very carefully, and adjust the dose accordingly.

ADULTS

The adult receiving antineoplastic drugs is confronted with many dilemmas that the nurse needs to address. Changes in body image are common, with loss of hair, skin changes, GI complaints, and weight loss. Fear of the diagnosis and the treatment is also common with these patients. Networking support systems and providing teaching, reassurance, and comfort can have a tremendous impact on the success of the drug therapy.

Pregnant and nursing women should not receive these drugs, which are toxic to the developing cells of the fetus. Pregnant women who are diagnosed with cancer are in a difficult situation: The drug therapy can have serious adverse effects on the fetus, and not using the drug therapy can be detrimental to the mother. Education, support, and referrals to appropriate specialists are important. Nursing women should find another method of feeding the baby to prevent the adverse effects to the fetus that occur when these drugs cross into breast milk. Use of barrier contraceptives is urged when these drugs are being used by women of childbearing age.

OLDER ADULTS

Older adults may be more susceptible to the CNS and GI effects of some of these drugs. Older patients should be monitored for hydration and nutritional status regularly. Safety precautions should be instituted if CNS effects occur, including increased lighting, assistance with ambulation, and use of supports.

Many older patients have decreased renal and/or hepatic function. Many of these drugs depend on the liver and kidney for metabolism and excretion. Renal and liver function tests should be done before (baseline) and periodically during the use of these drugs, and dose should be adjusted accordingly.

Protecting these patients from exposure to infection and injury is a very important aspect of their nursing care. Older patients are naturally somewhat immunosuppressed because of age, and giving drugs that further depress the immune system can lead to infections that are serious and difficult to treat. Monitor blood counts carefully, and arrange for rest or reduced dose as indicated.

gastrointestinal (GI) tract and those in hair follicles, skin, and bone marrow. These cells complete the cell cycle every few days. Cells that proceed very slowly through the cell cycle include those in the breasts, testicles, and ovaries. Some cells take weeks, months, or even years to complete the cycle.

Cancer cells tend to move through the cell cycle at about the same rate as their cells of origin. Malignant cells that remain in a dormant phase for long periods are difficult to destroy. These cells can emerge long after cancer treatment has finished—after weeks, months, or years—to begin their division and growth cycle all over again. For this reason, antineoplastic agents are often given in sequence over periods of time, in the hope that the drugs will affect the cancer cells as they emerge from dormancy or move into a new phase of the cell cycle. A combination of antineoplastic agents targeting different phases of the cell cycle is frequently most effective in treating many cancers.

The goal of cancer therapy, much like that of anti-infective therapy, is to limit the offending cells to the degree that the immune system can then respond without causing too much toxicity to the host. However, this is a particularly difficult task when using antineoplastic drugs because, for the most part, these agents are not specific to mutant cells, and affect normal human cells as well. In most cases, antineoplastic drugs primarily affect human cells that are rapidly multiplying with many cells in many phases of the cell cycle (e.g., those in the hair follicles, GI tract, and bone marrow). Much research is being done to develop drugs that will affect only the abnormal cells. Imatinib, released in 2001, was the first of a growing number of drugs to target the enzymes used by very specific abnormal cells. Other agents that affect only the mechanisms of cancer cells have been marketed. It is anticipated that many more such drugs will be released in the future.

Antineoplastic drugs are associated with many adverse effects, with specific adverse effects occurring with particular drugs. These effects are often unpleasant and debilitating. Some antineoplastic drugs exert toxic effects on ova and sperm production, affecting the person's fertility. These agents are also usually selective for rapidly growing cells, posing a danger to the developing fetus during pregnancy. Consequently, pregnancy is a contraindication to the use of antineoplastic drugs. These agents also jeopardize the immune system by causing **bone marrow suppression**, inhibiting the blood-forming components of the bone marrow and interfering with the body's normal protective actions against abnormal cells. The patient's hematological profile must always be assessed for toxic effects. Patients also need to understand the importance of returning every few weeks to go through the chemotherapy, with its adverse effects, over and over again. Many patients experience nausea and vomiting, a direct effect of the toxic drug as well as the body's response to the elements of cell death circulating in the bloodstream. Patients may also experience hair and/or skin effects as these cells are rapidly turning over cells and may be especially susceptible to the effects of the antineoplastic drugs.

Many antineoplastic drugs often result in another adverse effect, cancer itself. Cell death due to these agents increases the need for cellular growth, placing the person at increased risk for mutant cell development. Bone marrow is suppressed by the drug therapy, making the immune system very weak and less effective which might allow mutant cells to progress.

Most cancer patients are not considered to be "cured" until they have been cancer-free for a period of 5 years due to the possibility that cancer cells will emerge from dormancy to cause new tumors or problems. Some experts now consider cancer a chronic disease, the possibility of dormant cells emerging and becoming active again always being present. No cells have yet been identified that can remain dormant for longer than 5 years, so the chance of the emergence of one after that time is very slim.

A cancerous mass may be so large that no therapy can arrest its growth without killing the host. In such cases, antineoplastic agents are used as palliative therapy to shrink the size of the tumor and alleviate some of the signs and symptoms of the cancer, decreasing pain and increasing function. Here the goal of drug therapy is not to cure the disease but to try to improve the patient's quality of life in a situation in which there is no cure. Some emerging antineoplastic agents are discussed in Box 14.2.

Alkylating Agents

Because alkylating agents can affect cells even in the resting phase, these drugs are said to be non–cell cycle specific (Figure 14.4). They are most useful in the treatment of slow-growing cancers, which have many cells in the resting phase. Alkylating agents (Table 14.1) include the following drugs: altretamine (*Hexalen*), bendamustine (*Treanda*), busulfan (*Busulfex, Myleran*), carboplatin (generic), carmustine (*BiCNU, Gliadel*), chlorambucil (*Leukeran*), cisplatin (*Platinol, Platinol-AQ*), cyclophosphamide (generic), dacarbazine (*DTIC-Dome*), ifosfamide (*Ifex*), lomustine (*CeeNU*), mechlorethamine (*Mustargen*), melphalan (*Alkeran*), oxaliplatin (*Eloxatin*), procarbazine (*Matulane*), streptozocin (*Zanosar*), and temozolomide (*Temodar*).

Therapeutic Actions and Indications

Alkylating agents produce their cytotoxic effects by reacting chemically with portions of the RNA, DNA, or other cellular proteins, being most potent when they bind with cellular DNA. The oldest drugs in this class are the nitrogen mustards, and modifications of the structure of these drugs have led to the development of the nitrosoureas.

These drugs are most useful in the treatment of slow-growing cancers such as various lymphomas, leukemias, myelomas; some ovarian, testicular, and breast cancers; and some pancreatic cancers. See Table 14.1 for usual indications for each of the alkylating agents. These agents are not used interchangeably.

Pharmacokinetics

The alkylating agents vary in their degree of absorption, and little is known about their distribution in the tissues. They are metabolized and sometimes activated in the liver,

BOX 14.2 FOCUS ON The Evidence

New Drugs for the Battle Against Cancer

Arsenic trioxide (*Trisenox*), known as a poison in forensic medicine, has been approved for the induction and remission of promyelocytic leukemia (PML) in patients whose disease is refractory to conventional therapy and whose leukemia is characterized by t(15;17) translocation of PML/RAR-α (retinoic acid receptor alpha) gene expression. It is given intravenously at a rate of 0.15 mg/kg/d until bone marrow remission occurs and then 0.15 mg/kg/d starting 3 to 6 weeks after induction. The patient needs to be screened carefully for toxic reactions.

Other drugs are under development that target specific areas of the human genome. In the future, antineoplastic drugs may be able to target abnormal cells and not affect the healthy cells. This could relieve the suffering of many patients undergoing cancer chemotherapy.

Several familiar drugs are being studied for their ability to block angiogenesis. By blocking the development of new blood vessels to feed the tumor the growing cells in the tumor will lack nutrition and oxygen and will not be able to survive. Celecoxib (*Celebrex*), an anti-inflammatory drug, is being studied in various cancer combination drug trials for this effect. Some low-molecular-weight heparins, such as dalteparin (*Fragmin*), are also being studied for this effect.

A new approach to cancer chemotherapy dosing is gaining acceptance in many areas. Metronomic chemotherapy uses lower doses of drugs at shorter intervals without extended rest periods, treating cancer like a chronic disease, not an acute disorder. This protects the noncancerous cells in the body, so fewer of the adverse effects are seen, and has an effect on malignant cells as soon as they come out of the rest phase. This approach also seems to be very effective in blocking angiogenesis. It is a very different approach than traditional dosing, but much promising research is being done.

Table 14.1 *Drugs in Focus:* Alkylating Agents

Drug Name	Dosage/Route	Usual Indications
altretamine (*Hexalen*)	260 mg/m²/d PO for 14–21 consecutive days of a 28-d cycle	Palliative treatment of persistent or recurrent ovarian cancer after failure of first line therapy *Special considerations:* Premedicate with antiemetic; monitor blood counts and central nervous system status regularly
bendamustine (*Treanda*)	100 mg/m² IV over 30 min on days 1 and 2 of a 28-d cycle for up to 6 cycles	Treatment of chronic lymphocytic leukemia *Special considerations:* Dosing may need to be adjusted based on blood counts; monitor for infection, skin reactions
busulfan (*Busulfex, Myleran*)	*Induction:* 4–8 mg/d PO *Maintenance:* 1–3 mg/d PO *Injection:* 0.8 mg/kg as a 2-h IV infusion q6h for 4 d via a central venous catheter	Palliative treatment of chronic myelogenous leukemia, other myeloproliferative disorders. *Special considerations:* Dosing monitored by effects on bone marrow; always push fluids to decrease toxic renal effects; alopecia is common
carboplatin (generic)	360 mg/m² IV on day 1 every 4 wk; reduce dose as needed based on blood counts and with renal impairment	Palliative or initial treatment of ovarian cancer; may be useful in several other cancers *Special considerations:* Dose and timing determined by bone marrow response; alopecia is common
carmustine (*BiCNU, Gliadel*)	150–200 mg/m² IV every 6 wk as a single dose or divided daily injections; wafers implanted into brain at time of surgery	Treatment of brain tumors, Hodgkin disease, and multiple myelomas; available in implantable wafer form for treatment of glioblastoma *Special considerations:* Dose determined by bone marrow toxicity; do not repeat for 6 wk because of delayed toxicity; often used in combination therapy
chlorambucil (*Leukeran*)	0.1–0.2 mg/kg/d PO for 3–6 wk; or 0.4 mg/kg PO every 2 wk with maintenance dose of 0.03–0.1 mg/kg/d PO	Palliative treatment of lymphomas and leukemias including Hodgkin disease and CLL; being considered for the treatment of rheumatoid arthritis and other conditions *Special considerations:* Toxic to liver and bone marrow; dosing based on bone marrow response; carcinogenic, avoid use in pregnancy
cisplatin (*Platinol-AQ*)	20–50 mg/m²/d IV, once every 3 wk used in combination with other antineoplastic agents	Combination therapy for metastatic testicular or ovarian tumors, advanced bladder cancers *Special considerations:* Neurotoxic, nephrotoxic, and can cause serious hypersensitivity reactions
cyclophosphamide (generic)	*Induction:* 40–50 mg/kg/d IV over 2–5 d *or* 1–5 mg/kg/d *PO maintenance:* 1–5 mg/kg/d PO, or 10–15 mg/kg IV q7–10d	Treatment of lymphoma, myelomas, leukemias, and other cancers in combination with other drugs *Special considerations:* Hemorrhagic cystitis is a potentially fatal side effect; alopecia is common
dacarbazine (*DTIC-Dome*)	2–4.5 mg/kg/d IV for 10 d, repeat at 4-wk intervals *or* 150–250 mg/m²/d IV for 5 d in combination with other drugs	Treatment of metastatic malignant melanoma and as second-line therapy with other drugs for the treatment of Hodgkin disease. *Special considerations:* Bone marrow depression, GI toxicity, severe photosensitivity are common; extravasation can cause tissue necrosis or cellulitis—use extreme care, and monitor injection sites regularly
ifosfamide (*Ifex*)	1.2 g/m²/d IV for 5 consecutive days; repeat every 3 wk	Combination therapy as a third-line agent in treating germ cell testicular cancers, bone and soft tissue sarcomas *Special considerations:* Alopecia is common; monitor for bone marrow depression; push fluids to help prevent bladder toxicity
lomustine (*CeeNU*)	130 mg/m² PO as a single dose every 6 wk; adjust dose based on blood counts	Palliative combination therapy for Hodgkin disease and primary and metastatic brain tumors *Special considerations:* Immune suppression and GI effects are common
mechlorethamine (*Mustargen*)	0.4 mg/kg IV for each course; usually repeated every 3–6 wk; intracavity 0.2–0.4 mg/kg	Nitrogen mustard; palliative treatment in Hodgkin disease, leukemia, bronchial carcinoma, other cancers; injected for treatment of effusions secondary to cancer metastases *Special considerations:* GI toxicity, bone marrow suppression, and impaired fertility are common; handle with precautions; monitor for extravasation

(table continues on page 220)

Table 14.1 *Drugs in Focus:* Alkylating Agents *(continued)*

Drug Name	Dosage/Route	Usual Indications
melphalan (*Alkeran*)	*Multiple myeloma:* 6 mg/d PO for 2–3 wk, then a rest period *or* 16 mg/m² IV at 2-wk intervals for four doses, then at 4-wk intervals *Ovarian cancer:* 0.2 mg/kg/d PO for 5 d; repeat course every 4–5 wk	Nitrogen mustard; treatment for multiple myeloma, ovarian cancers *Special considerations:* Oral route is preferred; pulmonary fibrosis, bone marrow suppression, and alopecia are common
oxaliplatin (*Eloxatin*)	85 mg/m² IV with leucovorin, followed by fluorouracil (5-FU) at 2-wk cycles *or* 1,000 mg/m² IV at weekly intervals	Treatment of metastatic carcinoma of the colon or rectum when disease progresses after standard therapy; used in combination therapy *Special considerations:* Premedicate with antiemetics and dexamethasone; monitor for potentially dangerous anaphylactic reactions
procarbazine (*Matulane*)	*Adult:* 2–6 mg/kg/d PO; base the dose on bone marrow response *Pediatric:* 50 mg/m²/d; adjust the dose based on bone marrow response	Used in combination therapy for treatment of stages III and IV of Hodgkin disease *Special considerations:* Bone marrow toxicity; GI toxicity and skin lesions also limit use in some patients; severity of adverse effects regulates the dose of the drug
streptozocin (*Zanosar*)	500 mg/m² IV for 5 consecutive days, usually given every week *or* 1,000 mg/m³ IV at weekly intervals	Treatment of metastatic islet cell carcinoma of the pancreas *Special considerations:* GI and renal toxicity are common; causes infertility; wear rubber gloves to avoid drug contact with the skin—if contact occurs, wash with soap and water
temozolomide (*Temodar*)	75 mg/m²/d PO with radiation	Treatment of refractory astrocytoma or glioblastoma in patients refractory to other treatments *Special considerations:* Monitor bone marrow closely; especially toxic in women and the elderly

CLL, chronic lymphocytic leukemia.

with many of these agents using the cytochrome P450 systems. They are excreted in the urine.

Contraindications and Cautions

Alkylating agents are contraindicated during pregnancy and lactation *due to their potential for severe effects on the fetus and neonate.* Caution is necessary when giving alkylating agents to any individual with a known allergy to any of them; with bone marrow suppression, *which is often the index for redosing and dosing levels*; or with suppressed renal or hepatic function, *which may interfere with metabolism or excretion of these drugs and often indicates a need to change the dose.*

Adverse Effects

Adverse effects frequently encountered with the use of these alkylating agents are listed below; see Table 14.1 for a list of adverse effects specific to each agent. Amifostine (*Ethyol*) and mesna (*Mesnex*) are cytoprotective (cell-protecting) drugs that may be given to limit certain effects of cisplatin and ifosfamide, respectively (Box 14.3).

Hematological effects include bone marrow suppression, with leukopenia, thrombocytopenia, anemia, and pancytopenia, secondary to the effects of the drugs on the rapidly multiplying cells of the bone marrow. GI effects include nausea, vomiting, anorexia, diarrhea, and mucous membrane deterioration, all of which are related to the drugs'effects on the rapidly multiplying cells of the GI tract. Hepatic toxicity and renal toxicity may occur, depending on the exact mechanism of action. **Alopecia**, or hair loss, related to effects on the hair follicles, may also occur. All drugs that cause cell death can cause a potentially toxic increase in uric acid levels. Allopurinol has been used to help alleviate this problem and in 2004, a new drug, rasburicase, was introduced to manage uric acid levels in pediatric patients receiving antineoplastics resulting in tumor lysis and elevated uric acid levels (Box 14.4).

Clinically Important Drug–Drug Interactions

Alkylating agents that are known to cause hepatic or renal toxicity should be used cautiously with any other drugs that have similar effects. In addition, drugs that are toxic to the liver may adversely affect drugs that are metabolized in the liver or that act in the liver (e.g., oral anticoagulants). Always check for specific drug–drug interactions for each agent in a nursing drug guide.

KEY POINTS

- Alkylating agents affect cellular RNA, DNA, or other cellular proteins, are cell cycle nonspecific, and are most effective against slow-growing tumors.
- Patients receiving alkylating agents may experience alopecia, nausea, and vomiting and need to be monitored for bone marrow suppression and CNS toxicity.

BOX 14.3

Drugs that are Used as Adjuncts in Antineoplastic Chemotherapy

Amifostine (*Ethyol*) is a cytoprotective (cell-protecting) drug that preserves healthy cells from the toxic effects of cisplatin. It is thought to react to the specific acidity and vascularity of nontumor cells to protect them, and it may also act as a scavenger of free radicals released by cells that have been exposed to cisplatin. Amifostine is given at a dose of 910 mg/m^2 4 times a day as a 15-min IV infusion starting within 30 minutes after starting cisplatin therapy; timing is very important to its effectiveness. Now approved for use to prevent the renal toxicity associated with the use of cisplatin in patients with advanced ovarian cancer, amifostine is under investigation as an agent for protecting lung fibroblasts from the effects of paclitaxel. Because amifostine is associated with severe nausea and vomiting, concurrent administration of an antiemetic is recommended. It also can cause hypotension, and patients should be monitored closely for this condition.

Mesna (*Mesnex*) is a cytoprotective agent that is used to reduce the incidence of hemorrhagic cystitis caused by ifosfamide or cyclophosphamide. Mesna, which is known to react chemically with urotoxic metabolites of ifosfamide, is given intravenously at the time of the ifosfamide injection at a dose that is 20% of the ifosfamide dose and is repeated 4 and 8 hours afterward. Because mesna has been associated with nausea and vomiting an antiemetic may be useful.

Dexrazoxane (*Totect*) is approved for the treatment of extravasation resulting from IV antineoplastic antibiotic chemotherapy. It is given as an IV infusion over 1 to 2 hours once daily for 3 days. Dosage is as follows: day 1, 1,000 mg/m^2, maximum dose 2,000 mg; day 2, 1,000 mg m^2, maximum dose 2,000 mg; day 3,500 mg m^2, maximum dose 1,000 mg. The mechanism of action that allows this drug to protect cells from damage related to extravasation is not understood but it may block certain enzymes affected by the drugs. Dose should be reduced in patients with renal failure.

Ⓟ Prototype Summary: Chlorambucil

Indications: Palliative treatment of chronic lymphocytic leukemia, malignant lymphomas, and Hodgkin disease.

Actions: Alkylates cellular DNA, interfering with the replication of susceptible cells.

Pharmacokinetics:

Route	Onset	Peak	Duration
Oral	Varies	1 h	15–20 h

$T_{1/2}$: 60 to 90 minutes, metabolized in the liver and excreted in the urine.

Adverse Effects: Tremors, muscle twitching, confusion, nausea, hepatotoxicity, bone marrow suppression, sterility, cancer.

BOX 14.4

Drugs to Manage Rising Uric Acid Levels Associated with Tumor Lysis

Allopurinol (*Aloprim, Zyloprim*) inhibits the enzyme that allows the conversion of purines to uric acid, which is toxic to the body. It is used to help manage patients with leukemia, lymphoma, or other malignancies that result in elevated levels of serum and urinary uric acid levels. It lowers the level of uric acid to protect the kidneys and tissues. It is given orally at doses of 600 to 800 mg a day for 2 to 3 days with high fluid intake, maintenance doses are then determined based on the patient's response and serum uric acid levels.

Rasburicase (*Elitek*) is approved for the management of plasma uric acid levels in patients with leukemia, lymphoma, and solid tumor malignancies who are receiving antineoplastic therapy associated with tumor lysis and subsequent elevated serum uric acid levels. It is administered as a single daily IV infusion of 0.15 to 0.2 mg/kg over 30 minutes for 5 days. Chemotherapy should be started 4 to 24 hours after the first dose of rasburicase. Uric acid levels should be monitored frequently, using prechilled, heparinized vials that are kept in an ice-water bath. This analysis should be done within 4 hours of each rasburicase dose.

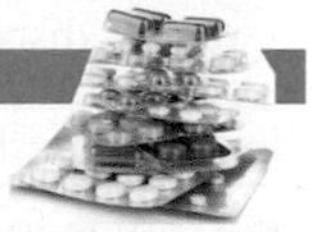

Nursing Considerations for Patients Receiving Alkylating Agents

Assessment: History and Examination

- Assess for contraindications or cautions: History of allergy to any of the alkylating agents *to avoid hypersensitivity reactions*; bone marrow suppression *to prevent further suppression*; renal or hepatic dysfunction *that might interfere with drug metabolism and excretion*; and current status related to pregnancy or lactation *to prevent potentially serious adverse effects on the fetus or nursing baby.*
- Perform a physical assessment *to establish baseline data for determining the effectiveness of the drug and the occurrence of any adverse effects associated with drug therapy.*
- Assess orientation and reflexes *to evaluate any central nervous system (CNS) effects*; respiratory rate and adventitious sounds *to monitor the disease* and *to evaluate for respiratory or hypersensitivity effects*; pulse, rhythm, and auscultation *to monitor for systemic or cardiovascular effects*; and bowel sounds and mucous membrane status *to monitor for GI effects.*

(continues on page 222)

- Monitor the results of laboratory tests such as complete blood count with differential *to identify possible bone marrow suppression and toxic drug effects and establish appropriate dosing for the drug*; and renal and liver function tests to determine need for *possible dose adjustment and identify toxic drug effects.*

Nursing Diagnoses

Nursing diagnoses related to drug therapy might include the following:

- Acute pain related to GI, CNS, and skin effects of the drug
- Disturbed body image related to alopecia, skin effects, impaired fertility
- Imbalanced nutrition, less than body requirements
- Risk for infection
- Fear, anxiety related to diagnosis and treatment
- Deficient knowledge regarding drug therapy

Planning

- The patient will receive the best therapeutic effect from the drug therapy.
- The patient will have limited adverse effects to the drug therapy.
- The patient will have an understanding of the drug therapy, adverse effects to anticipate. and measures to relieve discomfort and improve safety

Implementation with Rationale

- Arrange for blood tests before, periodically during, and for at least 3 weeks after therapy *to monitor bone marrow function to aid in determining the need for a change in dose or discontinuation of the drug* (see Box 14.5).
- Administer medication according to scheduled protocol and in combination with other drugs as indicated *to improve effectiveness.*
- Ensure that the patient is well hydrated *to decrease risk of renal toxicity.*
- Protect the patient from exposure to infection; limit invasive procedures *when bone marrow suppression limits the patient's immune/inflammatory responses.*
- Provide small, frequent meals, frequent mouth care, and dietary consultation as appropriate *to maintain nutrition when GI effects are severe.* Anticipate the need for antiemetics if necessary (see Box 14.6).
- Arrange for proper head covering at extremes of temperature if alopecia occurs; a wig, scarf, or hat *is important for maintaining body temperature.*
- Provide patient teaching about the following:
  - Follow the appropriate dosage regimen, including dates to return for further doses.
  - Cover the head at extremes of temperature.
  - Maintain nutrition if GI effects are severe.
  - Avoid exposure to infection.
  - Plan for appropriate rest periods because fatigue and weakness are common effects of the drugs.
  - Consult with a health care provider, if appropriate, related to the possibility of impaired fertility.
  - Use barrier contraceptives to reduce the risk of pregnancy during therapy.

Evaluation

- Monitor patient response to the drug (alleviation of cancer being treated, palliation of signs and symptoms of cancer).
- Monitor for adverse effects (bone marrow suppression, GI toxicity, neurotoxicity, alopecia, renal or hepatic dysfunction).
- Evaluate the effectiveness of the teaching plan (patient can name the drug, dosage, possible adverse effects to watch for, and specific measures to help avoid adverse effects).

Antimetabolites

Antimetabolites (Table 14.2) are drugs that have chemical structures similar to those of various natural metabolites that are necessary for the growth and division of rapidly growing neoplastic cells and normal cells. Antimetabolites include capecitabine (*Xeloda*), cladribine (generic), clofarabine (*Clolar*), cytarabine (*DepoCyt, Tarabine PFS*), floxuridine (generic), fludarabine (generic), fluorouracil (*Carac, Efudex, Fluoroplex*), gemcitabine (*Gemzar*), mercaptopurine (generic), methotrexate (*Rheumatrex, Trexall*), pemetrexed (*Alimta*), pentostatin (*Nipent*), pralatrexate (*Folotyn*), and thioguanine (generic).

Therapeutic Actions and Indications

Antimetabolites inhibit DNA production in cells that depend on certain natural metabolites to produce their DNA. They replace these needed metabolites and thereby prevent normal cellular function. Many of these agents inhibit thymidylate synthetase, DNA polymerase, or folic acid reductase, all of which are needed for DNA synthesis. They are considered to be S phase specific in the cell cycle. They are most effective in rapidly dividing cells, preventing cell replication, and leading to cell death (Figure 14.5). The antimetabolites are indicated for the treatment of various leukemias and some GI and basal cell cancers (see Table 14.2 for Usual Indications for each agent). Use of these drugs has been somewhat limited because neoplastic cells rapidly develop resistance to these agents. For this reason, these drugs are usually administered as part of a combination therapy.

BOX 14.5

Dealing with Bone Marrow Suppression

Bone marrow suppression is a frequently encountered adverse effect of antineoplastic chemotherapy. The cells in the bone marrow are rapidly turning over cells, constantly stimulated to produce blood components and so they are more likely to be affected by drugs that kill cells. The patient may experience a low red blood cell (RBC) count (anemia), low platelet counts, and low white blood cell (WBC) counts. The nurse is in the position to help the patient cope with these effects and prevent serious complications that occur. There are also drugs available that are often used to help stimulate the bone marrow.

Decreased Red Blood Cells

The patient with a low RBC count will experience fatigue. The patient should be counseled to space activities during the day and incorporate rest periods into their daily schedule. Sometimes just knowing that this is a normal response is helpful to the patient. Epoetin alfa (*Epogen, Procrit*) or darbepoetin (*Aranesp*) (see Chapter 49) is often used to stimulate RBC production. These drugs act like endogenous erythropoietin to directly stimulate the cells in the bone marrow to make RBCs. Caution must be used to closely monitor the patient's hemoglobin level as levels over 11 g/dL have been associated with more rapid cancer growth and cardiac events. These drugs must be injected and the patient's lab values followed closely.

Decreased Platelets

Platelet aggregation is the first step in preventing blood loss when a blood vessel is injured (see Chapter 48). When platelet levels are low the patient is at increased risk of blood loss. Patients should be alert for increased bruising, bleeding while brushing their teeth, or increased bleeding with any injury. Protection is the best approach for these patients. Using a soft bristled toothbrush, using an electric razor, avoiding sports or activities that could lead to injury are key teaching points.

Decreased White Blood Cells

The neutrophils are the first WBCs stimulated with any injury or infection. They are phagocytes that are called to an injured area to remove damage and prevent further injury. A patient with low WBC counts is at high risk for infection and even cancer development. Protection is a key teaching point for these patients: Avoid crowded areas, don't visit sick friends or hospitals, avoid people who are known to be ill, avoid activities that could cause injury, and don't dig in the dirt without protective gloves (many pathogens live in the soil). Drugs called colony-stimulating agents may be used to stimulate WBC production when it falls dangerously low. Filgrastim (*Neupogen*), which comes in prefilled syringes for patients to use at home, pegfilgrastim (*Neulasta*), and tbo-filgrastim (*Granix*) (see Chapter 17) are administered by subcutaneous injection, with the patient's blood counts followed closely to determine dosing and duration of treatment.

BOX 14.6

Antiemetics and Cancer Chemotherapy

Antineoplastic drugs can directly stimulate the chemoreceptor trigger zone (CTZ) in the medulla to induce nausea and vomiting. These drugs also cause cell death, which releases many toxins into the system, which in turn stimulate the CTZ. Because patients expect nausea and vomiting with the administration of antineoplastic agents the higher cortical centers of the brain can stimulate the CTZ to induce vomiting just at the thought of the chemotherapy.

A variety of antiemetic agents have been used in the course of antineoplastic therapy. Sometimes a combination of drugs is most helpful. It should also be remembered that an accepting environment, plenty of comfort measures (e.g., environmental control, mouth care, ice chips), and support for the patient can help to decrease the discomfort associated with the emetic effects of these drugs. Antihistamines to decrease secretions and corticosteroids to relieve inflammation are useful as adjunctive therapies.

Drugs that are known to help in treating antineoplastic chemotherapy–induced nausea and vomiting include the following:

- Dronabinol (*Marinol*) and nabilone (*Cesamet*) are synthetic derivatives of delta-9-tetrahydrocannabinol, the active ingredient in marijuana; this is not usually a first-line drug because of associated CNS effects. The usual dosage for dronabinol is 5 mg m^2 PO 1 to 3 hours before chemotherapy and repeated every 2 to 4 hours after chemotherapy. Nabilone is given orally as 1 to 2 mg PO twice daily initially, then daily during the cycle, and for 48 hours after the last dose of chemotherapy.
- Ondansetron (*Zofran*), granisetron (*Kytril*), and palonosetron (*Aloxi*), which is approved for use in children 1 mo–17 years, block serotonin receptors in the CTZ and are among the most effective antiemetics, especially if combined with a corticosteroid such as dexamethasone. The usual dosage is three 0.15-mg/kg doses IV or 8 mg PO three times a day starting 30 minutes before chemotherapy (ondansetron), or 10 mg/kg IV or 1 mg PO twice a day (granisetron), or 0.25 mg IV over 30 seconds, starting 30 minutes before chemotherapy (palonosetron). A combination oral product with netupitat (a human substance P/neurokin receptor blocker) and palonosetron (*Akynzeo*) is available for added effects.
- Aprepitant (*Emend*) blocks human substance P/neurokinin 1 receptors in the CNS, blocking the nausea and vomiting caused by severely emetogenic antineoplastic drugs without

(*continued*)

BOX 14.6

Antiemetics and Cancer Chemotherapy *(continued)*

effects on dopamine, serotonin, or norepinephrine. The usual dosage is 125 mg PO 1 hour before chemotherapy (day 1) and 80 mg PO once daily in the morning on days 2 and 3; given in combination with 12-mg dexamethasone PO on day 1 and 8-mg dexamethasone PO on days 2 to 4, and 32-mg ondansetron IV on day 1 only.

- Two benzodiazepines—alprazolam (*Xanax*), 0.5 mg PO four times a day, and lorazepam (*Ativan*), 2 to 6 mg/d PO—seem to be effective in directly blocking the CTZ to relieve nausea and vomiting caused by cancer chemotherapy; they are especially effective when combined with a corticosteroid.
- Haloperidol (*Haldol*), 0.5 to 2.0 mg PO four times a day, or 2 to 25 mg IM or IV, is a dopaminergic blocker that also is believed to have direct CTZ effects.
- Metoclopramide (*Reglan*), 2 mg/kg IV over at least 30 minutes, calms the activity of the GI tract; it is especially effective if combined with a corticosteroid, an antihistamine, and a centrally acting blocker such as haloperidol or lorazepam.
- Prochlorperazine (generic), 5 to 10 mg PO three to four times a day, or 5 to 10 mg IM, is a phenothiazine that has been found to have strong antiemetic action in the CNS; it can be given by a variety of routes.

Nausea and vomiting are unavoidable aspects of many chemotherapeutic regimens. However, treating the patient as the chemotherapy begins, using combination regimens, and providing plenty of supportive and comforting nursing care can help to alleviate some of the distress associated with these adverse effects.

Table 14.2 ***Drugs in Focus:* Antimetabolites**

Drug Name	Dosage/Route	Usual Indications
capecitabine (*Xeloda*)	2,500 mg/m^2/d PO in two divided doses for 2 wk, then 1 wk of rest, for three cycles *Dukes C colon cancer:* 1,250 mg/m^2 PO b.i.d. for 2 wk, then 1 wk of rest for a total of eight 3-wk cycles	Treatment of metastatic breast cancer with resistance to paclitaxel or anthracyclines; treatment of metastatic colorectal cancer as first-line therapy treatment of breast cancer with docetaxel in patients with metastatic disease; postsurgery Dukes C colon cancer *Special considerations:* Severe diarrhea can occur—monitor hydration and nutrition; monitor for bone marrow suppression; severe to fatal bleeding if combined with warfarin
cladribine (generic)	0.09 mg/kg/d IV for 7 consecutive days	Treatment of active hairy cell leukemia *Special considerations:* severe bone marrow depression can occur—monitor patient closely and reduce dose as needed; fever is common, especially early in treatment
clofarabine (*Clolar*)	52 mg/m^2 by IV infusion over 2 h daily for 5 d; repeat every 2–6 wk, based on baseline function	Treatment of patients 1–21 y of age with ALL after at least two relapses on other regimens *Special considerations:* GI toxicity, bone marrow suppression, and infection are common
cytarabine (*DepoCyt, Tarabine PFS*)	200 mg/m^2 per/d by continuous IV infusion for 5 d, repeat every 2 wk; intrathecal use, 30 mg/m^2 every 4 d	Treatment of meningeal and myelocytic leukemias; used in combination with other agents; lymphomatous meningitis *Special considerations:* GI toxicity and cytarabine syndrome (fever, myalgia, bone pain, chest pain, rash, conjunctivitis, and malaise) are common—this syndrome sometimes responds to corticosteroids; alopecia may occur; monitor for bone marrow suppression
floxuridine (generic)	0.1–0.6 mg/kg/d via intraarterial line	Palliative management of GI adenocarcinoma metastatic to the liver in patients who are not candidates for surgery *Special considerations:* Administer by intraarterial line only; bone marrow suppression, GI toxicity, neurotoxicity, and alopecia are common
fludarabine (generic)	25 mg/m^2/d IV for 5 d; repeat every 28 d	Treatment of CLL; unresponsive B cell CLL with no progress with at least one other treatment *Special considerations:* CNS toxicity can be severe; GI toxicity, respiratory complications, renal failure, and a tumor lysis syndrome are common
fluorouracil (*Adrucil, Carac, Efudex, Fluoroplex*)	12 mg/kg/d IV on days 1–4, then 6 mg/kg IV on days 6, 8, 10, and 12	Palliative treatment of various GI cancers; topical treatment of basal cell carcinoma and actinic and solar keratoses *Special considerations:* GI toxicity, bone marrow suppression, alopecia, and skin rash are common; avoid occlusive dressings with topical forms; wash hands thoroughly after coming in contact with drug

Drug Name	Dosage/Route	Usual Indications
gemcitabine (*Gemzar*)	1,000–1,250 mg/m² IV over 30 min once a week; timing based on other therapies and patient response	Treatment of locally advanced or metastatic adenocarcinoma of the pancreas; given with cisplatin for the treatment of inoperable non–small cell lung cancer; metastatic breast cancer, ovarian cancer after failure of a platinum-based therapy *Special considerations:* Can cause severe bone marrow depression, GI toxicity, pain, alopecia, interstitial pneumonitis
mercaptopurine (generic)	2.5 mg/kg/d PO for 4 wk; then reevaluate	Remission induction and maintenance therapy in acute leukemias *Special considerations:* bone marrow toxicity and GI toxicity are common; hyperuricemia is a true concern—ensure that the patient is well hydrated during therapy
methotrexate (*Rheumatrex*, *Trexall*)	Dose varies with route and disease being treated; 15–30 mg PO or IM is common	Treatment of leukemias, psoriasis, rheumatoid arthritis, and choriocarcinomas *Special considerations:* Hypersensitivity reactions can be severe; liver toxicity and GI complications are common; monitor for bone marrow suppression and increased susceptibility to infections; dose pack available for the oral treatment of psoriasis and rheumatoid arthritis
pemetrexed (*Alimta*)	500 mg/m² IV over 10 min on day 1 with 75 mg/m² cisplatin IV over 2 h; repeat cycle every 21 d	Treatment of malignant mesothelioma in patients whose disease is unresectable or who are not candidates for surgery; locally advanced or metastatic non–small cell lung cancer as a single agent after other chemotherapy *Special considerations:* pretreat with corticosteroids, folic acid, and vitamin B_{12}; monitor for bone marrow suppression and GI effects
pentostatin (*Nipent*)	4 mg/m² IV every other week	Hairy cell leukemia in adults if refractory to interferon-alpha therapy *Special considerations:* Associated with severe renal, hepatic, CNS, and pulmonary toxicities—monitor patient closely and reduce dose accordingly; 3–6 mo of interferon-alpha therapy should be tried before using pentostatin
pralatrexate (*Folotyn*)	30 mg/m² IV push over 2–5 min once weekly for 6 wk in a 7-wk cycle	Treatment of relapsed or refractory peripheral T-cell lymphoma *Special considerations:* Bone marrow suppression common; severe mucositis can occur—patient should receive vitamin B_{12} 1 mg IM every 8–10 wk and folic acid 1–1.25 mg/d PO
thioguanine (generic)	2 mg/kg/d PO for 4 wk; then dose may be increased if tolerated well	Remission induction and maintenance of acute leukemias alone or as part of combination therapy *Special considerations:* Bone marrow suppression, GI toxicity, miscarriage, and birth defects have been reported; monitor bone marrow status to determine dose and redosing; ensure that the patient is well hydrated during therapy to minimize hyperuricemia—patient may respond to allopurinol and urine alkalinization

ALL, acute lymphocytic leukemia; CLL, chronic lymphocytic leukemia.

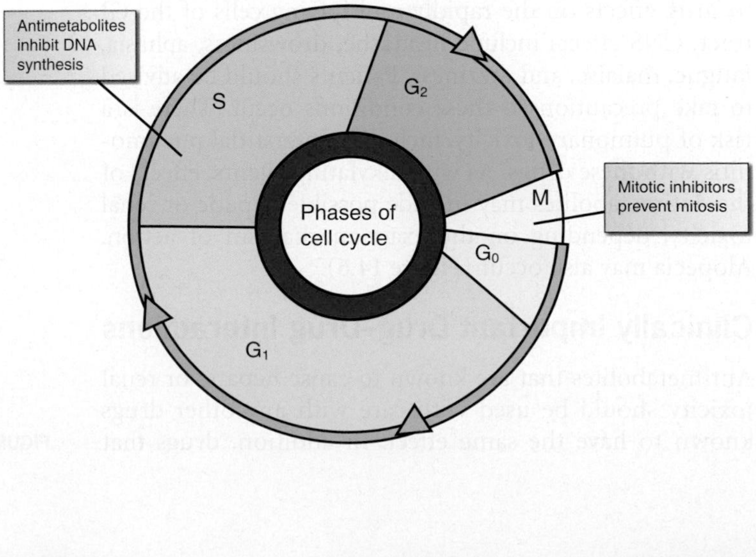

FIGURE 14.5 Sites of action of cell cycle–specific antineoplastic agents.

Pharmacokinetics

Methotrexate is absorbed well from the GI tract and is excreted unchanged in the urine. Patients with renal impairment may require reduced dose and increased monitoring when taking methotrexate. Methotrexate readily crosses the blood–brain barrier. Cytarabine, clofarabine, floxuridine, fluorouracil, gemcitabine, pemetrexed, and pralatrexate are not absorbed well from the GI tract and need to be administered parenterally. They are metabolized in the liver and excreted in the urine, necessitating close monitoring of patients with hepatic or renal impairment who are receiving these drugs. Mercaptopurine and thioguanine are absorbed slowly from the GI tract and are metabolized in the liver and excreted in the urine.

Contraindications and Cautions

Antimetabolites are contraindicated for use during pregnancy and lactation *because of the potential for severe effects on the fetus and neonate.* Caution is necessary when administering antimetabolites to any individual with a known allergy to any of them *to prevent hypersensitivity reactions*; with bone marrow suppression, *which is often the index for redosing and dosing levels*; with renal or hepatic dysfunction, *which might interfere with the metabolism or excretion of these drugs and often indicates a need to change the dose*; and with known GI ulcerations or ulcerative diseases *that might be exacerbated by the effects of these drugs.*

Adverse Effects

Adverse effects frequently encountered with the use of the antimetabolites are listed here. To counteract the effects of treatment with one antimetabolite—methotrexate—the drug leucovorin or its isomer levoleucovorin is sometimes given (Box 14.7).

Hematological effects include bone marrow suppression, with leukopenia, thrombocytopenia, anemia, and pancytopenia, secondary to the effects of the drugs on the rapidly multiplying cells of the bone marrow. Toxic GI effects include nausea, vomiting, anorexia, diarrhea, and mucous membrane deterioration, all of which are related to drug effects on the rapidly multiplying cells of the GI tract. CNS effects include headache, drowsiness, aphasia, fatigue, malaise, and dizziness. Patients should be advised to take precautions if these conditions occur. There is a risk of pulmonary toxicity, including interstitial pneumonitis with these drugs. As with alkylating agents, effects of the antimetabolites may include possible hepatic or renal toxicity, depending on the exact mechanism of action. Alopecia may also occur (Figure 14.6).

Clinically Important Drug–Drug Interactions

Antimetabolites that are known to cause hepatic or renal toxicity should be used with care with any other drugs known to have the same effect. In addition, drugs that

BOX 14.7

A Drug that Protects against an Antimetabolite

Leucovorin (generic) is an active form of folic acid that is used to "rescue" normal cells from the adverse effects of methotrexate therapy in the treatment of osteosarcoma. This drug is also used to treat folic acid deficiency conditions such as sprue, nutritional deficiency, pregnancy, and lactation. Leucovorin is given orally or intravenously at the time of methotrexate therapy and for the next 72 hours at a dose of 12 to 15 g/m^2 PO or IV followed by 10 mg/m^2 PO q6h for 72 hours. Use of this drug has been associated with pain at the injection site.

In 2008, levoleucovorin (*Fusilev*), an isomer of leucovorin, was also approved to diminish the toxicity and counteract the effects of impaired methotrexate elimination and of inadvertent overdose of folic acid antagonists after high-dose methotrexate therapy in osteosarcoma. The drug is given IV for up to 4 days, and dose is determined by the serum methotrexate level of the patient. There are high calcium levels in the solution, and the drug needs to be given slowly.

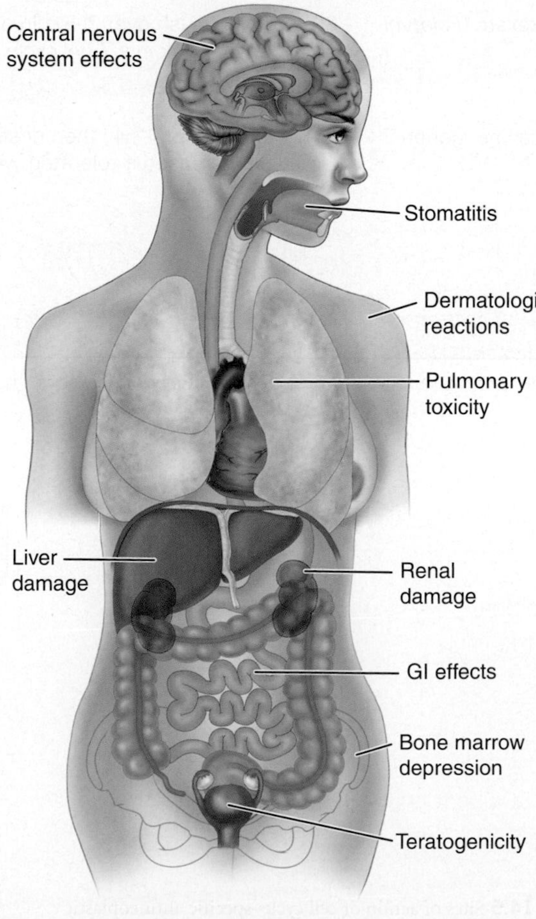

FIGURE 14.6 Common adverse effects associated with antineoplastic agents.

are toxic to the liver may adversely affect drugs that are metabolized in the liver or that act in the liver (e.g., oral anticoagulants). Check for specific drug–drug interactions for each agent in a nursing drug guide.

Ⓟ Prototype Summary: Methotrexate

Indications: Treatment of gestational choriocarcinoma; chorioadenoma destruens; hydatidiform, meningeal leukemia; symptomatic control of severe psoriasis; rheumatoid arthritis; juvenile rheumatoid arthritis.

Actions: Inhibits folic acid reductase, leading to inhibition of DNA synthesis and inhibition of cellular replication; affects the most rapidly dividing cells.

Pharmacokinetics:

Route	Onset	Peak
Oral	Varies	1–4 h
Intravenous	Rapid	0.5–2 h

$T_{1/2}$: 2 to 4 hours, excreted unchanged in the urine.

Adverse Effects: Fatigue, malaise, rashes, alopecia, ulcerative stomatitis, hepatic toxicity, severe bone marrow suppression, interstitial pneumonitis, chills, fever, anaphylaxis.

Nursing Considerations for Patients Receiving Antimetabolites

Assessment: History and Examination

- Assess for contraindications and cautions: history of allergy to the specific antimetabolite *to avoid hypersensitivity reactions*; bone marrow suppression *to prevent further suppression*; renal or hepatic dysfunction *that might interfere with drug metabolism and excretion*; current status related to pregnancy or lactation *to prevent potentially serious effects to the fetus or nursing baby*; and a history of GI ulcerative disease, *which could be exacerbated with the use of these drugs*.
- Perform a physical assessment *to establish baseline data for determining the effectiveness of the drug and the occurrence of any adverse effects associated with drug therapy*.
- Assess orientation and reflexes *to evaluate any CNS effects*; respiratory rate and adventitious sounds *to monitor the disease and to evaluate for respiratory or hypersensitivity* effects; pulse, rhythm, and cardiac auscultation *to monitor for systemic or cardiovascular effects*; and bowel sounds and mucous membrane status *to monitor for GI effects*.
- Monitor the results of laboratory tests such as complete blood count with differential to identify possible bone marrow suppression and toxic drug effects; and renal and liver function tests *to determine the need for possible dose adjustment and toxic drug effects*.

Nursing Diagnoses

Nursing diagnoses related to drug therapy might include the following:

- Acute pain related to GI, CNS, or skin effects of the drug
- Disturbed body image related to alopecia, skin effects, impaired fertility
- Fear, anxiety related to diagnosis and treatment
- Imbalanced nutrition, less than body requirements
- Risk for infection
- Deficient knowledge regarding drug therapy

Planning

- The patient will receive the best therapeutic effect from the drug therapy.
- The patient will have limited adverse effects to the drug therapy.
- The patient will have an understanding of the drug therapy, adverse effects to anticipate, and measures to relieve discomfort and improve safety.

Implementation with Rationale

- Arrange for blood tests to monitor bone marrow function before, periodically during, and for at least 3 weeks after therapy *to arrange to discontinue the drug or reduce the dose as needed* (see Box 14.5).
- Administer medication according to the scheduled protocol and in combination with other drugs as indicated *to improve the effectiveness of drug therapy*.
- Ensure that the patient is well hydrated *to decrease the risk of renal toxicity*.
- Provide small, frequent meals, frequent mouth care, and dietary consultation as appropriate *to maintain nutrition when GI effects are severe*. Anticipate the use of antiemetics as necessary (see Box 14.4).
- Arrange for proper head covering at extremes of temperature if alopecia occurs; a wig, scarf, or hat *is important for maintaining body temperature*. If alopecia is an anticipated effect of drug therapy, advise the patient to obtain a wig or head covering before the condition occurs.
- Protect the patient from exposure to infections *because bone marrow suppression will limit immune/inflammatory responses*.
- Provide support and encouragement *to help the patient cope with the diagnosis and the effects of drug therapy*.
- Provide the following patient teaching:
  - Follow the appropriate dosage regimen, including dates to return for further doses. Patients need to be reminded to report all other drugs and alternative therapies that they might be using. Box 14.8 discusses alternative therapies often used by cancer patients that could interact with their drug regimen.

(continues on page 228)

- Maintain nutrition if GI effects are severe.
- Cover the head at extremes of temperature if alopecia is anticipated.
- Plan for appropriate rest periods because fatigue and weakness are common effects of the drugs.
- Avoid situations that might lead to infection, including crowded places, sick people, and working in the soil.
- Use safety measures such as not driving or using dangerous equipment, due to possible dizziness, headache, and drowsiness.
- Think about consulting with a health care provider, if appropriate, due to the possibility of impaired fertility.
- Use barrier contraceptives to reduce the risk of pregnancy during therapy.

Evaluation

- Monitor patient response to the drug (alleviation of cancer being treated, palliation of signs and symptoms of cancer, palliation of rheumatoid arthritis or psoriasis).
- Monitor for adverse effects (bone marrow suppression, GI toxicity, neurotoxicity, alopecia, renal or hepatic dysfunction).
- Evaluate the effectiveness of the teaching plan (patient can name the drug, dosage, possible adverse effects to watch for, and specific measures to help avoid adverse effects).
- Monitor the effectiveness of comfort and safety measures and compliance with the regimen.

KEY POINTS

- Antimetabolites inhibit DNA production by inhibiting metabolites needed for the synthesis of DNA in susceptible cells.
- Antimetabolites are S-phase cell cycle specific and are used for some leukemias, as well as some GI and basal cell cancers.
- Bone marrow suppression, alopecia, and toxic GI effects are common adverse effects of antimetabolites.

Antineoplastic Antibiotics

Antineoplastic antibiotics (Table 14.3), although selective for bacterial cells, are also toxic to human cells. Because these drugs tend to be more toxic to cells that are multiplying rapidly, they are more useful in the treatment of certain cancers. Antineoplastic antibiotics include bleomycin (generic), dactinomycin (*Cosmegen*), daunorubicin (*DaunoXome*), doxorubicin (*Doxil*), epirubicin (*Ellence*), idarubicin (*Idamycin PFS*), mitomycin (generic), mitoxantrone (generic), and valrubicin (*Valstar*).

BOX 14.8 FOCUS ON Cultural Considerations

Alternative Therapies and Cancer

The diagnosis of cancer and the sometimes devastating effects of cancer treatment often drive patients to seek out alternative therapies, either as adjuncts to traditional cancer therapy or sometimes instead of traditional therapy. Because Asian Americans and Pacific Islanders often see drug therapy and other cancer therapies as part of a "yin/yang" belief system, they may turn to a variety of herbal therapies to "balance" their systems.

The nurse should be aware of some potential interactions that may occur when alternative therapies are used:

- *Echinacea*—may be hepatotoxic; increases the risk of hepatotoxicity when taken with antineoplastics that are hepatotoxic
- *Ginkgo*—inhibits blood clotting, which can cause problems after surgery or with bleeding neoplasms
- *Saw palmetto*—may increase the effects of various estrogen hormones and hormone modulators; advise patients taking such drugs to avoid this herb
- *St. John's wort*—can greatly increase photosensitivity, which can cause problems with patients who have received radiation therapy or are taking drugs that cause other dermatological effects; has been shown to interfere with the effectiveness of some antineoplastic agents

If a patient has an unexpected reaction to a drug, ask about whether he or she is using alternative therapies. Many of these agents are untested, and interactions and adverse effects are not well documented.

FOCUS ON Safe Medication Administration

Name confusion has occurred between daunorubicin, doxorubicin, epirubicin, idarubicin, valrubicin. These are very different drugs with different indications, dosages and the potential for serious adverse effects. If using any drug that ends in "rubicin" be aware that there are several of these dangerous drugs and check the orders carefully to make sure you are giving the right drug to the right patient.

Therapeutic Actions and Indications

Some antineoplastic antibiotics break up DNA links, and others prevent DNA synthesis.

The antineoplastic antibiotics are cytotoxic and interfere with cellular DNA synthesis by inserting themselves between base pairs in the DNA chain. This, in turn, causes a mutant DNA molecule, leading to cell death (Figure 14.4). See Table 14.3 for Usual Indications for each antineoplastic antibiotic. Like other antineoplastics the main adverse effects of these drugs are seen in cells that multiply rapidly, such as those in the bone marrow, GI tract, and skin. Their potentially serious adverse effects may limit their usefulness in patients with preexisting diseases and in those who are debilitated and, therefore, more susceptible to these effects.

Table 14.3 *Drugs in Focus:* Antineoplastic Antibiotics

Drug Name	Dosage/Route	Usual Indications
bleomycin (generic)	0.25–0.5 units/kg IM, IV, or subcutaneous once or twice weekly	Palliative treatment of squamous cell carcinomas, testicular cancers, and lymphomas; used to treat malignant pleural effusion *Special considerations:* GI toxicity, severe skin reactions, and hypersensitivity reactions may occur; pulmonary fibrosis can be a serious problem—baseline and periodic chest radiographs and pulmonary function tests are necessary
dactinomycin (*Cosmegen*)	*Adult:* 0.5 mg/d IV for up to 5 days *Pediatric:* 0.015 mg/kg/d IV for up to 5 d or a total dose of 2.5 mg/m²/wk	Part of combination drug regimen in the treatment of a variety of sarcomas and carcinomas; potentiates the effects of radiation therapy *Special considerations:* Bone marrow suppression and GI toxicity, which may be severe, limit the dose; effects may not appear for 1–2 wk; local extravasation can cause necrosis and should be treated with injectable corticosteroids, ice to the area, and restarting of the IV line in a different vein
daunorubicin (*DaunoXome*)	40 mg/m² IV, infused over 1 h; repeat every 2 wk	First-line treatment of advanced HIV infection and associated Kaposi sarcoma *Special considerations:* Complete alopecia is common, and GI toxicity and bone marrow suppression may also occur; severe necrosis may occur at sites of local extravasation—immediate treatment with corticosteroids, normal saline, and ice may help; if ulcerations occur, a plastic surgeon should be called
doxorubicin (*Doxil*)	60–75 mg/m² as a single IV dose; repeat every 21 d *Liposomal form:* 30–50 mg/m² IV over 1 h once every 2–4 wk	Treatment of a number of leukemias and cancers; used to induce regression; available in a liposomal form for treatment of AIDS-associated Kaposi sarcoma *Special considerations:* Complete alopecia is common; GI toxicity and bone suppression may occur; severe necrosis may occur at sites of local extravasation—immediate treatment with corticosteroids, normal saline, and ice may help; if ulcerations occur a plastic surgeon should be called; toxicity is dose related—an accurate record of each dose received is important in determining dose; severe pulmonary toxicity, alopecia, and injection site and GI toxicity occur
epirubicin (*Ellence*)	100–120 mg/m² IV given in repeated 3–4-wk cycles all on day 1 or divided on days 1 and 8	Adjunctive therapy in patients with evidence of axillary node tumor involvement after resection of primary breast cancer *Special considerations:* May cause cardiotoxicity and delayed cardiomyopathy; monitor for myelosuppression and hyperuricemia; severe local cellulitis and tissue necrosis can occur with extravasation
idarubicin (*Idamycin PFS*)	12 mg/m²/d IV for 3 d with cytarabine	Combination therapy for treatment of acute myeloid leukemia in adults *Special considerations:* May cause severe bone marrow suppression, which regulates dose; associated with cardiac toxicity, which can be severe; GI toxicity and local necrosis with extravasation are also common; severe necrosis may occur at sites of local extravasation—immediate treatment with corticosteroids, normal saline, and ice may help; if ulcerations occur a plastic surgeon should be called; it is essential to monitor heart and bone marrow function to protect the patient from potentially fatal adverse effects
mitomycin (generic)	20 mg/m² IV as a single dose at 6–8-wk intervals	Palliative treatment of disseminated adenocarcinoma of the stomach and pancreas *Special considerations:* Severe pulmonary toxicity, alopecia, and injection site and GI toxicity occur
mitoxantrone (generic)	12 mg/m²/d IV for 1–3 d *Multiple sclerosis:* 12 mg/m² IV as a short infusion every 3 mo	Part of combination therapy in the treatment of adult leukemias; treatment of bone pain in advanced prostatic cancer; reduction of neurological disability and frequency of relapses in chronic, progressive, relapsing multiple sclerosis *Special considerations:* Severe bone marrow suppression may occur and limits dose; alopecia, GI toxicity, and congestive heart failure often occur; avoid direct skin contact with the drug—use gloves and goggles; monitor bone marrow activity and cardiac activity to adjust dose or discontinue drug as needed
valrubicin (*Valstar*)	800 mg intravesically once a week for 6 wk	Intravesical therapy for carcinoma in situ of the bladder if refractory to bacillus Calmette-Guérin therapy (orphan drug) *Special considerations:* Use goggles and gloves when handling, avoid contact with eyes; severe bladder spasms have occurred; use caution with history of irritable bowel syndrome; do not clamp bladder catheter in place

Pharmacokinetics

The antineoplastic antibiotics are not absorbed well from the GI tract. They are given IV or injected into specific sites. They are metabolized in the liver and excreted in the urine at various rates. Many of them have very long half-lives (e.g., 45 hours for idarubicin; more than 5 days for mitoxantrone). Daunorubicin and doxorubicin do not cross the blood–brain barrier, but they are widely distributed in the body and are taken up by the heart, lungs, kidneys, and spleen. This can lead to toxic effects in these organs.

Contraindications and Cautions

All of these agents are contraindicated for use during pregnancy and lactation *because of the potential risk to the fetus and neonate.* Use caution when giving antineoplastic antibiotics to an individual with a known allergy to the antibiotic or related antibiotics, *to prevent hypersensitivity reactions.* Care is necessary when administering these agents to patients with the following conditions: bone marrow suppression, *which is often the index for redosing and dosing levels*; suppressed renal or hepatic function, *which might interfere with the metabolism or excretion of these drugs and often indicates a need to change the dose*; known GI ulcerations or ulcerative diseases, *which may be exacerbated by the effects of these drugs*; pulmonary problems with bleomycin or mitomycin, or cardiac problems with idarubicin or mitoxantrone, *which are specifically toxic to these organ systems.*

Adverse Effects

Adverse effects frequently encountered with the use of these antibiotics include bone marrow suppression, with leukopenia, thrombocytopenia, anemia, and pancytopenia, secondary to the effects of the drugs on the rapidly multiplying cells of the bone marrow. Toxic GI effects include nausea, vomiting, anorexia, diarrhea, and mucous membrane deterioration, all of which are related to drug effects on the rapidly multiplying cells of the GI tract. As with the alkylating agents and antimetabolites, effects of antineoplastic antibiotics may include renal or hepatic toxicity, depending on the exact mechanism of action. Alopecia may also occur. Specific antineoplastic antibiotics are toxic to the heart and lungs. Box 14.9 discusses a cardioprotective drug that interferes with the effects of doxorubicin.

Clinically Important Drug–Drug Interactions

Antimetabolites that are known to cause hepatic or renal toxicity should be used with care with any other drugs known to have the same effect. Drugs that result in toxicity to the heart or lungs should be used with caution with any other drugs that produce that particular toxicity. Check for specific drug–drug interactions for each agent in a nursing drug guide.

BOX 14.9

A Cardioprotective Drug

Dexrazoxane (*Zinecard*), a powerful intracellular chelating agent, is a cardioprotective drug that interferes with the cardiotoxic effects of doxorubicin. The associated adverse effects are difficult to differentiate from those attributable to doxorubicin. This agent is approved for use to prevent the cardiomyopathy associated with doxorubicin in doses greater than 300 mg/m^2 in women with metastatic breast cancer. Dexrazoxane is given intravenously in a dose proportional to (10 times greater than) the doxorubicin dose 30 minutes before the doxorubicin is administered.

Prototype Summary: Doxorubicin

Indications: To produce regression in acute lymphoblastic lymphoma, acute myeloblastic leukemia, Wilms tumor, neuroblastoma, soft tissue and bone sarcoma, breast carcinoma, ovarian carcinoma, thyroid carcinoma, Hodgkin and non-Hodgkin lymphomas, bronchogenic carcinoma; also to treat AIDS-related Kaposi sarcoma.

Actions: Binds to DNA and inhibits DNA synthesis in susceptible cells, causing cell death.

Pharmacokinetics:

Route	Onset	Peak	Duration
IV	Rapid	2 h	24–36 h

$T_{1/2}$: 12 minutes, then 3.3 hours, then 29.6 hours; metabolized in the liver and excreted in the bile, feces, and urine.

Adverse Effects: Cardiac toxicity, complete but reversible alopecia, nausea, vomiting, mucositis, red urine, myelosuppression, fever, chills, rash.

Nursing Considerations for Patients Receiving Antineoplastic Antibiotics

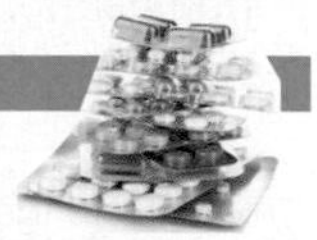

Assessment: History and Examination

- Assess for contraindications and cautions: History of allergy to the antibiotic in use *to avoid hypersensitivity reactions*; bone marrow suppression *to prevent further suppression*; renal or hepatic dysfunction *that might interfere with drug metabolism and excretion*; respiratory or cardiac disease *that could be further aggravated by the toxic effects of these drugs*; current status related to pregnancy or lactation *to prevent potentially serious adverse effects to the fetus or nursing baby*; and GI ulcerative disease, *which could be exacerbated by these drugs.*

- Perform a physical assessment *to establish baseline data for determining the effectiveness of the drug and the occurrence of any adverse effects associated with drug therapy.*
- Assess orientation and reflexes *to evaluate any CNS effects*; respiratory rate and adventitious sounds *to monitor the disease and evaluate for respiratory or hypersensitivity effects*; pulse, rhythm, cardiac auscultation, and baseline electrocardiogram *to monitor for systemic or cardiovascular effects*; and bowel sounds and mucous membrane status *to monitor for GI effects*.
- Monitor the results of laboratory tests such as complete blood count with differential to identify possible bone marrow suppression and toxic drug effects, as well as renal and liver function tests, *to determine the need for possible dose adjustment*.

Nursing Diagnoses

Nursing diagnoses related to drug therapy might include the following:

- Acute pain related to GI, CNS, or local effects of the drug
- Disturbed body Image related to alopecia or skin effects
- Imbalanced nutrition, less than body requirements
- Risk for infection
- Fear, anxiety related to diagnosis and treatment
- Deficient knowledge regarding drug therapy

Planning

- The patient will receive the best therapeutic effect from the drug therapy.
- The patient will have limited adverse effects to the drug therapy.
- The patient will have an understanding of the drug therapy, adverse effects to anticipate, and measures to relieve discomfort and improve safety.

Implementation with Rationale

- Arrange for blood tests to monitor bone marrow function before, periodically during, and for at least 3 weeks after therapy *to arrange to discontinue the drug or reduce the dose as needed* (see Box 14.5).
- Monitor cardiac and respiratory function, as well as clotting times as appropriate for the drug being used, *to arrange to discontinue the drug or reduce the dose as needed.*
- Protect the patient from exposure to infection *because bone marrow suppression will decrease immune/inflammatory reactions.*
- Administer medication according to scheduled protocol and in combination with other drugs as indicated *to improve the effectiveness of drug therapy*.
- Ensure that the patient is well hydrated *to decrease the risk of renal toxicity*.
- Provide small, frequent meals, frequent mouth care, and dietary consultation appropriate *to maintain nutrition when GI effects are severe.* Anticipate the need for antiemetics as necessary (see Box 14.4).
- Arrange for proper head covering at extremes of temperature if alopecia occurs; a wig, scarf, or hat *is important for maintaining body temperature.* If alopecia is an anticipated effect of drug therapy, advise the patient to obtain a wig or head covering before the condition occurs *to promote self-esteem and a positive body image.*
- Provide the following patient teaching:
  - Follow the appropriate dosage regimen, including dates to return for further doses.
  - Maintain nutrition if GI effects are severe.
  - Cover the head at extremes of temperature if alopecia is anticipated.
  - Plan for appropriate rest periods because fatigue and weakness are common effects of the drugs.
  - Avoid exposure to possible infection, including avoiding crowded places, sick people, and working in soil.
  - Use safety measures such as avoiding driving or using dangerous equipment to prevent injury due to possible dizziness, headache, and drowsiness.
  - Consult with a health care provider, if appropriate, regarding possibility of impaired fertility.
  - Use barrier contraceptives to reduce the risk of pregnancy during therapy.

Evaluation

- Monitor patient response to the drug (alleviation of cancer being treated and palliation of signs and symptoms of cancer).
- Monitor for adverse effects (bone marrow suppression, GI toxicity, neurotoxicity, alopecia, renal or hepatic dysfunction, and cardiac or respiratory dysfunction).
- Evaluate the effectiveness of the teaching plan (patient can name the drug, dosage, possible adverse effects to watch for, and specific measures to help avoid adverse effects).

KEY POINTS

- Antineoplastic antibiotics are toxic to rapidly dividing cells.
- These drugs are cell cycle specific, affecting the S phase.
- Bone marrow suppression, alopecia, and toxic GI effects are common adverse effects of antineoplastic antibiotics.

Mitotic Inhibitors

Mitotic inhibitors (Table 14.4) are drugs that kill cells as the process of mitosis begins (see *Figure* 14.5). These cell cycle–specific agents inhibit DNA synthesis. Like other antineoplastics the main adverse effects of the mitotic inhibitors occur with cells that rapidly multiply: Those in the bone marrow, GI tract, and skin. Mitotic inhibitors include cabazitaxel (*Jevtana*), docetaxel (*Taxotere*), eribulin (*Halaven*), etoposide (generic), ixabepilone (*Ixempra*), paclitaxel (*Abraxane*, *Onxol*, *Taxol*), teniposide (*Vumon*), vinblastine (generic), vincristine (generic), and vinorelbine (*Navelbine*).

Table 14.4 *Drugs in Focus:* Mitotic Inhibitors

Drug Name	Dosage/Route	Usual Indications
cabazitaxel (*Jevtana*)	25 mg/m² IV as a 1-h infusion every 3 wk	In combination with oral prednisone for the treatment of patients with hormone refractory metastatic prostate cancer previously treated with a docetaxel-containing regimen *Special considerations:* Serious to life-threatening hypersensitivity reactions have occurred; serious to life-threatening neutropenia can occur; monitor neutrophil count and withhold drug as needed; patient may experience GI disturbances, renal or hepatic failure—elderly patients are more susceptible to adverse effects, monitor accordingly.
docetaxel (*Taxotere*)	60–100 mg/m² IV over 1 h every 3 wk	Treatment of breast cancer and non–small cell lung cancer; androgen-dependent prostate cancer; gastric adenocarcinoma *Special considerations:* monitor patient closely—deaths have occurred during use; severe fluid retention can occur—premedicate with corticosteroids and monitor for weight gain; skin rash and nail disorders are usually reversible; monitor patients and bone marrow function closely during use
eribulin (*Halaven*)	1.4 mg/m² IV over 2–5 min on days 1 and 8 of 21-d course	Treatment of metastatic breast cancer in patients with at least two previous chemotherapy regimens *Special considerations:* Risk of prolonged QT interval, monitor ECG; risk of bone marrow suppression; peripheral neuropathy; alopecia may occur
etoposide (generic)	35–100 mg/m²/d IV for 4–5 d	Treatment of testicular cancers refractory to other agents; non–small cell lung carcinomas *Special considerations:* Fatigue, GI toxicity, bone marrow depression, and alopecia are common side effects; avoid direct skin contact with the drug; use protective clothing and goggles; monitor bone marrow function to adjust dose; rapid fall in blood pressure can occur during IV infusion—monitor patient carefully
ixabepilone (*Ixempra*)	40 mg/m² IV over 3 h every 3 wk	In combination with capecitabine for the treatment of patients with metastatic or locally advanced breast cancer *Special considerations:* Peripheral neuropathies are common; monitor for bone marrow suppression and hepatic impairment; dose will need to be adjusted based on these tests
paclitaxel (*Abraxane, Onxol Taxol*)	135–175 mg/m²/d IV over 3 h every 3 wk	Treatment of advanced ovarian cancer, breast cancer, non–small cell lung cancer, and AIDS-related Kaposi sarcoma *Special considerations:* Anaphylaxis and severe hypersensitivity reactions have occurred—monitor very closely during administration; also monitor for bone marrow suppression; cardiovascular toxicity and neuropathies have occurred
teniposide (*Vumon*)	165–250 mg/m² IV weekly in combination with other drugs	In combination with other drugs for induction therapy in childhood acute lymphoblastic leukemia *Special considerations:* GI toxicity, CNS effects, bone marrow suppression, and alopecia are common effects; avoid direct skin contact with the drug—use protective clothing and goggles; monitor bone marrow function to adjust dose; rapid fall in blood pressure can occur during IV infusion—monitor patient carefully
vinblastine (generic)	*Adult:* 3.7 mg/m² IV once weekly *Pediatric:* 2.5 mg/m² IV once weekly—dose may then be increased based on leukocyte count and patient response	Palliative treatment of various lymphomas and sarcomas; advanced Hodgkin disease; alone or as part of combination therapy for the treatment of advanced testicular germ cell cancers *Special considerations:* GI toxicity, CNS effects, and total loss of hair are common; antiemetics may help; avoid contact with drug; monitor injection sites for reactions
vincristine (generic)	*Adult:* 1.4 mg/m² IV at weekly intervals *Pediatric:* 1.5–2 mg/m² IV once weekly	Treatment of acute leukemia, various lymphomas, and sarcomas *Special considerations:* Extensive CNS effects are common, GI toxicity, local irritation at injection IV site, and hair loss commonly occur; syndrome of inappropriate secretion of antidiuretic hormone has been reported—monitor urine output and arrange for fluid restriction and diuretics as needed
vinorelbine (*Navelbine*)	30 mg/m² IV once weekly, based on granulocyte count	First-line treatment of unresectable advanced non–small cell lung cancer; stage IV non–small cell lung cancer and stage III non–small cell lung cancer with cisplatin *Special considerations:* GI and CNS toxicity are common; total loss of hair, local reaction at injection site, and bone marrow depression also occur; prepare a calendar with return dates for the series of injections; avoid extravasation but arrange for hyaluronidase infusion if it occurs; antiemetics may be helpful if reaction is severe

Therapeutic Actions and Indications

The mitotic inhibitors interfere with the ability of a cell to divide; they block or alter DNA synthesis, thus causing cell death. They work in the M phase of the cell cycle. These drugs are used for the treatment of a variety of tumors and leukemias. See Table 14.4 for Usual Indications for each of these agents.

FOCUS ON Safe Medication Administration

OSHA (Occupational Safety and Health Administration) and the CDC (Centers for Disease Control and Prevention) warn health care providers about the risk of exposure to antineoplastic agents. The list of hazardous drugs was updated in 2014 and includes drugs that could cause cancer, fetal death, reproductive toxicity , organ toxicity at low doses and genotoxicity. Antineoplastics generally fall into this category. Special care needs to be taken when administering these drugs. Some of these drugs must be prepared in a special setting using a hood that cuts down lung exposure. The nurse should avoid any skin, eye, or mucous membrane contact with these drugs that involves always wearing gloves when exposed to the drug, oral or injected, and may involve using protective goggles, a mask or respirator to protect the lungs, depending on the drug being used. Protecting other people is also an issue. Placing used syringes, etc. in a yellow box for biohazard disposal; double flushing patient wastes; if the patient is taking the drug at home the proper disposal of the drug and administration materials need to be stressed. Nurses working in cancer centers that do a great deal of antineoplastic drug administration receive special training to reduce the risk of exposure and to protect the health care providers and others from the potentially dangerous effects of these drugs.

Pharmacokinetics

Generally, these drugs are given intravenously because they are not well absorbed from the GI tract. They are metabolized in the liver and excreted primarily in the feces, making them safer for use in patients with renal impairment than the antineoplastics that are cleared through the kidney.

Contraindications and Cautions

These drugs should not be used during pregnancy or lactation *because of the potential risk to the fetus or neonate.* Use caution when giving these drugs to anyone with a known allergy to the drug or related drugs *to decrease the risk of serious hypersensitivity reactions.* Care is necessary for patients with the following conditions: Bone marrow suppression, *which is often the index for redosing and dosing levels*; renal or hepatic dysfunction, *which could interfere with the metabolism or excretion of these drugs and often indicates a need to change the dose*; and known GI ulcerations or ulcerative diseases, *which may be exacerbated by the effects of these drugs*; prolonged QT interval when using eribulin *which may prolong the QT interval leading to potentially serious arrhythmias.*

Adverse Effects

Adverse effects frequently encountered with the use of mitotic inhibitors include bone marrow suppression, with leukopenia, thrombocytopenia, anemia, and pancytopenia, secondary to the effects of the drugs on the rapidly multiplying cells of the bone marrow. GI effects include nausea, vomiting, anorexia, diarrhea, and mucous membrane deterioration. Eribulin is associated with prolonged QT intervals. As with the other antineoplastic agents, effects of the mitotic inhibitors may include possible hepatic or renal toxicity, depending on the exact mechanism of action. Alopecia may also occur. These drugs also cause necrosis and cellulitis if extravasation occurs, so it is necessary to regularly monitor injection sites and take appropriate action as needed.

FOCUS ON Safe Medication Administration

Preventing and Treating Extravasation

When an IV antineoplastic drug extravasates, or infiltrates into the surrounding tissue, serious tissue damage can occur. These drugs are toxic to cells, and the resulting tissue injury can result in severe pain, scarring, nerve and muscle damage, infection, and in very severe cases even amputation of the limb.

Prevention is the best way to deal with extravasation. Interventions that can help to prevent extravasation include the following: Use a distal vein, and avoid small veins on the wrist or digits; never use an existing line unless it is clearly open and running well; start the infusion with plain 5% dextrose in water (D5W) and monitor for any sign of extravasation; check the site frequently and ask the patient to report any discomfort in the area; and, if at all possible, do not use an infusion pump to administer one of these drugs because it will continue to deliver the drug under pressure and can cause severe extravasation.

If extravasation occurs, there are specific antidotes to use with some antineoplastic drugs. The antidote is usually administered through the IV line to allow it to infiltrate the same tissue, but if the line has been pulled, a tuberculin syringe can be used to inject the antidote subcutaneously into the tissue surrounding the infiltrated area.

Drug	Antidote and Suggested Dosage
etoposide teniposide vinblastine vincristine	Hyaluronidase (generic), 0.2 mL subcutaneously; then apply heat to disperse the drug and alleviate pain
daunorubicin doxorubicin vinblastine vincristine	8.4% Sodium bicarbonate, 5 mL; flush area with normal saline, apply cold compress; local infiltration with corticosteroids may also be ordered at 25–50 mg/mL of extravasate; if ulceration occurs, a plastic surgery consultation should be obtained
mechlorethamine	Isotonic sodium thiosulfate (1/6 M), 10 mL infused immediately, then apply an ice compress for 6–12 h
dactinomycin	50-mg Ascorbic acid injection; flush area with normal saline and apply cold compresses; consider the use of an injectable corticosteroid if reaction is severe

Clinically Important Drug–Drug Interactions

Mitotic inhibitors that are known to be toxic to the liver or the CNS should be used with care with any other drugs known to have the same adverse effect. Check specific drug–drug interactions for each agent in a nursing drug guide.

Ⓟ Prototype Summary: Vincristine

Indications: Acute leukemia, Hodgkin disease, non-Hodgkin lymphoma, rhabdomyosarcoma, neuroblastoma, Wilms tumor.

Actions: Arrests mitotic division at the stage of metaphase; the exact mechanism of action is not understood.

Pharmacokinetics:

Route	Onset	Peak
IV	Varies	15–30 min

$T_{1/2}$: 5 minutes, then 2.3 hours, then 85 hours; metabolized in the liver and excreted in the feces and urine.

Adverse Effects: Ataxia, cranial nerve manifestations, neuritic pain, muscle wasting, constipation, leukopenia, weight loss, loss of hair, death.

Nursing Considerations for Patients Receiving Mitotic Inhibitors

Assessment: History and Examination

- Assess for contraindications or cautions: History of allergy to the drug used (or related drugs) *to avoid hypersensitivity reactions*; bone marrow suppression *to prevent further suppression*; renal or hepatic dysfunction *that might interfere with drug metabolism and excretion*; current status of pregnancy or lactation *to prevent potentially serious adverse effects on the fetus or nursing baby*; and GI ulcerative disease, *which could be exacerbated by these drugs*; QT prolongation with eribulin *which could further prolong QT intervals.*
- Perform a physical assessment *to establish baseline data for determining the effectiveness of the drug and the occurrence of any adverse effects associated with drug therapy.*
- Assess orientation and reflexes *to evaluate any CNS effects*; skin *to evaluate for lesions*; hair and hair distribution *to monitor for adverse effects*; respiratory rate and adventitious sounds *to monitor the disease and to evaluate for respiratory or hypersensitivity effects*; and bowel sounds and mucous membrane status *to monitor for GI effects*; baseline ECG with eribulin *to monitor QT interval.*
- Monitor the results of laboratory tests such as complete blood count with differential *to identify possible bone marrow suppression and toxic drug effects*; and renal and liver function tests *to determine the need for possible dose adjustment as needed and to evaluate toxic drug effects.*
- Regularly inspect IV insertion sites *for signs of extravasation or inflammation, which need to be treated quickly.*

Nursing Diagnoses

Nursing diagnoses related to drug therapy might include the following:

- Acute pain related to GI, CNS, or local effects of the drug
- Disturbed body image related to alopecia, skin effects
- Risk for injury
- Fear, anxiety related to diagnosis and treatment
- Deficient knowledge regarding drug therapy

Planning

- The patient will receive the best therapeutic effect from the drug therapy.
- The patient will have limited adverse effects to the drug therapy.
- The patient will have an understanding of the drug therapy, adverse effects to anticipate, and measures to relieve discomfort and improve safety

Implementation with Rationale

- Arrange for blood tests to monitor bone marrow function before, periodically during, and for at least 3 weeks after therapy *to arrange to discontinue the drug or reduce the dose as needed* (see Box 14.5). Arrange for baseline and periodic ECG if using eribulin *to monitor the QT interval which could become prolonged.*
- Avoid direct skin or eye contact with the drug. Wear protective clothing and goggles while preparing and administering the drug *to prevent toxic reaction to the drug.*
- Administer medication according to scheduled protocol and in combination with other drugs as indicated *to improve the effectiveness of drug therapy.*
- Ensure that the patient is well hydrated *to decrease the risk of renal toxicity.*
- Monitor injection sites *to arrange appropriate treatment for extravasation, local inflammation, or cellulitis.*
- Protect the patient from exposure to infection *because bone marrow suppression will decrease immune/inflammatory responses.*
- Provide small, frequent meals, frequent mouth care, and dietary consultation as appropriate *to maintain nutrition if GI effects are severe.* Anticipate the need for antiemetics as necessary (see Box 14.4).
- Arrange for proper head covering at extremes of temperature if alopecia or epilation occurs; a wig, scarf, or hat *is important for maintaining body temperature.* If alopecia is an anticipated effect of drug therapy, advise

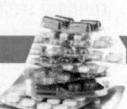

the patient to obtain a wig or head covering before the condition occurs *to promote self-esteem and a positive body image.*

- Provide the following patient teaching:
  - Follow the appropriate dosage regimen, including dates to return for further doses.
  - Maintain nutrition if GI effects are severe.
  - Cover the head at extremes of temperature if alopecia is anticipated.
  - Plan for appropriate rest periods because fatigue and weakness are common effects of the drugs.
  - Avoid situations that might lead to infection, including crowded areas, sick people, and working in the soil.
  - Use safety measures such as avoiding driving or using dangerous equipment, due to possible dizziness, headache, and drowsiness.
  - Consult with a health care provider, as appropriate, related to the possibility of impaired fertility.
  - Use barrier contraceptives to reduce the risk of pregnancy during therapy.

Evaluation

- Monitor patient response to the drug (alleviation of cancer being treated and palliation of signs and symptoms of cancer).
- Monitor for adverse effects (bone marrow suppression, GI toxicity, neurotoxicity, alopecia, renal or hepatic dysfunction, prolonged QT interval, and local reactions at the injection site).
- Evaluate the effectiveness of the teaching plan (patient can name the drug, dosage, possible adverse effects to watch for, and specific measures to help avoid adverse effects).

KEY POINTS

- Mitotic inhibitors kill cells during the M phase and are used to treat a variety of cancers.
- These drugs are usually given intravenously. Extravasation could be a serious problem
- Bone marrow suppression, alopecia, and toxic GI effects are common adverse effects of mitotic inhibitors.

Hormones and Hormone Modulators

Some cancers, particularly those involving the breast tissue, ovaries, uterus, prostate, and testes, are sensitive to estrogen stimulation. Estrogen receptor sites on the tumor react with circulating estrogen, and this reaction stimulates the tumor cells to grow and divide. Several antineoplastic agents are used to block or interfere with these receptor sites to prevent growth of the cancer and in some situations to actually cause cell death. Some hormones are used to block the release of gonadotropic hormones in breast or prostate cancer if the tumors are responsive to gonadotropic hormones. Others may block androgen receptor sites directly and are useful in the treatment of advanced prostate cancers. Hormones and hormone modulators include abiraterone (*Zytiga*), anastrazole (*Arimidex*), bicalutamide (*Casodex*), degarelix (*Firmagon*), enzalutamide (*Xtandi*), estramustine (*Emcyt*), exemestane (*Aromasin*), flutamide (generic), fulvestrant (*Faslodex*), goserelin (*Zoladex*), histrelin (*Vantas*), letrozole (*Femara*), leuprolide (*Lupron, Eligard*), megestrol (*Megace*), mitotane (*Lysodren*), nilutamide (*Nilandron*), tamoxifen (*Soltamox*), toremifene (*Fareston*), and triptorelin pamoate (*Trelstar*) (Table 14.5).

Therapeutic Actions and Indications

The hormones and hormone modulators used as antineoplastics are receptor site specific or hormone specific to block the stimulation of growing cancer cells that are sensitive to the presence of that hormone (see Figure 14.4). These drugs are indicated for the treatment of breast cancer in postmenopausal women or in other women without ovarian function. Some drugs are indicated for the treatment of prostatic cancers that are sensitive to hormone manipulation. Table 14.5 shows Usual Indications for each of the hormones and hormone modulators.

Pharmacokinetics

These drugs are readily absorbed from the GI tract, metabolized in the liver, and excreted in the urine. Caution must be used with any patient who has hepatic or renal impairment. These drugs cross the placenta and enter into breast milk.

Contraindications and Cautions

These drugs are contraindicated during pregnancy and lactation *because of toxic effects on the fetus and neonate.* Hypercalcemia is a contraindication to the use of toremifene, *which is known to increase calcium levels.* Use caution when giving hormones and hormone modulators to anyone with a known allergy to any of these drugs *to prevent hypersensitivity reactions.* Care is necessary in patients with bone marrow suppression, *which is often the index for redosing and dosing levels,* and in those with renal or hepatic dysfunction, *which could interfere with the metabolism or excretion of these drugs and often indicates a need to change the dose.*

Adverse Effects

Adverse effects frequently encountered with the use of these drugs involve the effects that are seen when estrogen is blocked or inhibited. Menopause-associated effects include hot flashes, vaginal spotting, vaginal dryness, moodiness, and depression. Other effects include bone marrow suppression and GI toxicity, including hepatic dysfunction. Hypercalcemia is also encountered as the calcium is pulled out of the bones without estrogen activity to promote calcium deposition. Many of these drugs increase the risk for cardiovascular disease because of their effects on the body. Abiraterone can increase the risk of adrenocortical insufficiency.

Table 14.5 *Drugs in Focus:* **Hormones and Hormone Modulators**

Drug Name	Dosage/Route	Usual Indications
abiraterone (*Zytiga*)	1,000 mg/d PO with 5-mg prednisone	Treatment of metastatic, castration-resistant prostate cancer in men who have received prior chemotherapy *Actions:* Androgen biosynthesis inhibitor *Special considerations:* Risk of mineral corticoid excess and cardiovascular events; liver toxicity; must be taken on an empty stomach; GI effects common
anastrazole (*Arimidex*)	1 mg/d PO	Treatment of advanced breast cancer in postmenopausal women after tamoxifen therapy; first-line and adjunctive treatment of postmenopausal women with locally advanced breast cancer *Actions:* Antiestrogen drug; blocks estradiol production without effects on adrenal hormones *Special considerations:* GI effects, signs and symptoms of menopause—hot flashes, mood swings, edema, vaginal dryness and itching—as well as bone pain and back pain, treatable with analgesics, may occur; monitor lipid concentrations in patients at risk for high cholesterol level
bicalutamide (*Casodex*)	50 mg/d PO	In combination with a luteinizing hormone for the treatment of advanced prostate cancer *Actions:* Antiandrogen drug that competitively binds androgen receptor sites *Special considerations:* Gynecomastia and breast tenderness occur in 33% of patients; GI complaints are common; pregnancy category X
degarelix (*Firmagon*)	240 mg by subcutaneous injection given in two 120-mg injections, then 80 mg subcutaneous every 28 d for maintenance	Treatment of patients with advanced prostate cancer *Actions:* Gonadotropin-releasing hormone receptor site antagonist, leads to decreased follicle-stimulating hormone and luteinizing hormone and decreased testosterone levels *Special considerations:* Pregnancy category X; risk of prolonged QT interval; injection site reactions, hot flashes, increased weight are common
enzalutamide (*Xtandi*)	160 mg/d PO	Treatment of metastatic, castration-resistant prostate cancer in men who have received prior chemotherapy *Actions:* Androgen receptor inhibitor *Special considerations:* Swallow capsules whole; pregnancy category X; GI effects, spinal cord compression, hypertension, anxiety, dizziness; reacts with many drugs, check drug regimen carefully
estramustine (*Emcyt*)	10–16 mg/kg/d PO in three to four divided doses for 30–90 d, then reevaluate	Palliative for treatment of metastatic and progressive prostate cancer *Actions:* Binds to estrogen steroid receptors, causing cell death *Special considerations:* GI toxicity, rash, bone marrow depression, breast tenderness, and cardiovascular toxicity are common adverse effects; 30–90 d of therapy may be required before effects are seen; monitor cardiovascular, liver, and bone marrow function throughout therapy
exemestane (*Aromasin*)	25 mg/d PO with meals	Treatment of advanced, metastatic breast cancer in postmenopausal women whose disease has progressed after tamoxifen therapy; adjunct treatment of postmenopausal women who have receptor-positive early breast cancer who have received tamoxifen for 2–3 y to finish 5-y course *Actions:* Inactivates steroid aromatase, lowering circulating estrogen levels and preventing the conversion of androgens to estrogen *Special considerations:* Avoid use in premenopausal women or in patients with liver or renal dysfunction; hot flashes, headache, GI upset, anxiety, and depression are common
flutamide (generic)	250 mg PO t.i.d. given 8 h apart	With a luteinizing hormone for treatment of locally confined and metastatic prostate cancer *Actions:* Antiestrogenic drug, inhibits androgen uptake and binding on target cells *Special considerations:* May cause liver toxicity, so liver function should be monitored regularly; associated with impaired fertility and cancer development; urine may become greenish; protect patient from exposure to the sun—photosensitivity is common

Drug Name	Dosage/Route	Usual Indications
fulvestrant (*Faslodex*)	250 mg IM at 1-mo intervals	Treatment of hormone receptor–positive metastatic breast cancer in postmenopausal women with disease progression after antiestrogen therapy *Actions:* Competitively binds to estrogen receptors, downregulating the estrogen receptor protein in breast cancer cells *Special considerations:* Pregnancy category X; hot flashes, depression, headache, and GI upset are common; mark calendar with monthly injection dates; injection site reactions may occur
goserelin (*Zoladex*)	3.6–10.8-mg implant, subcutaneous, every 28 d to 12 wk, varies with diagnosis	Treatment of advanced prostatic and breast cancers; management of endometriosis *Actions:* Synthetic luteinizing hormone that inhibits pituitary release of gonadotropic hormones *Special considerations:* A 3.6-mg dose is effective in decreasing the signs and symptoms of endometriosis; associated with hypercalcemia and bone density loss—monitor serum calcium levels regularly; impairs fertility and is carcinogenic; monitor male patients for possible ureteral obstruction, especially during month 1
histrelin (*Vantas*)	50-mg implant every 12 mo	Palliative treatment of advanced prostate cancer *Actions:* Inhibits gonadotropic secretion; decreases follicle-stimulating hormone and luteinizing hormone levels and testosterone levels *Special considerations:* Must be surgically implanted and removed; hot flashes very common; monitor implantation site
letrozole (*Femara*)	2.5 mg/d PO	Treatment of advanced breast cancer in postmenopausal women with disease after antiestrogen therapy; postsurgery adjunct for postmenopausal women with early hormone receptor–positive breast cancer who have had 5 y of tamoxifen *Actions:* Prevents the conversion of precursors to estrogens in all tissues *Special considerations:* GI toxicity, bone marrow depression, alopecia, hot flashes, and CNS depression are common effects; discontinue drug at any sign that the cancer is progressing
leuprolide (*Lupron*, *Eligard*)	3.7–30 mg by injection, implant, or depot every 1–4 mo, depending on preparation used	Treatment of advanced prostate cancer; also used to treat precocious puberty and endometriosis; depot form for uterine leiomyomata *Actions:* A natural luteinizing hormone that blocks the release of gonadotropic hormones *Special considerations:* Monitor cancer patient's prostate-specific antigen levels periodically; monitor bone density and serum calcium levels; warn patient that he may have difficulty voiding the first few weeks and may experience bone pain, hot flashes, and pain at injection site
megestrol (*Megace*)	*Breast cancer:* 160 mg/d PO *Endometrial cancer:* 40–320 mg/d *PO* *appetite stimulant:* 400–800 mg/d suspension PO	Palliative treatment of advanced breast or endometrial cancer; appetite stimulant for HIV patients *Actions:* Blocks luteinizing hormone release; efficacy not understood *Special considerations:* Monitor for thromboembolic events and weight gain; not for use during pregnancy
mitotane (*Lysodren*)	2–6 mg PO in divided doses t.i.d. to q.i.d.; maximum dose 9–10 g/d	Treatment of inoperable adrenocortical carcinoma *Actions:* Cytotoxic to corticosteroid-forming cells of the adrenal gland *Special considerations:* Can cause GI toxicity, CNS toxicity with vision and behavioral changes, adrenal insufficiency; monitor adrenal function, and arrange for replacement therapy as indicated
nilutamide (*Nilandron*)	300 mg/d PO for 30 d, then 150 mg/d PO	With surgical castration for treatment of metastatic prostate cancer *Actions:* Antiestrogenic drug, inhibits androgen uptake and binding on target cells *Special considerations:* May cause liver toxicity, and liver function test results should be monitored regularly; associated with interstitial pneumonitis—baseline and periodic chest radiographs should be obtained and drug discontinued at first sign of dyspnea

(table continues on page 238)

Table 14.5 ***Drugs in Focus:* Hormones and Hormone Modulators (*continued*)**

Drug Name	Dosage/Route	Usual Indications
tamoxifen (*Soltamox*)	20–40 mg/d PO	In combination therapy with surgery to treat breast cancer; treatment of advanced breast cancer in men and women; first drug approved for the prevention of breast cancer in women at high risk for breast cancer *Actions:* Antiestrogen, competes with estrogen for receptor sites in target tissues *Special considerations:* Signs and symptoms of menopause are common effects; CNS depression, bone marrow depression, and GI toxicity are also common; can change visual acuity and cause corneal opacities and retinopathy—pretherapy and periodic ophthalmic examinations are indicated
toremifene (*Fareston*)	60 mg/d PO	Treatment of advanced breast cancer in women with estrogen receptor–positive disease *Actions:* Binds to estrogen receptors and prevents growth of breast cancer cells *Special considerations:* Signs and symptoms of menopause are common effects; CNS depression and GI toxicity are also common
triptorelin pamoate (*Trelstar Depot*)	3.75 mg IM depot monthly *or* 11.25 mg IM depot every 3 mo *or* 22.5 mg IM depot every 6 mo	Treatment of advanced prostatic cancer *Actions:* Analogue of luteinizing hormone–releasing hormone; causes a decrease in follicle-stimulating hormone and luteinizing hormone levels, leading to a suppression of testosterone production. *Special considerations:* Monitor prostate-specific antigen and testosterone levels regularly; sexual dysfunction, urinary tract symptoms, bone pain, and hot flashes are common; schedule depot injections and mark calendars for patient

Clinically Important Drug–Drug Interactions

If hormones and hormone modulators are taken with oral anticoagulants, there is often an increased risk of bleeding. Care is also necessary when administering these agents with any drugs that might increase serum lipid levels.

Ⓟ Prototype Summary: Tamoxifen

Indications: Treatment of metastatic breast cancer, reduction of risk of invasive breast cancer in women with ductal carcinoma in situ, reduction in occurrence of contralateral breast cancer in patients receiving adjuvant tamoxifen therapy, reduction in incidence of breast cancer in women at high risk for breast cancer, treatment of McCune-Albright syndrome, and treatment of precocious puberty in female patients 2 to 10 years of age.

Actions: Competes with estrogen for binding sites in target tissues, such as the breast; a potent antiestrogenic agent.

Pharmacokinetics:

Route	Onset	Peak
Oral	Varies	4–7 h

$T_{1/2}$: 7 to 14 days; metabolized in the liver and excreted in the feces.

Adverse Effects: Hot flashes, rash, nausea, vomiting, vaginal bleeding, menstrual irregularities, edema, pain, cerebrovascular accident, pulmonary emboli.

Nursing Considerations for Patients Receiving Hormones and Hormone Modulators

Assessment: History and Examination

- Assess for contraindications or cautions: History of allergy to the drug in use or any related drugs *to avoid hypersensitivity reactions*; bone marrow suppression *to prevent further suppression*; renal or hepatic dysfunction *that might interfere with drug metabolism and excretion*; current status of pregnancy or lactation *to prevent potentially serious adverse effects on the fetus or nursing baby*; history of hypercalcemia and hypercholesterolemia *to avoid further increases in levels.*
- Perform a physical assessment *to establish baseline data for determining the effectiveness of the drug and the occurrence of any adverse effects associated with drug therapy.*
- Assess orientation and reflexes *to evaluate any CNS effects*; skin *to evaluate for lesions*; hair and hair distribution *to monitor for adverse drug effects*; blood pressure, pulse, and perfusion *to evaluate the status of the cardiovascular system and monitor for adverse drug effects*; and bowel sounds and mucous membrane status *to monitor for GI effects.*
- Monitor the results of laboratory tests such as complete blood count with differential to identify bone marrow suppression and toxic drug effects, serum calcium

levels to evaluate for hypercalcemia, and renal and liver function tests *to determine the need for possible dose adjustment to evaluate toxic drug effects.*

See the Critical Thinking Scenario for a full discussion of assessing and evaluating antineoplastic therapy for a patient with breast cancer.

Nursing Diagnoses

Nursing diagnoses related to drug therapy might include the following:

- Acute pain related to GI, CNS, or menopausal effects of the drug
- Disturbed body image related to antiestrogen effects, virilization
- Fear, anxiety related to diagnosis and treatment
- Deficient knowledge regarding drug therapy

Planning

- The patient will receive the best therapeutic effect from the drug therapy.
- The patient will have limited adverse effects to the drug therapy.
- The patient will have an understanding of the drug therapy, adverse effects to anticipate, and measures to relieve discomfort and improve safety.

Implementation with Rationale

- Arrange for blood tests to monitor bone marrow function before and periodically during therapy *to discontinue the drug or reduce the dose as needed* (see Box 14.5)
- Provide small, frequent meals, frequent mouth care, and dietary consultation as appropriate *to maintain nutrition when GI effects are severe.*
- Provide comfort measures *to help the patient cope with menopausal signs and symptoms* such as hygiene measures, temperature control, and stress reduction. Expect to reduce the dose if these effects become severe or intolerable.
- Advise the patient of the need to use barrier contraceptive measures while taking these drugs *to avert serious fetal harm.*
- Provide the following patient teaching:
  - Follow the appropriate dosage regimen, including dates to return for further doses.
  - Maintain nutrition even if GI effects are severe.
  - Use barrier contraceptives to prevent pregnancy during therapy
  - Try using comfort measures such as staying in a cool environment.
  - Perform hygiene and skin care and use measures to reduce stress to help cope with menopausal effects.
  - You may need to have periodic blood tests to monitor the effects of this drug on your body.

Evaluation

- Monitor patient response to the drug (alleviation of cancer being treated and palliation of signs and symptoms of cancer being treated).
- Monitor for adverse effects (bone marrow suppression, GI toxicity, menopausal signs and symptoms, hypercalcemia, and cardiovascular effects).
- Evaluate the effectiveness of the teaching plan (patient can name the drug, dosage, possible adverse effects to watch for, and specific measures to help avoid adverse effects).

KEY POINTS

- Hormones and hormonal agents are used to treat specific cancers that respond to hormone stimulation such as breast cancer or prostate cancer.
- The adverse effects of hormones and hormonal agent used to treat cancers are increased or decreased effects of the hormones on the body: Virilization, increased risk of cardiovascular disease, increased calcium levels.

Cancer Cell–Specific Agents

The goal of much of the current antineoplastic drug research is directed at finding drugs that are cancer cell specific. These drugs would not have the devastating effects on healthy cells in the body and would be more effective against particular cancer cells. Drugs that are available for cancer cell–specific actions include protein tyrosine kinase inhibitors, an epidermal growth factor inhibitor, and a proteasome inhibitor (Table 14.6). Many monoclonal antibodies have also been developed for specific cancers. These drugs are discussed in Chapter 17.

Protein Tyrosine Kinase Inhibitors

The protein kinase inhibitors (Table 14.6) act on specific enzymes that are needed for protein building by specific tumor cells. Blocking these enzymes inhibits tumor cell growth and division.

Each drug that has been developed inhibits a very specific protein kinase and acts on very specific tumors. They do not affect healthy human cells, so the patient does not experience the numerous adverse effects associated with antineoplastic chemotherapy. Imatinib (*Gleevec*), the first drug approved in this class, is given orally and is approved to treat chronic myelocytic leukemia (CML), several GI stromal tumors, various myeloproliferative disorders, aggressive systemic mastocytosis, and unresectable dermatofibrosarcoma protuberans. When the drug was first introduced patients who had CML and who had been switched to imatinib after traditional chemotherapy were

Table 14.6 ***Drugs in Focus:* Cancer Cell–Specific Agents**

Drug Name	Dosage/Route	Usual Indications
Protein Tyrosine Kinase Inhibitors		
afatinib (*Gilotrif*)	40 mg/d PO at least 1 h before or 2 h after a meal	Treatment of metastatic non–small cell lung cancer in tumors with epidermal growth factor receptor exon 19 deletion or exon 21 substitution *Special considerations:* Monitor liver and renal function; severe GI effects possible; risk of dehydration; not for use in pregnancy
Axitinib (*Inlyta*)	5 mg PO b.i.d., 12 h apart with a full glass of water	Treatment of advanced renal cell cancer after failure of one prior therapy *Special considerations:* GI perforation, hemorrhage, hepatic injury, hypertensive crisis, thrombotic events, renal injury possible
bosutinib (*Bosulif*)	500–600 mg/d PO	Treatment of accelerated blast cell–phase Philadelphia chromosome–positive CML with resistance to other therapy *Special considerations:* Severe GI toxicity; bone marrow suppression, hepatotoxicity, and fluid retention are possible
cabozantinib (*Cometriq*)	140 mg/d PO	Treatment of progressive, metastatic medullary thyroid cancer *Special considerations:* Thrombotic events, osteonecrosis of the jaw, hypertension, wound complications; monitor patient carefully
ceretinib (*Zykadia*)	750 mg/d PO on an empty stomach	Treatment of anaplastic lymphoma kinase–positive metastatic non–small cell lung cancer who have progressed after crizotinib therapy *Special considerations:* Severe GI toxicity, dose modification may be required; hepatotoxicity, interstitial lung disease, prolonged QT interval, hyperglycemia, bradycardia possible; not for use in pregnancy
crizotinib (*Xalkori*)	250 mg PO bid	Treatment of anaplastic lymphoma kinase–positive metastatic non–small cell lung cancer *Special considerations:* Hepatic toxicity, potentially fatal pneumonitis, prolonged QT interval; ensure proper use of drug
dabrafenib (*Tafinlar*)	100 mg/d PO on an empty stomach	Treatment of locally advanced non–small cell lung cancer; pancreatic cancer *Special considerations:* Bleeding, hemolytic anemia, GI perforation, hepatic toxicity, interstitial pneumonitis, exfoliative skin disorders; monitor patient very carefully
everolimus (*Afinitor*)	5–10 mg/d PO with food *Pediatric with tuberous sclerosis:* 4.5 mg/m²/day PO	Treatment of patients with advanced renal cell carcinoma after failure of treatment with sunitinib or sorafenib; treatment of tuberous sclerosis complex with brain tumor *Special considerations:* Pneumonitis, serious to fatal infections, oral ulcerations, and elevations in blood glucose, lipid, and creatinine levels may occur; monitor patient very closely; do not use in pregnancy
ibrutinib (*Imbruvica*)	560 mg/d PO	Treatment of mantle cell lymphoma after at least one other regimen *Special considerations:* Bone marrow suppression, secondary malignancy; monitor bone marrow function; screen for cancers
idelalisib (*Zydelig*)	150 mg PO b.i.d.	Treatment of relapsed CLL, relapsed follicular B-cell non-Hodgkin lymphoma, relapsed small lymphocytic lymphoma *Special considerations:* Serious cutaneous reactions, anaphylaxis; monitor blood counts, not for use in pregnancy
imatinib (*Gleevec*)	*Chronic-phase CML:* 400 mg/d PO, may be increased to 600 mg/d if needed *Blast-crisis CML:* 600 mg/d PO, may be increased to 400 mg PO b.i.d. *First-line CML treatment:* 400 mg/d PO *GI stromal tumors:* 400–600 mg/d PO *Aggressive systemic mastocytosis:* 400 mg/day PO *Dermatofibrosarcoma protuberans:* 800 mg/d PO	Treatment of CML patients in blast crisis or in chronic phase after interferon-alpha therapy; treatment of patients with Kit-positive malignant GIST; first-line treatment of CML; aggressive systemic mastocytosis; dermatofibrosarcoma protuberans *Special considerations:* Administer with a meal and a full glass of water; arrange for small, frequent meals if GI upset is a problem; provide analgesics for headache and muscle pain; monitor complete blood count and for edema to arrange for dose reduction if needed; patient should receive consultation to deal with high cost of drug
lapatinib (*Tykerb*)	*Advanced or metastatic breast cancer:* 1,250 mg (5 tablets) orally once daily on days 1–21 in combination with capecitabine 2,000 mg/m²/d PO in 2 doses approximately 12 h apart on days 1–14; give in a repeating 21-d cycle; reduce dose to 750 mg/d PO with severe hepatic dysfunction *Hormone receptor positive metastatic breast cancer:* 1,500 mg/d PO with letrozole 2.5 mg/d PO	In combination with capecitabine for the treatment of patients with advanced or metastatic breast cancer whose tumors overexpress HER2 and who have received prior treatment including anthracycline, taxane, and trastuzumab; treatment of HER2-positive metastatic breast cancer with letrozole *Special considerations:* Monitor heart function closely and decrease dose as needed; monitor for rash, GI toxicity; avoid grapefruit juice; many drug–drug interactions are possible

Drug Name	Dosage/Route	Usual Indications
Protein Tyrosine Kinase Inhibitors		
nilotinib (*Tasigna*)	400 mg PO b.i.d., approximately 12 h apart without food	Treatment of chronic-phase and accelerated-phase Philadelphia chromosome–positive chronic myelogenous leukemia in adult patients resistant or intolerant to prior therapy that included imatinib *Special considerations:* Monitor for prolonged QT interval, bone marrow suppression, and possible liver toxicity
palbociclib (*Ibrance*)	125 mg/d PO for 21 days with food, followed by 7 days of rest	Treatment of postmenopausal, ER-positive, HER2-negative advanced breast cancer with letrozole *Special considerations:* Monitor for infections, bone marrow suppression; interacts with many drugs; not for use in pregnancy
pazopanib (*Votrient*)	800 mg/d PO without food; reduce dose with hepatic impairment	Treatment of advanced renal cell carcinoma *Special considerations:* Monitor for prolonged QT interval; fatal hemorrhagic events have been reported; GI perforation and fistulas, hypertension, hypothyroidism have been reported; common effects include diarrhea, depigmentation of hair, and GI upset
ponatinib (*Iclusig*)	45 mg/d PO with food, adjust dose based on toxicity	Treatment of T3151-positive CML, T3151-positive ALL *Special considerations:* Hepatotoxicity, heart failure possible; monitor closely; not for use in pregnancy or breastfeeding
regorafenib (*Stivarga*)	160 mg/d PO for first 21 d of 28-d cycle with low-fat breakfast	Treatment of previously treated metastatic colorectal cancer; treatment of unresectable GI stromal tumors *Special considerations:* Risk of GI perforation, hepatotoxicity, MI, arrhythmias, dermatological toxicity; reacts with many drugs and grapefruit juice; stop 24 h before any surgery; not for use in pregnancy or breastfeeding
ruxolitinib (*Jakafi*)	20–25 mg PO b.i.d.	Treatment of intermittent, high-risk myelofibrosis *Special considerations:* Stop after 6 mo if no sign of spleen reduction; monitor for infections; safety precautions if dizziness is an issue
sorafenib (*Nexavar*)	400 mg PO b.i.d. on an empty stomach	Treatment of patients with advanced renal cell carcinoma and unresectable hepatocellular carcinoma *Special considerations:* Monitor for skin reactions, hand–foot syndrome, hypertension
sunitinib (*Sutent*)	50 mg/d PO for 4 wk, followed by 2 wk of rest; repeat cycle *Pancreatic tumors:* 37.5 mg/d PO continuously	Treatment of GIST, advanced renal cell cancer, progressive neuroendocrine cancerous pancreatic tumors *Special considerations:* Monitor for GI disturbances, bone marrow suppression; adjust dose as needed
temsirolimus (*Torisel*)	25 mg IV, infused over 30–60 min once per week, given 30 min after diphenhydramine 25–50 mg IV	Treatment of advanced renal cell carcinoma *Special considerations:* Monitor lung function, blood glucose, renal function; may experience slowed healing; avoid grapefruit juice, St. John's wort
trametinib (*Mekinist*)	2 mg/d PO, 1 h before or 2 h after a meal	Treatment of unresectable or metastatic melanoma with BRAF V600E or V600K mutations *Special considerations:* Ensure regular ophthalmic exams; serious vision changes to blindness possible; monitor LV function at least every 3 mo as serious cardiomyopathy can occur; interstitial pneumonitis possible; serious to fatal dermatological reactions.
vemurafenib (*Zelboraf*)	960 mg PO b.i.d., 12 h apart	Treatment of unresectable or metastatic melanoma with appropriate BRAF mutations *Special considerations:* Serious ophthalmologic damage; dermatologic toxicity with risk of Stevens-Johnson syndrome; new malignant melanoma; squamous cell carcinoma; liver toxicity; prolonged QT interval; assure proper use; monitor closely
ziv-aflibercept (*Zaltrap*)	4 mg/kg IV over 1 h every 2 wk	Treatment of metastatic colon cancer to oxaliplatin as part of combo therapy *Special considerations:* GI toxicity; thrombotic events; proteinuria; bone marrow suppression; do not use within 4 wk of surgery; contraceptive use during and for 3 mo after therapy
Epidermal Growth Factor Inhibitor		
erlotinib (*Tarceva*)	150 mg/d PO, 1 h before or 2 h after meal	Treatment of unresectable metastatic melanoma with BRAF V600E mutations *Special considerations:* Cutaneous malignancies, hemolytic anemia, tumor progression; loss of hair is possible

(table continues on page 242)

Table 14.6 Drugs in Focus: Cancer Cell–Specific Agents (continued)

Drug Name	Dosage/Route	Usual Indications
Proteasome Inhibitor		
bortezomib (*Velcade*)	1.3 mg/m² as a 3–5 s IV bolus or subcutaneously for nine 6-d cycles on days 1, 4, 8, 11, then 10 days of rest, 22, 25, 29, and 32	Treatment of multiple myeloma in patients with disease progression after two other therapies *Special considerations:* May cause peripheral neuropathies, hypotension, and bone marrow suppression; do not use during pregnancy

CML, chronic myelocytic leukemia; CLL, chronic lymphocytic leukemia; GIST, gastrointestinal stromal tumor; HER2, human epidermal receptor 2; ALL, acute lymphocytic leukemia; MI, myocardial infarction; BRAF, a gene on chromosome 7q34.

amazed at how good they felt and how much they recovered from the numerous adverse effects of the traditional chemotherapy. However, long-term effects include development of new cancers, cardiac toxicity, and bone marrow suppression. Unfortunately, this drug is expensive. It is estimated that 1 year of treatment with the drug (which needs to be taken continually) costs the patient between $30,000 and $35,000. Novartis, the drug company that manufactures *Gleevec*, has set up a patient assistance program with a sliding-scale price reduction based on income. They do not want patients to have to pay more than 20% of their annual income for the drug. Patients prescribed this drug may need support and assistance in obtaining financial help. Because they are relatively new to the market, all of the kinase inhibitors are relatively expensive. The protein tyrosine kinase inhibitors that are available include afatinib (*Gilotrif*), axitinib (*Inlyta*), bosutinib (*Bosulif*), cabozantinib (*Cometriq*), ceretinib (*Zykadia*), crizotinib (*Xalkori*), dabrafenib (*Tafinlar*), everolimus (*Afinitor*), ibrutinib (*Imbruvica*), idelalisib (*Zydeliq*), imatinib (*Gleevec*), lapatinib (*Tykerb*), nilotinib (*Tasigna*), palbociclib (*Ibrance*), pazopanib (*Vorient*), ponatinib (*Iclusig*), regorafenib (*Stivarga*), ruxolitinib (*Jakafi*), sorafenib (*Nexavar*), sunitinib (*Sutent*), and temsirolimus (*Torisel*), trametinib (*Mekinist*), vemurafenib (*Zelboraf*), and ziv-aflibercept (*Zaltrap*).

CRITICAL THINKING SCENARIO

Antineoplastic Therapy and Breast Cancer

THE SITUATION

B.P., a 34-year-old white woman, is a school teacher with two young daughters. She noticed a slightly painful lump under her arm when showering. About 2 weeks later, she found a mass in her right breast. Initial patient assessment found that she had no other underlying medical problems, had no allergies, and took no medications. Her family history was most indicative: Many of the women in her family—her mother, two grandmothers, three aunts, two older sisters, and one younger sister—died of breast cancer when they were in their early 30s. All data from the initial examination, including an evaluation of the lump in the upper outer quadrant of her breast and the presence of a fixed axillary node, were recorded as baseline data for further drug therapy and treatment. B.P. underwent a radical mastectomy with biopsy report for grade IV infiltrating ductal carcinoma (28 of 35 lymph nodes were positive for tumor) and then radiation therapy. Then she began a 1-year course of doxorubicin, cyclophosphamide, and paclitaxel (AC/paclitaxel/sequential).

CRITICAL THINKING

What are the important nursing implications for B.P.? *Think about the outlook for B.P., based on her biopsy results and her family history.*

What are the effects of high levels of stress on the immune system and the body's ability to fight cancer?

What impact will this disease have on B.P.'s job and her family? *Think about the adverse drug effects that can be anticipated.*

How can good patient teaching help B.P. to anticipate and cope with these many changes and unpleasant effects?

What future concerns should be addressed or at least approached at this point in the treatment of B.P.'s disease?

What are the implications for her two daughters?

How may a coordinated health team work to help the daughters cope with their mother's disease, as well as the prospects for their future?

DISCUSSION

The extent of B.P.'s disease, as evidenced by the biopsy results, does not signify a very hopeful prognosis. In this case the overall nursing care plan should take into account not only the acute needs related to surgery and drug therapy, but also future needs related to potential debilitation and even the prospect of death. Immediate needs include comfort and teaching measures to help B.P. deal with the mastectomy and

Antineoplastic Therapy and Breast Cancer (continued)

recovery from the surgery. She should be given an opportunity to vent her feelings and thoughts in a protected environment. Efforts should be made to help her to organize her life and plans around her radiation therapy and chemotherapy.

The adverse effects associated with the antineoplastic agents she will be given should be explained and possible ways to cope should be discussed. These effects include the following:

Alopecia. B.P. should be reassured that her hair will grow back, but she will need to cover her head in extremes of temperature. Purchasing a wig before the hair loss begins may be a good alternative to trying to remember later what her hair was like.

Nausea and vomiting. These effects will most often occur immediately after the drugs are given. Antiemetics may be ordered, but they are frequently not very effective.

Bone marrow suppression. This will make B.P. more susceptible to disease, which could be a problem for a teacher and a mother with young children. Ways to avoid contact and infection, as well as warning signs to report immediately, should be discussed.

Mouth sores. Stomatitis and mucositis are common problems. Frequent mouth care is important. The patient should be encouraged to maintain fluid intake and nutrition.

Because the antineoplastic therapy will be a long-term regimen, it might help to prepare a calendar of drug dates for use in planning other activities and events. All of B.P.'s treatment should be incorporated into a team approach that helps B.P. and her family deal with the impact of this disease and its therapy, as well as with the potential risk to her daughters. B.P.'s daughters are in a very high–risk group for this disease, so the importance of frequent examinations as they grow up needs to be stressed. In some areas of the country, health care providers are encouraging prophylactic mastectomies for women in this very high–risk group.

NURSING CARE GUIDE FOR B.P.: ANTINEOPLASTIC AGENTS

Assessment: History and Examination

Allergies to any of these drugs, renal or hepatic dysfunction, pregnancy or lactation, bone marrow suppression, or GI ulceration.

Concurrent use of ketoconazole, diazepam, verapamil, quinidine, dexamethasone, cisplatin, cyclosporine, teniposide, etoposide, vincristine, testosterone, digoxin which could interact with these drugs.

Local: Evaluation of injection site.

CNS: Orientation, affect, reflexes.

Skin: Color, lesions, texture.

GI: Abdominal, liver evaluation.

Laboratory tests: Complete blood count with differential; renal and hepatic function tests.

Nursing Diagnoses

Acute pain related to GI, CNS, or skin effects

Imbalanced nutrition: Less than body requirements related to GI effects

Disturbed body image related to diagnosis, therapy, adverse effects

Deficient knowledge regarding drug therapy

Risk for infection

Fear related to diagnosis and effects of drug treatment

Planning

The patient will receive the best therapeutic effect from the drug therapy.

The patient will have limited adverse effects to the drug therapy.

The patient will have an understanding of the drug therapy, adverse effects to anticipate, and measures to relieve discomfort and improve safety.

Implementation

Ensure safe administration of the drug.

Provide comfort and safety measures: Mouth and skin care, rest periods, safety precautions, antiemetics as needed, maintenance of nutrition, and head covering.

Provide support and reassurance to deal with drug effects, body image changes, discomfort, and diagnosis.

Provide patient teaching regarding drug name, dosage, adverse effects, precautions to take, signs and symptoms to report, and comfort measures to observe.

Evaluation

Evaluate drug effects: Resolution of cancer.

Monitor for adverse effects: GI toxicity, bone marrow suppression, CNS changes, renal and hepatic damage, alopecia, extravasation of drug.

Monitor for drug–drug interactions as listed.

Evaluate effectiveness of patient-teaching program.

Evaluate effectiveness of comfort and safety measures.

PATIENT TEACHING FOR B.P.

Antineoplastic agents work to destroy cells at various phases of their life cycle. The drugs are given in combination to affect the cells at these various stages. These drugs are prescribed to kill cancer cells that are growing in the body. Because these drugs also affect normal cells, they sometimes cause many adverse effects. Your drug combination includes doxorubicin, cyclophosphamide, and paclitaxel.

- These drugs are given in a 21-day cycle, followed by a rest period. You will need to mark your calendar with the treatment days and rest days. You will need to have regular blood tests to follow the effects of these drugs on your blood cells.

(continues on page 244)

Antineoplastic Therapy and Breast Cancer (continued)

- Common adverse effects of these drugs include the following:
  - *Nausea and vomiting.* Antiemetic drugs and sedatives may help. Your health care provider will be with you to help if these effects occur.
  - *Loss of appetite.* It is very important to keep up your strength. Tell people if there is something that you would be interested in eating—anything that appeals to you. Alert someone if you feel hungry, regardless of the time of day.
  - *Loss of hair.* Your hair will grow back, although its color or consistency may be different from what it was originally. It may help to purchase a wig before you lose your hair so that you can match appearance if you would like to. Hats and scarves may also be worn. It is very important to keep your head covered in extremes of temperature and to protect yourself from sun, heat, and cold. Because much of the body's heat can be lost through the head, not protecting yourself could cause serious problems.
  - *Mouth sores.* Frequent mouth care is very helpful. Try to avoid very hot or spicy foods.
  - *Fatigue, malaise.* Frequent rest periods and careful planning of your day's activities can be very helpful.
  - *Bleeding.* You may bruise more easily than you normally do, and your gums may bleed while you are brushing your teeth. Special care should be taken when shaving or brushing your teeth. Avoid activities that might cause an injury, and avoid medications that contain aspirin.
  - *Susceptibility to infection.* Avoid people with infections or colds, and avoid crowded, public places. In some cases the people who are caring for you may wear gowns and masks to protect you from their germs. Avoid working in your garden because soil is full of bacteria.
- Report any of the following to your health care provider: Bruising and bleeding, fever, chills, sore throat, difficulty breathing, flank pain, and swelling in your ankles or fingers.
- Take the full course of your prescription. It is very important to take the complete regimen that has been ordered for you. Cancer cells grow at different rates, and they go through rest periods during which they are not susceptible to the drugs. The disease must be attacked over time to eradicate the problem.
- Tell any doctor, nurse, or other health care provider that you are taking this drug.
- Try to maintain a balanced diet while you are taking this drug. Drink 10 to 12 glasses of water each day during the drug therapy.
- For the time that these drugs are being taken, you are urged to use a barrier contraceptive. These drugs can cause serious effects to a developing fetus, and precautions must be taken to avoid pregnancy. If you think that you are pregnant, consult your health care provider immediately.
- You need to have periodic blood tests and examinations while you are taking this drug. These tests help to guard against serious adverse effects and may be needed to determine the next dose of your drug.

Epidermal Growth Factor Inhibitor

In late 2004 the U.S. Food and Drug Administration (FDA) approved erlotinib (*Tarceva*), a drug that inhibits cell epidermal growth factor receptors. This growth factor is found on normal and cancerous cells but is more abundant on rapidly growing cells.

Proteasome Inhibitor

In 2003 the FDA approved bortezomib (*Velcade*) for the treatment of multiple myeloma in patients whose disease had progressed after two other standard therapies. This drug inhibits proteasome in human cells, a large protein complex that works to maintain cell homeostasis and protein production. Without it the cell loses homeostasis and dies. This drug was shown to delay growth in selected tumors.

Therapeutic Actions and Indications

Imatinib is an oral antineoplastic drug, a protein tyrosine kinase inhibitor that selectively inhibits the Bcr-Abl tyrosine kinase created by the Philadelphia chromosome abnormality in CML. Blocking this enzyme inhibits proliferation and induces cell division in Bcr-Abl–positive cell lines, as well as in new leukemic cells, thereby inhibiting tumor growth in CML patients in blast crisis. It also inhibits a specific receptor site in GI stromal tumor patients. Because of its specific effects on these tumor cells, it is not associated with adverse effects on normal human cells.

All of the other kinase inhibitors work by inhibiting various kinases in specific cancer cells. Table 14.6 shows Usual Indications for all protein tyrosine kinase inhibitors.

FOCUS ON Safe Medication Administration

Erlotinib is an oral drug that inhibits enzymes associated with epidermal growth factor. It is approved for the treatment of non–small cell lung cancer and for first-line treatment of pancreatic cancer when used in combination with gemcitabine.

Bortezomib blocks a large protein complex that is necessary for maintaining cell homeostasis, leading to cell death. It must be given IV and is approved for the treatment of mantle cell lymphoma and multiple myeloma.

Pharmacokinetics

Imatinib is slowly absorbed from the GI tract, reaching peak levels in 2 to 4 hours. It is extensively metabolized in the liver, with a half-life of 18 and then 40 hours. Each of the many kinase inhibitors is metabolized in the liver; the absorption and pharmacokinetics vary with kinase inhibitor.

Erlotinib is well absorbed orally from the GI tract, reaching peak levels in 4 hours. It is metabolized in the liver with a half-life of 36 hours.

Bortezomib, given IV, reaches peak effects at the end of the infusion. It is metabolized in the liver and has a half-life of 40 to 193 hours.

Contraindications and Cautions

All of these drugs are in pregnancy category D. For the time that these drugs are being taken, women of childbearing age should be advised to use barrier contraceptives. It can enter breast milk, and it should be used during lactation only if the benefits to the mother clearly outweigh the risks to the baby. Several of the drugs are contraindicated with patients who have or who are at risk for prolonged QT intervals (hypokalemia, hypomagnesia, or taking another drug that prolongs the QT interval) because they prolong the QT interval, and sudden deaths could occur. These drugs should not be given to anyone who has a history of hypersensitivity to any component of the drug being given.

Adverse Effects

The adverse effects associated with imatinib include GI upset, muscle cramps, heart failure, fluid retention, and skin rash. The severe bone marrow suppression, alopecia, and severe GI effects associated with more traditional antineoplastic therapy do not occur. Several of these drugs prolong the QT interval and need to be used with caution in patients with cardiac problems. Erlotinib and bortezomib are associated with cardiovascular events and pulmonary toxicity. Bortezomib has also been associated with peripheral neuropathy and liver and kidney impairment.

Clinically Important Drug–Drug Interactions

Use caution when administering these drugs with other drugs affected by the cytochrome P450 enzyme system. In addition, St. John's wort decreases the effectiveness of many of these drugs and should be avoided. It is also important to avoid any other drugs that are known to prolong the QT interval.

Ⓟ Prototype Summary: Imatinib

Indications: Treatment of adults with CML who are in blast crisis, accelerated phase, or chronic phase after failure with interferon-alpha therapy. It has since also been approved for use in the treatment of patients with CD117-positive unresectable or metastatic gastrointestinal stromal tumor (GIST), various myeloproliferative disorders, aggressive systemic mastocytosis, and unresectable dermatofibrosarcoma protuberans.

Actions: Tyrosine kinase inhibitor that selectively inhibits the Bcr-Abl tyrosine kinase created by the Philadelphia chromosome abnormality in CML and certain tumor cells present in GIST; blocking this enzyme inhibits proliferation and induces cell division.

Pharmacokinetics:

Route	Onset	Peak
Oral	Slow	2–4 h

$T_{1/2}$: 18 to 40 hours; metabolized in the liver and excreted in the feces.

Adverse Effects: Nausea, vomiting, bone marrow suppression, heart failure, headache, dizziness, edema, rash.

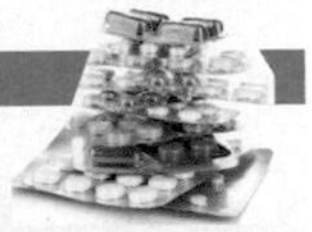

Nursing Considerations for Patients Receiving Cancer Cell–Specific Agents

These are similar to nursing care considerations for patients receiving alkylating agents.

KEY POINTS

- Cancer cell–specific drugs have been developed to target processes that occur in cancer cells but not in healthy cells. This specificity results in fewer toxic effects than with traditional antineoplastic therapy.
- Protein tyrosine kinase inhibitors, epidermal growth factor inhibitors, and proteasome inhibitors have been developed to target cancer cells specifically.

Miscellaneous Antineoplastics

Many other agents that do not fit into one of the previously discussed groups are used as antineoplastics to cause cell death. These drugs are used for treating a wide variety of cancers. Table 14.7 lists the unclassified antineoplastic

Table 14.7 *Drugs in Focus:* Miscellaneous Antineoplastics

Drug Name	Dosage/Route	Usual Indications
arsenic trioxide (*Trisenox*)	*Induction:* 0.15 mg/kg/d IV until remission *Consolidation:* Continue 3–6 wk after inducting for up to 25 doses	Induction and consolidation in patients with APL who are refractory to or relapsed from standard therapy *Actions:* Causes damage to fusion proteins and DNA failure, leading to cell death *Special considerations:* Monitor for cardiac toxicity; do not use during pregnancy
asparaginase *Erwinia chrysanthemi* (*Erwinaze*)	25,000 units/m² IM as part of a specific combination regimen	As part of combination therapy in treatment of ALL in patients with sensitivity to asparaginase or pegaspargase *Actions:* An enzyme that hydrolyzes the amino acid asparagine, which is needed by malignant cells for protein synthesis; inhibits cell proliferation; most effective in G_1 phase of the cell cycle *Special considerations:* Coagulation disorders; hyperglycemia hypersensitivity reactions to this drug are common, and patients should be tested and desensitized, if necessary, before using the drug; monitor blood tests regularly
azacitidine (*Vidaza*)	75 mg/m²/d subcutaneous for 7 d q4wk	Treatment of patients with myelodysplastic syndrome *Action:* Causes demethylation of DNA *Special considerations:* Premedicate for nausea; monitor for bone marrow suppression; patient should avoid pregnancy and fathering children while on drug
belinostat (*Beleodaq*)	1,000 mg/m²/d IV over 30 min on days 1–5 of a 21-d cycle	Treatment of relapsed or refractory T cell lymphoma *Actions:* Histone deacetylase inhibitor which induces cell cycle arrest and/or apoptosis in some transformed cells *Special considerations:* Bone marrow suppression may limit dosing; serious to fatal infections; hepatotoxicity possible; monitor for tumor lysis syndrome
bexarotene (*Targretin*)	300–400 mg/m² PO daily	Treatment of cutaneous manifestations of cutaneous T cell lymphoma in patients refractory to at least one other systemic therapy *Actions:* Binds and activates retinoid receptors *Special considerations:* Risk of serious pancreatitis, hepatic toxicity; photosensitivity
decitabine (*Dacogen*)	15 mg/m² IV over 3 h q8h for 3 d; repeat q6wk for at least 4 cycles	Treatment of patients with myelodysplastic syndromes *Action:* Affects DNA and inhibits DNA transfer *Special considerations:* Premedicate with antiemetics; monitor for bone marrow suppression
hydroxyurea (*Hydrea*)	80 mg/kg PO every third day; 20–30 mg/kg PO daily for continual therapy	Inhibits enzymes essential for the synthesis of DNA, causing cell death *Actions:* Treatment of melanoma, ovarian cancer, CML; in combination therapy for primary squamous cell cancers of the head and neck; also used in the treatment of sickle cell anemia *Special considerations:* Can cause bone marrow depression, headache, rash, GI toxicity, and renal dysfunction; encourage patient to drink 10–12 glasses of water each day while taking this drug
irinotecan (*Camptosar*)	125 mg/m² IV over 90 min, once a week for 4 wk, followed by 2 wk of rest; repeat every 6 wk	Treatment of metastatic colon or rectal cancer after treatment with 5-FU or given with 5-FU *Actions:* Disrupts DNA strands during DNA synthesis, causing cell death *Special considerations:* Can cause severe bone marrow depression, which regulates dose of the drug; causes GI toxicity, dyspnea, and alopecia
nelarabine (*Arranon*)	*Adult:* 1,500 mg/m² IV over 2 h on days 1, 3, and 5; repeat every 21 d *Pediatric:* 650 mg/m²/d IV over 1 h for 5 consecutive days; repeat every 21 d	Treatment of T cell acute lymphoblastic leukemia and T cell lymphoblastic lymphoma when disease has progressed after standard therapy *Actions:* Inhibits DNA synthesis and causes cell death *Special considerations:* Watch for neurological toxicities, including neuropathies and demyelination disorders; bone marrow suppression is common
omacetaxine (*Synribo*)	1.25 mg/m² subcutaneously b.i.d. for 14 consecutive days of a 28-d cycle then 1.25 mg/m² subcutaneously for 7 consecutive days of a 28-d cycle	Treatment of accelerated, resistant CML *Actions:* Protein synthesis inhibitor, causing cell death *Special considerations:* Monitor for severe bone marrow suppression or bleeding

Drug Name	Dosage/Route	Usual Indications
pegaspargase (*Oncaspar*)	2,500 IU/m² IM or IV q14d	Treatment of ALL *Actions:* An enzyme that hydrolyzes the amino acid asparaginase, which is needed by malignant cells for protein synthesis; inhibits cell proliferation; most effective in G_1 phase of the cell cycle *Special considerations:* Can cause potentially fatal hyperthermia, bone marrow depression, renal toxicity, and pancreatitis; monitor patient regularly, and arrange decreased dose as appropriate if toxic effects occur
porfimer (*Photofrin*)	2 mg/kg IV over 3–5 min; laser treatment must follow in 40–50 h and again in 96–120 h	Photosensitizing agent that is used with laser light to decrease tumor size in patients with obstructive esophageal cancers not responsive to laser treatment alone; transitional cell carcinoma in situ of urinary bladder; endobronchial non–small cell lung cancer; high-grade dysplasia or Barrett's esophagus *Actions:* Taken up by cells, causing radical reactions when cells are exposed to laser light, causing cell death *Special considerations:* Has been associated with pleural effusion and fistula; associated with GI and cardiac toxicity; must be given in conjunction with scheduled laser treatment, with at least 30 d between treatments; protect patient from exposure to light with protective clothing for 30 d after treatment (sunscreens are not effective); avoid direct contact with the drug—protective clothing and goggles are suggested
romidepsin (*Istodax*)	14 mg/m² IV over 4 h on days 1, 8, 15 of a 28-d cycle; repeat every 28 d	Treatment of cutaneous, peripheral T cell lymphoma progressing after other therapy *Actions:* Histone deacetylase inhibitor, causing cell death *Special considerations:* Severe bone marrow depression, QT prolongation, tumor lysis syndrome; mark calendar for treatment days; monitor patient closely
sipuleucel-T (*Provenge*)	3 doses IV over 60 min, administer over 3 wk	Autologous cellular immunotherapy used to induce an immune response to antigens found in most prostate cancers; treatment of asymptomatic or minimally symptomatic metastatic hormone refractory prostate cancer *Special considerations:* Premedicate with oral acetaminophen and an antihistamine; universal precautions are required; severe infusion reactions possible; monitor closely during administration; patient may experience fever, headache, nausea, joint pain
talc powder (*Sclerosol*)	4–8-g spray through open thoracotomy or during thoracoscopy	Prevention of recurrence of malignant pleural effusion *Actions:* Induces the inflammatory response, promoting adhesion of the pleura and preventing accumulation of fluid *Special considerations:* Monitor for cardiac and respiratory effects; no actual antineoplastic actions
topotecan (*Hycamtin*)	1.5 mg/m²/d IV for 5 d; as part of a 21-d course; minimum of four courses	Treatment of patients with metastatic ovarian cancer, small-cell lung cancer, persistent cervical cancer *Actions:* Damages DNA strand, causing cell death during cell division *Special considerations:* Can cause severe bone marrow depression, which regulates the dose of the drug; total alopecia, GI toxicity, and CNS effects may also limit the use of the drug; analgesics may be helpful
tretinoin (*Vesanoid*)	45 mg/m²/d PO for 30 d	Used to induce remission in APL; can cause severe respiratory and cardiac toxicity, including MI and cardiac arrest *Actions:* Promotes cell differentiation and repopulation of the bone marrow with normal cells in patients with APL *Special considerations:* GI toxicity, pseudotumor cerebri (papilledema, headache, nausea, vomiting, visual changes), skin rash, and fragility may limit use in some patients; discontinue drug at first sign of toxic effects; use for induction of remission only—then other chemotherapeutic agents should be used
vismodegib (*Erivedge*)	150 mg/d PO	Treatment of metastatic basal cell carcinoma in patients not candidates for surgery or radiation *Actions:* Inhibits the hedgehog signaling pathway in cancer cells leading to cell death *Special considerations:* Not for use in pregnancy or breastfeeding; cannot donate blood during and for 7 mo after treatment; hair loss possible
vorinostat (*Zolinza*)	400 mg/d PO with food	Treatment of cutaneous manifestations in patients with cutaneous T cell lymphoma *Action:* Histone deacetylase inhibitor *Special considerations:* Monitor for increased bleeding; excessive nausea and vomiting may occur; encourage fluid intake to prevent dehydration

APL, acute promyelocytic leukemia; ALL, acute lymphocytic leukemia; CML, chronic myelocytic leukemia; 5-FU, fluorouracil.

drugs, their indications, and any special considerations associated with the drug. Specific information about each drug may be obtained in a nursing drug guide (see Figure 14.4 for sites of action of miscellaneous antineoplastic agents).

SUMMARY

- Cancers arise from a single abnormal cell that multiplies and grows.
- Cancers can manifest as diseases of the blood and lymph tissue or as growth of tumors arising from epithelial cells (carcinomas) or from mesenchymal cells and connective tissue (sarcomas).
- Cancer cells lose their normal function (anaplasia), develop characteristics that allow them to grow in an uninhibited way (autonomy), have the ability to travel to other sites in the body that are conducive to their growth (metastasis), and can stimulate the production of blood vessels to bring nutrients to the growing tumor (angiogenesis).
- Antineoplastic drugs affect both normal cells and cancer cells by disrupting cell function and division at various points in the cell cycle; new drugs are being developed, such as protein kinase inhibitors, to target cancer cell–specific functions.
- Cancer drugs are usually most effective against cells that multiply rapidly (i.e., proceed through the cell cycle quickly). These cells include most neoplasms, bone marrow cells, cells in the GI tract, and cells in the skin or hair follicles.
- The goal of cancer chemotherapy is to decrease the size of the neoplasm so that the human immune system can deal with it.
- Antineoplastic drugs are often given in combination so that they can affect cells in various stages of the cell cycle, including cells that are emerging from rest or moving to a phase of the cycle that is disrupted by these drugs.
- Adverse effects associated with antineoplastic therapy include effects caused by damage to the rapidly multiplying cells, such as bone marrow suppression, which may limit the drug use; GI toxicity, with nausea, vomiting, mouth sores, and diarrhea; and alopecia (hair loss).
- Chemotherapeutic agents should not be used during pregnancy or lactation because they may result in potentially serious adverse effects on the rapidly multiplying cells of the fetus and neonate.
- The newest drugs developed as antineoplastic agents target very specific enzyme systems or processes used by the cancer cells but not by healthy human cells. These drugs are not as toxic to the patient as traditional antineoplastic drugs.

CHECK YOUR UNDERSTANDING

Answers to the questions in this chapter can be found in Answers to Check Your Understanding Questions on thePoint®.

MULTIPLE CHOICE

Select the best answer to the following.

1. Some properties of neoplastic cells are the same as the properties of normal cells, including
   a. anaplasia.
   b. metastasis.
   c. mitosis.
   d. autonomy.

2. Carcinomas are tumors that originate in
   a. mesenchyme.
   b. bone marrow.
   c. striated muscle.
   d. epithelial cells.

3. The goal of traditional antineoplastic drug therapy is to
   a. reduce the size of abnormal cell mass for immune system destruction.
   b. eradicate all of the abnormal cells that have developed.
   c. destroy all cells of the originating type.
   d. stimulate the immune system to destroy the neoplastic cells.

4. Cancer can be a difficult disease to treat because
   a. cells no longer progress through the normal cell cycle.
   b. cells can develop resistance to drug therapy.

c. cells remain dormant, emerging months to years later.
d. the exact cause of cancer is not known.

5. Antineoplastic drugs destroy human cells. They are most likely to cause cell death among healthy cells that
a. have poor cell membranes.
b. are rapidly turning over.
c. are in dormant tissues.
d. are across the blood–brain barrier.

6. Cancer treatment usually occurs in several different treatment phases. In assessing the appropriateness of another round of chemotherapy for a particular patient the nurse would evaluate which of the following as most important?
a. Hair loss
b. Bone marrow function
c. Anorexia
d. Heart rate

7. It is important to explain to women that chemotherapeutic agents should not be used during pregnancy because
a. the tendency to cause nausea and vomiting will be increased.
b. of potential serious adverse effects on the rapidly multiplying cells of the fetus.
c. bone marrow toxicity could alter hormone levels.
d. patients may be weakened by the drug regimen.

8. Cancer drugs are given in combination and over a period of time because it is difficult to affect
a. slowly growing cells.
b. cells in the dormant phase of the cell cycle.
c. cells that multiply rapidly and go through the cell cycle quickly.
d. cells that have moved from their normal site in the body

MULTIPLE RESPONSE

Select all that apply.

1. Which of the following points would be most important for the nurse to stress when developing a patient-teaching plan for a patient receiving antineoplastic therapy?
a. The importance of keeping the head covered at extremes of temperature.
b. The need to use barrier contraceptives because of the risk of serious fetal effects.
c. The importance of avoiding exposure to infection because the ability to heal or to fight infection is impaired.
d. The importance of avoiding food if nausea or vomiting is a problem.
e. The importance of avoiding digging in the dirt without protective coverings because of the many pathogens that live in the dirt that could cause infection.
f. The importance of taking periodic rest periods during the day because you will feel tired when your red blood cell count falls.

2. Hair loss, or alopecia, is an adverse effect of many antineoplastic agents. If a client is receiving a drug that usually causes alopecia, it is important that the nurse do which of the following?
a. Warn the patient that alopecia will occur.
b. Encourage the patient to arrange for an appropriate head covering at extremes of temperature.
c. Advise the patient to lie with the legs elevated and head low to promote circulation and prevent hair loss.
d. Encourage the patient to arrange for a wig or other head covering before the hair loss occurs.
e. Advise the patient that people will stare and can be rude when hair loss occurs.
f. Make arrangements for the patient to attend a support group before hair loss happens.

BIBLIOGRAPHY AND REFERENCES

Brunton, L., Chabner, B., & Knollman, B. (2011). *Goodman and Gilman's the pharmacological basis of therapeutics* (12th ed.). New York: McGraw-Hill.

Chabner, B. A., & Roberts, T. G. (2005). Timeline: Chemotherapy and the war on cancer. *Nature Reviews Cancer, 5*, 65–72.

DeVita, V. T., Hellman, S., & Rosenberg, S. A. (2011). *Cancer: Principles and practice of oncology* (9th ed.). Philadelphia, PA: Lippincott Williams & Wilkins.

Facts and Comparisons. (2015). *Drug facts and comparisons.* St. Louis, MO: Author.

Facts and Comparisons. (2015). *Professional's guide to patient drug facts.* St. Louis, MO: Author.

Grochow, L. B., & Ames, M. M. (1998). *A clinician's guide to chemotherapy, pharmacokinetics, and pharmacodynamics*. Baltimore, MD: Williams & Wilkins.

Karch, A. M. (2014). *Lippincott's nursing drug guide*. Philadelphia, PA: Lippincott Williams & Wilkins.

Meric-Bernstam, F., & Hung, M. (2006). Advances in targeting human epidermal growth factor receptor-2 signaling for cancer therapy. *Clinical Cancer Research, 12*, 6326–6334.

NIOSH. (2014). *NIOSH List of Antineoplastic and Other Hazardous Drugs in Healthcare Settings, 2014 (DHHS Publication 2014-138)*. Washington, D.C.: National Institute for Occupational Safety and Health.

Porth, C. M. (2013). *Pathophysiology: Concepts of altered health states* (9th ed.). Philadelphia, PA: Lippincott Williams & Wilkins.

Schulmeister, L. (2009). Vesicant chemotherapy—the management of extravasation. *Cancer Nursing Practice, 8*(3), 34–37.

Torimura, T., Iwamoto, H., Nakamura, T. (2013). Metronomic chemotherapy: Possible clinical application to advanced hepatocellular carcinoma. *Translational Oncology, 6*(5), 511–519.

PART 3

DRUGS ACTING ON THE IMMUNE SYSTEM

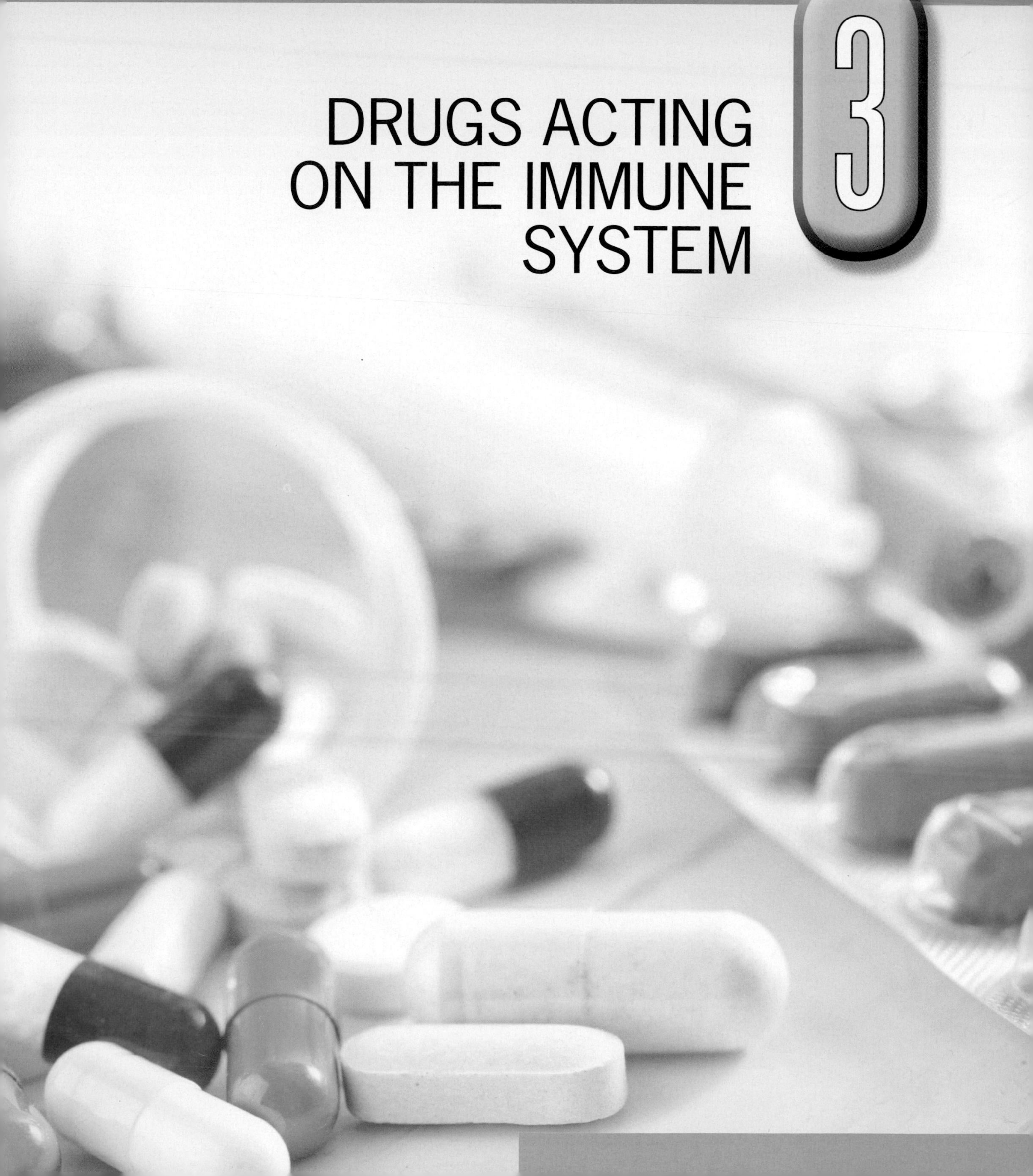

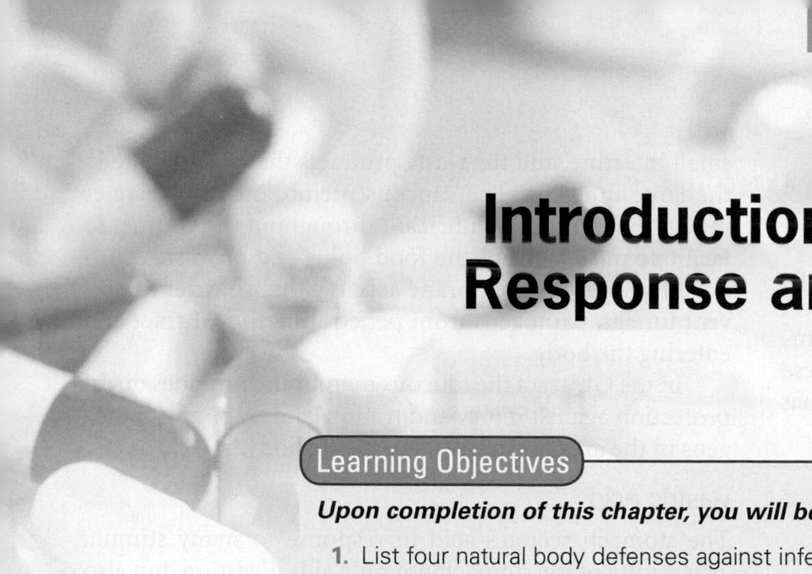

15 Introduction to the Immune Response and Inflammation

Learning Objectives

Upon completion of this chapter, you will be able to:

1. List four natural body defenses against infection.
2. Describe the cells associated with the body's fight against infection and their basic functions.
3. Outline the sequence of events in the inflammatory response.
4. Correlate the events in the inflammatory response with the clinical picture of inflammation.
5. Outline the sequence of events in an antibody-related immune reaction and correlate these events with the clinical presentation of such a reaction.

Glossary of Key Terms

antibodies: immunoglobulins; produced by B cell plasma cells in response to a specific protein; react with that protein to cause its destruction directly or through activation of the inflammatory response

antigen: foreign protein

arachidonic acid: released from injured cells to stimulate the inflammatory response through activation of various chemical substances

autoimmune disease: a disorder that occurs when the body responds to specific self-antigens to produce antibodies or cell-mediated responses against its own cells

B cells: lymphocytes programmed to recognize specific proteins; when activated, these cells cause the production of antibodies to react with that protein

calor: heat, one of the four cardinal signs of inflammation; caused by activation of the inflammatory response

chemotaxis: property of drawing neutrophils to an area

complement proteins: series of cascading proteins that react with the antigen–antibody complex to destroy the protein or stimulate an inflammatory reaction

dolor: pain, one of the four cardinal signs of inflammation; caused by activation of the inflammatory response

Hageman factor: first factor activated when a blood vessel or cell is injured; starts the cascading reaction of the clotting factors, activates the conversion of plasminogen to plasmin to dissolve clots, and activates the kinin system responsible for activation of the inflammatory response

interferon: tissue hormone that is released in response to viral invasion; blocks viral replication

interleukins: chemicals released by white blood cells (WBCs) to communicate with other WBCs and to support the inflammatory and immune reactions

kinin system: system activated by Hageman factor as part of the inflammatory response; includes bradykinin

leukocytes: white blood cells; can be neutrophils, basophils, or eosinophils

lymphocytes: white blood cells with large, varied nuclei; can be T cells or B cells

macrophages: mature leukocytes that are capable of phagocytizing an antigen (foreign protein); also called monocytes or mononuclear phagocytes

major histocompatibility complex: the genetic identification code carried on a chromosome; produces several proteins or antigens that allow the body to recognize cells as being self-cells

mast cells: fixed basophils found in the respiratory and gastrointestinal tracts and in the skin, which release chemical mediators of the inflammatory and immune responses when they are stimulated by local irritation

myelocytes: leukocyte-producing cells in the bone marrow that can develop into neutrophils, basophils, eosinophils, monocytes, or macrophages

phagocytes: neutrophils that are able to engulf and digest foreign material

phagocytosis: the process of engulfing and digesting foreign pyrogens

pyrogen: fever-causing substance

rubor: redness, one of the four cardinal signs of inflammation; caused by activation of the inflammatory response

T cells: lymphocytes programmed in the thymus gland to recognize self-cells; may be effector T cells, helper T cells, or suppressor T cells

tumor: swelling, one of the four cardinal signs of inflammation; caused by activation of the inflammatory response

The body has many defense systems in place to keep it intact and to protect it from external stressors. These stressors can include bacteria, viruses, other foreign pathogens or nonself-cells, trauma, and exposure to extremes of environmental conditions. The same defense systems that protect the body also help to repair it after cellular trauma or damage. Understanding the basic mechanisms involved in these defense systems helps to explain the actions of the drugs that affect the immune system and inflammation.

Body Defenses

The body's defenses include barrier defenses, cellular defenses, the inflammatory response, and the immune response. Each of these defenses plays a major role in maintaining homeostasis and preventing disease.

Barrier Defenses

Certain anatomical barriers exist to prevent the entry of foreign pathogens and to serve as important lines of defense in protecting the body. These barriers include the skin and mucous membranes, gastric acid, and the major histocompatibility complex (MHC).

Skin

The skin is the first line of defense. The skin acts as a physical barrier to protect the internal tissues and organs of the body. Glands in the skin secrete chemicals that destroy or repel many pathogens. The top layer of the skin falls off daily, which makes it difficult for any pathogen to colonize on the skin. In addition, the normal bacterial flora of the skin help to destroy many disease-causing pathogens.

Mucous Membranes

Mucous membranes line the areas of the body that are exposed to external influences but do not have the benefit of skin protection. These body areas include the respiratory tract, which is exposed to air; the gastrointestinal (GI) tract, which is exposed to anything ingested by mouth; and the genitourinary (GU) tract, which is exposed to many pathogens from the perineal and rectal area. Like the skin, the mucous membrane acts as a physical barrier to invasion. It also secretes a sticky mucus capable of trapping invaders and inactivating them for later destruction and removal by the body.

In the conducting airways of the respiratory tract the mucous membrane is lined with tiny, hair-like processes called cilia. The cilia sweep any captured pathogens or foreign materials upward toward the mouth, where they will be swallowed. The cilia also can move the captured material to an area causing irritation, which leads to removal by coughing or sneezing.

In the GI tract the mucous membrane serves as a protective coating, preventing erosion of GI cells by the acidic environment of the stomach, the digestive enzymes of the small intestine, and the waste products that accumulate in the large intestine. The mucous membrane also secretes mucus that serves as a lubricant throughout the GI tract to facilitate movement of the food bolus and of waste products. The mucous membrane acts as a thick barrier to prevent foreign pathogens from penetrating the GI tract and entering the body.

In the GU tract the mucous membrane provides direct protection against injury and trauma and traps any pathogens in the area for destruction by the body.

Gastric Acid

The stomach secretes acid in response to many stimuli. The acidity of the stomach not only aids digestion, but also destroys many would-be pathogens that are either ingested or swallowed after removal from the respiratory tract.

Major Histocompatibility Complex

The body's last barrier of defense is the ability to distinguish between self-cells and foreign cells. All of the cells and tissues of each person are marked for identification as part of that individual's genetic code. No two people have exactly the same code. In humans the genetic identification code is carried on a chromosome and is called the **major histocompatibility complex**. The MHC produces several proteins called histocompatibility antigens, or human leukocyte antigens (HLAs). These **antigens** (proteins) are located on the cell membrane and allow the body to recognize cells as being self-cells. Cells that do not have these proteins are identified as foreign and are targeted for destruction by the body.

Cellular Defenses

Any foreign pathogen that manages to get past the barrier defenses will encounter the human inflammatory and immune systems, or the mononuclear phagocyte system (MPS). Previously called the reticuloendothelial system the MPS is composed primarily of leukocytes, lymphocytes, lymphoid tissues, and numerous chemical mediators.

Stem cells in the bone marrow produce two types of white blood cells or **leukocytes**: The lymphocytes and the myelocytes. The **lymphocytes** are the key components of the immune system and consist of T cells, B cells, and natural killer cells (see later discussion of the Immune Response). The **myelocytes** can develop into a number of different cell types that are important in both the basic inflammatory response and the immune response. Myelocytes include neutrophils, basophils, eosinophils, and monocytes, or macrophages (Figure 15.1).

Neutrophils

Neutrophils are polymorphonuclear leukocytes that are capable of moving outside of the bloodstream (diapedesis) and engulfing and digesting foreign material (**phagocytosis**). When the body is injured or invaded by a pathogen, neutrophils are rapidly produced and move to the site of the insult to attack the foreign substance. Because neutrophils

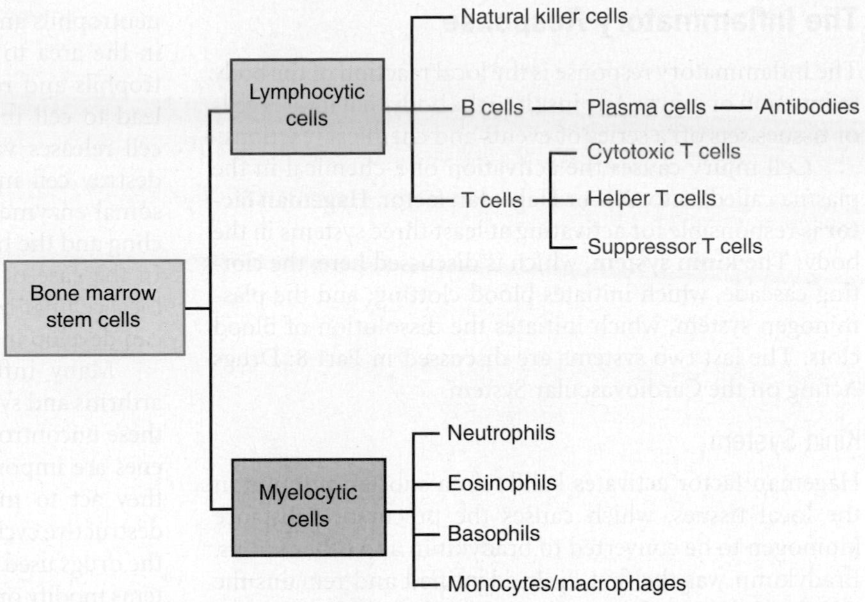

FIGURE 15.1 Types of white blood cells, or leukocytes, produced by the body.

are able to engulf and digest foreign material, they are called **phagocytes.** Phagocytes are able to identify nonself-cells by use of the MHC, and they can engulf these cells or mark them for destruction by cytotoxic T lymphocytes.

Basophils

Basophils are myelocytic leukocytes that are not capable of phagocytosis. They contain chemical substances or mediators that are important for initiating and maintaining an immune or inflammatory response. These substances include histamine, heparin, and other chemicals used in the inflammatory response.

Basophils that are fixed and do not circulate are called **mast cells.** They are found in the respiratory and GI tracts and in the skin. They release many of the chemical mediators of the inflammatory and immune responses when they are stimulated by local irritation.

Eosinophils

Eosinophils are circulating myelocytic leukocytes whose exact function is not understood. They are often found at the site of allergic reactions and may be responsible for removing the proteins and active components of the immune reaction from the site of an allergic response.

Monocytes/Macrophages

Monocytes or mononuclear phagocytes are also called **macrophages.** They are mature leukocytes that are capable of phagocytizing an antigen. Macrophages help to remove foreign material from the body, including pathogens, debris from dead cells, and necrotic tissue from injury sites, so that the body can heal. They also can process antigens and present them to active lymphocytes for destruction.

Macrophages can circulate in the bloodstream or they can be fixed in specific tissues, such as the Kupffer cells in the liver, the cells in the alveoli of the respiratory tract, and the microglia in the central nervous system (CNS), GI, circulatory, and lymph tissues. As active phagocytes, macrophages release chemicals that are necessary to elicit a strong inflammatory reaction. These cells also respond to chemical mediators released by other cells that are active in the inflammatory and immune responses to increase the intensity of a response and to facilitate the body's reaction.

Lymphoid Tissues

Lymphoid tissues that play an important part in the cellular defense system include the lymph nodes, spleen, thymus gland (a bipolar gland located in the middle of the chest, which becomes smaller with age), bone marrow, and lymphoid tissue throughout the respiratory and GI tracts. The bone marrow and the thymus gland are important for creation of the cellular components of the MPS. The bone marrow has a role in the differentiation of these cellular components. The thymus gland is responsible for the final differentiation of the T cells and for regulating the actions of the immune system. The lymph nodes and lymphoid tissue store concentrated populations of neutrophils, basophils, eosinophils, and lymphocytes in areas of the body that facilitate their surveillance for and destruction of foreign proteins. Other cells travel through the cardiovascular and lymph systems to search for foreign proteins or to reach the sites of injury or pathogen invasion.

KEY POINTS

- The body has several defense mechanisms in place to protect it from injury or foreign invasion.
- Barrier defenses include the skin, mucous membranes, normal flora, and gastric acid.
- Cellular defenses include blood cells such as the lymphocytes (T and B cells) and the myelocytes (neutrophils, eosinophils, basophils, and macrophages).

The Inflammatory Response

The inflammatory response is the local reaction of the body to invasion or injury. Any insult to the body that injures cells or tissues sets off a series of events and chemical reactions.

Cell injury causes the activation of a chemical in the plasma called factor XII or Hageman factor. **Hageman factor** is responsible for activating at least three systems in the body: The **kinin system**, which is discussed here; the clotting cascade, which initiates blood clotting; and the plasminogen system, which initiates the dissolution of blood clots. The last two systems are discussed in Part 8: Drugs Acting on the Cardiovascular System.

Kinin System

Hageman factor activates kallikrein a substance found in the local tissues, which causes the precursor substance kininogen to be converted to bradykinin and other kinins. Bradykinin was the first kinin identified and remains the one that is best understood.

Bradykinin causes local vasodilation, which brings more blood to the injured area and allows white blood cells to escape into the tissues. It also stimulates nerve endings to cause pain, which alerts the body to the injury.

Bradykinin also causes the release of arachidonic acid from the cell membrane. **Arachidonic acid** is the precursor to many substances called autocoids, including cyclooxygenase, prostacyclin, and thromboxane. These substances act like local hormones that cause an effect in the immediate area and then are broken down. These autocoids include the following:

- Prostaglandins, some of which augment the inflammatory reaction and some of which block it.
- Cyclooxygenase, which is involved in inflammation and various protective actions in the body.
- Leukotrienes, some of which can cause vasodilation and increased capillary permeability, and some of which can block the reactions.
- Thromboxanes, which cause local vasoconstriction and facilitate platelet aggregation and blood coagulation.

Histamine Release

While this series of Hageman factor–initiated events is proceeding, another locally mediated response is occurring. Injury to a cell membrane causes the local release of histamine. Histamine causes vasodilation, which brings more blood and blood components to the area. It also alters capillary permeability, making it easier for neutrophils and blood chemicals to leave the bloodstream and enter the injured area. In addition, histamine stimulates pain perception. The vasodilation and changes in capillary permeability bring neutrophils to the area to engulf and get rid of the invader or to remove the cell that has been injured.

Chemotaxis

Some leukotrienes activated by arachidonic acid have a property called **chemotaxis**, which is the ability to attract neutrophils and to stimulate them and other macrophages in the area to be very aggressive. Activation of the neutrophils and release of other chemicals into the area can lead to cell injury and destruction. When destroyed the cell releases various lysosomal enzymes that dissolve or destroy cell membranes and cellular proteins. The lysosomal enzymes are an important part of biological recycling and the breakdown of once-living tissues after death. In the case of an inflammatory reaction, they can cause local cellular breakdown and further inflammation, which can develop into a vicious cycle leading to cell death.

Many inflammatory diseases, such as rheumatoid arthritis and systemic lupus erythematosus, are examples of these uncontrolled cycles. The prostaglandins and leukotrienes are important to the inflammatory response because they act to moderate the reaction, thus preventing this destructive cycle from happening on a regular basis. Many of the drugs used to affect the inflammatory and immune systems modify or interfere with these inflammatory reactions.

Clinical Presentation

Activation of the inflammatory response produces a characteristic clinical picture. The Latin words *calor*, *tumor*, *rubor*, and *dolor* describe a typical inflammatory reaction. **Calor**, or heat, occurs because of the increased blood flow to the area. **Tumor**, or swelling, occurs because of the fluid that leaks into the tissues as a result of the change in capillary permeability. **Rubor**, or redness, is related again to the increase in blood flow caused by the vasodilation. **Dolor**, or pain, comes from the activation of pain fibers by histamine and the kinin system. These signs and symptoms occur any time a cell is injured (Figure 15.2). For example, if you scratch the top of your hand and wait for about a minute, the direct line of the scratch will be red (rubor) and raised (tumor). If you feel it gently, it will be warmer than the surrounding area (calor). You should also experience a burning sensation or discomfort at the site of the scratch (dolor). Invasion of the lungs by bacteria can produce pneumonia. If the lungs could be examined closely, they would also show the signs and symptoms of inflammation. They would be red from increased blood flow; fluid would start to leak out of the capillaries (often this can be heard as rales); the patient would complain of chest discomfort; and the increased blood flow to the area of infection would make it appear hot or very active on a scan. No matter what the cause of the insult, the body's local response is the same.

Once the inflammatory response is under way and neutrophils become active, engulfing and digesting injured cells or the invader, they release a chemical that is a natural **pyrogen**, or fever-causing substance. This pyrogen resets specific neurons in the hypothalamus to maintain a higher body temperature, seen clinically as a fever. The higher temperature acts as a catalyst to many of the body's chemical reactions, making the inflammatory and immune responses more effective. Treating fevers remains a controversial subject because lowering a

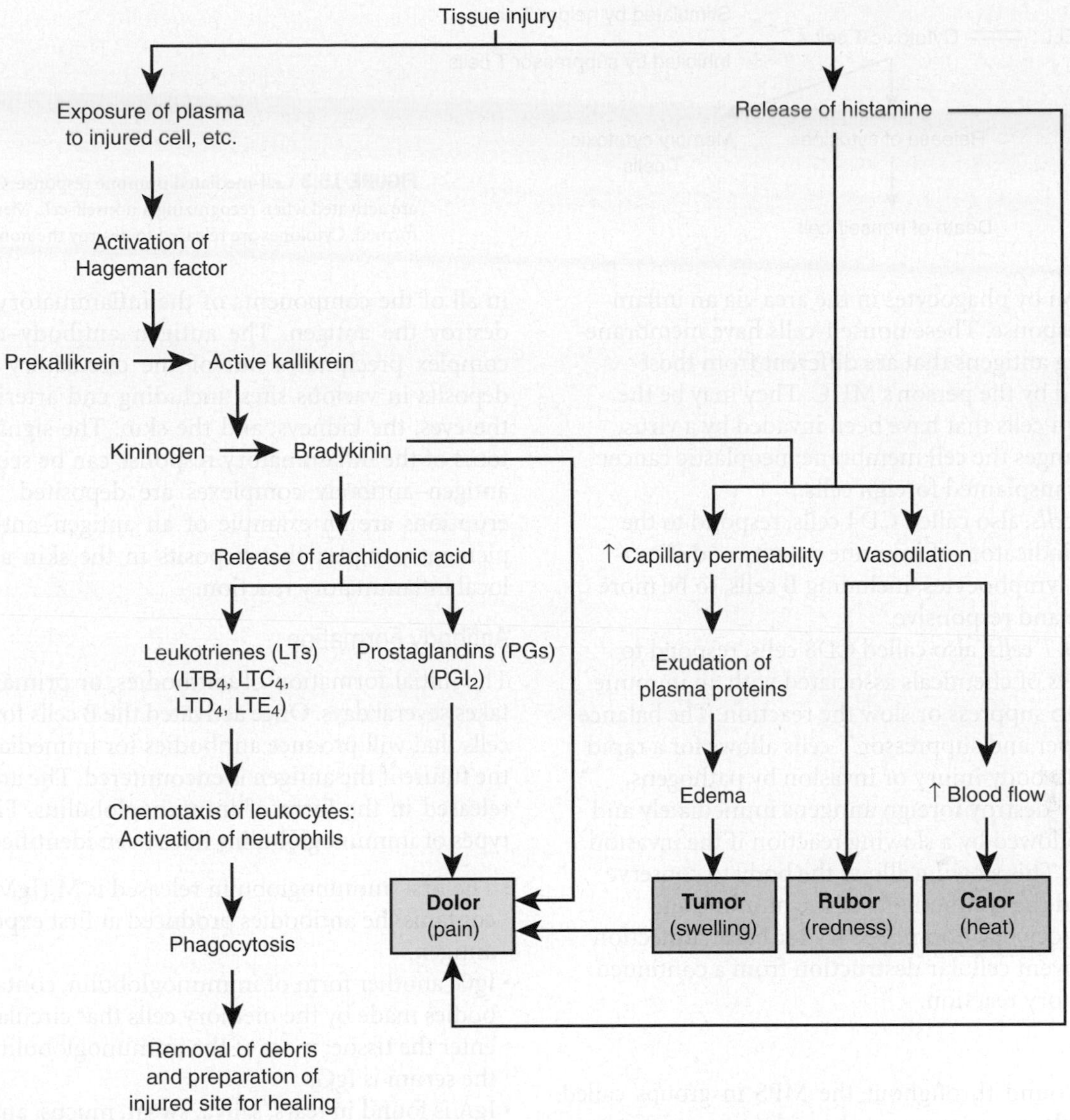

FIGURE 15.2 The inflammatory response in relation to the four cardinal signs of inflammation.

fever decreases the efficiency of the immune and inflammatory responses.

The leukotrienes (autocoids activated through the kinin system) affect the brain to induce slow-wave sleep, which is believed to be an important energy conservation measure for fighting the invader. They also cause myalgia and arthralgia (muscle and joint pain)—common signs and symptoms of various inflammatory diseases—which also cause reduced activity and save energy. All of these chemical responses make up the total clinical picture of an inflammatory reaction.

The Immune Response

More specific invasion can stimulate a more specific response through the immune system. As mentioned previously, stem cells in the bone marrow produce lymphocytes that can develop into T lymphocytes (so named because they migrate from the bone marrow to the thymus gland for activation and maturation) or B lymphocytes (so named because they are activated in the bursa of Fabricius in the chicken, although the specific point of activation in humans has not been identified). Other identified lymphocytes include natural killer cells and lymphokine-activated killer cells. Both of these cells are aggressive against neoplastic or cancer cells and promote rapid cellular death. They do not seem to be programmed for specific identification of cells.

Research in the area of lymphocyte identification is relatively new and continues to grow. There may be other lymphocytes with particular roles in the immune response that have not yet been identified.

T Cells

T cells are programmed in the thymus gland and provide what is called cell-mediated immunity (Figure 15.3). T cells develop into at least three different cell types:

1. *Effector or cytotoxic T cells* are found throughout the body. These T cells are aggressive against nonself-cells, releasing cytokines, or chemicals, that can either directly destroy a foreign cell or mark it for aggressive

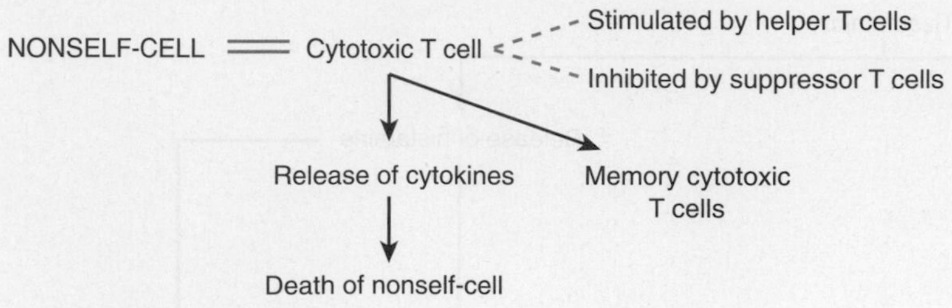

FIGURE 15.3 Cell-mediated immune response. Cytotoxic T cells are activated when recognizing a nonself-cell. Memory T cells are formed. Cytokines are released to destroy the nonself-cell.

destruction by phagocytes in the area via an inflammatory response. These nonself-cells have membrane-identifying antigens that are different from those established by the person's MHC. They may be the body's own cells that have been invaded by a virus, which changes the cell membrane; neoplastic cancer cells; or transplanted foreign cells.

2. *Helper T cells*, also called CD4 cells, respond to the chemical indicators of immune activity and stimulate other lymphocytes, including B cells, to be more aggressive and responsive.
3. *Suppressor T cells*, also called CD8 cells, respond to rising levels of chemicals associated with an immune response to suppress or slow the reaction. The balance of the helper and suppressor T cells allows for a rapid response to body injury or invasion by pathogens, which may destroy foreign antigens immediately and then be followed by a slowing reaction if the invasion continues. This slowing allows the body to conserve energy and the components of the immune and inflammatory reaction necessary for basic protection and to prevent cellular destruction from a continued inflammatory reaction.

B Cells

B cells are found throughout the MPS in groups called clones. B cells are programmed to identify specific proteins, or antigens. They provide what is called humoral immunity (Figure 15.4). When a B cell reacts with its specific antigen, it changes to become a plasma cell. Plasma cells produce **antibodies**, or immunoglobulins, which circulate in the body and react with this specific antigen when it is encountered. This is a direct chemical reaction. When the antigen and antibody react, they form an antigen–antibody complex. This new structure reveals a new receptor site on the antibody that activates a series of plasma proteins in the body called complement proteins.

Complement Proteins

Complement proteins react in a cascade fashion to form a ring around the antigen–antibody complex. The complement can destroy the antigen by altering the membrane, allowing an osmotic inflow of fluid that causes the cell to burst. They also induce chemotaxis (attraction of phagocytic cells to the area), increase the activity of phagocytes, and release histamine. Histamine release causes vasodilation, which increases blood flow to the area and brings in all of the components of the inflammatory reaction to destroy the antigen. The antigen–antibody–complement complex precipitates out of the circulatory system and deposits in various sites, including end arteries in joints, the eyes, the kidneys, and the skin. The signs and symptoms of the inflammatory response can be seen where the antigen–antibody complexes are deposited. Chickenpox eruptions are an example of an antigen–antibody–complement complex that deposits in the skin and causes a local inflammatory reaction.

Antibody Formation

The initial formation of antibodies, or primary response, takes several days. Once activated the B cells form memory cells that will produce antibodies for immediate release in the future if the antigen is encountered. The antibodies are released in the form of immunoglobulins. Five different types of immunoglobulins have been identified:

- The first immunoglobulin released is M (IgM), which contains the antibodies produced at first exposure to the antigen.
- IgG, another form of immunoglobulin, contains antibodies made by the memory cells that circulate and enter the tissue; most of the immunoglobulin found in the serum is IgG.
- IgA is found in tears, saliva, sweat, mucus, and bile. It is secreted by plasma cells in the GI and respiratory tracts and in epithelial cells. These antibodies react with specific pathogens that are encountered in exposed areas of the body.
- IgE is present in small amounts and seems to be related to allergic responses and to the activation of mast cells.
- IgD is another identified immunoglobulin whose role has not been determined.

This process of antibody formation, called acquired or active immunity, is a lifelong reaction. For example, a person exposed to chickenpox will have a mild respiratory reaction when the virus (varicella) first enters the respiratory tract. There will then be a 2-to 3-week incubation period as the body is forming IgM antibodies and preparing to attack any chickenpox virus that appears. The chickenpox virus enters a cell and multiplies. The cell eventually ruptures and ejects more viruses into the system. When this happens the body responds with the immediate release of antibodies, and a full-scale antigen–antibody response is seen throughout the body. Fever, myalgia, arthralgia,

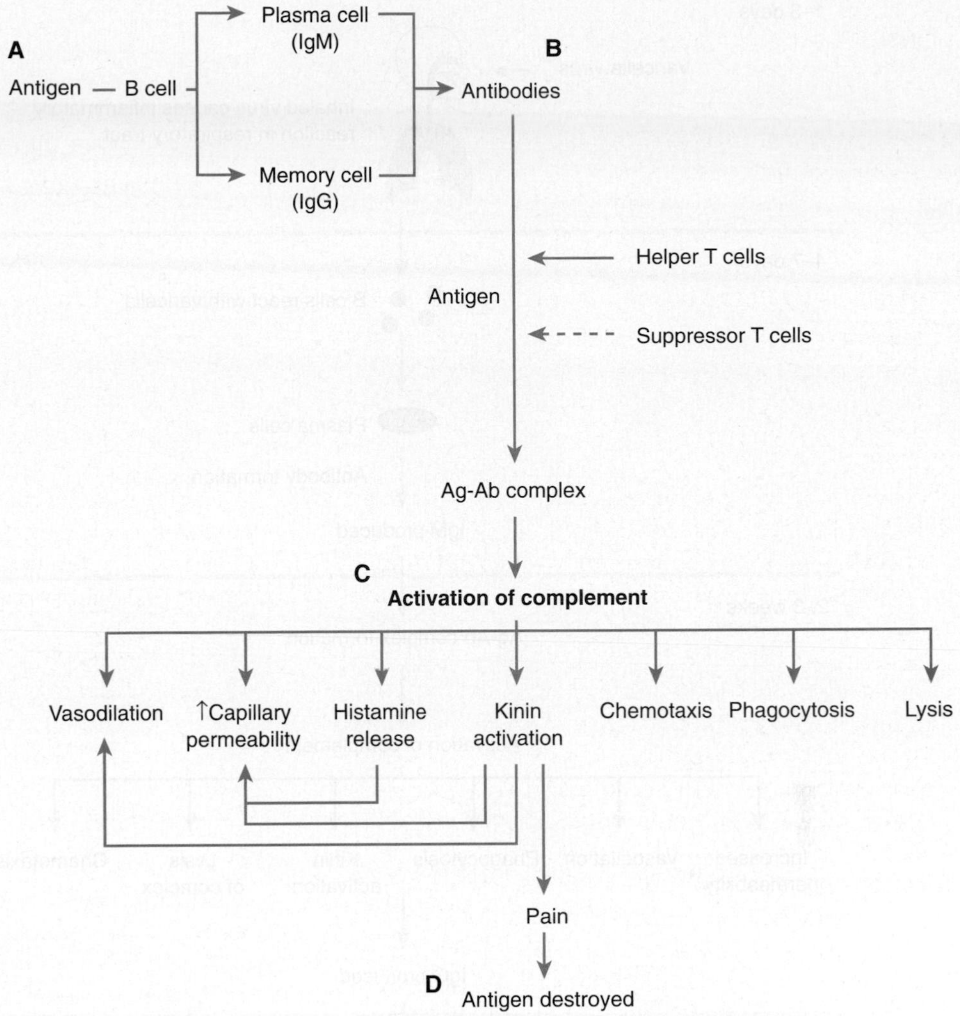

FIGURE 15.4 The humoral immune response. **(A)** A B cell reacts with a specific antigen to form plasma cells and memory cells, which produce antibodies. **(B)** Circulating antibodies react with the antigen to form an antigen–antibody (Ag-Ab) complex. This process is facilitated by helper T cells and suppressed by suppressor T cells. **(C)** The Ag-Ab complex activates circulating complement, which facilitates aggressive inflammatory reactions. **(D)** This process destroys the antigen.

and skin lesions are all part of the immune response to the virus. Once all of the invading chickenpox viruses have been destroyed or have entered the CNS to safely hibernate away from the antibodies the clinical signs and symptoms resolve. (Varicella can enter the CNS and stay dormant for many years. The antibodies are not able to cross into the CNS, and the virus remains unaffected while it stays there.)

The B memory cells will continue to make a supply of immunoglobulin, IgG, for use on future exposure to the chickenpox virus. That exposure usually does not evolve into a clinical case because the viruses are destroyed immediately on entering the body and do not have a chance to multiply. Older patients with weakened immune systems, people who are immunosuppressed, and individuals who have depleted their immune system fighting an infection are at risk for development of shingles if they had chickenpox earlier in their lives. The dormant virus, which has aged and changed somewhat, is able to leave the CNS along a nerve root because the immunosuppressed body is slow to respond. The antibodies do eventually respond to the varicella, and the signs and symptoms of shingles occur as the virus is attacked along the nerve root. Figure 15.5 outlines this entire process.

B clones cluster in areas where they are most likely to encounter the specific antigen that they have been programmed to recognize. For example, pathogens or antigens that are introduced into the body via the respiratory tract will meet up with the B cells in the tonsils and upper respiratory tract; antigens that enter the body through the GI tract will meet their B cells situated in the esophagus and GI tract. Theorists believe that the B cells are programmed genetically and are formed by the time of birth. Clones of B cells contain similar cells. The introduction of an antigen to which there are no preprogrammed B cells could result in widespread disease because the body would have no way of responding. A major concern about space travel has always been the introduction of a completely new antigen to Earth; for this reason, long periods of decontamination have been used after rocks or debris are brought back to Earth. Germ warfare research is ongoing in some countries to develop an antigen that has not been seen before and to which people would have no response.

Other Mediators

Several other factors also play an important role in the immune reaction. **Interferons** are chemicals that are

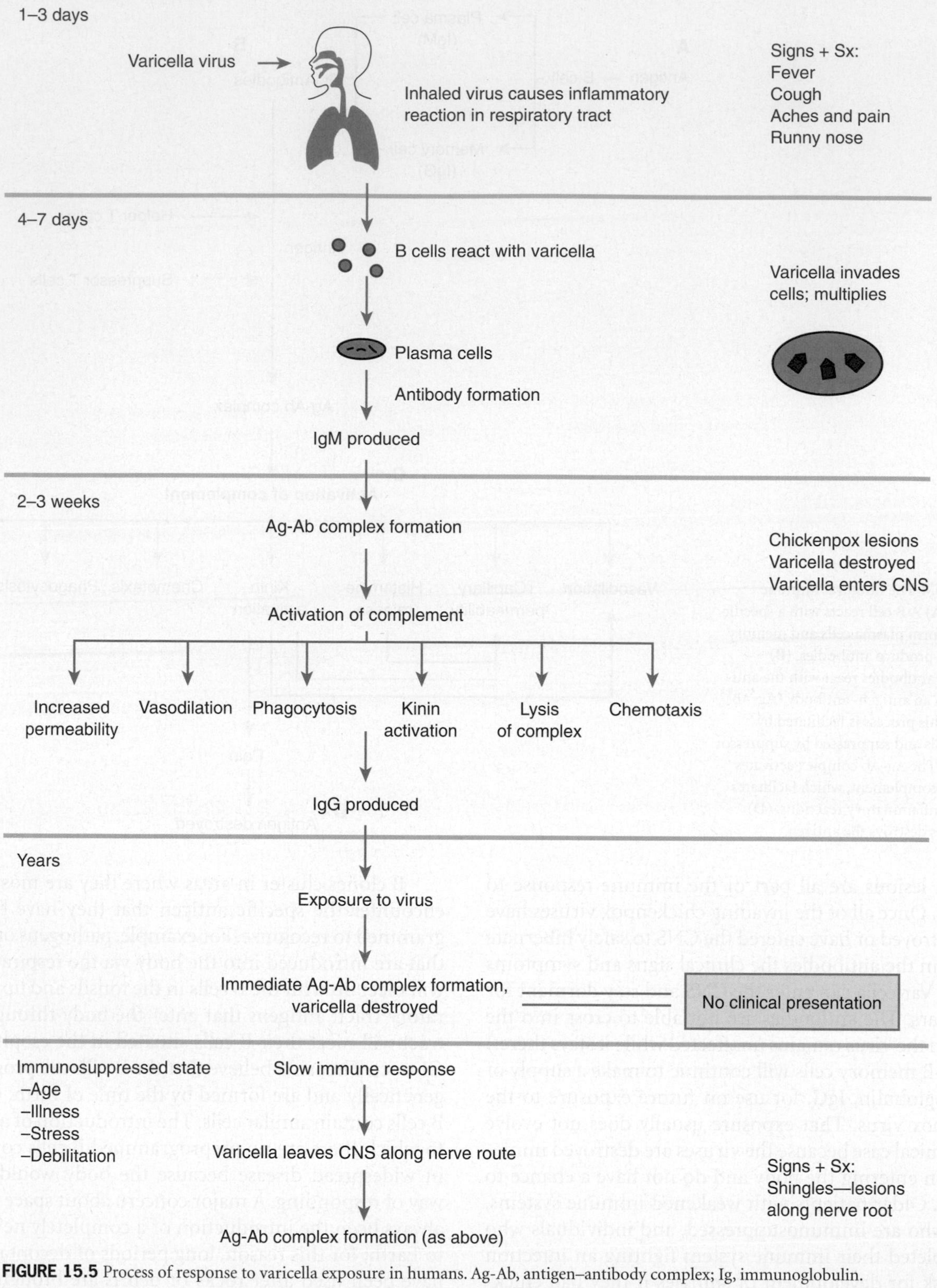

FIGURE 15.5 Process of response to varicella exposure in humans. Ag-Ab, antigen–antibody complex; Ig, immunoglobulin.

secreted by cells that have been invaded by viruses and possibly by other stimuli. The interferons prevent viral replication and also suppress malignant cell replication and tumor growth.

Interleukins are chemicals secreted by active leukocytes to influence other leukocytes. Interleukin 1 (IL-1) stimulates T and B cells to initiate an immune response. IL-2 is released from active T cells to stimulate the production of more T cells and to increase the activity of B cells, cytotoxic cells, and natural killer cells. Interleukins also cause fever, arthralgia, myalgia, and slow-wave sleep induction—all things that help the body to conserve

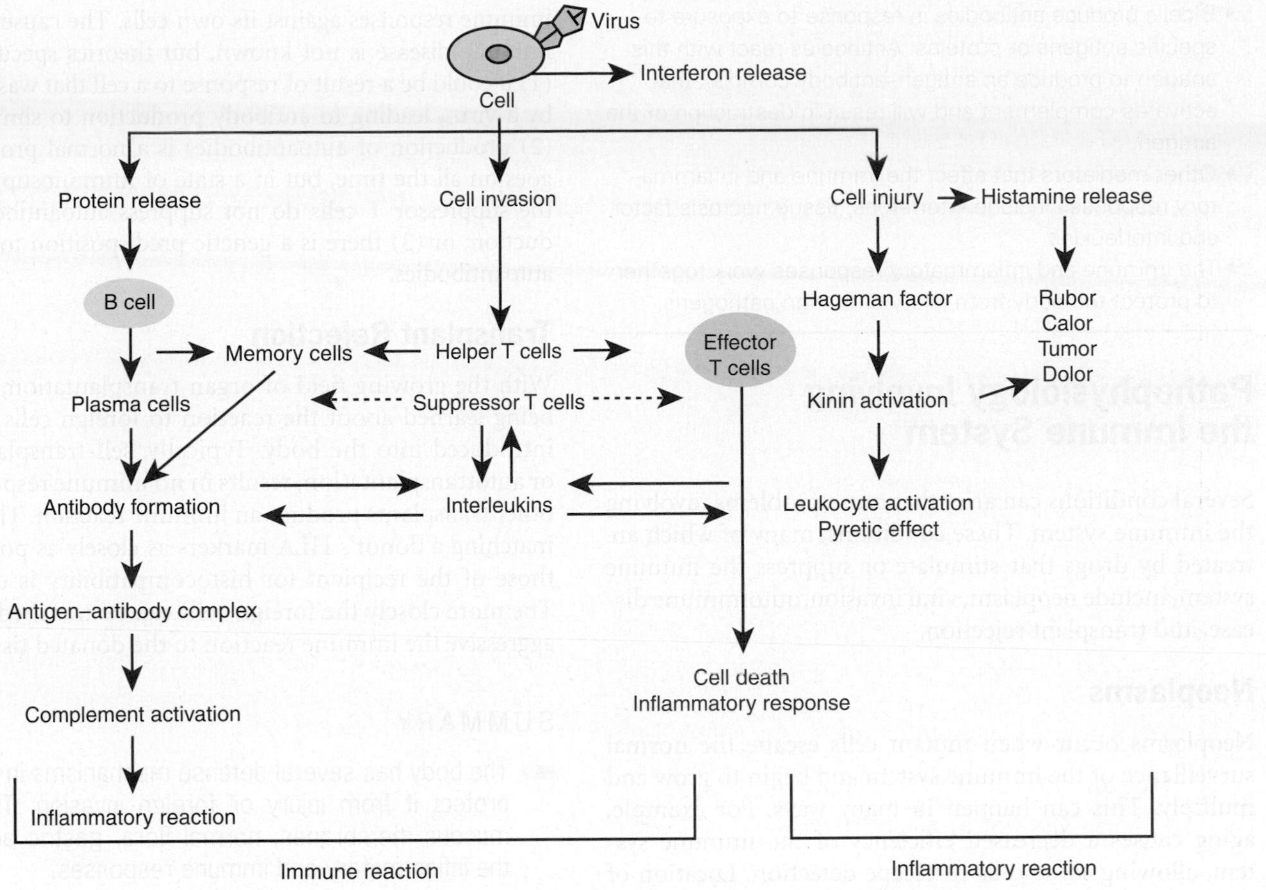

FIGURE 15.6 Interrelationship of immune and inflammatory reactions.

energy for use in fighting off the invader. Several other factors released by lymphocytes and basophils have been identified. These include interleukins such as B cell growth factor, macrophage-activating factor, macrophage-inhibiting factor, platelet-activating factor, eosinophil-chemotactic factor, and neutrophil-chemotactic factor.

The thymus gland also releases a number of hormones that aid in the maturation of T cells and that circulate in the body to stimulate and communicate with T cells. Thymosin, a thymus hormone that has been replicated, is important in the maturation of T cells and cell-mediated immunity. Research is ongoing on the use of thymosin in certain leukemias and melanomas to stimulate the immune response.

Tumor necrosis factor (TNF), a cytokine, is a chemical released by macrophages that inhibits tumor growth and can actually cause tumor regression. It also works with other chemicals to make the inflammatory and immune responses more aggressive and efficient. Research is ongoing to determine the therapeutic effectiveness of TNF. TNF receptor sites are now available for injection into patients with acute rheumatoid arthritis. These receptor sites react with TNF released by the macrophages in this inflammatory disease. All of these chemicals act as communication factors within the immune system, allowing coordination of the immune response.

Interrelationship of the Immune and Inflammatory Responses

The immune and inflammatory responses work together to protect the body and to maintain a level of homeostasis within the body. Helper T cells stimulate the activity of B cells and effector T cells. Suppressor T cells monitor the chemical activity in the body and act to suppress B cell and T cell activity when the foreign antigen is under control. Both B cells and T cells ultimately depend on an effective inflammatory reaction to achieve the end goal of destruction of the foreign protein or cell (Figure 15.6).

KEY POINTS

- The response to the inflammatory stimuli involves local vasodilation, increased capillary permeability, and the stimulation of pain fibers. These reactions alert the person to the injury and bring an increased blood flow to the area.
- The immune response provides a specific reaction to foreign cells or proteins.
- T cells can be cytotoxic, destroying nonself-cells; helper, augmenting an immune reaction; or suppressor, dampening the immune response to save energy and prevent cell damage.

(continued)

- B cells produce antibodies in response to exposure to specific antigens or proteins. Antibodies react with this antigen to produce an antigen–antibody complex that activates complement and will result in destruction of the antigen.
- Other mediators that affect the immune and inflammatory responses include interferons, tissue necrosis factor, and interleukins.
- The immune and inflammatory responses work together to protect the body from injury or foreign pathogens.

Pathophysiology Involving the Immune System

Several conditions can arise that cause problems involving the immune system. These conditions, many of which are treated by drugs that stimulate or suppress the immune system, include neoplasm, viral invasion, autoimmune disease, and transplant rejection.

Neoplasms

Neoplasms occur when mutant cells escape the normal surveillance of the immune system and begin to grow and multiply. This can happen in many ways. For example, aging causes a decreased efficiency of the immune system, allowing some cells to escape detection. Location of the mutant cells can make it difficult for lymphocytes to get to an area to respond. Mutant cells in breast tissue, for example, are not well perfused with blood and may escape detection until they are quite abundant. Sometimes cells are able to avoid detection by the T cells until the growing mass of cells is so large that the immune system cannot deal with it. Tumors also can produce blocking antibodies that cover the antigen receptor sites on the tumor and prevent recognition by cytotoxic T cells. In addition, a weakly antigenic tumor may develop; such a tumor elicits a mild response from the immune system and somehow tricks the T cells into allowing it to survive.

Viral Invasion of Cells

Viruses are parasites that can survive only by invading a host cell that provides the nourishment necessary for viral replication. Invasion of a cell alters the cell membrane and the antigenic presentation of the cell (the MHC). This change can activate cellular immunity, or it can be so subtle that the immune system's response to the cell is mild or absent. In some cases the response activates a cellular immune reaction to normal cells similar to the one that was invaded. This is one theory for the development of autoimmune disease.

Autoimmune Disease

Autoimmune disease occurs when the body responds to specific self-antigens to produce antibodies or cell-mediated immune responses against its own cells. The cause of autoimmune disease is not known, but theories speculate that (1) it could be a result of response to a cell that was invaded by a virus, leading to antibody production to similar cells; (2) production of autoantibodies is a normal process that goes on all the time, but in a state of immunosuppression, the suppressor T cells do not suppress autoantibody production; or (3) there is a genetic predisposition to develop autoantibodies.

Transplant Rejection

With the growing field of organ transplantation, more is being learned about the reaction to foreign cells that are introduced into the body. Typically, self-transplantation, or autotransplantation, results in no immune response. All other transplants produce an immune reaction. Therefore, matching a donor's HLA markers as closely as possible to those of the recipient for histocompatibility is essential. The more closely the foreign cells can be matched the less aggressive the immune reaction to the donated tissue.

SUMMARY

- The body has several defense mechanisms in place to protect it from injury or foreign invasion: The skin, mucous membranes, normal flora, gastric acid, and the inflammatory and immune responses.
- The inflammatory response is a general response to any cell injury and involves activation of Hageman factor to stimulate the kinin system and release of histamine from injured cells to generate local inflammatory responses.
- The clinical presentation of an inflammatory reaction is heat (calor), redness (rubor), swelling (tumor), and pain (dolor).
- The inflammatory response is a nonspecific reaction to any cellular injury and involves the activation of various chemicals and neutrophil activity. The immune response is specific to an antigen or protein that has entered the body and involves B cells, antibodies, and T cells.
- Several types of T cells exist: Effector or cytotoxic T cells, helper T cells, and suppressor T cells. Effector or cytotoxic T cells immediately destroy foreign cells. Helper T cells stimulate the immune and inflammatory reactions. Suppressor T cells dampen the immune and inflammatory responses to conserve energy and prevent cellular damage.
- B cells are programmed to recognize specific proteins or foreign antigens. Once in contact with that protein the B cell produces antibodies (immunoglobulins) that react directly with the protein.
- Reaction of an antibody with the specific receptor site on the protein activates the complement cascade of proteins and lyses the associated protein or precipitates an aggressive inflammatory reaction around it.

- Other chemicals are involved in communication among parts of the immune system and in local response to invasion. Any of these chemicals has the potential to alter the immune response.
- The T cells, B cells, and inflammatory reaction work together to protect the body from invasion, limit the response to that invasion, and return the body to a state of homeostasis.
- Patient problems that occur within the immune system include the development of neoplasms, viral invasions of cells that trigger immune responses, autoimmune diseases, and rejections of transplanted organs.

CHECK YOUR UNDERSTANDING

Answers to the questions in this chapter can be found in Answers to Check Your Understanding Questions on thePoint®.

MULTIPLE CHOICE

Select the best answer to the following.

1. Antibodies
- **a.** are carbohydrates.
- **b.** are secreted by activated T cells.
- **c.** are not found in circulating gamma globulins.
- **d.** are effective only against specific antigens.

2. B and T cells are similar in that they both
- **a.** secrete antibodies.
- **b.** play important roles in the immune response.
- **c.** are activated in the thymus gland.
- **d.** release cytotoxins to destroy cells.

3. Which of the following is not a cytokine?
- **a.** Interleukin 2
- **b.** Antibody
- **c.** Tumor necrosis factor
- **d.** Interferon

4. As part of the nonspecific defense against infection,
- **a.** blood flow and vascular permeability to proteins increase throughout the circulatory system.
- **b.** particles in the respiratory tract are engulfed by phagocytes.
- **c.** B cells are released from the bone marrow.
- **d.** neutrophils release lysosomes, heparin, and kininogen into the extracellular fluid.

5. B cells respond to an initial antigen challenge by
- **a.** reducing in size.
- **b.** immediately producing antigen-specific antibodies.
- **c.** producing a large number of cells that are unlike the original B cell.
- **d.** producing new cells that become plasma cells and memory cells.

6. Treating fevers remains a controversial subject because
- **a.** fevers make people feel ill.
- **b.** higher temperatures act as catalysts to many of the body's chemical reactions.
- **c.** higher temperatures can suppress the body's normal metabolism.
- **d.** higher temperatures can alter the body's hormone levels, particularly that of progesterone.

7. After describing the function of T cells the nurse would identify the need for additional teaching if the patient stated that T cells become which of the following?
- **a.** Cytotoxic T cells
- **b.** Helper T cells
- **c.** Suppressor T cells
- **d.** Antibody-secreting T cells

8. Interleukins are
- **a.** chemicals released when a virus enters a cell.
- **b.** chemicals secreted by activated leukocytes.
- **c.** part of the kinin system.
- **d.** activated by arachidonic acid.

(continues on page 264)

MULTIPLE RESPONSE

Select all that apply.

1. Which of the following statements could be used to describe a neutrophil?
   a. They possess the property of phagocytosis.
   b. When activated, they release a pyrogen that causes fever.
   c. When the body is injured, they are produced rapidly and in large numbers.
   d. They are not capable of movement outside the circulatory system.
   e. They are most often seen in response to an allergic reaction.
   f. They float around in the blood and release chemicals in response to injury.

2. The inflammatory response is activated whenever cell injury occurs. An inflammatory response would involve which of the following activities?
   a. Activation of Hageman factor.
   b. Vasodilation in the area of the injury.
   c. Generalized edema and tumor development.
   d. Changes in capillary permeability to allow proteins to leak out of the capillaries.
   e. Activation of complement.
   f. Production of interferon.

BIBLIOGRAPHY AND REFERENCES

Abbas, A., & Lichtman, A. (2012). *Basic immunology* (4th ed.). Philadelphia, PA: W.B. Saunders.

Brunton, L., Chabner, B., & Knollman, B. (2011). *Goodman and Gilman's the pharmacological basis of therapeutics* (12th ed.). New York: McGraw-Hill.

Doan, T., Melvold, R., Viselli, S., & Waltenbaugh, C. (2007). *Lippincott's illustrated reviews: Immunology*. Philadelphia, PA: Lippincott Williams & Wilkins.

Ganong, W. (2014). *Review of medical physiology* (24th ed.). Norwalk, CT: Appleton & Lange.

Guyton, A., & Hall, J. (2015). *Textbook of medical physiology* (13th ed.). Philadelphia, PA: W.B. Saunders.

Karch, A. M. (2014). *Lippincott's nursing drug guide*. Philadelphia, PA: Lippincott Williams & Wilkins.

Peakman, M., & Vergani, D. (2009). *Basic and clinical immunology* (2nd ed.). New York: Churchill-Livingstone.

Porth, C. M. (2013). *Pathophysiology: Concepts of altered health states* (9th ed.). Philadelphia, PA: Lippincott Williams & Wilkins.

Sompayrac, L. (2011). *How the immune system works* (4th ed.). Malden, MA: Blackwell Science.

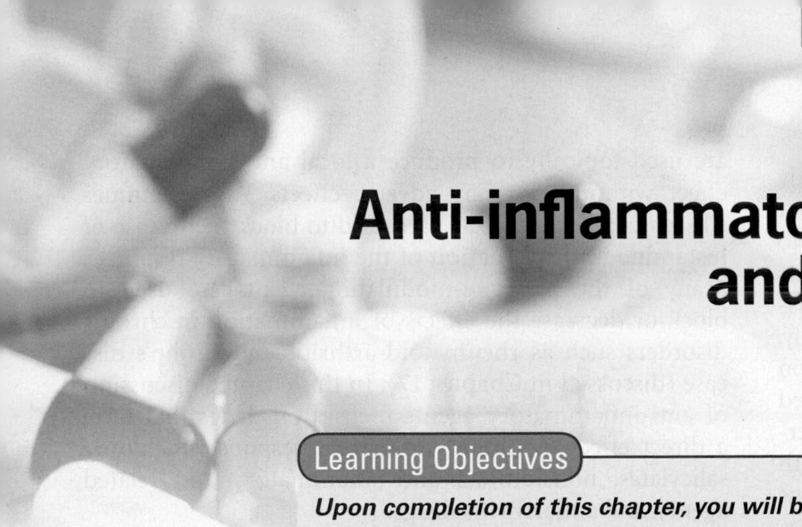

16 Anti-inflammatory, Antiarthritis, and Related Agents

Learning Objectives

Upon completion of this chapter, you will be able to:

1. Describe the sites of action of the various anti-inflammatory agents.
2. Describe the therapeutic actions, indications, pharmacokinetics, contraindications, most common adverse reactions, and important drug–drug interactions associated with each class of anti-inflammatory agents.
3. Discuss the use of anti-inflammatory drugs across the lifespan.
4. Compare and contrast the prototype drugs for each class of anti-inflammatory drugs with the other drugs in that class.
5. Outline the nursing considerations and teaching needs for patients receiving each class of anti-inflammatory agents.

Glossary of Key Terms

analgesic: compounds with pain-blocking properties, capable of producing analgesia

anti-inflammatory agents: drugs that block the effects of the inflammatory response

antipyretic: blocking fever, often by direct effects on the thermoregulatory center in the hypothalamus or by blockade of prostaglandin mediators

chrysotherapy: treatment with gold salts; gold is taken up by macrophages, which then inhibit phagocytosis; it is reserved for use in patients who are unresponsive to conventional therapy, and can be very toxic

inflammatory response: the body's nonspecific response to cell injury, resulting in pain, swelling, heat, and redness in the affected area

nonsteroidal anti-inflammatory drugs (NSAIDs):: drugs that block prostaglandin synthesis and act as anti-inflammatory, antipyretic, and analgesic agents

salicylates: salicylic acid compounds, used as anti-inflammatory, antipyretic, and analgesic agents; they block the prostaglandin system

salicylism: syndrome associated with high levels of salicylates—dizziness, ringing in the ears, difficulty hearing, nausea, vomiting, diarrhea, mental confusion, and lassitude

Drug List

Salicylates
- (P) aspirin
- balsalazide
- choline magnesium trisalicylate
- diflunisal
- mesalamine
- olsalazine
- salsalate

Nonsteroidal Anti-inflammatory and Related Agents

Nonsteroidal Anti-Inflammatory Agents (NSAIDs)

Propionic Acids
- fenoprofen
- flurbiprofen
- (P) ibuprofen
- ketoprofen
- naproxen
- oxaprozin

Acetic Acids
- diclofenac
- etodolac
- indomethacin
- ketorolac
- nabumetone
- sulindac
- tolmetin

Fenamates
- meclofenamate
- mefenamic acid

Oxicam Derivatives
- meloxicam
- piroxicam

Cyclooxygenase-2 Inhibitor
- celecoxib

Related Agent
- (P) acetaminophen

Antiarthritis Agents

Gold Compounds
- auranofin
- gold sodium thiomalate

Tumor Necrosis Factor Blockers
- adalimumab
- certolizumab
- etanercept
- golimumab
- infliximab

Other Antiarthritis Drugs
- anakinra
- hyaluronidase derivatives
- leflunomide
- penicillamine
- sodium hyaluronate
- tofacitinib

The **inflammatory response** is designed to protect the body from injury and pathogens. It employs a variety of potent chemical mediators to produce the reaction that helps to destroy pathogens and promote healing. As the body reacts to these chemicals, it produces signs and symptoms of disease, such as swelling, fever, aches, and pains. Occasionally, the inflammatory response becomes a chronic condition and can result in damage to the body, leading to increased inflammatory reactions. **Anti-inflammatory agents** generally block or alter the chemical reactions associated with the inflammatory response to stop one or more of the signs and symptoms of inflammation.

Anti-inflammatory, Antiarthritis, and Related Agents

Several different types of drugs are used as anti-inflammatory agents. Corticosteroids (discussed in Chapter 36) are used systemically to block the inflammatory and immune systems. Blocking these important protective processes may produce many adverse effects, including decreased resistance to infection and neoplasms. Corticosteroids also are used topically to produce a local anti-inflammatory effect without as many adverse effects. Antihistamines (discussed in Chapter 54) are used to block the release of histamine in the initiation of the inflammatory response. Many of the immune-modulating agents are used to block or decrease the effects of inflammation in chronic disorders such as rheumatoid arthritis and Crohn's disease (discussed in Chapter 17). In this chapter, discussion of anti-inflammatory agents focuses on drugs that have a direct effect on the inflammatory response, including salicylates, nonsteroidal anti-inflammatory and related agents, and antiarthritis drugs.

Because many anti-inflammatory drugs are available over the counter (OTC), there is a potential for abuse and overdosing. In addition, patients may take these drugs and block the signs and symptoms of a present illness, thus potentially causing the misdiagnosis of a problem. Patients also may combine these drugs and unknowingly induce toxicity. All of these drugs have adverse effects that can be dangerous if toxic levels of drug circulate in the body. See Box 16.1 for information on using these drugs with various age groups and Box 16.2 for problems that some African Americans have with anti-inflammatory drugs.

BOX 16.1 FOCUS ON **Drug Therapy Across the Lifespan**

Anti-inflammatory Agents

CHILDREN

Children are more susceptible to the GI and CNS effects of these drugs. Care must be taken to make sure that the child receives the correct dose of any anti-inflammatory agent. This can be a problem because many of these drugs are available in OTC pain, cold, flu, and combination products. Parents need to be taught to read the label to find out the ingredients and the dose they are giving the child.

Aspirin and choline magnesium trisalicylate are the only salicylates recommended for children. They should not be used when any risk of Reye syndrome exists: Children who have had a viral infection (influenza, chickenpox, etc.); who become febrile, lethargic; who have personality changes.

Ibuprofen, naproxen, tolmetin, meloxicam, and, in some cases, indomethacin are the NSAIDs approved for use in children.

Acetaminophen is the most used analgesic/antipyretic drug for children. Care must be taken to avoid overdose, which can cause severe hepatotoxicity. Dosages available in OTC products have been reduced; parents need to be cautioned about combining products.

Children with arthritis may receive treatment with gold salts or etanercept; they must be monitored very closely for toxic effects.

ADULTS

Adults need to be cautioned about the presence of these drugs in many OTC products and taught to be aware of exactly what they are taking to avoid serious toxic effects. They should also be cautioned to report OTC drug use to their health care provider when they are receiving any other prescription drug to avoid possible drug–drug interactions and the masking of signs and symptoms of disease.

Pregnant and nursing women should not use these drugs unless the benefit clearly outweighs the potential risk to the fetus or neonate. Salicylates, NSAIDs, and gold products have potentially severe adverse effects on the neonate and possibly the mother. Acetaminophen can be used cautiously if a pain preparation or antipyretic is needed. Nondrug measures should be taken when at all possible to decrease the potential risk. These women also need to be urged to avoid OTC drugs unless they are suggested by their health care providers.

OLDER ADULTS

Older patients may be more susceptible to the CNS and GI effects of some of these drugs. Dose adjustment is not needed for many of these agents. Geriatric warnings have been associated with naproxen, ketorolac, and ketoprofen because of reports of increased toxicity when they are used by older patients. These NSAIDs should be avoided if possible.

Gold salts, used to treat arthritis, which is more common in older patients, are particularly toxic for geriatric patients. Accumulations in tissues can lead to increased renal, GI, and even liver problems. If gold is used in this group the dose should be reduced and the patient monitored very closely for toxic effects.

BOX 16.2 FOCUS ON Cultural Considerations

Sensitivity to Anti-inflammatory Drugs

African Americans have a documented decreased sensitivity to the pain-relieving effects of many of the anti-inflammatory drugs. They do, however, have an increased risk of developing GI adverse effects to these drugs, including acetaminophen. This should be taken into consideration when using these drugs as analgesics. Increased doses may be needed to achieve a pain-blocking effect, but the increased dose will put these patients at an even greater risk for development of the adverse GI effects associated with these drugs. Monitor these patients closely, and use nondrug measures to decrease pain, such as positioning, environmental control, physical therapy, warm soaks, and so on. If African American patients are prescribed anti-inflammatory drugs, provide teaching about the signs and symptoms of GI bleeding and what to report, and monitor regularly for any adverse reactions to these drugs.

Salicylates

Salicylates (Table 16.1) are popular anti-inflammatory agents not only because of their ability to block the inflammatory response, but also because of their **antipyretic** (fever-blocking) and **analgesic** (pain-blocking) properties. Salicylates are some of the oldest anti-inflammatory drugs used. They were extracted from willow bark, poplar trees, and other plants by ancient peoples to treat fever, pain, and what we now call inflammation. They are generally available without prescription and are relatively nontoxic when used as directed. Aspirin (*Bayer*, *Empirin*, and others), which is available OTC, is one of the most widely used drugs for treating inflammatory conditions. Additional synthetic salicylates include balsalazide (*Colazal*), choline magnesium trisalicylate (*Tricosal*), diflunisal (generic), mesalamine (*Pentasa* and others), olsalazine (*Dipentum*), and salsalate (generic). A person who does not respond to one salicylate may respond to a different one.

Therapeutic Actions and Indications

Salicylates inhibit the synthesis of prostaglandin, an important mediator of the inflammatory reaction (Figure 16.1). The antipyretic effect of salicylates may be related to blocking of a prostaglandin mediator of pyrogens (chemicals that cause an increase in body temperature and that are released by active white blood cells) at the thermoregulatory center of the hypothalamus. At low levels, aspirin also affects platelet aggregation by inhibiting the synthesis of thromboxane A_2, a potent vasoconstrictor that normally increases platelet aggregation and blood clot formation. At higher levels, aspirin inhibits the synthesis of prostacyclin, a vasodilator that inhibits platelet aggregation.

Salicylates are indicated for the treatment of mild to moderate pain, fever, and numerous inflammatory conditions, including rheumatoid arthritis and osteoarthritis. (See Box 16.3 and the Critical Thinking Scenario for more on rheumatoid arthritis.) See *Table 16.1* for Usual Indications for each type of salicylate.

Table 16.1 *Drugs in Focus:* Salicylates

Drug Name	Dosage/Route	Usual Indications
aspirin (*Bayer*, *Empirin*, others)	*Adult:* 325–650 mg PO or PR q4h *MI:* 300–325 mg PO *Pediatric:* 65–100 mg/kg/d PO or PR in four to six divided doses; if <2 y of age, consult with prescriber	Treatment of fever, pain, inflammatory conditions; at low dose to prevent the risk of death and MI in patients with history of MI, prevention of transient ischemic attacks
balsalazide (*Colazal*)	Three 750-mg capsules PO t.i.d. for 8 wk	Treatment of mildly to moderately acute ulcerative colitis in adults
choline magnesium trisalicylate (*Tricosal*)	*Adult:* 1.5–3 g/d PO in two to three divided doses *Pediatric:* 50 mg/kg/d PO in two divided doses	Relief of mild pain, fevers; treatment of arthritis
diflunisal (generic)	500–1,000 mg/d PO in two divided doses	Treatment of moderate pain, arthritis in adults
mesalamine (*Pentasa*, others)	800 mg PO t.i.d. for 6 wk *or* 4 g/60 mL rectal suspension daily at bedtime *or* 500 mg suppository PR, retained for 1–3 h b.i.d.	Treatment of ulcerative colitis and other inflammatory bowel disease in adults
olsalazine (*Dipentum*)	1 g/d PO in two divided doses	Treatment of ulcerative colitis and other inflammatory bowel disease in adults
salsalate (generic)	3,000 mg/d PO in divided doses	Treatment of pain, fever, inflammation in adults

MI, myocardial infarction.

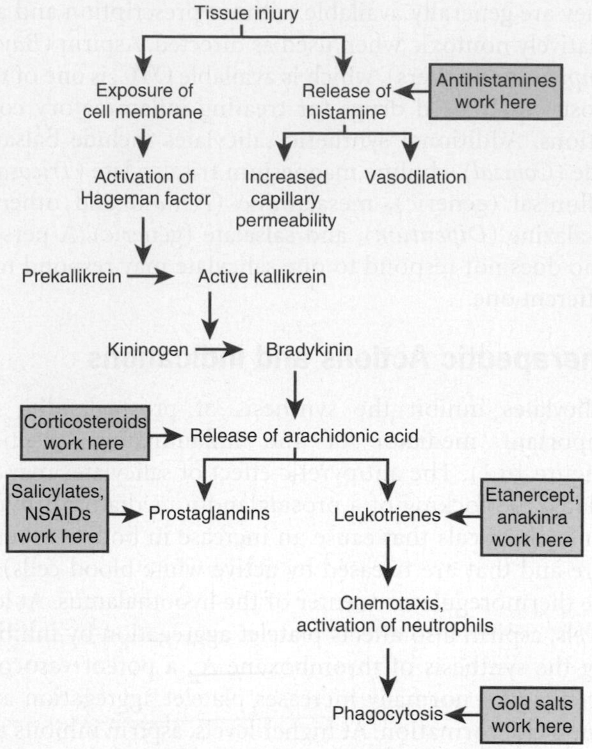

FIGURE 16.1 Sites of action of anti-inflammatory agents.

BOX 16.3

Pathophysiology of Rheumatoid Arthritis

Rheumatoid arthritis is a chronic, systemic disease that affects people of all ages. It is considered to be an autoimmune disease. Patients with rheumatoid arthritis have high levels of rheumatoid factor (RF), an antibody to immunoglobulin G (IgG). RF interacts with circulating IgG to form immune complexes, which tend to deposit in the synovial fluid of joints, as well as in the eye and other small vessels. The formation of the immune complex activates complement and precipitates an inflammatory reaction and release of TNF. During the immune reaction, lysosomal enzymes are released that destroy the tissues surrounding the joint. This destruction of normal tissue causes a further inflammatory reaction, and a cycle of destruction and inflammation ensues. Over time, the joint becomes severely damaged and the synovial space fills with scar tissue.

CRITICAL THINKING SCENARIO

Aspirin and Rheumatoid Arthritis

THE SITUATION

G.T. is an 82-year-old man on a fixed income with a 14-year history of rheumatoid arthritis. He is seen in the clinic for evaluation of his arthritis and to address his complaint that his medicines are not helping him. On examination, it is found that G.T.'s range of motion (ROM), physical examination of joints, and overall presentation have not changed since his last visit. G.T. states that he had been taking aspirin, as prescribed, for his arthritis. But he read that aspirin can cause severe stomach problems, so he had switched to *Ecotrin* (an aspirin and antacid combination). This drug was much more expensive than he could handle on his fixed income, so he had started taking the drug only once every 3 days.

CRITICAL THINKING

Think about the pathophysiology of rheumatoid arthritis and how the drugs ordered act on the inflammatory process:

How can the nurse best explain the disease and the drug regimen to this patient?

What could be contributing to G.T.'s perception that his condition has worsened?

What nursing interventions would be appropriate to help G.T. cope with his disease and his need for medication?

DISCUSSION

G.T. should be offered encouragement and support to deal with his progressive disease and the drug regimen required. The fact that his physical status has not changed but he perceives that the disease is worse may reflect other underlying problems that are making it more difficult for him to cope with chronic pain and limitations. The nurse should explore his social situation, any changes in his living situation, and support services. An examination should be done to determine whether other physical problems have emerged that could be adding to his sense that things are getting worse. The actions of aspirin on the arthritic process should be reviewed in basic terms, with emphasis on the importance of preventing further damage and maintaining high enough levels of aspirin to control the arthritis signs and symptoms. Pictures of the process involved in rheumatoid arthritis may help—the simpler the better in most cases.

G.T. also should be taught that all aspirin is the same, so it is acceptable to buy the cheapest generic aspirin. He can check the expiration date to make sure that the drug is fresh and still therapeutic and check that it does not smell like vinegar. Tell G.T. that the expensive combination product that G.T. has been using has not been proven to be any more effective at helping arthritis or at decreasing adverse effects than generic aspirin.

Aspirin and Rheumatoid Arthritis (continued)

If G.T. has been having gastrointestinal (GI) complaints with the aspirin, he can be encouraged to take the drug with food and to have small, frequent meals to keep stomach acid levels at a more steady state. If G.T. has not been having any GI complaints, he should be asked to report any immediately.

The importance of the placebo effect cannot be overlooked with this patient. Many patients actually state that they feel better when they are using well-recognized, brand name products. With support and encouragement, G.T. can be helped to follow his prescribed drug regimen and delay further damage from his arthritis.

NURSING CARE GUIDE FOR G.T.: ASPIRIN AND RHEUMATOID ARTHRITIS

Assessment: History and Examination

Allergies to aspirin; renal or hepatic impairment; ulcerative GI disease, peptic ulcer, hearing impairment, blood dyscrasias

Concurrent use of anticoagulants, steroids, ascorbic acid, alcohol, furosemide, acetazolamide, methazolamide, antacids, methotrexate, valproic acid, sulfonylureas, insulin, captopril, beta-adrenergic blockers, probenecid, spironolactone, nitroglycerin

Neurologic: Orientation, reflexes, affect

Musculoskeletal system: ROM, joint assessment

Skin: Color, lesions

Cardiovascular: Pulse, cardiac auscultation, blood pressure, perfusion

GI: Liver evaluation, bowel sounds

Lab tests: Complete blood count, liver and renal function tests

Nursing Diagnoses

Acute pain related to GI effects, headache

Disturbed sensory perception (auditory, kinesthetic) related to central nervous system (CNS) effects

Deficient knowledge regarding drug therapy

Planning

The patient will receive the best therapeutic effect from the drug therapy.

The patient will have limited adverse effects to the drug therapy.

The patient will have an understanding of the drug therapy, adverse effects to anticipate, and measures to relieve discomfort and improve safety.

Implementation

Ensure proper administration of the drug.

Administer with food if GI upset occurs.

Provide support and comfort measures to deal with adverse effects: Small, frequent meals; safety measures if CNS effects occur; measures for headache; bowel training as needed.

Provide patient teaching regarding drug name, dosage, side effects, precautions, and warnings to report; supplementary measures to help decrease arthritis pain.

Evaluation

Evaluate drug effects: Decrease in signs and symptoms of inflammation.

Monitor for adverse effects: CNS changes, rash, GI upset, GI bleeding

Monitor for drug–drug interactions as listed.

Evaluate effectiveness of patient-teaching program.

Evaluate effectiveness of comfort/safety measures.

PATIENT TEACHING FOR G.T.

- Your doctor has prescribed aspirin to help relieve the signs and symptoms of your rheumatoid arthritis. Aspirin works as an anti-inflammatory drug. It works in the body to decrease inflammation and to relieve the signs and symptoms of inflammation, such as pain, swelling, heat, tenderness, and redness. It does not cure your arthritis, but will help you to live with it more comfortably.
- Take your aspirin exactly as prescribed, every day. It is important to take the drug every day so that the blood levels of the aspirin are high enough to be effective. Do not use any aspirin that has a vinegar odor.
- Some of the following adverse effects may occur:
- Nausea, vomiting, abdominal discomfort: Taking the drug with food or eating small, frequent meals may help. If these effects persist, consult with your health care provider.
- Diarrhea, constipation: These effects may decrease over time; ensure ready access to bathroom facilities and consult with your health care provider for possible treatment.
- Drowsiness, dizziness, blurred vision: Avoid driving or performing tasks that require alertness if you experience any of these problems.
- Headache: If this becomes a problem, consult with your health care provider. Do not self-treat with more aspirin or other analgesics.
- Tell any health care provider who is taking care of you that you are taking this drug.
- Avoid using other OTC preparations while you are taking this drug. If you feel that you need one of these drugs, consult with your health care provider for the most appropriate choice. Many of these drugs may also contain aspirin and could cause an overdose.
- Report any of the following to your health care provider: fever, rash, GI pain, nausea, itching, or black or tarry stools.
- Keep this drug and all medications out of the reach of children.

Pharmacokinetics

Salicylates are readily absorbed directly from the stomach, reaching peak levels within 5 to 30 minutes. They are metabolized in the liver and excreted in the urine, with a half-life of 15 minutes to 12 hours, depending on the salicylate. Salicylates cross the placenta and enter breast milk; they are not indicated for use during pregnancy or lactation because of the potential adverse effects on the neonate and associated bleeding risks for the mother.

Contraindications and Cautions

Salicylates are contraindicated in the presence of known allergy to salicylates, other nonsteroidal anti-inflammatory drugs (NSAIDs) (more common with a history of nasal polyps, asthma, or chronic urticaria), or tartrazine (a dye that has a cross-sensitivity with aspirin) *because of the risk of allergic reaction*; bleeding abnormalities *because of the changes in platelet aggregation associated with these drugs*; impaired renal function *because the drug is excreted in the urine*; chickenpox or influenza *because of the risk of Reye syndrome in children and teenagers*; surgery or other invasive procedures scheduled within 1 week *because of the risk of increased bleeding*; and pregnancy or lactation *because of the potential adverse effects on the neonate or mother*.

Adverse Effects

The adverse effects associated with salicylates may be the result of direct drug effects on the stomach (nausea, dyspepsia, heartburn, epigastric discomfort) and on clotting systems (blood loss, bleeding abnormalities). **Salicylism** can occur with high levels of aspirin; dizziness, ringing in the ears, difficulty hearing, nausea, vomiting, diarrhea, mental confusion, and lassitude can occur. Acute salicylate toxicity may occur at doses of 20 to 25 g in adults or 4 g in children. Signs of salicylate toxicity include hyperpnea, tachypnea, hemorrhage, excitement, confusion, pulmonary edema, convulsions, tetany, metabolic acidosis, fever, coma, and cardiovascular (CV), renal, and respiratory collapse.

Clinically Important Drug–Drug Interactions

The salicylates interact with many other drugs, primarily because of alterations in absorption, effects on the liver, or extension of the therapeutic effects of the salicylate or the interacting drug (or both). The list of interacting drugs in each drug monograph in a nursing drug guide should be consulted and the prescriber consulted before adding or removing a salicylate from any drug regimen.

Ⓟ Prototype Summary: Aspirin

Indications: Treatment of mild to moderate pain, fever, inflammatory conditions; reduction of risk of transient ischemic attack or stroke; reduction of risk of myocardial infarction.

Actions: Inhibits the synthesis of prostaglandins; blocks the effects of pyrogens at the hypothalamus; inhibits platelet aggregation by blocking thromboxane A2.

Pharmacokinetics:

Route	Onset	Peak	Duration
Oral	5–30 min	0.25–2 h	3–6 h
Rectal	1–2 h	4–5 h	6–8 h

$T_{1/2}$: 15 minutes to 12 hours; metabolized in the liver and excreted in the urine.

Adverse Effects: Nausea, vomiting, heartburn, epigastric discomfort, occult blood loss, dizziness, tinnitus, acidosis.

Nursing Considerations for Patients Receiving Salicylates

Assessment: History and Examination

- Assess for contraindications or cautions: History of allergy to any salicylate or tartrazine *to avoid hypersensitivity reactions*; renal disease *because these drugs are excreted through the urine*; bleeding disorders *because of the drug effects on blood clotting*; chickenpox or influenza in children *to avoid the risk of Reye syndrome*; and pregnancy or lactation *to avoid adverse effects on the fetus or baby and risk of bleeding in the mother*.
- Perform physical assessment to establish baseline status before beginning therapy and to *monitor for any potential adverse effects*.
- Assess for the presence of any skin lesions *to monitor for dermatological effects*.
- Monitor temperature *to evaluate the drug's effectiveness in lowering temperature*.
- Evaluate CNS status—orientation, reflexes, eighth cranial nerve function, and affect—*to assess CNS effects of the drug*.
- Monitor pulse, blood pressure, and perfusion *to assess for bleeding effects or cardiovascular effects of the drug*.
- Evaluate respirations and adventitious sounds *to detect hypersensitivity reactions*.
- Perform a liver evaluation and monitor bowel sounds *to detect hypersensitivity reactions, bleeding, and GI effects of the drug*.
- Monitor laboratory tests for complete blood count (CBC), liver and renal function tests, urinalysis, stool guaiac, and clotting times *to detect bleeding or other*

adverse effects of the drug and changes in function that could interfere with drug metabolism and excretion.

Nursing Diagnoses

Nursing diagnoses related to drug therapy might include the following:

- Acute pain related to CNS and GI effects.
- Ineffective breathing pattern if toxic effects occur.
- Disturbed sensory perception (auditory, kinesthetic) if toxic effects occur.
- Deficient knowledge regarding drug therapy.

Planning

- The patient will receive the best therapeutic effect from the drug therapy.
- The patient will have limited adverse effects to the drug therapy.
- The patient will have an understanding of the drug therapy, adverse effects to anticipate, and measures to relieve discomfort and improve safety.

Implementation with Rationale

- Administer with food if GI upset is severe; provide small, frequent meals *to alleviate GI effects.*
- Administer drug as indicated; check all drugs being taken for possible salicylate ingredients; monitor dose *to avoid toxic levels.*
- Monitor for severe reactions *to avoid problems and provide emergency procedures* (gastric lavage, induction of vomiting, administration of charcoal) if they occur.
- Arrange for supportive care and comfort measures (rest, environmental control) *to decrease body temperature or to alleviate inflammation.*
- Ensure that the patient is well hydrated during therapy *to decrease the risk of toxicity.*
- Provide thorough patient teaching, including measures to avoid adverse effects and warning signs of problems, as well as proper administration, *to increase knowledge about drug therapy and to increase compliance with the drug regimen.*
- Offer support and encouragement *to deal with the drug regimen.*

Evaluation

- Monitor patient response to the drug (improvement in condition being treated, relief of signs and symptoms of inflammation).
- Monitor for adverse effects (GI upset, CNS changes, bleeding).
- Evaluate the effectiveness of the teaching plan (patient can name drug, dosage, adverse effects to watch for, specific measures to avoid adverse effects).
- Monitor the effectiveness of comfort measures and compliance with the drug regimen.

KEY POINTS

- Salicylates block prostaglandin activity, which decreases the inflammatory response and relieves the signs and symptoms of inflammation.
- Salicylates can cause GI irritation, eighth cranial nerve stimulation, and salicylism—ringing in the ears, acidosis, nausea, vomiting, diarrhea, mental confusion, and lassitude.

Nonsteroidal Anti-inflammatory and Related Agents

Nonsteroidal anti-inflammatory drugs (NSAIDs) provide strong anti-inflammatory and analgesic effects without the adverse effects associated with the corticosteroids (Table 16.2). Acetaminophen (*Tylenol*) is a related drug and a widely used agent. It has antipyretic and analgesic properties but does not have the anti-inflammatory effects of the salicylates or the NSAIDs. It is discussed in this chapter because it is used for many of the same reasons that NSAIDs are used, and the nurse needs to understand the similarities and differences of these drugs.

Nonsteroidal Anti-inflammatory Drugs

The NSAIDs are a drug class that has become one of the most commonly used drug types in the United States. Following unanticipated study results linking drugs in this class to an increased risk of CV events and death as well as increased bleeding in the GI tract a black box warning was added to all of these drugs pointing out the CV and GI risks associated with taking them.

This group of drugs includes propionic acids, acetic acids, fenamates, oxicam derivatives, and cyclooxygenase-2 (COX-2) inhibitors. The classes are defined by chemical structural differences, but clinically the NSAIDs are all-inclusive. See Table 16.2 for a list of these drugs by group, as well as their specific indications. The choice of NSAID depends on personal experience and the patient's response to the drug. A patient may have little response to one NSAID and a huge response to another. It may take several trials to determine the drug of choice for any particular patient (Box 16.4).

Therapeutic Actions and Indications

The anti-inflammatory, analgesic, and antipyretic effects of the NSAIDs are largely related to inhibition of prostaglandin synthesis (see Figure 16.1). The NSAIDs block two enzymes, known as COX-1 and COX-2. COX-1 is present in all tissues and seems to be involved in many body functions, including blood clotting, protecting the stomach

Table 16.2 Drugs in Focus: Nonsteroidal Anti-inflammatory Drugs (NSAIDs) and Related Agents

Drug Name	Dosage/Route	Usual Indications
NSAID Propionic Acids		
fenoprofen (*Nalfon*)	200–600 mg PO t.i.d. or q.i.d.	Treatment of pain, arthritis in adults
flurbiprofen (*Ansaid*)	200–300 mg PO in divided doses; ophthalmic solution: 1 drop (gtt) q30 min beginning 2 h after surgery	Long-term management of arthritis; topically to manage pain after eye surgery in adults
ibuprofen (*Motrin, Advil, Caldolor* IV, others)	*Adult:* 400–800 PO t.i.d. to q.i.d. 400–800 mg IV over 30 min every 6 h for pain; 400 mg IV over 30 min for fever followed by 400 mg every 4–6 h *or* 100–200 mg every 4 h to control fever *Pediatric:* 30–40 mg/kg/d PO in three to four divided doses for arthritis; 5–10 mg/kg PO q6–8 h for fever	Treatment of pain, arthritis, dysmenorrhea, juvenile arthritis
ketoprofen (*Orudis*)	25–75 mg PO t.i.d. to q.i.d.; reduce dose with hepatic or renal impairment; SR form: 200 mg/d PO	Short-term management of pain; long-term management of arthritis (SR form); ophthalmic form to relieve ocular itching
naproxen (*Naprosyn*)	*Adult:* 250–500 mg PO b.i.d.; do not give >200 mg q12 h for geriatric patients *Pediatric:* 10 mg/kg/d PO in two divided doses for juvenile arthritis; do not give OTC versions to children <12 y without consulting health care provider	Treatment of pain, arthritis, dysmenorrhea, juvenile arthritis
oxaprozin (*Daypro*)	1,200 mg PO daily	Treatment of arthritis in adults
Acetic Acids		
diclofenac (*Voltaren, Cataflam, Flector*)	100–200 mg/d PO; 25–50 mg b.i.d. to q.i.d. PO *Topical:* Apply one patch b.i.d. to most painful area	Treatment of acute and chronic pain associated with inflammatory conditions in adults
etodolac (*Lodine*)	800–1,200 mg/d PO in divided doses; 200–400 mg q6–8 h PO for pain management	Treatment of arthritis pain in adults; management of chronic pain (extended release formulation)
indomethacin (*Indocin*)	*Adult:* 75–150 mg/d PO in three to four divided doses *Pediatric (>2 y):* In special circumstances, 2 mg/kg/d PO in divided doses	Relief of moderate to severe pain in PO, topical, and PR forms; closure of patent ductus arteriosus in premature infants (given IV)
ketorolac (*Toradol*)	10 mg PO q4–6 h *or* 30–60 mg IM, switching to oral form as soon as possible, *or* 30 mg IV as a single dose *Ophthalmic:* 1 gtt to affected eye q.i.d.; reduce dose with renal impairment and in patients >65 y	Short-term management of pain in adults; topically to relieve ocular itching
nabumetone (*Relafen*)	1,000 mg/d PO as a single dose	Treatment of acute and chronic arthritis pain in adults
sulindac (*Clinoril*)	150–200 mg PO b.i.d.	Treatment of various inflammatory conditions in adults
tolmetin (*Tolectin*)	*Adult:* 400 mg PO t.i.d.; 600–800 mg/d in three to four doses for maintenance *Pediatric:* 20 mg/kg/d PO in three to four divided doses	Treatment of acute flares of rheumatoid and juvenile arthritis
Fenamates		
meclofenamate	100–400 mg/d PO	Treatment of mild to moderate pain, primary dysmenorrhea, rheumatoid arthritis, osteoarthritis
mefenamic acid (*Ponstel*)	500 mg PO, then 250 mg PO q6h as needed	Short-term treatment of pain in adults and children >14 y; primary dysmenorrhea
Oxicam Derivative		
meloxicam (*Mobic*)	*Adult:* 7.5 mg/d PO to a maximum of 15 mg/d *Pediatric:* 0.125 mg/kg/d PO to a maximum of 7.5 mg/d	Treatment of osteoarthritis, rheumatoid arthritis, and juvenile arthritis
piroxicam (*Feldene*)	20 mg/d PO as a single dose	Treatment of acute and chronic arthritis in adults

Drug Name	Dosage/Route	Usual Indications
Cyclooxygenase-2 Inhibitor		
celecoxib (*Celebrex*)	Initially 100–200 mg PO b.i.d; acute pain 400 mg PO; then 200 mg PO b.i.d. for FAP	Treatment of acute and chronic arthritis in adults; acute pain; primary dysmenorrhea; reduction of the number of colorectal polyps in FAP; ankylosing spondylitis
Related Agent		
acetaminophen (*Tylenol*)	*Adult:* 1,000 mg PO t.i.d. to q.i.d. *or* 325–650 mg PR q4–6 h *Pediatric:* Adjust dose based on age	Relief of pain and fever in a variety of situations

SR, sustained release; OTC, over the counter; FAP, familial adenomatous polyposis.

BOX 16.4 FOCUS ON The Evidence

Cyclooxygenase-2 Inhibitors

In late 2004 Merck voluntarily withdrew their COX-2 inhibitor, rofecoxib (*Vioxx*), from the market following release of a midstudy finding that the use of the drug over an 18-month period led to a significant increase in CV mortality in those taking the drug compared with a placebo group. The study, called the APPROVE study (Adenomatous Polyp Prevention on *Vioxx*), was targeted at testing whether the blocking of such growth factors as angiogenesis could decrease cancer risk in a specific population. The study participants took 25 mg of *Vioxx* each day for 18 months (the halfway point in the study) when the finding of increased CV events was announced and the study was stopped. The CV outcomes were not noted earlier than 18 months. Interestingly, other studies, including a 4-year study of the effects on Alzheimer's disease, did not show a significant difference in CV events between the placebo and drug groups. Yet, in the VIGOR (*Vioxx* Gastrointestinal Outcomes Research) study, in which rofecoxib was compared with naproxen (another NSAID) for 12 months, increased CV events were noted in the rofecoxib group after only 2 months.

The U.S. Food and Drug Administration (FDA) formed a committee to study the COX-2 inhibitors and then all of the NSAIDs on the market to see if there were any problems in oversight of drug safety and to make recommendations about the future use of these drugs.

Valdecoxib (*Bextra*) was withdrawn from the market at FDA request after the committee reviewed data. A small study did show an increase in CV events, including death, when *Bextra* was used immediately in postoperative patients recovering from coronary artery bypass graft (CABG) surgery. The drug was not proven to be especially more effective than other NSAIDs for relieving pain, and already had a black box warning about the increased possibility of severe skin reactions, including Stevens-Johnson syndrome. With those facts in mind and the possibility of a COX-2 link to increased CV events the FDA believed that the benefits of marketing the drug did not outweigh the potential risks for using the drug.

Celecoxib (*Celebrex*) remains on the market. The APC (Adenoma Prevention with Celecoxib) study did show a two- to threefold increase in CV events among patients using the drug compared with placebo over 33 months. There did seem to be a dose correlation, with more events in the group using a higher dose. A nearly identical study, the PreSAP (Prevention of Spontaneous Adenomatous Polyps) trial, showed no increase in CV events in the group using celecoxib. The Alzheimer's Disease Anti-Inflammatory Prevention Trial (ADAPT) did not appear to show an increase in CV events in the patients in that small study.

The media helped to fuel a real concern about the safety of any anti-inflammatory medication. The questions remain: Were the CV events related to dosage, length of drug use, or the underlying conditions of the patients being studied? Were the CV events a direct effect of the COX-2 inhibitor? Would these same events have occurred if the drug were used at the dosages approved and for the approved length of time? More long-term, controlled studies are needed to answer these questions. In the meantime, the FDA has recommended that valdecoxib and rofecoxib stay off the market until appropriate guidelines and controls are in place for their return; that all NSAID packaging information include warnings that there is potential risk for increased CV events as well as the risk of GI bleeding, and that health care providers use caution in recommending these drugs to anyone with an established CV risk; that all prescription NSAIDs be contraindicated in patients immediately after CABG surgery; and that the prescribing information for celecoxib include a black box warning referencing the available data about increased CV risk. Other COX-2 inhibitors, lumiracoxib and etoricoxib, are available in other countries, but have not been approved for sale in the United States related to very strict standards in proving efficacy and safety.

Specialists treating patients with chronic pain have petitioned to have the FDA return rofecoxib and valdecoxib to the market, citing patients who could only obtain relief using those drugs. Some patients only respond to these particular NSAIDs, and these specialists feel that the patients should have a choice, being informed of the risks, to continue their use to relieve pain. Clearly, more long-term studies are needed. The nurse may be asked about this controversy and what recommendations are in place by patients who want relief from pain but really want to understand the risks to their health. To get a complete summary of the research, the report to the FDA, and current recommendations and research, go to www.fda.gov and click on NSAIDs under Hot Topics on the right side of the page. This site is updated regularly and offers information geared to patients and to health care professionals.

lining, and maintaining sodium and water balance in the kidney. COX-1 turns arachidonic acid into prostaglandins as needed in a variety of tissues. COX-2 is active at sites of trauma or injury when more prostaglandins are needed, but it does not seem to be involved in the other tissue functions. By interfering with this part of the inflammatory reaction, NSAIDs block inflammation before all of the signs and symptoms can develop. Most NSAIDs also block various other functions of the prostaglandins, including protection of the stomach lining, regulation of blood clotting, and water and salt balance in the kidney. The COX-2 inhibitors are thought to act only at sites of trauma and injury to more specifically block the inflammatory reaction.

The adverse effects associated with most NSAIDs are related to blocking of both of these enzymes and changes in the functions that they influence—GI integrity, blood clotting, and sodium and water balance. The COX-2 inhibitors are designed to affect only the activity of COX-2, the enzyme that becomes active in response to trauma and injury. They do not interfere with COX-1, which is needed for normal functioning of these systems. Consequently, these drugs should not have the associated adverse effects seen when both COX-1 and COX-2 are inhibited. Experience has shown that the COX-2 inhibitors still have some effect on these other functions, and patients should still be evaluated for GI effects, changes in bleeding time, and water retention. Recent studies suggest that they may block some protective responses in the body, such as vasodilation and inhibited platelet clumping, which is protective if vessel narrowing or blockage occurs; blocking this effect could lead to CV problems. Box 16.5 summarizes the actions and adverse effects of the COX-1 and COX-2 enzymes.

The NSAIDs are indicated for relief of the signs and symptoms of rheumatoid arthritis and osteoarthritis, for relief of mild to moderate pain, for treatment of primary dysmenorrhea, and for fever reduction.

BOX 16.5

Comparison of Cyclooxygenase (COX) Receptors

COX-1	COX-2
Site of action	**Site of action**
Found in many tissues, important for homeostasis	Induced by inflammatory stimuli at the site of inflammation
Effects	**Effects**
• Converts arachidonic acid to inflammatory prostaglandins • Maintains renal function • Provides for gastric mucosa integrity • Promotes vascular hemostasis, increases bleeding • Autocrine effects causing fever	• Increases pain, inflammation • Vasodilates • Blocks platelet clumping
Effects of blocking	**Effects of blocking**
• Decreases swelling, pain, inflammation • Sodium retention, edema, increased blood pressure • GI erosion, bleeding • Decreases fever	• Decreases pain, inflammation • Prevents protective vasodilation, allows platelet clumping, which can lead to MI, cerebrovascular accident • Myriad of skin reactions, including Stevens-Johnson syndrome

Pharmacokinetics

The NSAIDs are rapidly absorbed from the GI tract, reaching peak levels in 1 to 3 hours. They are metabolized in the liver and excreted in the urine. NSAIDs cross the placenta and cross into breast milk. Therefore, they are not recommended during pregnancy and lactation because of the potential adverse effects on the fetus or neonate.

Contraindications and Cautions

The NSAIDs are contraindicated in the presence of allergy to any NSAID or salicylate, and celecoxib is also contraindicated in the presence of allergy to sulfonamides. Additional contraindications are CV dysfunction or hypertension *because of the varying effects of the prostaglandins*; peptic ulcer or known GI bleeding *because of the potential to exacerbate the GI bleeding*; and pregnancy or lactation *because of potential adverse effects on the neonate or mother*. Caution should be used with renal or hepatic dysfunction, *which could alter the metabolism and excretion of these drugs*, and with any other known allergies, *which indicate increased sensitivity*.

Adverse Effects

Patients receiving NSAIDs often experience nausea, dyspepsia, GI pain, constipation, diarrhea, or flatulence caused by direct GI effects of the drug. The potential for GI bleeding often is a cause of discontinuation of the drug. Headache, dizziness, somnolence, and fatigue also occur frequently and could be related to prostaglandin activity in the CNS. Bleeding, platelet inhibition, hypertension, and even bone marrow depression have been reported with chronic use and probably are related to the blocking of prostaglandin activity. Rash and mouth sores may occur, and anaphylactoid reactions ranging up to fatal anaphylactic shock have been reported in cases of severe hypersensitivity.

Clinically Important Drug–Drug Interactions

There often is a decreased diuretic effect when these drugs are taken with loop diuretics; there is a potential for decreased antihypertensive effect of beta-blockers if these drugs are combined; and there have been reports of lithium toxicity, especially when combined with ibuprofen. Patients who receive these combinations should be monitored closely, and appropriate dose adjustments should be made by the prescriber.

Prototype Summary: Ibuprofen

Indications: Relief of the signs and symptoms of rheumatoid arthritis and osteoarthritis; relief of mild to moderate pain; treatment of primary dysmenorrhea; fever reduction.

Actions: Inhibits prostaglandin synthesis by blocking COX-1 and COX-2 receptor sites, leading to an anti-inflammatory effect, analgesia, and antipyretic effects.

Pharmacokinetics:

Route	Onset	Peak	Duration
Oral	30 min	1–2 h	4–6 h
IV	Start of infusion	Minutes	4–6 h

$T_{1/2}$: 1.8 to 2.5 hours; metabolized in the liver and excreted in the urine.

Adverse Effects: Headache, dizziness, somnolence, fatigue, rash, nausea, dyspepsia, bleeding, constipation.

Acetaminophen

Acetaminophen (*Tylenol*) is used to treat moderate to mild pain and fever and often is used in place of the NSAIDs or salicylates. It has been the most frequently used drug for managing pain and fever in children. It is widely available OTC and is found in many combination products. It can be extremely toxic. It causes severe liver toxicity that can lead to death when taken in high doses. Every year children die from inadvertent acetaminophen overdose when parents give their child more than one OTC drug containing acetaminophen or administer a high dose of acetaminophen. The U.S. Food and Drug Administration and drug manufacturers have joined forces to produce mass media ads warning parents about this possibility and to limit the amount of acetaminophen that can be in each OTC product.

Therapeutic Actions and Indications

Acetaminophen acts directly on the thermoregulatory cells in the hypothalamus to cause sweating and vasodilation; this in turn causes the release of heat and lowers fever. The mechanism of action related to the analgesic effects of acetaminophen has not been identified.

Acetaminophen is indicated for the treatment of pain and fever associated with a variety of conditions, including influenza; for the prophylaxis of children receiving diphtheria–pertussis–tetanus immunizations (aspirin may mask Reye syndrome in children); and for the relief of musculoskeletal pain associated with arthritis (see Table 16.2).

Pharmacokinetics

Acetaminophen is rapidly absorbed from the GI tract, reaching peak levels in 0.5 to 2 hours. It is extensively metabolized in the liver and excreted in the urine, with a half-life of about 2 hours. Caution should be used in patients with hepatic or renal impairment, which could interfere with metabolism and excretion of the drug, leading to toxic levels. Acetaminophen crosses the placenta and enters breast milk; it should be used cautiously during pregnancy or lactation because of the potential adverse effects on the fetus or neonate.

Contraindications and Cautions

Acetaminophen is contraindicated in the presence of allergy to acetaminophen *because of the risk of hypersensitivity reactions.* It should be used cautiously in pregnancy or lactation *because of the potential for adverse effects on the fetus or baby* and in hepatic dysfunction or chronic alcoholism *because of associated toxic effects on the liver.*

Adverse Effects

Adverse effects associated with acetaminophen use include headache, hemolytic anemia, renal dysfunction, skin rash, and fever. Hepatotoxicity is a potentially fatal adverse effect that is usually associated with chronic use and overdose and is related to direct toxic effects on the liver. The dose that could prove toxic varies with the age of the patient, other drugs that the patient might be taking, and the underlying hepatic function of that patient. When overdose occurs, acetylcysteine can be used as an antidote. Life support measures may also be necessary.

Clinically Important Drug–Drug Interactions

There is an increased risk of bleeding with oral anticoagulants because of effects on the liver; of toxicity with chronic ethanol ingestion because of toxic effects on the liver; and of hepatotoxicity with barbiturates, carbamazepine, hydantoins, or rifampin. These combinations should be avoided, but if they must be used, appropriate dose adjustment should be made and the patient should be monitored closely.

Ⓟ Prototype Summary: Acetaminophen

Indications: Treatment of mild to moderate pain, fever, or signs and symptoms of the common cold or flu; musculoskeletal pain associated with arthritis and rheumatic disorders.

Actions: Acts directly on the hypothalamus to cause vasodilation and sweating, which will reduce fever; mechanism of action as an analgesic is not understood.

Pharmacokinetics:

Route	Onset	Peak	Duration
Oral	Varies	0.5–2 h	3–6 h

$T_{1/2}$: 1 to 3 hours; metabolized in the liver and excreted in the urine.

Adverse Effects: Rash, fever, chest pain, liver toxicity and failure, bone marrow suppression.

Nursing Considerations for Patients Receiving NSAIDs and Related Agents

Assessment: History and Examination

(Refer to Salicylates for nursing diagnoses, planning, implementation with rationale, and evaluation.)

- Assess for *contraindications or cautions*: Known allergies to any salicylates, NSAIDs, or tartrazine; pregnancy or lactation; hepatic or renal disease; CV dysfunction; hypertension; and GI bleeding or peptic ulcer.
- Assess for *baseline status before beginning therapy and for any potential adverse effects*: Presence of any skin lesions; temperature; orientation, reflexes, and affect; pulse, blood pressure, and perfusion; respirations and adventitious sounds; liver evaluation; bowel sounds; and CBC, liver and renal function tests, urinalysis, stool guaiac, and serum electrolytes.

KEY POINTS

- NSAIDs block prostaglandin synthesis at the COX-1 and COX-2 sites. This blocks inflammation but also blocks protection of the stomach lining, as well as the kidneys' regulation of water.
- There are many different NSAIDs. If one does not work for a particular patient, another one might.
- Acetaminophen causes vasodilation and heat release, lowering fever and working to relieve pain.
- Acetaminophen can cause liver failure. It is found in many OTC products. Teach patients to avoid toxic doses of acetaminophen.

Antiarthritis Agents

Other drugs that are used to block the inflammatory process include the antiarthritis drugs. Arthritis is a potentially debilitating inflammatory process in the joints that causes pain and bone deformities. Antiarthritis drugs include the gold compounds, which are used to prevent and suppress arthritis in selected patients with rheumatoid arthritis. The other antiarthritis drugs are specifically used to block the inflammation and tissue damage of rheumatoid arthritis (see Table 16.3).

Gold Compounds

Some patients with rheumatic inflammatory conditions do not respond to the usual anti-inflammatory therapies, and their conditions worsen despite weeks or months of standard pharmacological treatment. Some of these patients respond to treatment with gold salts, also known as **chrysotherapy**, in which gold is taken up by macrophages, which then inhibit phagocytosis; it is reserved for use in patients who are unresponsive to conventional therapy and can be very toxic. The gold salts available for use include auranofin (*Ridaura*) and gold sodium thiomalate (*Aurolate*).

Therapeutic Actions and Indications

Chrysotherapy results in inhibition of phagocytosis (see Figure 16.1). Because phagocytosis is blocked the release of lysosomal enzymes is inhibited and tissue destruction is decreased. This action allows gold salts to suppress and prevent some arthritis and synovitis. Gold salts are indicated to treat selected cases of rheumatoid and juvenile rheumatoid arthritis in patients whose disease has been unresponsive to standard therapy (see Table 16.3 for Usual Indications). These drugs do not repair damage; they prevent further damage and so are most effective if used early in the disease.

Pharmacokinetics

The gold salts are absorbed at varying rates, depending on their route of administration. They are widely distributed throughout the body but seem to concentrate in the hypothalamic–pituitary–adrenocortical system and in the adrenal and renal cortices. The gold salts are excreted in urine and feces. These drugs cross the placenta and cross into breast milk. They have been shown to be teratogenic in animal studies and should not be used during pregnancy or lactation. Barrier contraceptives should be recommended to women of childbearing age, and another method of feeding the baby should be used if gold therapy is needed in a lactating woman.

Table 16.3 *Drugs in Focus:* Antiarthritis Agents

Drug Name	Dosage/Route	Usual Indications
Gold Compounds		
auranofin (*Ridaura*)	*Adult:* 6 mg/d PO; monitor geriatric patients carefully *Pediatric:* 0.1–0.15 mg/kg/d PO	Oral agent for long-term therapy of rheumatic disorders
gold sodium thiomalate (*Aurolate*)	*Adult:* 10 mg IM, then 25 mg IM every other week; use caution in geriatric patients *Pediatric:* 10 mg IM, then 1 mg/kg IM every other week	Injected drug for early treatment of rheumatic disorders
Tumor Necrosis Factor Blockers		
adalimumab (*Humira*)	*Adult:* 40 mg subcutaneous every other week *Pediatric:* 20–40 mg subcutaneous every other week	Reduction of signs and symptoms of rheumatoid arthritis, psoriatic arthritis, ankylosing spondylitis, plaque psoriasis, juvenile idiopathic arthritis, Crohn's disease, ulcerative colitis
certolizumab (*Cimzia*)	*Adult:* 400 mg/wk subcutaneous (Crohn's), 200 mg/wk subcutaneous (arthritis)	Reduction of signs and symptoms of rheumatoid arthritis, Crohn's disease
etanercept (*Enbrel*)	*Adult:* 25 mg subcutaneous two times per week *or* 50 mg subcutaneous once a week *Pediatric (4–17 y):* 0.4 mg/kg subcutaneous two times per week with 72–96 h between doses; not recommended for patients <4 y	Reduction of signs and symptoms of severe rheumatoid arthritis in patients whose disease is unresponsive to other therapy; prevention of damage early in the disease; ankylosing spondylosis; psoriatic arthritis
golimumab (*Simponi*)	*Adult:* 50 mg/month subcutaneous *or* 2 mg/kg IV over 30 min at weeks 0, 4 then q8 wk	Treatment of active rheumatoid arthritis, psoriatic arthritis, alkylosing spondylosis
infliximab (*Remicade*)	*Adult:* 3 mg IV at weeks 0, 2, 6, then q8 wk (rheumatoid arthritis) *Adult and child:* 5 mg IV at weeks 0, 2, 6, then 5 mg/kg IV q8 wk (Crohn's disease, ulcerative colitis, ankylosing spondylosis, psoriatic arthritis, plaque psoriasis)	Treatment of Crohn's disease, ulcerative colitis, ankylosing spondylosis, rheumatoid arthritis, psoriatic arthritis, plaque psoriasis
Other Antiarthritis Drugs		
anakinra (*Kineret*)	*Adult:* 100 mg/d subcutaneous	Reduction of signs and symptoms of rheumatoid arthritis in patients ≥18 y if one or more other arthritis agents have failed
hyaluronidase derivatives (hylan G-F 20, *Synvisc*)	2 mL once a week for 3 wk injected into the affected knee	Relief of pain in the knees of arthritis patients whose disease is unresponsive to conventional treatment
leflunomide (*Arava*)	100 mg PO daily for 3 d, then 20 mg PO daily	Treatment of active rheumatoid arthritis, to relieve signs and symptoms and to slow the progression of disease in adults
penicillamine (*Depen*)	125–250 mg PO daily	Treatment of severe, active rheumatoid arthritis in adults whose disease is unresponsive to conventional therapy
sodium hyaluronate (*Hyalgan*)	2 mg once a week for 5 wk injected into the affected knee	Relief of pain in the knees of arthritis patients whose disease is unresponsive to conventional treatment
tofacitinib (*Xeljanz*)	*Adult:* 5 mg PO b.i.d.	Treatment of adults with moderate to severe active arthritis intolerant to other therapies

Contraindications and Cautions

Gold salts can be quite toxic and are contraindicated in the presence of any known allergy to gold, severe diabetes, congestive heart failure, severe debilitation, renal or hepatic impairment, hypertension, blood dyscrasias, recent radiation treatment, history of toxic levels of heavy metals, and pregnancy or lactation.

Adverse Effects

A variety of adverse effects is common with the use of gold salts, and they are probably related to their deposition in the tissues and effects at that local level: Stomatitis, glossitis, gingivitis, pharyngitis, laryngitis, colitis, diarrhea, and other GI inflammation; gold bronchitis and interstitial pneumonitis; bone marrow depression; vaginitis and nephrotic syndrome; dermatitis, pruritus, and exfoliative dermatitis; and allergic reactions ranging from flushing, fainting, and dizziness to anaphylactic shock.

Clinically Important Drug–Drug Interactions

These drugs should not be combined with penicillamine, antimalarials, cytotoxic drugs, or immunosuppressive agents other than low-dose corticosteroids because of the potential for severe toxicity.

Ⓟ Prototype Summary: Auranofin

Indications: Treatment of selected adults with rheumatoid arthritis, who have insufficient response to or intolerance to NSAIDs

Actions: Taken up by macrophages, which inhibits phagocytosis and release of lysosomal enzymes that cause damage associated with inflammation.

Pharmacokinetics:

Route	Onset	Peak
Oral	Slow	4–6 h

$T_{1/2}$: 3 to 7 days; excreted in the urine and feces.

Adverse Effects: Bone marrow suppression, renal toxicity, dermatitis, nausea, vomiting, stomatitis.

Disease-Modifying Antirheumatic Drugs

Other antiarthritis drugs, called disease-modifying antirheumatic drugs (DMARDs), are available for treating arthritis and aggressively affect the process of inflammation. Many rheumatologists are selecting DMARDs early in the diagnosis, before damage to the joints has occurred, because they alter the course of the inflammatory process. Two types of DMARDs discussed include tumor necrosis factor (TNF) blockers and other disease-modifying antirheumatic drugs. The adverse effects associated with these drugs (see Adverse Effects) can be severe to life-threatening because they alter the ability of the body to initiate or carry on an inflammatory reaction.

Tumor Necrosis Factor Blockers

Tumor necrosis factor (TNF) blockers are often the first class used with progressing arthritis. These drugs are discussed in Chapter 17 with immune modulators, but because of their increasing use in treating the various forms of arthritis, they will also be discussed in depth here. These drugs include adalimumab (*Humira*), certolizumab (*Cimzia*), etanercept (*Enbrel*), golimumab (*Simponi*), and infliximab (*Remicade*).

Therapeutic Actions and Indications

TNF blockers act to decrease the local effects of TNF, a locally released cytokine that can cause the death of tumor cells and stimulate a wide range of proinflammatory activities. The actions of this cytokine when inflammation occurs within a joint capsule can lead to the destruction of bone and the malformation of joints that is associated with arthritis. Drugs that block that action of TNF slow the inflammatory response and the joint damage associated with it. These drugs are indicated for the treatment of rheumatoid arthritis, polyarticular juvenile arthritis, psoriatic arthritis, plaque psoriasis, and ankylosing spondylitis. Adalimumab, certolizumab, and infliximab are also used in Crohn's disease and ulcerative colitis. See the Critical Thinking Scenario for a case study about DMARDs and psoriatic arthritis.

CRITICAL THINKING SCENARIO

DMARDs and Psoriatic Arthritis

THE SITUATION

J.G is a 46-year-old, former semipro baseball player. He has had progressive difficulty walking, opening jars, moving things and has attributed it to years of athletic training and what he describes as "body abuse." He is seen in the clinic for evaluation after severe joint pain and loss of ROM forced him to try to find some help. Examination reveals swollen red patches on the skin, and thick, silver scaly lesions on arms and legs, markedly decreased ROM, the worse being the right shoulder, swollen feet, walking with a marked limp, and complaints of severe joint pain which is worse in the morning. Blood tests show an elevated sedimentation rate, no elevation in rheumatoid factor, and the presence of the HLA-B27 genetic marker. A bone scan reveals bone loss. The diagnosis is made of psoriatic arthritis. After consulting with family and discovering several cousins with the same diagnosis, one of whom is in a wheelchair, J.G. asked for aggressive treatment. Numerous blood tests are ordered, including tests for HIV and hepatitis B, a tuberculin (TB) test, an order for a colonoscopy and gluten sensitivity. When all the tests come in, he is prescribed adalimumab (*Humira*).

CRITICAL THINKING

Think about the pathophysiology of psoriatic arthritis and how the drug ordered acts on the inflammatory process.

DMARDs and Psoriatic Arthritis (continued)

How can the nurse best explain the disease and the drug regimen to this patient?

How can the nurse explain the numerous tests required before using these drugs and the need for continued follow-up?

What nursing interventions would be appropriate to help J.G. deal with his disease?

DISCUSSION

Psoriatic arthritis is different than rheumatoid arthritis. It is an autoimmune disease that often runs in families and often expresses a particular genetic marker, the HLA-B27 allele. People with this often also have gluten sensitivity, and efforts are usually made to bring that under control with diet if it is a concurrent issue. The joints of these patients are slowly destroyed by the body's response to antigen–antibody deposits and the fingers and toes are often more involved than in rheumatoid arthritis. Since J.G. has had this progressive arthritis for many years without seeking medical help, it was decided to start out with a DMARD. Adalimumab is a TNF inhibitor, which will slow the destruction of the joints and also help to alleviate the dermal reaction that causes the skin lesions. It is hoped that this will alleviate pain and slow the destruction and remodeling of the joint and improve J.G.'s quality of life. The nurse needs to explain this process and then educate J.G. about the overall role of TNF in the immune response and the risks involved when this protective mechanism is gone. He will be at increased risk for infections and cancers. The many blood tests ordered will ensure that he doesn't have an infection already. The colonoscopy will screen for any GI cancers and establish a baseline that can be followed. He will need to learn how to administer a subcutaneous injection and the proper disposal of needles and syringes, signs of infection to be aware of, dietary changes if he does have gluten sensitivity, and exercises that will be beneficial in keeping him active and helping the joints.

NURSING CARE GUIDE FOR J.G.: DMARDS AND PSORIATIC ARTHRITIS

Assessment: History and Examination

Assess for tuberculosis, hepatitis B, HIV, travel exposure to fungal infections, cancers, active infection, heart failure, demyelinating diseases

Concurrent use of other tumor necrosis factor blockers, live vaccines

Neurologic: Orientation, reflexes, affect

Musculoskeletal system: ROM, joint assessment

Skin: color, lesions

Cardiovascular: pulse, cardiac auscultation, blood pressure, perfusion

GI: Liver evaluation

Lab tests: CBC, liver, and renal function tests, tests for HIV, hepatitis B, sedimentation rate

Nursing Diagnoses

Acute pain related to injection site recations, headache

Disturbed sensory perception (auditory, kinesthetic) related to CNS effects

Deficient knowledge regarding drug therapy

Planning

The patient will receive the best therapeutic effect from the drug therapy.

The patient will have limited adverse effects to the drug therapy.

The patient will have an understanding of the drug therapy, adverse effects to anticipate, and measures to relieve discomfort and improve safety.

Implementation

Ensure proper administration of the drug; teach patient proper administration of subcutaneous injections; proper disposal of needles and syringes; rotation of injection sites.

Provide support and comfort measures to deal with adverse effects: Safety measures if CNS effects occur; measures for headache; treatment of injection site reactions.

Provide patient teaching regarding drug name, dosage, proper administration, side effects, precautions, and warnings to report; supplementary measures to help decrease arthritis pain.

Evaluation

Evaluate drug effects: Decrease in signs and symptoms of inflammation; stopping progression of joint deterioration.

Monitor for adverse effects: CNS changes, headache, infections, cancer

Monitor for drug–drug interactions as listed.

Evaluate effectiveness of patient-teaching program.

Evaluate effectiveness of comfort/safety measures.

PATIENT TEACHING FOR J.G.

- Your doctor has prescribed adalimumab to help relieve the signs and symptoms of your psoriatic arthritis. This drug works to block part of your body's normal response to injury. It works in the body to decrease inflammation and to relieve the signs and symptoms of inflammation, such as pain, swelling, heat, tenderness, and redness. It does not cure your arthritis, but will help you to live with it more comfortably and will delay the damage to the joints that occurs with this disease.

(continues on page 280)

DMARDs and Psoriatic Arthritis (continued)

- You must administer this drug by subcutaneous injection every other week. Mark your calendar with the days you will need the injection. You will learn the proper administration of a subcutaneous injection. You must properly dispose of the needle and syringes as we have discussed.
- Some of the following adverse effects may occur:
- *Drowsiness, dizziness, blurred vision:* Avoid driving or performing tasks that require alertness if you experience any of these problems.
- *Headache:* If this becomes a problem, consult with your health care provider. Do not self-treat with more aspirin or other analgesics.
- *Infections:* You will be more susceptible to infections, you should avoid people with known illnesses, use mask and gloves if digging in the dirt, wash your hands frequently.
- *Cancer is more likely to occur:* You should have all the routine cancer screening that is recommended, skin evaluation, colonoscopy, prostate exam. Early detection is the best response.
- Tell any health care provider who is taking care of you that you are taking this drug.
- Avoid using other OTC preparations while you are taking this drug. If you feel that you need one of these drugs, consult with your health care provider for the most appropriate choice.
- Report any of the following to your health care provider: Fever, worsening rash, blurred vision, numbness or tingling in the extremities, extreme fatigue.
- Keep this drug and all medications out of the reach of children.

Pharmacokinetics

TNF blockers must be given subcutaneously, with the exception of infliximab which is given IV. They have a slow onset, usually peaking in 48–72 hours. They are primarily excreted in the tissues and have very long half-lives ranging from 115 hours to 2 weeks. They cross the placenta and may enter breast milk, so use in pregnancy and breastfeeding should be discouraged.

Contraindications and Cautions

These drugs cannot be used in anyone with an acute infection, cancer, sepsis, tuberculosis, hepatitis, myelosuppression or demyelinating disorders *because they block the body's immune/inflammatory response and serious reactions could occur.* Etanercept cannot be used with a history of allergy to Chinese hamster ovary products *because it is made from these products.* They should not be used in pregnancy or breastfeeding *because of the potential effects on the fetus or neonate.* Caution should be used with renal or hepatic disorders, heart failure, and latex allergies *to prevent adverse reactions.*

Adverse Effects

TNF blockers come with black box warnings about the risk of serious to fatal infections and the development of lymphomas and other cancers. Patients need to be screened and monitored accordingly. Demyelinating disorders have occurred, including multiple sclerosis and various neuritis conditions. Myocardial infarction (MI), heart failure, and hypotension are also reported with the use of these drugs. Irritation at the injection site can also occur.

Clinically Important Drug–Drug Interactions

Use of any other immune suppressant drugs with TNF blockers increases the risk of serious infections and cancer. Live vaccines should not be given while on these drugs.

Ⓟ Prototype Summary: Etanercept

Indications: Reduction of signs and symptoms, and improvement of function with rheumatoid arthritis, polyarticular juvenile idiopathic arthritis, psoriatic arthritis, ankylosing spondylitis, and plaque psoriasis.

Actions: Genetically engineered TNF receptors react with and deactivate TNF released by active leukocytes, keeping the inflammatory response in check.

Pharmacokinetics:

Route	Onset	Peak
Subcutaneous	Slow	72 h

$T_{1/2}$: 115 hours; metabolized in the tissues and excreted in the tissues.

Adverse Effects: Serious to fatal infections, lymphoma and other cancers, demyelinating disorders, MI, heart failure, injection site reactions.

Other Disease-Modifying Antirheumatic Drugs

Other DMARDs discussed in this chapter include drugs used when patients do not respond to conventional therapy—

anakinra (*Kineret*), leflunomide (*Arava*), tofacitinib (*Xeljanz*) and penicillamine (*Depen*)—and drugs used to directly decrease pain in joints affected by arthritis, including hyaluronidase derivative (*Synvisc*) and sodium hyaluronate (*Hyalgan*). Additional drugs also used to modify the disease process in rheumatoid arthritis include the antineoplastic drug methotrexate (see Chapter 14), the T cell suppressor abatacept (*Orencia*) (see Chapter 17), certain antimalarial drugs (see Chapter 12), some additional antineoplastic drugs such as cyclophosphamide (see Chapter 14), and the immune modulators cyclosporine A and azathioprine (Chapter 17).

Therapeutic Actions and Indications

Anakinra is one of the newer of the antiarthritis drugs. This drug is an interleukin-1 receptor antagonist. It blocks the increased interleukin-1, which is responsible for the degradation of cartilage in rheumatoid arthritis. This drug must be given each day by subcutaneous injection and is often used in combination with other antiarthritis drugs.

See Table 16.3 for Usual Indications.

Hyaluronidase derivatives, such as hylan G-F 20 and sodium hyaluronate, have elastic and viscous properties. These drugs are injected directly into the joints of patients with severe rheumatoid arthritis of the knee. They seem to cushion and lubricate the joint and relieve the pain associated with degenerative arthritis. They are given weekly for 3 to 5 weeks.

Leflunomide directly inhibits an enzyme, dihydroorotate dehydrogenase, that is active in the autoimmune process that leads to rheumatoid arthritis, relieving signs and symptoms of inflammation and blocking the structural damage this inflammation can cause, slowing disease progression.

Penicillamine lowers the immunoglobulin M rheumatoid factor levels in patients with acute rheumatoid arthritis, relieving the signs and symptoms of inflammation. It may take 2 to 3 months of therapy before a response is noted.

Tofacitinib is a kinase inhibitor that blocks signaling pathways within immune cells to prevent their activity. It is an oral agent and is reserved for patients who have not responded to traditional therapies.

Pharmacokinetics

Anakinra is slowly absorbed from the subcutaneous tissue, reaching peak levels in 3 to 7 hours. It is metabolized in the tissues and excreted in the urine. It has a half-life of 4 to 6 hours. The hyaluronidase derivatives are not absorbed systemically. Leflunomide is slowly absorbed from the GI tract, reaching peak levels in 6 to 12 hours. It undergoes hepatic metabolism and excretion in the urine. The half-life of leflunomide is 14 to 18 days.

Penicillamine is an oral drug that reaches peak levels in 1 to 3 hours after administration. It is extensively metabolized in the liver and excreted in the urine with a half-life of 2 to 3 hours. Tofacitinib is absorbed quickly, reaching peak levels in 0.5 to 1 hour, it is metabolized in the liver and excreted in the urine with a half-life of 3 hours.

Contraindications and Cautions

These drugs are contraindicated in the presence of allergy to the drugs or to the animal products from which they were derived (chicken products in hylan G-F 20 and sodium hyaluronate) *to avoid hypersensitivity reactions*; pregnancy or lactation *because of the potential for adverse effects on the fetus or neonate*; acute infection *because of the blocking of normal inflammatory pathways*; and liver or renal impairment, *which could be exacerbated by these drugs*.

Adverse Effects

A variety of adverse effects are common with the use of these drugs, including local irritation at injection sites (anakinra, etanercept, hyaluronidase derivatives, and sodium hyaluronate), pain with injection, and increased risk of infection. Leflunomide is associated with potentially fatal hepatic toxicity and rashes. Penicillamine is associated with a potentially fatal myasthenic syndrome, bone marrow depression, and assorted hypersensitivity reactions. Leflunomide has been associated with severe hepatic toxicity, hence the patient's liver function needs to be monitored closely. Tofacitinib has a black box warning outlining the risk of serious to fatal infections and the development of lymphomas and other cancers.

Clinically Important Drug–Drug Interactions

Hyaluronidase derivatives such as sodium hyaluronate should not be injected at the same time as local anesthetics.

Because leflunomide can cause severe liver dysfunction if it is combined with other hepatotoxic drugs, this combination should be avoided.

The absorption of penicillamine is decreased if it is taken with iron salts or antacids; if these are both being given, they should be separated by at least 2 hours.

Anakinra and tofacitinib should not be used with other immune suppressants because of an increased risk of serious infections.

Nursing Considerations for Patients Receiving DMARDs

Patients receiving DMARDs have moderate to severe arthritis or other immune conditions. These drugs alter the disease process by altering the patient's immune response to slow or block inflammation and damage that occurs with chronic inflammatory states. Details related to each individual drug can be found in the specific drug monograph in your nursing drug guide.

(continues on page 282)

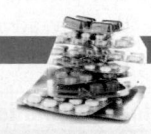

Assessment: History and Examination

- Assess for contraindications or cautions: History of allergy to any components of the drug, Chinese hamster ovary products (etanercept), chicken products (hyaluronidase) *to avoid hypersensitivity reactions*; active infections or cancers *because these drugs drugs alter the immune response and these conditions could become worse*; pregnancy or lactation *to avoid adverse effects on the fetus or baby.*
- Perform physical assessment to establish baseline status before beginning therapy and to *monitor for any potential adverse effects.*
- Assess lesions, temperature, any sign of infection *to monitor for adverse effects.*
- Evaluate CNS status—orientation, reflexes, eighth cranial nerve function, and affect—*to assess CNS effects of the drug.*
- Arrange for required cancer screening *to evaluate potential adverse effects of the drug.*
- Monitor range of motion, movement, pain levels *to evaluate effectiveness of drug therapy.*
- Evaluate respirations and adventitious sounds *to detect signs of infection.*
- Monitor laboratory tests for CBC, liver and renal function tests, TB test *to establish baseline and monitor for adverse effects of the drug.*

Nursing Diagnoses

Nursing diagnoses related to drug therapy might include the following:

- Acute pain related to CNS, disease process.
- Risk for infection related to drug effects
- Anxiety related to disease process and drug effects
- Deficient knowledge regarding drug therapy.

Planning

- The patient will receive the best therapeutic effect from the drug therapy.
- The patient will have limited adverse effects to the drug therapy.
- The patient will have an understanding of the drug therapy, adverse effects to anticipate, and measures to relieve discomfort and improve safety

Implementation with Rationale

- Teach patient proper preparation, administration of subcutaneous injections, and safe disposal of needles and syringes *to ensure therapeutic effectiveness and safety.*
- Monitor for immune suppression reactions *to avoid problems and provide emergency care as needed.*
- Monitor for CNS toxicity *to evaluate toxicity and provide appropriate interventions of drug discontinuation.*
- Arrange for continuation of nondrug therapies to deal with arthritis *to improve quality of life and enhance therapeutic effectiveness of drug therapy.*
- Ensure that the patient has routine cancer screening and regular follow-up *to avoid serious adverse effects and manage them quickly if they occur.*
- Provide thorough patient teaching, including measures to avoid adverse effects and warning signs of problems, as well as proper administration, *to increase knowledge about drug therapy and to increase compliance with the drug regimen.*
- Offer support and encouragement *to deal with the drug regimen and diagnosis.*

Evaluation

- Monitor patient response to the drug (improvement in condition being treated, relief of signs and symptoms of arthritis).
- Monitor for adverse effects (infections, cancer development, CNS toxicity).
- Evaluate the effectiveness of the teaching plan (patient can name drug, dosage, administration, adverse effects to watch for, specific measures to avoid adverse effects).
- Monitor the effectiveness of and compliance with the drug regimen.

KEY POINTS

- Gold salts prevent macrophage phagocytosis, lysosomal release, and tissue damage because the gold salts are taken up by phagocytes, which then are not able to function in the normal way.
- Gold salts are deposited in the tissues and cause an assortment of inflammatory reactions, including stomatitis, glossitis, gingivitis, pharyngitis, laryngitis, colitis, diarrhea, and other GI inflammation; gold bronchitis and interstitial pneumonitis; bone marrow depression; vaginitis and nephrotic syndrome; dermatitis, pruritus, and exfoliative dermatitis; and allergic reactions ranging from flushing, fainting, and dizziness to anaphylactic shock.
- Drugs used to alter the inflammatory process involved in arthritis are called disease-modifying antirheumatic drugs (DMARDs) and can be associated with serious to potentially fatal infections. If used early in the disease, they can prevent or slow down the damage caused to the joints.
- TNF blockers prevent the actions of TNF in the inflammatory/immune process. This relieves the signs and symptoms of arthritis and helps to slow bone breakdown and damage, but also makes the patient prone to serious infections and the development of cancers.
- The DMARDs can cause local irritation at the injection site, liver impairment, and a variety of CNS problems, including demyelinating disorders.

SUMMARY

- The inflammatory response, which is important for protecting the body from injury and invasion, produces many of the signs and symptoms associated with disease, including fever, aches and pains, and lethargy.
- Chronic or excessive activity by the inflammatory response can lead to the release of lysosomal enzymes and tissue destruction.
- Anti-inflammatory drugs block various chemicals associated with the inflammatory reaction. Anti-inflammatory drugs also may have antipyretic (fever-blocking) and analgesic (pain-blocking) activities.
- Salicylates block prostaglandin activity. NSAIDs block prostaglandin synthesis. Acetaminophen causes vasodilation and heat release, lowering fever and working to relieve pain. Gold salts prevent macrophage phagocytosis, lysosomal release, and tissue damage. DMARDs alter the course of the inflammatory process and treat arthritis by aggressively affecting the process of inflammation.
- Salicylates can cause acidosis and eighth cranial nerve damage. NSAIDs are most associated with GI irritation and bleeding. Acetaminophen can cause serious liver toxicity. The gold salts cause many systemic inflammatory reactions. Other antiarthritis drugs are associated with local injection site irritation and increased susceptibility to infection; leflunomide is associated with severe hepatic toxicity.
- Many anti-inflammatory drugs are available OTC, and care must be taken to prevent abuse or overuse of these drugs.
- DMARDs affect the immune response to slow inflammation and joint damage. They are associated with serious to potentially fatal injections and the development of cancers.

CHECK YOUR UNDERSTANDING

Answers to the questions in this chapter can be found in Answers to Check Your Understanding Questions on thePoint®.

MULTIPLE CHOICE

Select the best answer to the following.

1. A drug could be classified as an analgesic if it
- **a.** reduces fever.
- **b.** reduces swelling.
- **c.** reduces redness.
- **d.** reduces pain.

2. An antipyretic is a drug that can
- **a.** block pain.
- **b.** block swelling.
- **c.** block fever.
- **d.** block inflammation.

3. A nurse might not see a salicylate used as an anti-inflammatory if a drug was needed for its
- **a.** antipyretic properties.
- **b.** analgesic properties.
- **c.** OTC availability.
- **d.** parenteral availability.

4. The nonsteroidal NSAIDs affect the COX-1 and COX-2 enzymes. By blocking COX-2 enzymes the NSAIDs block inflammation and the signs and symptoms of inflammation at the site of injury or trauma. By blocking COX-1 enzymes, these drugs block
- **a.** fever regulation.
- **b.** prostaglandins that protect the stomach lining.
- **c.** swelling in the periphery.
- **d.** liver function.

5. Your patient has been receiving ibuprofen for many years to relieve the pain of osteoarthritis. Assessment of the patient should include
- **a.** an electrocardiogram.
- **b.** CBC with differential.
- **c.** respiratory auscultation.
- **d.** renal evaluation.

(continues on page 284)

6. Patients taking NSAIDs should be taught to avoid the use of OTC medications without checking with their prescriber because
   a. many of the OTC preparations contain NSAIDs, and inadvertent toxicity could occur.
   b. no one should take more than one type of pain reliever at a time.
   c. increased GI upset could occur.
   d. there is a risk of Reye syndrome.

7. Chronic or excessive activity by the inflammatory response can lead to
   a. loss of white blood cells.
   b. coagulation problems.
   c. release of lysosomal enzymes and tissue destruction.
   d. adrenal suppression.

8. A patient with rheumatoid arthritis who is on a fixed income and who is being treated with aspirin should be advised
   a. to use only brand name aspirin.
   b. to use only enteric-coated aspirin.
   c. to use generic aspirin.
   d. to switch to one of the NSAIDs.

MULTIPLE RESPONSE

Select all that apply.

1. A client is being treated for severe rheumatoid arthritis. The nurse could anticipate treatment with which of the following:
   a. Etanercept—TNF blocker
   b. Gold therapy
   c. Hylan G-F 20—hylans with elastic properties
   d. Ketoprofen
   e. Interferon beta-2a
   f. Methotrexate

2. The nurse notes an order for oxaprozin (*Daypro*) for the treatment of arthritis. Before administering the drug the nurse would assess the patient for which problems that could be cautions or contraindications?
   a. Headaches
   b. Dysmenorrhea
   c. Active peptic ulcer disease
   d. Chronic obstructive pulmonary disease
   e. Renal impairment
   f. Bleeding disorders

BIBLIOGRAPHY AND REFERENCES

Bresalier, R. S., Sandler, R. E., Quan, H., et al. (2005). Cardiovascular events associated with rofecoxib in a colorectal adenoma chemoprevention trial. *New England Journal of Medicine, 352*, 1092–1102.

Brunton, L., Chabner, B., & Knollman, B. (2011). *Goodman and Gilman's the pharmacological basis of therapeutics* (12th ed.). New York: McGraw-Hill.

Facts and Comparisons. (2015). *Drug facts and comparisons*. St. Louis, MO: Author.

Fitzgerald, G. A. (2004). Coxibs and cardiovascular disease. *New England Journal of Medicine, 351*, 1709–1711.

Heard, K., Bui, A., Mlynarchek, S.L., et al. (2014). Toxicity from repeated doses of acetaminophen in children: Assessment of causality and dose in reported cases. *American Journal of Therapeutics, 21*(3), 174–183.

Her, M., & Kavanaugh, A. (2012). Patient-reported outcomes in rheumatoid arthritis. *Current Opinion in Rheumatology, 24*(3), 327–334.

Karch, A. M. (2014). *Lippincott's nursing drug guide*. Philadelphia, PA: Lippincott Williams & Wilkins.

Kuehn, B. (2009). New pain guidelines for older patients: Avoid NSAIDs, consider opioids. *Journal of the American Medical Association, 302*(1), 19.

Lavonas, E., Reynolds, K., & Dart, R. (2010). Therapeutic acetaminophen is not associated with liver injury in children: A systematic review. *Pediatrics, 126*, 1430–1444.

Porth, C. M. (2013). *Pathophysiology: Concepts of altered health states* (9th ed.). Philadelphia, PA: Lippincott Williams & Wilkins.

Ruderman, E. (2012). Overview of safety of non-biologic and biologic DMARDs. *Rheumatology, 51*(6), vi37–vi43.

The Medical Letter. (2015). *Medical letter on drugs and therapeutics*. New Rochelle, NY: Author.

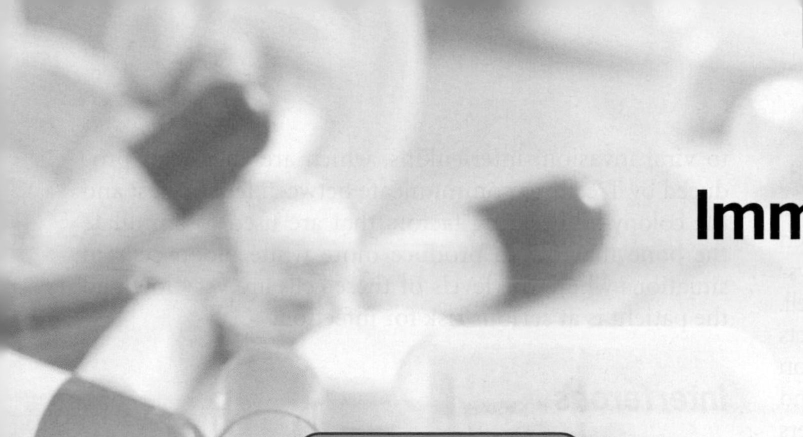

17 Immune Modulators

Learning Objectives

Upon completion of this chapter, you will be able to:

1. Describe the sites of actions of the various immune modulators.
2. Describe the therapeutic actions, indications, pharmacokinetics, contraindications, most common adverse effects, and important drug–drug interactions associated with each class of immune stimulants and immune suppressants.
3. Discuss the use of immune modulators across the lifespan.
4. Compare and contrast the prototype drugs for each class of immune modulators with the other drugs in that class and with drugs in other classes.
5. Outline the nursing considerations and teaching needs for patients receiving each class of immune modulators.

Glossary of Key Terms

immune stimulant: drug used to energize the immune system when it is exhausted from fighting prolonged invasion or needs help fighting a specific pathogen or cancer cell

immune suppressant: drug used to block or suppress the actions of the T cells and antibody production; used to prevent transplant rejection and to treat autoimmune diseases

monoclonal antibodies: specific antibodies produced by a single clone of B cells to react with a very specific antigen

recombinant DNA technology: use of bacteria to produce chemicals normally produced by human cells

Drug List

Immune Stimulants

Interferons

Ⓟ interferon alfa-2b
interferon beta-1a
interferon beta-1b
interferon gamma-1b
peginterferon alfa-2a
peginterferon alfa-2b

Interleukins

Ⓟ aldesleukin
oprelvekin

Colony-Stimulating Factors

Ⓟ filgrastim
pegfilgrastim
sargramostim
tbo-filgrastim

Immune Suppressants

Immune modulators

apremilast
dimethyl fumarate
fingolimod
lenalidomide
pomalidomide
teriflunomide
thalidomide

T and B Cell Suppressors

abatacept
alefacept
azathioprine
belatacept
cyclosporine
Ⓟ glatiramer acetate
mycophenolate
pimecrolimus
sirolimus
tacrolimus

Interleukin Receptor Antagonist

anakinra

Monoclonal Antibodies

adalimumab
alemtuzumab
basiliximab
belimumab
bevacizumab
blinatumomab
brentuximab
canakinumab
certolizumab
cetuximab
daclizumab
denosumab
eculizumab
golimumab
ibritumomab
infliximab
ipilimumab
Ⓟ natalizumab
nivolumab
obintuzumab
ofatumumab
omalizumab
palivizumab
pegaptanib
pembrolizumab
ramucirumab
ranibizumab
raxibacumab
rituximab
siltuximab
tocilizumab
tositumomab
trastuzumab
ustekinumab
vedolizumab

As the name implies, immune modulators are used to modify the actions of the immune system. **Immune stimulants** are used to energize the immune system when it is exhausted from fighting prolonged invasion or when the immune system needs help fighting a specific pathogen or cancer cell. **Immune suppressants** are used to block the normal effects of the immune system in cases of organ transplantation (in which nonself-cells are transplanted into the body and destroyed by the immune reaction), in autoimmune disorders (in which the body's defenses recognize self-cells as foreign and work to destroy them), and in some cancers. Each group acts at various sites within the immune response (Figure 17.1).

The knowledge base about the actions and components of the immune system is continually growing and changing. As new discoveries are made and the actions and interactions of the various components of the system become better understood, new applications will be found for modulating the immune system in a variety of disorders. Box 17.1 discusses the use of immune modulators across the lifespan. Box 17.2 discusses use of these agents during pregnancy.

Immune Stimulants

Immune stimulants (Table 17.1) include the interferons, which are naturally released from human cells in response to viral invasion; interleukins, which are chemicals produced by T cells to communicate between leukocytes; and the colony-stimulating factors that are used to stimulate the bone marrow to produce more white blood cells in situations where the levels of these cells are very low and the patient is at serious risk for infection.

Interferons

Interferons are substances naturally produced and released by human cells that have been invaded by viruses. They may also be released from cells in response to other stimuli, such as cytotoxic T cell activity. A number of interferons are available for use. Several are produced by **recombinant DNA technology**, including interferon alfa-2b (*Intron-A*), peginterferon alfa-2a (*Pegasys*), peginterferon alfa-2b (*Peg-Intron*), and interferon beta-1b (*Betaseron*). Interferon alfa-n3 (*Alferon N*) is produced by harvesting human leukocytes. Interferon beta-1a (*Avonex*) is produced from Chinese hamster ovary cells. Interferon gamma-1b (*Actimmune*) is produced by *Escherichia coli* bacteria. The interferon of choice depends on the condition being treated (see Table 17.1).

Therapeutic Actions and Indications

Interferons act to prevent virus particles from replicating inside cells. They also stimulate interferon receptor sites on

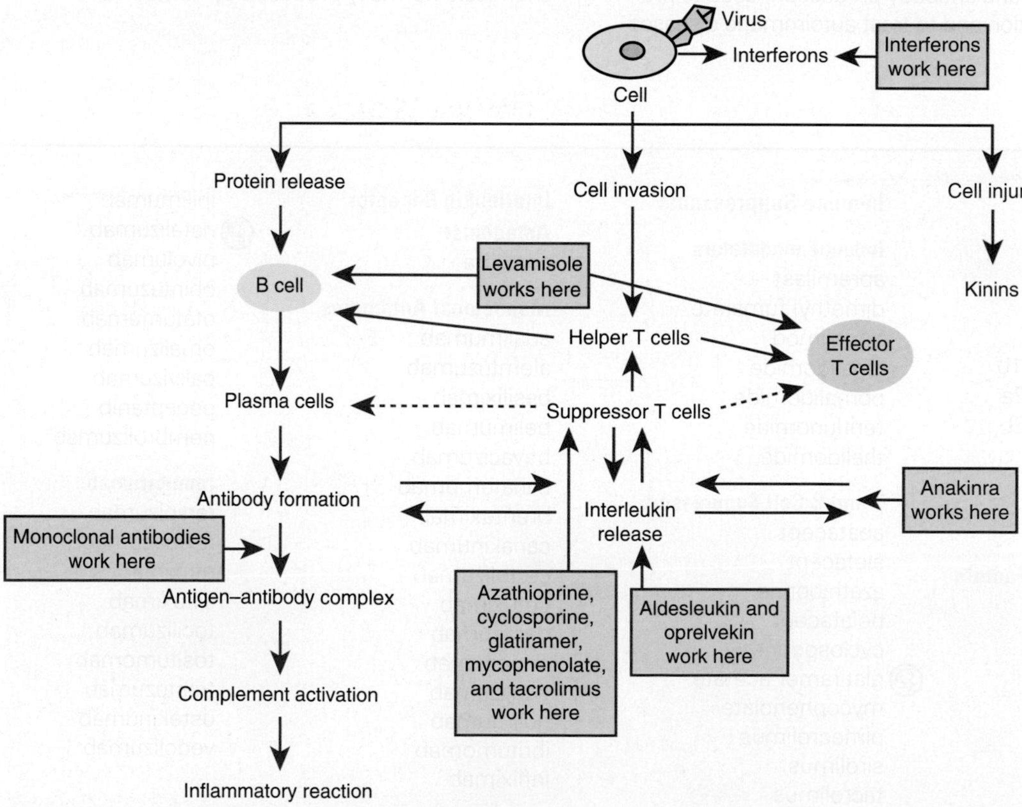

FIGURE 17.1 Sites of action of the immune modulators.

BOX 17.1 FOCUS ON Drug Therapy Across the Lifespan

Immune Modulators

CHILDREN

Most of the drugs that affect the immune system are not recommended for use in children or have not been tested in children. The exceptions—interferon alfa-2b, azathioprine, raxibacumab, cyclosporine, tacrolimus, and palivizumab—should be used cautiously, monitoring the child frequently for infection, GI, renal, hematological, or CNS effects.

The immune suppressants (azathioprine, cyclosporine, and tacrolimus) are usually needed in higher doses for children than for adults to achieve the same therapeutic effect.

Protecting the child from infection and injury is a very important part of the care of a child taking an immune modulator. This can be a great challenge with an active child.

ADULTS

Both the adult patient who is receiving a parenteral immune modulator and a significant other should learn the proper technique for injection, disposal of needles, and special storage precautions for the drug. It is important to stress ways to avoid exposure to infection and injury to prevent further complications. The patient should be encouraged to seek regular follow-up and medical care.

Immune modulators are contraindicated during pregnancy and lactation because of the potential for adverse effects on the fetus or neonate and complications for the mother. Women of childbearing age should be advised to use barrier contraceptives while taking these drugs and, if breastfeeding, should be counseled to find another method of feeding the baby. Some of these drugs impair fertility, and the patient should be advised of this fact before taking the drug.

OLDER ADULTS

Older patients may be more susceptible to the effects of the immune modulators, partly because the aging immune system is less efficient and less responsive.

These patients need to be monitored closely for infection, GI, renal, hepatic, and CNS effects. Baseline renal and liver function tests can help to determine whether a decreased dosage will be needed before beginning therapy.

Because these patients are more susceptible to infection, they need to receive extensive teaching about ways to avoid infection and injury sites on noninvaded cells to produce antiviral proteins, which prevent viruses from entering the cell. In addition, interferons have been found to inhibit tumor growth and replication, to stimulate cytotoxic T cell activity, and to enhance the inflammatory response. Of interest, interferon gamma-1b also acts like an interleukin, stimulating phagocytes to be more aggressive. See Table 17.1 for Usual Indications for each interferon.

noninvaded cells to produce antiviral proteins, which prevent viruses from entering the cell. In addition, interferons have been found to inhibit tumor growth and replication, to stimulate cytotoxic T cell activity and to enhance the inflammatory response. Of interest, interferon gamma-1b also acts like an interleukin, stimulating phagocytes to be more aggressive (see Table 17.1 for Usual Indications of each interferon).

BOX 17.2 FOCUS ON Gender Considerations

Immune Modulators and Pregnancy

Generally, immune modulators are contraindicated for use during pregnancy and lactation, largely because these drugs have been associated with fetal abnormalities, increased maternal and fetal infections, and suppressed immune responses in nursing babies. Female patients should be informed of the risk of using these drugs during pregnancy and receive counseling in the use of barrier contraceptives. (The use of barrier contraceptives is advised because the effects of oral contraceptives may be altered by liver changes or by changes in the body's immune response, potentially resulting in unexpected pregnancy.)

If a patient taking immune modulators becomes pregnant or decides that she wants to become pregnant, she should discuss this with her health care provider and review the risks associated with use of the drug or drugs being taken. The monoclonal antibodies should be used with caution during pregnancy and lactation. Because long-term studies of most of these drugs are not yet available, it may be prudent to advise patients taking these drugs to avoid pregnancy if possible.

Pharmacokinetics

The interferons are generally well absorbed after subcutaneous or intramuscular injection. They have a rapid onset of action and peak within 3 to 8 hours, with a half-life ranging from 3 to 8 hours, with the exception of interferon beta-1a, which has an onset of action of 12 hours and reaches peak levels in 48 hours, with a half-life of 10 hours. They are broken down in the liver and kidneys and seem to be excreted primarily through the kidneys.

Contraindications and Cautions

The use of interferons is contraindicated in the presence of known allergy to any interferon or product components *to prevent hypersensitivity reactions.* Many of the interferons are teratogenic in animals and therefore should not be used during pregnancy. Use of barrier contraceptives is advised for women of childbearing age. It is not known whether these drugs cross into breast milk, but *because of the potential adverse effects on the baby*, it is advised that the drugs not be used during lactation unless the benefits to the mother clearly

Table 17.1 *Drugs in Focus:* Immune Stimulants

Drug Name	Dosage/Route	Usual Indications
Interferons		
interferon alfa-2b (*Intron-A*)	*Adult:* Dose varies widely based on indication *Pediatric:* For hepatitis B, adjust adult dose to weight	Treatment of leukemias, Kaposi sarcoma, warts, hepatitis B, malignant melanoma
interferon alfa-n3 (*Alferon N*)	250,000 IU intralesionally twice per week for 8 wk	Intralesional treatment of warts, AIDS-related complex, AIDS orphan drug indication
interferon beta-1a (*Avonex*)	30 mcg IM once a week	Treatment of multiple sclerosis in adults
interferon beta-1b (*Betaseron*)	0.25 mg subcutaneous every other day, discontinue if disease is unremitting >6 mo	Treatment of multiple sclerosis in adults
interferon gamma-1b (*Actimmune*)	50 mcg/m² subcutaneous three times per week	Treatment of serious, chronic granulomatous disease in adults; delaying time to disease progression in severe, malignant osteopetrosis
peginterferon alfa-2b (*Peg-Intron*)	1 mcg/kg subcutaneous once a week for 1 y	Treatment of chronic hepatitis C in adults
Interleukins		
aldesleukin (*Proleukin*)	Two 5-d cycles of 600,000 IU/kg IV q8 h given over 15 min	Treatment of specific renal carcinomas in adults; also, drug is being investigated for use in the treatment of AIDS and AIDS-related disorders
oprelvekin (*Neumega*)	50 mcg/kg/d subcutaneous starting 1 d after chemotherapy and continuing for 14–21 d	Prevention of severe thrombocytopenia (an abnormal decrease in the number of platelets) after myelosuppressive chemotherapy
Colony-Stimulating Factors		
filgrastim (*Neupogen*)	4–8 mcg/kg/d subcutaneously or IV	Reduction of incidence of infection and reduction of time to neutrophil recovery in patients with nonmyeloid malignancies receiving antineoplastic chemotherapy and following bone marrow transplant
pegfilgrastim (*Neulasta*)	6 mg subcutaneously as a single dose once per chemotherapy cycle	Reduction of the incidence of infection in patients with nonmyeloid malignancies receiving bone marrow–suppressing antineoplastic drugs
sargramostim (*Leukine*)	250 mcg/m²/d as a 2 h IV infusion	Myeloid reconstitution following bone marrow transplantation, treatment of neutropenia following bone marrow transplantation failure, induction chemotherapy with AML
tbo-filgrastim (*Granix*)	5 mcg/kg/d subcutaneously; administer first dose no earlier than 24 h after chemotherapy, do not administer within 24 h of chemotherapy	Reduction in the duration of severe neutropenia in nonmyeloid malignancies being treated with myelosuppressive anti-cancer drugs

AML, acute myeloid leukemia.

outweigh any risks to the baby. Caution should be used in the presence of known cardiac disease *because hypertension and arrhythmias have been reported with the use of these drugs*, with myelosuppression *because these drugs may further suppress the bone marrow*, and with central nervous system (CNS) dysfunction of any kind *because of the potential for CNS depression and personality changes that have been reported.*

Adverse Effects

The adverse effects associated with the use of interferons are related to the immune or inflammatory reaction that is being stimulated (stimulating the immune and inflammatory response causes a flu-like syndrome with lethargy, myalgia, arthralgia, anorexia, nausea). Other commonly seen adverse effects include headache, dizziness, bone marrow depression, depression and suicidal ideation, photosensitivity, and liver impairment.

Prototype Summary: Interferon Alfa-2b

Indications: Hairy cell leukemia, malignant melanoma, AIDS-related Kaposi sarcoma, chronic hepatitis B and C, follicular lymphoma, intralesional treatment of condylomata acuminata in patients 18 years of age or older.

Actions: Inhibits the growth of tumor cells and enhances the immune response.

Pharmacokinetics:

Route	Onset	Peak
IM, subcutaneous	Rapid	3–12 h
IV	Rapid	End of infusion

$T_{1/2}$: 2 to 3 hours, metabolized in the kidney, excretion is unknown.

Adverse Effects: Dizziness, confusion, rash, dry skin, anorexia, nausea, bone marrow suppression, flu-like syndrome.

Clinically Important Drug–Drug Interactions

There are no reported clinically important drug–drug interactions with the interferons.

Interleukins

Interleukins are synthetic compounds much like the interferons; they communicate between lymphocytes, which stimulate cellular immunity and inhibit tumor growth. Interleukin-2 stimulates cellular immunity by increasing the activity of natural killer cells, platelets, and cytokines. Two interleukin preparations are available for use. Aldesleukin (*Proleukin*) is a human interleukin produced by recombinant DNA technology using *Escherichia coli* bacteria. Oprelvekin (*Neumega*) is a newer agent that is also produced by DNA technology (see Table 17.1).

Therapeutic Actions and Indications

Natural interleukin-2 is produced by various lymphocytes to activate cellular immunity and inhibit tumor growth by increasing lymphocyte numbers and their activity. When interleukins are administered, there are increases in the numbers of natural killer cells and lymphocytes, in cytokine activity, and in the number of circulating platelets. See Table 17.1 for Usual Indications.

Pharmacokinetics

The interleukins are rapidly distributed after injection. Aldesleukin, given IV, reaches peak levels in 13 minutes and has a half-life of 85 minutes. Oprelvekin, which is given subcutaneously, reaches peak levels in 3 to 5 hours and has a half-life of 7 to 8 hours. They are primarily cleared from the body by the kidneys.

Contraindications and Cautions

Interleukins are contraindicated in the presence of any allergy to an interleukin or *Escherichia coli*–produced product *to prevent hypersensitivity reactions. Because they were shown to be embryocidal and teratogenic in animal studies,* they should not be used during pregnancy. Use of barrier contraceptives is recommended for women of childbearing age who require one of these drugs. It is not clear whether the drugs cross into breast milk, but it is recommended that they not be used during lactation; if they must be used, another method of feeding the baby must be chosen *because of the potential for adverse effects in the baby.* Caution should be used with renal, liver, or cardiovascular impairment *because of the adverse effects of the drugs.*

Adverse Effects

The adverse effects associated with the interleukins can be attributed to their effect on the body during inflammation (flu-like effects: lethargy, myalgia, arthralgia, fatigue, fever). Respiratory difficulties, CNS changes, and cardiac arrhythmias also have been reported, and the patient should be monitored for these effects and the drug stopped if they do occur. Oprelvekin has been associated with severe hypersensitivity reactions, and patients should be closely watched when beginning therapy and encouraged to report any difficulty breathing or swallowing, chest tightness, or swelling.

Clinical Important Drug–Drug Interactions

There are no reported drug–drug interactions with the interleukins.

Prototype Summary: Aldesleukin

Indications: Metastatic renal cell carcinoma in adults, treatment of metastatic melanomas.

Actions: Activates human cellular immunity and inhibits tumor growth through increases in lymphocytes, platelets, and cytokines.

Pharmacokinetics:

Route	Onset	Peak	Duration
IV	5 min	13 min	3–4 h

$T_{1/2}$: 85 minutes, metabolized in the kidney and excreted in the urine.

Adverse Effects: Mental status changes, dizziness, hypotension, sinus tachycardia, arrhythmias, pruritus, nausea, vomiting, diarrhea, anorexia, gastrointestinal bleed, bone marrow suppression, respiratory difficulties, fever, chills, pain.

Colony-Stimulating Factors

The colony-stimulating factors are produced by recombinant DNA technology. Filgrastim (*Neupogen*), pegfilgrastim (*Neulasta*), and tbo-filgrastim increase the production of neutrophils in the bone marrow with little effect on other hematopoietic cells. Sargramostim (*Leukine*) increases the proliferation and differentiation of hematopoietic progenitor cells and can activate mature granulocytes and monocytes. The colony-stimulating factor of choice will depend on the condition being treated (see Table 17.1).

Therapeutic Actions and Indications

By increasing the production of white cells, the colony-stimulating factors can be used to reduce the incidence of infection in patients with bone marrow suppression, to decrease the neutropenia associated with bone marrow transplants and chemotherapy, and to help in the treatment of various blood-related cancers. See Table 17.1 for Usual Indications.

Pharmacokinetics

Filgrastim can be given IV or by subcutaneous injection, reaching peak levels in 2 hours IV or 8 hours subcutaneously; it has a half-life of about 220 minutes and a duration of 4 days; its metabolism and excretion are not known. Pegfilgrastim is only given by subcutaneous injection with similar onset but has a much longer half-life, 15 to 80 hours, than filgrastim. Tbo-filgrastim is only given subcutaneously, reaches peak levels in 4 to 6 hours and has a half-life of 3.5 hours. Sargramostim can be given IV or subcutaneously with a duration of 6 hours (IV) or 12 hours subcutaneously. It has a half-life of 1 to 3 hours; its metabolism and excretion are not known.

Contraindications and Cautions

Interleukins are contraindicated in the presence of any allergy to any component of the drug or to *Escherichia coli*–produced products *to prevent hypersensitivity reactions.* Sargramostim is contraindicated in neonates *because of benzyl alcohol in the solution* and with excessive leukemic myeloid blasts in the bone marrow or peripheral blood, *which could be worsened by the drug.* These drugs should be used with caution in pregnancy and lactation *because the potential effects on the fetus or neonate are not known.* Sargramostim should also be used with caution in hepatic or renal failure *which could alter the pharmacokinetics of the drug,* during or immediately after radiation or chemotherapy *because of a potential loss of effectiveness.*

Adverse Effects

The adverse effects associated with colony-stimulating factors are gastrointestinal (GI) effects (nausea, vomiting, diarrhea, constipation, anorexia), headache, fatigue, generalized weakness, alopecia and dermatitis, and generalized pain and bone pain. The effects are thought to be associated with the drug effects on the bone marrow cells and their increased activity.

Clinically Important Drug–Drug Interactions

The only reported drug–drug interactions associated with these drugs is an increase in the myeloproliferative effects of sargramostim when combined with lithium or corticosteroids; these combinations should be used with caution.

Ⓟ Prototype Summary: Filgrastim

Indications: Reduction of the incidence of infection and reduction in time to neutrophil recovery with myelosuppressive chemotherapy, leukemia, bone marrow transplants.

Actions: Increases the production of neutrophils in the bone marrow.

Pharmacokinetics:

Route	Peak	Duration
IV	2 h	4 d
Subcutaneous	8 h	4 d

$T_{1/2}$: 210 to 231 minutes, metabolism and excretion unknown.

Adverse Effects: Headache, fatigue, alopecia, rash, nausea, vomiting, diarrhea, stomatitis, anorexia, bone pain, cough, generalized pain.

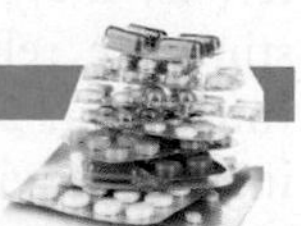

Nursing Considerations for Patients Receiving Immune Stimulants

Assessment: History and Examination

- Assess for contraindications and cautions: Known allergies to any of these drugs or their components *to prevent hypersensitivity reactions*, current status related to pregnancy or lactation *to avoid serious adverse effects on the fetus or baby*, and history of hepatic, renal, or cardiac disease; bone marrow depression; leukemic states; and CNS disorders, including seizures, *all of which could be exacerbated by the effects of these drugs.*
- Perform a physical assessment to determine *baseline status before beginning therapy and for any potential adverse effects*: Inspect for the presence of any skin lesions *to detect early dermatological effects*, obtain weight *to monitor for fluid retention*, monitor temperature to *detect any infection*, check heart rate and rhythm and blood pressure *to monitor for any cardiac effects of the drug*, and assess level of orientation and reflexes *to evaluate CNS effects of the drug.*

- Obtain a baseline electrocardiogram if appropriate *to evaluate cardiac function and monitor adverse effects of the drugs.*
- Assess patient's renal and liver function, including renal and liver function tests, *to determine the appropriateness of therapy* and *to determine the need for possible dose adjustment and toxic drug effects.*
- Monitor the results of laboratory tests such as complete blood count (CBC) *to identify changes in bone marrow function.*

Nursing Diagnoses

Nursing diagnoses related to drug therapy might include the following:

- Acute pain related to CNS, GI, and flu-like effects
- Imbalanced nutrition: Less than body requirements related to flu-like effects
- Anxiety related to diagnosis and drug therapy
- Deficient knowledge regarding drug therapy

Planning

- The patient will receive the best therapeutic effect from the drug therapy.
- The patient will have limited adverse effects to the drug therapy.
- The patient will have an understanding of the drug therapy, adverse effects to anticipate, and measures to relieve discomfort and improve safety.

Implementation with Rationale

- Arrange for laboratory tests before and periodically during therapy, including CBC and differential, *to monitor for drug effects and adverse effects.*
- Administer drug as indicated; instruct the patient and a significant other if injections are required *to ensure that the drug will be given even if the patient is not able to administer it.*
- Monitor for severe reactions, such as severe hypersensitivity reactions, and *arrange to discontinue the drug immediately if they occur.*
- Arrange for supportive care and comfort measures for flu-like symptoms (e.g., rest, environmental control, acetaminophen) *to help the patient cope with the drug effects.* Ensure that the patient is well hydrated during therapy *to prevent severe adverse effects.*
- Instruct female patients in the use of barrier contraceptives *to avoid pregnancy during therapy because of the potential for adverse effects on the fetus.*
- Offer support and encouragement *to deal with the diagnosis and the drug regimen.*
- Provide patient teaching about measures to avoid adverse effects, warning signs of problems, and proper administration technique.

Evaluation

- Monitor patient response to the drug (improvement in condition being treated).
- Monitor for adverse effects (flu-like symptoms, GI upset, CNS changes, bone marrow depression).
- Evaluate the effectiveness of the teaching plan (patient can name drug, dosage, adverse effects to watch for, specific measures to avoid adverse effects).
- Monitor the effectiveness of comfort measures and compliance with the regimen.

KEY POINTS

- Immune stimulants assist the immune system to fight specific pathogens or cancer cells; in doing so, they cause flu-like symptoms (lethargy, muscle and joint aches and pains, anorexia, nausea).
- Interferons are used to treat various cancers and warts.
- Interleukins stimulate cellular immunity and inhibit tumor growth.

Immune Suppressants

Immune suppressants (Table 17.2) often are used in conjunction with corticosteroids, which block the inflammatory reaction and decrease initial damage to cells. They are especially beneficial in cases of organ transplantation and in the treatment of autoimmune diseases. The immune suppressants include the immune modulators, T and B cell suppressors, an interleukin receptor antagonist, and **monoclonal antibodies**—antibodies produced by a single clone of B cells that react with specific antigens. There is a new drug, belatacept (*Nulojix*) (Box 17.3), that was approved for the prevention of acute transplant rejection in adults with kidney transplants.

Immune Modulators

The immune modulators block the release of various cytokines involved in the inflammatory response and activation of lymphocytes, decreasing immune activity. The result of blocking these chemicals is immune suppression. The immune modulators are a relatively new class of drugs and include fingolimod (*Gilenya*), lenalidomide (*Revlimid*), and thalidomide (*Thalomid*), an old drug with new uses, apremilast (*Otezla*), dimethyl fumarate (*Tecfidera*), pomalidomide (*Pomalyst*), and teriflunomide (*Aubagio*).

Therapeutic Actions and Indications

The immune modulators have a number of effects on the inflammatory system; lenalidomide and thalidomide

Table 17.2 *Drugs in Focus:* Immune Suppressants

Drug Name	Dosage/Route	Usual Indications
Immune Modulators		
fingolimod (*Gilenya*)	0.5 mg/d PO	Treatment of patients with relapsing forms of multiple sclerosis to reduce frequency of exacerbations and delay accumulation of physical disability
lenalidomide (*Revlimid*)	10 mg/d PO with water, 25 mg/d PO on days 1–21 of a 28-d cycle for multiple myeloma	Treatment of patients with transfusion-dependent anemia, treatment of multiple myeloma in patients who have received at least one other therapy
thalidomide (*Thalomid*)	100–300 mg/d PO for at least 2 wk, taper	Treatment of erythema nodosum following treatment for leprosy, newly diagnosed multiple myeloma, brain tumors, Crohn's disease, HIV wasting syndrome, graft vs. host reaction in bone marrow transplant
T and B Cell Suppressors		
abatacept (*Orencia*)	*<60 kg:* 500 mg IV repeated at 2 and 4 wk, then every 4 wk*60–100 kg:* 750 mg IV, repeated at 2 and 4 wk, then every 4 wk*>100 kg:* 1 g IV, repeated at 2 and 4 wk, then every 4 wk	Reduction of the signs and symptoms and slowing structural damage in adults with rheumatoid arthritis who have inadequate response to other drugs
alefacept (*Amevive*)	7.5-mg IV bolus once a week or 15 mg IM once a week, in 12-wk cycles	Treatment of adults with moderate to severe chronic plaque psoriasis who are candidates for systemic therapy
azathioprine (*Imuran*)	*Adult:* 3–5 mg/kg/d PO for prevention of rejection *Maintenance:* 1–3 mg/kg/d PO *Rheumatoid arthritis:* 1–2.5 mg/kg/d PO, reduce dose with renal impairment *Pediatric:* 3–5 mg/kg/d IV or PO to prevent rejection *Maintenance:* 1–3 mg/kg/d PO	Prevention of rejection in renal homotransplants, treatment of rheumatoid arthritis
cyclosporine (*Sandimmune*)	15 mg/kg PO as a single oral dose 4–12 h before transplantation, then 5–10 mg/kg/d PO *Pediatric:* Larger doses may be needed to achieve therapeutic levels	Suppression of rejection in a variety of transplant situations
(*Neoral*)	9–15 mg/kg PO as a single oral dose 4–12 h before transplantation, then 5–10 mg/kg/d PO—titrate down *Rheumatoid arthritis:* 2.5 mg/kg/d PO in two divided doses *Psoriasis:* 2.5 mg/kg PO b.i.d.	Treatment of rheumatoid arthritis, psoriasis
glatiramer acetate (*Copaxone*)	20 mg/d subcutaneous	Reduction of the number of relapses in multiple sclerosis in adults
mycophenolate (*CellCept*)	1–1.5 mg PO b.i.d.; may be started IV during transplantation, with switch to oral route as soon as possible	Prevention of rejection after renal, hepatic, or heart transplantation in adults; not for use in pregnancy
pimecrolimus (*Elidel*)	Topical, apply a thin layer over affected area twice daily	Treatment of atopic dermatitis; limit length of use, may be associated with skin malignancies
sirolimus (*Rapamune*)	6 mg PO as soon after transplant as possible, then 2 mg/d PO *Pediatric <13 yr:* 3 mg/m² PO loading dose, then 1 mg/m²/d PO	Prevention of rejection after renal transplantation
tacrolimus (*Prograf*)	0.075–0.2 mg/kg/d PO divided every 12 h *or* 0.01–0.05 mg/kg/d IV as a continuous infusion, topical apply thin layer to affected area b.i.d.	Prophylaxis for organ injection in liver, kidney, or heart transplants; topical treatment of atopic dermatitis

Drug Name	Dosage/Route	Usual Indications
Interleukin Receptor Antagonist		
anakinra (*Kineret*)	0.10–0.2 mg/kg/d PO in two divided doses, may begin as continuous IV infusion of 0.03–0.05 mg/kg/d, with switch to oral form as soon as possible *Pediatric:* May require higher doses to achieve therapeutic levels 100 mg/d subcutaneous	Prevention of rejection after renal or liver transplantation, reduction of the signs and symptoms and slowing structural damage in adults with rheumatoid arthritis who have inadequate response to other drugs
Monoclonal Antibodies		
adalimumab (*Humira*)	40 mg subcutaneous every other week; if also taking methotrexate, may require 40 mg subcutaneous once a week	Reduction of signs and symptoms and inhibition of structural damage in adults who have moderate to severe rheumatoid arthritis and who have not responded to other drugs
alemtuzumab (*Campath*)	3 mg/d IV as a 2-h infusion, increase slowly to maintenance dose of 30 mg/d IV three times per week for up to 12 wk	Treatment of B cell chronic lymphocytic leukemia in patients who have been treated with alkylating agents and have failed fludarabine therapy
basiliximab (*Simulect*)	20 mg IV twice—first dose within 24 h of transplantation, then at 4 d	Prevention of renal transplant rejection
belimumab (*Benlysta*)	10 mg/kg IV over 1 h, at 2-wk intervals for the first three doses, then every 4 wk	Treatment of adult patients with active, autoantibody-positive systemic lupus erythematosus
bevacizumab (*Avastin*)	5–15 mg/kg as an IV infusion	Treatment of metastatic colon cancer, renal cancer, non–small cell lung cancer, HER2 negative breast cancer; glioblastoma multiforme in combination with other drugs; constipation can be severe
blinatumomab (*Blincyto*)	28-d cycle, continuous IV infusion, 9 mcg/d days 1-7, 28 mcg/d days 8-28 then 2-wk rest	Treatment of Philadelphia chromosome negative acute lymphocytic leukemia
brentuximab (*Adcetris*)	1.8 mg/kg IV over 30 min every 3 wk	Treatment of Hodgkin's lymphoma, anaplastic large cell lymphoma
canakinumab (*Ilaris*)	***Cryopyrin-associated periodic syndrome:*** *Over 40 kg:* 150 mg subcutaneously every 8 wk *15–40 kg:* 2 mg/kg subcutaneously every 8 wk *Juvenile arthritis:* 4 mg/kg subcutaneously every 4 wk	Treatment of cryopyrin-associated periodic syndromes; juvenile idiopathic arthritis
certolizumab (*Cimzia*)	400 mg subcutaneously, repeated at weeks 2 and 4, then every 4 wk	Reduction of the signs and symptoms of Crohn's disease in adults with moderate to severe disease not controlled by standard therapy
cetuximab (*Erbitux*)	400 mg/m² IV over 120 min, then 250 mg/m² IV weekly	Treatment of advanced colon cancer, advanced squamous cell carcinoma of the head and neck; premedicate with antihistamine before infusion
daclizumab (*Zenapax*)	1 mg/kg IV for five doses, the first within 24 h of transplantation and the last within 14 d after transplantation	Prevention of renal transplant rejection
denosumab (*Prolia*)	60 mg subcutaneously every 6 mo	Treatment of postmenopausal women with osteoporosis at high risk for fracture
eculizumab (*Soliris*)	600 mg IV every 7 d for 4 wk, then 900 mg every 7 d, followed by 900 mg every 14 d	Treatment of paroxysmal nocturnal hemoglobinuria, a rare genetic condition in which patients have generations of abnormal blood cells that are lysed by the body, to reduce hemolysis

(table continues on page 294)

Table 17.2 *Drugs in Focus:* Immune Suppressants (continued)

Drug Name	Dosage/Route	Usual Indications
golimumab (*Simponi*)	50 mg subcutaneously once per month	Treatment of rheumatoid arthritis, psoriatic arthritis, ankylosing spondylitis; risk of severe infections
ibritumomab (*Zevalin*)	2 mg of antibody labeled with 0.3 or 0.4 mCi/kg of yttrium-90 IV	Treatment of B cell non-Hodgkin lymphoma in conjunction with rituximab
infliximab (*Remicade*)	5 mg/kg IV over 2 h, may be repeated at 2 and 6 wk	Decreases signs and symptoms of Crohn's disease in patients who do not respond to other therapy, treatment of fistulating Crohn's disease, also approved for use with methotrexate in the treatment of progressing moderate to severe rheumatoid arthritis
ipilimumab (*Yervoy*)	3 mg/kg IV over 90 min every 3 wk for a total of four doses	Treatment of unresectable or metastatic melanoma, risk of severe to fatal immune-mediated reactions
natalizumab (*Tysabri*)	300 mg IV once every 4 wk	Treatment of relapsing–remitting multiple sclerosis, Crohn's disease, risk of progressive multifocal leukoencephalopathy
nivolumab (*Opdivo*)	3 mg/kg IV over 60 min every 2 wk	Unresectable metastatic multiple myeloma; squamous non–small cell lung cancer
obintuzumab (*Gazyva*)	100 mg IV on day 1, 900 mg IV day 2, 1,000 mg IV on days 8 and 15 of a 28-d cycle, then 1,000 mg IV on day 1 of cycles 2–6	Treatment of previously untreated chronic lymphocytic leukemia with chlorambucil
ofatumumab (*Arzerra*)	300 mg IV, 1 wk later 2,000 mg IV a week for seven doses, followed 4 wk later by 2,000 mg every 4 wk for four doses	Treatment of chronic lymphocytic leukemia in patients refractory to fludarabine and alemtuzumab
omalizumab (*Xolair*)	0.15 mg/kg/d subcutaneous	Treatment of asthma with a very strong allergic component and seasonal allergic rhinitis not well controlled with traditional medications
palivizumab (*Synagis*)	15 mg/kg IM as a single dose at the start of RSV season	Prevention of serious RSV infection in high-risk children
pegaptanib (*Macugen*)	Injected into the intravitreal fluid of the eye once every 6 wk	Treatment of neovascular (wet) age-related macular degeneration
pembrolizumab (*Keytruda*)	2 mg/kg IV over 30 min every 3 wk	Treatment of metastatic or unresectable multiple myeloma
ramucirumab (*Cyramza*)	*Gastric cancer:* 8 mg/kg IV every 2 wk *Lung cancer:* 10 mg/kg IV on day one of a 21-d cycle	Treatment of advanced gastric or gastroesophageal adenocarcinoma; treatment of small-cell lung cancer
ranibizumab (*Lucentis*)	0.5 mg by intravitreal injection once a month	Treatment of macular degeneration (wet), treatment of macular edema following retinal vein occlusion
raxibacumab	*Over 50 kg:* 40 mg/kg IV over 1.25 hours *15–50 kg:* 60 mg/kg IV over 1.25 hours *15 kg or less:* 80 mg/kg IV over 1.25 hours	Treatment of adults and children with inhalational anthrax exposure with appropriate antibiotic therapy
rituximab (*Rituxan*)	375 mg/m² IV once weekly for four doses	Treatment of relapsed follicular B cell non-Hodgkin lymphoma
siltuximab (*Sylvant*)	11 mg/kg IV over 1 hour every 3 wk	Treatment of multicentric Castleman's disease
tocilizumab (*Actemra*)	4–8 mg/kg IV every 4 wk, with methotrexate	Relief of signs and symptoms of moderate to severe rheumatoid arthritis in adults
tositumomab with iodine-131 tositumomab (*Bexxar*)	450 mg IV in 50 mL of 0.9% sodium chloride over 60 min, then 35 mg of iodine-131 tositumomab over 30 min; repeat based on response	CD20-positive follicular non-Hodgkin lymphoma when disease is refractory to rituximab and relapsed following chemotherapy

Drug Name	Dosage/Route	Usual Indications
trastuzumab (*Herceptin*)	4 mg/kg IV over 90 min, then 2 mg/kg IV once a week over at least 30 min	Treatment of metastatic breast cancer with tumors that overexpress HER2
ustekinumab (*Stelara*)	45–90 mg by subcutaneous injection once a week, progressing to once a month, then once every 3 mo as determined by patient condition and response	Treatment of recalcitrant plaque psoriasis, psoriatic arthritis in adults not responsive to traditional therapy
vedolizumab (*Entyvio*)	300 mg IV over 30 min weeks 0, 2 and 6, then every 8 wk	Treatment of ulcerative colitis and Crohn's disease in patients with lack of response to TNF blockers and corticosteroids

HER2, human epidermal growth factor receptor 2; RSV, respiratory syncytial virus; CD20, a protein expressed on the surface of B cells; TNF, tumor necrosis factor.

inhibit the secretion of proinflammatory cytokines and increase the secretion of anti-inflammatory cytokines from monocytes and have varying effects on cell proliferation. Fingolimod inhibits the release of lymphocytes from lymph nodes into the peripheral blood so they cannot migrate to activate immune and inflammatory reactions. Fingolimod is the first oral agent for the treatment of relapsing forms of multiple sclerosis. Lenalidomide is used in treating multiple myeloma and myelodysplastic syndromes. Thalidomide is also used for treating multiple myeloma and erythema nodosum leprosum. The newer agent apremilast is used for adults with psoriatic arthritis. Dimethyl fumarate and teriflunomide are used to treat multiple sclerosis; pomalidomide is a thalidomide analog that is used in treating multiple myeloma.

BOX 17.3

New Immunosuppressive Agent

In 2011 belatacept (*Nulojix*) was approved for the prevention of acute transplant rejection in adults with kidney transplants. This immunosuppressive is in a new class of drugs; it is a T cell costimulation blocker. It inhibits T cell proliferation and the production of interleukins and blocks this first step in the immunologic reaction. In testing, this prolonged graft survival and decreased the production of antidonor antibodies. It is given as an IV infusion over 30 min the day prior to transplant and on day 5 posttransplant, then at the end of week 2, 4, 8, 16, and then once every 4 wk. Patients who receive this have an increased risk for posttransplant lymphoproliferative disorder. This happens most frequently in patients who were never exposed to Epstein-Barr virus, so it is recommended that it only be used in patients who have been previously exposed to Epstein-Barr virus. Patients should be advised to limit sun exposure because of the risk of skin cancer when the T cells are suppressed. Live vaccines should also be avoided when on this drug. All cancer screenings should be done with these patients because of the increased risk of cancer development.

Pharmacokinetics

Fingolimod is slowly absorbed from the GI tract, reaching peak levels in 12 to 16 hours. It is metabolized in the liver and excreted through the kidneys with a half-life of 6 to 9 days. Lenalidomide is absorbed quickly from the GI tract, reaching peak levels in 30 to 90 minutes. It is excreted unchanged in the urine with a half-life of 3 hours. Thalidomide is very slowly absorbed from the GI tract, reaching peak levels in 3 to 6 hours. The metabolism of thalidomide is not known; it is excreted in the urine with a half-life of 12 to 24 hours. Pomalidomide is absorbed from the GI tract, reaching peak levels in 2 to 3 hours. It is metabolized in the liver and excreted in the urine with a half-life of 7.5 to 9.5 hours. Apremilast is absorbed from the GI tract with peak levels reached in 2.5 hours. It is also metabolized in the liver with excretion in both urine and feces. Apremilast has a half life of 6 to 9 hours. Dimethyl fumarate is absorbed from the GI tract with peak levels occurring within 2 to 2.5 hours. It is metabolized by esterases throughout the body with the main excretion occurring as CO_2 through the lungs. The half-life of this drug is about an hour. Oral teriflunomide reaches peak levels in 1 to 4 hours; it is excreted unchanged in the bile. Most of the drug is eliminated from the body within 21 days.

Contraindications and Cautions

All of these drugs are contraindicated during pregnancy *because their effects on cells can cause serious fetal harm*; women of childbearing age should be advised to use barrier contraceptives when using this drug, and proof that the patient is not pregnant needs to be documented in the chart before beginning therapy and periodically during therapy. Teriflunomide is also contraindicated with severe hepatic impairment *which could become more severe due to the drug effects.*

T and B Cell Suppressors

Several T and B cell immune suppressors are available for use. Of the numerous agents available, cyclosporine is the most commonly used immune suppressant. Additional agents include abatacept (*Orencia*), alefacept (*Amevive*), azathioprine (*Imuran*), cyclosporine (*Sandimmune, Neoral*), glatiramer (*Copaxone*), mycophenolate (*CellCept*), pimecrolimus (*Elidel*), sirolimus (*Rapamune*), and tacrolimus (*Prograf*).

Therapeutic Actions and Indications

The exact mechanism of action of the T and B cell suppressors is not clearly understood. It has been shown that they block antibody production by B cells, inhibit suppressor and helper T cells, and modify the release of interleukins and of T cell growth factor (see Figure 17.1).

The T and B cell suppressors are indicated for the prevention and treatment of specific transplant rejections. See Table 17.2 for Usual Indications of each agent.

Pharmacokinetics

Cyclosporine is well absorbed from the GI tract, reaching peak levels in 1 to 2 hours. It is extensively metabolized in the liver by the cytochrome P450 system and is primarily excreted in the bile. The half-life of the drug is about 19 hours for *Sandimmune* and 8.4 hours for *Neoral*. It is available as an oral solution that can be mixed with milk, chocolate milk, or orange juice for ease of administration. Abatacept must be given as a 30-minute infusion every 2 to 4 weeks, depending on the patient's response. Peak levels are reached at the end of the infusion. Abatacept has a half-life of 12 to 23 days and usually reaches a steady state by 60 days of treatment. The drug is cleared from the body by the kidneys.

Alefacept is rapidly absorbed and can be given IM or IV. It reaches peak levels in 4 to 6 hours and has a half-life of 270 hours.

Azathioprine is rapidly absorbed from the GI tract, reaching peak levels in 1 to 2 hours. This drug is catabolized in the liver and red blood cells.

Little is known about the pharmacokinetics of glatiramer. Some of it is immediately hydrolyzed on injection, some enters the lymph system, and some may actually reach the systemic circulation.

Mycophenolate is readily absorbed and immediately metabolized to its active metabolite. Most of the metabolized drug is then excreted in the urine.

Sirolimus is rapidly absorbed from the GI tract, reaching peak levels in 1 hour. It is extensively metabolized in the liver, partly by the cytochrome P450 system. The drug is then excreted primarily in the feces.

Tacrolimus is rapidly absorbed from the GI tract, reaching peak levels in 1.5 to 3.5 hours. It is extensively metabolized in the liver by the cytochrome P450 system and is excreted in the urine.

Contraindications and Cautions

The use of T and B cell suppressors is contraindicated in the presence of any known allergy to the drug or its components *to prevent hypersensitivity reactions* and during pregnancy and lactation *because of the potential serious adverse effects on the fetus or neonate.* Caution should be used with renal or hepatic impairment, *which could interfere with the metabolism or excretion of the drug,* and in the presence of known neoplasms, *which potentially could spread with immune system suppression.*

Adverse Effects

Patients receiving these drugs are at increased risk for infection and for the development of neoplasms due to their blocking effect on the immune system. Other potentially dangerous adverse effects include hepatotoxicity, renal toxicity, renal dysfunction, and pulmonary edema. Patients may experience headache, tremors, secondary infections such as acne, GI upset, diarrhea, and hypertension.

Clinically Important Drug–Drug Interactions

There is an increased risk of toxicity if these drugs are combined with other drugs that are hepatotoxic or nephrotoxic. Extreme care should be used if such combinations are necessary. Other reported drug–drug interactions are drug specific; consult a drug guide or drug handbook.

Prototype Summary: Cyclosporine

Indications: Prophylaxis for organ rejection in kidney, liver, and heart transplants (used with corticosteroids); treatment of chronic rejection in patients previously treated with other immune suppressants; treatment of rheumatoid arthritis and recalcitrant psoriasis.

Actions: Reversibly inhibits immunocompetent lymphocytes; inhibits T helper cells and T suppressor cells, lymphokine production, and release of interleukin-2 and T-cell growth factor.

Pharmacokinetics:

Route	Onset	Peak
PO	Varies	3.5 h
IV	Rapid	1–2 h

$T_{1/2}$: 19 to 27 hours, metabolized in the liver and excreted in the bile and urine.

Adverse Effects: Tremor, hypertension, gum hyperplasia, renal dysfunction, diarrhea, hirsutism, acne, bone marrow suppression, interleukin receptor antagonist.

Interleukin Receptor Antagonist

An interleukin receptor antagonist works to block the activity of the interleukins that are released in an inflammatory or immune response. The only available interleukin receptor antagonist is anakinra (*Kineret*). See Table 17.2 for additional information about this drug.

Therapeutic Actions and Indications

Anakinra specifically antagonizes human interleukin-1 receptors, blocking the activity of interleukin-1. Interleukin-1 levels are elevated in response to inflammation or immune reactions and are thought to be responsible for the degradation of cartilage that occurs in rheumatoid arthritis. Anakinra is used to reduce the signs and symptoms of moderately to severely active rheumatoid arthritis in patients 18 years of age and older who have not responded to the traditional antirheumatic drugs.

Pharmacokinetics

The recommended dosage is 100 mg/d by subcutaneous injection. Anakinra is administered by subcutaneous injection and is absorbed slowly, reaching peak effects in 3 to 7 hours. It is metabolized in the tissues with a 4- to 6-hour half-life and is excreted in the urine.

Contraindications and Cautions

Anakinra is contraindicated with any known allergy to *Escherichia coli*–produced products or to anakinra itself *to prevent hypersensitivity reactions.* It should be used with caution during pregnancy and lactation *because the drug may cross the placenta and enter breast milk.* It is also used cautiously in patients with renal impairment, immunosuppression, or any active infection *because these could be exacerbated by the effects of the drug.* There is an increased risk of infection whenever this drug is used, and the patient needs to be protected from exposure to infections and monitored closely after any invasive procedures. Immunizations cannot be given while the patient is on this drug.

Adverse Effects

Headache, sinusitis, nausea, diarrhea, upper respiratory and other infections, and injection site reactions are among the most common adverse effects.

Clinically Important Drug–Drug Interactions

Patients who are also receiving etanercept (*Enbrel*) must be monitored very closely because severe and even life-threatening infections have occurred. Anakinra should not be combined with abatacept because of the potential for serious infections.

Monoclonal Antibodies

Antibodies that attach to specific receptor sites are being developed to respond to very specific situations. Every year, several new monoclonal antibodies are marketed, showing the rapid pace with which these agents are being developed and approved for clinical use. Monoclonal antibodies include adalimumab (*Humira*), alemtuzumab (*Campath*), basiliximab (*Simulect*), belimumab (Benlysta), bevacizumab (*Avastin*), blinatumomab (*Blincyto*), brentuxumab (*Adcetris*), canakinumab (*Ilaris*), certolizumab (*Cimzia*), cetuximab (*Erbitux*), daclizumab (*Zenapax*), denosumab (Prolia), eculizumab (*Soliris*), erlotinib (*Tarceva*), golimumab (Simponi), ibritumomab (*Zevalin*), infliximab (*Remicade*), ipilimumab (*Yervoy*), natalizumab (*Tysabri*), nivolumab (*Opdivo*), obintuzumab (*Gavyza*), ofatumumab (*Arzerra*), omalizumab (*Xolair*), palivizumab (*Synagis*), pegaptanib (*Macugen*), pembrolizumab (*Keytruda*), ramucirumab (*Cyramza*), ranibizumab (*Lucentis*), raxibacumab (generic), rituximab (*Rituxan*), siltuximab (Sylvant), tocilizumab (*Actemra*), tositumomab combined with iodine-131 tositumomab (*Bexxar*), trastuzumab (*Herceptin*), ustekinumab (*Stelara*), and vedolizumab (*Entyvio*).

Therapeutic Actions and Indications

Muromonab-CD3, the first monoclonal antibody approved for use, is a T cell–specific antibody that was available as an IV agent. It reacted as an antibody to human T cells, disabling the T cells and acting as an immune suppressor (see Figure 17.1). Muromonab was withdrawn from the market in 2014 when other treatments became more readily available.

Adalimumab, certolizumab, golimumab, and infliximab are antibodies specific for human tumor necrosis factor. they keep the inflammatory reaction in check by reacting with and deactivating the free-floating tumor necrosis factor released by active leukocytes. They are used for treating various forms of arthritis, Crohn's disease and ulcerative colitis. These drugs are discussed in Chapter 16.

Alemtuzumab is an antibody specific for lymphocyte receptor sites.

Basiliximab and daclizumab are specific to interleukin-2 receptor sites on activated T lymphocytes; they react with those sites and block cellular response to allograft transplants. Canakinumab is a specific interleukin-6 blocker and is used for cryopyrin-associated periodic syndromes and juvenile arthritis.

Cetuximab is an antibody specific to epidermal growth factor receptor sites. Trastuzumab also reacts with human epidermal growth factor receptor 2 (HER2), a genetic defect that is seen in certain metastatic breast cancers. It is used in the treatment of metastatic breast cancer in tumors that overexpress HER2.

Blinatumomab, brentuximab, and obintuzumab are specific T cell antibodies, altering their function.

Eculizumab binds to complement proteins and prevents the formation of the complement complex.

Ranibizumab binds to sites of active forms of vascular endothelial growth factor, preventing new vascular growth in the area of injection. Ramucirumab and ranibizumab also inhibit endothelial growth receptors. Ramucirumab is effective in gastric and lung cancers. Ranibizumab is used for treating macular edema and macular degeneration.

Erlotinib, bevacizumab, pegaptanib, and tositumomab combined with iodine-131 tositumomab are effective against specific malignant receptor sites.

Ibritumomab, ofatumumab, and rituximab are antibodies specific to sites on activated B lymphocytes.

Natalizumab is an antibody specific to surface receptors on all leukocytes except neutrophils.

Nivolumab and pembrolizumab are antibodies to programmed death receptor-1 sites and are used for treating specific cancers.

Omalizumab is an antibody to immunoglobulin E, an important factor in allergic reactions. It has not had a great deal of success because of related respiratory adverse effects but is now approved for chronic urticaria conditions.

Palivizumab is specific to the antigenic site on respiratory syncytial virus (RSV); it inactivates that virus. It is used to prevent RSV disease in high-risk children.

Tocilizumab, siltuximab, and ustekinumab are antibodies specific to interleukins.

Belimumab, which is a specific inhibitor of B lymphocyte stimulator which inhibits the survival of B lymphocytes and their differentiation into immunoglobulin-producing cells.

It is used for adult patients with active, autoantibody-positive systemic lupus erythematosus who are receiving standard therapy.

Ipilimumab is a human cytotoxic T cell antigen-4–blocking antibody. By blocking this site, T cells are activated and proliferate at a faster rate. It is used to treat patients with unresectable or metastatic melanoma. It is associated with potentially fatal immune-mediated reactions, and its use must be carefully evaluated.

Vedolizumab is an integrin blocker that inhibits the movement of T cells across the gastric mucosa. It is used for treating ulcerative colitis and Crohn's disease in patients who do not respond to traditional therapies.

Pharmacokinetics

With the exception of erlotinib (an oral agent), all of the monoclonal antibodies have to be injected. They can be given IV, IM, or subcutaneously. Because antibodies are proteins, they are rapidly broken down in the GI tract. They are processed by the body like naturally occurring antibodies.

Contraindications and Cautions

Monoclonal antibodies are contraindicated in the presence of any known allergy to the drug or to murine products *to prevent hypersensitivity reactions* and in the presence of fluid overload, *which could be exacerbated.* They should be used cautiously with fever (treat the fever before beginning therapy) and in patients who have had previous administration of the monoclonal antibody (*serious hypersensitivity reactions can occur with repeat administration*). Because of the potential for adverse effects, they should not be used during pregnancy or lactation unless the benefit clearly outweighs the potential risk to the fetus or neonate.

Adverse Effects

The most serious adverse effects associated with the use of monoclonal antibodies are acute pulmonary edema (dyspnea, chest pain, wheezing), which is associated with severe fluid retention, and cytokine release syndrome (flu-like symptoms that can progress to third-spacing of fluids and shock). Other adverse effects that can be anticipated include fever, chills, malaise, myalgia, nausea, diarrhea, vomiting, and increased susceptibility to infection and cancer development (Figure 17.2).

Eculizumab can lead to intravascular hemolysis with resultant fatigue, pain, dark urine, shortness of breath, and blood clots.

Bevacizumab is associated with GI perforation, hemorrhage, and impaired healing.

Erlotinib is reserved for patients whose disease has progressed after other therapies.

The manufacturer of natalizumab stopped marketing the drug weeks after its release because of reports of CNS complications. It was returned to the market in June 2006 with warnings about the potential for CNS complications.

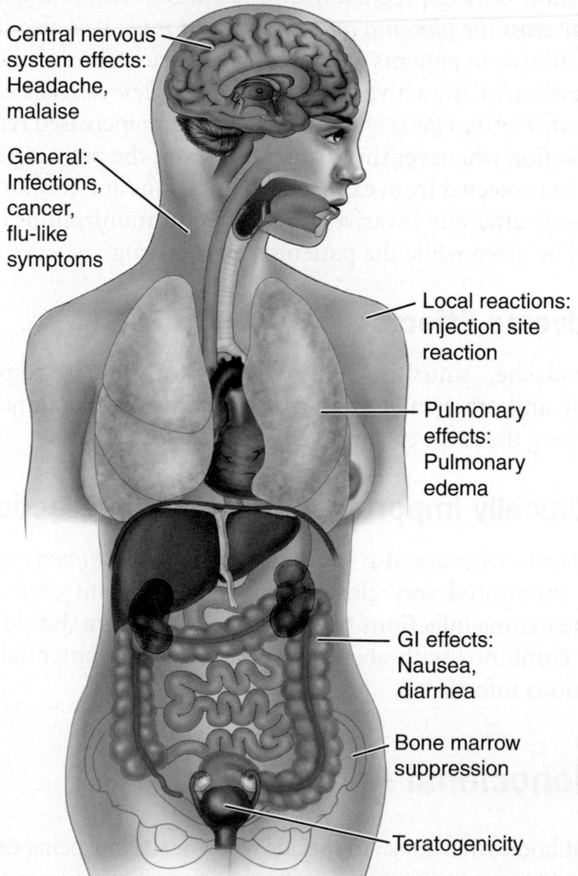

FIGURE 17.2 Variety of adverse effects and toxicities associated with immune modulators.

Blinatumomab is associated with potentially life-threatening cytokine release syndrome and life-threatening neurological toxicities.

Brentuximab and obinutuzumab are associated with progressive multifocal leukoencephalopathy.

Ramucirumab is associated with potentially life-threatening hemorrhage.

Belimumab is associated with CNS effects including an increased risk for depression and suicidality. There is also a risk of hypersensitivity reactions during the IV infusion, and patients should be premedicated before each infusion.

Ipilimumab has been associated with severe to fatal immune-mediated reactions due to the activation and proliferation of T cells. It has a black box warning about the possibility and suggests baseline thyroid and liver function tests and exams of the skin, neurological function, and GI function.

Clinically Important Drug–Drug Interactions

Use caution and arrange to reduce the dose if a monoclonal antibody is combined with any other immunosuppressant drug because severe immune suppression with increased infections and neoplasms can occur.

Ⓟ Prototype Summary: Bevacizumab

Indications: Treatment of metastatioc colorectal cancer, non-squamous cell non-small cell lung cancer, glioblastoma, renal cell carcinoma, cervical cancer, ovarian cancer.

Actions: Monoclonal antibody that binds to and inhibits vascular endothelial growth factor leading to decreased angiogensis and cell proliferation.

Pharmacokinetics:

Route	Onset	Peak	Duration
IV	Minutes	2–7 d	7–10 days

$T_{1/2}$: 20 days, metabolized in the tissues.

Adverse Effects: Headache, back pain, hypertension, GI perforation, hemorrhage, surgery and wound complications, thrombotic events.

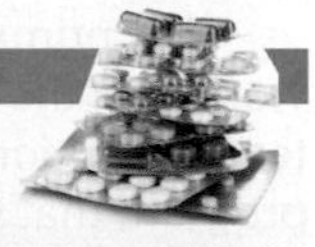

Nursing Considerations for Patients Receiving Immune Suppressants

Assessment: History and Examination

- Assess for contraindications and cautions: Any known allergies to any of these drugs or their components *to prevent hypersensitivity reactions*, current status related to pregnancy or lactation *because of the potential risk to the fetus or baby*, history of renal or hepatic impairment *that might interfere with drug metabolism and excretion*, and history of neoplasm, *which could be exacerbated with the use of these drugs.*
- Perform a physical assessment *to determine baseline status before beginning therapy and for any potential adverse effects*: Inspect the skin *to detect the presence of any lesions*, obtain weight *to monitor for fluid retention*, monitor temperature *to monitor for potential infection*, monitor pulse and blood pressure *to assess the cardiac effects of these drugs*, and assess level of orientation and reflexes *to monitor for any CNS changes associated with drug use.*
- Obtain a baseline electrocardiogram *to evaluate cardiac function.*
- Assess the patient's renal and liver function, including renal and liver function tests, *to determine the appropriateness of therapy and determine the need for possible dose adjustment and toxic drug effects.*
- Monitor the results of laboratory tests such as (CBC *to identify changes in bone marrow function.*

Nursing Diagnoses

Nursing diagnoses related to drug therapy might include:

- Acute pain related to CNS, GI, and flu-like effects
- Risk for infection related to immune suppression
- Imbalanced nutrition: Less than body requirements, related to nausea and vomiting
- Deficient knowledge regarding drug therapy

Planning

- The patient will receive the best therapeutic effect from the drug therapy.
- The patient will have limited adverse effects to the drug therapy.
- The patient will have an understanding of the drug therapy, adverse effects to anticipate, and measures to relieve discomfort and improve safety.

Implementation with Rationale

- Arrange for laboratory tests before and periodically during therapy, including CBC, differential, and liver and renal function tests, *to monitor for drug effects and adverse effects.*
- Administer the drug as indicated; instruct the patient and a significant other if injections are required *to ensure proper administration of the drug.*
- Protect the patient from exposure to infections and maintain a strict aseptic technique for any invasive procedures *to prevent infections during immunosuppression.*
- Arrange for supportive care and comfort measures for flu-like symptoms (rest, environmental control, acetaminophen) *to decrease patient discomfort and increase therapeutic compliance.*
- Monitor nutritional status during therapy; provide small, frequent meals, mouth care, and nutritional consultation as necessary *to ensure adequate nutrition.*

(continues on page 300)

- Instruct female patients in the use of barrier contraceptives *to avoid pregnancy during therapy because of the risk of adverse effects to the fetus.*
- Suggest another method of feeding the baby if a woman is nursing while on these drugs *because of the potential for adverse effects on the baby.*
- Offer support and encouragement *to help the patient deal with the diagnosis and the drug regimen.*
- Provide thorough patient teaching, including measures to avoid adverse effects, warning signs of problems, and proper administration, *to increase knowledge about drug therapy and to increase compliance with the drug regimen.*
- Offer support and encouragement *to help the patient deal with the diagnosis and the drug regimen.*

Evaluation

- Monitor patient response to the drug (prevention of transplant rejection, improvement in autoimmune disease or cancer, prevention of RSV disease, improvement in signs and symptoms of Crohn's disease or rheumatoid arthritis).
- Monitor for adverse effects (flu-like symptoms, GI upset, increased infections, neoplasms, fluid overload).
- Evaluate the effectiveness of the teaching plan (patient can name drug, dosage, adverse effects to watch for, specific measures to avoid adverse effects, proper administration technique).
- Monitor the effectiveness of comfort measures and compliance to the regimen (see Critical Thinking Scenario).

CRITICAL THINKING SCENARIO

Holistic Care for a Heart Transplant Patient

THE SITUATION

After waiting on a transplant list for 4 years, T.B. received a human heart transplant to replace his heart, which had been severely damaged by cardiomyopathy. Before getting the transplant, T.B. was bedridden, on oxygen, and near death. The transplant has given T.B. a "new lease on life," and he is determined to do everything possible to stay healthy and improve his activity and lifestyle. Currently, he is being maintained on cyclosporine, mycophenolate, and corticosteroids.

CRITICAL THINKING

What important teaching facts would help T.B. to achieve his goal? *Think about the psychological impact of the heart transplant and the "new lease on life."*

What activity, dietary, and supportive guidelines should be outlined for T.B.?

What impact will T.B.'s drug regimen have on his plans?

How can all of the aspects of his condition and medical care be coordinated to give T.B. the best possible advantages for the future?

DISCUSSION

T.B.'s medical regimen will include a very complicated combination of rehabilitation, nutrition, drug therapy, and prevention. T.B. should know the risks of transplant rejection and the measures that will be used to prevent it. He should also know the names of his medications and when to take them, the signs and symptoms of rejection to watch for, and what to do if they occur. T.B. must understand the need to prevent exposure to infections and the precautions required, such as avoiding crowded areas and people with known diseases, avoiding injury, and taking steps to maintain cleanliness and avoid infection if an injury occurs.

The medications that T.B. is taking may cause him to experience flu-like symptoms, which can be quite unpleasant. A restful, quiet environment may help to decrease his stress. Acetaminophen may be ordered to help alleviate the fever, aches, and pains.

T.B. may also experience GI upset, nausea, and vomiting related to drug effects. A nutritional consultation may be requested to help T.B. maintain a good nutritional state. Frequent mouth care and small, frequent meals may help. Proper nutrition will help T.B. to recover, heal, and maintain his health.

T.B.'s primary health care provider will need to work with the transplantation surgeon, rehabilitation team, nutritionist, and cardiologist to coordinate a total program that will help T.B. avoid problems and make the most of his transplanted heart.

NURSING CARE GUIDE FOR T.B.: CYCLOSPORINE, MYCOPHENOLATE, AND CORTICOSTEROIDS

Assessment: History and Examination

- Assess for history of allergies to any immunosuppressant; renal or hepatic impairment; history of neoplasm; concurrent use of cholestyramine,

Holistic Care for a heart Transplant Patient (continued)

theophylline, phenytoin, other nephrotoxic drugs, digoxin, lovastatin, diltiazem, metoclopramide, nicardipine, amiodarone, androgens, azole antifungals, or macrolides; grapefruit juice.

- Review physical examination findings, including orientation, reflexes, affect (neurological); temperature and weight (general); pulse, cardiac auscultation, blood pressure, edema, electrocardiogram (cardiovascular); liver evaluation (GI); and laboratory test results (CBC, liver and renal function tests, condition being treated).

Nursing Diagnoses

Acute pain related to CNS, GI, flu-like symptoms
Risk for infection related to immune suppression
Imbalanced nutrition: Less than body requirements related to GI effects
Activity intolerance related to fatigue, drug effects
Deficient knowledge regarding drug therapy

Planning

The patient will receive the best therapeutic effect from the drug therapy.
The patient will have limited adverse effects to the drug therapy.
The patient will have an understanding of the drug therapy, adverse effects to anticipate, and measures to relieve discomfort and improve safety

Implementation

Arrange for laboratory tests before and periodically during therapy.
Administer drug as indicated.
Protect patient from exposure to infection.
Provide supportive and comfort measures to deal with adverse effects.
Monitor nutritional status and intervene as needed.
Provide patient teaching regarding the drugs and their dosage, adverse effects, precautions, and warning signs to report to care provider.

Evaluation

Evaluate drug effects: Prevention of transplant rejection, improvement of autoimmune disease.
Monitor for adverse effects: Infection, flu-like symptoms, GI upset, fluid overload, neoplasm.
Monitor for drug–drug interactions and drug–food interactions.
Evaluate effectiveness of patient-teaching program and of comfort and safety measures.

PATIENT TEACHING FOR T.B.: CYCLOSPORINE, MYCOPHENOLATE, AND CORTICOSTEROIDS

- You will need to take a combination of drugs to prevent your body from rejecting your new organ. These drugs include cyclosporine, mycophenolate, and corticosteroids. They suppress the activity of your immune system and prevent your body from rejecting any transplanted tissue.
- You should never stop taking your drugs without consulting your health care provider. If your prescription is low or you are unable to take the medication for *any* reason, notify your health care provider.
- You should not take your cyclosporine with grapefruit juice.
- Some of the following adverse effects may occur:
  - *Nausea, vomiting*: Taking the drug with food and eating small frequent meals may help. It is very important that you maintain good nutrition. A consult with a nutritionist may be needed to help you if these GI problems are severe.
  - *Diarrhea*: This may not decrease; ensure ready access to bathroom facilities.
  - *Flu-like symptoms*: Rest and a cool, peaceful environment may help; acetaminophen may be ordered to help relieve discomfort.
  - *Rash, mouth sores*: Frequent skin and mouth care may ease these effects.
- You will be more susceptible to infection because your body's normal defenses will be decreased. You should avoid crowded places, people with known infections, and working in soil. If you notice any signs of illness or infection, notify your health care provider immediately.
- Tell any doctor, nurse, or other health care provider involved in your care that you are taking these drugs.
- You will need to schedule periodic blood tests and perhaps biopsies while you are being treated with these drugs.
- Report any of the following to your health care provider: Unusual bleeding or bruising, fever, sore throat, mouth sores, fatigue, and any other signs of infection or injury.
- Keep your medications safely out of the reach of children and pets and do not share medications with anyone else.

KEY POINTS

- Immune suppressants are used to depress the immune system when needed to prevent transplant rejection or severe tissue damage associated with autoimmune disease. Research is ongoing to extend the use of various immune suppressants to other situations, including various autoimmune disorders.
- Increased susceptibility to infection and increased risk of neoplasm are potentially dangerous effects associated with the use of immune suppressants. Patients need to be protected from infection, injury, and invasive procedures.

SUMMARY

- Immune stimulants boost the immune system when it is exhausted from fighting off prolonged invasion or needs help to fight a specific pathogen or cancer cell. They include interferons and interleukins.
- Interferons are naturally released from cells in response to viral invasion; they are used to treat various cancers and warts.
- Interleukins stimulate cellular immunity and inhibit tumor growth; they are used to treat very specific cancers.
- Adverse effects seen with immune stimulants are related to the immune response (flu-like symptoms, including fever, myalgia, lethargy, arthralgia, and fatigue).
- Immune suppressants are used to depress the immune system when needed to prevent transplant rejection or severe tissue damage associated with autoimmune disease. Research is ongoing to extend the use of various immune suppressants to other situations, including various autoimmune disorders.
- Increased susceptibility to infection and increased risk of neoplasm are potentially dangerous effects associated with the use of immune suppressants. Patients need to be protected from infection, injury, and invasive procedures.

CHECK YOUR UNDERSTANDING

Answers to the questions in this chapter can be found in Answers to Check Your Understanding Questions on thePoint®.

MULTIPLE CHOICE

Select the best answer to the following.

1. In which situation would the nurse least likely expect to administer an immune suppressant?
   a. Treatment of transplant rejection
   b. Treatment of autoimmune disease
   c. Reduction of number of relapses in multiple sclerosis
   d. Treatment of aggressive cancers

2. The nurse would expect to administer interferon alfa-n3 (*Alferon N*) as the drug of choice for
   a. treatment of leukemias.
   b. treatment of multiple sclerosis.
   c. intralesional treatment of warts.
   d. treatment of Kaposi sarcoma.

3. Patient teaching for a patient receiving an interferon would include
   a. proper use of oral contraceptives.
   b. use of aspirin to control adverse effects.
   c. importance of cardiovascular workouts.
   d. proper methods injecting the drug.

4. Patients who are receiving an immune stimulant may experience any of the clinical signs of immune response activity, including
   a. flu-like symptoms.
   b. diarrhea.
   c. constipation.
   d. headache.

5. Organ transplants are often rejected by the body because the T cells recognize the transplanted cells as foreign and try to destroy them. Treatment with an immune suppressant would
   a. activate antibody production.
   b. stimulate interleukin release.
   c. stimulate thymus secretions.
   d. block the initial damage to the transplanted cells.

6. You might use a monoclonal antibody in treating
   a. warts.
   b. herpes zoster.
   c. tumors that overexpress HER2.
   d. Kaposi sarcoma.

MULTIPLE RESPONSE

Select all that apply.

1. The nurse is assigned to care for a client who is receiving immune suppressants. The nurse would continually assess the client for which of the following anticipated adverse effects?
- **a.** Development of cancers
- **b.** Increased risk of infection
- **c.** Cardiac standstill
- **d.** Development of secondary infections
- **e.** Increased bleeding tendencies
- **f.** Hepatomegaly

2. Teaching points that the nurse would incorporate into the care of a client receiving cyclosporine would include which of the following?
- **a.** Use barrier contraceptives to avoid pregnancy.
- **b.** If mouth sores occur, try to restrict eating as much as possible.
- **c.** Dilute the solution with milk, chocolate milk, or orange juice and drink immediately.
- **d.** Avoid drinking grapefruit juice when on this drug.
- **e.** Stop taking the drug if GI upset or fever occurs.
- **f.** Refrigerate the oral solution.

BIBLIOGRAPHY AND REFERENCES

Brunton, L., Chabner, B., & Knollman, B. (2011). *Goodman and Gilman's the pharmacological basis of therapeutics* (12th ed.). New York: McGraw-Hill.

Dimitrov, A. (Ed.). (2009). *Therapeutic antibodies; methods and protocols.* New York. Humana Press.

Facts and Comparisons. (2015). *Drug facts and comparisons.* St. Louis, MO: Author.

Fox, D. (2010). *New insights into rheumatoid arthritis.* Philadelphia, PA: Saunders.

Hashkes, P. J., & Laxer, R. M. (2005). Medical treatment of juvenile idiopathic arthritis. *Journal of the American Medical Association, 294,* 1671–1684.

Karch, A. M. (2014). *Lippincott's nursing drug guide.* Philadelphia, PA: Lippincott Williams & Wilkins.

Mitka, M. (2010). Targeted therapies take aim against lung cancer and melanoma. *Journal of the American Medical Association, 304*(6), 624–626.

Porth, C. M. (2013). *Pathophysiology: Concepts of altered health states* (9th ed.). Philadelphia, PA: Lippincott Williams & Wilkins.

Slomski, A. (2013). Monoclonal antibody may be helpful for inflammatory bowel disease. *Journal of the American Medical Association, 310*(16), 1665.

The Medical Letter. (2015). *Medical letter on drugs and therapeutics.* New Rochelle, NY: Author.

Weisman, M., Weinblatt, M., Louie, J. (2010). *Targeted treatment of the rheumatic diseases.* Philadelphia, PA: Saunders/Elsevier.

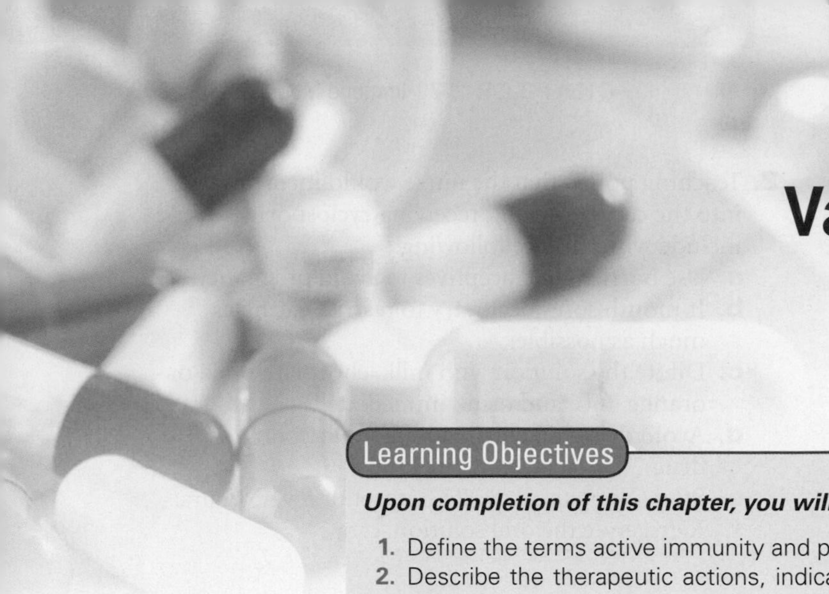

18 Vaccines and Sera

Learning Objectives

Upon completion of this chapter, you will be able to:

1. Define the terms active immunity and passive immunity.
2. Describe the therapeutic actions, indications, pharmacokinetics, contraindications, most common adverse effects, and important drug–drug interactions associated with each vaccine, immune serum, antitoxin, and antivenin.
3. Discuss the use of vaccines and sera across the lifespan, including recommended immunization schedules.
4. Compare and contrast the prototype drugs for each class of vaccine and immune serum with others in that class.
5. Outline the nursing considerations and teaching needs for patients receiving a vaccine or immune serum.

Glossary of Key Terms

active immunity: the formation of antibodies secondary to exposure to a specific antigen; leads to the formation of plasma cells, antibodies, and memory cells to immediately produce antibodies if exposed to that antigen in the future; imparts lifelong immunity

antitoxins: immune sera that contain antibodies to specific toxins produced by invaders; may prevent the toxin from adhering to body tissues and causing disease

antivenins: immune sera that contain antibodies to specific venins produced by poisonous snakes or spiders; may prevent the venom from causing cell death

biological: vaccines, immune sera, and antitoxins that are used to stimulate the production of antibodies, to provide preformed antibodies to facilitate an immune reaction, or to react specifically with the toxins produced by an invading pathogen

immune sera: preformed antibodies found in immune globulin from animals or humans who have had a specific disease and developed antibodies to it

immunization: the process of stimulating active immunity by exposing the body to weakened or less toxic proteins associated with specific disease-causing organisms; the goal is to stimulate immunity without causing the full course of a disease

passive immunity: the injection of preformed antibodies into a host at high risk for exposure to a specific disease; immunity is limited by the amount of circulating antibody

serum sickness: reaction of a host to injected antibodies or foreign sera; host cells make antibodies to the foreign proteins, and a massive immune reaction can occur

vaccine: immunization containing weakened or altered protein antigens to stimulate a specific antibody formation against a specific disease; refers to a product used to stimulate active immunity

Drug List

Vaccines

Bacterial Vaccines

bacille Calmette-Guérin (BCG)
Haemophilus influenzae b conjugate vaccine
Haemophilus influenzae b conjugate vaccine and hepatitis B surface antigen
meningococcal polysaccharide vaccine
meningococcal vaccine, serotype B
pneumococcal vaccine, polyvalent
pneumococcal 13-valent conjugate vaccine
typhoid vaccine

Toxoids

diphtheria and tetanus toxoids, absorbed
diphtheria and tetanus toxoids and acellular pertussis vaccine, absorbed

- diphtheria and tetanus toxoids and acellular pertussis and *Haemophilus influenzae* b conjugate vaccines
- diphtheria and tetanus toxoids and acellular pertussis and inactivated poliovirus vaccine
- diphtheria and tetanus toxoids and acellular pertussis, absorbed, and hepatitis B (recombinant) and inactivated poliovirus vaccines, combined

Viral Vaccines

- H5N1 influenza vaccine
- hepatitis A vaccine, inactivated
- hepatitis A vaccine, inactivated, with hepatitis B recombinant vaccine
- hepatitis B vaccine
- human papillomavirus recombinant vaccine, bivalent types 16 and 18
- human papillomavirus recombinant vaccine, quadrivalent
- influenza A (H5N1) vaccine
- influenza A (H5N1) vaccine adjuvanted
- influenza virus vaccine
- influenza virus vaccine, intranasal
- Japanese encephalitis vaccine
- (P) measles, mumps, rubella vaccine, live
- measles, mumps, rubella, varicella virus vaccine, live
- poliovirus vaccine, inactivated
- rabies vaccine
- rotavirus vaccine, live, oral
- varicella virus vaccine, live
- yellow fever vaccine
- zoster vaccine, live

Immune Sera

- antithymocyte immune globulin
- botulism immune globulin
- cytomegalovirus immune globulin
- hepatitis B immune globulin
- (P) immune globulin, intramuscular
- immune globulin, intravenous
- immune globulin, subcutaneous
- lymphocyte immune globulin
- rabies immune globulin
- RHO immune globulin
- RHO immune globulin, microdose
- tetanus immune globulin
- vaccinia immune globulin IV
- varicella zoster immune globulin

Antitoxins and Antivenins

- antivenin (*Micrurus fulvius*)
- black widow spider antivenin (*Latrodectus mactans*)
- botulism antitoxin
- centruroides (scorpion) immune fab
- crotalidae polyvalent immune fab

Vaccines and immune sera, including antivenins and antitoxins, are usually referred to as **biologicals**. They are used to stimulate the production of antibodies, to provide preformed antibodies to facilitate an immune reaction, or to react specifically with the toxins produced by an invading pathogen or venins injected by poisonous snakes or spiders. Stimulating the production of antibodies to specific antigens with vaccines provides the person with immunity to that antigen. Vaccines are frequently called immunizations because they stimulate immunity. Many diseases that were once devastating or fatal can now be prevented by stimulating an immune response and the development of antibodies without the need for the patient to actually contract the disease. Prudent, preventative medical care requires the routine administration of certain vaccines to prevent diseases. The immune sera provide treatments for specific antigens, toxins, or venins and are used after exposure to antigens or toxins or after bites from poisonous snakes or spiders to make diseases less invasive and aggressive or to prevent clinical problems from developing at all. Box 18.1 discusses the use of biologicals among various age groups.

Immunity

Immunity is a state of relative resistance to a disease that develops after exposure to the specific disease-causing agent. People are not born with immunity to diseases, so they must acquire immunity by stimulating B cell clones to form plasma cells and then antibodies.

Active immunity occurs when the body recognizes a foreign protein and begins producing antibodies to react with that specific protein or antigen. After plasma cells are formed to produce antibodies, specific memory cells that produce the same antibodies are created. If the specific foreign protein is introduced into the body again, these memory cells react immediately to release antibodies. This type of immunity was always thought to be lifelong, but it was discovered that patients who had been immunized against smallpox often had no antibodies to smallpox after many years. It is thought that the eradication of the disease has resulted in no stimulation of the memory cells, and after a prolonged period with no stimulation, perhaps the memory cells no longer produce antibodies.

Passive immunity occurs when preformed antibodies are injected into the system and react with a specific antigen. These antibodies come from animals that have been infected with the disease or from humans who have had the disease and have developed antibodies. The circulating antibodies act in the same manner as those produced from plasma cells, recognizing the foreign protein and attaching to it, rendering it harmless. Unlike active immunity, passive immunity is limited. It lasts only as long as the circulating antibodies last because the body does not produce its own antibodies.

In some cases the host human responds to the circulating injected antibodies, which are foreign proteins to

BOX 18.1 FOCUS ON Drug Therapy Across the Lifespan

Biologicals

CHILDREN

Routine immunization for children has become a standard of care in the United States. Parents should receive written records of immunizations given to their children to assure continuity of care. The parent should be asked to report adverse reactions to any immunization. Sensitive children may receive divided doses of their immunizations to help prevent adverse reactions.

Simple comfort measures—warm soaks at the injection site, acetaminophen to reduce fever or aches and pains, and comfort from parents or caregivers—will help the child to deal with the immunization experience.

Parent education is a very important aspect of the immunization procedure. Parents may need reassurance and educational materials when concerns about the safety of immunizations arise.

Immune sera are used for specific exposures. Botulism immune globulin is specific for treatment of infants younger than 1 year of age with botulism.

ADULTS

There are a number of reasons adults should receive certain immunizations. For example, adults who are traveling to areas with high risk for particular diseases—and who may not have previously been exposed to those diseases—are advised to be immunized.

In addition, all adults are advised to be immunized yearly with an influenza vaccine and once with a pneumococcal pneumonia vaccine and the pneumococcal 13-valent vaccine. These vaccines provide some protection against diseases that can prove dangerous for people with chronic lung, CV, or endocrine disorders. The influenza vaccine changes yearly, depending on predictions of which flu strain might be emergent in that year. The pneumonia vaccine contains 23 strains and is believed to offer lifetime protection.

Tetanus shots also are recommended for adults every 10 years or with any injury that potentially could precipitate a tetanus infection and is currently given with a pertussis booster to help protect children from this exposure.

Immune sera are used for specific exposures.

OLDER ADULTS

Older patients are at greater risk for severe illness from influenza and pneumococcal infections. The yearly flu shot and the pneumococcal and pneumococcal 13-valent vaccines should be stressed for this group.

A tetanus booster every 10 years will also help to protect older adults from exposure to that illness. Ask the patient about any adverse reaction to previous tetanus boosters and weigh the risk against the possible exposure to tetanus.

If an older patient is traveling to an area where a particular disease is endemic and the risk of exposure is great, the Centers for Disease Control and Prevention (http://www.cdc.gov) should be contacted to determine whether the appropriate vaccine is acceptable for use in the older patient.

Immune sera are used for specific exposures. Older adults are at increased risk for severe reactions and should be monitored closely.

the host's body, by producing its own antibodies to the injected antibodies. This results in **serum sickness**, a massive immune reaction manifested by fever, arthritis, flank pain, myalgia, and arthralgia.

Immunization

Immunization is the process of artificially stimulating active immunity by exposing the body to weakened or less toxic proteins associated with specific disease-causing organisms. The proteins could be a weakened bacterial cell membrane, the protein coat of a virus, or a virus (protein coat with the genetic fragment that makes up the virus) that has been chemically weakened so that it cannot cause disease. The goal is to cause an immune response without having the patient suffer the full course of a disease. Adults may require immunizations in certain situations: Exposure, travel to an area endemic for a disease they have not had and have not been immunized against, and occupations that are considered high risk (Figure 18.1). Children are routinely immunized against many infections that were once quite devastating (Figure 18.2; Box 18.2). For example, smallpox was one of the first diseases against which children were immunized. Today, smallpox is considered to be eradicated worldwide. Concerns over biological terrorism have renewed interest in this disease, and smallpox vaccine is now available to the military to provide help for people who might be at high risk for exposure to a potential attack by terrorists using smallpox.

Diphtheria, pertussis, tetanus, *Haemophilus influenzae* b, hepatitis B, hepatitis A, chickenpox, poliovirus, meningitis, measles, mumps, rotavirus, and rubella are all standard childhood immunizations today. The bacille Calmette-Guérin vaccine for tuberculosis is widely used throughout the world in countries with a high incidence of tuberculosis to limit the spread of the disease. However, it is not routinely used in the United States because the incidence of tuberculosis is relatively low, and it can induce false-positive tuberculin skin test results. The human papillomavirus (HPV) vaccine is now recommended to protect against several of the viruses that cause many cervical or anal cancers.

The use of vaccines is not without controversy. Severe reactions, although rare, have occurred, resulting in concerns about the safety of vaccines and their administration, especially in children (Box 18.3). The

Recommended adult immunization schedule, by vaccine and age group [1]

VACCINE ▼ AGE GROUP ►	19–21 years	22–26 years	27–49 years	50–59 years	60–64 years	≥ 65 years
Influenza*,2	1 dose annually					
Tetanus, diphtheria, pertussis (TD/TDap)*,3	Substitute 1-time dose of Tdap for Td booster; then boost with Td every 10 yrs					
Varicella*,4	2 doses					
Human papillomavirus (HPV): Female*,5	3 doses					
Human papillomavirus (HPV): Male*,5	3 doses					
Zoster6					1 dose	
Measles, mumps, rubella (MMR)*,7	1 or 2 doses					
Pneumococcal 13-valent conjugate (PCV13)*,8						1-time dose
Pneumococcal polysaccharide (PPSV23)8	1 or 2 doses					1 dose
Meningococcal*,9	1 or more doses					
Hepatitis A*,10	2 doses					
Hepatitis B*,11	3 doses					
Haemophilus influenzae type b (Hib)*,12	1 or 3 doses					

*Covered by the Vaccine Injury Compensation Program

For all persons in this category who meet the age requirements and who lack documentation of vaccination or have no evidence of previous infection; zoster vaccine recommended regardless of prior episode of zoster

Recommended if some other risk factor is present (e.g., on the basis of medical, occupational, lifestyle, or other indications)

No recommendation

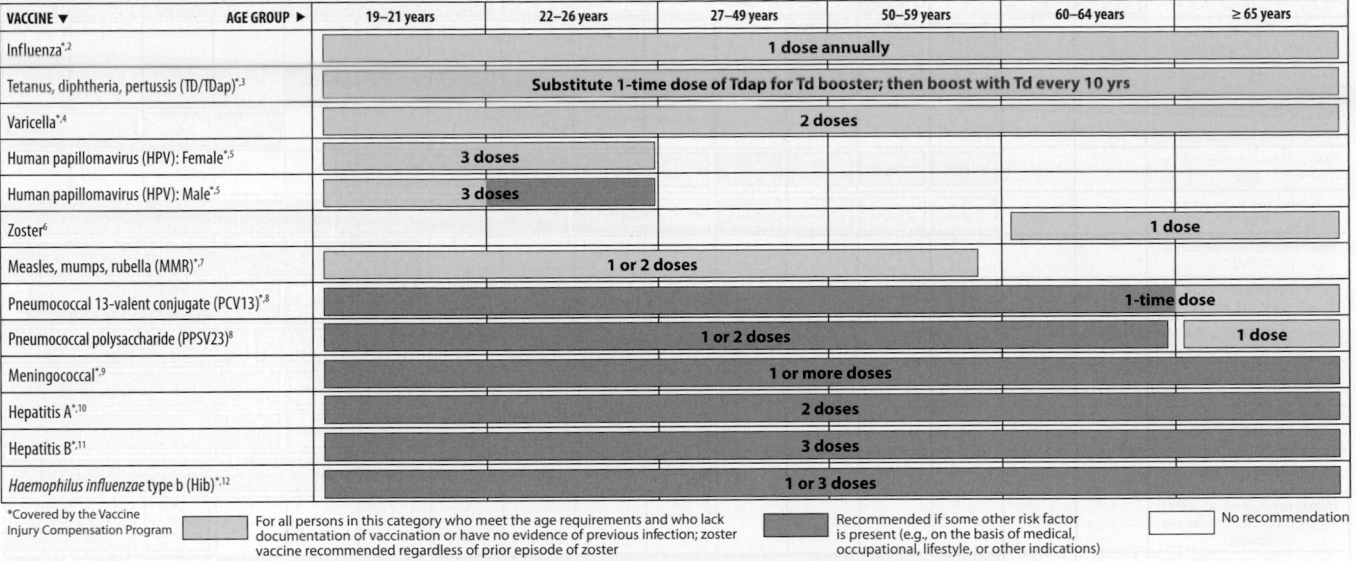

Vaccines that might be indicated for adults based on medical and other indications [1]

VACCINE ▼ INDICATION ►	Pregnancy	Immuno-compromising conditions (excluding human immunodeficiency virus [HIV]) 4,6,7,8,13	HIV infection CD4+ T lymphocyte count 4,6,7,8,13 < 200 cells/μL	HIV infection CD4+ T lymphocyte count ≥ 200 cells/μL	Men who have sex with men (MSM)	Kidney failure, end-stage renal disease, receipt of hemodialysis	Heart disease, chronic lung disease, chronic alcoholism	Asplenia (including elective splenectomy and persistent complement component deficiencies) 8,12	Chronic liver disease	Diabetes	Healthcare personnel
Influenza*,2	1 dose IIV annually				1 dose IIV or LAIV annually	1 dose IIV annually					1 does IIV or LAIV annually
Tetanus, diphtheria, pertussis (Td/Tdap)*,3	1 dose Tdap each pregnancy	Substitute 1-time dose of Tdap for Td booster; then boost with Td every 10 yrs									
Varicella*,4	Contraindicated			2 doses							
Human papillomavirus (HPV) Female*,5		3 doses through age 26 yrs				3 doses through age 26 yrs					
Human papillomavirus (HPV) Male*,5		3 doses through age 26 yrs				3 doses through age 21 yrs					
Zoster6	Contraindicated				1 dose						
Measles, mumps, rubella (MMR)*,7	Contraindicated			1 or 2 doses							
Pneumococcal 13-valent conjugate (PCV13)*,8		1 dose									
Pneumococcal polysaccharide (PPSV23)8	1 or 2 doses										
Meningococcal*,9	1 or more doses										
Hepatitis A*,10	2 doses										
Hepatitis B*,11	3 doses										
Haemophilus influenzae type b (Hib)*,12		post-HSCT recipients only	1 or 3 doses								

*Covered by the Vaccine Injury Compensation Program

For all persons in this category who meet the age requirements and who lack documentation of vaccination or have no evidence of previous infection; zoster vaccine recommended regardless of prior episode of zoster

Recommended if some other risk factor is present (e.g., on the basis of medical, occupational, lifestyle, or other indications)

No recommendation

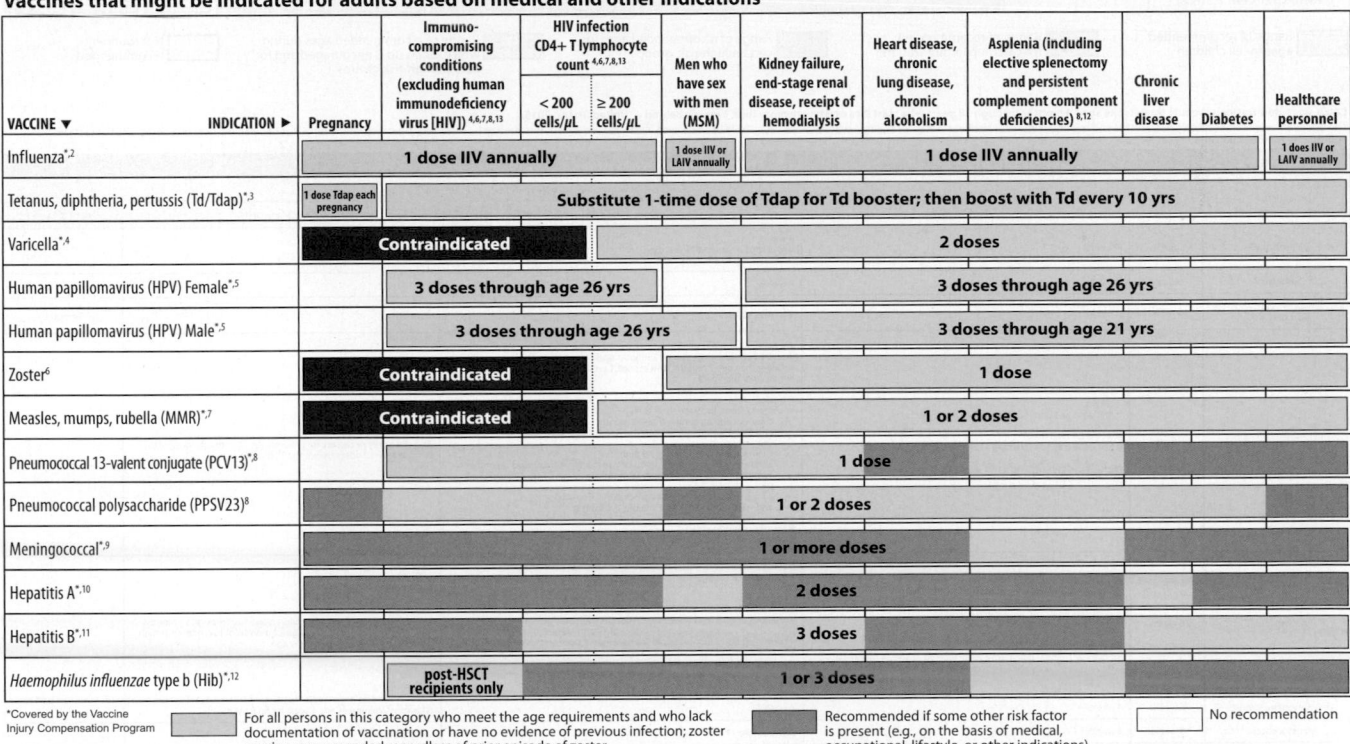

FIGURE 18.1 Recommended vaccines for adults. (Source: Centers for Disease Control and Prevention and the American Academy of Pediatrics, 2016.)

central reporting of adverse effects or suspected adverse effects may help to clarify concerns about reactions to immunizations.

Antigens are also processed and injected to help some people who have severe allergic reactions. People who receive allergy shots to help them cope with the signs and symptoms of allergic reactions are receiving antigenic proteins that stimulate antibody production to prevent the allergic response by stimulating production of another antibody in the body.

Recommended immunization schedule for persons aged 0 through 18 years – United States, 2015.

Vaccine	Birth	1 mo	2 mos	4 mos	6 mos	9 mos	12 mos	15 mos	18 mos	19–23 mos	2-3 yrs	4-6 yrs	7-10 yrs	11-12 yrs	13–15 yrs	16–18 yrs
Hepatitis B[1] (HepB)	1st dose	←------ 2nd dose -----→			←------------ 3rd dose ------------→											
Rotavirus[2] (RV) RV1 (2-dose series); RV5 (3-dose series)			1st dose	2nd dose	See footnote 2											
Diphtheria, tetanus, & acellular pertussis[3] (DTaP: <7 yrs)			1st dose	2nd dose	3rd dose			←----- 4th dose -----→				5th dose				
Tetanus, diphtheria, & acellular pertussis[4] (Tdap: ≥7 yrs)														(Tdap)		
Haemophilus influenzae type b[5] (Hib)			1st dose	2nd dose	See footnote 5		←---3rd or 4th dose, See footnote 5---→									
Pneumococcal conjugate[6] (PCV13)			1st dose	2nd dose	3rd dose		←----- 4th dose -----→									
Pneumococcal polysaccharide[6] (PPSV23)																
Inactivated poliovirus[7] (IPV: <18 yrs)			1st dose	2nd dose	←------------ 3rd dose ------------→							4th dose				
Influenza[8] (IIV; LAIV) 2 doses for some: See footnote 8					Annual vaccination (IIV only) 1 or 2 doses						Annual vaccination (LAIV or IIV) 1 or 2 doses		Annual vaccination (LAIV or IIV) 1 dose only			
Measles, mumps, rubella[9] (MMR)					See footnote 9		←----- 1st dose -----→					2nd dose				
Varicella[10] (VAR)							←----- 1st dose -----→					2nd dose				
Hepatitis A[11] (HepA)							←-------2-dose series, See footnote 11--------→									
Human papillomavirus[12] (HPV2: females only; HPV4: males and females)														(3-dose series)		
Meningococcal[13] (Hib-MenCY ≥ 6 weeks; MenACWY-D ≥9 mos; MenACWY-CRM ≥ 2 mos)			See footnote 13											1st dose		Booster

- Range of recommended ages for all children
- Range of recommended ages for catch-up immunization
- Range of recommended ages for certain high-risk groups
- Range of recommended ages during which catch-up is encouraged and for certain high-risk groups
- Not routinely recommended

Catch-up immunization schedule for persons aged 4 months through 18 years who start late or who are more than 1 month behind — United States, 2015.
The figure below provides catch-up schedules and minimum intervals between doses for children whose vaccinations have been delayed. A vaccine series does not need to be restarted, regardless of the time that has elapsed between doses. Use the section appropriate for the child's age.

Vaccine	Minimum Age for Dose 1	Minimum Interval Between Doses: Dose 1 to Dose 2	Dose 2 to Dose 3	Dose 3 to Dose 4	Dose 4 to Dose 5
Children age 4 months through 6 years					
Hepatitis B[1]	Birth	4 weeks	8 weeks *and* at least 16 weeks after first dose. Minimum age for the final dose is 24 weeks.		
Rotavirus[2]	6 weeks	4 weeks	4 weeks[2]		
Diphtheria, tetanus, and acellular pertussis[3]	6 weeks	4 weeks	4 weeks	6 months	6 months[3]
Haemophilus influenzae type b[5]	6 weeks	4 weeks if first dose was administered before the 1st birthday. 8 weeks (as final dose) if first dose was administered at age 12 through 14 months. No further doses needed if first dose was administered at age 15 months or older.	4 weeks[5] if current age is younger than 12 months **and** first dose was administered at younger than age 7 months, **and** at least 1 previous dose was PRP-T (ActHib, Pentacel) or unknown. 8 weeks *and* age 12 through 59 months (as final dose)[5] • if current age is younger than 12 months **and** first dose was administered at age 7 through 11 months; OR • if current age is 12 through 59 months **and** first dose was administered before the 1st birthday, **and** second dose administered at younger than 15 months; OR • if both doses were PRP-OMP (PedvaxHIB; Comvax) **and** were administered before the 1st birthday. No further doses needed if previous dose was administered at age 15 months or older.	8 weeks (as final dose) This dose only necessary for children age 12 through 59 months who received 3 doses before the 1st birthday.	
Pneumococcal[6]	6 weeks	4 weeks if first dose administered before the 1st birthday. 8 weeks (as final dose for healthy children) if first dose was administered at the 1st birthday or after. No further doses needed for healthy children if first dose administered at age 24 months or older.	4 weeks if current age is younger than 12 months and previous dose given at <7months old. 8 weeks (as final dose for healthy children) if previous dose given between 7-11 months (wait until at least 12 months old); OR if current age is 12 months or older and at least 1 dose was given before age 12 months. No further doses needed for healthy children if previous dose administered at age 24 months or older.	8 weeks (as final dose) This dose only necessary for children aged 12 through 59 months who received 3 doses before age 12 months or for children at high risk who received 3 doses at any age.	
Inactivated poliovirus[7]	6 weeks	4 weeks[7]	4 weeks[7]	6 months[7] (minimum age 4 years for final dose).	
Meningococcal[13]	6 weeks	8 weeks[13]	See footnote 13	See footnote 13	
Measles, mumps, rubella[9]	12 months	4 weeks			
Varicella[10]	12 months	3 months			
Hepatitis A[11]	12 months	6 months			
Children and adolescents age 7 through 18 years					
Tetanus, diphtheria; tetanus, diphtheria, and acellular pertussis[4]	7 years[4]	4 weeks	4 weeks if first dose of DTaP/DT was administered before the 1st birthday. 6 months (as final dose) if first dose of DTaP/DT was administered at or after the 1st birthday.	6 months if first dose of DTaP/DT was administered before the 1st birthday.	
Human papillomavirus[12]	9 years	Routine dosing intervals are recommended.[12]			
Hepatitis A[11]	Not applicable (N/A)	6 months			
Hepatitis B[1]	N/A	4 weeks	8 weeks **and** at least 16 weeks after first dose.		
Inactivated poliovirus[7]	N/A	4 weeks	4 weeks[7]	6 months[7]	
Meningococcal[13]	N/A	8 weeks[13]			
Measles, mumps, rubella[9]	N/A	4 weeks			
Varicella[10]	N/A	3 months if younger than age 13 years. 4 weeks if age 13 years or older.			

FIGURE 18.2 Recommended immunization schedule for children. (Source: Centers for Disease Control and Prevention and the American Academy of Pediatrics, 2016.)

Catch-up immunization schedule for persons aged 4 months through 18 years who start late or who are more than 1 month behind — The figure below provides catch-up schedules and minimum intervals between doses for children whose vaccinations have been delayed. A vaccine series does not need to be restarted, regardless of the time that has elapsed between doses. Use the section appropriate for the child's age.

Persons aged 4 months through 6 years					
Vaccine	Minimum Age for Dose 1	Minimum Interval Between Doses			
		Dose 1 to dose 2	Dose 2 to dose 3	Dose 3 to dose 4	Dose 4 to dose 5
Hepatitis B	Birth	4 weeks	8 weeks and at least 16 weeks after first dose; minimum age for the final dose is 24 weeks		
Rotavirus[1]	6 weeks	4 weeks	4 weeks[1]		
Diphtheria, tetanus, pertussis[2]	6 weeks	4 weeks	4 weeks	6 months	6 months[2]
Haemophilus influenzae type b[3]	6 weeks	4 weeks if first dose administered at younger than age 12 months 8 weeks (as final dose) if first dose administered at age 12–14 months No further doses needed if first dose administered at age 15 months or older	4 weeks[3] if current age is younger than 12 months 8 weeks (as final dose)[3] if current age is 12 months or older and first dose administered at younger than age 12 months and second dose administered at younger than 15 months No further doses needed if previous dose administered at age 15 months or older	8 weeks (as final dose) This dose only necessary for children aged 12 months through 59 months who received 3 doses before age 12 months	
Pneumococcal[4]	6 weeks	4 weeks if first dose administered at younger than age 12 months 8 weeks (as final dose for healthy children) if first dose administered at age 12 months or older or current age 24 through 59 months No further doses needed for healthy children if first dose administered at age 24 months or older	4 weeks if current age is younger than 12 months 8 weeks (as final dose for healthy children) if current age is 12 months or older No further doses needed for healthy children if previous dose administered at age 24 months or older	8 weeks (as final dose) This dose only necessary for children aged 12 months through 59 months who received 3 doses before age 12 months or for children at high risk who received 3 doses at any age	
Inactivated poliovirus[5]	6 weeks	4 weeks	4 weeks	6 months[5] minimum age 4 years for final dose	
Meningococcal[6]	9 months	8 weeks[6]			
Measles, mumps, rubella[7]	12 months	4 weeks			
Varicella[8]	12 months	3 months			
Hepatitis A	12 months	6 months			
Persons aged 7 through 18 years					
Tetanus, diphtheria/ tetanus, diphtheria, pertussis[9]	7 years[9]	4 weeks	4 weeks if first dose administered at younger than age 12 months 6 months if first dose administered at 12 months or older	6 months if first dose administered at younger than age 12 months	
Human papillomavirus[10]	9 years	Routine dosing intervals are recommended[10]			
Hepatitis A	12 months	6 months			
Hepatitis B	Birth	4 weeks	8 weeks (and at least 16 weeks after first dose)		
Inactivated poliovirus[5]	6 weeks	4 weeks	4 weeks[5]	6 months[5]	
Meningococcal[6]	9 months	8 weeks[6]			
Measles, mumps, rubella[7]	12 months	4 weeks			
Varicella[8]	12 months	3 months if person is younger than age 13 years 4 weeks if person is aged 13 years or older			

FIGURE 18.2 (*Continued*)

BOX 18.2

Patient Teaching

Pediatric Immunization

It is well documented that by preventing potentially devastating diseases, society prevents unneeded suffering and death and saves valuable citizens for the future. Pediatric immunization has helped to greatly decrease the incidence of most childhood diseases and has prevented associated complications. In the United States, routine immunization is considered standard medical practice. The 2015 outbreak of measles stemming from the very popular theme park Disney World was a real reminder of the severity and danger of these diseases that one seldom sees when all children are vaccinated.

Ensuring that every child has the opportunity to receive the recommended immunizations has become a political as well as a social issue. The cost of preventing a disease that most people have never even seen may be difficult to justify to families who have trouble putting food on the table. Widespread campaigns to provide free immunizations and health screening to all children have addressed this problem but have not been totally successful.

In addition, periodic reports of severe or even fatal reactions to standard immunizations alarm many parents about the risks of immunizations. These parents need facts as well as reassurance about modern efforts to prevent and screen for these reactions.

Public education efforts should be directed at providing parents with information about pediatric immunization and encouraging them to act on that information. Nurses are often in the ideal position to provide this information, during prenatal visits, while screening for other problems, or even standing in line at a grocery store. It is important for nurses to be well versed on the need for standard immunizations and screening to prevent severe reactions. The Centers for Disease Control and Prevention (http://www.cdc.gov) offers current information and updates for health care providers, as well as patient-teaching materials that can be printed for easy reference.

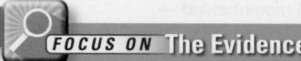

BOX 18.3 FOCUS ON The Evidence

Studies Find No Link between MMR Vaccine and Autism

The Immunization Safety Review Committee Board of Health Promotion and Disease Prevention of the Institute of Medicine under the auspices of the Centers for Disease Control and Prevention and the National Institutes of Health has concluded that there is no evidence to support a linkage between the use of MMR vaccine and the development of autism (a psychiatric neurological impairment affecting children and marked by deficits in communication and social attachment). The original research by Andrew Wakefield supporting a link was published in the *British Medical Journal* in 1996. With more study since that time the *BMJ* has disclaimed this study as fraud and continues to report, as late as 2011, more evidence of fraudulent information that was published in that original article. The media, however, continue to pursue this possible connection, raising concerns for parents about the use of vaccines in children.

Among materials studied by the Institute of Medicine were questionnaires about reported symptoms and the timing of the vaccination and Vaccine Adverse Event Reporting System reports. The information obtained will help determine a need for other research, and it will also be used to educate parents. Parents can be referred to www.cdc.gov; click on vaccine safety to get current information and to review the research that has been done.

Source: Immunization Safety Review Committee. (2004). *Immunization safety review: Vaccines and autism.* Washington, DC: National Academies Press.

FOCUS ON Safe Medication Administration

Use of Allergenic Extracts

Many people receive "allergy shots" or injections of allergenic extracts. These extracts contain various antigens based on specific standardizations. The exact action of these extracts is not completely understood, but it has been shown that after injection, specific immunoglobulin G (IgG) antibodies appear in the serum. These antibodies compete with immunoglobulin E (IgE) for the receptor site on a specific antigen that is the cause of the allergy (IgE is the immune globulin that is associated with allergic reactions; these antibodies react with mast cells, causing the release of histamine and other inflammatory chemicals when they have combined with the antigen). After repeated exposure to the antigens the levels of IgG antibodies increase and the circulating levels of IgE seem to decrease, leading to less allergic response. It may take 4 to 6 months of subcutaneous injections of the allergenic extract every 3 to 14 days to achieve relief from the symptoms of the allergic reaction. The IgG levels remain high for weeks or sometimes months, but the individual response varies widely. Many people are maintained with a weekly injection once the desired response has been achieved.

In 2014 three sublingual allergen extracts were approved. These are thought to work in the same way that the injections work, but avoid the need for injections and visits to the health care facility. Ragweed pollen extract (Ragwitek), Timothy grass pollen extract (Grastek), and grass pollen extract (Oralair) are administered sublingually and rapidly absorbed into the bloodstream. The patient needs to be observed for at least 30 min following the first dose because of a risk of anaphylactic reaction. Once it is determined that the patient can tolerate the drug, it is taken daily, staring 12–16 weeks before the allergen season begins and continuing throughout the season. The patient should also be prescribed an Epi-pen to have on hand in case a severe allergic response develops.

Vaccines

The word **vaccine** comes from the Latin word for smallpox, *vaccinia.* Vaccines are immunizations containing weakened or altered protein antigens that stimulate the formation of antibodies against a specific disease (Figure 18.3). They are used to promote active immunity (see Table 18.1).

Due to recent events and the fear of terrorist activities, concern has risen about the use of various diseases as biological weapons. Box 18.4 discusses vaccines and the use of biological weapons.

Vaccines can be made from chemically inactivated microorganisms or from live or weakened viruses or bacteria. Toxoids are vaccines that are made from the toxins produced by the microorganism. The toxins are altered so that they are no longer poisonous but still have the recognizable protein antigen that will stimulate antibody production.

The particular vaccine that is used depends on the possible exposure a person will have to a particular disease and the age of the person. Some vaccines are used only in children, and some cannot be used in infants. Some vaccines require booster doses—doses that are given a few months after the initial dose to further stimulate antibody production. For example, Box 18.5 discusses the HPV vaccine, which protects young women from many cervical cancers and young men from genital warts and anal cancer. This vaccine is given in a series of three injections to achieve full protection. In many cases, antibody titers (levels of the antibody in the serum) can be used to evaluate a person's response to an immunization and determine the need for a booster dose.

Therapeutic Actions and Indications

Vaccines stimulate active immunity in people who are at high risk for development of a particular disease. The vaccine needed for a patient depends on the exposure that person will have to the pathogen. Exposure is usually determined by where the person lives and his or her travel plans and work or family environment exposures. Vaccines are thought to provide lifelong immunity to the

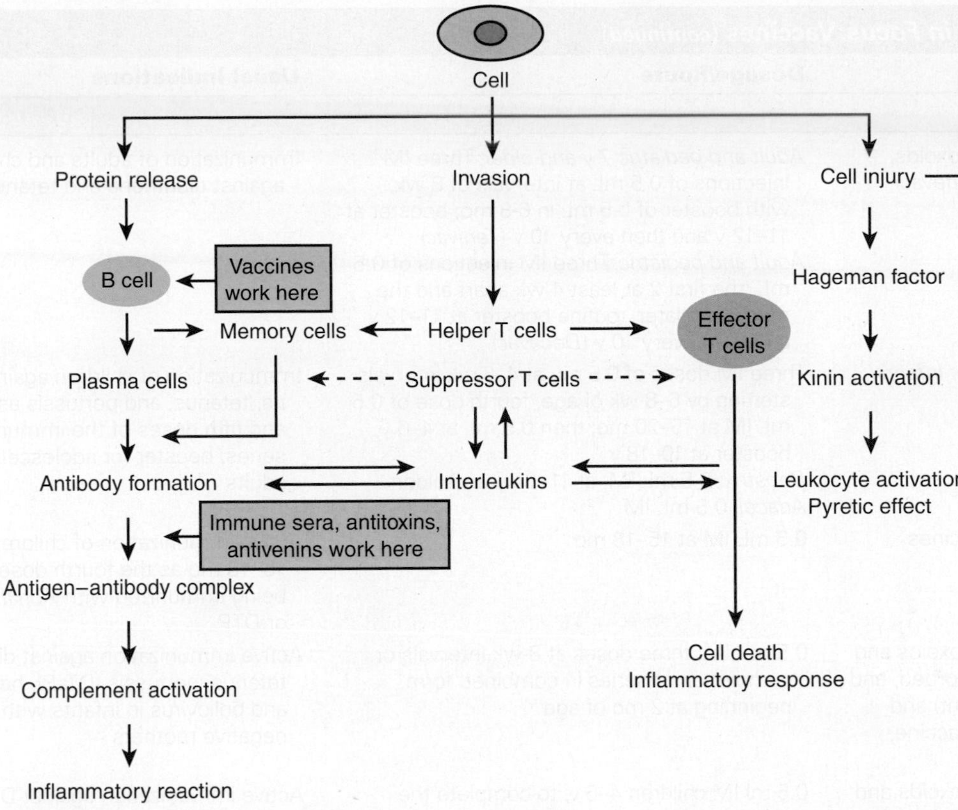

FIGURE 18.3 Sites of action of biologicals.

Table 18.1 ***Drugs in Focus:* Vaccines**

Drug Name	Dosage/Route	Usual Indications
Bacterial Vaccines		
bacille Calmette-Guérin (*TICE*)	0.2–0.3 mL percutaneously	Prevention of tuberculosis with high risk of exposure
Haemophilus influenzae b conjugate vaccine (*HibTITER, Liquid PedvaxHIB, ActHIB*)	0.5 mL IM; ages vary with preparation	Active immunization against *Haemophilus influenzae* type b infection in infants and children
Haemophilus influenzae b conjugate vaccine and hepatitis B surface antigen (*Comvax*)	Three 0.5-mL IM injections at 2, 4, and 6 mo, with 0.5-mL booster at 15–18 mo	Immunization of children against *H. influenzae* type b and hepatitis B infections
meningococcal polysaccharide vaccine (*Menomune-A/C/Y/W-135, Menactra, Menveo*)	0.5 mL IM	Immunization against meningococcal infections for patients 9 months–55 y of age
meningococcal vaccine serotype B (*Bexsero, Trumenba*)	Two 0.5-mL IM doses at least a month apart (*Bexsero*) Three 0.5-mL doses at months 0, 2, and 6 (*Trumenba*)	Immunization against meningococcal infections, serotype B in patients 10–25 y of age
pneumococcal vaccine, polyvalent (*Pneumovax 23*)	0.5 mL subcutaneous or IM, not recommended for children <2 y of age	Immunization against pneumococcal infections
pneumococcal 13-valent conjugate vaccine (*Prevnar-13*)	*7–11 mo:* Three 0.5-mg IM doses at least 4 wk apart and the last one at >1 y *12–23 mo:* Two 0.5-mg IM doses 2 mo apart *24 mo–9 y:* One 0.5-mg IM dose *50 y and older:* One 0.5-mg IM dose	Prevention of invasive pneumococcal disease in infants and children and adults over 50 y of age
typhoid vaccine (*Vivotif Berna Typhim VI*)	Two doses of 0.5 mL subcutaneous at intervals of ≥4 wk with booster given every 3 y *or* one capsule PO on days 1, 3, 5, and 7	Immunization against typhoid fever

(table continues on page 312)

Table 18.1 ***Drugs in Focus:* Vaccines *(continued)***

Drug Name	Dosage/Route	Usual Indications
Toxoids		
diphtheria and tetanus toxoids, adsorbed (*Decavac, Tenevac*)	*Adult and pediatric 7 y and older:* Three IM injections of 0.5 mL at intervals of 8 wk, with booster of 0.5 mL in 6-8 mo; booster at 11–12 y and then every 10 y (*Tenivac*) *Adult and pediatric:* Three IM injections of 0.5 mL, the first 2 at least 4 wk apart and the third 6 mo later, routine booster at 11–12 y and then every 10 y (*Decavac*)	Immunization of adults and children against diphtheria and tetanus
DTaP, adsorbed (*Tripedia, Infanrix, Adacel, Boostrix*)	Three IM doses of 0.5 mL at 4–6 wk intervals starting by 6–8 wk of age; fourth dose of 0.5 mL IM at 15–20 mo; then 0.5 mL at 4–6 y; booster at 10–18 y *Boostrix*: 0.5 mL IM; at 11–65 y and older *Adacel*: 0.5 mL IM	Immunization of children against diphtheria, tetanus, and pertussis as the fourth and fifth doses of the immunization series; booster for adolescents and adults
DTaP-HIB conjugate vaccines (*TriHIBit*)	0.5 mL IM at 15–18 mo	Active immunization of children aged 15–18 mo as the fourth dose when being immunized with *ActHIB*, DTaP, or DTP
diphtheria and tetanus toxoids and acellular pertussis, adsorbed, and hepatitis B (recombinant) and inactivated poliovirus vaccine, combined (*Pediarix*)	0.5 mL IM, three doses at 8-wk intervals or completion of series in combined form, beginning at 2 mo of age	Active immunization against diphtheria, tetanus, pertussis (DTaP), hepatitis B, and poliovirus in infants with HBsAg-negative mothers
diphtheria and tetanus toxoids and acellular pertussis, absorbed, and poliovirus vaccine (*Kinrix*)	0.5 ml IM children 4–6 y, to complete the series started with *Infanrix* or *Pediarix*	Active immunization against DTaP, and poliovirus in children needing to complete the series
Viral Vaccines		
H5N1 influenza vaccine	*Patients 18–64 y:* 1 mL IM, then 1 mL IM 21–35 d later	Active immunization of patients 18–64 y of age at increased risk for exposure to avian flu
hepatitis A vaccine, inactivated (*Havrix, Vaqta*)	*Adult:* 1 mL IM with a booster dose in 6–12 mo *Pediatric:* 0.5 mL IM with a repeat dose in 6–12 mo	Immunization of adults and children against hepatitis A infection
hepatitis A vaccine, inactivated, with hepatitis B recombinant vaccine (*Twinrix*)	1 mL IM followed by booster doses at 1 and 6 mo	Immunization against hepatitis A and hepatitis B infections in people ≥18 y of age
hepatitis B vaccine (*Engerix-B, Recombivax HB*)	0.5–1 mL IM, followed by 0.5–1 mL IM at 1 and 6 mo	Immunization against hepatitis B infections in susceptible people and in infants born to mothers with hepatitis B
HPV recombinant vaccine, bivalent types 16 and 18 (*Cervarix*)	Three doses of 0.5 mL IM given at 0, 1, and 6 mo	Prevention of diseases caused by oncogenic HPV types 16 and 18 in females ages 10–25 y
HPV, recombinant, quadrivalent (*Gardasil*)	*9–26 y:* 0.5 mL IM, then 0.5 mL IM 2 mo later, followed by 0.5 mL IM 6 mo after the first dose	Active immunization against HPV responsible for causing genital warts and cervical cancer, prevention of genital warts in males, prevention of anal cancer and associated precancerous lesions in patients 9–26 y
influenza A (H5N1) vaccine	0.5 mL IM yearly	Active immunization against influenza virus in patients 6 mo and older
influenza virus types A and B vaccine (*Afluria, Fluarix, Fluzone, Fluvirin, Fluzone High Dose*)	*Adult:* 0.5 mL IM *Pediatric:* 0.25–0.5 mL IM, repeated in 4 wk	Active immunization against influenza types A and B in all patients over 6 mo of age

Drug Name	Dosage/Route	Usual Indications
influenza virus types A and B vaccine, intranasal (*FluMist*)	*9–49 y:* 0.5 mL intranasal once each flu season *5–8 y not previously vaccinated with FluMist:* Two doses of 0.5 mL each intranasally given 60 d apart *5–8 y previously vaccinated with FluMist:* 0.5 mL intranasally once per flu season *2–8 y not previously vaccinated:* Two doses given as 0.1 mL in each nostril at least 1 month apart *2–8 y old previously vaccinated:* One dose of 0.1 mL in each nostril	Active immunization to prevent disease caused by influenza A and B viruses
Japanese encephalitis vaccine (*JE-VAX*)	1 mL subcutaneous on days 0, 7, and 30 *1–3 y:* 0.5 mL subcutaneous on days 0, 7, and 30	Immunization of persons >1 y of age who reside in or will travel to endemic areas
measles, mumps, rubella vaccine (*M-M-R-II*)	0.5 mL subcutaneous	Immunization against measles, mumps, and rubella in adults and children >15 mo of age
measles, mumps, rubella, varicella virus vaccine (*ProQuad*)	0.5 mL subcutaneous	Simultaneous immunization against measles, mumps, rubella, and varicella in children aged 12 mo–12 y
poliovirus vaccine, inactivated (*IPOL*)	0.5 mL subcutaneous at 2, 4, and 12–15 mo; booster when starting school *Adult:* 0.5 mL subcutaneous, two doses at intervals of 1–2 mo, with a third dose 6–12 mo later	Immunization against polio infections in adults and children
rabies vaccine (*Imovax Rabies, RabAvert*)	*Preexposure:* 1 mL IM on days 0, 7, 21, and 28 *Postexposure:* 1 mL IM on days 0, 3, 7, 21, and 28	Preexposure immunization against rabies for high-risk people; postexposure antirabies regimen with rabies immune globulin
rotavirus vaccine, live, oral pentavalent (*RotaTeq*)	Three doses of 2 mL PO starting at age 6–12 wk, with subsequent doses at 4–10-wk intervals (third dose should be given at 32 wk)	Prevention of rotavirus gastroenteritis in infants and children
varicella virus vaccine (*Varivax*)	0.5 mL subcutaneous, followed by 0.5 mL subcutaneous 4–8 wk later	Immunization against chicken pox infections in adults and children ≥12 mo of age
yellow fever vaccine (*YF-Vax*)	*Pediatric 1–12 y:* 0.5 mL subcutaneous; 0.5 mL subcutaneous booster every 10 y	Immunization of travelers to areas where yellow fever is endemic
zoster vaccine (*Zostavax*)	*Adults 50 y and older:* 0.5 mL by subcutaneous injection	Prevention of herpes zoster (shingles) in adults 50 y and older

DTaP, diphtheria and tetanus toxoids and acellular pertussis vaccine; DTaP-HIB, diphtheria and tetanus toxoids and acellular pertussis and *Haemophilus influenzae* type b; DTP, xxxx; HBsAg, hepatitis B surface antigen; HPV, human papillomavirus.

disease against which the patient is being immunized. Table 18.1 lists the various vaccines available along with usual indications.

Pharmacokinetics

There is no pharmacokinetic information on these biologicals, which are treated like endogenous antibodies in the body.

Contraindications and Cautions

The use of vaccines is contraindicated in the presence of immune deficiency *because the vaccine could cause disease and the body would not be able to respond as anticipated if it is in an immunodeficient state*, during pregnancy *because of potential effects on the fetus and on the success of the pregnancy*, in patients with known allergies to any of the components of the vaccine (refer to each individual vaccine for specifics, sometimes including eggs, where some pathogens are cultured), or in patients who are receiving immune globulin or who have received blood or blood products within the last 3 months *because a serious immune reaction could occur.*

Caution should be used any time a vaccine is given to a child with a history of febrile convulsions or cerebral injury, or in any condition in which a potential fever would

BOX 18.4

Vaccines and Biological Weapons

The events of September 11, 2001, and the subsequent war on terrorism have heightened awareness of several diseases that might be in development as biological weapons. Anthrax, plague, tularemia, smallpox, botulism, and a variety of viral hemorrhagic fevers are all considered to be likely biological warfare weapons.

Anthrax

A vaccine is available in the United States made from inactivated cell-free filtrate of an avirulent strain of the anthrax bacillus. It is available only for military use. Active production stopped in 1998, but production and supply issues were made high priorities. Ciprofloxacin and, in sensitive cases, doxycycline and penicillins are effective in treating postexposure cases. The vaccine is given and repeated in 2 and 4 weeks, along with the appropriate antibiotic, to patients who have been exposed. The monoclonal antibody , raxibacumab, was approved in 2014 and is specific to the anthrax bacillus and is used for treatment postexposure, along with standard antibiotic therapy.

Plague

Plague is easily spread from person to person and, without treatment, can progress rapidly to respiratory failure and death. There is currently no vaccine for plague; a whole-cell vaccine that was used for many years is no longer available. Research is ongoing using a pneumonic plague vaccine that has successfully protected animals. Several drugs have been found to be lifesaving with plague—streptomycin, doxycycline, ciprofloxacin, and chloramphenicol.

Smallpox

Smallpox was considered eradicated since no new cases had been seen in 20 years. Smallpox is highly transmissible and has a 30% mortality rate in unvaccinated people. Immunization against smallpox ended in the 1970s. There is now a vaccine, which is given to military personnel and people thought to be at high risk. It is currently thought that the vaccine is no longer effective after 20 years, although there is no definite evidence that previously vaccinated people have no protection. The smallpox vaccine uses live virus, placed in punctures made in the skin. After exposure, vaccination given within the first 3 to 4 days can prevent the disease. If it has been 7 days or longer since exposure the vaccine and a vaccinia immune globulin should be used, if any are available. So far, no drugs are thought to be effective in treating smallpox. Early studies have, however, shown cidofovir to be effective in vitro.

Tularemia

Tularemia in an aerosolized form can cause systemic and respiratory illness with a 35% mortality rate. It is not passed from person to person. There is no vaccine available, but doxycycline and ciprofloxacin can be used after exposure, and gentamicin has been effective after symptoms appear.

Botulism

Botulism, produced by *Clostridium botulinum*, can be aerosolized or used to contaminate food. The toxin it produces causes cranial nerve palsies that can result in muscle paralysis and respiratory failure. A botulinum toxoid is available through the Centers for Disease Control and Prevention for the military and high-risk workers. Antitoxin is also available for patients with specific exposures, and research is ongoing with an equine antitoxin effective against all seven serotypes of botulism that is thought to cause fewer hypersensitivity reactions than what is currently available.

Viral Hemorrhagic Fever

Lassa, Marburg, Junin, and Ebola viruses cause hemorrhagic fevers with mortality rates as high as 90%. No vaccines are currently available for these agents, although the United States Army has had success with a vaccine for Junin. Ribavirin has been effective in some cases of Lassa fever and has been effective orally for postexposure prophylaxis. It is being studied for effectiveness with these other viruses. Currently, there is no established treatment, and this area is one of the highest priorities for combating possible biological warfare. The outbreak of Ebola in Africa in 2014 and return of infected workers to the United States brought a great deal of attention to this problem. Many drug companies are working to find a treatment for these viral infections.

be dangerous. Caution also should be used in the presence of any acute infection.

Adverse Effects

Adverse effects of vaccines are associated with the immune or inflammatory reaction that is being stimulated: Moderate fever, rash, malaise, chills, fretfulness, drowsiness, anorexia, vomiting, and irritability. Pain, redness, swelling, and even nodule formation at the injection site are also common. In rare instances, severe hypersensitivity reactions have been reported.

Clinically Important Drug–Drug Interactions

Vaccines should not be given with any immunosuppressant drugs, including corticosteroids, which could alter the body's response to the vaccine.

BOX 18.5 FOCUS ON The Evidence

Vaccine to Protect Against Cervical Cancer

In 2006 the U.S. Food and Drug Administration approved the first vaccine to protect against cancer caused by a virus. HPV is the most common sexually transmitted infection in the United States. The Centers for Disease Control and Prevention estimates that 6 million Americans become infected with genital HPV each year and that half of sexually active men and women become infected at some time during their lifetime. Most of the time the body's defense system will clear the virus, but some types of HPV can be more virulent. There are many types of HPV; some cause genital warts, and others are known to cause abnormal cells on the lining of the cervix, which can lead to cervical cancer years later.

The vaccine *Gardasil* is effective against HPV types 16 and 18 (which account for 70% of cervical cancers) and against types 6 and 11 (which are responsible for 90% of genital warts). The vaccine is recommended for girls and women aged 9 to 26 years. Studies have shown that it is only effective if it is given before HPV infection occurs, so it is best given before the girl or woman becomes sexually active. The vaccine is given as a series of three injections. The second injection given about 2 months after the first, and the last injection given about 6 months later. Tests are being done to evaluate the effectiveness of the vaccine in males and to monitor the long-term effectiveness of the vaccine. Because it is new, it is not yet known whether a booster injection will be needed later and its effects if given inadvertently to a pregnant woman. Side effects that have been reported include the usual flu-like symptoms seen with immunization and pain at the injection site.

The vaccine is not without controversy. In 2007, it cost approximately $360 for the three-shot series, making it an expensive injection. In February 2007 the governor of Texas issued an executive order mandating that the vaccine be given to all schoolgirls entering the sixth grade. A group resenting the mandate for a vaccine sued, and the order was overruled. New Hampshire and Alaska have adopted voluntary programs that supply the vaccine free of charge to girls 11 to 18 years (New Hampshire) or 9 to 18 years (Alaska). Those debating the use of the drug cite the potential for preventing more than 9,700 new cases and 3,700 deaths from cervical cancer every year, whereas others question the long-term effects and effectiveness of the vaccine, stating that it is poor judgment to mandate something with such a short track record. Others fear that women who have had the vaccine will stop getting an annual pelvic exam and Pap smear, which is still needed because cervical cancer can be caused by other factors. Others fear that the protection offered by the vaccine will lead to earlier or more frequent sexual activity among women who have had the vaccination.

This is the first vaccine to protect against cancer, and it is hoped that more such vaccines will be developed in the future. The willingness of parents to listen to the pros and cons and accept the need for this vaccine will have a big impact on the success of this and other such vaccines.

Nursing Considerations for Patients Receiving Vaccines

Assessment: History and Examination

- Assess for contraindications or cautions: Known allergies to any vaccines or to the components of the one being used *to prevent hypersensitivity reactions*; current status related to pregnancy, *which is a contraindication to the use of vaccines*; recent administration of immune globulin or blood products, *which could alter the response to the vaccine*; history of immune deficiency, *which could alter immune reactions*; and evidence of acute infection, *which could be exacerbated by the introduction of other antigens.*
- Perform a physical assessment *to determine baseline status before beginning therapy and for any potential adverse effects*: Inspect for the presence of any skin lesions *to monitor for hypersensitivity reactions*; check temperature *to monitor for possible infection*; monitor pulse, respirations, and blood pressure; auscultate lungs for adventitious sounds; and assess level of orientation and affect *to monitor for hypersensitivity reactions to the vaccine.*
- Evaluate the range of motion of the extremity to be used for vaccine administration *to assure adequate blood flow to deal with the antigen and inflammatory reaction.*
- Assess tissue perfusion to establish a baseline *to monitor for potential hypersensitivity reactions.*

Nursing Diagnoses

Nursing diagnoses related to drug therapy might include the following:

- Acute pain related to injection, gastrointestinal (GI), and flu-like effects
- Ineffective tissue perfusion if severe reaction occurs
- Deficient knowledge regarding drug therapy

Planning

- The patient will receive the best therapeutic effect from the drug therapy.
- The patient will have limited adverse effects to the drug therapy.
- The patient will have an understanding of the drug therapy, adverse effects to anticipate, and measures to relieve discomfort and improve safety.

Implementation with Rationale

- Do not use to treat acute infection; *a vaccine is only used to prevent infection with future exposures.*
- Do not administer if the patient exhibits signs of acute infection or immune deficiency *because the vaccine can cause a mild infection and can exacerbate acute infections.*
- Do not administer if the patient has received blood, blood products, or immune globulin within the last 3 months *because a severe immune reaction could occur.*
- Arrange for proper preparation and administration of the vaccine; check on the timing and dose of each injection *because dose, preparation, and timing vary with individual vaccines.*
- Maintain emergency equipment on standby, including epinephrine, *in case of severe hypersensitivity reaction.*
- Arrange for supportive care and comfort measures for flu-like symptoms (rest, environmental control, acetaminophen) and for injection discomfort (local heat application, anti-inflammatories, resting arm) *to promote patient comfort.*
- Do not administer aspirin to children for the treatment of discomforts associated with the immunization. *Aspirin can mask warning signs of Reye's syndrome, a potentially serious disease.*
- Provide thorough patient teaching, including measures to avoid adverse effects, warning signs of problems, and the need to keep a written record of immunizations, *to increase knowledge about drug therapy and to increase compliance with the drug regimen.*
- Provide a written record of the immunization, including the need to return for booster immunizations and timing of the boosters, if necessary, *to increase patient compliance with medical regimens.*

Evaluation

- Monitor patient response to the drug (prevention of disease, appropriate antibody titer levels).
- Monitor for adverse effects (flu-like symptoms; GI upset; local pain, swelling, nodule formation at the injection site).
- Evaluate the effectiveness of the teaching plan (patient can name drug, dosage, adverse effects to watch for; has written record of immunizations; can state when to return for the next immunization or booster if needed).
- Monitor the effectiveness of comfort measures and adherence to the regimen.

See Critical Thinking Scenario for additional information on educating a parent about vaccines.

CRITICAL THINKING SCENARIO

Educating a Parent about Vaccines

THE SITUATION

S.D. is a 25-year-old, first-time mother who has brought her 2-month-old daughter to the well-baby clinic for a routine evaluation. The baby is found to be healthy, growing well, and within normal parameters for her age. At the end of the visit the nurse prepares to give the baby the first of her routine immunizations. S.D. becomes concerned and expresses fears about paralysis and infant deaths associated with immunizations.

CRITICAL THINKING

What information should S.D. be given about immunizations?

What nursing interventions would be appropriate at this time? *Think of ways to explain the importance of immunizations to S.D. while supporting her concerns for the welfare of her baby.*

How can this experience be incorporated into a teaching plan for S.D. and her baby?

DISCUSSION

S.D. should be reassured before the baby is immunized. The nurse can tell her that paralysis and infant deaths were reported in the past but that efforts continue to make the vaccines pure. Careful monitoring of the child and the child's response to each immunization can help avoid such problems. Reassure S.D. that the immunizations will prevent her daughter from contracting many, sometimes deadly, diseases. Praise S.D.'s efforts for researching information that might affect her baby and for asking questions that could have an impact on her child and her understanding of her care.

Educating a Parent about Vaccines (continued)

The recommended schedule of immunizations should be given to S.D. so that she is aware of what is planned and how the various vaccines are spaced and combined. She should be encouraged to monitor the baby after each injection for fever, chills, and flu-like reactions. When she gets home, she can medicate the baby with acetaminophen to avert many of these symptoms before they happen. (S.D. should be advised not to give the baby aspirin, which could cover up Reye's syndrome, a potentially serious disorder.) S.D. also should be told that the injection site might be sore, swollen, and red but that this will pass in a couple of days. S.D. can ease the baby's discomfort by applying warm soaks to the area for about 10 to 15 minutes every 2 hours.

S.D. should be encouraged to write down all of the immunizations that the baby has had and to keep this information handy for easy reference. She should also be encouraged to record any adverse effects that occur after each immunization. If reactions are uncomfortable, it is possible to split doses of future immunizations.

The nurse should give S.D. a chance to vent her concerns and fears. First-time parents may be more anxious than experienced ones when dealing with issues involving a new baby. To alleviate S.D.'s anxiety the nurse should provide a telephone number that S.D. can call if the baby seems to be having a severe reaction or if S.D. wants to discuss any questions or concerns. She should feel that support is available for any concern that she may have. Because this interaction is likely to form the basis for future interactions with S.D., it is important to establish a sense of respect and trust.

NURSING CARE GUIDE FOR S.D.'S BABY: VACCINES

Assessment: History and Examination

Allergies to the serum base, acute infection, immunosuppression

General: Temperature

Cardiovascular (CV): Pulse, cardiac auscultation, blood pressure, edema, perfusion

Respiratory: Respirations, adventitious sounds

Skin: Lesions

Joints: Range of motion

Nursing Diagnoses

Acute pain related to infection and flu-like symptoms

Ineffective tissue perfusion if severe reaction occurs

Deficient knowledge regarding drug therapy

Planning

The patient will receive the best therapeutic effect from the drug therapy.

The patient will have limited adverse effects to the drug therapy.

The patient will have an understanding of the drug therapy, adverse effects to anticipate, and measures to relieve discomfort and improve safety.

Implementation

Ensure proper preparation and administration of vaccine within appropriate time frame.

Provide supportive and comfort measures to deal with adverse effects: Anti-inflammatory/antipyretic, local heat application, small meals, rest, and a quiet environment.

Provide parent teaching regarding drug name, adverse effects and precautions, and warning signs to report.

Provide emergency life support if needed for acute reaction.

Evaluation

Evaluate drug effects: Serum titers reflecting immunization (if appropriate).

Monitor for adverse effects: pain, flu-like symptoms, local discomfort.

Evaluate effectiveness of parent-teaching program.

Evaluate effectiveness of comfort and safety measures.

Evaluate effectiveness of emergency measures if needed.

PATIENT TEACHING FOR S.D.

- This immunization will help your baby to develop antibodies to protect her against diphtheria, tetanus, and pertussis. The baby will develop antibodies to these diseases, and this will prevent the baby from contracting one of these potentially deadly diseases in the future.
- The injection site might be sore and painful. Heat applied to the area may help this discomfort and speed the baby's recovery.
- Adverse effects that the baby might experience include fever, muscle aches, joint aches, fatigue, malaise, crying, and fretfulness. Acetaminophen may help these discomforts; check with your health care provider for the correct dose to use for the baby. Rest, small meals, and a quiet environment may also help the baby to feel better.
- The adverse effects should pass within 2 to 3 days. If they seem to be causing undue discomfort or persist longer than a few days, notify your health care provider.
- Booster immunizations are required for this immunization. Your baby should receive a booster immunization at your next well-baby checkup. Keep a written record of this immunization.
- Please contact your health care provider if you have any questions or concerns.

Prototype Summary: Measles, Mumps, and Rubella Vaccine

Indications: Active immunization against measles, mumps, and rubella (MMR) in children older than 15 months and adults.

Actions: Attenuated MMR viruses produce a modified infection and stimulate an active immune reaction with the production of antibodies to these viruses.

Pharmacokinetics:

Route	Onset	Peak
IM	Rapid	3–12 h

$T_{1/2}$: Unknown; metabolized in the tissues, excretion is unknown.

Adverse Effects: Moderate fever, rash, or burning or stinging wheal or flare at the site of injection; rarely, febrile convulsions and high fever; Guillain-Barré syndrome, ocular palsies.

KEY POINTS

- Immunity is a state of relative resistance to a disease that develops only after exposure to the specific disease-causing agent.
- Vaccines provide active immunity by stimulating the production of antibodies to a specific protein, which may produce the signs and symptoms of a mild immune reaction but protects the person from the more devastating effects of disease.

Immune Sera

As explained earlier, passive immunity can be achieved by providing preformed antibodies to a specific antigen. These antibodies are found in immune sera, which may contain antibodies to toxins, venins, bacteria, viruses, or even red blood cell antigenic factors. The term **immune sera** is usually used to refer to sera that contain antibodies to specific bacteria or viruses. The term **antitoxin** refers to immune sera that have antibodies to very specific toxins that might be released by invading pathogens. The term **antivenin** is used to refer to immune sera that have antibodies to venom that might be injected through spider or snake bites. These drugs are used to provide early treatment following exposure to known antigens. They are very specific for antigens to which they can respond (see Table 18.2).

Therapeutic Actions and Indications

Immune sera are used to provide passive immunity to a specific antigen, which could be a pathogen, venom, or toxin. They also may be used as prophylaxis against specific diseases after exposure in patients who are immunosuppressed. In addition, immune sera may be used to lessen the severity of a disease after known or suspected exposure (see Figure 18.3 for sites of action of immune sera and antitoxins). Table 18.2 lists the various available immune sera, antitoxins, and antivenins, as well as Usual Indications.

Pharmacokinetics

No pharmacokinetic data are available for these biologicals.

Table 18.2 *Drugs in Focus:* Immune Sera

Drug Name	Dosage/Route	Usual Indications
Immune Sera		
antithymocyte immune globulin (*Thymoglobulin*)	1.5 mg/kg/d for 7–14 d as 6-h infusion for the first dose and ≥4 h for each subsequent dose	Treatment of renal transplant acute rejection in conjunction with immunosuppression
botulism immune globulin (*Baby BIG*)	*Pediatric <1 y:* 50 mg/kg IV as an infusion	Treatment of patients <1 y with infant botulism caused by toxin type A or B
cytomegalovirus immune globulin (*CytoGam*)	15 mg/kg IV over 30 min, increased to 30 mg/kg IV over 30 min, then 60 mg/kg IV to a max of 150 mg/kg; infuse at 72 h, at 2 wk, and then at 4, 6, 8, 12, and 16 wk after transplantation	Attenuation of primary cytomegalovirus disease after renal transplantation
hepatitis B immune globulin (*BayHep B, Nabi-HB*)	0.06 mL/kg IM, repeated at 3 and 6 mo	Postexposure prophylaxis against hepatitis B
immune globulin, intramuscular (*BayGam*, others)	Dose varies with exposure; check manufacturer's instructions	Prophylaxis after exposure to hepatitis A, measles, varicella, or rubella
immune globulin, intravenous (*Gamimune N, Octagam*, and others)	Dose varies with exposure; check manufacturer's instructions	Prophylaxis after exposure to hepatitis A, measles, varicella, or rubella; bone marrow and other transplants; Kawasaki disease; chronic lymphocytic leukemia; treatment of patients with immunoglobulin deficiency

Table 18.2 *Drugs in Focus:* Immune Sera (continued)

Drug Name	Dosage/Route	Usual Indications
immune globulin, subcutaneous (*Gamunex-C, Hizentra, Vivaglobin*)	100–200 mg/kg subcutaneously every week	Treatment of idiopathic thrombocytopenic purpura, chronic inflammatory demyelinating polyneuropathy
lymphocyte immune globulin (*Atgam*)	*Adult:* 10–30 mg/kg/d IV *Pediatric:* 5–25 mg/kg/d IV for aplastic anemia	Management of allograft rejection in renal transplantation; treatment of aplastic anemia
rabies immune globulin (*HyperRAB S/D, Imogam Rabies*)	20 IU/kg IM	Protection against rabies in nonimmunized patients exposed to rabies
RHO immune globulin (*BayRho-D Full Dose, RhoGAM*)	1 vial IM within 72 h after delivery	Prevention of sensitization to the Rh factor
RHO immune globulin, micro-dose (*BayRho-D Mini-Dose, MICRhoGAM*)	1 vial IV within 72 h after delivery	Prevention of sensitization to the Rh factor
tetanus immune globulin (*BayTet*)	250 units IM	Passive immunization against tetanus at time of injury
vaccinia immune globulin IV (*VIGIV*)	2 mL/kg (100 mg/kg) IV	Treatment and management of vaccinia infections
varicella zoster immune globulin (*Varizig*)	1.25 mL diluted IM *or* 2.5 mL diluted IV over 3–5 min	Reduction in the severity of chickenpox if used within 4 d of exposure
Antitoxins and Antivenins		
antivenin (*Micrurus fulvius*) (generic)	30–50 mL IV, flush with fluids after antivenin has infused	Neutralizes the venom of coral snakes
Black widow spider antivenin (generic)	25 mL IM or IV in 10–50-mL saline over 15 min	Treatment of symptoms of black widow spider bites
botulism antitoxin (*Botulism Antitoxin Heptavalent*)	IV, dose based on CDC protocol and exposure	Treatment of suspected or known exposure to all types of botulism neurotoxin, patients 1 y and older
centruroides immune fab (*Anascorp*)	3 vials IV over 10 min, then 1 vial at a time every 30–60 min until clinically stable	Treatment of scorpion stings
crotalidae polyvalent immune fab (*CroFab*)	4–6 vials IV given diluted over 60 min	Treatment of rattlesnake bites

CDC, Centers for Disease Control and Prevention.

Contraindications and Cautions

Immune sera are contraindicated in patients with a history of severe reaction to any immune sera or to products similar to the components of the sera *to prevent potential serious hypersensitivity reactions.* They should be used with caution during pregnancy *because of potential risk to the fetus,* in patients with coagulation defects or thrombocytopenia, or in patients with a known history of previous exposure to the immune sera *because increased risk of hypersensitivity reaction occurs with each use.*

Adverse Effects

Adverse effects can be attributed either to the effect of immune sera on the immune system (rash, nausea, vomiting, chills, fever) or to allergic reactions (chest tightness, falling blood pressure, difficulty breathing). Local reactions, such as swelling, tenderness, pain, or muscle stiffness at the injection site, are very common (Figure 18.4).

Clinically Important Drug–Drug Interactions

Caution should be used if these drugs are combined with any immune suppressant drugs, including corticosteroids. These can alter the body's response to the biologicals.

Ⓟ Prototype Summary: Immune Globulin, Intramuscular

Indications: Prophylaxis against hepatitis A, measles, varicella, rubella; prophylaxis for patients with immunoglobulin deficiency.

Actions: Provides preformed antibodies to hepatitis A, measles, varicella, rubella, and perhaps other antigens, providing a passive, short-term immunity.

Pharmacokinetics:

Route	Onset	Peak
IM	Slow	2–5 d

$T_{1/2}$: Unknown; metabolized in the tissues, excretion is unknown.

Adverse Effects: Tenderness, muscle stiffness at site of injection; urticaria, angioedema, nausea, vomiting, chills, fever, chest tightness.

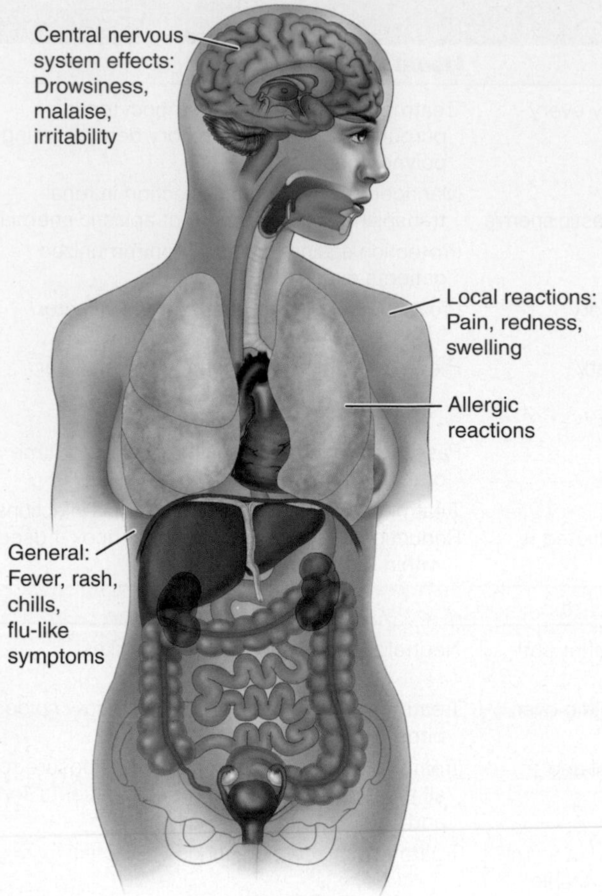

FIGURE 18.4 Variety of adverse effects and toxicities associated with vaccines and immune sera.

Nursing Considerations for Patients Receiving Immune Sera

Assessment: History and Examination

- Assess for contraindications or cautions: Any known allergies to any of these drugs or their components *to prevent hypersensitivity reactions*; current status related to pregnancy, *which would be a contraindication for immune sera*; previous exposure to the serum being used *because hypersensitivity reactions become worse with repeated exposure*; evidence of thrombocytopenia or coagulation disorders, *which could be exacerbated by the effects of immune sera*; and immunization history *to determine the potential for hypersensitivity reactions*.
- Perform a physical assessment *to determine baseline status before beginning therapy and for any potential adverse effects*: Inspect for the presence of any skin lesions *to monitor for hypersensitivity reactions*; check temperature *to monitor for possible infection*; monitor pulse, respirations, and blood pressure; auscultate lungs for adventitious sounds; and assess level of orientation and affect *to monitor for hypersensitivity reactions to the vaccine*.

Nursing Diagnoses

Nursing diagnoses related to drug therapy might include the following:

- Acute pain related to local, GI, and flu-like effects
- Ineffective tissue perfusion related to possible severe reactions
- Deficient knowledge regarding drug therapy

Planning

- The patient will receive the best therapeutic effect from the drug therapy.
- The patient will have limited adverse effects to the drug therapy.
- The patient will have an understanding of the drug therapy, adverse effects to anticipate, and measures to relieve discomfort and improve safety.

Implementation with Rationale

- Do not administer to any patient with a history of severe reaction to immune globulins or to the components of the drug being used *because severe immune reactions can occur.*
- Administer the drug as indicated. *Preparation varies with each product; always check the manufacturer's guidelines.*
- Monitor for severe reactions and have emergency equipment ready *to allow prompt intervention should a severe reaction occur.*
- Arrange for supportive care and comfort measures for flu-like symptoms (rest, environmental control, acetaminophen) and for the local reaction (heat to injection site, anti-inflammatories) *to promote patient comfort.*
- Provide thorough patient teaching, including measures to avoid adverse effects and warning signs of problems, *to improve patient compliance.*
- Provide a written record of immune sera use and encourage the patient or family to keep that information *to ensure proper medical treatment and to avert future reactions.*

Evaluation

- Monitor the patient's response to the drug (improvement in disease signs and symptoms, prevention of severe disease).
- Monitor for adverse effects (flu-like symptoms, GI upset, local inflammation, and pain).
- Evaluate the effectiveness of the teaching plan (patient can name drug, dosage, adverse effects to watch for, and specific measures to avoid adverse effects and to promote comfort and acknowledge the need to retain a written record of injection).
- Monitor the effectiveness of comfort measures and compliance with the regimen.

KEY POINTS

- Immune sera provide preformed antibodies to specific proteins for people who have been exposed to them or are at high risk for exposure.
- The term immune sera typically refers to sera that contain antibodies to specific bacteria or viruses.

SUMMARY

- Immunity (relative resistance to a disease) may be active or passive. Active immunity results from the body making antibodies against specific proteins for immediate release if that protein reenters the body. Passive immunity results from preformed antibodies to a specific protein, which offers protection against the protein only for the life of the circulating antibodies.
- Immunizations are given to stimulate active immunity in a person who is at high risk for exposure to specific diseases. Immunizations are a standard part of preventive medicine.
- Vaccines can be made from chemically inactivated microorganisms or from live, weakened viruses or bacteria. Toxoids are vaccines that are made from the toxins produced by the microorganism that are altered so that they are no longer poisonous but still have the recognizable protein antigen that will stimulate antibody production.
- Immune sera provide preformed antibodies to specific proteins for people who have been exposed to them or are at high risk for exposure.
- The term immune sera typically refers to sera that contain antibodies to specific bacteria or viruses. Antitoxins are immune sera that have antibodies to very specific toxins that might be released by invading pathogens. Antivenins are immune sera that have antibodies to venom that might be injected through spider or snake bites.
- Serum sickness—a massive immune reaction—occurs more frequently with immune sera than with vaccines. Patients need to be monitored for any history of hypersensitivity reactions, and emergency equipment should be available.
- Patients/parents should be advised to keep a written record of all immunizations or immune sera used. Booster doses for various vaccines may be needed to further stimulate antibody production.

CHECK YOUR UNDERSTANDING

Answers to the questions in this chapter can be found in Answers to Check Your Understanding Questions on thePoint®.

MULTIPLE CHOICE

Select the best answer to the following.

1. When preparing a presentation for a local parent group about vaccines the nurse would describe vaccines as being used to stimulate
   a. passive immunity to a foreign protein.
   b. active immunity to a foreign protein.
   c. serum sickness.
   d. a mild disease in healthy people.

2. After teaching a parent about common adverse effects associated with routine immunizations, which of the following, if stated by the parent, would indicate the need for additional teaching?
   a. Difficulty breathing and fainting
   b. Fever and rash
   c. Drowsiness and fretfulness
   d. Swelling and nodule formation at the site of injection

3. Which vaccine would the nurse be least likely to recommend for a 6-month-old child?
   a. Diphtheria, tetanus, pertussis vaccine
   b. *Haemophilus influenzae* b vaccine
   c. Poliovirus vaccine
   d. Chickenpox vaccine

4. It is now recommended that all people over the age of 6 months should receive a flu vaccine every fall based on the understanding that the vaccine is repeated because
   a. the immunity wears off after a year.
   b. the strains of virus predicted to cause the flu change every year.
   c. a booster shot will activate the immune system.
   d. flu shots do not produce good antibodies.

5. The nurse reviews a patient's record to make sure that tetanus booster shots have been given
   a. only with exposure to anaerobic bacteria.
   b. every 2 years.
   c. every 5 years.
   d. every 10 years.

6. A nurse suffers a needlestick after injecting a patient with suspected hepatitis B. The nurse should
   a. have repeated titers to determine whether she was exposed to hepatitis B and if she was have hepatitis immune globulin.
   b. immediately receive hepatitis immune globulin and begin hepatitis B vaccines if she has not already received them.
   c. start antibiotic therapy immediately.
   d. go on sick leave until all screening tests are negative.

7. A patient is to receive immune globulin after exposure to hepatitis A. The patient has a previous history of allergies to various drugs. Before giving the immune globulin the nurse should
   a. have emergency equipment readily available.
   b. premedicate the patient with aspirin.
   c. make sure all of the patient's vaccinations are up to date.
   d. make sure the patient has a ride home.

MULTIPLE RESPONSE

Select all that apply.

1. A public education campaign to stress the importance of childhood immunizations should include which of the following points?
   a. Prevention of potentially devastating diseases outweighs the discomfort and risks of immunization.
   b. Routine immunization is standard practice in the United States.
   c. The practice of routine immunizations has virtually wiped out many previously deadly or debilitating diseases.
   d. The risk of severe adverse reactions is on the rise and is not being addressed.
   e. If there is a family history of autism, that person should avoid immunizations.
   f. The temporary discomfort associated with the immunization can be treated with over-the-counter drugs.

2. A mother brings her child to his 18-month well-baby visit. The nurse would not give the child his routine immunizations in which of the following situations?
   a. He cried at his last immunization.
   b. He developed a fever or rash after his last immunization.
   c. He currently has a fever and symptoms of a cold.
   d. He is allergic to aspirin.
   e. He is currently taking oral corticosteroids.
   f. His siblings are all currently being treated for a viral infection.

3. When assessing the medical record of an older adult to evaluate the status of his immunizations the nurse would be looking for evidence of which of the following?
   a. Yearly pneumococcal vaccination
   b. Yearly flu vaccination
   c. Tetanus booster every 10 years
   d. Tetanus booster every 5 years
   e. Measles, mumps, rubella vaccine if the patient was born after 1957
   f. Varicella vaccine only if there is evidence that the patient had chickenpox as a child

BIBLIOGRAPHY AND REFERENCES

American Medical Association. (2015). *AMA drug evaluations.* Chicago, IL: Author.

Brunton, L., Chabner, B., & Knollman, B. (2011). *Goodman and Gilman's the pharmacological basis of therapeutics* (12th ed.). New York: McGraw-Hill.

Charo, R. (2007). Politics, parents and prophylaxis: Mandating HPV vaccinations. *New England Journal of Medicine, 356*, 1905–1908.

Cohn, A. C., MacNeil, J. R., Clark, T. A., et al. (2013). Prevention and control of meningococcal disease: Recommendations of the advisory committee on immunization practices. *Morbidity and Mortality Weekly Report, 62*(RRO2), 1–22.

Dunne, E., & Markowitz, L. (2014). Reducing the burden of HPV-associated cancer and disease CDC grand rounds [*Centers for Disease Control and Prevention*]. Available online at: http://www.cdc.gov/mmwr/preview/mmwrhtml/mm6304a1.htm

Facts and Comparisons. (2015). *Drug facts and comparisons.* St. Louis, MO: Author.

Guilano, A. R., Palesky, J. M., Goldstone, S., et al. (2011). Efficacy of quadrivalent HPV vaccine against HPV infection and disease in males. *New England Journal of Medicine, 364*, 401–411.

Immunization Safety Review Committee. (2004). *Immunization safety review: Vaccines and autism.* Washington, DC: National Academies Press.

Karch, A. M. (2014). *Lippincott's nursing drug guide.* Philadelphia, PA: Lippincott Williams & Wilkins.

Katz, S. L. (2005). A vaccine-preventable infectious disease kills half a million children a year. *Journal of Infectious Diseases, 192*, 1679–1680.

Porth, C. M. (2013). *Pathophysiology: Concepts of altered health states* (9th ed.). Philadelphia, PA: Lippincott Williams & Wilkins.

The Medical Letter. (2015). *Medical letter on drugs and therapeutics.* New Rochelle, NY: Author.

PART 4

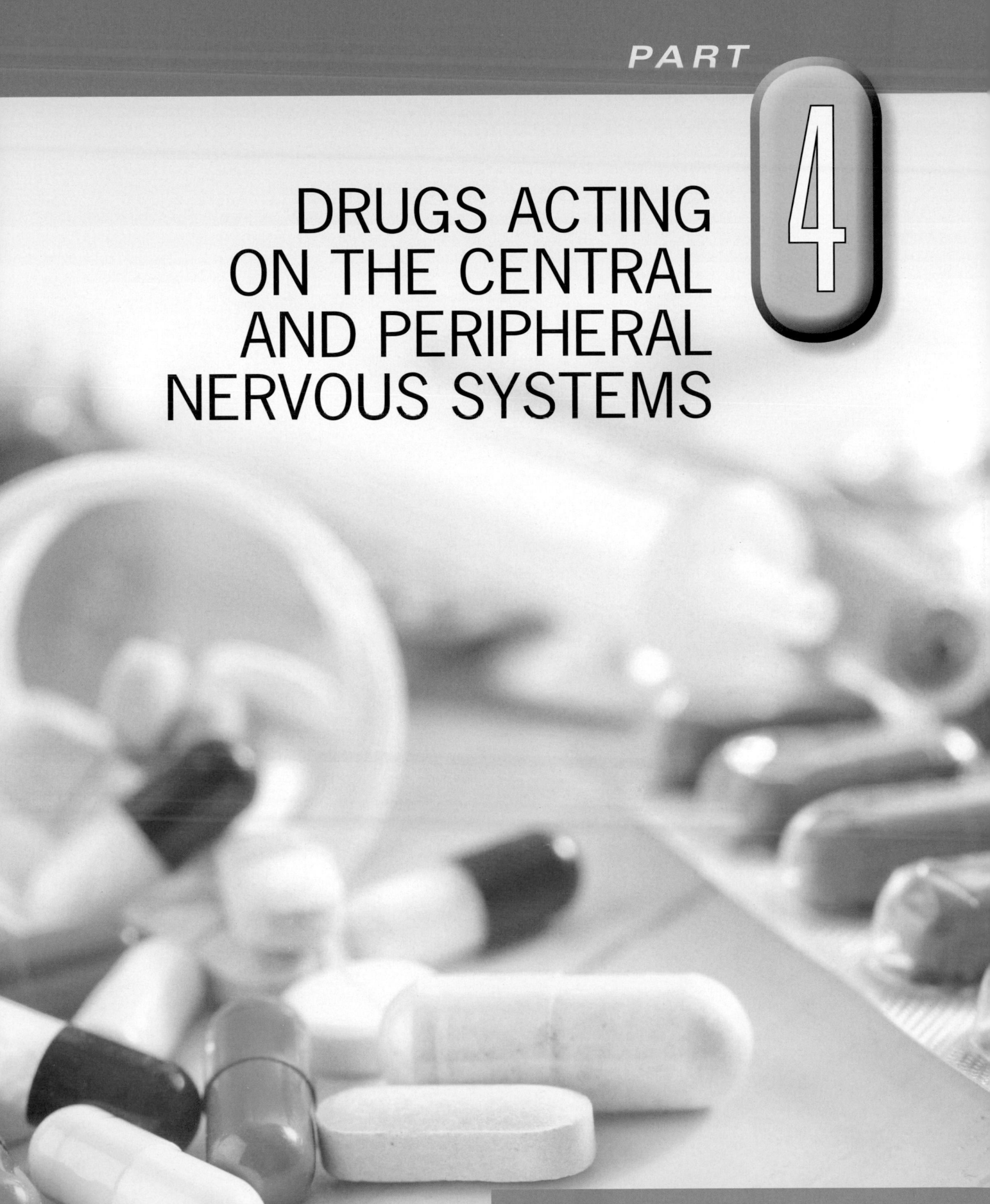

DRUGS ACTING ON THE CENTRAL AND PERIPHERAL NERVOUS SYSTEMS

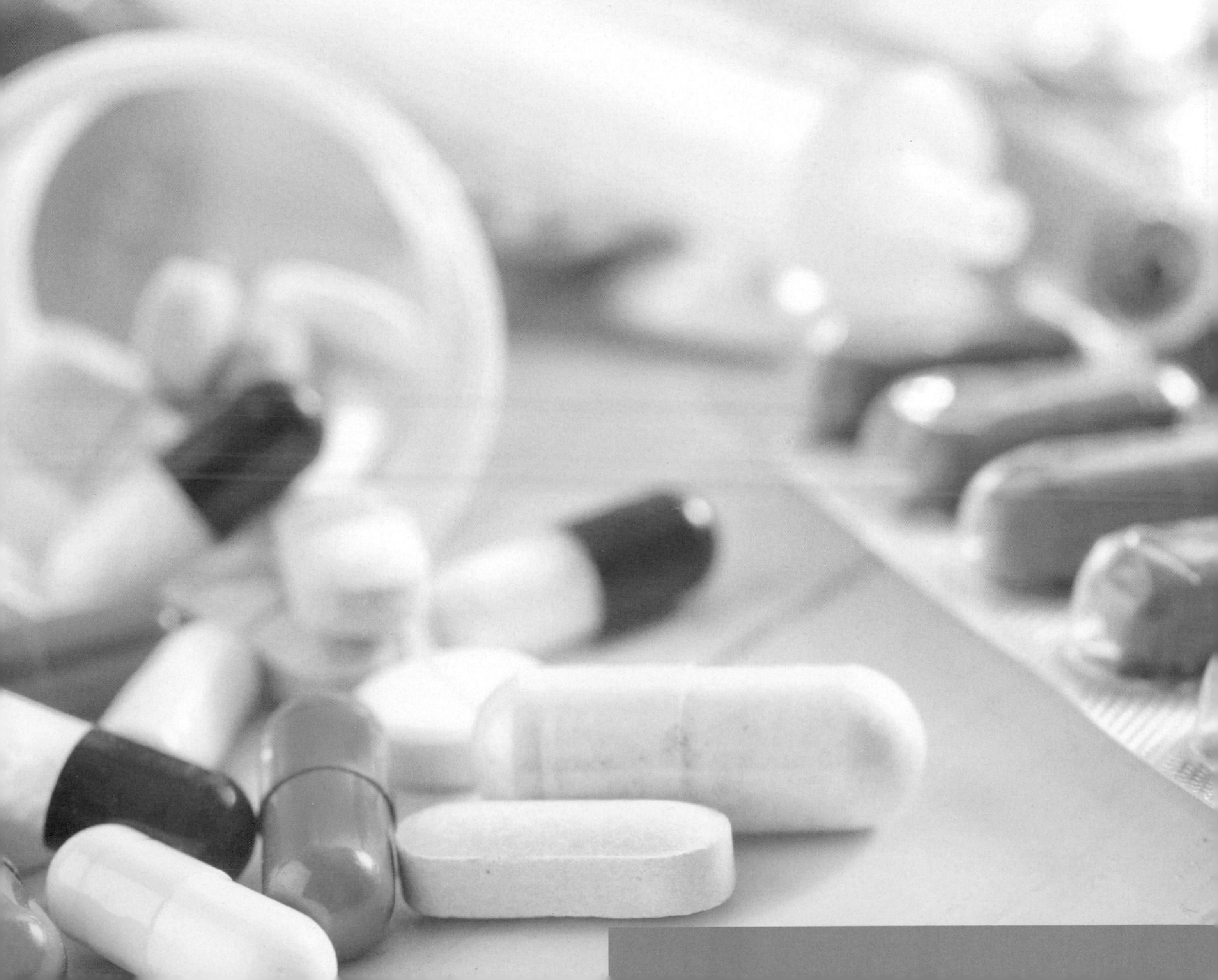

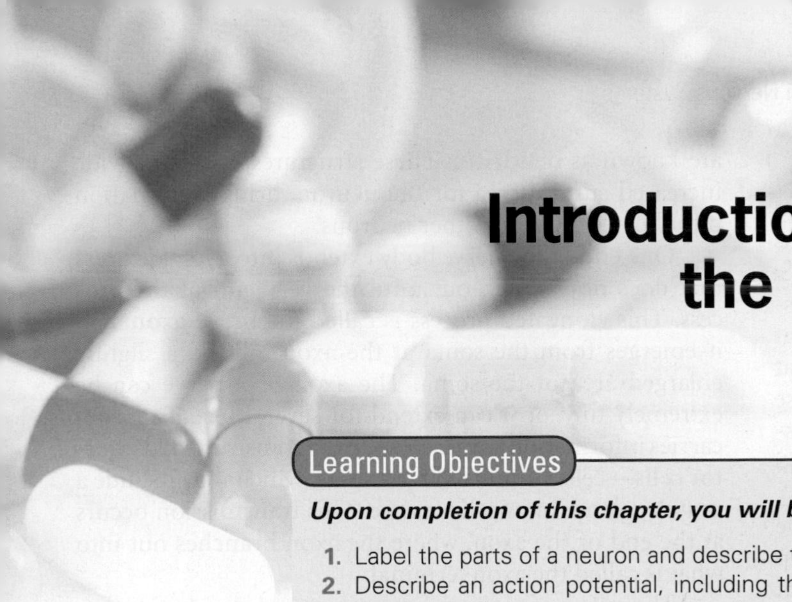

19 Introduction to Nerves and the Nervous System

Learning Objectives

Upon completion of this chapter, you will be able to:

1. Label the parts of a neuron and describe the functions of each part.
2. Describe an action potential, including the roles of the various electrolytes involved in the action potential.
3. Explain what a neurotransmitter is, including its origins and functions at the synapse.
4. Describe the function of the cerebral cortex, cerebellum, hypothalamus, thalamus, midbrain, pituitary gland, medulla, spinal cord, and reticular activating system.
5. Discuss what is known about learning and the impact of emotion on the learning process.

Glossary of Key Terms

action potential: sudden change in electrical charge of a nerve cell membrane; the electrical signal by which neurons send information

afferent: neurons or groups of neurons that bring information to the central nervous system; sensory nerve

axon: long projection from a neuron that carries information from one nerve to another nerve or effector

dendrite: short projection on a neuron that transmits information

depolarization: opening of the sodium channels in a nerve membrane to allow the influx of positive sodium ions, reversing the membrane charge so it is no longer polarized

effector cell: cell stimulated by a nerve; may be a muscle, a gland, or another nerve cell

efferent: neurons or groups of neurons that carry information from the central nervous system to an effector; motor neurons are efferent

engram: short-term memory made up of a reverberating electrical circuit of action potentials

forebrain: upper level of the brain; consists of the two cerebral hemispheres, where thinking and coordination of sensory and motor activity occur

ganglia: a group of nerve bodies

hindbrain: most primitive area of the brain, the brainstem; consists of the pons and medulla, which control basic, vital functions and arousal, and the cerebellum, which controls motor functions that regulate balance

limbic system: area in the midbrain that is rich in epinephrine, norepinephrine, and serotonin and seems to control emotions

midbrain: the middle area of the brain; it consists of the hypothalamus and thalamus and includes the limbic system

neuron: structural unit of the nervous system

neurotransmitter: chemical produced by a nerve and released when the nerve is stimulated; reacts with a specific receptor site to cause a reaction

repolarization: return of a membrane to a resting state, with more sodium ions outside the membrane and a relatively negative charge inside the membrane

Schwann cell: insulating cell found on nerve axons; allows "leaping" electrical conduction to speed the transmission of information and prevent tiring of the neuron

soma: cell body of a neuron; contains the nucleus, cytoplasm, and various granules

synapse: junction between a nerve and an effector; consists of the presynaptic nerve ending, a space called the synaptic cleft, and the postsynaptic cell

The nervous system is responsible for controlling the functions of the human body, analyzing incoming stimuli, and integrating internal and external responses. The nervous system is composed of the central nervous system (CNS; the brain and spinal cord) and the peripheral nervous system (PNS). The PNS is composed of sensory receptors that bring information into the CNS and motor nerves that carry information away from the CNS to facilitate response to stimuli. The autonomic nervous system, which is discussed in Chapter 29, uses components of the CNS and PNS to regulate automatic or unconscious responses to stimuli.

The structural unit of the nervous system is the nerve cell, or **neuron**. The billions of nerve cells that make up the nervous system are organized to allow movement realization of various sensations, response to internal and external stimuli, and learning, thinking, and emotion. The mechanisms that are involved in all of these processes are not clearly understood. The actions of drugs that are used to affect the functioning of the nerves and the responses that these drugs cause throughout the nervous system provide some of the current theories about the workings of the nervous system.

Physiology of the Nervous System

The nervous system operates through the use of electrical impulses and chemical messengers to transmit information throughout the body and to respond to internal and external stimuli. The properties and functions of the neuron provide the basis for all nervous system functions.

Neurons

As noted previously, the neuron is the structural unit of the nervous system. The human body contains about 14 billion neurons. About 10 billion of these are located in the brain, and the remainder make up the spinal cord and PNS.

Neurons have several distinctive cellular features (Figure 19.1). Each neuron is made up of a cell body, or **soma**, which contains the cell nucleus, cytoplasm, and various granules and other particles. Short, branch-like projections that cover most of the surface of a neuron are known as **dendrites**. These structures, which provide increased surface area for the neuron, bring information into the neuron from other neurons.

One end of the nerve body extends into a long process that does not branch out until the very end of the process. This elongated process is called the nerve **axon**, and it emerges from the soma at the axon hillock, a slightly enlarged area of the soma. The axon of a nerve can be extremely tiny, or it can extend for several feet. The axon carries information from a nerve to be transmitted to **effector cells**—cells stimulated by a nerve, which may include a muscle, gland, or another nerve. This transmission occurs at the end of the axon, where the axon branches out into what is called the axon terminal.

The axons of many nerves are packed closely together in the nervous system and look like cable or fiber tracts. **Afferent** fibers are nerve axons that run from peripheral receptors into the CNS. In contrast, **efferent** fibers are nerve axons that carry nerve impulses from the CNS to the periphery to stimulate muscles or glands. (An easy way to remember the difference between afferent and efferent is to recall that efferent fibers exit from the CNS.)

It is currently thought that neurons are unable to reproduce; so, if nerves are destroyed, they are lost. If dendrites and axons are lost, nerves regenerate those structures; however, for this regeneration to occur, the soma and the axon hillock must remain intact. For a clinical example, consider a person who has closed a car door on his or her finger. Sensation and movement may be lost or limited for a certain period, but because the nerve bodies for most of the nerves in the hand are located in **ganglia** (groups of nerve bodies) in the wrist, they are able to regenerate the damaged axon or dendrites. Over time, sensation and full movement should return.

Research on possible ways to stimulate the reproduction of nerves is under way. Although scientists have used nerve growth factor with fetal cell implants to stimulate some nerve growth, it is currently assumed that nerves in normal situations are unable to reproduce.

Action Potential

Nerves send messages by conducting electrical impulses called **action potentials**.

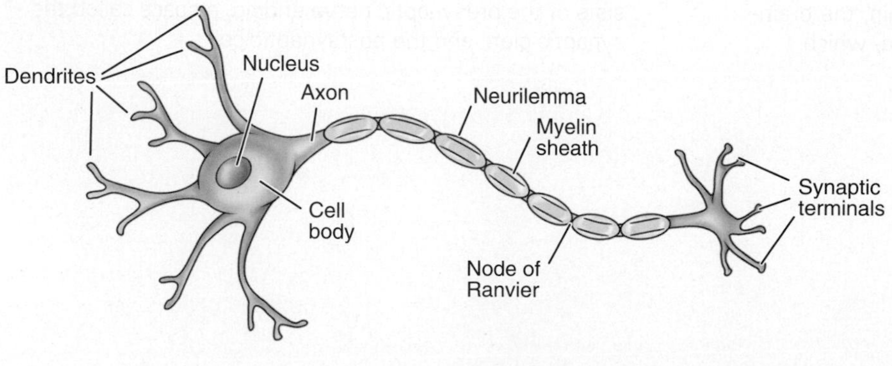

FIGURE 19.1 The neuron, functional unit of the nervous system.

Nerve membranes, which are capable of conducting action potentials along the entire membrane, send messages to nearby neurons or to effector cells that may be located inches to feet away via this electrical communication system. Like all cell membranes, nerve membranes have various channels or pores that control the movement of substances into and out of the cell. Some of these channels allow the movement of sodium, potassium, and calcium. When cells are at rest, their membranes are impermeable to sodium. However, the membranes are permeable to potassium ions.

The sodium–potassium pump that is active in the membranes of neurons is responsible for this property of the membrane. This system pumps sodium ions out of the cell and potassium ions into the cell. At rest, more sodium ions are outside the cell membrane, and more potassium ions are inside. Electrically, the inside of the cell is relatively negative compared with the outside of the membrane, which establishes an electrical potential along the nerve membrane. This membrane is polarized, the positive pole outside the membrane and the negative pole inside the membrane. When nerves are at rest, this is referred to as the resting membrane potential of the nerve.

Stimulation of a neuron causes **depolarization** of the nerve, which means that the sodium channels open in response to the stimulus, and sodium ions rush into the cell, following the established concentration gradient. If an electrical monitoring device is attached to the nerve at this point a positive rush of ions is recorded. The electrical charge on the inside of the membrane changes from relatively negative to relatively positive. The cell has become depolarized, losing the positive and negative poles. This sudden reversal of membrane potential, called the action potential (Figure 19.2), lasts less than a microsecond. Using the sodium–potassium pump the cell then returns that section of membrane to the resting membrane potential, a process called **repolarization**. The action potential generated at one point along a nerve membrane stimulates the generation of an action potential in adjacent portions of the cell membrane, and the stimulus travels the length of the cell membrane.

Nerves can respond to stimuli several hundred times per second, but for a given stimulus to cause an action potential it must have sufficient strength and must occur when the nerve membrane is able to respond—that is, when it has repolarized. A nerve cannot be stimulated again while it is depolarized. The balance of sodium and potassium across the cell membrane must be reestablished.

Nerves require energy (i.e., oxygen and glucose) and the correct balance of the electrolytes sodium and potassium to maintain normal action potentials and transmit information into and out of the nervous system. If an individual has anoxia or hypoglycemia the nerves might not be able to maintain the sodium–potassium pump, and that individual may become severely irritable or too stable (not responsive to stimuli).

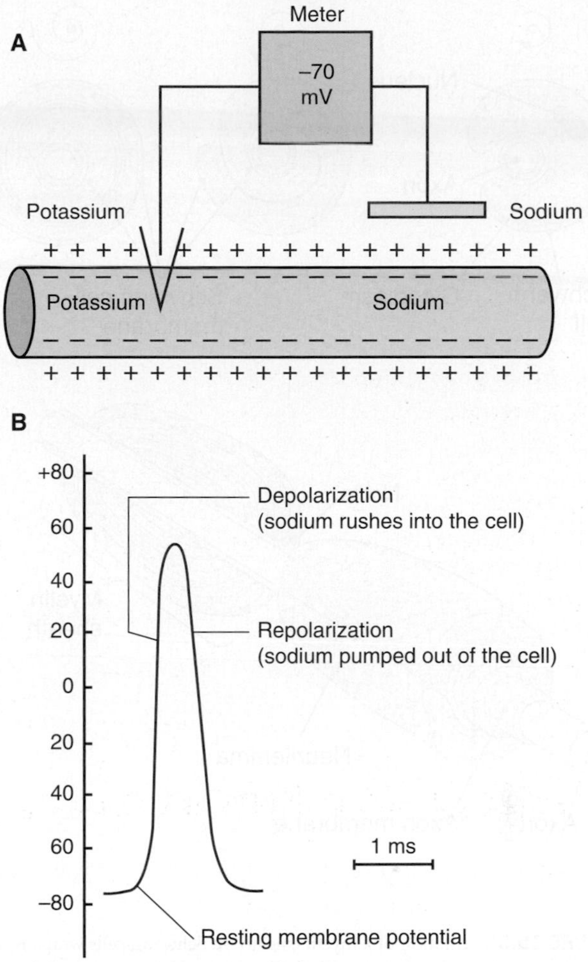

FIGURE 19.2 The action potential. **A.** Segment of an axon showing that, at rest, the inside of the membrane is relatively negatively charged and the outside is positively charged. A pair of electrodes placed as shown would record a potential difference of about –70 mV; this is the resting membrane potential. **B.** An action potential of about 1 ms that would be recorded if the axon shown in panel (A) were brought to threshold. At the peak of the action potential the charge on the membrane reverses polarity.

Long nerves are myelinated: They have a myelin sheath that speeds electrical conduction and protects the nerves from the fatigue that results from frequent formation of action potentials. Even though many of the tightly packed nerves in the brain do not need to travel far to stimulate another nerve, some of them are myelinated. The effect of this myelination is not understood.

Myelinated nerves have **Schwann cells**, located at specific intervals along nerve axons, that are very resistant to electrical stimulation (Figure 19.1). The Schwann cells wrap themselves around the axon in jelly roll fashion (Figure 19.3). Between the Schwann cells are areas of uncovered nerve membrane called the nodes of Ranvier. So-called "leaping" nerve conduction occurs along these exposed nerve fibers. An action potential excites one section of the nerve membrane, and the electrical impulse then "skips" from one node to the next, generating an action potential. Because the membrane is forming fewer

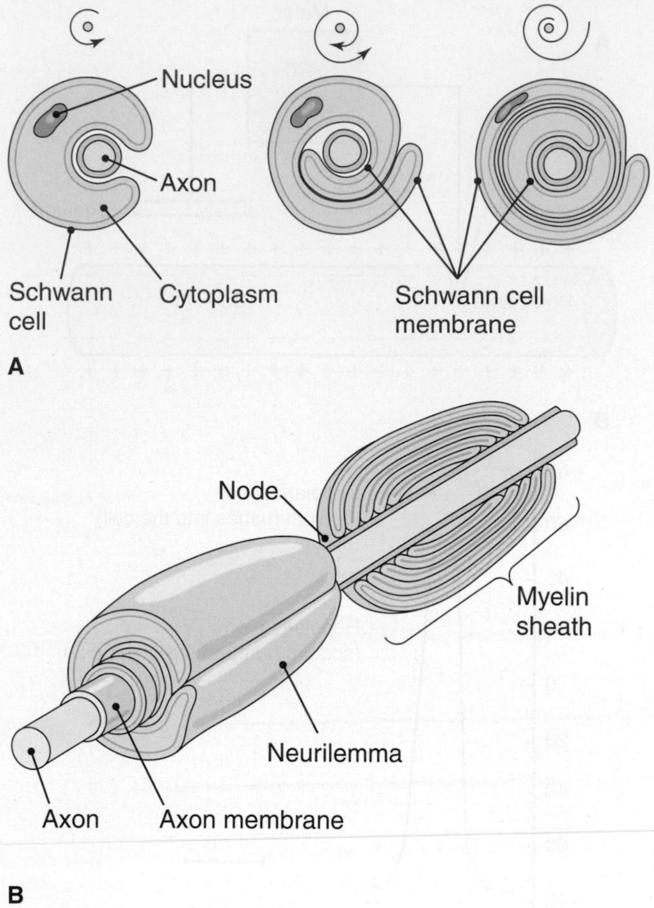

FIGURE 19.3 Formation of a myelin sheath. **A.** Schwann cells wrap around the axon, creating a myelin coating. **B.** The outermost layer of the Schwann cell forms the neurilemma. Spaces between the cells are the nodes of Ranvier.

action potentials the speed of conduction is much faster, and the nerve is protected from being exhausted or using up energy to form multiple action potentials. This node-to-node mode of conduction is termed *saltatory* or leaping *conduction* (Figure 19.1).

If the Schwann cells become enlarged or swollen and block the nodes of Ranvier, which is what occurs in the neuromuscular disease multiple sclerosis, conduction does not occur because the electrical impulse has a limited firing range. A stimulus may simply be "lost" along the nerve. Believed to be an autoimmune disorder that attacks Schwann cells and leads to swelling and scarring of these cells, multiple sclerosis is characterized by a progressive loss of nerve response and muscle function.

Nerve Synapse

When the electrical action potential reaches the end of an axon the electrical impulse comes to a halt. At this point the stimulus no longer travels at the speed of electricity. The transmission of information between two nerves or between a nerve and a gland or muscle is chemical. Nerves communicate with other nerves or effectors at the nerve **synapse** (Figure 19.4). The synapse is made up of a presynaptic nerve, the synaptic cleft, and the postsynaptic effector cell. The nerve axon, called the presynaptic nerve, releases a chemical called a **neurotransmitter** into the synaptic cleft, and the neurotransmitter reacts with a very specific receptor site on the postsynaptic cell to cause a reaction.

Neurotransmitters

Neurotransmitters stimulate postsynaptic cells either by exciting or by inhibiting them. The reaction that occurs when a neurotransmitter stimulates a receptor site depends on the specific neurotransmitter that it releases and the receptor site it activates. A nerve may produce only one type of neurotransmitter, using building blocks such as tyrosine or choline from the extracellular fluid, often absorbed from dietary sources. The neurotransmitter, packaged into vesicles, moves to the terminal membrane of the axon, and when the nerve is stimulated the vesicles contract and push the neurotransmitter into the synaptic cleft. The calcium channels in the nerve membrane are open during the action potential, and the presence of calcium causes the contraction. When the cell repolarizes, calcium leaves the cell, and the contraction stops. Once released into the synaptic cleft the neurotransmitter reacts with very specific receptor sites to cause a reaction.

To return the effector cell to a resting state so that it can be stimulated again, if needed, neurotransmitters must be inactivated. Neurotransmitters may be either reabsorbed by the presynaptic nerve in a process called reuptake (a recycling effort by the nerve to reuse the materials and save resources) or broken down by enzymes in the area (e.g., monoamine oxidase breaks down the catecholamine neurotransmitters; the enzyme acetylcholinesterase breaks down the neurotransmitter acetylcholine). Several neurotransmitters have been identified. As research continues, other neurotransmitters may be discovered, and the actions of known neurotransmitters will be better understood.

The following are selected neurotransmitters:

- *Acetylcholine*, which communicates between nerves and muscles, is also important as the preganglionic neurotransmitter throughout the autonomic nervous system and as the postganglionic neurotransmitter in the parasympathetic nervous system and in several pathways in the brain.
- *Norepinephrine* and *epinephrine* are catecholamines, which are released by nerves in the sympathetic branch of the autonomic nervous system and are classified as hormones when they are released from cells in the adrenal medulla. These neurotransmitters also occur in high levels in particular areas of the brain, such as the limbic system.
- *Dopamine*, which is found in high concentrations in certain areas of the brain, is involved in the coordination of impulses and responses, both motor and intellectual.

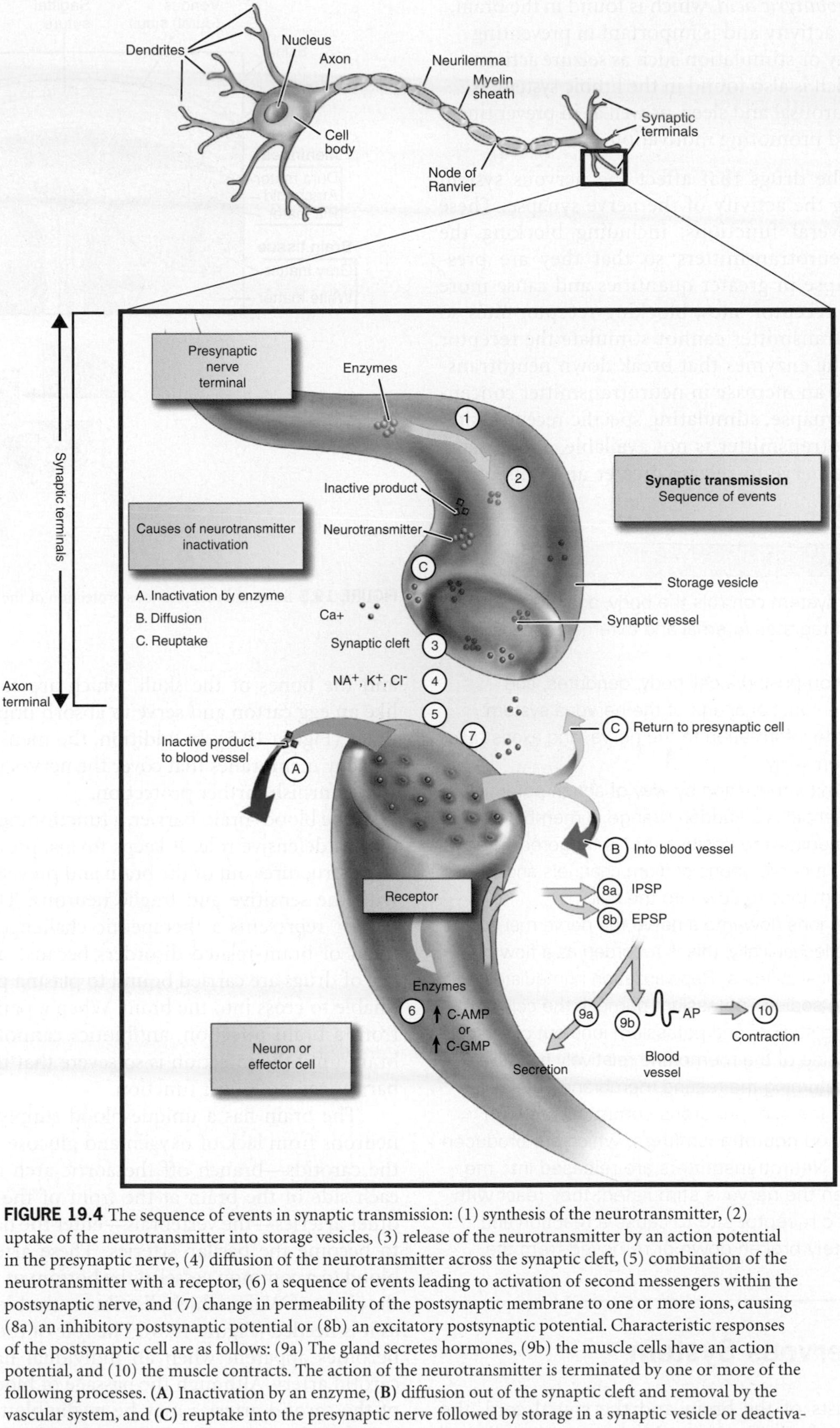

FIGURE 19.4 The sequence of events in synaptic transmission: (1) synthesis of the neurotransmitter, (2) uptake of the neurotransmitter into storage vesicles, (3) release of the neurotransmitter by an action potential in the presynaptic nerve, (4) diffusion of the neurotransmitter across the synaptic cleft, (5) combination of the neurotransmitter with a receptor, (6) a sequence of events leading to activation of second messengers within the postsynaptic nerve, and (7) change in permeability of the postsynaptic membrane to one or more ions, causing (8a) an inhibitory postsynaptic potential or (8b) an excitatory postsynaptic potential. Characteristic responses of the postsynaptic cell are as follows: (9a) The gland secretes hormones, (9b) the muscle cells have an action potential, and (10) the muscle contracts. The action of the neurotransmitter is terminated by one or more of the following processes. **(A)** Inactivation by an enzyme, **(B)** diffusion out of the synaptic cleft and removal by the vascular system, and **(C)** reuptake into the presynaptic nerve followed by storage in a synaptic vesicle or deactivation by an enzyme.

- *Gamma-aminobutyric acid*, which is found in the brain, inhibits nerve activity and is important in preventing overexcitability or stimulation such as seizure activity.
- *Serotonin*, which is also found in the limbic system, is important in arousal and sleep, as well as in preventing depression and promoting motivation.

Many of the drugs that affect the nervous system involve altering the activity of the nerve synapse. These drugs have several functions, including blocking the reuptake of neurotransmitters so that they are present in the synapse in greater quantities and cause more stimulation of receptor sites, blocking receptor sites so that the neurotransmitter cannot stimulate the receptor site, blocking the enzymes that break down neurotransmitters to cause an increase in neurotransmitter concentration in the synapse, stimulating specific receptor sites when the neurotransmitter is not available, and causing the presynaptic nerve to release greater amounts of the neurotransmitter.

KEY POINTS

- The nervous system controls the body, analyzes external stimuli, and integrates internal and external responses to stimuli.
- The neuron, comprising a cell body, dendrites, and an axon, is the functional unit of the nervous system. Dendrites route information to the nerve, and axons take the information away.
- Nerves transmit information by way of action potentials. An action potential is a sudden change in membrane charge from negative to positive that is triggered when stimulation of a nerve opens sodium channels and allows positive sodium ions to flow into the cell.
- When sodium ions flow into a nerve the nerve membrane depolarizes. Mechanically, this is recorded as a flow of positive electrical charges. Repolarization immediately follows, with the sodium–potassium pump in the cell membrane pumping sodium and potassium ions out of the cell, leaving the inside of the membrane relatively negative to the outside, returning the resting membrane potential.
- At the end of the axon, neurons communicate with chemicals called neurotransmitters, which are produced by the nerve. Neurotransmitters are released into the synapse when the nerve is stimulated; they react with a very specific receptor site to cause a reaction and are immediately broken down or removed from the synapse.

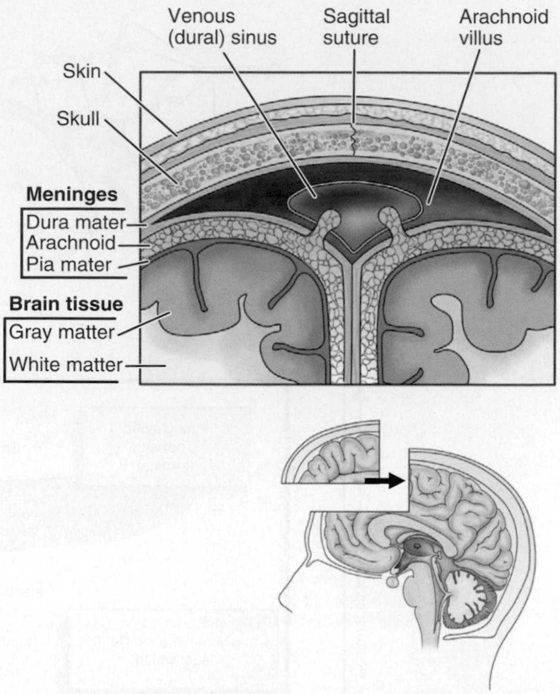

FIGURE 19.5 Bony and membranous protection of the brain.

Central Nervous System

The CNS consists of the brain and the spinal cord, the two parts of the body that contain the vast majority of nerves. The bones of the vertebrae protect the spinal cord, and the bones of the skull, which are corrugated much like an egg carton and serve to absorb impact, protect the brain (Figure 19.5). In addition, the meninges, which are stretchy membranes that cover the nerves in the brain and spine, furnish further protection.

The blood–brain barrier, a functioning boundary, also plays a defensive role. It keeps toxins, proteins, and other large structures out of the brain and prevents their contact with the sensitive and fragile neurons. The blood–brain barrier represents a therapeutic challenge to drug treatment of brain-related disorders because a large percentage of drugs are carried bound to plasma proteins and are unable to cross into the brain. When a patient is suffering from a brain infection, antibiotics cannot cross into the brain until the infection is so severe that the blood–brain barrier can no longer function.

The brain has a unique blood supply to protect the neurons from lack of oxygen and glucose. Two arteries—the carotids—branch off the aortic arch and go up into each side of the brain at the front of the head, and two other arteries—the vertebrals—enter the back of the brain to become the basilar arteries. These arteries all deliver blood to a common vessel at the bottom of the brain called the circle of Willis, which distributes the blood to the brain as it is needed (Figure 19.6). The role of the circle of Willis becomes apparent when an individual has an occluded carotid artery. Although the passage of blood through one of the carotid arteries may be negligible the areas of the brain on that side will still have a full blood supply because of the blood sent to those areas via the circle of Willis.

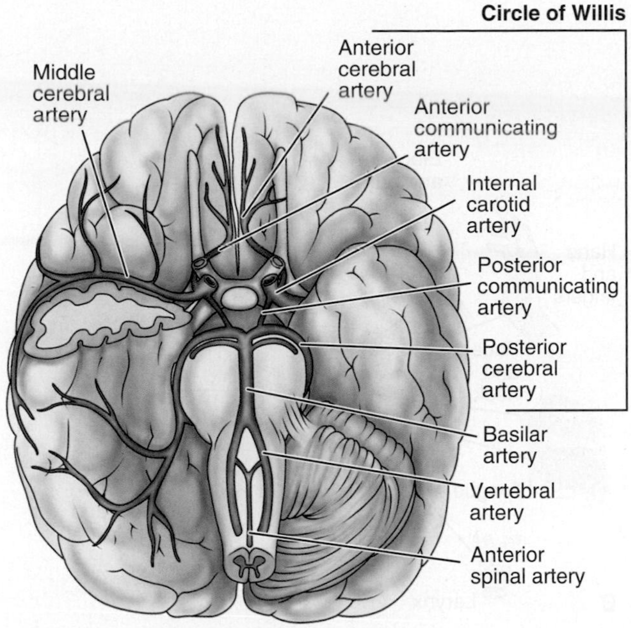

FIGURE 19.6 The protective blood supply of the brain: the carotid, vertebral, and basilar arteries join to form the circle of Willis.

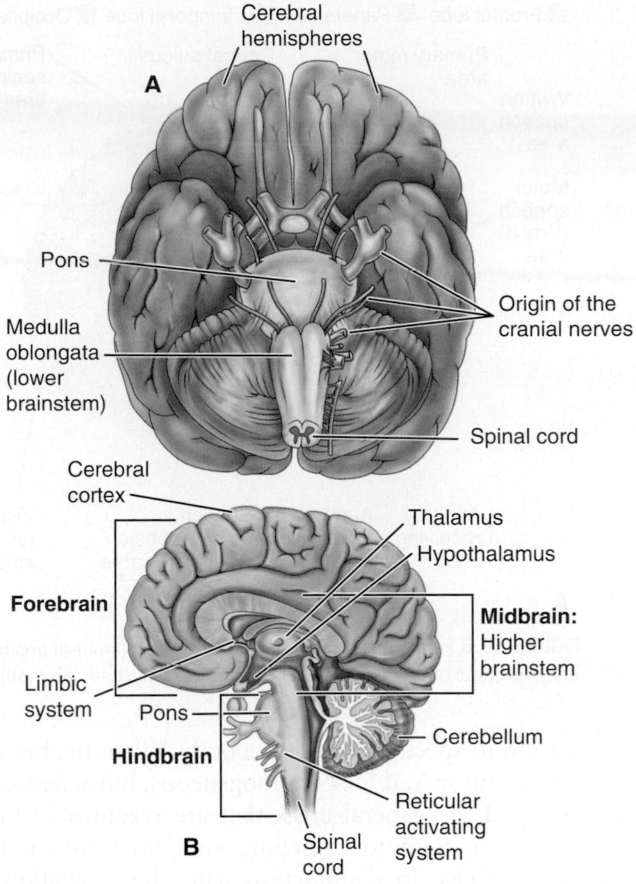

FIGURE 19.7 Anatomy of the brain. **A.** A view of the underside of the brain. **B.** The medial or midsagittal view of the brain.

Anatomy of the Brain

The brain has three major divisions: the hindbrain, the midbrain, and the forebrain (Figure 19.7).

The **hindbrain**, which runs from the top of the spinal cord into the midbrain, is the most primitive area of the brain and contains the brainstem, where the pons and medulla oblongata are located. These areas of the brain control basic, vital functions, such as the respiratory centers, which control breathing; the cardiovascular centers, which regulate blood pressure; the chemoreceptor trigger zone and emetic zone, which control vomiting; the swallowing center, which coordinates the complex swallowing reflex; and the reticular activating system (RAS), which controls arousal and awareness of stimuli and contains the sleep center. The RAS filters the billions of incoming messages, selecting only the most significant for response. When levels of serotonin become high in the RAS, the system shuts down and sleep occurs. The medulla absorbs serotonin from the RAS; when the levels are low enough, consciousness or arousal results.

The cranial nerves (see Figure 19.7), which also emerge from the hindbrain, involve *specific* senses (sight, smell, hearing, balance, taste) and some muscle activity of the head and neck (e.g., chewing, eye movement). The cerebellum—a part of the brain that looks like a skein of yarn and lies behind the other parts of the hindbrain—coordinates the motor function that regulates posture, balance, and voluntary muscle activity.

The **midbrain** contains the thalamus, the hypothalamus, and the limbic system (see Figure 19.7). The thalamus sends direct information into the cerebrum to transfer sensations, such as cold, heat, pain, touch, and muscle sense. The hypothalamus, which is poorly protected by the blood–brain barrier, acts as a major sensor for activities in the body. Areas of the hypothalamus are responsible for temperature control, water balance, appetite, and fluid balance. In addition, the hypothalamus plays a central role in the endocrine system and in the autonomic nervous system.

The **limbic system** is an area of the brain that contains high levels of three neurotransmitters: epinephrine, norepinephrine, and serotonin. Stimulation of this area, which appears to be responsible for the expression of emotions, may lead to anger, pleasure, motivation, stress, and so on. This part of the brain seems to be largely responsible for the "human" aspect of brain function. Drug therapy aimed at alleviating emotional disorders such as depression and anxiety often involves attempting to alter the levels of epinephrine, norepinephrine, and serotonin.

The **forebrain** is made up of two cerebral hemispheres joined together by an area called the corpus callosum. These two hemispheres contain the sensory neurons, which receive nerve impulses, and the motor neurons, which send them. They also contain areas that coordinate speech and communication and seem to be the area where learning takes place (see Figure 19.7). Different areas of the brain appear to be responsible for receiving and sending

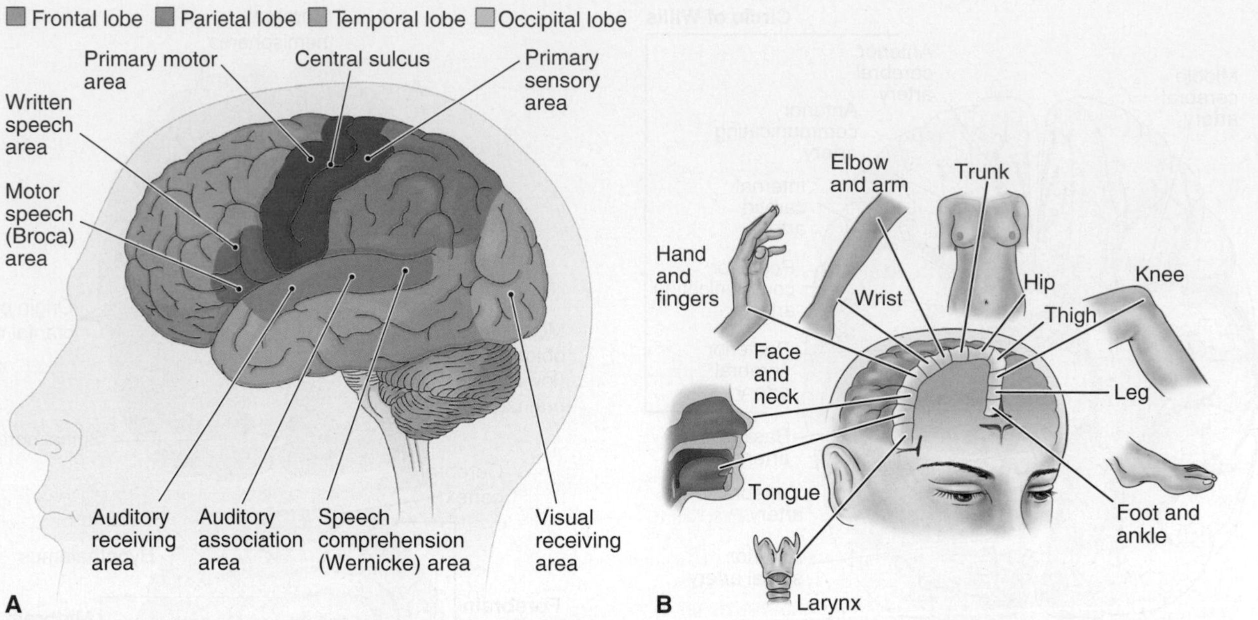

FIGURE 19.8 Functional areas of the brain. **A.** Topographical organization of functions of control and interpretation in the cerebral cortex. **B.** Areas of the brain that control specific areas of the body. Size indicates relative distribution of control.

information to specific areas of the body. When the brain is viewed at autopsy, it looks homogeneous, but scientists have mapped the general areas that are responsible for sensory response, motor function, and other functions (see Figure 19.8). In conjunction with the cerebellum, groups of ganglia or nerve cell bodies called the basal ganglia, located at the bottom of the brain, make up the extrapyramidal motor system. This system coordinates motor activity for unconscious activities such as posture and gait.

Anatomy of the Spinal Cord

The spinal cord is made up of 31 pairs of spinal nerves. Each spinal nerve has two components or roots. These mixed nerve parts include a sensory fiber (called the dorsal root) and a motor fiber (called the ventral root). The spinal sensory fibers bring information into the CNS from the periphery. The motor fibers carry information away from the brain and cause movement or reaction.

Functions of the Central Nervous System

The brain is responsible for coordinating reactions to the constantly changing external and internal environment. In all animals the function of this organ is essentially the same. The human component involving emotions, learning, and conscious response takes the human nervous system beyond a simple reflex system and complicates the responses seen to any stimulus.

Sensory Functions

Millions of sensory impulses are constantly streaming into the CNS from peripheral receptors. Many of these impulses go directly to specific areas of the brain designated to deal with input from particular areas of the body or from the senses. The responses that occur as a result of these stimuli can be altered by efferent neurons that respond to emotions through the limbic system, to learned responses stored in the cerebral cortex, or to autonomic input mediated through the hypothalamus.

The intricacies of the human brain can change the response to a sensation depending on the situation. People may react differently to the same stimulus. For example, if an individual drops a can on his or her foot, the physiological response is one of pain and a stimulation of the sympathetic branch of the autonomic nervous system. If the person is alone or in a very comfortable environment (e.g., fixing dinner at home), he or she may scream, swear, or jump around. However, if that person is in the company of other people (e.g., a cooking teacher working with a class), he or she may be much more dignified and quiet, even though the physiological effect on the body is the same.

Motor Functions

The sensory nerves that enter the brain react with related motor nerves to cause a reaction mediated by muscles or glands. The motor impulses that leave the cortex are further regulated or coordinated by the pyramidal system, which coordinates voluntary movement, and the extrapyramidal system, which coordinates unconscious motor activity that regulates control of position and posture. For example, some drugs may interfere with the extrapyramidal system and cause tremors, shuffling gait, and lack of posture and position stability. Motor fibers from the cortex cross to the other side of the spinal cord before emerging to interact with peripheral effectors. In this way, motor stimuli coming from the right side of the brain affect motor activity on the left side of the body. For example, an area of the left cortex may send an impulse down to the spinal cord that reacts with an interneuron, crosses to the other side of the spinal cord, and causes a finger on the right hand to twitch.

Intellectual and Emotional Functions

The way that the cerebral cortex uses sensory information is not clearly understood, but research has demonstrated that the two hemispheres of the brain process information in different ways. The right side of the brain is the more artistic side, concerned with forms and shapes, and the left side is more analytical, concerned with names, numbers, and processes. Why the two hemispheres are different and how they develop differently is not known.

When learning takes place, distinct layers of the cerebral cortex are affected, and an actual membrane change occurs in a neuron to store information in the brain permanently. Learning begins as an electrical circuit called an **engram**, a reverberating circuit of action potentials that eventually becomes a long-term, permanent memory in the presence of the proper neurotransmitters and hormones. Scientists do not understand exactly how this happens, but it is known that the nerve requires oxygen, glucose, and sleep to process an engram into a permanent memory, and during that processing, structural changes occur to the cells involved in the engram. This reverberating circuit is responsible for short-term memory. When patients have a decreased blood supply to the brain, short-term memory may be lost, and they are not able to remember new things. This happens because the engram requires a constant supply of oxygen and glucose to maintain that electrical circuit and if it cannot be maintained it is lost. Because they are unable to remember new things the brain falls back on long-term, permanent memory for daily functioning. For example, a patient may be introduced to a nurse and have no recollection of the nurse 2 hours later and yet be able to recall the events of several years ago vividly.

Several substances appear to affect learning. Antidiuretic hormone, which is released during reactions to stress, is one such substance. Although too much stress prevents learning, feeling slightly stressed may increase a person's ability to learn. A patient who is a little nervous about upcoming surgery, for example, seems to display a better mastery of facts about the surgery and postoperative procedures than a patient who is very stressed and scared or one who appears to show no interest or concern. Oxytocin is another substance that seems to increase actual learning. Because childbirth is the only known time that oxytocin levels increase the significance of this is not understood. Nurses who work with maternity patients should know that women in labor will very likely remember the smallest details about the whole experience and should use whatever opportunity is made available to do teaching.

In addition, the limbic system appears to play an important role in how a person learns and reacts to stimuli. The emotions associated with a memory as well as with the present have an impact on stimulus response. The placebo effect is a documented effect of the mind on drug therapy. If a person perceives that a drug will be effective, it is much more likely to actually be effective. This effect, which uses the actions of the cerebrum and the limbic system, can have a tremendous impact on drug response. Events that are perceived as stressful by some patients may be seen as positive by other patients.

KEY POINTS

- The CNS consists of the brain and spinal cord, which are protected by bone and meninges. To ensure blood flow to the brain if a vessel should become damaged the brain also has a protective blood supply moderated by the circle of Willis.
- The hindbrain, the most primitive area of the brain, contains the centers that control basic, vital functions. The pons, the medulla, and the RAS, which regulates arousal and awareness, are all located in the hindbrain. The cerebellum, which helps to coordinate motor activity, is found at the back of the hindbrain.
- The midbrain consists of the hypothalamus, the thalamus, and the limbic system. The limbic system is responsible for the expression of emotion, and the thalamus and hypothalamus coordinate internal and external responses and direct information into the cerebral cortex.
- The cerebral cortex consists of two hemispheres, which regulate the communication between sensory and motor neurons and are the sites of thinking and learning.

Clinical Significance of Drugs that Act on the Nervous System

The features of the human nervous system, including the complexities of the human brain, sometimes make it difficult to predict the exact reaction of a particular patient to a given drug. When a drug is used to affect the nervous system the occurrence of many systemic effects is always a possibility because the nervous system affects the entire body. The chapters in this part address the individual classes of drugs used to treat disorders of the nervous system, including their adverse effects. An understanding of the actions of specific drugs makes it easier to anticipate what therapeutic and adverse effects might occur. In addition, nurses should consider all of the learned, cultural, and emotional aspects of the patient's situation in an attempt to provide optimal therapeutic benefit and minimal adverse effects.

SUMMARY

- Although nerves do not reproduce, they can regenerate injured parts if the soma and axon hillock remain intact.
- Efferent nerves take information out of the CNS to effector sites; afferent nerves are sensory nerves that take information into the CNS.

- When the transmission of action potentials reaches the axon terminal, it causes the release of chemicals called neurotransmitters, which cross the synaptic cleft to stimulate an effector cell, which can be another nerve, a muscle, or a gland.
- A neurotransmitter must be produced by a nerve (each nerve can produce only one kind), it must be released into the synapse when the nerve is stimulated, it must react with a very specific receptor site to cause a reaction, and it must be immediately broken down or removed from the synapse so that the cell can be ready to be stimulated again.
- Much of the drug therapy in the nervous system involves receptor sites and the release or reuptake and breakdown of neurotransmitters.
- The CNS consists of the brain and spinal cord, which are protected by bone and meninges. To ensure blood flow to the brain if a vessel should become damaged the brain also has a protective blood supply moderated by the circle of Willis.
- The hindbrain, the most primitive area of the brain, contains the centers that control basic, vital functions. The pons, the medulla, and the RAS, which regulates arousal and awareness, are all located in the hindbrain. The cerebellum, which helps to coordinate motor activity, is found at the back of the hindbrain.
- The midbrain consists of the hypothalamus, the thalamus, and the limbic system. The limbic system is responsible for the expression of emotion, and the thalamus and hypothalamus coordinate internal and external responses and direct information into the cerebral cortex.
- The cerebral cortex consists of two hemispheres, which regulate the communication between sensory and motor neurons and are the sites of thinking and learning.
- The mechanisms of learning and processing learned information are not understood. Emotion-related factors influence the human brain, which handles stimuli and responses in complex ways.
- Much remains to be learned about the human brain and how drugs influence it. The actions of many drugs that have known effects on human behavior are not understood.

CHECK YOUR UNDERSTANDING

Answers to the questions in this chapter can be found in Answers to Check Your Understanding Questions on thePoint®.

MULTIPLE CHOICE

Select the best answer to the following.

1. The cerebellum
  a. initiates voluntary muscle movement.
  b. helps regulate the tone of skeletal muscles.
  c. if destroyed, would result in the loss of all voluntary skeletal activity.
  d. contains the centers responsible for the regulation of body temperature.

2. At those regions of the nerve membrane where myelin is present, there is
  a. low resistance to electrical current.
  b. high resistance to electrical current.
  c. high conductance of electrical current.
  d. energy loss for the cell.

3. The nerve synapse
  a. is not resistant to electrical current.
  b. cannot become exhausted.
  c. has a synaptic cleft.
  d. transfers information at the speed of electricity.

4. Which of the following could result in the initiation of an action potential?
  a. Depolarizing the membrane
  b. Decreasing the extracellular potassium concentration
  c. Increasing the activity of the sodium–potassium active transport system
  d. Stimulating the nerve with a threshold electrical stimulus during the absolute refractory period of the membrane

5. Neurotransmitters are
  a. produced in the muscle to communicate with nerves.
  b. the chemicals used to stimulate or suppress effectors at the nerve synapse.
  c. usually found in the diet.
  d. nonspecific in their action on various nerves.

6. The limbic system is an area of the brain that
  a. is responsible for coordination of movement.
  b. is responsible for the special senses.
  c. is responsible for the expression of emotions.
  d. controls sleep.

7. The most primitive area of the brain, the brainstem, contains areas responsible for
   a. vomiting, swallowing, respiration, arousal, and sleep.
   b. learning.
   c. motivation and memory.
   d. taste, sight, hearing, and balance.

8. A clinical indication of poor blood supply to the brain, particularly to the higher levels where learning takes place, would be
   a. loss of long-term memory.
   b. loss of short-term memory.
   c. loss of coordinated movement.
   d. insomnia.

MULTIPLE RESPONSE

Select all that apply.

1. In explaining the importance of a constant blood supply to the brain the nurse would tell the student which of the following?
   a. Energy is needed to maintain nerve membranes and cannot be produced without oxygen.
   b. Carbon dioxide must constantly be removed to maintain the proper pH.
   c. Little glucose is stored in nerve cells, so a constant supply is needed.
   d. The brain needs a constant supply of insulin and thyroid hormone.
   e. The brain swells easily and needs the blood supply to reduce swelling.
   f. Circulating aldosterone levels maintain the fluid balance in the brain.

2. The blood–brain barrier could be described by which of the following?
   a. It is produced by the cells that make up the meninges.
   b. It is regulated by the microglia in the CNS.
   c. It is weaker in certain parts of the brain.
   d. It is uniform in its permeability throughout the CNS.
   e. It is an anatomical structure that can be punctured.
   f. It is more likely to block the entry of proteins into the CNS.

BIBLIOGRAPHY AND REFERENCES

Barrett, K., Barman, S., Boitano, S., et al. (2014). *Ganong's review of medical physiology* (24th ed.). New York: McGraw-Hill.

Brunton, L., Chabner, B., & Knollman, B. (2011). *Goodman and Gilman's the pharmacological basis of therapeutics* (12th ed.). New York: McGraw-Hill.

Guyton, A., & Hall, J. (2015). *Textbook of medical physiology* (13th ed.). Philadelphia, PA: W. B. Saunders.

Karch, A. M. (2014). *Lippincott's nursing drug guide.* Philadelphia, PA: Lippincott Williams & Wilkins.

Noback, C., Strominger, N. L., Demarest, R. J., et al. (2012). *The human nervous system: Structure and function* (7th ed.). Totowa, NJ: Humana Press.

Parpura, V., & Hayden, P. (2009). *Astrocytes in the physiology of the nervous system.* New York: Springer.

Porth, C. M. (2013). *Pathophysiology: Concepts of altered health states* (9th ed.). Philadelphia, PA: Lippincott Williams & Wilkins.

Thibodeau, G., & Patton, K. (2012). *Anthony's textbook of anatomy and physiology* (20th ed.). St. Louis, MO: Mosby.

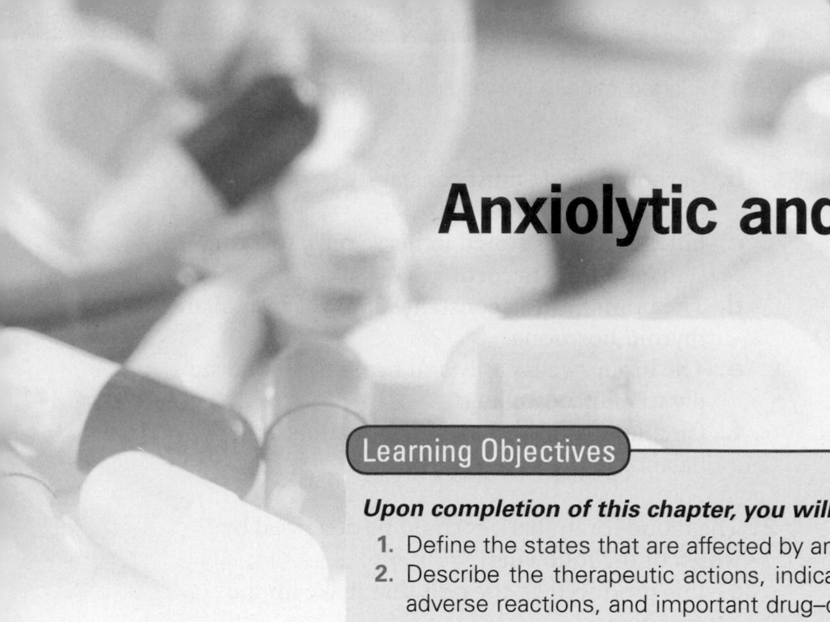

Anxiolytic and Hypnotic Agents 20

Learning Objectives

Upon completion of this chapter, you will be able to:

1. Define the states that are affected by anxiolytic or hypnotic agents.
2. Describe the therapeutic actions, indications, pharmacokinetics, contraindications, most common adverse reactions, and important drug–drug interactions associated with each class of anxiolytic or hypnotic agent.
3. Discuss the use of anxiolytic or hypnotic agents across the lifespan.
4. Compare and contrast the prototype drugs for each class of anxiolytic or hypnotic drug with the other drugs in that class.
5. Outline the nursing considerations and teaching needs for patients receiving each class of anxiolytic or hypnotic agent.

Glossary of Key Terms

anxiety: unpleasant feeling of tension, fear, or nervousness in response to an environmental stimulus, whether real or imaginary

anxiolytic: drug used to depress the central nervous system (CNS); prevents the signs and symptoms of anxiety

barbiturate: former mainstay drug used for the treatment of anxiety and for sedation and sleep induction; associated with potentially severe adverse effects and many drug–drug interactions, which makes it less desirable than some of the newer agents

benzodiazepine: drug that acts in the limbic system and the reticular activating system to make gamma-aminobutyric acid (GABA), an inhibitory neurotransmitter, more effective, causing interference with neuron firing; depresses CNS to block the signs and symptoms of anxiety; and may cause sedation and hypnosis in higher doses

hypnosis: extreme sedation resulting in CNS depression and sleep

hypnotic: drug used to depress the CNS; causes sleep

sedation: loss of awareness of and reaction to environmental stimuli

sedative: drug that depresses the CNS; produces a loss of awareness of and reaction to the environment

Drugs List

Benzodiazepines Used as Anxiolytic–Hypnotics
- alprazolam
- chlordiazepoxide
- clonazepam
- clorazepate
- (P) diazepam
- estazolam
- flurazepam
- lorazepam
- midazolam
- oxazepam
- quazepam
- temazepam
- triazolam

Barbiturates Used as Anxiolytic–Hypnotics
- amobarbital
- butabarbital
- pentobarbital
- (P) phenobarbital
- secobarbital

Other Anxiolytic and Hypnotic Drugs
- buspirone
- dexmedetomidine
- diphenhydramine
- eszopiclone
- meprobamate
- promethazine
- ramelteon
- suvorexant
- tasimelteon
- zaleplon
- zolpidem

The drugs discussed in this chapter are used to alter an individual's responses to environmental stimuli. They have been called **anxiolytics** because they can prevent feelings of tension or fear, **sedatives** because they can calm patients and make them unaware of their environment, **hypnotics** because they can cause sleep, and minor tranquilizers because they can produce a state of tranquility in anxious patients. In the past, a given drug would simply be used at different doses to yield each of these effects. Further research into how the brain reacts to outside stimuli has resulted in the increased availability of specific agents that produce particular goals and avoid unwanted adverse effects. Use of these drugs also varies across the lifespan (Box 20.1).

States Affected by Anxiolytic and Hypnotic Drugs

Anxiety

Anxiety is a feeling of tension, nervousness, apprehension, or fear that usually involves unpleasant reactions to a stimulus, whether actual or unknown. Anxiety is often accompanied by signs and symptoms of the sympathetic stress reaction (see Chapter 29), which may include sweating, fast heart rate, rapid breathing, and elevated blood pressure. Mild anxiety, a not uncommon reaction, may serve as a stimulus or motivator in some situations. A person who feels anxious about being alone in a poorly lit parking lot at night may be motivated to take extra safety precautions. When anxiety becomes overwhelming or severe, it can interfere with the activities of daily living and lead to medical problems related to chronic stimulation of the sympathetic nervous system. A severely anxious person may, for example, be afraid to leave the house or to interact with other people. In these cases, treatment is warranted. Anxiolytic drugs are drugs that are used to lyse or break the feeling of anxiety.

Sedation

The loss of awareness and reaction to environmental stimuli is termed **sedation**. This condition may be desirable in patients who are restless, nervous, irritable, or overreacting to stimuli. Although sedation is anxiolytic, it may frequently lead to drowsiness. For example, sedative-induced drowsiness is a concern for outpatients who need to be alert and responsive in their normal lives. On the other hand, this tiredness may be desirable for patients who are

BOX 20.1 FOCUS ON Drug Therapy Across the Lifespan

Anxiolytic and Hypnotic Agents

CHILDREN

Use of anxiolytic and hypnotic drugs with children is challenging. The response of the child to the drug may be unpredictable; inappropriate aggressiveness, crying, irritability, and tearfulness are common. Using good sleep hygiene measures is the preferred approach to insomnia in children.

Of the benzodiazepines, only chlordiazepoxide, clonazepam, clorazepate, and diazepam have established pediatric dosages. Some of the others are used in pediatric settings; dosage may be calculated using age and weight.

The barbiturates, being older drugs, have established pediatric dosages. These drugs must be used with caution because of the often unexpected responses. Children must be monitored very closely for CNS depression and excitability.

The antihistamines diphenhydramine and promethazine are more popular for use in helping to calm children and to induce rest and sleep. Care must be taken to assess for possible dried secretions and effects on breathing. Dosage must be calculated carefully.

ADULTS

Adults using these drugs for the treatment of insomnia need to be cautioned that they are for short-term use only. The reason for the insomnia should be sought (e.g., medical, hormonal, or anxiety problems). Other methods for helping to induce sleep—established routines, quiet activities before bed, a back rub, or warm bath—should be encouraged before drugs are prescribed. Adults receiving anxiolytics also may need referrals for counseling and diagnosis of possible causes. Adults should be advised to avoid driving and making legal decisions when taking these drugs.

Liver function should be evaluated before and periodically during therapy.

These drugs are contraindicated during pregnancy and lactation because of the potential for adverse effects on the fetus and possible sedation of the baby. The antihistamines, which have not been associated with congenital malformations, may be the safest to use, with caution, if an anxiolytic or hypnotic drug must be used.

OLDER ADULTS

Older patients may be more susceptible to the adverse effects of these drugs, from unanticipated CNS effects to increased sedation, dizziness, and even hallucinations. This is a major safety concern with this group. Dosages of all of these drugs should be reduced, and the patient should be monitored very closely for toxic effects and to provide safety measures if CNS effects do occur.

Baseline liver and renal function tests should be performed, and these values should be monitored periodically for any changes that would indicate a need to decrease dosage further or to stop the drug.

Nondrug measures to reduce anxiety and to help induce sleep are important with older patients. The patient should be screened for physical problems, neurological deterioration, or depression, which could contribute to the insomnia or anxiety.

about to undergo surgery or other procedures and who are receiving medical support. The choice of an anxiolytic drug depends on the situation in which it will be used, keeping the related adverse effects in mind.

Hypnosis

Extreme sedation results in further central nervous system (CNS) depression and sleep, or **hypnosis**. Hypnotics are used to help people fall asleep by causing sedation. Drugs that are effective hypnotics act on the reticular activating system (RAS) and block the brain's response to incoming stimuli. Hypnosis, therefore, is the extreme state of sedation, in which the person no longer senses or reacts to incoming stimuli.

Benzodiazepines Used as Anxiolytic–Hypnotics

Benzodiazepines, the most frequently used anxiolytic drugs, prevent anxiety without causing much associated sedation. In addition, they are less likely to cause physical dependence than many of the older sedative–hypnotics that are used to relieve anxiety. Table 20.1 lists the available benzodiazepines, including common indications and specific information about each drug. The benzodiazepines used as anxiolytics include alprazolam (*Xanax*), chlordiazepoxide (*Librium*), clonazepam (*Klonopin*), clorazepate (*Tranxene*), diazepam (*Valium*), estazolam (generic), flurazepam (generic), lorazepam (*Ativan*), midazolam

Table 20.1 ***Drugs in Focus:*** **Benzodiazepines Used as Anxiolytics***

Drug Name	Dosage/Route	Usual Indications
alprazolam (*Xanax*)	0.25–0.5 mg PO t.i.d. up to 1–10 mg/d PO have been used, reduced dosage in elderly	Anxiety, panic attacks *Onset:* 30 min *Duration:* 4–6 h *Special considerations:* Taper after long-term therapy
chlordiazepoxide (*Librium*)	*Adult:* 5–25 mg PO t.i.d. to q.i.d. *or* 50–100 mg IV or IM, may be repeated; reduce dosage with older patients *Pediatric (>6 y):* 5 mg PO b.i.d. to q.i.d., 25–50 mg IV or IM	Anxiety, alcohol withdrawal, preoperative anxiolytic *Onset:* 10–15 min *Duration:* 2–3 d *Special considerations:* Monitor injection sites
clonazepam (*Klonopin*)	*Adult:* 0.25 mg PO b.i.d., titrate to 1 mg/d PO *Pediatric:* 0.01–0.03 mg/kg/d PO given in 2–3 doses, do not exceed 0.05 mg/kg/d	Panic disorders, restless leg syndrome, seizure disorders *Onset:* Slow *Duration:* 1–6 wk *Special considerations:* Monitor for suicidal ideation, liver function and blood counts with long-term therapy, taper after long-term therapy
clorazepate (*Tranxene*)	*Adult:* 15–60 mg/d in divided doses, 7.5–15 mg/d PO for elderly patients *Pediatric (9–12 y):* 7.5 mg PO b.i.d. as adjunct therapy for epilepsy	Anxiety, alcohol withdrawal, partial seizures *Onset:* Rapid *Duration:* Days *Special considerations:* Taper dosage
diazepam (*Valium*)	*Adult:* 2–10 mg PO b.i.d. to q.i.d. *or* 0.2 mg/kg PR, 2–2.5 mg PO b.i.d. for elderly patients *Pediatric:* 1–2.5 mg PO t.i.d. to q.i.d., 0.3–0.5 mg/kg PR	Anxiety, alcohol withdrawal, muscle relaxant, preoperative anxiolytic *Onset:* 5–60 min *Duration:* 3 h *Special considerations:* Taper after long-term therapy
estazolam (generic)	1 mg PO at bedtime, start with 0.5 mg for elderly or debilitated patient	Hypnotic, treatment of insomnia *Onset:* 45–60 min *Duration:* 2 h *Special considerations:* Monitor liver and renal function, CBC if used long-term
flurazepam (generic)	30 mg PO at bedtime, 15 mg PO at bedtime for elderly or debilitated patients	Hypnotic, treatment of insomnia *Onset:* Varies *Duration:* 30–60 min *Special considerations:* Monitor liver and renal function, CBC in long-term use

Drug Name	Dosage/Route	Usual Indications
lorazepam (*Ativan*)	2–6 mg/d PO in divided doses *or* 0.05 mg/kg IM *or* 0.044 mg/kg IV	Anxiety, preanesthesia anxiolytic *Onset:* 1–30 min *Duration:* 12–24 h *Special considerations:* Monitor injection sites, reduce dosage of narcotics given with this drug
midazolam (generic)	*Adult:* Sedation—5 mg IM; conscious sedation for short procedures—1–2.5 mg IV, maintenance dose 25% of initial dose; sedation in critical care—10–50 mcg/kg IV as a loading dose, repeat every 10–15 min until desired effect is seen, infusion of 20–100 mcg/kg/h maintenance *Pediatric:* Sedation—0.1–0.015 mg/kg IM or PO; conscious sedation for short procedures 50–100 mcg/kg IV; sedation in critical care—30–200 mcg/kg IV as a loading dose, maintenance infusion of 60–120 mcg/kg/h	Sedation, anxiety, conscious sedation for short procedures; continuous sedation of intubated or mechanically ventilated patients *Onset:* 3–15 min *Duration:* 2–6 h *Special considerations:* Do not administer intraarterially; keep resuscitation equipment nearby, be prepared to breathe for the patient as needed
oxazepam (generic)	10–15 mg PO t.i.d. to q.i.d.	Anxiety, alcohol withdrawal *Onset:* Slow *Duration:* 2–4 h *Special considerations:* Preferred for elderly
quazepam (*Doral*)	15 mg PO at bedtime	Hypnotic, treatment of insomnia *Onset:* Varies *Duration:* 4–6 h *Special considerations:* Monitor liver and renal function, CBC if used for long-term therapy; taper after long-term therapy
temazepam (*Restoril*)	15–30 mg PO at bedtime	Hypnotic, treatment of insomnia *Onset:* Varies *Duration:* 4–6 h *Special considerations:* Taper after long-term therapy
triazolam (*Halcion*)	0.125–0.5 mg PO at bedtime	Hypnotic, treatment of insomnia *Onset:* Varies *Duration:* 2–4 h *Special considerations:* Monitor liver and renal function, CBC; taper after long-term therapy

*Onset of action and duration are important in selecting the correct drug for a particular use.
CBC, complete blood count.

(generic), oxazepam (generic), quazepam (*Doral*), temazepam (*Restoril*), and triazolam (*Halcion*). Box 20.2 provides an exercise in calculating dose for a pediatric patient receiving a sedative/hypnotic.

Therapeutic Actions and Indications

The benzodiazepines are indicated for the treatment of the following conditions: Anxiety disorders, alcohol withdrawal, hyperexcitability and agitation, and preoperative relief of anxiety and tension to aid in balanced anesthesia. These drugs act in the limbic system and the RAS to make gamma-aminobutyric acid (GABA) more effective, causing interference with neuron firing (Figure 20.1). GABA stabilizes the postsynaptic cell. This leads to an anxiolytic effect at doses lower than those required to induce sedation and hypnosis. The exact mechanism of action is not clearly understood.

Pharmacokinetics

The benzodiazepines are well absorbed from the gastrointestinal (GI) tract, with peak levels achieved in 30 minutes to 2 hours. They are lipid soluble and well distributed throughout the body, crossing the placenta and entering breast milk. The benzodiazepines are metabolized extensively in the liver. Patients with liver disease must receive a smaller dose and be monitored closely. Excretion is primarily through the urine.

BOX 20.2 FOCUS ON Calculations

Your 3-year-old patient, weighing 10 kg, is prescribed phenobarbital as a hypnotic at bedtime. The order reads: 6 mg/kg PO at bedtime. The drug comes in an elixir 24 mg/mL. How much of the elixir would you give at bedtime?

First, figure out what the correct dose would be:

$$6 \text{ mg/kg} \times 10 \text{ kg} = 60 \text{ mg}$$

Set up the equation using available form = prescribed dose:

$$4 \text{ mg/mL} = 60 \text{ mg/dose}$$

Then, cross-multiply:

$$4 \text{ mg (dose)} = 60 \text{ mg (mL)}$$
$$\text{dose} = 60 \text{ mg (mL)}/4 \text{ mg}$$
$$\text{dose} = 15 \text{ mL}$$

Because this is a child, it is good practice to ask another nurse to calculate the correct dosage and then compare your work, so you can double-check the accuracy of your calculations.

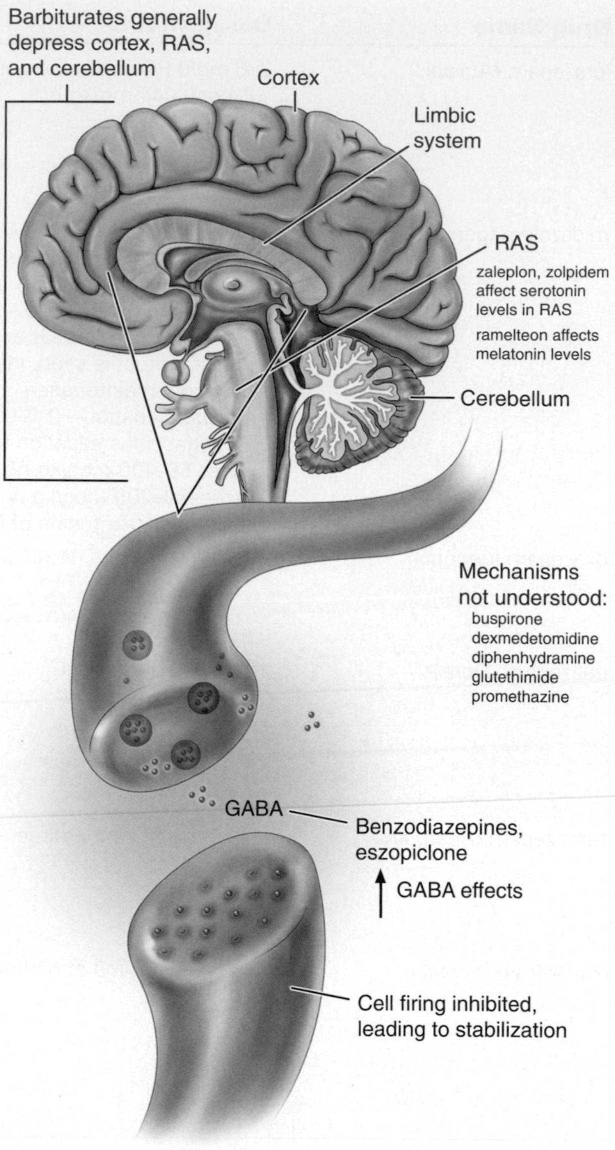

FIGURE 20.1 Sites of action of the benzodiazepines, barbiturates, and other anxiolytics. GABA, gamma-aminobutyric acid; RAS, reticular activating system.

Contraindications and Cautions

Contraindications to benzodiazepines include allergy to any benzodiazepine *to prevent hypersensitivity reactions*; psychosis, *which could be exacerbated by sedation*; and acute narrow-angle glaucoma, shock, coma, or acute alcoholic intoxication, *all of which could be exacerbated by the depressant effects of these drugs*.

In addition, these sedative–hypnotics are contraindicated in pregnancy *because a predictable syndrome of cleft lip or palate, inguinal hernia, cardiac defects, microcephaly, or pyloric stenosis occurs when they are taken in the first trimester*. Neonatal withdrawal syndrome may also result. Breastfeeding is also a contraindication *because of potential adverse effects on the neonate (e.g., sedation)*.

Use with caution in elderly or debilitated patients *because of the possibility of unpredictable reactions* and in cases of renal or hepatic dysfunction, *which may alter the metabolism and excretion of these drugs, resulting in direct toxicity*. Dose adjustments usually are needed for such patients. Box 20.3 provides information about the effect of benzodiazepines in African American patients.

Adverse Effects

The adverse effects of benzodiazepines are associated with the impact of these drugs on the central and peripheral nervous systems. Nervous system effects include sedation, drowsiness, depression, lethargy, blurred vision, "sleep driving" and other complex behaviors, headaches, apathy, light-headedness, amnesia, and confusion. In addition, mild paradoxical excitatory reactions may occur during the first 2 weeks of therapy.

Several other kinds of adverse effects may occur. GI conditions such as dry mouth, constipation, nausea,

BOX 20.3 FOCUS ON Cultural Considerations

Benzodiazepine Levels

Special care should be taken when anxiolytic or hypnotic drugs are given to African Americans. About 15% to 20% of African Americans are genetically predisposed to delayed metabolism of benzodiazepines. As a result, they may develop high serum levels of these drugs, with increased sedation and an increased incidence of adverse effects.

If an anxiolytic or hypnotic agent is the drug of choice for an African American individual the smallest possible dose should be used, and the patient should be monitored very closely during the first week of treatment. Dosage adjustments are necessary to achieve the most effective dose with the fewest adverse effects.

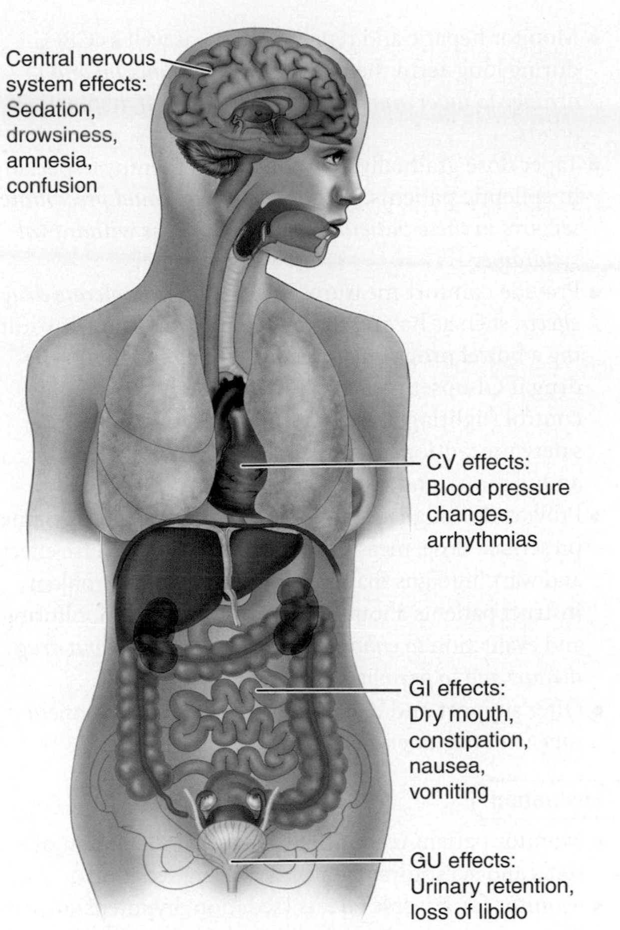

FIGURE 20.2 Variety of adverse effects and toxicities associated with anxiolytics and hypnotics.

vomiting, and elevated liver enzymes may result. Cardiovascular problems may include hypotension, hypertension, arrhythmias, palpitations, and respiratory difficulties. Hematological conditions such as blood dyscrasias and anemia are possible. Genitourinary effects include urinary retention and hesitancy, loss of libido, and changes in sexual functioning. Because phlebitis, local reactions, and thrombosis may occur at local injection sites, such sites should be monitored. Abrupt cessation of these drugs may lead to a withdrawal syndrome characterized by nausea, headache, vertigo, malaise, and nightmares (Figure 20.2).

Clinically Important Drug–Drug Interactions

The risk of CNS depression increases if benzodiazepines are taken with alcohol or other CNS depressants, so such combinations should be avoided. In addition, the effects of benzodiazepines increase if they are taken with cimetidine, oral contraceptives, or disulfiram. If any of these drugs is used with benzodiazepines, patients should be monitored and the appropriate dose adjustments made.

Finally, the impact of benzodiazepines may be decreased if they are given with theophyllines or ranitidine. If either of these drugs is used, dose adjustment may be necessary.

Ⓟ Prototype Summary: Diazepam

Indications: Management of anxiety disorders, acute alcohol withdrawal, muscle relaxation. preoperative relief of anxiety and tension.

Actions: Acts in the limbic system and reticular formation to potentiate the effects of GABA, an inhibitory neurotransmitter; may act in spinal cord and supraspinal sites to produce muscle relaxation.

Pharmacokinetics:

Route	Onset	Peak	Duration
Oral	30–60 min	1–2 h	3 h
Rectal	Rapid	1.5 h	3 h

$T_{1/2}$: 20 to 80 hours; metabolized in the liver, excreted in urine.

Adverse Effects: Mild drowsiness, depression, lethargy, apathy, fatigue, restlessness, bradycardia, tachycardia, constipation, diarrhea, incontinence, urinary retention, changes in libido, drug dependence with withdrawal syndrome.

Nursing Considerations for Patients Receiving Benzodiazepines

Assessment: History and Examination

- Assess for contraindications or cautions: Known allergies to benzodiazepines *to prevent hypersensitivity reactions*; impaired liver or kidney function, *which could alter the metabolism and excretion of a particular drug*; any condition *that might be exacerbated by the depressant effects of the drugs* (e.g., glaucoma, coma, psychoses, shock, acute alcohol intoxication); and pregnancy and lactation.
- Assess for baseline status before beginning therapy *to check for occurrence of any potential adverse effects.* Assess for the following: Temperature and weight; skin color and lesions; affect, orientation, reflexes, and vision; pulse, blood pressure, and perfusion; respiratory rate, adventitious sounds, and presence of chronic pulmonary disease; and bowel sounds on abdominal examination.
- Perform laboratory tests, including renal and liver function tests and complete blood count (CBC).

Refer to the Critical Thinking Scenario for a full discussion of nursing care for a patient dealing with anxiety.

Nursing Diagnoses

Nursing diagnoses related to drug therapy might include the following:

- Disturbed thought processes and disturbed sensory perception (visual, kinesthetic) related to CNS effects
- Risk for injury related to CNS effects
- Disturbed sleep pattern related to CNS effects
- Deficient knowledge regarding drug therapy

Planning

- The patient will receive the best therapeutic effect from the drug therapy.
- The patient will have limited adverse effects to the drug therapy.
- The patient will have an understanding of the drug therapy, adverse effects to anticipate, and measures to relieve discomfort and improve safety.

Implementation with Rationale

- Do not administer intraarterially *because serious arteriospasm and gangrene could occur.* Monitor injection sites carefully for local reactions to institute treatment as soon as possible.
- Do not mix IV drugs in solution with any other drugs *to avoid potential drug–drug interactions.*
- Give parenteral forms only if oral forms are not feasible or available and switch to oral forms, *which are safer and less likely to cause adverse effects,* as soon as possible.
- Give IV drugs slowly *because these agents have been associated with hypotension, bradycardia, and cardiac arrest.*
- Arrange to reduce the dose of narcotic analgesics in patients receiving a benzodiazepine *to decrease potentiated effects and sedation.*
- Maintain patients who receive parenteral benzodiazepines in bed for a period of at least 3 hours. Do not permit ambulatory patients to operate a motor vehicle after an injection *to ensure patient safety.*
- Monitor hepatic and renal function, as well as CBC, during long-term therapy *to detect dysfunction and to arrange to taper and discontinue the drug if dysfunction occurs.*
- Taper dose gradually after long-term therapy, especially in epileptic patients. *Acute withdrawal could precipitate seizures in these patients. It may also cause withdrawal syndrome.*
- Provide comfort measures *to help patients tolerate drug effects,* such as having them void before dosing, instituting a bowel program as needed, giving food with the drug if GI upset is severe, providing environmental control (lighting, temperature, stimulation), taking safety precautions (use of side rails, assistance with ambulation), and aiding orientation.
- Provide thorough patient teaching, including drug name, prescribed dose, measures for avoidance of adverse effects, and warning signs that may indicate possible problems. Instruct patients about the need for periodic monitoring and evaluation *to enhance patient knowledge about drug therapy and to promote compliance.*
- Offer support and encouragement *to help the patient cope with the diagnosis and the drug regimen.*

Evaluation

- Monitor patient response to the drug (alleviation of signs and symptoms of anxiety; sleep; sedation).
- Monitor for adverse effects (sedation, hypotension, cardiac arrhythmias, hepatic or renal dysfunction, blood dyscrasias).
- Evaluate the effectiveness of the teaching plan (patient can give the drug name, dosage, possible adverse effects to watch for, specific measures to help avoid adverse effects, and the importance of continued follow-up).
- Monitor the effectiveness of comfort measures and compliance with the regimen.

CRITICAL THINKING SCENARIO

Benzodiazepines

THE SITUATION

P.P., a 43-year-old mother of three teenage sons, comes to the outpatient department for a routine physical examination. Results are unremarkable except for blood pressure of 145/90, pulse rate of 98, and apparent tension—she is jittery, avoids eye contact, and sometimes appears teary eyed. She says that she is having some problems dealing with "life in general." Her sons present many stresses, and her husband, who is busy with his career, has little time to deal with issues at home. When he *is* home, he is very demanding. In addition, she thinks she is beginning menopause and is having trouble coping with the idea of menopause as well as with some of the symptoms. Overall, she feels lonely and has no outlet for her anger, tension, or stress. A health care provider, who reassures P.P. that this problem is common in women of her age, prescribes the benzodiazepine diazepam (*Valium*) to help P.P. deal with her anxiety.

Benzodiazepines (continued)

CRITICAL THINKING

What sort of crisis intervention would be most appropriate for P.P.?
What nursing interventions are helpful at this point?
What nondrug interventions might be helpful?
What other support systems could be used to help P.P. deal with all that is going on in her life?
Think about the overwhelming problems that P.P. has to deal with on a daily basis and how the anxiolytic effects of diazepam might change her approach to these problems. Could the problems actually get worse?
Develop a care plan for the long-term care of P.P.

DISCUSSION

Anxiolytics are useful for controlling the unpleasant signs and symptoms of anxiety. The diazepam prescribed for P.P. may provide some immediate relief, enabling her to survive the "crisis" period and plan changes in her life in general. However, the associated drowsiness and sedation may make coping with the problems in her life even more difficult. She should be taught the adverse effects of diazepam, the warning signs of serious adverse effects, and the health problems to report.

A follow-up evaluation should be scheduled. Additional meetings with the same health care provider are important for the long-term solution to P.P.'s anxiety. Her need for drug therapy should be reevaluated once she can discover other support systems and develop other ways of coping. Although anxiolytic therapy may be beneficial initially, it will not solve the problems that are causing anxiety, and in this case the causes for the anxiety are specific. Anxiolytic therapy should be considered only as a short-term aid.

Unlike P.P., many patients in severe crisis do not consciously identify the many causes of stress, or stressors. However, P.P. has identified a list of factors that makes her life stressful. This facilitates the development of coping strategies. She may find the following support systems helpful:

- Referral to a counselor and involvement of the entire family in identifying problems and ways to deal with them
- Support groups for women in various stages of life (e.g., entering menopause, mothers of children who are entering the teens). Just having the opportunity to discuss problems and explore ways of dealing with them helps many people.

NURSING CARE GUIDE FOR P.P.: DIAZEPAM

Assessment: History and Examination

Allergies to diazepam, psychoses, acute narrow-angle glaucoma, acute alcohol intoxication, impaired liver or kidney function, pregnancy, breastfeeding, concurrent use of alcohol, omeprazole, cimetidine, disulfiram, oral contraceptives, theophylline, ranitidine
Cardiovascular: Blood pressure, pulse, perfusion
CNS: Orientation, affect, reflexes, vision
Skin: Color, lesions, texture
Respiratory: Respiration, adventitious sounds
GI: Abdominal examination, bowel sounds
Laboratory tests: Hepatic and renal function tests, CBC

Nursing Diagnoses

Disturbed thought processes and disturbed sensory perception (visual, kinesthetic) related to CNS effects
Risk for injury related to CNS effects
Disturbed sleep patterns related to CNS effects
Deficient knowledge regarding drug therapy

Planning

The patient will receive the best therapeutic effect from the drug therapy.
The patient will have limited adverse effects to the drug therapy.
The patient will have an understanding of the drug therapy, adverse effects to anticipate, and measures to relieve discomfort and improve safety.

Implementation

Provide comfort and safety measures, small meals, drugs with food if GI upset occurs, bowel program as needed; taper dosage after long-term use; reduce dosage if other medications include narcotics; lower dose with renal or hepatic impairment.
Provide support and reassurance to deal with drug effects.
Provide patient teaching regarding drug, dosage, adverse effects, safety precautions, and unusual symptoms to report.

Evaluation

Evaluate drug effects: Relief of signs and symptoms of anxiety.
Monitor for adverse effects, particularly sedation, dizziness, insomnia, blood dyscrasia, GI upset, hepatic or renal dysfunction, and cardiovascular effects.
Monitor for drug–drug interactions.
Evaluate effectiveness of patient-teaching program.
Evaluate effectiveness of comfort and safety measures.

(continues on page 344)

Benzodiazepines (continued)

PATIENT TEACHING FOR P.P.

- The drug that has been prescribed for you is called diazepam, or *Valium.* It belongs to a class of drugs called benzodiazepines, which are used to relieve tension and nervousness. Exactly how the drug works is not completely understood, but it does relax muscle spasms, relieve insomnia, and promote calm. Common side effects of this drug include:
  - *Dizziness and drowsiness:* Avoid driving or performing hazardous or delicate tasks that require concentration if these effects occur.
  - *Nausea, vomiting, and weight loss:* Small, frequent meals may help to relieve nausea. If weight loss occurs, monitor the loss; if the loss is extensive, consult your health care provider. Do not take this drug with antacids.
  - *Constipation or diarrhea:* These reactions usually pass with time. If they do not, consult with your health care provider for appropriate therapy.
  - *Vision changes, slurred speech, and unsteadiness:* These effects also subside with time. Take extra care in your activities for the first few days. If these reactions do not go away after 3 or 4 days, consult your health care provider.
- Report any of the following conditions to your health care provider: Rash, fever, sore throat, insomnia, depression, clumsiness, or nervousness.
- Tell any doctor, nurse, or other health care provider involved in your care that you are taking this drug.
- Keep this drug and all medications safely away from children or pets.
- Avoid the use of over-the-counter medications or herbal therapies while you are taking this drug. If you think that you need one of these products, consult with your health care provider about the best choice because many of these products can interfere with your medication.
- Avoid alcohol while you are taking this drug. Combining alcohol and a benzodiazepine can cause serious problems.
- If you have been taking this drug for a prolonged time, do not stop taking it suddenly. Your body will need time to adjust to the loss of the drug, and the dosage will need to be reduced gradually to prevent serious problems. When discontinuing use of this drug, tell your health care provider if the following occurs: Trembling, muscle cramps, sweating, irritability, confusion, or seizures.

KEY POINTS

- Anxiety is a feeling of tension, nervousness, apprehension, or fear. In the extreme, anxiety may produce physiological manifestations and may interfere with activities of daily life. Anxiolytic drugs, such as the benzodiazepines, depress the CNS to diminish these feelings.
- CNS depressants, such as sedatives, block the awareness of and reaction to environmental stimuli. They induce drowsiness, as do hypnotic drugs, which also depress the CNS and inhibit neuronal arousal.
- Hypnotics react with GABA-inhibitory sites to depress the CNS. They can cause drowsiness, lethargy, and other CNS effects.

Barbiturates Used as Anxiolytic–Hypnotics

Barbiturates were once the sedative–hypnotic drugs of choice. Not only is the likelihood of sedation and other adverse effects greater with these drugs than with newer sedative–hypnotic drugs but the risk of addiction and dependence is also greater. For these reasons, newer anxiolytic drugs have replaced the barbiturates in most instances.

The barbiturates used as anxiolytic–hypnotics include amobarbital (*Amytal Sodium*), butabarbital (*Butisol*), pentobarbital (*Nembutal Sodium*), phenobarbital (generic), and secobarbital (*Seconal*). Table 20.2 lists the available barbiturates, including common indications and specific information about each drug.

Therapeutic Actions and Indications

Barbiturates are general CNS depressants that inhibit neuronal impulse conduction in the ascending RAS, depress the cerebral cortex, alter cerebellar function, and depress motor output (see Figure 20.1). Thus, they can cause sedation, hypnosis, anesthesia, and in extreme cases coma. In general, barbiturates are indicated for the relief of the signs and symptoms of anxiety and for sedation, insomnia, preanesthesia, and the treatment of seizures (Table 20.2). Parenteral forms, which reach peak levels faster and have a faster onset of action, may be used for the treatment of acute manic reactions and many forms of seizures (see Chapter 23).

Pharmacokinetics

Barbiturates are absorbed well, reaching peak levels in 20 to 60 minutes. They are metabolized in the liver to varying degrees, depending on the drug, and excreted in the

Table 20.2 *Drugs in Focus:* Barbiturates Used as Anxiolytic–Hypnotics*

Drug Name	Dosage/Route	Usual Indications
amobarbital (*Amytal Sodium*)	*Adult:* 65–500 mg IM or IV; reduce dosage with older patients *Pediatric (6–12 y):* 65–500 mg IM or IV, monitor very closely	Sedative–hypnotic, convulsions, manic reactions *Onset:* 15–60 min *Duration:* 3–8 h *Special considerations:* Monitor carefully if administered by IV
butabarbital (*Butisol*)	*Adult:* 15–30 mg PO t.i.d. to q.i.d., 50–100 mg PO at bedtime for sedation; reduce dosage in elderly *Pediatric:* 7.5–30 mg PO based on age and weight	Short-term sedative–hypnotic *Onset:* 45–60 min *Duration:* 6–8 h *Special considerations:* Taper gradually after long-term use; use caution in children, may produce aggressiveness, excitability
pentobarbital (*Nembutal*)	*Adult:* 20 mg PO t.i.d. to q.i.d., 100 mg at bedtime for insomnia, 120–200 mg PR, 150–200 mg IM or 100 mg IV; reduce dosage in elderly patients *Pediatric:* 2–6 mg/kg/d, adjust dosage based on age and weight	Sedative–hypnotic, preanesthetic *Onset:* 10–15 min *Duration:* 2–4 h *Special considerations:* Taper gradually after long-term use, give IV slowly, monitor injection sites
phenobarbital (generic)	*Adult:* 30–120 mg/d PO, IM, or IV; reduce dosage in elderly patients *Pediatric:* 1–3 mg/kg IV or IM	Sedative–hypnotic, control of seizures, preanesthetic *Onset:* 10–60 min *Duration:* 4–16 h *Special considerations:* Taper gradually after long-term use, give IV slowly, monitor injection sites
secobarbital (*Seconal*)	*Adult:* 100–300 mg PO; reduce dosage in elderly patients *Pediatric:* 2–6 mg/kg PO	Preanesthetic sedation, convulsive seizures of tetanus *Onset:* Rapid *Duration:* 1–4 h *Special considerations:* Taper gradually after long-term use

*Onset of action and duration are important in selecting the correct drug for a particular use.

urine. The longer-acting barbiturates tend to be metabolized slower and excreted to a greater degree unchanged in the urine. They are known to induce liver enzyme systems, increasing the metabolism of the barbiturate broken down by that system, as well as that of any other drug that may be metabolized by that enzyme system. Patients with hepatic or renal dysfunction require lower doses of the drug to avoid toxic effects and should be monitored closely. Barbiturates are lipid soluble; they readily cross the placenta and enter breast milk.

Contraindications and Cautions

Contraindications to barbiturates include allergy to any barbiturate *to avoid hypersensitivity reactions* and a previous history of addiction to sedative–hypnotic drugs *because the barbiturates are more addicting than most other anxiolytics.* Other contraindications are latent or manifest porphyria, *which may be exacerbated*; marked hepatic impairment or nephritis, *which may alter the metabolism and excretion of these drugs*; and respiratory distress or severe respiratory dysfunction, *which could be exacerbated by the CNS depression caused by these drugs.* Pregnancy is a contraindication *because of potential adverse effects on the fetus*; congenital abnormalities have been reported with barbiturate use.

Use with caution in patients with acute or chronic pain *because barbiturates can cause paradoxical excitement, masking other symptoms*; with seizure disorders *because abrupt withdrawal of a barbiturate can precipitate status epilepticus*; and with chronic hepatic, cardiac, or respiratory diseases, *which could be exacerbated by the depressive effects of these drugs.* Care should be taken with lactating women *because of the potential for adverse effects on the infant.*

Adverse Effects

As previously stated, the adverse effects caused by barbiturates are more severe than those associated with other, newer sedative–hypnotics. For this reason, barbiturates are no longer considered the mainstay for the treatment of anxiety. In addition, the development of physical tolerance and psychological dependence is more likely with the barbiturates than with other anxiolytics.

The most common adverse effects are related to general CNS depression. CNS effects may include drowsiness, somnolence, lethargy, ataxia, vertigo, a feeling of a "hangover," thinking abnormalities, paradoxical excitement, anxiety, and hallucinations. GI signs and symptoms such as nausea, vomiting, constipation, diarrhea, and epigastric pain may occur. Associated cardiovascular effects may include bradycardia, hypotension (particularly with IV administration), and syncope. Serious hypoventilation may occur, and respiratory depression and laryngospasm may also result, particularly with IV administration. Hypersensitivity reactions, including rash, serum sickness, and Stevens-Johnson syndrome, which is sometimes fatal, may also occur.

Clinically Important Drug–Drug Interactions

Increased CNS depression results if these agents are taken with other CNS depressants, including alcohol, antihistamines, and other tranquilizers. If other CNS depressants are used, dose adjustments are necessary.

There often is an altered response to phenytoin if it is combined with barbiturates; evaluate the patient frequently if this combination cannot be avoided. If barbiturates are combined with monoamine oxidase (MAO) inhibitors, increased serum levels and effects occur. If the older sedative–hypnotics are combined with MAO inhibitors, patients should be monitored closely and necessary dose adjustments made.

In addition, because of an enzyme induction effect of barbiturates in the liver the following drugs may not be as effective as desired: Oral anticoagulants, digoxin, tricyclic antidepressants, corticosteroids, oral contraceptives, estrogens, acetaminophen, metronidazole, carbamazepine, beta-blockers, griseofulvin, phenylbutazones, theophyllines, quinidine, and doxycycline. If these agents are given in combination with barbiturates, patients should be monitored closely; frequent dose adjustments may be necessary to achieve the desired therapeutic effect.

Ⓟ Prototype Summary: Phenobarbital

Indications: Sedation, short-term treatment of insomnia, long-term treatment of tonic–clonic seizures and cortical focal seizures, emergency control of certain acute convulsive episodes, preanesthetic.

Actions: Inhibits conduction in the ascending RAS; depresses the cerebral cortex; alters cerebellar function; depresses motor output; can produce excitation, sedation, hypnosis, anesthesia, and deep coma; and has anticonvulsant activity.

Pharmacokinetics:

Route	Onset	Onset	Peak
Oral	15 min	30–60 min	10–16 h
IM, subcutaneous		10–30 min	4–6 h
IV	Up to 15 min	5 min	4–6 h

$T_{1/2}$: 79 hours; metabolized in the liver, excreted in urine.

Adverse Effects: Somnolence, agitation, confusion, hyperkinesias, ataxia, vertigo, CNS depression, hallucinations, bradycardia, hypotension, syncope, nausea, vomiting, constipation, diarrhea, hypoventilation, apnea, withdrawal syndrome, rash, Stevens-Johnson syndrome.

Nursing Considerations for Patients Receiving Barbiturates

Assessment: History and Examination

- Assess for contraindications or cautions: Known allergies to barbiturates *to prevent hypersensitivity reactions* or a history of addiction to sedative–hypnotic drugs *to avert a similar problem with these drugs*; impaired hepatic or renal function *that could alter the metabolism and excretion of the drug;* cardiac dysfunction or respiratory dysfunction; seizure disorders, *which could be exacerbated by these drugs*; acute or chronic pain disorders, *which should be evaluated before using these drugs*; and pregnancy or lactation, *which would indicate a need for caution when using these drugs.*
- Assess for baseline status *before beginning therapy and for the occurrence of any potential adverse effects.* Assess the following: Temperature and weight; blood pressure and pulse, including perfusion; skin color and lesions; affect, orientation, and reflexes; respiratory rate and adventitious sounds; and bowel sounds.

Nursing Diagnoses

Nursing diagnoses related to drug therapy might include the following:

- Disturbed thought processes and disturbed sensory perception (visual, auditory, kinesthetic, tactile) related to CNS effects
- Risk for injury related to CNS effects
- Impaired gas exchange related to respiratory depression
- Deficient knowledge regarding drug therapy

Planning

- The patient will receive the best therapeutic effect from the drug therapy.
- The patient will have limited adverse effects to the drug therapy.
- The patient will have an understanding of the drug therapy, adverse effects to anticipate, and measures to relieve discomfort and improve safety.

Implementation with Rationale

- Do not administer these drugs intraarterially *because serious arteriospasm and gangrene could occur.* Monitor injection sites carefully *for local reactions.*
- Do not mix IV drugs in solution with any other drugs *to avoid potential drug–drug interactions.*
- Give parenteral forms only if oral forms are not feasible or available, and switch to oral forms as soon as possible *to avoid serious reactions or adverse effects.*
- Give IV medications slowly *because rapid administration may cause cardiac problems.*

- Provide standby life support facilities *in case of severe respiratory depression or hypersensitivity reactions.*
- Taper dose gradually after long-term therapy, especially in patients with epilepsy. Acute withdrawal *may precipitate seizures or cause withdrawal syndrome in these patients.*
- Provide comfort measures *to help patients tolerate drug effects,* including small, frequent meals; access to bathroom facilities; bowel program as needed; consuming food with the drug if GI upset is severe; and environmental control, safety precautions, orientation, and appropriate skin care as needed.
- Provide thorough patient teaching, including drug name, prescribed dosage, measures for avoidance of adverse effects, and warning signs that may indicate possible problems. Instruct patients about the need for periodic monitoring and evaluation *to enhance patient knowledge about drug therapy and to promote compliance.*
- Offer support and encouragement *to help the patient cope with the diagnosis and the drug regimen.*

Evaluation

- Monitor patient response to the drug (alleviation of signs and symptoms of anxiety, sleep, sedation, reduction in seizure activity).
- Monitor for adverse effects (sedation, hypotension, cardiac arrhythmias, hepatic or renal dysfunction, skin reactions, dependence).
- Evaluate the effectiveness of the patient-teaching plan (patient can give the drug name, dosage, possible adverse effects to watch for, specific measures to help avoid adverse effects, and the importance of continued follow-up).
- Monitor the effectiveness of comfort measures and compliance with the regimen.

KEY POINTS

- Barbiturates are an older class of drugs used as anxiolytics, sedatives, and hypnotics. Because they are associated with potentially serious adverse effects and interact with many other drugs, they are less desirable than the benzodiazepines or other anxiolytics.

Other Anxiolytic and Hypnotic Drugs

Other drugs are used to treat anxiety or to produce hypnosis that do not fall into either the benzodiazepine or the barbiturate group. See Table 20.3 for a list of other anxiolytic–hypnotic drugs, including usual indications and special considerations. Such medications include the following:

- Antihistamines (promethazine [generic], diphenhydramine [*Benadryl*]) can be very sedating in some people. They are used as preoperative medications and postoperatively to decrease the need for narcotics.
- Buspirone, a newer antianxiety agent, has no sedative, anticonvulsant, or muscle-relaxant properties, and its mechanism of action is unknown. However, it reduces the signs and symptoms of anxiety without many of the CNS effects and severe adverse effects associated with other anxiolytic drugs. It is rapidly absorbed from the GI tract, metabolized in the liver, and excreted in urine.
- Dexmedetomidine (*Precedex*) is given IV at a starting dose of 1 mcg/kg over 10 minutes and then a controlled infusion for up to 24 hours. It is used for the sedation of newly intubated and mechanically ventilated patients in an intensive care unit.
- Eszopiclone (*Lunesta*) is a newer agent used to treat insomnia. It is thought to react with GABA sites near benzodiazepine receptors. It is rapidly absorbed, metabolized in the liver, and excreted in the urine. It has been associated with "sleep driving" and other complex behaviors as well as next day sedation, memory loss, and loss of coordination. Because of these concerns the recommended starting dosage has been decreased.
- Meprobamate (generic) is an older drug that is used to manage acute anxiety for up to 4 months. It works in the limbic system and thalamus and has some anticonvulsant properties and CNS muscle-relaxing effects. It is rapidly absorbed and is metabolized in the liver and excreted in urine.
- Ramelteon (*Rozerem*) is the first of a new class of sedative–hypnotics, the melatonin receptor agonists. This drug stimulates melatonin receptors, which are thought to be involved in the maintenance of circadian rhythm and the sleep–wake cycle. Ramelteon is used for the treatment of insomnia characterized by difficulty with sleep onset. It is rapidly absorbed, with peak levels in 30 to 90 minutes. It is metabolized in the liver and excreted in the feces and urine.
- Suvorexant (*Belsomra*) was approved in 2014 and is one of a new class of drugs called orexin receptor antagonists. The orexin signaling system is thought to be a central promoter of wakefulness, and blocking these sites is thought to suppress the drive to wake up. It is absorbed quickly from the GI tract, reaching peak levels in 30 minutes to 2 hours. It is metabolized in the liver and excreted in the feces with a half-life of about 12 hours. It has been associated with "sleep driving" and other complex behaviors. The patient should be in bed within 30 minutes of taking the drug and plan to stay in bed for 7 hours, to decrease the safety risks of the CNS effects. It is used to treat insomnia.
- In 2014, tasimelteon (*Hetlioz*), another melatonin receptor agonist, was approved for the treatment on non–24-hour sleep–wake disorder, a common problem in patients with complete blindness who are not able

Table 20.3 *Drugs in Focus:* Other Anxiolytic/Hypnotic Drugs

Drug Name	Usual Indications/Dosage
buspirone (generic)	Oral drug for anxiety disorders, off-label use, signs and symptoms of premenstrual syndrome. Initially 7.5 mg PO b.i.d., titrate to usual range of 20–30 mg/d. *Special considerations:* May cause dry mouth, headache; use with caution in patients with hepatic or renal impairment and in elderly patients
dexmedetomidine (*Precedex*)	IV drug used for newly intubated and mechanically ventilated patients in the intensive care unit. 1 mcg/kg IV over 10 min then 0.2–0.7 mcg/kg/h IV using controlled infusion device for up to 24 h. *Special considerations:* Do not use longer than 24 h; monitor patient continually
diphenhydramine (*Benadryl*)	PO, IM, or IV for sleep aid, motion sickness, allergic rhinitis; oral drug for short-term treatment of insomnia (up to 1 wk). Oral, 25–50 mg PO q4–6 h; IV or IM, 10–50 mg; max 400 mg/d *Special considerations:* Antihistamine, drying effects common; monitor patients for thickened respiratory secretions and breathing difficulties, a problem that can cause concern after anesthesia
eszopiclone (*Lunesta*)	Oral drug for the treatment of insomnia 1 mg PO immediately before bed; max dose 3 mg *Special considerations:* Tablet must be swallowed whole; instruct the patient to take this drug just before bed and allow 8 h for sleep
meprobamate (generic)	Oral drug used for the short-term management of anxiety disorders. 1,200–1,600 mg/d PO in 3–4 divided doses *Special considerations:* Supervise dose in patients who are addiction prone, withdraw gradually over 2 wk if patient has been maintained on the drug for weeks or months
promethazine (*Phenergan*)	PO, IM, or IV use to decrease the need for postoperative pain relief and for preoperative sedation. 50 mg PO, IV, or IM *Special considerations:* An antihistamine; monitor injection sites carefully; monitor patients for thickened respiratory secretions and breathing difficulties, a problem that can cause concern after anesthesia
ramelteon (*Rozerem*)	Oral drug for the treatment of insomnia characterized by difficulty falling asleep. 8 mg PO within 30 min of bed *Special considerations:* Patient should take 30 min before bed and allow 8 h for sleep, monitor for depression and suicidal ideation
suvorexant (*Belsomra*)	Oral drug for treatment of insomnia with difficulty in sleep onset and/or sleep maintenance. 10 mg PO, max 20 mg/d *Special considerations:* Take only once a night; should be in bed within 30 min of dose and plan to stay there for 7 h. Safety issues during night of use and the next day as somnolence may persist.
tasimelteon (*Hetlioz*)	Oral drug for treatment of non–24-hour sleep–wake disorder. 20 mg/d PO at bedtime. *Special considerations:* Take at bedtime, the same time each night; can impair mental alertness, safety precautions required; may cause fetal harm
zaleplon (*Sonata*)	Oral drug for the short-term treatment of insomnia. 10 mg/d PO at bedtime. *Special considerations:* Patient should take before bed and devote 4–8 h to sleep; use with caution in patients with hepatic or renal impairment; elderly patients are especially sensitive to these drugs—administer a lower dose and monitor these patients carefully
zolpidem (*Ambien*)	Oral drug for short-term treatment of insomnia. 10 mg/d PO at bedtime *Special considerations:* Dispense the least amount possible to depressed and/or suicidal patients; withdraw gradually if used for prolonged period; patient should take before bed and devote 4–8 h to sleep; use with caution in patients with hepatic or renal impairment; elderly patients are especially sensitive to these drugs—administer a lower dose and monitor these patients carefully

to maintain circadian rhythm and the sleep–wake cycle because the retina does not experience light exposure. It is absorbed rapidly with peak levels in 30 to 180 minutes. It is metabolized in the tissues with a half-life of about 1.5 hours and is excreted in the urine.

- Zaleplon (*Sonata*) and zolpidem (*Ambien*), both of which cause sedation, are used for the short-term treatment of insomnia. They are thought to work by affecting serotonin levels in the sleep center near the RAS. These drugs are metabolized in the liver and excreted in the urine. They are also associated with "sleep driving" and other complex behaviors, and carry a warning about safety issues associated with these CNS effects.

SUMMARY

- Anxiolytics, or minor tranquilizers, are drugs used to treat anxiety by depressing the CNS. When given at higher doses, these drugs may be sedatives or hypnotics.
- Sedatives block the awareness of and reaction to environmental stimuli, resulting in associated CNS depression that may cause drowsiness, lethargy, and other effects. This action can be beneficial when a patient is very excited or afraid.
- Hypnotics further depress the CNS, particularly the RAS, to inhibit neuronal arousal and induce sleep.

- Benzodiazepines are a group of drugs used as anxiolytics. They react with GABA-inhibitory sites to depress the CNS. They can cause drowsiness, lethargy, and other CNS effects.
- Barbiturates are an older class of drugs used as anxiolytics, sedatives, and hypnotics. Because they are associated with potentially serious adverse effects and interact with many other drugs, they are less desirable than the benzodiazepines or other anxiolytics.
- Buspirone, another anxiolytic drug, does not cause sedation or muscle relaxation. Because of the absence of CNS effects, it is much preferred in certain circumstances (e.g., when a person must drive, go to work, or maintain alertness).
- Newer hypnotic agents act in the RAS to affect serotonin levels (zaleplon and zolpidem), affect melatonin levels in the brain (ramelteon, tasimelteon), or block orexin receptors (suvorexant).

CHECK YOUR UNDERSTANDING

Answers to the questions in this chapter can be found in Answers to Check Your Understanding Questions on thePoint®.

MULTIPLE CHOICE

Select the best answer to the following.

1. Drugs that are used to alter a patient's response to the environment are called
   a. hypnotics.
   b. sedatives.
   c. antiepileptics.
   d. anxiolytics.

2. The benzodiazepines are the most frequently used anxiolytic drugs because
   a. they are anxiolytic at doses much lower than those needed for sedation or hypnosis.
   b. they can also be stimulating.
   c. they are more likely to cause physical dependence than older anxiolytic drugs.
   d. they do not affect any neurotransmitters.

3. Barbiturates cause liver enzyme induction, which could lead to
   a. rapid metabolism and loss of effectiveness of other drugs metabolized by those enzymes.
   b. increased bile production.
   c. CNS depression.
   d. the need to periodically lower the barbiturate dose to avoid toxicity.

4. A person who could benefit from an anxiolytic drug for short-term treatment of insomnia would not be prescribed
   a. zolpidem.
   b. zaleplon.
   c. buspirone.
   d. meprobamate.

5. Anxiolytic drugs block the awareness of and reaction to the environment. This effect would not be beneficial
   a. to relieve extreme fear.
   b. to moderate anxiety related to unknown causes.
   c. in treating a patient who must drive a vehicle for a living.
   d. in treating a patient who is experiencing a stress reaction.

6. Mr. Jones is the chief executive officer of a large company and has been experiencing acute anxiety attacks. His physical examination was normal, and he was diagnosed with anxiety. Considering his occupation and his need to be alert and present to large groups on a regular basis the following anxiolytic would be a drug of choice for Mr. Jones:
   a. phenobarbital
   b. diazepam
   c. clorazepate
   d. buspirone

7. The benzodiazepines react with
   a. GABA receptor sites in the RAS to cause inhibition of neural arousal.
   b. norepinephrine receptor sites in the sympathetic nervous system.
   c. acetylcholine receptor sites in the parasympathetic nervous system.
   d. monoamine oxidase to increase norepinephrine breakdown.

8. A pediatric patient is prescribed phenobarbital preoperatively to relieve anxiety and produce sedation. After giving the injection, you should assess the patient for
a. acute Stevens-Johnson syndrome.
b. bone marrow depression.
c. paradoxical excitement.
d. withdrawal syndrome.

MULTIPLE RESPONSE

Select all that apply.

1. In assessing a client who is experiencing anxiety the nurse would expect to find which of the following?
a. Rapid breathing
b. Rapid heart rate
c. Fear and apprehension
d. Constricted pupils
e. Decreased abdominal sounds
f. Hypotension

2. Your client has a long history of anxiety and has always responded well to diazepam. She has just learned that she is pregnant and feels very anxious. She would like a prescription for diazepam to get her through her early anxiety. What rationale would the nurse use in explaining why this is not recommended?
a. This drug is known to cause a predictable syndrome of birth defects, including cleft lip and pyloric stenosis.
b. Babies born to mothers taking benzodiazepines may progress through a neonatal withdrawal syndrome.
c. Cardiac defects and small-brain development may occur if this drug is taken in the first trimester.
d. This drug almost always causes loss of the pregnancy.
e. The hormones the body produces during pregnancy will make you unresponsive to diazepam.
f. This drug could have adverse effects on your baby; we should explore nondrug measures to help you deal with the anxiety.

BIBLIOGRAPHY AND REFERENCES

Bemda, L., & Scates, A. (2010). Melatonin treatment for insomnia in pediatric patients with ADHD. *Annals of Pharmacotherapy, 44*, 185–191.

Brunton, L., Chabner, B., & Knollman, B. (2011). *Goodman and Gilman's the pharmacological basis of therapeutics* (12th ed.). New York: McGraw-Hill.

Facts and Comparisons. (2015). *Drug facts and comparisons*. St. Louis, MO: Author.

Facts and Comparisons. (2015). *Professional's guide to patient drug facts*. St. Louis, MO: Author.

Gotter, A. L., Garson, S. L., Stevens, J., et al. (2014). Differential sleep-promoting effects of dual orexin antagonists and GABA A receptor modulators. *BMC Neuroscience, 15*, 109.

Karch, A. M. (2014). *Lippincott's nursing drug guide*. Philadelphia, PA: Lippincott Williams & Wilkins.

Porth, C. M. (2013). *Pathophysiology: Concepts of altered health states* (9th ed.). Philadelphia, PA: Lippincott Williams & Wilkins.

Roy-Byrne, P., Craske, M., Sullivan, G., et al. (2010). Delivery of evidenced based treatment for multiple anxiety disorders in primary care. *Journal of the American Medical Association, 303*(19), 1921–1928.

Sangal, R. B., Bluhm, J. L., Lankford, D. A., et al. (2014). Eszopiclone for insomnia associated with ADHD. *Pediatrics, 134*(4), 1095–1103.

Sobonsky, J. (2015). Overview and management of anxiety disorders. *US Pharmacist, 39*(11), 56–62.

Torpy, J., Burke, A., & Golub, R. (2011). Generalized anxiety disorders. *Journal of the American Medical Association, 305*(5), 522.

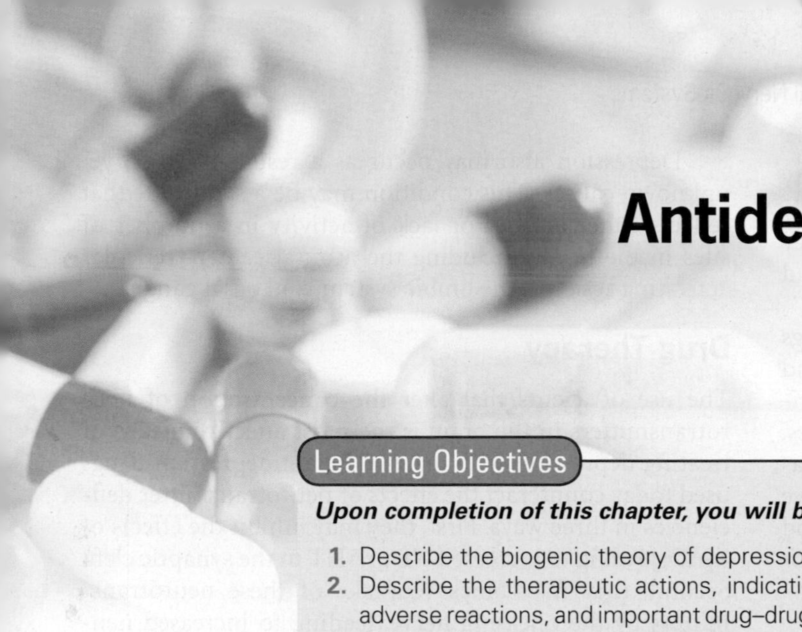

Antidepressant Agents 21

Learning Objectives

Upon completion of this chapter, you will be able to:

1. Describe the biogenic theory of depression.
2. Describe the therapeutic actions, indications, pharmacokinetics, contraindications, most common adverse reactions, and important drug–drug interactions associated with each class of antidepressant.
3. Discuss the use of antidepressants across the lifespan.
4. Compare and contrast the prototype drugs for each class of antidepressant with the other drugs in that class and with drugs in the other classes of antidepressants.
5. Outline the nursing considerations and teaching needs for patients receiving each class of antidepressant.

Glossary of Key Terms

affect: feeling that a person experiences when he or she responds emotionally to the environment

biogenic amine: one of the neurotransmitters norepinephrine, serotonin, or dopamine; it is thought that a deficiency of these substances in key areas of the brain results in depression

depression: affective disorder in which a person experiences sadness that is much more severe and longer lasting than is warranted by the event that seems to have precipitated it, with a more intense mood; the condition may not even be traceable to a specific event or stressor

monoamine oxidase inhibitor (MAOI): drug that prevents the enzyme monoamine oxidase from breaking down norepinephrine (NE), leading to increased NE levels in the synaptic cleft; relieves depression and also causes sympathomimetic effects

selective serotonin reuptake inhibitor (SSRI): drug that specifically blocks the reuptake of serotonin and increases its concentration in the synaptic cleft; relieves depression and is not associated with anticholinergic or sympathomimetic adverse effects

tricyclic antidepressants (TCAs): drug that blocks the reuptake of norepinephrine and serotonin; relieves depression and has anticholinergic and sedative effects

tyramine: an amine found in food that causes vasoconstriction and raises blood pressure; ingesting foods high in tyramine while taking an MAOI poses the risk of a severe hypertensive crisis

Drug List

Tricyclic Antidepressants
amitriptyline
amoxapine
clomipramine
desipramine
doxepin
(P) imipramine
maprotiline
nortriptyline
protriptyline
trimipramine

Monoamine Oxidase Inhibitors
isocarboxazid
(P) phenelzine
tranylcypromine

Selective Serotonin Reuptake Inhibitors
citalopram
escitalopram
(P) fluoxetine
fluvoxamine
paroxetine
sertraline
vilazodone
vortioxetine

Other Antidepressants
bupropion
desvenlafaxine
duloxetine
levomilnacipran
milnacipran
mirtazapine
nefazodone
selegiline
trazodone
venlafaxine

When you ask people how they feel, they may say "pretty good" or "not so great." People's responses are usually appropriate to what is happening in their lives, and they describe themselves as being in a good mood or a bad mood. Some days are better than others.

Affect is a term that is used to refer to people's feelings in response to their environment, whether positive and pleasant or negative and unpleasant. All people experience different affective states at various times in their lives. These states of mind, which change in particular situations, usually do not last very long and do not often involve extremes of happiness or depression. If a person's mood goes far beyond the usual normal "ups and downs," he or she is said to have an affective disorder.

Depression and Antidepressants

Depression is a very common affective disorder involving feelings of sadness that are much more severe and longer lasting than the suspected precipitating event, and the mood of affected individuals is much more intense. The depression may not even be traceable to a specific event or stressor (i.e., there are no external causes). Patients who are depressed may have little energy, sleep disturbances, a lack of appetite, limited libido, and inability to perform activities of daily living. They may describe overwhelming feelings of sadness, despair, hopelessness, and disorganization.

In many cases, the depression is never diagnosed, and the patient is treated for physical manifestations of the underlying disease, such as fatigue, malaise, obesity, anorexia, or alcoholism and drug dependence. Clinical depression is a disorder that can interfere with a person's family life, job, and social interactions. Left untreated, it can produce multiple physical problems that can lead to further depression or, in extreme cases, even suicide.

Biogenic Amine Theory of Depression

Research on the development of the drugs known to be effective in relieving depression led to formulation of the current hypothesis regarding the cause of depression. Scientists have theorized that depression results from a deficiency of **biogenic amines** in key areas of the brain; these biogenic amines include norepinephrine (NE), dopamine, and serotonin (5HT). Both NE and 5HT are released throughout the brain by neurons that react with multiple receptors to regulate arousal, alertness, attention, moods, appetite, and sensory processing. Deficiencies of these neurotransmitters may develop for three known reasons. First, monoamine oxidase (MAO) may break them down to be recycled or restored in the neurons. Second, rapid fire of the neurons may lead to their depletion. Third, the number or sensitivity of postsynaptic receptors may increase, thus depleting neurotransmitter levels.

Depression also may occur as a result of other, yet unknown causes. This condition may be a syndrome that reflects either activity or lack of activity in a number of sites in the brain, including the arousal center (reticular activating system), the limbic system, and basal ganglia.

Drug Therapy

The use of agents that alter the concentration of neurotransmitters in the brain is the most effective means of treating depression with drugs. The antidepressant drugs used today counteract the effects of neurotransmitter deficiencies in three ways. First, they may inhibit the effects of MAO, leading to increased NE or 5HT in the synaptic cleft. Second, they may block reuptake of these neurotransmitters by the releasing nerve, leading to increased neurotransmitter levels in the synaptic cleft. Third, they may regulate receptor sites and the breakdown of neurotransmitters, leading to an accumulation of neurotransmitter in the synaptic cleft.

Antidepressants may be classified into three groups: the tricyclic antidepressants (TCAs), the monoamine oxidase inhibitors (MAOIs), and the selective serotonin reuptake inhibitors (SSRIs). Other drugs that are used as antidepressants similarly increase the synaptic cleft concentrations of these neurotransmitters (Figure 21.1). For information on how antidepressants affect people from young to old see Box 21.1.

Tricyclic Antidepressants

The **tricyclic antidepressants (TCAs)**, including the amines, secondary amines, and tetracyclics, all reduce the reuptake of 5HT and NE into nerves. Because all TCAs are similarly effective the choice of TCA depends on individual response to the drug and tolerance of adverse effects. A patient who does not respond to one TCA may respond to another drug from this class. TCAs that are available include the amines amitriptyline (generic), amoxapine (generic), clomipramine (*Anafranil*), doxepin (generic), imipramine (*Tofranil*), and trimipramine (*Surmontil*); the secondary amines desipramine (*Norpramin*), nortriptyline (*Pamelor*), and protriptyline (*Vivactil*); and the tetracyclic drug maprotiline (generic). Table 21.1 shows the relative frequency of the occurrence of adverse effects by specific type of TCA.

Therapeutic Actions and Indications

The TCAs inhibit presynaptic reuptake of the neurotransmitters 5HT and NE, which leads to an accumulation of these neurotransmitters in the synaptic cleft and increased stimulation of the postsynaptic receptors. The exact mechanism of action in decreasing depression is not known but is thought to be related to the accumulation of NE and 5HT in certain areas of the brain.

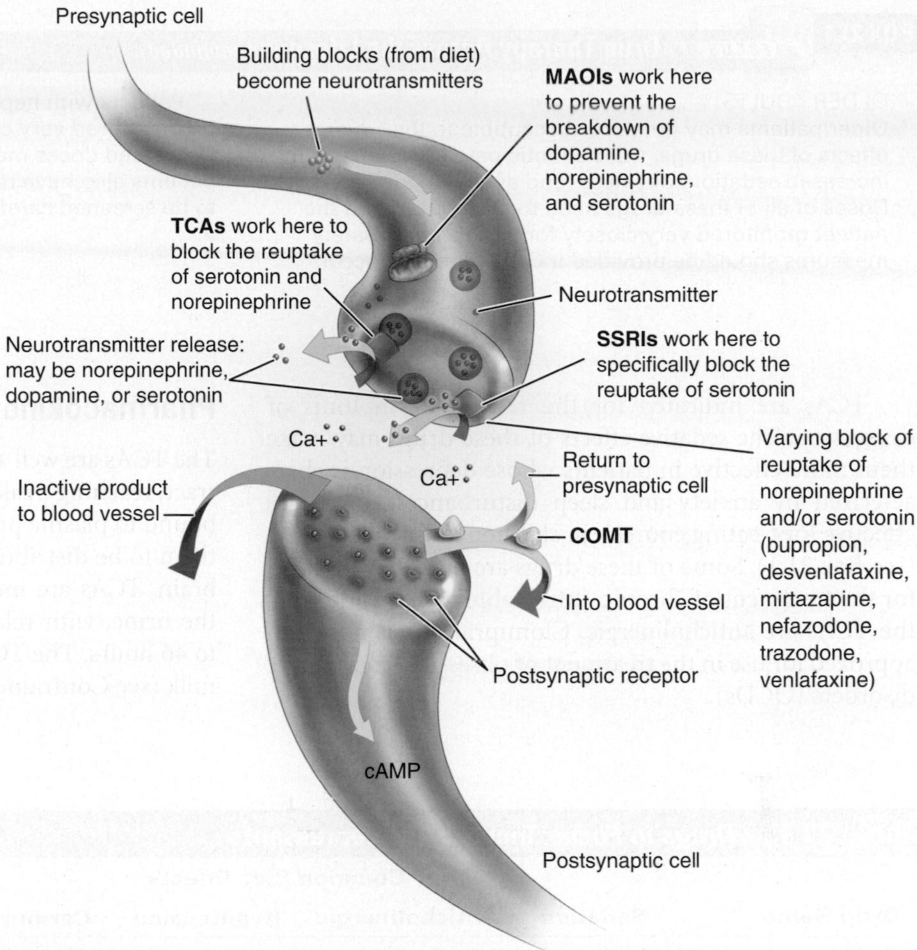

FIGURE 21.1 Sites of action for the antidepressants: monoamine oxidase inhibitors (MAOIs), tricyclic antidepressants (TCAs), selective serotonin reuptake inhibitors (SSRIs), and other agents. cAMP, cyclic adenosine monophosphate; COMT, catecholamine-*O*-methyltransferase.

BOX 21.1 FOCUS ON **Drug Therapy Across the Lifespan**

Antidepressant Agents

CHILDREN

Use of antidepressant drugs with children poses a challenge. The response of the child to the drug may be unpredictable, and the long-term effects of many of these agents are not clearly understood. Studies have not shown efficacy in using these drugs to treat depression in children and also indicate that there may be an increase in suicidal ideation and suicidal behavior when antidepressants are used to treat depression in children.

Of the tricyclic drugs (TCAs), clomipramine, imipramine, nortriptyline, and trimipramine have established pediatric doses in children older than 6 years. Children should be monitored closely for adverse effects, and dose changes should be made as needed.

MAOIs should be avoided in children if at all possible because of the potential for drug–food interactions and the serious adverse effects.

The SSRIs can cause serious adverse effects in children. Fluvoxamine and sertraline have established pediatric dose guidelines for the treatment of OCDs. Fluoxetine is widely used to treat depression in adolescents, and a 2000 survey of off-label uses of drugs showed that it was being used in children as young as 6 months. Dosage regimens must be established according to the child's age and weight, and a child receiving an antidepressant should be monitored very carefully. Underlying medical reasons for the depression should be ruled out before antidepressant therapy is begun. Again, these children should be monitored for any suicidal ideation.

ADULTS

Adults using these drugs should have medical causes for their depression ruled out before therapy is begun. Thyroid disease, hormonal imbalance, and CV disorders can all lead to the signs and symptoms of depression.

The patient needs to understand that the effects of drug therapy may not be seen for 4 weeks and that it is important to continue the therapy for at least that long.

These drugs should be used very cautiously during pregnancy and lactation because of the potential for adverse effects on the fetus and possible neurological, cardiac, and respiratory effects on the baby. Use should be reserved for situations in which the benefits to the mother far outweigh the potential risks to the neonate.

(continues on page 354)

BOX 21.1 FOCUS ON **Drug Therapy Across the Lifespan** *(continued)*

OLDER ADULTS

Older patients may be more susceptible to the adverse effects of these drugs, from unanticipated CNS effects to increased sedation, dizziness, and even hallucinations. Doses of all of these drugs need to be reduced and the patient monitored very closely for toxic effects. Safety measures should be provided if CNS effects do occur.

Patients with hepatic or renal impairment should be monitored very closely while taking these drugs. Decreased doses may be needed. Because many older patients also have renal or hepatic impairment, they need to be screened carefully.

TCAs are indicated for the relief of symptoms of depression. The sedative effects of these drugs may make them more effective in patients whose depression is characterized by anxiety and sleep disturbances. Some are effective for treating enuresis in children older than 6 years (see Box 21.1). Some of these drugs are being investigated for the treatment of chronic, intractable pain. In addition, the TCAs are anticholinergic. Clomipramine is now also approved for use in the treatment of obsessive–compulsive disorders (OCDs).

Pharmacokinetics

The TCAs are well absorbed from the gastrointestinal (GI) tract, reaching peak levels in 2 to 4 hours. They are highly bound to plasma proteins and are lipid soluble; this allows them to be distributed widely in the tissues, including the brain. TCAs are metabolized in the liver and excreted in the urine, with relatively long half-lives, ranging from 8 to 46 hours. The TCAs cross the placenta and enter breast milk (see Contraindications and Cautions).

Table 21.1 ***Drugs in Focus:*** **Tricyclic Antidepressants**

	Common Side Effects				
Drug Name	**Sedation**	**Anticholinergic**	**Hypotension**	**Cardiovascular**	**Usual Dosage**
Amines					
amitriptyline (generic)	+ + + +	+ + + +	+ + + +	+ +	75–150 mg/d PO
amoxapine (generic)	+	+	+ +	+ +	50–100 mg PO b.i.d. to t.i.d.
clomipramine (*Anafranil*)	+ + +	+ + +	+ + +	+ + +	*Adult:* 25–50 mg PO q.i.d. *Pediatric:* 25 mg PO q.i.d. to a maximum of 3 mg/kg/d
doxepin (generic)	+ + +	+ + +	+ +	+ +	25–50 mg PO t.i.d.
imipramine (*Tofranil*)	+ +	+ +	+ + +	+ +	*Adult:* 50–200 mg/d PO *Pediatric:* 30–40 mg/d PO
trimipramine (*Surmontil*)	+ + +	+ +	+ +	+ +	*Adult:* 75–150 mg/d PO *Pediatric:* 50 mg/d PO *Geriatric:* 50–100 mg/d PO
Secondary Amines					
desipramine (*Norpramin*)	+	+	+ +	+ +	100–200 mg/d PO
nortriptyline (*Aventyl, Pamelor*)	+	+	+	+	*Adult:* 25–50 mg PO t.i.d. to q.i.d. *Pediatric:* 30–50 mg/d PO in divided doses *Geriatric:* 30–50 mg/d PO in divided doses
protriptyline (*Vivactil*)	+	+ + +	+	+	15–40 mg/d PO in three or four divided doses, 5 mg PO t.i.d. for elderly patients
Tetracyclic					
maprotiline (generic)	+ +	+	+ +	+ +	75–150 mg/d PO, reduce dose in elderly patients

+ + + +, marked effects; + + +, moderate effects; + +, mild effects; +, negligible effects.

Contraindications and Cautions

One contraindication to the use of TCAs is the presence of allergy to any of the drugs in this class *because of the risk of hypersensitivity reactions*. Other contraindications include recent myocardial infarction *because of the potential occurrence of reinfarction or extension of the infarct with the cardiac effects of the drug*, myelography within the previous 24 hours or in the next 48 hours *because of a possible drug–drug interaction with the dyes used in these studies*, and concurrent use of an MAOI *because of the potential for serious adverse effects or toxic reactions*. In addition, pregnancy and lactation are contraindications *because of the potential for adverse effects in the fetus and neonate*; TCAs should not be used unless the benefit to the mother clearly outweighs the potential risk to the neonate.

TCAs should be used with caution in patients with preexisting cardiovascular (CV) disorders *because of the cardiac stimulatory effects of the drug* and with *any condition that would be exacerbated by the anticholinergic effects*, such as angle-closure glaucoma, urinary retention, prostate hypertrophy, or GI or genitourinary (GU) surgery. Care should also be taken with psychiatric patients, *who may exhibit a worsening of psychoses or paranoia*, and with manic–depressive patients, *who may shift to a manic stage*. There is a black box warning on all of the TCAs bringing attention to a risk of suicidality, especially in children, adolescents, and young adults; caution should be used, and the amount of drug dispensed at any given time should be limited with potentially suicidal patients. In addition, caution is necessary in patients with a history of seizures *because the seizure threshold may be decreased secondary to stimulation of the receptor sites* and in elderly patients. The presence of hepatic or renal disease, *which could interfere with metabolism and excretion of these drugs and lead to toxic levels*, also necessitates caution and the need for a lower dose of the drug.

Adverse Effects

The adverse effects of TCAs are associated with the effects of the drugs on the central nervous system (CNS) (Figure 21.2) and on the peripheral nervous system. Sedation, sleep disturbances, fatigue, hallucinations, disorientation, visual disturbances, difficulty in concentrating, weakness, ataxia, and tremors may occur.

Use of TCAs may lead to GI anticholinergic effects, such as dry mouth, constipation, nausea, vomiting, anorexia, increased salivation, cramps, and diarrhea. Resultant GU effects may include urinary retention and hesitancy, loss of libido, and changes in sexual functioning. CV effects such as orthostatic hypotension, hypertension, arrhythmias, myocardial infarction, angina, palpitations, and stroke may also pose problems. Miscellaneous reported effects include alopecia, weight gain or loss, flushing, chills, and nasal congestion.

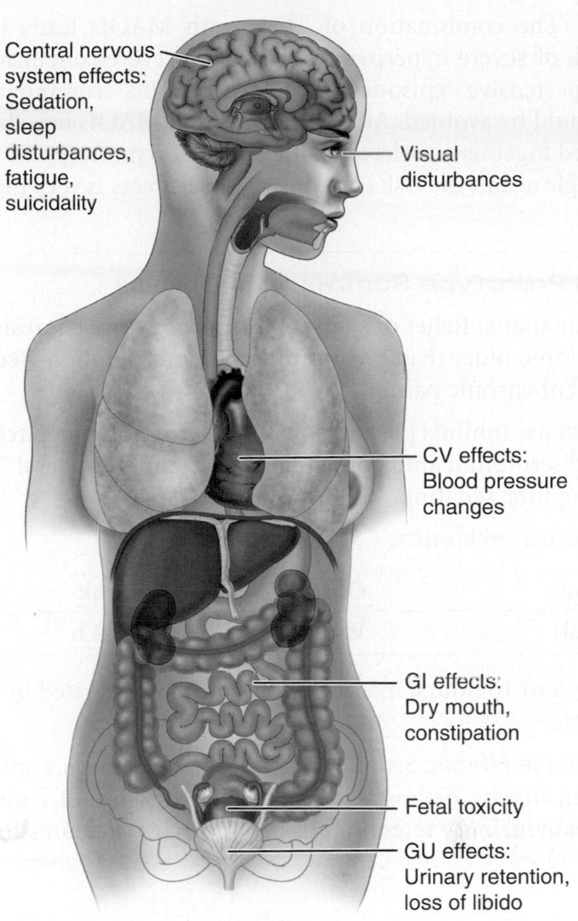

FIGURE 21.2 Variety of adverse effects and toxicities associated with antidepressants.

These adverse effects may be intolerable to some patients, who then stop taking the particular TCA. Abrupt cessation of all TCAs causes a withdrawal syndrome characterized by nausea, headache, vertigo, malaise, and nightmares.

Clinically Important Drug–Drug Interactions

If TCAs are given with cimetidine, fluoxetine, or ranitidine an increase in TCA levels results, with an increase in both therapeutic and adverse effects, especially anticholinergic conditions. Patients should be monitored closely, and appropriate dose reductions should be made.

Other drug combinations may also pose problems. The combination of TCAs and oral anticoagulants leads to higher serum levels of the anticoagulants and increased risk of bleeding. Blood tests should be done frequently, and appropriate dose adjustments in the oral anticoagulant should be made.

If TCAs are combined with sympathomimetics or clonidine the risk of arrhythmias and hypertension is increased. This combination should be avoided, especially in patients with underlying CV disease.

The combination of TCAs with MAOIs leads to a risk of severe hyperpyretic crisis with severe convulsions, hypertensive episodes, and death. This combination should be avoided. Although TCAs and MAOIs have been used together in selected patients who do not respond to a single agent, the risk of severe adverse effects is very high.

Ⓟ Prototype Summary: Imipramine

Indications: Relief of symptoms of depression; enuresis in children older than 6 years, off-label consideration—control of chronic pain.

Actions: Inhibits presynaptic reuptake of norepinephrine and serotonin; anticholinergic at CNS and peripheral receptors; sedating.

Pharmacokinetics:

Route	Onset	Peak
Oral	Varies	2–4 h

$T_{1/2}$: 8 to 16 hours; metabolized in the liver, excreted in the urine.

Adverse Effects: Sedation, anticholinergic effects, confusion, anxiety, orthostatic hypotension, dry mouth, constipation, urinary retention, rash, bone marrow depression.

Nursing Considerations for Patients Receiving Tricyclic Antidepressants

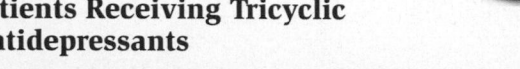

Assessment: History and Examination

- Assess for any known allergies to these drugs *to avoid hypersensitivity reactions*; impaired liver or kidney function, *which could alter metabolism and excretion of the drug*; glaucoma, benign prostatic hypertrophy, cardiac dysfunction, GI obstruction, surgery, or recent myocardial infarction, *all of which could be exacerbated by the effects of the drug*; and pregnancy or lactation *to avoid potential adverse effects on the fetus or baby*.
- Assess whether the patient has a history of seizure disorders or a history of psychiatric problems or suicidal thoughts, or myelography within the past 24 hours or in the next 48 hours, or is taking a MAOI, *to avoid potentially serious adverse reactions*.
- Assess temperature and weight; skin color and lesions; affect, orientation, and reflexes; vision; blood pressure, including orthostatic blood pressure; pulse and perfusion; respiratory rate and adventitious sounds; and bowel sounds on abdominal examination. *This determines baseline status before beginning therapy and for any potential adverse effects.* Also obtain an electrocardiogram as well as renal and liver function tests.

Nursing Diagnoses

Nursing diagnoses related to drug therapy might include the following:

- Acute pain related to anticholinergic effects, headache, and CNS effects
- Decreased cardiac output related to CV effects
- Disturbed thought processes and disturbed sensory perception (visual, auditory, kinesthetic, tactile, or olfactory) related to CNS effects
- Risk for injury related to CNS effects
- Deficient knowledge regarding drug therapy

Planning

- The patient will receive the best therapeutic effect from the drug therapy, relief of depression.
- The patient will have limited adverse effects to the drug therapy.
- The patient will have an understanding of the drug therapy, adverse effects to anticipate, and measures to relieve discomfort and improve safety.

Implementation with Rationale

- Limit drug access if the patient is suicidal *to decrease the risk of overdose to cause harm.*
- Maintain the initial dose for 4 to 8 weeks *to evaluate the therapeutic effect.*
- Administer parenteral forms of the drug only if oral forms are not feasible or available; switch to an oral form, *which is less toxic and associated with fewer adverse effects*, as soon as possible.
- Administer a major portion of the dose at bedtime if drowsiness and anticholinergic effects are severe *to decrease the risk of patient injury. Elderly patients may not be able to tolerate larger doses.*
- Reduce dose if minor adverse effects occur and discontinue the drug slowly if major or potentially life-threatening adverse effects occur *to ensure patient safety.*
- Provide comfort measures *to help the patient tolerate drug effects*. These measures may include voiding before dosing, instituting a bowel program as needed, taking food with the drug if GI upset is severe, and environmental control (lighting, temperature, stimuli).
- Provide thorough patient teaching, including drug name, prescribed dosage, measures for avoidance of adverse effects, and warning signs that may indicate possible problems. Instruct the patient about the need for periodic monitoring and evaluation *to enhance patient knowledge about drug therapy and to promote compliance.*

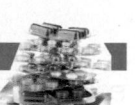

- Offer support and encouragement to help the patient cope with the diagnosis and the drug regimen.

Evaluation

- Monitor patient response to the drug (alleviation of signs and symptoms of depression).
- Monitor for adverse effects (sedation, anticholinergic effects, hypotension, cardiac arrhythmias, suicidal thoughts).
- Evaluate the effectiveness of the teaching plan (patient can give the drug name, dosage, possible adverse effects to watch for, specific measures to help avoid adverse effects, and importance of continued follow-up).
- Monitor the effectiveness of comfort measures and compliance with the regimen.

KEY POINTS

- Affect is a term that refers to the feelings that people experience when they respond emotionally.
- Depression is an affective disorder characterized by inappropriate sadness, despair, and hopelessness.
- According to the biogenic amine theory, depression is caused by a brain deficiency of the biogenic amines. Antidepressant drugs are thought to raise the level of the biogenic amines.

Monoamine Oxidase Inhibitors

Monoamine oxidase inhibitors (MAOIs) (Table 21.2) irreversibly inhibits MAO, an enzyme found in nerves and other tissues (including the liver), to break down the biogenic amines NE, dopamine, and 5HT and relieve depression. At one time, MAOIs were used more often, but now they are used rarely because they require a specific dietary regimen to prevent toxicity. There are some patients, however, who only seem to respond to these particular drugs, so they remain available. Agents still in use include isocarboxazid (*Marplan*), phenelzine (*Nardil*), and tranylcypromine (*Parnate*). The choice of an MAOI depends on the prescriber's experience and individual response. A patient who does not respond to one MAOI may respond to another.

Table 21.2 ***Drugs in Focus:* Monoamine Oxidase Inhibitors**

Drug Name	Dosage/Route	Usual Indications
isocarboxazid (*Marplan*)	10 mg PO b.i.d., may reach a maximum of 40 mg/d	Treatment of depression not responsive to other agents
phenelzine (*Nardil*)	15 mg PO t.i.d., maintenance 15 mg/d PO	Treatment of depression not responsive to other agents
tranylcypromine (*Parnate*)	30 mg/d PO in divided doses, maximum 60 mg/d	Treatment of adult reactive depression

Therapeutic Actions and Indications

Blocking the breakdown of the biogenic amines NE, dopamine, and 5HT allows these amines to accumulate in the synaptic cleft and in neuronal storage vesicles, causing increased stimulation of the postsynaptic receptors. It is thought that this increased stimulation of the receptors causes relief of depression. The MAOIs are generally indicated for treatment of the signs and symptoms of depression in patients who cannot tolerate or do not respond to other, safer antidepressants (see Table 21.2).

Pharmacokinetics

The MAOIs are well absorbed from the GI tract, reaching peak levels in 2 to 3 hours. They are metabolized in the liver primarily by acetylation and are excreted in the urine. Patients with liver or renal impairment and those known as "slow acetylators" may require lowered doses to avoid exaggerated effects of the drugs. The MAOIs cross the placenta and enter breast milk (see Contraindications and Cautions).

Contraindications and Cautions

Contraindications to the use of MAOIs include allergy to any of these antidepressants because of the risk of hypersensitivity reactions; pheochromocytoma because the sudden increases in NE levels could result in severe hypertension and CV emergencies; CV disease, including hypertension, coronary artery disease, angina, and congestive heart failure, which could be exacerbated by increased NE levels; and known abnormal CNS vessels or defects because the potential increase in blood pressure and vasoconstriction associated with higher NE levels could precipitate a stroke. A history of headaches may also be a contraindication.

Other contraindications include renal or hepatic impairment, *which could alter the metabolism and excretion of these drugs and lead to toxic levels*, and myelography within the past 24 hours or in the next 48 hours *because of the risk of severe reaction to the dye used in myelography*.

In addition, caution should be used with psychiatric patients, who could be overstimulated or shift to a manic phase as a result of the stimulation associated with MAOIs, and in patients with seizure disorders or hyperthyroidism, both of which could be exacerbated by the stimulation of these drugs. There is a black box warning on all drugs of this class to bring awareness to a possible risk of suicidality in

Table 21.3 Tyramine-Containing Foods

Foods High in Tyramine	Foods with Moderate Amounts of Tyramine	Foods with Low Amounts of Tyramine
Aged cheeses: cheddar cheese, blue cheese, Swiss cheese, Camembert Aged or fermented meats, fish, or poultry: Chicken paté, beef liver paté, caviar Brewer's yeast Fava beans Red wines: Chianti, burgundy, sherry, vermouth Smoked or pickled meats, fish, or poultry: Herring, sausage, corned beef, salami, pepperoni Soy sauce	Meat extracts: Consommé, bouillon Pasteurized light and pale beer Avocados	Distilled liquors: Vodka, gin, Scotch, rye Cheeses: American, mozzarella, cottage cheese, cream cheese Chocolate Fruits: Figs, raisins, grapes, pineapple, oranges Sour cream Yogurt

patients using these drugs, especially with children, adolescents, and young adults. Care should also be taken with patients who are soon to undergo elective surgery because of the potential for unexpected effects with NE accumulation during the stress reaction and with female patients who are pregnant or breastfeeding because of potential adverse effects on the fetus and neonate; these drugs should be used during pregnancy and lactation only if the benefit to the mother clearly outweighs the potential risk to the neonate.

Adverse Effects

The MAOIs are associated with some adverse effects, more of which are fatal, than most other antidepressants. The effects relate to the accumulation of NE in the synaptic cleft. Dizziness, excitement, nervousness, mania, hyperreflexia, tremors, confusion, insomnia, agitation, and blurred vision may occur.

MAOIs can cause liver toxicity. Other GI effects can include nausea, vomiting, diarrhea or constipation, anorexia, weight gain, dry mouth, and abdominal pain. Urinary retention, dysuria, incontinence, and changes in sexual function may also occur. CV effects can include orthostatic hypotension, arrhythmias, palpitations, angina, and the potentially fatal hypertensive crisis. This last condition is characterized by occipital headache, palpitations, neck stiffness, nausea, vomiting, sweating, dilated pupils, photophobia, tachycardia, and chest pain. It may progress to intracranial bleeding and fatal stroke.

Clinically Important Drug–Drug Interactions

Drug interactions of MAOIs with other antidepressants include hypertensive crisis, coma, and severe convulsions with TCAs, and a potentially life-threatening serotonin syndrome with SSRIs. A period of 6 weeks should elapse after stopping an SSRI before beginning therapy with an MAOI.

If MAOIs are given with other sympathomimetic drugs (e.g., methyldopa), sympathomimetic effects increase. Combinations with insulin or oral antidiabetic agents result in additive hypoglycemic effects. Patients who receive these combinations must be monitored closely, and appropriate dose adjustments should be made.

Clinically Important Drug–Food Interactions

Tyramine and other pressor amines that are found in food, which are normally broken down by MAO enzymes in the GI tract, may be absorbed in high concentrations in the presence of MAOIs, resulting in increased blood pressure. In addition, tyramine causes the release of stored NE from nerve terminals, which further contributes to high blood pressure and hypertensive crisis. Patients who take MAOIs should avoid the tyramine-containing foods listed in Table 21.3.

Prototype Summary: Phenelzine

Indications: Treatment of patients with depression who are unresponsive to other antidepressive therapy or in whom other antidepressive therapy is contraindicated.

Actions: Irreversibly inhibits MAO, allowing norepinephrine, 5HT, and dopamine to accumulate in the synaptic cleft; this accumulation is thought to be responsible for the clinical effects.

Pharmacokinetics:

Route	Onset	Duration
Oral	Slow	48–96 h

$T_{1/2}$: Unknown; metabolized in the liver, excreted in the urine.

Adverse Effects: Dizziness, vertigo, headache, overactivity, hyperreflexia, tremors, mania, weakness, drowsiness, fatigue, sweating, orthostatic hypotension, constipation, diarrhea, dry mouth, edema, anorexia, potential for hypertensive crisis.

Nursing Considerations for Patients Receiving Monoamine Oxidase Inhibitors

Assessment: History and Examination

- Assess for any known allergies to these drugs to avoid hypersensitivity reactions; impaired liver or kidney function that could alter the metabolism and excretion of the drug; cardiac dysfunction; GI or GU obstruction, which could be exacerbated by the drug; surgery, including elective surgery, because the effects of changes in norepinephrine levels are unpredictable following surgery; seizure disorders; psychiatric conditions or suicidality; and occurrence of myelography within the past 24 hours or in the next 48 hours to avoid the possibility of severe reactions.
- Determine whether female patients are pregnant or breastfeeding because these drugs should not be used during pregnancy or lactation.
- Assess temperature and weight; skin color and lesions; affect, orientation, and reflexes; vision; blood pressure, including orthostatic blood pressure; pulse and perfusion; respiratory rate and adventitious sounds; and bowel sounds on abdominal examination *to determine baseline status and for any potential adverse effects before beginning therapy*. Also obtain an electrocardiogram and renal and liver function tests.

Nursing Diagnoses

Nursing diagnoses related to drug therapy might include the following:

- Acute pain related to sympathomimetic effects, headache, and CNS effects
- Decreased cardiac output related to CV effects
- Disturbed thought processes and disturbed sensory perception (visual, kinesthetic) related to CNS effects
- Risk for injury related to CNS effects
- Deficient knowledge regarding drug therapy

Planning

- The patient will receive the best therapeutic effect from the drug therapy, relief of depression.
- The patient will have limited adverse effects to the drug therapy.
- The patient will have an understanding of the drug therapy, adverse effects to anticipate, and measures to relieve discomfort and improve safety

Implementation with Rationale

- Limit drug access to a potentially suicidal patient *to decrease the risk of overdose.*
- Monitor the patient for 2 to 4 weeks to ascertain the onset of the full therapeutic effect.
- Monitor blood pressure and orthostatic blood pressure carefully to arrange for a slower increase in dose as needed for patients who show a tendency toward hypotension.
- Monitor liver function before and periodically during therapy and *arrange to discontinue the drug at the first sign of liver toxicity.*
- Discontinue drug and monitor the patient carefully at any complaint of severe headache *to decrease the risk of severe hypertension and cerebrovascular effects.*
- Have phentolamine or another adrenergic blocker on standby *as treatment in case of hypertensive crisis.*
- Provide comfort measures *to help the patient tolerate drug effects.* These include voiding before dosing, instituting a bowel program as needed, taking food with the drug if GI upset is severe, and environmental control (lighting, temperature, decreased stimulation).
- Provide a list of potential drug–food interactions that can cause severe toxicity *to decrease the risk of a serious drug–food interaction.* Provide a diet that is low in tyramine-containing foods.
- Provide thorough patient teaching, including drug name, prescribed dosage, measures for avoidance of adverse effects, and warning signs that may indicate possible problems. Instruct the patient about the need for periodic monitoring and evaluation *to enhance patient knowledge about drug therapy and to promote compliance.*
- Offer support and encouragement to help the patient cope with the disease and the drug regimen.

Evaluation

- Monitor patient response to the drug (alleviation of signs and symptoms of depression).
- Monitor for adverse effects (sedation, sympathomimetic effects, hypotension, cardiac arrhythmias, GI disturbances, hypertensive crisis).
- Evaluate the effectiveness of the teaching plan (patient can give the drug name, dosage, possible adverse effects to watch for, specific measures to help avoid adverse effects, importance of continued follow-up, and importance of avoiding foods high in tyramine).
- Monitor the effectiveness of comfort measures and compliance with the regimen.

KEY POINTS

- The MAOIs prevent the breakdown of NE and 5HT by MAO, leading to an increased level of these biogenic amines in the synaptic cleft. This accumulation of the amines is thought to relieve the signs and symptoms of depression.
- Patients taking MAOIs need to avoid foods high in tyramine to prevent serious increases in blood pressure and hypertensive crises.

Selective Serotonin Reuptake Inhibitors

Selective serotonin reuptake inhibitors (SSRIs) (Table 21.4), the newest group of antidepressant drugs, specifically block the reuptake of 5HT, with little to no known effect on NE. Because SSRIs do not have the many adverse effects associated with TCAs and MAOIs, they are a better choice for many patients. SSRIs include fluoxetine (*Prozac*), the first SSRI; citalopram (*Celexa*); escitalopram (*Lexapro*); fluvoxamine (*Luvox*); paroxetine (*Paxil*); sertraline (*Zoloft*); vilazodone (*Viibryd*); and vortioxetine (*Brintellix*).

Therapeutic Actions and Indications

The action of SSRIs blocking the reuptake of 5HT increases the levels of 5HT in the synaptic cleft and may contribute to the antidepressant and other effects attributed to these drugs.

SSRIs are indicated for the treatment of depression, OCDs, panic attacks, bulimia, premenstrual dysphoric disorder (PMDD), posttraumatic stress disorders, social phobias, and social anxiety disorders. A period of up to 4 weeks is necessary for realization of the full therapeutic effect. Patients may respond well to one SSRI and yet show little or no response to another one. The choice of drug depends on the indications and individual response. Box 21.2 provides more information. Ongoing investigations are focusing on the use of these antidepressant drugs in the treatment of other psychiatric disorders (see Table 21.4).

Pharmacokinetics

The SSRIs are well absorbed from the GI tract, metabolized in the liver, and excreted in the urine and feces. The half-life varies widely with the drug being used.

Contraindications and Cautions

The SSRIs are contraindicated in the presence of allergy to any of these drugs *because of the risk of hypersensitivity reactions.* Caution should be used in patients with impaired renal or hepatic function *that could alter the metabolism and excretion of the drug, leading to toxic effects*, or with diabetes, *which could be exacerbated by the stimulating effects of these drugs.* Caution should also be used with severely depressed or suicidal patients, especially children, adolescents, and young adults *because of a risk of increased*

Table 21.4 ***Drugs in Focus:* Selective Serotonin Reuptake Inhibitors**

Drug Name	Dosage/Route	Usual Indications
citalopram (*Celexa*)	20 mg/d PO b.i.d., up to 40 mg/d may be needed	Treatment of depression in adults has also been used to treat panic disorder, PMDD, OCDs, social phobias, trichotillomania, and posttraumatic stress disorders
escitalopram (*Lexapro*)	10 mg/d PO as a single dose, 10–20 mg/d PO maintenance	Treatment of major depressive disorder, maintenance of patients with major depressive disorder and generalized anxiety disorder
fluoxetine (Prozac, Sarafem)	20 mg/d PO in the AM; do not exceed 60 mg/d; reduce dose with hepatic impairment; also available in a 90-mg, once-a-week formulation	Treatment of depression, bulimia, OCDs, panic disorders, PMDD in adults; also under investigation for treatment of other psychiatric disorders, including obesity, alcoholism, chronic pain, and various neuropathies
fluvoxamine (*Luvox*)	*Adult:* 50 mg PO at bedtime to a maximum of 300 mg/d; reduce dose with hepatic impairment *Pediatric (8–17 y):* 25 mg PO at bedtime; do not exceed 250 mg/d	Treatment of OCDs; also under investigation for treatment of depression, bulimia, panic disorder, and social phobia
paroxetine (*Paxil*)	10–20 mg/d PO, do not exceed 50 mg/d, *or* 62.5 mg/d controlled release tablets; reduce dose in hepatic or renal dysfunction and with the elderly	Treatment of depression, OCDs, PMDD, posttraumatic stress reaction, social anxiety disorders, general anxiety disorders, and various panic disorders in adults; also under investigation for treatment of chronic headache, diabetic neuropathy, and hot flashes
sertraline (*Zoloft*)	*Adult:* 25–50 mg/d PO; reduce dose with hepatic dysfunction, OCD *Pediatric:* 25–50 mg/d PO based on age and severity of OCD	Treatment of depression, OCDs, social anxiety disorder, posttraumatic stress disorder, panic disorders, PMDD
vilazodone (*Viibryd*)	10 mg/d PO for 7 d, followed by 20 mg/d for 7 d, then the maintenance dose of 40 mg/d PO taken with food	Treatment of adult patients with major depressive disorder
vortioxetine (*Brintellix*)	10–20 mg/d PO as tolerated	Treatment of adult patients with major depressive disorder

PMDD, premenstrual dysphoric disorder; OCDs, obsessive–compulsive disorders.

BOX 21.2 FOCUS ON Cultural Considerations

The Popularity of Prozac

A rise in the diagnosis of depression began in the 1990s, with that decade's fast-paced lifestyle, high-stress jobs, explosion of information, and rapid change. Many people who have high expectations of both themselves and others are overworked and overstimulated to a point at which they become clinically depressed.

There is now a selection of relatively safe and nontoxic drugs that can be used to treat depression—SSRIs. For several years, the SSRIs remained in the top-selling category of prescription drugs. Fluoxetine (*Prozac*), in particular, has been the subject of numerous talk shows, books, and movies. In many ways, *Prozac* was the "in" drug of the 1990s. This societal phenomenon put pressure on health care providers to prescribe a drug even if it was not appropriate to a given patient's situation. In some instances, patients just wanted the drug that helped their friend. They may not have been willing to listen to their health care provider or to take the time to be properly diagnosed; they just wanted an SSRI. *Prozac* is not the solution to everyone's problem, and it is often difficult to explain this fact to a patient. It also may be hard to get the patient to understand that this drug is not a quick fix; it takes 4 to 6 weeks to achieve full therapeutic effectiveness. Fortunately, the SSRIs have the least adverse effects of the antidepressants, and such fads usually pass in a few years.

It is important to remember the powerful effects of the media on health care–seeking behavior. As more and more drugs are advertised in magazines and on television, patients are becoming aware of options and "cures" that they might like to try. Patient education is a tricky yet important part of any health care intervention and an extremely important aspect of health care in our society.

suicidality. The *SSRIs have been associated with congenital abnormalities in animal studies* and should be used during pregnancy only if the benefits to the mother clearly outweigh the potential risks to the fetus. Recent reports have linked use of SSRIs during pregnancy with pulmonary and cardiac problems in the newborn. The SSRIs enter breast milk and can cause adverse effects in the baby, so a different method of feeding the baby should be selected if an SSRI is required by the mother.

Adverse Effects

The adverse effects associated with SSRIs, which are related to the effects of increased 5HT levels, include CNS effects such as headache, drowsiness, dizziness, insomnia, anxiety, activation of mania/hypomania, tremor, agitation, and seizures. GI effects such as nausea, vomiting, diarrhea, dry mouth, anorexia, constipation, and changes in taste often occur, as do GU effects, including painful menstruation, cystitis, sexual dysfunction, urgency, and impotence. Respiratory changes may include cough, dyspnea, upper respiratory infections, and pharyngitis. SSRIs may also cause serious intraocular pressure changes if used in patients with untreated narrow-angle glaucoma. Other reported effects are sweating, rash, fever, and pruritus. Recent studies have linked the incidence of suicidal ideation and suicide attempts to the use of these drugs in pediatric patients and adolescents (see Box 21.3).

Clinically Important Drug–Drug Interactions

Because of the risk of serotonin syndrome if SSRIs are used with MAOIs, this combination should be avoided,

BOX 21.3 FOCUS ON The Evidence

Childhood Suicide and Antidepressants

The Food and Drug Administration (FDA) issued a talk paper in late spring 2003 after reports from the British press cited an increase in suicidal behavior in children being treated with paroxetine (*Paxil*). The FDA compiled a review of reports for eight different antidepressant drugs—citalopram, fluoxetine, fluvoxamine, mirtazapine, nefazodone, paroxetine, sertraline, and venlafaxine—that were being studied for use in pediatric populations.

The data from these studies did not clearly establish a link between increased suicidal ideation and the use of these antidepressants, but the data also did not establish effectiveness in major depressive disorder in children for any of the drugs, except fluoxetine. Many journals and news reports have discussed an increase in suicide attempts and completed suicides in pediatric patients being treated with antidepressants. Many anecdotal reports have been submitted to MedWatch reporting the same events. The FDA points out, however, that these reports are hard to interpret and, without a control group, it is difficult to know whether these effects are also seen in this age group of children even when they are not being treated with antidepressants. In 20 placebo-controlled studies involving these eight drugs and more than 4,100 pediatric patients, there were no reports of completed suicides.

In fall 2004 the FDA issued an advisory to all prescribers noting the studies that had been done and concluding that there was not enough evidence at that point that suicidal ideation was inherent to many major depressive disorders. In 2006 a black box warning was added to all antidepressants bringing attention to the increase in suicidality, especially in children and adolescents, when these drugs were used. All of these drugs should be used with caution, prescriptions should be written in the smallest quantity feasible, and parents should be educated about the warning signs of suicide. Continued research is being carried out to study the actual cause-and-effect relation. The FDA has issued guidelines based on a review of all studies. See http://www.drugwatch.com/ssri/fda-warnings/

Box 21.4 FOCUS ON Herbal and Alternative Therapies

Patients being treated with SSRIs are at an increased risk of developing a severe reaction, including serotonin syndrome, as well as an increased sensitivity to light if they are also taking St. John's wort. Because this herbal therapy is often used to self-treat depression, it is important to forewarn any patient who is taking an SSRI not to combine it with taking St. John's wort.

Also caution patients that there is an increased risk of seizures if evening primrose is used with antidepressants, and patients should be cautioned against this combination. Interactions have also been reported when antidepressants are combined with ginkgo, ginseng, and valerian. Patients should be cautioned against using these herbs while taking antidepressants.

and at least 2 to 4 weeks should be allowed between use of the two types of drugs if switching from one to the other. In addition, the use of SSRIs with TCAs results in increased therapeutic and toxic effects. If these combinations are used, patients should be monitored closely, and appropriate dose adjustments should be made. Serotonin syndrome, a serious to potentially fatal reaction, can occur if these drugs are combined with any drug or herb that increases 5HT levels—other SSRIs, serotonin–norepinephrine reuptake inhibitors (SNRIs), St. John's wort, triptans. There is an increased risk of bleeding if these drugs are combined with aspirin, nonsteroidal anti-inflammatory drugs (NSAIDs), antiplatelet drugs, or drugs that affect coagulation. For more information see Box 21.4.

Ⓟ Prototype Summary: Fluoxetine

Indications: Treatment of depression, OCDs, bulimia, premenstrual dysphoric disorder, panic disorders; off-label uses include chronic pain, alcoholism, neuropathies, obesity.

Actions: Inhibits CNS neuronal reuptake of 5HT, with little effect on NE and little affinity for cholinergic, histaminic, or alpha-adrenergic sites.

Pharmacokinetics:

Route	Onset	Peak
Oral	Slow	6–8 h

$T_{1/2}$: 2 to 4 weeks; metabolized in the liver, excreted in the urine and feces.

Adverse Effects: Headache, nervousness, insomnia, drowsiness, anxiety, tremor, dizziness, sweating, rash, nausea, vomiting, diarrhea, dry mouth, anorexia, sexual dysfunction, upper respiratory infections, weight loss, fever.

Nursing Considerations for Patients Receiving Selective Serotonin Reuptake Inhibitors

Assessment: History and Examination

- Assess for any known allergies to SSRIs *to avoid hypersensitivity reactions*; severe depression or suicidality, angle-closure glaucoma, bipolar disorder, *which could be exacerbated by these drugs*; impaired liver or kidney function, *which could alter metabolism and excretion of the drug*; and diabetes mellitus. Find out whether female patients are pregnant or breastfeeding *because caution should be used in these situations and drug use limited.*
- Assess temperature and weight; skin color and lesions; affect, orientation, and reflexes; vision; blood pressure and pulse; respiratory rate and adventitious sounds; and bowel sounds on abdominal examination *for baseline status before beginning therapy and for any potential adverse effects.* Also obtain renal and liver function tests.

Refer to Critical Thinking Scenario for a full discussion of nursing care for a patient who is dealing with depression.

Nursing Diagnoses

Nursing diagnoses related to drug therapy might include the following:

- Acute pain related to GI, GU, and CNS effects
- Disturbed thought processes and disturbed sensory perception (kinesthetic, tactile) related to CNS effects
- Imbalanced nutrition related to GI effects
- Deficient knowledge regarding drug therapy

Planning

- The patient will receive the best therapeutic effect from the drug therapy, relief of depression.
- The patient will have limited adverse effects to the drug therapy.
- The patient will have an understanding of the drug therapy, adverse effects to anticipate, and measures to relieve discomfort and improve safety

Implementation with Rationale

- Arrange for lower dose in elderly patients and in those with renal or hepatic impairment *because of the potential for severe adverse effects.*
- Monitor the patient for up to 4 weeks to ascertain the onset of full therapeutic effect before adjusting dose.
- Establish suicide precautions for severely depressed patients and limit the quantity of the drug dispensed *to decrease the risk of overdose to cause harm.*
- Administer the drug once a day in the morning *to achieve optimal therapeutic effects.* If dose is increased

or if the patient is having severe GI effects the dose can be divided. Serious name confusion has been reported with some of the SSRIs.

- Suggest that the patient use barrier contraceptives to prevent pregnancy while taking this drug because serious fetal abnormalities can occur.
- Provide comfort measures *to help the patient tolerate drug effects.* These may include voiding before dosing, instituting a bowel program as needed, taking food with the drug if GI upset is severe, or environmental control (lighting, temperature, stimuli).
- Provide thorough patient teaching, including the drug name, prescribed dosage, measures for avoidance of adverse effects, and warning signs that may indicate possible problems. Instruct patients about the need for periodic monitoring and evaluation *to enhance patient knowledge about drug therapy and to promote compliance.*
- Offer support and encouragement to help the patient cope with the disease and the drug regimen.

Evaluation

- Monitor patient response to the drug (alleviation of signs and symptoms of depression, OCD, bulimia, panic disorder).
- Monitor for adverse effects (sedation, dizziness, GI upset, respiratory dysfunction, GU problems, skin rash).
- Evaluate the effectiveness of the teaching plan (patient can give the drug name, dosage, possible adverse effects to watch for, specific measures to help avoid adverse effects, importance of continued follow-up, and importance of avoiding pregnancy).
- Monitor the effectiveness of comfort measures and compliance with the regimen.

CRITICAL THINKING SCENARIO

Selective Serotonin Reuptake Inhibitors

THE SITUATION

D.J., a 46-year-old married woman, complains of weight gain, malaise, fatigue, sleeping during the day, loss of interest in daily activities, and bouts of crying for no apparent reason. On examination, she weighs 8 pounds more than the standard weight for her height; all other findings are within normal limits. In conversation with a nurse, D.J. says that in the past 10 months several events have occurred. She lost both of her parents, her only child graduated from high school and went away to college, her nephew died of renal failure, her one sister learned she had metastatic breast cancer, and she lost her job as a day care provider when the client family moved out of town. In addition, the family cat of 17 years was diagnosed with terminal leukemia. D.J. is prescribed fluoxetine (*Prozac*) and is given an appointment with a counselor.

Critical Thinking

What nursing interventions are appropriate at this time?

What sort of crisis intervention would be most appropriate? Balance the benefits of pointing out all of the losses and points of grief that you detect in D.J.'s story with the risks of upsetting her strained coping mechanisms.

What can D.J. expect to experience as a result of the SSRI therapy?

How can you help D.J. cope during the lengthy period it takes to reach therapeutic effects?

What other future interventions should be planned with D.J.?

DISCUSSION

Many patients in severe crisis do not consciously identify the many things that are causing them stress. They have developed coping mechanisms to help them survive and cope with their day-to-day activities. However, D.J. seems to have reached her limit, and she exhibits many of the signs and symptoms of depression. However, it is important to make sure that she does not have some underlying medical condition that could be contributing to her complaints. Because of her age, she may also be perimenopausal, which could account for some of her problems.

It is hoped that the fluoxetine, an SSRI, will enable D.J. to regain her ability to cope and her normal affect. The drug should give her brain a chance to reach a new biochemical balance. Before she begins taking the fluoxetine, she should receive a written sheet listing the pertinent drug information, adverse effects to watch for, warning signs to report, and a telephone number to call in case she has questions later or just needs to talk. The written information is especially important because she may not remember drug-related discussions or instructions clearly.

(continues on page 364)

Selective Serotonin Reuptake Inhibitors (continued)

Once the SSRI reaches therapeutic levels, which can take as long as 4 weeks, D.J. may start to feel like her "old self" and may be strong enough to begin dealing with all her grief. She may recover from her need for the SSRI over time and use of the medication can then be discontinued.

NURSING CARE GUIDE FOR D.J.: FLUOXETINE

Assessment: History and Examination

Allergies to fluoxetine or any other antidepressant SSRI, renal or hepatic dysfunction, pregnancy or lactation, diabetes

Concurrent use of tricyclic antidepressants, cyproheptadine, lithium, MAOIs, benzodiazepines, alcohol, other SSRIs

CV: Blood pressure, pulse

CNS: Orientation, affect, reflexes, vision

Skin: Color, lesions, texture

Respiratory: Respiration, adventitious sounds

GI: Abdominal examination, bowel sounds

Laboratory tests: Hepatic and renal function tests

Nursing Diagnoses

Acute pain related to GI, GU, CNS effects

Disturbed thought processes related to CNS effects

Imbalanced nutrition related to GI effects

Deficient knowledge regarding drug therapy

Planning

The patient will receive the best therapeutic effect from the drug therapy.

The patient will have limited adverse effects to the drug therapy.

The patient will have an understanding of the drug therapy, adverse effects to anticipate, and measures to relieve discomfort and improve safety.

Implementation

Administer drug in morning; divide doses if GI upset occurs.

Provide comfort, safety measures; small meals; void before dosing; side rails; pain medication as needed; suggest barrier contraceptive; limit dosage with potentially suicidal patients; lower dose with renal or hepatic impairment.

Provide support and reassurance to help D.J. deal with drug effects (4-week delay in full effectiveness).

Provide patient teaching regarding drug dosage, adverse effect conditions to report, and the need to use barrier contraceptives.

Evaluation

Evaluate drug effects: Relief of signs and symptoms of depression.

Monitor for adverse effects: Sedation, dizziness, insomnia; respiratory dysfunction; GI upset; GU problems; rash.

Monitor for drug–drug interactions.

Evaluate effectiveness of patient-teaching program.

Evaluate effectiveness of comfort and safety measures.

PATIENT TEACHING FOR D.J.

- The drug that has been prescribed is called a selective serotonin reuptake inhibitor, or SSRI. SSRIs change the concentration of 5HT in specific areas of the brain. An increase in 5HT level is believed to relieve depression.
- The drug should be taken once a day in the morning. If your dosage has been increased or if you are having stomach upset the dose may be divided.
- It may take as long as 4 weeks before you feel the full effects of this drug. Continue to take the drug every day during that time so that the concentration of the drug in your body eventually reaches effective levels.
- Common side effects of SSRIs include the following:
  - *Dizziness, drowsiness, nervousness, and insomnia*: If these effects occur, avoid driving or performing hazardous or delicate tasks that require concentration.
  - *Nausea, vomiting, and weight loss*: Small frequent meals may help. Monitor your weight loss; if it becomes excessive, consult your health care provider.
  - *Sexual dysfunction and flu-like symptoms*: These effects may be temporary. Consult with your health care provider if these conditions become bothersome.
  - Report any of the following conditions to your health care provider: Rash mania, seizures, and severe weight loss, increasing depression or thoughts of suicide.
- Tell your doctors, nurses, and other health care providers that you are taking this drug. Keep this drug and all medications out of the reach of children and pets. Do not take this drug during pregnancy because severe fetal abnormalities could occur. The use of barrier contraceptives is recommended while you are taking this drug. If you think that you are pregnant or would like to become pregnant, consult with your health care provider.

KEY POINTS

- The SSRIs prevent the reuptake of serotonin into the presynaptic nerve, leading to an accumulation of these biogenic amines in the synaptic cleft. This accumulation causes increased stimulation of the postsynaptic nerve and may be responsible for the antidepressant effects of these drugs.
- The SSRIs are not associated with many of the CNS, CV, and anticholinergic effects of other antidepressants.
- Combination of SSRIs with other SSRIs or with other drugs that are known to increase 5HT levels increase the risk of serotonin syndrome.
- Increased bleeding is possible with these drugs since they affect 5HT, a key component in platelet activity. Caution should be used if any of these drugs is combined with other drugs known to affect bleeding.

Other Antidepressants

Some other effective antidepressants do not fit into any of the three groups that have been discussed in this chapter. These drugs have varying effects on NE, 5HT, and dopamine. Although it is not known how their actions are related to clinical efficacy, these agents may be most effective in treating depression in patients who do not respond to other antidepressants. They may even be used before MAOIs or TCAs, which have many more adverse effects. As with the other antidepressants, these drugs have a black box warning to be alert for the possibility of increased suicidality, especially in children, adolescents, and young adults, whenever the drugs are used. Other antidepressants include the following (see Table 21.5 for Usual Indications):

Bupropion (*Wellbutrin*, *Zyban*) weakly blocks the reuptake of NE, 5HT, and dopamine. At lower doses, this drug is effective in smoking cessation. It is well absorbed from the GI tract, metabolized in the liver, and excreted in the urine. There are no adequate studies done in pregnancy, and the drug should be used during pregnancy only if the benefits to the mother clearly outweigh the potential risks to the fetus. Bupropion does enter breast milk and should not be used by nursing mothers. The drug is available in a sustained release formulation as well as an extended release formula, which some patients find to be more convenient.

Desvenlafaxine (*Pristiq*) is the newest of the SSRIs. It blocks the reuptake of NE and 5HT. It is readily absorbed from the GI tract, reaching peak levels in 7.5 hours. It is metabolized in the liver and excreted through urine within about 72 hours. It passes into breast milk and should not be used by nursing mothers. As with other SSRIs, it should

Table 21.5 ***Drugs in Focus:* Other Antidepressants**

Drug Name	Dosage/Route	Usual Indications
bupropion (Wellbutrin, Wellbutrin SR, Wellbutrin XL, Zyban)	300 mg/d PO given in three doses *or* 150 mg PO b.i.d. in sustained release form *or* 150–300 mg/d as a single dose of extended release form	Treatment of depression in adults, smoking cessation
desvenlafaxine (*Pristiq*)	50 mg/d PO with or without food, range 50–400 mg/d	Treatment of major depressive disorder in adults
duloxetine (*Cymbalta*)	20 mg/d PO b.i.d., up to 60 mg/d may be needed	Treatment of major depressive disorder, neuropathic pain, fibromyalgia
milnacipran (*Savella*)	12.5 mg/d PO, increase over a week to 50 mg PO b.i.d., up to 200 mg/d has been used	Management of fibromyalgia in adults
mirtazapine (*Remeron*)	15 mg/d PO, may be increased to a maximum of 45 mg/d; reduce dose in elderly patients and those with renal or hepatic dysfunction	Treatment of depression in adults
nefazodone (generic)	100 mg PO b.i.d., to a maximum of 600 mg/d; reduce dose in elderly	Treatment of depression in adults
selegiline (*Emsam*)	Initially, one 6-mg/24-h transdermal system applied to dry, intact skin on the upper thigh, upper torso, or upper arm; may be increased to a maximum 12-mg/24-h system; geriatric patients, maximum 6 mg/2 h	Treatment of major depressive disorder
trazodone (*Desyrel*)	150 mg/d PO in divided doses; up to 600 mg/d, reduce dose with the elderly *Pediatric:* 1.5–2 mg/kg/d PO in divided doses; do not exceed 6 mg/kg/d	Treatment of depression in adults and children 6–18 y
venlafaxine (Effexor, Effexor XR)	75 mg/d PO in divided doses to 375 mg/d; 75 mg/d PO sustained release formulation to a maximum 225 mg/d; reduce dose with hepatic and renal impairment	Treatment and prevention of depression in generalized anxiety disorder; social anxiety disorder; decreases addictive behavior

be used in pregnancy only if the benefit clearly outweighs the risk. It is taken orally, once a day.

Duloxetine (*Cymbalta*) blocks the reuptake of NE and 5HT. It is rapidly absorbed from the GI tract, metabolized in the liver, and excreted in the feces and urine. It has a half-life of 8 to 17 hours. It is used for treating major depressive disorders, neuropathic pain, generalized anxiety disorder, and fibromyalgia. This drug must be swallowed whole—not cut, crushed, or chewed. Patients should be monitored for liver toxicity. Use in pregnancy and during lactation is not recommended. This drug should be tapered when it is discontinued to decrease adverse effects.

Levomilnacipran (*Fetzima*) is a new drug approved in 2013 that blocks the reuptake of both NE and 5HT. It is used to treat major depressive disorder in adults. It is taken once a day and can be increased to achieve the desired result. It has a 12-hour half-life and is metabolized in the liver and excreted in the urine. It has a black box warning about the risk of suicidality, and is associated with serotonin syndrome when combined with other drugs that affect 5HT levels.

Milnacipran (*Savella*) is a drug that selectively blocks the reuptake of NE and 5HT. It is absorbed rapidly from the GI tract, metabolized in the liver, and excreted in the urine with a half-life of 6 to 8 hours. It is only approved for use in the treatment of adults with fibromyalgia. Use in pregnancy and lactation is not recommended. Patients should be monitored for suicidality.

Mirtazapine (*Remeron*) is rapidly absorbed from the GI tract, extensively metabolized in the liver, and excreted in the urine. Mirtazapine has a half-life of 20 to 40 hours. How its many anticholinergic effects relate to its antidepressive effects is not known. Little is known about its effects in pregnancy and lactation, and it should be used during those times only if the benefit to the mother clearly outweighs the potential risk to the neonate.

Nefazodone (generic) has a short half-life of 2 to 4 hours. It is well absorbed from the GI tract, metabolized in the liver, and excreted in the urine. It has been associated with severe liver toxicity in some patients, and because of this its use has become limited. Little is known about its effects in pregnancy and breastfeeding, and it should be used during those times only if the benefit to the mother clearly outweighs the potential risk to the fetus or neonate.

Selegiline (*Emsam*) is a MAO type B inhibitor that has been used for many years in the treatment of Parkinson's disease and is now available as a transdermal system, *Emsam*, for the treatment of major depressive disorder. The drug is slowly absorbed into the bloodstream over 24 hours. It is metabolized in the liver and excreted through urine. The drug does cross the placenta and enters breast milk, so it should only be used during pregnancy and lactation if the benefit outweighs the potential risk to the neonate. This drug is associated with CNS effects as well as GI effects including nausea, vomiting, dry mouth, and abdominal pain. Patients need to be taught to apply the patch to dry, intact skin on the upper torso, upper thigh, or upper arm. They should always remove the old patch before applying a new one to avoid inadvertent overdose.

Trazodone (*Desyrel*), which blocks 5HT and some 5HT precursor reuptake, is effective in some forms of depression but has many CNS effects associated with its use. It is readily absorbed from the GI tract, extensively metabolized in the liver, and excreted in the urine and feces. Trazodone caused fetal abnormalities in animal studies and crosses into breast milk. It should be used during pregnancy and lactation only if the benefits to the mother clearly outweigh the potential risks to the fetus. A black box warning has been added to this drug, cautioning about the need to limit the quantity of the drug to depressed patients, the risk for low blood pressure, and a risk for priapism. Because of these warnings the use of this drug has also become limited.

Venlafaxine (*Effexor*) mildly blocks the reuptake of NE, 5HT, and dopamine and has fewer adverse CNS effects than trazodone. Its popularity has increased with the introduction of an extended release form that does away with the multiple daily doses that are required with the regular form. Venlafaxine is readily absorbed from the GI tract, extensively metabolized in the liver, and excreted in the urine. Adequate studies have not been done in pregnancy and lactation, and it should be used during those times only if the benefit to the mother clearly outweighs the potential risk to the neonate.

FOCUS ON Smoking Cessation

The effects of smoking on morbidity and mortality have been in the headlines for many years. Multimedia campaigns to illustrate the detrimental effects of smoking are having an impact on smokers and health care providers. The Agency for Health Care Policy and Research (AHCPR) has published guidelines for health care providers to promote smoking cessation as a regular and vital part of any health care visit. Nicotine is very addictive and those who try to quit smoking have to struggle to succeed. The AHCPR has developed multiple programs and offers free access to consumers to help in the process. A real desire to quit is essential for any success, so counseling, talking to the patient, offering insights, and even statistics about the detrimental effects should be a basic part of the patient interaction. Nicotine patches and nicotine gum are available by prescription to help the patient ease off the effects of nicotine that are so addicting. Buproprion, an antidepressant, is approved under the brand name ***Zyban*** *to help with smoking cessation as well as alleviate some of the depression that may occur as nicotine is removed from the body. Varenicline (****Chantix****) is a nicotine receptor agonist which binds to the nicotine*

FOCUS ON Smoking Cessation (Continued)

receptors in the CNS and prevents nicotine from binding and stimulating the receptors. The patient should pick a date to stop smoking, begin the drug one week before that date, and should quit smoking between days 8 to 35 of the treatment plan. The drug therapy should be part of a complete support and education program. If the patient has not been able to stop smoking in 12 weeks the drug should be stopped. The factors that prevented success should be addressed and the treatment regimen can be restarted. This drug has a black box warning for potentially serious mental health events, including behavioral changes, depression, hostility, aggression, and suicidality. It is also associated with potentially dangerous CV events. Weighing the health risks of smoking versus the adverse effects of the drug is an important part of the decision to try this approach. Patients who opt to use varenicline should be monitored closely for these effects. Log on to therealcost.betobaccofree.hhs.gov/costs/health-costs/index.html to access the smoking cessation information available for health care providers and consumers.

SUMMARY

- Depression is a very common affective disorder; it is associated with many physical manifestations and is often misdiagnosed. It could be that depression is caused by a series of events that are not yet understood.
- Antidepressant drugs—TCAs, MAOIs, and SSRIs—increase the concentrations of the biogenic amines in the brain.
- Selection of an antidepressant depends on individual drug response and tolerance of associated adverse effects. The adverse effects of TCAs are sedating and anticholinergic; those of MAOIs are CNS related and sympathomimetic. The adverse effects of SSRIs are fewer, but they do cause CNS changes.
- Other antidepressants with unknown mechanisms of action are also effective in treating depression.
- All of these drugs have a black box warning of the risk of suicidality, particularly in children, adolescents, and young adults.

CHECK YOUR UNDERSTANDING

Answers to the questions in this chapter can be found in Answers to Check Your Understanding Questions on thePoint®.

MULTIPLE CHOICE

Select the best answer to the following.

1. The biogenic amine theory of depression states that depression is a result of
  a. an unpleasant childhood.
  b. gamma-aminobutyric acid (GABA) inhibition.
  c. deficiency of NE, dopamine, or 5HT in key areas of the brain.
  d. blockages within the limbic system, which controls emotions and affect.

2. When teaching a patient receiving TCAs, it is important to remember that TCAs are associated with many anticholinergic adverse effects. Teaching about these drugs should include anticipation of
  a. increased libido and increased appetite.
  b. polyuria and polydipsia.
  c. urinary retention, arrhythmias, and constipation.
  d. hearing changes, cataracts, and nightmares.

3. Adverse effects may limit the usefulness of TCAs with some patients. Nursing interventions that could alleviate some of the unpleasant aspects of these adverse effects include
  a. always administering the drug when the patient has an empty stomach.
  b. reminding the patient not to void before taking the drug.
  c. increasing the dose to override the adverse effects.
  d. taking the major portion of the dose at bedtime to avoid experiencing drowsiness and the unpleasant anticholinergic effects.

4. You might question an order for a MAOI as a first step in the treatment of depression, remembering that these drugs are reserved for use in cases in which there has been no response to other agents because
  a. MAOIs can cause hair loss.
  b. MAOIs are associated with potentially serious drug–food interactions.
  c. MAOIs are mostly recommended for use in surgical patients.
  d. MAOIs are more expensive than other agents.

(continues on page 368)

5. Your patient is being treated for depression and is started on a regimen of *Prozac* (fluoxetine). She calls you 10 days after the drug therapy has started to report that nothing has changed and she wants to try a different drug. You should
   a. tell her to try sertraline (*Zoloft*) because some patients respond to one SSRI and not another.
   b. ask her to try a few days without the drug to see whether there is any difference.
   c. add an MAOI to her drug regimen to get an increased antidepressant effect.
   d. encourage her to keep taking the drug as prescribed because it usually takes up to 4 weeks to see the full antidepressant effect.

6. The drug of choice for a patient with a documented OCD who is also suffering from depression and occasional panic disorder would be
   a. Celexa.
   b. Paxil.
   c. Luvox.
   d. Prozac.

7. Venlafaxine (*Effexor*) is an antidepressant that might be very effective for use in patients who
   a. have proven to be responsive to other antidepressants.
   b. can tolerate multiple side effects.
   c. are reliable at taking multiple daily dosings.
   d. have not responded to other antidepressants and would benefit from once-a-day dosing.

8. Depression is an affective disorder that is
   a. always precipitated by a specific event.
   b. most common in patients with head injuries.
   c. characterized by overwhelming sadness, despair, and hopelessness.
   d. very evident and easy to diagnose in the clinical setting.

MULTIPLE RESPONSE

Select all that apply.

1. Depression is a very common affective disorder that strikes many people. In assessing a client who might be suffering from depression the nurse would expect to find which of the following?
   a. Lack of energy
   b. Hyperactivity
   c. Sleep disturbances
   d. Libido problems
   e. Confusion
   f. Decreased reflexes

2. A client reports that he thinks he is taking an antidepressant, but he is not sure. In reviewing his medication history, which of the following drugs would be considered antidepressants?
   a. Tetracyclic drugs
   b. Cholinergics
   c. SSRIs
   d. MAOIs
   e. Angiotensin II receptor blockers
   f. Benzodiazepine

BIBLIOGRAPHY AND REFERENCES

American Psychiatric Association. (2010). *Practice guideline for the treatment of patients with major depressive disorders* (3rd ed.). Washington, DC: Author.

Brunton, L., Chabner, B., & Knollman, B. (2011). *Goodman and Gilman's the pharmacological basis of therapeutics* (12th ed.). New York: McGraw-Hill.

Facts & Comparisons. (2015). *Drug facts and comparisons*. St. Louis, MO: Author.

Facts & Comparisons. (2015). *Professional's guide to patient drug facts*. St. Louis, MO: Author.

Hauser, W., Bernardy, K., Uceyler, N., et al. (2009). Treatment of fibromyalgia syndrome with antidepressants: A meta-analysis. *Journal of the American Medical Association, 301*(2), 198–209.

Karch, A. M. (2014). *Lippincott's nursing drug guide*. Philadelphia, PA: Lippincott Williams & Wilkins.

Nischal, A., Tripathi, A., Nischal, A., et al. (2012). Suicide and antidepressants: What current evidence indicates. *Mens Sana Monographs, 10*(1), 33–44.

Porth, C. M. (2013). *Pathophysiology: Concepts of altered health states* (9th ed.). Philadelphia, PA: Lippincott Williams & Wilkins.

Rey, J., & Birmach, B. (Eds.). (2009). *Treating childhood and adolescent depression*. New York: Lippincott William & Wilkins.

Robinson, D. (2009). Antidepressant treatment and pregnancy: An update. *Primary Psychiatry, 16*(7), 19–22.

U.S. Food and Drug Administration. (2003). FDA Public Health Advisory. Subject: Reports of suicidality in pediatric patients being treated with antidepressants for major depressive disorder (MDD) [*Food and Drug Administration*]. Available online at: http://www.fda.gov/CDER/drug/advisory/mdd.htm

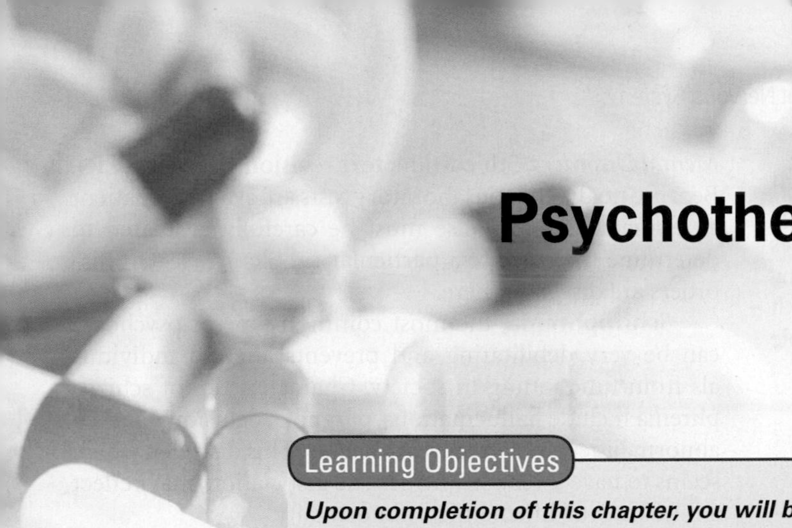

Psychotherapeutic Agents 22

Learning Objectives

Upon completion of this chapter, you will be able to:

1. Define the term psychotherapeutic agent and list conditions that the psychotherapeutic agents are used to treat.
2. Describe the therapeutic actions, indications, pharmacokinetics, contraindications, most common adverse reactions, and important drug–drug interactions associated with each class of psychotherapeutic agent.
3. Discuss the use of psychotherapeutic agents across the lifespan.
4. Compare and contrast the prototype drugs for each class of psychotherapeutic agent with other drugs in that class and with drugs in the other classes of psychotherapeutic agents.
5. Outline the nursing considerations and teaching needs for patients receiving each class of psychotherapeutic agents.

Glossary of Key Terms

antipsychotic: drug used to treat disorders involving thought processes; dopamine receptor blocker that helps affected people to organize their thoughts and respond appropriately to stimuli

attention deficit disorder: behavioral syndrome characterized by an inability to concentrate for longer than a few minutes and excessive activity

bipolar disorder: behavioral disorder that involves extremes of depression alternating with hyperactivity and excitement

major tranquilizer: former name of antipsychotic drugs; the name is no longer used because it implies that the primary effect of these drugs is sedation, which is no longer thought to be the desired therapeutic action

mania: state of hyperexcitability; one phase of bipolar disorders, which alternate between periods of severe depression and mania

narcolepsy: mental disorder characterized by daytime sleepiness and periods of sudden loss of wakefulness

neuroleptic: a drug with many associated neurological adverse effects that is used to treat disorders that involve thought processes (e.g., schizophrenia)

schizophrenia: the most common type of psychosis; characteristics include hallucinations, paranoia, delusions, speech abnormalities, and affective problems

Drug List

Antipsychotic/Neuroleptic Drugs

Typical Antipsychotics

(P) chlorpromazine
fluphenazine
haloperidol
loxapine
perphenazine
pimozide
prochlorperazine
thioridazine
thiothixene
trifluoperazine

Atypical Antipsychotics

aripiprazole
asenapine
(P) clozapine
iloperidone
lurasidone
olanzapine
paliperidone
quetiapine
risperidone
ziprasidone

Drugs for Bipolar Disorders

aripiprazole
lamotrigine
(P) lithium
olanzapine
quetiapine
ziprasidone

Central Nervous System Stimulants

armodafinil
atomoxetine
dexmethylphenidate
dextroamphetamine
guanfacine
(P) lisdexamfetamine
methylphenidate
modafinil

The drugs discussed in this chapter are used to treat psychoses—perceptual and behavioral disorders. These psychotherapeutic agents are targeted at thought processes rather than affective states. Although they do not cure any psychotic disorders, psychotherapeutic agents do help both adult and pediatric patients to function in a more acceptable manner and carry on activities of daily living (Box 22.1).

Mental Disorders and their Classification

Mental disorders were once attributed to environmental influences and life experiences such as poor parenting or trauma. Mental disorders are now thought to be caused by some inherent dysfunction within the brain that leads to abnormal thought processes and responses. Most theories attribute these disorders to some sort of chemical imbalance in specific areas within the brain. Diagnosis of a mental disorder is often based on distinguishing characteristics as described in the *Diagnostic and Statistical Manual of Mental Disorders*, 5th edition, text revision (DSM-IV-TR). Because no diagnostic laboratory tests are available, patient assessment and response must be carefully evaluated to determine the basis of a particular problem. Selected disorders are discussed here.

Schizophrenia, the most common type of psychosis, can be very debilitating and prevents affected individuals from functioning in society. Characteristics of schizophrenia include hallucinations, paranoia, delusions, speech abnormalities, and affective problems. This disorder, which seems to have a very strong genetic association, may reflect a fundamental biochemical abnormality.

Bipolar disorder involves extremes of depression alternating with hyperactivity and excitement. This condition may reflect a biochemical imbalance followed by overcompensation on the part of neurons and their inability to reestablish stability.

Narcolepsy is characterized by daytime sleepiness and sudden periods of loss of wakefulness. This disorder may reflect problems with stimulation of the brain by the reticular activating system (RAS) or problems with response to that stimulation.

BOX 22.1 FOCUS ON Drug Therapy Across the Lifespan

Psychotherapeutic Agents

CHILDREN

Many of these agents are used in children, often in combination with other CNS drugs in an attempt to control symptoms and behavior. Long-term effects of many of these agents are not known, and parents should be informed of this fact.

Of the antipsychotics, chlorpromazine, haloperidol, pimozide, prochlorperazine, risperidone, thioridazine, and trifluoperazine are the only ones with established pediatric regimens. Aripiprazole has doses for children 13–17 years of age. The dose is often higher than that required for adults. The child should be monitored carefully for adverse effects and developmental progress.

Lithium does not have a recommended pediatric dose, and the drug should not ordinarily be used in children. If it is used, the dose should be carefully calculated from the child's age and weight, and the child should be monitored very closely for renal, CNS, CV, and endocrine function.

The CNS stimulants are often used in children to manage various attention deficit disorders. Caution should be used with extended release preparations because they differ markedly in timing and effectiveness. A baseline ECG should be done to rule out congenital heart problems. The child should be assessed carefully and challenged periodically for the necessity of continuing the drug. Treatment should be part of an interdisciplinary approach.

ADULTS

Adults using these drugs should be under regular care and should be monitored regularly for adverse effects. The QTc interval should be evaluated before thioridazine or ziprasidone is prescribed and periodically during use.

Patients receiving lithium should be encouraged to maintain hydration and salt intake. They need to understand the importance of periodic monitoring of serum lithium levels.

These drugs should be used very cautiously during pregnancy and lactation because of the potential for adverse effects on the fetus or neonate. A woman maintained on one of these drugs needs to be counseled about the risk to the fetus versus the risk of returning symptoms if the drug is stopped. Use should be reserved for situations in which the benefits to the mother far outweigh the potential risks to the neonate. Women of childbearing age who need to take lithium should be advised to use barrier contraceptives while taking the drug because of the potential for serious congenital abnormalities.

OLDER ADULTS

Older patients may be more susceptible to the adverse effects of these drugs. All doses need to be reduced and patients monitored very closely for toxic effects and to provide safety measures if CNS effects do occur. They should not be used to control behavior with dementia.

Patients with renal impairment should be monitored very closely while taking lithium. Decreased doses may be needed. Because many older patients may also have renal impairment, they need to be screened carefully. They should be urged to maintain hydration and salt intake, which can be a challenge with some older patients.

Prolongation of the QTc interval—associated with use of thioridazine or ziprasidone—may be a concern in elderly patients with coronary disease. Careful screening and monitoring should be done if these drugs are needed for such patients.

Attention deficit disorders involve various conditions characterized by an inability to concentrate on one activity for longer than a few minutes and a state of hyperkinesis. These conditions are usually diagnosed in school-aged children but can occur in adults.

Antipsychotic/Neuroleptic Drugs

The **antipsychotic** drugs, which are essentially dopamine receptor blockers, are used to treat disorders that involve thought processes. Because of their associated neurological adverse effects, these medications are also called **neuroleptic** agents. At one time, these drugs were known as **major tranquilizers**. However, that name is no longer used because the primary action of these drugs is not sedation but a change in neuron stimulation and response (Figure 22.1).

Antipsychotics are classified as either typical or atypical. Typical antipsychotics include chlorpromazine (*Thorazine*), fluphenazine (*Prolixin*), haloperidol (*Haldol*), loxapine (*Loxitane*), perphenazine (*Trilafon*), pimozide (*Orap*), prochlorperazine (generic), thiothixene (*Navane*), and trifluoperazine (*generic*). Atypical antipsychotics include aripiprazole (*Abilify*), asenapine (Saphris), clozapine (*Clozaril*), iloperidone (*Fanapt*), lurasidone (*Latuda*), olanzapine (*Zyprexa, Zyprexa Zydis*), paliperidone (*Invega*), quetiapine (*Seroquel, Seroquel XR*), risperidone (*Risperdal, Risperdal Conta*), and ziprasidone (*Geodon*). Table 22.1 lists both typical and antipsychotic agents, including the specific type and the occurrence of sedation and other adverse effects.

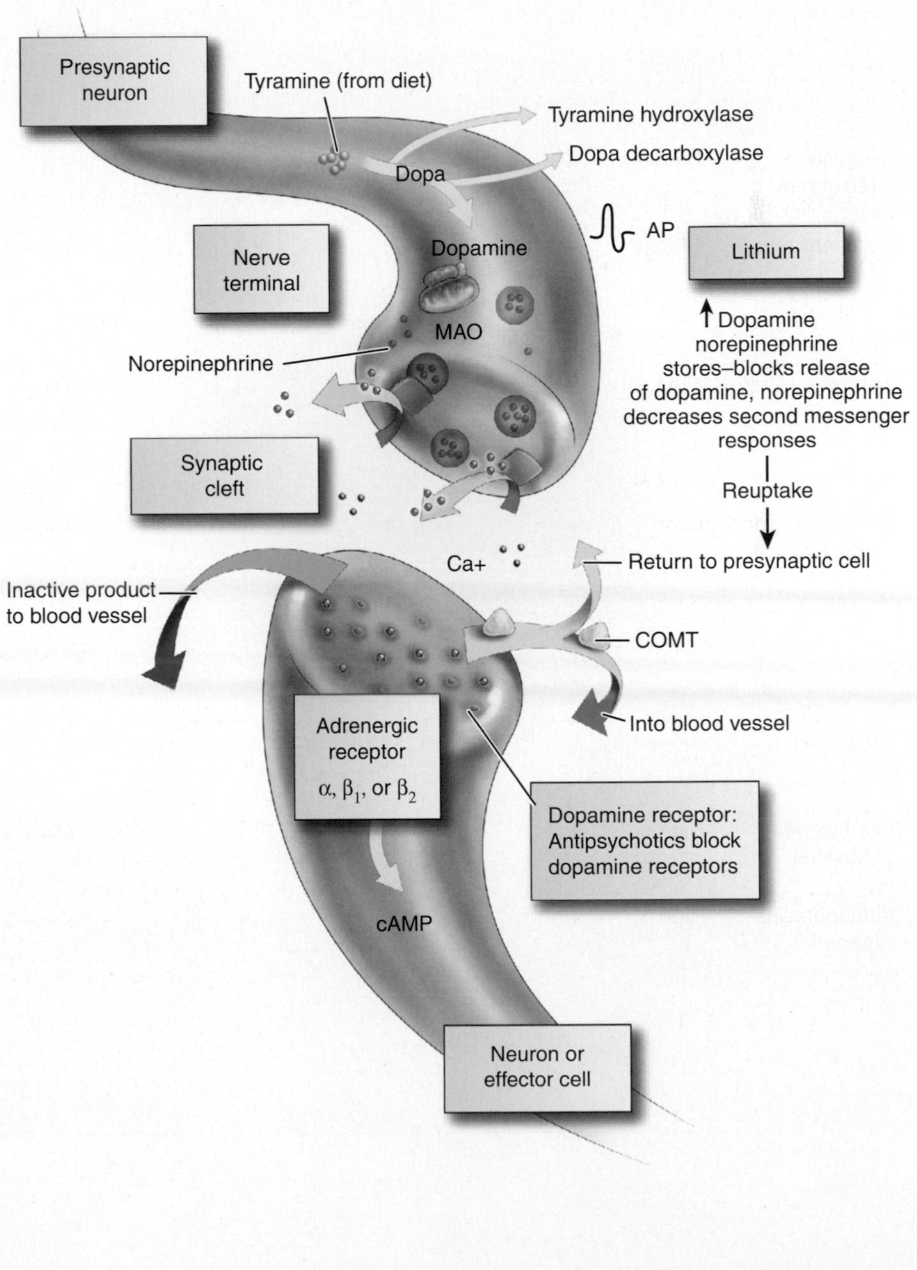

FIGURE 22.1 Sites of action of the drugs used to treat mental disorders: Antipsychotics, central nervous system stimulants, lithium.

Table 22.1 Drugs in Focus: Antipsychotic/Neuroleptic Drugs

		Common Side Effects				
Drug Name	**Potency**	**Sedation**	**Anticholinergic**	**Hypotension**	**Extrapyramidal**	**Usual Dosage**
Typical Antipsychotics						
chlorpromazine (generic)	Low	+ + + +	+ + +	+ + +	+ +	*Adult:* 25 mg IM for acute episode, may be repeated; switch to 25–50 mg PO t.i.d. *Pediatric:* 0.5–1 mg/kg q4–8 h PO, IM, or PR
fluphenazine (*Prolixin*)	High	+	+	+	+ + + +	*Adult:* 0.5–10 mg/d PO in divided doses; 1.25–10 mg/d IM in divided doses *Geriatric:* 1–2.5 mg/d PO, adjust dose based on response
haloperidol (*Haldol*)	High	+	+/–	+	+ + + +	*Adult:* 0.5–2 mg PO t.i.d. *or* 2–5 mg IM, may be repeated in 1 h, 4–8 h more common *Geriatric:* Reduce dose *Pediatric (3–12 y):* 0.5 mg/d PO; 0.05–0.075 mg/kg/d PO for Tourette syndrome and behavioral syndromes
loxapine (*Loxitane*)	Medium	+ + +	+ +	+ +	+ + +	*Adult:* 20–60 mg/d PO; 12.5–50 mg IM or IV for acute states
perphenazine (*Trilafon*)	Medium	+ +	+	+ +	+ + +	*Adult:* 4–8 mg PO t.i.d. *or* 5–10 mg IM q6 h; switch to oral as soon as possible *Geriatric:* 1/2–1/3 of adult dose
pimozide (*Orap*)	High	+	+	+ +	+ + +	*Adult:* 1–2 mg/d PO in divided doses *Pediatric (>12 y):* 0.05 mg/kg PO at bedtime; do not exceed 10 mg/d
prochlorperazine (generic)	Low	+	+ +	+	+ + +	*Adult:* 5–10 mg PO t.i.d. to q.i.d.; 10–20 mg IM for acute states *Geriatric:* Reduce dose *Pediatric:* 2.5 mg PO t.i.d.; 0.03 mg/kg IM for acute states; 20–25 mg/d PR
thioridazine (*generic*)	Low	+ + + +	+ + +	+ + +	+	*Adult:* 50–100 mg PO t.i.d., monitor QTc intervals *Pediatric:* Up to 3 mg/kg/d PO
thiothixene (*Navane*)	High	+	+	+	+ + + +	*Adult:* 2 mg PO t.i.d.; up to a maximum 60 mg/d in severe cases
trifluoperazine (generic)	High	+	+	+	+ + + +	*Adult:* 2–5 mg PO b.i.d.; 1–2 mg IM q4–6 h in severe cases *Geriatric:* Reduce dose *Pediatric (6–12 y):* 1 mg PO daily or b.i.d.: 1 mg IM daily or b.i.d. for severe cases

		Common Side Effects				
Drug Name	**Potency**	**Sedation**	**Anticholinergic**	**Hypotension**	**Extrapyramidal**	**Usual Dosage**
Typical Antipsychotics						
aripiprazole (*Abilify*)	Medium	+	+	+ +	+	*Adult:* 10–15 mg/d PO *Pediatric (13–17 y):* 10–30 mg/d PO
clozapine (*Clozaril*)	Low	+ + + +	+ +	+ + +	+/–	*Adult:* Initially 25 mg PO b.i.d. to t.i.d.; up to 500 mg/d; available only through the *Clozaril* Patient Management System, which monitors white blood cell count and compliance issues, only 1-wk supply given at a time
lurasidone (*Latuda*)	Low	+ +	+ +	+	+	*Adult:* 40 mg/d PO with food, titrated to a maximum 80 mg/d, do not exceed 40 mg/d with renal or hepatic dysfunction
olanzapine (*Zyprexa, Zyprexa Zydis*)	High	+ + + +	+ +	+ + +	+	*Adult:* 5–10 mg/d PO, up to 20 mg/d PO for bipolar mania; available in disintegrating tablets, which can be taken without swallowing
paliperidone (*Invega*)	Medium	+	+	+ +	+ +	*Adult:* 6 mg/d PO; maximum dose 12 mg/d *Renal impairment:* Maximum dose 6 mg/d with moderate impairment, maximum dose 3 mg/d with severe impairment
quetiapine (*Seroquel, Seroquel XR*)	Medium	+ + + +	+ +	+ +	+/–	*Adult:* Initially 25 mg PO b.i.d., up to 300–400 mg/d; 400–900 mg/d PO (XR) *Geriatric, hepatic impairment, or hypotensives:* Reduce dose and titrate very slowly
risperidone (*Risperdal, Risperdal Conta*)	High	+ + +	+	+ +	+ +	*Adult:* 1 mg PO b.i.d. up to 8 mg/d *or* 25 mg IM once every 2 wk *Pediatric* *10–17 y:* 0.5–6 mg/d PO (bipolar disorders) *13–17 y:* 1–6 mg/d PO (schizophrenia) *Geriatric, renal impaired, or hypotensives:* 0.5 mg PO b.i.d. initially, titrate slowly
ziprasidone (*Geodon*)	Medium	+ + +	+ +	+	+	*Adult:* 20–80 mg PO b.i.d.; rapid control of as-stated behavior 10–20 mg IM (maximum dose 40 mg/d IM); monitor QTc intervals

Each plus sign indicates increased incidence of the given adverse effect.
XR, extended release.

FOCUS ON Safe Medication Administration

Name confusion has been reported between chlorpromazine (an antipsychotic) and chlorpropamide (an antidiabetic agent). Serious adverse effects have occurred. Manufacturers of these two drugs have been working to make the labels of the drugs very distinctive to help eliminate some of these errors. If your patient is prescribed chlorpromazine, make sure the patient is aware of the name of the drug, its intended use, and what it should look like.

FOCUS ON Safe Medication Administration

*Name confusion has occurred between **Risperdal** (risperidone) and **Requip** (ropinirole) with some patients experiencing serious adverse effects. If you have a patient receiving either of these medications, it is a good idea to double-check what was ordered and what is being given.*

Therapeutic Actions and Indications

The typical antipsychotic drugs block dopamine receptors, preventing the stimulation of the postsynaptic neurons by dopamine. They also depress the RAS, limiting the stimuli coming into the brain. They also have anticholinergic, antihistamine, and alpha-adrenergic blocking effects, all related to the blocking of the dopamine receptor sites. Newer atypical antipsychotics block both dopamine and serotonin receptors. This dual action may help to alleviate some of the unpleasant neurological effects and depression associated with the typical antipsychotics (see Table 22.1).

The antipsychotics are indicated for schizophrenia and for manifestations of other psychotic disorders, including hyperactivity, combative behavior, and severe behavioral problems in children (short-term control); some of them are also approved for the treatment of bipolar disorder. Chlorpromazine, one of the older antipsychotics, is also used to decrease preoperative restlessness and apprehension, to treat intermittent porphyria, as an adjunct in the treatment of tetanus, and to control nausea, vomiting, and intractable hiccups. Haloperidol is frequently used to treat acute psychiatric situations and is available for IV use when prolonged parenteral therapy is required because of swallowing difficulties or the acuity of the behavioral problems.

Prochlorperazine is also frequently used to control severe nausea and vomiting associated with surgery and chemotherapy. It has the advantage of being available in oral, rectal, and parenteral forms. Aripiprazole, one of the newer atypical antipsychotics, has been found to be effective in treating schizophrenia, major depressive disorder, and bipolar disorders and has been used parenterally for the treatment of acute agitation associated with these disorders. Lurasidone, the newest of the atypical antipsychotics, is used for adults with schizophrenia. Olanzapine and ziprasidone are also used for bipolar disorders and parenterally to treat acute agitation. Quetiapine is also approved for short-term treatment of acute manic episodes associated with bipolar disease. Risperidone is used frequently to treat irritability and aggression associated with autistic disorders in children and adolescents, as well as for acute manic episodes of bipolar disease. Paliperidone is now also approved for treatment of schizoaffective disorders. Any of these drugs may be effective in a particular patient; the selection of a specific drug depends on the desired potency and patient tolerance of the associated adverse effects. A patient who does not respond to one drug may react successfully to another agent. Responses may also vary because of cultural issues (Box 22.2). To determine the best therapeutic regimen for a particular patient, it may be necessary to try more than one drug.

BOX 22.2 FOCUS ON Cultural Considerations

Antipsychotic Drugs and Drugs for Bipolar Disorders

The ways in which patients in certain cultural groups respond to antipsychotic drugs—either physiologically or emotionally—may vary. Therefore, when a pharmacological regimen is incorporated into overall patient care, health care providers must consider and respect an individual patient's cultural beliefs and needs.

- African Americans respond more rapidly to antipsychotic medications and have a greater risk for development of disfiguring adverse effects, such as tardive dyskinesia. Consequently, these patients should be started off at the lowest possible dose and monitored closely. African Americans also display a higher red blood cell plasma lithium ratio than Caucasians do, and they report more adverse effects from lithium therapy. These patients should be monitored closely because they have a higher potential for lithium toxicity at standard therapeutic ranges.
- Patients in Asian countries, such as India, Turkey, Malaysia, China, Japan, and Indonesia, receive lower doses of neuroleptics and lithium to achieve the same therapeutic response as seen in patients in the United States. This may be related to these individuals' lower body mass as well as metabolic differences, and it may have implications for dosing protocols for patients in these ethnic groups who undergo therapy in the United States.
- Arab American patients metabolize antipsychotic medications more slowly than Asian Americans do and may require lower doses to achieve the same therapeutic effects as in Caucasians.
- Individuals in some cultures use herbs and other folk remedies, and the use of herbs may interfere with the metabolism of Western medications. The nurse should carefully assess for herbal use and be aware of potential interactions.

Pharmacokinetics

The antipsychotics are erratically absorbed from the gastrointestinal (GI) tract, depending on the drug and the preparation of the drug. IM doses provide four to five times the active dose as oral doses, and caution is required if one is switching between routes. The antipsychotics are widely distributed in the tissues and are often stored there, being released for up to 6 months after the drug is stopped. They are metabolized in the liver and excreted through the bile and urine. Children tend to metabolize these drugs faster than do adults, and elderly patients tend to metabolize them more slowly, making it necessary to carefully monitor these patients and adjust doses as needed. Clinical effects may not be seen for several weeks, and patients should be encouraged to continue taking the drugs even if they see no immediate effectiveness. The antipsychotics cross the placenta and enter breast milk (see Contraindications and Cautions).

Contraindications and Cautions

Antipsychotic drugs are contraindicated in the presence of underlying diseases *that could be exacerbated by the dopamine-blocking effects of these drugs.* They are also contraindicated in the following conditions, *which can be exacerbated by the drugs*: central nervous system (CNS) depression, circulatory collapse, Parkinson's disease, coronary disease, severe hypotension, bone marrow suppression, and blood dyscrasias. Prolongation of the QTc interval is a contraindication to the use of mesoridazine, thioridazine, and ziprasidone, all of which can further prolong the QTc interval, *leading to increased risk of serious cardiac arrhythmias.* Antipsychotics are contraindicated for use in elderly patients with dementia *because this use is associated with an increased risk of cardiovascular (CV) events and death.* In 2005 the U.S. Food and Drug Administration issued a public health advisory regarding the use of antipsychotics after postmarketing studies showed that when these drugs were used to control behavioral symptoms of dementia in older adults the patients being treated experienced increased CV events and death. None of these drugs is approved for this use, but it was common practice in many settings to use them, off-label, to establish behavioral control of patients with dementia. The manufacturers of all of these drugs sent out "Dear Health Care Provider" letters to remind health care providers that this is not an approved use and to alert them of the risk for death if they used the drug in this way. Antipsychotics now have a black box warning on the prescribing information outlining this safety information and contraindication.

Caution should be used in the presence of medical conditions *that could be exacerbated by the anticholinergic effects of the drugs*, such as glaucoma, peptic ulcer, and urinary or intestinal obstruction. In addition, care should be taken in patients with seizure disorders *because the threshold for seizures could be lowered*, in patients with thyrotoxicosis *because of the possibility of severe neurosensitivity*, and in patients with active alcoholism *because of potentiation of the CNS depression.*

Other situations that warrant caution include myelography within the last 24 hours or scheduled within the next 48 hours *because severe neuron reaction to the dye used in these tests can occur* and pregnancy or lactation *because of the potential of adverse effects on the fetus or neonate*; antipsychotic agents should be used only if the benefit to the mother clearly outweighs the potential risk to the fetus or baby. Because children are more apt to develop dystonia from the drugs, *which could confuse the diagnosis of Reye's syndrome*, caution should be used with children younger than 12 years of age who have a CNS infection or chickenpox. *The use of antipsychotics may result in bone marrow suppression, leading to blood dyscrasias*, so care should be taken with patients who are immunosuppressed and those who have cancer.

Adverse Effects

The adverse effects associated with the antipsychotic drugs are related to their dopamine-blocking, anticholinergic, antihistamine, and alpha-adrenergic activities. The most common CNS effects are sedation, weakness, tremor, drowsiness, extrapyramidal side effects, pseudoparkinsonism, dystonia, akathisia, tardive dyskinesia, and potentially irreversible neuroleptic malignant syndrome (Box 22.3) (Figure 22.2). Anticholinergic effects include dry mouth, nasal congestion, flushing, constipation, urinary retention, impotence, glaucoma, blurred vision, and photophobia. Blocking of dopamine leads to an increase in prolactin levels and subsequent gynecomastia (breast development and occasionally milk production). This can be a concern especially for male patients taking these drugs and they should be advised of that possibility. CV effects, which are probably related to the dopamine-blocking effects, include hypotension, orthostatic hypotension, cardiac arrhythmias, congestive heart failure, and pulmonary edema. Several of these agents (thioridazine, mesoridazine, ziprasidone) are associated with prolongation of the QTc interval, which could lead to serious or even

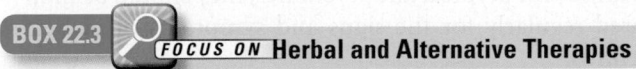

BOX 22.3 FOCUS ON **Herbal and Alternative Therapies**

Evening Primrose

Patients with schizophrenia should be advised to avoid the use of evening primrose. This herb has been associated with increased symptoms and CNS hyperexcitability.

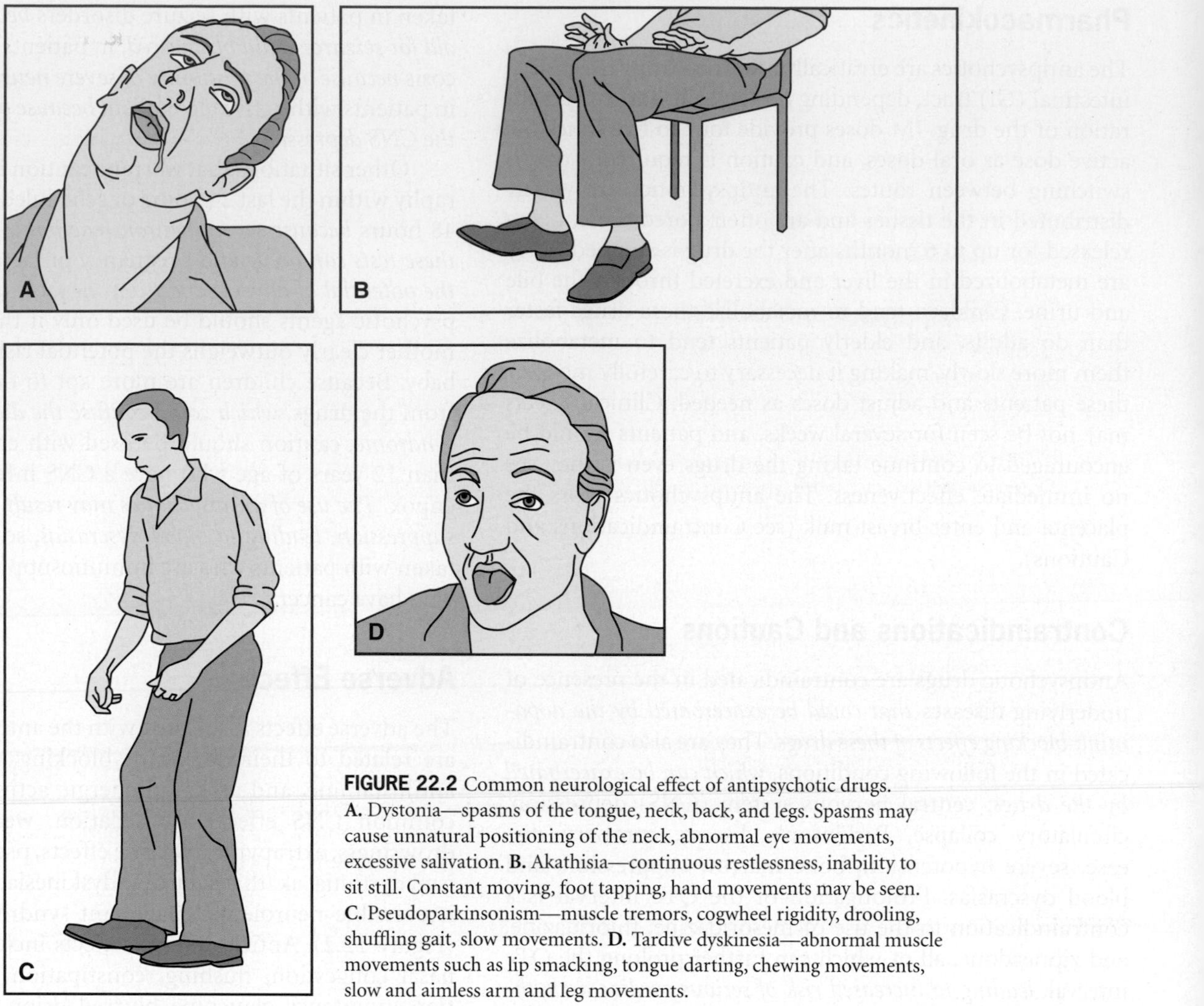

FIGURE 22.2 Common neurological effect of antipsychotic drugs. **A.** Dystonia—spasms of the tongue, neck, back, and legs. Spasms may cause unnatural positioning of the neck, abnormal eye movements, excessive salivation. **B.** Akathisia—continuous restlessness, inability to sit still. Constant moving, foot tapping, hand movements may be seen. **C.** Pseudoparkinsonism—muscle tremors, cogwheel rigidity, drooling, shuffling gait, slow movements. **D.** Tardive dyskinesia—abnormal muscle movements such as lip smacking, tongue darting, chewing movements, slow and aimless arm and leg movements.

fatal cardiac arrhythmias. Patients receiving these drugs should have a baseline and periodic electrocardiogram (ECG) during therapy. All of the atypical antipsychotics include warnings that there is a risk for the development of diabetes mellitus and weight gain when these drugs are used (Figure 22.3). Ziprasidone has been associated with serious to fatal skin reactions and the systemic symptoms of DRESS (drug reaction with eosinophilia and systemic symptoms). Consequently, when patients are maintained on any of the atypical antipsychotics, they should be monitored regularly for the signs and symptoms of diabetes mellitus.

Respiratory effects such as laryngospasm, dyspnea, and bronchospasm may also occur. The phenothiazines (chlorpromazine, fluphenazine, prochlorperazine, promethazine, and thioridazine) often turn the urine pink to reddish-brown as a result of their excretion. Although this effect may cause great patient concern, it has no clinical significance. In addition, bone marrow suppression is a possibility with some antipsychotic agents.

Clinically Important Drug–Drug Interactions

Because the combination of antipsychotics with beta-blockers may lead to an increase in the effect of both drugs, this combination should be avoided if possible. Antipsychotic–alcohol combinations result in an increased risk of CNS depression, and antipsychotic–anticholinergic combinations lead to increased anticholinergic effects, so dose adjustments are necessary. Patients who take either of these combinations should be monitored closely for adverse effects, and supportive measures should be provided. Patients should not take thioridazine or ziprasidone with any other drug that is associated with prolongation of the QTc interval.

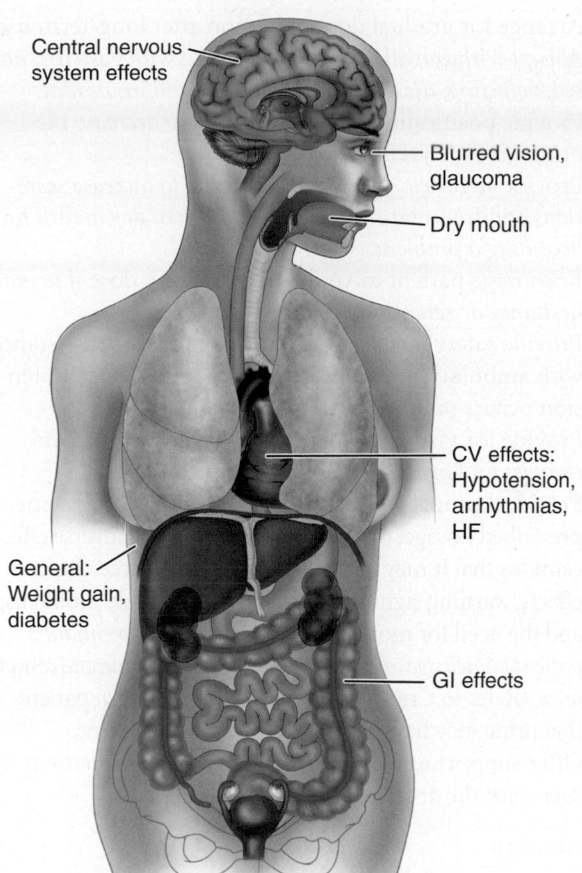

FIGURE 22.3 Adverse effects and toxicities associated with psychotherapeutic agents.

Prototype Summary: Chlorpromazine

Indications: Management of manifestations of psychotic disorders, relief of preoperative restlessness, adjunctive treatment of tetanus, acute intermittent porphyria, severe behavioral problems in children, and control of hiccups, nausea, and vomiting.

Actions: Blocks postsynaptic dopamine receptors in the brain, depresses those parts of the brain involved in wakefulness and emesis, anticholinergic, antihistaminic, alpha-adrenergic blocking.

Pharmacokinetics:

Route	Onset	Peak	Duration
Oral	30–60 min	2–4 h	4–6 h
Intramuscular	10–15 min	15–20 min	4–6 h

$T_{1/2}$: 2 hours, then 30 hours; metabolized in the liver, excreted in the urine.

Adverse Effects: Drowsiness, insomnia, vertigo, extrapyramidal symptoms, orthostatic hypotension, photophobia, blurred vision, dry mouth, nausea, vomiting, anorexia, urinary retention, photosensitivity.

Prototype Summary: Clozapine

Indications: Management of severely ill patients with schizophrenia who are unresponsive to standard drugs; reduction of risk of recurrent suicidal behavior in patients with schizophrenia or schizoaffective disorder.

Actions: Blocks dopamine and serotonin receptors, depresses the RAS, anticholinergic, antihistaminic, alpha-adrenergic blocking.

Pharmacokinetics:

Route	Onset	Peak	Duration
Oral	Varies	1–6 h	Weeks

$T_{1/2}$: 4 to 12 hours; metabolized in the liver, excreted in the urine and feces.

Adverse Effects: Drowsiness, sedation, seizures, dizziness, syncope, headache, tachycardia, nausea, vomiting, fever, neuroleptic malignant syndrome.

Nursing Considerations for Patients Receiving Antipsychotic/Neuroleptic Drugs

Assessment: History and Examination

- Assess for *contraindications or cautions for the use of the drug* including any known allergies to these drugs, severe CNS depression, circulatory collapse, coronary disease including prolonged QTc interval, brain damage, severe hypotension, glaucoma, respiratory depression, diabetes, urinary or intestinal obstruction, thyrotoxicosis, seizure disorder, bone marrow suppression, pregnancy or lactation, and myelography within the last 24 hours or scheduled in the next 48 hours. In children younger than 12 years of age, screen for CNS infections.
- Assess temperature; skin color and lesions; CNS orientation, affect, reflexes, and bilateral grip strength; bowel sounds and reported output; pulse, auscultation, and blood pressure, including orthostatic blood pressure; respiration rate and adventitious sounds; and urinary output *to determine baseline status before beginning therapy and for any potential adverse effects.* Also obtain liver and renal function tests, blood glucose levels, thyroid function tests, electrocardiogram if appropriate, and complete blood count (CBC).

Refer to the Critical Thinking Scenario for a full discussion of nursing care for a patient who is prescribed antipsychotic drugs.

(continues on page 378)

Nursing Diagnoses

Nursing diagnoses related to drug therapy might include the following:

- Impaired physical mobility related to extrapyramidal effects.
- Decreased cardiac output related to hypotensive effects.
- Risk for injury related to CNS effects and sedation.
- Impaired urinary elimination related to anticholinergic effects.
- Deficient knowledge regarding drug therapy.

Planning

- The patient will receive the best therapeutic effect from the drug therapy.
- The patient will have limited adverse effects to the drug therapy.
- The patient will have an understanding of the drug therapy, adverse effects to anticipate, and measures to relieve discomfort and improve safety.

Implementation with Rationale

- Do not allow patient to crush or chew sustained release capsules, *which will speed up their absorption and may cause toxicity.*
- If administering parenteral forms, keep patient recumbent for 30 minutes *to reduce the risk of orthostatic hypotension.*
- Consider warning the patient or the patient's guardians about the risk of development of tardive dyskinesias with continued use, *so they are prepared for that neurological change.*
- Caution patient/guardians about the risk of gynecomastia when using these drugs, *to prevent undue stress.*
- Monitor CBC *to arrange to discontinue the drug at signs of bone marrow suppression.*
- Monitor blood glucose levels with long-term use *to detect the development of glucose intolerance.*
- Arrange for gradual dose reduction after long-term use. *Abrupt withdrawal has been associated with gastritis, nausea, vomiting, dizziness, arrhythmias, and insomnia.*
- Provide positioning of legs and arms *to decrease the discomfort of dyskinesias.*
- Provide sugarless candy and ice chips *to increase secretions* and frequent mouth care *to prevent dry mouth from becoming a problem.*
- Encourage patient to void before taking a dose *if urinary hesitancy or retention is a problem.*
- Provide safety measures such as side rails and assistance with ambulation if CNS effects or orthostatic hypotension occurs *to prevent patient injury.*
- Provide for vision examinations *to determine ocular changes and arrange appropriate dose change.*
- Provide thorough patient teaching, including drug name, prescribed dosage, measures for avoidance of adverse effects, cautions that it may take weeks to see the desired clinical effects, warning signs that may indicate possible problems, and the need for monitoring and evaluation *to enhance patient knowledge about drug therapy and to promote compliance.* (Refer to Critical Thinking Scenario.) Warn patient that urine may have a pink to reddish-brown color.
- Offer support and encouragement *to help the patient to cope with the drug regimen.*

Evaluation

- Monitor patient response to the drug (decrease in signs and symptoms of psychotic disorder).
- Monitor for adverse effects (sedation, anticholinergic effects, hypotension, extrapyramidal effects, bone marrow suppression).
- Evaluate the effectiveness of the teaching plan (patient can give the drug name and dosage, possible adverse effects to watch for, specific measures to prevent adverse effects, and warning signs to report).
- Monitor the effectiveness of comfort measures and compliance with the regimen.

CRITICAL THINKING SCENARIO

Antipsychotic Drugs

THE SITUATION

B.A., a 36-year-old, single, professional woman, was diagnosed with chronic schizophrenia when she was a senior in high school. Her condition has been well controlled with chlorpromazine (generic), and she is able to maintain steady employment, live in her own home, and carry on a fairly active social life. At her last evaluation, she appeared to be developing bone marrow suppression, and her physician decided to try to taper the drug dosage. As the dosage was being lowered, B.A. became withdrawn and listless, missed several days of work, and canceled most of her social engagements. Afraid of interacting with people, she stayed in bed most of the time. She reported having thoughts of death and paranoid ideation about her neighbors that she was beginning to think might be true.

CRITICAL THINKING

What nursing interventions are appropriate at this time?

What supportive measures might be useful to help B.A. cope with this crisis and allow her to function normally again?

Antipsychotic Drugs (continued)

What happens to brain chemistry after long-term therapy with phenothiazines?
What drug options should be tried?
Are there any other options that might be useful?

DISCUSSION

Schizophrenia is not a disorder that can be resolved simply with proper counseling. B.A., an educated woman with a long history of taking phenothiazines, realizes the necessity of drug therapy to correct the chemical imbalance in her brain. She may need a high-potency antipsychotic to return her to the level of functioning she had reached before experiencing this setback. Her knowledge of her individual responses can be used to help select an appropriate drug and dosage. Her experiences may also facilitate her care planning and new drug regimen.

B.A. will need support to cope with problems at work—from her inability to go in to work, to coping with feelings about not meeting her social obligations, to finding the motivation to get up and become active again. She might do well with behavior modification techniques that give her some control over her activities and allow her to use her knowledge and experience with her own situation to her advantage in forming a new medical regimen. She may need support in explaining her problem to her employer and her social contacts in ways that will help her avoid the prejudice associated with mental illness and will allow her every opportunity to return to her regular routine as soon as she can.

Because it may take several months to find the drug or drugs that will bring B.A. back to a point of stabilization, it is important to have a consistent, reliable health care team in place to support her through this stabilization period. She should have a reliable contact person to call when she has questions and when she needs support.

NURSING CARE GUIDE FOR B.A.: ANTIPSYCHOTIC/NEUROLEPTIC DRUGS

Assessment: History and Examination

Allergies to any of these drugs, CNS depression, CV disease, pregnancy or lactation, myelography, glaucoma, hypotension, thyrotoxicosis, seizures
Concurrent use of anticholinergics, barbiturate anesthetics, alcohol, meperidine, beta-blockers, epinephrine, norepinephrine
CV: Blood pressure, pulse, orthostatic blood pressure
CNS: Orientation, affect, reflexes, vision
Skin: Color, lesions, texture
Respiratory: Respiration, adventitious sounds
GI: Abdominal examination, bowel sounds
Laboratory tests: Thyroid, liver, and renal function tests and CBC

Nursing Diagnoses

Impaired physical mobility related to extrapyramidal effects
Risk for injury related to CNS effects
Decreased cardiac output related to CV effects
Impaired urinary elimination related to anticholinergic effects
Deficient knowledge regarding drug therapy

Planning

The patient will receive the best therapeutic effect from the drug therapy.
The patient will have limited adverse effects to the drug therapy.
The patient will have an understanding of the drug therapy, adverse effects to anticipate, and measures to relieve discomfort and improve safety.

Implementation

Give drug in evening; do not allow patient to chew or crush sustained release capsules.
Provide comfort and safety measures: Void before dosing; raise side rails; provide sugarless lozenges, mouth care; institute safety measures if CNS effects occur; position patient to relieve dyskinesia discomfort; taper dosage after long-term therapy.
Provide support and reassurance to help patient cope with drug effects.
Teach patient about drug, dosage, adverse effects, conditions to report, and precautions.

Evaluation

Evaluate drug effects: Relief of signs and symptoms of psychotic disorders.
Monitor for adverse effects: Sedation, dizziness, insomnia; anticholinergic effects; extrapyramidal effects; bone marrow suppression; skin rash.
Monitor for drug–drug interactions as listed.
Evaluate effectiveness of patient-teaching program.
Evaluate effectiveness of comfort and safety measures.

PATIENT TEACHING FOR B.A.

- The drugs that are useful for treating schizophrenia are called antipsychotic or neuroleptic drugs. These drugs affect the activities of certain chemicals in your brain and are used to treat certain mental disorders.
- Drugs in this group should be taken exactly as prescribed. Because these drugs affect many body systems, it is important that you have medical checkups regularly.
- Common effects of these drugs include:
- *Dizziness, drowsiness, and fainting:* Avoid driving or performing hazardous tasks or delicate tasks that

(continues on page 380)

Antipsychotic Drugs (continued)

require concentration if these occur. Change position slowly. The dizziness usually passes after 1–2 weeks of drug use.

- *Pink or reddish urine (with phenothiazines):* These drugs sometimes cause urine to change color. Do not be alarmed by this change; it does not mean that your urine contains blood.
- *Sensitivity to light:* Bright light might hurt your eyes and sunlight might burn your skin more easily. Wear sunglasses and protective clothing when you must be out in the sun.
- *Constipation:* Consult with your health care provider if this becomes a problem.
- Report any of the following conditions to your health care provider: *Sore throat, fever, rash, tremors, weakness, and vision changes.*
- Tell any doctor, nurse, or other health care provider that you are taking this drug.
- Keep this drug and all medications out of the reach of children.
- Avoid the use of alcohol or other depressants while you are taking this drug. You also may want to limit your use of caffeine if you feel very tense or cannot sleep.
- Avoid the use of over-the-counter drugs while you are on this drug. Many of them contain ingredients that could interfere with the effectiveness of your drug. If you feel that you need one of these preparations, consult with your health care provider about the most appropriate choice.
- Take this drug exactly as prescribed. If you run out of medicine or find that you cannot take your drug for any reason, consult your health care provider. After this drug has been used for a period of time, additional adverse effects may occur if it is suddenly stopped. This drug dosage will need to be tapered over time.

KEY POINTS

- Mental disorders are thought process disorders that may be caused by some inherent dysfunction within the brain. A psychosis is a thought disorder, and schizophrenia is the most common psychosis in which delusions and hallucinations are hallmarks.
- Antipsychotic drugs are generally dopamine receptor blockers that are effective in helping people to organize thought patterns and to respond appropriately to stimuli.
- Antipsychotics can cause hypotension, anticholinergic effects, sedation, and extrapyramidal effects, including parkinsonism, ataxia, and tremors.

Drugs for Bipolar Disorders

Mania, at the opposite pole from depression, occurs in individuals with bipolar disorder who experience a period of depression followed by a period of mania. The cause of mania is not understood, but it is thought to be an overstimulation of certain neurons in the brain. The mainstay for treatment of mania has always been lithium (*Lithobid*). Today, many other drugs are used successfully in treating bipolar disorders, including aripiprazole (*Abilify*), olanzapine (*Zyprexa, Zyprexa Zydis*), quetiapine (*Seroquel*), and ziprasidone (*Geodon*), which are atypical antipsychotics, and lamotrigine (*Lamictal*), an antiepileptic agent discussed in greater detail in Chapter 23. These new approvals were the first advances since the 1970s in the treatment of bipolar disorder (see Table 22.2).

Table 22.2 ***Drugs in Focus:* Drugs for Bipolar Disorders**

Drug Name	Dosage/Route	Usual Indications
aripiprazole (*Abilify*)	30 mg/d PO	Treatment of acute manic and mixed episodes of bipolar disorders
lamotrigine (*Lamictal*)	25 mg/d PO	Long-term maintenance of patients with bipolar disorders; decreases occurrence of acute mood episodes
lithium salts (*Lithobid*)	600 mg PO t.i.d. for acute episodes; 300 mg PO t.i.d. to q.i.d. for maintenance; reduce dose with elderly patients	Treatment of manic episodes of manic-depressive or bipolar illness; maintenance therapy to prevent or diminish the frequency and intensity of future manic episodes; currently being studied for improvement of neutrophil counts in patients with cancer chemotherapy—induced neutropenia and as prophylaxis of cluster headaches and migraine headaches; not recommended for children <12 y
olanzapine (*Zyprexa, Zyprexa Zydis*)	10 mg/d PO; range 5–20 mg/d	Management of acute manic episodes associated with bipolar disorder, in combination with lithium or valproate, or as monotherapy
quetiapine (*Seroquel*)	50 mg PO b.i.d., titrate to a maximum 800 mg/d	Adjunct or monotherapy for the treatment of manic episodes associated with bipolar disorder
ziprasidone (*Geodon*)	40 mg PO b.i.d. with food; maximum 80 mg b.i.d.	Treatment of acute manic and mixed episodes of bipolar disorders

Lithium salts (*Lithobid*) are taken orally for the management of manic episodes and prevention of future episodes. These very toxic drugs can cause severe CNS, renal, and pulmonary problems that may lead to death. Despite the potential for serious adverse effects, lithium is used with caution because it is consistently effective in the treatment of mania. The therapeutically effective serum level is 0.6 to 1.2 mEq/L.

Therapeutic Actions and Indications

Lithium functions in several ways. It alters sodium transport in nerve and muscle cells; inhibits the release of norepinephrine and dopamine, but not serotonin, from stimulated neurons; increases the intraneuronal stores of norepinephrine and dopamine slightly; and decreases intraneuronal content of second messengers. This last mode of action may allow it to selectively modulate the responsiveness of hyperactive neurons that might contribute to the manic state. Although the biochemical actions of lithium are known the exact mechanism of action in decreasing the manifestations of mania are not understood.

Pharmacokinetics

Lithium is readily absorbed from the GI tract, reaching peak levels in 30 minutes to 3 hours. It follows the same distribution pattern in the body as water. It slowly crosses the blood–brain barrier. Lithium is excreted from the kidney, although about 80% is reabsorbed. During periods of sodium depletion or dehydration, the kidney reabsorbs more lithium into the serum, often leading to toxic levels. Therefore, patients must be encouraged to maintain hydration while taking this drug. Lithium crosses the placenta and enters breast milk and has been associated with congenital abnormalities (see Contraindications and Cautions).

Contraindications and Cautions

Lithium is contraindicated in the presence of hypersensitivity to lithium *to prevent hypersensitivity reactions*. In addition, it is contraindicated in the following conditions: Significant renal or cardiac disease *that could be exacerbated by the toxic effects of the drug*; a history of leukemia; metabolic disorders, including sodium depletion; dehydration; and diuretic use *because lithium depletes sodium reabsorption, and severe hyponatremia may occur*. (Hyponatremia leads to lithium retention and toxicity.)

Pregnancy and lactation are also contraindications *because of the potential for adverse effects on the fetus or neonate*; breastfeeding should be discontinued while using lithium, and women of childbearing age should be advised to use birth control while taking this drug. Caution should be used in any condition *that could alter sodium levels*, such as protracted diarrhea or excessive sweating; with suicidal or impulsive patients; and in patients who have infection with fever, *which could be exacerbated by the toxic effects of the drug*.

Adverse Effects

The adverse effects associated with lithium are directly related to serum levels of the drug.

- *Serum levels of <1.5 mEq/L:* CNS problems, including lethargy, slurred speech, muscle weakness, and fine tremor; polyuria, which relates to renal toxicity; and beginning of gastric toxicity, with nausea, vomiting, and diarrhea.
- *Serum levels of 1.5 to 2 mEq/L:* Intensification of all of the foregoing reactions, with ECG changes.
- *Serum levels of 2 to 2.5 mEq/L:* Possible progression of CNS effects to ataxia, clonic movements, hyperreflexia, and seizures; possible CV effects such as severe ECG changes and hypotension; large output of dilute urine secondary to renal toxicity; fatalities secondary to pulmonary toxicity.
- *Serum levels >2.5 mEq/L:* Complex multiorgan toxicity, with a significant risk of death.

Clinically Important Drug–Drug Interactions

Some drug–drug combinations should be avoided. A lithium–haloperidol combination may result in an encephalopathic syndrome, consisting of weakness, lethargy, confusion, tremors, extrapyramidal symptoms, leukocytosis, and irreversible brain damage. See Box 22.4 for a serious lithium-herbal interaction.

If lithium is given with carbamazepine, increased CNS toxicity may occur, and a lithium–iodide salt combination results in an increased risk of hypothyroidism. Patients who receive either of these combinations should be monitored carefully. In addition, a thiazide diuretic–lithium combination increases the risk of lithium toxicity because of the loss of sodium and increased retention of lithium. If this combination is used the dose of lithium should be decreased and the patient should be monitored closely.

In the following instances the serum lithium level should be monitored closely and appropriate dose adjustments made. With the combination of lithium and some urine-alkalinizing drugs, including antacids and tromethamine, there is a possibility of decreased effectiveness of lithium. If lithium is combined with indomethacin or with some nonsteroidal anti-inflammatory drugs, higher plasma levels of lithium occur.

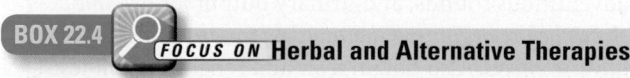

BOX 22.4 FOCUS ON Herbal and Alternative Therapies

Psyllium

Patients being treated with lithium should be encouraged not to use the herbal therapy psyllium, which is used to treat constipation and to lower cholesterol levels. If this agent is combined with lithium the absorption of the lithium may be blocked, and the patient will not receive therapeutic levels. If the patient feels a need for a drug to relieve constipation or is concerned about cholesterol levels, he or she should be encouraged to discuss alternative measures with the health care provider.

Ⓟ Prototype Summary: Lithium

Indications: Treatment of manic episodes of bipolar disorder and maintenance treatment of bipolar disorder.

Actions: Alters sodium transport in nerve and muscle cells; inhibits the release of norepinephrine and dopamine, but not serotonin, from stimulated neurons; increases the intraneuronal stores of norepinephrine and dopamine slightly; and decreases the intraneuronal content of second messengers.

Pharmacokinetics:

Route	Onset	Peak	Duration
Oral	Unknown	0.5–3 h	8–12 h
Oral, extended release	Unknown	4–12 h	12–18 h

$T_{1/2}$: 24 hours; excreted in the urine.

Adverse Effects: CNS problems, including lethargy, slurred speech, muscle weakness, and fine tremor; polyuria, gastric toxicity, with nausea, vomiting, and diarrhea progressing; CV collapse, coma; adverse effects are related to serum drug levels.

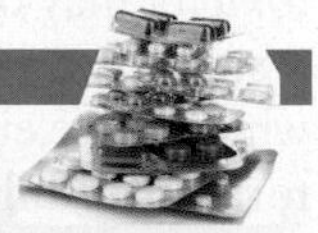

Nursing Considerations for Patients Receiving Lithium

Assessment: History and Examination

- Assess for *contraindications or cautions for the use of the drug*, including any known allergies to lithium; renal or CV disease; dehydration; sodium depletion, use of diuretics, protracted sweating, or diarrhea; suicidal or impulsive patients with severe depression; pregnancy or lactation; and infection with fever.
- Assess temperature; skin color and lesions; CNS orientation, affect, and reflexes; bowel sounds and reported output; pulse, auscultation, and blood pressure, including orthostatic blood pressure; respiration rate and adventitious sounds; and urinary output *for baseline status before beginning therapy and for any potential adverse effects*. Also obtain liver and renal function tests, thyroid function tests, CBC, and baseline ECG, and obtain serum lithium levels as appropriate.

Nursing Diagnoses

Nursing diagnoses related to drug therapy might include the following:

- Acute pain related to GI, CNS, and vision effects.
- Risk for injury related to CNS effects.
- Impaired urinary elimination related to renal toxic effects.
- Disturbed thought processes related to CNS effects.
- Deficient knowledge regarding drug therapy.

Planning

- The patient will receive the best therapeutic effect from the drug therapy.
- The patient will have limited adverse effects to the drug therapy.
- The patient will have an understanding of the drug therapy, adverse effects to anticipate, and measures to relieve discomfort and improve safety.

Implementation with Rationale

- Administer drug cautiously, with daily monitoring of serum lithium levels, to patients with significant renal or CV disease, dehydration, or debilitation, as well as those taking diuretics, *to monitor for toxic levels and to arrange for appropriate dose adjustment.*
- Administer drug with food or milk *to alleviate GI irritation if GI upset is severe.*
- Arrange to decrease dose after acute manic episodes. *Lithium tolerance is greatest during acute episodes and decreases when the acute episode is over.*
- Ensure that the patient maintains adequate intake of salt and fluid *to decrease toxicity.*
- Monitor patient's clinical status closely, especially during the initial stages of therapy, *to provide appropriate supportive management as needed.*
- Arrange for small, frequent meals; sugarless lozenges to suck; and frequent mouth care *to increase secretions and decrease discomfort as needed.*
- Provide safety measures such as side rails and assistance with ambulation if CNS effects occur *to prevent patient injury.*
- Provide thorough patient teaching, including drug name, prescribed dosage, measures for avoidance of adverse effects, cautions that it may take time to see the desired therapeutic effects, warning signs that may indicate possible problems, and the need to avoid pregnancy while taking lithium *to enhance patient knowledge about drug therapy and to promote compliance.*
- Offer support and encouragement *to help the patient to cope with the drug regimen.*

Evaluation

- Monitor patient response to the drug (decreased manifestations and frequency of manic episodes).
- Monitor for adverse effects (CV toxicity, renal toxicity, GI upset, respiratory complications).
- Evaluate effectiveness of the teaching plan (patient can give the drug name and dosage and describe the possible adverse effects to watch for, specific measures to help avoid adverse effects, warning signs to report, and the need to avoid pregnancy).
- Monitor effectiveness of comfort measures and compliance with the regimen.

KEY POINTS

- Lithium, a membrane stabilizer, is the standard antimanic drug. Because it is a very toxic salt, serum levels must be carefully monitored to prevent severe toxicity.
- Many other CNS drugs, including many of the atypical antipsychotics, are now approved for use in bipolar disorder. Many patients respond to a combination of these drugs to control their bipolar signs and symptoms.

Central Nervous System Stimulants

CNS stimulants are used clinically to treat both attention deficit disorders and narcolepsy. Paradoxically, these drugs calm hyperkinetic children and help them to focus on one activity for a longer period. They also redirect and excite the arousal stimuli from the RAS (Figure 22.4; see also Figure 22.1). The CNS stimulants that are used to treat attention deficit disorder and narcolepsy include: methylphenidate (*Ritalin*, *Concerta*, and others); dexmethylphenidate (*Focalin*), an isomer of methylphenidate used in lower doses than methylphenidate; dextroamphetamine (*Dexedrine*); lisdexamfetamine (*Vyvanse*), an amphetamine; modafinil (*Provigil*), which is not associated with many of the systemic stimulatory effects of some of the other CNS stimulants; and three other drugs—armodafinil (*Nuvigil*), which is thought to act through dopaminergic mechanisms but it is not associated with the cardiac and systemic stimulatory effects seen with other CNS stimulants; atomoxetine (*Strattera*), which is a selective norepinephrine reuptake inhibitor with anticholinergic effects but without the CV and stimulatory effects, making it preferable in patients who cannot tolerate the systemic stimulatory effects; and guanfacine (*Intuniv*), a centrally acting alpha-adrenergic stimulator that has been used for treating hypertension for many years. It was recently approved to treat attention deficit hyperactivity disorder (ADHD) and does not have any of the cardiac and blood pressure effects seen with the other drugs used to treat this disorder (see Table 22.3).

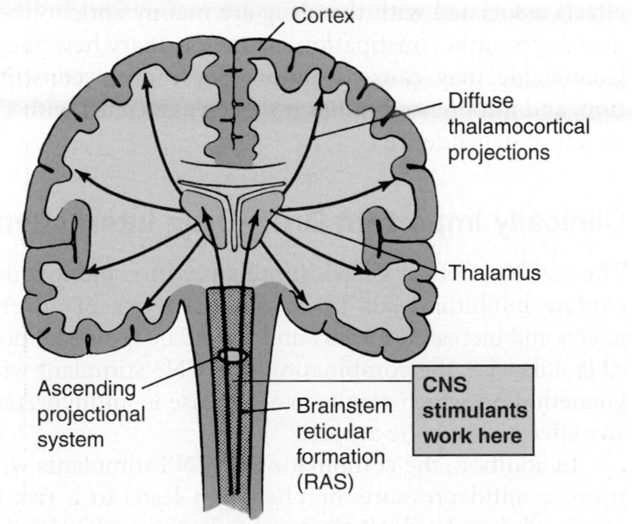

FIGURE 22.4 Site of action of the central nervous system (CNS) stimulants in the reticular activating system (RAS).

Therapeutic Actions and Indications

The CNS stimulants act as cortical and RAS stimulants, possibly by increasing the release of catecholamines from presynaptic neurons, leading to an increase in stimulation of the postsynaptic neurons. The paradoxical effect of calming hyperexcitability through CNS stimulation seen in attention deficit syndrome is believed to be related to increased stimulation of an immature RAS, which leads to the ability to be more selective in response to incoming stimuli.

The CNS stimulants are indicated, as part of a comprehensive treatment program, for the treatment of attention deficit syndromes, including behavioral syndromes characterized by hyperactivity and distractibility, as well as for narcolepsy and improvement of wakefulness in people with various sleep disorders. Most of these drugs are controlled substances, and it is important to include that point in the teaching plan; the drugs should be secured at home to prevent inappropriate use or distribution. In 2015 lisdexamfetamine was also approved for the treatment of binge-eating disorders in adults; it carries a black box warning that it is not approved as a weight loss agent.

Pharmacokinetics

These drugs are rapidly absorbed from the GI tract, reaching peak levels in 2 to 4 hours. They are metabolized in the liver and excreted in the urine, with half-lives ranging from 2 to 15 hours, depending on the drug. Safety for use during pregnancy and lactation has not been established; during those periods, these drugs should be used only if the benefit to the mother clearly outweighs the potential risk to the fetus or neonate.

Contraindications and Cautions

The CNS stimulants are contraindicated in the presence of known allergy to the drug, *which could lead to hypersensitivity reactions*. Other contraindications include the following conditions: Marked anxiety, agitation, or tension and severe fatigue or glaucoma, *which could be exacerbated by the CNS stimulation caused by these drugs*; cardiac disease, *which could be aggravated by the stimulatory effects of these drugs, making it important to rule out congenital heart problems*; and pregnancy and

Table 22.3 ***Drugs in Focus:* Central Nervous System Stimulants**

Drug Name	Dosage/Route	Usual Indications
armodafinil (*Nuvigil*)	150–250 mg/d PO as a single dose in the morning *Shift work sleep disorder:* 150 mg/d PO at 1 h before the start of shift	Management of patients with obstructive sleep disorders (including sleep apnea), narcolepsy, and shift work sleep disorders to improve wakefulness
atomoxetine (*Strattera*)	*Adults and children >70 kg:* 40 mg/d PO, slowly increase to a target daily dose of 80 mg *Children ≤70 kg:* 0.5 mg/kg/d, increase to a target daily dose of 1.2 mg/kg/d *Hepatic impairment:* decrease dose by 50%	Treatment of attention deficit/hyperactivity disorders as part of a total treatment program
dexmethylphenidate (*Focalin*)	2.5–5 mg PO b.i.d.; do not exceed 10 mg PO b.i.d.	Treatment of attention deficit/hyperactivity disorder in patients aged ≥6 y
dextroamphetamine (*Dexedrine*)	*Narcolepsy:* 5–60 mg/d PO in divided doses *Attention deficit disorders:* 2.5–5 mg/d PO taken in the morning *Obesity:* 5–30 mg/d PO (not recommended for children <12 y)	Treatment of narcolepsy, attention deficit disorders, behavioral syndromes, exogenous obesity
guanfacine (*Intuniv*)	*Children 6–17 y:* 1 mg/d PO, ER tablet, may be titrated to maximum 4 mg/d	Treatment of ADHD in ER tablet form; taper when discontinuing
lisdexamfetamine (*Vyvanse*)	*Pediatric (6–12 y):* 30 mg/d PO; maximum dose 70 mg/d	Treatment of attention deficit/hyperactivity disorder in children 6–12 y of age
methylphenidate (*Ritalin, Concerta,* and others)	*Adult:* 10–60 mg/d PO in divided doses, depending on preparation *Pediatric:* 5 mg PO b.i.d.; increase gradually, do not exceed 60 mg/d	Treatment of attention deficit disorders and other behavioral syndromes associated with hyperactivity, as well as narcolepsy; currently available in various forms allowing for dosing one, two, or three times a day
modafinil (*Provigil*)	200 mg/d PO as a single dose; reduce dose with hepatic impairment and in the elderly	Treatment of narcolepsy in adults, for improving wakefulness in various sleep disorders, and for improving wakefulness in people with obstructive sleep apnea/hypopnea syndrome

ER, extended release; ADHD, attention deficit hyperactivity disorder.

lactation *because of the potential for adverse effects on the fetus or neonate.*

Caution should be used in patients with a history of seizures, *which could be potentiated by the CNS stimulation*; in patients with a history of drug dependence, including alcoholism, *because these drugs may result in physical and psychological dependence*; and in patients with hypertension, *which could be exacerbated by the stimulatory effects of these drugs.*

Adverse Effects

The adverse effects associated with these drugs are related to the CNS stimulation they cause. CNS effects can include nervousness, insomnia, dizziness, headache, blurred vision, and difficulty with accommodation. GI effects such as anorexia, nausea, and weight loss may occur. CV effects can include hypertension, arrhythmias, and angina. Sudden cardiac death has been associated with the use of these drugs. Studies showed that the majority of these deaths occurred in children with undocumented cardiac defects; because of this a baseline ECG should be done before beginning therapy. Skin rashes are a common reaction to some of these drugs. Physical and psychological dependence may also develop. Because CNS stimulants have this effect the drugs are controlled substances. Atomoxetine, which does not show dependence development, is not a controlled substance. The adverse effects associated with this drug are mainly anticholinergic (dry mouth, constipation, nausea, urinary hesitancy). Guanfacine may cause sedation, dry mouth, constipation, and impotence but has not been associated with CV effects of dependence.

Clinically Important Drug–Drug Interactions

The combination of a CNS stimulant with a monoamine oxidase inhibitor leads to an increased risk of adverse effects and increased toxicity and should be avoided if possible. Likewise, the combination of a CNS stimulant with guanethidine, which results in a decrease in antihypertensive effects, should be avoided.

In addition, the combination of CNS stimulants with tricyclic antidepressants or phenytoin leads to a risk of increased drug levels. Patients who receive such a combination should be monitored for toxicity.

Ⓟ Prototype Summary: Methylphenidate

Indications: Narcolepsy and attention deficit disorder

Actions: Mild cortical stimulant with CNS actions similar to those of amphetamines.

Pharmacokinetics:

Route	Onset	Peak	Duration
Oral	Varies	1–3 h	4–6 h

$T_{1/2}$: 1 to 3 hours; metabolized in the liver, excreted in the urine.

Adverse Effects: Nervousness, insomnia, increased or decreased pulse rate and blood pressure, tachycardia, loss of appetite, nausea, and abdominal pain.

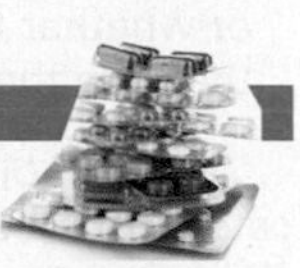

Nursing Considerations for Patients Receiving Central Nervous System Stimulants

Assessment: History and Examination

- Assess for *contraindications or cautions for the use of the drug*, including any known allergies to the drug; glaucoma, anxiety, tension, fatigue, or seizure disorder; cardiac disease and hypertension; pregnancy or lactation; a history of leukemia; and a history of drug dependency, including alcoholism.
- Assess temperature; skin color and lesions; CNS orientation, affect, and reflexes; ophthalmic examination; bowel sounds and reported output; pulse, auscultation, and blood pressure, including orthostatic blood pressure; respiration rate and adventitious sounds; and urinary output *to determine baseline status before beginning therapy and for any potential adverse effects.* Also obtain a CBC.

Nursing Diagnoses

Nursing diagnoses related to drug therapy might include the following:

- Disturbed thought processes related to CNS effects of the drug.
- Decreased cardiac output related to CV effects of the drug.
- Risk for injury related to CNS and visual effects of the drug.
- Deficient knowledge regarding drug therapy.

Planning

- The patient will receive the best therapeutic effect from the drug therapy.
- The patient will have limited adverse effects to the drug therapy.
- The patient will have an understanding of the drug therapy, adverse effects to anticipate, and measures to relieve discomfort and improve safety.

Implementation with Rationale

- Ensure proper diagnosis of behavioral syndromes and narcolepsy *because these drugs should not be used until underlying medical causes of the problem are ruled out.*
- Arrange to interrupt the drug periodically in children who are receiving the drug for behavioral syndromes *to determine whether symptoms recur and therapy should be continued.*
- Arrange to dispense the least amount of drug possible *to minimize the risk of overdose and abuse.*
- Administer drug before 6 PM *to reduce the incidence of insomnia.*
- Monitor weight, CBC, and ECG *to ensure early detection of adverse effects and proper interventions.*
- Consult with the school nurse or counselor *to ensure comprehensive care of school-aged children receiving CNS stimulants* (Box 22.5).
- Provide safety measures such as side rails and assistance with ambulation if CNS effects occur *to prevent patient injury.*
- Provide thorough patient teaching, including drug name, prescribed dosage, the need to secure the drug as a controlled substance, measures for avoidance of adverse effects, warning signs that may indicate possible problems, and the need for monitoring and evaluation *to enhance patient knowledge about drug therapy and to promote compliance.* Offer support and encouragement to help the patient to cope with the drug regimen.

Evaluation

- Monitor patient response to the drug (decrease in manifestations of behavioral syndromes, decrease in daytime sleep and narcolepsy).
- Monitor for adverse effects (CNS stimulation, CV effects, rash, physical or psychological dependence, GI dysfunction).
- Evaluate effectiveness of the teaching plan (patient can give the drug name and dosage, name possible adverse effects to watch for and specific measures to help avoid adverse effects, and describe the need for follow-up and evaluation).
- Monitor effectiveness of comfort measures and compliance with the regimen.

KEY POINTS

- An attention deficit disorder is a behavioral syndrome characterized by hyperactivity and a short attention span.
- Narcolepsy is a disorder characterized by daytime sleepiness and sudden loss of wakefulness.
- CNS stimulants, which stimulate cortical levels and the RAS to increase RAS activity, are used to treat attention deficit disorders and narcolepsy. These drugs improve concentration and the ability to filter and focus incoming stimuli.

BOX 22.5 FOCUS ON The Evidence

School Nursing and Ritalin Administration

In the last several years the number of schoolchildren receiving diagnoses of attention deficit disorder or minimal brain dysfunction and being prescribed methylphenidate (*Ritalin*) has increased dramatically. Because this drug needs to be given two or three times each day, it has become the responsibility of the school nurse to dispense the drug during the day. Some school nurses reportedly spend between 50% and 70% of their time administering these drugs and completing the necessary paperwork. In 2000–2001, several long-acting formulations of methylphenidate became available.

Concerta, previously available in an extended release tablet in 18- and 36-mg strengths, is now also available in a 54-mg strength. This form is suggested for every-12-hours dosing. *Metadate CD* is approved as a 20-mg extended release capsule that is suggested as a once-daily treatment for children with attention deficit disorder. *Ritalin SR* is another extended release formulation that is designed to be given every 8 hours. These extended release forms are not interchangeable, and the instructions that come with the drug that is prescribed should be checked carefully. The advantage of these extended release forms is expected to be a decrease in the number of students who must see the nurse for medication during the school day and, perhaps, a decrease in the stigma that may be associated with needing this drug.

The school nurse has additional responsibilities besides administering the drug. The school nurse is responsible for assessing children's response to the drug and for coordinating the teacher's and health care provider's input into each individual case, including the incidence of adverse effects and the appropriateness of the drug therapy.

The nurse should:

- Ensure that the proper diagnosis is made before supporting the use of the drug.
- Constantly evaluate and work with the primary health care provider to regularly challenge children without the drug to see whether the drug is doing what is expected or whether the child is maturing and no longer needs the drug therapy.

The school nurse needs to be prepared to be an advocate for the best therapeutic intervention for a particular child. Because long-term methylphenidate therapy is associated with many adverse effects, use of the drug should not be taken lightly.

SUMMARY

- Schizophrenia, the most common psychosis, is characterized by delusions, hallucinations, and inappropriate responses to stimuli.
- Bipolar disorder is a behavioral disorder that involves extremes of depression alternating with hyperactivity and excitement.
- An attention deficit disorder is a behavioral syndrome characterized by hyperactivity and a short attention span.
- Narcolepsy is a disorder characterized by daytime sleepiness and sudden loss of wakefulness.
- Lithium, a membrane stabilizer, is the standard antimanic drug. Because it is a very toxic salt, serum levels must be carefully monitored to prevent severe toxicity. Many other CNS drugs are now approved for use in bipolar disorder.
- CNS stimulants, which stimulate cortical levels and the RAS to increase RAS activity, are used to treat attention deficit disorders and narcolepsy. These drugs improve concentration and the ability to filter and focus incoming stimuli.

CHECK YOUR UNDERSTANDING

Answers to the questions in this chapter can be found in Answers to Check Your Understanding Questions on thePoint®.

MULTIPLE CHOICE

Select the best answer to the following.

1. Mental disorders are now thought to be caused by some inherent dysfunction within the brain that leads to abnormal thought processes and responses. They include
   a. depression.
   b. anxiety.
   c. seizures.
   d. schizophrenia.
2. Antipsychotic drugs are basically
   a. serotonin reuptake inhibitors.
   b. norepinephrine blockers.
   c. dopamine receptor blockers.
   d. acetylcholine stimulators.
3. Adverse effects associated with antipsychotic drugs are related to the drugs' effects on receptor sites and can include
   a. insomnia and hypertension.
   b. dry mouth, hypotension, and glaucoma.

c. diarrhea and excessive urination.
d. increased sexual drive and improved concentration.

4. Lithium toxicity can be dangerous. Patient assessment to evaluate for appropriate lithium levels would look for
a. serum lithium levels >3 mEq/L.
b. b serum lithium levels >4 mEq/L.
c. serum lithium levels <1.5 mEq/L.
d. undetectable serum lithium levels.

5. Your patient, a 6-year-old boy, is starting a regimen of *Ritalin* (methylphenidate) to control an attention deficit disorder. Family teaching should include which of the following?
a. This drug can be shared with other family members who might seem to need it.
b. This drug may cause insomnia, weight loss, and GI upset.
c. Do not alert the school nurse to the fact that this drug is being taken because the child could have problems later on.
d. This drug should not be stopped for any reason for several years.

6. Antipsychotic drugs are also known as neuroleptic drugs because
a. they cause numerous neurological effects.
b. they frequently cause epilepsy.
c. they are also minor tranquilizers.
d. they are the only drugs known to directly affect nerves.

7. Attention deficit disorders (the inability to concentrate or focus on an activity) and narcolepsy (sudden episodes of sleep) are both most effectively treated with the use of
a. neuroinhibitors.
b. dopamine receptor blockers.
c. major tranquilizers.
d. CNS stimulants.

8. Haloperidol (*Haldol*) is a potent antipsychotic that is associated with
a. severe extrapyramidal effects.
b. severe sedation.
c. severe hypotension.
d. severe anticholinergic effects.

MULTIPLE RESPONSE

Select all that apply.

1. Before administering lithium to a client the nurse should check for the concomitant use of which of the following drugs, which could cause serious adverse effects?
a. ibuprofen
b. haloperidol
c. thiazide diuretics
d. antacids
e. ketoconazole
f. theophylline

2. Dyskinesias are a common side effect of antipsychotic drugs. Nursing interventions for the patient receiving antipsychotic drugs should include which of the following?
a. Positioning to decrease discomfort of dyskinesias
b. Implementing safety measures to prevent injury
c. Encouraging the patient to chew tablets to prevent choking
d. Careful teaching to alert the patient and family about this adverse effect
e. Applying ice to the joints to prevent damage
f. Pureeing all food to decrease the risk of aspiration

BIBLIOGRAPHY AND REFERENCES

American Psychiatric Association. (2013). *Diagnostic and statistical manual of mental disorders* (5th ed., text revision). Washington, DC: Author.

Brown, T. E. (2013 *A new understanding of ADHD in children and adults*. New York: Routledge.

Brunton, L., Chabner, B., & Knollman, B. (2011). *Goodman and Gilman's the pharmacological basis of therapeutics* (12th ed.). New York: McGraw-Hill.

Facts and Comparisons. (2015). *Drug facts and comparisons*. St. Louis, MO: Author.

Facts and Comparisons. (2015). *Professional's guide to patient drug facts*. St. Louis, MO: Author.

Karch, A. M. (2014). *Lippincott's nursing drug guide*. Philadelphia, PA: Lippincott Williams & Wilkins.

Kuehn, B. (2008). Antipsychotics risky for the elderly. *Journal of the American Medical Association, 300*(4), 379–380.

Porth, C. M. (2013). *Pathophysiology: Concepts of altered health states* (9th ed.). Philadelphia, PA: Lippincott Williams & Wilkins.

Sikich, L., Frazier, J., Mcclellan, J., et al. (2008). Children and antipsychotics. *American Journal of Psychiatry,* 10.1176/appi.ajp.2008.08050756.

Tiihonen, J., Haukka, J., Taylor, M., et al. (2011). A nationwide cohort study of oral and depot antipsychotics after first hospitalization or schizophrenia. *American Journal of Psychiatry, 168*(6), 603–609, 10.1176/appi.ajp.2011.10081224.

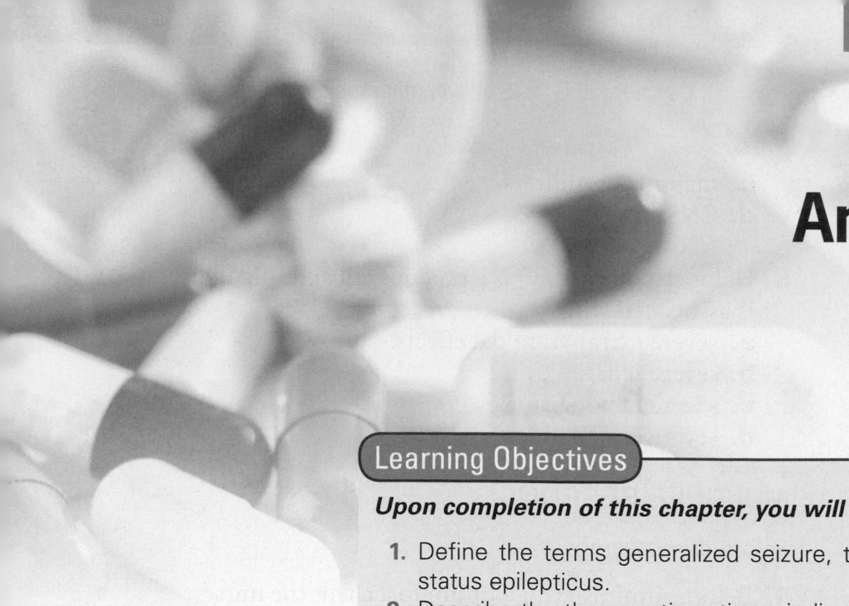

Antiseizure Agents 23

Learning Objectives

Upon completion of this chapter, you will be able to:

1. Define the terms generalized seizure, tonic–clonic seizure, absence seizure, partial seizure, and status epilepticus.
2. Describe the therapeutic actions, indications, pharmacokinetics, contraindications, most common adverse reactions, and important drug–drug interactions associated with each class of antiseizure agents.
3. Discuss the use of antiepileptic drugs across the lifespan.
4. Compare and contrast the prototype drugs for each class of antiepileptic drug with the other drugs in that class and with drugs from the other classes.
5. Outline the nursing considerations and teaching needs for patients receiving each class of antiepileptic agents.

Glossary of Key Terms

absence seizure: type of generalized seizure that is characterized by sudden, temporary loss of consciousness, sometimes with staring or blinking for 3 to 5 seconds; formerly known as a petit mal seizure

antiepileptic: drug used to treat the abnormal and excessive energy bursts in the brain that are characteristic of epilepsy

convulsion: tonic–clonic muscular reaction to excessive electrical energy arising from nerve cells in the brain

epilepsy: collection of various syndromes, all of which are characterized by seizures

generalized seizure: seizure that begins in one area of the brain and rapidly spreads throughout both hemispheres

partial seizures: also called focal seizures; seizures involving one area of the brain that do not spread throughout the entire organ

seizure: sudden discharge of excessive electrical energy from nerve cells in the brain

status epilepticus: state in which seizures rapidly recur; most severe form of generalized seizure

tonic–clonic seizure: type of generalized seizure that is characterized by serious clonic–tonic muscular reactions and loss of consciousness, with exhaustion and little memory of the event on awakening; formerly known as a grand mal seizure

Drug List

Drugs for Treating Generalized Seizures

Hydantoins
ethotoin
fosphenytoin
(P) phenytoin

Barbiturates and Barbiturate-like Drugs
(P) phenobarbital
primidone

Benzodiazepines
clobazam
clonazepam
(P) diazepam

Succinimides
(P) ethosuximide
methsuximide

Drugs that Modulate the Inhibitory Neurotransmitter GABA
acetazolamide
(P) valproic acid
zonisamide

Drugs for Treating Partial Seizures
(P) carbamazepine
clorazepate
egozabine
felbamate
gabapentin
lacosamide
lamotrigine
levetiracetam
oxcarbazepine
pregabalin
rufinamide
tiagabine
topiramate
vigabatrin

Epilepsy, the most prevalent of the neurological disorders, is not a single disease but a collection of different syndromes characterized by the same feature: Sudden discharge of excessive electrical energy from nerve cells located within the brain, which leads to a **seizure**. In some cases, this release stimulates motor nerves, resulting in convulsions, with tonic–clonic muscle contractions that have the potential to cause injury, tics, or spasms. Other discharges may stimulate autonomic or sensory nerves and cause very different effects, such as a barely perceptible, temporary lapse in consciousness or a sympathetic reaction. Because epilepsy involves a loss of control, it can be very frightening to patients when they are first diagnosed (Box 23.1).

The treatment of epilepsy varies widely, depending on the exact problem and its manifestations. The drugs that are used to manage epilepsy are called **antiepileptics**, or antiseizure agents, and are sometimes referred to as anticonvulsants; however, because not all types of epilepsy involve **convulsions**, this term is not generally applicable. The drug of choice for any given situation depends on the type of epilepsy, patient age (Box 23.2), specific patient characteristics such as cultural variations (Box 23.3), and patient tolerance for associated adverse effects. Drugs can be used to treat more than one type of seizure. Table 23.1 lists drugs and the types of seizures that they can be used to treat.

Nature of Seizures

The form that a particular seizure takes depends on the location of the cells that initiate the electrical discharge and the neural pathways that are stimulated by the initial volley of electrical impulses. For the most part, epilepsy seems to be caused by abnormal neurons that are very sensitive to stimulation or overrespond for some reason. They do not appear to be different from other neurons in any other way. Seizures caused by these abnormal cells are called primary seizures because no underlying cause can be identified. In some cases, however, outside factors—head injury, drug overdose, environmental exposure, and so on—may precipitate seizures. Such seizures are often referred to as secondary seizures.

Classification of Seizures

Accurate diagnosis of seizure type is very important for determining the correct medication to prevent future seizures while causing the fewest problems and adverse effects. Seizures were formerly categorized as grand mal (tonic–clonic seizures) or petit mal (absence seizures), but the International Classification of Seizures currently refers to seizures in a more systematic approach (based on the description of symptoms and characteristics), grouping them into two main categories: Generalized or partial seizures. Each of these categories can be further subdivided (see Figure 23.1).

BOX 23.1 *FOCUS ON* **Patient and Family Teaching**

Teaching and Counseling Patients with Epilepsy

Epilepsy, with its stigma, is frightening to people who know little about the disease. This condition has long been associated with some sort of brain dysfunction or possession by the devil or evil spirits. In some eras, exorcism was the first choice of treatment for a person with a seizure disorder. A person who receives a diagnosis of epilepsy must deal with this stigma as well as the significance of the diagnosis. What does having epilepsy mean? Individuals who are newly diagnosed with epilepsy must consider restrictions on their independence as well as the prospect of chronic therapy for control of this problem.

In our society the ability to be readily mobile—to drive to appointments, work, or religious obligations—is very important to many people. Most states require physicians to report new diagnoses of epilepsy. In most cases the driving privileges of affected individuals are revoked, at least temporarily. The conditions for recovering the license vary with the diagnosis and the laws of each state.

The person who is newly diagnosed with epilepsy has to cope not only with the stigma of epilepsy but also with the loss of a driver's license. The nurse may be in the best position to help the patient adjust to both of these problems through patient education and referrals to community resources. Thorough patient teaching should include the following:

- Explanations of old stigmas
- Ways in which people may react to the diagnosis
- Ways in which patients can educate family, friends, and employers about the realities of the condition and its treatment
- Actions to take if a seizure happens so that no injuries occur and no panic develops
- Information about the availability of public transportation
- The importance of encouraging patients with epilepsy to carry or wear a MedicAlert identification to alert any emergency caregivers to their condition and to what drugs they are taking if they are not able to speak for themselves
- Contact information regarding other community support services

Many communities have epilepsy support groups that can supply information on valuable resources as well as updated facts about the laws in each area. While patients are first adjusting to epilepsy and its implications, it may help to put them in contact with such organizations. The local chapter of the Epilepsy Foundation of America may be able to offer support groups, lists of resources, and support. Individuals with epilepsy should have several options for getting around without feeling that they are being a burden or an imposition.

BOX 23.2 FOCUS ON Drug Therapy Across the Lifespan

Antiseizure Agents

CHILDREN

Antiepileptic drugs can have an impact on a child's learning and social development. Children may also be more sensitive to the sedating effects of some of these drugs. Children should be monitored very closely and often require a switch to a different agent or dosage adjustments based on their response.

Newborns (1–10 days of age) respond best to intramuscular phenobarbital if an antiepileptic is needed.

Older children (2 months–6 years of age) absorb and metabolize many of these drugs more quickly than adults do and require a larger dosage per kilogram to maintain therapeutic levels. Careful calculation of drug dosage using both weight and age are important in helping the child to receive the best therapeutic effect with the least toxicity. After the age of 10–14 years, many of these drugs can be given in the standard adult dose.

Parents of children receiving these drugs should receive consistent support and education about the seizure disorder and the medications being used to treat it. Many communities have local support groups that can offer lots of educational materials and support programs. It is a very frightening experience to watch your child have a tonic–clonic seizure, and parents should be supported with this in mind.

ADULTS

Adults using these drugs should be under regular care and should be monitored regularly for adverse effects. They should be encouraged to carry or wear a MedicAlert identification to alert emergency personnel that antiepileptic drugs are being taken. Adults also need education and support to deal with the old stigma of seizures as well as the lifestyle changes and drug effects that they may need to cope with.

Most of these drugs have been associated with fetal abnormalities in animal studies. Some of them are clearly associated with predictable congenital effects in humans. Women of childbearing age should be encouraged to use contraceptives while taking these drugs. If a pregnancy does occur, or if a woman taking one of these drugs desires to become pregnant, the importance of the drug to the mother should be weighed against the potential risk to the fetus. Stopping an antiepileptic can precipitate seizures that could cause anoxia and its related problems for the mother and the baby. Women who are nursing should be encouraged to find another way of feeding the baby to avoid the sedating and CNS effects that the drugs can have on the infant.

OLDER ADULTS

Older patients may be more susceptible to the adverse effects of these drugs. Dosages of all of these drugs may need to be reduced, and the patient should be monitored very closely for toxic effects and to provide safety measures if CNS effects do occur.

Patients with renal or hepatic impairment should be monitored very closely. Baseline renal and liver function tests should be done and dosages adjusted as appropriate. Serum levels of the drug should be monitored closely in such cases to prevent serious adverse effects.

The older patient should also be encouraged to wear or carry a MedicAlert identification in case there is an emergency and the patient is not able to communicate information about the drug or disorder.

Generalized Seizures

Generalized seizures begin in one area of the brain and rapidly spread throughout both hemispheres of the brain. Patients who have a generalized seizure usually experience a loss of consciousness resulting from this massive electrical activity throughout the brain.

BOX 23.3 FOCUS ON Cultural Considerations

Altered Metabolism of Antiseizure Agents

Because of differences in liver enzyme functioning among Arab Americans and Asian Americans, patients in these ethnic groups may not metabolize antiseizure agents in the same way as patients in other ethnic groups. They may require not only lower doses to achieve the same therapeutic effects but also frequent dose adjustment.

Nurses need to be aware that the therapeutic range for patients in these ethnic groups may differ from standard norms and that these patients may be more apt to show adverse or toxic reactions to antiepileptic drugs at lower doses. As with all medications the lowest possible dose should be used. Serum drug levels should be closely monitored and titrated carefully and slowly to achieve the maximum benefits with the fewest adverse effects.

Generalized seizures are further classified into the following five types:

1. **Tonic–clonic seizures** involve dramatic tonic–clonic muscle contractions (involuntary muscle contraction followed by relaxation appearing as an aggressive spasm), loss of consciousness, and a recovery period characterized by confusion and exhaustion.
2. **Absence seizures** involve abrupt, brief (3- to 5-second) periods of loss of consciousness. Absence seizures occur commonly in children, starting at about 3 years of age, and frequently disappear by puberty. Absence seizures do not usually involve muscle contractions.
3. Myoclonic seizures involve short, sporadic periods of muscle contractions that last for several minutes. They are relatively rare and are often secondary seizures.
4. Febrile seizures are related to very high fevers and usually involve tonic–clonic seizures. Febrile seizures most frequently occur in children; they are usually self-limited and do not reappear.

Table 23.1 Antiepileptic Drug Therapy Grouped by Seizure Class

Partial Seizures	Generalized Seizures (Except Status Epilepticus)	Status Epilepticus
carbamazepine	carbamazepine	diazepam
clobazam	clonazepam	fosphenytoin
clonazepam	ethosuximide	lorazepam
clorazepate	ethotoin	midazolam
cthotoin	felbamate (Lennox-Gastaut syndrome)	pentobarbital
celbamate	lamotrigine	phenobarbital
ezogabine	levetiracetam	phenytoin
gabapentin	methsuximide	propofol
lacosamide	oxcarbazepine	
lamotrigine	phensuximide	
levetiracetam	phenytoin	
oxcarbazepine	topiramate	
phenytoin	valproic acid	
pregabalin	zonisamide	
rufinamide		
tiagabine		
topiramate		
valproic acid		
vigabatrin		
zonisamide		

Adopted from Aschenbrenner, D. S., & Venable, S.J. (2011). *Drug therapy in nursing* (4th ed.). Philadelphia, PA: Lippincott Williams & Wilkins.

5. Jacksonian seizures are seizures that begin in one area of the brain and involve one part of the body, and then progressively spread to other parts of the body; they can develop into generalized tonic–clonic seizures.
6. Psychomotor seizures are complex seizures that involve sensory, motor, and psychic components. They usually begin with a loss of consciousness, and patients have no memory of the event. Patients may exhibit automatic movements, emotional outbursts, and motor or psychological disturbances.
7. **Status epilepticus**, potentially the most dangerous of seizure conditions, is a state in which seizures rapidly recur again and again with no recovery between seizures.

Partial Seizures

Partial seizures, or focal seizures, are so called because they involve one area of the brain, usually originate from one site or focus, and do not spread throughout the entire organ. The presenting symptoms depend on exactly where in the brain the excessive electrical discharge is occurring. Partial seizures can be further classified as follows:

- Simple partial seizures, which occur in a single area of the brain and may involve a single muscle movement or sensory alteration
- Complex partial seizures, which involve a series of reactions or emotional changes and complex sensory changes such as hallucinations, mental distortion, changes in personality, loss of consciousness, and loss of social inhibitions. Motor changes may include involuntary urination, chewing motions, diarrhea, and so on. The onset of complex partial seizures usually occurs by the late teens.

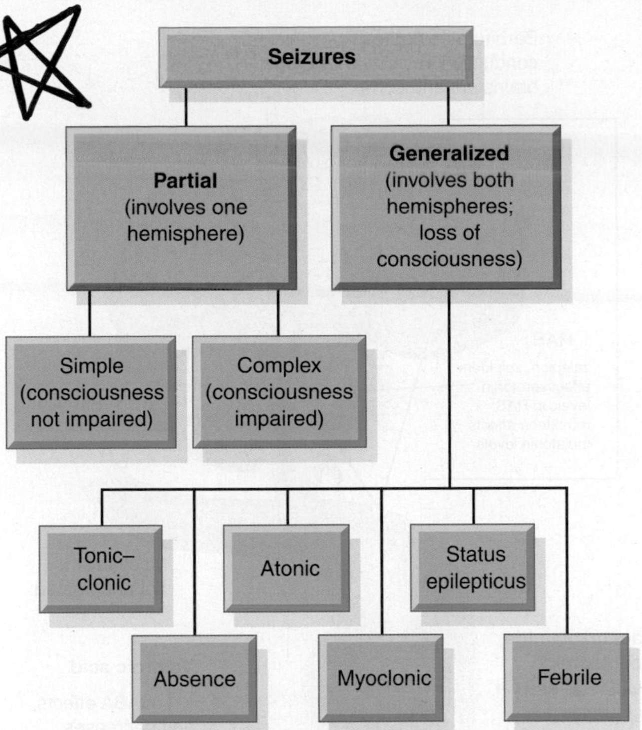

FIGURE 23.1 Classification of seizures. (From Aschenbrenner, D. S., & Venable, S. J. (2011). *Drug therapy in nursing* (3rd ed.). Philadelphia, PA: Lippincott Williams & Wilkins.)

KEY POINTS

- Epilepsy is characterized by seizures that result from sudden discharge of excessive electrical energy from nerve cells in the brain.
- There are two major categories of seizures: Generalized and partial seizures.
- Generalized seizures include the following types: Tonic–clonic, absence, myoclonic, febrile, Jacksonian, psychomotor, and rapid recurring (status epilepticus).
- Partial seizures may be simple or complex.

Drugs for Treating Generalized Seizures

Drugs typically used to treat generalized seizures stabilize the nerve membranes by blocking channels in the cell membrane or altering receptor sites. Because they work generally on the central nervous system (CNS), sedation and other CNS effects often result. Various drugs are used to treat generalized seizures, including hydantoins, barbiturates, barbiturate-like drugs, benzodiazepines, and succinimides. These drugs affect the entire brain and reduce the chance of sudden electrical outburst. Associated adverse effects are often related to total brain stabilization (Figure 23.2).

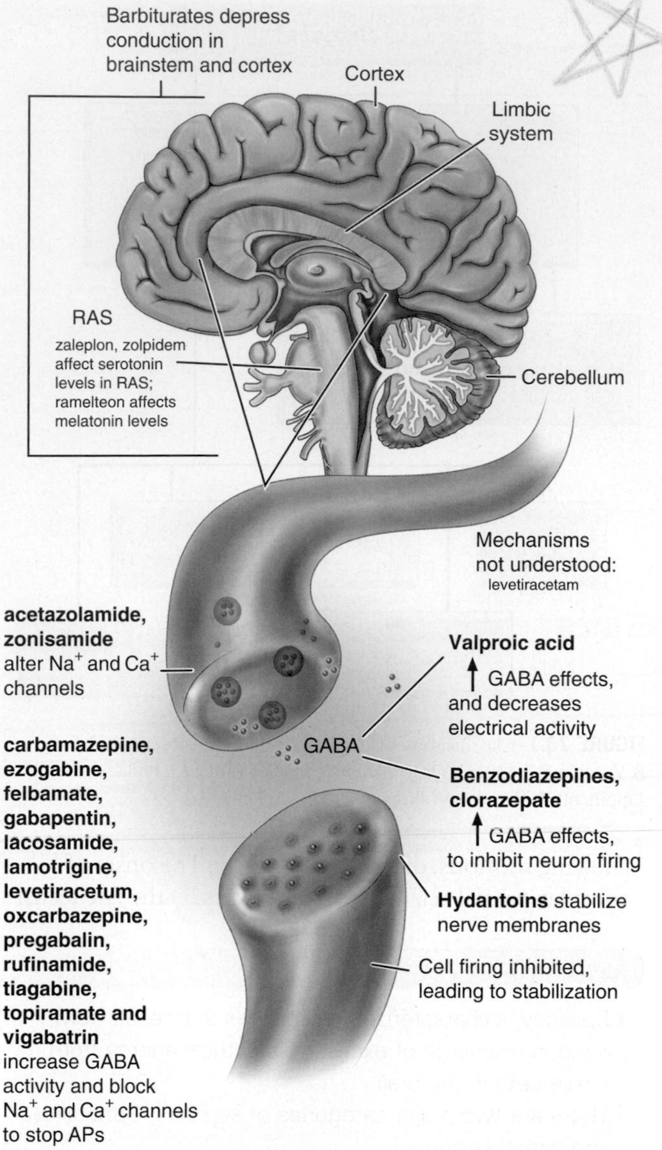

FIGURE 23.2 Sites of action of drugs used to treat various types of epilepsy. AP, action potential; GABA, gamma-aminobutyric acid; RAS, reticular activating system.

Absence seizures, another type of generalized seizure, may require drugs that are different than those used to treat or prevent other types of generalized seizures. The succinimides and drugs that modulate the inhibitory neurotransmitter gamma-aminobutyric acid (GABA) are most frequently used (see Table 23.2).

Hydantoins

Hydantoins include ethotoin (*Peganone*), fosphenytoin (*Cerebyx*), and phenytoin (*Dilantin*). Because hydantoins are generally less sedating than many other antiepileptics, they may be the drugs of choice for patients who are not willing to tolerate sedation and drowsiness. They do have significant adverse effects; thus, less toxic drugs, such as benzodiazepines, have replaced them in many situations.

> **FOCUS ON Safe Medication Administration**
>
> *Be aware that name confusion has been reported among* ***Cerebyx*** *(fosphenytoin),* ***Celebrex*** *(celecoxib; a nonsteroidal anti-inflammatory agent),* ***Celexa*** *(citalopram, a selective serotonin reuptake inhibitor antidepressant), and* ***Xanax*** *(alprazolam, an antianxiety drug). Because these drugs have sound-alike, look-alike names, if your patient is prescribed any of these drugs, make sure you know what the drug is being used for and that the patient is getting the correct prescribed drug.*

Therapeutic Actions and Indications

The hydantoins stabilize nerve membranes throughout the CNS directly by influencing ionic channels in the cell membrane, thereby decreasing excitability and hyperexcitability to stimulation. By decreasing conduction through nerve pathways, they reduce the tonic–clonic, muscular, and emotional responses to stimulation. See Table 23.2 for Usual Indications.

Pharmacokinetics

Phenytoin and ethotoin are well absorbed from the gastrointestinal (GI) tract, metabolized in the liver, and excreted in the urine. Therapeutic serum phenytoin levels range from 10 to 20 mcg/mL. The therapeutic serum levels of ethotoin are from 15 to 50 mcg/mL. Fosphenytoin is given intramuscularly or intravenously. It is metabolized in the liver and excreted in the urine. The therapeutic serum levels peak about 10 to 20 minutes after the infusion. Phenytoin is available in oral and parenteral forms.

Contraindications and Cautions

Hydantoins are generally contraindicated in the presence of allergy to any of these drugs *to avoid hypersensitivity reactions. Many of these agents are associated with specific birth defects* and should not be used in pregnancy or lactation unless the risk of seizures outweighs the potential risk to the fetus. In such cases the mother should be informed of the potential risks. The risk of taking a woman with a seizure disorder off an antiepileptic drug that has stabilized her condition may be greater than the risk of the drug to the fetus. Discontinuing the drug could result in status epilepticus, which has a high risk of hypoxia for the mother and the fetus. Research has not been able to show the effects of even a minor seizure during pregnancy on the fetus, making it important to prevent seizures during pregnancy if at all possible. Women of childbearing age should be urged to use barrier contraceptives while taking these drugs. If a pregnancy does occur, the woman should receive educational materials and counseling.

Caution should be used with elderly or debilitated patients, *who may respond adversely to the CNS depression,* and with patients who have impaired renal or liver function *that may interfere with drug metabolism and excretion.* Patients with hepatic impairment are at risk for increased

Table 23.2 ***Drugs in Focus:* Drugs for Treating Generalized Seizures**

Drug Name	Dosage/Route	Usual Indications
Hydantoins		
ethotoin (*Peganone*)	*Adult:* 2–3 g/d PO in four to six divided doses *Pediatric:* 500 mg–1 g/d PO; consider age and weight	Treatment of tonic–clonic and psychomotor seizures
fosphenytoin (*Cerebyx*)	*Adult:* Loading dose, 15–20 mg PE/kg IV given as 100–150 mg PE per minute; maintenance, 4–6 mg PE/kg/d; reduce dose with renal or hepatic impairment	Short-term control of status epilepticus, prevention of seizures after neurosurgery
phenytoin (*Dilantin*)	*Adult:* 100 mg PO t.i.d., up to 300–400 mg/d; 10–15 mg/kg IV *Pediatric:* 5–8 mg/kg/d PO; 5–10 mg/kg IV in divided doses	Treatment of tonic–clonic seizures, prevention of status epilepticus, and treatment of seizures after neurosurgery
Barbiturates and Barbiturate-Like Drugs		
phenobarbital (*Solfoton, Luminal*)	*Adult:* 60–100 mg/d PO; 200–320 mg IM or IV for acute episodes, may be repeated in 6 h; reduce dose with elderly and with renal or hepatic impairment *Pediatric:* 3–6 mg/kg/d PO; 4–6 mg/kg/d IM or IV; 15–20 mg/kg IV over 10–15 min for status epilepticus	Long-term treatment of tonic–clonic seizures localized in the cortex; treatment of cortical focal seizures, simple partial seizures, febrile seizures; used as a sedative/hypnotic; emergency control of status epilepticus and acute seizures associated with eclampsia, tetanus, and other conditions
primidone (*Mysoline*)	*Adult:* 250 mg PO five to six times per day *Pediatric (>8 y):* 250 mg PO five to six times per day *Pediatric (<8 y):* 125–250 mg PO t.i.d.	Alternative choice in treatment of tonic–clonic, partial, febrile, and refractory seizures; may be combined with other agents to treat seizures that cannot be controlled by any other antiseizure agents
Benzodiazepines		
clobazam (*Onfi*)	*Adult and pediatric (2 y and older):* 5 mg per day PO, then 5–10 mg PO b.i.d.	Adjunct treatment of seizures associated with Lennox-Gastaut syndrome
clonazepam (*Klonopin*)	*Adult:* Initially 1.5 mg/d PO in three divided doses, up to a maximum 20 mg/d *Pediatric (>10 y):* 0.01–0.03 mg/kg/d PO initially, then up to 0.1–0.2 mg/kg/d PO	Treatment of absence and myoclonic seizures; administered to patients who do not respond to succinimides; being studied for use in the treatment of panic attacks, restless leg movements during sleep, hyperkinetic dysarthria, acute manic episodes, multifocal tic disorders, and neuralgias and as an adjunct in the treatment of schizophrenia
diazepam (*Valium*)	*Adult:* 2–10 mg PO b.i.d. to q.i.d. *or* 0.2 mg/kg PR, may repeat in 4–12 h *Geriatric or debilitated patients:* 2–2.5 mg PO daily to b.i.d *Pediatric:* 1–2.5 mg PO t.i.d. to q.i.d. *or* 0.3–0.5 mg/kg PR with a repeat in 4–12 h if needed	Treatment of severe convulsions, clonic–tonic seizures, status epilepticus; treatment of alcohol withdrawal and tetanus; relieves tension, preoperative anxiety; being studied for use in treatment of panic attacks; this drug is no longer used for long-term management of epilepsy
Succinimides		
ethosuximide (*Zarontin*)	*Adult and pediatric (>6 y):* 500 mg/d PO *Pediatric (3–6 y):* 250 mg/d PO, increase cautiously as needed	Drug of choice for treatment of absence seizures
methsuximide (*Celontin*)	*Adult:* 300 mg/d PO, up to 1.2 g/d *Pediatric:* Determine dose by age and weight considerations	Treatment of absence seizures refractory to other agents
Drugs that Modulate the Inhibitory Neurotransmitter Gamma-Aminobutyric Acid		
acetazolamide (*Diamox*)	8–30 mg/kg/d PO regardless of age; 250 mg PO daily if used with other antiepileptics	Treatment of absence seizures, especially in children; open-angle and secondary glaucoma; to decrease edema associated with heart failure and drug use; and as a prophylaxis and for mountain sickness
valproic acid (*Depakene*)	*Adult:* 10–15 mg/kg/d PO up to a maximum 60 mg/kg/d *Pediatric:* Use extreme caution, determine dose by age and weight	Drug of choice for myoclonic seizures; second-choice drug for treatment of absence seizures; also effective in mania, migraine headaches, and complex partial seizures
zonisamide (*Zonegran*)	*Adults (>16 y):* 100 mg PO daily up to 600 mg/d	Adjunct for treatment of absence seizures

PE, phenytoin sodium equivalent.

toxicity from phenytoin. Caution should be used when giving ethotoin to diabetic patients and patients with severe cardiovascular problems. Patients receiving fosphenytoin intravenously require careful monitoring of their cardiovascular status during the infusion period. Some potentially serious name confusion has occurred with fosphenytoin (see prior Focus on Safe Medication Administration). Other contraindications include coma, depression, or psychoses, *which could be exacerbated by the generalized CNS depression.*

Adverse Effects

The most common adverse effects relate to CNS depression and its effects on body function: Depression, confusion, drowsiness, lethargy, fatigue, constipation, dry mouth, anorexia, cardiac arrhythmias and changes in blood pressure, urinary retention, and loss of libido.

Specifically, the hydantoins may cause severe liver toxicity, bone marrow suppression, gingival hyperplasia, potentially serious dermatological reactions (e.g., hirsutism, Stevens-Johnson syndrome), and frank malignant lymphoma, all of which are directly related to cellular toxicity (Figure 23.3).

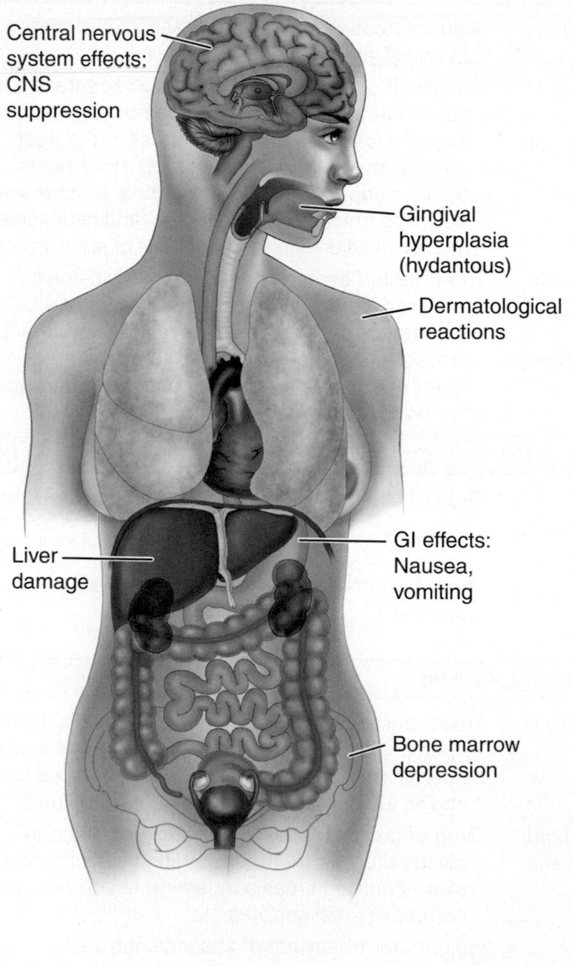

FIGURE 23.3 Common adverse effects associated with antiseizure agents. CNS, central nervous system, GI, gastrointestinal.

BOX 23.4 FOCUS ON Herbal and Alternative Therapies

Patients being treated for epilepsy should be advised not to use the herb evening primrose because it increases the risk of having seizures. Patients being treated with barbiturates or phenytoin should be advised not to use ginkgo, which could cause serious adverse effects.

Clinically Important Drug–Drug Interactions

Because the risk of CNS depression is increased with hydantoins taken with alcohol, patients should be advised not to drink alcohol while they are taking these agents. Always consult a drug reference before any drug is added to or withdrawn from a therapeutic regimen that involves any of these agents. Box 23.4 describes a hazardous drug–herbal therapy interaction associated with antiepileptic medications.

Prototype Summary: Phenytoin

Indications: Control of tonic–clonic and psychomotor seizures, prevention of seizures during neurosurgery, control of status epilepticus.

Actions: Stabilizes neuronal membranes and prevents hyperexcitability caused by excessive stimulation; limits the spread of seizure activity from an active focus; has cardiac antiarrhythmic effects similar to those of lidocaine.

Pharmacokinetics:

Route	Onset	Peak	Duration
Oral	Slow	2–12 h	6–12 h
IV	1–2 h	Rapid	12–24 h

$T_{1/2}$: 6 to 24 hours; metabolized in the liver, excreted in the urine.

Adverse Effects: Nystagmus, ataxia, dysarthria, slurred speech, mental confusion, dizziness, fatigue, tremor, headache, dermatitis, Stevens-Johnson syndrome, nausea, gingival hyperplasia, liver damage, hematopoietic complications, sometimes fatal.

Barbiturates and Barbiturate-like Drugs

Barbiturates and barbiturate-like drugs include phenobarbital (*Solfoton, Luminal*), and primidone (*Mysoline*). These drugs are associated with significant CNS depression.

Therapeutic Actions and Indications

The barbiturates and barbiturate-type drugs inhibit impulse conduction in the ascending reticular activating system (RAS), depress the cerebral cortex, alter cerebellar function, and depress motor nerve output. They stabilize nerve membranes throughout the CNS directly by influencing ionic channels in the cell membrane, thereby decreasing excitability and hyperexcitability to stimulation. By decreasing conduction through nerve pathways, they reduce the tonic–clonic, muscular, and emotional responses to stimulation. Phenobarbital depresses conduction in the lower brainstem and the cerebral cortex and depresses motor conduction. See Table 23.2 for Usual Indications for each of these agents.

Pharmacokinetics

Phenobarbital, which is available in oral and parenteral forms, is well absorbed from the GI tract, metabolized in the liver, and excreted in the urine. This drug has very low lipid solubility, giving it a slow onset and a very long duration of activity. The therapeutic serum level range is 15 to 40 mcg/mL.

Primidone, available only as an oral agent, is well absorbed from the GI tract, metabolized in the liver to phenobarbital metabolites, and excreted in the urine. It tends to have a longer half-life than phenobarbital. The therapeutic serum levels are 5 to 12 mcg/mL.

Contraindications and Cautions

Contraindications and cautions for barbiturates are the same as those discussed for hydantoins.

Adverse Effects

The most common adverse effects associated with barbiturates relate to CNS depression and its effects on body function: Depression, confusion, drowsiness, lethargy, fatigue, constipation, dry mouth, anorexia, cardiac arrhythmias and changes in blood pressure, urinary retention, and loss of libido. Because barbiturates and barbiturate-like drugs depress nerve function, they can produce sedation, hypnosis, anesthesia, and deep coma. The degree of depression is dose related. At doses below those needed to cause hypnosis, these drugs block seizure activity.

In addition, phenobarbital may be associated with physical dependence and withdrawal syndrome. The drug has also been linked to severe dermatological reactions and the development of drug tolerance related to changes in drug metabolism over time.

Clinically Important Drug–Drug Interactions

Because the risk of CNS depression is increased when barbiturates are taken with alcohol, patients should be advised not to drink alcohol while they are taking these agents. Always consult a drug reference before any drug is added to or withdrawn from a therapeutic regimen that involves any of these agents.

Ⓟ Prototype Summary: Phenobarbital

Indications: Long-term treatment of generalized tonic–clonic and cortical focal seizures, emergency control of certain acute convulsive episodes (status epilepticus, tetanus, eclampsia, meningitis), and anticonvulsant treatment of generalized tonic–clonic seizures and focal seizures (parenteral).

Actions: General CNS depressant, inhibits impulse conduction in the ascending RAS, depresses the cerebral cortex, alters cerebellar function, depresses motor output, and can produce excitation, sedation, hypnosis, anesthesia, and deep coma.

Pharmacokinetics:

Route	Onset	Duration
Oral	30–60 min	10–16 h
IM, subcutaneous	10–30 min	4–6 h
IV	5 min	4–6 h

$T_{1/2}$: 79 hours; metabolized in the liver, excreted in the urine.

Adverse Effects: Somnolence, insomnia, vertigo, nightmares, lethargy, nervousness, hallucinations, insomnia, anxiety, dizziness, bradycardia, hypotension, syncope, nausea, vomiting, constipation, diarrhea, hypoventilation, respiratory depression, tissue necrosis at injection site, withdrawal syndrome.

Benzodiazepines

Some benzodiazepines are used as antiepileptic agents. These include clobazam (*Onfi*), clonazepam (*Klonopin*), and diazepam (*Valium*).

Therapeutic Actions and Indications

The benzodiazepines may potentiate the effects of GABA, an inhibitory neurotransmitter that stabilizes nerve cell membranes. These drugs, which appear to act primarily in the limbic system and the RAS, also cause muscle relaxation and relieve anxiety without affecting cortical functioning substantially. The benzodiazepines stabilize nerve membranes throughout the CNS to decrease excitability and hyperexcitability to stimulation. By decreasing conduction through nerve pathways, they reduce the tonic–clonic, muscular, and emotional responses to stimulation. In general, these drugs have limited toxicity and are well tolerated by most people. (See Chapter 20 for the use of benzodiazepines as sedatives and anxiolytics.) See Table 23.2 for Usual Indications for each of these agents. Clonazepam may lose its effectiveness within 3 months (affected patients may respond to dose adjustment). Clobazam, the newest drug in this class, is indicated for adjunct treatment of seizures associated with Lennox-Gastaut syndrome in patients 2 years of age and older.

Pharmacokinetics

Diazepam is available in oral and rectal forms. Clonazepam is now available in an orally disintegrating tablet, making it a good choice for patients who have difficulty swallowing capsules or tablets. Clobazam is available in oral form only. These agents are well absorbed from the GI tract, metabolized in the liver, and excreted in the urine. They have a long half-life of 18 to 50 hours.

Contraindications and Cautions

Contraindications for benzodiazepines are the same as those discussed for hydantoins.

Adverse Effects

The most common adverse effects associated with benzodiazepines relate to CNS depression and its effects on body function: Depression, confusion, drowsiness, lethargy, fatigue, constipation, dry mouth, anorexia, cardiac arrhythmias, and changes in blood pressure, urinary retention, and loss of libido. Benzodiazepines may be associated with physical dependence and withdrawal syndrome, especially with rapid reduction in dose.

Clinically Important Drug–Drug Interactions

Because the risk of CNS depression is increased when benzodiazepines are taken with alcohol, patients should be advised not to drink alcohol while they are taking these agents. Always consult a drug reference before any drug is added to or withdrawn from a therapeutic regimen that involves any of these agents.

Ⓟ Prototype Summary: Diazepam

Indications: Management of anxiety disorders, acute alcohol withdrawal; muscle relaxant, treatment of tetanus, adjunct in status epilepticus and severe recurrent convulsive seizures, preoperative relief of anxiety and tension, management of epilepsy in patients who require intermittent use to control bouts of increased seizure activity.

Actions: Acts in the limbic system and reticular formation, potentiates the effects of GABA, has little effect on cortical function.

Pharmacokinetics:

Route	Onset	Peak	Duration
Oral	30–60 min	1–2 h	3 h
IM	15–30 min	30–45 min	3 h
IV	1–5 min	30 min	15–60 min
Recta	Rapid	1.5 h	3 h

$T_{1/2}$: 20 to 80 hours; metabolized in the liver, excreted in the urine.

Adverse Effects: Drowsiness, sedation, depression, lethargy, apathy, fatigue, disorientation, bradycardia, tachycardia, paradoxical excitatory reactions, constipation, diarrhea, incontinence, urinary retention, drug dependence with withdrawal syndrome.

Succinimides

The succinimides include ethosuximide (*Zarontin*) and methsuximide (*Celontin*). The succinimides are most frequently used to treat absence seizures, a form of generalized seizure.

Therapeutic Actions and Indications

Although the exact mechanism of action is not understood the succinimides suppress the abnormal electrical activity in the brain that is associated with absence seizures. The action may be related to activity in inhibitory neural pathways in the brain (see Figure 23.2).

Ethosuximide and methsuximide are indicated for the control of absence seizures (see Table 23.2). Ethosuximide should be tried first; methsuximide should be reserved for the treatment of seizures that are refractory to other agents because it is associated with more severe adverse effects.

Pharmacokinetics

Ethosuximide and methsuximide are available for oral use. These drugs cross the placenta and enter breast milk (see Contraindications and Cautions). The succinimides are readily absorbed from the GI tract, reaching peak levels in 1 to 7 hours, depending on the drug. They are metabolized in the liver and excreted in the urine. The half-life of ethosuximide is 30 hours in children and 60 hours in adults; the half-life of methsuximide is 2.6 to 4 hours. The established therapeutic serum level for ethosuximide is 40 to 100 mcg/mL.

Contraindications and Cautions

The succinimides are contraindicated in the presence of allergy to any of these drugs *to avoid hypersensitivity reactions.* Caution should be used with succinimides in patients with intermittent porphyria, *which could be exacerbated by the adverse effects of these drugs,* and those with renal or hepatic disease, *which could interfere with the metabolism and excretion of these drugs and lead to toxic levels.* Use during pregnancy should be discussed with the woman *because of the potential for adverse effects on the fetus.* Another method of feeding the baby should be used if one of these drugs is needed during lactation *because of the potential for adverse effects on the baby.*

Adverse Effects

Ethosuximide has relatively few adverse effects compared with many other antiepileptic drugs. Many of the adverse effects associated with the succinimides are related to their depressant effects in the CNS. These may include depression, drowsiness, fatigue, ataxia, insomnia, headache, and blurred vision. Decreased GI activity with nausea, vomiting, anorexia, weight loss, GI pain, and constipation or diarrhea may also occur. Bone marrow suppression, including potentially fatal pancytopenia, and dermatological reactions such as pruritus, urticaria, alopecia, and Stevens-Johnson syndrome may occur as a result of direct chemical irritation of the skin and bone marrow.

Clinically Important Drug–Drug Interactions

Use of succinimides with primidone may cause a decrease in serum levels of primidone. Patients should be monitored and appropriate dose adjustments made if these two agents are used together.

Prototype Summary: Ethosuximide

Indications: Control of absence seizures.

Actions: May act in inhibitory neuronal systems, suppresses the electroencephalographic pattern associated with absence seizures, reduces frequency of attacks.

Pharmacokinetics:

Route	Peak
Oral	3–7 h

$T_{1/2}$: 30 hours (children), 60 hours (adults); metabolized in the liver, excreted in the urine and bile.

Adverse Effects: Drowsiness, ataxia, dizziness, irritability, nervousness, headache, blurred vision, pruritus, Stevens-Johnson syndrome, nausea, vomiting, epigastric pain, anorexia, diarrhea, and pancytopenia.

Other Drugs for Treating Absence Seizures

Three other drugs that are used in the treatment of absence seizures do not fit into a specific drug class (Table 23.2). These include acetazolamide (*Diamox*), valproic acid (*Depakene*), and zonisamide (*Zonegran*).

Therapeutic Actions and Indications

Valproic acid reduces abnormal electrical activity in the brain and may also increase GABA activity at inhibitory receptors. It has been used for migraine prevention and has a pregnancy category X rating when used for that purpose. Acetazolamide—a sulfonamide—alters electrolyte movement, stabilizing nerve cell membranes. Another sulfonamide—zonisamide—is a newer agent that inhibits voltage-sensitive sodium and calcium channels, thus stabilizing nerve cell membranes and modulating calcium-dependent presynaptic release of excitatory neurotransmitters. See Table 23.2 for Usual Indications related to these drugs.

Pharmacokinetics

Valproic acid, available for oral and IV use, is readily absorbed from the GI tract, reaching peak levels in 1 to 4 hours. It is metabolized in the liver and excreted in the urine with a half-life of 6 to 16 hours.

Acetazolamide, which can be given orally, IM, or IV, is readily absorbed from the GI tract and is excreted unchanged in the urine with a half-life of 2.5 to 6 hours.

Zonisamide, an oral drug, is well absorbed from the GI tract, reaching peak levels in 2 to 6 hours. It is primarily excreted unchanged in the urine, with a half-life of 63 hours.

Contraindications and Cautions

These drugs are contraindicated with known allergy to any component of the drug. The sulfonamides are also contraindicated with known allergy to antibacterial sulfonamides and thiazide diuretics *to avoid hypersensitivity reactions.* When it is discontinued, zonisamide should be tapered over 2 weeks *because of a risk of precipitating seizures.* Patients who take this drug should be very well hydrated *due to risk of renal calculi development.*

Caution should be used in patients with hepatic or renal impairment, *which could alter metabolism and excretion of the drug.* These drugs should not be used during pregnancy or lactation unless the benefit clearly outweighs the risk to the fetus or neonate *because of the potential for serious adverse effects on the baby.*

Adverse Effects

Valproic acid is associated with liver toxicity. All of these drugs cause CNS effects related to CNS suppression—weakness, fatigue, drowsiness, dizziness, and paresthesias. Acetazolamide and zonisamide may cause rash and dermatological changes. Zonisamide is associated with bone marrow suppression, renal calculi development, and GI upset.

Clinically Important Drug–Drug Interactions

Acetazolamide increases the serum levels of quinidine, tricyclic antidepressants, and amphetamines and may increase salicylate toxicity when given with salicylates. Valproic acid can increase serum levels and potential toxicity of phenobarbital, ethosuximide, diazepam, primidone, and zidovudine. If any of these drugs are used in combination the patient should be monitored carefully and doses adjusted appropriately. Breakthrough seizures have been reported when valproic acid is combined with phenytoin, and extreme care should be taken if this combination must be used. Zonisamide levels and toxicity are increased if it is combined with carbamazepine, and the patient should be monitored and zonisamide dose reduced as needed.

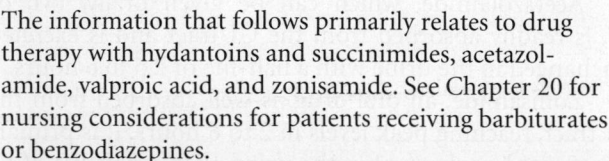

Nursing Considerations for Patients Receiving Drugs for Treating Generalized Seizures

The information that follows primarily relates to drug therapy with hydantoins and succinimides, acetazolamide, valproic acid, and zonisamide. See Chapter 20 for nursing considerations for patients receiving barbiturates or benzodiazepines.

Assessment: History and Examination

- Assess for contraindications or cautions to the use of hydantoins, including known history of allergy to hydantoins *to avoid hypersensitivity reactions*; cardiac arrhythmias, hypotension, diabetes, coma, or psychoses, *which could be exacerbated by the use of the drug*; history of renal or hepatic dysfunction *that might interfere with drug metabolism or excretion*; and current status related to pregnancy and lactation.
- Assess for contraindications or cautions to the use of succinimides, including any known allergies to these drugs; history of intermittent porphyria, *which could be exacerbated by these drugs*; history of renal or hepatic dysfunction *that might interfere with drug metabolism or excretion*; and current status related to pregnancy or lactation *because of the potential risks to the fetus or baby.*
- Obtain a description of seizures, including onset, aura, duration, and recovery, *to determine type of seizure and establish a baseline.*
- Perform a physical assessment to establish baseline data *for determining the effectiveness of therapy and the occurrence of any potential adverse effect.*
- Inspect the skin for color and lesions *to determine evidence of possible skin effects*; assess pulse and blood pressure and auscultate heart *to evaluate for possible cardiac effects*; assess level of orientation, affect, reflexes, and bilateral grip strength *to evaluate any CNS effects*; monitor bowel sounds and urine output to determine possible GI or genitourinary (GU) effects; and evaluate gums and mucous membranes *to establish baseline and monitor changes associated with adverse effects.*
- Obtain a baseline electroencephalogram if appropriate *to evaluate brain function.*
- Assess the patient's renal and liver function, including renal and liver function tests, *to determine appropriateness of therapy and determine the need for possible dose adjustment.*

Refer to the Critical Thinking Scenario for a full discussion of nursing care for a patient who is being prescribed antiepileptic drugs.

Nursing Diagnoses

Nursing diagnoses related to drug therapy might include the following:

- Acute discomfort related to GI, CNS, and GU effects
- Disturbed thought processes related to CNS effects
- Risk for infection related to bone marrow suppression (succinimides, zonisamide)
- Risk for injury related to CNS effects or toxic drug levels
- Impaired skin Integrity related to dermatological effects
- Deficient knowledge regarding drug therapy

Planning

- The patient will receive the best therapeutic effect from the drug therapy.
- The patient will have limited adverse effects to the drug therapy.
- The patient will have an understanding of the drug therapy, adverse effects to anticipate, and measures to relieve discomfort and improve safety.

Implementation with Rationale

- Discontinue the drug at any sign of hypersensitivity reaction, liver dysfunction, or severe skin rash *to limit reaction and prevent potentially serious reactions.*
- Administer the drug with food *to alleviate GI irritation if GI upset is a problem.*
- Monitor for adverse effects and provide appropriate supportive care as needed *to help the patient cope with these effects.*
- Monitor complete blood count (CBC) before and periodically during therapy *to detect bone marrow suppression early and provide appropriate interventions.*
- Discontinue the drug if skin rash, bone marrow suppression, or unusual depression or personality changes occur *to prevent the development of more serious adverse effects.*
- Discontinue the drug slowly, and never withdraw the drug quickly, *because rapid withdrawal may precipitate absence seizures.*
- Monitor for drug–drug interactions *to arrange to adjust doses appropriately if any drug is added to or withdrawn from the drug regimen.*

- Arrange for counseling for women of childbearing age who are taking these drugs. *Because these drugs have the potential to cause serious damage to the fetus*, women should understand the risk of birth defects and use barrier contraceptives to avoid pregnancy.
- Offer support and encouragement *to help the patient cope with the drug regimen and diagnosis.*
- Provide thorough patient teaching, including drug name and prescribed dosage, as well as measures for avoidance of adverse effects and warning signs that may indicate possible problems *to enhance patient knowledge about drug therapy and to promote compliance*; and the need for periodic blood tests *to evaluate blood counts to reduce the risk for infection and for drug levels to evaluate therapeutic effectiveness and minimize the risk for toxicity*.
- Suggest the wearing or carrying of a MedicAlert bracelet *to alert emergency workers and health care providers about the use of an antiepileptic drug.*

Evaluation

- Monitor patient response to the drug (decrease in incidence or absence of seizures; serum drug levels within the therapeutic range); evaluate for therapeutic blood levels (40 to 100 mcg/mL) for ethosuximide *to ensure the most appropriate dose of the drug.*
- Monitor for adverse effects (CNS changes, GI depression, urinary retention, arrhythmias, blood pressure changes, liver toxicity, bone marrow suppression, severe dermatological reactions).
- Evaluate the effectiveness of the teaching plan (patient can give the drug name and dosage and name possible adverse effects to watch for and specific measures to prevent them; patient is aware of the risk of birth defects and the need to carry information about the diagnosis and use of this drug).
- Monitor the effectiveness of comfort measures and compliance with the regimen.

CRITICAL THINKING SCENARIO

Antiepileptic Drugs

THE SITUATION

J.M., an athletic, 18-year-old, high-school senior, suffered his first seizure during math class. He seemed attentive and alert, and then he suddenly slumped to the floor and suffered a full tonic–clonic (grand mal) seizure. The other students were frightened and did not know what to do. Fortunately, the teacher was familiar with seizures and quickly reacted to protect J.M. from hurting himself and to explain what was happening.

J.M. was diagnosed with idiopathic generalized epilepsy with tonic–clonic (grand mal) seizures. The combination of phenytoin and phenobarbital that he began taking made him quite drowsy during the day. These drugs were unable to control the seizures, and he suffered three more seizures in the next month—one at school and two at home. J.M. is now undergoing reevaluation for possible drug adjustment and counseling.

CRITICAL THINKING

What teaching implications should be considered when meeting with J.M.? *Consider his age and the setting of his first seizure.*

What problems might J.M. encounter in school and in athletics related to the diagnosis and the prescribed medication? *Consider measures that may help him avoid some of the unpleasant side effects related to this particular drug therapy. Driving a car may be a central social focus in the life of a high-school senior.*

What problems can be anticipated and confronted before they occur concerning laws that forbid individuals with newly diagnosed epilepsy from driving?

Develop a teaching protocol for J.M. How will you involve the entire family in the teaching plan?

DISCUSSION

On their first meeting, it is important for the nurse to establish a trusting relationship with J.M. and his family. J.M., who is at a sensitive stage of development, requires a great deal of support and encouragement to cope with the diagnosis of epilepsy and the need for drug therapy. He may need to ventilate his feelings and concerns and discuss how he can reenter school without worrying about having a seizure in class. The nurse should implement a thorough drug teaching program, including a description of warning signs to watch for that should be reported to a health care professional. J.M. should be encouraged to take the following preventive measures:

- Have frequent oral hygiene to protect the gums.
- Avoid operating dangerous machinery or performing tasks that require alertness while drowsy and confused.
- Pace activities as much as possible to help deal with any fatigue and malaise.
- Take the drugs with meals if GI upset is a problem.

(continues on page 400)

Antiepileptic Drugs (continued)

This information should be given to both J.M. and his family in written form for future reference, along with the name of a health care professional and a telephone number to call with questions or comments. The importance of continuous medication to suppress the seizures should be stressed. The adverse effects of many of these drugs make it difficult for some patients to remain compliant with their drug regimen.

After the discussion with J.M. the nurse should meet with his family members, who also need support and encouragement to deal with his diagnosis and its implications. They need to know what seizures are, how the prescribed antiepileptic drugs affect the seizures, what they can do when seizures occur, and complete information about the drugs he must take and their anticipated drug effects. In addition, it is important to work with family members to determine whether any particular thing precipitated the seizures. In other words, was there any warning or aura? This may help with adjustment of drug dosages or avoidance of certain situations or stimuli that precipitate seizures. Family members should be encouraged to report and record any seizure activity that occurs.

Most states do not permit individuals with newly diagnosed epilepsy to drive, and states have varying regulations about the return of the driver's license after a seizure-free interval. If driving makes up a major part of J.M.'s social activities, this news may be even more unacceptable than his diagnosis. J.M. and his family should be counseled and helped to devise other ways of getting to places and coping with this restriction. J.M. may be interested in referral to a support group for teens with similar problems, where he can share ideas, support, and frustrations.

J.M. 's condition is a chronic one that will require continual drug therapy and evaluation. He will need periodic reteaching and should have the opportunity to ask additional questions and to ventilate his feelings. J.M. should be encouraged to wear or carry a MedicAlert tag so that emergency medical personnel are aware of his diagnosis and the medications he is taking.

NURSING CARE GUIDE FOR J.M.: ANTIEPILEPTIC AGENTS

Assessment: History and Examination

Allergies to any of these drugs; hypotension; arrhythmias; bone marrow suppression; coma; psychoses; pregnancy or lactation; hepatic or renal dysfunction

Concurrent use of valproic acid, cimetidine, disulfiram, isoniazid, phenacemide, sulfonamides, diazoxide, folic acid, rifampin, sucralfate, theophylline, primidone, acetaminophen

Cardiovascular: Blood pressure, pulse, peripheral perfusion

CNS: Orientation, reflexes, affect, strength, electroencephalograph (EEG)

Skin: Color, lesions, texture, temperature

GI: Abdominal evaluation, bowel sounds

Respiratory: Respiration, adventitious sounds

Laboratory tests: CBC, liver and renal function tests

Nursing Diagnoses

Acute pain related to GI, CNS, and GU effects

Risk for injury related to CNS effects

Disturbed thought processes related to CNS effects

Deficient knowledge regarding drug therapy

Impaired skin integrity related to dermatological effects

Planning

The patient will receive the best therapeutic effect from the drug therapy.

The patient will have limited adverse effects to the drug therapy.

The patient will have an understanding of the drug therapy, adverse effects to anticipate, and measures to relieve discomfort and improve safety.

Implementation

Discontinue drug at first sign of liver dysfunction or skin rash.

Provide comfort and safety measures: Positioning, give with meals, skin care.

Provide support and reassurance to cope with diagnosis, restrictions, and drug effects.

Provide patient teaching regarding drug name, dosage, side effects, symptoms to report, and the need to wear MedicAlert information; other drugs to avoid.

Evaluation

Evaluate drug effects: Decrease in incidence and frequency of seizures; serum drug levels within therapeutic range.

Monitor for adverse effects: CNS effects (multiple); bone marrow suppression; rash, skin changes; GI effects—nausea, anorexia; arrhythmias.

Monitor for drug–drug interactions: Increased depression with CNS depressants, alcohol, drugs as listed.

Evaluate effectiveness of patient-teaching program.

Evaluate effectiveness of comfort/safety measures.

Antiepileptic Drugs (continued)

PATIENT TEACHING FOR J.M.

- The drugs that are being evaluated for you are called antiepileptic agents. They are used to stabilize abnormal cells in the brain that have been firing excessively and causing seizures.
- The timing of these doses is very important. To be effective, this drug must be taken regularly.
- Do not stop taking this drug suddenly. If for any reason you are unable to continue taking the drug, notify your health care provider at once. This drug must be slowly withdrawn when its use is discontinued.
- Common effects of these drugs include:
  - *Fatigue, weakness, and drowsiness:* Try to space activities evenly throughout the day and allow rest periods to avoid these effects. Take safety precautions and avoid driving or operating dangerous machinery if these conditions occur.
  - *Headaches and difficulty sleeping:* These usually disappear as your body adjusts to the drug. If they persist and become too uncomfortable, consult with your health care provider.
  - *GI upset, loss of appetite, and diarrhea or constipation:* Taking the drug with food or eating small, frequent meals may help alleviate this problem.
- Report any of the following conditions to your health care provider: *skin rash, severe nausea and vomiting, impaired coordination, yellowing of the eyes or skin, fever, sore throat, personality changes, and unusual bleeding or bruising.*
- It is advisable to wear or carry a MedicAlert warning so that any person who takes care of you in an emergency will know that you are taking this drug.
- Tell any doctor, nurse, or other health care provider involved in your care that you are taking this drug.
- Keep this drug and all medications out of the reach of children.
- Do not take any other drug, including over-the-counter medications and alcohol, without consulting with your health care provider. Many of these preparations interact with the drug and could cause adverse effects.
- Report and record any seizure activity that you have while you are taking this drug.
- Take this drug exactly as prescribed. Regular medical follow-up, which may include blood tests, will be necessary to evaluate the effects of this drug on your body.

KEY POINTS

- Drugs used to treat generalized seizures include the hydantoins, barbiturates, and benzodiazepines.
- Drugs used to treat absence seizures—a particular type of generalized seizure—include the hydantoins, succinimides, acetazolamide, valproic acid, and zonisamide.
- All of these drugs stabilize nerve membranes throughout the CNS to decrease excitability and hyperexcitability to stimulation.
- Adverse effects associated with these drugs reflect the CNS depression—lethargy, somnolence, fatigue, dry mouth, constipation, and dizziness. Serious liver, bone marrow, and dermatological problems can occur with specific drugs.

Drugs for Treating Partial Seizures

Partial seizures may be simple (involving only a single muscle or reaction) or complex (involving a series of reactions or emotional changes). Drugs used in the treatment of partial seizures include carbamazepine (*Tegretol*, *Epitol*, and others), clorazepate (*Tranxene*, *Gen-Xene*, and others), ezogabine (*Potiga*), felbamate (*Felbatol*), gabapentin (*Neurontin*), lacosamide (*Vimpat*), lamotrigine (*Lamictal*), levetiracetam (*Keppra*), oxcarbazepine (*Trileptal*), pregabalin (*Lyrica*), rufinamide (*Banzel*), tiagabine (*Gabitril*), topiramate (*Topamax*), and vigabatrin (*Sabril*) (see Table 23.3). Some of the drugs used to treat generalized seizures have also been found to be useful in treating partial seizures (see Table 23.1).

FOCUS ON Safe Medication Administration

Name confusion has been reported between ***Keppra*** *(levetiracetam) and* ***Kaletra*** *(lopinavir/ritonavir), an HIV antiviral combination drug. Both drugs come in a liquid form, and confusion has been reported in the administration of the two drugs, causing serious adverse effects. Use extreme caution when administering these drugs.*

Therapeutic Actions and Indications

The drugs used to control partial seizures stabilize nerve membranes in either of two ways—directly, by altering sodium and calcium channels, or indirectly, by increasing the activity of GABA, an inhibitory neurotransmitter, and thereby decreasing excessive activity (see Figure 23.2). Carbamazepine, felbamate, and oxcarbazepine are used as monotherapy, and the remaining drugs are used as adjunctive therapy (see Table 23.3 for Usual Indications for each

Table 23.3 ***Drugs in Focus:* Drugs for Treating Partial Seizures**

Drug Name	Dosage/Route	Usual Indications
carbamazepine (*Tegretol, Epitol*)	*Adult:* 800–1,200 mg/d PO in divided doses q6–8 h *Pediatric (>12 y):* Adult doses, do not exceed 1,000 mg/d *Pediatric (6–12 y):* 20–30 mg/kg/d PO in divided doses t.i.d. to q.i.d. *Pediatric (<6 y):* 35 mg/kg/d PO	Drug of choice for treatment of partial seizures and tonic–clonic seizures; treatment of trigeminal neuralgia, bipolar disorder
clorazepate (*Tranxene, Gen-Xene*)	*Adult:* 7.5 mg PO t.i.d., up to 90 mg/d *Pediatric (9–12 y):* 7.5 mg PO b.i.d., up to 60 mg/d	Used as adjunct for treatment of partial seizures; also used for anxiety disorders, acute symptoms of alcohol withdrawal
ezogabine (*Potiga*)	100 mg PO t.i.d. initially, titrate to maintenance dose of 200–400 mg PO t.i.d.	Adjunct treatment of adult patients with partial seizures when other measures have failed.
felbamate (*Felbatol*)	*Adult and pediatric >14 y:* 2,600 mg/d PO *Pediatric (2–14 y):* 15 mg/kg/d PO in divided doses three to four times per day	Used as monotherapy or adjunctive therapy for treatment of partial seizures; adjunctive therapy for Lennox-Gastaut syndrome in children; however, drug is reserved for those cases that are unresponsive to other therapies due to its risks for severe adverse effects
gabapentin (*Neurontin*)	*Adult:* 900–1,800 mg/d PO in divided doses t.i.d. *Pediatric (3–12 y):* 10–15 mg/kg per day PO in divided doses	Used as adjunct in treating partial seizures; treatment of post-herpetic pain in adults and children aged 3–12 y; has orphan drug status for the treatment of ALS; migraines, bipolar disorders, tremors of multiple sclerosis, and nerve-generated pain states
lacosamide (*Vimpat*)	*Adult:* Initially 50 mg PO b.i.d., titrate to maintenance dose of 200–400 mg/d PO, IV dose is the same; decrease dose with renal or hepatic impairment	Adjunctive therapy for adults with partial onset seizures, reserve IV use for short term when oral is not possible
lamotrigine (*Lamictal*)	*Adult:* 300–500 mg/d PO in divided doses b.i.d. *Pediatric (2–12 y):* 1–5 mg/kg/d PO in divided doses b.i.d. *Pediatric (>12 y):* 100–400 mg/d PO in divided doses b.i.d.	Used as adjunct or for monotherapy in treating partial seizures and in treatment of seizures associated with Lennox-Gastaut syndrome in adults and children ≥2 years of age; long-term treatment of bipolar disorders
levetiracetam (*Keppra*)	*Adult:* 500 mg PO b.i.d. up to 3,000 mg/d *Pediatric (4–16 y):* 10 mg/kg PO b.i.d. to a maximum of 1,500–3,000 mg/d	Newer drug approved for adjunctive treatment of partial seizures in adults and children ≥4 years of age; in 2007 it was also approved for the treatment of primary generalized tonic–clonic seizures in adults and treatment of children ≥6 years of age with idiopathic generalized epilepsy; being studied for use in absence seizures, myoclonic seizures, and drug-resistant seizures of multiple types
oxcarbazepine (*Trileptal*)	*Adult:* 600 mg PO b.i.d. *Pediatric (4–16 y):* 8–10 mg/kg per day PO	Used for monotherapy or adjunctive therapy in treatment of partial seizures in adults and children 4–16 y of age; also being studied as an alternate treatment of bipolar disease
pregabalin (*Lyrica*)	150–600 mg/d PO in divided doses *Neuropathic pain:* 100 mg PO t.i.d. *Post-herpetic neuralgia:* 75–150 mg PO t.i.d.	Used for adjunctive treatment of adults with partial onset seizures; management of neuropathic pain associated with diabetic peripheral neuropathy and post-herpetic neuralgia; fibromyalgia
rufinamide (*Banzel*)	*Adult:* Initially 400–800 mg/day PO, titrate to a target dose of 3,200 mg/d *Pediatric (4 and older):* 10 mg/kg/d PO in divided doses, titrate to a target dose of 45 mg/kg/d or 3,200 mg/d whichever is less	Adjunctive treatment of seizures associated with Lennox-Gastaut syndrome
tiagabine (*Gabitril*)	*Adult:* 4 mg PO daily up to 56 mg/d in two to four divided doses *Pediatric (12–18 y):* 4 mg PO daily up to a maximum 32 mg/d in two to four divided doses	Used as adjunct in treating partial seizures in adults and in children 12–18 y of age

Drug Name	Dosage/Route	Usual Indications
topiramate (*Topamax*)	*Adult:* 400 mg PO daily in two divided doses; reduce dose in renal impairment *Pediatric (2–16 y):* 5–9 mg/kg/d PO in two divided doses	Used as adjunct in treating partial seizures in adults and children 2–16 y of age; also approved for treatment of tonic–clonic seizures, for prevention of migraine headaches, and as adjunct therapy in Lennox-Gastaut syndrome; being studied for use in cluster headaches, infantile spasms, alcohol dependence, bulimia nervosa, and weight loss
vigabatrin (*Sabril*)	*Adult:* 500 mg PO b.i.d. to a maximum of 1.5 g PO b.i.d. with other antiepileptics *Pediatric (1 mo–2 y):* 50 mg/kg PO b.i.d. of oral solution to a maximum 150 mg/kg PO b.i.d.	Monotherapy for children 1 mo–2 y for infantile spasm; adjunctive therapy for adults with complex partial seizures not controlled by other therapy

ALS, amyotrophic lateral sclerosis.

agent). Each of the drugs used for treating partial seizures has a slightly different mechanism of action:

Carbamazepine is chemically related to the tricyclic antidepressants. It has the ability to inhibit polysynaptic responses and to block sodium channels to prevent the formation of repetitive action potentials in the abnormal focus.

Clorazepate and felbamate are thought to potentiate the effects of the inhibitory neurotransmitter GABA.

Gabapentin inhibits polysynaptic responses and blocks stimulus increases in certain situations. Gabapentin is also approved to be used in the treatment of amyotrophic lateral sclerosis (ALS), post-herpetic neuralgia, and restless leg syndrome. It has many off-label uses and is often seen as a drug in the polypharmacy needed to achieve therapeutic results with psychiatric patients.

The newer drugs lacosamide and rufinamide inhibit voltage-sensitive sodium channels, which results in a stabilization of nerve membranes and an inhibition of neuronal firing.

Ezogabine is a neuronal potassium channel opener, blocking repolarization and inhibiting neuronal firing.

Lamotrigine may inhibit voltage-sensitive sodium and calcium channels, stabilize nerve cell membranes, and modulate calcium-dependent presynaptic release of excitatory neurotransmitters. Levetiracetam is a newer drug, and its mechanism of action is not understood; its antiepileptic action does not seem to be associated with any known mechanisms of inhibitory or excitatory neurotransmission. (See also the Focus on Safe Medication Administration for information about potentially serious name confusion that has occurred with levetiracetam.)

Oxcarbazepine's exact mechanism of action is also unknown. It inhibits voltage-sensitive sodium channels, stabilizing hyperexcited nerve cell membranes. It also increases potassium conductance and modulates calcium-dependent presynaptic release of excitatory neurotransmitters. Any or all of these effects may be responsible for the antiseizure effects of the drug.

Pregabalin, which was introduced in the United States in 2005, has a high binding affinity for voltage-gated calcium channels in the cerebrovascular system. It seems to modulate the calcium function in these neurons, leading to a decreased release of neurotransmitters into the synaptic cleft and a decrease in cell activity. In 2007 pregabalin became the first drug approved in the United States for the treatment of fibromyalgia.

Tiagabine binds to GABA reuptake receptors, causing an increase in GABA levels in the brain. Because GABA is an inhibitory neurotransmitter the result is a stabilizing of nerve membranes and a decrease in excessive activity.

Topiramate is another newer drug that blocks sodium channels in neurons with sustained depolarization and increases GABA activity, inhibiting nerve activity.

Vigabatrin blocks the enzyme GABAase, which leads to more GABA at the nerve synapse, leading to more stabilization of the nerve.

Pharmacokinetics

These drugs are all given orally. Levetiracetam and lacosamide are also available for IV use.

Carbamazepine is absorbed from the GI tract and metabolized in the liver by the cytochrome P450 system. It is excreted in the urine with a half-life of 25 to 65 hours.

Clorazepate is rapidly absorbed from the GI tract, reaching peak levels in 1 to 2 hours. After metabolism in the liver, it is excreted in the urine with a half-life of 30 to 100 hours.

Ezogabine is absorbed rapidly from the GI tract, reaching peak levels in 30 minutes to 2 hours. After being metabolized in the liver, it is excreted in the urine with a half-life of 7 to 11 hours.

Felbamate is absorbed well from the GI tract and is primarily excreted unchanged in the urine with a half-life of 20 to 23 hours.

Gabapentin is well absorbed from the GI tract and widely distributed in the body. It is excreted unchanged in the urine with a half-life of 5 to 7 hours.

Lacosamide is well absorbed from the GI tract, reaching peak levels in 1 to 4 hours; if given IV, peak levels are achieved at the end of the infusion. It is metabolized in the liver with a 13-hour half-life and is excreted in the urine.

Lamotrigine is rapidly absorbed from the GI tract, metabolized in the liver, and primarily excreted in the urine. The half-life of lamotrigine is approximately 25 hours.

Levetiracetam is rapidly absorbed from the GI tract, reaching peak levels in 1 hour. It goes through very little metabolism, with most of the drug being excreted unchanged in the urine with a half-life of 6 to 8 hours.

Oxcarbazepine is completely absorbed from the GI tract and extensively metabolized in the liver. It is excreted in the urine with a half-life of 2 and then 9 hours.

Pregabalin is rapidly absorbed orally, reaching peak levels in 1.5 hours. It is not metabolized but is eliminated unchanged in the urine with a half-life of 6.3 hours.

Rufinamide is well absorbed from the GI tract with peak levels in 4 to 6 hours, metabolized in the liver and excreted in the urine; it has a half-life of 6 to 10 hours.

Tiagabine is rapidly absorbed from the GI tract, reaching peak levels in 45 minutes. It is metabolized in the liver by the cytochrome P450 system. It is excreted in the urine with a half-life of 4 to 7 hours.

Topiramate is rapidly absorbed from the GI tract, reaching peak levels in 2 hours. It is widely distributed and is excreted unchanged in the urine.

Vigabatrin is completely absorbed from the GI tract, does not undergo metabolism, and is excreted in the urine with a half-life of 7.5 hours.

Contraindications and Cautions

Contraindications to the drugs used to control partial seizures include the following conditions: Presence of any known allergy to the drug *to avoid hypersensitivity reactions*; bone marrow suppression, *which could be exacerbated by the drug effects*; and severe hepatic dysfunction, *which could be exacerbated and could interfere with the metabolism of the drugs.*

Carbamazepine, clorazepate, ezogabine, gabapentin, and oxcarbazine have been shown to be dangerous to a fetus and should not be used during pregnancy. Women of childbearing age should be advised to use contraception. These drugs enter breast milk and can cause serious adverse effects in the baby. If any of these drugs is needed during lactation, another method of feeding the baby should be used.

There are no clear studies about the effects of felbamate, lacosamide, lamotrigine, levetiracetam, pregabalin, rufinamide, tiagabine, topiramate, or vigabatrin use during pregnancy and lactation. Therefore, these drugs should not be used during pregnancy or lactation unless the benefits to the mother clearly outweigh potential adverse effects in the fetus or neonate. Men considering fathering a child should be advised that in animal studies, males receiving pregabalin had decreased fertility and associated birth defects in offspring.

Caution should also be used in the following situations: With renal or hepatic dysfunction, *which could alter the metabolism and excretion of the drugs*, and with renal stones, *which could be exacerbated by the effects of some of these agents.*

Adverse Effects

The most frequently occurring adverse effects associated with the drugs used for partial seizures relate to the CNS depression that results. The following conditions may occur: Drowsiness, fatigue, weakness, confusion, headache, and insomnia; GI depression, with nausea, vomiting, and anorexia; and upper respiratory infections. These antiepileptics can also be directly toxic to the liver and the bone marrow, causing dysfunction. The exact effects of each drug vary. All of these drugs have a black box warning about the potential for increased suicidality when on these drugs. These drugs should also be tapered when discontinued because of the risk for precipitating seizures with sudden withdrawal.

Felbamate has been associated with severe liver failure and aplastic anemia. Lamotrigine has been associated with very serious to life-threatening rashes, and the drug should be discontinued at the first sign of any rash. Patients with renal dysfunction are more likely to experience toxic effects of levetiracetam, and the dose for these patients needs to be decreased accordingly.

The adverse effects most commonly seen with pregabalin are related to CNS depression—tremor, dizziness, somnolence, and visual changes. This drug does have a controlled substance rating as Category V. It can cause feelings of well-being and euphoria. Because of this, its use should be limited in patients who have a history of abuse of medications or alcohol.

A reduced dose of topiramate is recommended for patients with renal impairment. The drug also has been associated with marked CNS depression. Tiagabine has also been associated with serious skin rash.

Vigabatrin is associated with a loss of vision, and the patient should be monitored before and during treatment. If vision changes begin to occur the drug should be stopped.

Clinically Important Drug–Drug Interactions

If any of these drugs is taken with other CNS depressants or alcohol a potential for increased CNS depression exists. Caution patients to avoid alcohol while taking drugs for partial seizures or to take extreme precautions if such combinations cannot be avoided.

In addition, numerous drug–drug interactions are associated with carbamazepine. Always consult a drug reference whenever a drug is added to or withdrawn from a carbamazepine-containing regimen. Dose adjustments may be necessary.

Hormonal contraceptives may lose effectiveness if combined with rufinamide. Women needing a contraceptive when on rufinamide should consider a barrier contraceptive.

Ⓟ Prototype Summary: Carbamazepine

Indications: Treatment of seizure disorders, including partial seizures with complex patterns; tonic–clonic seizures; mixed seizures; trigeminal neuralgia.

Actions: Inhibits polysynaptic responses and blocks posttetanic potentiations; mechanism of action is not understood; related to the tricyclic antidepressants.

Pharmacokinetics:

Route	Onset	Peak
Extended release	Slow	4–5 h
	Slow	3–12 h

$T_{1/2}$: 25 to 65 hours, then 12 to 17 hours; metabolized in the liver, excreted in the urine and feces.

Adverse Effects: Drowsiness, ataxia, dizziness, nausea, vomiting, cardiovascular (CV) complications, hepatitis, hematological disorders, Stevens-Johnson syndrome.

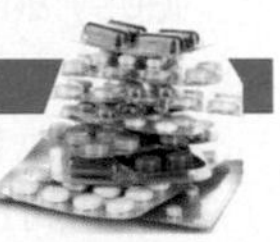

Nursing Considerations for Patients Receiving Drugs to Treat Partial Seizures

Assessment: History and Examination

- Assess for contraindications and cautions: Any known allergies to these drugs *to avoid hypersensitivity reactions*; history of bone marrow suppression or renal stones, *which could be exacerbated by these drugs*; history of renal or hepatic dysfunction *that might interfere with drug metabolism and excretion*; and current status of pregnancy or lactation, *which are contraindicated or require caution when using these drugs.*
- Perform a physical assessment to establish baseline data for determining the effectiveness of therapy and the occurrence of any *potential adverse effects.*
- Inspect the skin for color and lesions *to determine evidence of possible skin effects*; assess pulse and blood pressure and auscultate heart *to evaluate for possible cardiac effects*; assess level of orientation, affect, reflexes, and bilateral grip strength *to evaluate any CNS effects*; monitor bowel sounds and urine output *to determine possible GI or GU effects.*
- Obtain a baseline EEG if appropriate *to evaluate brain function.*
- Assess the patient's renal and liver function, including renal and liver function tests, *to determine the appropriateness of therapy and determine the need for possible dose adjustment.*
- Monitor the results of laboratory tests such as urinalysis and CBC with differential *to identify changes in bone marrow function.*

Nursing Diagnoses

Nursing diagnoses related to drug therapy might include the following:

- Acute pain related to GI and CNS effects
- Disturbed thought processes related to CNS effects
- Risk for injury related to CNS effects
- Risk for infection related to bone marrow suppression effects
- Deficient knowledge regarding drug therapy

Planning

- The patient will receive the best therapeutic effect from the drug therapy.
- The patient will have limited adverse effects to the drug therapy.
- The patient will have an understanding of the drug therapy, adverse effects to anticipate, and measures to relieve discomfort and improve safety.

Implementation with Rationale

- Administer the drug with food *to alleviate GI irritation if GI upset is a problem.*
- Monitor CBC before and periodically during therapy *to detect and prevent serious bone marrow suppression.*
- Protect the patient from exposure to infection *if bone marrow suppression occurs.*
- Discontinue the drug if skin rash, bone marrow suppression, unusual depression, or personality changes occur *to prevent further serious adverse effects.*
- Discontinue the drug slowly, and never withdraw the drug quickly, *because rapid withdrawal may precipitate seizures.*
- Arrange for counseling for women of childbearing age who are taking these drugs. *Because these drugs have the potential to cause serious damage to the fetus*, women should understand the risk of birth defects and use barrier contraceptives to avoid pregnancy.
- Evaluate for therapeutic blood levels of carbamazepine (4 to 12 mcg/mL) *to ensure that the most effective dose is being used.*
- Provide safety measures to protect the patient from injury or falls *if CNS changes occur.*
- Provide patient teaching, including drug name and prescribed dosage, as well as measures for avoidance of

(continues on page 406)

adverse effects, warning signs that may indicate possible problems, and the need for periodic laboratory testing and monitoring and evaluation *to enhance patient knowledge about drug therapy and to promote compliance.*
- Suggest that the patient wear or carry a MedicAlert bracelet *to alert emergency workers and health care providers about the use of an antiepileptic drug.*
- Offer support and encouragement *to help the patient cope with the drug regimen and diagnosis.*

Evaluation

- Monitor patient response to the drug (decrease in incidence or absence of seizures).
- Monitor for adverse effects (CNS changes, GI depression, bone marrow suppression, severe dermatological reactions, liver toxicity, renal stones).
- Evaluate the effectiveness of the teaching plan (patient can give the drug name and dosage and name possible adverse effects to watch for and specific measures to prevent them; patient is aware of the risk of birth defects and the need to carry information about the diagnosis and use of this drug)

KEY POINTS

- Drugs used in the treatment of partial seizures include drugs that stabilize the nerve membrane by altering electrolyte movement or increasing GABA activity.
- Some of the drugs used to treat generalized seizures have also been found to be useful in treating partial seizures.
- Adverse effects associated with the use of drugs used in treating partial seizures include CNS depressive effects and dermatological disorders.

SUMMARY

- Epilepsy is a collection of different syndromes, all of which have the same characteristic: A sudden discharge of excessive electrical energy from nerve cells located within the brain. This event is called a seizure.
- Seizures can be divided into two groups: Generalized and partial (focal).
- Generalized seizures can be further classified as tonic–clonic (grand mal); absence (petit mal); myoclonic; febrile; and rapidly recurrent (status epilepticus).
- Partial (focal) seizures can be further classified as simple or complex.
- Drug treatment depends on the type of seizure that the patient has experienced and the toxicity associated with the available agents.
- Drug treatment is directed at stabilizing the overexcited nerve membranes and/or increasing the effectiveness of GABA, an inhibitory neurotransmitter.
- Adverse effects associated with antiepileptics (e.g., insomnia, fatigue, confusion, GI depression, bradycardia) reflect the CNS depression caused by the drugs.
- Patients being treated with an antiepileptic should be advised to wear or carry a MedicAlert notification to alert emergency medical professionals to their epilepsy and their use of antiepileptic drugs.
- Patients being treated with an antiepileptic are often on long-term therapy, which requires compliance with their drug regimen and restrictions associated with their disorder and the drug effects.

CHECK YOUR UNDERSTANDING

Answers to the questions in this chapter can be found in Answers to Check Your Understanding Questions on thePoint®.

MULTIPLE CHOICE

Select the best answer to the following.

1. When teaching a group of students about epilepsy, which of the following should the nurse include?
   a. Always characterized by grand mal seizures
   b. Only a genetic problem
   c. The most prevalent neurological disorder
   d. The name given to one brain disorder

2. Which of the following would the nurse be least likely to include as a type of generalized seizure?
   a. Petit mal seizures
   b. Febrile seizures
   c. Grand mal seizures
   d. Complex seizures

3. Which instruction would the nurse encourage a patient receiving an antiepileptic drug to do?
   a. Give up his or her driver's license.
   b. Wear or carry a MedicAlert identification.
   c. Take antihistamines to help dry up secretions.
   d. Keep the diagnosis a secret to avoid prejudice.

4. Drugs that are commonly used to treat grand mal seizures include
   a. barbiturates, benzodiazepines, and hydantoins.
   b. barbiturates, antihistamines, and local anesthetics.
   c. hydantoins, phenobarbital, and phensuximide.
   d. benzodiazepines, phensuximide, and valproic acid.

5. The drug of choice for the treatment of absence seizures is
   a. valproic acid.
   b. methsuximide.
   c. phensuximide.
   d. ethosuximide.

6. Focal or partial seizures
   a. start at one point and spread quickly throughout the brain.
   b. are best treated with benzodiazepines.
   c. involve only part of the brain.
   d. are easily diagnosed and recognized.

7. One drug that is used alone in the treatment of partial seizures is
   a. carbamazepine.
   b. topiramate.
   c. lamotrigine.
   d. gabapentin.

8. Treatment of epilepsy is directed at
   a. blocking the transmission of nerve impulses into the brain.
   b. stabilizing overexcited nerve membranes.
   c. blocking peripheral nerve terminals.
   d. thickening the meninges to dampen brain electrical activity.

MULTIPLE RESPONSE

Select all that apply.

1. A client has been stabilized on phenytoin (*Dilantin*) for several years and has not experienced a grand mal seizure in more than 3 years. The client decides to stop the drug because it no longer seems to be needed. In counseling the client the nurse should include which of the following points?
   a. He will always need this drug.
   b. This drug needs to be slowly tapered to avoid potentially serious adverse effects.
   c. He is probably correct and the drug is not needed.
   d. The drug should not be stopped until appropriate blood tests are done.
   e. Stopping the drug suddenly could precipitate seizures because the nerves will be more sensitive.
   f. His insurance company 'won't cover any problems that might occur if he stops the drug without physician approval.

2. The most common adverse effects associated with antiepileptic therapy reflect the depression of the CNS. In assessing a client on antiepileptic therapy the nurse would monitor the patient for which of the following?
   a. Hypertension
   b. Insomnia
   c. Confusion
   d. GI depression
   e. Increased salivation
   f. Tachycardia

BIBLIOGRAPHY AND REFERENCES

Brunton, L., Chabner, B., & Knollman, B. (2011). *Goodman and Gilman's the pharmacological basis of therapeutics* (12th ed.). New York: McGraw-Hill.

Chang, G. B., Buchhalter, J., & Mullan, B. (2004). Mechanism of disease: Epilepsy. *New England Journal of Medicine, 349*, 1257–1266.

Delanty, N. (2010). *Seizures: Medical causes and management.* New York: Humana Press.

Facts and Comparisons. (2015). *Drug facts and comparisons.* St. Louis, MO: Author.

Facts and Comparisons. (2015). *Professional's guide to patient drug facts.* St. Louis, MO: Author.

Karch, A. M. (2014). *Lippincott's nursing drug guide.* Philadelphia, PA: Lippincott Williams & Wilkins.

Pandolfo, M. (2011). Genetics of epilepsy. *Seminars in Neurology, 31*(5), 506–518.

Porth, C. M. (2013). *Pathophysiology: Concepts of altered health states* (9th ed.). Philadelphia, PA: Lippincott Williams & Wilkins.

Wyllie, E., Cascino, G. D., Gidal, B. E., et al. (2010). *Treatment of epilepsy: Principles and practice.* Philadelphia, PA: Lippincott Williams & Wilkins.

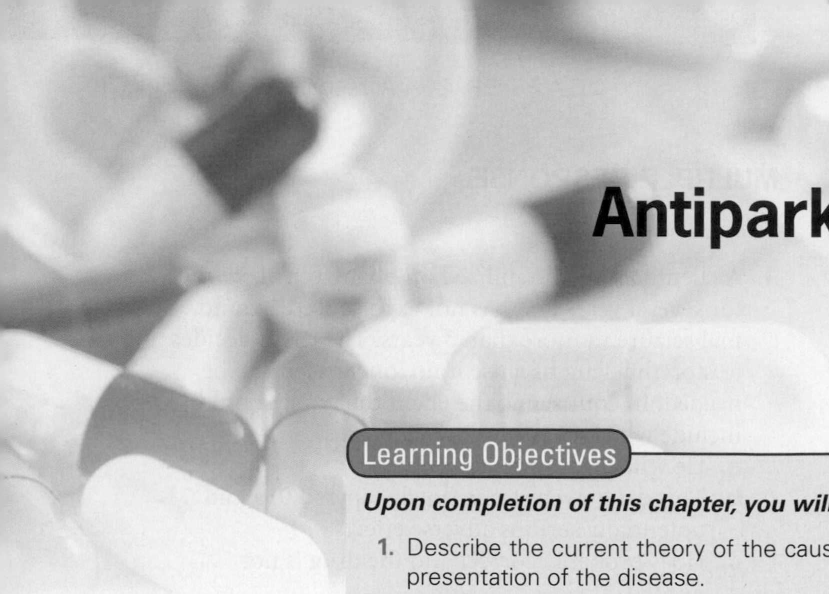

24 Antiparkinsonism Agents

Learning Objectives

Upon completion of this chapter, you will be able to:

1. Describe the current theory of the cause of Parkinson's disease and correlate this with the clinical presentation of the disease.
2. Describe the therapeutic actions, indications, pharmacokinetics, contraindications, most common adverse reactions, and important drug–drug interactions associated with antiparkinsonism agents.
3. Discuss the use of antiparkinsonism agents across the lifespan.
4. Compare and contrast the prototype drugs for each class of antiparkinsonism agents with the other drugs in that class and with drugs from the other classes used to treat the disease.
5. Outline the nursing considerations and teaching needs for patients receiving each class of antiparkinsonism agents.

Glossary of Key Terms

anticholinergic: drug that opposes the effects of acetylcholine at acetylcholine receptor sites

bradykinesia: difficulty in performing intentional movements and extreme slowness and sluggishness; characteristic of Parkinson's disease

corpus striatum: part of the brain that reacts with the substantia nigra to maintain a balance of suppression and stimulation

dopaminergic: drug that increases the effects of dopamine at receptor sites

Parkinson's disease: debilitating disease, characterized by progressive loss of coordination and function, which results from the degeneration of dopamine-producing cells in the substantia nigra

parkinsonism: Parkinson's disease–like extrapyramidal symptoms that are adverse effects associated with particular drugs or brain injuries

substantia nigra: a part of the brain rich in dopamine and dopamine receptors; site of degenerating neurons in Parkinson's disease

Drug List

Dopaminergic Agents
amantadine
apomorphine
bromocriptine
carbidopa–levodopa
(P) levodopa
pramipexole
rasagiline
ropinirole

Anticholinergic Agents
(P) benztropine
diphenhydramine
trihexyphenidyl

Adjunctive Agents
entacapone
selegiline
tolcapone

In the 1990s several prominent figures—former heavyweight boxing champion Muhammad Ali, former US Attorney General Janet Reno, and actor Michael J. Fox—revealed that they had **Parkinson's disease**, a progressive, chronic neurological disorder. In general, Parkinson's disease may develop in people of any age, but it usually affects those who are past middle age and entering their 60s or even later years. Therefore, the occurrence of Parkinson's disease in these well-known individuals who were relatively young at the time of diagnosis is that much more interesting. The cause of the condition is not known.

At this time, there is no cure for Parkinson's disease. Therapy is aimed at management of signs and symptoms to provide optimal functioning for as long as possible.

Parkinson's Disease and Parkinsonism

Lack of coordination is characteristic of Parkinson's disease. Rhythmic tremors develop, insidiously at first. In some muscle groups these tremors lead to rigidity, and in others weakness. Affected patients may have trouble maintaining position or posture, and they may develop the condition known as **bradykinesia**, marked by difficulties in performing intentional movements and extreme slowness or sluggishness.

As Parkinson's disease progresses, walking becomes a problem; a shuffling gait is a hallmark of the condition. In addition, patients may drool, and their speech may be slow and slurred. As the cranial nerves are affected, they may develop a mask-like expression. Difficulty swallowing, often leading to aspiration pneumonia, is a major issue as the disease progresses. It may be difficult to safely administer oral drugs to these patients. Parkinson's disease does not affect the higher levels of the cerebral cortex, so a very alert and intelligent person may be trapped in a progressively degenerating body.

Parkinsonism is a term used to describe the Parkinson's disease–like extrapyramidal symptoms that are adverse effects associated with particular drugs or brain injuries. Patients typically exhibit tremors and bradykinesia.

Pathophysiology

Although the cause of Parkinson's disease is not known, it is known that the signs and symptoms of the disease relate to damaged neurons in the basal ganglia of the brain. Theories about the cause of the degeneration of these neurons range from viral infection, blows to the head, brain infection, atherosclerosis, and exposure to certain drugs and environmental factors.

Even though the actual cause is not known the mechanism that causes the signs and symptoms of Parkinson's disease is understood. In a part of the brain called the **substantia nigra**, a dopamine-rich area, nerve cell bodies begin to degenerate. This process results in a reduction of the number of impulses sent to the **corpus striatum** in the basal ganglia. This area of the brain, in conjunction with the substantia nigra, helps to maintain muscle tone not related to any particular movement. The corpus striatum is connected to the substantia nigra by a series of neurons that use gamma-aminobutyric acid, an inhibitory neurotransmitter. The substantia nigra sends nerve impulses back into the corpus striatum using the inhibitory neurotransmitter dopamine. The two areas then mutually inhibit activity in a balanced manner.

Higher neurons originating in the cerebral cortex secrete acetylcholine (an excitatory neurotransmitter) in the area of the corpus striatum to coordinate intentional movements of the body. When dopamine decreases in the area a chemical imbalance occurs that allows the cholinergic or excitatory cells to dominate. This affects the functioning of the basal ganglia and of the cortical and cerebellar components of the extrapyramidal motor system. The extrapyramidal system is one that provides coordination for unconscious muscle movements, including those that control position, posture, and movement. The result of this imbalance in the motor system is apparent as the manifestations of Parkinson's disease (Figure 24.1).

Treatment

At this time, there is no treatment that arrests the neuron degeneration of Parkinson's disease and the eventual decline in patient function. Surgical procedures involving the basal ganglia have been tried with varying success at prolonging the degeneration caused by this disease. Drug therapy remains the primary treatment.

Therapy is aimed at restoring the balance between the declining levels of dopamine, which has an inhibitory effect on the neurons in the basal ganglia, and the now-dominant cholinergic neurons, which are excitatory.

This may help to reduce the signs and symptoms of parkinsonism and restore normal function for a time (Figure 24.2).

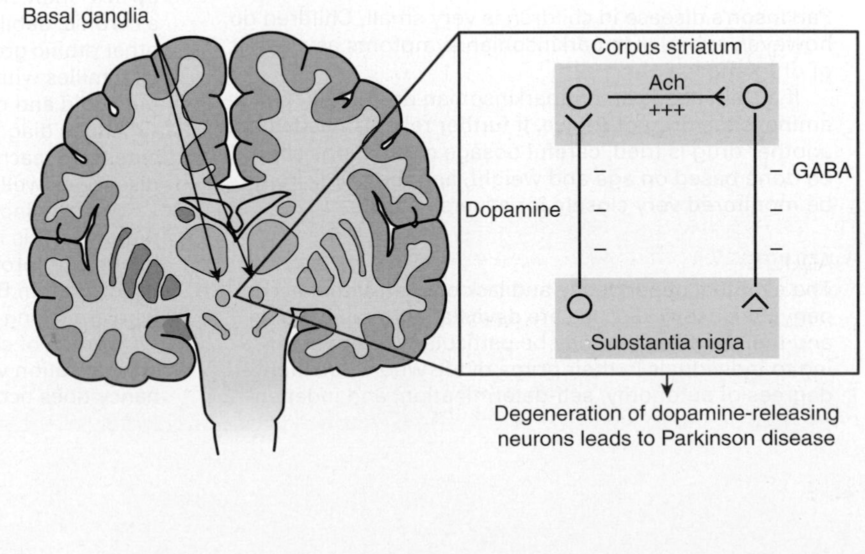

FIGURE 24.1 Schematic representation of the degeneration of neurons that leads to Parkinson's disease. Cells in the corpus striatum send impulses to the substantia nigra using gamma-aminobutyric acid (GABA) to inhibit activity. In turn, the substantia nigra sends impulses to the corpus striatum, using dopamine, to inhibit activity. Cortical areas use acetylcholine (Ach) to stimulate intentional movements.

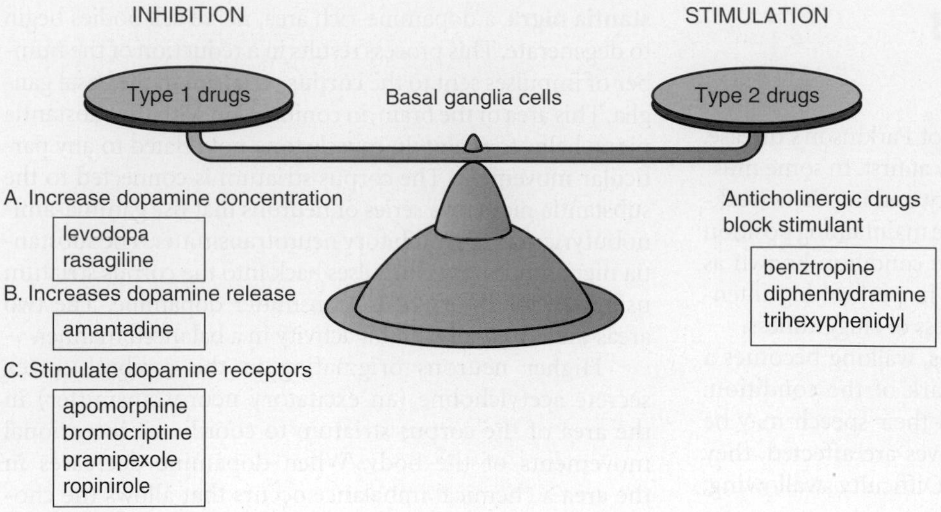

FIGURE 24.2 Drug therapy in treating Parkinson's disease is aimed at achieving a balance between the stimulating cholinergic effects and the inhibitory effects of dopamine in the basal ganglia. Type 1 drugs affect dopamine and are inhibitory. Type 2 drugs block cholinergic effects, preventing stimulation.

Total management of patient care in individuals with Parkinson's disease presents a challenge. Patients should be encouraged to be as active as possible, to perform exercises to prevent the development of skeletal deformities, and to attend to their own care as long as they can. When swallowing becomes an issue a speech therapist may be helpful in teaching the patient to swallow safely, and thickening agents may be needed to help facilitate swallowing. Both the patient and family need instruction about following drug protocols and monitoring adverse effects, as well as encouragement and support for coping with the progressive nature of the disease (Box 24.1). Because of the degenerative effects of this disease, patients may experience episodes of depression or be emotionally upset. Psychological support, as well as physical support, is a crucial aspect of care.

KEY POINTS

- Parkinson's disease is a progressive nervous system disease characterized by tremors, changes in posture and gait, and a mask-like facial expression.
- The loss of dopamine-secreting cells results in a loss of the inhibitory dopamine effect and is thought to be responsible for Parkinson's disease.

BOX 24.1 *FOCUS ON* **Drug Therapy Across the Lifespan**

Antiparkinsonism Agents

CHILDREN

The safety and effectiveness of most of these drugs has not been established in children. The incidence of Parkinson's disease in children is very small. Children do, however, experience parkinsonian symptoms as a result of drug effects.

If a child needs an antiparkinsonian drug, diphenhydramine is the drug of choice. If further relief is needed and another drug is tried, careful dosage calculations should be done based on age and weight, and the child should be monitored very closely for adverse effects.

ADULTS

The eventual dependence and lack of control that accompany Parkinson's disease are devastating to all patients and their families but may be particularly overwhelming to individuals in their prime of life who value high degrees of autonomy, self-determination, and independence. Although these characteristics are not associated with any particular ethnic group, they are valued more highly among certain cultures than others. For example, Latinos—who traditionally have strong extended family ties—may not have the same problems adjusting to a chronic, debilitating illness in a relative as members of other ethnic groups. It is important for the nurse to assess all families with sensitivity to determine what convictions they hold and plan nursing care accordingly.

Adults diagnosed with Parkinson's disease require extensive teaching and support and help coping with the disease as well as with the effects of the drugs.

With the increasing interest in herbal and alternative therapies, it is important to stress the need to inform the health care provider about any other treatment being used. Vitamin B_6 can pose a serious problem for patients who are taking some of these drugs.

Women of childbearing age should be advised to use contraception when they are on these drugs. If a pregnancy does occur, or is desired, they need counseling

BOX 24.1 FOCUS ON Drug Therapy Across the Lifespan (continued)

about the potential for adverse effects. Women who are nursing should be encouraged to find another method of feeding the baby because of the potential for adverse drug effects on the baby.

OLDER ADULTS

Although Parkinson's disease may affect individuals of any age, gender, or nationality, the frequency of the disease increases with age. This debilitating condition, which affects more men than women, may be one of many chronic problems associated with aging.

The drugs that are used to manage Parkinson's disease are associated with more adverse effects in older people with long-term problems. Both anticholinergic and dopaminergic drugs aggravate glaucoma, benign prostatic hypertrophy, constipation, cardiac problems, and chronic obstructive pulmonary diseases. Special precautions and frequent follow-up visits are necessary for older patients with Parkinson's disease, and their drug dosages may need to be adjusted frequently to avoid serious problems. In many cases, other agents are given to counteract the effects of these drugs, and patients then have complicated drug regimens with many associated adverse effects and problems. Consequently, it is essential for these patients to have extensive written drug-teaching protocols.

Dopaminergic Agents

Dopaminergics—drugs that increase the effects of dopamine at receptor sites—have been proven to be even more effective than anticholinergics in the treatment of parkinsonism (see Table 24.1). Dopaminergic agents include amantadine (generic), apomorphine (*Apokyn*), bromocriptine (*Parlodel*), levodopa (generic), carbidopa–levodopa (*Sinemet*), pramipexole (*Mirapex*), rasagiline (*Azilect*), ropinirole (*Requip*), and rotigotine (*Neupro*).

Therapeutic Actions and Indications

Dopamine does not cross the blood–brain barrier. Therefore, other drugs that act like dopamine or increase dopamine concentrations indirectly must be used to

Table 24.1 *Drugs in Focus:* Dopaminergic Agents

Drug Name	Dosage/Route	Usual Indications
amantadine (generic)	100 mg PO b.i.d., up to 400 mg/d has been used	Antiviral, treatment of idiopathic and drug-induced parkinsonism in adults
apomorphine (*Apokyn*)	2–6 mg subcutaneous t.i.d., given with trimethobenzamide: 300 mg PO t.i.d.	Intermittent treatment of hypomobility "off" episodes of advanced Parkinson's disease
bromocriptine (*Parlodel*)	1.25 mg PO b.i.d., titrate up to 10–40 mg/d	Treatment of idiopathic Parkinson's disease, may be beneficial in later stages when response to levodopa decreases
carbidopa–levodopa (*Sinemet*)	100-mg levodopa with 10–25-mg carbidopa PO t.i.d.	Treatment of idiopathic Parkinson's disease
levodopa (*Dopar*)	0.5–1 g/d PO in two divided doses, titrate up to 8 g/d, most often given in combination with carbidopa as *Sinemet:* 25-mg carbidopa/100-mg levodopa PO t.i.d.	Treatment of idiopathic Parkinson's disease
pramipexole (*Mirapex*)	0.125 mg PO t.i.d., titrate up to 1.5 mg PO t.i.d.	Treatment of idiopathic Parkinson's disease
rasagiline (*Azilect*)	1 mg/d PO, 0.5 mg/d PO if used with levodopa	Initial monotherapy and as adjunct to levodopa to treat idiopathic Parkinson's disease
ropinirole (*Requip*)	0.25 mg PO t.i.d., titrate up to maximum dose of 24 mg/d	Treatment of idiopathic Parkinson's disease in early stages and in later stages when combined with levodopa, treatment of restless legs syndrome
Rotigotine (*Neupro*)	2–8-mg/24-h transdermal patch, based on patient response and tolerance; 1–3-mg/24-h patch for restless leg syndrome	Treatment of all stages of Parkinson's disease, combined with other drugs; treatment of restless leg syndrome

increase dopamine levels in the substantia nigra or to directly stimulate the dopamine receptors in that area. This action helps to restore the balance between the inhibitory and stimulating neurons. Dopaminergic agents are effective as long as enough intact neurons remain in the substantia nigra to respond to increased levels of dopamine. After the neural degeneration has progressed beyond a certain point, these agents are no longer effective.

The dopaminergics are indicated for the relief of the signs and symptoms of idiopathic Parkinson's disease (see Table 24.1 for Usual Indications for each of these agents). Levodopa is the mainstay of treatment for Parkinson's disease. This precursor of dopamine crosses the blood–brain barrier and is converted into dopamine. In this way, it acts like a replacement therapy. Although levodopa is almost always given in combination form with carbidopa as a fixed combination drug (*Sinemet*), other drugs besides carbidopa may be used (see Adjunctive Agents). When used with carbidopa the enzyme dopa decarboxylase is inhibited in the periphery, diminishing the metabolism of levodopa in the gastrointestinal (GI) tract and in peripheral tissues, thereby leading to higher levels crossing the blood–brain barrier. Because the carbidopa decreases the amount of levodopa needed to reach a therapeutic level in the brain the dose of levodopa can be decreased, which reduces the incidence of adverse side effects.

In 2015 an extended release combination of levodopa/carbidopa (*Rytary*) was approved for use in Parkinson's disease, postencephalitic parkinsonism and post–carbon monoxide poisoning parkinsonism.

Amantadine is an antiviral drug that also seems to increase the release of dopamine, being effective as long as there is a possibility of more dopamine release.

Apomorphine is a newer adjunctive therapy for Parkinson's disease that directly binds with postsynaptic dopamine receptors. Similar to apomorphine, bromocriptine, pramipexole, and rotigotine act as direct dopamine agonists on dopamine receptor sites in the substantia nigra. Because bromocriptine does not depend on cells in the area to biotransform it or to increase the release of already produced dopamine, it may be effective longer than levodopa or amantadine.

Ropinirole is a newer drug that directly stimulates dopamine receptors. It is also used to treat restless leg syndrome.

Rotigotine is the newest of the dopamine agonists. It is only available in a transdermal form, which is very helpful when swallowing is an issue; and it is also used to treat restless leg syndrome.

Rasagiline is another newer dopamine agonist that increases dopamine in the nerve synapse, particularly in areas of the brain responsible for controlling movement and coordination. It inhibits monoamine oxidase (MAO) type B, which is found primarily in the central nervous system (CNS). Because this drug works on an enzyme found mostly inside the CNS, it has fewer peripheral adverse effects. It can be used as initial monotherapy or as an adjunct therapy with levodopa.

Pharmacokinetics

The dopaminergics are usually given orally and are generally well absorbed from the GI tract and widely distributed in the body. Apomorphine, however, must be given subcutaneously and rotigotine is given transdermally. The dopaminergics are metabolized in the liver and peripheral cells and excreted in the urine. They cross the placenta and enter breast milk.

Contraindications and Cautions

The dopaminergics are contraindicated in the presence of any known allergy to the drug or drug components *to prevent hypersensitivity reactions* and in angle-closure glaucoma, *which could be exacerbated by these drugs.* Dopaminergics enter breast milk and should not be used during lactation *because of the potential for adverse effects in the baby*. In addition, levodopa is contraindicated in patients with a history or presence of suspicious skin lesions *because this drug has been associated with the development of melanoma.*

Administer dopaminergic agents cautiously with patients who have *any condition that could be exacerbated by dopamine receptor stimulation,* such as cardiovascular disease, including myocardial infarction, arrhythmias, and hypertension; bronchial asthma; history of peptic ulcers; urinary tract obstruction; and psychiatric disorders. Care also is necessary during pregnancy *because these drugs cross the placenta and could adversely affect the fetus* and in patients with renal and hepatic disease, *which could interfere with the metabolism and excretion of the drug.* Closely monitor cardiac status in patients receiving apomorphine *because of the associated risk for hypotension and prolonged QT interval.*

Adverse Effects

The adverse effects associated with the dopaminergics usually result from stimulation of dopamine receptors. CNS effects may include anxiety, nervousness, headache, malaise, fatigue, confusion, mental changes, blurred vision, muscle twitching, and ataxia. Peripheral effects may include anorexia, nausea, vomiting, dysphagia, and constipation or diarrhea; cardiac arrhythmias, hypotension, and palpitations; bizarre breathing patterns; urinary retention; and flushing, increased sweating, and hot flashes. Bone marrow depression and hepatic dysfunction have also been reported (Figure 24.3).

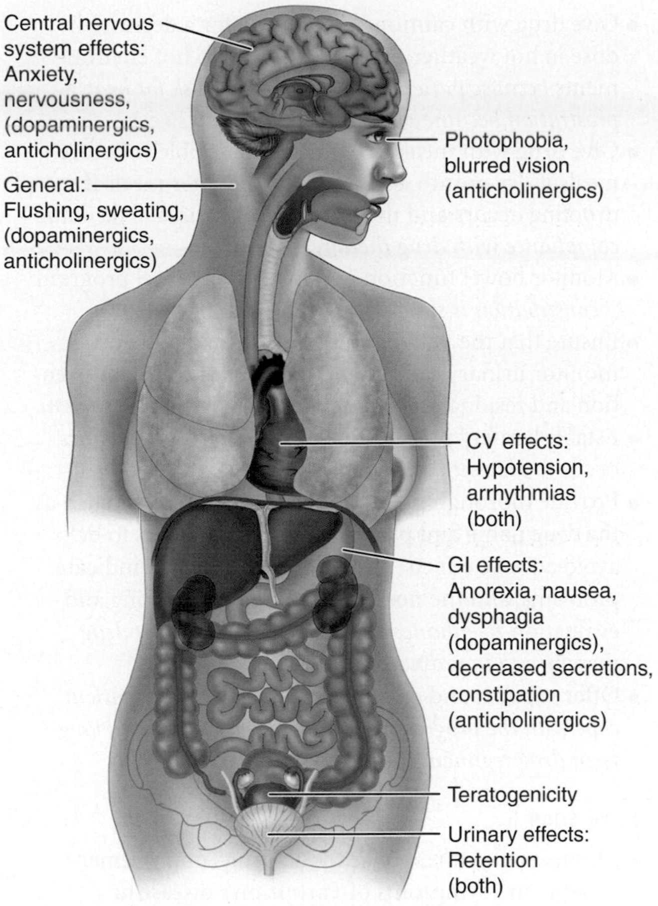

FIGURE 24.3 Common adverse effects and toxicities associated with antiparkinsonism agents.

Clinically Important Drug–Drug Interactions

If dopaminergics are combined with monoamine oxidase inhibitors (MAOIs), therapeutic effects increase and a risk of hypertensive crisis exists. The MAOI should be stopped 14 days before beginning therapy with a dopaminergic.

The combination of levodopa with vitamin B_6 or with phenytoin may lead to decreased efficacy of the levodopa (see Critical Thinking Scenario). Reduced effectiveness of both drugs may also result if dopaminergics are combined with dopamine antagonists. In addition, patients who take dopaminergics should be cautioned to avoid over-the-counter vitamins; if such medications are used the patient should be monitored closely because a decrease in dopaminergic effectiveness can result.

Patients using rasagiline should avoid tyramine-containing foods, as well as St. John's wort, meperidine, and other analgesics, to avoid potentially serious reactions.

Ⓟ Prototype Summary: Levodopa

Indications: Treatment of parkinsonism and Parkinson's disease.

Actions: Precursor of dopamine, which is deficient in parkinsonism; crosses the blood–brain barrier, where it is converted to dopamine and acts as a replacement neurotransmitter; effective for 2 to 5 years in relieving the symptoms of Parkinson's disease.

Pharmacokinetics:

Route	Onset	Peak	Duration
Oral	Varies	0.5–2 h	5 h

$T_{1/2}$: 1 to 3 hours; metabolized in the liver, excreted in the urine.

Adverse Effects: Adventitious movements, ataxia, increased hand tremor, dizziness, numbness, weakness, agitation, anxiety, anorexia, nausea, dry mouth, dysphagia, urinary retention, flushing, cardiac irregularities.

Nursing Considerations for Patients Receiving Anticholinergic Agents

Assessment: History and Examination

- Assess for contraindications or cautions: Any known allergies to these drugs *to avoid hypersensitivity reactions*; GI depression or obstruction, urinary hesitancy or obstruction, benign prostatic hypertrophy, or glaucoma, *which may be exacerbated by the peripheral anticholinergic effect of the drug*; cardiac arrhythmias, hypertension, or hypotension, *which may be increased due to the dominance of sympathetic stimulatory activity due to blockage of parasympathetic activity*; myasthenia gravis, *which may be exacerbated by blockage of acetylcholine receptors*; current status related to pregnancy or lactation *due to risk of fetal or infant adverse effects*; hepatic dysfunction, *which could interfere with drug metabolism and increase risk for toxicity*; and exposure to a hot environment, *which may block the individual's reflex sweating.*
- Perform a physical assessment *to determine baseline data for determining the effectiveness of the drug and the occurrence of adverse effects associated with drug therapy.*
- Assess level of orientation and neurological status, including affect, reflexes, bilateral grip strength, gait, tremors, and spasticity, *to evaluate any CNS effects.*
- Monitor pulse, blood pressure, and cardiac output *to evaluate for possible adverse effects related to blocking of suppressive action on the heart.*

(*continues on page 414*)

- Auscultate bowel sounds *to evaluate GI motility and detect possible indications of paralytic ileus.*
- Assess urine output and palpate bladder to determine adequate renal and bladder function.
- Monitor the results of laboratory tests such as renal and liver function tests *to determine the need for possible dose adjustment and identify potential toxic effects.*

Nursing Diagnoses

Nursing diagnoses related to drug therapy might include the following:

- Impaired oral mucous membranes related to anticholinergic effects
- Risk for impaired thermoregulation related to anticholinergic effects
- Impaired urinary elimination related to genitourinary effects
- Constipation related to GI effects
- Disturbed thought processes related to CNS effects
- Risk for injury related to CNS effects
- Deficient knowledge regarding drug therapy

Planning

- The patient will receive the best therapeutic effect from the drug therapy.
- The patient will have limited adverse effects to the drug therapy.
- The patient will have an understanding of the drug therapy, adverse effects to anticipate, and measures to relieve discomfort and improve safety

Implementation with Rationale

- Arrange to decrease dose or discontinue the drug *if dry mouth becomes so severe that swallowing becomes difficult.* Provide sugarless lozenges to suck and frequent mouth care to help with this problem.
- Give drug with caution and arrange for a decrease in dose in hot weather or with exposure to hot environments *because patients are at increased risk for heat prostration because of decreased ability to sweat.*
- Give drug with meals if GI upset is a problem, before meals if dry mouth is a problem, and after meals if drooling occurs and the drug causes nausea *to facilitate compliance with drug therapy.*
- Monitor bowel function and institute a bowel program *if constipation is severe.*
- Ensure that the patient voids before taking the drug; monitor urinary output and palpate for bladder distention and residual urine *if urinary retention is a problem.*
- Establish safety precautions if CNS or vision changes occur *to prevent patient injury.*
- Provide thorough patient teaching about topics such as the drug name and prescribed dose, measures to help avoid adverse effects, warning signs that may indicate problems, and the need for periodic monitoring and evaluation *to enhance patient knowledge about drug therapy and to promote compliance.*
- Offer support and encouragement *to help the patient cope with the progressive nature of the disease and long-term drug regimen.*

Evaluation

- Monitor patient response to the drug (improvement in signs and symptoms of Parkinson's disease or parkinsonism).
- Monitor for adverse effects (CNS changes, urinary retention, GI slowing, tachycardia, decreased sweating, flushing).
- Evaluate the effectiveness of the teaching plan (patient can give the drug name and dosage, name possible adverse effects to watch for and specific measures to prevent them, and discuss the importance of continued follow-up).
- Monitor the effectiveness of support measures and compliance with the regimen.

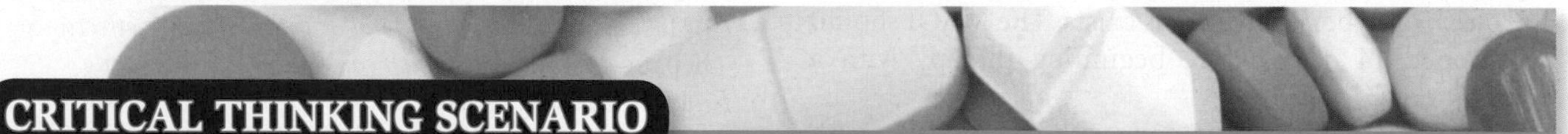

CRITICAL THINKING SCENARIO

Effects of Vitamin B_6 Intake on Levodopa Levels

THE SITUATION

S.S., a 58-year-old man with well-controlled Parkinson's disease, presents with severe nausea, anorexia, fainting spells, and heart palpitation. He has been maintained on levodopa for the Parkinson's disease, and he claims to have followed his drug regimen religiously.

According to S.S., the only change in his lifestyle has been the addition of several health foods and vitamins. His daughter, who recently returned from her freshman year in college, has begun a new health regimen, including natural foods and plenty of supplemental vitamins. She was so enthusiastic about her new approach that everyone in the family agreed to give this diet a try.

Effects of Vitamin B_6 Intake on Levodopa Levels (continued)

CRITICAL THINKING

Based on S.S.'s signs and symptoms, what has probably occurred?

In Parkinson's disease is it possible to differentiate a deterioration of illness from a toxic reaction to a drug?

What nursing implications should be considered when teaching S.S. and his family about the effects of vitamin B_6 on levodopa levels?

In what ways can the daughter cope with her role in this crisis?

Develop a new care plan for S.S. that involves all family members and that includes drug teaching.

DISCUSSION

The presenting symptoms reflect an increase in Parkinson symptoms as well as an increase in peripheral dopamine reactions (e.g., palpitations, fainting, anorexia, nausea). It is necessary to determine whether the problem involves a further degeneration in the neurons in the substantia nigra or the particular medication that S.S. has been taking. In many patients, responsiveness to levodopa is lost as neural degeneration continues.

The explanation of the new lifestyle—full of grains, natural foods, and vitamins—alerted the nurse to the possibility of excessive vitamin B_6 intake. In reviewing the vitamin bottles and some of the food packages supplied by S.S., it seemed that too much vitamin B_6, which speeds the conversion of levodopa to dopamine before it can cross the blood–brain barrier, might be the reason the patient's symptoms recurred.

The status of S.S.'s Parkinson's disease should be evaluated, and then he can be restarted on levodopa. The smallest dose possible should be used initially, with gradual increases to achieve the maximum benefit with the fewest side effects. It would be wise to consider combining the drug with carbidopa to prevent some of the patient's recent problems.

In addition, S.S. should receive thorough drug teaching in written form for future reference. The need to avoid vitamin B_6 should be emphasized. The entire family should be involved in an explanation of what happened and how this situation can be avoided in the future. Because the daughter may feel guilty about her role, she should have the opportunity to discuss her feelings and explore the positive impact of healthy food on nutrition and quality of life. This situation can serve as a good teaching example for staff as well as present them with an opportunity to review drug therapy in Parkinson's disease and the risks and benefits of more extreme diets.

NURSING CARE GUIDE FOR S.S.: LEVODOPA

Assessment: History and Examination

Allergies to levodopa; chronic obstructive pulmonary disease; dysrhythmias, hypotension, hepatic or renal dysfunction; psychoses; peptic ulcer; glaucoma

Concurrent use of MAOIs, phenytoin, pyridoxine, papaverine, or tricyclic antidepressants

Focus physical examination on:

CV: Blood pressure, pulse rate, peripheral perfusion, electrocardiogram results

CNS: Orientation, affect, reflexes, grip strength

Renal: Output, bladder palpation

GI: Abdominal examination, bowel sounds

Respiratory: Respiration, adventitious sounds

Laboratory tests: Renal and liver function tests, complete blood count

Nursing Diagnoses

Risk for injury related to CNS effects

Disturbed thought processes related to CNS effects

Deficient knowledge regarding drug therapy

Constipation related to GI effects

Planning

The patient will receive the best therapeutic effect from the drug therapy.

The patient will have limited adverse effects to the drug therapy.

The patient will have an understanding of the drug therapy, adverse effects to anticipate, and measures to relieve discomfort and improve safety.

Implementation

Ensure safe and appropriate administration of drug.

Provide comfort and safety: Slow positioning changes; assess orientation, provide pain medication as needed; give drug with food; administer with carbidopa; have patient void before each dose.

Provide support and reassurance to deal with disease and drug effects.

Instruct the patient regarding drug dose, effects, and adverse symptoms to report.

Evaluation

Evaluate drug effects: Relief of signs and symptoms of Parkinson's disease.

Monitor for adverse effects: CNS effects; renal changes, urinary retention; GI effects (constipation); increased sweating or flushing.

(continues on page 416)

Effects of Vitamin B_6 Intake on Levodopa Levels (continued)

Monitor for drug–drug interactions: Hypertensive crisis with MAOIs, decreased effects with vitamin B_6 or phenytoin.

Evaluate the effectiveness of the patient-teaching program.

Evaluate the effectiveness of comfort and safety measures.

PATIENT TEACHING FOR S.S.

- The drug that has been prescribed is called levodopa. It increases the levels of dopamine in the central areas of the brain and helps to reduce the signs and symptoms of Parkinson's disease.
- Often, this drug is combined with carbidopa, which allows the correct levels of levodopa to reach the brain.
- People who take this drug must have their individual dose needs adjusted over time. Common effects of this drug include:
  - *Fatigue, weakness, and drowsiness*: Try to space activities evenly through the day; allow rest periods to avoid these side effects. Take safety precautions, and avoid driving or operating dangerous machinery if these conditions occur.
  - *Dizziness, fainting*: Change position slowly to avoid dizzy spells.
  - *Increased sweating, darkened urine*: This is a normal reaction. Avoid very hot environments.
  - *Headaches, difficulty sleeping*: These usually pass as the body adjusts to the drug. If they become too uncomfortable and persist, consult with your health care provider.
- Report any of the following to your health care provider: *Uncontrolled movements of any body part, chest pain or palpitations, depression or mood changes, difficulty in voiding, or severe or persistent nausea and vomiting.*
- Be aware that vitamin B_6 interferes with the effects of levodopa. If you feel that you need a vitamin product, consult with your health care provider about using an agent that does not contain vitamin B_6.
- Avoid eating large quantities of health foods that contain vitamin B_6, such as grains and brans. If you are taking a carbidopa–levodopa combination, these precautions are not as important.
- Tell any doctor, nurse, or other health care provider involved in your care that you are taking this drug.
- Keep this drug and all medications out of the reach of children.
- Do not overexert yourself when you begin to feel better. Pace yourself.
- Take this drug exactly as directed, and schedule regular medical checkups to evaluate its effects.

KEY POINTS

- Dopaminergic drugs are used to increase the effects of dopamine at receptor sites, restoring the balance of neurotransmitters in the basal ganglia.
- The adverse effects associated with these drugs are related to the systemic effects of dopamine, increased heart rate, increased blood pressure, decreased GI activity, and urinary retention.
- Levodopa is the standard dopaminergic used to treat parkinsonism and Parkinson's disease. Several other dopaminergics are now used as adjuncts to levodopa to increase the dopamine effects as long as possible.

Anticholinergic Agents

Anticholinergics (Table 24.2) are drugs that oppose the effects of acetylcholine at receptor sites in the substantia nigra and the corpus striatum, thus helping to restore chemical balance in the area. Anticholinergics used to treat Parkinson's disease include benztropine (*Cogentin*), diphenhydramine (*Benadryl*), and trihexyphenidyl (generic).

Therapeutic Actions and Indications

The anticholinergics used to treat parkinsonism are synthetic drugs that have been developed to have a greater affinity for cholinergic receptor sites in the CNS than for those in the peripheral nervous system. However, they still block to some extent the cholinergic receptors that are responsible for stimulation of the parasympathetic nervous system's postganglionic effectors. This blockage is associated with the adverse effects (see Chapter 33), including slowed GI motility and secretions, with dry mouth and constipation, urinary retention, blurred vision, and dilated pupils.

Anticholinergic drugs are indicated for the treatment of parkinsonism, whether idiopathic, atherosclerotic, or postencephalitic, and for the relief of symptoms of extrapyramidal disorders associated with the use of some drugs, including phenothiazines. Although these drugs are not as effective as levodopa in the treatment of advancing cases of the disease, they may be useful as adjunctive therapy and for patients who no longer respond to levodopa. See Table 24.2 for Usual Indications.

Pharmacokinetics

The anticholinergic drugs are variably absorbed from the GI tract, reaching peak levels in 1 to 4 hours. They are

Table 24.2 *Drugs in Focus:* Anticholinergic Agents

Drug Name	Dosage/Route	Usual Indications
benztropine (*Cogentin*)	0.5–6 mg/d PO may be needed, 1–2 mg IM or IV; reduce dose in older patients	Adjunctive treatment of parkinsonism and drug-induced parkinsonism resulting from drug effects of phenothiazines
diphenhydramine (*Benadryl*)	*Adult:* 25–50 mg PO t.i.d. to q.i.d.; 10–50 mg IM or IV, maximum dose 400 mg/d *Pediatric:* 12.5–25 mg PO t.i.d. to q.i.d.; do not exceed 300 mg/d, 5 mg/kg/d IM or IV divided into four equal doses, maximum daily dose 300 mg	Adjunctive agent for treatment of Parkinson's disease; treatment of parkinsonism, including drug-induced disease particularly in the elderly and in patients at the early stages of disease
trihexyphenidyl (generic)	1–2 mg PO daily initially, titrate up to 6–10 mg/d; up to 15 mg/d may be needed	Adjunct to levodopa in treatment of parkinsonism, can be used alone for the control of drug-induced extrapyramidal disorders

metabolized in the liver and excreted by cellular pathways. All of them cross the placenta and enter breast milk (see Contraindications and Cautions). Benztropine and diphenhydramine are available in oral and intramuscular/intravenous forms. Trihexyphenidyl is only available in an oral form.

Contraindications and Cautions

Anticholinergics are contraindicated in the presence of allergy to any of these agents *to avoid hypersensitivity reactions.* In addition, they are contraindicated in narrow-angle glaucoma, GI obstruction, genitourinary (GU) obstruction, and prostatic hypertrophy, *all of which could be exacerbated by the peripheral anticholinergic effects of these drugs,* and in myasthenia gravis, *which could be exacerbated by the blocking of acetylcholine receptor sites at neuromuscular synapses.* The safety and efficacy for use in children have not been established.

Administer these agents cautiously in the following conditions: Tachycardia and other dysrhythmias and hypertension or hypotension *because the blocking of the parasympathetic system may cause a dominance of sympathetic stimulatory activity* and hepatic dysfunction, *which could interfere with the metabolism of the drugs and lead to toxic levels.* They should be used during pregnancy and lactation only if the benefit to the mother clearly outweighs the potential risk to the fetus or neonate. In addition, use caution in individuals who work in hot environments *because reflex sweating may be blocked, placing the individuals at risk for heat prostration.*

Adverse Effects

The use of anticholinergics for Parkinson's disease and parkinsonism is associated with CNS effects that relate to the blocking of central acetylcholine receptors, such as disorientation, confusion, and memory loss. Agitation, nervousness, delirium, dizziness, light-headedness, and weakness may also occur.

Anticipated peripheral anticholinergic effects include dry mouth, nausea, vomiting, paralytic ileus, and constipation related to decreased GI secretions and motility. In addition, other adverse effects may occur, including the tachycardia, palpitations, and hypotension related to the blocking of the suppressive cardiac effects of the parasympathetic nervous system; urinary retention and hesitancy related to a blocking of bladder muscle activity and sphincter relaxation; blurred vision and photophobia related to pupil dilation and blocking of lens accommodation; and flushing and reduced sweating related to a blocking of the cholinergic sites that stimulate sweating and blood vessel dilation in the skin.

Clinically Important Drug–Drug Interactions

When these anticholinergic drugs are used with other drugs that have anticholinergic properties, including the tricyclic antidepressants and the phenothiazines, there is a risk of potentially fatal paralytic ileus and an increased risk of toxic psychoses. If such combinations must be given, monitor patients closely and implement supportive measures. Dose adjustments often are necessary. In addition, when antipsychotic drugs are combined with anticholinergics a risk for decreased antipsychotic therapeutic effectiveness may occur, possibly as a result of a central antagonism of the two agents.

Ⓟ Prototype Summary: Benztropine

Indications: Adjunctive therapy for Parkinson's disease, relief of symptoms of extrapyramidal disorders (parkinsonism) that accompany neuroleptic therapy.

Actions: Acts as an anticholinergic, principally in the CNS, returning balance to the basal ganglia and reducing the severity of rigidity, akinesia, and tremors; peripheral anticholinergic effects help to reduce drooling and other secondary effects of parkinsonism.

Pharmacokinetics:

Route	Onset	Peak	Duration
Oral	1 h	Unknown	6–10 h
IM, IV	15 min	Unknown	6–10 h

$T_{1/2}$: Unknown, metabolized in the liver.

Adverse Effects: Disorientation, confusion, memory loss, nervousness, light-headedness, dizziness, depression, blurred vision, mydriasis, dry mouth, constipation, urinary retention, urinary hesitation, flushing, decreased sweating.

Nursing Considerations for Patients Receiving Dopaminergic Agents

Assessment: History and Examination

- Assess for contraindications or cautions: Any known allergies to these drugs *to avoid hypersensitivity reactions*; GI depression or obstruction, urinary hesitancy or obstruction, benign prostatic hypertrophy, or glaucoma, *which may be exacerbated by these drugs*; cardiac arrhythmias, hypertension, or respiratory disease, *which may be exacerbated by dopamine receptor stimulation;* current status of pregnancy or lactation, *which are cautions or contraindications to use of the drug*; and renal or hepatic dysfunction, *which could interfere with the drug's excretion or metabolism.*
- Perform a physical assessment *to determine baseline status before beginning therapy, to determine the effectiveness of drug therapy, and to monitor for any potential adverse effects.*
- Inspect the skin for evidence of skin lesions or history of melanoma if the patient is to receive levodopa, *which could cause or exacerbate melanoma.*
- Assess level of orientation and neurological status, including affect, reflexes, bilateral grip strength, gait, tremors, and spasticity, *to evaluate any CNS effects.*
- Auscultate lungs and assess respiratory status *to evaluate for changes that could be exacerbated by the drug's effect.*
- Monitor pulse, blood pressure, and cardiac output *to evaluate for possible adverse effects.*
- Auscultate bowel sounds to evaluate GI motility *to assess for adverse effects.*
- Assess urine output and palpate bladder *to determine adequate bladder and renal function.*
- Monitor the results of laboratory tests, such as liver and renal function studies, *to determine need for possible dose adjustment*, and complete blood count with differential *to evaluate for possible bone marrow suppression.*

Nursing Diagnoses

Nursing diagnoses related to drug therapy might include the following:

- Disturbed thought processes related to CNS effects
- Risk for urinary retention related to dopaminergic effects
- Constipation related to dopaminergic effects
- Risk for injury related to CNS effects and incidence of orthostatic hypertension
- Deficient knowledge regarding drug therapy

Planning

- The patient will receive the best therapeutic effect from the drug therapy.
- The patient will have limited adverse effects to the drug therapy.
- The patient will have an understanding of the drug therapy, adverse effects to anticipate, and measures to relieve discomfort and improve safety

Implementation with Rationale

- Arrange to decrease the dose of the drug if therapy has been interrupted for any reason *to prevent systemic dopaminergic effects.*
- Evaluate disease progress and signs and symptoms periodically and record *for reference of disease progress and drug response.*
- Give the drug with meals *to alleviate GI irritation if GI upset is a problem.*
- Monitor bowel function and institute a bowel program *if constipation is severe.*
- Ensure that the patient voids before taking the drug *if urinary retention is a problem.*
- Monitor urinary output, palpate bladder, and check for residual urine *if urinary retention becomes a problem.*
- Establish safety precautions if CNS or vision changes occur *to prevent patient injury.*
- Monitor hepatic, renal, and hematological tests periodically during therapy *to detect early signs of dysfunction and consider reevaluation of drug therapy.*
- Provide support services and comfort measures as needed *to improve patient compliance.*
- Provide thorough patient teaching about topics such as the drug name and prescribed dose, measures to help avoid adverse effects, warning signs that may indicate problems, and the need for periodic monitoring and evaluation *to enhance patient knowledge about drug therapy and to promote compliance.*
- Offer support and encouragement to help the patient cope with the disease and drug regimen.

Evaluation

- Monitor patient response to the drug (improvement in signs and symptoms of Parkinson's disease).
- Monitor for adverse effects (CNS changes, urinary retention, GI depression, tachycardia, increased sweating, flushing).
- Evaluate the effectiveness of the teaching plan (patient can give the drug name and dosage, name possible adverse effects to watch for and specific measures to prevent them, and discuss the importance of continued follow-up).
- Monitor the effectiveness of support measures and compliance with the regimen.

Table 24.3 *Drugs in Focus:* Adjunctive Antiparkinsonism Drugs

Drug Name	Dosage/Route	Usual Indications
entacapone (*Comtan*)	200 mg PO taken with levodopa–carbidopa, maximum of eight doses per day	Adjunctive treatment of idiopathic Parkinson's disease with levodopa–carbidopa for patients who are experiencing "wearing off" of drug effects
tolcapone (*Tasmar*)	100 mg PO t.i.d., maximum daily dose 600 mg	Adjunctive treatment of idiopathic Parkinson's disease with levodopa–carbidopa
selegiline (*Eldepryl*)	5 mg PO b.i.d. (at breakfast and lunch); attempt to decrease levodopa–carbidopa dose after 2–3 d *Orally disintegrating tablet:* 1.25 mg/d PO with breakfast	Adjunctive treatment of idiopathic Parkinson's disease with levodopa–carbidopa in patients whose response to that therapy has decreased

KEY POINTS

- Anticholinergic agents are used to suppress the stimulatory effects of acetylcholine in the substantia nigra, bringing balance into the control of movement.
- The adverse effects associated with the anticholinergic drugs are related to blocking of the acetylcholine in the parasympathetic nervous system—dry mouth, constipation, urinary retention, increased heart rate, and decreased sweating.

Adjunctive Agents

Adjunctive agents used to improve patient response to traditional therapy include entacapone (*Comtan*), tolcapone (*Tasmar*), and selegiline (*Eldepryl*). See Table 24.3 for additional information.

Entacapone is used with carbidopa–levodopa to increase the plasma concentration and duration of action of levodopa. It is available in fixed combination tablets containing levodopa, carbidopa, and entacapone called *Stalevo.* It does this by inhibiting catecholamine-*O*-methyl transferase (COMT), a naturally occurring enzyme that eliminates catecholamines, including dopamine. It is given with the carbidopa–levodopa at a dose of 200 mg PO, with a maximum of eight doses a day. It is readily absorbed from the GI tract, metabolized in the liver, and excreted in the urine and feces. Women of childbearing age should be encouraged to use barrier contraceptives while taking this drug, which crosses the placenta and could have adverse effects on the fetus.

Tolcapone works in a similar way with carbidopa–levodopa to further increase plasma levels of levodopa. Tolcapone also blocks the enzyme COMT, which is responsible for the breakdown of dopamine. Because this drug has been associated with fulminant and potentially fatal liver damage, it is contraindicated in the presence of liver disease. Tolcapone is reserved for use in later stages of Parkinson's disease, when carbidopa–levodopa is losing its effectiveness. It undergoes hepatic metabolism after GI absorption and is excreted in the urine and feces. It is given in doses of 100 or 200 mg PO three times a day, up to a maximum of 600 mg/d. Women of childbearing age should be encouraged to use barrier contraceptives while taking this drug, which crosses the placenta and could have adverse effects on the fetus.

Selegiline is used with carbidopa–levodopa after patients have shown signs of deteriorating response to this treatment. Its mechanism of action is not understood. It does irreversibly inhibit MAO, which has an important role in the breakdown of catecholamines, including dopamine. It is also approved in a dermal system for the treatment of depression. The maximum daily dose of the drug is 10 mg, and the dose of levodopa needs to be reduced when this drug is started. It is well absorbed from the GI tract, extensively metabolized in the liver, and excreted in the urine. It is not known whether this drug crosses the placenta, but it should be used in pregnancy only if the benefits to the mother clearly outweigh any potential risks to the fetus. Because of the risk of MAOI-induced hypertensive effects, patients should be urged to immediately report severe headache and any other unusual symptoms that they have not experienced before.

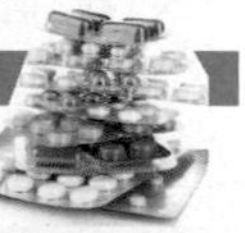

Nursing Considerations for Patients Receiving Adjunctive Agents

Nursing considerations for patients receiving the drugs listed in this section are similar to those for patients receiving the dopaminergic drugs. Details related to each individual drug can be found in the specific drug monograph in your nursing drug guide.

KEY POINTS

- Adjunctive drugs are used to increase the responsiveness of the cells to dopamine. They act to decrease the breakdown of dopamine, leaving it on the receptor for longer periods of time.
- Adjunctive drugs are only used in combination with carbidopa–levodopa and are usually reserved for use when the patient stops responding adequately to traditional therapy.

SUMMARY

- Parkinson's disease is a progressive, chronic neurological disorder for which there is no cure.
- Loss of dopamine-secreting neurons in the substantia nigra is characteristic of Parkinson's disease. Destruction of dopamine-secreting cells leads to an imbalance between excitatory cholinergic cells and inhibitory dopaminergic cells.
- Signs and symptoms of Parkinson's disease include tremor, changes in posture and gait, slow and deliberate movements (bradykinesia), and eventually drooling and changes in speech.
- Drug therapy for Parkinson's disease is aimed at restoring the dopamine–acetylcholine balance. The signs and symptoms of the disease can be managed until the degeneration of neurons is so extensive that a therapeutic response no longer occurs.
- Anticholinergic drugs are used to block the excitatory cholinergic receptors, and dopaminergic drugs are used to increase dopamine levels or to directly stimulate dopamine receptors.
- Many adverse effects are associated with the drugs used for treating Parkinson's disease, including CNS changes, anticholinergic effects when using the anticholinergics (atropine-like or parasympathetic blocking effects), and dopamine stimulation (sympathetic-type effects) in the peripheral nervous system when using the dopaminergics.

CHECK YOUR UNDERSTANDING

Answers to the questions in this chapter can be found in Answers to Check Your Understanding Questions on thePoint®.

MULTIPLE CHOICE

Select the best answer to the following.

1. Parkinson's disease is a progressive, chronic neurological disorder that is usually
a. associated with severe head injury.
b. associated with chronic diseases.
c. associated with old age.
d. known to affect people of all ages with no known cause.

2. Parkinson's disease reflects an imbalance between inhibitory and stimulating activity of nerves in the
a. reticular activating system.
b. cerebellum.
c. basal ganglia.
d. limbic system.

3. The main underlying problem with Parkinson's disease seems to be a decrease in the neurotransmitter
a. acetylcholine.
b. norepinephrine.
c. dopamine.
d. serotonin.

4. Anticholinergic drugs are effective in early Parkinson's disease. They act to
a. block stimulating effects of acetylcholine in the brain to bring activity back into balance.
b. block the signs and symptoms of the disease, making it more acceptable.
c. inhibit dopamine effects in the brain and increase neuron activity.
d. increase the effectiveness of the inhibitory neurotransmitter gamma-aminobutyric acid.

5. A patient receiving an anticholinergic drug for Parkinson's disease is planning a winter trip to Tahiti. The temperature in Tahiti is 70 degrees warmer than at home. What precautions should the patient be urged to take?
a. Take the drug with plenty of water to stay hydrated.
b. Reduce dose and take precautions to reduce the risk for heat stroke.
c. Wear sunglasses and use sunscreen because of photophobia that will develop.
d. Avoid drinking the water to prevent gastric distress.

6. Replacing dopamine in the brain would seem to be the best treatment for Parkinson's disease. This is difficult because dopamine
a. is broken down in gastric acid.
b. is not available in drug form.
c. cannot cross the blood–brain barrier.
d. is used peripherally before reaching the brain.

7. A patient taking levodopa and over-the-counter megavitamins might experience
a. cure from Parkinson's disease.
b. return of Parkinson's symptoms.
c. improved health and well-being.
d. a resistance to viral infections.

8. A patient who has been diagnosed with Parkinson's disease for many years and whose symptoms were controlled using *Sinemet* has started to exhibit increasing signs of the disease. Possible treatment might include
   a. increased exercise program.
   b. addition of diphenhydramine to the drug regimen.
   c. combination therapy with an anticholinergic drug.
   d. changes in diet to eliminate vitamin B6.

MULTIPLE RESPONSE

Select all that apply.

1. A client asks the nurse to explain parkinsonism to him. Which of the following possible causes of parkinsonism might be included in the explanation?
   a. Adverse effect of drug therapy
   b. Brain injury
   c. Viral infection
   d. Dementia
   e. Bacterial infection
   f. Birth defect
2. No therapy is available that will stop the loss of neurons and the eventual decline of function in clients with Parkinson's disease. As a result, nursing care should involve which of the following interventions?
   a. Regular exercises to slow loss of function
   b. Supportive education as drugs fail and new therapy is needed
   c. Community and family support networking
   d. Discontinuation of drug therapy to test for a cure
   e. Special vitamin therapy to slow the loss of the neurons
   f. Explanations of the adjunctive drug therapy that may be used.

BIBLIOGRAPHY AND REFERENCES

Bjorklund, A., & Cenci-Nilsson, A. (2010). *Recent advances in Parkinson's disease: Part 1 Basic research.* St. Louis, MO: Elsevier.

Bjorklund, A., & Cenci-Nilsson, A. (2010). *Recent advances in Parkinson's disease: Part 2 Translational and clinical research.* St. Louis, MO: Elsevier.

Bjorklund, A. (2013). Cell therapy for Parkinson's disease: What next? *Movement Disorders, 28*(1), 110–115

Brunton, L., Chabner, B., & Knollman, B. (2011). *Goodman and Gilman's the pharmacological basis of therapeutics* (12th ed.). New York: McGraw-Hill.

Facts and Comparisons. (2015). *Drug facts and comparisons.* St. Louis, MO: Author.

Facts and Comparisons. (2015). *Professional's guide to patient drug facts.* St. Louis, MO: Author.

Hanin, I., Nitsch, R., Windisch, M., et al. (Eds.). (2013). Alzheimer's and Parkinson's diseases: Mechanisms, clinical strategies, and promising treatments of neurodegenerative diseases. *Neurodegenerative Diseases, 11*(suppl. 1).

Karch, A. M. (2014). *Lippincott's nursing drug guide.* Philadelphia, PA: Lippincott Williams & Wilkins.

Leader, L., Leader, G., & Miller, N. (2009). *Parkinson's disease: Dopamine metabolism and applied biochemistry.* London, UK: Denor Press.

Nitsch, R. M., Fisher, A., Windisch, M., et al. (Eds.). (2011). *Alzheimer's and Parkinson's disease: Advances, concept and new challenges.* Unionville, CT: S. Karger Pub.

Porth, C. M. (2013). *Pathophysiology: Concepts of altered health states* (9th ed.). Philadelphia, PA: Lippincott Williams & Wilkins.

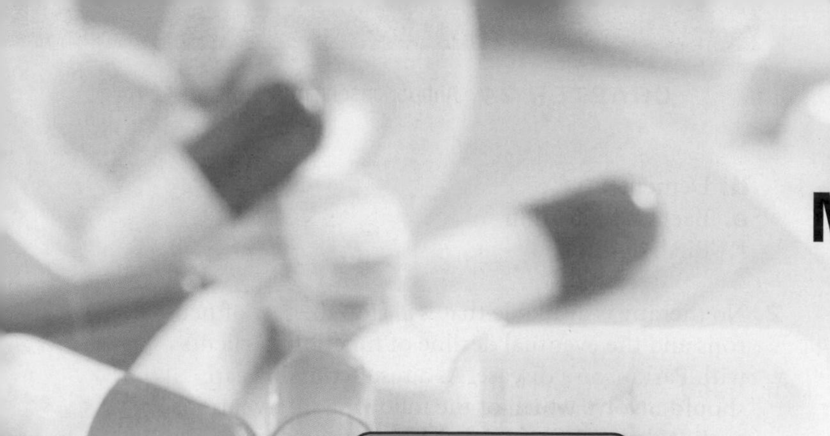

Muscle Relaxants 25

Learning Objectives

Upon completion of this chapter, you will be able to:

1. Describe a spinal reflex and discuss the pathophysiology of muscle spasm and muscle spasticity.
2. Describe the therapeutic actions, indications, pharmacokinetics, contraindications, most common adverse reactions, and important drug–drug interactions associated with the centrally acting and the direct-acting skeletal muscle relaxants.
3. Discuss the use of muscle relaxants across the lifespan.
4. Compare and contrast the prototype drugs baclofen and dantrolene with other muscle relaxants in their classes.
5. Outline the nursing considerations, including important teaching points for patients receiving muscle relaxants as adjuncts to anesthesia.

Glossary of Key Terms

basal ganglia: lower area of the brain, associated with coordination of unconscious muscle movements that involve movement and position

cerebellum: lower portion of the brain, associated with coordination of muscle movements, including voluntary motion, as well as extrapyramidal control of unconscious muscle movements

extrapyramidal tract: cells from the cortex and subcortical areas, including the basal ganglia and the cerebellum, which coordinate unconsciously controlled muscle activity; allows the body to make automatic adjustments in posture or position and balance

hypertonia: state of excessive muscle response and activity

interneuron: neuron in the CNS that communicates with other neurons, not with muscles or glands

pyramidal tract: fibers within the CNS that control precise, intentional movement

spasticity: sustained muscle contractions

spindle gamma loop system: simple reflex arcs that involve sensory receptors in the periphery that respond to stretch and spinal motor nerves and cause muscle fiber contraction: Responsible for maintaining muscle tone and keeping an upright position against the pull of gravity

Drug List

Centrally Acting Skeletal Muscle Relaxants

- (P) baclofen
- carisoprodol
- chlorzoxazone
- cyclobenzaprine
- metaxalone
- methocarbamol
- orphenadrine
- tizanidine

Direct-Acting Skeletal Muscle Relaxants

- (P) dantrolene
- incobotulinum toxin A
- onabotulinum toxin A
- rimabotulinum toxin type B

Many injuries and accidents result in local damage to muscles or the skeletal anchors of muscles. These injuries may lead to muscle spasm and pain, which may be of long duration and may interfere with normal functioning. The perception of pain and response to pain is a very individual response, as discussed in Chapter 26. In a situation where muscle spasm is causing pain, relaxing the muscle can often remove the physiologilcal stimulus for pain. Damage to central nervous system (CNS) neurons may cause a permanent state of muscle **spasticity**—sustained muscle contractions—as a result of loss of nerves that help to maintain balance in controlling muscle activity.

Neuron damage, whether temporary or permanent, may be treated with skeletal muscle relaxants. Most skeletal muscle relaxants work in the brain and spinal cord, where they interfere with the cycle of muscle spasm and pain. However, botulinum toxins and dantrolene enter muscle fibers directly. See Box 25.1 for discussion of the use of these muscle relaxants in various age groups.

Nerves and Movement

Posture, balance, and movement are the result of a constantly fluctuating sequence of muscle contraction and relaxation. The nerves that regulate these actions are the spinal motor neurons. These neurons are influenced by higher level brain activity in the lower areas of the brain: The **cerebellum** (associated with conscious muscle movements) and **basal ganglia** (associated with unconscious muscle movements). This brain activity provides coordination of contractions, and the cerebral cortex allows conscious thought to regulate movement.

Spinal Reflexes

The spinal reflexes are the simplest nerve pathways that monitor movement and posture (Figure 25.1). Spinal reflexes can be simple, involving an incoming sensory neuron and an outgoing motor neuron, or more complex, involving **interneurons** that communicate with the related

BOX 25.1 FOCUS ON **Drug Therapy Across the Lifespan**

Skeletal Muscle Relaxants

CHILDREN

The safety and effectiveness of most of these drugs have not been established in children. If a child older than 12 years of age requires a skeletal muscle relaxant after an injury, metaxalone has an established pediatric dosage. Other agents have been used, with adjustments to the adult dosage based on the child's age and weight.

Baclofen is often used to relieve the muscle spasticity associated with cerebral palsy. A caregiver needs intensive education in the use of the intrathecal infusion pump and how to monitor the child for therapeutic as well as adverse effects.

Methocarbamol is the drug of choice if a child needs to be treated for tetanus.

Dantrolene is used to treat upper motor neuron spasticity in children. The dosage is based on body weight and increases over time. The child should be screened regularly for CNS and GI (including hepatic) toxicity.

Botulinum toxins are not approved for use in children. The use of these neurotoxins in children has been associated with the development of botulism.

ADULTS

Adults being treated for acute musculoskeletal pain should be cautioned to avoid driving and to take safety precautions against injury because of the related CNS effects, including dizziness and drowsiness. Rest of the muscle, heat, massage, physical therapy are key components to recovery from any muscular injury or pain.

Adults complaining of muscle spasm pain that may be related to anxiety often respond very effectively to diazepam, which is a muscle relaxant and anxiolytic.

Women of childbearing age should be advised to use contraception when they are taking these drugs. If a pregnancy does occur, or is desired, they need counseling about the potential for adverse effects. Women who are nursing should be encouraged to find another method of feeding the baby because of the potential for adverse drug effects on the baby.

Premenopausal women are also at increased risk for the hepatotoxicity associated with dantrolene and should be monitored very closely for any change in hepatic function and given written information about the prodrome syndrome that often occurs with the hepatic toxicity.

OLDER ADULTS

Older patients are more likely to experience the adverse effects associated with these drugs—CNS, GI, and cardiovascular. Because older patients often also have renal or hepatic impairment, they are also more likely to have toxic levels of the drug related to changes in metabolism and excretion.

Carisoprodol is the centrally acting skeletal muscle relaxant of choice for older patients and for those with hepatic or renal impairment.

If dantrolene is required for an older patient, lower doses and more frequent monitoring are needed to assess for potential cardiac, respiratory, and liver toxicity.

Older women who are receiving hormone replacement therapy are at the same risk for development of hepatotoxicity as premenopausal women and should be monitored accordingly.

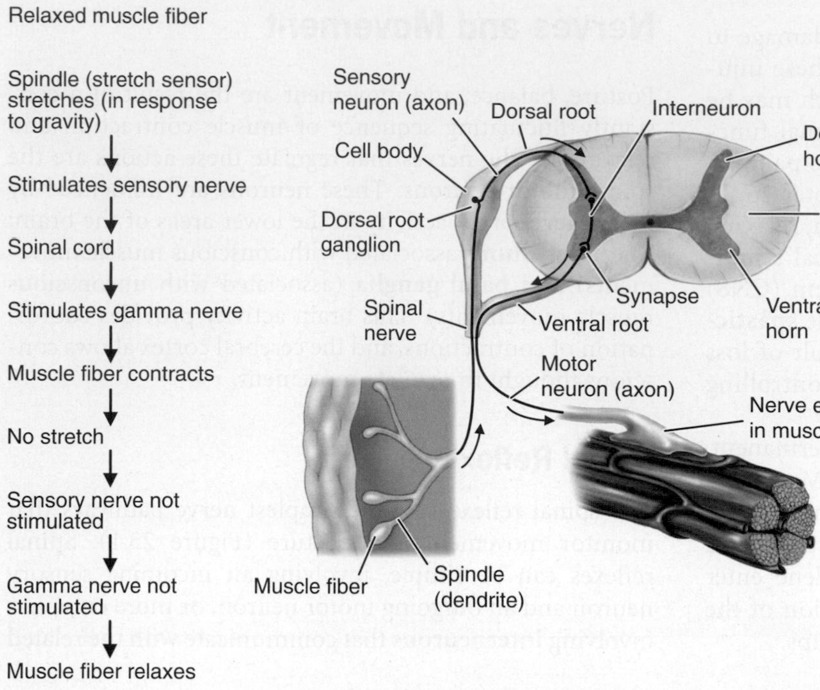

FIGURE 25.1 Reflex arc showing the pathway of impulses. The spindle gamma loop reflex arc: the relaxing and contracting of muscle fibers causes muscle tone and ability to stand upright and promotes venous return.

centers in the brain. Simple reflex arcs involve sensory receptors in the periphery and spinal motor nerves. Such reflex arcs make up what is known as the **spindle gamma loop system**; they respond to stretch receptors or spindles on muscle fibers to cause a muscle fiber contraction that relieves the stretch. In this system, nerves from stretch receptors form a synapse with gamma nerves in the spinal cord, which send an impulse to the stretched muscle fibers to stimulate their contraction. These reflexes are responsible for maintaining muscle tone and keeping an upright position against the pull of gravity and are important in helping venous return when the contracting muscle fibers massage veins to help move the blood toward the heart. Other spinal reflexes may involve synapses with interneurons within the spinal cord, which adjust movement and response based on information from higher brain centers to coordinate movement and position.

Brain Control

Many areas within the brain influence the spinal motor nerves. Areas of the brainstem, the basal ganglia, and the cerebellum modulate spinal motor nerve activity and help to coordinate activity among various muscle groups, thereby allowing coordinated movement and control of body muscle motions. Nerve areas within the cerebral cortex allow conscious, or intentional, movement. Nerves within the cortex send signals down the spinal cord, where they cross to the opposite side of the spinal cord before sending out nerve impulses to cause muscle contraction. In this way, each side of the cortex controls muscle movement on the opposite side of the body.

Different fibers control different types of movements. Those fibers that control precise, intentional movement make up the **pyramidal tract** within the CNS. The **extrapyramidal tract** is composed of cells from the cerebral cortex, as well as those from several subcortical areas, including the basal ganglia and the cerebellum. This tract modulates or coordinates unconsciously controlled muscle activity, and it allows the body to make automatic adjustments in posture or position and balance. The extrapyramidal tract controls lower level, or crude, movements. Many are now not using the terms pyramidal and extrapyramidal tracts to describe movement since so many movements can't be clearly classified into one or the other tract.

Neuromuscular Abnormalities

All of the areas mentioned work together to allow for a free flow of impulses into and out of the CNS to coordinate posture, balance, and movement. When injuries, diseases, and toxins affect the normal flow of information into and out of the CNS motor pathways, many clinical signs and symptoms may develop, ranging from simple muscle spasms to spasticity—or sustained muscle spasm—and paralysis.

Muscle Spasm

Muscle spasms often result from injury to the musculoskeletal system—for example, overstretching a muscle, wrenching a joint, or tearing a tendon or ligament. These injuries can cause violent and painful involuntary muscle

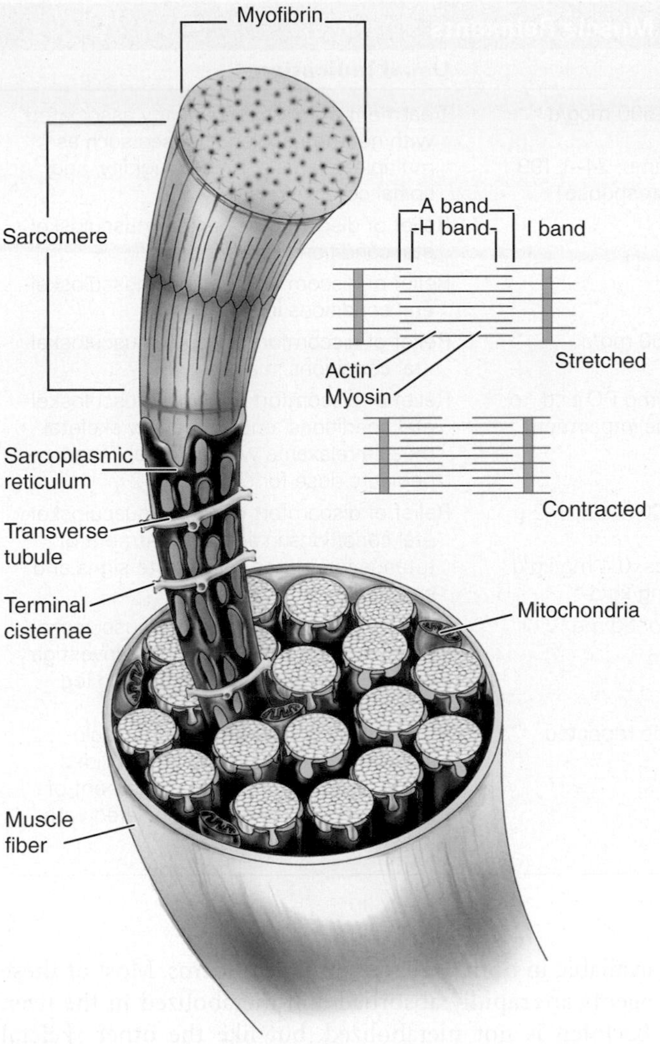

FIGURE 25.2 When stimulation stops, calcium ions are actively transported back into the sarcoplasmic reticulum, resulting in decreased calcium ions in the sarcoplasm. The removal of calcium ions restores the inhibitory action of troponin–tropomyosin; crossbridge action is impossible in this state.

contractions. It is thought that these spasms are caused by the flood of sensory impulses coming to the spinal cord from the injured area. These impulses can be passed through interneurons to spinal motor nerves, which stimulate an intense muscle contraction. The contraction cuts off blood flow to the muscle fibers in the injured area, causing lactic acid to accumulate and resulting in pain. The new flood of sensory impulses caused by the pain may lead to further muscle contraction, and a vicious cycle may develop (Figure 25.2).

Muscle Spasticity

Muscle spasticity is the result of damage to neurons within the CNS rather than injury to peripheral structures. Because the spasticity is caused by nerve damage in the CNS, it is a permanent condition. Spasticity may result from an increase in excitatory influences or a decrease in inhibitory influences within the CNS. The interruption in the balance among all of these higher influences within the CNS may lead to excessive stimulation of muscles, or **hypertonia**, in opposing muscle groups at the same time, a condition that may cause contractures and permanent structural changes. This control imbalance also results in a loss of coordinated muscle activity.

For example, the signs and symptoms of cerebral palsy and paraplegia are related to the disruption in the nervous control of the muscles. The exact presentation of any chronic neurological disorder depends on the specific nerve centers and tracts that are damaged and how the control imbalance is manifested.

KEY POINTS

- Movement and muscle control are regulated by spinal reflexes and the upper CNS, including the basal ganglia, cerebellum, and cerebral cortex.
- Spinal reflexes can be simple, involving an incoming sensory neuron and an outgoing motor neuron, or more complex, involving interneurons that communicate with the related centers in the brain.
- The pyramidal tract in the cerebellum coordinates intentional muscle movement, and the extrapyramidal tract in the cerebellum and basal ganglia coordinates involuntary muscle activity.
- Muscle or skeletal damage may send a multitude of stimuli to the spinal cord and result in muscle spasms or extended contraction.
- Damaged motor neurons can cause muscle spasticity and impaired movement and coordination.

Centrally Acting Skeletal Muscle Relaxants

Centrally acting skeletal muscle relaxants (Table 25.1) include baclofen (*Lioresal*), carisoprodol (*Soma*), chlorzoxazone (*Parafon*), cyclobenzaprine (*Amrix*), metaxalone (*Skelaxin*), methocarbamol (*Robaxin*), orphenadrine (*Banflex, Flexon*), and tizanidine (*Zanaflex*). Diazepam (*Valium*), a drug widely used as an anxiety agent (see Chapter 20), also has been shown to be an effective centrally acting skeletal muscle relaxant. It may be advantageous in situations in which anxiety may be precipitating the muscle spasm.

Other measures in addition to these drugs should be used to alleviate muscle spasm and pain. Such modalities as rest of the affected muscle, heat applications to increase blood flow to the area to remove the pain-causing chemicals, physical therapy to return the muscle to normal tone and activity, and anti-inflammatory agents—including nonsteroidal anti-inflammatory drugs (NSAIDs)—if the underlying problem is related to injury or inflammation may help.

Table 25.1 ***Drugs in Focus:* Centrally Acting Skeletal Muscle Relaxants**

Drug Name	Dosage/Route	Usual Indications
baclofen (*Lioresal*)	*Adult:* 40–80 mg PO daily, 12–1,500 mcg/d per intrathecal infusion pump *Pediatric:* Intrathecal infusion pump, 24–1,199 mcg/d—base dose on patient response	Treatment of muscle spasticity associated with neuromuscular diseases such as multiple sclerosis, muscle rigidity, and spinal cord injuries
carisoprodol (*Soma*)	350 mg PO t.i.d. to q.i.d.	Relief of discomfort of acute musculoskeletal conditions in adults
chlorzoxazone (*Parafon*)	250 mg PO t.i.d. to q.i.d.	Relief of discomfort of acute musculoskeletal conditions in adults
cyclobenzaprine (*Amrix*)	10 mg PO t.i.d., do not exceed 60 mg/d	Relief of discomfort of acute musculoskeletal conditions in adults
metaxalone (*Skelaxin*)	*Adult and pediatric (>12 y):* 800 mg PO t.i.d. to q.i.d.; reduce dose with hepatic impairment	Relief of discomfort of acute musculoskeletal conditions, one of the few skeletal muscle relaxants with an established pediatric dose for children >12 y
methocarbamol (*Robaxin*)	*Adult:* 1.5 g PO q.i.d., up to 30–60 mg/d; 1–2 g IV or IM for tetanus *Pediatric:* 15 mg/kg IV for tetanus, 0.4 mg/kg/d PO initially, maintenance 0.2 mg/kg/d	Relief of discomfort of acute musculoskeletal conditions in adults, treatment of tetanus in children to alleviate signs and symptoms of tetanus
orphenadrine (*Banflex, Flexon*)	100 mg PO, AM and at bedtime *or* 60 mg IV or IM q12 h	Relief of discomfort of acute musculoskeletal conditions in adults, under investigation for relief of quinidine-induced leg cramps
tizanidine (*Zanaflex*)	8 mg PO as a single dose may be repeated q6–8 h as needed	Relief of discomfort of acute musculoskeletal conditions in adults, provides acute and intermittent management of increased muscle tone associated with spasticity

Therapeutic Actions and Indications

The centrally acting skeletal muscle relaxants work in the CNS to interfere with the reflexes that are causing the muscle spasm. Because these drugs lyse or destroy spasm, they are often referred to as spasmolytics. Although the exact mechanism of action of these skeletal muscle relaxants is not known, it is thought to involve action in the upper or spinal interneurons. Tizanidine is an alpha-adrenergic agonist and is thought to increase inhibition of presynaptic motor neurons in the CNS. The primary indication for the use of centrally acting skeletal muscle agents is the relief of discomfort associated with acute, painful musculoskeletal conditions as an adjunct to rest, physical therapy, and other measures. Because these drugs work in the upper levels of the CNS, possible depression must be anticipated with their use. See Table 25.1 for Usual Indications for each of these agents.

Pharmacokinetics

Baclofen is available in oral and intrathecal forms and can be administered via a delivery pump for the treatment of central spasticity. Cyclobenzaprine is available in a controlled release oral form for continual control of the discomfort without repeated dosings. Methocarbamol is available in both oral and parenteral forms. Most of these agents are rapidly absorbed and metabolized in the liver. Baclofen is not metabolized, but like the other skeletal muscle relaxants it is excreted in the urine.

Contraindications and Cautions

Centrally acting skeletal muscle relaxants are contraindicated in the presence of any known allergy to any of these drugs *to prevent hypersensitivity reactions* and with skeletal muscle spasms resulting from rheumatic disorders, *which would not benefit from these drugs.* In addition, baclofen should not be used to treat any spasticity that contributes to locomotion, upright position, or increased function. *Blocking this spasticity results in loss of these functions.* All centrally acting skeletal muscle relaxants should be used cautiously in the following circumstances: With a history of epilepsy *because the CNS depression and imbalance caused by these drugs may exacerbate the seizure disorder*; with cardiac dysfunction *because muscle function may be depressed*; with any condition marked by muscle weakness, *which the drugs could make much worse*; and with hepatic or renal dysfunction (especially with metaxalone and tizanidine), *which could interfere with the metabolism and excretion of the drugs, leading to toxic levels.* Carisoprodol may be safer than the other spasmolytics in older patients and in patients with renal or hepatic dysfunction. *No good studies exist regarding the effects of these agents during pregnancy and lactation*; therefore, use should be limited to those situations in which the benefit to the mother clearly outweighs any potential risk to the fetus or neonate.

Adverse Effects

The most frequently seen adverse effects associated with these drugs relate to the associated CNS depression: drowsiness, fatigue, weakness, confusion, headache, and insomnia. Gastrointestinal (GI) disturbances, which may be linked to CNS depression of the parasympathetic reflexes, include nausea, dry mouth, anorexia, and constipation. In addition, hypotension and arrhythmias may occur, again as a result of depression of normal reflex arcs. Urinary frequency, enuresis, and feelings of urinary urgency reportedly may occur. Chlorzoxazone may discolor the urine, becoming orange to purplish-red when metabolized and excreted. Patients should be warned about this effect to prevent any fears of blood in the urine. Tizanidine has been associated with liver toxicity and hypotension in some patients (Figure 25.3).

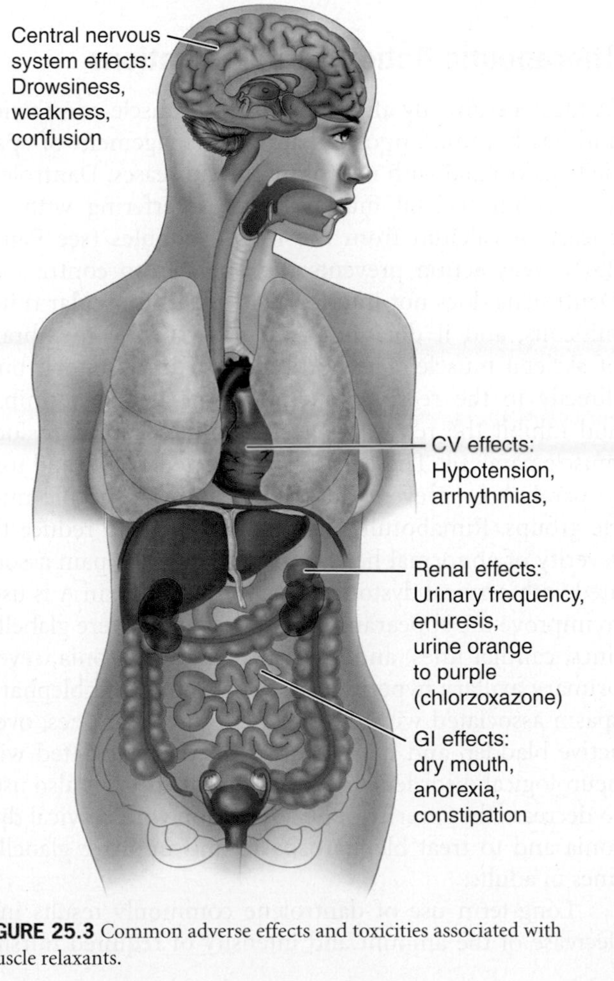

FIGURE 25.3 Common adverse effects and toxicities associated with muscle relaxants.

Clinically Important Drug–Drug Interactions

If any of the centrally acting skeletal muscle relaxants are taken with other CNS depressants or alcohol, CNS depression may increase. Patients should be cautioned to avoid alcohol while taking these muscle relaxants; if this combination cannot be avoided, they should take extreme precautions.

Prototype Summary: Baclofen

Indications: Alleviation of signs and symptoms of spasticity, may be of use in spinal cord injuries or spinal cord diseases.

Actions: Gamma-aminobutyric acid analogue, exact mechanism of action is not understood, inhibits monosynaptic and polysynaptic spinal reflexes, CNS depressant.

Pharmacokinetics:

Route	Onset	Peak	Duration
Oral	1 h	2 h	4–8 h
Intrathecal	30–60 min	4 h	4–8 h

$T_{1/2}$: 3 to 4 hours; not metabolized, excreted in the urine.

Adverse Effects: Transient drowsiness, dizziness, weakness, fatigue, constipation, headache, insomnia, hypotension, nausea, urinary frequency.

Nursing Considerations for Patients Receiving Centrally Acting Skeletal Muscle Relaxants

Assessment: History and Examination

- Assess for *contraindications or cautions for the use of the drug*, including any known allergies, *to prevent hypersensitivity reactions*; cardiac depression, epilepsy, muscle weakness, or rheumatic disorder, *which could be exacerbated by the effects of these drugs*; pregnancy or lactation, *which would be contraindications to use of the drugs*; and renal or hepatic dysfunction, *which alter metabolism and excretion of the drugs.*
- Assess temperature; skin color and lesions; CNS orientation, affect, reflexes, bilateral grip strength, and spasticity evaluation; bowel sounds and reported output; and liver and renal function tests *to determine baseline status before beginning therapy and for any potential adverse effects.*

Nursing Diagnoses

Nursing diagnoses related to drug therapy might include the following:

- Acute pain related to GI and CNS effects
- Disturbed thought processes related to CNS effects

(continues on page 428)

- Risk for injury related to CNS effects
- Deficient knowledge regarding drug therapy

Planning

- The patient will receive the best therapeutic effect from the drug therapy, relaxation of muscle and relief of discomfort.
- The patient will have limited adverse effects to the drug therapy.
- The patient will have an understanding of the drug therapy, adverse effects to anticipate, and measures to relieve discomfort and improve safety.

Implementation with Rationale

- Provide additional measures to relieve discomfort—heat, rest for the muscle, NSAIDs, and positioning—*to augment the effects of the drug at relieving the musculoskeletal discomfort.*
- Discontinue drug at any sign of hypersensitivity reaction or liver dysfunction *to prevent severe toxicity.*
- If using baclofen, taper the drug slowly over 1 to 2 weeks *to prevent the development of psychoses and hallucinations.* Use baclofen cautiously in patients whose spasticity contributes to mobility, posture, or balance *to prevent loss of this function.*
- If patient is receiving baclofen through a delivery pump the patient should understand the pump, the reason for frequent monitoring, and how to adjust the dose and program the unit *to enhance patient knowledge and promote compliance.*
- Monitor respiratory status *to evaluate adverse effects and arrange for appropriate dose adjustment or discontinuation of the drug.*
- Provide thorough patient teaching, including drug name, prescribed dosage, measures for avoidance of adverse effects, warning signs that may indicate possible problems, and the need for monitoring and evaluation *to enhance patient knowledge about drug therapy and to promote compliance.*
- Offer support and encouragement *to help the patient cope with the drug regimen.*

Evaluation

- Monitor patient response to the drug (improvement in muscle spasm and relief of pain; improvement in muscle spasticity).
- Monitor for adverse effects (CNS changes, GI depression, urinary urgency).
- Evaluate the effectiveness of the teaching plan (patient can give the drug name and dosage, name possible adverse effects to watch for and specific measures to prevent them, and describe, if necessary, proper intrathecal administration).
- Monitor the effectiveness of comfort measures and compliance with the regimen.

KEY POINTS

- The centrally acting skeletal muscle relaxants interfere with the reflexes that are causing the muscle spasm.
- The centrally acting skeletal muscle relaxants cause CNS depression, and the adverse effects associated with them are related to the CNS depression (insomnia, dizziness, confusion, anticholinergic effects).
- The centrally acting muscle relaxants are used for the relief of discomfort associated with acute, painful musculoskeletal conditions as an adjunct to rest, physical therapy, and other measures.

Direct-Acting Skeletal Muscle Relaxants

The direct-acting skeletal muscle relaxants enter the muscle to prevent muscle contraction directly. Direct-acting skeletal muscle relaxants (Table 25.2) include dantrolene (*Dantrium*), onabotulinumtoxin A (*Botox, Botox Cosmetic*) incobotulinumtoxin A (*Xeomin*), and rimabotulinumtoxin B (*Myobloc*).

Refer to the Critical Thinking Scenario for a full discussion of nursing care for a patient who is receiving *Botox* to treat migraines.

Therapeutic Actions and Indications

Dantrolene directly affects peripheral muscle contraction and has become important in the management of spasticity associated with neuromuscular diseases. Dantrolene acts within skeletal muscle fibers, interfering with the release of calcium from the muscle tubules (see Figure 25.2). This action prevents the fibers from contracting. Dantrolene does not interfere with neuromuscular transmissions, and it does not affect the surface membrane of skeletal muscle. The botulinum toxins A and B bind directly to the receptor sites of motor nerve terminals and inhibit the release of acetylcholine, leading to local muscle paralysis. These drugs are injected locally and used to paralyze or prevent the contractions of specific muscle groups. Rimabotulinumtoxin B is used to reduce the severity of abnormal head position and neck pain associated with cervical dystonia. Onabotulinumtoxin A is used to improve the appearance of moderate to severe glabellar lines, canthal lines, and to treat cervical dystonia, severe primary axillary hyperhidrosis, strabismus and blepharospasm associated with dystonia, chronic migraines, overactive bladder, and detrusor overactivity associated with neurological disorders. Incobotulinumtoxin A is also used to decrease the severity of head position with cervical dystonia and to treat blepharospasm and improve glabellar lines in adults.

Long-term use of dantrolene commonly results in a decrease of the amount and intensity of required nursing

Table 25.2 *Drugs in Focus:* Direct-Acting Skeletal Muscle Relaxants

Drug Name	Dosage/Route	Usual Indications
dantrolene (*Dantrium*)	*Adult:* Initially 25 mg PO, increase based on spinal cord injuries, prevention and management of response to a maximum 400 mg/d for spasticity *Prevention of malignant hyperthermia:* 4–8 mg/kg/d PO for 1–2 d before surgery *or* 2.5 mg/kg IV over 1 h, given 1 h before surgery; postcrisis, 4–8 mg/kg/d PO for 1–3 d *Pediatric:* Initially 0.5 mg/kg/d PO b.i.d., titrate to a maximum 100 mg PO q.i.d. for spasticity; for malignant hyperthermia, follow adult dose	Management of upper motor neuron–associated muscle spasticity such as spinal cord injury, myasthenia gravis, cerebral palsy, multiple sclerosis, muscular dystrophy, polio, tetanus, quadriplegia, and amyotrophic lateral sclerosis; prevention or treatment of malignant hyperthermia—a state of intense muscle contraction and resulting hyperpyrexia; used orally as preoperative prophylaxis in susceptible patients who must undergo anesthesia and after acute episodes to prevent recurrence
incobotulinumtoxin A (*Xeomin*)	*Cervical dystonia:* 120 units per session in selected muscles *Blepharospasm:* 5.6 units per injection, up to 6 injections per eye *Glabellar lines:* 5 injections of 4 units each per session, may repeat in 3 mo	Treatment of cervical dystonia; treatment of blepharospasm in adult previously treated with onobutulinumtoxin A; improvement in appearance of glabellar lines with corrugator or procerus muscle activity in adults
onabotulinumtoxin A (*Botox, Botox Cosmetic*)	*Adult:* 20 units (0.5-mL solution) injected as divided doses of 0.1 mL (4 units) into each of five sites (two in each corrugator muscle and one in the procerus muscle) repeated every 3–4 mo, local injection associated with particular disorder—see manufacturer's guidelines *Cervical dystonia:* 120 units per treatment session in selected muscles *Blepharospasm:* 5.6 units per injection with up to 6 injections per eye *Bladder overactivity:* 100 units across 20 sites into the detrusor muscle *Detrusor overactivity due to neurological disease:* 100 units across 30 sites into the detrusor *Chronic migraine:* 155 units per site across 6–7 head, neck muscles	Improvement of appearance in glabellar (frown) lines associated with corrugator or procerus muscle activity in adults, canthal lines, treatment of cervical dystonia, treatment of strabismus and blepharospasm associated with dystonia in patients ≥12 y of age, treatment of severe primary axillary hyperhidrosis (sweating) when injected into the axillary area Treatment of overactive bladder, detrusor overactivity associated with neurological conditions Treatment of chronic migraine
rimabotulinumtoxin B (*Myobloc*)	2,500–5,000 units IM injected locally into affected muscles	Reduction of severity of abnormal head position and neck pain associated with cervical dystonia

care. Continued long-term use is justified as long as the drug reduces painful and disabling spasticity. This agent is not used for the treatment of muscle spasms associated with musculoskeletal injury or rheumatic disorders. Table 25.2 presents additional information about these agents, including Usual Indications.

Pharmacokinetics

Dantrolene is used in oral or parenteral forms. Dantrolene is slowly absorbed from the GI tract and metabolized in the liver with a half-life of 4 to 8 hours. Excretion is through the urine. Dantrolene crosses the placenta and was found to be embryotoxic in animal studies. Use should be reserved for those situations in which the benefit to the mother clearly outweighs the risk to the fetus. Dantrolene enters breast milk and is contraindicated for use during lactation. Safety for use in children younger than 5 years of age has not been established; because the long-term effects are not known, careful consideration should be given to use of the drug in children. The botulinum toxins are not generally absorbed systemically, and there is no pharmacokinetic information available.

Contraindications and Cautions

Dantrolene is contraindicated in the presence of any known allergy to the drug *to prevent hypersensitivity reactions*. It is also contraindicated in the following conditions: Spasticity that contributes to locomotion, upright position, or increased function, *which would be lost if that spasticity were blocked*; active hepatic disease, *which might interfere with metabolism of the drug and because of known liver toxicity*; and lactation *because the drug may cross into breast milk and cause adverse effects in the infant*. The botulinum toxins are contraindicated in the presence of allergy to any component of the drug *to prevent hypersensitivity reactions* or with active infection at the site of the injection *because injecting the drug could aggravate the infection.*

Caution should be used with dantrolene in the following circumstances: In women and in all patients older than 35 years *because of increased risk of potentially fatal hepatocellular disease* (Box 25.2); in patients with a history of liver disease or previous dysfunction, *which could make the liver more susceptible to cellular toxicity*; in patients with respiratory depression, *which could be exacerbated by muscular weakness*; in patients with cardiac disease *because cardiac muscle depression may be a risk*; and during pregnancy *because of the potential for adverse effects on the fetus.* Caution should be used with the botulinum toxins with any peripheral neuropathic disease; with neuromuscular disorders, *which could be exacerbated by the effects of the drug*; in children *because it is not approved for use in children and severe effects including botulism have been reported*; with pregnancy and lactation *because the potential effects on the fetus or baby are not known*; and with any known cardiovascular disease *because of the potential changes in tissue perfusion and risk of systemic absorption.*

BOX 25.2 FOCUS ON **Gender Considerations**

Understanding the Risks of Liver Damage with Dantrolene

Dantrolene (*Dantrium*) is associated with potentially fatal hepatocellular injury. When liver damage begins to occur, patients often experience a prodrome, or warning syndrome, which includes anorexia, nausea, and fatigue. The incidence of such hepatic injury is greater in women and in patients older than 35 years of age.

In women, a combination of dantrolene and estrogen seems to affect the liver, thus posing a greater risk. Women of all ages may be at increased risk because those entering menopause may be taking hormone replacement therapy. Patients older than 35 years of age are at increasing risk of liver injury because of the changing integrity of the liver cells that comes with age and exposure to toxins over time.

If a particular woman needs dantrolene for relief of spasticity, she should not be taking any estrogens (e.g., birth control pills, hormone replacement therapy), and she should be monitored closely for any sign of liver dysfunction. For safer relief of spasticity in these patients, baclofen may be helpful.

CRITICAL THINKING SCENARIO

Direct-Acting Muscle Relaxant: Incobotulinumtoxin A

THE SITUATION

M.D. is a 38-year-old teacher with a long history of chronic migraines. She reports that she has tried everything but still has migraines 15–20 days a month. This continuous problem has caused her to take a leave of absence from her teaching job. She saw an ad for *Botox* for chronic migraines and has come to the clinic to see if that is an option for her. She reports that she knows several people who go to *Botox* parties and was wondering if this is the same drug and if it can be given at one of these parties. She has some concerns about *Botox* treatments that did not seem to have good results.

CRITICAL THINKING

What basic principles must be included in the nursing care plan for M.D. *Think about the action of this drug and the potential problems that could occur. Since M.D. associates the drug with Botox parties, what other information does she need to know?*

What therapeutic goals might the nurse set for M.D.?

What additional drug-related information needs to be shared with M.D. to make her comfortable with any treatment choice that she might make?

DISCUSSION

Botox (incobotulinumtoxin A) has a strong reputation in the media for giving people instant "face lifts" and helping people to look younger. There are places where these injections are given in homes or beauty salons and, consequently, the drug may not be seen as having any potential adverse effects. The drug is a neurotoxin and paralyzes muscles by blocking nerve transmission. When used for improving the appearance of lines on the face the drug is injected into the affected areas and must be repeated every 3 months. The muscles can no longer move so any folds seem to disappear. People have reported visual changes, lopsided response, or no response. When used to treat chronic migraines the drug is injected into 12–14 sites on the head, neck, and shoulders. The muscles used are injected bilaterally. This injection sequence is repeated every 12 weeks.

Direct-Acting Muscle Relaxant: Incobotulinumtoxin A (continued)

Patients have reported head and neck pain as the most common adverse effect. The drug does carry a black box warning that there is possibility of the toxin spreading from the injection sites and has caused botulism. The studies done on this use of the drug found that some people began to feel better very quickly and overall all patients had fewer headache days; but with all pain treatments, the actual response is very individual.

The patient should be praised for taking the initiative to come in and explore this option for treatment. The nurse would need to review all of M.D.'s history and various methods that have been used to treat her migraines. Her neurologist should be brought into the discussion to weigh the pros and cons of this approach. When a patient has a chronic problem that traditional methods don't seem to be able to help, it is important to support her search for possible treatments. Other nontraditional approaches might include acupuncture, massage, herbal therapies, or stimulus reduction. In M.D.'s case, after careful consideration of her status, it was decided to try the incobotulinumtoxin A injections to relieve her chronic migraines. The nurse needs to explain the series of injections that will need to be done in a medical facility and not at a *Botox* party. This will allow the health care professionals to ensure safe injections, decrease the risk of infection, and keep careful records of each site used for the repeat injections.

NURSING CARE GUIDE FOR M.D.: INCOBOTULINUMTOXIN A

Assessment: History and Examination

Obtain a full history of migraine incidence, treatments, and response to treatment.

Assess for any active infection, known allergy to any ingredient in the drug, difficulty swallowing, history of anaphylactic reactions.

Perform a physical assessment:

CV: Arrhythmias, hypertension

CNS: Orientation, affect,

Skin: Color, lesions in head, neck area

Respiratory: Respiration, adventitious sounds

Nursing Diagnoses

Acute pain related to injection effects

Risk for infection related to repeated injections

Deficient knowledge regarding drug therapy

Planning

The patient will receive the best therapeutic effect from the drug therapy.

The patient will have limited adverse effects to the drug therapy.

The patient will have an understanding of the drug therapy, adverse effects to anticipate, and measures to relieve discomfort and improve safety.

Implementation

Ensure ready access to ephinephrine in case of anaphylactic reaction to injections.

Mark chart with sites of each injection given.

Ensure there is no sign of infection or open areas near injection sites.

Provide comfort and safety measures, positioning, pain medication as needed.

Provide support and reassurance to encourage M.D.

Teach L.G. about drug, drug effects, and symptoms of reportable serious adverse effects.

Evaluation

Evaluate drug effects: Relief of migraine frequency, relief of migraine pain

Monitor for adverse effects: Headache, infection at injection sites , potential for botulism (difficulty breathing and/or swallowing).

Evaluate effectiveness of patient-teaching program.

PATIENT TEACHING FOR L.G.

- The drug prescribed for you is a direct-acting muscle relaxant called *Botox* (incobotulinumtoxin A). This drug stops muscles from moving. It is not really understood how the many injections into your head and neck actually help relieve migraines, but it is thought to be related to the muscle relaxation and changes in certain chemicals in the area.
- Common side effects of this drug include:
  - *Pain at the injection sites:* Report this to your provider
  - *Headache:* An analgesic may be ordered to help.
- Report any of the following to your health care provider: *Fever, chills, appearance of any signs of infection at your injection sites; difficulty breathing or swallowing.*
- You will need to return for another series of injections in 12 weeks; if your migraines become worse in that time, call your health care provider.

Adverse Effects

The most frequently seen adverse effects associated with dantrolene relate to drug-caused CNS depression: Drowsiness, fatigue, weakness, confusion, headache and insomnia, and visual disturbances. GI disturbances may be linked to direct irritation or to alterations in smooth muscle function caused by the drug-induced calcium effects. Such adverse GI effects may include GI irritation, diarrhea, constipation, and abdominal cramps. Dantrolene may also cause direct hepatocellular damage and hepatitis that can be fatal. Urinary frequency, enuresis, and feelings of urinary urgency reportedly occur, and crystalline urine with pain or burning on urination may result. In addition, several unusual adverse effects may occur, including acne, abnormal hair growth, rashes, photosensitivity, abnormal sweating, chills, and myalgia.

The botulinum toxins have been associated with anaphylactic reactions; with headache, dizziness, muscle pain, and paralysis; and with redness and edema at the injection site. Adverse effects associated with use of botulinumtoxin A for cosmetic purposes include headache, respiratory infections, flu-like syndrome, and droopy eyelids in severe cases. Pain, redness, and muscle weakness also have been reported. Children treated with these drugs have reportedly developed botulism. The reactions tended to be temporary, but there have been reports of reactions that lasted several months. The U.S. Food and Drug Administration strongly reminds providers that this is a prescription drug and should be used only under close medical supervision and not injected at trendy "Botox parties."

Clinically Important Drug–Drug Interactions

If dantrolene is combined with estrogens the incidence of hepatocellular toxicity is apparently increased. If possible, this combination should be avoided. If the botulinum toxins are used with other drugs that interfere with neuromuscular transmission—neuromuscular junction blockers, lincosamides, quinidine, magnesium sulfate, anticholinesterases, succinylcholine, or polymyxin—or with aminoglycosides, there is a risk of additive effects. If any of these must be given in combination, extreme caution should be used.

Prototype Summary: Dantrolene

Indications: Control of clinical spasticity resulting from upper motor neuron disorders, preoperatively to prevent or attenuate the development of malignant hyperthermia in susceptible patients, IV for management of fulminant malignant hyperthermia.

Actions: Interferes with the release of calcium from the sarcoplasmic reticulum within skeletal muscles, preventing muscle contraction; does not interfere with neuromuscular transmission.

Pharmacokinetics:

Route	Onset	Peak	Duration
Oral	Slow	4–6 h	8–10 h
IV	Rapid	5 h	6–8 h

$T_{1/2}$: 9 hours (oral), 4 to 8 hours (IV); excreted in the urine.

Adverse Effects: Drowsiness, dizziness, weakness, fatigue, diarrhea, hepatitis, myalgia, tachycardia, transient blood pressure changes, rash, urinary frequency.

Nursing Considerations for Patients Receiving Centrally Acting Skeletal Muscle Relaxants

Assessment: History and Examination

- Assess for *contraindications or cautions for the use of the drug* including any known allergies *to prevent hypersensitivity reactions*; cardiac depression; epilepsy; muscle weakness; respiratory depression, *which could be exacerbated by the effects of these drugs*; pregnancy and lactation, *which require cautious use*; renal or hepatic dysfunction, *which could alter the metabolism and excretion of the drug*; and local infections (if using the botulinum toxins) *to prevent exacerbation of the infections.*
- Assess temperature; skin color and lesions; CNS orientation, affect, reflexes, bilateral grip strength, and spasticity; respiration and adventitious sounds; pulse, electrocardiogram, and cardiac output; bowel sounds and reported output; and liver and renal function tests *to determine baseline status before beginning therapy and for any potential adverse effects.*

Refer to the Critical Thinking Scenario for a full discussion of nursing care for a patient who is receiving a direct-acting skeletal muscle relaxant.

Nursing Diagnoses

Nursing diagnoses related to drug therapy might include the following:

- Acute pain related to GI and CNS effects
- Disturbed thought processes related to CNS effects
- Risk for injury related to CNS effects
- Deficient knowledge regarding drug therapy

Planning

- The patient will receive the best therapeutic effect from the drug therapy.
- The patient will have limited adverse effects to the drug therapy.
- The patient will have an understanding of the drug therapy, adverse effects to anticipate, and measures to relieve discomfort and improve safety.

Implementation with Rationale

- Discontinue the drug at any sign of liver dysfunction. *Early diagnosis of liver damage may prevent permanent dysfunction. Arrange for the drug to be discontinued if signs of liver damage appear.* A prodrome, with nausea, anorexia, and fatigue, is present in 60% of patients with evidence of hepatic injury.

- Do not administer botulinum toxins into any area with an active infection *because of the risk of exacerbation of the infection.*
- Monitor intravenous access sites of dantrolene for potential extravasation *because the drug is alkaline and very irritating to tissues.*
- Institute other supportive measures (e.g., ventilation, anticonvulsants as needed, cooling blankets) for the treatment of malignant hyperthermia *to support the patient through the reaction.*
- Periodically discontinue dantrolene for 2 to 4 days *to monitor therapeutic effectiveness.* A clinical impression of exacerbation of spasticity indicates a positive therapeutic effect and justifies continued use of the drug.
- Establish a therapeutic goal before beginning oral therapy with dantrolene (e.g., to gain or enhance the ability to engage in a therapeutic exercise program, to use braces, to accomplish transfer maneuvers) *to promote patient compliance and a sense of success with therapy.*
- Discontinue dantrolene if diarrhea becomes severe *to prevent dehydration and electrolyte imbalance.* The drug may be restarted at a lower dose.
- Provide thorough patient teaching, including drug name, prescribed dosage, measures for avoidance of adverse effects, warning signs that may indicate possible problems, and the need for monitoring and evaluation *to enhance patient knowledge about drug therapy and to promote compliance.*
- Offer support and encouragement to help the patient cope with the drug regimen.

Evaluation

- Monitor patient response to the drug (improvement in spasticity, improvement in movement and activities; improvement in continence, migraines, dystonia, facial lines, sweating with botulinum toxins).
- Monitor for adverse effects (CNS changes, diarrhea, liver toxicity, urinary urgency).
- Evaluate the effectiveness of the teaching plan (patient can give the drug name and dosage, possible adverse effects to watch for and specific measures to prevent adverse effects, and therapeutic goals).
- Monitor the effectiveness of comfort measures and compliance with the regimen.

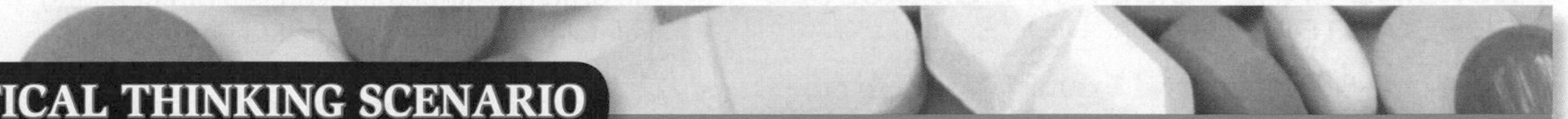

CRITICAL THINKING SCENARIO

Skeletal Muscle Relaxants for Cerebral Palsy

THE SITUATION

L.G. is 26 years old. He was diagnosed with cerebral palsy shortly after his birth. He lives in the community in a group home with six other affected people. Two adult caregivers provide supervision. In the past few months, L.G.'s spasticity has progressed severely, making it impossible for him to carry on his daily activities without extensive assistance.

Following a clinical evaluation, his health care team suggests trying a course of dantrolene therapy. After learning about the risks of dantrolene-related hepatic dysfunction, L.G. decides that the benefits of dantrolene therapy are more important to him than the risks of hepatotoxicity. The health care team proceeds with a complete physical examination, including liver enzyme analysis. Therapy begins and a clinic staff member schedules L.G. for a visit by a public health nurse in 4 days.

CRITICAL THINKING

What basic principles must be included in the nursing care plan for L.G. for the visiting nurses? *Think about the importance of including the adult caregivers in any teaching or evaluation programs. Consider specific problems that could develop that L.G. would be unable to handle on his own.*

What therapeutic goals might the nurse set with L.G. and his caregiver? How might these be evaluated?

What additional drug-related information should be posted in the group home and reviewed with L.G. and his caregivers?

DISCUSSION

In the first visit to the home, the nurse needs to establish a relationship with L.G. and his caregivers. They should all realize that drug therapy, and other measures, are needed to help L.G. attain his full potential and make use of his existing assets. Step-by-step therapeutic goals should be established and written down for future reference. Small reachable goals, such as partially dressing himself, walking to the table for meals, and managing parts of his daily hygiene routine are best at the beginning. Written goals provide a good basis for future evaluation when drug therapy is stopped briefly to determine its therapeutic effectiveness. It also helps L.G. to see progress and improvement.

In addition, the nurse should perform a complete examination to obtain baseline data. The patient should

(continues on page 434)

Skeletal Muscle Relaxants for Cerebral Palsy (continued)

be asked about any noticeable changes or problems since starting the drug. If improvement appears to have occurred the dosage may be slowly increased until the optimal level of functioning has been achieved. The nurse is in a position to evaluate this and report it to the primary caregiver.

While in the home, the nurse can also evaluate resources and environmental limitations and suggest improvements (e.g., use of leg braces). L.G. and his caregivers should receive a drug teaching card that includes a telephone number to call with questions or concerns, warning signs of liver disease, and a list of findings to report. The nurse should discuss anticipated appointments for liver function tests to ensure that L.G. can keep the appointments. The health care team should work closely with L.G. to maximize his involvement in his care and to minimize unnecessary problems and confusion. Because the treatment involves a long-term commitment a good working relationship among all members of the health care team is important to ensure continuity of care and optimal results.

NURSING CARE GUIDE FOR L.G.: MUSCLE RELAXANTS

Assessment: History and Examination

Concentrate the health history on allergies to any skeletal muscle relaxants, respiratory depression, muscle weakness, hepatic or renal dysfunction, and concurrent use of verapamil or alcohol.

Focus the physical examination on the following:

CV: Blood pressure pulse rate, peripheral perfusion, electrocardiogram

CNS: Orientation, affect, reflexes, grip strength

Skin: Color, lesions, texture, temperature

GI: Abdominal examination, bowel sounds

Respiratory: Respiration, adventitious sounds

Laboratory tests: Renal and hepatic function

Nursing Diagnoses

Acute pain related to GI, GU, and CNS effects

Risk for injury related to CNS effects

Disturbed thought processes related to CNS effects

Deficient knowledge regarding drug therapy

Planning

The patient will receive the best therapeutic effect from the drug therapy.

The patient will have limited adverse effects to the drug therapy.

The patient will have an understanding of the drug therapy, adverse effects to anticipate, and measures to relieve discomfort and improve safety.

Implementation

Discontinue drug at first sign of liver dysfunction.

Provide comfort and safety measures: Positioning, orientation, safety measures, pain medication as needed.

Provide support and reassurance to help L.G. deal with spasticity and drug effects.

Teach L.G. about drug, dosage, drug effects, and symptoms of reportable serious adverse effects.

Evaluation

Evaluate drug effects: Relief of spasticity, improved daily function.

Monitor for adverse effects: Multiple CNS effects, respiratory depression, rash, skin changes, GI problems (diarrhea, hepatotoxicity), urinary urgency, or weakness.

Monitor for drug–drug interactions: Myocardial suppression with verapamil or alcohol.

Evaluate effectiveness of patient-teaching program.

PATIENT TEACHING FOR L.G.

- The drug prescribed for you is a direct-acting skeletal muscle relaxant called dantrolene (*Dantrium*). This drug makes spastic muscles relax. Because this drug may cause liver damage, it is important that you have regular medical checkups.
- Common side effects of skeletal muscle relaxants, such as dantrolene, include:
  - *Fatigue, weakness, and drowsiness:* Try to pace activities evenly throughout the day and allow rest periods to avoid discouraging side effects. If they become too severe, consult your health care provider.
  - *Dizziness and fainting:* Change position slowly to avoid dizzy spells. If these effects should occur, avoid activities that require coordination and concentration.
  - *Diarrhea:* Be sure to be near bathroom facilities if this occurs. This effect usually subsides after a few weeks.
- Report any of the following to your health care provider: *Fever, chills, rash, itching, changes in the color of your urine or stool, or a yellowish tint to the eyes or skin.*
- Keep this drug and all medications out of the reach of children.
- Do not overexert yourself when you begin to feel better. Pace yourself.
- Take this drug exactly as directed and schedule regular medical checkups to evaluate the effects of this drug on your body.

KEY POINTS

- Centrally acting skeletal muscle relaxants are used to relieve the effects of muscle spasm. Dantrolene, a direct-acting skeletal muscle relaxant, is used to control spasticity and prevent malignant hyperthermia.
- The rimabotulinumtoxin B is used to reduce the severity of abnormal head position and neck pain associated with cervical dystonia. Onabotulinumtoxin A is used to improve the appearance of moderate to severe glabellar lines, canthal lines, and to treat cervical dystonia; severe primary axillary hyperhidrosis; strabismus and blepharospasm associated with dystonia; chronic migraines; overactive bladder and detrusor overactivity associated with neurological disorders. Incobotulinumtoxin A is also used to decrease the severity of head position with cervical dystonia, to treat blepharospasm, and improve glabellar lines in adults.

SUMMARY

- Upper level controls of muscle activity include the pyramidal tract in the cerebellum, which regulates coordination of intentional muscle movement, and the extrapyramidal tract in the cerebellum and basal ganglia, which coordinates crude movements related to unconscious muscle activity.
- Damage to a muscle or anchoring skeletal structure may result in the arrival of a flood of impulses to the spinal cord. Such overstimulation may lead to a muscle spasm or a state of increased contraction.
- Damage to motor neurons can cause muscle spasticity, with a lack of coordination between muscle groups and loss of coordinated activity, including the ability to perform intentional tasks and maintain posture, position, and locomotion.
- Centrally acting skeletal muscle relaxants are used to relieve the effects of muscle spasm. Dantrolene, a direct-acting skeletal muscle relaxant, is used to control spasticity and prevent malignant hyperthermia.
- The rimabotulinumtoxin B is used to reduce the severity of abnormal head position and neck pain associated with cervical dystonia. Onabotulinumtoxin A is used to improve the appearance of moderate to severe glabellar lines and to treat cervical dystonia, severe primary axillary hyperhidrosis, and strabismus and blepharospasm associated with dystonia. Incobotulinumtoxin A is also used to decrease the severity of head position with cervical dystonia and to treat blepharospasm in adults previously treated with botulinum A.

CHECK YOUR UNDERSTANDING

Answers to the questions in this chapter can be found in Answers to Check Your Understanding Questions on thePoint®.

MULTIPLE CHOICE

Select the best answer to the following.

1. A muscle spasm often results from
a. damage to the basal ganglia.
b. CNS damage.
c. injury to the musculoskeletal system.
d. chemical imbalance within the CNS.

2. Muscle spasticity is the result of
a. direct damage to a muscle cell.
b. overstretching of a muscle.
c. tearing of a ligament.
d. damage to neurons within the CNS.

3. Signs and symptoms of tetanus, which includes severe muscle spasm, are best treated with
a. baclofen.
b. diazepam.
c. carisoprodol.
d. methocarbamol.

4. The drug of choice for a patient experiencing severe muscle spasms and pain precipitated by anxiety is
a. methocarbamol.
b. baclofen.
c. diazepam.
d. carisoprodol.

5. Dantrolene (*Dantrium*) differs from the other skeletal muscle relaxants because
a. it acts in the highest levels of the CNS.
b. it is used to treat muscle spasms as well as muscle spasticity.
c. it cannot be used to treat neuromuscular disorders.
d. it acts directly within the skeletal muscle fiber and not within the CNS.

(continues on page 436)

6. The use of neuromuscular junction blockers may sometimes cause a condition known as malignant hyperthermia. The drug of choice for prevention or treatment of this condition is
   a. baclofen.
   b. diazepam.
   c. dantrolene.
   d. methocarbamol.

7. Dantrolene is associated with potentially fatal cellular damage. If your patient's condition is being managed with dantrolene, the patient should
   a. have repeated complete blood counts during therapy.
   b. have renal function tests done monthly.
   c. be monitored for signs of liver damage and have liver function tests done regularly.
   d. have a thorough eye examination before and periodically during therapy.

MULTIPLE RESPONSE

Select all that apply.

1. Spasmolytics, or centrally acting muscle relaxants, block the reflexes in the CNS that lead to spasm. While a patient is taking one of these drugs, which of the following interventions should be implemented?
   a. Rest for the affected muscle
   b. Heat to the affected area
   c. Ice packs to the affected area
   d. Use of anti-inflammatory agents
   e. Body temperature check every 2 hours to watch for malignant hyperthermia
   f. Positioning to decrease pain and spasm

2. Muscle relaxants would be used in which of the following circumstances?
   a. To treat spasticity related to spinal cord injury
   b. To treat spasticity that contributes to locomotion, upright position, or increase in function
   c. To treat spasticity that is related to toxins, such as tetanus
   d. To treat spasticity that is a result of neuromuscular degeneration
   e. To reduce the severity of head position associated with cervical dystonia
   f. To reduce the appearance of frown lines (glabellar lines)

BIBLIOGRAPHY AND REFERENCES

Albanese, A. (2011). Terminology for preparations of botulinum neurotoxins: What a difference a name makes. *Journal of the American Medical Association, 305*(1), 89–90.

Brunton, L., Chabner, B., & Knollman, B. (2011). *Goodman and Gilman's the pharmacological basis of therapeutics* (12th ed.). New York: McGraw-Hill.

Delgado, M. R., Hirtz, S., Alsen, M., et al. (2010). Practice parameter: Pharmacologic treatment of spasticity in children and adolescents with cerebral palsy. *Neurology, 74*(4), 336–343.

Facts and Comparisons. (2015). *Drug facts and comparisons.* St. Louis, MO: Author.

Facts and Comparisons. (2015). *Professional's guide to patient drug facts.* St. Louis, MO: Author.

Karch, A. M. (2015). *Lippincott's nursing drug guide.* Philadelphia, PA: Lippincott Williams & Wilkins.

Kuehn, B. (2008). Botulinum toxins may have effects beyond injection site. *Journal of the American Medical Association, 299*(1), 2261–2263.

Litman, R. S., & Rosenberg, N. (2005). Malignant hyperthermia: Update on susceptibility testing. *Journal of the American Medical Association, 293*(23), 2918–2924.

Porth, C. M. (2013). *Pathophysiology: Concepts of altered health states* (9th ed.). Philadelphia, PA: Lippincott Williams & Wilkins.

Rossler, R., Donath, L., Verhagen, E., et al. (2014). Exercise-based injury prevention in child and adolescent sport: A systemic review. *Sports Medicine, 44*(12), 1733–1748.

26

Narcotics, Narcotic Antagonists, and Antimigraine Agents

Learning Objectives

Upon completion of this chapter, you will be able to:

1. Outline the gate theory of pain and explain therapeutic ways to block pain using the gate theory.
2. Describe the therapeutic actions, indications, pharmacokinetics, contraindications, most common adverse reactions, and important drug–drug interactions associated with narcotics and antimigraine agents.
3. Discuss the use of the different classes of narcotics, narcotic antagonists, and antimigraine agents across the lifespan.
4. Compare and contrast the prototype drugs morphine, pentazocine, naloxone, ergotamine, and sumatriptan with other drugs in their respective classes.
5. Outline the nursing considerations, including important teaching points, for patients receiving a narcotic, a narcotic antagonist, or an antimigraine drug.

Glossary of Key Terms

A fibers: large-diameter nerve fibers that carry peripheral impulses associated with touch and temperature to the spinal cord

A-delta fibers: small-diameter nerve fibers that carry peripheral impulses associated with pain to the spinal cord

C fibers: unmyelinated, slow-conducting fibers that carry peripheral impulses associated with pain to the spinal cord

ergot derivative: drug that causes a vascular constriction in the brain and the periphery; relieves or prevents migraine headaches but is associated with many adverse effects

gate control theory: theory that states that the transmission of a nerve impulse can be modulated at various points along its path by descending fibers from the brain that close the "gate" and block transmission of pain information and by A fibers that are able to block transmission in the dorsal horn by closing the gate for transmission for the A-delta and C fibers

migraine headache: headache characterized by severe, unilateral, pulsating head pain associated with systemic effects, including gastrointestinal (GI) upset and sensitization to light and sound; related to a hyperperfusion of the brain from arterial dilation

narcotics: drugs, originally derived from opium, that react with specific opioid receptors throughout the body

narcotic agonists: drugs that react at opioid receptor sites to stimulate the effects of the receptors

narcotic agonists–antagonists: drugs that react at some opioid receptor sites to stimulate their activity and at other opioid receptor sites to block activity

narcotic antagonists: drugs that block the opioid receptor sites; used to counteract the effects of narcotics or to treat an overdose of narcotics

opioid receptors: receptor sites on nerves that react with endorphins and enkephalins, which are receptive to narcotic drugs

pain: a sensory and emotional experience associated with actual or potential tissue damage

spinothalamic tract: nerve pathway from the spine to the thalamus along which pain impulses are carried to the brain

triptan: selective serotonin receptor blocker that causes a vascular constriction of cranial vessels; used to treat acute migraine attacks

Drug List

Narcotics

Narcotic Agonists
- codeine
- fentanyl
- hydrocodone
- hydromorphone
- levorphanol
- meperidine
- methadone
- Ⓟ morphine
- opium
- oxycodone
- oxymorphone
- remifentanil
- sufentanil
- tapentadol
- tramadol

Narcotic Agonists–Antagonists
- buprenorphine
- butorphanol
- nalbuphine
- Ⓟ pentazocine

Narcotic Antagonists
- Ⓟ naloxone
- naltrexone

Antimigraine Agents

Ergot Derivatives
- dihydroergotamine
- Ⓟ ergotamine

Triptans
- almotriptan
- eletriptan
- frovatriptan
- naratriptan
- rizatriptan
- Ⓟ sumatriptan
- zolmitriptan

Pain, by definition, is a sensory and emotional experience associated with actual or potential tissue damage. The perception of pain is part of the clinical presentation in many disorders and is one of the hardest sensations for patients to cope with during the course of a disease or dysfunction. The drugs involved in the management of severe pain, whether acute or chronic, are discussed in this chapter. These agents all work in the central nervous system (CNS)—the brain and the spinal cord—to alter the way that pain impulses arriving from peripheral nerves are processed. These agents can change the perception and tolerance of pain. Two major types of drugs are considered here: The narcotics—the opium derivatives that are used to treat many types of pain; and the antimigraine drugs, which are reserved for the treatment of migraine headache, a type of severe headache. Narcotic antagonists, which are used to block the effects of the narcotics in cases of overdose, also are discussed.

Pain

Pain is described as an unpleasant sensation and emotional experience. In many ways it is a subjective experience. The physiological processes that cause pain are perceived and reacted to in different ways because of learned experiences, cultural differences, and environmental stimuli. Pain occurs whenever tissues are damaged. The injury to cells releases many chemicals, including kinins and prostaglandins, which stimulate specific sensory nerves. Pain can be acute or chronic. Acute pain occurs in response to recent tissue damage or injury. This type of pain makes a person aware of an injury and should lead to measures to care for the injury and teaches the person to avoid similar situations that could cause this pain. Chronic pain is constant or intermittent pain that keeps occurring long past the time the injured area would be expected to heal. Chronic pain can cause a stress reaction, interrupt much-needed sleep, and interfere with all of the activities of daily living. Pain can also be classified by location. "Where does it hurt?" is a common question in assessing pain. Sometimes the location of the pain is a direct indicator of where the tissue damage has occurred. In some cases, so-called referred pain occurs. A person experiencing pain from damage to heart muscle may actually feel the pain in the neck or jaw. The sensation of pain is experienced in a different area of the body. Referred pain often follows predictable pathways, which helps health care providers figure out where the injury has occurred. Pain can be further classified by originating source as nociceptive, neuropathic, or psychogenic. Nociceptive pain is caused by a direct stimulus to a pain receptor. Neuropathic pain is caused by nerve injury. Psychogenic pain is pain that is associated with emotional, psychological, or behavioral stimuli.

Pain Impulse Transmission and Perception

Two small-diameter sensory nerves, called the **A-delta** and **C fibers**, respectively, respond to stimulation by generating nerve impulses that produce pain sensations. The A-delta fibers are small, myelinated fibers that respond quickly to acute pain. The C fibers are unmyelinated and are slow conducting. Pain impulses from the skin, subcutaneous tissues, muscles, and deep visceral structures are conducted to the dorsal, or posterior, horn of the spinal cord on these fibers. In the spinal cord, these nerves form synapses with spinal cord nerves that then send impulses to the brain (Figure 26.1).

In addition, large-diameter sensory nerves enter the dorsal horn of the spinal cord. These so-called **A fibers** do not transmit pain impulses; instead, they transmit sensations associated with touch and temperature. The A fibers, which are larger and conduct impulses more rapidly than do the smaller fibers, can actually block the ability of the smaller fibers to transmit their signals to the secondary neurons in the spinal cord. The dorsal horn, therefore, can be both excitatory and inhibitory with regard to pain impulses that are transmitted from the periphery.

The impulses reaching the dorsal horn are transmitted upward toward the brain by a number of specific ascending nerve pathways. These pathways run from the

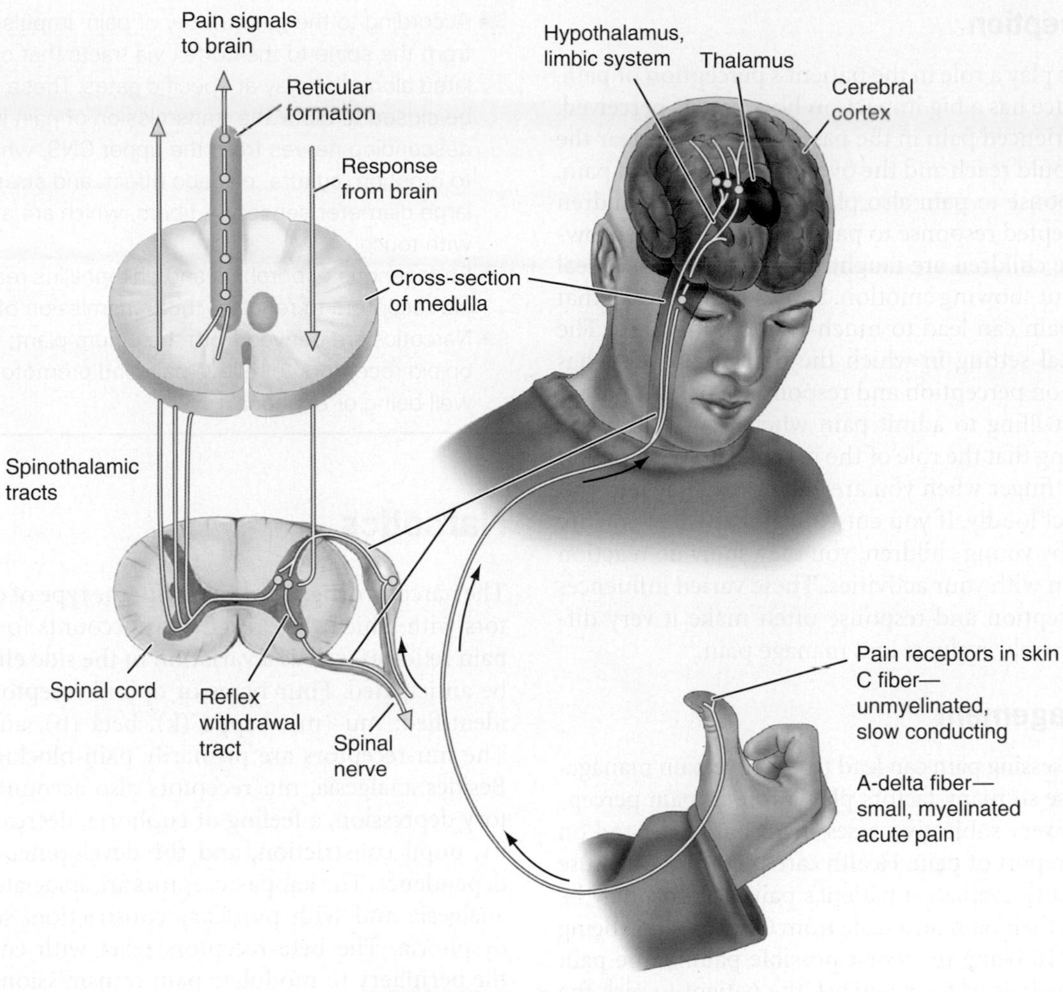

FIGURE 26.1 Neural pathways of pain.

spinal cord into the thalamus, where they form synapses with various nerve cells that transmit the information to the cerebral cortex, along the **spinothalamic tracts**. According to the **gate control theory** the transmission of these impulses can be modulated or adjusted all along these tracts. All along the spinal cord the interneurons can act as "gates" by blocking the ascending transmission of pain impulses. It is thought that the gates can be closed by stimulation of the larger A fibers and by descending impulses coming down the spinal cord from higher levels in such areas as the cerebral cortex, the limbic system, and the reticular activating system.

The inhibitory influence of the higher brain centers on the transmission of pain impulses helps to explain much of the mystery associated with pain. Several factors, including learned experiences, cultural expectations, individual tolerance, and the placebo effect, can activate the descending inhibitory nerves coming from the upper CNS. These other factors need to be considered and incorporated into pain management strategies, which usually involve the use of drugs. For example, the placebo effect, stress reduction, acupuncture, and back rubs (which stimulate the A fibers) all can play important roles in the effective management of pain.

Pain Receptors

Opioid receptors are receptor sites that respond to naturally occurring peptides: The endorphins and the enkephalins. These receptor sites are found in the CNS, on nerves in the periphery, and on cells in the gastrointestinal (GI) tract. In the brainstem, opioid receptors help to control blood pressure, pupil diameter, GI secretions, and the chemoreceptor trigger zone (CTZ) that regulates nausea and vomiting, cough, and respiration. In the spinal cord and thalamus, these receptors help to integrate and relate incoming information about pain. The endorphins and enkephalins normally modulate the pain information coming into the brain. Endorphins are released during stress to block the sensation of pain. Professional athletes may be injured during an important game and have no sensation of pain or injury because their stress reaction is highly activated, and the endorphins are blocking pain transmission into the brain. In the hypothalamus, stimulation of the opioid receptors may interrelate the endocrine and neural responses to pain. In the limbic system the receptors incorporate emotional aspects of pain and response to pain. At peripheral nerve sites, they may block the release of neurotransmitters that are related to pain and inflammation.

Pain Perception

Many factors play a role in the patient's perception of pain. Past experience has a big impact on how pain is perceived. Having experienced pain in the past a patient may fear the intensity it could reach and the overall impact of that pain. Learned response to pain also plays a large role. Children learn the accepted response to painful stimuli when growing up. Some children are taught to ignore pain and deal with it without showing emotion. Some children learn that reacting to pain can lead to much-wanted attention. The environmental setting in which the pain occurs also has an influence on perception and response to pain. A parent may not be willing to admit pain when the children are present, feeling that the role of the parent is to be strong. If you cut your finger when you are alone, you may perceive pain and react loudly. If you cut your finger when you are surrounded by young children, you may show no reaction and just go on with your activities. These varied influences on pain perception and response often make it very difficult to effectively evaluate and manage pain.

Pain Management

Accurately assessing pain can lead to effective pain management. Because so many factors play a role in pain perception and it is very subjective, assessment has to depend on the patient's report of pain. Health care providers often use a scale system to evaluate a patient's pain. Patients may be asked to rank their pain on a scale from 0 to 10, with 0 being no pain and 10 being the worst possible pain. Some pain scales use drawings of faces and ask the patient to pick the face that most reflects the pain they feel. Numerous methods, both nonpharmacological and pharmacological, may be used to manage pain. Nonpharmacological treatments can include warmth, massage, positioning, acupuncture, or meditation. Pharmacological methods often include the use of nonsteroidal anti-inflammatory drugs or acetaminophen (Chapter 15) for tissue-related pain or atypical antipsychotics or other CNS depressants for the treatment of neurogenic pain. These methods can be used individually or in combination. The goal is to achieve maximum pain relief.

One major method of pain management involves the use of narcotics. The **narcotics**, or opioids, were first derived from the opium plant. Although most narcotics are now synthetically prepared, their chemical structure resembles that of the original plant alkaloids. All drugs in this class are similar, in that they occupy specific opioid receptors in the CNS. Their actions in the body are related to the stimulation of the various opioid receptors that they occupy.

KEY POINTS

- When tissue is injured, various chemicals are released and pain results.
- A-delta and C fibers carry pain impulses to the spinal cord.
- According to the gate theory of pain, impulses travel from the spine to the cortex via tracts that can be modulated along the way at specific gates. These gates can be closed to block the transmission of pain impulses by descending nerves from the upper CNS, which relate to emotion, culture, placebo effect, and stress, and by large-diameter sensory A fibers, which are associated with touch.
- Endogenous endorphins and enkephalins react with opioid receptors to regulate the transmission of pain.
- Narcotics are derived from the opium plant; they bind to opioid receptors to relieve pain and promote feelings of well-being or euphoria.

Narcotics

The narcotic drugs used vary with the type of opioid receptors with which they react. This accounts for a change in pain relief, as well as a variation in the side effects that can be anticipated. Four types of opioid receptors have been identified: mu (m), kappa (k), beta (b), and sigma (s). The mu-receptors are primarily pain-blocking receptors. Besides analgesia, mu-receptors also account for respiratory depression, a feeling of euphoria, decreased GI activity, pupil constriction, and the development of physical dependence. The kappa-receptors are associated with some analgesia and with pupillary constriction, sedation, and dysphoria. The beta-receptors react with enkephalins in the periphery to modulate pain transmission. The sigma-receptors cause pupillary dilation and may be responsible for the hallucinations, dysphoria, and psychoses that can occur with narcotic use. The administration of narcotics requires specific considerations related to age (Box 26.1).

Narcotic Agonists

The **narcotic agonists** (Table 26.1) are drugs that react with the opioid receptors throughout the body to cause analgesia, sedation, or euphoria (Figure 26.2). Anticipated effects other than analgesia are mediated by the types of opioid receptors affected by each drug. Because of the potential for the development of physical dependence while taking these drugs the narcotic agonists are classified as controlled substances. The degree of control is determined by the relative ability of each drug to cause physical dependence. With the rising problem of addiction to and abuse of prescription drugs, measures are being taken to help to better control these drugs. Hydrocodone and oxycodone have moved to C-II, providing more restrictions on their use and sale. In addition, manufacturers are working to develop tamper resistant and abuse resistant tablets. Narcotic agonists include codeine, fentanyl (*Actiq, Duragesic*), hydrocodone (*Hysingla ER, Zohydro ER*), hydromorphone (*Dilaudid*), levorphanol (generic),

BOX 26.1 FOCUS ON Drug Therapy Across the Lifespan

Narcotics

CHILDREN

The safety and effectiveness of many of these drugs have not been established in children. If a narcotic is used the dose should be calculated very carefully, and the child should be monitored closely for the adverse effects associated with narcotic use.

Narcotics that have an established pediatric dose include codeine, fentanyl (but not transdermal fentanyl), hydrocodone, meperidine, and morphine. Narcotics that are not recommended for children are levorphanol, oxymorphone, and oxycodone

Methadone is not recommended as an analgesic in children. If a child older than 13 years of age requires a narcotic agonist–antagonist, buprenorphine is the drug of choice. Naloxone is the drug of choice for reversal of narcotic effects and narcotic overdose in children.

ADULTS

Adults being treated for acute pain should be reassured that the risk of addiction to a narcotic during treatment is remote. They should be encouraged to ask for pain medication before the pain is acute to get better coverage for their pain. Many institutions allow patients to self-regulate intravenous drips to control their pain postoperatively.

The narcotics are contraindicated or should only be used with caution during pregnancy because of the potential for adverse effects on the fetus. These drugs enter breast milk and can cause opioid effects in the baby, so caution should be used during lactation. Morphine, meperidine, and oxymorphone are often used for analgesia during labor. The mother should be monitored closely for adverse reactions, and if the drug is used over a prolonged labor the newborn infant should be monitored for opioid effects.

OLDER ADULTS

Elderly patients should be specifically asked whether they require pain medication. Because many older patients can recall a time when nurses were able to spend more time with patients, they may tend to believe that the nurse will meet their needs.

Older patients are more likely to experience the adverse effects associated with these drugs, including CNS, GI, and CV effects. Older adults who tolerated narcotics well at a younger age may have a very different response with age. These patients should be monitored when the drugs are started to evaluate response and toxicity.

Because older patients often have renal or hepatic impairment, they are also more likely to have toxic levels of the drug related to changes in metabolism and excretion. The older patient should have safety measures in effect—side rails, call light, assistance to ambulate—when receiving one of these drugs in the hospital setting.

meperidine (*Demerol*), methadone (*Dolophine*), morphine (*Roxanol, Astramorph*), opium (*Paregoric*), oxycodone (*OxyContin*), oxymorphone (generic), remifentanil (*Ultiva*), sufentanil (*Sufental*), tapentadol (*Nucynta*), and tramadol (*Ultram*).

Therapeutic Actions and Indications

The narcotic agonists act at specific opioid receptor sites in the CNS to produce analgesia, sedation, and a sense of well-being. They also are used as antitussives and as adjuncts to general anesthesia to produce rapid analgesia, sedation, and respiratory depression. Indications for narcotic agonists include relief of severe acute or chronic pain, preoperative medication, analgesia during anesthesia, and specific individual indications, depending on their receptor affinity (see Table 26.1 for Usual Indications for each narcotic agonist). Accurate calculation of a dose is crucial to prevent overdosing patients. Box 26.2 describes how to calculate dose for one narcotic agonist.

In deciding which narcotic to use in any particular situation, it is important to consider all of these aspects of the patient's condition and to select the drug that will be most effective in each situation with the fewest adverse effects for the patient. Each patient is different, and his or her response to a drug also is different (Box 26.3). For instance, if an analgesic that is long acting but not too sedating is desired for an outpatient, hydrocodone might fit those objectives. Fentanyl, which is available for injection, is also available as a lozenge for treating breakthrough pain, as a buccal tablet, as a transdermal patch, and as a sublingual tablet or nasal spray to be used as needed for treating breakthrough pain in cancer patients. See the Critical Thinking Scenario for information about using morphine to relieve pain.

Pharmacokinetics

IV administration is the most reliable way to achieve therapeutic levels of narcotics. IM and subcutaneous administration offer varying rates of absorption, and absorption is slower in female than in male patients because of the normal fat content of female muscles and tissue. These drugs undergo hepatic metabolism and are generally excreted in the urine and bile. Half-life periods vary widely, depending on the drug being used. These agents cross the placenta and are known to enter breast milk.

Contraindications and Cautions

The narcotic agonists are contraindicated in the following conditions: Presence of any known allergy to any narcotic

Table 26.1 *Drugs in Focus:* Narcotics

Drug Name	Dosage/Route	Usual Indications
Narcotic Agonists		
codeine (generic)	*Adult:* 15–60 mg PO, IM, IV, or subcutaneous q4–6 h; 10–20 mg PO q4–6 h for cough *Pediatric:* 0.5 mg/kg PO, IM, or subcutaneous q4–6 h; 2.5–10 mg PO q4–6 h for cough	Relief of mild to moderate pain; relief of coughing induced by mechanical or chemical irritation of the respiratory tract
fentanyl (*Actiq, Duragesic*)	*Adult:* 0.05–0.1 mg IM, 30–60 min before surgery; 0.002 mg/kg IV or IM during surgery; 0.05–0.1 mg postoperatively; 5 mcg/kg transmucosally; for transdermal patch, calculate the previous day's narcotics need and use table to convert to patch strength; sublingual tablet or nasal spray—initially a dose of100 mcg to a maximum of 800 mcg sublingually or as a nasal spray in one nostril for treatment of breakthrough cancer pain *Pediatric (>2 y):* 2–3 mcg/kg IM or IV; base transmucosal dose on weight and do not exceed 400 mcg	For analgesia before, during, and after surgery; transdermal patch for management of chronic pain; control of breakthrough pain
hydrocodone (*Hysingla ER, Zohydro ER*)	*Adult:* 10 mg PO q12 h in combination products for pain; may increase in 10-mg increments as needed	Relief of pain requiring continuous analgesia for prolonged periods
hydromorphone (*Dilaudid*)	2–4 mg PO q4–6 h *or* 3 mg PR q6–8 h *or* 1–4 mg subcutaneous or IM q4–6 h	Relief of moderate to severe pain in adults
levorphanol (generic)	1 mg IV by slow injection *or* 1–2 mg IM or subcutaneous q6–8 h *or* 2 mg PO q6–8 h	Management of moderate to severe pain in adults; postoperative pain in adults
meperidine (*Demerol*)	*Adult:* 50–150 mg PO, IM, or subcutaneous q3–4 h; during labor, 100 mg IM or subcutaneous q1–3 h *Pediatric:* 1–1.8 mg/kg IM, subcutaneous, or PO q3–4 h	Relief of moderate to severe pain, preoperative analgesia and support of anesthesia, and obstetrical analgesia
methadone (*Dolophine*)	2.5–10 mg IM, subcutaneous, or PO q3–4 h for pain; 15–20 mg PO for withdrawal, then 20 mg PO q4–8 h for maintenance treatment	Relief of severe pain; detoxification and temporary maintenance treatment of narcotic addiction in adults
morphine (*Roxanol, Astramorph*)	*Adult:* 10 to 20-mg solution PO *or* 15- to 30-mg tablets PO q4 h *or* 10 mg subcutaneous or IM q4 h *or* 2–10 mg/70 kg IV over 4–5 min *or* 10–20 mg PR q4 h *Pediatric:* 0.1–0.2 mg/kg IM or subcutaneous q4 h	Relief of moderate to severe chronic and acute pain; preoperatively and postoperatively and during labor
opium (*Paregoric*)	*Adult:* 0.6 mL liquid PO q.i.d. *or* 5–10 mL camphorated tincture one to four times per day PO *Pediatric:* 0.005–0.02 mg/kg PO q3–4 h *or* 0.25–0.5 mL/kg PO q1–4h of camphorated tincture	Treatment of diarrhea, relief of moderate pain
oxycodone (*OxyContin, Oxecta*)	10–30 mg PO q4 h as needed	Relief of moderate to severe pain in adults
oxymorphone (*Numorphan*)	0.5 mg IV initially; 1–1.5 mg IM or subcutaneous q4–6 h as needed; 0.5–1 mg IM for labor; 5 mg PR q4–6 h	Relief of moderate to severe pain in adults; preoperative medication; obstetrical analgesia
remifentanil (*Ultiva*)	*Adult and pediatric (>2 y):* Dose determined by general anesthetic being used	Analgesic for use during general anesthesia *Special considerations:* Must be under the direct supervision of anesthesia practitioner
sufentanil (*Sufental*)	*Adult:* 1–2 mcg/kg IV with general anesthesia *Pediatric:* 10–25 mcg/kg IV	Analgesic for use during general anesthesia; used as an epidural agent in labor and delivery *Special considerations:* Must be under the direct supervision of anesthesia practitioner
tapentadol (*Nucynta*)	50–100 mg PO every 4–6 h	Relief of moderate to severe pain in patients 18 y and older *Special considerations:* Risk of serious serotonin syndrome if combined with SSRIs, MAOIs, TCAs, St. John's wort
tramadol (*Ultram*)	*Adults:* Rapid relief of pain—50–100 mg PO q4–6 h to a maximum 400 mg/d; chronic pain—25 mg/d PO titrated slowly to a maximum 400 mg/d	Relief of moderate to moderately severe pain *Special considerations:* Limit use in patients with a history of addictions

Drug Name	Dosage/Route	Usual Indications
Narcotic Agonists–Antagonists		
buprenorphine (*Buprenex*)	*Adult and pediatric (>13 y):* 0.3 mg IM or slow IV q6 h as needed	Treatment of mild to moderate pain
butorphanol (generic)	*Adult:* 0.5–2 mg IV q3–4h *or* 1–4 mg IM q3–4 h; 1 mg nasal spray, repeated in 60–90 min, then in 3–4 h as needed *Geriatric:* Use one-half of the adult dose at twice the usual interval *Pediatric:* Not recommended for children <18 y	Used as preoperative medication to relieve moderate to severe pain; treatment of migraine headaches, with fewer peripheral adverse effects than many of the traditional antimigraine drugs
nalbuphine (generic)	10 mg/70 kg IM, subcutaneous, or IV q3–6 h as needed; do not exceed 160 mg/d	Relief of pain during labor and delivery; used as adjunct to general anesthesia; treatment of moderate to severe pain in adults
pentazocine (*Talwin*)	*Adult and pediatric (>12 y):* 30 mg IM, subcutaneous, or IV q3–4 h as needed *or* 50 mg PO q3–4 h as needed; do not exceed 360 mg/d; 30 mg IM most common for labor	Relief of moderate to severe pain during labor and delivery; treatment of postpartum pain; used as adjunct to general anesthesia
Narcotic Antagonists		
naloxone (*Evzia*)	*Adult:* for overdose, 0.4–2 mg IV, may repeat at 2- to 3-min intervals; for reversal of opioid effects, 0.1–0.2 mg IV, may repeat at 2- to 3-min intervals *Pediatric:* For overdose, 0.01 mg/kg IV, repeat as needed; for reversal of opioid effects, 0.005–0.01 mg IV at 2- to 3-min intervals *Adult and pediatric:* 0.4 mg/0.4 mL using prefilled auto-injector IM or subcutaneously	Diagnosis of narcotic overdose, reversal of opioid effects
naltrexone (*ReVia*)	*Adult:* 50 mg/d PO	Adjunct treatment of alcohol or narcotic dependence in adults

SSRI, selective serotonin reuptake inhibitor; MAOI, monoamine oxidase inhibitor; TCA, tricyclic antidepressant.

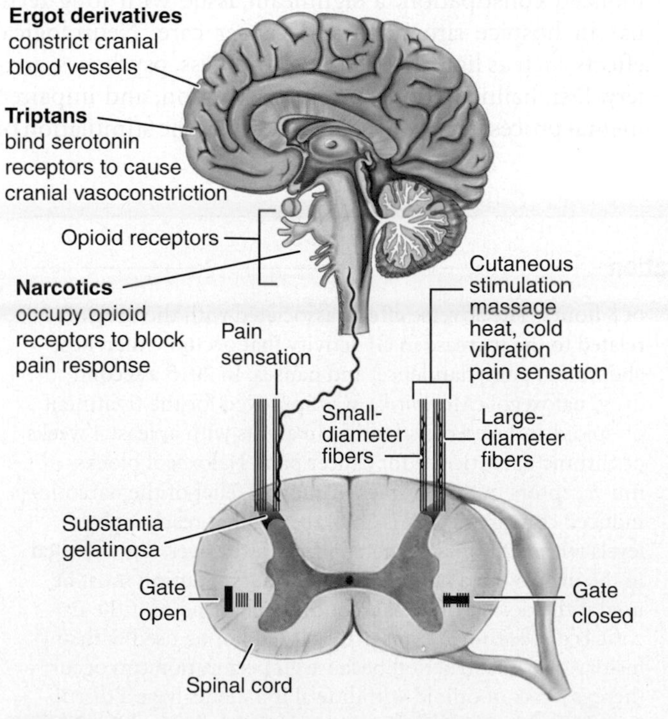

FIGURE 26.2 Sites of action. Narcotics occupy opioid receptors to block pain response. Ergot derivatives constrict cranial blood vessels, and triptans bind serotonin receptors to cause cranial vasoconstriction.

agonist *to avoid hypersensitivity reactions*; diarrhea caused by toxic poisons *because depression of GI activity could lead to increased absorption and toxicity*; and after biliary surgery or surgical anastomoses *because of the adverse effects associated with slowed GI activity due to narcotics.*

BOX 26.2 FOCUS ON Calculations

You are taking care of a 4-year-old child after surgery. An order has been written for 1.5 mg/kg meperidine IM q3–4 h as needed. The child is waking up and crying, so you decide to start the pain medication. The meperidine is available as 10 or 50 mg/mL. You note that the child weighs 20 kg. How much meperidine would you inject?

20 kg × 1.5 mg/kg = 30 mg needed

You could give 3 mL of the 10-mg/mL preparation:

(x mL/30 mg = 1 mL/10 mg; $x = 3$)

Or you could give 0.6 mL of the 50-mg/mL preparation:

(x mL/30 mg = 1 mL/50 mg; x = 0.6 mL)

In this case, you might prefer to give the child the smaller volume, using 0.6 mL of the 50-mg/mL solution to deliver the 30 mg of meperidine.

BOX 26.3 FOCUS ON **Cultural Considerations**

Differences in Responses to Narcotic Therapy

Because of physical and cultural differences among various ethnic groups, patients from certain groups respond differently to particular medications. Nurses should keep in mind that patients in some ethnic groups are genetically predisposed to metabolize medications differently. For example, Arab Americans may not achieve the same pain relief from narcotics as patients in other ethnic groups; their inborn differences in metabolism may require larger doses to achieve therapeutic effects.

Some African American patients seem to have a decreased sensitivity to the pain-relieving qualities of some narcotics, although the reason for this is unknown. Moreover, increasing the dosage of these medications may not increase the level of pain relief and actually may be toxic. In such cases, another class of medication might be used to "boost" the pain-relieving qualities of the narcotic.

Among some immigrant and first-generation Asian Americans, it may not be socially acceptable to show strong emotion, such as that associated with pain. The sensitive nurse will frequently ask such patients if they are comfortable or require additional medication.

Oxycodone is classified as pregnancy category B, whereas all of the other narcotic agonists are in category C, so it might be the drug of choice if one is needed during pregnancy. Extended release oxycodone (*OxyContin*) has been associated with abuse because when the tablet is cut, crushed, or chewed the entire dose of the drug is released at once. In 2011 *Oxecta,* a new form of extended release oxycodone, was approved. It is in a new aversion technology that makes it difficult to swallow if cut, crushed, or chewed and is thought to discourage abuse of this form of the drug. It cannot be used in nasogastric (NG) or feeding tubes because of its makeup. Pregnant women must be cautioned not to cut, crush, or chew these tablets if they are prescribed this drug. Many sources recommend waiting 4 to 6 hours after receiving a narcotic before breastfeeding the baby if a narcotic is needed for pain control.

Caution should be used in patients with respiratory dysfunction, *which could be exacerbated by the respiratory depression caused by these drugs*; recent GI or genitourinary (GU) surgery, acute abdomen or ulcerative colitis, *which could become worse with the GI depressive effects of the narcotics*; head injuries, alcoholism, delirium tremens, or cerebral vascular disease, *which could be exacerbated by the CNS effects of the drugs*; liver or renal dysfunction, *which could alter the metabolism and excretion of the drugs*; and during pregnancy, labor, or lactation *because of potential adverse effects on the fetus or neonate, including respiratory depression.*

Adverse Effects

The most frequently seen adverse effects associated with narcotic agonists relate to their effects on various opioid receptors. Respiratory depression with apnea, cardiac arrest, and shock may result from narcotic-induced respiratory center depression. Orthostatic hypotension is commonly seen with some narcotics. GI effects such as nausea, vomiting, constipation, and biliary spasm may occur as a result of CTZ stimulation and negative effects on GI motility. Box 26.4 discusses drugs approved to treat opioid-induced constipation, a significant issue with long-term use in hospice situations and cancer care. Neurological effects such as light-headedness, dizziness, psychoses, anxiety, fear, hallucinations, pupil constriction, and impaired mental processes may occur as a result of the stimulation of

BOX 26.4

Laxatives for Dealing with Narcotic-Induced Constipation

One of the most uncomfortable side effects of narcotic use is constipation. Frequently, when ordering a narcotic for pain a prescriber will also order a laxative to avert serious constipation discomfort. When a patient is on long-term narcotics for controlling pain in cases of cancer or in hospice settings where palliative care uses narcotics to make patients comfortable, constipation can be a real problem. In 2008 methylnaltrexone bromide (*Relistor*) was approved for the treatment of opioid-induced constipation in patients who are receiving palliative care and who no longer respond to traditional laxatives. *Relistor* is a peripherally acting, mu-specific opioid antagonist. It blocks the mu-receptors responsible for constipation related to opioid use. *Relistor* is given by subcutaneous injection once each day. It is rapidly absorbed from the tissues, reaching peak levels in 30 minutes. It is excreted primarily unchanged in the urine with a half-life of 8 hours. The adverse effects associated with the drug are related to the increase in GI activity that occurs—diarrhea, abdominal pain, flatulence, and nausea. In 2015 a second drug, naloxegol (*Movantik*), was approved for the treatment of opioid-induced constipation in adults with at least 4 weeks of chronic narcotic use for cancer pain. Naloxegol blocks mu-receptors in the GI track leading to relief of the narcotic-induced constipation. It is an oral drug that reaches peak levels within 2 hours, is metabolized in the liver, and excreted in the urine with a half life of 6–11 hours. Caution must be used if the dosage of the narcotics are changed or if the narcotic is discontinued. This drug should not be used with any history of GI obstruction because GI perforation can occur; there is a risk of opioid withdrawal if patients have a disruption in the blood–brain barrier and are using this drug. This laxative has the advantage of being an oral drug.

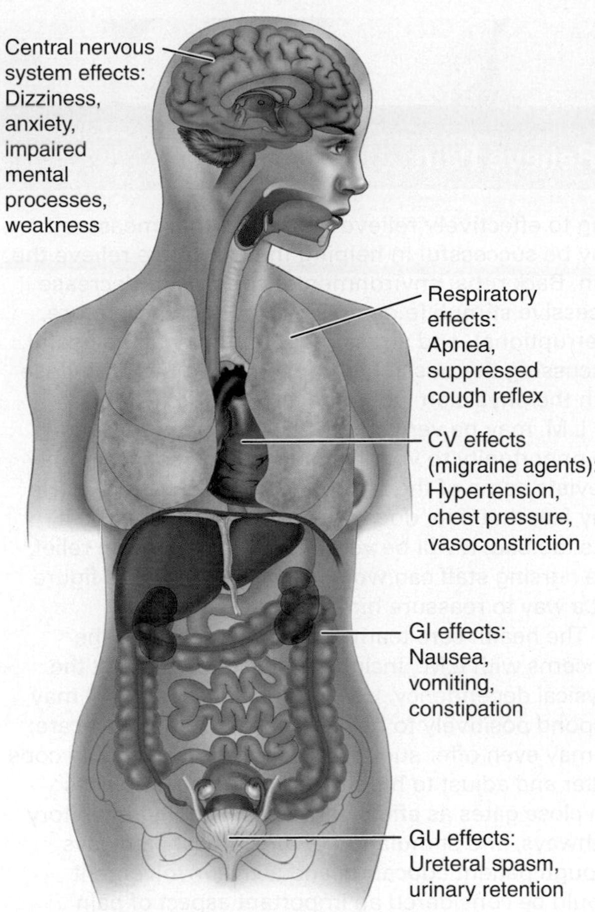

FIGURE 26.3 Common adverse effects and toxicities associated with narcotics, antimigraine agents.

CNS opioid receptors in the cerebrum, limbic system, and hypothalamus (Figure 26.3). GU effects, including ureteral spasm, urinary retention, hesitancy, and loss of libido, may be related to direct receptor stimulation or to CNS activation of sympathetic pathways. In addition, sweating and dependence (both physical and psychological) are possible, more so with some agents than with others.

Clinically Important Drug–Drug Interactions

When narcotic agonists are given with barbiturate general anesthetics or with some phenothiazines and monoamine oxidase inhibitors (MAOIs), the likelihood of respiratory depression, hypotension, and sedation or coma is increased. If these drug combinations cannot be avoided, patients should be monitored closely and appropriate supportive measures taken. Tapentadol, the newest of these drugs, also blocks norepinephrine reuptake in the CNS and patients taking this drug should avoid selective serotonin re-uptake inhibitors (SSRIs), MAOIs, tricyclic antidepressants (TCAs), and St. John's wort because of the increased risk of potentially life-threatening serotonin syndrome.

Ⓟ Prototype Summary: Morphine

Indications: Relief of moderate to severe acute or chronic pain; preoperative medication; component of combination therapy for severe chronic pain; intraspinal to reduce intractable pain.

Actions: Acts as an agonist at specific opioid receptors in the CNS to produce analgesia, euphoria, and sedation.

Pharmacokinetics:

Route	Onset	Peak	Duration
Oral	Varies	60 min	5–7 h
PR	Rapid	20–60 min	5–7 h
Subcutaneous	Rapid	50–90 min	5–7 h
IM	Rapid	30–60 min	5–6 h
IV	Immediate	20 min	5–6 h

$T_{1/2}$: 1.5 to 2 hours; metabolized in the liver, excreted in the urine and bile.

Adverse Effects: Light-headedness, dizziness, sedation, nausea, vomiting, dry mouth, constipation, ureteral spasm, respiratory depression, apnea, circulatory depression, respiratory arrest, shock, cardiac arrest.

Narcotic Agonists–Antagonists

The **narcotic agonists–antagonists** (Table 26.1) stimulate certain opioid receptors but block other such receptors. These drugs, which have less abuse potential than the pure narcotic agonists, exert a similar analgesic effect as morphine. Like morphine, they may cause sedation, respiratory depression, and constipation. They have also been associated with more psychotic-like reactions, and they may even induce a withdrawal syndrome in patients who have been taking narcotics for a long period.

Available narcotic agonists–antagonists include buprenorphine (*Buprenex*), butorphanol (generic), nalbuphine (generic), and pentazocine (*Talwin*).

Therapeutic Actions and Indications

The narcotic agonists–antagonists act at specific opioid receptor sites in the CNS to produce analgesia, sedation, euphoria, and hallucinations. In addition, they block opioid receptors that may be stimulated by other narcotics. These drugs have three functions: (1) relief of moderate to severe pain, (2) adjuncts to general anesthesia, and (3) relief of pain during labor and delivery. See Table 26.1 for Usual Indications for each narcotic agonist–antagonist agent.

CRITICAL THINKING SCENARIO

Using Morphine to Relieve Pain

THE SITUATION

L.M., a 25-year-old businessman, was in a car crash and suffered a fractured pelvis, a fractured left tibia, a fractured right humerus, and multiple contusions and abrasions. For the first 2 days after surgery to reduce the fractures, L.M. was heavily sedated. As healing progressed, he was taught to use a patient-controlled analgesia (PCA) system using morphine. PCA provides a baseline, constant infusion of morphine and gives the patient control of the system to add bolus doses of morphine if he feels that pain is not being controlled. The system prevents overdose by locking out extra doses until a specific period of time has elapsed. L.M. became agitated when he was not able to give himself a bolus because the appropriate time between boluses had not elapsed. The nurse working with L.M. noted an increase in blood pressure, pulse, and respirations. L.M. had no fever. He did seem very anxious and rated his pain at 10. The nurse tried several nonpharmacological measures to alleviate the pain and spent time talking with L.M. and reassuring him. By day 5, L.M. was switched to an oral morphine and plans were made to wean him from narcotics.

CRITICAL THINKING

What basic principles must be included in the nursing care plan for this patient? *Think about the difficult position the floor nurse is in when L.M. begins demanding pain relief before the prescribed time limit.*

What implications will L.M.'s agitation have on the way that the staff responds to him and on other patients in the area?

What other nursing measures could be used to help relieve pain and make the narcotic more effective?

What plans could the health team make with L.M. to give him more control over his situation and increase the chances that the pain relief will be effective?

DISCUSSION

In assessing L.M.'s response to drug therapy, you suspect that the morphine was not providing the desired therapeutic effect. Numerous research studies have shown that, in general, the dose of narcotics prescribed for acute pain relief provides inadequate analgesic coverage. It could be that the dose of morphine ordered for L.M. was just not sufficient to relieve his pain. This patient has many causes of acute pain and will heal more quickly if the pain is managed better. He has requested more drugs because the dose is too small or the intervals between doses are too long to effectively relieve his pain. Other measures may be successful in helping the morphine relieve the pain. Back rubs, environmental controls to decrease excessive stimuli (e.g., noise, lighting, temperature, interruptions), and stress reduction may all be useful. Discussing the possibility of increasing the drug dose with the physician would be appropriate.

L.M. may be very anxious about his injuries, and the opportunity to vent his feelings and concerns may alleviate some of the tension associated with pain. He may fear that if he does not cover the pain before it gets too bad, it will be very hard to get any pain relief. The nursing staff can work on this concern and figure out a way to reassure him.

The health care team should try to discuss the concerns with L.M., including the concern about the physical dependency. L.M. is a businessman and may respond positively to having some input into his care; he may even offer suggestions as to how he could cope better and adjust to his situation. Cortical impulses can close gates as effectively as descending inhibitory pathways, and stimulation of the cortical pathways through patient education and active involvement should be considered an important aspect of pain relief. Because L.M.'s injuries are extensive a long-term approach should be taken to his care. The sooner that L.M. can be involved the better the situation will be for everyone involved.

NURSING CARE GUIDE FOR L.M.: NARCOTICS

Assessment: History and Examination

Assess history of allergies to any narcotic drug, respiratory depression, GI or biliary surgery, hepatic or renal dysfunction, alcoholism, or convulsive disorders.

Focus the physical examination on the following:

Cardiovascular (CV): Blood pressure, pulse rate, peripheral perfusion, electrocardiogram

CNS: Orientation, affect, reflexes, grip strength

Skin: Color, lesions, texture, temperature

GI: Abdominal examination, bowel sounds

Respiratory: Respiration, adventitious sounds

Laboratory tests: Renal and liver function tests

Nursing Diagnoses

Acute pain related to injuries, GI, CNS, GU effects

Disturbed sensory perceptions (visual, auditory, kinesthetic) related to CNS effects

Impaired gas exchange related to respiratory depression

Deficient knowledge regarding drug therapy

Using Morphine to Relieve Pain (continued)

Anxiety related to injuries, drug regimen
Constipation

Planning

The patient will receive the best therapeutic effect from the drug therapy.

The patient will have limited adverse effects to the drug therapy.

The patient will have an understanding of the drug therapy, adverse effects to anticipate, and measures to relieve discomfort and improve safety.

Implementation

Provide a narcotic antagonist, facilities for assisted ventilation during intravenous administration.

Provide comfort and safety measures: Orientation, accurate timing of doses, monitoring for extravasation, and additional measures for pain relief to increase effects.

Provide support and reassurance to deal with drug effects and addiction potential.

Provide patient teaching about the drug, dosage, drug effects, and symptoms of serious reactions to report.

Evaluation

Evaluate drug effects: Relief of pain, sedation.

Monitor for adverse effects: CNS effects (multiple), respiratory depression, rash, skin changes, GI depression, constipation.

Monitor drug–drug interactions: Increased respiratory depression, sedation, coma with barbiturate anesthetics, MAOIs, phenothiazines, SSRIs, TCAs.

Evaluate the effectiveness of the patient-teaching program.

Evaluate the effectiveness of comfort and safety measures.

PATIENT TEACHING FOR L.M.

- A narcotic is used to relieve pain. Do not hesitate to take this drug if you feel uncomfortable. Remember that it is important to use the drug before the pain becomes severe and thus more difficult to treat.
- Common effects of these drugs include:
  - *Constipation*: Your health care provider will suggest appropriate measures to alleviate this common problem.
  - *Dizziness, drowsiness, and visual changes*: If any of these occur, avoid driving, operating complex machinery, or performing delicate tasks. If these effects occur in the hospital the side rails on the bed may be raised for your protection.
  - *Nausea and loss of appetite*: Taking the drug with food may help. Lying quietly until these sensations pass may also help to alleviate this problem.
- Report any of the following to your health care provider: *severe nausea or vomiting, skin rash, or shortness of breath or difficulty breathing.*
- Avoid the use of alcohol, antihistamines, and other over-the-counter drugs while taking this drug. Many of these drugs could interact with this narcotic.
- Tell any doctor, nurse, dentist, or other health care provider involved in your care that you are taking this drug.
- Keep this drug and all medications out of the reach of children.
- Do not take any leftover medication for other disorders, and do not let anyone else take your medication.
- Take this drug exactly as prescribed. Regular medical follow-up is necessary to evaluate the effects of this drug on your body

Pharmacokinetics

Narcotic agonists–antagonists are readily absorbed after IM administration and reach peak levels rapidly when given IV. They are metabolized in the liver and are excreted in the urine or feces. They are known to cross the placenta and enter breast milk.

Buprenorphine is available for use in IM and IV forms. Butorphanol is available for IM or IV administration and as a nasal spray. Nalbuphine is administered parenterally (subcutaneous, IM, or IV). Pentazocine is available in parenteral and oral forms, making it the preferred drug for patients who will be switched from parenteral to oral forms after surgery or labor.

Contraindications and Cautions

Narcotic agonists–antagonists are contraindicated in the presence of any known allergy to any narcotic agonist–antagonist *to avoid hypersensitivity reactions.*

Nalbuphine should not be given to patients who are allergic to sulfites *to avoid a cross-hypersensitivity reaction.*

Caution should be used in cases of physical dependence on a narcotic *because a withdrawal syndrome may be precipitated*; the narcotic antagonistic properties can block the analgesic effect and intensify the pain. Narcotic agonists–antagonists may be desirable for relieving chronic pain in patients who are susceptible to narcotic dependence, but extreme care must be used if patients are switched directly from a narcotic agonist to one of these drugs.

Caution should also be exercised in the following conditions: Chronic obstructive pulmonary disease or other respiratory dysfunction, *which could be exacerbated by respiratory depression*; acute myocardial infarction (MI), documented coronary artery disease (CAD), or hypertension, *which could be exacerbated by the cardiac stimulatory effects of these drugs*; and renal or hepatic dysfunction, *which could interfere with the metabolism and excretion of the drug.*

Pentazocine must be administered cautiously to patients with known heart disease *because the drug may cause cardiac stimulation, including arrhythmias, hypertension, and increased myocardial oxygen consumption, which could lead to angina, MI, or heart failure.*

There are no adequate studies regarding their effects during pregnancy. They should be used during pregnancy only if the benefit to the mother clearly outweighs the risk to the fetus *because of potential adverse effects on the neonate, including respiratory depression.* They are used to relieve pain during labor and delivery, which provides a short-term exposure to the fetus. They are known to enter breast milk and should be used with caution during lactation *because of the potential for adverse effects on the baby.*

Adverse Effects

The most frequently seen adverse effects associated with narcotic agonists–antagonists relate to their effects on various opioid receptors. Respiratory depression with apnea and suppression of the cough reflex is associated with the respiratory center depression. Nausea, vomiting, constipation, and biliary spasm may occur as a result of CTZ stimulation and the negative effects on GI motility. Light-headedness, dizziness, psychoses, anxiety, fear, hallucinations, and impaired mental processes may occur as a result of the activation of CNS opioid receptors in the cerebrum, limbic system, and hypothalamus. GU effects, including ureteral spasm, urinary retention, hesitancy, and loss of libido, may be related to direct receptor stimulation or to CNS activation of sympathetic pathways. Although sweating and dependence, both physical and psychological, are possible, their occurrence is considered less likely than with narcotic agonists.

Clinically Important Drug–Drug Interactions

When narcotic agonists–antagonists, like narcotic agonists, are given with barbiturate general anesthetics the likelihood of respiratory depression, hypotension, and sedation or coma increases. If this combination cannot be avoided, patients should be monitored closely and appropriate supportive measures taken.

Use of narcotic agonists–antagonists in patients who have previously received any narcotic puts these patients at risk for increased adverse effects, including respiratory depression. When such a sequence of drugs is used, patients require support and monitoring.

Pentazocine has been abused in combination with tripelennamine (T's and Blues) because of the hallucinogenic, euphoric effect of the two drugs, with potentially fatal complications.

Ⓟ Prototype Summary: Pentazocine

Indications: Relief of moderate to severe pain; preanesthetic medication and a supplement to surgical anesthesia.

Actions: An agonist at specific opioid receptors in the CNS, producing analgesia and sedation; an agonist at sigma opioid receptors, causing dysphoria and hallucinations; acts at mu-receptors to antagonize the analgesia and euphoria.

Pharmacokinetics:

Route	Onset	Peak	Duration
PO, IM, subcutaneous	15–30 min	1–3 h	3 h
IV	2–3 min	15 min	3 h

$T_{1/2}$: 2 to 3 hours; metabolized in the liver, excreted in the urine and bile.

Adverse Effects: Light-headedness, dizziness, sedation, euphoria, nausea, vomiting, constipation, tachycardia, palpitations, sweating, ureteral spasm, physical dependence.

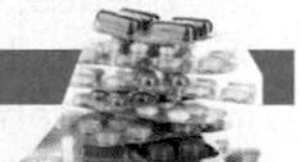

Nursing Considerations for Patients Receiving Narcotic Agonists and Narcotic Agonists–Antagonists

Assessment: History and Examination

- Assess *for contraindications or cautions*: Any known allergies to these drugs or to sulfites if using nalbuphine *to avoid hypersensitivity reactions*; respiratory dysfunction, *which may be exacerbated by the respiratory depression caused by these drugs*; MI or CAD, *which could be exacerbated by the effects of these drugs*; renal or hepatic dysfunction, *which might interfere with drug metabolism or excretion*; current status of pregnancy and lactation, *which require cautious use of the drugs*; history of heart disease if administering pentazocine *to reduce the risk of potential cardiac stimulation*; diarrhea caused by toxic poisons *because depression of GI activity could lead to increased absorption and toxicity*; and after biliary surgery or surgical anastomoses *because of the adverse effects associated with slowed GI activity due to narcotics.*

- Perform a pain assessment with the patient *to establish baseline and evaluate the effectiveness of drug therapy.*
- Perform a physical assessment to *establish baseline status before beginning therapy, determine drug effectiveness, and evaluate for any potential adverse effects.*
- Assess orientation, affect, reflexes, and pupil size to evaluate any central CNS effects; monitor respiratory rate and auscultate lungs for adventitious sounds *to evaluate respiratory effects.*
- Monitor pulse, blood pressure, and cardiac output *to evaluate for cardiac effects.*
- Palpate abdomen for distention and auscultate bowel sounds *to monitor for GI effects*; assess urine output and palpate for bladder distention *to evaluate for GU effects.*
- Monitor the results of laboratory tests such as liver and renal function tests *to determine the need for possible dose adjustment and identify toxic drug effects*; obtain an electrocardiogram *to evaluate for possible cardiac stimulation and arrhythmias secondary to pentazocine administration.*

Nursing Diagnoses

Nursing diagnoses related to drug therapy might include the following:

- Disturbed sensory perception (visual, auditory, kinesthetic) related to CNS effects
- Constipation related to GI effects
- Impaired gas exchange related to respiratory depression
- Risk for injury related to CNS effects of the drug

Planning

- The patient will receive the best therapeutic effect from the drug therapy.
- The patient will have limited adverse effects to the drug therapy.
- The patient will have an understanding of the drug therapy, adverse effects to anticipate, and measures to relieve discomfort and improve safety.

Implementation with Rationale

- Perform baseline and periodic pain assessments with the patient *to monitor drug effectiveness and provide appropriate changes in pain management protocol as needed.*
- Have a narcotic antagonist and equipment for assisted ventilation readily available when administering the drug IV *to provide patient support in case of severe reaction.*
- Monitor injection sites for irritation and extravasation *to provide appropriate supportive care if needed.*
- Monitor timing of analgesic doses. *Prompt administration may provide a more acceptable level of analgesia and lead to quicker resolution of the pain.*
- Use extreme caution when injecting these drugs into any body area that is chilled or has poor perfusion or shock *because absorption may be delayed, and after repeated doses an excessive amount is absorbed all at once.*
- Use additional measures to relieve pain (e.g., back rubs, stress reduction, hot packs, ice packs) *to increase the effectiveness of the narcotic being given and reduce pain.*
- Monitor respiratory status before beginning therapy and periodically during therapy *to monitor for potential respiratory depression.*
- Institute comfort and safety measures, such as side rails and assistance with ambulation, *to ensure patient safety*; bowel program as needed *to treat constipation*; environmental controls *to decrease stimulation*; and small, frequent meals *to relieve GI distress if GI upset is severe.*
- Reassure patients that the risk of addiction is minimal. *Most patients who receive these drugs for medical reasons do not develop dependency syndromes.*
- Offer support and encouragement *to help the patient cope with the drug regimen.*
- Provide thorough patient teaching, including drug name, prescribed dose, and schedule of administration; measures for avoidance of adverse effects; warning signs that may indicate possible problems; safety measures such as avoiding driving, getting assistance with ambulation, avoiding making important decisions or signing important papers; and the need for monitoring and evaluation *to enhance patient knowledge about drug therapy and to promote compliance.*

Evaluation

- Monitor patient response to the drug (relief of pain, sedation).
- Monitor for adverse effects (CNS changes, GI depression, respiratory depression, arrhythmias, hypertension).
- Evaluate the effectiveness of the teaching plan (the patient can give the drug name and dosage and describe possible adverse effects to watch for, specific measures to prevent them, and warning signs to report).
- Monitor the effectiveness of comfort measures and compliance with the regimen.

Narcotic Antagonists

The **narcotic antagonists** (Table 26.1) are drugs that bind strongly to opioid receptors but do not activate them. They block the effects of the opioid receptors and are often used to block the effects of too many opioids in the system. The narcotic antagonists in use include naloxone (*Evzio*) and naltrexone (*ReVia*).

Therapeutic Actions and Indications

The narcotic antagonists block opioid receptors and reverse the effects of opioids, including respiratory depression, sedation, psychomimetic effects, and hypotension.

These agents are indicated for reversal of the adverse effects of narcotic use, including respiratory depression and sedation, and for treatment of narcotic overdose (see Table 26.1 for Usual Indications for each narcotic antagonist agent). The narcotic antagonists do not have an appreciable effect in most people, but individuals who are addicted to narcotics experience the signs and symptoms of withdrawal when receiving these drugs rapidly. In 2014 naloxone was released in an autoinjector (*Evzio*) for use by first responders, family members of known narcotic users who could be at risk for overdose, and emergency care workers. It is thought that rapid response to overdose can save many lives.

Pharmacokinetics

Narcotic antagonists may be administered parenterally (subcutaneous, IM, or IV) or orally. These drugs are well absorbed after injection and are widely distributed in the body. They undergo hepatic metabolism and are excreted primarily in the urine.

Contraindications and Cautions

Narcotic antagonists are contraindicated in the presence of any known allergy to any narcotic antagonist *to avoid hypersensitivity reactions.* Caution should be used in the following circumstances: During pregnancy and lactation *because of potential adverse effects on the fetus and neonate*; with narcotic addiction *because of the precipitation of a withdrawal syndrome*; and with CV disease, *which could be exacerbated by the reversal of the depressive effects of narcotics.*

Adverse Effects

The most frequently seen adverse effects associated with these drugs relate to the blocking effects of the opioid receptors. The most common effect is an acute narcotic abstinence syndrome that is characterized by nausea, vomiting, sweating, tachycardia, hypertension, tremulousness, and feelings of anxiety. A naloxone challenge should be administered before giving naltrexone to help to avoid acute reactions.

CNS excitement and reversal of analgesia are especially common after surgery. CV effects related to the reversal of the opioid depression can include tachycardia, blood pressure changes, dysrhythmias, and pulmonary edema.

Clinically Important Drug–Drug Interactions

To reverse the effects of buprenorphine, butorphanol, nalbuphine, or pentazocine, larger doses of narcotic antagonists may be needed.

Prototype Summary: Naloxone

Indications: Complete or partial reversal of narcotic depression; diagnosis of suspected opioid overdose.

Actions: Pure narcotic antagonist; reverses the effects of the opioids, including respiratory depression, sedation, and hypotension.

Pharmacokinetics:

Route	Peak	Onset	Duration
IV	Unknown	2 min	4–6 h
IM, subcutaneous	Unknown	3–5 min	4–6 h

$T_{1/2}$: 30 to 81 minutes; metabolized in the liver, excreted in the urine.

Adverse Effects: Acute narcotic abstinence syndrome (nausea, vomiting, sweating, tachycardia, fall in blood pressure), hypotension, hypertension, pulmonary edema.

Nursing Considerations for Patients Receiving Narcotic Antagonists

Assessment: History and Examination

- Assess *for contraindications or cautions*: Any known allergies to these drugs *to avoid hypersensitivity reactions*; history of narcotic addition, *which may lead to narcotic abstinence syndrome*; history of MI or CAD, *which may be exacerbated by the reversal of opioid depression*; and current status of pregnancy and lactation, *which require cautious use of these drugs.*
- Perform a physical assessment to establish *baseline status before beginning therapy and for any potential adverse effects.*
- Assess the patient's neurological status, including level of orientation, affect, reflexes, and pupil size, *to evaluate CNS effects*; monitor respiratory rate and auscultate lungs for adventitious sounds *to evaluate respiratory status.*
- Monitor vital signs, including pulse and blood pressure, *to identify changes and risks to the CV system.*
- Obtain an electrocardiogram as appropriate *to evaluate for cardiac effects.*

Nursing Diagnoses

Nursing diagnoses related to drug therapy might include the following:

- Acute pain related to withdrawal and CV effects
- Decreased cardiac output related to CV effects
- Risk for injury related to CNS effects
- Deficient knowledge regarding drug therapy

Planning

- The patient will receive the best therapeutic effect from the drug therapy.
- The patient will have limited adverse effects to the drug therapy.
- The patient will have an understanding of the drug therapy, adverse effects to anticipate, and measures to relieve discomfort and improve safety.

Implementation with Rationale

- Maintain open airway and provide artificial ventilation and cardiac massage as needed *to support the patient.* Administer vasopressors as needed *to manage narcotic overdose.*
- Administer naloxone challenge before giving naltrexone *because of the serious risk of acute withdrawal.*
- Provide continuous monitoring of the patient, *adjusting the dose as needed, during treatment of acute overdose.*
- Provide comfort and safety measures *to help the patient cope with the withdrawal syndrome.*
- Ensure that patients receiving naltrexone have been narcotic free for 7 to 10 days *to prevent severe withdrawal syndrome.* Check urine opioid levels if there is any question.
- If the patient is receiving naltrexone as part of a comprehensive narcotic or alcohol withdrawal program, advise the patient to wear or carry a MedicAlert warning *so that medical personnel know how to treat the patient in an emergency.*
- Institute comfort and safety measures, such as side rails and assistance with ambulation, *to ensure patient safety;* institute bowel program as needed *for treatment of constipation*; use environmental controls *to decrease stimulation*; and provide, small frequent meals *to relieve GI irritation if GI upset is severe.*
- Offer support and encouragement *to help the patient cope with the effects of the drug regimen.*
- Provide thorough patient teaching, including drug name and prescribed dosage; measures to avoid adverse effects; warning signs to report immediately that may indicate possible problems; safety measures such as avoiding driving, avoiding making important decisions, and having a responsible person available for assistance; and the importance of continued monitoring and evaluation *to enhance patient knowledge about drug therapy and to promote compliance.*

Evaluation

- Monitor patient response to the drug (reversal of opioid effects, treatment of alcohol dependence).
- Monitor for adverse effects (CV changes, arrhythmias, hypertension).
- Evaluate the effectiveness of the teaching plan (patient can give the drug name and dosage and describe possible adverse effects to watch for, specific measures to prevent them, and warning signs to report).
- Monitor the effectiveness of comfort measures and compliance with the regimen.

KEY POINTS

- Narcotic agonists react with opioid receptor sites to stimulate their activity.
- Narcotic agonists–antagonists react with some opioid receptor sites to stimulate activity and block other opioid receptor sites.
- Narcotic antagonists are used to treat narcotic overdose or to reverse unacceptable adverse effects.

Migraine Headaches

The term **migraine headache** is used to describe several different syndromes, all of which include severe, throbbing headaches on one side of the head. This pain can be so severe that it can cause widespread disturbances, affecting GI and CNS function, including mood and personality changes.

Migraine headaches should be distinguished from cluster headaches and tension headaches (Box 26.5). Cluster headaches usually begin during sleep and involve sharp, steady eye pain that lasts 15 to 90 minutes, with sweating, flushing, tearing, and nasal congestion. Tension headaches, which usually occur at times of stress, feel like a dull band of pain around the entire head and last from 30 minutes to 1 week. They are accompanied by anorexia, fatigue, and a mild intolerance to light or sound.

Migraines generally are classified as common or classic. Common migraines, which occur without an aura, cause

BOX 26.5 FOCUS ON **Gender Considerations**

Headache Distribution

Headaches are distributed in the general population in a definite gender-related pattern. For example:

- Migraine headaches are three times more likely to occur in women than men.
- Cluster headaches are more likely to occur in men than in women.
- Tension headaches are more likely to occur in women than in men.

There is some speculation that the female predisposition to migraine headaches may be related to the vascular sensitivity to hormones. Some women can directly plot migraine occurrence to periods of fluctuations in their menstrual cycle. The introduction of the triptan class of antimigraine drugs has been beneficial for many of these women.

severe, unilateral, pulsating pain that is frequently accompanied by nausea, vomiting, and sensitivity to light and sound. Such migraine headaches are often aggravated by physical activity. Classic migraines are usually preceded by an aura—a sensation involving sensory or motor disturbances—that usually occurs about 1/2 hour before the pain begins. The pain and adverse effects are the same as those of the common migraine.

It is believed that the underlying cause of migraine headaches is arterial dilation. Headaches accompanied by an aura are associated with hypoperfusion of the brain during the aura stage, followed by reflex arterial dilation and hyperperfusion. The underlying cause and continued state of arterial dilation are not clearly understood, but they may be related to the release of bradykinins, serotonin, or a response to other hormones and chemicals.

Antimigraine Agents

For many years the one standard treatment for migraine headaches was acute analgesia, often involving a narcotic, together with control of lighting and sound and the use of **ergot derivatives**. In the late 1990s a new class of drugs, the **triptans**, was found to be extremely effective in treating migraine headaches without the adverse effects associated with ergot derivative use. Because these agents are associated with many systemic adverse effects, their usefulness is limited in some patients (Box 26.6). Other classes of drugs have been used with some success in the prevention of migraines, including the beta adrenergic blockers, angiotensin-converting enzyme inhibitors, and various carbonic anhydrase inhibitors. Table 26.2 includes additional information about each class of antimigraine agents.

Ergot Derivatives

The ergot derivatives cause constriction of cranial blood vessels and decrease the pulsation of cranial arteries. As a result, they reduce the hyperperfusion of the basilar artery vascular bed.

Available ergot derivatives include dihydroergotamine (*Migranal, D.H.E. 45*) and ergotamine (*Ergomar*).

Therapeutic Actions and Indications

The ergot derivatives block alpha-adrenergic and serotonin receptor sites in the brain to cause a constriction of cranial vessels, a decrease in cranial artery pulsation, and a decrease in the hyperperfusion of the basilar artery bed (see Figure 26.2). These drugs are indicated for the prevention or abortion of migraine or vascular headaches. Ergotamine, the prototype drug in this class, was the mainstay of migraine headache treatment before the development of triptans (see Table 26.2 for Usual Indications for each drug). In 2003 dihydroergotamine in the parenteral form was also approved for the treatment of cluster headaches.

Pharmacokinetics

The ergot derivatives are rapidly absorbed from many routes, with an onset of action ranging from 15 to 30 minutes. They are metabolized in the liver and primarily excreted in the bile.

Dihydroergotamine is available as a nasal spray or for IM or IV administration. This agent is the drug of choice if the oral route of administration is not possible.

Ergotamine is administered sublingually for rapid absorption. *Cafergot*, the very popular oral form, combines ergotamine with caffeine to increase its absorption from the GI tract.

BOX 26.6 FOCUS ON **Drug Therapy Across the Lifespan**

Antimigraine Agents

CHILDREN

None of the drugs used to treat migraines are recommended for use in children. The ergot derivatives can have many adverse effects in children, and there is not enough clinical experience with triptans to recommend them for use in children. In 2015 topiramate (*Topamax*), an antiseizure medication, was approved for migraine prevention and treatment in patients 12 and older, so would be the drug of choice if one was needed.

ADULTS

Adults requesting treatment for migraine headaches should be carefully evaluated before one of the antimigraine drugs is used to ensure that the headache being treated is of the type that can benefit from these drugs.

The ergots and the triptans are contraindicated during pregnancy because of the potential for adverse effects in the mother and fetus. Women of childbearing age should be advised to use contraception while they are taking these drugs. Women who are nursing should be encouraged to find another method of feeding the baby because of the potential for adverse drug effects on the baby.

OLDER ADULTS

Older adults are more likely to have chronic diseases such as CV disease or renal or hepatic impairment that would be exacerbated by the antimigraine drugs. They should be used with extreme caution in older adults. The older adult should be encouraged to take the least amount of the drug possible and should be monitored closely for any sign of chest pain, MI, or acute vascular changes. Safety measures are extremely important with the older adult. If the patient is in an institutional setting, side rails, assistance with moving, and careful monitoring should be used.

Table 26.2 Drugs in Focus: Antimigraine Agents

Drug Name	Dosage/Route	Usual Indications
Ergot Derivatives		
dihydroergotamine (*Migranal, D.H.E. 45*)	One spray (0.5 mg) in each nostril, may repeat in 15 min for a total of four sprays *or* 1 mg IM at first sign of headache, repeat in 1 h for a total of 3 mg or 2 mg IV, do not exceed 6 mg/wk	Rapid treatment of acute attacks of migraines in adults
ergotamine (*Ergomar*)	One tablet sublingually at the first sign of headache, repeat at 30-min intervals for a total of three tablets *or* one inhalation at first sign of headache, repeat in 5 min to a total of six inhalations per day	Prevention and abortion of migraine attacks in adults
Triptans		
almotriptan (*Axert*)	6.25–12.5 mg PO at onset of aura or symptoms	Treatment of acute migraines in adults
eletriptan (*Relpax*)	20–40 mg PO; may repeat in 2 h if needed; do not exceed 80 mg/d	Treatment of acute migraines in adults
frovatriptan (*Frova*)	2.5 mg PO as a single dose at first sign of headache; may repeat in 2 h; do not exceed three doses in 24 h	Treatment of acute migraines (with or without aura) in adults
naratriptan (*Amerge*)	1–2.5 mg PO with fluid; may repeat in 4 h if needed	Treatment of acute migraines in adults
rizatriptan (*Maxalt, Maxalt-MLT*)	5–10 mg PO; may repeat in 2 h; do not exceed 30 mg/d	Treatment of acute migraines in adults; orally disintegrating tablet may be useful if there is difficulty swallowing
sumatriptan (*Imitrex*)	50–100 mg PO at first sign of headache, may repeat in 2 h; by nasal spray in one nostril, may repeat in 2 h; do not exceed 40 mg/d	Treatment of acute migraines, cluster headaches in adults
zolmitriptan (*Zomig, Zomig-ZMT*)	2.5 mg PO; may repeat in 2 h; do not exceed 10 mg/d	Treatment of acute migraines in adults; orally disintegrating tablet may be useful if there is difficulty swallowing

Contraindications and Cautions

Ergot derivatives are contraindicated in the following circumstances: Presence of allergy to ergot preparations *to avoid hypersensitivity reactions*; CAD, hypertension, or peripheral vascular disease, *which could be exacerbated by the CV effects of these drugs*; impaired liver function, *which could alter the metabolism and excretion of these drugs*; and pregnancy or lactation *because of the potential for adverse effects on the fetus and neonate.* Ergotism (vomiting, diarrhea, and seizures) has been reported in affected infants.

Caution should be used in two instances: With pruritus, *which could become worse with drug-induced vascular constriction,* and with malnutrition *because ergot derivatives stimulate the CTZ and can cause severe GI reactions, possibly worsening malnutrition.*

Adverse Effects

The adverse effects of ergot derivatives can be related to the drug-induced vascular constriction. CNS effects include numbness, tingling of extremities, and muscle pain; CV effects such as pulselessness, weakness, chest pain, arrhythmias, localized edema and itching, and MI may also occur. In addition, the direct stimulation of the CTZ can cause GI upset, nausea, vomiting, and diarrhea. Ergotism, a syndrome associated with the use of these drugs, causes nausea, vomiting, severe thirst, hypoperfusion, chest pain, blood pressure changes, confusion, drug dependency (with prolonged use), and a drug withdrawal syndrome.

Clinically Important Drug–Drug Interactions

If these drugs are combined with beta-blockers the risk of peripheral ischemia and gangrene is increased. Such combinations should be avoided.

Ⓟ Prototype Summary: Ergotamine

Indications: Prevention or abortion of vascular headaches.

Actions: Constricts cranial blood vessels, decreases pulsation of cranial arteries, and decreases hyperperfusion of the basilar artery vascular bed; mechanism of action is not understood.

Pharmacokinetics:

Route	Onset	Peak
Sublingual	Rapid	0.5–3 h

$T_{1/2}$: 2.7 hours, then 21 hours; metabolized in the liver, excreted in the feces.

Adverse Effects: Numbness, tingling in the fingers and toes, muscle pain in the extremities, pulselessness or weakness in the legs, precordial distress, tachycardia, bradycardia, ergotism (nausea, vomiting, diarrhea, severe thirst, hypoperfusion, chest pain, confusion).

Triptans

The triptans are a class of drugs that cause cranial vascular constriction and relief of migraine headache pain in many patients. These drugs are not associated with the vascular and GI effects of the ergot derivatives. The triptan of choice for a particular patient depends on personal experience and other preexisting medical conditions. A patient may have a poor response to one triptan and respond well to another (Box 26.5).

Available triptans include almotriptan (*Axert*), eletriptan (*Relpax*), frovatriptan (*Frova*), naratriptan (*Amerge*), rizatriptan (*Maxalt, Maxalt-MLT*), sumatriptan (*Imitrex*), and zolmitriptan (*Zomig, Zomig-ZMT*).

Therapeutic Actions and Indications

The triptans bind to selective serotonin receptor sites to cause vasoconstriction of cranial vessels, relieving the signs and symptoms of migraine headache (see Figure 26.2). They are indicated for the treatment of acute migraine and are not used for prevention of migraines (see Table 26.2 for Usual Indications for each of the triptans).

Sumatriptan, the first drug of this class, is used for the treatment of acute migraine attacks and for the treatment of cluster headaches in adults. It can be given orally, subcutaneously, or by nasal spray.

Naratriptan, rizatriptan, zolmitriptan, and eletriptan are used orally only for the treatment of acute migraines. Rizatriptan and zolmitriptan are also available as fast-dissolving tablets.

CRITICAL THINKING SCENARIO

Relieving Migraine Pain

THE SITUATION

B.F., a 32-year-old financial planner, was experiencing severe headaches that she attributed to long hours at the computer and eye fatigue related to screen use. When standard NSAID therapy and rest periods did not seem to help, she began keeping a log of what she experienced, how she felt, and what was going on in her environment. After watching a TV documentary, she became very concerned that she may have a brain tumor so she made an appointment to see her health care provider. Her provider reviewed her logs and did a complete physical exam, including a brief neuro exam. She came to the conclusion that B.F was actually having migraine headaches. The pain was on one side of her head, she was often nauseous, had visual disturbances, and on several occasions had to stay in bed and call in sick to work because she just could not function. The headaches occurred about every 3 weeks and did not seem to be related to her menstrual cycle. B.F. requested a CAT (computed tomography) scan to make sure she did not have a brain tumor. It was explained that her physical findings were otherwise normal and she agreed to try zolmitriptan the next time she felt a headache coming on to see what happened.

CRITICAL THINKING

What basic principles must be included in the nursing care plan for this patient? *Think about the patient's fears, the impact of the multimedia on health care decisions, and the impact of the loss of work and function on a young woman.*

What other nursing measures could be used to help relieve pain and ease the patient's anxiety? *What measures can be used to relax the patient and relieve her anxiety?*

What teaching points need to be covered to help facilitate a safe and therapeutic response to the drug therapy prescribed? *Think about timing of doses, adverse effects that could occur, and other nondrug measures to help alleviate pain and discomfort.*

DISCUSSION

The patient suffered from headaches for quite some time before seeking medical assistance. This may reflect a lack of confidence in the health care system or a fear of what was really going on in her head. The impact of the TV documentary was impressive, and caused a great deal of concern and anxiety for the patient. These responses are known to activate the sympathetic nervous system, which could further add to discomfort and headache pain. The nurse working with this patient needs to listen to her fears, try to explain what the patient saw on TV, and work to provide support, assurance, and develop trust with the patient

Although the physical exam was negative, it is still important to discuss with the patient what that means. She should be praised for keeping her detailed log surrounding her headaches and encouraged to continue to log them when they occur. It will be important to explain what a migraine headache is, what happens in the brain, and the reasons for the various responses that she experienced. She will need thorough teaching about the timing of zolmitriptan administration, the use of

Relieving Migraine Pain (continued)

the disintegrating tablet, as well as the adverse effects that she might experience. Numbness and tingling may cause added concerns for her, so warning her that this may occur is very important. Environmental controls should also be discussed, as controlling them can make the drug therapy more effective and the patient will be more comfortable, leading to decreased anxiety, which will further help relieve the situation.

NURSING CARE GUIDE FOR B.F.: TRIPTANS

Assessment: History and Examination

Assess history of allergies to zolmitritan, active CAD or angina, pregnancy or breastfeeding.
Focus the physical examination on the following:
CV: Blood pressure, pulse rate, peripheral perfusion, reflexes
CNS: Orientation, affect
Skin: Color, lesions, texture, temperature
Laboratory tests: Renal tests

Nursing Diagnoses

Disturbed sensory perceptions (visual, auditory, kinesthetic) related to CNS effects
Deficient knowledge regarding drug therapy
Anxiety related to diagnosis, drug regimen

Planning

The patient will receive the best therapeutic effect from the drug therapy.
The patient will have limited adverse effects to the drug therapy.
The patient will have an understanding of the drug therapy, adverse effects to anticipate, and measures to relieve discomfort and improve safety.

Implementation

Administer drug at onset of headache, not for prevention; may repeat in 2 hours if pain persists.
Place orally disintegrating tablet on tongue, let it dissolve, and then have patient swallow.
Monitor blood pressure if any risk of CAD or angina.
Provide comfort and safety measures: Monitor lighting, sound, room temperature, positioning
Provide safety measures if dizziness, vertigo, or visual changes occur.
Provide patient teaching about the drug, dosage, drug effects, and symptoms of serious reactions to report.

Evaluation

Evaluate drug effects: Relief of pain.
Monitor for adverse effects: CNS effects, numbness or tingling, blood pressure changes.
Monitor drug–drug interactions: Severe effects with MAOIs, increased vasoactive reactions with ergots, cimetidine, hormonal contraceptives; serotonin syndrome with sibutramine; prolonged QT interval with other QT-prolonging drugs.
Evaluate the effectiveness of the patient-teaching program.
Evaluate the effectiveness of comfort and safety measures.

PATIENT TEACHING FOR B.F.

- The drug prescribed for your migraine headaches is called a triptan. This drug works to constrict the blood vessels in your brain to prevent the vasodilation that occurs and causes migraines.
- Take this drug exactly as prescribed, at the onset of your headache. Place the disintegrating tablet on your tongue and let it dissolve, then swallow. You should lower the lights, turn off noise, regulate the room temperature, and try to relax while the drug works. If the headache persists after 2 hours, you can take another tablet. Do not take more than two per day. If the headache still persists, call your health care provider.
- Common effects of these drugs include:
  - *Dizziness, drowsiness, and visual changes:* If any of these occur, avoid driving, operating complex machinery, or performing delicate tasks.
  - *Numbness, tingling, feelings of pressure or heaviness:* The drug causes blood vessels to constrict so you may feel like your arms or legs have "gone to sleep," this will pass when the drug wears off.
- Report any of the following to your health care provider: *Feelings of heat, flushing, nausea, chest pain or pressure, swelling of the lips or eyelids*
- Tell any doctor, nurse, dentist, or other health care provider involved in your care that you are taking this drug.
- Keep this drug and all medications out of the reach of children.
- Do not use this drug if you think you are pregnant or want to become pregnant, consult with your health care provider.

Pharmacokinetics

The triptans are rapidly absorbed from many sites; they are metabolized in the liver (sumatriptan by monoamine oxidase) and are primarily excreted in the urine. They cross the placenta and have been shown to be toxic to the fetus in animal studies. They also enter breast milk. The safety and efficacy of use in children have not been established.

Contraindications and Cautions

Triptans are contraindicated with any of the following conditions: Allergy to any triptan *to avoid hypersensitivity reactions*; pregnancy *because of the possibility of severe adverse effects on the fetus*; and active CAD, *which could be exacerbated by the vessel-constricting effects of these drugs.* These drugs should be used with caution in elderly patients *because of the possibility of underlying vascular disease*; in patients with risk factors for CAD; in lactating women *because of the possibility of adverse effects on the infant*; and in patients with renal or hepatic dysfunction, *which could alter the metabolism and excretion of the drug*. Rizatriptan seems to have more angina-related effects, and it is not recommended for patients with a history of CAD, *which could be exacerbated by its cardiac effects*.

Adverse Effects

The adverse effects associated with the triptans are related to the vasoconstrictive effects of the drugs. CNS effects may include numbness, tingling, burning sensation, feelings of coldness or strangeness, dizziness, weakness, myalgia, and vertigo. GI effects such as dysphagia and abdominal discomfort may occur. CV effects can be severe and include blood pressure alterations and tightness or pressure in the chest. Almotriptan is reported to have fewer side effects than the other triptans, and it is also thought that the longer half-life of this drug will prevent the rebound headaches that may be seen with other triptans.

Clinically Important Drug–Drug Interactions

Combining triptans with ergot-containing drugs results in a risk of prolonged vasoactive reactions.

There is a risk of severe adverse effects if these drugs are used within 2 weeks after discontinuation of a MAOI *because of the increased vasoconstrictive effects that occur*. If triptans are to be given, it is imperative that the patient has not received an MAOI in more than 2 weeks.

Ⓟ Prototype Summary: Sumatriptan

Indications: Treatment of acute migraine; treatment of cluster headaches (subcutaneous route).

Actions: Binds to serotonin receptors to cause vasoconstrictive effects on cranial blood vessels.

Pharmacokinetics:

Route	Onset	Peak	Duration
Nasal spray	Varies	5–20 min	Unknown
Oral	1–1.5 h	2–4 h	Up to 24 h
Subcutaneous	Rapid	1–5 h	Up to 24 h

$T_{1/2}$: 115 minutes; metabolized in the liver, excreted in the urine.

Adverse Effects: Dizziness, vertigo, weakness, myalgia, blood pressure alterations, tightness or pressure in the chest, injection site discomfort, tingling, burning sensations, numbness.

Nursing Considerations for Patients Receiving Antimigraine Agents

Assessment: History and Examination

- Assess for contraindications or cautions: Any known allergies to any component of the drugs *to avoid hypersensitivity reactions*; history of MI, CAD, or hypertension, *which may be exacerbated by the drug*; hepatic or renal dysfunction, *which could alter the metabolism and excretion of the drug*; pruritus or malnutrition, *which could be exacerbated by ergot derivatives*; and current status of pregnancy and lactation, *which would be cautions to the use of these drugs*.
- Perform a physical assessment to establish *baseline status before beginning therapy, determine drug effectiveness, and evaluate for any potential adverse effects*.
- Assess the patient's neurological status, including level of orientation, affect, and reflexes, *to evaluate CNS effects of the drugs*.
- Monitor for complaints of extremity numbness and tingling *to identify effects on vascular constriction*.
- Inspect the skin for localized edema, itching, or breakdown with ergot derivatives *to evaluate potential dermatological effects*.
- Assess vital signs, including pulse rate and blood pressure; obtain an electrocardiogram as appropriate *to evaluate cardiac status for changes*.
- Monitor the results of laboratory tests, including liver and renal function tests, *to determine the need for dose adjustment and identify possible toxic effects*.

Nursing Diagnoses

Nursing diagnoses related to drug therapy might include the following:

- Acute pain related to CV and vasoconstrictive effects
- Decreased cardiac output related to CV effects
- Disturbed sensory perception (visual, auditory, kinesthetic, and tactile) related to CNS effects
- Risk for injury related to changes in peripheral sensation, CNS effects
- Deficient knowledge regarding drug therapy

Planning

- The patient will receive the best therapeutic effect from the drug therapy.
- The patient will have limited adverse effects to the drug therapy.
- The patient will have an understanding of the drug therapy, adverse effects to anticipate, and measures to relieve discomfort and improve safety.

Implementation with Rationale

- Administer the drug to relieve acute migraines; *these drugs are not used for prevention.*
- Administer at the first sign of a headache and do not wait until it is severe *to improve therapeutic effectiveness.*
- Arrange for safety precautions if CNS or visual changes occur *to prevent patient injury.*
- Provide comfort and safety measures, such as environmental controls and stress reduction, *for the relief of headache.* Provide additional pain relief as needed.
- Monitor the blood pressure of any patient with a history of CAD, and discontinue the drug if any sign of angina or prolonged hypertension occurs, *to prevent severe vascular effects.*
- Offer support and encouragement *to help the patient cope with the disorder and associated drug regimen.*
- Provide thorough patient teaching, including drug name, prescribed dose, and schedule for administration; measures to avoid adverse effects; warning signs that may indicate possible problems; signs of ergotism if taking ergot derivatives; safety measures such as avoiding driving and avoiding overdose; and importance of follow-up monitoring and evaluation *to enhance patient knowledge about drug therapy and to promote compliance.*

Evaluation

- Monitor patient response to the drug (relief of acute migraine headaches).
- Monitor for adverse effects (CV changes, arrhythmias, hypertension, CNS changes).
- Evaluate the effectiveness of the teaching plan (patient can give the drug name and dosage and describe possible adverse effects to watch for, specific measures to prevent them, and warning signs to report).
- Monitor the effectiveness of comfort measures and compliance with the regimen.

KEY POINTS

- Migraine headaches are severe, throbbing headaches on one side of the head that may be associated with an aura or warning syndrome. These headaches are thought to be caused by arterial dilation and hyperperfusion of the cerebral vessels.
- Treatment of migraines may involve either ergot derivatives or triptans. Ergot derivatives cause vasoconstriction and are associated with sometimes severe systemic vasoconstrictive effects, whereas triptans are a class of selective serotonin receptor blockers, cause CNS vasoconstriction, but are not associated with as many adverse systemic effects.

SUMMARY

- Pain occurs any time that tissue is injured and various chemicals are released. The pain impulses are carried to the spinal cord by small-diameter A-delta and C fibers, which form synapses with interneurons in the dorsal horn of the spinal cord.
- Opioid receptors found throughout various tissues in the body react with endogenous endorphins and enkephalins to modulate the transmission of pain impulses.
- Narcotics, derived from the opium plant, react with opioid receptors to relieve pain. In addition, they lead to constipation, respiratory depression, sedation, and suppression of the cough reflex; they also stimulate feelings of well-being or euphoria.
- Because narcotics of all kinds are associated with the development of physical dependency, they are controlled substances.
- The effectiveness and adverse effects associated with specific narcotics are associated with their particular affinity for various types of opioid receptors.
- Narcotic agonists react with opioid receptor sites to stimulate their activity.
- Narcotic agonists–antagonists react with some opioid receptor sites to stimulate activity and block other opioid receptor sites. These drugs are not as addictive as pure narcotic agonists.
- Narcotic antagonists, which work to reverse the effects of narcotics, are used to treat narcotic overdose or to reverse unacceptable adverse effects.
- Migraine headaches are severe, throbbing headaches on one side of the head that may be associated with an aura or warning syndrome. These headaches are thought to be caused by arterial dilation and hyperperfusion of the brain vessels.
- Treatment of migraines may involve either ergot derivatives or triptans. Ergot derivatives cause vasoconstriction and are associated with sometimes severe systemic vasoconstrictive effects, whereas triptans, a newer class of selective serotonin receptor blockers, cause CNS vasoconstriction but are not associated with as many adverse systemic effects.

CHECK YOUR UNDERSTANDING

Answers to the questions in this chapter can be found in Answers to Check Your Understanding Questions on thePoint®.

MULTIPLE CHOICE

Select the best answer to the following.

1. According to the gate control theory, pain
   a. is caused by gates in the CNS.
   b. can be blocked or intensified by gates in the CNS.
   c. is caused by gates in peripheral nerve sensors.
   d. cannot be affected by learned experiences.

2. Opioid receptors are found throughout the body
   a. only in people who have become addicted to opiates.
   b. in increasing numbers with chronic pain conditions.
   c. to incorporate pain perception and blocking.
   d. to initiate the release of endorphins.

3. Most narcotics are controlled substances because they
   a. are very expensive.
   b. can cause respiratory depression.
   c. can be addictive.
   d. can be used only in a hospital setting.

4. Injecting a narcotic into an area of the body that is chilled can be dangerous because
   a. an abscess will form.
   b. the injection will be very painful.
   c. an excessive amount may be absorbed all at once.
   d. narcotics are inactivated in cold temperatures.

5. Proper administration of an ordered narcotic
   a. can lead to addiction.
   b. should be done promptly to prevent increased pain and the need for larger doses.
   c. would include holding the drug as long as possible until the patient really needs it.
   d. should rely on the patient's request for medication.

6. Migraine headaches
   a. occur during sleep and involve sweating and eye pain.
   b. occur with stress and feel like a dull band around the entire head.
   c. often occur when drinking coffee.
   d. are throbbing headaches on one side of the head.

7. The triptans are a class of drugs that bind to selective serotonin receptor sites and cause
   a. cranial vascular dilation.
   b. cranial vascular constriction.
   c. clinical depression
   d. nausea and vomiting.

8. The only triptan that has been approved for use in treating cluster headaches as well as migraines is
   a. naratriptan.
   b. rizatriptan.
   c. sumatriptan.
   d. zolmitriptan.

MULTIPLE RESPONSE

Select all that apply.

1. Narcotics are drugs that react with opioid receptors throughout the body. Which of the following would the nurse expect to find when assessing a patient who was taking a narcotic?
   a. Hypnosis
   b. Sedation
   c. Analgesia
   d. Euphoria
   e. Orthostatic hypotension
   f. Increased salivation

2. The nurse would expect to administer a narcotic as the analgesic of choice for which patients?
   a. A patient with severe postoperative pain
   b. A patient with severe chronic obstructive pulmonary disease and difficulty breathing
   c. A patient with severe, chronic pain
   d. A patient with ulcerative colitis
   e. A patient with recent biliary surgery
   f. A cancer patient with severe bone pain

BIBLIOGRAPHY AND REFERENCES

Beaulieu, P., Lussier, D., Porreca, F., et al. (2010). *Pharmacology of pain.* Seattle, WA: IASP Press.

Brunton, L., Chabner, B., & Knollman, B. (2011). *Goodman and Gilman's the pharmacological basis of therapeutics* (12th ed.). New York: McGraw-Hill.

Facts and Comparisons. (2015). *Drug facts and comparisons.* St. Louis, MO: Author.

Facts and Comparisons. (2015). *Professional's guide to patient drug facts.* St. Louis, MO: Author.

Karch, A. M. (2014). *Lippincott's nursing drug guide.* Philadelphia, PA: Lippincott Williams & Wilkins.

Lipton, R., Bigal, M., Steiner, T., et al. (2004). Classification of primary headaches. *Neurology, 63,* 427–435.

Miaskowski, C. (2005). Patient controlled modalities for acute postoperative pain management. *Journal of PeriAnesthesia Nursing, 20,* 255–267.

Porth, C. M. (2013). *Pathophysiology: Concepts of altered health states* (9th ed.). Philadelphia, PA: Lippincott Williams & Wilkins.

Stannard, C., Kalso, E., & Ballantyne, J. (Eds.). (2010). *Evidence-based clinical pain management.* Hoboken, NJ: Wiley-Blackwell.

Vadivelu, N., Urman, R. D., & Hines, R. L. (Eds.). (2011). *Essentials of pain management.* New York. Springer.

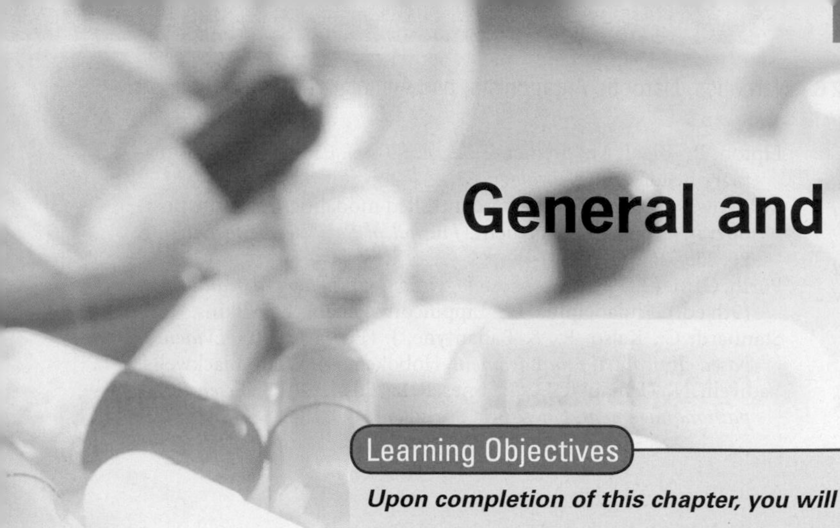

27 General and Local Anesthetic Agents

Learning Objectives

Upon completion of this chapter, you will be able to:

1. Describe the concept of balanced anesthesia.
2. Describe the actions and uses of local anesthesia.
3. Describe the therapeutic actions, indications, pharmacokinetics, contraindications, most common adverse reactions, and important drug–drug interactions associated with general and local anesthetics.
4. Outline the preoperative and postoperative needs of a patient receiving general or local anesthesia.
5. Compare and contrast the prototype drugs methohexital, midazolam, nitrous oxide, desflurane, and lidocaine with other drugs in their respective classes.
6. Outline the nursing considerations, including important teaching points, for patients receiving general and local anesthetics.

Glossary of Key Terms

amnesia: loss of memory of an event or procedure

analgesia: loss of pain sensation

anesthetic: drug used to cause complete or partial loss of sensation

balanced anesthesia: use of several different types of drugs to achieve the quickest, most effective anesthesia with the fewest adverse effects

general anesthesia: use of drugs to induce a loss of consciousness, amnesia, analgesia, and loss of reflexes to allow performance of painful surgical procedures

induction: time from the beginning of anesthesia until achievement of surgical anesthesia

local anesthesia: use of powerful nerve blockers that prevents depolarization of nerve membranes, blocking the transmission of pain stimuli and, in some cases, motor activity

plasma esterase: enzyme found in plasma that immediately breaks down ester-type local anesthetics

unconsciousness: loss of awareness of one's surroundings

volatile liquid: liquid that is unstable at room temperature and releases vapors; used as an inhaled general anesthetic, usually in the form of a halogenated hydrocarbon

Drug List

General Anesthetic Agents

Barbiturate Anesthetics
(P) methohexital

Nonbarbiturate General Anesthetics
droperidol
etomidate
ketamine
(P) midazolam
propofol

Anesthetic Gases
(P) nitrous oxide

Volatile Liquids
(P) desflurane
enflurane
isoflurane
sevoflurane

Local Anesthetic Agents

Esters
benzocaine
chloroprocaine
tetracaine

Amides
bupivacaine
dibucaine
(P) lidocaine
mepivacaine
prilocaine
ropivacaine

Other
pramoxine

Anesthetics are drugs that are used to cause complete or partial loss of sensation. The anesthetics can be subdivided into general and local anesthetics, depending on their site of action. General anesthetics are central nervous system (CNS) depressants used to produce loss of pain sensation and consciousness. Local anesthetics are drugs used to cause loss of pain sensation and feeling in a designated area of the body without the systemic effects associated with severe CNS depression. This chapter discusses various general and local anesthetics. Box 27.1 highlights information about using anesthetics with various age groups.

General Anesthesia

General anesthesia involves the administration of a combination of several different general anesthetic agents to achieve the following goals: **analgesia**, or loss of pain perception; **unconsciousness**, or loss of awareness of one's surroundings; and **amnesia**, or inability to recall what took place. Ideally, the drugs are combined to achieve the best effects with the fewest adverse effects. In addition, general anesthesia also blocks the body's reflexes. Blockage of autonomic reflexes prevents involuntary reflex response to bodily injury that might compromise a patient's cardiac, respiratory, gastrointestinal (GI), and immune status. Blockage of muscle reflexes prevents jerking movements that might interfere with the success of the surgical procedure.

Risk Factors Associated with General Anesthesia

Widespread CNS depression, which is not without risks, occurs with general anesthesia. In addition, all other body systems are affected. Because of the wide systemic effects, patients must be evaluated for factors that may increase their risk. These factors include the following:

- *CNS factors:* Underlying neurological disease (e.g., epilepsy, stroke, myasthenia gravis) that presents a risk for abnormal reaction to the CNS-depressing and muscle-relaxing effects of these drugs.

BOX 27.1 FOCUS ON Drug Therapy Across the Lifespan

Anesthetic Agents

CHILDREN

Children are at greater risk for complications after anesthesia—laryngospasm, bronchospasm, aspiration, and even death. They require very careful monitoring and support, and the anesthetist needs to be very skilled at calculating dosage and balance during the procedure. Propofol is widely used for diagnostic tests and short procedures in children older than 3 years of age because of its rapid onset and metabolism and generally smooth recovery. Sevoflurane has a minimal impact on intracranial pressure and allows a very rapid induction and recovery with minimal sympathetic reaction. It is still quite expensive, however, which may limit its use. The dosage of anesthetics may need to be higher in children, and that factor will be considered by the anesthetist.

Nursing care after general anesthesia should include support and reassurance; assessment of the child for any skin breakdown related to immobility; and safety precautions until full recovery has occurred.

Local anesthetics are used in children in much the same way that they are used in adults.

Bupivacaine and tetracaine do not have established doses for children younger than 12 years of age. Benzocaine should not be used in children younger than 1 year of age.

When topically applying a local anesthetic, it is important to remember that there is greater risk of systemic absorption and toxicity with infants.

Tight diapers can act like occlusive dressings and increase systemic absorption. Children need to be cautioned not to bite themselves when receiving dental anesthesia.

ADULTS

Adults require a considerable amount of teaching and support when receiving anesthetics, including what will happen, what they will feel, how it will feel when they recover, and the approximate time to recovery.

Adults should be monitored closely until fully recovered from general anesthetics and should be cautioned to prevent injury when receiving local anesthetics. It is important to remember to reassure and talk to adults who may be aware of their surroundings yet unable to speak.

Most of the general anesthetics are not recommended for use during pregnancy because of the potential risk to the fetus. Short-onset and local anesthetics are frequently used at delivery. Use of a regional or other local anesthetic is usually preferred if surgery is needed during pregnancy. During lactation, it is recommended that the mother wait 4 to 6 hours to feed the baby after the anesthetic is used.

OLDER ADULTS

Older patients are more likely to experience the adverse effects associated with these drugs, including CNS, CV, and dermatological effects. Thinner skin and the possibility of decreased perfusion to the skin make them especially susceptible to skin breakdown during immobility. Because older patients often also have renal or hepatic impairment, they are also more likely to have toxic levels of the drug related to changes in metabolism and excretion. The older patient should have safety measures in effect, such as side rails, a call light, and assistance to ambulate; special efforts to provide skin care to prevent skin breakdown are especially important with older skin. The older patient may require longer monitoring and regular orienting and reassuring. After general anesthesia, it is very important to promote vigorous pulmonary toilet to decrease the risk of pneumonia.

- *Cardiovascular (CV) factors:* Underlying vascular disease, coronary artery disease, or hypotension, which put patients at risk for severe reactions to anesthesia, such as hypotension and shock, dysrhythmias, and ischemia.
- *Respiratory factors:* Obstructive pulmonary disease (e.g., asthma, chronic obstructive pulmonary disease, bronchitis), which can complicate the delivery of gas anesthetics, as well as the intubation and mechanical ventilation that must be used in most cases of general anesthesia.
- *Renal and hepatic function:* Conditions that interfere with the metabolism and excretion of anesthetics (e.g., acute renal failure, hepatitis) and could result in prolonged anesthesia and the need for continued support during recovery. Toxic reactions to the accumulation of abnormally high levels of anesthetic agents may even occur.

Balanced Anesthesia

With the wide variety of drugs available the therapeutic effects required need to be balanced with the potential for adverse effects. This is accomplished by **balanced anesthesia**—the combining of several drugs, each with a specific effect, to achieve analgesia, muscle relaxation, unconsciousness, and amnesia rather than using one drug. Balanced anesthesia commonly involves the following agents:

- *Preoperative medications*, which may include the use of anticholinergics that decrease secretions to facilitate intubation and prevent bradycardia associated with neural depression.
- *Sedative–hypnotics* to relax the patient, facilitate amnesia, and decrease sympathetic stimulation.
- *Antiemetics* to decrease the nausea and vomiting associated with the slowing of GI activity.
- *Antihistamines* to decrease the chance of allergic reaction and help to dry up secretions.
- *Narcotics* to aid analgesia and sedation.

Many of these drugs are given before the general anesthetic is administered to facilitate the process. Some are continued during surgery to aid the general anesthetic, allowing therapeutic effects at lower doses. For example, patients may receive a neuromuscular junction (NMJ) blocker (Chapter 28) to stop muscle activity and a rapid-acting intravenous general anesthetic to induce anesthesia, and then a gas general anesthetic to balance the anesthetic effect during the procedure and allow for easier recovery. Careful selection of appropriate general anesthetic agents, along with monitoring and support of the patient, helps to alleviate many problems.

Administration of General Anesthesia

General anesthesia is delivered by a physician or nurse anesthetist trained in the delivery of these potent drugs along with intubation, mechanical ventilation, and full life support. During the delivery of anesthesia, the patient can go through predictable stages (Figure 27.1), referred to as the depth of anesthesia:

Stage 1, the analgesia stage, refers to the loss of pain sensation, with the patient still conscious and able to communicate.

Stage 2, the excitement stage, is a period of excitement and often combative behavior, with many signs of sympathetic stimulation (e.g., tachycardia, increased respirations, blood pressure changes).

Stage 3, surgical anesthesia, involves relaxation of skeletal muscles, return of regular respirations, and progressive loss of eye reflexes and pupil dilation. Surgery can be safely performed in stage 3.

Stage 4, medullary paralysis, is very deep CNS depression with loss of respiratory and vasomotor center stimuli, in which death can occur rapidly. If a patient reaches this level the anesthesia has become too intense and the situation is critical.

General anesthesia administration also is divided into three phases: Induction, maintenance, and recovery.

Induction

Induction is the period from the beginning of anesthesia until stage 3, or surgical anesthesia, is reached. The

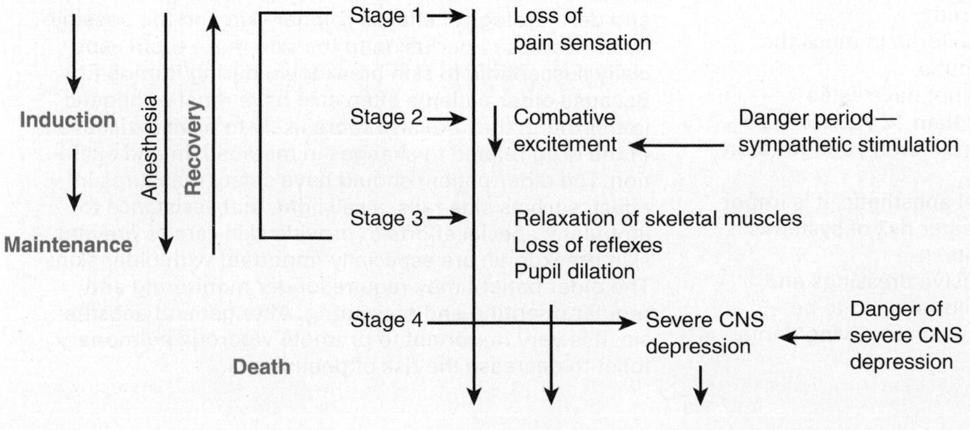

FIGURE 27.1 Stages of general anesthesia.

danger period for many patients during induction is stage 2 because of the systemic stimulation that occurs. Often a rapid-acting anesthetic is used to move quickly through this phase and into stage 3. NMJ blockers may be used during induction to facilitate intubation, which is necessary to support the patient with mechanical ventilation during anesthesia (see Chapter 28).

Maintenance

Maintenance is the period from stage 3 until the surgical procedure is complete. A slower, more predictable anesthetic, such as a gas anesthetic, may be used to maintain the anesthesia once the patient is in stage 3.

Recovery

Recovery is the period from discontinuation of the anesthetic until the patient has regained consciousness, movement, and the ability to communicate. During recovery the patient requires continuous monitoring for any adverse effects of the drugs used, and ensure support of the patient's vital functions as necessary.

KEY POINTS

- General anesthesia produces analgesia, amnesia, and unconsciousness.
- General anesthesia places the patient at risk for problems because of its extensive CNS depression and widespread effects on other body systems.
- Balanced anesthesia involves the administration of several drugs rather than a single drug to achieve analgesia, muscle relaxation, unconsciousness, and amnesia.
- Induction of anesthesia is the period ranging from administration of the anesthetic to the point of surgical anesthesia.

General Anesthetic Agents

Several different types of drugs are used as general anesthetics. These include barbiturate and nonbarbiturate anesthetics, gas anesthetics, and volatile liquids. See Table 27.1 for a listing of general anesthetic agents along with the anticipated adverse effects of these drugs.

Table 27.1 ***Drugs in Focus:* General Anesthetic Agents**

				Systems Alert[a]					
Drug Name	**Onset**	**Recovery**	**Analgesia**	***CV***	***Resp.***	***CNS***	***GI***	***Renal***	***Hepatic***
Barbiturate Anesthetics									
methohexital (*Brevital*)	10–30 s	3–4 min	None	—	+++	—	—	—	—
Nonbarbiturate General Anesthetics									
droperidol (*Inapsine*)	3–10 min	2–4 h	—	++	—	+	—	+	+
etomidate (*Amidate*)	1 min	3–5 min	—	—		+	++	—	
ketamine (*Ketalar*)	30 s	45 min	+	++	—	+++	—	—	—
midazolam (*generic*)	15 min	30 min	+	—	+++	—	++	—	—
propofol (*Diprivan*)	30–60 s	25–100 min	+	++	+	++	—	—	—
Anesthetic Gases									
nitrous oxide (*Blue*)	1–2 min	Rapid	++++	+++	+		—	—	—
Volatile Liquids									
desflurane (*Suprane*)	1–2 min	15–20 min	+	—	++++		—	—	—
enflurane (*Ethrane*)	1–2 min	15–20 min	+	+	+		—	++	
isoflurane (*generic*)	1–2 min	15–20 min	+	++	+	—	+	—	—
sevoflurane (*Ultane*)	30 s	10 min	+	—	++	—	—	—	—

[a]Systems alert indicates physiological systems with anticipated adverse effects to these drugs. When drugs are selected, the patient's condition and potential for serious problems with these adverse effects should be considered.
—, no effect; +, mild effect, ++, moderate effect; +++, strong effect; ++++, powerful effect; CV, cardiovascular; Resp., respiratory; CNS, central nervous system; GI, gastrointestinal.

Barbiturate Anesthetics

Barbiturate anesthetics (Table 27.1) are intravenous drugs used to induce rapid anesthesia, they are then maintained with an inhaled drug. Methohexital (*Brevital*) is the only drug remaining in this class (see Box 27.2, Focus on The Evidence: The Loss of Thiopental).

Therapeutic Actions and Indications

Methohexital lacks analgesic properties, and the patient may require postoperative analgesics.

Pharmacokinetics

Methohexital has a rapid onset of action and a recovery period that is usually 3 to 4 minutes. This drug is lipophilic. It is dissolved and rapidly absorbed through the lipid blood–brain barrier and diffuses into the brain very rapidly.

Contraindications and Cautions

Methohexital cannot come in contact with silicone (rubber stoppers and disposable syringes often contain silicone) *because it will cause an immediate breakdown of the silicone*. As a result, it poses special problems, and special precautions must be taken. This drug should not be used until the anesthesiologist and staff are ready and equipped for intubation and respiratory support *because of the rapid onset and because these drugs can cause respiratory depression and apnea*. This drug should not be used during pregnancy or lactation unless the benefit clearly outweighs the potential risk to the fetus or neonate *because of the CNS-depressive effects of these drugs*.

Adverse Effects

The adverse effects associated with these drugs are related to the suppression of the CNS with decreased pulse, hypotension, suppressed respirations, and decreased GI activity. Nausea and vomiting after recovery are common.

Clinically Important Drug–Drug Interactions

Caution must be used when these drugs are used with any other CNS suppressants. Barbiturates can cause decreased effectiveness of theophylline, oral anticoagulants, beta-blockers, corticosteroids, hormonal contraceptives, phenylbutazones, metronidazole, quinidine, and carbamazepine. Combinations of barbiturate anesthetics and narcotics may produce apnea more commonly than occurs with other analgesics.

Prototype Summary: Methohexital

Indications: Induction of anesthesia, maintenance of anesthesia; induction of a hypnotic state.

Actions: Depresses the CNS to produce hypnosis and anesthesia without analgesia.

Pharmacokinetics:

Route	Onset	Duration
IV	30 s	3–4 min
IM	2–10 min	20–30 min
Rectal	5–15 min	20–30 min

$T_{1/2}$: 3 to 8 hours; metabolized in the liver, excreted in the urine.

Adverse Effects: Emergence delirium, headache, restlessness, anxiety, CV depression, respiratory depression, apnea, salivation, hiccups, skin rashes.

BOX 27.2 FOCUS ON The Evidence

The Loss of Thiopental

In recent years thiopental (*Pentothal*) became very hard to find and now is no longer available in the United States. Many anesthesiologists are very concerned about this loss of a really good drug for people needing anesthesia. The problem revolved around the use of thiopental as part of a three-drug cocktail used for lethal injection. In states where death by lethal injection is an approved capital punishment a combination of first thiopental, which would cause unconsciousness and relaxation; followed by a paralytic, usually a neuromuscular junction blocker (Chapter 28), which could cause total muscle flaccidity and stop the jerking and muscle spasms that occur in response to high potassium levels and death; and then IV potassium, which would rapidly cause cardiac death. The rapid onset of action of the drugs and the relaxed state of the patient were considered acceptable as not causing unusual pain and suffering. The manufacturers of thiopental slowly stopped producing the drug, as a protest to the use of the death penalty. States still using lethal injection had to find other combinations to use. Several lawsuits have followed because a good alternative is not yet available. The use of only midazolam and hydromorphone resulted in a drawn-out struggle which included gasping for air, muscle spasms and twitching. Other combinations are being tried with varying success. In 2010 the American Nurses Association (ANA) issued a position statement on the role of the nurse in capital punishment situations. The ANA is strongly opposed to any nurse participation in any part of the process. This procedure, it stated, is against the established ethical principles that govern the profession of nursing. In the meantime, patients no longer have access to a very good anesthetic agent and anesthesiologists work to find the best combination for use in surgery.

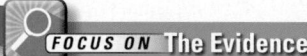

Nonbarbiturate Anesthetics

The other parenteral drugs used for intravenous administration in anesthesia are nonbarbiturates with a wide variety of effects. Such anesthetics include droperidol (*Inapsine*), etomidate (*Amidate*), ketamine (*Ketalar*), midazolam (well known as *Versed* but only available in a generic form as that brand name has been retired), and propofol (*Diprivan*) (see Table 27.1).

Therapeutic Action and Indications

Midazolam is the prototype nonbarbiturate anesthetic. It is a very potent amnesiac. These drugs are thought to act in the reticular activating system and limbic system to potentiate the effects of gamma-aminobutyric acid. Midazolam's amnesiac effects occur at doses below those needed to cause sedation. It is widely used to produce amnesia or sedation for many diagnostic, therapeutic, and endoscopic procedures. Midazolam can also be used to induce anesthesia and to provide continuous sedation for intubated and mechanically ventilated patients. Droperidol produces marked sedation and produces a state of mental detachment. It also has antiemetic effects, reducing the incidence of nausea and vomiting in surgical and diagnostic procedures. Etomidate is used as a general anesthetic and is sometimes used to sedate patients receiving mechanical ventilation. Ketamine has been associated with a bizarre state of unconsciousness in which the patient appears to be awake but is unconscious and cannot feel pain. This drug, which causes sympathetic stimulation with increase in blood pressure and heart rate, may be helpful in situations when cardiac depression is dangerous. Propofol often is used for short procedures because it has a very rapid clearance and produces much less of a hangover effect and allows for quick recovery. It is also used to maintain patients on mechanical ventilation.

Pharmacokinetics

Midazolam has a rapid onset but does not reach peak effectiveness for 30 to 60 minutes. Droperidol has an onset of action within 3 minutes and an ultrashort recovery period. Etomidate has an onset within 1 minute and a rapid recovery period within 3 to 5 minutes. Ketamine has an onset of action within 30 seconds and a very slow recovery period (45 minutes). Propofol is a very short-acting anesthetic with a rapid onset of action of 30 to 60 seconds.

Contraindications and Cautions

Midazolam is more likely to cause nausea and vomiting than are some of the other anesthetics, and so it should be used with caution in any patient who could be compromised by vomiting. It has been associated with respiratory depression and respiratory arrest, and so life support equipment should be readily available whenever it is used. Droperidol should be used with caution in patients with renal or hepatic failure and should be used with extreme care in patients with prolonged QT intervals or who are at risk for prolonged QT intervals. Etomidate is not recommended for use in children younger than 10 years of age.

Adverse Effects

Patients receiving any general anesthetic are at risk for skin breakdown because they will not be able to move. Care must be taken to prevent decubitus ulcer formation. Patients receiving midazolam should be monitored for respiratory depression and CNS suppression (Figure 27.2). During the recovery period, droperidol may cause hypotension, chills, hallucinations, and drowsiness. It may also cause QT prolongation, which puts the patient at risk for serious cardiac arrhythmias. During the recovery period with etomidate, many patients experience myoclonic and tonic movements, as well as nausea and vomiting. Ketamine crosses the blood–brain barrier and can cause hallucinations, dreams, and psychotic episodes. Propofol often causes local burning on injection. It can cause bradycardia, hypotension, and in extreme cases pulmonary edema.

Clinically Important Drug–Drug Interactions

Droperidol should not be used with other drugs that prolong the QT interval. If this combination is necessary the patient should be monitored continuously. Ketamine may also potentiate the muscular blocking of NMJ blockers, and the patient may require prolonged periods of respiratory support. Midazolam is associated with increased

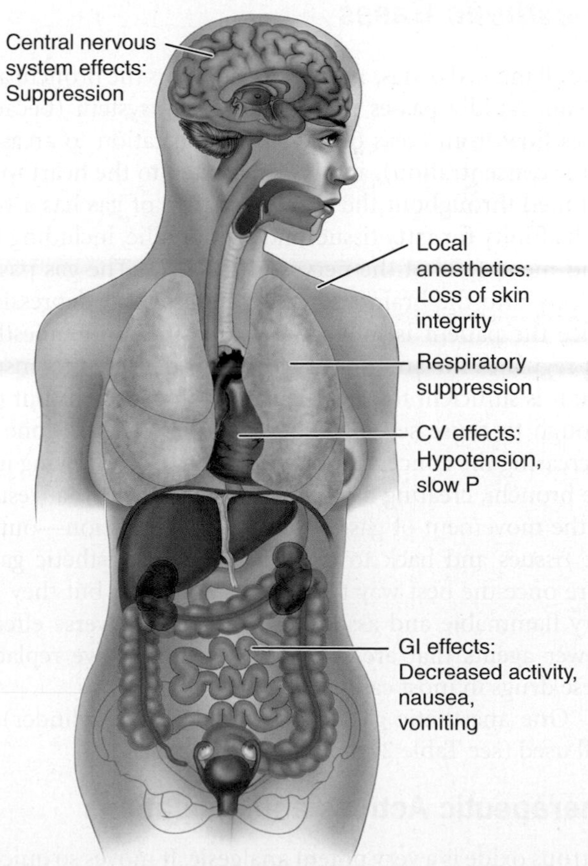

FIGURE 27.2 Common adverse effects associated with anesthetic agents.

toxicity and length of recovery when used in combination with inhaled anesthetics, other CNS depressants, narcotics, or propofol. If any of these agents are used in combination, careful balancing of drug doses is necessary.

Prototype Summary: Midazolam

Indications: Sedation, anxiolysis, and amnesia before diagnostic, therapeutic, or endoscopic procedures; induction of anesthesia; continuous sedation of intubated patients.

Actions: Acts mainly at the limbic system and reticular activating system; potentiates the effects of gamma-aminobutyric acid; has little effect on cortical function; exact mechanism of action is not understood.

Pharmacokinetics:

Route	Onset	Peak	Duration
Oral	30–60 min	12 h	2–6 h
IM	15 min	30 min	2–6 h
IV	3–5 min	<30 min	2–6 h

$T_{1/2}$: 1.8 to 6.8 hours; metabolized in the liver, excreted in the urine.

Adverse Effects: Transient drowsiness, sedation, drowsiness, lethargy, apathy, fatigue, disorientation, restlessness, constipation, diarrhea, incontinence, urinary retention, bradycardia, tachycardia, phlebitis at IV injection site.

Anesthetic Gases

Like all inhaled drugs, anesthetic gas enters the bronchi and alveoli, rapidly passes into the capillary system (because gases flow from areas of higher concentration to areas of lower concentration), and is transported to the heart to be pumped throughout the body. This type of gas has a very high affinity for fatty tissue, and is lipophilic, including the lipid membrane of the nerves in the CNS. The gas passes quickly into the brain and causes severe CNS depression. Once the patient is in stage 3 of anesthesia the anesthetist regulates the amount of gas that is delivered to ensure that it is sufficient to keep the patient unconscious but not enough to cause severe CNS depression. This is done by decreasing the concentration of the gas that is flowing into the bronchi, creating a concentration gradient that results in the movement of gas in the opposite direction—out of the tissues and back to expired air. The anesthetic gases were once the best way to achieve anesthesia, but they are very flammable and associated with toxic adverse effects. Newer agents that are safer and less toxic have replaced these drugs in most cases.

One anesthetic gas, nitrous oxide (blue cylinder), is still used (see Table 27.1).

Therapeutic Actions and Indications

Nitrous oxide is a very potent analgesic. It moves so quickly in and out of the body that it can actually accumulate and cause pressure in closed body compartments such as the sinuses. Because nitrous oxide is such a potent analgesic, it is used frequently for dental surgery. It does not cause muscle relaxation. Nitrous oxide is usually combined with other agents for anesthetic use.

Pharmacokinetics

Nitrous oxide has a rapid onset of action, usually within 1 to 2 minutes, and a rapid recovery period. Timing of recovery depends on the other drugs being used.

Contraindications and Cautions

Nitrous oxide can block the reuptake of oxygen after surgery and cause hypoxia. Because of this reaction, it is always given in combination with oxygen. Susceptible patients should be monitored for signs of hypoxia, chest pain, and stroke. This drug should not be used during pregnancy unless the benefit clearly outweighs the potential risk to the fetus. Nursing mothers should wait 4 hours before nursing a baby when they have been administered nitrous oxide.

Adverse Effects

As with other general anesthetics, patients need to be monitored for skin integrity when they are not able to move for periods of time. Nitrous oxide can cause acute sinus and middle-ear pain, bowel obstruction, and pneumothorax because it so rapidly moves into and accumulates in closed spaces. Because nitrous oxide inactivates vitamin B_{12}, patients should also be monitored for low vitamin B_{12} levels, including neurological, immune, and hematological complications.

Clinically Important Drug–Drug Interactions

Caution should be used if these drugs are combined with any other drug that causes CNS depression. If these agents must be used together the patient should be monitored closely.

Prototype Summary: Nitrous Oxide

Indications: Induction and maintenance of anesthesia.

Actions: Depresses the CNS to produce anesthesia and analgesia.

Pharmacokinetics:

Route	Onset	Duration
Inhalation	1–2 min	20 min

$T_{1/2}$: Minutes; not metabolized, excreted in the lungs.

Adverse Effects: CV depression, respiratory depression, apnea, earache, sinus pain, vomiting, malignant hyperthermia.

Volatile Liquids

Inhaled anesthetics also can be **volatile liquids**—liquids that are unstable at room temperature and release gases. These gases are then inhaled by the patient. Therefore, volatile liquids act like gas anesthetics.

Most of the volatile liquids in use are halogenated hydrocarbons such as desflurane (*Suprane*), enflurane (*Ethrane*), isoflurane (*Forane*), and sevoflurane (*Ultane*) (see Table 27.1).

Therapeutic Actions and Indications

Desflurane is widely used in outpatient surgery because of its rapid onset and quick recovery time. Isoflurane is widely used to maintain anesthesia after inductions. It can cause muscle relaxation. Sevoflurane is used in outpatient surgery as an induction agent and is rapidly cleared for quick recovery.

Pharmacokinetics

Desflurane, enflurane, and isoflurane have a rapid onset—also within 1 to 2 minutes—and rapid recovery—usually within 15 to 20 minutes. Sevoflurane, the newest of the volatile liquids, has a very rapid onset of action—within 30 seconds—and a very rapid clearance—lasting only about 10 minutes. These drugs are all cleared through the lungs.

Contraindications and Cautions

Desflurane use should be avoided in patients with respiratory problems and in those with increased sensitivity *because of its irritation to the airways and tendency to cause respiratory depression.* In addition, it is not recommended for induction in pediatric patients *because of its irritation of the airways.* Enflurane should not be used in patients with known cardiac or respiratory disease or renal dysfunction *because it is associated with renal toxicity, cardiac arrhythmias, and respiratory depression.* Isoflurane and sevoflurane should be used with caution in patients with respiratory depression *to avoid severe respiratory depression.* All of these drugs have the potential to trigger malignant hyperthermia and should be used with caution in any patient at high risk for developing it *to avoid development of malignant hyperthermia.* Dantrolene, the preferred treatment for malignant hyperthermia, should be readily available whenever any of these drugs is used. These drugs should be avoided in pregnancy and lactation unless the benefit clearly outweighs the risk to the fetus or baby *because of the CNS-depressive effects of the drugs.*

Adverse Effects

Desflurane is associated with a collection of respiratory reactions, including cough, increased secretions, and laryngospasm. Isoflurane is associated with hypotension, hypercapnia, muscle soreness, and a bad taste in the mouth, but it does not cause cardiac arrhythmias or respiratory irritation as do some other volatile liquids. Enflurane may cause renal impairment. Adverse effects of sevoflurane are thought to be minimal.

Clinically Important Drug–Drug Interactions

Caution should be used when any of these drugs is combined with other CNS suppressants.

Prototype Summary: Desflurane

Indications: Induction and maintenance of general anesthesia.

Actions: Depresses the CNS, causing anesthesia; relaxes muscles; sensitizes the myocardium to the effects of norepinephrine and epinephrine.

Pharmacokinetics:

Route	Onset	Peak	Duration
Inhaled	Rapid	Rapid	End of inhalation

$T_{1/2}$: Unknown; metabolized in the liver, excreted in the urine.

Adverse Effects: Transient drowsiness, sedation, lethargy, apathy, fatigue, disorientation, restlessness, bradycardia, tachycardia, hypoxia, acidosis, apnea, cough, laryngospasm.

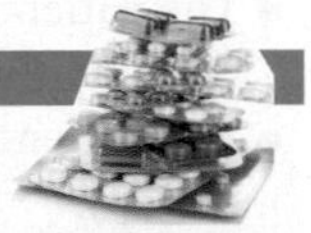

Nursing Considerations for Patients Receiving General Anesthetic Agents

Assessment: History and Examination

- Assess for *contraindications or cautions*: Any known allergies to general anesthetics *to avoid hypersensitivity reactions*; impaired liver or kidney function, *which might interfere with drug metabolism and excretion*; myasthenia gravis or cardiac or respiratory disease, *which may be exacerbated by the depressive effects of the drug*; personal or family history of malignant hyperthermia, *which may be triggered by the use of general anesthetics.*
- Perform a physical assessment, including weighing the patient, *to determine the appropriate dosing of the drug and to establish a baseline status before beginning therapy and evaluate for any potential adverse effects.*
- Assess the patient's neurological status, including level of consciousness, affect, reflexes, and pupil size and reaction, and evaluate muscle tone and response, *to monitor CNS depression and provide appropriate support as needed.*

(continues on page 468)

- Monitor vital signs, including temperature, pulse, and blood pressure, for changes, and auscultate lung and heart sounds *to monitor for adverse effects of the drugs.*
- Obtain an electrocardiogram (ECG) *to evaluate for underlying cardiac problems that may be exacerbated by the drug.*
- Assess skin color and lesions *to monitor for potential skin breakdown resulting from patient paralysis and immobility while under anesthesia.*
- Auscultate abdomen for bowel sounds *to evaluate GI motility.*
- Monitor the results of laboratory tests, including renal and liver function tests, *to determine the possible need for a reduction in dose and evaluate for possible toxicity.*

Nursing Diagnoses

Nursing diagnoses related to drug therapy might include the following:

- Impaired gas exchange related to respiratory depression.
- Impaired skin integrity related to immobility secondary to effects of positioning during anesthesia and immobility.
- Risk for injury related to CNS-depressive effects of the drug.
- Disturbed thought processes and disturbed sensory perception related to CNS depression.
- Deficient knowledge regarding drug therapy.

Planning

- The patient will receive the best therapeutic effect from the drug therapy.
- The patient will have limited adverse effects to the drug therapy.
- The patient will have an understanding of the drug therapy, adverse effects to anticipate, and measures to relieve discomfort and improve safety.

Implementation with Rationale

- Keep in mind that the drug must be administered by trained personnel (usually an anesthesiologist) *because of the potential risks associated with its use.*
- Have emergency equipment to maintain airway and provide mechanical ventilation readily available *when patient is not able to maintain respiration because of CNS depression.*
- Monitor temperature *for prompt detection and treatment of malignant hyperthermia.* Maintain dantrolene on standby.
- Monitor pulse, respiration, blood pressure, ECG, and cardiac output continually during administration *to assess systemic response to CNS depression and provide appropriate support as needed.*
- Monitor temperature and reflexes because *dose adjustment may be needed to alleviate potential problems and to maximize overall benefit with the least toxicity.*
- Institute safety precautions, such as side rails, and monitor patient until the recovery phase is complete and the patient is conscious and able to move and communicate *to ensure patient safety.*
- Provide comfort measures *to help the patient tolerate drug effects.* Provide pain relief as appropriate, along with reassurance and support, *to deal with the effects of anesthesia and loss of control;* skin care and turning *to prevent skin breakdown;* and supportive care *for conditions such as hypotension and bronchospasm.*
- Offer support and encouragement *to help the patient cope with the procedure and the drugs being used.*
- Provide preoperative patient teaching, *realizing that most patients who receive the drug will be unconscious or will be receiving teaching about a particular procedure:*
  - Information about the anesthetic (e.g., what to expect, rate of onset, time to recovery)
  - Medications that may be used preoperatively
  - Effects of the medication on the patient preoperatively
  - Measures to maintain the patient's safety preoperatively and during recovery
  - How the patient will feel during the recovery phase
  - Signs and symptoms to report during recovery and afterward

Evaluation

- Monitor patient response to the drug (analgesia, loss of consciousness).
- Monitor for adverse effects (respiratory depression, hypotension, bronchospasm, slowed GI activity, skin breakdown, malignant hyperthermia).
- Evaluate the effectiveness of the teaching plan (patient can relate anticipated effects of the drug and the recovery process).
- Monitor the effectiveness of comfort and safety measures.

KEY POINTS

- General anesthetics must be administered by physicians or nurse anesthetists trained in their administration and prepared to provide constant monitoring and life support measures to assist the patient when the CNS is depressed.
- General anesthetics include barbiturates and nonbarbiturate drugs, which are administered parenterally, and anesthetic gases and volatile liquids, which are administered through inhalation.
- Patients receiving general anesthetics must be constantly monitored because the CNS depression can cause respiratory arrest, CV reactions including hypotension, and alterations in GI activity that can lead to nausea and vomiting.

Local Anesthesia

Local anesthesia refers to a loss of sensation in limited areas of the body. Local anesthesia can be achieved by several different methods: Topical administration, infiltration, field block, nerve block, and intravenous regional anesthesia.

Topical Administration

Topical local anesthesia involves the application of a cream, lotion, ointment, or drop of a local anesthetic to traumatized skin to relieve pain. It can also involve applying these forms to the mucous membranes in the eye, nose, throat, mouth, urethra, anus, or rectum to relieve pain or to anesthetize the area to facilitate a medical procedure. Although systemic absorption is rare with topical application, it can occur if there is damage or breakdown of the tissues in the area.

Infiltration

Infiltration local anesthesia involves injecting the anesthetic directly into the tissues to be treated (e.g., sutured, drilled, cut). This injection brings the anesthetic into contact with the nerve endings in the area and prevents them from transmitting nerve impulses to the brain.

Field Block

Field block local anesthesia involves injecting the anesthetic all around the area that will be affected by the procedure or surgery. This is more intense than infiltration anesthesia because the anesthetic agent comes in contact with all of the nerve endings surrounding the area. This type of block is often used for tooth extractions.

Nerve Block

Nerve block local anesthesia involves injecting the anesthetic at some point along the nerve or nerves that run to and from the region in which the loss of pain sensation or muscle paralysis is desired. These blocks are performed not in the surgical field, but at some distance from the field. They involve a greater area with potential for more adverse effects. Several types of nerve blocks are possible:

- *Peripheral nerve block:* Blockage of the sensory and motor aspects of a particular nerve for relief of pain or for diagnostic purposes.
- *Central nerve block:* Injection of anesthetic into the roots of the nerves in the spinal cord.
- *Epidural anesthesia:* Injection of the drug into the epidural space where the nerves emerge from the spinal cord.
- *Caudal block:* Injection of anesthetic into the sacral canal, below the epidural area.
- *Spinal anesthesia:* Injection of anesthetic into the spinal subarachnoid space.

Intravenous Regional Local Anesthesia

Intravenous regional local anesthesia involves carefully draining all of the blood from the patient's arm or leg, securing a tourniquet to prevent the anesthetic from entering the general circulation, and then injecting the anesthetic into the vein of the arm or leg. This technique is used for very specific surgical procedures.

Local Anesthetic Agents

Local anesthetic agents (Table 27.2) are used primarily to prevent the patient from feeling pain for varying periods of time after the agents have been administered in the peripheral nervous system. In increasing concentrations, local anesthetics can also cause loss of the following sensations (in this sequence): Temperature, touch, proprioception (position sense), and skeletal muscle tone. If these other aspects of nerve function are progressively lost, recovery occurs in the reverse order of the loss.

The local anesthetics are very powerful nerve blockers, and it is very important that their effects be limited to a particular area of the body. They should not be absorbed systemically. Systemic absorption could produce toxic effects on the nervous system and the heart (e.g., severe CNS depression, cardiac arrhythmias).

Local anesthetics are classified as esters or amides. The agent of choice depends on the method of administration, the length of time for which the area is to be anesthetized, and consideration of potential adverse effects. Esters include benzocaine (*Dermoplast, Lanacane, Unguentine*), chloroprocaine (*Nesacaine*) and tetracaine (*Pontocaine*). Amides include bupivacaine (*Marcaine, Sensorcaine*), dibucaine (*Nupercainal*), lidocaine (*Dilocaine, Solarcaine, Xylocaine, Lidoderm, Octocaine*), mepivacaine (*Carbocaine, Isocaine, Polocaine*), prilocaine (*Citanest Dental*), and ropivacaine (*Naropin*). Pramoxine (*Tronothane, PrameGel, Itch-X, Prax*) is a local anesthetic agent that does not fit into either of these classes.

Therapeutic Actions and Indications

Local anesthetics work by causing a temporary interruption in the production and conduction of nerve impulses. They affect the permeability of nerve membranes to sodium ions, which normally infuse into the cell in response to stimulation. By preventing the sodium ions from entering the nerve, they stop the nerve from depolarizing. A particular section of the nerve cannot be stimulated, and nerve impulses directed toward that section are lost when they reach that area.

The way in which a local anesthetic is administered helps to increase its effectiveness by delivering it directly to the area that is causing or will cause the pain, thereby decreasing systemic absorption and related toxic effects (Figure 27.3). Local anesthetics are indicated for

Table 27.2 ***Drugs in Focus:*** **Local Anesthetic Agents**

Drug name	Onset	Duration	Administration	Special Considerations
Esters				
benzocaine (*Dermoplast, Lanacane, Unguentine*)	1 min	30–60 min	Skin, mucous membranes	Avoid tight bandages with skin preparation
chloroprocaine (*Nesacaine*)	6–15 min	15–75 min	Nerve block, caudal, epidural	Do not use with subarachnoid administration
tetracaine (*Pontocaine*)	15–30 min	2–25 h	Spinal, prolonged spinal, skin	Monitor skin condition if immobile; provide reassurance if prolonged; keep supine to avoid headache after spinal
Amides				
bupivacaine (*Marcaine, Sensorcaine*)	5–20 min	2–7 h	Local, epidural, dental, caudal, subarachnoid, sympathetic, retrobulbar	Do not use Bier block—deaths have occurred
dibucaine (*Nupercainal*)	<15 min	3–4 h	Skin, mucous membranes	Monitor for local reactions
lidocaine (*Dilocaine, Solarcaine, Xylocaine, Lidoderm, Octocaine*)	5–15 min	30–90 min	Caudal, epidural, spinal, cervical, dental, skin, mucous membrane, topical patch	Short acting, preferred for short procedures; danger if absorbed systemically
mepivacaine (*Carbocaine, Isocaine, Polocaine*)	3–15 min	45–90 min	Nerve block, obstetric, cervical, epidural, dental, local infiltration	Caution with renal impairment
prilocaine (*Cilanest*)	1–15 min	0.5–3 h	Nerve block, dental	Advise patients not to bite themselves
ropivacaine (*Naropin*)	1–5 min	2–6 h	Nerve block, epidural, caudal	Avoid rapid infusion; offers good pain management postop and obstetrics
Other				
pramoxine (*Tronothane, PrameGel, Itch-X, Prax*)	3–5 min	<60 min	Skin, mucous membranes	Do not cover with tight bandages; protect patient from injury

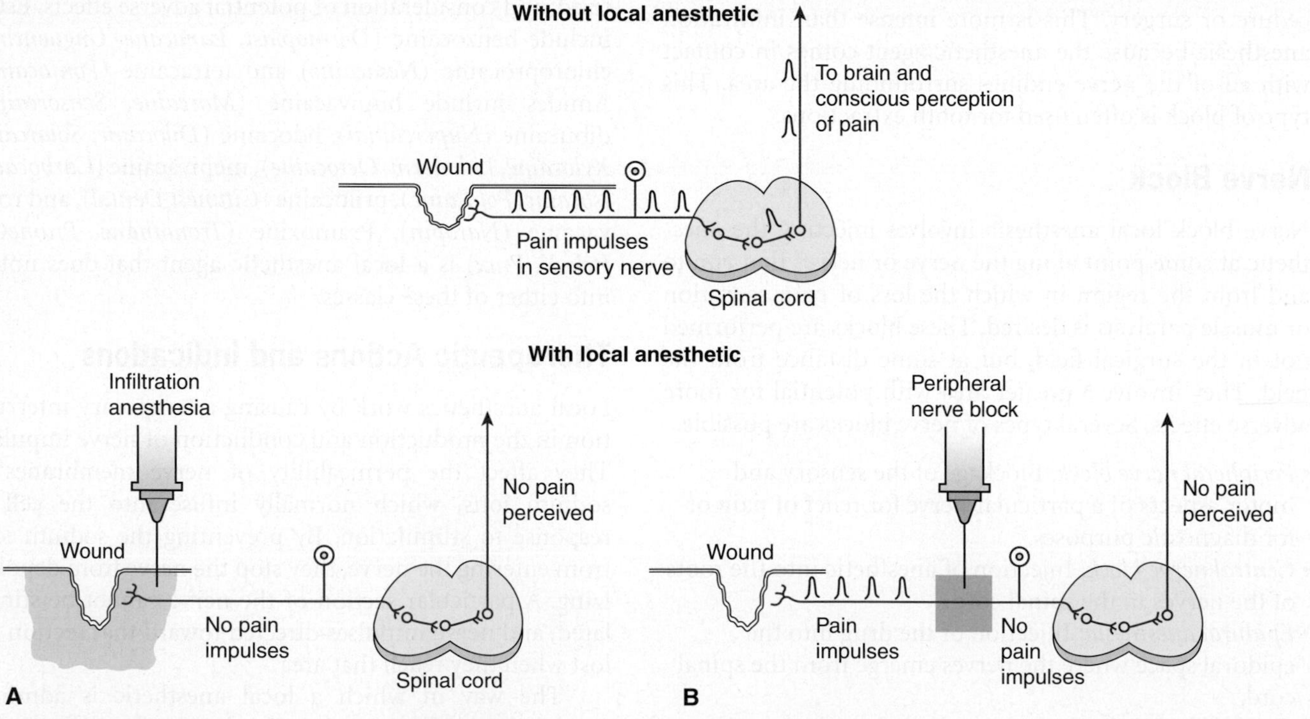

FIGURE 27.3 Mechanism of action of local anesthetics.(**Top**) An injury produces pain impulses (action potentials) that are conducted and transmitted in an area of the brain in which pain is perceived. **A:** Conduction of the pain impulse has been blocked by infiltration anesthetics at the site of the injury. **B:** A nerve block at some distance from the injury. Local anesthetics block the movement of sodium into the nerve and prevent nerve depolarization, stopping the transmission of the pain impulse.

infiltration anesthesia, peripheral nerve block, spinal anesthesia, and the relief of local pain. In 2005 the U.S. Food and Drug Administration approved a local anesthetic product that combines lidocaine and tetracaine in a dermal patch, called *Synera* (see Focus on Safe Medication Administration, under Contraindications and Cautions, for more information about this drug.)

Pharmacokinetics

The ester local anesthetics are broken down immediately in the plasma by enzymes known as **plasma esterases**. The amide local anesthetics are metabolized more slowly in the liver, and serum levels of these drugs can increase and lead to toxicity.

Contraindications and Cautions

The local anesthetics are contraindicated with any of the following conditions: History of allergy to any one of these agents or to parabens *to avoid hypersensitivity reactions*; heart block, *which could be greatly exacerbated with systemic absorption*; shock, *which could alter the local delivery and absorption of these drugs*; and decreased plasma esterases, *which could result in toxic levels of the ester-type local anesthetics*.

They should be used during pregnancy and lactation only if the benefit outweighs any potential risk to the fetus or neonate if the drug is inadvertently absorbed systemically *because of the suppressive effects on nerves*.

FOCUS ON Safe Medication Administration

Combination Local Anesthetic

***Synera**, a local anesthetic product that is a combination of lidocaine and tetracaine and is available in a dermal patch was approved for use on intact skin to provide local dermal anesthesia when doing venipunctures or inserting IV cannulae or for superficial dermatological procedures that could cause discomfort for the patient. When using it for venipunctures or inserting an IV, one patch is applied 20 to 30 minutes before the procedure. If a superficial dermatological procedure is being performed, one patch is applied to the area 30 minutes before the procedure. The patch must be removed if the patient is undergoing a magnetic resonance imaging scan to prevent burning related to the dermal patch. The site should be monitored for any local irritation.*

Adverse Effects

The adverse effects of these drugs may be related to their local blocking of sensation (e.g., skin breakdown, self-injury, biting oneself). Loss of skin integrity is always a problem if the patient is unable to move, and care must be taken to prevent skin breakdown. Other problematic effects are associated with the route of administration and the amount of drug that is absorbed systemically. These effects are related to the blockade of nerve depolarization throughout the system. Effects that may occur include CNS effects such as headache (especially with epidural and spinal anesthesia), restlessness, anxiety, dizziness, tremors, blurred vision, and backache; GI effects such as nausea and vomiting; CV effects such as peripheral vasodilation, myocardial depression, arrhythmias, and blood pressure changes, all of which may lead to fatal cardiac arrest; and respiratory arrest.

Clinically Important Drug–Drug Interactions

When local anesthetics and succinylcholine are given together, increased and prolonged neuromuscular blockade occurs. There is also less risk of systemic absorption and increased local effects if these drugs are combined with epinephrine.

Prototype Summary: Lidocaine

Indications: Infiltration anesthesia, peripheral and sympathetic nerve blocks, central nerve blocks, spinal and caudal anesthesia, topical anesthetic for skin or mucous membrane disorders

Actions: Blocks the generation and conduction of action potentials in sensory nerves by reducing sodium permeability, reducing the height and rate of rise of the action potential, increasing the excitation threshold, and slowing the conduction velocity

Pharmacokinetics:

Route	Onset	Peak	Duration
IM	5–10 min	5–15 min	2 h
Topical	Not generally absorbed systemically		

$T_{1/2}$: 10 minutes, then 1.5 to 3 hours; metabolized in the liver, excreted in the urine

Adverse Effects: Headache, backache, hypotension, urinary retention, urinary incontinence, pruritus, seizures; when locally applied: Burning, stinging, swelling, tenderness.

Nursing Considerations for Patients Receiving Local Anesthetic Agents

Assessment: History and Examination

- Assess for *contraindications and cautions*: Any known allergies to these drugs or to parabens *to avoid hypersensitivity reactions*; impaired liver function, *which could alter metabolism and clearance of the drug*; low plasma esterases, *which could lead to toxicity of esters*; heart

(continues on page 472)

block, *which could be exacerbated by the drug effects*; shock *to prevent altered local delivery and absorption*; and current status of pregnancy or lactation, *which are cautions to the use of the drug.*
- Perform a physical assessment to establish a *baseline status before beginning therapy and for any potential adverse effects.*
- Inspect site for local anesthetic application *to ensure integrity of the skin and to prevent inadvertent systemic absorption of the drug.*
- Assess the patient's neurological status, including level of orientation, reflexes, pupil size and reaction, muscle tone and response, and sensation *to evaluate the effectiveness of the drug and monitor for potential toxic neurological effects.*
- Monitor vital signs, including temperature, pulse, and blood pressure, and assess respiratory rate and auscultate lungs *for adventitious sounds to identify changes and possible systemic absorption.*
- Monitor laboratory test results, such as liver function tests and plasma esterases (if appropriate), *to determine possible need for dose adjustment.*

Refer to the Critical Thinking Scenario for a full discussion of nursing care for a patient who is receiving local anesthesia.

Nursing Diagnoses

Nursing diagnoses related to drug therapy might include the following:

- Disturbed sensory perception (kinesthetic, tactile) related to local anesthetic effect
- Impaired skin integrity related to immobility caused by actions of the drug
- Risk for injury related to loss of sensation and mobility
- Deficient knowledge regarding drug therapy

Planning

- The patient will receive the best therapeutic effect from the drug therapy.
- The patient will have limited adverse effects to the drug therapy.
- The patient will have an understanding of the drug therapy, adverse effects to anticipate, and measures to relieve discomfort and improve safety

Implementation with Rationale

- Have emergency equipment readily available *to maintain airway and provide mechanical ventilation if needed.*
- Ensure that drugs for managing hypotension, cardiac arrest, and CNS alterations are readily available *in case of severe reaction and toxicity.*
- Ensure that patients receiving spinal anesthesia or epidural anesthesia are well hydrated and remain lying down for up to 12 hours after the anesthesia *to minimize headache.*
- Establish safety precautions *to prevent injury during the time that the patient has a loss of sensation and/or mobility.*
- Provide meticulous skin care to the site of administration *to reduce the risk of breakdown.*
- Provide comfort measures *to help the patient tolerate drug effects.* Provide pain relief, as well as skin care and turning *to prevent skin breakdown*, and supportive care for hypotension *to prevent shock or serious hypoxia.*
- Offer support and encouragement *to help the patient cope with the procedure and drugs being used.*
- Provide thorough patient teaching, including anesthetic to be given, method for administration, activities involved with administering and monitoring the drug, and safety precautions.

Evaluation

- Monitor patient response to the drug (loss of feeling in designated area).
- Monitor for adverse effects (respiratory depression, blood pressure changes, arrhythmias, GI upset, skin breakdown, injury, CNS alterations).
- Evaluate the effectiveness of the teaching plan (the patient can relate the anticipated effects of the drug and the recovery process).

CRITICAL THINKING SCENARIO

Local Anesthesia

THE SITUATION

A.M., a 32-year-old male athlete with a history of asthma (which could indicate pulmonary dysfunction), was admitted to the hospital for an inguinal hernia repair. At the patient's request the surgeon elected to use a local anesthetic employing spinal anesthesia. Because the extent of the repair was unknown (A.M. had undergone two previous repairs), bupivacaine, a long-acting anesthetic, was selected. He remained alert (blood pressure 120/64 mm Hg, pulse 62 beats/

Local Anesthesia (continued)

min, respiration rate 10/min) and stable throughout the procedure. Two hours after the conclusion of the procedure, A.M. appeared agitated (blood pressure 154/68 mm Hg, pulse 88 beats/min, respiration rate 12/min). Although he did not complain of discomfort, he did state that he still had no feeling and had only limited movement of his legs.

CRITICAL THINKING

What safety precautions need to be taken?
What nursing interventions should be done at this point?
How could the patient be reassured? *Think about the anxiety level of the patient—an athlete who elected to have local anesthesia may have a problem with control and feel somewhat invincible. Consider the anxiety that loss of mobility and sensation in the legs may cause in a person who makes his living as an athlete.*
In addition, consider the expected duration of action of bupivacaine and the rate of return of function.

DISCUSSION

Bupivacaine is a long-acting anesthetic with effects that may persist for several hours. The timing of the drug's effects should be explained to A.M., and he should be monitored for a period of time to determine whether his agitated state and slightly elevated vital signs are a result of anxiety or an unanticipated reaction to the surgery or the drug. Life support equipment should be on standby in case his condition is a toxic drug reaction or some unanticipated problem occurring after surgery.

The nurse is in the best position to perform the following interventions: Explaining the effects of the drug and the anticipated recovery schedule; keeping the patient as flat as possible to decrease the headache usually associated with spinal anesthesia; encouraging the patient to turn from side to side periodically to allow skin care to be performed and to alleviate the risk of pressure sore development; and staying with the patient as much as possible to reassure him, to answer his questions, and to encourage him to talk about his feelings and reaction.

If the agitated state is caused by a stress reaction the patient should return to normal; comfort measures, teaching, and reassurance should be provided. An elevated systolic pressure with a normal diastolic pressure often is an indication of a sympathetic stress response. An athlete is more likely than most people to suffer great anxiety and fear if his legs become numb and he is unable to move them. Teaching and comfort measures may be all that is needed to relieve the anxiety and ensure a good recovery.

NURSING CARE GUIDE FOR A.M.: LOCAL ANESTHESIA

Assessment: History and Examination

Assess for allergies to local anesthetics or to parabens, cardiac disorders, vascular problems, hepatic dysfunction; also assess for concurrent use of succinylcholine.
Focus physical examination on the following:
CV: Blood pressure, pulse, peripheral perfusion, ECG
CNS: Orientation, affect, reflexes, vision
Skin: Color, lesions, texture, sweating
Respiratory: Respiration, adventitious sounds
Laboratory tests: Liver function tests, plasma esterases

Nursing Diagnoses

Disturbed sensory perception (kinesthetic, tactile) related to anesthesia
Anxiety related to drug effects
Impaired skin integrity related to immobility
Risk for injury related to loss of sensation and mobility
Deficient knowledge regarding drug therapy

Planning

The patient will receive the best therapeutic effect from the drug therapy.
The patient will have limited adverse effects to the drug therapy.
The patient will have an understanding of the drug therapy, adverse effects to anticipate, and measures to relieve discomfort and improve safety.

Implementation

Provide comfort and safety measures: Positioning, skin care, side rails, pain medication as needed, maintain airway, antidotes on standby.
Provide support and reassurance to deal with loss of sensation and mobility.
Provide patient teaching about procedure being performed and what to expect.
Provide life support as needed.

Evaluation

Evaluate drug effects: Loss of sensation, loss of movement.
Monitor for adverse effects: CV effects (blood pressure changes, arrhythmias), respiratory depression, GI upset, CNS alterations, skin breakdown, anxiety, and fear.
Monitor for drug–drug interactions as indicated for each drug.
Evaluate the effectiveness of the patient-teaching program and comfort and safety measures.

(continues on page 474)

Local Anesthesia (continued)

Constantly monitor vital signs and muscular function and sensation as it returns.

PATIENT TEACHING FOR A.M.

Teaching about local anesthetics is usually incorporated into the overall teaching plan about the procedure that the patient will undergo. Things to highlight with the patient would include the following:

- Discussion of the overall procedure:
  - What it will feel like (any numbness, tingling, inability to move, pressure, pain, choking?)
  - Any anticipated discomfort
  - How long it will last
  - Concerns during the procedure: Report any discomfort and ask any questions as they arise
- Discussion of the recovery:
  - How long it will take
  - Feelings to expect: Tingling, numbness, pressure, itching
  - Pain that will be felt as the anesthesia wears off
  - Measures to reduce pain in the area
  - Signs and symptoms to report (e.g., pain along a nerve route, palpitations, feeling faint, disorientation)

KEY POINTS

- Local anesthetics block the depolarization of nerve membranes, preventing the transmission of pain sensations and motor stimuli.
- Local anesthetics are administered to deliver the drug directly to the desired area and to prevent systemic absorption, which could lead to serious interruption of nerve impulses and response.
- Ester-type local anesthetics are immediately destroyed by plasma esterases. Amide local anesthetics are destroyed in the liver and have a greater risk of accumulation and systemic toxicity.

SUMMARY

- General anesthetics result in analgesia, amnesia, and unconsciousness; they also block muscle reflexes that could interfere with a surgical procedure or put the patient at risk for harm.
- The use of general anesthetics involves a widespread CNS depression that could be harmful, especially in patients with underlying CNS, CV, or respiratory diseases.
- Anesthesia proceeds through four predictable stages from loss of sensation to total CNS depression and death.
- Induction of anesthesia is the period of time from the beginning of anesthesia administration until the patient reaches surgical anesthesia.
- Balanced anesthesia involves giving a variety of drugs, including anticholinergics, rapid intravenous anesthetics, inhaled anesthetics, NMJ blockers, and narcotics.
- Patients receiving general anesthetics should be monitored for any adverse effects; they need reassurance and safety measures until the recovery of sensation, mobility, and ability to communicate.
- Local anesthetics block the depolarization of nerve membranes, preventing the transmission of pain sensations and motor stimuli.
- Local anesthetics are administered to deliver the drug directly to the desired area and to prevent systemic absorption, which could lead to serious interruption of nerve impulses and response.
- Ester-type local anesthetics are immediately destroyed by plasma esterases. Amide local anesthetics are destroyed in the liver and have a greater risk of accumulation and systemic toxicity.
- Nursing care of patients receiving general or local anesthetics should include safety precautions to prevent injury and skin breakdown; support and reassurance to deal with the loss of sensation and mobility; and patient teaching regarding what to expect, to decrease stress and anxiety.

CHECK YOUR UNDERSTANDING

Answers to the questions in this chapter can be found in Answers to Check Your Understanding Questions on thePoint®.

MULTIPLE CHOICE

Select the best answer to the following.

1. The most dangerous period for many patients undergoing general anesthesia is during which stage?
- **a.** Stage 1, when communication becomes difficult
- **b.** Stage 2, when systemic stimulation occurs
- **c.** Stage 3, when skeletal muscles relax
- **d.** There is no real danger during general anesthesia

2. Recovery after a general anesthetic refers to the period of time
- **a.** from the beginning of the anesthesia until the patient is ready for surgery.
- **b.** during the surgery when anesthesia is maintained at a certain level.
- **c.** from discontinuation of the anesthetic until the patient has regained consciousness, movement, and the ability to communicate.
- **d.** when the patient is in the most danger of CNS depression.

3. While a patient is receiving a general anesthetic, he or she must be continually monitored because
- **a.** the patient has no pain sensation.
- **b.** generalized CNS depression affects all body functions.
- **c.** the patient cannot move.
- **d.** the patient cannot communicate.

4. The nursing instructor determines that teaching about general anesthetics was successful when the students identify which person as being most qualified to administer general anesthetics?
- **a.** Nursing supervisor
- **b.** Graduate nurse
- **c.** Trained physician
- **d.** Surgeon

5. Local anesthetics are used to block feeling in specific body areas. If given in increasing concentrations, local anesthetics can cause loss, in order, of the following:
- **a.** Temperature sensation, touch sensation, proprioception, and skeletal muscle tone
- **b.** Touch sensation, skeletal muscle tone, temperature sensation, and proprioception
- **c.** Proprioception, skeletal muscle tone, touch sensation, and temperature sensation
- **d.** Skeletal muscle tone, touch sensation, temperature sensation, and proprioception

MULTIPLE RESPONSE

Select all that apply.

1. Comfort measures that are important for a patient receiving a local anesthetic would include which of the following?
- **a.** Skin care and turning
- **b.** Reassurance over loss of control and sensation
- **c.** Use of antihypertensive agents
- **d.** Use of analgesics as needed
- **e.** Ice applied to the area involved
- **f.** Safety precautions to prevent injury

2. A nurse would anticipate the use of general anesthetics for which of the following reasons?
- **a.** To produce analgesia
- **b.** To produce amnesia
- **c.** To activate the reticular activating system
- **d.** To block muscle reflexes
- **e.** To cause unconsciousness
- **f.** To prevent nausea

3. Balanced anesthesia combines different classes of drugs to achieve the best effects with the fewest adverse effects. Balanced anesthesia usually involves the use of which of the following?
- **a.** Anticholinergics
- **b.** Narcotics
- **c.** Sedative/hypnotics
- **d.** Adrenergic beta-blockers
- **e.** Dantrolene
- **f.** Neuromuscular blocking agents

BIBLIOGRAPHY AND REFERENCES

Barash, P. G., Cullen, B. F., Stoelting, R. K., et al. (2015). *Clinical anesthesia fundamentals*. Philadelphia, PA: Wolters Kluwer.

Brunton, L., Chabner, B., & Knollman, B. (2011). *Goodman and Gilman's the pharmacological basis of therapeutics* (12th ed.). New York: McGraw-Hill.

Clifford, T. (2011). Peripheral nerve blocks. *Journal of Perianesthesia Nursing, 26*(2), 120–121.

Facts and Comparisons. (2015). *Drug facts and comparisons*. St. Louis, MO: Author.

Facts and Comparisons. (2015). *Professional's guide to patient drug facts*. St. Louis, MO: Author.

Fleisher, L., & Roizen, M. (2011). *Essence of anesthesia practice: Expert consultant*. Philadelphia, PA: Saunders.

Karch, A. M. (2014). *Lippincott's nursing drug guide*. Philadelphia, PA: Lippincott Williams & Wilkins.

Meier, G., & Buettner, J. (2009). *Peripheral regional anesthetics*. New York: Thieme.

Pine, M., Holt, K. D., & Lou, Y. (2003). Surgical mortality and type of anesthesia provider. *American Association of Nurse Anesthetists Journal, 71*, 109–116.

Porth, C. M. (2013). *Pathophysiology: Concepts of altered health states* (9th ed.). Philadelphia, PA: Lippincott Williams & Wilkins.

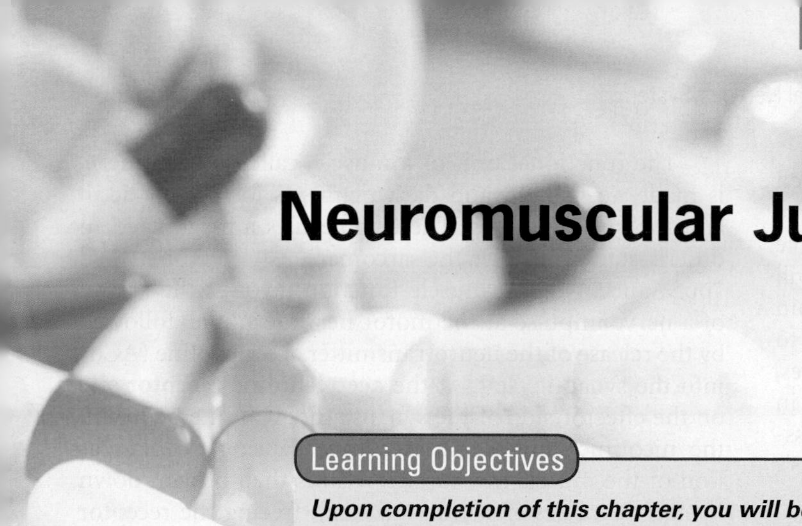

28 Neuromuscular Junction Blocking Agents

Learning Objectives

Upon completion of this chapter, you will be able to:

1. Draw and label a neuromuscular junction.
2. Describe the therapeutic actions, indications, pharmacokinetics, contraindications, most common adverse reactions, and important drug–drug interactions associated with the depolarizing and nondepolarizing neuromuscular junction blockers.
3. Discuss the use of neuromuscular junction blockers across the lifespan.
4. Compare and contrast the prototype drugs pancuronium and succinylcholine with other neuromuscular junction blockers.
5. Outline the nursing considerations, including important teaching points, for patients receiving a neuromuscular junction blocker.

Glossary of Key Terms

acetylcholine receptor site: area on the muscle cell membrane where acetylcholine (ACh) reacts with a specific receptor site to cause stimulation of the muscle in response to nerve activity

depolarizing neuromuscular junction (NMJ) blocker: stimulation of a muscle cell, causing it to contract, with no allowance for repolarization and restimulation of the muscle; characterized by contraction and then paralysis

malignant hyperthermia: reaction to some NMJ drugs in susceptible individuals; characterized by extreme muscle rigidity, severe hyperpyrexia, acidosis, and in some cases death

neuromuscular junction (NMJ): the synapse between a nerve and a muscle cell

nondepolarizing neuromuscular junction (NMJ) blocker: no stimulation or depolarization of the muscle cell; prevents depolarization and stimulation by blocking the effects of acetylcholine

paralysis: lack of muscle function

sarcomere: functional unit of a muscle cell, composed of actin and myosin molecules arranged in layers to give the unit a striped or striated appearance

sliding filament theory: theory explaining muscle contraction as a reaction of actin and myosin molecules when they are freed to react by the inactivation of troponin after calcium is allowed to enter the cell during depolarization

Drug List

Neuromuscular Junction Blocking Agents

Nondepolarizing NMJs
- atracurium
- cisatracurium
- (P) pancuronium
- rocuronium
- vecuronium

Depolarizing NMJ
- (P) succinylcholine

Nerves communicate with muscles at a synapse called the neuromuscular junction (NMJ). At this point, a nerve stimulates a muscle to contract. If the nerve is not able to communicate with the muscle cell, the muscle will not be able to contract, and paralysis will result. Certain clinical situations require that a patient not be able to move muscles, including surgery, diagnostic procedures, and mechanical ventilation. Anesthetics (discussed in Chapter 27) can prevent muscle movement by suppressing function through the central nervous system (CNS), with many systemic complications from this depression. The NMJ blocking drugs are used to prevent the nerve stimulation at the muscle cell and cause paralysis of the muscle directly without total CNS depression and its many systemic effects.

The Neuromuscular Junction

The **neuromuscular junction** is the point at which a motor neuron communicates with a skeletal muscle fiber. The end result is muscular contraction. NMJ blocking agents affect the normal functioning of muscles by interfering with the normal processes that occur at the junction of nerve and muscle cell.

The functional unit of a muscle, called a **sarcomere**, is made up of light and dark filaments formed by actin and myosin molecules. These molecules are arranged in orderly stacks that give the sarcomere a striated or striped appearance. Normal muscle function involves the arrival of a nerve impulse at the motor nerve terminal, followed by the release of the neurotransmitter acetylcholine (ACh) into the synaptic cleft. At the **acetylcholine receptor site** on the effector side of the synapse the ACh interacts with the nicotinic cholinergic receptors, causing depolarization of the muscle membrane. ACh is then broken down by acetylcholinesterase (an enzyme), freeing the receptor for further stimulation. With stimulation, this depolarization allows the release of calcium ions, stored in tubules, into the cell. The calcium binds to troponin, a chemical found throughout the sarcomere. This binding of troponin releases the actin- and myosin-binding sites, allowing them to react with each other. The actin and myosin molecules react with each other again and again, sliding along the filament and making it shorter. This is a contraction of the muscle fiber according to the **sliding filament theory** (Figure 28.1). As the calcium is removed from the cell during repolarization of the muscle membrane the troponin is freed and once again prevents the actin and myosin from reacting with each other. The muscle filament then relaxes or slides back to the resting position.

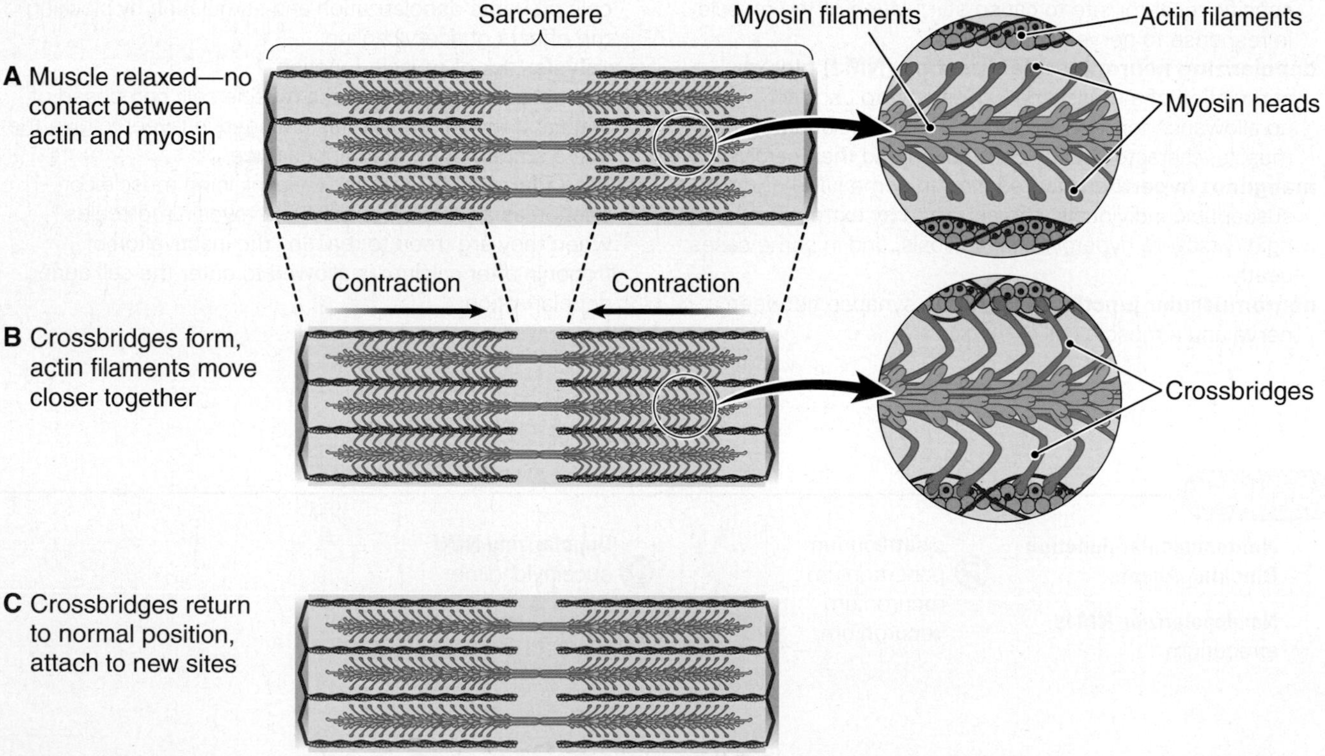

FIGURE 28.1 Sliding filament mechanism of skeletal muscle contraction. **A:** Muscle is relaxed, and there is no contact between the actin and myosin filaments. **B:** Cross-bridges form, and the actin filaments are moved closer together as the muscle fiber contracts. **C:** The cross-bridges return to their original position and attach to new sites to prepare for another pull on the actin filaments and further contraction.

A dynamic balance of excitatory and inhibitory impulses to the muscle results in muscle tone. However, if ACh cannot react with the cholinergic muscle receptor or if the muscle cells cannot repolarize to allow new stimulation and muscle contraction, muscle **paralysis**, or loss of muscle function, occurs.

KEY POINTS

- The nerves and muscles communicate at the NMJ.
- ACh acts as the neurotransmitter at the NMJ.
- NMJ blockers interfere with muscle function.

Neuromuscular Junction Blocking Agents

Drugs that affect the NMJ can be divided into two groups. One group, the **nondepolarizing neuromuscular junction blockers**, includes those agents that act as antagonists to ACh at the NMJ and prevent depolarization of muscle cells. The other group, the **depolarizing neuromuscular junction blockers** (of which there is one drug), act as an ACh agonist at the junction, causing stimulation of the muscle cell and staying on the receptor site, preventing it from repolarizing, which results in muscle paralysis with the muscle in a constant, contracted state. Both of these types of drugs are used to cause paralysis for the performance of surgical procedures, endoscopic diagnostic procedures, or facilitation of mechanical ventilation. Table 28.1 lists these drugs, their preferred uses, and potential problems. Box 28.1 highlights information about using NMJ blockers with various age groups (see also the Critical Thinking Scenario for nursing care related to an elderly patient receiving an NMJ).

Nondepolarizing Neuromuscular Junction Blockers

The first NMJ blocker to be discovered was curare, a poison used on the tips of arrows or spears by hunters to paralyze their game. Animals died when their respiratory muscles became paralyzed. Because the poison was destroyed by the cooking process or by gastric acid if the meat were eaten raw, it was safe for humans. Curare was first purified for clinical use as the NMJ blocker tubocurarine, which has since been replaced with more refined drugs that can control onset and duration of effect.

Nondepolarizing NMJ blockers include atracurium (generic), cisatracurium (*Nimbex*), pancuronium (generic), rocuronium (generic), and vecuronium (generic).

Therapeutic Actions and Indications

Nondepolarizing NMJ blockers are used when clinical situations require or desire muscle paralysis (see Table 28.1 for preferred uses). Therapeutically, nondepolarizing NMJ blockers:

Table 28.1 ***Drugs in Focus:*** **Neuromuscular Junction (NMJ) Blockers**

Drug Name	Preferred Uses	Special Considerations
NMJ Blockers		
atracurium (generic)	Mechanical ventilation; long duration of action; surgical procedures	Has no effect on pain perception or consciousness; do not use before induction of anesthesia; bradycardia is more common with this drug; reduce dose in renal failure
cisatracurium (*Nimbex*)	Intermediate action; used for surgical procedures and to facilitate intubation	No known effect on pain perception or consciousness; contains benzyl alcohol, avoid use in neonates
pancuronium (generic)	Surgical procedures; mechanical ventilation	Vagolytic effect, associated with increased heart rate; long-term use for mechanical ventilation, monitor for prolonged adverse effects
rocuronium (generic)	Rapid onset; preferred for rapid intubation; short outpatient surgical procedures	No known effect on pain perception or consciousness; may be associated with pulmonary hypertension; use caution with hepatic impairment
vecuronium (generic)	Short surgical procedures; intubation; mechanical ventilation	May contain benzyl alcohol; avoid use in neonates, can cause fatalities in premature infants; monitor with long-term use during ventilation; if response does not occur with first twitch test, discontinue, may be associated with permanent muscle damage
Depolarizing NMJ Blocker		
succinylcholine (*Anectine, Quelicin*)	Surgical procedures; intubation; mechanical ventilation	May cause myalgia secondary to muscle contraction; associated with increased intraocular pressure; increased intragastric pressure, which may cause vomiting; more likely to cause malignant hyperthermia

BOX 28.1 FOCUS ON Drug Therapy Across the Lifespan

NMJ Blocking Agents

CHILDREN

Children require very careful monitoring and support after the use of NMJ blockers. These agents are used by anesthetists who are skilled in their use and with full support services available.

The nondepolarizing NMJs are preferable because of the lack of muscle contraction with its resultant discomfort on recovery. Succinylcholine is usually preferred when a very short-acting, rapid-onset blocker is needed (e.g., for intubation).

ADULTS

Adults need to be monitored closely for full return of muscle function. If succinylcholine is used, they need to be told that they will experience muscle pain and discomfort when the procedure is over.

The NMJs are used during pregnancy and lactation only if the benefit to the mother outweighs the potential risk to the fetus or neonate.

OLDER ADULTS

Because older patients often also have renal or hepatic impairment, they are more likely to have toxic levels of the drug related to changes in metabolism and excretion. The older patient should receive special efforts to provide skin care to prevent skin breakdown, which is more likely with older skin. The older patient may require longer monitoring and regular orienting and reassuring.

- Serve as an adjunct to general anesthetics during surgery when reflex muscle movement could interfere with the surgical procedure or the delivery of gas anesthesia.
- Facilitate mechanical intubation by preventing resistance to passing of the endotracheal tube and in situations in which patients "fight" or resist the respirator.
- Facilitate various endoscopic diagnostic procedures when reflex muscle reaction could interfere with the procedure.
- Facilitate electroconvulsive therapy when intense skeletal muscle contractions as a result of electric shock could cause the patient broken bones or other injury.

Pharmacokinetics

All nondepolarizing NMJ blockers are similar in structure to ACh and compete with ACh for the muscle Ach receptor site (Figure 28.2). As a result, they occupy the muscular cholinergic receptor site and do not allow stimulation to occur. These agents do not cause the activation of muscle cells, and consequently muscle contraction does not occur. Because they are not broken down by acetylcholinesterase, their effect is longer lasting than that of ACh. The nondepolarizing NMJ blockers are hydrophilic instead of lipophilic, so they do not readily cross the blood–brain barrier and have little effect on the ACh receptors in the brain.

Nondepolarizing NMJs are metabolized in the serum, although metabolism is dependent on the liver to produce the needed plasma cholinesterases. Most of the metabolites are excreted in the urine.

Each nondepolarizing NMJ blocker differs in terms of time of onset and duration (Figure 28.3). The drug of choice in any given situation is determined by the procedure being performed, including the estimated time involved.

Contraindications and Cautions

Nondepolarizing NMJ blockers are contraindicated in the following conditions: Known allergy to any of these drugs *to prevent hypersensitivity reactions*; myasthenia gravis *because blocking of the ACh cholinergic receptors aggravates the neuromuscular disease* (which results from destruction of the ACh receptor sites) *and increases the muscular effects* (see Chapter 32); renal or hepatic disease, *which could interfere with the metabolism or excretion of these drugs, leading to toxic effects*; and pregnancy.

Caution should be used in patients with any family or personal history of **malignant hyperthermia**, a serious adverse effect associated with these drugs that is characterized by extreme muscle rigidity, severe hyperpyrexia (fever), acidosis, and death in some cases, *because malignant hyperthermia can occur with the use of these drugs.* Caution should also be used in the following circumstances: Pulmonary or cardiovascular (CV) dysfunction, *which could be exacerbated by the paralysis of the respiratory muscles and resulting changes in perfusion and respiratory function*; altered fluid and electrolyte imbalance, *which could affect membrane stability and subsequent muscular function*; some respiratory conditions *that could be made worse by the histamine release associated with some of these agents*; and lactation *because of the potential for adverse effects on the baby.*

Adverse Effects

The adverse effects related to the use of nondepolarizing NMJ blockers are associated with the paralysis of muscles. Profound and prolonged muscle paralysis is always possible, and patients must be supported until they are able to resume voluntary and involuntary muscle movement. When the respiratory muscles are paralyzed, depressed

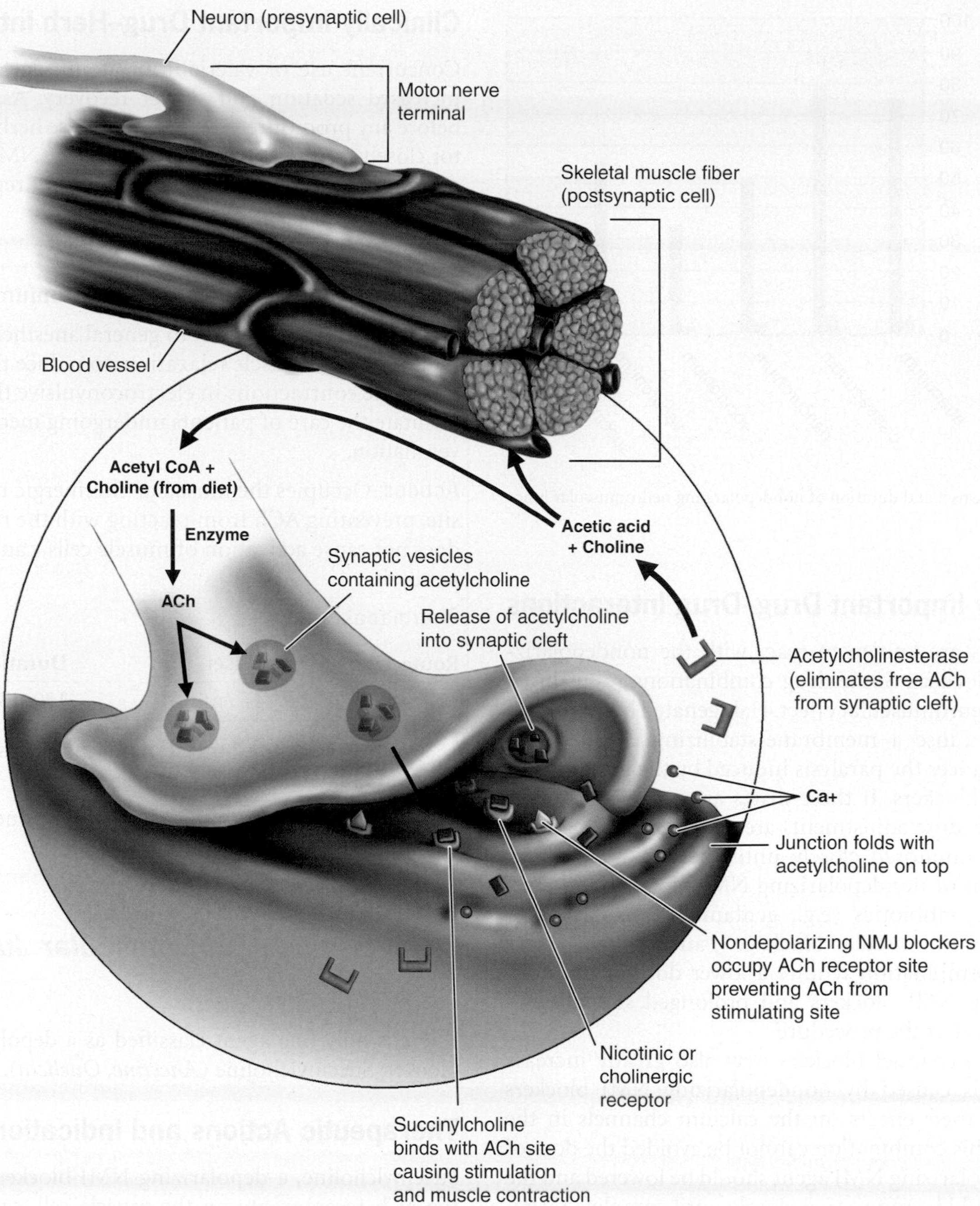

FIGURE 28.2 Sites of action of neuromuscular junction blockers.

respiration, bronchospasm, and apnea are anticipated adverse effects. These agents are never used without an anesthesiologist or nurse anesthetist present who can provide assisted ventilatory measures and deliver oxygen under positive pressure. Intubation is an anticipated procedure with these drugs.

The histamine release associated with many of the depolarizing NMJ blockers can cause respiratory obstruction with wheezing and bronchospasm. Hypotension and cardiac arrhythmias may occur in patients who do not adapt to the drugs effectively, use the drugs for prolonged periods, have certain underlying conditions, or take certain drugs (e.g., vecuronium) that are known to affect CV receptors. Prolonged drug use may also result in gastrointestinal (GI) dysfunction related to paralysis of the muscles in the GI tract; constipation, vomiting, regurgitation, and aspiration may occur. Pressure ulcers may develop because the patient loses reflex muscle movement that protects the body. Hyperkalemia may occur as a result of muscle membrane alterations.

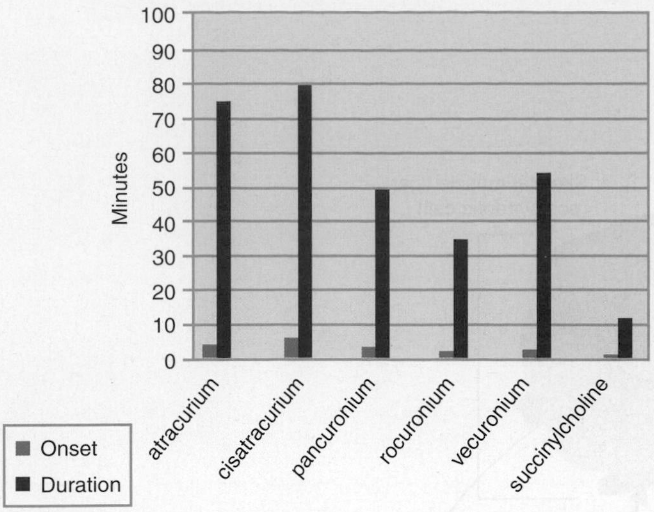

FIGURE 28.3 Onset and duration of nondepolarizing neuromuscular junction blockers.

Clinically Important Drug–Drug Interactions

Many drugs are known to react with the nondepolarizing NMJ blockers. Some drug combinations result in an increased neuromuscular effect. Halogenated hydrocarbon anesthetics cause a membrane-stabilizing effect, which greatly enhances the paralysis induced by the nondepolarizing NMJ blockers. If these drugs are used together for a procedure, dose adjustments are necessary, and patients should be monitored closely until they recover fully. A combination of nondepolarizing NMJ blockers and aminoglycoside antibiotics (e.g., gentamicin) also leads to increased neuromuscular blockage. Patients who receive this drug combination require a lower dose of the nondepolarizing NMJ blockers and prolonged support and monitoring after the procedure.

Calcium-channel blockers may also greatly increase the paralysis caused by nondepolarizing NMJ blockers because of their effects on the calcium channels in the muscle. If this combination cannot be avoided the dose of the nondepolarizing NMJ agent should be lowered and the patient should be monitored closely until complete recovery occurs.

If nondepolarizing NMJ blockers are combined with cholinesterase inhibitors the effectiveness of the nondepolarizing NMJ blockers is decreased because of a buildup of ACh in the synaptic cleft.

Combination with xanthines (e.g., theophylline, aminophylline) could result in reversal of the neuromuscular blockage. Patients receiving this combination of drugs should be monitored very closely during the procedure for the potential of early arousal and return of muscle function.

Do not mix the drug with any alkaline solutions such as barbiturates because a precipitate may form, making it inappropriate for use.

Clinically Important Drug–Herb Interactions

Concurrent use of valerian, melatonin, kava may cause increased sedation and slower recovery. Assess patients before any procedure for the use of these herbs and monitor closely during and after the use of the NMJ blocker for any potential recovery issues if the patient reports the use of these herbs.

Ⓟ Prototype Summary: Pancuronium

Indications: As an adjunct to general anesthesia; to induce skeletal muscle relaxation; to reduce the intensity of muscle contractions in electroconvulsive therapy; to facilitate the care of patients undergoing mechanical ventilation.

Actions: Occupies the muscular cholinergic receptor site, preventing ACh from reacting with the receptor; does not cause activation of muscle cells; causes a flaccid paralysis.

Pharmacokinetics:

Route	Onset	Duration
IV	4–6 min	120–180 min

$T_{1/2}$: 89 to 161 minutes; metabolized in the tissues, excreted unchanged in the urine.

Adverse Effects: Respiratory depression, apnea, bronchospasm, cardiac arrhythmias.

Depolarizing Neuromuscular Junction Blocker

There is only one agent classified as a depolarizing NMJ blocker: Succinylcholine (*Anectine*, *Quelicin*).

Therapeutic Actions and Indications

Succinylcholine, a depolarizing NMJ blocker, attaches to the ACh receptor site on the muscle cell, causing a prolonged depolarization of the muscle. This depolarization causes stimulation of the muscle and muscle contraction (seen as twitching) and then flaccid paralysis. Both effects cause muscles to stop responding to stimuli, and paralysis occurs.

Succinylcholine has a rapid onset and a short duration of action because it is broken down by cholinesterase in the plasma. Unlike endogenous ACh, however, succinylcholine is not broken down instantly. The result is a prolonged contraction of the muscle, which cannot be restimulated. Eventually, a gradual repolarization occurs as continually stimulated channels in the cell membrane close. Certain ethnic groups may have a genetic predisposition for a prolongation of paralysis (Box 28.2).

BOX 28.2 FOCUS ON **Cultural Considerations**

Succinylcholine and Paralysis

Succinylcholine is broken down in the body by cholinesterase, an enzyme found in the plasma. Several conditions may cause the body to produce less of this enzyme, including cirrhosis, metabolic disorders, carcinoma, burns, dehydration, malnutrition, hyperpyrexia, thyrotoxicosis, collagen diseases, and exposure to neurotoxic insecticides. If plasma cholinesterase levels are low the serum levels of succinylcholine remain elevated and the paralysis can last much longer than anticipated. These patients need support and ventilation for long periods after surgery.

There is also a genetic predisposition to low plasma cholinesterase levels. Patients should be asked whether they or any family member has a history of either low plasma cholinesterase levels or prolonged recovery from anesthetics. Alaskan Eskimos belong to such a genetic group, and they are especially likely to suffer prolonged paralysis and inability to breathe for several hours after succinylcholine has been used for surgery. If there is no other drug of choice for these patients, special care must be taken to monitor their response and ensure their breathing for an extended postoperative period.

Pharmacokinetics

Succinylcholine, like the nondepolarizing NMJ blockers, is metabolized in the serum, although metabolism is dependent on the liver to produce the needed plasma cholinesterases. Patients with hepatic impairment may experience prolonged effects of this drug. Onset of action is usually within 1 minute, and duration of effect is 10 to 12 minutes. Most of the metabolites are excreted in the urine. Patients with renal impairment may be at risk for increased toxicity from the drugs. Succinylcholine crosses the placenta. Effects on lactation are not known.

Contraindications and Cautions

The contraindications and cautions for succinylcholine are the same as for nondepolarizing NMJ blockers. Succinylcholine is often used during cesarean sections, but accurate timing is necessary to prevent serious effects on the fetus. In addition, succinylcholine should be used with caution in patients with fractures *because the muscle contractions it causes might lead to additional trauma*; in patients with narrow-angle glaucoma or penetrating eye injuries *because intraocular pressure increases*; and in patients with paraplegia or spinal cord injuries, *which could cause loss of potassium from the overstimulated cells and hyperkalemia.* Extreme caution is necessary in the presence of genetic or disease-related conditions causing low plasma cholinesterase levels, such as cirrhosis, metabolic disorders, carcinoma, burns, dehydration, malnutrition, hyperpyrexia, thyroid toxicosis, collagen diseases, and exposure to neurotoxic insecticides. *Low plasma cholinesterase levels may result in a very prolonged paralysis because succinylcholine is not broken down in the plasma and continues to stimulate the receptor site, leading to a need for prolonged support after use of the drug is discontinued.*

Adverse Effects

The adverse effects of succinylcholine are the same as those for nondepolarizing NMJ blockers. In addition, succinylcholine is associated with muscle pain related to the initial muscle contraction reaction. A nondepolarizing NMJ blocker may be given first to prevent some of these contractions and the associated discomfort. Aspirin also alleviates much of this pain after the procedure. Malignant hyperthermia, which may occur in susceptible patients, is a very serious condition characterized by massive muscle contraction, sharply elevated body temperature, severe acidosis, and if uncontrolled death (Figure 28.4). This reaction is most likely with succinylcholine, and treatment involves dantrolene (see Chapter 25) to inhibit the muscle effects of the NMJ blocker.

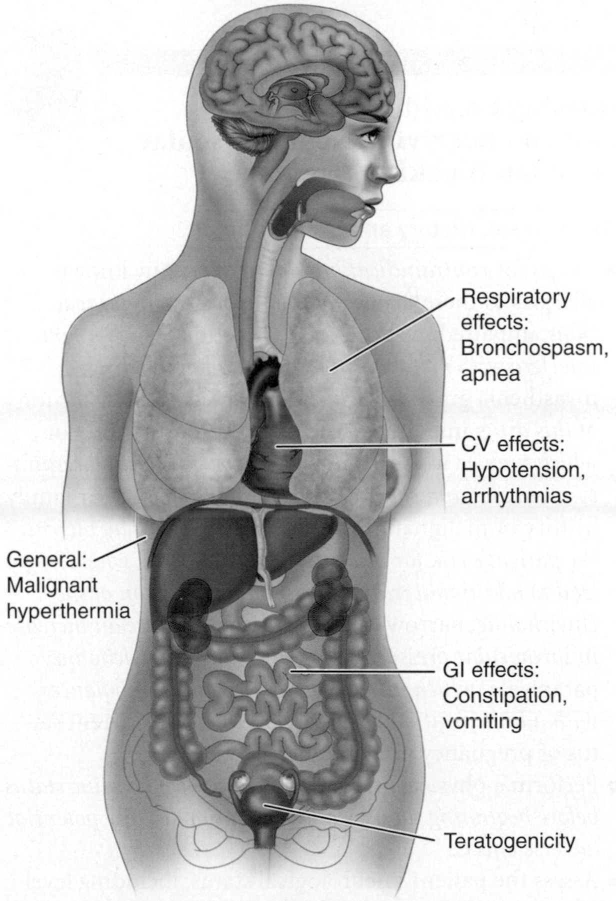

FIGURE 28.4 Common adverse effects associated with neuromuscular junction blockers.

Clinically Important Drug–Drug Interactions

Potential drug–drug interactions for succinylcholine are the same as for the nondepolarizing NMJ blockers.

Ⓟ Prototype Summary: Succinylcholine

Indications: As an adjunct to general anesthesia; to facilitate endotracheal intubation; to induce skeletal muscle relaxation during surgery or mechanical ventilation.

Actions: Combines with ACh receptors at the motor endplate to produce depolarization; this inhibits neuromuscular transmission, causing a flaccid paralysis.

Pharmacokinetics:

Route	Onset	Duration
IV	30–60 s	4–6 min

$T_{1/2}$: 2 to 3 minutes; metabolized in the tissues, excreted unchanged in the urine.

Adverse Effects: Muscle pain, related to the contraction of the muscles as a first reaction; respiratory depression, apnea.

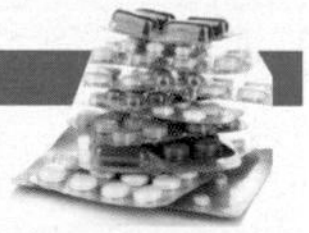

Nursing Considerations for Patients Receiving Neuromuscular Junction Blocking Agents

Assessment: History and Examination

- Assess for *contraindications or cautions*: Any known allergies to these drugs *to avoid hypersensitivity reactions*; impaired liver or kidney function, *which might interfere with metabolism or excretion of the drug*; myasthenia gravis, *which may be exacerbated by the use of this drug*; impaired cardiac or respiratory function, *which may be worsened due to the drug's effect on respiratory muscles and changes in perfusion*; personal or family history of malignant hyperthermia, *which may increase the patient's risk for this condition*; fractures, *which might lead to additional trauma with administration of succinylcholine*; narrow-angle glaucoma *because an increase in intraocular pressure can occur with succinylcholine*; paraplegia, *which might lead to potassium imbalance with administration of succinylcholine*; and current status of pregnancy or lactation.
- Perform a physical assessment *to establish baseline status before beginning therapy and evaluation for any potential adverse effects.*
- Assess the patient's neurological status, including level of orientation, affect, reflexes, pupil size and reactivity, and muscle tone and response, *to monitor drug effects and recovery.*
- Monitor respiratory rate and auscultate lung sounds for evidence of adventitious sounds *to evaluate effects on respiratory muscles and monitor for adverse reactions.*
- Monitor vital signs, including temperature, pulse rate, and blood pressure, *to identify changes.*
- Auscultate the abdomen for evidence of bowel sounds *to monitor effects on GI muscles and recovery.*
- Inspect the skin for color and evidence of pressure areas or breakdown, *which could result when movement ceases.*
- Monitor the results of laboratory tests, including liver function tests, *to determine the need for possible dose adjustment and serum electrolyte levels to determine potential cautions to the use of the drugs.*

Refer to the Critical Thinking Scenario for a full discussion of nursing care for an elderly patient who is receiving succinylcholine.

Nursing Diagnoses

Nursing diagnoses related to drug therapy may include the following:

- Impaired gas exchange related to depressed respirations
- Impaired skin integrity related to immobility from prolonged drug effects
- Impaired verbal communication related to effects on muscle activity
- Fear related to paralysis
- Risk of injury related to loss of muscle control
- Pain related to prolonged muscle contraction with succinylcholine use
- Deficient knowledge regarding drug therapy

Planning

- The patient will receive the best therapeutic effect from the drug therapy.
- The patient will have limited adverse effects to the drug therapy.
- The patient will have an understanding of the drug therapy, adverse effects to anticipate, and measures to relieve discomfort and improve safety.

Implementation with Rationale

- Be aware that administration of the drug should be performed by trained personnel (usually an anesthesiologist) *because of the potential for serious adverse effects and the need for immediate ventilatory support.*
- Ensure that emergency supplies and equipment are readily available *to maintain airway and provide mechanical ventilation.*
- Do not mix the drug with any alkaline solutions such as barbiturates *because a precipitate may form, making it inappropriate for use.*
- Test patient response and recovery periodically if the drug is being given over a long period to maintain

mechanical ventilation. *Discontinue the drug if response does not occur or is greatly delayed.*

- Monitor patient temperature *for prompt detection and treatment of malignant hyperthermia*; have dantrolene readily available *for treatment of malignant hyperthermia if it should occur.*
- Arrange for a small dose of a nondepolarizing NMJ blocker before the use of succinylcholine *to reduce the adverse effects associated with muscle contraction.*
- Ensure that a cholinesterase inhibitor is readily available *to overcome excessive neuromuscular blockade caused by nondepolarizing NMJ blockers.*
- Have a peripheral nerve stimulator on standby *to assess the degree of neuromuscular blockade, if appropriate.*
- Provide comfort measures *to help the patient tolerate drug effects,* such as pain relief as appropriate; reassurance, support, and orientation *for conscious patients unable to move or communicate*; skin care and turning *to prevent skin breakdown*; and supportive care *for emergencies such as hypotension and bronchospasm.*
- Monitor patient response closely (blood pressure, temperature, pulse, respiration, reflexes) to determine effectiveness; expect dose adjustment *to ensure the greatest therapeutic effect with minimal risk of toxicity.*
- Provide thorough patient preoperative teaching about this drug *because most patients who receive the drug will be receiving teaching about a particular procedure and will be unconscious when the drug is given.* Teaching includes drug to be given, method for administration, effects of the drug (i.e., what to expect), and safety precautions.
- Offer support and encouragement to help the patient to cope with drug effects.

Evaluation

- Monitor patient response to the drug (adequate muscle paralysis).
- Monitor for adverse effects (respiratory depression, hypotension, bronchospasm, GI slowdown, skin breakdown, fear related to helplessness and inability to communicate).
- Evaluate effectiveness of the teaching plan (the patient can relate anticipated effects of the drug and the recovery process).
- Monitor the effectiveness of comfort measures and compliance with the regimen.

KEY POINTS

- Nondepolarizing NMJ blockers prevent ACh from exciting the muscle, and paralysis ensues because the muscle cannot respond.
- Depolarizing NMJ blockers cause muscle paralysis by acting like ACh. They excite (depolarize) the muscle and prevent repolarization and further stimulation. There is only one drug available in this class.

CRITICAL THINKING SCENARIO

Using Succinylcholine in an Elderly Patient

THE SITUATION

S.N., an 82-year-old white woman in very good health, has been admitted to the hospital for an exploratory laparotomy to evaluate a probable abdominal mass. On admission, health care practitioners learned that she had a history of mild hypertension that was well regulated by diuretic therapy. She received a baseline physical examination and preoperative instruction. On the morning of the surgery, it was noted that the anesthesiologist planned to give her a general anesthetic and succinylcholine to ensure muscle paralysis.

CRITICAL THINKING

What areas must be considered for S.N.? Consider the patient's age and associated chronic problems that often occur with aging. Also consider the support that she has available and potential physical and emotional support that she might need before and after this procedure. Use of an NMJ blocker in elderly presents brings some nursing challenges that may not be seen with younger patients.

What particular nursing care activities should be considered with S.N.? Because S.N. has been maintained on long-term diuretic therapy, she is at special risk for electrolyte imbalance.

What, if any, complications could arise if S.N. has electrolyte disturbances before surgery?

DISCUSSION

Before surgery, the preoperative teaching protocol should be reviewed with the patient. S.N. should be advised that she may experience back and neck pain secondary to the muscle contractions caused by succinylcholine and throat pain after the procedure. Reassure her that this is normal and that medication will be made available to alleviate the discomfort. Review deep breathing and coughing; she may need

(continues on page 486)

Using Succinylcholine in an Elderly Patient (continued)

encouragement to clear secretions from her lungs and ensure full inflation. This is usually easier to do if it is a familiar activity. S.N.'s serum electrolytes should be evaluated before surgery because potassium imbalance can cause unexpected effects with succinylcholine. Renal and hepatic function tests also should be performed to ensure that the dose of the NMJ blocker is not excessive.

During the procedure, S.N.'s cardiac and respiratory status should be monitored carefully for any potential problems; such effects are more common in people with underlying physical problems. Because of S.N.'s age and potential circulatory problems, she should receive meticulous skin care and turning as soon as the procedure allows this kind of movement. She should be turned frequently during the recovery period, and her skin should be checked for any breakdown. Nursing personnel must remain close by the patient until she has regained muscle control and the ability to communicate. She should be evaluated for the need for pain medication and position adjustments.

S.N. will require additional teaching about her diagnosis and potential treatment. This should wait until she has regained full ability to communicate and is able to respond and participate in any discussion that may be held. At that time, she may require emotional support and encouragement. It may be necessary to contact available family or social service agencies regarding her physical and medical needs.

NURSING CARE GUIDE FOR S.N.: SUCCINYLCHOLINE

Assessment: History and Examination

Assess allergies to the drug, and assess for history of respiratory or cardiac disorders, myasthenia gravis, hepatic or renal dysfunction, fractures, and glaucoma

Concurrent use of aminoglycosides or calcium channel blockers

Focus the physical examination on the following:

CV: Blood pressure, pulse rate, peripheral perfusion, and electrocardiogram

CNS: Orientation, affect, reflexes, and vision

Skin: color, lesions, texture, and sweating

Genitourinary: Urinary output and bladder tone

GI: Abdominal examination

Respiratory: Respirations and adventitious sounds

Nursing Diagnoses

Impaired gas exchange related to depressed respirations

Risk for impaired skin integrity related to immobility

Pain related to prolonged muscle contractions with succinylcholine use

Deficient knowledge regarding drug therapy

Impaired verbal communication due to fear related to paralysis and inability to communicate

Planning

The patient will receive the best therapeutic effect from the drug therapy.

The patient will have limited adverse effects to the drug therapy.

The patient will have an understanding of the drug therapy, adverse effects to anticipate, and measures to relieve discomfort and improve safety.

Implementation

Provide comfort and safety measures: Positioning, skin care, temperature control, pain medication as needed, maintain airway, ventilate patient, have antidotes on standby.

Provide support and reassurance to deal with paralysis and inability to communicate.

Provide patient teaching about procedure being performed and what to expect.

Assist with life support as needed.

Evaluation

Evaluate drug effects: Muscle paralysis.

Monitor for adverse effects: CV effects (tachycardia, hypotension, respiratory distress, increased respiratory secretions), GI effects (constipation, nausea), skin breakdown, anxiety, fear.

Monitor for drug–drug interactions as indicated.

Evaluate the effectiveness of the patient-teaching program and comfort and safety measures.

Constantly monitor vital signs and watch for return of normal muscular function.

PATIENT TEACHING FOR S.N.

- Before the surgery is performed, you will be given a drug to paralyze your muscles called a neuromuscular blocking agent. It is important that your muscles do not move at this time because it could interfere with the procedure.
- Common effects of these drugs include complete paralysis:
  - You will not be able to move or to speak while you are receiving this drug.
  - You will not be able to breathe on your own, and you will receive assistance in breathing.
- This drug may not affect your level of consciousness, and it can be very frightening to be unable to communicate with anyone around you. Someone will be with you, will try to anticipate your needs, and will explain what is going on at all times.

Using Succinylcholine in an Elderly Patient (continued)

- This drug may have no effect on your pain perception. Every effort will be made to make sure that you do not experience pain.
- You will be receiving succinylcholine; with this drug, you may experience back and throat pain related to muscle contractions that occur. You will be able to take aspirin to relieve this discomfort, and a warm compress may also help.
- Recovery of your muscle function may take 2 to 3 hours, and someone will be nearby at all times until you have recovered from the paralysis.

SUMMARY

- The nerves communicate with muscles at a point called the NMJ, using ACh as the neurotransmitter.
- NMJ blockers interfere with muscle function. The two groups of NMJ blockers are nondepolarizing and depolarizing agents.
- The nondepolarizing NMJs include those agents that act as antagonists to ACh at the NMJ and prevent depolarization of muscle cells. The depolarizing NMJs act as an ACh agonist at the junction, causing stimulation of the muscle cell and then preventing it from repolarizing.
- NMJ blockers are primarily used as adjuncts to general anesthesia to facilitate endotracheal intubation, to facilitate mechanical ventilation, and to prevent injury during electroconvulsive therapy.
- Adverse effects of NMJ blockers, such as prolonged paralysis, inability to breathe, weakness, muscle pain and soreness, and effects of immobility, are related to muscle function blocking.
- Care of patients receiving NMJ blockers must include support and reassurance because communication is decreased with paralysis; vigilant maintenance of airways and respiration; prevention of skin breakdown; and monitoring for return of function.

CHECK YOUR UNDERSTANDING

Answers to the questions in this chapter can be found in Answers to Check Your Understanding Questions on thePoint®.

MULTIPLE CHOICE

Select the best answer to the following.

1. Nondepolarizing NMJ blockers
  a. antagonize ACh to prevent depolarization of muscle cells.
  b. act as agonists of ACh, leading to depolarization of muscle cells.
  c. prevent the repolarization of muscle cells.
  d. are associated with painful muscle contractions on administration.

2. Curare is used as a poison on arrow tips in some cultures. Curare
  a. is a depolarizing NMJ blocker.
  b. causes muscle paralysis in the brain.
  c. is not affected by cooking.
  d. has no clinical use today.

3. Succinylcholine has a more rapid onset of action and a shorter duration of activity than the nondepolarizing NMJ blockers because it
  a. does not bind well to receptor sites.
  b. rapidly crosses the blood–brain barrier and is lost.
  c. is broken down by acetylcholinesterase that is found in the plasma.
  d. is very unstable.

4. When planning the care of a patient who is to receive an NMJ blocker the nurse would expect which of the following about the patient?
  a. Transfer to an intensive care unit would be essential.
  b. Intubation would be necessary to maintain respirations.
  c. He would have no memory of any events.
  d. No adverse effects would occur after the drug is stopped.

(continues on page 488)

5. Malignant hyperthermia can occur with any NMJ blocker, but it most often occurs with succinylcholine. The nurse would expect to see which drug ordered?
   a. Phenobarbital
   b. Pancuronium
   c. Dantrolene
   d. Diazepam

6. Patient recovery from an NMJ blocker
   a. is predictable, based on the drug given.
   b. can be affected by genetic enzyme deficiency.
   c. can always be ensured because of the drug half-life.
   d. can be shortened by administration of oxygen.

7. When preparing NMJ blockers for administration, it is important that they
   a. are not mixed in with any alkaline solutions.
   b. are not exposed to light.
   c. are not mixed with any other drug.
   d. are not mixed with heparin.

MULTIPLE RESPONSE

Select all that apply.

1. The nurse would expect administration of an NMJ blocker as the drug of choice to accomplish which of the following?
   a. Facilitate endotracheal intubation
   b. Facilitate mechanical ventilation
   c. Prevent injury during electroconvulsive therapy
   d. Relieve pain during labor and delivery
   e. Treat myasthenia gravis
   f. Treat a patient with a history of malignant hyperthermia

BIBLIOGRAPHY AND REFERENCES

Brunton, L., Chabner, B., & Knollman, B. (2011). *Goodman and Gilman's the pharmacological basis of therapeutics* (12th ed.). New York: McGraw-Hill.

Facts and Comparisons. (2015). *Drug facts and comparisons*. St. Louis, MO: Author.

Facts and Comparisons. (2015). *Professional's guide to patient drug facts*. St. Louis, MO: Author.

Gibbs, N. M. (2012). Risks of anesthesia and surgery in elderly patients. *Journal of Anesthesia and Intensive Care, 40*(1), 14–16.

Karch, A. M. (2014). *Lippincott's nursing drug guide*. Philadelphia, PA: Lippincott Williams & Wilkins.

Miller, R. D., & Pardo, M. (2011). *Basics of anesthesia* (6th ed.). New York: Saunders.

Nagelhout, J. J., & Plaus, K. (2013). *Nurse anesthesia* (5th ed.). New York: Saunders.

Porth, C. M. (2013). *Pathophysiology: Concepts of altered health states* (9th ed.). Philadelphia, PA: Lippincott Williams & Wilkins.

Rosenberg, H., Davis, M., James, D., et al. (2007). Malignant hyperthermia. *Orphanet Journal of Rare Diseases, 2*(21), 21.

Wadlund, D. L. (2006). Prevention, recognition and management of nursing complications in the intraoperative and postoperative surgical patient. *Nursing Clinics of North America, 41*, 219–229.

PART 5

DRUGS ACTING ON THE AUTONOMIC NERVOUS SYSTEM

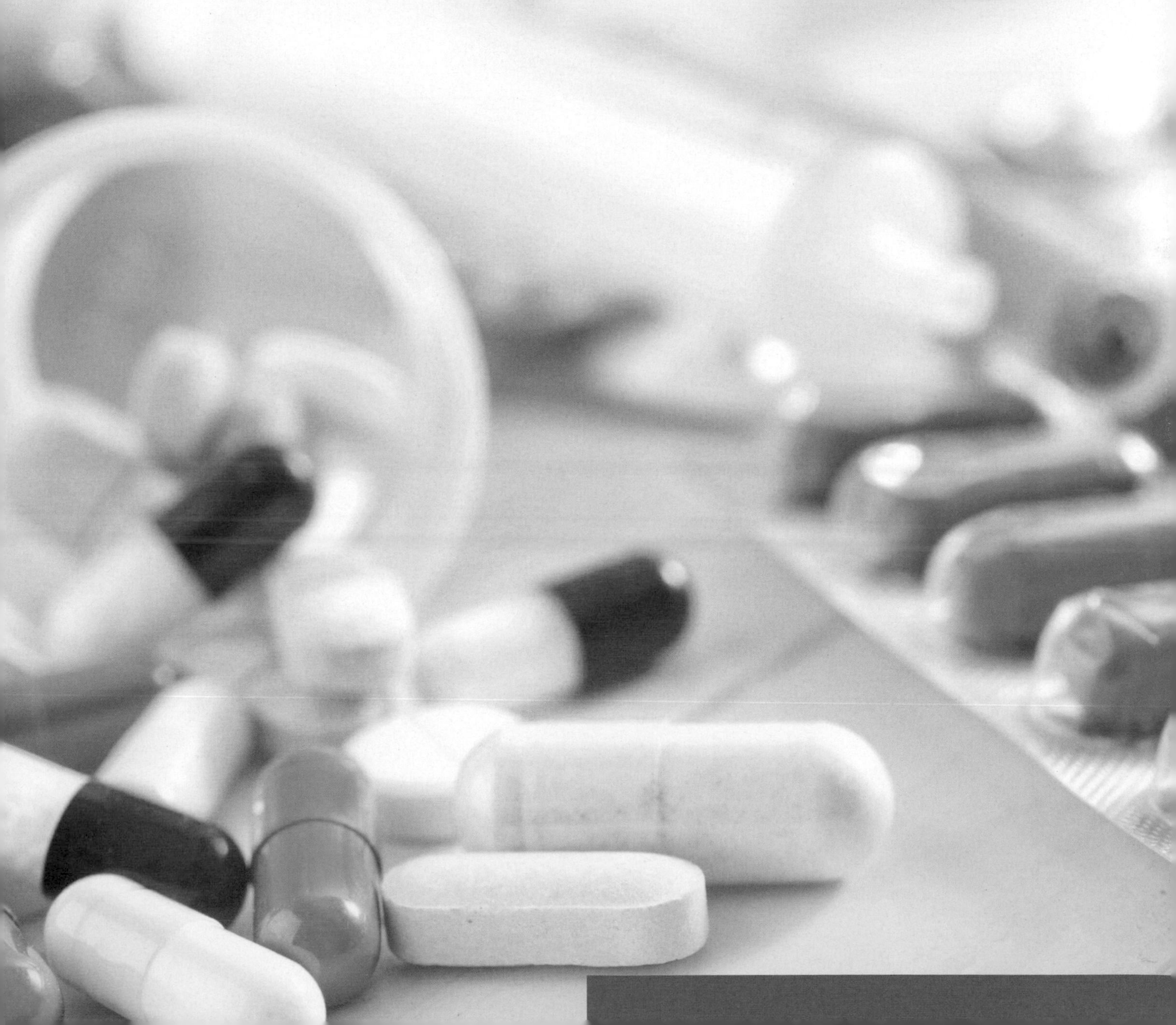

Introduction to the Autonomic Nervous System 29

Learning Objectives

Upon completion of this chapter, you will be able to:

1. Describe how the autonomic nervous system differs anatomically from the rest of the nervous system.
2. Outline a sympathetic response and the clinical manifestation of this response.
3. Describe the alpha- and beta-receptors found within the sympathetic nervous system by sites and actions that follow the stimulation of each kind of receptor.
4. Outline the events that occur with stimulation of the parasympathetic nervous system.
5. Define the terms muscarinic receptor and nicotinic receptor, giving an example of each.

Glossary of Key Terms

acetylcholinesterase: enzyme responsible for the immediate breakdown of acetylcholine when released from the nerve ending; prevents overstimulation of cholinergic receptor sites

adrenergic receptors: receptor sites on effectors that respond to norepinephrine/epinephrine

alpha-receptors: adrenergic receptors that are found in smooth muscles

autonomic nervous system: portion of the central and peripheral nervous systems that, with the endocrine system, functions to maintain internal homeostasis

beta-receptors: adrenergic receptors that are found in the heart, lungs, and vascular smooth muscle

cholinergic receptors: receptor sites on effectors that respond to acetylcholine

ganglia: groups of closely packed nerve cell bodies

monoamine oxidase (MAO): enzyme that breaks down norepinephrine to make it inactive

muscarinic receptors: cholinergic receptors that also respond to stimulation by muscarine

nicotinic receptors: cholinergic receptors that also respond to stimulation by nicotine

parasympathetic nervous system: "rest-and-digest" response mediator that contains central nervous system (CNS) cells from the cranium or sacral area of the spinal cord, long preganglionic axons, ganglia near or within the effector tissue, and short postganglionic axons that react with cholinergic receptors

sympathetic nervous system: "fight-or-flight" response mediator; composed of CNS cells from the thoracic or lumbar areas, short preganglionic axons, ganglia near the spinal cord, and long postganglionic axons that react with adrenergic receptors

The **autonomic nervous system** (ANS) is sometimes called the involuntary or visceral nervous system because it mostly functions with the person having little conscious awareness of its activity. Working closely with the endocrine system the ANS helps to regulate and integrate the body's internal functions within a relatively narrow range of normal on a minute-to-minute basis. The ANS integrates parts of the central nervous system (CNS) and peripheral nervous system to automatically react to changes in the internal and external environments (Figure 29.1).

Structure and Function of the Autonomic Nervous System

The main nerve centers for the ANS are located in the hypothalamus, the medulla, and the spinal cord. Nerve impulses that arise in peripheral structures are carried to these centers by afferent nerve fibers. These integrating centers in the CNS respond by sending out efferent impulses along the autonomic nerve pathways. These impulses adjust the functioning of various internal organs in ways that keep the body's internal environment constant, or homeostatic.

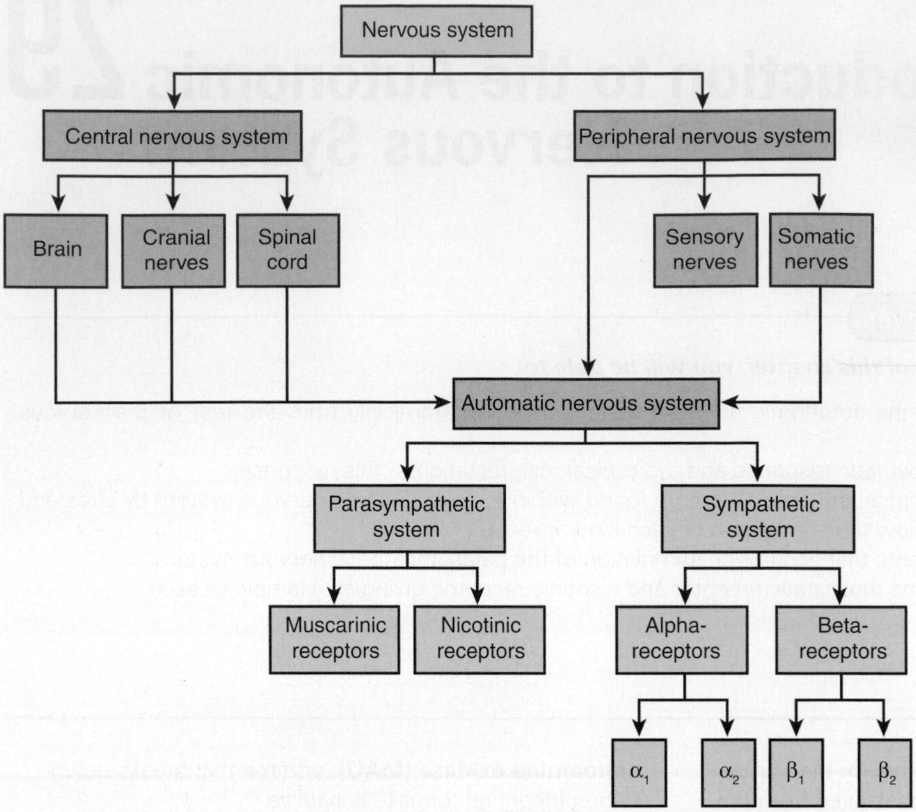

FIGURE 29.1 Organization of the nervous system.

Nerve Impulse Transmission

Throughout the ANS, nerve impulses are carried from the CNS to the outlying organs by way of a two-neuron system. In most peripheral nervous system activities the CNS nerve body sends an impulse directly to an effector organ or muscle. The ANS does not send impulses directly to the periphery. Instead, axons from CNS neurons end in **ganglia**, or groups of nerve bodies that are packed together, located outside of the CNS. These ganglia receive information from the preganglionic neuron that started in the CNS and relay that information along postganglionic neurons. The postganglionic neurons transmit impulses to the neuroeffector cells—muscles, glands, and organs.

Functions

The ANS works to regulate blood pressure, heart rate, respiration, body temperature, water balance, urinary excretion, and digestive functions, among other things. This system exerts minute-to-minute control of body responses, which is balanced by the two divisions of the ANS.

Divisions

The ANS is divided into two branches: The **sympathetic nervous system** (SNS) and the **parasympathetic nervous system**. These two branches differ in three basic ways: (1) the location of the originating cells in the CNS, (2) the location of the nerve ganglia, and (3) the preganglionic and postganglionic neurons (Table 29.1 and Figure 29.2).

Table 29.1 Comparison of the Sympathetic and Parasympathetic Nervous Systems

Characteristic	Sympathetic	Parasympathetic
CNS nerve origin	Thoracic, lumbar spinal cord	Cranium, sacral spinal cord
Preganglionic neuron	Short axon	Long axon
Preganglionic neurotransmitter	ACh	ACh
Ganglia location	Next to spinal cord	Within or near effector organs
Postganglionic neuron	Long axon	Short axon
Postganglionic neurotransmitter	Norepinephrine, epinephrine	ACh
Neurotransmitter terminator	MAO, COMT	Acetylcholinesterase
General response	Fight or flight	Rest and digest

CNS, central nervous system; ACh, acetylcholine; MAO, monoamine oxidase; COMT, catechol-*O*-methyl transferase.

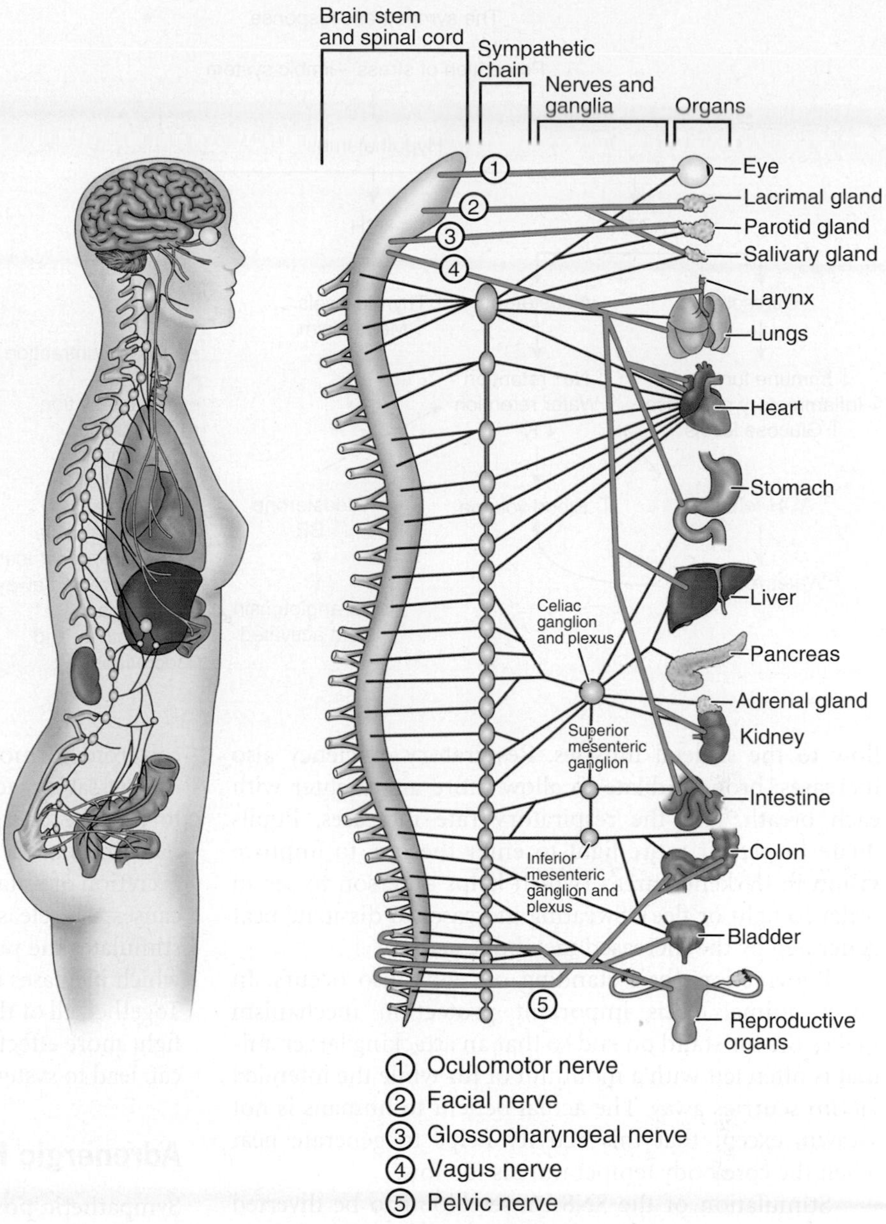

FIGURE 29.2 The autonomic nervous system. The sympathetic, or thoracolumbar, division sends relatively short preganglionic fibers to the chains of paravertebral ganglia and to certain outlying ganglia. The second cell, or postganglionic cell, sends relatively long postganglionic fibers to the organs it innervates. The parasympathetic, or craniosacral, division sends long preganglionic fibers that synapse with a second nerve cell in ganglia located close to or within the organs that are then innervated by short postganglionic fibers.

Sympathetic Nervous System

The SNS is sometimes referred to as the "fight-or-flight" system, or the system responsible for preparing the body to respond to stress. Stress can be either internal, such as cell injury or death, or external, such as a perceived or learned reaction to various external situations or stimuli. For the most part the SNS acts much like an accelerator, speeding things up for action.

Structure and Function

The SNS is also called the thoracolumbar system because the CNS cells that originate impulses for this system are located in the thoracic and lumbar sections of the spinal cord. These cells send out short preganglionic fibers that synapse or communicate with nerve ganglia located in chains running alongside the spinal cord. Acetylcholine (ACh) is the neurotransmitter released by these preganglionic nerves. The nerve ganglia, in turn, send out long postganglionic fibers that synapse with neuroeffectors, using norepinephrine or epinephrine as the neurotransmitter. One of the sympathetic ganglia, on either side of the spinal cord, does not develop postganglionic axons but produces norepinephrine and epinephrine, which are secreted directly into the bloodstream. These ganglia have evolved into the adrenal medullae. When the SNS is stimulated the chromaffin cells of the adrenal medullae secrete epinephrine and norepinephrine directly into the bloodstream.

When stimulated the SNS prepares the body to flee or to turn and fight (Figure 29.3). Cardiovascular activity increases, as do blood pressure, heart rate, and blood

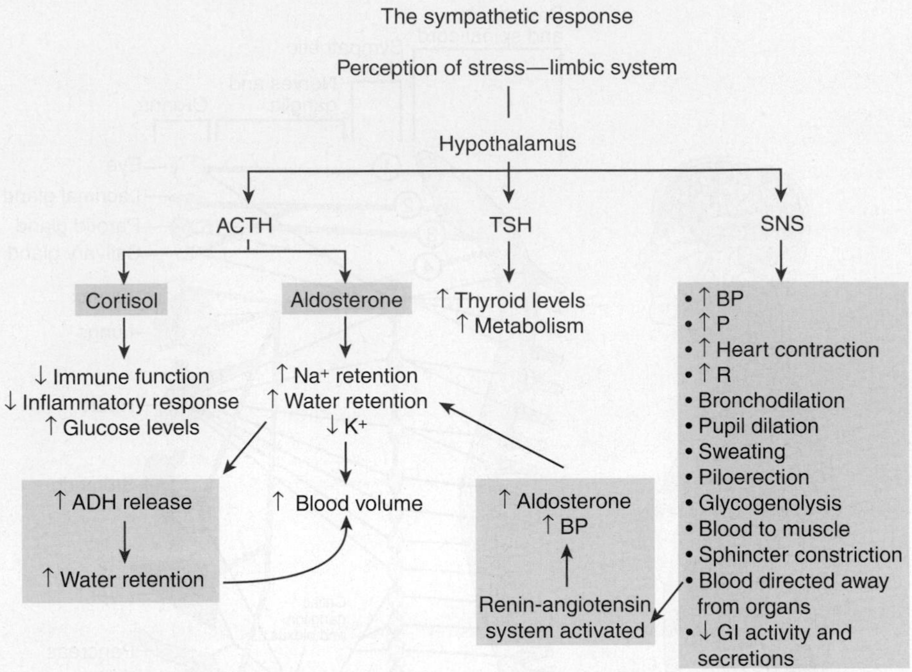

FIGURE 29.3 The "fight-or-flight" response. The sympathetic stress reaction. ACTH, adrenocorticotropic hormone; ADH, antidiuretic hormone; BP, blood pressure; GI, gastrointestinal; P, pulse; R, respiratory rate; SNS, sympathetic nervous system; TSH, thyroid-stimulating hormone.

flow to the skeletal muscles. Respiratory efficiency also increases; bronchi dilate to allow more air to enter with each breath, and the respiratory rate increases. Pupils dilate to permit more light to enter the eye, to improve vision in darkened areas (which helps a person to see in order to fight or flee). Sweating increases to dissipate heat generated by the increased metabolic activity.

Piloerection (hair standing on end) also occurs. In lower animals, this important protection mechanism makes the fur stand on end so that an attacking larger animal is often left with a mouthful of fur while the intended victim scurries away. The actual benefit to humans is not known, except that this activity helps to generate heat when the core body temperature is too low.

Stimulation of the SNS causes blood to be diverted away from the gastrointestinal (GI) tract because there is no real need to digest food during a flight-or-fight situation. Subsequently, bowel sounds decrease and digestion slows dramatically; sphincters are constricted, and bowel evacuation does not occur. Blood is also diverted away from other internal organs, including the kidneys, resulting in activation of the renin–angiotensin system (Chapter 42) and a further increase in blood pressure and blood volume as water is retained by the kidneys. Sphincters in the urinary bladder are also constricted, precluding urination.

Several other metabolic activities occur that prepare the body to fight or flee. For example, glucose is formed by glycogenolysis to increase blood glucose levels and provide energy. The hypothalamus causes the secretion of adrenocorticotropic hormone, leading to a release of the adrenal hormones, including cortisol, which suppresses the immune and inflammatory reactions to preserve energy that otherwise might be used by these activities. The corticosteroid hormones also block protein production, another energy-saving activity, and increase the release of glucose to provide energy. Aldosterone, also released with adrenal stimulation, retains sodium and water and causes the excretion of potassium in the urine. The hypothalamus also causes the release of thyroid-stimulating hormone, which stimulates the production and release of thyroid hormone, which increases metabolism and the efficient use of energy. Together, all of these activities prepare the body to flee or to fight more effectively. When overstimulated, however, they can lead to system overload and a variety of disorders.

Adrenergic Response

Sympathetic postganglionic nerves that synthesize, store, and release norepinephrine are referred to as adrenergic nerves. Adrenergic nerves are also found within the CNS. The chromaffin cells of the adrenal medulla also are adrenergic because they synthesize, store, and release norepinephrine, as well as epinephrine.

Norepinephrine Synthesis and Storage

Norepinephrine belongs to a group of structurally related chemicals called catecholamines that also includes dopamine, serotonin, and epinephrine. Norepinephrine is made by the nerve cells using tyrosine, which is obtained in the diet. Dihydroxyphenylalanine (DOPA) is produced by a nerve, using tyrosine from the diet and other chemicals. With the help of the enzyme DOPA decarboxylase the DOPA is converted to dopamine, which in turn is converted to norepinephrine in adrenergic cells. The norepinephrine then is stored in granules or storage vesicles within the cell. These vesicles move down the nerve axon

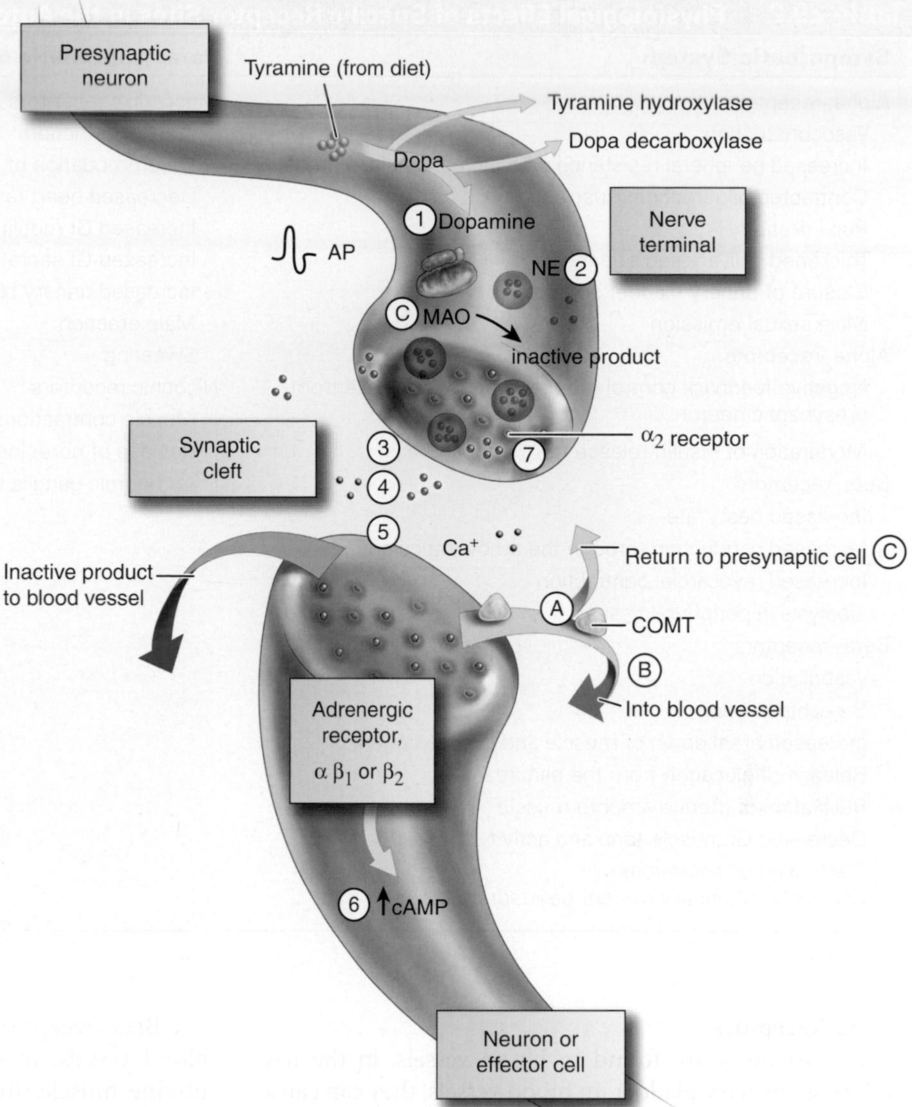

FIGURE 29.4 Sequence of events at an adrenergic synapse. **(1)** Dopamine, a precursor of norepinephrine (NE), is synthesized from tyrosine in several steps. **(2)** Dopamine is taken into the storage vesicle and converted to NE. **(3)** Release of neurotransmitter by an action potential (AP) in the presynaptic nerve. **(4)** Diffusion of neurotransmitter across synaptic cleft. **(5)** Combination of neurotransmitter with receptor. The events resulting from NE's occupying of receptor sites depend on the nature of the postsynaptic cell. **(6)** Interaction of NE with many beta-receptors leads to increased synthesis of cyclic adenosine monophosphate (cAMP). **(7)** Feedback control at alpha$_2$-receptor leads to decreased NE relapse from presynaptic neuron. Deactivation of NE occurs by breakdown of NE by the enzyme COMT **(A)** or more importantly by reuptake into the presynaptic neuron **(C)** where it may be reused or inactivated by another enzyme, monoamine oxidase (MAO). Some of the neurotransmitter may also diffuse away from the synaptic cleft **(B)**.

to the terminals of the axon, where they line up along the cell membrane. To be an adrenergic nerve the nerve must contain all of the enzymes and building blocks necessary to produce norepinephrine (Figure 29.4).

Norepinephrine Release

When the nerve is stimulated the action potential travels down the nerve axon and arrives at the axon terminal (see Chapter 19). The action potential then depolarizes the axon membrane. This action allows calcium into the nerve, causing the membrane to contract and the storage vesicles to fuse with the cell membrane, releasing their load of norepinephrine into the synaptic gap or cleft. The norepinephrine travels across the very short gap to very specific adrenergic receptor sites on the effector cell on the other side of the synaptic gap.

Adrenergic Receptors

Adrenergic receptors can be stimulated by the neurotransmitter released from the axon in the immediate vicinity, and they can be further stimulated by circulating norepinephrine and epinephrine secreted directly into the bloodstream by the adrenal medulla. The receptor sites that react with neurotransmitters at adrenergic sites have been classified as **alpha-receptors** and **beta-receptors.** These receptors are further classified as alpha$_1$-, alpha$_2$-, beta$_1$-, and beta$_2$-receptors (Table 29.2). It is thought that receptors may respond to different concentrations of norepinephrine or different ratios of norepinephrine and epinephrine. Different drugs that are known to affect the SNS may affect parts of the sympathetic response but not all of it, because they are designed to stimulate specific adrenergic receptors.

Table 29.2 Physiological Effects of Specific Receptor Sites in the Autonomic Nervous System

Sympathetic System	Parasympathetic System
$Alpha_1$-receptors	Muscarinic receptors
Vasoconstriction	Pupil constriction
Increased peripheral resistance with increased blood pressure	Accommodation of the lens
Contracted piloerection muscles	Decreased heart rate
Pupil dilation	Increased GI motility
Thickened salivary secretions	Increased GI secretions
Closure of urinary bladder sphincter	Increased urinary bladder contraction
Male sexual emission	Male erection
$Alpha_2$-receptors	Sweating
Negative feedback control of norepinephrine release from presynaptic neuron	Nicotinic receptors
	Muscle contractions
Moderation of insulin release from the pancreas	Release of norepinephrine from the adrenal medulla
$Beta_1$-receptors	Autonomic ganglia stimulation
Increased heart rate	
Increased conduction through the atrioventricular node	
Increased myocardial contraction	
Lipolysis in peripheral tissues	
$Beta_2$-receptors	
Vasodilation	
Bronchial dilation	
Increased breakdown of muscle and liver glycogen	
Release of glucagon from the pancreas	
Relaxation of uterine smooth muscle	
Decreased GI muscle tone and activity	
Decreased GI secretions	
Relaxation of urinary bladder detrusor muscle	

GI, gastrointestinal.

Alpha-Receptors

$Alpha_1$-receptors are found in blood vessels, in the iris, and in the urinary bladder. In blood vessels, they can cause vasoconstriction and increase peripheral resistance, thus raising blood pressure. In the iris, they cause pupil dilation. In the urinary bladder, they cause the increased closure of the internal sphincter.

$Alpha_2$-receptors are located on nerve membranes and act as modulators of norepinephrine release. When norepinephrine is released from a nerve ending, it crosses the synaptic cleft to react with its specific receptor site. Some of it also flows back to react with the alpha-receptor on the nerve membrane. This causes a reflex decrease in norepinephrine release. In this way the $alpha_2$-receptor helps to prevent overstimulation of effector sites. These receptors are also found on the beta cells in the pancreas, where they help to moderate the insulin release stimulated by SNS activation.

Beta-Receptors

$Beta_1$-receptors are found in cardiac tissue, where they can stimulate increased myocardial activity and increased heart rate. They are also responsible for increased lipolysis or breakdown of fat for energy in peripheral tissues.

$Beta_2$-receptors are found in the smooth muscle in blood vessels, in the bronchi, in the periphery, and in uterine muscle. In blood vessels, $beta_2$ stimulation leads to vasodilation. $Beta_2$-receptors also cause dilation in the bronchi. In the periphery, they can cause increased muscle and liver breakdown of glycogen and increased release of glucagon from the alpha cells of the pancreas. Stimulation of $beta_2$-receptors in the uterus results in relaxed uterine smooth muscle.

$Beta_3$-receptors are found in the kidney and help to stimulate the renin–angiotensin–aldosterone system. These receptors in the urinary bladder also cause relaxation of the bladder.

Termination of Response

Once norepinephrine has been released into the synaptic cleft, stimulation of the receptor site is terminated and disposal of any extra norepinephrine, as well as the neurotransmitter that has reacted with the receptor site, must occur. Most of the free norepinephrine molecules are taken up by the nerve terminal that released them in a process called reuptake. This neurotransmitter is then repackaged into vesicles to be released later with nerve stimulation. This is an effective recycling effort by the nerve. Enzymes are also in the area, as well as in the liver, to metabolize or biotransform any remaining norepinephrine or any norepinephrine that is absorbed into circulation. These enzymes are **monoamine oxidase (MAO)** and catechol-*O*-methyl transferase (COMT).

KEY POINTS

- The ANS, which is divided into two branches—the SNS and the parasympathetic nervous system—works with the endocrine system to regulate internal functioning and maintain homeostasis.
- The SNS is responsible for the fight-or-flight response.
- The SNS is composed of CNS cells arising in the thoracic or lumbar area of the spinal cord and long postganglionic axons that react with effector cells. The neurotransmitter used by the preganglionic cells is ACh; the neurotransmitter used by the postganglionic cells is norepinephrine.
- SNS adrenergic receptors are classified as alpha$_1$-, alpha$_2$-, beta$_1$-, or beta$_2$-receptors.

Parasympathetic Nervous System

In many areas the parasympathetic nervous system works in opposition to the SNS. This allows the autonomic system to maintain a fine control over internal homeostasis. For example, the SNS increases heart rate, whereas the parasympathetic system decreases it. Thus, the ANS can influence heart rate by increasing or decreasing sympathetic activity or by increasing or decreasing parasympathetic activity. This is very much like controlling the speed of a car by moving between the accelerator and the brake or combining the two. Whereas the SNS is associated with the stress reaction and expenditure of energy, the parasympathetic system is associated with activities that help the body to store or conserve energy, a "rest-and-digest" response (Table 29.3).

Structure and Function

The parasympathetic system is sometimes called the craniosacral system because the CNS neurons that originate parasympathetic impulses are found in the cranium (one of the most important being the vagus or tenth cranial nerve) and in the sacral area of the spinal cord

Table 29.3 Comparing the Effects of Autonomic Stimulation

Effector Site	Sympathetic Reaction	Parasympathetic Reaction
Eye Structures		
Iris radial muscle	Contraction (pupil dilates)	—
Iris sphincter muscle	—	Contraction (pupil constricts)
Ciliary muscle	—	Contraction (lens accommodates for near vision)
Lacrimal glands		↑ Secretions
Heart	↑ Rate, contractility ↑ Atrioventricular conduction	↓ Rate ↓ Atrioventricular conduction
Blood Vessels		
Skin, mucous membranes	Constriction	—
Skeletal muscle	Dilation	—
Bronchial muscle	Relaxation (dilation)	Constriction
GI System		
Muscle motility and tone	↓ Activity	↑ Activity
Sphincters	Contraction	Relaxation
Secretions	↓ Secretions	↑ Activity
Salivary glands	Thick secretions	Copious, watery secretions
Gallbladder	Relaxation	Contraction
Liver	Glyconeogenesis	—
Urinary Bladder		
Detrusor muscle	Relaxation	Contraction
Trigone muscle and sphincter	Contraction	Relaxation
Sex Organs		
Male	Emission	Erection (vascular dilation)
Female	Uterine relaxation	—
Skin Structures		
Sweat glands	↑ Sweating	—
Piloerector muscles	Contracted (goose bumps)	—

—, no reaction or response; GI, gastrointestinal.

(see Figure 29.1). The terms cholinergic, muscarinic, and vagal are often used interchangeably when discussing the parasympathetic system. It has long preganglionic axons that meet in ganglia located close to or within the organ to be affected. The postganglionic axon is very short, going directly to the effector cell. The neurotransmitter used by both the preganglionic and postganglionic neurons is ACh.

Parasympathetic system stimulation results in the following actions:

- Increased motility and secretions in the GI tract to promote digestion and absorption of nutrients.
- Decreased heart rate and contractility to conserve energy and provide rest for the heart.
- Constriction of the bronchi, with increased secretions.
- Relaxation of the GI and urinary bladder sphincters, allowing evacuation of waste products.
- Pupillary constriction, which decreases the light entering the eye and decreases stimulation of the retina.

These activities are aimed at increasing digestion, absorption of nutrients, and building of essential proteins, as well as a general conservation of energy.

Cholinergic Response

Neurons that use ACh as their neurotransmitter are called cholinergic neurons. There are four basic kinds of cholinergic nerves:

1. All preganglionic nerves in the ANS, both sympathetic and parasympathetic
2. Postganglionic nerves of the parasympathetic system and a few SNS nerves, such as those that reenter the spinal cord and cause general body reactions such as sweating
3. Motor nerves on skeletal muscles
4. Cholinergic nerves within the CNS

Acetylcholine Synthesis and Storage

ACh is an ester of acetic acid and an organic alcohol called choline. Cholinergic nerves use choline, obtained in the diet, to produce ACh. The last step in the production of the neurotransmitter involves choline acetyltransferase, an enzyme that is also produced within cholinergic nerves. Just like norepinephrine the ACh is produced in the nerve and travels to the end of the axons, where it is packaged into vesicles. To be a cholinergic nerve the nerve must contain all of the enzymes and building blocks necessary to produce ACh.

Acetylcholine Release

The vesicles full of ACh move to the nerve membrane; when an action potential reaches the nerve terminal, calcium entering the cell causes the membrane to contract and secrete the neurotransmitter into the synaptic cleft. The ACh travels across the synaptic cleft and reacts with very specific cholinergic receptor sites on the effector cell (Figure 29.5).

Cholinergic Receptors

Cholinergic receptors or ACh receptors are found on organs and muscles. They have been classified as muscarinic receptors and nicotinic receptors. This classification is based on very early research of the ANS that used muscarine (a plant alkaloid from mushrooms) and nicotine (a plant alkaloid found in tobacco plants) to study the actions of the parasympathetic system.

Muscarinic Receptors

As the name implies, **muscarinic receptors** are receptors that can be stimulated by muscarine. They are found in visceral effector organs, such as the GI tract, bladder, and heart, in sweat glands, and in some vascular smooth muscle. Stimulation of muscarinic receptors causes pupil constriction, increased GI motility and secretions (including saliva), increased urinary bladder contraction, and a slowing of the heart rate.

Nicotinic Receptors

Nicotinic receptors are located in the CNS, the adrenal medulla, the autonomic ganglia, and the neuromuscular junction. Stimulation of nicotinic receptors causes skeletal muscle contractions, autonomic responses such as signs and symptoms of a stress reaction, and release of norepinephrine and epinephrine from the adrenal medulla.

Termination of Response

Once the effector cell has been stimulated by ACh, stimulation of the receptor site must be terminated and destruction of any ACh must occur. The destruction of ACh is carried out by the enzyme **acetylcholinesterase**. This enzyme reacts with the ACh to form a chemically inactive compound. The breakdown of the released ACh is accomplished in 1/1,000 second, and the receptor is vacated, allowing the effector membrane to repolarize and be ready for the next stimulation.

KEY POINTS

- The parasympathetic system, when stimulated, acts as a rest-and-digest response. It increases the digestion, absorption, and metabolism of nutrients and slows metabolism and function to save energy.
- The parasympathetic system comprises CNS cells that arise in the cranium and sacral region of the spinal cord, long preganglionic axons that secrete ACh, ganglia located very close to or within the effector tissue, and short postganglionic axons that also secrete ACh.
- ACh is made by choline from the diet and packaged into storage vesicles to be released by the cholinergic nerve into the synaptic cleft. ACh is broken down to an inactive form almost immediately by acetylcholinesterase.
- Parasympathetic system receptors are classified as muscarinic or nicotinic, depending on what response they have to these plant alkaloids.

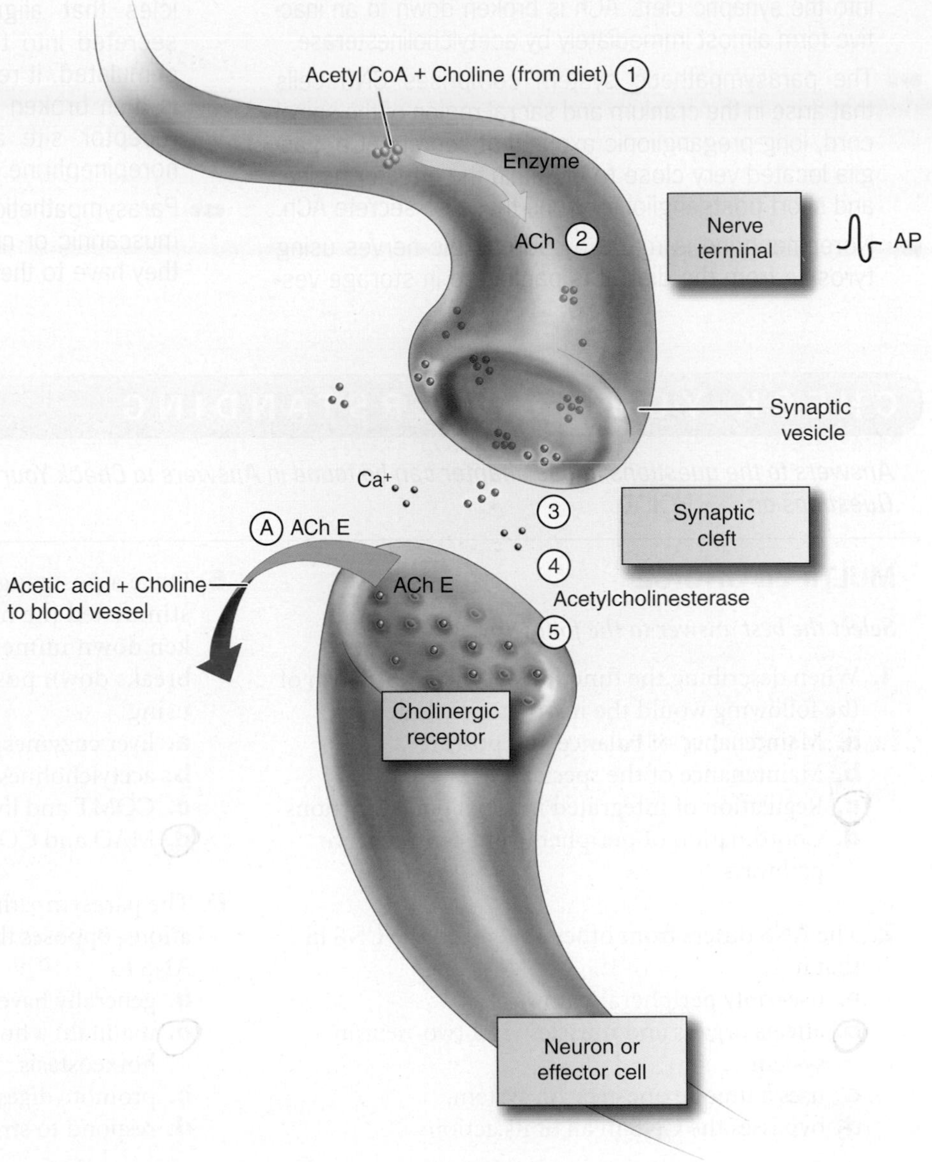

FIGURE 29.5 Sequence of events at a cholinergic synapse. **(1)** Synthesis of acetylcholine (ACh) from choline (a substance in the diet) and a cofactor (the enzyme is choline acetyltransferase, CoA). **(2)** Uptake of neurotransmitter into storage (synaptic) vesicle. **(3)** Release of neurotransmitter by an action potential (AP) in the presynaptic nerve. **(4)** Diffusion of neurotransmitter across the synaptic cleft. **(5)** Combination of neurotransmitter with receptor. The events resulting from Ach's occupation of receptor sites depend on the nature of the postsynaptic cell. ACh excites some cells and inhibits others. An enzyme, acetylcholinesterase (AChE), found in the tissues and on the postsynaptic cell, inactivates ACh **(A)**. Some of the products diffuse into the circulation, but most of the choline formed is taken up and reused by the cholinergic neuron.

SUMMARY

- The ANS works with the endocrine system to regulate internal functioning and maintain homeostasis.
- The two branches of the ANS, the SNS and the parasympathetic nervous system, work in opposition to maintain minute-to-minute regulation of the internal environment and to allow rapid response to stress situations.
- The SNS, when stimulated, is responsible for the fight-or-flight response. It prepares the body for immediate reaction to stressors by increasing metabolism, diverting blood to big muscles, and increasing cardiac and respiratory function.
- The parasympathetic system, when stimulated, acts as a rest-and-digest response. It increases the digestion, absorption, and metabolism of nutrients and slows metabolism and function to save energy.
- The SNS is composed of CNS cells arising in the thoracic or lumbar area of the spinal cord, short preganglionic axons, ganglia located near the spinal cord, and long postganglionic axons that react with effector cells. The neurotransmitter used by the preganglionic cells is ACh; the neurotransmitter used by the postganglionic cells is norepinephrine.
- One SNS ganglion on either side of the spinal cord does not develop postganglionic axons but instead secretes norepinephrine directly into the bloodstream to travel throughout the body to react with adrenergic receptor sites. These ganglia evolve into the adrenal medulla.
- SNS adrenergic receptors are classified as being alpha$_1$-, alpha$_2$-, beta$_1$-, or beta$_2$-receptors based on the effectors that they stimulate.
- ACh is made by choline from the diet and packaged into storage vesicles to be released by the cholinergic nerve

into the synaptic cleft. ACh is broken down to an inactive form almost immediately by acetylcholinesterase.

- The parasympathetic system comprises CNS cells that arise in the cranium and sacral region of the spinal cord, long preganglionic axons that secrete ACh, ganglia located very close to or within the effector tissue, and short postganglionic axons that also secrete ACh.
- Norepinephrine is made by adrenergic nerves using tyrosine from the diet. It is packaged in storage vesicles that align on the axon membrane and is secreted into the synaptic cleft when the nerve is stimulated. It reacts with specific receptor sites and is then broken down by MAO or COMT to relax the receptor site and recycle the building blocks of norepinephrine.
- Parasympathetic system receptors are classified as muscarinic or nicotinic, depending on what response they have to these plant alkaloids.

CHECK YOUR UNDERSTANDING

Answers to the questions in this chapter can be found in Answers to Check Your Understanding Questions on thePoint®.

MULTIPLE CHOICE

Select the best answer to the following.

1. When describing the functions of the ANS, which of the following would the instructor include?
- **a.** Maintenance of balance and posture
- **b.** Maintenance of the special senses
- **c.** Regulation of integrated internal body functions
- **d.** Coordination of peripheral and central nerve pathways

2. The ANS differs from other systems in the CNS in that it
- **a.** uses only peripheral pathways.
- **b.** affects organs and muscles via a two-neuron system.
- **c.** uses a unique one-neuron system.
- **d.** bypasses the CNS in all of its actions.

3. If you suspect that a person is very stressed and is experiencing a sympathetic stress reaction, you would expect to find
- **a.** increased bowel sounds and urinary output.
- **b.** constricted pupils and warm, flushed skin.
- **c.** slow heart rate and decreased systolic blood pressure.
- **d.** dilated pupils and elevated systolic blood pressure.

4. The nurse determines that the beta$_2$-receptors in the SNS have been stimulated by which finding?
- **a.** Increased heart rate
- **b.** Increased myocardial contraction
- **c.** Bronchial dilation
- **d.** Uterine contraction

5. Once a postganglionic receptor site has been stimulated the neurotransmitter must be broken down immediately. The sympathetic system breaks down postganglionic neurotransmitters by using
- **a.** liver enzymes and acetylcholinesterase.
- **b.** acetylcholinesterase and MAO.
- **c.** COMT and liver enzymes.
- **d.** MAO and COMT.

6. The parasympathetic nervous system, in most situations, opposes the actions of the SNS, allowing the ANS to
- **a.** generally have no effect.
- **b.** maintain a fine control over internal homeostasis.
- **c.** promote digestion.
- **d.** respond to stress most effectively.

7. Cholinergic neurons, those using ACh as their neurotransmitter, would be least likely found in
- **a.** motor nerves on skeletal muscles.
- **b.** preganglionic nerves in the sympathetic and parasympathetic systems.
- **c.** postganglionic nerves in the parasympathetic system.
- **d.** the adrenal medulla.

8. Stimulation of the parasympathetic nervous system would cause
- **a.** slower heart rate and increased GI secretions.
- **b.** faster heart rate and urinary retention.
- **c.** vasoconstriction and bronchial dilation.
- **d.** pupil dilation and muscle paralysis.

MULTIPLE RESPONSE

Select all that apply.

1. The SNS
- **a.** is called the thoracolumbar system.
- **b.** is called the fight-or-flight system.
- **c.** is called the craniosacral system.
- **d.** uses ACh as its sole neurotransmitter.
- **e.** uses epinephrine as its sole neurotransmitter.
- **f.** is active during a stress reaction.

2. The sympathetic system uses catecholamines at the postganglionic receptors. Which of the following are considered to be catecholamines?
- **a.** Dopamine
- **b.** Norepinephrine
- **c.** ACh
- **d.** Epinephrine
- **e.** MAO
- **f.** Serotonin

BIBLIOGRAPHY AND REFERENCES

Barnett, K., Barnam, S., Boitano, S., et al. (2012). *Ganong's review of medical physiology* (24th ed.). New York: McGraw-Hill.

Brunton, L., Chabner, B., & Knollman, B. (2011). *Goodman and Gilman's the pharmacological basis of therapeutics* (12th ed.). New York: McGraw-Hill.

Edwards, D., & Burnard, P. (2003). A systemic review of stress and stress management for mental health nurses. *Journal of Advanced Nursing, 42*, 169–200.

Hall, J. (2015). *Guyton and Hall textbook of medical physiology* (13th ed.). Philadelphia, PA: W. B. Saunders.

Janig, W. (2008). *Integrative action of the autonomic nervous system.* New York: Cambridge University Press.

Mortzer, S. A., & Hertig, V. (2004). Stress, stress response, and health. *Nursing Clinics of North America, 39*, 1–17.

Porth, C. M. (2013). *Pathophysiology: Concepts of altered health states* (9th ed.). Philadelphia, PA: Lippincott Williams & Wilkins.

Rider, S. H. (2004). Psychological distress: Concept analysis. *Journal of Advanced Nursing, 45*, 536–545.

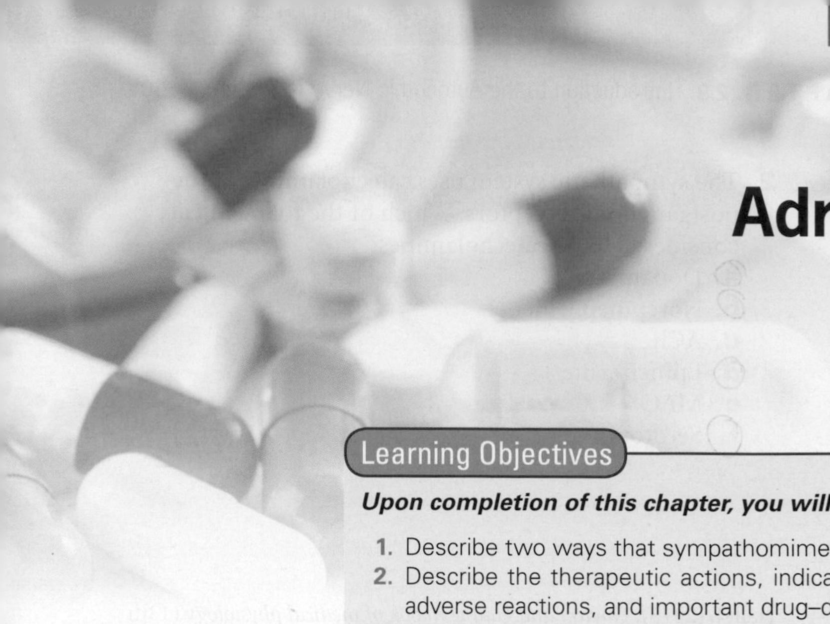

Adrenergic Agonists 30

Learning Objectives

Upon completion of this chapter, you will be able to:

1. Describe two ways that sympathomimetic drugs act to produce effects at adrenergic receptors.
2. Describe the therapeutic actions, indications, pharmacokinetics, contraindications, most common adverse reactions, and important drug–drug interactions associated with adrenergic agonists.
3. Discuss the use of adrenergic agents across the lifespan.
4. Compare and contrast the prototype drugs dopamine, phenylephrine, and isoproterenol with other adrenergic agonists.
5. Outline the nursing considerations, including important teaching points, for patients receiving an adrenergic agent.

Glossary of Key Terms

adrenergic agonist: a drug that stimulates the adrenergic receptors of the sympathetic nervous system, either directly (by reacting with receptor sites) or indirectly (by increasing norepinephrine levels)

alpha-agonist: specifically stimulating to the alpha-receptors within the sympathetic nervous system, causing body responses seen when the alpha-receptors are stimulated

beta-agonist: specifically stimulating to the beta-receptors within the sympathetic nervous system, causing body responses seen when the beta-receptors are stimulated

glycogenolysis: breakdown of stored glucose to increase the blood glucose levels

sympathomimetic: drug that mimics the sympathetic nervous system (SNS) with the signs and symptoms seen when the SNS is stimulated

Drug List

Alpha-and Beta-Adrenergic Agonists
dobutamine
dopamine
ephedrine
(P) epinephrine
norepinephrine

Alpha-Specific Adrenergic Agonists
clonidine (alpha2-specific)
midodrine
(P) phenylephrine

Beta-Specific Adrenergic Agonists (Also See Beta-Adrenergic Agonists in Chapter 55)
albuterol
arformoterol
formoterol
indacaterol
(P) isoproterenol
levalbuterol
metaproterenol
olodaterol
salmeterol
terbutaline

An **adrenergic agonist** is also called a **sympathomimetic** drug because it mimics the effects of the sympathetic nervous system (SNS). The therapeutic and adverse effects associated with these drugs are related to their stimulation of adrenergic receptor sites. That stimulation can be either direct, by occupation of the adrenergic receptor, or indirect, by modulation of the release of neurotransmitters from the axon. Some drugs act in both ways. Adrenergic agonists also can affect both the alpha- and beta-receptors, or they can act at specific receptor sites.

The use of adrenergic agonists varies from ophthalmic preparations for dilating pupils to systemic preparations used to support individuals experiencing shock. They are used in patients of all ages (Box 30.1).

BOX 30.1 FOCUS ON Drug Therapy Across the Lifespan

Adrenergic Agonists

CHILDREN

Children are at greater risk for complications associated with the use of adrenergic agonists, including tachycardia, hypertension, tachypnea, and GI complications. The dosage for these agents needs to be calculated from the child's body weight and age. It is good practice to have a second person check the dosage calculation before administering the drug to avoid potential toxic effects. Children should be carefully monitored and supported during the use of these drugs.

Phenylephrine is often found in OTC allergy and cold preparations, and parents need to be instructed to be very careful with the use of these drugs—they should check the labels for ingredients, monitor the recommended dose, and avoid combining drugs that contain similar ingredients.

ADULTS

Adults being treated with adrenergic agonists for shock or shock-like states require constant monitoring and dosage adjustments based on their response. Patients who may be at increased risk for cardiac complications should be monitored very closely and started on a lower dose.

Adults using these agents for glaucoma or for seasonal rhinitis need to be cautioned about the use of OTC drugs and alternative therapies that might increase the drug effects and cause serious adverse effects.

Many of these drugs are used in emergency situations and may be used during pregnancy and lactation. In general, there are no adequate studies about their effects during pregnancy and lactation, and in those situations they should be used only if the benefit to the mother is greater than the risk to the fetus or neonate.

OLDER ADULTS

Older patients are more likely to experience the adverse effects associated with these drugs—CNS, CV, GI, and respiratory. Because older patients often have renal or hepatic impairment, they are also more likely to have toxic levels of the drug related to changes in metabolism and excretion. Older patients should be started on lower doses of the drugs and should be monitored very closely for potentially serious arrhythmias or blood pressure changes.

They also should be cautioned about the use of OTC drugs and complementary therapies that could increase drug effects and cause serious adverse reactions.

FOCUS ON Safe Medication Administration

Administering Ophthalmic Medications

Some of the adrenergic agonists are applied in the eye; it is important to review the administration technique. First, wash hands thoroughly. Do not touch the dropper to the eye or to any other surfaces. Have the patient tilt his or her head back or lie down and stare upward. Gently grasp the lower eyelid and pull the eyelid away from the eyeball. Instill the prescribed number of drops into the lower conjunctival sac and then release the lid slowly (Figure 30.1). Have the patient close the eye and look downward. Apply gentle pressure to the inside corner of the eye for 3 minutes. Do not rub the eyeball, and do not rinse the dropper. If more than one type of eyedrop is being used, wait 5 minutes before administering the next one.

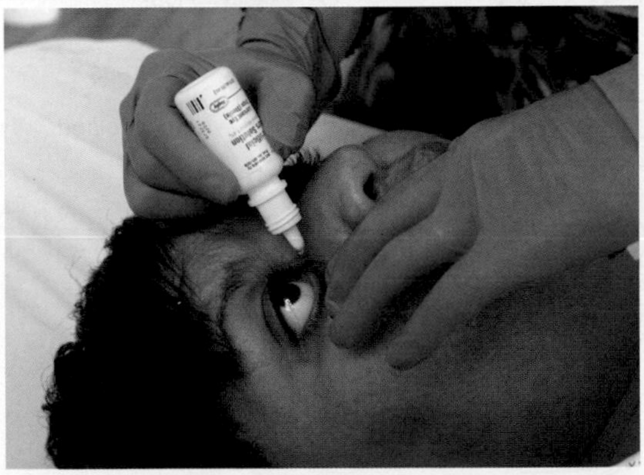

FIGURE 30.1 After gently exposing the lower conjunctival sac the nurse administers an eyedrop. (From Lynn, P. (2006). *Taylor's clinical nursing skills: A nursing process approach* (2nd ed., p. 244). Philadelphia, PA: Lippincott Williams & Wilkins, Figure 4.)

Alpha- and Beta-Adrenergic Agonists

Drugs that are generally sympathomimetic (Figure 30.2) are called **alpha-agonists** (stimulate alpha-receptors) and **beta-agonists** (stimulate beta-receptors). These agonists stimulate all of the adrenergic receptors; that is, they affect both alpha- and beta-receptors (Table 30.1). Agents that affect both alpha- and beta-receptor sites include dobutamine (generic), dopamine (generic), ephedrine (generic), epinephrine (*Adrenalin*, *Adrenaclick*), and norepinephrine (*Levophed*). Some of these drugs are naturally occurring catecholamines.

Therapeutic Actions and Indications

The effects of the sympathomimetic drugs are mediated by the adrenergic receptors in target organs: Heart rate increases with increased myocardial contractility; bronchi dilate and respirations increase in rate and depth; blood vessels constrict, causing an increase in blood pressure; intraocular pressure decreases; **glycogenolysis** (breakdown of glucose stores so that the glucose can be used as energy) occurs throughout the body; pupils dilate; and sweating can increase (see Figure 30.2). These drugs generally are indicated for the treatment of hypotensive states or shock, bronchospasm, and some types of asthma. Table 30.1 discusses Usual Indications for each of these agents.

Dopamine, a naturally occurring catecholamine, is the sympathomimetic of choice for the treatment of shock. It stimulates the heart and blood pressure but also causes a renal and splanchnic arteriole dilation that increases blood flow to the kidneys, preventing the diminished renal

Table 30.1 ***Drugs in Focus:* Alpha- and Beta-Adrenergic Agonists**

Drug Name	Dosage/Route	Usual Indications
dobutamine (generic)	2.5–10 mcg/kg/min IV with dose adjusted based on patient response	Treatment of heart failure
dopamine (generic)	Initially 5–10 mcg/kg/min IV with incremental increases up to 20–50 mcg/kg/min based on patient response	Treatment of shock
ephedrine (generic)	*Adult:* 25–50 mg IM, subcutaneous, or IV for acute treatment; 25–50 mg PO for asthma maintenance *Pediatric:* 25–100 mg/m^2 IM or subcutaneous in four to six divided doses; 3 mg/kg/d in four to six divided doses PO, subcutaneous, or IV for bronchodilation	Treatment of hypotensive episodes
epinephrine (*Adrenalin, Adrenaclick*)	*Adult:* 0.5–1.0 mg IV for acute treatment; 0.3–0.5 mg subcutaneous or IM for respiratory distress; may be used in a nebulizer or as topical nasal drops *Pediatric:* 0.005–0.01 mg/kg IV, base dose on age, weight, and response; do not repeat more than q6 h; topical nasal drops for children >6 y as needed	Treatment of shock when increased blood pressure and heart contractility are essential; to prolong effects of regional anesthetic; primary treatment for bronchospasm; to produce a local vasoconstriction that prolongs the effects of local anesthetics
norepinephrine (*Levophed*)	8–12 mcg base/min IV; base rate and dose on patient response	Treatment of shock; used during cardiac arrest to get sympathetic activity

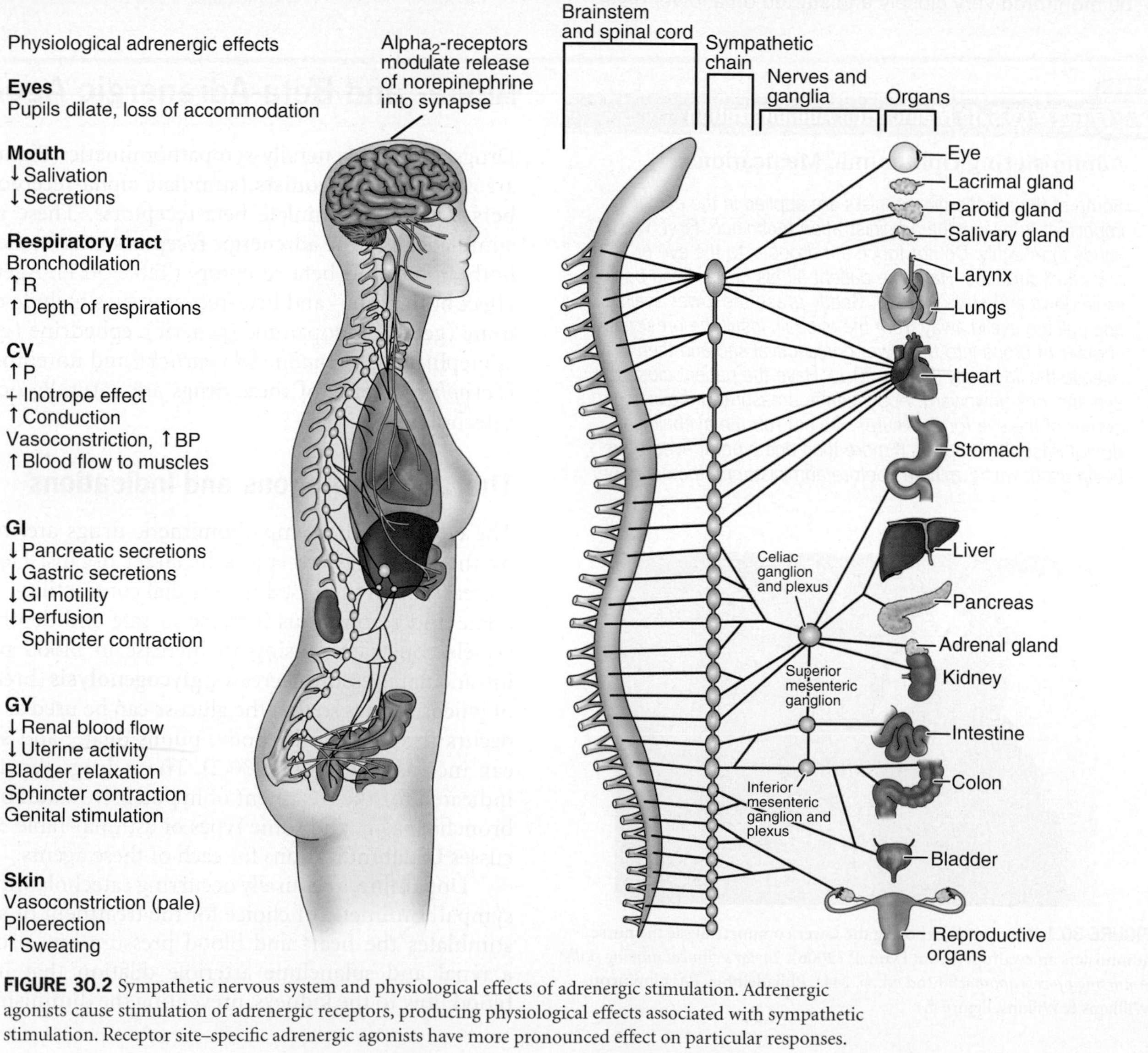

FIGURE 30.2 Sympathetic nervous system and physiological effects of adrenergic stimulation. Adrenergic agonists cause stimulation of adrenergic receptors, producing physiological effects associated with sympathetic stimulation. Receptor site–specific adrenergic agonists have more pronounced effect on particular responses.

blood supply and possible renal shutdown that can occur with epinephrine or norepinephrine, which are also naturally occurring catecholamines that interact with both alpha- and beta-adrenergic receptors and are used for the treatment of shock and to stimulate the body after cardiac arrest and for immediate relief of anaphylaxis (see Table 30.1 for additional indications for epinephrine and norepinephrine).

Dobutamine and ephedrine are synthetic catecholamines. Dobutamine, although it acts at both receptor sites, has a slight preference for beta$_1$-receptor sites. It is used in the treatment of heart failure because it can increase myocardial contractility without much change in rate and does not increase the oxygen demand of the cardiac muscle, an advantage over all of the other sympathomimetic drugs.

Ephedrine stimulates the release of norepinephrine from nerve endings and acts directly on adrenergic receptor sites. Although ephedrine was once used for situations ranging from the treatment of shock to chronic management of asthma and allergic rhinitis, its use in many areas is declining because of the availability of less toxic drugs with more predictable onset and action.

FOCUS ON Safe Medication Administration

***Ephedra**, an herb that acts like ephedrine, has been in headlines in recent years because people who were using the herb to promote weight loss died suddenly. Several states have limited its sale—the U.S. Food and Drug Administration (FDA) is studying the herb, an isomer of epinephrine—and are pushing for the authority to regulate the product. The FDA has banned **ephedra** as a drug, but many states still allow the sale of the herb. Patients should be taught about the potential danger of this product. Any patient who is at risk for serious reactions to the stimulatory effects of a sympathomimetic—patients with narrow-angle glaucoma, dehydration, cerebral or peripheral vascular disease, cardiac disease or arrhythmias, hypertension, renal dysfunction, thyroid disease, diabetes, prostatic disorders, pregnancy, or lactation—should receive direct teaching about the dangers of this product. To review the FDA warnings in preparing your teaching protocol, go to http://nccam.nih.gov/health/alerts/ephedra/consumeradvisory.htm.*

Many over-the-counter (OTC) cold products contain ephedrine or pseudoephedrine. These products can be used to produce methamphetamine, an often-abused street drug. By law the sale of these products is now restricted. The products are found behind the counter at pharmacies, not on open shelves, and the amount that can be purchased at any given time is limited.

Pharmacokinetics

These drugs are generally absorbed rapidly after injection or passage through mucous membranes. They are metabolized in the liver and excreted in the urine. When used in emergency situations, they are given IV to achieve rapid onset of action.

Contraindications and Cautions

The alpha- and beta-agonists are contraindicated in patients with known hypersensitivity to any component of the drug *to prevent hypersensitivity reactions*; pheochromocytoma *because the systemic overload of catecholamines could be fatal*; with tachyarrhythmias or ventricular fibrillation *because the increased heart rate and oxygen consumption usually caused by these drugs could exacerbate these conditions*; with hypovolemia, *for which fluid replacement would be the treatment for the associated hypotension*; and with halogenated hydrocarbon general anesthetics, *which sensitize the myocardium to catecholamines and could cause serious cardiac effects.* Caution should be used with any kind of peripheral vascular disease (e.g., atherosclerosis, Raynaud disease, diabetic endarteritis), *which could be exacerbated by systemic vasoconstriction.* Because the sympathomimetic drugs stimulate the SNS, they should be used during pregnancy and lactation only if the benefits to the mother clearly outweigh any potential risks to the fetus or neonate.

Adverse Effects

The adverse effects associated with the use of alpha- and beta-adrenergic agonists may be associated with the drugs' effects on the SNS: Arrhythmias, hypertension, palpitations, angina, and dyspnea related to the effects on the heart and cardiovascular (CV) system; nausea, vomiting, and constipation related to the depressant effects on the gastrointestinal (GI) tract; and headache, sweating, feelings of tension or anxiety, and piloerection related to sympathetic stimulation (Figure 30.3). Hypokalemia can occur as a result of the release of aldosterone that occurs with sympathetic stimulation and the resultant loss of potassium. Patients may present with muscle cramps related to the shift in potassium. Because all of these drugs cause vasoconstriction, care must be taken to avoid extravasation of any infused drug. The vasoconstriction in the area of extravasation can lead to necrosis and cell death in that area.

Clinically Important Drug–Drug Interactions

Increased effects of tricyclic antidepressants (TCAs) and monoamine oxidase inhibitors (MAOIs) can occur because of the increased norepinephrine levels or increased receptor stimulation that occurs with both drugs. There is an increased risk of hypertension if alpha- and beta-adrenergic agonists are given with any other drugs that cause hypertension, including herbal therapies and OTC preparations (Box 30.2). Any adrenergic agonist will lose effectiveness if combined with any adrenergic antagonist. Monitor the patient's drug regimen for appropriate use of the drugs.

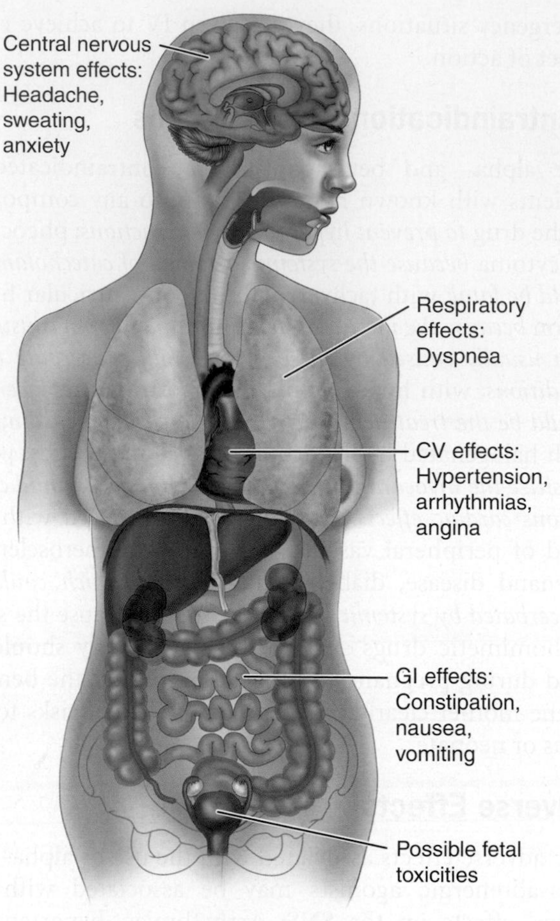

FIGURE 30.3 Common adverse effects associated with adrenergic agonists.

Ⓟ Prototype Summary: Dopamine

Indications: Correction of hemodynamic imbalances present in shock.

Actions: Acts directly and by the release of norepinephrine from sympathetic nerve terminals; mediates dilation of vessels in the renal and splanchnic beds to maintain renal perfusion while stimulating the sympathetic response.

Pharmacokinetics:

Route	Onset	Peak	Duration
IV	1–2 min	10 min	Length of infusion

$T_{1/2}$: 2 minutes; metabolized in the liver, excreted in the urine.

Adverse Effects: Tachycardia, ectopic beats, anginal pain, hypotension, dyspnea, nausea, vomiting, headache.

BOX 30.2 FOCUS ON Herbal and Alternative Therapies

Patients being treated with any adrenergic agonists who are also taking ma huang, guarana, or caffeine are at increased risk for overstimulation, including increased blood pressure, stroke, and death. Counsel patients to avoid these combinations.

Nursing Considerations for Patients Receiving Alpha- and Beta-Adrenergic Agonists

Assessment: History and Examination

Assess for contraindications or cautions: Any known allergies to these drugs *to avoid hypersensitivity reactions*; pheochromocytoma, *which could lead to fatal reactions due to systemic overload of catecholamines*; tachyarrhythmias or ventricular fibrillation, *which could be exacerbated by these drugs*; hypovolemia, *which would require fluid replacement as treatment for the associated hypotension*; general anesthesia with halogenated hydrocarbon anesthetics, *which could lead to serious cardiac effects*; the presence of vascular disease, *which could be exacerbated with the use of these drugs*; and *current status of pregnancy and lactation*:

- Perform a physical assessment to establish baseline status *before beginning therapy, and during therapy, to evaluate for any potential adverse effects and to determine the effectiveness of therapy.*
- Assess vital signs, especially pulse and blood pressure, *to monitor for possible excess stimulation of the cardiac system*; obtain an electrocardiogram (ECG) *to evaluate for possible arrhythmias.*
- Note respiratory rate and auscultate lungs for adventitious sounds *to evaluate effects on bronchi and respirations.*
- Monitor urine output *to evaluate perfusion of the kidneys and therapeutic effects.*
- Monitor the results of laboratory tests, such as renal and liver function tests, *to determine the need for possible dose adjustment*, and serum electrolyte levels to *evaluate fluid loss and appropriateness of therapy.*

Refer to Critical Thinking Scenario for a full discussion of nursing care for a patient who is experiencing adrenergic agonist toxicity.

Nursing Diagnoses

Nursing diagnoses related to drug therapy may include the following:

- Decreased cardiac output related to CV effects
- Ineffective tissue perfusion related to CV effects or possible extravasation
- Deficient knowledge regarding drug therapy

Planning

- The patient will receive the best therapeutic effect from the drug therapy.
- The patient will have limited adverse effects to the drug therapy.
- The patient will have an understanding of the drug therapy, adverse effects to anticipate, and measures to relieve discomfort and improve safety

Implementation with Rationale

- Use extreme caution in calculating and preparing doses of these drugs *because even small errors could have serious effects.* Always dilute a parenteral drug before use if it is not prediluted *to prevent tissue irritation on injection.*
- Use proper, aseptic technique when administering ophthalmic or nasal agents *to prevent injection and assure the therapeutic effectiveness of the drug.*
- Monitor patients receiving the drug ophthalmically or nasally for all of the systemic effects associated with parenteral administration *to prevent potentially serious adverse effects if the drug is absorbed systemically.*
- Monitor patient response closely (blood pressure, ECG, urine output, cardiac output) and adjust dose accordingly *to ensure the most benefit with the least amount of toxicity.*
- Maintain phentolamine on standby *in case extravasation occurs*; infiltration of the site with 10 mL of saline containing 5 to 10 mg of phentolamine is usually effective in saving the area.
- Offer support and encouragement *to deal with the drug regimen.*
- Provide comfort measures to help the patient cope with sympathomimetic effects of the drug.
- Monitor light exposure *to prevent sensitivity to light caused by pupil dilation*, encourage voiding before giving the drug *to alleviate urinary retention caused by sphincter contraction*, monitor bowel function and provide assistance as needed *to deal with GI suppression*, and offer support and relaxation measures *to deal with feelings of tension and anxiety.*
- Provide the following patient teaching to patients using these drugs orally or ophthalmically. Most of these drugs are given in emergency situations and teaching will be based on the patient's condition and awareness. Teaching includes:
  - Drug name, prescribed dosage, and schedule for administration
  - Rationale for the drug
  - Proper technique for administration
  - Measures to prevent or avoid adverse effects
  - Need to check with prescriber before taking any OTC medication
  - Warning signs that might indicate a problem
  - Importance of avoiding intake of caffeine-containing products
  - Need for follow-up monitoring and evaluation

Evaluation

- Monitor the patient response to the drug (improvement in blood pressure, ocular pressure, bronchial airflow).
- Monitor for adverse effects (CV changes, decreased urine output, headache, GI upset).
- Monitor the effectiveness of comfort measures and compliance with the regimen.
- Evaluate the effectiveness of the teaching plan (patient can name the drug, dosage, adverse effects to watch for, and specific measures to avoid them).

CRITICAL THINKING SCENARIO

Adrenergic Agonist Toxicity

THE SITUATION

M.C. is a 26-year-old man who has recently moved to the northeastern United States from New Mexico. He has been suffering from sinusitis, runny nose, and cold-like symptoms for 2 weeks. He appears at an outpatient clinic with complaints of headache, "jitters," inability to sleep, loss of appetite, and a feeling of impending doom. He states that he feels "on edge" and has not been productive in his job as a watch repairman and jewelry maker. According to his history, M.C. has been treated with several different drugs for nocturnal enuresis, a persisting childhood problem. Only ephedrine, which he has been taking for 2 years, has been successful (an off-label use of the drug). He has no other significant health problems. He denies any side effects from the use of ephedrine but does admit to self-medicating his nagging cold with OTC preparations—a nasal spray used four times a day and a combination decongestant–pain reliever. A physical examination reveals a pulse of 104 beats/min, blood pressure 154/86 mm Hg, and respiration 16/min. The patient appears flushed and slightly diaphoretic.

CRITICAL THINKING

What are the important nursing implications for M.C.? *Think about the problems that confront a patient in a new area seeking health care for the first time.*

Adrenergic Agonist Toxicity (continued)

What could be causing the problems that M.C. presents with? *The diagnosis of ephedrine overdose was eventually made based on the patient history of OTC drug use and the presenting signs and symptoms.*

Keeping in mind that this diagnosis means that M.C. has an overstimulated sympathetic stress reaction, what other physical problems can be anticipated? *Overwhelming feelings of anxiety and stress are influencing M.C.'s response to work and health care.*

Given this fact, how may the nurse best deal with explaining the problem and how it could have happened—without making the patient feel uninformed or that the practice of his former health care provider is being questioned?

What treatment should be planned and what teaching points should be covered for M.C.?

DISCUSSION

The first step in caring for M.C. is establishing a trusting relationship to help alleviate some of the anxiety he is feeling. Being in a new state and seeking health care in a new setting can be very stressful for patients under normal circumstances. In M.C.'s case the sympathomimetic effects of the drugs that he has been taking make him feel even more anxious and jittery.

A careful patient history will help to determine whether there are any underlying medical problems that could be exacerbated by these drug effects. A review of M.C.'s nocturnal enuresis and the treatments that have been tried will enhance understanding of his former health care and suggest possible implications for further study. This questioning will also reassure M.C. that he is an important member of the health team and that the information he has to offer is valued.

A careful review of the OTC drugs that M.C. has been using will be informative for the patient, as well as for the health care providers, who have not actually checked OTC drugs for those specific ingredients, but combining them to ease signs and symptoms often results in toxic levels and symptoms of overdose. Many of these preparations contain sympathomimetics, such as phenylephrine, which will have additive effects to the ephedrine. M.C. will need a full teaching program about the effects of his ephedrine and which OTC drugs to avoid. The treatment for his current problems involves withdrawal of the OTC drugs; when these drug levels fall the signs and symptoms will disappear. M.C. may also wish to avoid nicotine and caffeine because these stimulants could increase his "jitters."

To build trust and ensure that the underlying cause of the problem was drug toxicity, M.C. should receive written patient instructions that highlight warning signs to report, including chest pain, palpitations, and difficulty voiding. He also should be given the health care provider's telephone number with instructions to call the next day and report on his health status. Finally, specimens of nasal discharge should be cultured and antibiotic treatment prescribed, if appropriate.

NURSING CARE GUIDE FOR M.C.: ADRENERGIC AGONIST TOXICITY

Assessment: History and Examination

Assess the patient's history of drug allergies, CV dysfunction, pheochromocytoma, narrow-angle glaucoma, prostatic hypertrophy, thyroid disease, or diabetes, as well as concurrent use of MAOIs, TCAs, reserpine, ephedrine, or urinary alkalinizers.

Focus the physical examination on the following:

CV: Blood pressure, pulse rate, peripheral perfusion, and ECG

Central nervous system (CNS): Orientation, affect, reflexes, peripheral sensation, and vision

Skin: Color and temperature

GI: Abdominal examination

Genitourinary (GU): Urine output, bladder percussion, and prostate palpation

Respiratory: Respiratory rate and adventitious sounds

Nursing Diagnoses

Decreased cardiac output related to CV effects

Acute pain related to CV and systemic effects

Impaired tissue perfusion related to CV effects

Deficient knowledge regarding drug therapy

Planning

The patient will receive the best therapeutic effect from the drug therapy.

The patient will have limited adverse effects to the drug therapy.

The patient will have an understanding of the drug therapy, adverse effects to anticipate, and measures to relieve discomfort and improve safety.

Implementation

Ensure safe and appropriate administration of the drug.

Provide comfort and safety measures: Temperature and lighting control (patient may have pupil dilation secondary to sympathetic effects), mouth care, and skin care.

Monitor blood pressure, pulse rate, and respiratory status throughout drug therapy.

Provide support and reassurance to deal with drug therapy and drug effects.

Provide patient teaching about drug name, dosage, side effects, precautions, and warning signs to report.

Adrenergic Agonist Toxicity (continued)

Evaluation

Evaluate drug effects: Relief of enuresis.

Monitor for adverse effects: CV effects, dizziness, confusion, headache, rash, difficulty voiding, sweating, flushing, and pupillary dilation.

Monitor for drug–drug interactions as indicated.

Evaluate the effectiveness of the patient-teaching program and comfort and safety measures.

PATIENT TEACHING FOR M.C.

- The drug that you have been taking is ephedrine. It is called an adrenergic agonist (or a sympathomimetic drug). Ephedrine acts by mimicking the effects of the SNS, which is the part of your nervous system that is responsible for your response to fear or danger (this is called the "fight-or-flight" response). Because this drug triggers many effects in the body, you may experience some undesired adverse effects. It is crucial to discuss the effect of the drug with your health care provider and to try to make the effect as tolerable as possible.
- If the drug is in a solution, check it before each use. If the solution is pink, brown, or black, discard it.
- If you have diagnosed prostate problems, it might help to void before taking each dose of the drug.
- Some of the following adverse effects may occur:
  - *Restlessness or shaking:* If these occur, avoid driving, operating machinery, or performing delicate tasks.
  - *Flushing or sweating:* Avoid warm temperatures and heavy clothing; frequent washing with cool water may help.
  - *Heart palpitations:* If you feel that your heart is beating too fast or skipping beats, sit down for a while and rest. If the feeling becomes too uncomfortable, notify your health care provider.
  - *Sensitivity to light:* Avoid glaring lights or wear sunglasses if you are in bright light. Be careful when moving between extremes of light because your vision may not adjust quickly.
  - Report any of the following to your health care provider: *Difficulty voiding, chest pain, difficulty breathing, dizziness, headache, or changes in vision.*
- Do not stop taking this drug suddenly; make sure that you have enough of your prescription. This drug dose should be reduced gradually over 2 to 4 days when you are instructed to discontinue it by your health care provider.
- Avoid OTC medications, including cold and allergy remedies and diet pills. If you feel that you need one of these, check with your health care provider first.
- Tell any health care provider who takes care of you that you are taking this drug.
- Keep this drug and all medications out of the reach of children. Do not share this drug with other people.

KEY POINTS

- Adrenergic agonists (sympathomimetics) stimulate the adrenergic receptors in the SNS.
- Alpha- and beta-adrenergic agonists stimulate all of the adrenergic receptors in the SNS. They induce a fight-or-flight response and are frequently used to treat shock.

Alpha-Specific Adrenergic Agonists

Alpha-specific adrenergic agonists (Table 30.2), or alpha-agonists, are drugs that bind primarily to alpha-receptors rather than to beta-receptors. Three drugs belong to this class: Clonidine (*Catapres*), midodrine (generic), and phenylephrine (*Neo-Synephrine*, and others).

Therapeutic Actions and Indications

Therapeutic effects of the alpha-specific adrenergic agonists result from the stimulation of alpha-receptors within the SNS (see Figure 30.2). The uses are varied, depending on the specific drug and the route of administration (Table 30.2).

Phenylephrine, a potent vasoconstrictor and alpha$_1$-agonist with little or no effect on the heart or bronchi, is used in many combination cold and allergy products. Parenterally, it is used to treat shock or shock-like states, to overcome paroxysmal supraventricular tachycardia, to prolong local anesthesia, and to maintain blood pressure during spinal anesthesia. Topically, it is used to treat allergic rhinitis and to relieve the symptoms of otitis media. Ophthalmically, it is used to dilate the pupils for eye examination, before surgery, or to relieve elevated eye pressure associated with glaucoma. Phenylephrine is found in many cold and allergy products because it is so effective in constricting topical vessels and decreasing the swelling, signs, and symptoms of rhinitis. (See Box 30.3 regarding brimonidine, a topical drug approved in 2013 for treating rosacea.)

Midodrine is an oral drug that is used to treat orthostatic hypotension in patients who do not respond to traditional therapy. It activates alpha$_1$-adrenergic receptors, leading to peripheral vasoconstriction and an increase in vascular tone and blood pressure. This effect can cause a serious supine hypertension. Patients need to be monitored in the standing, sitting, and supine positions to determine whether this will be a problem.

Table 30.2 ***Drugs in Focus:* Alpha-Specific Adrenergic Agonists**

Drug Name	Dosage/Route	Usual Indications
clonidine (*Catapres*)	0.1 mg PO b.i.d. initially up to a maximum 2.4 mg/d if needed; transdermal system may increase from 0.1 to 0.3 mg/d	Treatment of essential hypertension; chronic pain; to ease opiate withdrawal; used only for adults
midodrine (generic)	10 mg PO t.i.d. during daytime hours when patient is upright	Treatment of orthostatic hypotension
phenylephrine (generic)	1–10 mg PO subcutaneous or IV *or* 0.1–0.5 mg IV as a starting dose; 0.5 mg IV by rapid injection to convert tachycardias; 1–2 gtt in affected eye(s) for glaucoma	Cold and allergies; shock and shock-like states; supraventricular tachycardias; glaucoma; allergic rhinitis; otitis media

BOX 30.3

Alpha-Agonist Approved for Treatment of Rosacea

Mirvaso (brimonidine) was approved in late 2013 as a topical treatment for rosacea. Rosacea is a persistent facial erythema or redness, which might be related to a vascular sensitivity in certain patients. In the past, topical steroids were often used to help patients with this disorder, but the use of corticosteroids often made the condition worse. Brimonidine is an alpha-agonist and causes a local vasoconstriction at the site of application, decreasing the redness associated with vasodilation and improving the appearance of the skin. It is applied in pea-size amounts each day to the head, chin, nose, and each check. The eyes and lips are avoided. It is not for oral, ophthalmic, or intravaginal use. Patients are advised to wash their hands immediately after applying the gel and to avoid application to any area that is eroded or has open skin. In some cases, vascular insufficiency can occur, so the area should be monitored closely. Since the drug is not generally absorbed systemically, there are few systemic effects.

Rapid Response for Anaphylaxis

Epinephrine is available in a number of different autoinjectors for use in the emergency treatment of acute allergic reactions including anaphylaxis. Dosing varies between adults and children and it is important to make sure the correct injector is being used. The traditional *EpiPen* (0.3 mg/0.3 mL) and *EpiPen Jr.* (0.15 mg/0.15 mL) are well known to people. *Adrenaclick* comes in the same solutions but provides color-coded use for immediate injection into the upper thigh. In 2014 an updated *Auvi-Q* injector was introduced which has a protective carrying case, easy use ability to inject subcutaneously or IM through clothing, and a voice instruction system to assure proper use and actual injection. Any patient at risk for anaphylaxis should be carefully instructed in the carrying and use of these autoinjectors. They are for emergency use only and the patient should seek immediate medical care following use. Proper disposal of the autoinjector varies with the injector and should be part of the instructional session. Patients should know that they may experience sweating, tremors, anxiety, fast heart rate, weakness, dizziness, or GI upset following the use of this drug.

Midodrine is a grandfathered drug that had never gone through rigorous testing. In 2010, when the drug was tested, its effectiveness was not clear and the manufacturer was required to put the drug through testing to establish effectiveness. So far, that testing has not been done and it is not clear how long the drug will be available. (See Box 30.4 regarding droxidopa, a drug approved in 2014 for treating orthostatic hypotension.)

Clonidine specifically stimulates CNS alpha$_2$-receptors. This leads to decreased sympathetic outflow from the CNS because the alpha$_2$-receptors moderate the release of norepinephrine from the nerve axon. Clonidine is available in oral and transdermal forms for use to control hypertension and as an injection for epidural infusion to control pain in cancer patients. Because of its centrally acting effects, clonidine is associated with many more CNS effects (bad dreams, sedation, drowsiness, fatigue, headache) than other sympathomimetics. It can also cause

BOX 30.4

Droxidopa for Orthostatic Hypotension

In 2014 droxidopa (*Northera*) was approved for the treatment of orthostatic hypotension, dizziness, and lightheadedness in adults with symptomatic neurogenic orthostatic hypotension caused by primary autonomic failure, dopamine beta-hydroxylase deficiency, and nondiabetic autonomic neuropathy. Droxidopa is a synthetic amino acid precursor of norepinephrine. It is metabolized to norepinephrine in the tissues throughout the body. It is not completely understood how that affects orthostatic hypotension but the conversion to norepinephrine in the tissues is thought to cause vasoconstriction leading to a higher blood pressure. The efficacy of the drug beyond 2 weeks of use has not been reported. *Northera* has a black box warning that there is a risk of supine hypertension and CV risk; it is also associated with fever and confusion, headache, dizziness, and fatigue. With the fate still unknown for midodrine, for many years the only drug for orthostatic hypotension, the introduction of this new option for treating orthostatic hypotension offers an acceptable option.

extreme hypotension, heart failure, and bradycardia due to its decreased effects of the sympathetic outflow from the CNS.

Pharmacokinetics

These drugs are generally well absorbed from all routes of administration and reach peak levels in a short period—20 to 45 minutes. They are widely distributed in the body, metabolized in the liver, and primarily excreted in the urine. The transdermal form of clonidine is slow release and has a 7-day duration of effects, so it only needs to be replaced once a week. Phenylephrine can be given IM, subcutaneously, IV, orally, and as a nasal or an ophthalmic solution.

Contraindications and Cautions

The alpha-specific adrenergic agonists are contraindicated in the presence of allergy to the specific drug *to avoid hypersensitivity reactions*; severe hypertension or tachycardia *because of possible additive effects*; and narrow-angle glaucoma, *which could be exacerbated by arterial constriction. There are no adequate studies about use during pregnancy and lactation*, so use should be reserved for situations in which the benefit to the mother outweighs any potential risk to the fetus or neonate.

They should be used with caution in the presence of CV disease or vasomotor spasm *because these conditions could be aggravated by the vascular effects of the drug*; thyrotoxicosis or diabetes *because of the thyroid-stimulating and glucose-elevating effects of sympathetic stimulation*; or renal or hepatic impairment, *which could interfere with metabolism and excretion of the drug.*

Adverse Effects

Patients receiving these drugs often experience adverse effects that are extensions of the therapeutic effects or other sympathetic stimulatory reactions. CNS effects include feelings of anxiety, restlessness, depression, fatigue, strange dreams, and personality changes. Blurred vision and sensitivity to light may occur because of the pupil dilation that occurs when the sympathetic system is stimulated. CV effects can include arrhythmias, ECG changes, blood pressure changes, and peripheral vascular problems. Nausea, vomiting, and anorexia can occur, related to the depressant effects of the SNS on the GI tract. GU effects can include decreased urinary output, difficulty urinating, dysuria, and changes in sexual function related to the sympathetic stimulation of these systems. These drugs should not be stopped suddenly; adrenergic receptors will be very sensitive to catecholamines, and sudden withdrawal can lead to tachycardia, hypertension, arrhythmias, flushing, and even death. Avoid these effects by tapering the drug over 2 to 4 days when it is being discontinued. As with other sympathomimetics, if phenylephrine is given IV, care should be taken to avoid extravasation. The vasoconstricting effects of the drug can lead to necrosis and cell death in the area of extravasation.

Clinically Important Drug–Drug Interactions

Phenylephrine combined with MAOIs can cause severe hypertension, headache, and hyperpyrexia; this combination should be avoided. Increased sympathomimetic effects occur when phenylephrine is combined with TCAs; if this combination must be used the patient should be monitored very closely.

Clonidine has a decreased antihypertensive effect if taken with TCAs, and a paradoxical hypertension occurs if it is combined with propranolol. If these combinations are used, the patient response should be monitored closely and dose adjustment made as needed.

Midodrine can precipitate increased drug effects of digoxin, beta-blockers, and many antipsychotics. Such combinations should be avoided.

Any adrenergic agonist will lose effectiveness if combined with any adrenergic antagonist. Monitor the patient's drug regimen for appropriate use of the drugs.

Prototype Summary: Phenylephrine

Indications: Treatment of vascular failure in shock or drug-induced hypotension to overcome paroxysmal supraventricular tachycardia and to prolong spinal anesthesia; as a vasoconstrictor in regional anesthesia to maintain blood pressure during anesthesia; topically, for symptomatic relief of nasal congestion and as adjunctive therapy in middle ear infections; ophthalmically to dilate pupils and as a decongestant to provide temporary relief of eye irritation.

Actions: Powerful postsynaptic alpha-adrenergic receptor stimulant causing vasoconstriction and raising systolic and diastolic blood pressure with little effect on the beta-receptors in the heart.

Pharmacokinetics:

Route	Onset	Duration
IV	Immediate	15–20 min
IM, subcutaneous	10–15 min	30–120 min
Topically	Very little systemic absorption occurs	

$T_{1/2}$: 47 to 100 hours; metabolized in the tissues and liver; excreted in the urine and bile.

Adverse Effects: Fear, anxiety, restlessness, headache, nausea, decreased urine formation, pallor.

Nursing Considerations for Patients Receiving Alpha-Specific Adrenergic Agonists

Assessment: History and Examination

- Assess for contraindications or cautions: Any known allergies to the drug *to avoid hypersensitivity reactions*; presence of any CV diseases, *which could be exacerbated by the vascular effects of these drugs*; thyrotoxicosis or diabetes, *which would lead to an increase in thyroid stimulation or glucose elevation*; chronic renal failure, *which could be exacerbated by drug use*; renal or hepatic impairment, *which could interfere with drug excretion or metabolism;* and current status of pregnancy and lactation.
- Perform a physical assessment to establish *baseline status before beginning therapy to determine effectiveness and during therapy to evaluate for any potential adverse effects.*
- Assess level of orientation, affect, reflexes, and vision *to monitor for CNS changes related to drug therapy.*
- Monitor blood pressure and pulse, assess peripheral perfusion, and obtain ECG, if indicated, *to determine drug effectiveness and evaluate for adverse CV effects.*
- Assess urinary output *to evaluate renal function and monitor for adverse effects of the drug.*
- Evaluate patient for nausea and constipation *to assess adverse effects of the drug and establish appropriate interventions.*
- Monitor laboratory test results, such as renal and liver function tests, *to determine drug effects on renal and hepatic systems.*

Nursing Diagnoses

Nursing diagnoses related to drug therapy might include the following:

- Disturbed sensory perception (visual, kinesthetic, tactile) related to CNS effects
- Discomfort related to GI and GU effects of the drug and pupil dilation causing sensitivity to light
- Risk for injury related to CNS or CV effects of the drug and potential for extravasation
- Decreased cardiac output related to blood pressure changes, arrhythmias, or vasoconstriction
- Deficient knowledge regarding drug therapy

Planning

- The patient will receive the best therapeutic effect from the drug therapy.
- The patient will have limited adverse effects to the drug therapy.
- The patient will have an understanding of the drug therapy, adverse effects to anticipate, and measures to relieve discomfort and improve safety.

Implementation with Rationale

- Do not discontinue the drug abruptly *because sudden withdrawal can result in rebound hypertension, arrhythmias, flushing, and even hypertensive encephalopathy and death*; taper drug over 2 to 4 days.
- Do not discontinue the drug before surgery; mark the patient's chart and monitor blood pressure carefully during surgery. *Sympathetic stimulation may alter the normal response to anesthesia, as well as recovery from anesthesia.*
- Monitor blood pressure, orthostatic blood pressure, pulse, rhythm, and cardiac output regularly, even with ophthalmic preparations, *to adjust dose or discontinue the drug if CV effects are severe.*
- When giving phenylephrine intravenously, ensure that an alpha-blocking agent is readily available to counteract the effects *in case severe reaction occurs*; infiltrate any area of extravasation with phentolamine within 12 hours after extravasation *to preserve tissue.*
- Arrange for supportive care and comfort measures, including rest and environmental control, *to decrease CNS irritation*; analgesics for headache *to relieve discomfort*; safety measures, such as use of side rails and assistance with ambulation if CNS effects occur, *to protect the patient from injury*; and protective measures *if CNS effects are severe.*
- Provide thorough patient teaching about drug name, dose, and schedule for administration; technique for administration if appropriate; measures to prevent potential adverse effects such as voiding before taking the drug and use of bowel-training activities if constipation is a problem; safety measures such as avoiding driving and operating dangerous machinery if CNS effects occur and getting up and down slowly if orthostatic hypotension is an issue; warning signs of problems; and importance of monitoring and follow-up *to improve compliance and ensure safe and effective use of the drug.*

Evaluation

- Monitor patient response to the drug (improvement in condition being treated).
- Monitor for adverse effects (GI upset, CNS, and CV changes).
- Monitor the effectiveness of comfort measures and compliance with the regimen.
- Evaluate the effectiveness of the teaching plan (patient can name drug, dosage, adverse effects to watch for, and specific measures to avoid them).

KEY POINTS

- Alpha-specific adrenergic agonists, such as phenylephrine, midodrine, and clonidine, stimulate only the alpha-receptors within the SNS. Clonidine specifically stimulates alpha$_2$-receptors and is used to treat hypertension because its action blocks the release of norepinephrine from nerve axons.
- Care must be taken to prevent extravasation when used IV; the vasoconstrictive properties of the drug can cause necrosis and cell death in the area of extravasation.
- These drugs should be tapered over 2 to 4 days when discontinued because the adrenergic receptors will be very sensitive, and rebound hypertension, tachycardia, arrhythmias, and even death can occur.

Beta-Specific Adrenergic Agonists

Most of the drugs that belong to the class of beta-specific adrenergic agonists (Table 30.3), or beta-agonists, are beta$_2$-specific agonists and are used to manage and treat bronchial spasm, asthma, and other obstructive pulmonary conditions. These drugs, including albuterol (*Proventil HFA, Ventolin*), arformoterol (*Brovana*), formoterol (*Foradil, Perforomist*), indacaterol (*Arcapta*), levalbuterol (*Xopenex*), metaproterenol (generic), olodaterol (*Striverdi Respimat*), salmeterol (*Serevent*), and terbutaline (generic), are discussed at length in Chapter 55, which deals with drugs used to treat obstructive pulmonary diseases. Beta$_3$-agonists act to relax the bladder and are used to help treat overactive bladder as discussed in Chapter 52.

Table 30.3 ***Drugs in Focus:* Beta-Specific Adrenergic Agonists**

Drug Name	Dosage/Route	Usual Indications
albuterol (*Proventil, Ventolin*)	*Adult:* 2–4 mg t.i.d.–q.i.d. PO, or 1–2 inhalations every 4–6 h *Pediatric:* 2 mg t.i.d.–q.i.d. PO *or* 1.25–2.5 mg b.i.d. by inhalation	Treatment and prevention of bronchospasm; treatment of acute bronchospasm and exercise-induced bronchospasm when used by inhalation
arformoterol (*Brovana*)	*Adult:* 15 mcg b.i.d by nebulization, do not exceed 30 mcg/d	Long-term maintenance treatment of bronchospasm in adult patients with chronic obstructive pulmonary disease
formoterol (*Foradil, Perforomist*)	*Adult:* Oral inhalation of 12 mcg every 12 h *or* 20 mcg/2 mL by oral inhalation using a jet nebulizer twice daily *Pediatric (12 y and older for exercise-induced bronchospasm):* Oral inhalation 12 mcg 15 min before exercise *Pediatric (5 y and older for maintenance treatment of asthma):* Oral inhalation *or* 12 mcg every 12 h	Long-term maintenance treatment of asthma in adults and children 5 y and older; prevention of exercise-induced bronchospasm
indacaterol (*Arcapta*)	*Adult:* Oral inhalation, 75 mcg inhaled once a day	Long-term maintenance treatment of bronchospasm in adult patients with chronic obstructive pulmonary disease
isoproterenol (*Isuprel*)	*Adult:* IV injection, 0.02–0.06 mg; IV infusion, 5 mcg/min; 0.2 mg IM or subcutaneous *Pediatric:* 0.1–1.0 mcg/kg/min IV has been used	Treatment of shock, cardiac arrest, and certain ventricular arrhythmias; treatment of heart block in transplanted hearts; prevention of bronchospasm during anesthesia, treatment of acute hyperkalemia in the hospital setting
levalbuterol (*Xopenex*)	*Adult and pediatric (12 y and older):* 0.63 mg t.i.d. by nebulization *Pediatric (6–11 y):* 0.31 mg t.i.d. by nebulization *Pediatric (4 y and older):* Two inhalations every 4–6 h	Treatment and prevention of bronchial asthma and reversible bronchospasm in patients 4 y and older
metaproterenol (generic)	*Adult and pediatric (12 y and older):* 2–3 inhalations every 3–4 h; 2.5 mL by nebulization; 20 mg PO t.i.d.–q.i.d. *Pediatric (6–9 y):* 10 mg PO t.i.d.–q.i.d.; 0.1–0.2 mL in saline by nebulization	Treatment of bronchial asthma and reversible bronchospasm; by inhalation, treatment of acute asthma attacks in children 6 y and older
olodaterol (*Striverdi Respimat*)	*Adult:* 2 oral inhalations once daily at the same time each day: 2.5 mcg/inhalation	Long-term maintenance treatment of bronchospasm in adult patients with chronic obstructive pulmonary disease
salmeterol (*Serevent Diskus*)	*Adult and pediatric (12 y and older):* 1 inhalation b.i.d.; 30 min before exercise with exercise-induced bronchospasm	Treatment and prevention of bronchial asthma and reversible bronchospasm, including exercise-induced bronchospasm (patients 4 y and older)
terbutaline (generic)	*Adult and pediatric (15 y and older):* 5 mg PO t.i.d.; 0.25 mg subcutaneous, may be repeated in 15 min to a maximum of 0.5 mg/4 h *Pediatric (12–15 y):* 2.5 mg PO t.i.d.	Treatment and prevention of bronchial asthma and reversible bronchospasm

This chapter specifically addresses isoproterenol (*Isuprel*), which is used as a sympathomimetic for its overall stimulatory properties.

Therapeutic Actions and Indications

Therapeutic effects of isoproterenol are related to its stimulation of all beta-adrenergic receptors. Desired effects of the drug include increased heart rate, conductivity, and contractility; bronchodilation; increased blood flow to skeletal muscles and splanchnic beds; and relaxation of the uterus. Its use has decreased over the years as more specific drugs with less toxicity have been developed to treat the cardiac problems isoproterenol was developed to treat. Some research has shown that isoproterenol exerts a "coronary steal" effect, diverting blood away from injured or hypoxic areas of the heart muscle, an effect that can increase the size and extent of an evolving myocardial infarction, further decreasing its usefulness in the clinical setting. There are some emergency situations, however, that respond well to isoproterenol. See Table 30.3 for Usual Indications.

Pharmacokinetics

Isoproterenol is rapidly distributed after injection; it is metabolized in the liver and excreted in the urine. The half-life is relatively short—less than 1 hour.

Contraindications and Cautions

Isoproterenol is contraindicated in the presence of allergy to the drug or any components of the drug *to avert hypersensitivity reactions*; with pulmonary hypertension, *which could be exacerbated by the effects of the drug*; during anesthesia with halogenated hydrocarbons, *which sensitize the myocardium to catecholamines and could cause a severe reaction*; with eclampsia, uterine hemorrhage, and intrauterine death, *which could be complicated by uterine relaxation or increased blood pressure*; and during pregnancy and lactation *because of potential effects on the fetus or neonate.* Caution should be used with diabetes, thyroid disease, vasomotor problems, degenerative heart disease, or history of stroke, *all of which could be exacerbated by the sympathomimetic effects of the drug*, and with severe renal impairment, *which could alter excretion of the drug.*

Adverse Effects

Patients receiving isoproterenol often experience adverse effects related to the stimulation of sympathetic adrenergic receptors. CNS effects include restlessness, anxiety, fear, tremor, fatigue, and headache. CV effects can include tachycardia, angina, myocardial infarction, and palpitations. Pulmonary effects can be severe, ranging from difficulty breathing, coughing, and bronchospasm to severe pulmonary edema. GI upset, nausea, vomiting, and anorexia can occur as a result of the slowing of the GI tract with SNS stimulation. Hypokalemia can occur as a result of the release of aldosterone that occurs with sympathetic stimulation and the resultant loss of potassium. Other anticipated effects can include sweating, pupil dilation, rash, and muscle cramps which occur as a result of the potassium shift.

Clinically Important Drug–Drug Interactions

Increased sympathomimetic effects can be expected if this drug is taken with other sympathomimetic drugs. Decreased therapeutic effects can occur if this drug is combined with beta-adrenergic blockers.

Prototype Summary: Isoproterenol

Indications: Management of bronchospasm during anesthesia; vasopressor during shock; adjunct in the management of cardiac standstill and arrest, as well as serious ventricular arrhythmias that require increased inotropic action.

Actions: Acts on beta-adrenergic receptors to produce increased heart rate, positive inotropic effect, bronchodilation, and vasodilation.

Pharmacokinetics:

Route	Onset	Duration
IV	Immediate	1–2 min

$T_{1/2}$: Unknown; metabolized in the tissues.

Adverse Effects: Restlessness, apprehension, anxiety, fear, cardiac arrhythmias, tachycardia, nausea, vomiting, heartburn, respiratory difficulties, coughing, pulmonary edema, sweating, pallor.

Nursing Considerations for Patients Receiving Beta-Specific Adrenergic Agonists

Assessment: History and Examination

- Assess for contraindications or cautions: Any known allergies to any drug or any components of the drug *to avoid possible hypersensitivity reactions*; pulmonary hypertension, which *could be exacerbated by the effects of the drug*; anesthesia with halogenated hydrocarbons, *which sensitize the myocardium to catecholamines and could cause severe reaction*; eclampsia, uterine hemorrhage, and intrauterine death, *which could be complicated by uterine relaxation or increased blood pressure*; diabetes, thyroid disease, vasomotor problems, degenerative heart disease, or history of stroke, *all of which could be exacerbated by the sympathomimetic effects of the drugs*; severe renal impairment, *which could interfere with the excretion of the drug*; and current status of pregnancy and lactation.

- Perform a physical assessment to establish a *baseline before beginning therapy and during therapy to determine the drug's effectiveness and identify any potential adverse effects.*
- Assess CV status, including pulse rate and blood pressure, *to evaluate for any CV effects associated with SNS stimulation*; obtain an ECG *to evaluate for changes indicating excessive SNS stimulation.*
- Assess respiratory status and listen for adventitious sounds *to monitor drug effects and assess for any adverse effects.*
- Monitor urine output *to evaluate renal function and kidney perfusion.*
- Monitor laboratory test results, including thyroid function tests, blood glucose levels, and renal function, *to monitor drug effects and potential adverse effects.*

Nursing Diagnoses

Nursing diagnoses related to drug therapy might include the following:

- Acute pain related to CV and systemic effects
- Decreased cardiac output related to CV effects
- Ineffective tissue perfusion related to CV effects
- Deficient knowledge regarding drug therapy

Planning

- The patient will receive the best therapeutic effect from the drug therapy.
- The patient will have limited adverse effects to the drug therapy.
- The patient will have an understanding of the drug therapy, adverse effects to anticipate, and measures to relieve discomfort and improve safety

Implementation with Rationale

- Monitor pulse and blood pressure carefully during administration *to arrange to discontinue the drug at any sign of toxicity.*
- Ensure that a beta-adrenergic blocker is readily available when giving parenteral isoproterenol *in case severe reaction occurs.*
- Use minimal doses of isoproterenol needed to achieve desired effects *to prevent adverse effects and maintain patient safety.*
- Arrange for supportive care and comfort measures, including rest and environmental control, *to relieve CNS effects*; provide analgesics for headache and safety measures if CNS effects occur *to provide comfort and prevent injury*; and avoid overhydration *to prevent pulmonary edema.*
- Provide thorough patient teaching, including drug name, dosage, and frequency of administration; rationale for administration; monitoring required; anticipated adverse effects, measures to reduce these, and warning signs of problems to report immediately *to improve compliance and ensure safe and effective use of the drug.*

Evaluation

- Monitor patient response to the drug (improvement in condition being treated, stabilization of blood pressure, prevention of preterm labor, cardiac stimulation).
- Monitor for adverse effects (GI upset, CNS changes, respiratory problems).
- Evaluate the effectiveness of the teaching plan (patient can name drug, dosage, adverse effects to watch for, and specific measures to reduce them).
- Monitor the effectiveness of comfort measures and compliance with the regimen.

KEY POINTS

- Most of the beta$_2$-specific adrenergic agonists are used to manage and treat asthma, bronchospasm, and other obstructive pulmonary diseases.
- Isoproterenol, a nonspecific beta-specific adrenergic agent, is used for its sympathomimetic effects to treat shock, cardiac standstill, and certain arrhythmias when used systemically; it is especially effective in the treatment of heart block in transplanted hearts.
- Because of its many adverse effects, isoproterenol is reserved for use in emergency situations that do not respond to other, safer therapies.

SUMMARY

- Adrenergic agonists, also called sympathomimetics, are drugs that mimic the effects of the SNS and are used to stimulate the adrenergic receptors within the SNS. The adverse effects associated with these drugs are usually also a result of sympathetic stimulation.
- Adrenergic agonists include alpha- and beta-adrenergic agonists, which stimulate both types of adrenergic receptors in the SNS, and alpha-specific and beta-specific adrenergic agonists, which stimulate only alpha-receptors or only beta-receptors, respectively.
- Alpha-specific adrenergic agonists, such as phenylephrine, midodrine, and clonidine, stimulate only the alpha-receptors within the SNS. Clonidine specifically stimulates alpha$_2$-receptors and is used to treat hypertension because its action blocks the release of norepinephrine from nerve axons.
- Many of the beta$_2$-specific adrenergic agonists are used to manage and treat asthma, bronchospasm, and other obstructive pulmonary diseases.
- Isoproterenol, a nonspecific beta-specific adrenergic, is used to treat shock, cardiac standstill, and certain arrhythmias when used systemically; it is especially effective in the treatment of heart block in transplanted hearts.

CHECK YOUR UNDERSTANDING

Answers to the questions in this chapter can be found in Answers to Check Your Understanding Questions on thePoint®.

MULTIPLE CHOICE

Select the best answer to the following.

1. The instructor determines that teaching about adrenergic drugs has been successful when the class identifies the drugs as also being called
   a. sympatholytic agents.
   b. cholinergic agents.
   c. sympathomimetic agents.
   d. anticholinergic agents.

2. The adrenergic agent of choice for treating the signs and symptoms of allergic rhinitis is
   a. norepinephrine.
   b. phenylephrine.
   c. dobutamine.
   d. dopamine.

3. An adrenergic agent being used to treat shock infiltrates into the tissue with intravenous administration. Which action by the nurse would be most appropriate?
   a. Watch the area for any signs of necrosis and report it to the physician.
   b. Notify the physician and decrease the rate of infusion.
   c. Remove the IV and prepare phentolamine for administration to the area.
   d. Apply ice and elevate the arm.

4. Phenylephrine, an alpha-specific agonist, is found in many cold and allergy preparations. The nurse instructs the patient to be alert for which adverse effects?
   a. Urinary retention and pupil constriction
   b. Hypotension and slow heart rate
   c. Personality changes and increased appetite
   d. Cardiac arrhythmias and difficulty urinating

5. Adverse effects associated with adrenergic agonists are related to the generalized stimulation of the SNS and could include
   a. slowed heart rate.
   b. constriction of the pupils.
   c. hypertension.
   d. increased GI secretions.

6. A patient has elected to take an OTC cold preparation that contains phenylephrine. The nurse would advise the patient not to take that drug if the patient has
   a. thyroid or CV disease.
   b. a cough and runny nose.
   c. chronic obstructive pulmonary disease.
   d. hypotension.

MULTIPLE RESPONSE

Select all that apply.

1. Isoproterenol is a nonspecific beta-agonist. The nurse might expect to administer this drug for which of the following conditions?
   a. Preterm labor
   b. Bronchospasm
   c. Cardiac standstill
   d. Shock
   e. Heart block in transplanted hearts
   f. Heart failure

2. A nurse would question the order for an adrenergic agonist for a patient who is also receiving which of the following:
   a. Anticholinergic drugs
   b. Halogenated hydrocarbon anesthetics
   c. Beta-blockers
   d. Benzodiazepines
   e. MAOIs
   f. TCAs

BIBLIOGRAPHY AND REFERENCES

American Association of Critical Care Nurses. (2009). *Core curriculum for progressive nursing care.* St. Louis, MO: Saunders/Elsevier.

Brunton, L., Chabner, B., & Knollman, B. (2011). *Goodman and Gilman's the pharmacological basis of therapeutics* (12th ed.). New York: McGraw-Hill.

Facts and Comparisons. (2015). *Drug facts and comparisons.* St. Louis, MO: Author.

Facts and Comparisons. (2015). *Professional's guide to patient drug facts.* St. Louis, MO: Author.

Gheorghiade, M., Filippatos, G. S., & Felker, G. M. (2011). Diagnosis and management of acute failure syndromes. In R. O. Bonow, D. L. Mann, D. P. Zipes, et al. (Eds.), *Braunwald's heart disease:*

A textbook of cardiovascular medicine (9th ed.). Philadelphia, PA: Saunders; chap 27.

Hasdai, D., Berger, P., Battler, A., et al. (Eds.). (2010). *Cardiogenic shock*. Totowa, NJ: Humana Press.

Karch, A. M. (2014). *Lippincott's nursing drug guide*. Philadelphia, PA: Lippincott Williams & Wilkins.

National Center for Complementary and Alternative Medicine. (2004). Consumer advisory: Ephedra [National Institutes of Health]. Available online at: http://nccam.nih.gov/health/alerts/ephedra/consumeradvisory.htm

Porth, C. M. (2013). *Pathophysiology: Concepts of altered health states* (9th ed.). Philadelphia, PA: Lippincott Williams & Wilkins.

31 Adrenergic Antagonists

Learning Objectives

Upon completion of this chapter, you will be able to:

1. Describe the effects of adrenergic blocking agents on adrenergic receptors, correlating these effects with their clinical effects.
2. Describe the therapeutic actions, indications, pharmacokinetics, contraindications and cautions, most common adverse reactions, and important drug–drug interactions associated with adrenergic blocking agents.
3. Discuss the use of adrenergic blocking agents across the lifespan.
4. Compare and contrast the prototype drugs labetalol, phentolamine, doxazosin, propranolol, and atenolol with other adrenergic blocking agents.
5. Outline the nursing considerations, including important teaching points, for patients receiving an adrenergic blocking agent.

Glossary of Key Terms

adrenergic-receptor-site specificity: a drug's affinity for only adrenergic receptor sites; certain drugs may have specific affinity for only alpha- or only beta-adrenergic receptor sites

alpha$_1$-selective adrenergic blocking agents: drugs that block the postsynaptic alpha$_1$-receptor sites, causing a decrease in vascular tone and a vasodilation that leads to a fall in blood pressure; these drugs do not block the presynaptic alpha$_2$-receptor sites, and therefore the reflex tachycardia that accompanies a fall in blood pressure does not occur

beta-adrenergic blocking agents: drugs that, at therapeutic levels, selectively block the beta-receptors of the sympathetic nervous system

beta$_1$-selective adrenergic blocking agents: drugs that, at therapeutic levels, specifically block the beta$_1$-receptors in the sympathetic nervous system while not blocking the beta$_2$-receptors and resultant effects on the respiratory system

bronchodilation: relaxation of the muscles in the bronchi, resulting in a widening of the bronchi; an effect of sympathetic stimulation

pheochromocytoma: a tumor of the chromaffin cells of the adrenal medulla that periodically releases large amounts of norepinephrine and epinephrine into the system with resultant severe hypertension and tachycardia

sympatholytic: a drug that lyses, or blocks, the effects of the sympathetic nervous system

Drug List

Nonselective Adrenergic Blocking Agents

amiodarone
carvedilol
(P) labetalol

Nonselective Alpha-Adrenergic Blocking Agents

(P) phentolamine

Alpha$_1$-Selective Adrenergic Blocking Agents

alfuzosin
(P) doxazosin
prazosin
tamsulosin
terazosin

Nonselective Beta-Adrenergic Blocking Agents

carteolol
metipranolol
nadolol
nebivolol
(P) propranolol
sotalol
timolol

Beta1-Selective Adrenergic Blocking Agents

acebutolol
(P) atenolol
betaxolol
bisoprolol
esmolol
metoprolol

Adrenergic antagonists or adrenergic blocking agents are also called **sympatholytic** drugs because they lyse, or block, the effects of the sympathetic nervous system (SNS). The therapeutic and adverse effects associated with these drugs are related to their **adrenergic-receptor-site specificity**; that is, the ability to react with specific adrenergic receptor sites without activating them, thus preventing the typical manifestations of SNS activation. By occupying the adrenergic receptor site, they prevent norepinephrine released from the nerve terminal or from the adrenal medulla from activating the receptor, thus blocking the SNS effects.

The adrenergic blockers have varying degrees of specificity for the adrenergic receptor sites. For example, some can interact with both alpha- and beta-receptors. Some are specific to alpha-receptors, with some being even more specific to just alpha$_1$-receptors. Other adrenergic blockers interact with both beta$_1$- and beta$_2$-receptors, whereas others interact with just either beta$_1$- or beta$_2$-receptors. This specificity allows the clinician to select a drug that will have the desired therapeutic effects without the undesired effects that occur when the entire SNS is blocked. In general, however, the specificity of adrenergic blocking agents depends on the concentration of drug in the body. Most specificity is lost with higher serum drug levels (Figure 31.1).

The effects of the adrenergic blocking agents vary with the age of the patient (Box 31.1). Various alternative and herbal remedies also can affect these drugs (Box 31.2).

Nonselective Adrenergic Blocking Agents

Drugs that block both alpha- and beta-adrenergic receptors are primarily used to treat cardiac-related conditions. These drugs include amiodarone (*Cordarone*), carvedilol (*Coreg*), and labetalol (*Trandate*) (see Table 31.1).

Therapeutic Actions and Indications

Adrenergic blocking agents competitively block the effects of norepinephrine at alpha-and beta-receptors throughout the SNS. Subsequently, this results in lower blood pressure, slower pulse rate, and increased renal perfusion with decreased renin levels. Most of these drugs are indicated to treat essential hypertension, alone or in combination with diuretics.

Labetalol is used IV and orally to treat hypertension. It also can be used with diuretics and has been used to treat hypertension associated with **pheochromocytoma** (tumor of the chromaffin cells of the adrenal medulla, which periodically releases large amounts of norepinephrine and epinephrine into the system) and clonidine withdrawal. Amiodarone, which is available in oral and IV forms, is saved for serious emergencies and only used as an antiarrhythmic (see Chapter 45). Carvedilol is only available orally and is used to treat hypertension, as well as heart failure (HF) and left ventricular dysfunction after myocardial infarction (MI). Table 31.1 shows Usual Indications for each of these agents.

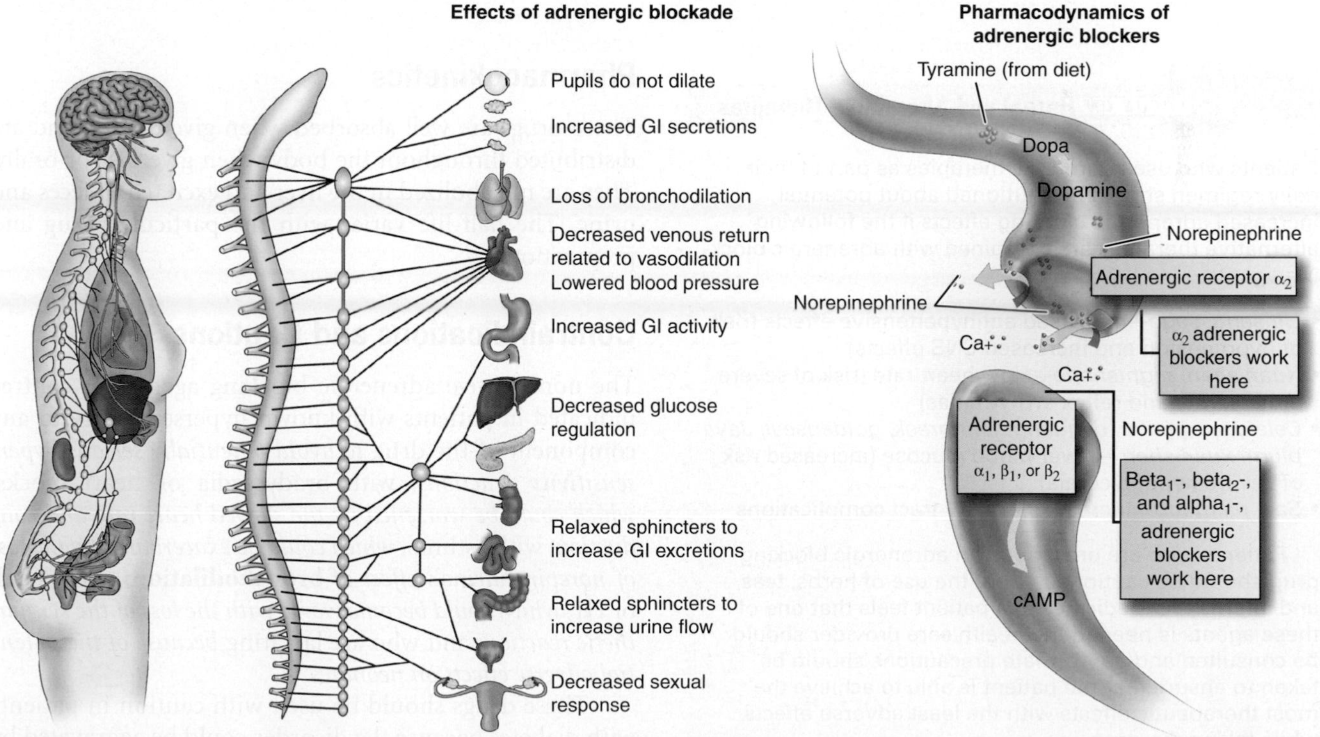

FIGURE 31.1 Site of action of adrenergic receptors and resultant physiological responses. These responses are blocked by adrenergic blockers.

BOX 31.1 FOCUS ON **Drug Therapy Across the Lifespan**

Adrenergic Blocking Agents

CHILDREN

Children are at greater risk for complications associated with the use of adrenergic blocking agents, including bradycardia, difficulty breathing, and changes in glucose metabolism. The safety and efficacy for use of these drugs has not been established for children younger than 18 years of age. If one of these drugs is used the dose for these agents needs to be calculated from the child's body weight and age. It is good practice to have a second person check the dose calculation before administering the drug to avoid potential toxic effects. Three adrenergic blocking agents have established pediatric doses, and they might be the drugs to consider when one is needed: Prazosin is used to treat hypertension, and phentolamine, which is used during surgery for pheochromocytoma. Children should be carefully monitored and supported when these drugs are given. Propranolol as an oral solution form is used for the treatment of proliferating infantile hemoangioma in children 5 weeks to 5 months of age

ADULTS

Adults being treated with adrenergic blocking agents should be cautioned about the many adverse effects associated with the drugs. Patients with diabetes need to be reeducated about ways to monitor themselves for hyperglycemia and hypoglycemia because the sympathetic reaction (sweating, feeling tense, increased heart rate, rapid breathing) usually alerts patients that there is a problem with their glucose levels. Patients with severe thyroid disease are also at high risk for serious adverse effects when taking these drugs, and if one of them is needed the patient should be monitored very closely. Propranolol and metoprolol are associated with more CNS adverse effects than other adrenergic blockers, and patients who have CNS complications already or who develop CNS problems while taking an adrenergic blocker might do better with a different agent.

In general, there are no adequate studies about the effects of adrenergic blockers during pregnancy and lactation, and they should be used only in those situations in which the benefit to the mother is greater than the risk to the fetus or neonate. Adrenergic blockers can affect labor, and babies born to mothers taking these drugs may exhibit adverse CV, respiratory, and CNS effects. Many of these drugs were teratogenic in animal studies. Because of a similar risk of adverse reactions on the baby, nursing mothers should find another way to feed the baby if an adrenergic blocking drug is needed.

OLDER ADULTS

Older patients are more likely to experience the adverse effects associated with these drugs—CNS, CV, GI, and respiratory effects. Because older patients often also have renal or hepatic impairment, they are more likely to have toxic levels of the drug related to changes in metabolism and excretion. The older patient should be started on lower doses of the drugs and should be monitored very closely for potentially serious arrhythmias or blood pressure changes. Bisoprolol is often a drug of choice for older patients who require an adrenergic blocker for hypertension because it is not associated with as many problems in the elderly and regular dosing profiles can be used.

BOX 31.2 FOCUS ON **Herbal and Alternative Therapies**

Patients who use alternative therapies as part of their daily regimen should be cautioned about potential increased adrenergic blocking effects if the following alternative therapies are combined with adrenergic blocking agents:

- *Ginseng, sage*—increased antihypertensive effects (risk of hypotension and increased CNS effects)
- *Xuan shen, nightshade*—slow heart rate (risk of severe bradycardia and reflex arrhythmias)
- *Celery, coriander, di huang, fenugreek, goldenseal, Java plum, xuan shen*—lower blood glucose (increased risk of severe hypoglycemia)
- *Saw palmetto*—increased urinary tract complications

Patients who are prescribed an adrenergic blocking drug should be cautioned about the use of herbs, teas, and alternative medicines. If a patient feels that one of these agents is needed the health care provider should be consulted and appropriate precautions should be taken to ensure that the patient is able to achieve the most therapeutic effects with the least adverse effects while taking the drug.

Pharmacokinetics

These drugs are well absorbed when given orally and are distributed throughout the body when given IV or orally. They are metabolized in the liver and excreted in feces and urine. The half-life varies with the particular drug and preparation.

Contraindications and Cautions

The nonselective adrenergic blocking agents are contraindicated in patients with known hypersensitivity to any component of the drug *to avoid potentially serious hypersensitivity reactions*; with bradycardia or heart blocks, *which could be worsened by the slowed heart rate and conduction*; with asthma, *which could be exacerbated by the loss of norepinephrine's effect of* **bronchodilation**; with shock or HF, *which could become worse with the loss of the sympathetic reaction*; and who are lactating *because of the potential adverse effects on neonates.*

These drugs should be used with caution in patients with diabetes because the disorder could be aggravated by the blocked sympathetic response and because the usual

Table 31.1 ***Drugs in Focus:* Nonselective Adrenergic Blocking Agents**

Drug Name	Dosage/Route	Usual Indications
amiodarone (*Cordarone*)	800–1,600 mg/d PO, reduce to 400 mg/d for maintenance; 1,000 mg IV over 24 h; for maintenance 540 mg IV over 18 h	Treatment of life-threatening ventricular arrhythmias
carvedilol (*Coreg*)	6.25–12.5 mg PO b.i.d. for hypertension; 3.125–6.25 mg PO b.i.d. for HF	Treatment of hypertension and HF in adults, alone or as part of combination therapy
labetalol (*Normodyne, Trandate*)	100 mg PO b.i.d. initially, maintenance 200–400 mg PO b.i.d.; 20 mg IV, slowly with additional doses given at 10-min intervals to a maximum dose of 300 mg for severe hypertension	Treatment of hypertension, hypertension associated with pheochromocytoma, and clonidine withdrawal

HF, heart failure.

signs and symptoms of hypoglycemia and hyperglycemia are masked with the SNS blockade. Caution also should be used in patients with bronchospasm, which could progress to respiratory distress due to the loss of norepinephrine's bronchodilating actions; and in pregnancy because there are no well-defined studies to evaluate the potential risk to the fetus. The drugs should only be used if the benefit to the mother clearly outweighs the potential risk to the fetus.

Adverse Effects

The adverse effects associated with the use of nonselective adrenergic blocking agents are usually associated with the drug's effects on the SNS. These effects can include dizziness, paresthesias, insomnia, depression, fatigue, and vertigo, *which are related to the blocking of norepinephrine's effect in the central nervous system (CNS)*. Nausea, vomiting, diarrhea, anorexia, and flatulence are *associated with the loss of the balancing sympathetic effect on the gastrointestinal (GI) tract and increased parasympathetic dominance.* Cardiac arrhythmias, hypotension, HF, pulmonary edema, and cerebrovascular accident, or stroke, are *related to the lack of stimulatory effects and loss of vascular tone in the cardiovascular (CV) system.* Bronchospasm, cough, rhinitis, and bronchial obstruction are *related to loss of bronchodilation of the respiratory tract and vasodilation of mucous membrane vessels* (Figure 31.2). Other effects reported include decreased exercise tolerance, hypoglycemia, and rash *related to the sympathetic blocking effects.* Abruptly stopping these drugs after long-term therapy can result in MI, stroke, and arrhythmias *related to an increased hypersensitivity to catecholamines that develops when the receptor sites have been blocked.* Carvedilol has been associated with hepatic failure *related to its effects on the liver.*

Clinically Important Drug–Drug Interactions

There is increased risk of excessive hypotension if any of these drugs is combined with volatile liquid general anesthetics such as enflurane, halothane, or isoflurane. The effectiveness of diabetic agents is increased, leading to hypoglycemia when such agents are used with these drugs; patients should be monitored closely and dose adjustments made as needed. In addition, carvedilol has been associated with potentially dangerous conduction system disturbances when combined with verapamil or diltiazem; if this combination is used the patient requires continuous monitoring.

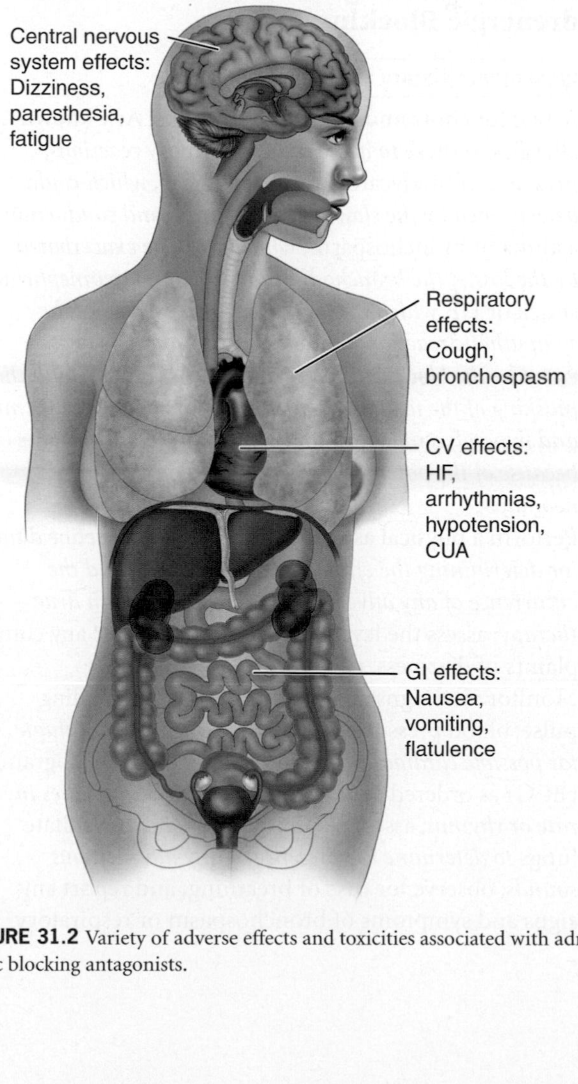

FIGURE 31.2 Variety of adverse effects and toxicities associated with adrenergic blocking antagonists.

Ⓟ Prototype Summary: Labetalol

Indications: Hypertension, alone or in combination with other drugs; off-label uses—control of blood pressure in pheochromocytoma, clonidine withdrawal hypertension.

Actions: Competitively blocks alpha- and beta-receptor sites in the SNS, leading to lower blood pressure without reflex tachycardia and decreased renin levels.

Pharmacokinetics:

Route	Onset	Peak	Duration
Oral	Varies	1–2 h	8–12 h
IM	Immediate	5 min	5.5 h

$T_{1/2}$: 6 to 8 hours; metabolized in the liver; excreted in the urine.

Adverse Effects: Dizziness, vertigo, fatigue, gastric pain, flatulence, impotence, bronchospasm, dyspnea, cough, decreased exercise tolerance.

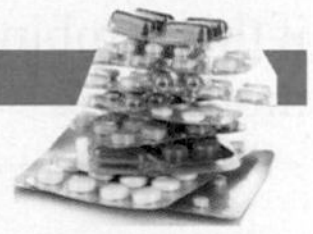

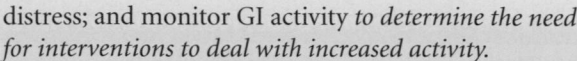

Nursing Considerations for Patients Receiving Nonselective Adrenergic Blocking Agents

Assessment: History and Examination

- Assess for contraindications or cautions: Any known allergies to these *to avoid hypersensitivity reactions*; presence of bradycardia or heart blocks, *which could be worsened by the slowing of heart rate and conduction*; asthma or bronchospasm, *which could be exacerbated by the loss of the bronchodilation effect of norepinephrine*; shock or HF, *which could worsen with the loss of the sympathetic reaction*; diabetes, *which could be aggravated by the blocking of the sympathetic response and the masking of the usual signs and symptoms of hypoglycemia and hyperglycemia*; and pregnancy or lactation status *because of the potential adverse effects on the fetus or neonate.*
- Perform a physical assessment *to establish baseline data for determining the effectiveness of the drug and the occurrence of any adverse effects associated with drug therapy*; assess the level of orientation and for any complaints of dizziness, paresthesias, or vertigo.
- Monitor vital signs and assess CV status, including pulse, blood pressure, and cardiac output, *to evaluate for possible cardiac effects*; obtain an electrocardiogram (ECG) as ordered *to assess for possible irregularities in rate or rhythm*; assess respiratory rate and auscultate lungs *to determine the presence of any adventitious sounds*; observe for ease of breathing, and report any signs and symptoms of bronchospasm or respiratory distress; and monitor GI activity *to determine the need for interventions to deal with increased activity.*
- Monitor the results of laboratory tests such as renal and liver function studies and electrolyte levels *to determine the need for possible dose adjustment*; monitor blood glucose levels *to evaluate for hyperglycemia or hypoglycemia.*

Nursing Diagnoses

Nursing diagnoses related to drug therapy might include the following:

- Decreased cardiac output related to CV effects
- Ineffective airway clearance related to lack of bronchodilating effects
- Risk for injury related to CNS effects
- Diarrhea related to increased parasympathetic activity
- Deficient knowledge regarding drug therapy

Planning

- The patient will receive the best therapeutic effect from the drug therapy.
- The patient will have limited adverse effects to the drug therapy.
- The patient will have an understanding of the drug therapy, adverse effects to anticipate, and measures to relieve discomfort and improve safety.

Implementation with Rationale

- Do not discontinue abruptly after chronic therapy *because hypersensitivity to catecholamines may develop and the patient could have a severe reaction*; taper drug slowly over 2 weeks, monitoring the patient.
- Consult with the physician about withdrawing the drug before surgery *because withdrawal is controversial; effects on the sympathetic system after surgery can cause problems.*
- Encourage the patient to adopt lifestyle changes, including diet, exercise, smoking cessation, and stress reduction, *to aid in lowering blood pressure.*
- Assess heart rate *for changes that might suggest arrhythmias.* Obtain blood pressure in various positions *to assess for orthostatic hypotension.*
- Institute safety precautions especially if the patient complains of dizziness, fatigue, or vertigo or if orthostatic hypotension occurs *to prevent injury to the patient.*
- Monitor GI function and need for increased access to bathroom facilities and need for increased fluid intake *related to diarrhea.*
- Monitor for any sign of liver failure *to arrange to discontinue the drug if this occurs* (this effect is more likely to happen with carvedilol).
- Offer support and encouragement *to help the patient deal with the drug regimen.*

- Provide thorough patient teaching, including drug name, dosage, and schedule for administration; measures to prevent adverse effects and warning signs of problems; the need to avoid herbal or alternative therapies unless allowed by the prescriber; and safety measures, such as changing position slowly and avoiding driving or operating hazardous machinery; and the need for monitoring and evaluation *to enhance patient knowledge about drug therapy and to promote compliance.*

Evaluation

- Monitor patient response to the drug (improvement in blood pressure and HF).
- Monitor for adverse effects (CV changes, headache, GI upset, bronchospasm, liver failure).
- Evaluate the effectiveness of the teaching plan (patient can name drug, dosage, adverse effects to watch for, specific measures to avoid adverse effects).
- Monitor the effectiveness of comfort measures and compliance with the regimen.

KEY POINTS

- Adrenergic blocking agents block the effects of the SNS.
- The nonselective adrenergic blocking agents block all receptors; that is, both alpha-and beta-receptors. Selective adrenergic blocking agents have specific affinity for alpha- or beta-receptors or for specific alpha$_1$-, beta$_1$-, or beta$_2$-receptor sites.
- Blocking all of the receptor sites within the SNS results in a lowering of blood pressure.

Nonselective Alpha-Adrenergic Blocking Agents

Some adrenergic blocking agents have a specific affinity for alpha-receptor sites. Their use is somewhat limited because of the development of even more specific and safer drugs. Only one of these drugs, phentolamine (*Regitine*), is still used (Table 31.2).

Therapeutic Actions and Indications

Phentolamine blocks the postsynaptic alpha$_1$-adrenergic receptors, decreasing sympathetic tone in the vasculature and causing vasodilation, which leads to a lowering of blood pressure. It also blocks presynaptic alpha$_2$-receptors, preventing the feedback control of norepinephrine release. The result is an increase in reflex tachycardia that occurs when blood pressure is lowered. Phentolamine is most frequently used to prevent cell death and tissue sloughing after extravasation of intravenous norepinephrine or dopamine, causing a local vasodilation and a return of blood flow to the area. Table 31.2 shows Usual Indications for each of these agents.

Pharmacokinetics

Phentolamine is rapidly absorbed after IV or IM injection and is excreted in the urine. There are few data on its metabolism and distribution.

Contraindications and Cautions

Phentolamine is contraindicated in the presence of allergy to this or similar drugs and in the presence of coronary artery disease or MI *because of the potential exacerbation of these conditions*; it should be used cautiously in pregnancy or lactation *because of the potential adverse effects on the fetus or neonate.*

Adverse Effects

Patients receiving phentolamine often experience extensions of the therapeutic effects, including hypotension, orthostatic hypotension, angina, MI, cerebrovascular accident, flushing, tachycardia, and arrhythmia—*all of which are related to vasodilation and decreased blood pressure.* Headache, weakness, and dizziness often occur *in response to hypotension.* Nausea, vomiting, and diarrhea may also occur.

Clinically Important Drug–Drug Interactions

Ephedrine and epinephrine may have decreased hypertensive and vasoconstrictive effects if they are taken concomitantly with phentolamine because these agents work in opposing ways in the body. Increased hypotension may occur if this drug is combined with alcohol, which is also a vasodilator.

Table 31.2 ***Drugs in Focus:*** **Nonselective Alpha-Adrenergic Blocking Agent**

Drug Name	Dosage/Route	Usual Indications
phentolamine (*Regitine*)	*Adult:* 5 mg IV or IM 1–2 h before surgery; 5–10 mg in 10 mL of saline injected into area of extravasation within 12 h after extravasation *Pediatric:* 1 mg IM or IV 1–2 h before surgery; treat extravasation as in the adult	Prevention of cell death and tissue sloughing after extravasation of IV norepinephrine or dopamine, and severe hypertension reactions caused by manipulation of the pheochromocytoma before and during surgery; diagnosis of pheochromocytoma

Prototype Summary: Phentolamine

Indications: Prevention or control of hypertensive episodes associated with pheochromocytoma; test for diagnosis of pheochromocytoma; prevention and treatment of dermal necrosis and sloughing associated with IV extravasation of norepinephrine or dopamine.

Actions: Competitively blocks postsynaptic $alpha_1$- and presynaptic $alpha_2$-receptors, causing a vasodilation and lowering of blood pressure, accompanied by increased reflex tachycardia.

Pharmacokinetics:

Route	Onset	Peak	Duration
Intramuscular	Rapid	20 min	30–45 min
IV	Immediate	2 min	15–30 min

$T_{1/2}$: Metabolism and excretion are unknown.

Adverse Effects: Acute and prolonged hypotensive episodes, MI, tachycardia, arrhythmias, nausea, flushing.

Nursing Considerations for Patients Receiving Nonselective Alpha-Adrenergic Blocking Agents

Assessment: History and Examination

- Assess for contraindications or cautions: Any known allergies to these drugs *to avoid hypersensitivity reactions*; presence of any CV diseases, *which may be exacerbated by the use of this drug*; and current status of pregnancy or lactation *because of the potential for adverse effects to the fetus or neonate.*
- Perform a physical assessment *to establish baseline data for determining the effectiveness of the drug and occurrence of any adverse effects.*
- Assess orientation, affect, and reflexes *to monitor for CNS changes related to drug therapy*; monitor CV status, including pulse, blood pressure, peripheral perfusion, and cardiac output, *to determine changes in function*, and urine output, *which will reflect perfusion of the kidney as another assessment of cardiac function.*

Nursing Diagnoses

Nursing diagnoses related to drug therapy might include the following:

- Risk for injury related to CNS and CV effects of the drug
- Decreased cardiac output related to blood pressure changes, arrhythmias, and vasodilation
- Deficient knowledge regarding drug therapy

Planning

- The patient will receive the best therapeutic effect from the drug therapy.
- The patient will have limited adverse effects to the drug therapy.
- The patient will have an understanding of the drug therapy, adverse effects to anticipate, and measures to relieve discomfort and improve safety

Implementation with Rationale

- Monitor heart rate and blood pressure closely and frequently for changes *to anticipate the need to discontinue the drug if adverse reactions are severe*; provide supportive management if needed.
- Inject phentolamine directly into the area of extravasation of epinephrine or dopamine *to prevent local cell death.*
- Arrange for supportive care and comfort measures, such as rest, environmental control, and other measures, *to decrease CNS irritation*; provide headache medication *to alleviate patient discomfort.*
- Institute safety measures *to prevent injury* if the patient experiences weakness, dizziness, or orthostatic hypotension.
- Provide thorough patient teaching, including drug name, dosage, and schedule for administration; potential adverse effects and measures to prevent them; and warning signs of problems *to enhance patient knowledge about drug therapy and to promote compliance.*
- Offer support and encouragement *to help the patient deal with the need for the drug.*

Evaluation

- Monitor patient response to the drug (improvement in signs and symptoms of pheochromocytoma, improvement in tissue condition after extravasation).
- Monitor for adverse effects (orthostatic hypotension, arrhythmias, CNS effects such as headache or dizziness)
- Evaluate the effectiveness of the teaching plan (patient can name drug, dosage, adverse effects to watch for, and specific measures to avoid them).
- Monitor the effectiveness of support measures.

KEY POINTS

- Nonselective alpha-adrenergic blocking agents are used to treat pheochromocytoma, a tumor of the adrenal medulla. A reflex tachycardia commonly occurs when the blood pressure falls.
- Phentolamine is a nonselective alpha-adrenergic blocker used most commonly for the prevention and treatment of dermal necrosis and sloughing associated with IV extravasation of norepinephrine or dopamine.

Table 31.3 ***Drugs in Focus:*** **Alpha$_1$-Selective Adrenergic Blocking Agents**

Drug Name	Dosage/Route	Usual Indications
alfuzosin (*Uroxatral*)	10 mg/d PO	Treatment of BPH
doxazosin (*Cardura*)	1 mg/d PO up to 16 mg/d PO for hypertension; 1–8 mg/d PO for BPH	Treatment of hypertension and BPH
prazosin (*Minipress*)	*Adult:* 1 mg PO b.i.d. to t.i.d. with maintenance at 6–15 mg/d PO in divided doses *Pediatric:* 0.5–7 mg PO t.i.d.	Treatment of hypertension, alone or in combination with other drugs
tamsulosin (*Flomax*)	0.4–0.8 mg/d PO 30 min after the same meal each day	Treatment of BPH
terazosin (generic)	1–5 mg/d PO, preferably at bedtime for hypertension; 10 mg/d PO for BPH	Treatment of hypertension and BPH

BPH, benign prostatic hypertrophy.

Alpha$_1$-Selective Adrenergic Blocking Agents

Alpha$_1$-selective adrenergic blocking agents are drugs that have a specific affinity for alpha$_1$-receptors. These drugs include alfuzosin (*Uroxatral*), doxazosin (*Cardura*), prazosin (*Minipress*), tamsulosin (*Flomax*), and terazosin (generic) (see Table 31.3).

Therapeutic Actions and Indications

The therapeutic effects of the alpha$_1$-selective adrenergic blocking agents come from their ability to block the postsynaptic alpha$_1$-receptor sites. This causes a decrease in vascular tone and vasodilation, which leads to a fall in blood pressure. Because these drugs do not block the presynaptic alpha$_2$-receptor sites the reflex tachycardia that accompanies a fall in blood pressure does not occur. They also block smooth muscle receptors in the prostate, prostatic capsule, prostatic urethra, and urinary bladder neck, which leads to a relaxation of the bladder and prostate and improved flow of urine in male patients with benign prostatic hypertrophy (BPH). These drugs are available in oral form and can be used to treat BPH (see Chapter 52 for further discussion on BPH) and hypertension. The drugs may be used alone or as part of a combination therapy. Table 31.3 shows Usual Indications for each of these agents.

Pharmacokinetics

The alpha$_1$-selective adrenergic blocking agents are well absorbed after oral administration and undergo extensive hepatic metabolism. They are excreted in the urine.

Contraindications and Cautions

The alpha$_1$-selective adrenergic blocking agents are contraindicated in the presence of allergy to any of these drugs *to avoid hypersensitivity reactions* and also with lactation *because the drugs cross into breast milk and could have adverse effects on the neonate.* They should be used cautiously in the presence of HF or renal failure *because their blood pressure–lowering effects could exacerbate these conditions* and with hepatic impairment, *which could alter the metabolism of these drugs.* Caution also should be used during pregnancy *because of the potential for adverse effects on the fetus.*

Adverse Effects

The adverse effects associated with the use of these drugs *are usually related to their effects of SNS blockage.* CNS effects include headache, dizziness, weakness, fatigue, drowsiness, and depression. Nausea, vomiting, abdominal pain, and diarrhea may occur *as a result of direct effects on the GI tract and sympathetic blocking.* Anticipated CV effects include arrhythmias, hypotension, edema, HF, and angina. The vasodilation caused by these drugs can also cause flushing, rhinitis, reddened eyes, nasal congestion, and priapism.

Clinically Important Drug–Drug Interactions

Increased hypotensive effects may occur if these drugs are combined with any other vasodilating or antihypertensive drugs, such as nitrates, calcium-channel blockers, drugs used for erectile dysfunction and angiotensin-converting enzyme inhibitors.

Ⓟ Prototype Summary: Doxazosin

Indications: Treatment of mild to moderate hypertension as monotherapy or in combination with other antihypertensives; treatment of BPH.

Actions: Reduces total peripheral resistance through alpha blockade; does not affect heart rate or cardiac output; increases high-density lipoproteins while lowering total cholesterol levels.

Pharmacokinetics:

Route	Onset	Peak	Duration
Oral	Varies	2–3 h	Not known

$T_{1/2}$: 22 hours; metabolized in the liver; excreted in the bile, feces, and urine.

Adverse Effects: Headache, fatigue, dizziness, postural dizziness, vertigo, tachycardia, edema, nausea, dyspepsia, diarrhea, sexual dysfunction.

Nursing Considerations for Patients Receiving $Alpha_1$-Selective Adrenergic Blocking Agents

Assessment: History and Examination

- Assess for contraindications or cautions: Any known allergies to either drug *to avoid hypersensitivity reactions*; heart failure or renal failure, *which could be exacerbated by drug use*; hepatic dysfunction, *which could alter the drug's metabolism*; and current status of pregnancy or lactation *because of unknown or adverse effects to the fetus or neonate.*
- Perform a physical assessment *to establish baseline data for determining the effectiveness of drug therapy and the occurrence of any adverse effects.*
- Monitor the level of orientation, affect, and reflexes *to monitor for CNS changes related to drug therapy.*
- Monitor vital signs and assess CV status, including pulse, blood pressure, peripheral perfusion, and cardiac output, *to evaluate for possible cardiac effects*; obtain an electrocardiogram as ordered *to assess for possible irregularities in rate or rhythm.*
- Assess renal function, including urinary output, *to evaluate effects on the renal system and assess BPH and its effects on urinary output.*
- Monitor renal and hepatic function tests *to evaluate potential need for dose adjustment.*

Nursing Diagnoses

Nursing diagnoses related to drug therapy might include the following:

- Acute pain related to headache, GI upset, flushing, nasal congestion
- Risk for injury related to CNS or CV effects of the drug
- Decreased cardiac output related to blood pressure changes, arrhythmias, vasodilation
- Deficient knowledge regarding drug therapy

Planning

- The patient will receive the best therapeutic effect from the drug therapy.
- The patient will have limited adverse effects to the drug therapy.
- The patient will have an understanding of the drug therapy, adverse effects to anticipate, and measures to relieve discomfort and improve safety.

Implementation with Rationale

- Monitor blood pressure, pulse, rhythm, and cardiac output regularly *to evaluate for changes that may indicate a need to adjust dose or discontinue the drug if CV effects are severe.*
- Establish safety precautions if CNS effects or orthostatic hypotension occurs *to prevent patient injury.*
- Arrange for small, frequent meals if GI upset is severe *to relieve discomfort and maintain nutrition.*
- Arrange for supportive care and comfort measures (rest, environmental control, other measures) *to decrease CNS effects*; provide headache medication *to alleviate patient discomfort*; arrange safety measures if CNS effects occur *to prevent patient injury.*
- Offer support and encouragement *to help the patient deal with the drug regimen.*
- Provide thorough patient teaching, including drug name, dosage, and administration; measures to prevent adverse effects and warning signs to report to prescriber; safety measures such as changing positions slowly and avoiding driving or operating hazardous machinery; the need to report the use of other drugs, including drugs for erectile dysfunction and dietary measures in conjunction with drug therapy *to promote blood pressure control* or alleviate GI upset *to enhance patient knowledge about drug therapy and to promote compliance.*
- Offer support and encouragement *to help the patient deal with the drug regimen.*

Evaluation

- Monitor patient response to the drug (lowering of blood pressure, improved urine flow with BPH).
- Monitor for adverse effects (GI upset, CNS, or CV changes).
- Evaluate effectiveness of the teaching plan (patient can name drug, dosage, adverse effects to watch for, and specific measures to avoid them).
- Monitor the effectiveness of comfort measures and compliance with the regimen.

KEY POINTS

- $Alpha_1$-selective adrenergic blocking agents decrease blood pressure by blocking the postsynaptic $alpha_1$-receptor sites, decreasing vascular tone, and promoting vasodilation.
- $Alpha_1$-selective adrenergic blocking agents are used to treat hypertension and are often used to treat BPH because of their relaxing effects on the bladder and prostate.

Nonselective Beta-Adrenergic Blocking Agents

The **beta-adrenergic blocking agents** (Table 31.4) are used to treat CV problems (hypertension, angina, migraine headaches) and to prevent reinfarction after MI. These drugs are widely used and include carteolol (generic),

Table 31.4 Drugs in Focus: Nonselective Beta-Adrenergic Blocking Agents

Drug Name	Dosage/Route	Usual Indications
carteolol (generic)		Treatment of chronic open-angle glaucoma
metipranolol (*OptiPranolol*)	One drop in affected eye(s) b.i.d.; 1–2 drops in affected eye(s) b.i.d.	Treatment of chronic open-angle glaucoma, ocular hypertension
nebivolol (*Bystolic*)	Initially 5 mg/d PO, increase at 2-wk intervals based on patient response; maximum dose 40 mg/d	Treatment of hypertension, alone or as part of combination therapy in adults
nadolol (*Corgard*)	*Angina:* 40–80 mg/d PO *Hypertension:* 40–80 mg/d PO, up to 320 mg/d may be needed; reduce dose in renal impairment	Treatment of hypertension, management of chronic angina in adults; drug of choice in an angina patient who is also hypertensive
propranolol (*Inderal, Hemangeol*)	Dose varies widely based on indication; check drug guide for specific information	Treatment of hypertension, angina, idiopathic hypertrophic subaortic stenosis–induced palpitations, angina and syncope, certain cardiac arrhythmias induced by catecholamines or digoxin, pheochromocytoma; prevention of reinfarction after MI; prophylaxis for migraine headache (which may be caused by vasodilation and is relieved by vasoconstriction, although the exact action is not clearly understood); prevention of stage fright (which is a sympathetic stress reaction to a particular situation); treatment of essential tremors; treatment of proliferating infantile hemangioma
sotalol (*Betapace, Betapace AF*)	*Betapace:* 80 mg PO b.i.d., up to 320 mg PO b.i.d. may be needed *Betapace AF:* 80 mg/d PO based on QT interval and patient response, up to 120 mg b.i.d. may be needed Reduce dose of both with renal impairment	Treatment of potentially life-threatening ventricular arrhythmias (*Betapace*); maintenance of normal sinus rhythm in patients with atrial fibrillation/flutter (*Betapace AF*)
timolol (*Timoptic*)	10 mg PO b.i.d., increases based on patient response; 1–2 drops (gtt) in affected eye(s) for glaucoma	Treatment of hypertension; prevention of reinfarction after MI; prophylaxis for migraine; in ophthalmic form, reduction of intraocular pressure in open-angle glaucoma

MI, myocardial infarction.

metipranolol (*OptiPranolol*), nadolol (*Corgard*), nebivolol (*Bystolic*), propranolol (*Inderal*), sotalol (*Betapace, Betapace AF*), and timolol (*Timoptic*). The prototype drug, propranolol, was in fact the most prescribed drug in the United States in the 1980s.

Therapeutic Actions and Indications

The therapeutic effects of these drugs are related to their competitive blocking of the beta-adrenergic receptors in the SNS. The blockade of the beta-receptors in the heart and in the juxtaglomerular apparatus of the nephron accounts for the majority of the therapeutic benefit. Decreased heart rate, contractility, and excitability, as well as a membrane-stabilizing effect, lead to a decrease in arrhythmias, decreased cardiac workload, and decreased oxygen consumption. The juxtaglomerular cells are not stimulated to release renin, which further decreases the blood pressure. These effects are useful in treating hypertension and chronic angina and can help to prevent reinfarction after an MI by decreasing cardiac workload and oxygen consumption. Sotalol is used exclusively for treating life-threatening ventricular arrhythmias and to maintain sinus rhythm in patients with atrial flutter or atrial fibrillation (see Chapter 45).

Propranolol is very effective in blocking all of the beta-receptors in the SNS and was one of the first drugs of the class (see Table 31.4 for Usual Indications). Since the introduction of propranolol, newer and more selective drugs have become available that are not associated with some of the adverse effects seen with total blockade of the SNS beta-receptors. In 2014 propranolol was approved in an oral solution form for the treatment of proliferating infantile hemoangioma in children 5 weeks to 5 months of age (*Hemangeol*). Nebivolol is the newest adrenergic blocker available and is not associated with the variety of adverse effects seen with propranolol use. Timolol has several recommended uses, which are listed in Table 31.4; timolol, carteolol, and metipranolol are available in an ophthalmic form of the drug for reduction of intraocular pressure in patients with open-angle glaucoma. When these drugs are used topically, eye muscle relaxation occurs. In addition, because they are applied topically, they are usually not absorbed systemically from this route.

Pharmacokinetics

These drugs are absorbed from the GI tract after oral administration and undergo hepatic metabolism. Food has been found to increase the bioavailability of propranolol, although this effect was not found with other beta-adrenergic blocking agents. Absorption of sotalol is decreased by the presence of food. Propranolol also crosses the blood–brain barrier, but nadolol, and sotalol do not, making them a better choice if CNS effects occur with propranolol. These drugs are all excreted in the urine. Carteolol and metipranolol are only available in an ophthalmic form and are not usually absorbed systemically.

Contraindications and Cautions

Nonselective beta-adrenergic blocking agents are contraindicated in the presence of allergy to any of these drugs or any components of the drug being used *to avoid hypersensitivity reactions*; with bradycardia or heart blocks, shock, or HF, *which could be exacerbated by the cardiac-suppressing effects of these drugs*; with bronchospasm, chronic obstructive pulmonary disease (COPD), or acute asthma, *which could worsen due to the blocking of sympathetic bronchodilation*; with pregnancy *because teratogenic effects have occurred in animal studies with all of these drugs except sotalol and because neonatal apnea, bradycardia, and hypoglycemia could occur*; and with lactation *because of the potential effects on the neonate, which could include slowed heart rate, hypotension, and hypoglycemia*. The safety and efficacy for use of these drugs in children have not been established.

These drugs should be used cautiously in patients with diabetes and hypoglycemia *because of the blocking of the normal signs and symptoms of hypoglycemia and hyperglycemia*; with thyrotoxicosis *because of the adrenergic blocking effects on the thyroid gland*; or with renal or hepatic dysfunction, *which could interfere with the excretion and metabolism of these drugs*.

Adverse Effects

Patients receiving these drugs often experience adverse effects *related to blockage of beta-receptors in the SNS*. CNS effects include headache, fatigue, dizziness, depression, paresthesias, sleep disturbances, memory loss, and disorientation. CV effects can include bradycardia, heart block, HF, hypotension, and peripheral vascular insufficiency. Pulmonary effects can range from difficulty breathing, coughing, and bronchospasm to severe pulmonary edema and bronchial obstruction. GI upset, nausea, vomiting, diarrhea, gastric pain, and even colitis can occur as a result of unchecked parasympathetic activity and the blocking of the sympathetic receptors. Genitourinary (GU) effects can include decreased libido, impotence, dysuria, and Peyronie disease. Other effects that can occur include decreased exercise tolerance (patients often report that their "get up and go" is gone), hypoglycemia or hyperglycemia, and liver changes. If these drugs are stopped abruptly after long-term use, there is a risk of angina, MI, hypertension, and stroke because the receptor sites become hypersensitive to catecholamines after being blocked by the drugs.

Clinically Important Drug–Drug Interactions

A paradoxical hypertension occurs when beta-blockers are given with clonidine, and an increased rebound hypertension with clonidine withdrawal may also occur. It is best to avoid this combination.

A decreased antihypertensive effect occurs when beta-blockers are given with nonsteroidal anti-inflammatory drugs (NSAIDs); if this combination is used the patient should be monitored closely and dose adjustment should be made to achieve the desired control of blood pressure.

An initial hypertensive episode followed by bradycardia may occur if these drugs are given with epinephrine. Peripheral ischemia may occur if the beta-blockers are taken in combination with ergot alkaloids.

When these drugs are given with insulin or other antidiabetic agents, there is a potential for change in blood glucose levels. The patient also will not display the usual signs and symptoms of hypoglycemia or hyperglycemia, which are caused by activation of the SNS. Because these effects are blocked the patient will need new indications to alert him or her to potential problems. If this combination is used the patient should monitor blood glucose levels frequently throughout the day and should be alert to new manifestations indicating glucose imbalance.

Ⓟ Prototype Summary: Propranolol

Indications: Treatment of hypertension, angina pectoris, idiopathic hypertrophic subaortic stenosis, supraventricular tachycardia, tremor; prevention of reinfarction after MI; adjunctive therapy in pheochromocytoma; prophylaxis of migraine headache; management of situational anxiety, treatment of proliferating infantile hemoangioma.

Actions: Competitively blocks beta-adrenergic receptors in the heart and juxtaglomerular apparatus; reduces vascular tone in the CNS.

Pharmacokinetics:

Route	Onset	Peak	Duration
Oral	20–30 min	60–90 min	6–12 h
IV	Immediate	1 min	4–6 h

$T_{1/2}$: 3 to 5 hours; metabolized in the liver; excreted in the urine.

Adverse Effects: Allergic reaction, bradycardia, heart failure, cardiac arrhythmias, cerebrovascular accident, pulmonary edema, gastric pain, flatulence, impotence, decreased exercise tolerance, bronchospasm.

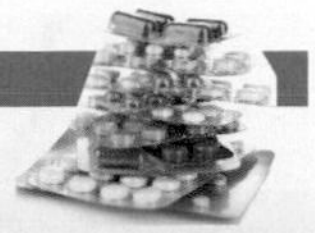

Nursing Considerations for Patients Receiving Nonselective Beta-Adrenergic Blocking Agents

Assessment: History and Examination

- Assess for contraindications or cautions: Known allergy to any drug or to any components of the drug *to avoid hypersensitivity reactions*; bradycardia or heart blocks, shock, or heart failure, *which could be exacerbated by the cardiac-suppressing effects of these drugs*; bronchospasm, chronic obstructive pulmonary disease, or acute asthma, *which could worsen with blocking of sympathetic bronchodilation*; diabetes or hypoglycemia, *which could lead to altered blood glucose levels*; thyrotoxicosis *because of adrenergic blocking effects on the thyroid gland*; renal or hepatic dysfunction, *which could interfere with the excretion or metabolism of these drugs*; and status of pregnancy and lactation *because of the potential effects on the fetus or neonate.*
- Perform a physical assessment to establish baseline data *for determining the effectiveness of the drug and the occurrence of any adverse effects.*
- Assess level of orientation and sensory function *to evaluate for possible CNS effects.*
- Monitor cardiopulmonary status, including pulse, blood pressure, and respiratory rate; auscultate lungs for adventitious breath sounds; obtain an ECG as ordered *to evaluate for changes in heart rate or rhythm;* check color, sensation, and capillary refill of extremities *to evaluate for possible peripheral vascular insufficiency.*
- Assess abdomen, including auscultating bowel sounds, *to monitor for GI effects.*
- Monitor the results of laboratory tests, such as electrolyte levels, to *monitor for risks for arrhythmias*; adrenal and hepatic function studies *to determine the need for possible dose adjustment.*

Refer to the Critical Thinking Scenario for a full discussion of nursing care for a patient who is receiving beta-adrenergic blocking agents.

Nursing Diagnoses

Nursing diagnoses related to drug therapy might include the following:

- Acute pain related to CNS, GI, and systemic effects
- Decreased cardiac output related to CV effects
- Ineffective tissue perfusion related to CV effects
- Risk for injury related to CNS effects
- Risk for activity intolerance related to suppression of the sympathetic system
- Deficient knowledge regarding drug therapy

Planning

- The patient will receive the best therapeutic effect from the drug therapy.
- The patient will have limited adverse effects to the drug therapy.
- The patient will have an understanding of the drug therapy, adverse effects to anticipate, and measures to relieve discomfort and improve safety

Implementation with Rationale

- Do not stop these drugs abruptly after chronic therapy, but taper gradually over 2 weeks *because long-term use of these drugs can sensitize the myocardium to catecholamines, and severe reactions could occur.*
- Continuously monitor any patient receiving an intravenous form of these drugs *to avert serious complications caused by rapid sympathetic blockade.*
- Monitor blood pressure, pulse, rhythm, and cardiac output regularly *to evaluate drug effectiveness and to monitor for changes that may indicate a need to adjust dose or discontinue the drug if CV effects are severe.*
- Arrange for supportive care and comfort measures (rest, environmental control, other measures) *to relieve CNS effects*; institute safety measures if CNS effects occur *to prevent patient injury*; provide small, frequent meals and mouth care *to help relieve the discomfort of GI effects*; establish daily activity program, spacing activities *to help the patient deal with activity intolerance.*
- Offer support and encouragement *to help the patient deal with the drug regimen.*
- Provide thorough patient teaching, including drug name, dose, and schedule of administration; use of drug with food or meals, if appropriate; possible adverse effects and measures to prevent them; warning signs to report; safety measures, such as changing position slowly, avoiding driving or using hazardous machinery, and pacing activities; and the need for follow-up evaluation and possible changes in dose to achieve therapeutic effectiveness *to enhance patient knowledge about drug therapy and to promote compliance.*

Evaluation

- Monitor patient response to the drug (lowering of blood pressure, decrease in anginal episodes, improvement in condition being treated).
- Monitor for adverse effects (GI upset, CNS changes, respiratory problems, CV effects, loss of libido, and impotence).
- Evaluate the effectiveness of the teaching plan (patient can name drug, dosage, adverse effects to watch for, and specific measures to avoid them).
- Monitor the effectiveness of comfort measures and compliance with the regimen.

CRITICAL THINKING SCENARIO

Nonselective Beta-Blockers (Propranolol)

THE SITUATION

M.R., a 59-year-old man, has been seen several times complaining of tremor in his hands that eventually made it very difficult for him to work as a computer programmer. A diagnosis of essential tremor was made, and he was prescribed propranolol (*Inderal*) 20 mg twice daily. M.R. had good effects with the drug and had no further problems until the following June, when acute respiratory distress developed while he was picnicking in a state park with his family. On the way to the emergency room, he suffered an apparent respiratory arrest. He was admitted to the hospital and placed in the respiratory intensive care unit. It was found that M.R. had a history of hay fever and allergic rhinitis during the pollen season but had never experienced such a severe reaction.

CRITICAL THINKING

Why did M.R. have such a severe reaction? What appropriate measures should be taken to ensure that M.R. recovers fully and does not reexperience this event?

What sort of support will M.R. and his family need after going through such a frightening experience? Think about the children who may have witnessed the respiratory arrest and how they should be reassured, depending on their ages. *Think about the support M.R.'s wife may need and the fear that may now be associated with M.R.'s condition. M.R. has been taking propranolol for several months and needs to decide whether he should continue the drug with modifications to his lifestyle or the addition of other drugs to deal with his respiratory issues.*

What kind of teaching program will need to be developed to help M.R. deal with this drug and its potential adverse effects?

DISCUSSION

Propranolol, a nonselective beta-blocker, was prescribed to decrease the tremor he was experiencing. The exact action of this drug to decrease the tremor is thought to be related to its membrane-stabilizing properties. The desired therapeutic effect is the reduction of the tremor, but all of the beta-blocking effects will occur and need to be monitored. He did well on the drug until pollen season arrived. That is because propranolol, a nonselective beta-blocker, prevented the compensatory bronchodilation that occurs when the SNS is stimulated. When the pollen reacted with M.R.'s airways, causing them to swell and become narrower, his swollen bronchial tubes were unable to allow air to flow through them. The result was bronchial constriction and respiratory distress that, in M.R.'s case, progressed to a respiratory arrest. Before he began taking propranolol, M.R. probably had been effectively compensating for the swelling of the bronchi through bronchodilation and had never experienced such a reaction. There are few other drugs for treating essential tremor. M.R. and his health care providers will need to decide whether the benefit that the drug has brought to him is worth the potential for adverse effects. They might be able to suggest additional drugs to deal with the seasonal allergic reactions to make the use of propranolol safer for this patient.

M.R. may want to discuss this frightening incident with his health care provider. He also may want to include his family in this discussion. It should be stressed that he did so well up to this point because he had not been exposed to pollen and therefore had not had the problem that brought him into the hospital this time. M.R. probably never reported the occurrence of hay fever to his health care provider when the drug was prescribed because it had never been a problem and probably did not seem significant to him. M.R. and his family should receive support and be encouraged to talk about what happened and how they reacted to it. It is normal to feel frightened and unsure when a loved one is in distress. They should be involved in the discussion of what medical regimen would be most appropriate for M.R. at this point.

NURSING CARE GUIDE FOR M.R.: PROPRANOLOL

Assessment: History and Examination

Review the patient's history for allergy to propranolol, HF, shock, bradycardia, heart block, hypotension, COPD, thyroid disease, diabetes, respiratory impairment, and concurrent use of barbiturates, NSAIDs, piroxicam, sulindac, lidocaine, cimetidine, phenothiazines, clonidine, theophylline, and rifampin.

Focus the physical examination on the following:

CV: Blood pressure, pulse, peripheral perfusion, ECG
CNS: Orientation, affect, reflexes, vision
Skin: Color, lesions, texture
GU: Urinary output, sexual function
GI: Abdominal, liver evaluation
Respiratory: Respirations, adventitious sounds

Nursing Diagnoses

Decreased cardiac output related to CV effects
Acute pain related to CNS, GI, systematic effects
Impaired tissue perfusion, related to CV effects
Deficient knowledge regarding drug therapy

Nonselective Beta-Blockers (Propranolol) (continued)

Planning

The patient will receive the best therapeutic effect from the drug therapy.

The patient will have limited adverse effects to the drug therapy.

The patient will have an understanding of the drug therapy, adverse effects to anticipate, and measures to relieve discomfort and improve safety.

Implementation

Ensure safe and appropriate administration of the drug.

Provide comfort and safety measures: Assistance/side rails; temperature control; rest periods; mouth care; small, frequent meals.

Monitor blood pressure, pulse, and respiratory status throughout drug therapy.

Taper the drug gradually if it is to be discontinued to decrease the risk of severe hypertension, MI, or stroke related to abrupt withdrawal.

Provide support and reassurance to deal with drug effects and discomfort, sexual dysfunction, and fatigue.

Provide patient teaching regarding drug name, dosage, side effects, precautions, and warning signs to report.

Evaluation

Evaluate drug effects: Blood pressure within normal limits, decrease in essential tremors, stabilized cardiac rhythm.

Monitor for adverse effects: CV effects; HF, block; dizziness, confusion; sexual dysfunction; GI effects; hypoglycemia; respiratory problems.

Monitor for drug–drug interactions as indicated.

Evaluate the effectiveness of the patient-teaching program.

Evaluate the effectiveness of comfort and safety measures.

PATIENT TEACHING FOR M.R.

- The drug that has been prescribed for you, propranolol, is a nonselective beta-adrenergic blocking agent. A beta-adrenergic blocking agent works to prevent certain stimulating activities that normally occur in the body in response to such factors as stress, injury, or excitement. It stabilizes certain nerve membranes, which helps to decrease your tremor.
- You should learn to take your pulse and monitor it daily, writing the pulse rate on the calendar. Your current pulse rate is 82 beats/min.
- Never discontinue this medication suddenly. If you find that your prescription is running low, notify your health care provider at once. This drug needs to be tapered over time to prevent severe reactions when its use is discontinued. Some of the following adverse effects may occur:
  - *Fatigue, weakness*: Try to stagger your activities throughout the day to allow rest periods.
  - *Dizziness, drowsiness*: If these should occur, take care to avoid driving, operating dangerous machinery, or doing delicate tasks. Change position slowly to avoid dizzy spells.
  - *Change in sexual function*: Be assured that this is a drug effect and discuss it with your health care provider.
  - *Nausea, diarrhea*: These GI discomforts often diminish with time. If they become too uncomfortable or do not improve, talk to your health care provider.
  - *Dreams, confusion*: These are drug effects. If they become too uncomfortable, discuss them with your health care provider.
- Report any of the following to your health care provider: Very slow pulse, need to sleep on more pillows at night, difficulty breathing, swelling in the ankles or fingers, sudden weight gain, mental confusion or personality change, fever, or rash.
- Avoid over-the-counter medications, including cold and allergy remedies and diet pills. Many of these preparations contain drugs that could interfere with this medication. If you feel that you need one of these, check with your health care provider first.
- Tell any doctor, nurse, or other health care provider that you are taking these drugs, keep all medications out of the reach of children, and do not share these drugs with other people.

KEY POINTS

- Beta-blockers are drugs used to block the beta-receptors within the SNS. These drugs are used for a wide range of conditions, including hypertension, stage fright, migraines, angina, and essential tremors.
- Nonselective blockade of all beta-receptors results in a loss of the reflex bronchodilation that occurs with sympathetic stimulation. This limits the use of these drugs in patients who smoke or have allergic or seasonal rhinitis, asthma, or COPD.

Beta$_1$-Selective Adrenergic Blocking Agents

Beta$_1$-selective adrenergic blocking agents (Table 31.5) have an advantage over the nonselective beta-blockers in some cases. Because they do not usually block beta$_2$-receptor sites, they do not block the sympathetic bronchodilation that is so important for patients with lung diseases or allergic rhinitis. Consequently, these drugs are preferred for patients who smoke or who have asthma, any other

Table 31.5 ***Drugs in Focus:* Beta$_1$-Selective Adrenergic Blocking Agents**

Drug Name	Dosage/Route	Usual Indications
acebutolol (*Sectral*)	400 mg/d PO, up to 1,200 mg/d may be used; decrease dose with the elderly and with renal and hepatic impairment	Treatment of hypertension and premature ventricular contractions in adults
atenolol (*Tenormin*)	Initially 50 mg/d PO, may be increased to 100 mg/d; reduce dose with renal impairment	Treatment of MI, chronic angina, hypertension in adults (atenolol is more widely used than the other drugs of this class for hypertension)
betaxolol (*Betoptic*)	10–20 mg/d PO; reduce to 5 mg/d PO with the elderly; 1–2 drops (gtt) in affected eye(s) for glaucoma	Treatment of hypertension in adults; available as ophthalmic agent for treatment of ocular hypertension, open-angle glaucoma
bisoprolol (*Zebeta*)	Initially 5 mg/d PO, up to 20 mg/d PO may be needed; reduce dose with renal or hepatic impairment	Treatment of hypertension in adults, alone or as part of combination therapy
esmolol (*Brevibloc*)	50–200 mcg/kg/min IV, with dose based on patient response	Treatment of supraventricular tachycardias (e.g., atrial flutter, atrial fibrillation) in adults, and noncompensatory tachycardia when the heart rate must be slowed (IV use only)
metoprolol (*Lopressor, Toprol XL*)	100–400 mg/d PO, based on patient response; XL preparation for treatment of angina: 50–200 mg/d PO based on patient response; acute MI: three IV bolus doses of 5 mg each at 2-min intervals; if tolerated start PO therapy 15 min after last IV dose	Treatment of hypertension; prevention of reinfarction after MI; early acute MI treatment; treatment of stable and symptomatic HF (extended release preparation only)

MI, myocardial infarction; HF, heart failure.

obstructive pulmonary disease, or seasonal or allergic rhinitis. These selective beta-blockers are also used for treating hypertension, angina, and some cardiac arrhythmias. Beta$_1$-selective adrenergic blocking agents include acebutolol (*Sectral*), atenolol (*Tenormin*), betaxolol (*Betoptic*), bisoprolol (*Zebeta*), esmolol (*Brevibloc*), and metoprolol (*Lopressor, Toprol XL*).

Therapeutic Actions and Indications

The therapeutic effects of these drugs are related to their ability to selectively block beta$_1$-receptors in the SNS at therapeutic doses. As a result, these drugs do not block the beta$_2$-receptors and therefore do not prevent sympathetic bronchodilation. However, the selectivity is lost with doses higher than the recommended range.

The blockade of the beta$_1$-receptors in the heart and in the juxtaglomerular apparatus accounts for most of the therapeutic benefits. Decreased heart rate, contractility, and excitability, as well as a membrane-stabilizing effect, lead to a decrease in arrhythmias, decreased cardiac workload, and decreased oxygen consumption. The juxtaglomerular cells are not stimulated to release renin, which further decreases blood pressure. These drugs are useful in treating cardiac arrhythmias, hypertension, and chronic angina and can help to prevent reinfarction after an MI by decreasing cardiac workload and oxygen consumption.

Beta$_1$-selective adrenergic blocking agents in ophthalmic form are used to decrease intraocular pressure and to treat open-angle glaucoma. The beta$_1$-selective blocker of choice depends on the condition or combination of conditions being treated and personal experience with the drugs. See Table 31.5 for Usual Indications for each drug.

Pharmacokinetics

The beta$_1$-selective adrenergic blockers are absorbed from the GI tract after oral administration, reach peak levels directly with IV infusion, and are not usually absorbed when given in ophthalmic form. The bioavailability of metoprolol is increased if it is taken *in the presence of* food. These drugs are metabolized in the liver and excreted in the urine. Metoprolol readily crosses the blood–brain barrier and may cause more CNS effects than acebutolol and atenolol, which do not cross the barrier.

Contraindications and Cautions

The beta$_1$-selective adrenergic blockers are contraindicated in the presence of allergy to the drug or any components of the drug *to avoid hypersensitivity reactions*; with sinus bradycardia, heart block, cardiogenic shock, HF, or hypotension, *all of which could be exacerbated by the cardiac-depressing and blood pressure–lowering effects of these drugs*; and with lactation *because of the potential adverse effects on the neonate.* They should be used with caution in patients with diabetes, thyroid disease, or COPD *because of the potential for adverse effects on these diseases with sympathetic blockade*; and in pregnancy *because of the potential for adverse effects on the fetus.* The safety and efficacy of the use of these drugs in children have not been established.

Adverse Effects

Patients receiving these drugs often experience adverse effects *related to the blocking of beta$_1$-receptors in the SNS.* CNS effects include headache, fatigue, dizziness, depression, paresthesias, sleep disturbances, memory loss, and disorientation. CV effects can include bradycardia, heart block,

HF, hypotension, and peripheral vascular insufficiency. Pulmonary effects ranging from rhinitis to bronchospasm and dyspnea can occur; these effects are not as likely to occur with these drugs as with the nonselective beta-blockers. GI upset, nausea, vomiting, diarrhea, gastric pain, and even colitis can occur as a result of unchecked parasympathetic activity and the blocking of the sympathetic receptors. GU effects can include decreased libido, impotence, dysuria, and Peyronie disease. Other effects that can occur include decreased exercise tolerance (patients often report that their "get up and go" is gone), hypoglycemia or hyperglycemia, and liver changes that are reflected in increased concentrations of liver enzymes. If these drugs are stopped abruptly after long-term use, there is a risk of severe hypertension, angina, MI, and stroke *because the receptor sites become hypersensitive to catecholamines after being blocked by the drug.*

Clinically Important Drug–Drug Interactions

A decreased hypertensive effect occurs if these drugs are given with clonidine, NSAIDs, rifampin, or barbiturates. If such a combination is used the patient should be monitored closely and dose adjustment made.

There is an initial hypertensive episode followed by bradycardia if these drugs are given with epinephrine. Increased serum levels and increased toxicity of intravenous lidocaine will occur if it is given with these drugs.

An increased risk for orthostatic hypotension occurs if these drugs are taken with prazosin. If this combination is used the patient must be monitored closely and safety precautions taken.

The selective $beta_1$-blockers have increased effects if they are taken with verapamil, cimetidine, methimazole, or propylthiouracil. The patient should be monitored closely and appropriate dose adjustment made.

Prototype Summary: Atenolol

Indications: Treatment of angina pectoris, hypertension, MI; off-label uses are prevention of migraine headaches, alcohol withdrawal syndrome, and supraventricular tachycardias.

Actions: Blocks $beta_1$-adrenergic receptors, decreasing the excitability of the heart, cardiac output, and oxygen consumption; decreases renin release, which lowers blood pressure.

Pharmacokinetics:

Route	Onset	Peak	Duration
Oral	Varies	2–4 h	24 h
IV	Immediate	5 min	24 h

$T_{1/2}$: 6 to 7 hours; excreted in the bile, feces, and urine.

Adverse Effects: Allergic reaction, dizziness, bradycardia, heart failure, arrhythmias, gastric pain, flatulence, impotence, bronchospasm, decreased exercise tolerance.

Nursing Considerations for Patients Receiving $Beta_1$-Selective Adrenergic Blocking Agents

Assessment: History and Examination

- Assess for contraindications or cautions: Known allergies to any drug or any components of the drug *to avoid hypersensitivity reactions*; bradycardia or heart blocks, shock, or heart failure, *which could be exacerbated by the cardiac-suppressing effects of these drugs*; diabetes, thyroid disease, or chronic obstructive pulmonary disease *to reduce risk of adverse effects on these conditions due to sympathetic blockade*; and current status of pregnancy or lactation *because of the potential effects on the fetus or neonate.*
- Perform a physical assessment to establish baseline status before beginning therapy *to determine the effectiveness of therapy and evaluate for any potential adverse effects.*
- Assess neurological status, including level of orientation and sensation, *to evaluate for CNS effects.*
- Monitor cardiac status, including pulse, blood pressure, and heart rate, *to identify changes*, and obtain an ECG as ordered *to evaluate for changes in heart rate or rhythm.*
- Assess pulmonary status, including respirations, and auscultate lungs for adventitious sounds *to monitor respiratory status.*
- Examine the abdomen and auscultate bowel sounds *to evaluate GI effects.*
- Monitor urine output *to monitor the effectiveness of cardiac output and any changes in renal perfusion.*
- Monitor the results of laboratory tests, including electrolyte levels, *to monitor for risk of arrhythmias*, and renal and hepatic function studies *to determine the need for possible dose adjustment.*

Nursing Diagnoses

Nursing diagnoses related to drug therapy might include the following:

- Acute pain related to CNS, GI, and systemic effects
- Decreased cardiac output related to CV effects
- Ineffective tissue perfusion related to CV effects
- Risk for injury related to CNS effects
- Activity intolerance related to sympathetic blocking
- Deficient knowledge regarding drug therapy

Planning

- The patient will receive the best therapeutic effect from the drug therapy.
- The patient will have limited adverse effects to the drug therapy.

(continues on page 534)

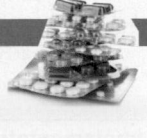

- The patient will have an understanding of the drug therapy, adverse effects to anticipate, and measures to relieve discomfort and improve safety.

Implementation with Rationale

- Do not stop these drugs abruptly after chronic therapy, but taper gradually over 2 weeks *to prevent the possibility of severe reactions.* Long-term use of these drugs can sensitize the myocardium to catecholamines, *and severe reactions could occur.*
- Consult with the physician about discontinuing these drugs before surgery *because withdrawal of the drug before surgery when the patient has been maintained on the drug is controversial.*
- Give oral forms of the metoprolol with food *to facilitate absorption.*
- Continuously monitor any patient receiving an IV form of these drugs *to detect severe reactions to sympathetic blockade and to ensure rapid response if these reactions occur.*
- Arrange for supportive care and comfort measures, including rest, environmental control, and other measures, *to relieve CNS effects*; safety measures if CNS effects occur *to protect the patient from injury*; small, frequent meals and mouth care *to relieve the discomfort of GI effects*; and an activity program and daily energy management ideas *to help to deal with activity intolerance.*
- Offer support and encouragement *to help the patient deal with the drug regimen.*
- Provide thorough patient teaching, including drug name, dosage, and schedule for administration; use of drug with food or meals if appropriate; technique for ophthalmic administration if indicated; potential adverse effects, measures to avoid drug-related problems, and warning signs of problems; safety measures such as changing position slowly and avoiding driving or operating hazardous machinery; and energy conservation measures as appropriate *to provide drug education and improve compliance to the drug regimen.*

Evaluation

- Monitor patient response to the drug (lowered blood pressure, fewer anginal episodes, lowered intraocular pressure).
- Monitor for adverse effects (GI upset, CNS changes, CV effects, loss of libido and impotence, potential respiratory effects).
- Evaluate the effectiveness of the teaching plan (patient can name drug, dosage, adverse effects to watch for, and specific measures to avoid them).
- Monitor the effectiveness of comfort measures and compliance with the regimen.

KEY POINTS

- $Beta_1$-selective adrenergic blocking agents do not block the $beta_1$-receptors that are responsible for bronchodilation and therefore are preferred in patients with respiratory problems.
- $Beta_1$-selective adrenergic blocking agents are used to treat hypertension and angina in extended release forms and to treat HF.
- All of the adrenergic blocking drugs must be tapered when they are discontinued after long-term use. The blocking of the receptor sites makes them hypersensitive to catecholamines, and extreme hypertension, angina, MI, or stroke could occur.

SUMMARY

- Adrenergic blocking agents, or sympatholytic drugs, lyse, or block, the effects of the SNS.
- Both the therapeutic and the adverse effects associated with these drugs are related to their blocking of the normal responses of the SNS.
- The alpha- and beta-adrenergic blocking agents block all of the receptor sites within the SNS, which results in lower blood pressure, slower pulse, and increased renal perfusion with decreased renin levels. These drugs are indicated for the treatment of essential hypertension. They are associated with many adverse effects, including the blocking of reflex bronchodilation, cardiac suppression, and diabetic reactions.
- Selective adrenergic blocking agents have been developed that, at therapeutic levels, have specific affinity for alpha- or beta-receptors or for specific $alpha_1$-, $beta_1$-, or $beta_2$-receptor sites. This specificity is lost at levels higher than the therapeutic range.
- Alpha-adrenergic drugs specifically block the alpha-receptors of the SNS. At therapeutic levels, they do not block beta-receptors.
- Nonspecific alpha-adrenergic blocking agents are used to treat pheochromocytoma, a tumor of the adrenal medulla.
- $Alpha_1$-selective adrenergic blocking agents block the postsynaptic $alpha_1$-receptor sites, causing a decrease in vascular tone and a vasodilation that leads to a fall in blood pressure without the reflex tachycardia that occurs when the presynaptic $alpha_2$-receptor sites are also blocked.
- Beta-blockers are drugs used to block the beta-receptors within the SNS. These drugs are used for a wide range of conditions, including hypertension, stage fright, migraines, angina, and essential tremors.

- Blockade of all beta-receptors results in a loss of the reflex bronchodilation that occurs with sympathetic stimulation. This limits the use of these drugs in patients who smoke or have allergic or seasonal rhinitis, asthma, or COPD.
- $Beta_1$-selective adrenergic blocking agents do not block the $beta_1$-receptors that are responsible for bronchodilation and therefore are preferred in patients with respiratory problems.

CHECK YOUR UNDERSTANDING

Answers to the questions in this chapter can be found in Answers to Check Your Understanding Questions on thePoint®.

MULTIPLE CHOICE

Select the best answer to the following.

1. Adrenergic blocking drugs, because of their clinical effects, are also known as
- **a.** anticholinergics.
- **b.** sympathomimetics.
- **c.** parasympatholytics.
- **d.** sympatholytics.

2. The nurse would anticipate administering drugs that generally block all adrenergic receptor sites to treat
- **a.** allergic rhinitis.
- **b.** COPD.
- **c.** cardiac-related conditions.
- **d.** premature labor.

3. Phentolamine (*Regitine*), an alpha-adrenergic blocker, is most frequently used
- **a.** to prevent cell death after extravasation of intravenous dopamine or norepinephrine.
- **b.** to treat COPD in patients with hypertension or arrhythmias.
- **c.** to treat hypertension and BPH in male patients.
- **d.** to block bronchoconstriction during acute asthma attacks.

4. A patient with which of the following would most likely be prescribed an $alpha_1$-selective adrenergic blocking agent?
- **a.** COPD and hypotension
- **b.** Hypertension and BPH
- **c.** Erectile dysfunction and hypotension
- **d.** Shock states and bronchospasm

5. The beta-blocker of choice for a patient who is hypertensive and has angina is
- **a.** nadolol.
- **b.** propranolol
- **c.** timolol.
- **d.** carteolol.

6. A nurse would question an order for $beta_1$-selective adrenergic blocker for a patient with
- **a.** cardiac arrhythmias.
- **b.** hypertension.
- **c.** cardiogenic shock.
- **d.** open-angle glaucoma.

7. A smoker who is being treated for hypertension with a beta-blocker is most likely receiving
- **a.** a nonspecific beta-blocker.
- **b.** an $alpha_1$-specific beta-blocker.
- **c.** beta- and alpha-blockers.
- **d.** a $beta_1$-specific blocker

8. You would caution a patient who is taking an adrenergic blocker
- **a.** to avoid exposure to infection.
- **b.** to stop the drug if he or she experiences flu-like symptoms.
- **c.** never to stop the drug abruptly.
- **d.** to avoid exposure to the sun.

MULTIPLE RESPONSE

Select all that apply.

1. A nurse would question an order for a beta-adrenergic blocker if the patient was also receiving what other drugs?
- **a.** Clonidine
- **b.** Ergot alkaloids
- **c.** Aspirin
- **d.** NSAIDs
- **e.** Triptans
- **f.** Epinephrine

2. The beta-adrenergic blocker propranolol is approved for a wide variety of uses. Which of the following are approved indications?
- **a.** Migraine headaches
- **b.** Stage fright
- **c.** Bronchospasm
- **d.** Reinfarction after an MI
- **e.** Erectile dysfunction
- **f.** Hypertension

BIBLIOGRAPHY AND REFERENCES

Andrews, M., & Boyle, J. (2011). *Transcultural concepts in nursing care* (6th ed.). Philadelphia, PA: Lippincott Williams & Wilkins.

Brunton, L., Chabner, B., & Knollman, B. (2011). *Goodman and Gilman's the pharmacological basis of therapeutics* (12th ed.). New York: McGraw-Hill.

Cleland, J. G. (2003). Beta blockers for heart failure: Why, which, when and where. *Medical Clinics of North America, 87*, 339–371.

Cruickshank, J. M. (2014). Beta blocker therapy for patients with hypertension. *Journal of the American Medical Association, 311*(8), 862.

Dakin, C. (2008). New approaches to heart failure in the ED. *American Journal of Nursing, 108*(3), 68–71.

Facts and Comparisons. (2015). *Drug facts and comparisons*. St. Louis, MO: Author.

Greenberg, B., Barnard, D., Narayan, S., et al. (2010). *Management of heart failure*. Hoboken, NJ: Wiley-Blackwell.

Karch, A. M. (2014). *Lippincott's nursing drug guide*. Philadelphia, PA: Lippincott Williams & Wilkins.

Medical Letter. (2015). *The medical letter on drugs and therapeutics*. New Rochelle, NY: Author.

Porth, C. M. (2013). *Pathophysiology: Concepts of altered health states* (9th ed.). Philadelphia, PA: Lippincott Williams & Wilkins.

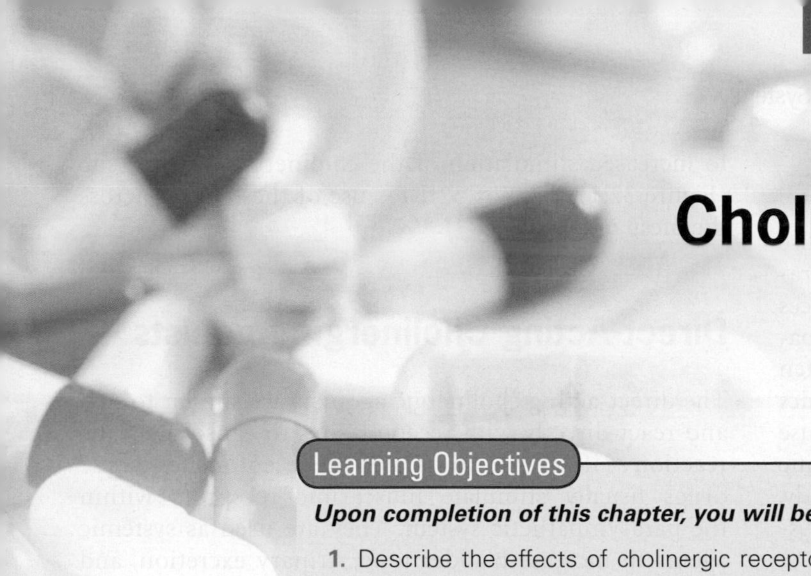

Cholinergic Agonists 32

Learning Objectives

Upon completion of this chapter, you will be able to:

1. Describe the effects of cholinergic receptors, correlating these effects with the clinical effects of cholinergic agonists.
2. Describe the therapeutic actions, indications, pharmacokinetics, contraindications and cautions, most common adverse reactions, and important drug–drug interactions associated with the direct- and indirect-acting cholinergic agonists.
3. Discuss the use of cholinergic agonists across the lifespan.
4. Compare and contrast the prototype drugs bethanechol, donepezil, and pyridostigmine with other cholinergic agonists.
5. Outline the nursing considerations, including important teaching points, for patients receiving a cholinergic agonist.

Glossary of Key Terms

acetylcholinesterase: enzyme responsible for the immediate breakdown of acetylcholine when released from the nerve ending; prevents overstimulation of cholinergic receptor sites

Alzheimer's disease: degenerative disease of the cortex with loss of acetylcholine-producing cells and cholinergic receptors; characterized by progressive dementia

cholinergic agonists: responding to acetylcholine; refers to receptor sites stimulated by acetylcholine, as well as neurons that release acetylcholine

miosis: constriction of the pupil; relieves intraocular pressure in some types of glaucoma

myasthenia gravis: autoimmune disease characterized by antibodies to cholinergic receptor sites, leading to destruction of the receptor sites and decreased response at the neuromuscular junction; it is progressive and debilitating, leading to paralysis

nerve gas: irreversible acetylcholinesterase inhibitor used in warfare to cause paralysis and death by prolonged muscle contraction and parasympathetic crisis

parasympathomimetic: mimicking the effects of the parasympathetic nervous system, leading to bradycardia, hypotension, pupil constriction, increased gastrointestinal secretions and activity, increased bladder tone, relaxation of sphincters, and bronchoconstriction

Drug List

Direct-Acting Cholinergic Agonists
(P) bethanechol
carbachol
cevimeline
pilocarpine

Indirect-Acting Cholinergic Agonists
Agents for Myasthenia Gravis
edrophonium
neostigmine
(P) pyridostigmine

Agents for Alzheimer's disease
(P) donepezil
galantamine
rivastigmine

Cholinergic agonists act at the same site as the neurotransmitter acetylcholine (ACh) and increase the activity of the ACh receptor sites throughout the body. Because these sites are found extensively throughout the parasympathetic nervous system, their stimulation produces a response similar to what is seen when the parasympathetic system is activated. As a result, these drugs are often called **parasympathomimetic** because their action mimics the action of the parasympathetic nervous system. Because the action of these drugs cannot be limited to a specific site, their effects can be widespread throughout the body, and they are usually associated with many undesirable systemic effects.

Cholinergic agonists work either directly or indirectly. Direct-acting cholinergic agonists occupy receptor sites for ACh on the membranes of the effector cells of the postganglionic cholinergic nerves, causing increased stimulation of the cholinergic receptor. In contrast, indirect-acting cholinergic agonists cause increased stimulation of the ACh receptor sites by reacting with the enzyme **acetylcholinesterase** and preventing it from breaking down the ACh that was released from the nerve. These drugs produce their effects indirectly by producing an increase in the level of ACh in the synaptic cleft, leading to increased stimulation of the cholinergic receptor site (Figure 32.1). See Box 32.1 for use of these drugs across the lifespan.

Direct-Acting Cholinergic Agonists

The direct-acting cholinergic agonists are similar to Ach and react directly with receptor sites to cause the same reaction as if Ach had stimulated the receptor sites. These drugs usually stimulate muscarinic receptors within the parasympathetic system. They are used as systemic agents to increase bladder tone, urinary excretion, and gastrointestinal (GI) secretions and as ophthalmic agents to induce miosis to relieve the increased intraocular pressure of glaucoma (see Table 32.1). Systemic absorption usually does not occur when these drugs are used ophthalmically.

Direct-acting cholinergic agonists include bethanechol (*Duvoid*, *Urecholine*), carbachol (*Miostat*), cevimeline (*Evoxac*), and pilocarpine (*Salagen*). These agents are used infrequently today because of their widespread parasympathetic activity. More specific and less toxic drugs are now available and preferred.

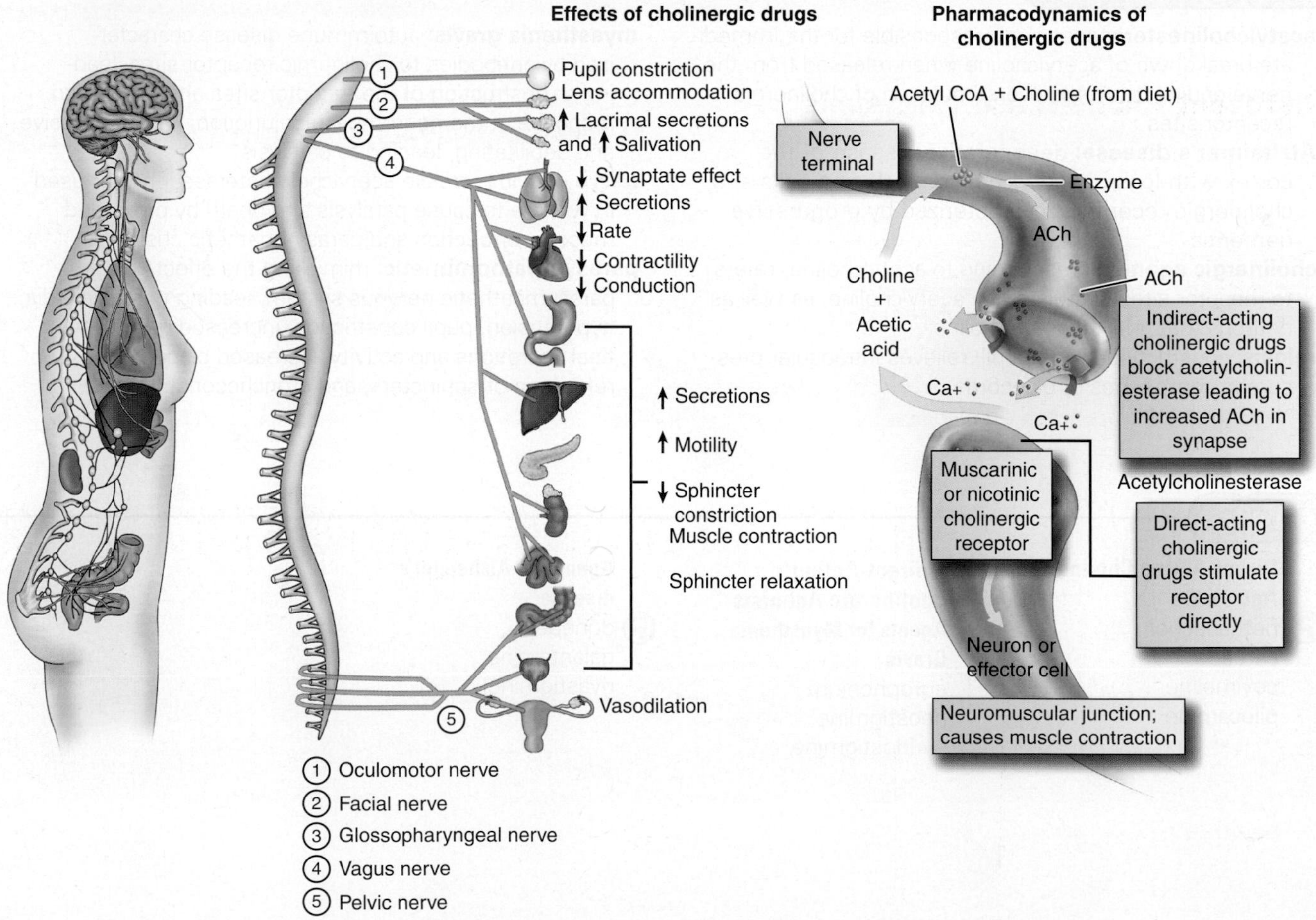

FIGURE 32.1 Pharmacodynamics of cholinergic drugs and associated physiological responses.

BOX 32.1 FOCUS ON Drug Therapy Across the Lifespan

Cholinergic Agonists

CHILDREN

Children may be more susceptible to the adverse effects associated with the cholinergic agonists, including GI upset, diarrhea, increased salivation that could lead to choking, and loss of bowel and bladder control, a problem that could cause stress in the child. Children should be monitored closely if these agents are used and should receive appropriate supportive care.

Bethanechol is approved for the treatment of neurogenic bladder in children older than 8 years of age. Neostigmine and pyridostigmine are used in the control of myasthenia gravis and for reversal of neuromuscular junction blocker effects in children. Care should be taken in determining the appropriate dose based on weight. Edrophonium is used for diagnosis of myasthenia gravis only.

ADULTS

Adults should be cautioned about the many adverse effects that can be anticipated when using a cholinergic agonist. Flushing, increased sweating, increased salivation and GI upset, and urinary urgency often occur. The patient also needs to be aware that dizziness, drowsiness, and blurred vision may occur and that driving and operating dangerous machinery should be avoided.

In general, there are no adequate studies about the effects of these drugs during pregnancy and lactation. Therefore, the cholinergic agonist should be used only in those situations in which the benefit to the mother is greater than the risk to the fetus or neonate. Nursing mothers who require one of these drugs should find another way to feed the baby.

OLDER ADULTS

Older patients are more likely to experience the adverse effects associated with these drugs—CNS, cardiovascular, GI, respiratory, and urinary effects. Because older patients often have renal or hepatic impairment, they are also more likely to have toxic levels of the drug related to changes in metabolism and excretion.

The older patient should be started on lower doses of the drugs and should be monitored very closely for potentially serious arrhythmias or hypotension. Safety precautions should be established if the drug causes dizziness or drowsiness. Special efforts may also be needed to help the patient maintain fluid intake and nutrition if the GI effects become uncomfortable. Taking the drug with food and eating several small meals throughout the day may alleviate some of these problems.

Therapeutic Actions and Indications

The direct-acting cholinergic agonists act at cholinergic receptors in the peripheral nervous system to mimic the effects of ACh and parasympathetic stimulation. These parasympathetic effects include slowed heart rate and decreased myocardial contractility, vasodilation, bronchoconstriction and increased bronchial mucus secretion, increased GI activity and secretions, increased bladder tone, relaxation of GI and bladder sphincters, and pupil constriction (see Figure 32.1).

The agent bethanechol, which has an affinity for the cholinergic receptors in the urinary bladder, is available for use orally and subcutaneously to treat nonobstructive postoperative and postpartum urinary retention and to treat neurogenic bladder atony. It directly increases detrusor muscle tone and relaxes the sphincters to improve bladder emptying. Because this drug is not destroyed by acetylcholinesterase, the effects on the receptor site are longer lasting than with stimulation by ACh. See Table 32.1 for additional indications.

Table 32.1 ***Drugs in Focus:*** **Direct-Acting Cholinergic Agonists**

Drug Name	Dosage/Route	Usual Indications
bethanechol (*Duvoid, Urecholine*)	10–50 mg PO b.i.d. to q.i.d.	Treatment of nonobstructive postoperative and postpartum urinary retention, neurogenic bladder atony in adults and children >8 y; diagnosis and treatment of reflux esophagitis in adults, and used orally in infants and children for treatment of esophageal reflux
carbachol (*Miostat*)	1–2 drops (gtt) in affected eye(s) as needed, up to three times a day	Induction of miosis to relieve increased intraocular pressure of glaucoma; allows surgeons to perform certain surgical procedures
cevimeline (*Evoxac*)	30 mg PO t.i.d.	Treatment of symptoms of dry mouth in patients with Sjögren's syndrome
pilocarpine (*Salagen*)	5–10 mg PO t.i.d. with meals if treating Sjögren's syndrome	Treatment of symptoms of dry mouth in patients with Sjögren's syndrome

Carbachol is available as an ophthalmic agent. It is used to induce **miosis**, or pupil constriction; to relieve the increased intraocular pressure of glaucoma; and to allow surgeons to perform certain surgical procedures.

Cevimeline and pilocarpine, which bind to muscarinic receptors throughout the system, are used to increase secretions in the mouth and GI tract and relieve the symptoms of dry mouth that are in seen in Sjögren's syndrome. They are approved for use in adults and are given three times a day, often with meals.

Pharmacokinetics

The direct-acting cholinergic agonists are generally well absorbed after oral administration and have relatively short half-lives, ranging from 1 to 6 hours. The metabolism and excretion of these drugs are not known but are believed to occur at the synaptic level using normal processes similar to the way that ACh is handled. Drugs used topically are not generally absorbed systemically.

Contraindications and Cautions

These drugs are used sparingly *because of the potential undesirable systemic effects of parasympathetic stimulation.* They are contraindicated with hypersensitivity to any component of the drug *to avoid hypersensitivity reaction* and in the presence of any condition that would be exacerbated by parasympathetic effects, such as bradycardia, hypotension, vasomotor instability, and coronary artery disease, *which could be made worse by the cardiac- and cardiovascular-suppressing effects of the parasympathetic system.* Peptic ulcer, intestinal obstruction, or recent GI surgery *could be negatively affected by the GI-stimulating effects of the parasympathetic nervous system.* Asthma *could be exacerbated by the increased parasympathetic effect, overriding the protective sympathetic bronchodilation.* Bladder obstruction or impaired healing of sites from recent bladder surgery *could be aggravated by the stimulatory effects on the bladder.* Epilepsy and parkinsonism *could be affected by the stimulation of ACh receptors in the brain.* Caution should be used during pregnancy and lactation *because of the potential adverse effects on the fetus or neonate.*

Adverse Effects

Patients should be cautioned about the potential adverse effects of these drugs. Even if the drug is being given as a topical ophthalmic agent, there is always a possibility that it can be absorbed systemically. The adverse effects associated with these drugs are related to parasympathetic nervous system stimulation. Cardiovascular effects can include bradycardia, heart block, hypotension, and even cardiac arrest related to the cardiac-suppressing effects of the parasympathetic nervous system. GI effects can include nausea, vomiting, cramps, diarrhea, increased salivation, and involuntary defecation related to the increase in GI secretions and activity (Figure 32.2). Swallowing difficulties leading to aspiration may occur with cevimeline or oral pilocarpine due to the increase in salivary secretions. Dehydration is possible due to the increase in GI motility and resultant diarrhea. Urinary tract effects can include a sense of urgency related to the stimulation of the bladder muscles and sphincter relaxation. Other effects may include flushing and increased sweating secondary to stimulation of the cholinergic receptors in the sympathetic nervous system.

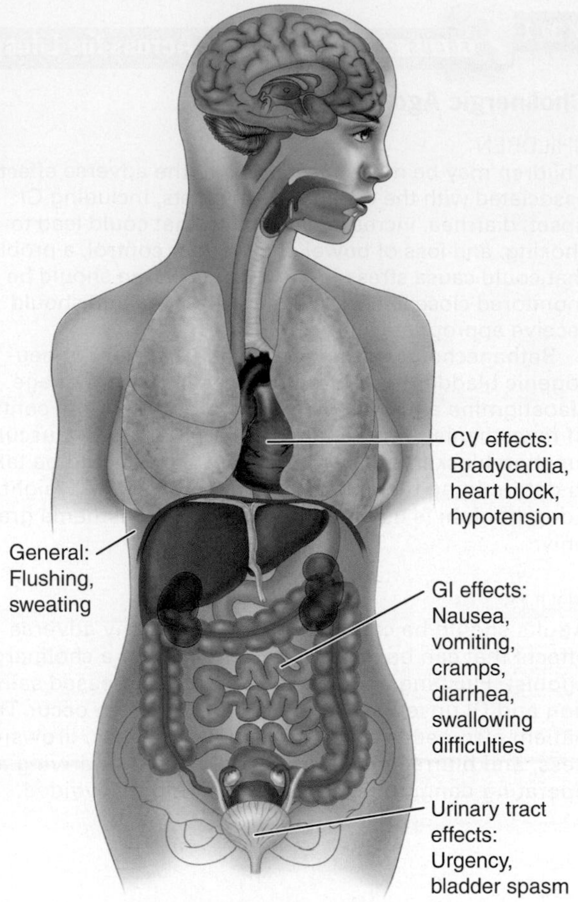

FIGURE 32.2 Variety of adverse effects and toxicities associated with cholinergic agonists.

Clinically Important Drug–Drug Interactions

There is an increased risk of cholinergic effects if these drugs are combined or given with acetylcholinesterase inhibitors, such as neostigmine. The patient should be monitored and appropriate dose adjustments made.

Prototype Summary: Bethanechol

Indications: Acute postoperative or postpartum nonobstructive urinary retention, neurogenic atony of the bladder with retention.

Actions: Acts directly on cholinergic receptors to mimic the effects of ACh, increases tone of detrusor muscles and causes emptying of the bladder.

Pharmacokinetics:

Route	Onset	Peak	Duration
Oral	30–90 min	60–90 min	1–6 h

$T_{1/2}$: Metabolism and excretion unknown, thought to be synaptic.

Adverse Effects: Abdominal discomfort, salivation, nausea, vomiting, sweating, flushing.

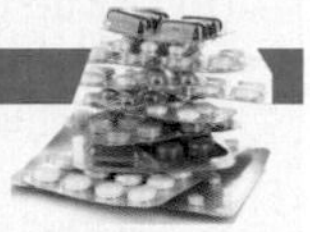

Nursing Considerations for Patients Receiving Direct-Acting Cholinergic Agonists

Assessment: History and Examination

- Assess for contraindications or cautions: Known allergies to these drugs *to avoid hypersensitivity reactions*; bradycardia, vasomotor instability, peptic ulcer, and obstructive urinary or GI diseases; recent GI or genitourinary (GU) surgery; asthma; parkinsonism or epilepsy, *which could be exacerbated or complicated by parasympathetic stimulation*; and current status of pregnancy and lactation *because of the potential for adverse effects on the fetus or neonate.*
- Perform a physical assessment *to establish a baseline status before beginning therapy, determine the effectiveness of therapy, and evaluate for any potential adverse effects.*
- Assess vital signs, including pulse and blood pressure, and cardiopulmonary status, including heart and lung sounds, *to evaluate for changes related to cardiovascular effects of parasympathetic activity*; obtain an electrocardiogram (ECG) as indicated *to evaluate heart rate and rhythm.*
- Assess abdomen, auscultating *for bowel sounds*; palpate bladder *for distention.*
- Monitor intake and output, noting any complaints of urinary urgency, *to monitor for drug effects on the urinary system.*

Nursing Diagnoses

Nursing diagnoses related to drug therapy might include the following:

- Acute pain related to GI effects
- Decreased cardiac output related to cardiovascular effects
- Impaired urinary elimination related to effects on the bladder
- Risk for injury related to blurred vision and changes in visual acuity
- Potential for diarrhea related to GI stimulatory effects
- Deficient knowledge regarding drug therapy

Planning

- The patient will receive the best therapeutic effect from the drug therapy.
- The patient will have limited adverse effects to the drug therapy.
- The patient will have an understanding of the drug therapy, adverse effects to anticipate, and measures to relieve discomfort and improve safety.

Implementation with Rationale

- Ensure proper administration of ophthalmic preparations *to increase the effectiveness of drug therapy and minimize the risk of systemic absorption.*
- Administer oral drug on an empty stomach *to decrease nausea and vomiting.*
- Monitor patient response closely, including blood pressure, ECG, urine output, and cardiac output, *and arrange to adjust dose accordingly to ensure the most benefit with the least amount of toxicity.* Maintain a cholinergic-blocking drug on standby such as atropine *to use as an antidote for excessive doses of cholinergic drugs* (see Focus on Safe Medication Administration in discussion of Agents for Myasthenia Gravis) *to reverse overdose or counteract severe reactions* (see Chapter 33 for further discussion of atropine).
- Provide safety precautions if the patient reports poor visual acuity in dim light *to prevent injury.*
- Monitor urinary output *to evaluate effects on the bladder*; ensure ready access to bathroom facilities *as needed with GI stimulation.*
- Provide thorough patient teaching, including drug name, dosage, and schedule of administration; administration of oral forms before meals or without food; proper administration for ophthalmic preparations as indicated; measures to prevent or minimize adverse effects; need for readily available access to toileting facilities; warning signs of problems; and importance of follow-up and evaluation , *to increase patient knowledge and improve compliance to drug regimen.*

Evaluation

- Monitor patient response to the drug (improvement in bladder function, increased salivation, miosis).

(continues on page 542)

- Monitor for adverse effects (cardiovascular changes, GI stimulation, urinary urgency, respiratory distress).
- Evaluate the effectiveness of the teaching plan (patient can name drug, dosage, adverse effects to watch for and specific measures to avoid them, proper administration of ophthalmic drugs).
- Monitor the effectiveness of comfort and safety measures and compliance with the regimen.

KEY POINTS

- Cholinergic agonists stimulate the parasympathetic nerves, some nerves in the brain, and the neuromuscular junction at the same site that ACh does.
- Cholinergic agonists are used topically in the eye to produce miosis (pupillary constriction) and treat glaucoma.
- Systemically, these agents are used to increase bladder tone (e.g., postoperative or postpartum) and to increase secretions to relieve dry mouth associated with Sjögren's syndrome.

Indirect-Acting Cholinergic Agonists

The indirect-acting cholinergic agonists do not react directly with ACh receptor sites; instead, they react chemically with acetylcholinesterase (the enzyme responsible for the breakdown of ACh) in the synaptic cleft to prevent it from breaking down ACh. As a result, the ACh that is released from the presynaptic nerve remains in the area and accumulates, stimulating the ACh receptors for a longer period of time than normally expected. These drugs work at all ACh receptors, in the parasympathetic nervous system, in the central nervous system (CNS), and at the neuromuscular junction. Most of these drugs bind reversibly to acetylcholinesterase, so their effects pass with time when the acetylcholinesterase is released and allowed to break down ACh. However, there are certain indirect-acting cholinergic agonists that irreversibly bind to acetylcholinesterase. These drugs are not used therapeutically; they are being developed as nerve gas to be used as weapons (Box 32.2). Because these drugs might be encountered in a war situation, it is important to have an antidote readily available to military personnel and any civilians who might be affected. Pralidoxime is the antidote developed for the irreversible indirect-acting cholinergic agonists and is also used to reverse poisoning associated with organophosphate pesticides (Box 32.3).

The reversible indirect-acting cholinergic agonists fall into two main categories: (1) agents used to treat myasthenia gravis and (2) agents used to treat Alzheimer's disease.

BOX 32.2

Nerve Gas: An Irreversible Indirect-Acting Cholinergic Agonist

Recent worldwide events and conflicts have made the potential use of nerve gas a major news story. Developed as a weapon, nerve gas is an irreversible acetylcholinesterase inhibitor. The drug is inhaled and quickly spreads throughout the body, where it permanently binds with acetylcholinesterase. This causes an accumulation of ACh at nerve endings and a massive cholinergic response. The heart rate slows and becomes ineffective, pupils and bronchi constrict, the GI tract increases activity and secretions, and muscles contract and remain that way. The muscle contraction soon immobilizes the diaphragm, causing breathing to stop. The bodies of people who are killed by nerve gas have a characteristic rigor of muscle contraction.

If an attack using nerve gas is expected, individuals who may be exposed are given intramuscular injections of atropine (to temporarily block cholinergic activity and to activate acetylcholine sites in the CNS) and pralidoxime (to free up the acetylcholinesterase to start breaking down acetylcholine). An autoinjection is provided to military personnel who may be at risk. The injector is used to give atropine and then pralidoxime. The injections are repeated in 15 minutes. If symptoms of nerve gas exposure exist after an additional 15 minutes the injections are repeated. If symptoms still persist after a third set of injections, medical help should be sought.

BOX 32.3

Pralidoxime: Antidote for Irreversible Indirect-Acting Cholinergic Agonists

Pralidoxime (*Protopam Chloride*), the antidote for irreversible acetylcholinesterase-inhibiting drugs, or nerve gas, is given IM or IV to reactivate the acetylcholinesterase that has been blocked by these drugs. Freeing up the acetylcholinesterase allows it to break down accumulated acetylcholine that has overstimulated ACh receptor sites, causing paralysis.

Pralidoxime does not readily cross the blood–brain barrier, and it is most useful for treating peripheral drug effects. It reacts within minutes after injection and should be available for any patient receiving indirect-acting cholinergic agonists to treat myasthenia gravis. The patient and a significant other should understand when to use the drug and how to administer it.

Pralidoxime is also used with atropine (which does cross the blood–brain barrier and will block the effects of accumulated acetylcholine at CNS sites) to treat organophosphate pesticide poisoning and nerve gas exposure (see Box 32.2), both of which cause inactivation of acetylcholinesterase.

Adverse effects associated with the use of pralidoxime include dizziness, blurred vision, diplopia, headache, drowsiness, hyperventilation, and nausea. These effects are also seen with exposure to nerve gas and organophosphate pesticides, so it can be difficult to differentiate drug effects from the effects of the poisoning.

Agents for Myasthenia Gravis

Myasthenia gravis is a chronic muscular disease caused by a defect in neuromuscular transmission. It is thought to be an autoimmune disease in which patients make antibodies to their ACh receptors. These antibodies cause gradual destruction of the ACh receptors, resulting in fewer and fewer receptor sites available for stimulation. ACh is the neurotransmitter that is used at the nerve–muscle synapse. If the ACh receptors are blocked and cannot be stimulated, muscle activity is decreased. The disease is marked by progressive weakness and lack of muscle control, with periodic acute episodes. Some patients have a very mild clinical presentation, such as drooping eyelids, and go into remission with no further signs and symptoms for several years. Other patients have a more severe course of the disease, with progressive skeletal muscle weakness that may confine them to a wheelchair. The disease can further progress to paralysis of the diaphragm, which interferes with breathing and would prove fatal without intervention. Often, during the course of the disease, the patient will experience a very intense phase of the disease, called a myasthenic crisis. Management of this crisis can be very challenging.

FOCUS ON Safe Medication Administration

Myasthenic Crisis versus Cholinergic Crisis

Myasthenia gravis is an autoimmune disease that runs an unpredictable course throughout the patient's life. Often, the disease goes through an intense phase called a myasthenic crisis, marked by extreme muscle weakness and respiratory difficulty.

Because of the variability of the disease and the tendency to have crises and periods of remission, management of the drug dose for a patient with myasthenia gravis is a nursing challenge. If a patient goes into remission a smaller dose is needed. If a patient has a crisis an increased dose is needed. To further complicate the clinical picture, the presentation of a cholinergic overdose or cholinergic crisis is similar to the presentation of a myasthenic crisis. The patient with a cholinergic crisis presents with progressive muscle weakness and respiratory difficulty as the accumulation of ACh at the cholinergic receptor site leads to reduced impulse transmission and muscle weakness. This is a crisis when the respiratory muscles are involved.

For a myasthenic crisis, the correct treatment is increased cholinergic drug. However, treatment of a cholinergic crisis requires withdrawal of the drug. The patient's respiratory difficulty usually necessitates acute medical attention. At this point the drug edrophonium can be used as a diagnostic agent to distinguish the two conditions. If the patient improves immediately after the edrophonium injection, the problem is a myasthenic crisis, which is improved by administration of the cholinergic drug. If the patient gets worse the problem is probably a cholinergic crisis, and withdrawal of the patient's cholinergic drug along with intense medical support is indicated. Atropine helps to alleviate some of the parasympathetic reactions to the cholinergic drug. However, because atropine is not effective at the neuromuscular junction, only time will reverse the drug toxicity.

The patient and a significant other will need support, teaching, and encouragement to deal with the tricky regulation of the cholinergic medication throughout the course of the disease. Nurses in the acute care setting need to be mindful of the difficulty in distinguishing drug toxicity from the need for more drug—and be prepared to respond appropriately.

The drugs used to help patients with this progressive disease are several indirect-acting cholinergic agonists that do not cross the blood–brain barrier and do not effect ACh transmission in the brain (see Table32.2). These drugs include edrophonium, (Enlon), neostigmine (generic), and pyridostigmine (Mestinon).

Agents for Alzheimer's Disease

Alzheimer's disease is a progressive disorder involving neural degeneration in the cortex that leads to a marked loss of memory and of the ability to carry on activities of daily living. Because of this, Alzheimer's disease can have very negative effects on the patient and his or her family (Box 32.4).

The cause of the disease is not yet known, but it is known that there is a progressive loss of ACh-producing neurons and their target neurons in the cortex of the brain. These neurons seem to be related to memory and associations between memories that allow connections between thoughts and stimuli (e.g., seeing a face and being able to know that it is a face and to name the person the face belongs to). There are three reversible indirect-acting cholinergic agonists available to slow the progression of this disease. These include galantamine (*Razadyne*), rivastigmine (*Exelon*), and donepezil (*Aricept*) (see Table 32.2). In late 2003 an *N*-methyl-D-aspartate (NMDA) receptor antagonist, memantine (*Namenda*), was also approved for use in the treatment of Alzheimer's disease. This drug works in a unique way to block various receptor sites in the brain and slow the buildup of plaque on the involved axons, which seems to slow the effects of this disease, and is the only drug of its class that is available (Box 32.5). In 2015 a combination of an extended release capsule containing memantine and donepezil (*Namzaric*) was approved for treatment of Alzheimer's disease, targeting two different sites of action.

Therapeutic Actions and Indications

The indirect-acting cholinergic agonists work by reversibly blocking acetylcholinesterase at the synaptic cleft. This blocking allows the accumulation of ACh released from the nerve endings and leads to increased and prolonged stimulation of ACh receptor sites at all of the postsynaptic cholinergic sites. Indirect-acting cholinergic agonists

Table 32.2 ***Drugs in Focus:* Indirect-Acting Cholinergic Agonists**

Drug Name	Dosage/Route	Usual Indications
Agents for Myasthenia Gravis		
edrophonium (*Enlon*)	*Diagnosis:* 2 mg IV over 15–30 s, then 8 mg IV if response was seen *or* 10 mg IM, repeat with 2 mg IM in 12 h to rule out false-negative results *Antidote:* 10 mg IV over 30–45 s, repeat as needed, maximum dose 40 mg *Pediatric (diagnosis only):* 0.5–2 mg IV based on weight *or* 2–5 mg IM	Diagnosis of myasthenia gravis (see Box 32.4); reversal of toxicity from nondepolarizing neuromuscular junction–blocking drugs, which are used to paralyze muscles during surgery (see Chapter 28)
neostigmine (generic)	*Adult:* 0.5 mg subcutaneous or IM for control; 0.022 mg/kg IM for diagnosis; 0.5–2 mg IV as antidote, maximum dose 5 mg *Pediatric:* 0.01–0.04 mg/kg/dose IM, IV, or subcutaneous for control q2–3 h; 0.04 mg/kg IM for diagnosis; 0.07–0.08 mg/kg IV, slowly, for antidote	Diagnosis and management of myasthenia gravis; reversal of toxicity from nondepolarizing neuromuscular junction–blocking drugs, which are used to paralyze muscles during surgery (see Chapter 28)
pyridostigmine (*Mestinon*)	*Adult:* Average, 180–540 mg daily PO for myasthenia gravis; 0.1–0.25 mg/kg IV for antidote; 30 mg q8 h starting several hours before exposure to nerve gas *Pediatric:* 7 mg/d PO in five or six divided doses for myasthenia gravis	Management of myasthenia gravis; antidote to neuromuscular junction blockers; increases survival after exposure to nerve gas
Agents for Alzheimer's Disease		
donepezil (*Aricept*)	5–10 mg PO daily at bedtime; available as an oral disintegrating tablet	Management of Alzheimer's dementia, including severe dementia
galantamine (*Razadyne*)	4–12 mg PO b.i.d.; reduce dose to 16 mg/d maximum with renal or hepatic impairment; available as an oral solution 4 mg/mL; range 16–32 mg/d; extended release tablets, range 16–24 mg/d taken as a single dose	Management of mild to moderate Alzheimer's dementia; delays progression of disease
rivastigmine (*Exelon*)	1.5–6 mg PO b.i.d., based on patient response and tolerance; transdermal system, one 4.6 mg/24 h patch placed once a day, maximum 9.5 mg/24 h	Management of mild to moderate Alzheimer's dementia; treatment of dementia related to Parkinson disease

work to relieve the signs and symptoms of myasthenia gravis and increase muscle strength by allowing ACh to accumulate in the synaptic cleft at neuromuscular junctions. Indirect-acting cholinergic agonists that more readily cross the blood–brain barrier and seem to affect mostly the cells in the cortex to increase ACh concentration in the area of the brain where ACh-producing cells are dying, affecting memory and the ability to access and link different memories, are used in the treatment of Alzheimer's disease. In addition to usual indications, pyridostigmine

BOX 32.4 ***FOCUS ON* Cultural Considerations**

Alzheimer's Disease

Alzheimer's disease is a chronic, progressive disease of the brain's cortex. Eventually it results in memory loss so severe that the patient may not remember how to perform basic activities of daily living and may not recognize close family members. Although Alzheimer's disease primarily strikes the elderly, it has a tremendous impact on family members of all ages. For example, adult children of Alzheimer's patients, many of whom are busy raising children of their own, may find themselves in the role of caregivers—in essence, becoming parents of their parent. This new role can put tremendous stress on individuals who are trying to struggle with work, family, and issues related to their parent's care.

When caring for an Alzheimer's patient and family the nurse must remember that the patient's cultural background can affect how the family copes. For instance, those who tend to have solid extended families or who are part of communities that offer strong social support and interdependence may be better equipped to deal with caring for the patient as the disease progresses. In contrast, families that are more goal and achievement oriented and who value autonomy and independence may find themselves overwhelmed by the patient's needs and may require more support and referrals to community resources.

The nurse is in the best position to evaluate the family situation. By approaching each situation as unique and striving to incorporate cultural and social norms into the considerations for care the nurse can help to ease the family's burden while also maintaining the dignity of the patient and the family through this difficult experience.

BOX 32.5

Another Treatment for Alzheimer's Disease

In late 2003 the U.S. Food and Drug Administration approved a new drug for treating Alzheimer's disease. The drug, memantine hydrochloride (*Namenda*), had been used in Europe for several years and had been reported to slow the memory loss of patients with moderate to severe dementia associated with Alzheimer's disease. Memantine has a low to moderate affinity for NMDA receptors with no effects on dopamine, gamma-aminobutyric acid, histamine, glycine, or adrenergic receptor sites. It is thought that persistent activation of the CNS NMDA receptors contributes to the symptoms of Alzheimer's disease. By blocking these sites, it is thought that the symptoms are reduced or delayed.

The drug is available in a tablet form and an oral solution and is started at 5 mg/d PO, increasing by 5 mg/d at weekly intervals. The target dose is 20 mg/d given as 10 mg twice daily. Dose reduction should be considered in patients with renal impairment. Headache, dizziness, fatigue, confusion, and constipation are common adverse effects. The drug should not be taken with anything that alkalinizes the urine. Patients and family members need to understand that this drug is not a cure but may offer some extended time with mild symptoms. The long-term effects of this drug have not been studied in the United States.

has also been approved for military personnel to increase survival after exposure to particular **nerve gases**—irreversible acetylcholinesterase inhibitors used in warfare to cause paralysis and death by prolonged muscle contraction and parasympathetic crisis—and to reverse the effects of nondepolarizing neuromuscular junction blockers used to cause paralysis in surgery. See Table 32.2 for Usual Indications for each drug.

Pharmacokinetics

Anticholinesterase inhibitors are well absorbed after oral administration and distributed throughout the body. The sites of metabolism and excretion for all of these drugs are not known. It is thought that they are metabolized at the nerve synapse or in the tissues.

Neostigmine is a synthetic drug that has a strong influence at the neuromuscular junction. Neostigmine has a duration of action of 2 to 4 hours and therefore must be given every few hours, based on patient response, to maintain a therapeutic level.

Pyridostigmine has a longer duration of action than neostigmine (3 to 6 hours) and is preferred in some cases for the management of myasthenia gravis because it does not need to be taken as frequently. Pyridostigmine is available in oral and parenteral forms; the latter can be used if the patient is having trouble swallowing.

Edrophonium is administered intravenously and has a very short duration of action (10 to 20 minutes).

The drugs used to treat Alzheimer's disease are well absorbed and distributed through the body. They are metabolized in the liver by the cytochrome P450 system, so caution must be used for patients with hepatic impairment and for cases in which many interacting drugs are used. The drugs used to treat Alzheimer's disease are excreted in the urine.

Galantamine is available in tablet and oral solution form. It has a half-life of 7 hours and is taken twice a day. An extended release form, recently available, can be taken just once a day. Rivastigmine is available in capsule and solution forms to help with patients who have swallowing difficulties, as well as a transdermal patch that is applied once a day. The duration of effects for rivastigmine is 12 hours. Donepezil, with a 70-hour half-life, is available in oral form, as tablets and as a rapidly dissolving tablet. It can be given in once-a-day dosing, which is advantageous with a disease that affects memory and the patient's ability to remember to take pills throughout the day. None of these drugs reverse the effects of the disorder. Studies show that they may somewhat delay the losses seen with the disease.

Contraindications and Cautions

Anticholinesterase inhibitors are contraindicated in the presence of allergy to any of these drugs *to avoid hypersensitivity reactions*; with bradycardia or intestinal or urinary tract obstruction, *which could be exacerbated by the stimulation of cholinergic receptors*; in pregnancy *because the uterus could be stimulated and labor induced*; and during lactation *because of the potential effects on the baby.*

Caution should be used with *any condition that could be exacerbated by cholinergic stimulation.* Although the effects of these drugs are generally more localized to the cortex and the neuromuscular junction the possibility of parasympathetic effects must be considered carefully in patients with asthma, coronary disease, peptic ulcer, arrhythmias, epilepsy, or parkinsonism, *which could be exacerbated by the effects of parasympathetic stimulation.* Drugs used to treat Alzheimer's disease are metabolized in the liver and excreted in the urine, so caution should be used in the presence of hepatic or renal dysfunction, *which could interfere with the metabolism and excretion of the drugs.*

Adverse Effects

The adverse effects associated with agents for treating myasthenia gravis or Alzheimer's disease are related to stimulation of the parasympathetic nervous system. GI effects can include nausea, vomiting, cramps, diarrhea, increased salivation, and involuntary defecation related to the increase in GI secretions and activity due to parasympathetic nervous system stimulation. Cardiovascular effects can include bradycardia, heart block, hypotension, and even cardiac arrest, related to the cardiac-suppressing effects of the parasympathetic nervous system. Urinary tract effects can include a sense of urgency related to stimulation of the bladder muscles and sphincter relaxation.

Miosis and blurred vision, headaches, dizziness, and drowsiness can occur related to CNS cholinergic effects. Other effects may include flushing and increased sweating secondary to stimulation of the cholinergic receptors in the sympathetic nervous system.

Clinically Important Drug–Drug Interactions

There may be an increased risk of GI bleeding if these drugs are used with nonsteroidal anti-inflammatory drugs (NSAIDs) because of the combination of increased GI secretions and the GI mucosal erosion associated with the use of NSAIDs. If this combination is used the patient should be monitored closely for any sign of GI bleeding. The effect of anticholinesterase drugs is decreased if they are taken in combination with any cholinergic drugs because these work in opposition to each other.

Ⓟ Prototype Summary: Pyridostigmine

Indications: Treatment of myasthenia gravis, antidote for nondepolarizing neuromuscular junction blockers, increased survival after exposure to nerve gas.

Actions: Reversible cholinesterase inhibitor that increases the levels of ACh, facilitating transmission at the neuromuscular junction.

Pharmacokinetics:

Route	Onset	Duration
Oral	35–45 min	3–6 h
IM	15 min	3–6 h
IV	5 min	3–6 h

$T_{1/2}$: 1.9 to 3.7 hours; metabolized in the liver and tissue; excreted in the urine.

Adverse Effects: Bradycardia, cardiac arrest, tearing, miosis, salivation, dysphagia, nausea, vomiting, increased bronchial secretions, urinary frequency, and incontinence.

Ⓟ Prototype Summary: Donepezil

Indications: Treatment of mild to moderate Alzheimer's disease.

Actions: Reversible cholinesterase inhibitor that causes elevated ACh levels in the cortex, which slows the neuronal degradation of Alzheimer's disease.

Pharmacokinetics:

Route	Onset	Peak
Oral	Varies	2–4 h

$T_{1/2}$: 70 hours; metabolized in the liver; excreted in the urine.

Adverse Effects: Insomnia, fatigue, rash, nausea, vomiting, diarrhea, dyspepsia, abdominal pain, muscle cramps.

Nursing Considerations for Patients Receiving Indirect-Acting Cholinergic Agonists

Assessment: History and Examination

- Assess for contraindications or cautions: Known allergies to any of these drugs *to avoid hypersensitivity reactions*; arrhythmias, coronary artery disease, hypotension, urogenital or GI obstruction, or peptic ulcer, *which could be exacerbated by cholinergic stimulation*; recent GI or GU surgery, *which could limit use of the drugs because of the stimulatory effects of the parasympathetic system, which could aggravate healing*; regular use of NSAIDs, cholinergic drugs, or theophylline, *which could cause a drug–drug interaction*; and current status of pregnancy and lactation *because of potential effects to the fetus or neonate.*
- Perform a physical assessment *to establish baseline status before beginning therapy and to determine any potential adverse effects*; assess orientation, affect, reflexes, ability to carry on activities of daily living (Alzheimer's drugs), and vision *to monitor for CNS changes related to drug therapy*; blood pressure, pulse, ECG, peripheral perfusion, and cardiac output *to monitor the parasympathetic effects on the vascular system*; and urinary output and renal and liver function tests *to monitor drug effects on the renal system and liver, which could change the metabolism and excretion of the drugs.*

Refer to the Critical Thinking Scenario for a full discussion of nursing care for a patient who is receiving indirect-acting cholinergic agonists.

Nursing Diagnoses

Nursing diagnoses related to drug therapy might include the following:

- Disturbed thought processes related to CNS effects
- Acute pain related to GI effects
- Decreased cardiac output related to blood pressure changes, arrhythmias, and vasodilation
- Deficient knowledge regarding drug therapy
- Risk for injury related to CNS effects
- Diarrhea related to GI stimulatory effects

Planning

- The patient will receive the best therapeutic effect from the drug therapy.
- The patient will have limited adverse effects to the drug therapy.
- The patient will have an understanding of the drug therapy, adverse effects to anticipate, and measures to relieve discomfort and improve safety.

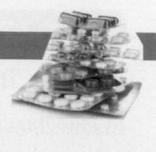

Implementation with Rationale

- If the drug is given intravenously, administer it slowly *to avoid severe cholinergic effects.*
- Maintain atropine sulfate on standby *as an antidote in case of overdose or severe cholinergic reaction.*
- Discontinue the drug if excessive salivation, diarrhea, emesis, or frequent urination becomes a problem *to decrease the risk of severe adverse reactions.*
- Administer the oral drug with meals *to decrease GI upset if it is a problem.*
- Mark the patient's chart and notify the surgeon if the patient is to undergo surgery *because prolonged muscle relaxation may occur if succinylcholine-type anesthetics are used.* The patient will require prolonged support and monitoring.
- Monitor the patient being treated for Alzheimer's disease for any progress *because the drug is not a cure and only slows progression*; refer families to supportive services.
- The patient who is being treated for myasthenia gravis and a significant other should receive instruction in drug administration, warning signs of drug overdose, and signs and symptoms to report immediately *to enhance patient knowledge about drug therapy and to promote compliance.*
- Arrange for supportive care and comfort measures, including rest, environmental control, and other measures, *to decrease CNS irritation*; headache medication *to relieve pain*; safety measures if CNS effects occur *to prevent injury*; protective measures if CNS effects are severe *to prevent patient injury*; and small, frequent meals if GI upset is severe *to decrease discomfort and maintain nutrition.*
- Provide thorough patient teaching, including dosage, adverse effects to anticipate and measures to avoid them, and warning signs of problems, as well as proper administration for each route used, *to enhance patient knowledge about drug therapy and to promote compliance.*
- Offer support and encouragement *to help the patient deal with the diagnosis and drug regimen.*

Evaluation

- Monitor patient response to the drug (improvement in condition being treated).
- Monitor for adverse effects (GI upset, CNS changes, cardiovascular changes, GU changes).
- Evaluate the effectiveness of the teaching plan (patient can name drug, dosage, adverse effects to watch for and specific measures to avoid them, and proper administration).
- Monitor the effectiveness of comfort measures and compliance with the regimen.

CRITICAL THINKING SCENARIO

Indirect-Acting Cholinergic Agonists

THE SITUATION

A.J., a 75-year-old man with an unremarkable medical history, is seen in the clinic for evaluation of memory loss and confusion. Three years ago, his wife began to notice memory gaps and confusion when A.J. was driving around town. He would get lost only a few blocks from home. The problem has gotten steadily worse. He was diagnosed with Alzheimer's disease after neurological tests and medical evaluation ruled out other causes for his problem. He did not want to take any drugs, but when he heard the diagnosis he became quite frightened and agreed to try medication. His wife states that she is somewhat concerned about giving him medication because he has sometimes had trouble swallowing and chokes on his food. She excitedly tells A.J. that once he starts the medication, his memory will return and things will be normal again. A.J. is placed on rivastigmine.

CRITICAL THINKING

What could be responsible for A.J.'s symptoms?

What modifications can be made to the prescription to ensure patient safety if A.J. is having trouble swallowing?

What important information about the disease and the effectiveness of drug therapy needs to be discussed with A.J. and his wife? *Will things return to normal?*

What potential adverse effects can be anticipated with rivastigmine, and how might these effects complicate the situation for this patient and his wife?

DISCUSSION

Alzheimer's disease is a chronic, progressive disease that involves the loss of neurons in the cortex of the brain that are responsible for making connections between different memories. A.J. has had the problem for at least 3 years, and his loss of memory and

(continues on page 548)

Indirect-Acting Cholinergic Agonists (continued)

confusion have gotten worse over that period of time. Unfortunately, there is nothing available at this time that can stop the loss of neurons or restore the function that has already been lost.

One of the problems that occur with Alzheimer's disease is difficulty swallowing. Swallowing is a complex CNS reflex that requires coordination of impulses, and with this disease the ability to swallow in a coordinated manner is often lost. This can lead to aspiration and pneumonia, which are often the underlying causes of death with Alzheimer's disease. Since A.J. already has some difficulty swallowing, it would be important to look into the forms in which rivastigmine is provided. In this case the drug is available in capsule form and as an oral solution. The oral solution might be suggested because it could be much easier to swallow. As the disease progresses the drug is available as a transdermal system, which would eliminate the need to swallow the drug. The status of A.J.'s swallowing should be evaluated before starting therapy and periodically as time goes on to determine how safe the dosage form of the drug is for his particular situation.

A.J. and his wife should receive information on Alzheimer's disease and its progression. The drugs available at this time do not reverse the memory loss and they do not cure the disease. A.J.'s wife may be encouraged to monitor A.J.'s behavior, ability to perform activities of daily living, and other significant markers of importance to them. The drug should slow the progression of the disease, and it might be helpful to monitor progress to see if the drug is being effective. She might also want to become involved in an Alzheimer's support group or organization, which could provide valuable support, educational materials, and access to community resources. This is an overwhelming diagnosis, and it might be necessary to approach these individuals over several visits to give them both time to adjust. It is important to always include a family member and provide information in writing for later reference when providing teaching to a patient with Alzheimer's disease.

Many of the adverse effects associated with the indirect-acting cholinergic agonists are a result of the parasympathetic stimulation caused by these drugs and may complicate A.J.'s care as his disease progresses. GI effects can include increased salivation, which may further add to his difficulty swallowing; nausea and vomiting, which could make it difficult to maintain nutrition; and cramps, diarrhea, and involuntary defecation related to the increase in GI secretions and activity, which could make toileting difficult and add to Mrs. J.'s home care burden. Cardiovascular effects can include bradycardia, heart block, and hypotension, which could lead to dizziness and weakness and further complicate safety issues. Urinary tract effects can include a sense of urgency related to stimulation of the bladder muscles and sphincter relaxation, which could lead to incontinence as the patient becomes less responsive to normal reflexes. Miosis and blurred vision, headaches, dizziness, and drowsiness can occur, further complicating safety issues. The benefits of slowing the progression of the disease often need to be weighed against all of the potential adverse effects that can complicate care and safety.

NURSING CARE GUIDE FOR A.J.: INDIRECT-ACTING CHOLINERGIC AGONISTS

Assessment: History and Examination

Assess for contraindications or cautions: Known allergies to any of components of this drug, arrhythmias, coronary artery disease, hypotension, urogenital or GI obstruction, peptic ulcer, recent GI or GU surgery, and regular use of NSAIDs, cholinergic drugs, or theophylline.

Focus the physical exam on the following:

CNS: Orientation, affect, reflexes, memory response, ability to carry out simple commands, vision

CV: Blood pressure, pulse, peripheral perfusion, electrocardiography

GI: Abdominal exam

GU: Urinary output, bladder tone

Respiratory: Respirations, adventitious sounds

Skin: Color, temperature, texture

Nursing Diagnoses

Decreased cardiac output related to CV effects

Impaired urinary elimination related to GU effects

Risk for injury related to CNS effects

Risk for diarrhea

Deficient knowledge regarding drug therapy

Planning

The patient will receive the best therapeutic effect from the drug therapy.

The patient will have limited adverse effects to the drug therapy.

The patient will have an understanding of the drug therapy, adverse effects to anticipate, and measures to relieve discomfort and improve safety.

Implementation

Ensure safe and appropriate administration of the drug; monitor the ability to swallow and the appropriateness of dosage form.

Provide comfort and safety measures (e.g., physical assistance, raising side rails on the bed); temperature control; pain relief; small, frequent meals.

Monitor cardiac status and urine output throughout drug therapy.

Indirect-Acting Cholinergic Agonists (continued)

Provide support and reassurance to deal with side effects, discomfort, and GI effects.

Provide patient and family teaching regarding drug name, dosage, side effects, precautions, and warning signs of serious adverse effects to report.

Evaluation

Evaluate drug effects: Slowing of progression of dementia.

Monitor for adverse effects: CV effects—bradycardia, heart block, hypotension; urinary problems; GI effects; respiratory problems.

Monitor for drug–drug interactions.

Evaluate the effectiveness of patient and teaching program and comfort and safety measures.

Patient/Family Teaching for A.J.

- The drug that was ordered for you is called rivastigmine. It is called a cholinergic agonist or a parasympathetic drug because it mimics the effects of the parasympathetic nervous system. Cholinergic drugs get this name because they act at certain nerve–nerve and nerve–muscle junctions in the body that are called cholinergic sites. They use a chemical called acetylcholine to carry out their functions. The nerves in your brain that are affected by Alzheimer's disease use acetylcholine to help you to remember things and make connections between memories. This drug will not reverse the losses of memory, but may slow the loss.
- Some of the following adverse effects may occur.
  - *Nausea, vomiting, diarrhea:* It is wise to be near bathroom facilities after taking your drug. If these symptoms become too severe, consult with your health care provider.
  - *Flushing, sweating:* Staying in a cool environment and wearing lightweight clothing may help.
  - *Increased salivation:* This may increase your difficulty in swallowing.
  - *Urgency to void:* Maintaining access to a bathroom may relieve some of this discomfort.
  - *Headache:* Aspirin or another headache medication (if not contraindicated in your particular case) will help to alleviate this pain.
  - *Changes in vision, dizziness:* These might lead to falls or more confusion.
- Report any of the following to your health care provider: *very slow pulse, light-headedness, fainting, excessive salivation, abdominal cramping or pain, weakness or confusion, blurring of vision, further signs of dementia.*
- Tell any doctor, nurse, or other health care provider involved in your care that you are taking this drug.

KEY POINTS

- Myasthenia gravis is an autoimmune disease characterized by antibodies to ACh receptors. This results in a loss of ACh receptors and eventual loss of response at the neuromuscular junction.
- Acetylcholinesterase inhibitors are used to treat myasthenia gravis because they allow the accumulation of ACh in the synaptic cleft, prolonging stimulation of any ACh sites that remain.
- Alzheimer's disease is a progressive dementia characterized by a loss of ACh-producing neurons and ACh receptor sites in the neurocortex.
- Acetylcholinesterase inhibitors that cross the blood–brain barrier are used to manage Alzheimer's disease by increasing ACh levels in the brain and slowing the progression of the disease.

SUMMARY

- Cholinergic drugs are chemicals that act at the same site as the neurotransmitter ACh, stimulating the parasympathetic nerves, some nerves in the brain, and the neuromuscular junction.
- Direct-acting cholinergic drugs react with the ACh receptor sites to cause cholinergic stimulation.
- Use of direct-acting cholinergic drugs is limited by the systemic effects of the drug. One drug is used to induce miosis and to treat glaucoma; one agent is available to treat neurogenic bladder and bladder atony postoperatively or postpartum, and another agent is available to increase GI secretions and relieve the dry mouth of Sjögren's syndrome.
- All indirect-acting cholinergic drugs are acetylcholinesterase inhibitors. They block acetylcholinesterase to prevent it from breaking down ACh in the synaptic cleft.
- Cholinergic stimulation by acetylcholinesterase inhibitors is due to an accumulation of the ACh released from the nerve ending.
- Myasthenia gravis is an autoimmune disease characterized by antibodies to the ACh receptors. This results in a loss of ACh receptors and eventual loss of response at the neuromuscular junction.
- Acetylcholinesterase inhibitors are used to treat myasthenia gravis because they allow the accumulation of ACh in the synaptic cleft, prolonging stimulation of any ACh sites that remain.
- Alzheimer's disease is a progressive dementia characterized by a loss of ACh-producing neurons and ACh receptor sites in the neurocortex.

- Acetylcholinesterase inhibitors that cross the blood–brain barrier are used to manage Alzheimer's disease by increasing ACh levels in the brain and slowing the progression of the disease.
- Side effects associated with the use of these drugs are related to stimulation of the parasympathetic nervous system (bradycardia, hypotension, increased GI secretions and activity, increased bladder tone, relaxation of GI and GU sphincters, bronchoconstriction, pupil constriction) and may limit the usefulness of some of these drugs.

CHECK YOUR UNDERSTANDING

Answers to the questions in this chapter can be found in Answers to Check Your Understanding Questions on thePoint®.

MULTIPLE CHOICE

Select the best answer to the following.

1. Indirect-acting cholinergic agents
   a. react with acetylcholine receptor sites on the membranes of effector cells.
   b. react chemically with acetylcholinesterase to increase acetylcholine concentrations.
   c. are used to increase bladder tone and urinary excretion.
   d. should be given with food to slow absorption.
2. A patient is to receive pilocarpine. The nurse understands that this drug would be most likely used to treat which of the following?
   a. Myasthenia gravis
   b. Neurogenic bladder
   c. Sjögren's disease dry mouth
   d. Alzheimer's disease
3. Myasthenia gravis is treated with indirect-acting cholinergic agents that
   a. lead to accumulation of acetylcholine in the synaptic cleft.
   b. block the GI effects of the disease, allowing for absorption.
   c. directly stimulate the remaining acetylcholine receptors.
   d. can be given only by injection because of problems associated with swallowing.
4. A patient with myasthenia gravis is no longer able to swallow. Which of the following would the nurse expect the physician to order?
   a. Rivastigmine
   b. Memantine
   c. Pyridostigmine
   d. Edrophonium
5. Alzheimer's disease is marked by a progressive loss of memory and is associated with
   a. degeneration of dopamine-producing cells in the basal ganglia.
   b. loss of acetylcholine-producing neurons and their target neurons in the CNS.
   c. loss of acetylcholine receptor sites in the parasympathetic nervous system.
   d. increased levels of acetylcholinesterase in the CNS.
6. The nurse would expect to administer donepezil to a patient with Alzheimer's disease who
   a. cannot remember family members' names.
   b. is mildly inhibited and can still follow medical dosing regimens.
   c. is able to carry on normal activities of daily living.
   d. has memory problems and would benefit from once-a-day dosing.
7. Adverse effects associated with the use of cholinergic drugs include
   a. constipation and insomnia.
   b. diarrhea and urinary urgency.
   c. tachycardia and hypertension.
   d. dry mouth and tachycardia.
8. Nerve gas is an irreversible acetylcholinesterase inhibitor that can cause muscle paralysis and death. An antidote to such an agent is
   a. atropine.
   b. propranolol.
   c. pralidoxime.
   d. neostigmine.

MULTIPLE RESPONSE

Select all that apply.

1. A nurse is explaining myasthenia gravis to a family. Which of the following points would be included in the explanation?

a. It is thought to be an autoimmune disease.
b. It is associated with destruction of acetylcholine receptor sites.
c. It is best treated with potent antibiotics.
d. It is a chronic and progressive muscular disease.
e. It is caused by demyelination of the nerve fiber.
f. Once diagnosed, it has a 5-year survival rate.

2. A nurse would question an order for a cholinergic drug if the patient was also taking which of the following?

a. Theophylline
b. NSAIDs
c. Cephalosporin
d. Atropine
e. Propranolol
f. Memantine

BIBLIOGRAPHY AND REFERENCES

Andrews, M., & Boyle, J. (2011). *Transcultural concepts in nursing care* (6th ed.). Philadelphia, PA: Lippincott Williams & Wilkins.

Brunton, L., Chabner, B., & Knollman, B. (2011). *Goodman and Gilman's the pharmacological basis of therapeutics* (12th ed.). New York: McGraw-Hill.

Facts and Comparisons. (2015). *Drug facts and comparisons*. St. Louis, MO: Author.

Iqbal, K., & Grundke-Iqbal, I. (2004). Inhibition of neurofibrillary degeneration: A promising approach to Alzheimer's disease and other tautopathies. *Current Drug Targets, 5*(6), 495–501.

Kaminski, H. (2011). *Myasthenia gravis and related disorders*. New York: Springer Publishing.

Karch, A. M. (2014). *Lippincott's nursing drug guide*. Philadelphia, PA: Lippincott Williams & Wilkins.

Medical Letter. (2015). *The medical letter on drugs and therapeutics*. New Rochelle, NY: Author.

Naylor, M. D., Stephen, C., Bowles, K. H., et al. (2005). Cognitively impaired older adults: From hospital to home. *American Journal of Nursing, 105*, 52–61.

Porth, C. M. (2013). *Pathophysiology: Concepts of altered health states* (9th ed.). Philadelphia, PA: Lippincott Williams & Wilkins.

Reisberg, B., Doody, R., Stöffler, A., et al. (2003). Memantine in moderate-to-severe Alzheimer's disease. *New England Journal of Medicine, 348*, 1333–1341.

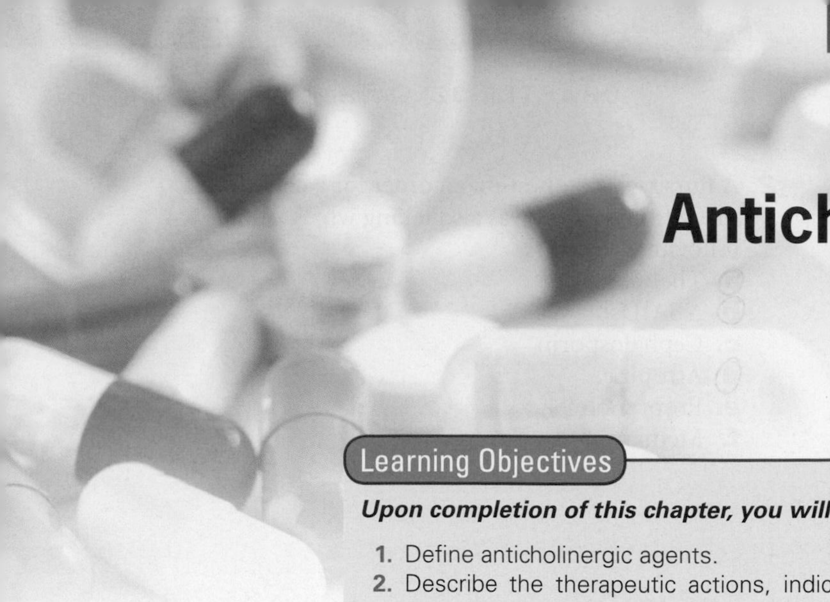

33 Anticholinergic Agents

Learning Objectives

Upon completion of this chapter, you will be able to:

1. Define anticholinergic agents.
2. Describe the therapeutic actions, indications, pharmacokinetics, contraindications and cautions, most common adverse reactions, and important drug–drug interactions of anticholinergic agents.
3. Discuss the use of anticholinergic agents across the lifespan.
4. Compare and contrast the prototype drug atropine with other anticholinergic agents.
5. Outline the nursing considerations, including important teaching points, for patients receiving anticholinergic agents.

Glossary of Key Terms

anticholinergic: drug that opposes the effects of acetylcholine at acetylcholine receptor sites

belladonna: a plant that contains atropine as an alkaloid; used to dilate the pupils as a fashion statement in the past; used in herbal medicine much as atropine is used today

cycloplegia: inability of the lens in the eye to accommodate to near vision, causing blurring and inability to see near objects

mydriasis: relaxation of the muscles around the pupil, leading to pupil dilation

parasympatholytic: lysing or preventing parasympathetic effects

Drug List

Anticholinergic Agents/Parasympatholytics

aclidinium
(P) atropine
darifenacin
dicyclomine
fesoterodine
flavoxate
glycopyrrolate
hyoscyamine
ipratropium
meclizine
methscopolamine
propantheline
scopolamine
solifenacin
tiotropium
toliterodine
trospium

Drugs that are used to block the effects of acetylcholine are called **anticholinergic** drugs. Because this action lyses, or blocks, the effects of the parasympathetic nervous system, they are also called **parasympatholytic** agents. This class of drugs was once very widely used to decrease gastrointestinal (GI) activity and secretions in the treatment of ulcers and to decrease other parasympathetic activities to allow the sympathetic system to become more dominant. Today, more specific and less systemically toxic drugs are available for many of the conditions that would benefit from these effects. Therefore, this class of drugs is less commonly used. Atropine is the only widely used anticholinergic drug. Box 33.1 discusses the use of anticholinergics across the lifespan.

Anticholinergics/Parasympatholytics

Anticholinergic agents include aclidinium (*Tudorza Pressair*), atropine (generic), darifenacin (*Enablex*), dicyclomine (generic), fesoterodine (*Toviaz*), flavoxate (generic), glycopyrrolate (*Robinul*), hyoscyamine (*Symax* and others), ipratropium (*Atrovent*), meclizine (*Bonine*), methscopolamine (*Pamine*), propantheline (generic), scopolamine

BOX 33.1 FOCUS ON Drug Therapy Across the Lifespan

Anticholinergic Agents/Parasympatholytics

CHILDREN

The anticholinergic agents are often used in children. Children are often more sensitive to the adverse effects of the drugs, including constipation, urinary retention, heat intolerance, and confusion. If a child is given one of these drugs the child should be closely watched and monitored for adverse effects, and appropriate supportive measures should be instituted. Dicyclomine is not recommended for use in children.

ADULTS

Adults need to be made aware of the potential for adverse effects associated with the use of these drugs. They should be encouraged to void before taking the medication if urinary retention or hesitancy is a problem. They should be encouraged to drink plenty of fluids and to avoid hot temperatures because heat intolerance can occur and it will be important to maintain hydration should this happen. Safety precautions may be needed if blurred vision and dizziness occur. The patient should be urged not to drive or perform tasks that require concentration and coordination.

These drugs should not be used during pregnancy because they cross the placenta and could cause adverse effects on the fetus. If the benefit to the mother clearly outweighs the potential risk to the fetus, they should be used with caution. Nursing mothers should find another method of feeding the baby if an anticholinergic drug is needed because of the potential for serious adverse effects on the baby.

OLDER ADULTS

Older adults are more likely to experience the adverse effects associated with these drugs; dose should be reduced, and the patient should be monitored very closely. Because older patients are more susceptible to heat intolerance owing to decreased body fluid and decreased sweating, extreme caution should be used when an anticholinergic drug is given. The patient should be urged to drink plenty of fluids and to avoid extremes of temperature on exertion in warm temperatures. The older adult is more likely to experience confusion, hallucinations, and psychotic syndromes when taking an anticholinergic drug. Safety precautions may be needed if CNS effects are severe. Older adults may also have renal impairment, making them more likely to have problems excreting these drugs. Further reduction in dose may be needed in the older patient who also has renal dysfunction.

(*Transderm Scop*), solifenacin (*VESIcare*), tiotropium (*Spiriva*), toliterodine (*Detrol*), and trospium (*Sanctura*) (see Table 33.1).

Therapeutic Actions and Indications

The anticholinergic drugs competitively block the acetylcholine receptors at the muscarinic cholinergic receptor sites that are responsible for mediating the effects of parasympathetic postganglionic impulses (Figure 33.1). Some are more specific to particular receptors in the respiratory, genitourinary (GU), or GI tracts, making them preferred for treating specific conditions, and others more generally depress the parasympathetic system. When the parasympathetic system is blocked the effects of the sympathetic system are more prominently seen. These drugs can be used to decrease secretions before anesthesia, to treat parkinsonism (by blocking the stimulating effects of acetylcholine), to restore cardiac rate and blood pressure after vagal stimulation during surgery, to relieve bradycardia caused by a hyperactive carotid sinus reflex, to relieve pylorospasm and hyperactive bowel, to prevent the signs and symptoms of motion sickness and vomiting, to relax biliary and ureteral colic, to relax bladder detrusor muscles and tighten sphincters, to help to control crying or laughing episodes in patients with brain injuries, to relax uterine hypertonicity, to help in the management of peptic ulcer, to control rhinorrhea associated with hay fever, as an antidote for cholinergic drugs and for poisoning by certain mushrooms, and as an ophthalmic agent to cause mydriasis or cycloplegia in acute inflammatory conditions (Table 33.1). Anticholinergic drugs also are thought to block the effects of acetylcholine in the central nervous system (CNS), which may account for their effectiveness in treating motion sickness and preventing nausea and vomiting.

Atropine, the prototype drug, has been used for many years and is derived from the plant **belladonna**. (Belladonna was once used by fashionable ladies of the European courts to dilate their pupils in an effort to make them more innocent looking and alluring.) Atropine is used to depress salivation and bronchial secretions and to dilate the bronchi, but it can thicken respiratory secretions (causing obstruction of airways). Atropine also is used to inhibit vagal responses in the heart, to relax the GI and GU tracts, to inhibit GI secretions, to cause **mydriasis** or relaxation of the pupil of the eye (also called a mydriatic effect; Box 33.2), and to cause **cycloplegia**, or inhibition of the ability of the lens in the eye to accommodate to near vision (also called a cycloplegic effect).

Both atropine and scopolamine work by blocking only the muscarinic effectors in the parasympathetic nervous system and the few cholinergic receptors in the sympathetic nervous system (SNS), such as those that control sweating. They act by competing with acetylcholine for the muscarinic acetylcholine receptor sites. They do not block the nicotinic receptors and therefore have little or no effect at the neuromuscular junction.

Table 33.1 *Drugs in Focus:* Anticholinergic Agents/Parasympatholytics

Drug Name	Dosage/Route	Usual Indications
aclidinium (*Tudzoa Pressair*)	400 mcg b.i.d. by oral inhalation	Long-term maintenance treatment of bronchospasm associated with COPD
atropine (generic)	0.4–0.6 mg IM, subcutaneous, or IV; use caution with older patients *Pediatric:* 0.1–0.4 mg IV, IM, or subcutaneous based on weight	Decrease secretions, bradycardia, pylorospasm, ureteral colic, relaxing of bladder, emotional lability with head injuries, antidote for cholinergic drugs, pupil dilation
darifenacin (*Enablex*)	7.5–15 mg/d PO	Treatment of overactive bladder with symptoms of urge urinary incontinence, urgency, and urinary frequency
dicyclomine (generic)	160 mg/d PO in four divided doses; 80 mg/d IM in four divided doses—do not give IV	Treatment of irritable or hyperactive bowel in adults
fesoterodine (*Toviaz*)	4–8 mg/d PO	Treatment of overactive bladder with symptoms of urge urinary incontinence, urgency, and urinary frequency
flavoxate (generic)	100–200 mg PO t.i.d. to q.i.d.	Symptomatic relief of dysuria, urgency, nocturia, suprapubic pain, frequency and incontinence associated with cystitis, prostatitis, urethritis, urethrocystitis, urethrotrigonitis
glycopyrrolate (*Robinul*)	*Adult:* 1–2 mg PO b.i.d. to t.i.d. for ulcers; 0.004 mg/kg IM 30–60 min before surgery, then 0.1 mg IV during surgery *Pediatric:* 0.002–0.004 mg/kg IM 30–60 min before surgery, then 0.004 mg/kg IV during surgery	Decrease secretions before anesthesia or intubation; used orally as an adjunct for treatment of ulcers (although not drug of choice); protects the patient from the peripheral effects of cholinergic drugs; reverses neuromuscular blockade
hyoscyamine (*Symax*, others)	0.125–0.25 mg t.i.d. to q.i.d. PO or sublingually; 0.25–0.5 mg b.i.d. to q.i.d. IM, IV or subcutaneous	Adjunctive therapy to treat peptic ulcer, overactive GI disorders; neurogenic bladder or cystitis; parkinsonism; biliary or renal colic; to decrease secretions preoperatively; treatment of partial heart block associated with vagal activity; treatment of rhinitis or anticholinesterase poisoning
ipratropium (*Atrovent*)	500 mcg t.i.d. to q.i.d. by inhalation; two inhalations by aerosol (do not exceed 12 inhalations per day)	Maintenance treatment of bronchospasm associated with COPD; nasal spray for symptomatic relief of perennial and seasonal rhinitis
meclizine (*Bonine, Antivert*)	25–100 mg PO daily in divided doses, for motion sickness begin 1 h before travel	Prevention and treatment of nausea, vomiting, and motion sickness; possibly effective for treatment of vertigo
methscopolamine (*Pamine*)	2.5 mg PO 30 min before meals and 2.5–5 mg PO at bedtime	Adjunctive therapy for the treatment of peptic ulcer
propantheline (*generic*)	*Adult:* 15 mg PO 30 min before meals and at bedtime *Pediatric:* As antisecretory agent, 1.5 mg/kg/d PO in divided doses t.i.d. to q.i.d. as antispasmodic, 2–3 mg/kg/d PO in divided doses q4–6 h and at bedtime	To decrease GI secretions and stop GI spasms in conditions that would benefit from these actions
scopolamine (*Transderm Scop*)	*Adult:* 0.32–0.65 mg subcutaneous or IM; 1–2 drops (gtt) in eye(s) for refraction; 1.5 mg transdermal every 3 d for motion sickness; use caution with older patients *Pediatric:* do not use PO or transdermal system with children; 0.006 mg/kg subcutaneous, IM, or IV	Decreases nausea and vomiting associated with motion sickness; decreases GI secretions; used to induce obstetric amnesia and relax the pregnant patient; relieves urinary problems; used as adjunctive for ulcers; used to dilate pupils to aid examination of the eye and pre and postoperatively with eye surgery
solifenacin (*VESIcare*)	5–10 mg/d PO	Treatment of overactive bladder with symptoms of urge urinary incontinence, urgency, and urinary frequency
tiotropium (*Spiriva*)	Inhalation of the contents of one capsule (18 mcg) each day using an inhalation device	Maintenance treatment of bronchospasm associated with COPD, for long-term use
toliterodine (*Detrol*)	2 mg PO b.i.d. or 4 mg/d PO extended release	Treatment of overactive bladder with symptoms of urge urinary incontinence, urgency, and urinary frequency
trospium (*Sanctura*)	20 mg PO b.i.d. or 60-mg extended release tablet PO once a day	Treatment of urinary incontinence, urgency, and frequency associated with overactive bladder
umeclidinium (*Incruse Ellipta*)	One inhalation/d (62.5 mcg)	Long-term, once-daily maintenance treatment of COPD

COPD, chronic obstructive pulmonary disease; GI, gastrointestinal.

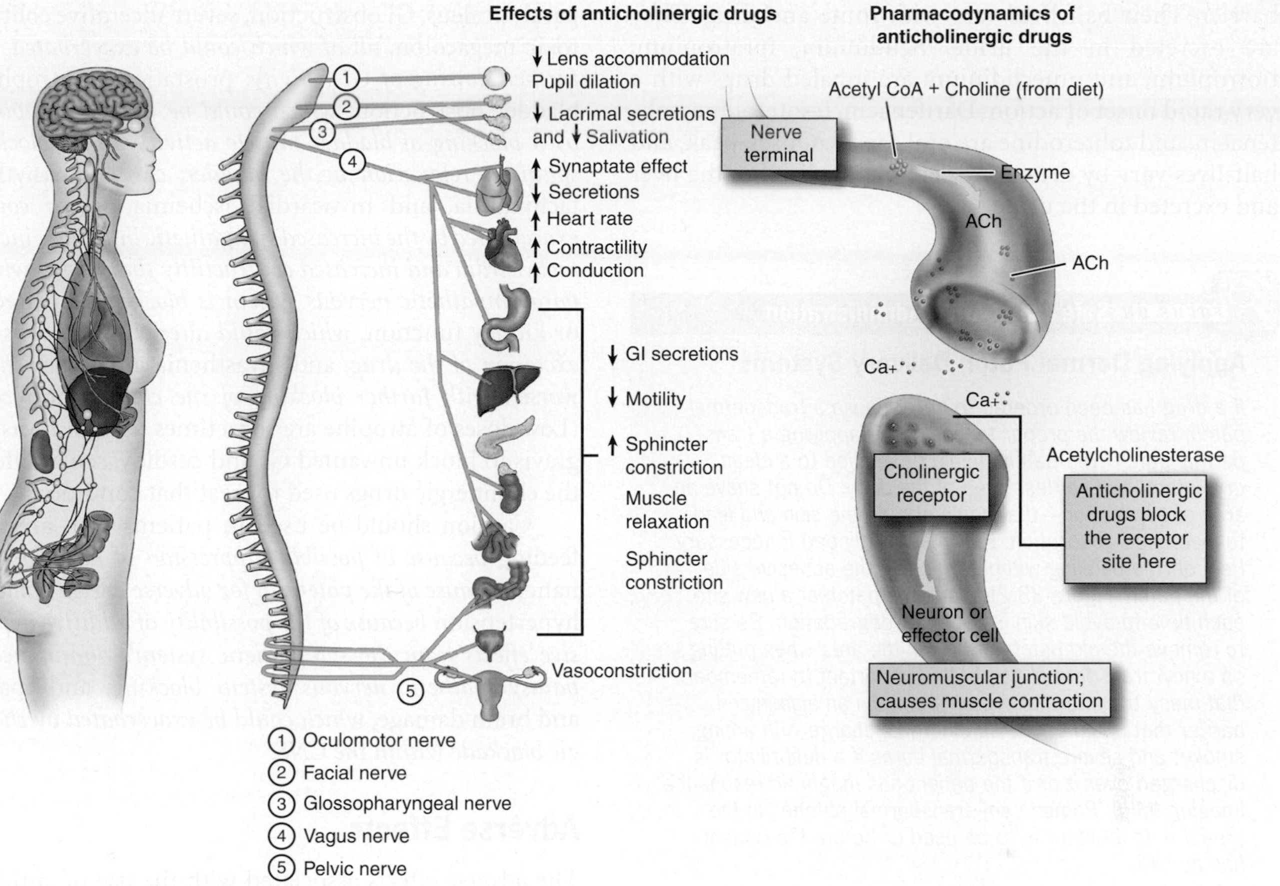

FIGURE 33.1 Pharmacodynamics of anticholinergic drugs and associated physiological responses.

Flavoxate and trospium act more specifically on the smooth muscle of the urinary tract to relax the bladder and ureter and are used to treat overactive bladder and bladder spasms; they are discussed in Chapter 52. Aclidinium, ipratropium, tiotropium, and umeclidinium act more specifically to decrease respiratory secretions and cause bronchodilation and are used as bronchodilators and to decrease symptoms of upper respiratory irritation. These agents are discussed in Chapter 55. Meclizine reduces the sensitivity of the labyrinthine apparatus and partially blocks the cholinergic receptors in the chemoreceptor trigger zone, helping to decrease the effects of motion sickness and preventing nausea and vomiting. Hyoscyamine and methscopolamine act more specifically on the receptors in the GI tract and are used as adjuncts in the treatment of peptic ulcers, irritable bowel syndrome, and GI disorders. These agents are discussed in Chapter 58. Darifenacin, fesoterodine, solifenacin, and toliterodine are used to treat overactive bladder with symptoms of urinary incontinence, urgency, and urinary frequency. See Chapter 52 for further discussion of these drugs.

BOX 33.2 *FOCUS ON* **Cultural Considerations**

Mydriatic Effects

Nurses working in eye clinics or administering preoperative medications for eye surgery should be aware that mydriatics (including atropine) are much less effective in African Americans than in the general population. Increased dose may be needed, and there may be a prolonged time to peak effect. This effect, although somewhat less pronounced, is seen in any individual with dark-pigmented eyes.

Pharmacokinetics

The anticholinergics are well absorbed after oral and parenteral administration. Atropine and scopolamine are administered through PO, IM, IV, subcutaneous, and ophthalmic routes. Scopolamine is also available as a transdermal system (see Focus on Safe Medication Administration: Applying Dermal Patch Delivery Systems). Meclizine, dicyclomine, and propantheline are oral drugs, although dicyclomine is also available in IM form. Glycopyrrolate is available through PO, IM, IV, and subcutaneous routes. These drugs are widely distributed throughout the body and cross the blood–brain barrier. Their half-lives vary with route and drug. They are excreted in the urine. Aclidinium, ipratropium, tiotropium, and umeclidinium are inhaled drugs with a very rapid onset of action. Darifenacin, fesoterodine, solifenacin, and toliterodine are oral agents. Onset, peak, and half-lives vary by drug. They are metabolized in the liver and excreted in the urine.

FOCUS ON Safe Medication Administration

Applying Dermal Patch Delivery Systems

If a drug has been ordered to be given via a transdermal patch, review the proper technique for applying a transdermal patch. The patch should be applied to a clean, dry, intact, and hairless area of the body. Do not shave an area of application—that could abrade the skin and lead to increased absorption. Hair may be clipped if necessary. Peel off the backing without touching the adhesive side of the patch (Figure 33.2). Place the patch at a new site each time to avoid skin irritation or degradation. Be sure to remove the old patch and clean the area when putting on a new transdermal patch. It is important to remember that many transdermal systems contain an aluminized barrier that could cause an electrical charge with arcing, smoke, and severe transdermal burns if a defibrillator is discharged over it or if the patient has magnetic resonance imaging (MRI). Remove any transdermal patches in the area if a defibrillator is to be used or before the patient has an MRI.

Contraindications and Cautions

Anticholinergics are contraindicated in the presence of known allergy to any of these drugs *to avoid hypersensitivity reactions*. They are also contraindicated with any condition that could be exacerbated by blockade of the parasympathetic nervous system. These conditions include glaucoma *because of the possibility of increased intraocular pressure with pupil dilation*; stenosing peptic ulcer, intestinal atony, paralytic ileus, GI obstruction, severe ulcerative colitis, and toxic megacolon, *all of which could be exacerbated with a further slowing of GI activity*; prostatic hypertrophy and bladder obstruction, *which could be further compounded by a blocking of bladder muscle activity and a blocking of sphincter relaxation in the bladder*; cardiac arrhythmias, tachycardia, and myocardial ischemia, *which could be exacerbated by the increased sympathetic influence, including tachycardia and increased contractility that occurs when the parasympathetic nervous system is blocked*; impaired liver or kidney function, *which could alter the metabolism and excretion of the drug*; and myasthenia gravis, *which could worsen with further blocking of the cholinergic receptors*. (Low doses of atropine are sometimes used in myasthenia gravis to block unwanted GI and cardiovascular effects of the cholinergic drugs used to treat that condition.)

Caution should be used in patients who are breastfeeding *because of possible suppression of lactation*; pregnancy *because of the potential for adverse effects to the fetus*; hypertension *because of the possibility of additive hypertensive effects from the sympathetic system's dominance with parasympathetic nervous system blocking*; and spasticity and brain damage, *which could be exacerbated by cholinergic blockade within the CNS*.

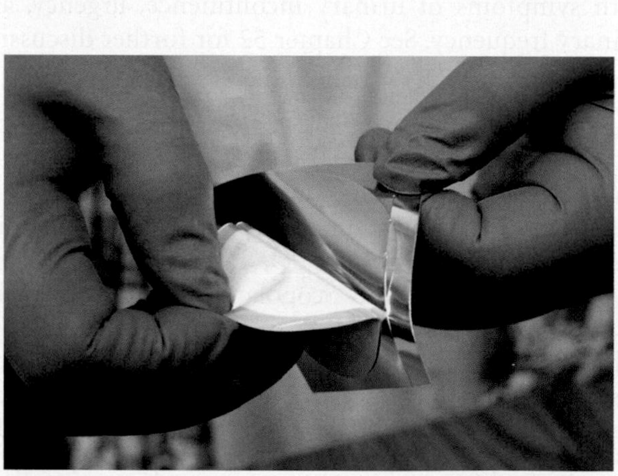

FIGURE 33.2 Carefully remove the backing from the patch without touching the adhesive.

Adverse Effects

The adverse effects associated with the use of anticholinergic drugs are caused by the systemic blockade of cholinergic receptors. What are adverse effects in some cases may be the desired therapeutic effects in others (Table 33.2). The intensity of adverse effects is related to drug dose: The more of the drug in the system the greater are the systemic effects. These adverse effects could include CNS effects, such as blurred vision, pupil dilation, and resultant photophobia, cycloplegia, and increased intraocular pressure, all of which are related to the blocking of the parasympathetic effects in the eye.

Weakness, dizziness, insomnia, mental confusion, and excitement are effects related to cholinergic receptor blockade within the CNS (Figure 33.3). Dry mouth results from the blocking of GI secretions. Altered taste perception, nausea, heartburn, constipation, bloated feelings, and paralytic ileus are related to a slowing of GI activity. Tachycardia and palpitations are possible effects related to blocking of the parasympathetic effects on the heart. Urinary hesitancy and retention are related to the blocking of bladder muscle activity and sphincter relaxation. Decreased sweating and an increased predisposition to heat prostration are related to the inability to cool the body by sweating, a result of blocking of the sympathetic cholinergic receptors responsible for sweating. Suppression of lactation is related to anticholinergic effects in the breasts and in the CNS. The severity of the adverse effects is related to the dose of the drug.

FOCUS ON Safe Medication Administration

Atropine Toxicity

Although atropine is used in a large variety of clinical settings (see Table 33.1 for Usual Indications), this drug can also be a poison, causing severe toxicity. Because it is found in many natural products, including the belladonna plant, and may be present in herbal or alternative therapy products, atropine toxicity can occur inadvertently. Atropine toxicity should be considered whenever a patient receiving an anticholinergic drug presents with a sudden onset of bizarre mental and neurological symptoms. Toxicity is dose related and usually progresses as follows:

0.5 mg atropine: Slight cardiac slowing, dryness of mouth, inhibition of sweating
1.0 mg atropine: Definite mouth and throat dryness, thirst, rapid heart rate, pupil dilation
2.0 mg atropine: Rapid heart rate, palpitations; marked mouth dryness; dilated pupils; some blurring of vision
5.0 mg atropine: All of the foregoing and marked speech disturbances; difficulty swallowing; restlessness, fatigue, and headache; dry and hot skin; difficulty voiding; reduced intestinal peristalsis
10.0 mg atropine: All of the foregoing symptoms, more marked; pulse rapid and weak; iris nearly gone; vision blurred; skin flushed, hot, dry, and scarlet; ataxia; restlessness and excitement; hallucinations; delirium; and coma

Treatment is as follows. If the poison was taken orally, immediate gastric lavage should be done to limit absorption. Physostigmine can be used as an antidote. A slow intravenous injection of 0.5 to 4 mg (depending on the size of the patient and the severity of the symptoms) usually reverses the delirium and coma of atropine toxicity. Physostigmine is metabolized rapidly, so the injection may need to be repeated every 1 to 2 hours until the atropine has been cleared from the system. A barbiturate can be used if an anticonvulsant is needed. Cool baths and alcohol sponging may relieve the fever and hot skin. In extreme cases, respiratory support may be needed. It is important to remember that the half-life of atropine is 2.5 hours; at extremely high doses, several hours may be needed to clear the atropine from the body.

Table 33.2 Effects of Parasympathetic Blockade and Associated Therapeutic Uses

Physiological Effect	Therapeutic Uses
Gastrointestinal	
Smooth muscle: Blocks spasm, blocks peristalsis *Secretory glands:* Decreases acid and digestive enzyme production	Decreases motility and secretory activity in peptic ulcer, gastritis, cardiospasm, pylorospasm, enteritis, diarrhea, hypertonic constipation
Urinary Tract	
Decreases tone and motility in the ureters and fundus of the bladder; increases tone in the bladder sphincter	Increases bladder capacity in children with enuresis, spastic paraplegics; decreases urinary urgency and frequency in cystitis; antispasmodic in renal colic and to counteract bladder spasm caused by morphine
Biliary Tract	
Relaxes smooth muscle, antispasmodic	Relief of biliary colic; counteracts spasms caused by narcotics
Bronchial Muscle	
Weakly relaxes smooth muscle	Aerosol form may be used in asthma; may counteract bronchoconstriction caused by drugs
Cardiovascular System	
Increases heart rate (may decrease heart rate at very low doses); causes local vasodilation and flushing	Counteracts bradycardia caused by vagal stimulation, carotid sinus syndrome, surgical procedures; used to overcome heart blocks following MI; used to counteract hypotension caused by cholinergic drugs
Ocular Effects	
Pupil dilation, cycloplegia	Allows ophthalmological examination of the retina, optic disk; relaxes ocular muscles and decreases irritation in iridocyclitis, choroiditis
Secretions	
Reduces sweating, salivation, respiratory tract secretions	Preoperatively before inhalation of anesthesia; reduces nasal secretions in rhinitis, hay fever; may be used to reduce excessive sweating in hyperhidrosis
Central Nervous System	
Decreases extrapyramidal motor activity; atropine may cause excessive stimulation, psychosis, delirium, disorientation; scopolamine causes depression, drowsiness	Decreases tremor in parkinsonism; helps to prevent motion sickness; scopolamine may be in OTC sleep aids

MI, myocardial infarction; OTC, over the counter.

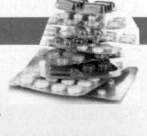

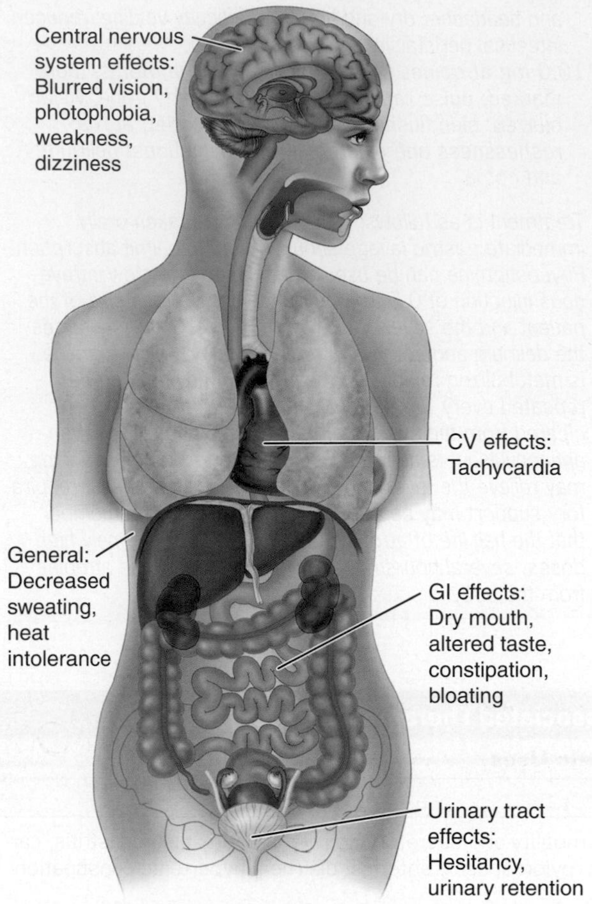

FIGURE 33.3 Variety of adverse effects and toxicities associated with anticholinergic agents.

Clinically Important Drug–Drug Interactions

The incidence of anticholinergic effects increases if these drugs are combined with any other drugs with anticholinergic activity, including antihistamines, antiparkinsonism drugs, monoamine oxidase inhibitors, and tricyclic antidepressants. If such combinations must be used the patient should be monitored closely and dose adjustments made. Patients should be advised to avoid over-the-counter products that contain these drugs. The effectiveness of phenothiazines decreases if they are combined with anticholinergic drugs, and the risk of paralytic ileus increases. This combination should be avoided. Anticholinergics also may interact with certain herbal therapies (see Box 33.3).

BOX 33.3 FOCUS ON Herbal and Alternative Therapies

The risk of anticholinergic effects can be exacerbated if anticholinergic agents are combined with burdock, rosemary, or turmeric used as herbal therapy. Advise patients who use herbal therapies to avoid these combinations.

KEY POINTS

- At cholinergic receptor sites, anticholinergic drugs block the effects of acetylcholine. Because they block the effects of the parasympathetic nervous system, they are also known as parasympatholytic drugs.
- When the parasympathetic system is blocked the pupils dilate, the heart rate rises, and GI activity and urinary bladder tone and function decrease.

Prototype Summary: Atropine

Indications: To decrease secretions before surgery, treatment of parkinsonism, restoration of cardiac rate and arterial pressure following vagal stimulation, relief of bradycardia and syncope due to hyperactive carotid sinus reflex, relief of pylorospasm, relaxation of the spasm of biliary and ureteral colic and bronchospasm, control of crying and laughing episodes associated with brain lesions, relaxation of uterine hypertonicity, management of peptic ulcer, control of rhinorrhea associated with hay fever, antidote for cholinergic overdose and poisoning from various mushrooms.

Actions: Competitively blocks acetylcholine muscarinic receptor sites, blocking the effects of the parasympathetic nervous system.

Pharmacokinetics:

Route	Onset	Peak	Duration
IM	10–15 min	30 min	4 h
IV	Immediate	2–4 min	4 h
Subcutaneous	Varies	1–2 h	4 h
Topical	5–10 min	30–40 min	7–14 d

$T_{1/2}$: 2.5 hours; metabolized in the liver; excreted in the urine.

Adverse Effects: Blurred vision, mydriasis, cycloplegia, photophobia, palpitations, bradycardia, dry mouth, altered taste perception, urinary hesitancy and retention, decreased sweating, and predisposition to heat prostration (see Focus on Safe Medication Administration: Atropine Toxicity).

Nursing Considerations for Patients Receiving Anticholinergic Agents

Assessment: History and Examination

- Assess for contraindications or cautions: Any known allergies to these drugs *to avoid hypersensitivity reactions*; glaucoma; stenosing peptic ulcer, intestinal atony, paralytic ileus, GI obstruction, severe ulcerative colitis, and toxic megacolon; prostatic hypertrophy and bladder obstruction; cardiac arrhythmias, tachycardia, and myocardial ischemia, *all of which could be exacerbated by parasympathetic blockade*; impaired liver or kidney function, *which could alter the metabolism and excretion of the drug*; myasthenia gravis, *which could worsen with further blocking of the cholinergic receptors*; pregnancy *because of the potential for adverse effects on the fetus*; lactation *because of possible suppression of lactation*; hypertension because of the possible additive hypertensive effects; and muscle spasticity and brain damage, *which could be exacerbated by cholinergic blockade.*

See the Critical Thinking Scenario to learn more about nursing care for the patient who has heart disease and is taking anticholinergic drugs.

- Perform a physical assessment, including a review of all body systems, *to establish baseline status before beginning therapy, determine drug effectiveness, and evaluate for any potential adverse effects.*
- Assess neurological status, including level of orientation, affect, reflexes, and papillary response, *to evaluate any CNS effects.*
- Monitor vital signs and cardiopulmonary status, including pulse, blood pressure, heart rate, and heart sounds; auscultate lung sounds. Obtain an electrocardiogram if ordered *to identify changes in heart rate or rhythm.*
- Assess abdomen; auscultate bowel sounds; evaluate bowel and bladder patterns; monitor urinary output; palpate bladder for possible distention *to evaluate for GI and GU adverse effects.*
- Monitor the results of laboratory tests, including renal function studies, *to determine need for possible dose adjustment and to identify potential toxicity.*

Nursing Diagnoses

Nursing diagnoses related to drug therapy might include the following:

- Acute pain related to GI, CNS, GU, and cardiovascular effects
- Decreased cardiac output related to cardiovascular effects
- Constipation related to GI effects
- Impaired urinary elimination related to bladder relaxation effects
- Risk for injury related to CNS effects
- Risk for hyperthermia related to decrease in ability to sweat
- Noncompliance related to adverse drug effects
- Deficient knowledge regarding drug therapy

Planning

- The patient will receive the best therapeutic effect from the drug therapy.
- The patient will have limited adverse effects to the drug therapy.
- The patient will have an understanding of the drug therapy, adverse effects to anticipate, and measures to relieve discomfort and improve safety.

Implementation with Rationale

- Ensure proper administration of the drug *to ensure effective use and decrease the risk of adverse effects* (see Focus on Safe Medication Administration: Atropine Toxicity).
- Provide comfort measures *to help the patient tolerate drug effects*; sugarless lozenges to suck and frequent mouth care *to alleviate problems associated with dry mouth*; lighting control *to alleviate photophobia*; small and frequent meals *to alleviate GI discomfort*; bowel program, including a high-fiber diet, *to alleviate constipation*; safety precautions, such as side rails if appropriate, assistance with ambulation, and advice to avoid driving or operating hazardous machinery *to prevent injury if CNS effects are severe*; analgesics *to relieve pain if headaches occur*; voiding before taking medication *if urinary retention is a problem* (commonly occurs with benign prostatic hyperplasia); and encouraging fluid intake and monitoring heat exposure *because the ability to sweat will be reduced.*
- Monitor patient response closely, including blood pressure, electrocardiogram, urine output, and cardiac output, *for changes that may indicate a need to adjust dose to ensure benefit with the least amount of toxicity.*
- Offer support and encouragement *to help the patient deal with the drug regimen.*
- Provide thorough patient teaching about drug name, dosage, and schedule for administration; proper technique for topical application, if appropriate (see Focus on Safe Medication Administration: Atropine Toxicity); measures to minimize or prevent adverse effects; safety measures such as avoiding driving, operating hazardous machinery, staying hydrated, and monitoring exposure to heat; dietary recommendations if appropriate; avoidance of over-the-counter medications, unless allowed by physician; warning signs of problems and the need to report these; and importance of follow-up monitoring and evaluation *to improve patient knowledge and help increase compliance to the drug regimen.*

Evaluation

- Monitor patient response to the drug (improvement in disorder being treated).
- Monitor for adverse effects (cardiovascular changes, GI problems, CNS effects, urinary hesitancy and retention, pupil dilation and photophobia, decrease in sweating, and heat intolerance).
- Evaluate the effectiveness of the teaching plan (patient can name drug, dosage, adverse effects to watch for and specific measures to avoid them, proper administration of ophthalmic drugs).
- Monitor the effectiveness of comfort measures and compliance with the regimen.

CRITICAL THINKING SCENARIO

Anticholinergic Drugs and Heart Disease

THE SITUATION

E.K., a 64-year-old woman with a long history of heart disease, has suffered from repeated bouts of cystitis. The course of her most current infection was marked by severe pain, frequency, urgency, and even nocturnal enuresis. She was treated with an antibiotic deemed appropriate after a urine culture and sensitivity test, and she was given atropine to relax her bladder spasms and alleviate some of the unpleasant side effects that she was experiencing. Within the next few days, she plans to travel to a warm climate for the winter and wants any information that she should have before she goes.

CRITICAL THINKING

E.K. presents many nursing care problems. What are the implications of giving an anticholinergic drug to a person with a long history of heart disease?

Repeated bouts of cystitis are not normal; what potential problems should be addressed in this area?

E.K. is about to leave for her winter home in the South; what teaching plans will be essential for her if she is taking atropine when she leaves?

What are the medical problems that can arise with people who live in different areas at different times of the year?

Considering her age, what written information should E.K. take with her as she travels?

DISCUSSION

E.K. is doing well with her cardiac problems at the moment, but she could develop problems as a result of the anticholinergic drug that has been prescribed. The anticipated adverse effect of tachycardia could tip the balance in a compensated heart, leading to heart failure or oxygen delivery problems. She will need to be carefully evaluated for the status of her heart disease and potential problems.

E.K. should be further evaluated for the cause of her repeated bouts with cystitis. Does she have a structural problem, a dietary problem, or a simple hygiene problem? She should receive instruction on ways to avoid bladder infections, such as wiping only from front to back, voiding after sexual intercourse, avoiding baths, avoiding citrus juices and other alkaline ash foods that decrease the acidity of the urine and promote bacterial growth, and pushing fluids as much as possible.

E.K. also should be evaluated to establish a baseline for vision, reflexes, the possibility of glaucoma, GI problems, and so on. She should receive thorough teaching about her atropine, especially adverse effects to anticipate, safety measures to take if vision changes occur, and a bowel program that she can follow to avoid constipation.

Because E.K. is leaving a cold climate and traveling to a warm climate, she will need to be warned that atropine decreases sweating. This means that she may be susceptible to heat stroke in the warmer climate. She should be encouraged to take precautions to avoid these problems.

It will be difficult to monitor E.K. while she is away. It should be anticipated that patients such as E.K. might have two sets of health care providers who may not communicate with each other. It is important to give E.K. written information about her current diagnosis, including test results; details about her drugs, including dosages; information about the adverse effects she may experience and ways to deal with them; and ways to avoid cystitis in the future. It may be useful to include a telephone number that E.K. can use or can give to her southern health care provider to use if further testing or follow-up is indicated.

NURSING CARE GUIDE FOR E.K.: HEART DISEASE

Assessment: History and Examination

Assess for a history of allergy to anticholinergic drugs, chronic obstructive pulmonary disease (COPD), narrow-angle glaucoma, myasthenia gravis, bowel or urinary obstruction, tachycardia, and recent GI or urinary surgery

Focus the physical examination on the following:

CV: Blood pressure, pulse rate, peripheral perfusion, electrocardiogram (ECG)

CNS: Orientation, affect, reflexes, vision

Skin: Color, lesions, texture, sweating

GU: Urinary output, bladder tone

GI: Abdominal exam

Respiratory: Respiratory rate, adventitious sounds

Nursing Diagnoses

Decreased cardiac output related to cardiovascular effects

Constipation related to GI effects

Impaired urinary elimination related to bladder relaxation effects

Risk for injury related to CNS effects

Risk for hyperthermia related to decrease in ability to sweat

Deficient knowledge regarding drug therapy

Anticholinergic Drugs and Heart Disease (continued)

Planning

The patient will receive the best therapeutic effect from the drug therapy.

The patient will have limited adverse effects to the drug therapy.

The patient will have an understanding of the drug therapy, adverse effects to anticipate, and measures to relieve discomfort and improve safety.

Implementation

Ensure safe and appropriate administration of drug.

Provide comfort and safety measures, including assistance/side rails; temperature control; dark glasses; small, frequent meals; artificial saliva, fluids; sugarless lozenges, mouth care; bowel program.

Provide support and reassurance to deal with drug effects, discomfort, and GI effects.

Provide patient teaching regarding drug name, dosage, adverse effects, precautions, and warnings to report.

Monitor blood pressure and pulse rate, and adjust dose as needed.

Evaluation

Evaluate drug effects: Pupil dilation, decrease in signs and symptoms being treated.

Monitor for adverse effects: CV effects—tachycardia, heart failure; CNS—confusion, dreams; urinary retention; GI effects—constipation; visual blurring, photophobia.

Monitor for drug–drug interactions as indicated for each drug.

Evaluate effectiveness of patient-teaching program and comfort and safety measures.

PATIENT TEACHING FOR E.K.

- Anticholinergics are drugs that block or stop the actions of a group of nerves that are part of the parasympathetic nervous system. These drugs may decrease the activity of your GI tract, dilate your pupils, or speed up your heart.
- Some of the following adverse effects may occur:
  - *Dry mouth, difficulty swallowing*: Frequent mouth care will help to remove dried secretions and keep the mouth fresh. Sucking on sugarless candies will help to keep the mouth moist. Taking lots of fluids with meals (unless you are on fluid restriction) will help swallowing.
  - *Blurred vision, sensitivity to light*: If your vision is blurred, avoid driving, operating hazardous machinery, or doing close work that requires attention to details until your vision returns to normal. Dark glasses will help to protect your eyes from the light.
  - *Retention of urine*: Take the drug just after you have emptied your bladder. Moderate your fluid intake while the drug's effects are the highest; if possible, take the drug before bedtime, when this effect will not be a problem.
  - *Constipation*: Include fluid and roughage in your diet, and follow any bowel regimen that you may have. Monitor your bowel movements so that appropriate laxatives can be taken if necessary.
  - *Flushing, intolerance to heat, decreased sweating*: This drug blocks sweating, which is your body's way of cooling off. This places you at increased risk for heat stroke. Avoid extremes of temperature, dress coolly on very warm days, and avoid exercise as much as possible.
  - Report any of the following to your health care provider: *Eye pain, skin rash, fever, rapid heartbeat, chest pain, difficulty breathing, agitation or mood changes* (a dose adjustment may help to alleviate this problem).
- Avoid the use of over-the-counter medications, especially for sleep and nasal congestion; avoid antihistamines, diet pills, and cold capsules. These products may contain drugs that cause similar anticholinergic effects, which could cause a severe reaction. Consult with your health care provider if you feel that you need medication for symptomatic relief.
- Tell any doctor, nurse, or other health care provider involved in your care that you are taking these drugs.
- Keep this drug, and all medications, out of the reach of children. Do not share these drugs with other people.

KEY POINTS

- Atropine is the most commonly used anticholinergic drug. It is indicated for a wide variety of conditions and is available in oral, parenteral, and topical forms.
- Patients receiving anticholinergic drugs must be monitored for dry mouth, difficulty swallowing, constipation, urinary retention, tachycardia, pupil dilation and photophobia, cycloplegia and blurring of vision, and heat intolerance caused by a decrease in sweating.

SUMMARY

- Anticholinergic drugs, also called parasympatholytic drugs, block the effects of acetylcholine at cholinergic receptor sites, thus blocking the effects of the parasympathetic nervous system.
- Parasympathetic nervous system blockade causes an increase in heart rate, decrease in GI activity, decrease in urinary bladder tone and function, and pupil dilation and cycloplegia.

- These drugs also block cholinergic receptors in the CNS and sympathetic postganglionic cholinergic receptors, including those that cause sweating.
- Many systemic adverse effects associated with the use of anticholinergic drugs are due to the systemic cholinergic blocking effects that also produce the desired therapeutic effect.
- Atropine is the most commonly used anticholinergic drug. It is indicated for a wide variety of conditions and is available in oral, parenteral, and topical forms.
- Patients receiving anticholinergic drugs must be monitored for dry mouth, difficulty swallowing, constipation, urinary retention, tachycardia, pupil dilation and photophobia, cycloplegia and blurring of vision, and heat intolerance caused by a decrease in sweating.

CHECK YOUR UNDERSTANDING

Answers to the questions in this chapter can be found in Answers to Check Your Understanding Questions on thePoint®.

MULTIPLE CHOICE

Select the best answer to the following.

1. Anticholinergic drugs are used
- **a.** to allow the sympathetic system to dominate.
- **b.** to block the parasympathetic system, which is commonly hyperactive.
- **c.** as the drugs of choice for treating ulcers.
- **d.** to stimulate GI activity.

2. Atropine and scopolamine work by blocking
- **a.** nicotinic receptors only.
- **b.** muscarinic and nicotinic receptors.
- **c.** muscarinic receptors only.
- **d.** adrenergic receptors to allow cholinergic receptors to dominate.

3. Which of the following suggestions would the nurse make to help a patient who is receiving an anticholinergic agent reduce the risks associated with decreased sweating?
- **a.** Covering the head and using sunscreen
- **b.** Ensuring hydration and temperature control
- **c.** Changing position slowly and protecting from the sun
- **d.** Monitoring for difficulty swallowing and breathing

4. Which of the following would the nurse be least likely to include when developing a teaching plan for a patient who is receiving an anticholinergic agent?
- **a.** Encouraging the patient to void before dosing
- **b.** Setting up a bowel program to deal with constipation
- **c.** Encouraging the patient to use sugarless lozenges to combat dry mouth
- **d.** Performing exercises to increase the heart rate

MULTIPLE RESPONSES

Select all that apply.

1. A nurse would expect atropine to be used for which of the following?
- **a.** To depress salivation
- **b.** To dry up bronchial secretions
- **c.** To increase the heart rate
- **d.** To promote uterine contractions
- **e.** To treat myasthenia gravis
- **f.** To treat Alzheimer's disease

2. Remembering that anticholinergics block the effects of the parasympathetic nervous system the nurse would question an order for an anticholinergic drug for patients with which of the following conditions?
- **a.** Ulcerative colitis
- **b.** Asthma
- **c.** Bradycardia
- **d.** Inner ear imbalance
- **e.** Glaucoma
- **f.** Prostatic hyperplasia

BIBLIOGRAPHY AND REFERENCES

Andrews, M., & Boyle, J. (2011). *Transcultural concepts in nursing care* (6th ed.). Philadelphia, PA: Lippincott Williams & Wilkins.

Brunton, L., Chabner, B., & Knollman, B. (2011). *Goodman and Gilman's the pharmacological basis of therapeutics* (12th ed.). New York: McGraw-Hill.

Facts and Comparisons. (2015). *Drug facts and comparisons*. St. Louis, MO: Author.

Karch, A. M. (2014). *Lippincott's nursing drug guide*. Philadelphia, PA: Lippincott Williams & Wilkins.

The Medical Letter. (2015). *The medical letter on drugs and therapeutics*. New Rochelle, NY: Author.

Porth, C. M. (2013). *Pathophysiology: Concepts of altered health states* (9th ed.). Philadelphia, PA: Lippincott Williams & Wilkins.

PART

6

DRUGS ACTING ON THE ENDOCRINE SYSTEM

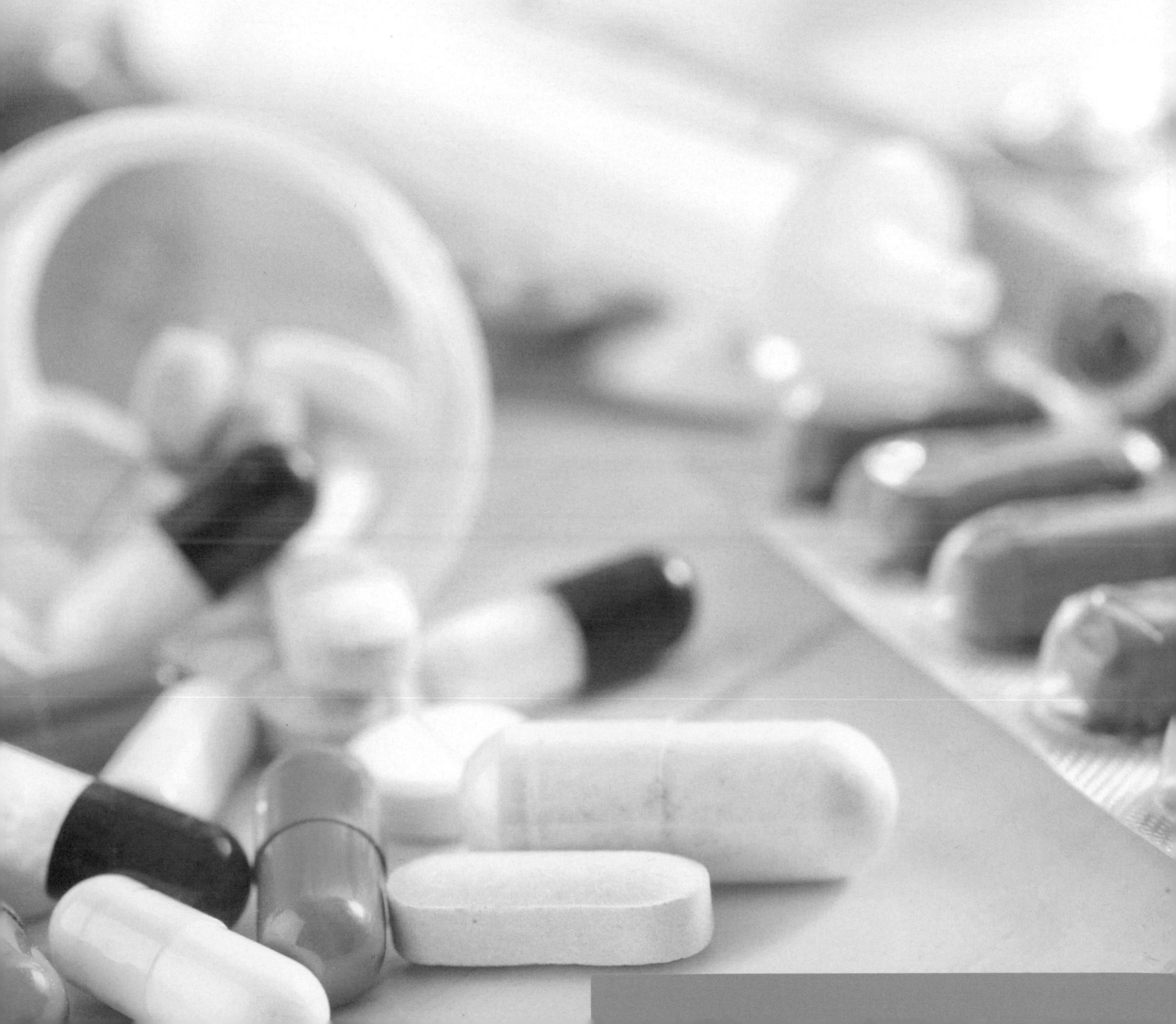

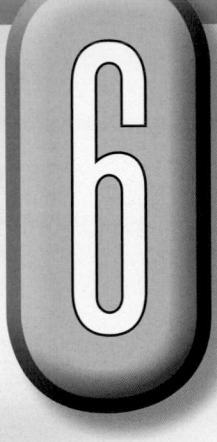

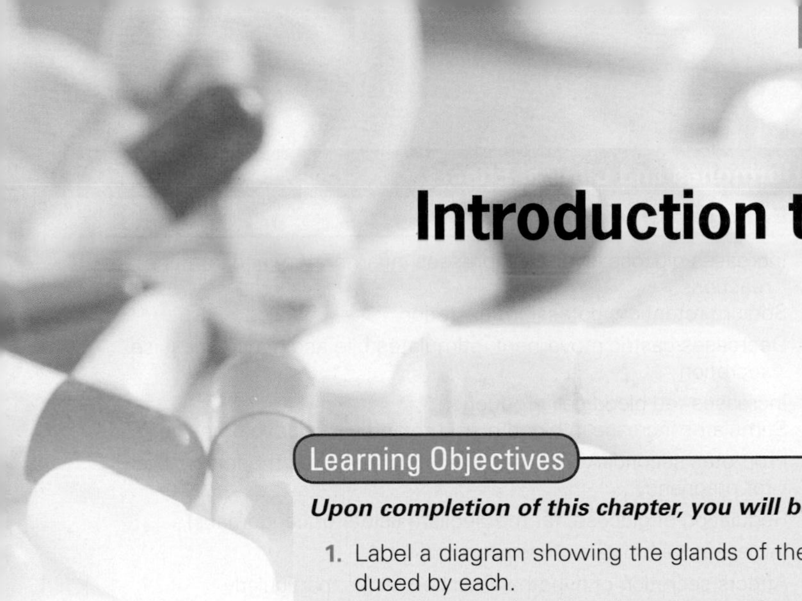

Introduction to the Endocrine System 34

Learning Objectives

Upon completion of this chapter, you will be able to:

1. Label a diagram showing the glands of the traditional endocrine system and list the hormones produced by each.
2. Describe two theories of hormone action.
3. Discuss the role of the hypothalamus as the master gland of the endocrine system, including influences on the actions of the hypothalamus.
4. Outline a negative feedback system within the endocrine system and explain the ways that this system controls hormone levels in the body.
5. Describe the hypothalamic–pituitary axis (HPA) and what would happen if a hormone level was altered within the HPA.

Glossary of Key Terms

anterior pituitary: lobe of the pituitary gland that produces stimulating hormones, as well as growth hormone, prolactin, and melanocyte-stimulating hormone

diurnal rhythm: response of the hypothalamus and then the pituitary and adrenals to wakefulness, sleeping, and light exposure

glands: organized groups of specialized cells that secrete hormones, or chemical messengers, directly into the bloodstream to communicate within the body

hormones: chemical messengers working within the endocrine system to communicate within the body

hypothalamic–pituitary axis: interconnection of the hypothalamus and pituitary to regulate the levels of certain endocrine hormones through a complex series of negative feedback systems

hypothalamus: "master gland" of the neuroendocrine system; regulates both nervous and endocrine responses to internal and external stimuli

negative feedback system: control system in which increasing levels of a hormone lead to decreased levels of releasing and stimulating hormones, leading to decreased hormone levels, which stimulates the release of releasing and stimulating hormones; allows tight control of the endocrine system

neuroendocrine system: the combination of the nervous and endocrine systems, which work closely together to maintain regulatory control and homeostasis in the body

pituitary gland: gland found in the sella turcica of the brain; produces hormones, endorphins, and enkephalins and stores two hypothalamic hormones

posterior pituitary: lobe of the pituitary that receives antidiuretic hormone and oxytocin via nerve axons from the hypothalamus and stores them to be released when stimulated by the hypothalamus

releasing hormones or factors: chemicals released by the hypothalamus into the anterior pituitary to stimulate the release of anterior pituitary hormones

The endocrine system, in conjunction with the nervous system, works to maintain internal homeostasis and to integrate the body's response to the external environment. Their activities and functions are so closely related that it is probably more correct to refer to them as the **neuroendocrine system.** However, this section deals with drugs affecting the "traditional" endocrine system, which includes **glands**—organized groups of specialized cells that produce and secrete **hormones**, or chemical messengers, directly into the bloodstream to communicate within the body.

Some organs function like endocrine glands, but they are not considered part of the traditional endocrine system. In addition, certain hormones that influence body functioning are not secreted by endocrine glands. For example, prostaglandins are tissue hormones produced in various tissues; they do not enter the bloodstream, but exert their effects right in the area where they are released. Moreover, neurotransmitters, such as norepinephrine and dopamine, can be classified as hormones because they are secreted directly into the bloodstream for dispersion

Table 34.1 Endocrine Glands with Associated Hormones and Clinical Effects

Gland	Hormones Produced	Principal Effects
Adrenal cortex	Cortisol Aldosterone	Increases glucose levels, suppresses inflammatory and immune reactions Sodium retention, potassium excretion
Intestine	Secretin, cholecystokinin	Decreases gastric movement, stimulates bile and pancreatic juice secretion
Kidney (juxtaglomerular cells)	Erythropoietin Renin	Increases red blood cell production Stimulates increase in blood pressure and vascular volume
Ovaries	Estrogen, progesterone	Promotes secondary sex characteristics, prepares the female body for pregnancy
Pancreas	Insulin, glucagon, somatostatin	Regulation of glucose, fat metabolism (islets of Langerhans)
Parathyroid glands	Parathyroid hormone	Increases serum calcium levels
Pineal gland	Melatonin	Affects secretion of hypothalamic hormones, particularly gonadotropin-releasing hormone
Placenta	Estrogens, progesterones	Maintains fetal growth and development, prepares the body for delivery
Stomach	Gastrin	Stimulates stomach acid production
Testes	Testosterone	Stimulates secondary sex characteristics in males
Thyroid	Thyroid hormone Calcitonin	Stimulates basal metabolic rate (how the body uses energy) Decreases serum calcium levels

throughout the body. There also are many gastrointestinal (GI) hormones that are produced in GI cells and act locally. All of these hormones are addressed in the chapters most related to their effects.[1]

Structure and Function of the Endocrine System

The endocrine system provides communication within the body and helps to regulate growth and development, reproduction, energy use, and electrolyte balance. The endocrine system is closely interconnected with the nervous system, and the two systems work to maintain homeostasis within the body to ensure maximum function and adequate response to various internal and external stressors.

Glands

The endocrine glands are collections of specialized cells that produce hormones that cause an effect at hormone receptor sites. These glands do not have ducts, so they secrete their hormones directly into the bloodstream.

[1]GI hormones are discussed in Part 11: Drugs Acting on the Gastrointestinal System. Neurotransmitters acting like hormones are discussed in Chapter 29: Introduction to the Autonomic Nervous System. The reproductive hormones are discussed in Chapter 39: Introduction to the Reproductive System. Hormones active in the inflammatory and immune response are discussed in Part 3: Drugs Acting on the Immune System. Specific traditional endocrine glands and hormones are discussed in Chapter 35 (hypothalamic and pituitary hormones), Chapter 36 (adrenocortical hormones), Chapter 37 (thyroid and parathyroid hormones), and Chapter 38 (pancreatic hormones).

There are many endocrine glands in the body. Table 34.1 lists the endocrine glands, the hormones that they produce, and the clinical effects that the hormones cause.

Hormones

Hormones are chemicals that are produced in the body and that meet specific criteria. All hormones:

- Are produced in very small amounts
- Are secreted directly into the bloodstream
- Travel through the blood to specific receptor sites throughout the body
- Act to increase or decrease the normal metabolic cellular processes when they react with their specific receptor sites
- Are immediately broken down

Hormones may act in two different ways. Some hormones react with specific receptor sites on a cell membrane to stimulate the nucleotide cyclic adenosine monophosphate (cyclic AMP) within the cell to cause an effect. For example, when insulin reacts with an insulin receptor site, it activates intracellular enzymes that cause many effects, including changing the cell membrane's permeability to glucose. Hormones such as insulin that do not enter the cell but react with specific receptor sites on the cell membrane act very quickly—often within seconds—to produce an effect.

Other hormones, such as estrogen, actually enter the cell and react with a receptor site inside the cell to change messenger RNA, which enters the cell nucleus to affect cellular DNA and thereby alters the cell's function. These hormones that enter the cell before they can cause an effect take quite a while to produce an effect. The full effects of estrogen may not be seen for months to years, as evidenced by the changes that occur at puberty. Because the neuroendocrine system tightly regulates the body's processes within a narrow range of normal limits, overproduction or underproduction of any hormone can affect the body's activities and other hormones within the system.

KEY POINTS

- The endocrine system and the nervous system regulate body functions and maintain homeostasis largely with the help of hormones, which are chemicals produced within the body. Hormones increase or decrease cellular activity.
- The endocrine system regulates growth and development, reproduction, energy use in the body, and electrolyte balance.
- Hormones can react with receptors on the cell membrane to cause an immediate effect on a cell by altering enzyme systems near the cell membrane or they may enter the cell and react with receptor sites on messenger RNA, which then enters the nucleus and alters cell function.

The Hypothalamus

The **hypothalamus** is the coordinating center for the nervous and endocrine responses to internal and external stimuli. The hypothalamus constantly monitors the body's homeostasis by analyzing input from the periphery and the central nervous system (CNS) and coordinating responses through the autonomic, endocrine, and nervous systems. In effect, it is the "master gland" of the neuroendocrine system. This title was once given to the pituitary gland because of its many functions and well-protected location (see The Pituitary Gland).

The hypothalamus has various neurocenters—areas specifically sensitive to certain stimuli—that regulate a number of body functions, including body temperature, thirst, hunger, water retention, blood pressure, respiration, reproduction, and emotional reactions. Situated at the base of the forebrain the hypothalamus receives input from virtually all other areas of the brain, including the limbic system, cerebral cortex, and the special senses that are controlled by the cranial nerves—smell, sight, touch, taste, and hearing. Because of its positioning the hypothalamus is able to influence, and be influenced by, emotions and thoughts. The hypothalamus also is located in an area of the brain that is poorly protected by the blood–brain barrier, so it is able to act as a sensor to various electrolytes, chemicals, and hormones that are in circulation and do not affect other areas of the brain.

The hypothalamus maintains internal homeostasis by sensing blood chemistries and by stimulating or suppressing endocrine, autonomic, and CNS activity. In essence, it can turn the autonomic nervous system and its effects on or off. The hypothalamus also produces and secretes a number of **releasing hormones or factors** that stimulate the pituitary gland, which in turn stimulates or inhibits various endocrine glands throughout the body (Figure 34.1). These releasing hormones include growth hormone–releasing hormone, thyrotropin-releasing hormone (TRH), gonadotropin-releasing hormone, corticotropin-releasing hormone, and prolactin-releasing hormone. The hypothalamus also produces two inhibiting factors that act as regulators to shut off the production of hormones when levels become too high: Growth hormone (GH) release–inhibiting factor (somatostatin) and prolactin (PRL)-inhibiting factor (PIF). Recent research has indicated that PIF may actually be dopamine, a neurotransmitter. Patients who are taking dopamine-blocking drugs often develop galactorrhea (inappropriate milk production) and breast enlargement, theoretically because PIF also is blocked and prolactin (PRL) levels continue to rise, stimulating breast tissue and milk production. Research is ongoing about the chemical structure of several of the releasing factors.

The hypothalamus is connected to the pituitary gland by two networks: A vascular capillary network carries the hypothalamic-releasing factors directly into the anterior pituitary, and a neurological network delivers two other hypothalamic hormones—antidiuretic hormone (ADH) and oxytocin—to the posterior pituitary to be stored. These hormones are released as needed by the body when stimulated by the hypothalamus.

KEY POINTS

- As the "master gland" of the neuroendocrine system the hypothalamus helps to regulate the central and autonomic nervous systems and the endocrine system to maintain homeostasis.
- The hypothalamus produces stimulating and inhibiting factors that travel to the anterior pituitary through a capillary system to stimulate the release of pituitary hormones or block the production of certain pituitary hormones when levels of target hormones get too high.
- The hypothalamus is connected to the posterior pituitary by a nerve network that delivers the hypothalamic hormones ADH and oxytocin to be stored in the posterior pituitary until the hypothalamus stimulates their release.

The Pituitary Gland

The **pituitary gland** is located in the skull in the bony sella turcica under a layer of dura mater. It is divided into three lobes: An anterior lobe, a posterior lobe, and an

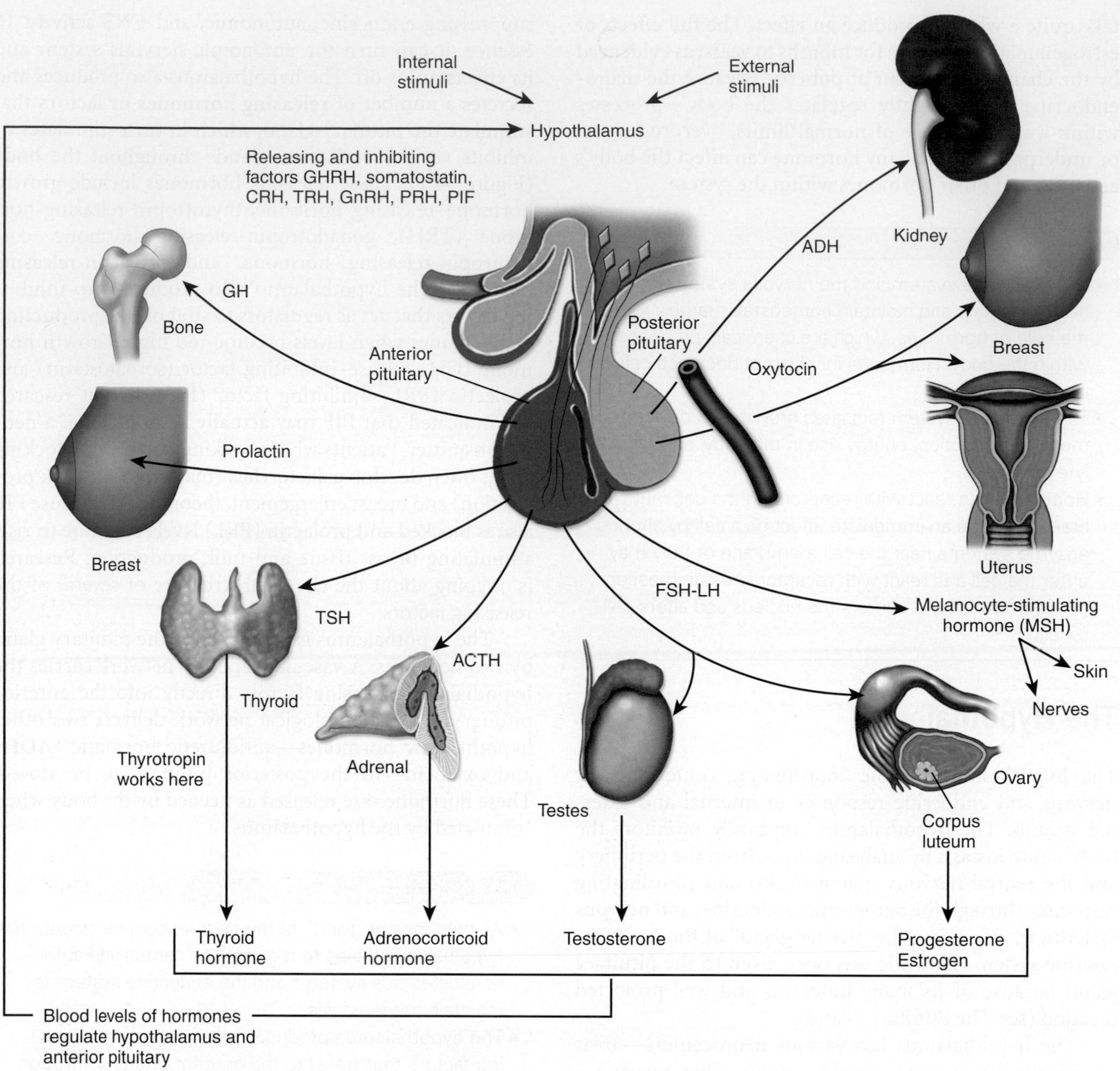

FIGURE 34.1 The traditional endocrine system. The hypothalamus secretes releasing factors to stimulate the pituitary gland to produce stimulating factors that enter the circulation and react with specific target glands, which produce endocrine hormones.

intermediate lobe. Traditionally, the anterior pituitary was known as the body's master gland because it has so many important functions and, through feedback mechanisms, regulates the function of many other endocrine glands. In addition, its unique and protected position in the brain led early scientists to believe that it must be the chief control gland. However, as knowledge of the endocrine system has grown, scientists now designate the hypothalamus as the master gland because it has even greater direct regulatory effects over the neuroendocrine system, including stimulation of the pituitary gland to produce its hormones.

The Anterior Pituitary

The **anterior pituitary** produces six major hormones: GH, adrenocorticotropic hormone (ACTH), follicle-stimulating hormone, luteinizing hormone, PRL, and thyroid-stimulating hormone (TSH, also called thyrotropin) (Table 34.2; see also Figure 34.1). These hormones are essential for the regulation of growth, reproduction, and some metabolic processes. Deficiency or overproduction of these hormones disrupts this regulation.

The anterior pituitary hormones are released in a rhythmic manner into the bloodstream. Their secretion

Table 34.2 Hypothalamic Hormones, Associated Anterior Pituitary Hormones, and Target Organ Response

Hypothalamus Hormones	Anterior Pituitary Hormones	Target Organ Response
Stimulating Hormones		
CRH	ACTH	Adrenal corticosteroid hormones
TRH	TSH	Thyroid hormone
GHRH	GH	Cell growth
GnRH	LH and FSH	Estrogen and progesterone (females), testosterone (males)
PRH	PRL	Milk production
	MSH	Melanin stimulation (color change in animals, nerve growth in humans)
Inhibiting Hormones		
Somatostatin (growth hormone–inhibiting factor)		Stops release of GH
PIF (prolactin-inhibiting factors)		Stops release of PRL

CRH, corticotropin-releasing hormone; ACTH, adrenocorticotropic hormone; TRH, thyroid-releasing hormone; TSH, thyroid-stimulating hormone; GHRH, growth hormone–releasing hormone; GH, growth hormone; GnRH, gonadotropin-releasing hormone; LH, luteinizing hormone; FSH, follicle-stimulating hormone; PRH, prolactin-releasing hormone; PRL, prolactin; MSH, melanocyte-stimulating hormone.

varies with time of day (often referred to as **diurnal rhythm**) or with physiological conditions such as exercise or sleep. Their release is affected by activity in the CNS, by hypothalamic hormones, by hormones of the peripheral endocrine glands, by certain diseases that can alter endocrine functioning, and by a variety of drugs, which can directly or indirectly upset the homeostasis in the body and cause an endocrine response. Normally, diurnal rhythm occurs when the hypothalamus begins secretion of corticotropin-releasing factor (CRF) in the evening, peaking at about midnight; adrenocortical peak response is between 6 and 9 AM; levels fall during the day until evening, when the low level is picked up by the hypothalamus and CRF secretion begins again.

The anterior pituitary also produces melanocyte-stimulating hormone (MSH) and various lipotropins. MSH plays an important role in animals that use skin color changes as an adaptive mechanism. It also might be important for nerve growth and development in humans. Lipotropins stimulate fat mobilization but have not been clearly isolated in humans.

The Posterior Pituitary

The **posterior pituitary** stores two hormones that are produced by the hypothalamus and deposited in the posterior lobe via the nerve axons where they are produced. These two hormones are ADH, also referred to as vasopressin, and oxytocin. ADH is directly released in response to increased plasma osmolarity or decreased blood volume (which often results in increased osmolarity). The osmoreceptors in the hypothalamus stimulate the release of ADH. Oxytocin stimulates uterine smooth muscle contraction in late phases of pregnancy and also causes milk release or "let-down" reflex in lactating women. Its release is stimulated by various hormones and neurological stimuli associated with labor and with lactation.

The Intermediate Lobe

The intermediate lobe of the pituitary produces endorphins and enkephalins, which are released in response to severe pain or stress and occupy specific endorphin receptor sites in the brainstem to block the perception of pain. These hormones are also produced in peripheral tissues and in other areas of the brain. They are released in response to overactivity of pain nerves, sympathetic stimulation, transcutaneous stimulation, guided imagery, and vigorous exercise.

KEY POINTS

The pituitary gland has three lobes:

- The anterior lobe produces stimulating hormones in response to hypothalamic stimulation.
- The posterior lobe of the pituitary stores ADH and oxytocin, which are two hormones produced by the hypothalamus.
- The intermediate lobe of the pituitary produces endorphins and enkephalins to modulate pain perception.

Endocrine Regulation

The production and release of hormones needs to be tightly regulated within the body. Hormones are released in small amounts to accomplish what needs to be done to maintain homeostasis within the body. The fine-tuning and regulation of hormone release through the hypothalamus are often regulated by a series of negative feedback systems. Other hormones are not controlled in this fashion but respond to other direct stimuli.

Hypothalamic–Pituitary Axis

Because of its position in the brain the hypothalamus is stimulated by many things, such as light, emotion, cerebral cortex activity, and a variety of chemical and hormonal stimuli. Together, the hypothalamus and the pituitary function closely to maintain endocrine activity along what is called the **hypothalamic–pituitary axis** (HPA) using a series of negative feedback systems.

A **negative feedback system** works much like the law of supply and demand in business. In business, when there is an adequate supply of a product, production of that product will slow down because there is an adequate supply and no current demand for it. When the supply is used up, demand will increase, and so production will pick up. Production continues until the supply is adequate and demand is reduced. When the hypothalamus senses a need for a particular hormone—for example, thyroid hormone—it secretes the releasing factor TRH directly into the anterior pituitary. In response to the TRH the anterior pituitary secretes TSH, which in turn stimulates the thyroid gland to produce thyroid hormone. When the hypothalamus senses the rising levels of thyroid hormone, it stops secreting TRH, resulting in decreased TSH production and subsequent reduced thyroid hormone levels. The hypothalamus, sensing the falling thyroid hormone levels, secretes TRH again. The negative feedback system continues in this fashion, maintaining the levels of thyroid hormone within a relatively narrow range of normal (Figure 34.2).

It is thought that this feedback system is more complex than once believed. The hypothalamus probably also senses TRH and TSH levels and regulates TRH secretion within a narrow range, even if thyroid hormone is not produced. The anterior pituitary may also be sensitive to TSH levels and thyroid hormone, regulating its own production of TSH. This complex system provides backup controls and regulation if any part of the HPA fails. This system also can create complications, especially when there is a need to override or interact with the total system, as is the case with hormone replacement therapy or the treatment of endocrine disorders. Supplying an exogenous hormone, for example, may increase the hormone levels in the body, but then may affect the HPA to stop production of releasing and stimulating hormones, leading to a decrease in the body's normal production of the hormone.

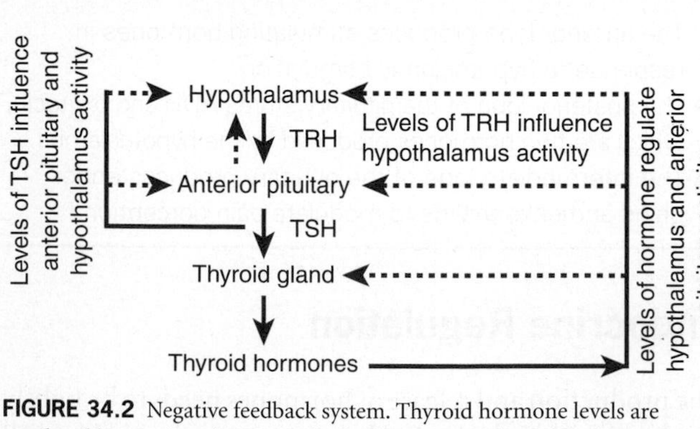

FIGURE 34.2 Negative feedback system. Thyroid hormone levels are regulated by a series of negative feedback systems influencing thyrotropin-releasing hormone (TRH), thyroid-stimulating hormone (TSH), and thyroid hormone levels.

Two of the anterior pituitary hormones (i.e., GH and PRL) do not have a target organ to produce hormones and so cannot be regulated by the same type of feedback mechanism. The hypothalamus in this case responds directly to rising levels of GH and PRL. When levels rise the hypothalamus releases the inhibiting factors somatostatin and PIF directly to inhibit the pituitary's release of GH and PRL, respectively. The HPA functions through negative feedback loops or the direct use of inhibiting factors to constantly keep these hormones regulated.

Other Forms of Regulation

Hormones other than stimulating hormones also are released in response to stimuli. For example, the pancreas produces and releases insulin, glucagon, and somatostatin from different cells in response to varying blood glucose levels and to stimulatory factors released by the GI tract. The parathyroid glands release parathyroid hormone, or parathormone, in response to local calcium levels. The juxtaglomerular cells in the kidney release erythropoietin and renin in response to decreased pressure or decreased oxygenation of the blood flowing into the glomerulus. GI hormones are released in response to local stimuli in areas of the GI tract, such as acid, proteins, or calcium. The thyroid gland produces and secretes another hormone, called calcitonin, in direct response to serum calcium levels. Many different prostaglandins are released throughout the body in response to local stimuli in the tissues that produce them. Activation of the sympathetic nervous system directly causes release of ACTH and the adrenocorticoid hormones to prepare the body for fight or flight. Aldosterone, an adrenocorticoid hormone, is released in response to ACTH but also is released directly in response to high potassium levels.

As more is learned about the interactions of the nervous and endocrine systems, new ideas are being formed about how the body controls its intricate homeostasis. When administering any drug that affects the endocrine or nervous systems, it is important for the nurse to remember how closely related all of these activities are. Expected or unexpected adverse effects involving areas of the endocrine and nervous systems often occur.

KEY POINTS

- The hypothalamus and pituitary operate by a series of negative feedback mechanisms called the HPA. The hypothalamus secretes releasing factors to cause the anterior pituitary to release stimulating hormones, which act with specific endocrine glands to cause the release of hormones.
- GH and PRL are released by the anterior pituitary and directly influence cell activity. These hormones are regulated by the release of the hypothalamic-inhibiting factors somatostatin and PIF in response to the levels of the pituitary hormones GH and PRL.
- Some hormones are not influenced by the HPA and are released in response to direct local stimulation.

SUMMARY

- The endocrine system is a regulatory system that communicates through the use of hormones.
- Because the endocrine and nervous systems are tightly intertwined in the regulation of body homeostasis, they are often referred to as the neuroendocrine system.
- A hormone is a chemical that is produced within the body, is needed in only small amounts, travels to specific receptor sites to cause an increase or decrease in cellular activity, and is broken down immediately.
- As the "master gland" of the neuroendocrine system the hypothalamus helps to regulate the central and autonomic nervous systems and the endocrine system to maintain homeostasis.
- The pituitary is made up of three lobes: Anterior, posterior, and intermediate. The anterior lobe produces stimulating hormones in response to hypothalamic stimulation. The posterior lobe stores two hormones produced by the hypothalamus—ADH and oxytocin. The intermediate lobe produces endorphins and enkephalins to modulate pain perception.
- The hypothalamus and pituitary operate by a series of negative feedback mechanisms called the HPA. The hypothalamus secretes releasing factors to cause the anterior pituitary to release stimulating hormones, which act with specific endocrine glands to cause the release of hormones or, in the case of GH and PRL, to stimulate cells directly. This stimulation shuts down the production of releasing factors, which leads to decreased stimulating factors and, subsequently, decreased hormone release.
- GH and PRL are released by the anterior pituitary and directly influence cell activity. These hormones are regulated by the release of hypothalamic-inhibiting factors in response to hormone levels or a cellular mediator.
- Some hormones are not influenced by the HPA and are released in response to direct local stimulation.
- When any drug that affects either the endocrine or the nervous system is given, adverse effects may occur throughout both systems because they are closely interrelated.

CHECK YOUR UNDERSTANDING

Answers to the questions in this chapter can be found in Answers to Check Your Understanding Questions on thePoint®.

MULTIPLE CHOICE

Select the best answer to the following.

1. Which of the following best describes aldosterone?
  a. It causes the loss of sodium and water from the renal tubules.
  b. It is under direct hormonal control from the hypothalamus.
  c. It is released into the bloodstream in response to angiotensin I.
  d. It is released into the bloodstream in response to high potassium levels.

2. When explaining the role of ADH to a group of students, which of the following would the instructor include?
  a. It is produced by the anterior pituitary.
  b. It causes the retention of water by the kidneys.
  c. It is released by the hypothalamus.
  d. It causes the retention of sodium by the kidneys.

3. The endocrine glands
  a. form part of the communication system of the body.
  b. cannot be stimulated by hormones circulating in the blood.

(continues on page 574)

c. cannot be viewed as integrating centers of reflex arcs.
d. are only controlled by the hypothalamus.

4. The hypothalamus maintains internal homeostasis and could be considered the master endocrine gland because
a. it releases stimulating hormones that cause endocrine glands to produce their hormones.
b. no hormone-releasing gland responds unless stimulated by the hypothalamus.
c. it secretes releasing hormones that are an important part of the HPA.
d. it regulates temperature control and arousal, as well as hormone release.

5. The posterior lobe of the pituitary gland
a. secretes a number of stimulating hormones.
b. produces endorphins to modulate pain perception.
c. has no function that has yet been identified.
d. stores ADH and oxytocin, which are produced in the hypothalamus.

6. After teaching a group of students about the negative feedback system, identification of which of the following as an example would indicate that the students have understood the teaching?
a. Growth hormone control
b. Prolactin control
c. Melanocyte-stimulating hormone control
d. Thyroid hormone control

7. Internal body homeostasis and communication are regulated by
a. the cardiovascular and respiratory systems.
b. the nervous and cardiovascular systems.
c. the endocrine and nervous systems.
d. the endocrine and cardiovascular systems.

MULTIPLE RESPONSE

Select all that apply.

1. Hormones exert their influence on human cells by influencing which of the following?
a. Enzyme-controlled reactions
b. Messenger RNA
c. Lysosome activity
d. Transcription RNA
e. Cellular DNA
f. Cyclic AMP activity

2. The specific criteria that define a hormone would include which of the following?
a. It is produced in very small amounts.
b. It is secreted directly into the bloodstream.
c. It is slowly metabolized in the liver and lungs.
d. It reacts with a very specific receptor set on a target cell.
e. A mechanism is always available to immediately destroy it.
f. It can change a cell's basic function.

3. Some endocrine glands do not respond to the HPA. These glands include the
a. thyroid gland.
b. ovaries.
c. parathyroid glands.
d. adrenal cortex.
e. endocrine pancreas.
f. GI gastrin-secreting cells

BIBLIOGRAPHY AND REFERENCES

Fauci, A. S., Braunwald, E., Kasper, D., et al. (2011). *Harrison's principles of internal medicine* (18th ed.). New York: McGraw-Hill.

Girard, J. (1992). *Endocrinology of puberty*. Farmington, NY: Karger.

Goldman, L., & Auseille, D. (Eds.). (2011). *Cecil's textbook of medicine* (24th ed.). Philadelphia, PA: W. B. Saunders.

Hall, J. (2015). *Guyton and Hall textbook of medical physiology* (13th ed.). Philadelphia, PA: W. B. Saunders.

Joseph, R. (1996). *Neuropsychiatry, neuropsychology and clinical neurosciences* (2nd ed.). Baltimore, MD: Lippincott Williams & Wilkins.

Karch, A. M. (2014). *Lippincott's nursing drug guide*. Philadelphia, PA: Lippincott Williams & Wilkins.

Kronenberg, H. M., Melmed, S., Polonsky, K. S., et al. (Eds.). (2011). *Williams textbook of endocrinology* (12th ed.). Philadelphia, PA: W. B. Saunders.

Melmed, S. (2002). *The pituitary*. Hoboken, NJ: Wiley-Blackwell.

Porth, C. (2013). *Pathophysiology: Concepts of altered health states* (9th ed.). Philadelphia, PA: Lippincott Williams & Wilkins.

35 Hypothalamic and Pituitary Agents

Learning Objectives

Upon completion of this chapter, you will be able to:

1. Describe the anatomical and physiological relationship between the hypothalamus and the pituitary gland and list the hormones produced by each.
2. Describe the therapeutic actions, indications, pharmacokinetics, contraindications, most common adverse reactions, and important drug–drug interactions associated with the hypothalamic and pituitary agents.
3. Discuss the use of hypothalamic and pituitary agents across the lifespan.
4. Compare and contrast the prototype drugs leuprolide, somatropin, bromocriptine mesylate, and desmopressin with other hypothalamic and pituitary agents.
5. Outline the nursing considerations and nursing care, including important teaching points, for patients receiving a hypothalamic or pituitary agent.

Glossary of Key Terms

acromegaly: thickening of bony surfaces in response to excess growth hormone after the epiphyseal plates have closed

diabetes insipidus: condition resulting from a lack of antidiuretic hormone, which results in the production of copious amounts of glucose-free urine

dwarfism: small stature, resulting from lack of growth hormone in children

gigantism: response to excess levels of growth hormone before the epiphyseal plates close; heights of 7 to 8 feet are not uncommon

hypopituitarism: lack of adequate function of the pituitary; reflected in many endocrine disorders

Drug List

Drugs Affecting Hypothalamic Hormones

Agonists
- goserelin
- histrelin
- (P) leuprolide
- nafarelin
- tesamorelin

Antagonists
- degarelix
- ganirelix

Drugs Affecting Anterior Pituitary Hormones

Growth Hormone Agonists
- (P) somatropin
- somatropin rDNA origin

Growth Hormone Antagonists
- (P) bromocriptine mesylate
- lanreotide
- octreotide acetate
- pegvisomant

Drugs Affecting Other Anterior Pituitary Hormones
- chorionic gonadotropin
- chorionic gonadotropin alpha
- cosyntropin
- thyrotropin alpha

Drugs Affecting Posterior Pituitary Hormones
- conivaptan
- (P) desmopressin
- tolvaptan

As described in Chapter 34 the endocrine system's main function is to maintain homeostasis. This is achieved through a complex balance of glandular activities that either stimulate or suppress hormone release. Too much or too little glandular activity disrupts the body's homeostasis, leading to various disorders and interfering with the normal functioning of other endocrine glands. The drugs presented in this chapter are those used to either replace or interact with the hormones or factors produced by the hypothalamus and pituitary. See Figure 35.1 for sites of action of hypothalamic and pituitary agents. Box 35.1 discusses the use of these drugs in various age groups.

Drugs Affecting Hypothalamic Hormones

The hypothalamus uses a number of hormones or factors to either stimulate or inhibit the release of hormones from the anterior pituitary. Factors that stimulate the release of hormones are growth hormone–releasing hormone, thyrotropin-releasing hormone, gonadotropin-releasing hormone (GnRH), corticotropin-releasing hormone, and prolactin-releasing hormone. Factors that inhibit the release of hormones are somatostatin (growth hormone–inhibiting factor) and prolactin-inhibiting factor. Not all

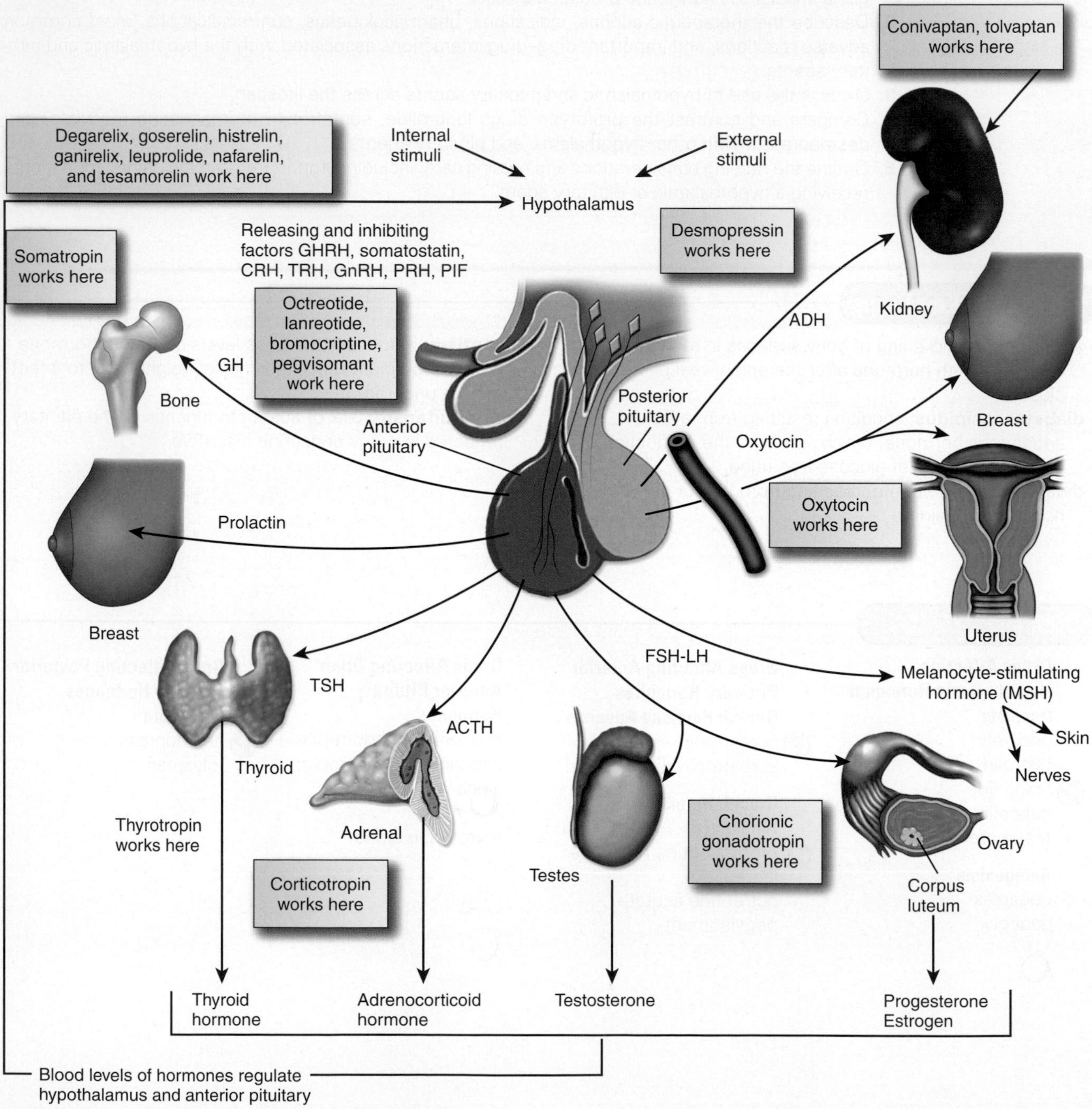

FIGURE 35.1 Sites of action of hypothalamic/pituitary agents.

BOX 35.1 FOCUS ON Drug Therapy Across the Lifespan

Hypothalamic and Pituitary Agents

CHILDREN

Children who receive any of the hypothalamic or pituitary agents need to be monitored closely for adverse effects associated with changes in overall endocrine function, particularly growth and development and metabolism. Periodic radiograph of the long bones, as well as monitoring of blood sugar levels and electrolytes, should be a standard part of the treatment plan. Children receiving growth hormone pose many challenges (see Box 35.2). Children who are using desmopressin for diabetes insipidus need to have the administration technique monitored and should have an adult responsible for the overall treatment protocol.

ADULTS

Adults also need frequent monitoring of electrolytes and blood sugar levels when receiving any of these agents. Adults using nasal forms of drugs to control diabetes insipidus should review the proper administration of the drug with the primary care provider periodically; inappropriate administration can lead to complications and lack of therapeutic effect. Adults receiving regular injections of these drugs should learn the proper storage, preparation, and administration of the drug, including rotation of injection sites.

These drugs should not be used during pregnancy or lactation unless the benefit to the mother clearly outweighs any risk to the fetus or neonate because of the potential for severe adverse effects associated with the use of these drugs.

OLDER ADULTS

Older adults may be more susceptible to the imbalances associated with alterations in the endocrine system. They should be evaluated periodically during treatment for hydration and nutrition, as well as for electrolyte balance. Proper administration technique should be reviewed, and nasal mucous membranes should be evaluated regularly because older patients are more apt to develop dehydrated membranes and possibly ulcerations, leading to improper dosing of drugs delivered nasally.

of these hormones are available for pharmacological use (see Table 34.1).

Available hypothalamic releasing hormones include goserelin (*Zoladex*) (synthetic GnRH), histrelin (*Vantas*) (a GnRH used as an antineoplastic agent), leuprolide (*Lupron*) and nafarelin (*Synarel*) (potent GnRH agonists which will actually block gonadotropin secretion with continuous use), and tesamorelin (*Egrifta*) (a GRH analogue used to stimulate the release of growth hormone [GH] from the pituitary). Available antagonists that block the effects of hypothalamic releasing hormones include degarelix (*Firmagon*) (blocks GnRH and is used as an antineoplastic agent) and ganirelix acetate (*Antagon*) (blocks GnRH). See Table 35.1 for a complete list of these drugs.

Table 35.1 *Drugs in Focus:* Drugs Affecting Hypothalamic Hormones

Drug Name	Dosage/Route	Usual Indications
Agonists		
goserelin (*Zoladex*)	3.6 mg subcutaneously every 28 d *or* 10.8 mg subcutaneously every 3 mo	Used as an antineoplastic agent for treatment of specific hormone-stimulated cancers
histrelin (*Vantas*)	One implant implanted subcutaneously every 12 mo	Palliative treatment of advanced prostate cancer
leuprolide (*Lupron*)	*Prostate cancer:* 1 mg/d subcutaneously or various depot preparations *Endometriosis:* 3.75 mg IM once a month *Precocious puberty:* 50 mcg/kg/d subcutaneously	Used as antineoplastic agent for treatment of specific cancers, treatment of endometriosis and precocious puberty that results from hypothalamic activity
nafarelin (*Synarel*)	400 mcg/d divided as one spray in left nostril AM or PM; one spray in right nostril AM or PM *Precocious puberty:* 1,600–1,800 mcg/d intranasally	Treatment of endometriosis and precocious puberty
tesamorelin (*Egrifta*)	2 mg subcutaneously once a day	Reduction of excessive abdominal fat in HIV-infected patients with lipodystrophy
Antagonists		
degarelix (*Firmagon*)	Initially 240 mg by subcutaneously injection of two 120-mg injections at separate sites; maintenance 80 mg subcutaneously every 28 d	Treatment of advanced prostate cancer
ganirelix (*Antagon*)	250 mcg subcutaneously on day 2 or 3 of the menstrual cycle	Inhibition of premature luteinizing hormone surge in women undergoing controlled ovarian stimulation as part of a fertility program

Therapeutic Actions and Indications

The hypothalamic hormones are found in such minute quantities that the actual chemical structures of all of these hormones have not been clearly identified. Not all of the hypothalamic hormones are used as pharmacological agents. A number of the hypothalamic-releasing hormones described here are used for diagnostic purposes only, and others are used primarily as antineoplastic agents. Tesamorelin is used to stimulate GH and its lipolytic effects, helping to decrease the excess abdominal fat in HIV-infected patients with lipodystrophy.

Agonists

Goserelin, histrelin, leuprolide, and nafarelin are analogues of GnRH. Following an initial burst of follicle-stimulating hormone (FSH) and/or luteinizing hormone (LH) release, they inhibit pituitary gonadotropin secretion, with a resultant drop in the production of sex hormones. Tesamorelin is an analogue of human GH–releasing factor that stimulates the release of GH from the pituitary. See Table 35.1 for Usual Indications for each of these agents.

Antagonists

Degarelix and ganirelix acetate are antagonists of GnRH. See Table 35.1 for Usual Indications for each of these agents.

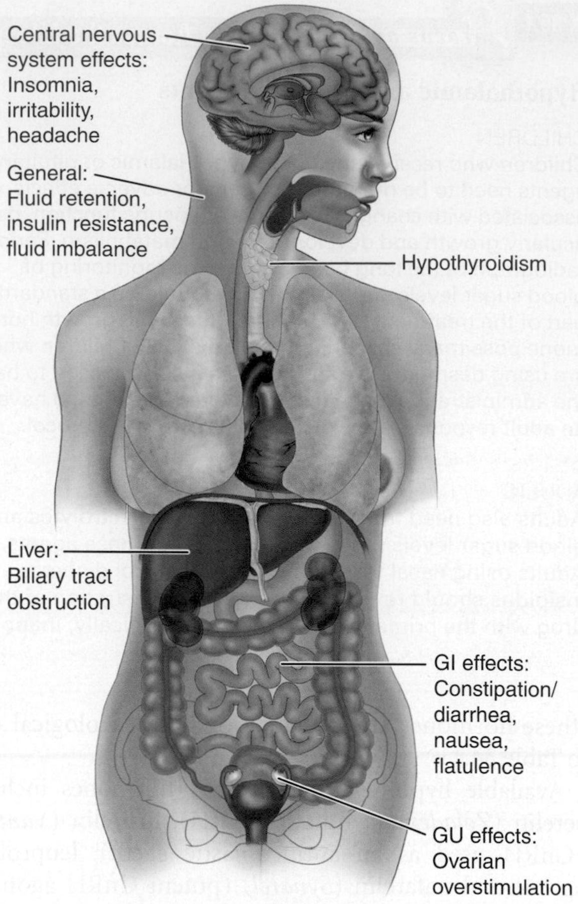

FIGURE 35.2 Variety of adverse effects and toxicities associated with hypothalamic and pituitary agents.

Pharmacokinetics

For the most part, these drugs are absorbed slowly when given IM, subcutaneously, or in depot form. They tend to have very long half-lives of days to weeks. Metabolism is not understood, but it is thought that they are metabolized by endogenous hormonal pathways. Because they are hormones or similar to hormones, they cross the placenta and cross into breast milk. Most of them are excreted in the urine. Nafarelin is given in a nasal form.

Contraindications and Cautions

These drugs are contraindicated with known hypersensitivity to any component of the drug *because of the risk of hypersensitivity reactions* and during pregnancy and lactation *because of the potential adverse effects to the fetus or baby.* Caution should be used with renal impairment, *which could interfere with excretion of the drug*; with peripheral vascular disorders, *which could alter the absorption of injected drug*; and with rhinitis when using nafarelin, *which could alter the absorption of the nasal spray.*

Adverse Effects

Adverse effects associated with these drugs are related to the stimulation or blocking of regular hormone control. Agonists can lead to increased release of sex hormones, leading to ovarian overstimulation, flushing, increased temperature and appetite, and fluid retention (Figure 35.2). Antagonists can lead to a decrease in testosterone levels, leading to loss of energy, decreased sperm count and activity, and potential alterations in secondary sex characteristics, or to a decrease in female sex hormones, leading to lack of menstruation, fluid and electrolyte changes, insomnia, and irritability.

Ⓟ Prototype Summary: Leuprolide

Indications: Treatment of advanced prostatic cancer, endometriosis, central precocious puberty, uterine leiomyomata.

Actions: GnRH agonist that occupies pituitary GnRH receptors and desensitizes them; causes an initial increase and then profound decrease in LH and FSH levels.

Pharmacokinetics:

Route	Onset	Peak	Duration
IM depot	4 h	Variable	1, 2, 3, or 4 mo

$T_{1/2}$: 3 hours; metabolism and excretion are unknown.

Adverse Effects: Dizziness, headache, pain, peripheral edema, myocardial infarction, nausea, vomiting, anorexia, constipation, urinary frequency, hematuria, hot flashes, increased sweating.

Nursing Considerations for Patients Receiving Drugs Affecting Hypothalamic Hormones

The specific nursing care of the patient who is receiving a hypothalamic-releasing factor is related to the hormone (or hormones) that the drug is affecting (see Chapters 40 and 41 for sex hormones). Drugs used for diagnostic purposes are short-lived; information about these agents should be included in any patient teaching about the diagnostic procedure. Nursing process guidelines for other agents can be found with the therapeutic drug class to which they belong (e.g., antineoplastic agents, Chapter 14).

KEY POINTS

- The hypothalamus releases hormones that act as releasing factors, stimulating the anterior pituitary to release specific stimulating factors and inhibiting factors that act to stop the production of specific anterior pituitary hormones.
- Not all of the hypothalamic hormones are available for pharmacological use; those that are available are used mostly for diagnostic testing, for treating some forms of cancer, or as adjuncts in fertility programs.

Drugs Affecting Anterior Pituitary Hormones

Agents that affect pituitary function are used mainly to mimic or antagonize the effects of specific pituitary hormones. They may be used either as replacement therapy for conditions resulting from a hypoactive pituitary or for diagnostic purposes. Antagonists are also available that may be used to block the effects of the anterior pituitary hormones (Table 35.2).

Growth Hormone Agonists

The anterior pituitary hormone that is most commonly used pharmacologically is GH. GH is responsible for

Table 35.2 *Drugs in Focus:* Drugs Affecting Anterior Pituitary Hormones

Drug Name	Dosage/Route	Usual Indications
Growth Hormone Agonists		
somatropin (*Nutropin, Saizen, Humatrope*)	Dose varies with each product, check manufacturer's instructions; must be given subcutaneously or IM	Treatment of children with growth failure due to lack of GH or to chronic renal failure; replacement of GH in patients with GH deficiency; long-term treatment of growth failure in children born small for gestational age who do not achieve catch-up growth by 2 y of age; treatment of short stature associated with Turner's syndrome or Prader-Willi's syndrome; also approved to increase protein production and growth in various AIDS-related states
somatropin rDNA origin (*Zorbtive*)	0.1 mg/kg subcutaneously for 4 wk	Reserved for use in treatment of adults with short bowel syndrome who are receiving specialized nutritional support
Growth Hormone Antagonists		
bromocriptine mesylate (*Parlodel*)	1.25–2.5 mg/d PO	Treatment of acromegaly in patients who are not candidates for or cannot tolerate other therapy, not recommended for children <15 y
lanreotide (*Somatuline Depot*)	Initially 90 mg subcutaneously every 4 wk for 3 mo; then adjust dose based on patient response	Long-term treatment of acromegaly in patients with inadequate response to or who cannot be treated with surgery or radiation
octreotide (*Sandostatin*)	100–500 mcg subcutaneously t.i.d.; adjust dose in elderly patients	Treatment of acromegaly in adults who are not candidates for or cannot tolerate other therapy
pegvisomant (*Somavert*)	40 mg subcutaneously as a loading dose, then 10 mg/d subcutaneously	Treatment of acromegaly in adults who are not candidates for or who cannot tolerate other therapy

(table continues on page 580)

Table 35.2 *Drugs in Focus:* Drugs Affecting Anterior Pituitary Hormones (*continued*)

Drug Name	Dosage/Route	Usual Indications
Drugs Affecting Other Anterior Pituitary Hormones		
chorionic gonadotropin (*Chorex*, others)	Dose varies with indication; 4,000–10,000 IU IM one to three times per week is not unusual	Treatment of male hypogonadism, to induce ovulation in females with functioning ovaries, for treatment of prepubertal cryptorchidism when there is no anatomical obstruction to testicular movement
chorionic gonadotropin alpha (*Ovidrel*)	250 mcg subcutaneously given 1 d after last dose of a FSH stimulator	Induction of ovulation in infertile females who have been pretreated with FSH
cosyntropin (*Cortrosyn*)	0.25–0.75 mg IV or IM	Diagnosis of adrenal function
thyrotropin alpha (*Thyrogen*)	0.9 mg IM, followed by 0.9 mg IM in 24 h	Adjunctive treatment for postradioiodine ablation of thyroid tissue in patients with near-total thyroidectomy and well-differentiated thyroid cancer without metastasis

GH, growth hormone; FSH, follicle-stimulating hormone.

linear skeletal growth, the growth of internal organs, protein synthesis, and the stimulation of many other processes that are required for normal growth. **Hypopituitarism** is often seen as GH deficiency before any other signs and symptoms occur. Hypopituitarism may occur as a result of developmental abnormalities or congenital defects of the pituitary, circulatory disturbances (e.g., hemorrhage, infarction), acute or chronic inflammation of the pituitary, and pituitary tumors. GH deficiency in children results in short stature (**dwarfism**). Adults with somatotropin deficiency syndrome (SDS) may have hypopituitarism as a result of pituitary tumors or trauma, or they may have been treated for GH deficiency as children, resulting in a shutdown of the pituitary production of somatotropin.

GH deficiency was once treated with GH injections extracted from the pituitary glands of cadavers. The supply of GH was therefore rather limited and costly (Box 35.2). Synthetic human GH is now available from recombinant DNA (rDNA) sources, using genetic engineering. Synthetic GH is expensive, but it is thought to be safer than cadaver GH and is being used increasingly to treat GH deficiencies. Somatropin (*Humatrope, Nutropin, Saizen, Genotropin, Serostim,* and others) and somatropin rDNA origin (*Zorbtive*) are used for GH replacement today. Box 35.3 discusses an alternate treatment for growth failure.

BOX 35.2

Growth Hormone Therapy

In the past, GH therapy was expensive and unsafe. The use of cadaver pituitaries resulted in unreliable hormone levels and, in many cases, hypersensitivity reactions to the proteins found in the drug. With the advent of genetic engineering and the development of safer, more reliable forms of GH, there has been a surge in use of the drug to treat children with short stature. Even so, the drug is still costly and not without adverse effects.

GH can be used to treat growth failure caused either by lack of GH or by renal failure. It also can help children with normal GH levels who are just genetically small. Before the drug is prescribed the child must undergo screening procedures and specific testing (including radiographs and blood tests) and must display a willingness to have regular injections. The child taking this drug will need to have pretherapy and periodic tests of thyroid function, blood glucose levels, glucose tolerance tests, and tests for GH antibodies (a risk that increases with the length of therapy). In addition, radiographs of the long bones will be taken to monitor for closure of the epiphyses, a sign that the drug must be stopped. Because the child who is taking GH may experience sudden growth, he or she will need to be monitored for nutritional needs, as well as psychological trauma that may occur with the sudden change in body image. Insulin therapy and replacement thyroid therapy may be needed, depending on the child's response to the drug. (See also Focus on Safe Medication Administration related to GH therapy.)

Therapeutic Actions and Indications

In clinical practice the agents that are used purely as a replacement for anterior pituitary hormones are those acting as GH—somatropin and somatropin rDNA origin. Both of these drugs are produced with the use of rDNA technology. See Table 35.2 for Usual Indications.

Pharmacokinetics

Somatropin is injected and reaches peak levels within 7 hours. Box 35.4 discusses a new delivery system for this drug. It is widely distributed in the body and localizes in highly perfused tissues, particularly the liver and kidney. Excretion occurs through the urine and feces. Patients with liver or renal dysfunction may experience reduced clearance and increased concentrations of the drug.

Contraindications and Cautions

Somatropin is contraindicated with any known allergy to the drug or ingredients in the drug *to avoid hypersensitivity reactions.* It is also contraindicated in the presence of closed epiphyses or with underlying cranial lesions *because*

BOX 35.3

New Treatment for Growth Failure in Children

In late 2005 the U.S. Food and Drug Administration approved two drugs that contain human insulin–like growth factor-1 (IGF-1) and human insulin–like growth factor–binding protein-3. These factors promote linear growth in children and also have anabolic effects, sensitize cells to insulin, and have insulin-like effects on metabolism. They do not directly alter GH levels. As more is learned about the intricate interrelationship of the various hormones, more-specific drugs may be developed to target very specific disorders. The drugs mecasermin (*Increlex*) and mecasermin rinfabate (*Iplex*) were approved for the long-term treatment of growth failure in children with severe primary IGF-1 deficiency or with GH gene depletion who have developed neutralizing antibodies to GH. Mecasermin has since been withdrawn from the market. *Increlex* is given by subcutaneous injection, initially 0.04–0.08 mg/kg (40–80 mcg/kg) b.i.d., and then increased by 0.04 mg/kg per dose to a maximum dose of 0.12 mg/kg b.i.d. When using this drug, hypoglycemia is common, and patients must be monitored to ensure that they eat after administration. Tonsillar hypertrophy is also common, and the child should be monitored appropriately.

FOCUS ON Safe Medication Administration

When receiving GH the child's family will need instructions on storage, preparation, and administration (see implementation in Nursing Considerations). They also must be advised to report any lack of growth, as well as signs of glucose intolerance (thirst, hunger, voiding pattern changes) or thyroid dysfunction (fatigue, thinning hair, slow pulse, puffy skin, intolerance to the cold).

The use of GH involves an interrelationship among many subspecialists and expensive and regular medical evaluation and care. The key to the success of this therapy may be the attitude and cooperation of the young patient.

BOX 35.4

New Delivery System for Growth Hormone

Saizen (somatropin) is a preparation of recombinant DNA–produced human GH that is used to treat children with growth failure due to lack of GH. The drug must be given by injection six or seven times a week. A new delivery form is now available to ease the discomfort and trauma of the frequent injections. The cool.click delivery system is a neon-colored, needle-free system that delivers the drug through the skin using a fine mist. Tests have shown the bioequivalency of this method with standard injection techniques, and the young patients who must use this drug are much less resistant to the dosing. Various drug companies anticipate similar delivery systems, which will provide a therapeutic dose of drugs without the associated discomfort of IM or subcutaneous injection.

of the risk of serious complications and with abdominal surgery and acute illness secondary to complications of open heart surgery *because of potential problems with healing.* It should be used with caution in pregnancy and lactation *because of the potential for adverse effects on the fetus.*

Adverse Effects

The adverse effects that most often occur when using GH include the development of antibodies to GH and subsequent signs of inflammation and autoimmune-type reactions, such as swelling and joint pain, and the endocrine reactions of hypothyroidism and insulin resistance.

Clinically Important Drug–Drug Interactions

Caution should be used when these agents are combined with any drugs using the cytochrome P450 liver enzyme system because of a risk for change in metabolism of the combined drugs.

Ⓟ Prototype Summary: Somatropin

Indications: Long-term treatment of children with growth failure associated with various deficiencies, girls with Turner's syndrome, AIDS wasting and cachexia, GH deficiency in adults, and treatment of growth failure in children of small gestational age who do not achieve catch-up growth by 2 years of age.

Actions: Replaces human GH; stimulates skeletal growth, growth of internal organs, and protein synthesis.

Pharmacokinetics:

Route	Onset	Peak
IM, subcutaneous	Varies	5–7.5 h

$T_{1/2}$: 15 to 50 minutes; metabolized in the liver and excreted in the urine and feces.

Adverse Effects: Development of antibodies to growth hormone, insulin resistance, swelling, joint pain, headache, injection-site pain.

Nursing Considerations for Patients Receiving Drugs Affecting Growth Hormone Agonists

Assessment: History and Examination

- Assess history of allergy to any GH or binder, presence of closed epiphyses or underlying cranial lesions, serious infection following open heart surgery, abdominal surgery, and pregnancy or lactation status *to determine contraindications to the use of the drug.*
- Assess height, weight, thyroid function tests, glucose tolerance tests, and GH levels *to determine baseline status before beginning therapy and for any potential adverse effects.*

(continues on page 582)

Nursing Diagnoses

Nursing diagnoses related to drug therapy might include the following:

- Imbalanced nutrition: Less than body requirements related to metabolic changes
- Acute pain related to need for injections
- Deficient knowledge regarding drug therapy

Planning

- The patient will receive the best therapeutic effect from the drug therapy.
- The patient will have limited adverse effects to the drug therapy.
- The patient will have an understanding of the drug therapy, adverse effects to anticipate, and measures to relieve discomfort and improve safety.

Implementation with Rationale

- Reconstitute the drug following manufacturer's directions *because individual products vary*; administer IM or subcutaneously *for appropriate delivery of drug.*
- Monitor response carefully when beginning therapy *to allow appropriate dose adjustments as needed.*
- Monitor thyroid function, glucose tolerance, and GH levels periodically *to monitor endocrine changes and to institute treatment as needed.*
- Provide thorough patient teaching, including measures to take to avoid adverse effects, warning signs of problems, and the need for regular evaluation (including blood tests) *to enhance patient knowledge about drug therapy and promote compliance.* Instruct a family member or caregiver in the following points:
  - Storage of the drug (refrigeration is required)
  - Preparation of the drug (the reconstitution procedure varies depending on the brand name product used)
  - Administration techniques (sterile technique, need to rotate injection sites, and need to monitor injection sites for atrophy or extravasation)

Evaluation

- Monitor patient response to the drug (return of GH levels to normal, growth and development).
- Monitor for adverse effects (hypothyroidism, glucose intolerance, nutritional imbalance).
- Evaluate the effectiveness of the teaching plan (patient can name drug, dosage, adverse effects to watch for, and specific measures to avoid them; family member can demonstrate proper technique for preparation and administration of the drug).
- Monitor the effectiveness of comfort measures and compliance with the regimen.

Growth Hormone Antagonists

GH hypersecretion is usually caused by pituitary tumors and can occur at any time of life. This is often referred to as hyperpituitarism. If hypopituitarism occurs before the epiphyseal plates of the long bones fuse, it causes an acceleration in linear skeletal growth, producing **gigantism** of 7 to 8 feet in height with fairly normal body proportions. In adults, after epiphyseal closure, linear growth is impossible. Instead, hypersecretion of GH causes enlargement in the peripheral parts of the body, such as the hands and feet, and the internal organs, especially the heart. **Acromegaly** is the term used to describe the onset of excessive GH secretion that occurs after puberty and epiphyseal plate closure.

Most conditions of GH hypersecretion are treated by radiation therapy or surgery. Drug therapy for GH excess can be used for those patients who are not candidates for surgery or radiation therapy. The drugs include a dopamine agonist (bromocriptine [*Parlodel*]), the prototype drug; two somatostatin analogues (octreotide acetate [*Sandostatin*] and lanreotide [*Somatuline Depot*]); and a GH analogue (pegvisomant [*Somavert*]).

Therapeutic Actions and Indications

Somatostatin is an inhibitory factor released from the hypothalamus. It is not used to decrease GH levels, although it does do that very effectively. Because it has multiple effects on many secretory systems (e.g., it inhibits release of gastrin, glucagon, and insulin) and a short duration of action, it is not desirable as a therapeutic agent. Analogues of somatostatin, octreotide acetate and lanreotide are considerably more potent in inhibiting GH release with less of an inhibitory effect on insulin release. Consequently, they are used instead of somatostatin.

Bromocriptine, a semisynthetic ergot alkaloid, is a dopamine agonist frequently used to treat acromegaly. It may be used alone or as an adjunct to irradiation. Dopamine agonists inhibit GH secretion in some patients with acromegaly; the opposite effect occurs in normal individuals. Bromocriptine's GH-inhibiting effect may be explained by the fact that dopamine increases somatostatin release from the hypothalamus.

Lanreotide, which acts like somatostatin, is given as a monthly depot subcutaneous injection. It also affects insulin growth factor levels and is used long term for patients with acromegaly who have had no response to or cannot be treated with surgery or radiation.

Pegvisomant is a GH analogue that was approved for the treatment of acromegaly in patients who do not respond to other therapies. It binds to GH receptors on cells, inhibiting GH effects. It must be given by daily subcutaneous injections. Table 35.2 shows Usual Indications for each of these agents.

Pharmacokinetics

Octreotide and lanreotide must be administered subcutaneously. Octreotide is rapidly absorbed and widely distributed throughout the body, and it is metabolized in the tissues with about 30% excreted unchanged in the urine. Lanreotide forms a depot in the subcutaneous tissue and is slowly released into circulation with a half-life of 25 to 30 days. It is metabolized in the tissues and excretion is not known.

Bromocriptine is administered orally and effectively absorbed from the gastrointestinal (GI) tract. The drug undergoes extensive first-pass metabolism in the liver and is primarily excreted in the bile.

Pegvisomant is given by subcutaneous injection and is slowly absorbed, reaching peak effects in 33 to 77 hours. It also clears from the body at a slow rate, with a half-life of 6 days. The drug is excreted in the urine.

Contraindications and Cautions

Bromocriptine should not be used during pregnancy or lactation *because of effects on the fetus and because it blocks lactation. Because there are no adequate studies of effects* of octreotide, lanreotide, and pegvisomant in pregnancy and during lactation, use of these drugs should be reserved for situations in which the benefits to the mother clearly outweigh any potential risks to the fetus or neonate. GH antagonists are contraindicated in the presence of any known allergy to the drug *to prevent hypersensitivity reactions.* They should be used cautiously in the presence of any other endocrine disorder (e.g., diabetes, thyroid dysfunction) *that could be exacerbated by the blocking of GH.*

Adverse Effects

Patients with renal dysfunction may accumulate higher levels of octreotide. GI complaints (e.g., constipation or diarrhea, flatulence, and nausea) are not uncommon because of the drug's effects on the GI tract. Octreotide and lanreotide have also been associated with the development of acute cholecystitis, cholestatic jaundice, biliary tract obstruction, and pancreatitis. Patients must be assessed for the possible development of any of these problems. Other less common adverse effects include headache, sinus bradycardia or other cardiac arrhythmias, and decreased glucose tolerance. Because octreotide and lanreotide are administered subcutaneously, they can be associated with discomfort and/or inflammation at injection sites.

Lanreotide is associated with changes in blood glucose levels and glucose should be followed carefully while on the drug.

Bromocriptine is also associated with GI disturbances. Because of its dopamine-blocking effects, it may cause drowsiness and postural hypotension. It blocks lactation and should not be used by nursing mothers.

Pegvisomant may cause pain and inflammation at the injection site (common). Increased incidence of infection, nausea, and diarrhea and changes in liver function may also occur.

Clinically Important Drug–Drug Interactions

Increased serum bromocriptine levels and increased toxicity occur if it is combined with erythromycin. This combination should be avoided.

The effectiveness of bromocriptine may decrease if it is combined with phenothiazines. If this combination is used the patient should be monitored carefully.

Patients receiving pegvisomant may require higher doses to receive adequate GH suppression if they are also taking opioids. The mechanism of action of this interaction is not understood.

Ⓟ Prototype Summary: Bromocriptine Mesylate

Indications: Treatment of Parkinson's disease, hyperprolactinemia associated with pituitary adenomas, female infertility associated with hyperprolactinemia, and acromegaly; short-term treatment of amenorrhea or galactorrhea.

Actions: Acts directly on postsynaptic dopamine receptors in the brain.

Pharmacokinetics:

Route	Onset	Peak	Duration
PO	Varies	1–3 h	14 h

$T_{1/2}$: 3 hours, then 45 to 50 hours; metabolized in the liver and excreted in the bile.

Adverse Effects: Dizziness, fatigue, light-headedness, nasal congestion, drowsiness, nausea, vomiting, abdominal cramps, constipation, diarrhea, headache.

Nursing Considerations for Patients Receiving Growth Hormone Antagonists

Assessment: History and Examination

- Assess for history of allergy to any GH antagonist or binder *to prevent hypersensitivity reactions*; other endocrine disturbances, *which could be exacerbated when blocking GH*; and pregnancy and lactation *because of the potential for adverse effects to the fetus and the blocking of lactation.*
- Assess orientation, affect, and reflexes; blood pressure, pulse, and orthostatic blood pressure; abdominal

(continues on page 584)

examination; glucose tolerance tests; and GH levels, *to determine baseline status before beginning therapy and for any potential adverse effects.*

Nursing Diagnoses

Nursing diagnoses related to drug therapy might include the following:

- Imbalanced nutrition: More than body requirements related to metabolic changes
- Acute pain related to need for injections (octreotide, pegvisomant)
- Deficient knowledge regarding drug therapy

Planning

- The patient will receive the best therapeutic effect from the drug therapy.
- The patient will have limited adverse effects to the drug therapy.
- The patient will have an understanding of the drug therapy, adverse effects to anticipate, and measures to relieve discomfort and improve safety

Implementation with Rationale

- Reconstitute octreotide and pegvisomant following manufacturer's directions; administer these drugs subcutaneously and rotate injection sites regularly *to prevent skin breakdown and to ensure proper delivery of the drug.*
- Inject lanreotide deep into the subcutaneous fat in the superior quadrant of the buttocks; alternate injection sites from right to left *to ensure proper delivery of the drug and prevent local reactions.*
- Monitor thyroid function, glucose tolerance, and GH levels periodically *to detect problems and to institute treatment as needed.*
- Arrange for baseline and periodic ultrasound evaluation of the gallbladder if using octreotide or lanreotide *to detect any gallstone development and to arrange for appropriate treatment.*
- Provide thorough patient teaching, including measures to avoid adverse effects, warning signs of problems, and need for regular evaluation (including blood tests), *to enhance patient knowledge about drug therapy and promote compliance.* Instruct a family member in proper preparation and administration techniques *to ensure that there is another responsible person to administer the drug if needed.*

Evaluation

- Monitor patient response to the drug (return of GH levels to normal, growth and development).
- Monitor for adverse effects (hypothyroidism, glucose intolerance, nutritional imbalance, GI disturbances, headache, dizziness, cholecystitis).
- Evaluate the effectiveness of the teaching plan (patient can name drug, dosage, adverse effects to watch for, and specific measures to avoid them; family member can demonstrate proper technique for preparation and administration of drug).
- Monitor the effectiveness of comfort measures and compliance with the regimen.

Drugs Affecting Other Anterior Pituitary Hormones

Drugs that affect GH are the most commonly used drugs affecting anterior pituitary hormones. There are several other anterior pituitary hormones that can now be affected by drugs. The other anterior pituitary hormones that are available for pharmacological use include chorionic gonadotropin (*Chorex*), chorionic gonadotropin alpha (*Ovidrel*), cosyntropin (*Cortrosyn*), and thyrotropin alpha (*Thyrogen*).

Chorionic gonadotropin acts like LH and stimulates the production of testosterone and progesterone. Usual Indications are presented in Table 35.2. (See Chapters 40 and 41 for nursing implications.) Chorionic gonadotropin alpha is used as a fertility drug to induce ovulation in women treated with FSH (see Chapters 40 and 41).

Cosyntropin is used for diagnostic purposes to test adrenal function and responsiveness. Cosyntropin has a rapid onset and a short duration of activity and therefore is not used for therapeutic purposes. (See Chapters 40 and 41 for nursing implications.)

Thyrotropin alpha is used as adjunctive treatment for radioiodine ablation of thyroid tissue remnants in patients who have undergone a near-total to total thyroidectomy for well-differentiated thyroid cancer and who do not have evidence of metastatic thyroid cancer.

KEY POINTS

- Hypothalamic-releasing factors stimulate the anterior pituitary to release hormones, which in turn stimulate endocrine glands or cell metabolism. The anterior pituitary hormones are mostly used for diagnostic testing, for treating some cancers, or in fertility programs.
- In children, deficiency of GH may be responsible for dwarfism; in adults it is associated with SDS.
- GH may be replaced by substances produced by rDNA processes, which are safer than replacement drugs used in the past.
- In cases of GH excess, drugs are used to block the effects of GH. Care must be taken to monitor these patients because of the systemic effects of the drugs.

Drugs Affecting Posterior Pituitary Hormones

The posterior pituitary stores two hormones produced in the hypothalamus: Antidiuretic hormone (ADH, also known as vasopressin) and oxytocin. Oxytocin stimulates milk ejection or "let down" in lactating women. In pharmacological doses, it can be used to initiate or improve uterine contractions in labor. Oxytocin is discussed in Chapter 40.

ADH possesses antidiuretic, hemostatic, and vasopressor properties. Posterior pituitary disorders can occur secondary to head trauma or surgery, metastatic cancer, lymphoma, disseminated intravascular coagulation (discussed in Chapter 48), or septicemia. Posterior pituitary disorders that are seen clinically involve ADH release and include diabetes insipidus, which results from insufficient secretion of ADH, and syndrome of inappropriate antidiuretic hormone (SIADH), which occurs with excessive secretion of ADH. Both conditions can now be treated pharmacologically. (See the Critical Thinking Scenario related to diabetes insipidus and posterior pituitary hormones.)

Diabetes insipidus is characterized by the production of a large amount of dilute urine containing no glucose. Blood becomes concentrated and blood glucose levels are higher than normal, and the patient presents with polyuria (lots of urine), polydipsia (lots of thirst), and dehydration. With this rare metabolic disorder, patients produce large quantities of dilute urine and are constantly thirsty. Diabetes insipidus is caused by a deficiency in the amount of posterior pituitary ADH and may result from pituitary disease or injury (e.g., head trauma, surgery, tumor). The condition can be acute and short in duration or it can be a chronic, lifelong problem.

SIADH presents with fluid retention, dilution of the blood and all of the blood elements, serious issues with water balance and fluid volume. This disorder is now treated with drugs that block the ADH or vasopressin receptors, so water is no longer retained and urine is produced, helping to restore water balance. Keeping the fluid balance in check can be very tricky and patients receiving these drugs need to be closely monitored in the hospital.

CRITICAL THINKING SCENARIO

Diabetes Insipidus and Posterior Pituitary Hormones (Desmopressin)

THE SITUATION

B.T. is a 56-year-old teacher with diabetes insipidus. Her condition was eventually regulated on desmopressin nasal spray, one or two sprays per nostril four times a day. B.T. seemed highly interested in her disease and therapy and learned to control her dose by symptom control. For several years, her symptoms were well controlled. Then, at her last clinical visit, it was noted that she had postnasal ulcerations and nasal rhinitis. She also complained of several GI symptoms, including upset stomach, abdominal cramps, and diarrhea.

CRITICAL THINKING

Think about the pathophysiology of diabetes insipidus. What are the effects of desmopressin on the body, and what adverse effects might occur if the drug was being absorbed inappropriately?

Because B.T. has used the drug for so many years, she may have forgotten some of the teaching points about her disease and drug administration. Outline a care plan for B.T. that includes necessary teaching points and takes into consideration her long experience with her disease and her drug therapy. Think about specific warning signs that should be highlighted for B.T. and ways to involve her in the teaching program that might make it more pertinent to her and her needs.

DISCUSSION

An essential aspect of the ongoing nursing process is continual evaluation of the effectiveness of the drug therapy. An evaluation of this situation shows that B.T.'s postnasal mucosa was ulcerated, possibly as a result of overexposure to the vasoconstrictive properties of the drug. B.T.'s GI tract also seemed to show evidence of increased ADH effects. These factors suggest that perhaps the drug was being administered incorrectly, resulting in excessive exposure of the nasal mucosa to the drug, increased absorption, and increased levels of the drug reaching the systemic circulation.

The nurse should watch B.T. administer a dose of the drug to herself, then discuss the signs and symptoms of problems that B.T. should watch for. In this case, B.T. remembered most of the details of her drug teaching. But when administering the drug, she tilted her head back, tipped the bottle upside down, and then squirted the drug into each nostril. When the nurse questioned B.T. about her technique, she explained

(continues on page 586)

Diabetes Insipidus and Posterior Pituitary Hormones (Desmopressin) (continued)

that she had seen an advertisement on TV about nasal sprays and realized that she had been doing it wrong all these years. The nurse explained the difference in the types of nasal sprays and reviewed the entire teaching plan with B.T. The drug was discontinued and B.T. was placed on subcutaneous ADH until the nasal ulcerations healed. As a patient becomes more familiar with drug therapy the details about the drug may be forgotten.

It is important to remember that patient teaching needs regular updating and evaluation. This point is often forgotten when dealing with patients who have been taking a drug for years. However, remembering to assess the patient's knowledge about the drug can prevent problems such as B.T.'s from developing. Because B.T. is a teacher, she might be interested in developing a teaching protocol that will meet her needs and serve as an appropriate reminder about the disease and drug therapy. If B.T. is actively involved in preparing such a plan, it will be more effective and might be remembered much longer.

NURSING CARE GUIDE FOR B.T.: DIABETES INSIPIDUS AND POSTERIOR PITUITARY HORMONES

Assessment: History and Examination

Assess for allergies to any anticholinergic agent and other drugs. Also assess for a history of chronic obstructive pulmonary disease, narrow-angle glaucoma, myasthenia gravis, bowel or urinary obstruction, pregnancy or lactation, tachycardia, and recent GI or urinary tract surgery.

Focus the physical assessment on the following:

Cardiovascular (CV): Blood pressure, pulse rate, peripheral perfusion, electrocardiogram

CNS: Orientation, affect, reflexes, vision

Skin: Color, lesions, texture, sweating

Genitourinary (GU): Urinary output, bladder tone

GI: Abdominal examination

Respiratory: Respiratory rate, adventitious sounds

Nursing Diagnoses

Decreased cardiac output related to CV effects

Acute pain related to GI, GU, CNS, CV effects

Constipation related to GI effects

Deficient knowledge regarding drug therapy

Noncompliance related to adverse effects

Planning

The patient will receive the best therapeutic effect from the drug therapy.

The patient will have limited adverse effects to the drug therapy.

The patient will have an understanding of the drug therapy, adverse effects to anticipate, and measures to relieve discomfort and improve safety.

Implementation

Ensure safe and appropriate administration of the drug.

Provide comfort and safety measures, such as physical assistance or raised side rails if B.T. is hospitalized; temperature control; dark eyeglasses; small, frequent meals; artificial saliva, fluids; sugarless lozenges, mouth care; and bowel program.

Provide support and reassurance to deal with drug effects, discomfort, and GI effects.

Teach patient about drug therapy, including drug name, dosage, adverse effects, precautions, and warning signs of serious adverse effects to report.

Monitor blood pressure and pulse rate and adjust dosage as needed.

Evaluation

Evaluate drug effects, including decrease in signs and symptoms being treated.

Monitor for adverse effects: CV effects—tachycardia, heart failure; CNS—confusion, dreams, visual blurring, photophobia; GU—urinary retention; GI effects—constipation.

Monitor for drug–drug interactions as indicated for each drug.

Evaluate the effectiveness of patient-teaching program and comfort and safety measures.

PATIENT TEACHING FOR B.T.

- The anterior pituitary hormone desmopressin or ADH acts to promote the reabsorption of water in your kidneys, replacing the ADH that you are missing in your body. This lack of ADH is the cause of your diabetes insipidus. This drug will replace the missing hormone. This drug also causes your blood vessels to contract and may increase the activity of your GI tract. Some of the following adverse effects may occur:
  - *Tremor, dizziness, vision changes:* If these occur, you should avoid driving a car, operating dangerous machinery, or performing any other tasks that require alertness.
  - *GI cramping, passing of gas:* Eating small, frequent meals may help.
  - *Nasal irritation, development of lesions:* Proper administration of the drug will decrease this effect.
- Use caution to administer the nasal solution correctly. Sit upright and press a finger over one nostril to close it. Hold the spray bottle upright and place the tip of the bottle about 1.5 cm into the open nostril. A firm squeeze on the bottle will deliver the drug. Do not use excessive force when squeezing

Diabetes Insipidus and Posterior Pituitary Hormones (Desmopressin) (continued)

the bottle. Do not tip your head back during administration.

- Tell any doctor, nurse, or other health care provider involved in your care that you are taking this drug.
- Watch for any signs of water intoxication (drowsiness, light-headedness, headache, seizures, coma) and report this to your health care provider immediately.
- Report any nasal pain or runny nose, which might indicate that you are not administering the drug correctly.
- Keep this drug, and all medications, out of the reach of children. Do not share this drug with other people.

ADH itself is never used as therapy for diabetes insipidus. Instead, synthetic preparations of ADH, which are purer and have fewer adverse effects, are used. Only one ADH preparation is currently available, desmopressin (*DDAVP, Stimate*) (see Table 35.3).

There are currently two drugs available that selectively block vasopressin or ADH receptors: conivaptan (*Vaprisol*) and tolvaptan (*Samsca*). These drugs are used to treat clinically significant hypervolemic or euvolemic hyponatremia, including patients with SIADH. By blocking the vasopressin receptors, they cause an increased excretion of water which results in an increase in serum sodium concentrations and a return to fluid balance.

Therapeutic Actions and Indications

ADH is released in response to increases in plasma osmolarity or decreases in blood volume. It produces its antidiuretic activity in the kidneys, causing the cortical and medullary parts of the collecting duct to become permeable to water, thereby increasing water reabsorption and decreasing urine formation. These activities reduce plasma osmolarity and increase blood volume.

The vasopressin blockers cause a loss of water through the urine and therefore increase in serum sodium levels as the water level decreases. They must be given under close supervision in the hospital to monitor fluid volume carefully. See Table 35.3 for Usual Indications for these drugs.

Pharmacokinetics

Desmopressin is rapidly absorbed and metabolized; it is excreted in the liver and kidneys. Desmopressin is available for oral, IV, subcutaneous, and nasal administration. Tolvaptan is given orally, is readily absorbed, and has a half-life of 12 hours. Conivaptan is given by continuous IV infusion, the half-life of the drug is 5 hours, and it is excreted in the urine and feces.

FOCUS ON Safe Medication Administration

Administering a Nasal Spray

Instruct the patient to sit upright and press a finger over one nostril to close it. Then, with the spray bottle held upright, have the patient place the tip of the bottle about 1.5 cm (1/2 in.) into the open nostril. A firm squeeze should deliver the drug to the desired mucosal area for absorption. Caution the patient not to use excessive force and not to tip the head back because these actions could result in ineffective administration.

Contraindications and Cautions

Drugs affecting the anterior pituitary hormones are contraindicated with any known allergy to the drug or its components *to avoid potential hypersensitivity reactions* or with severe renal dysfunction, *which could alter the effects*

Table 35.3 ***Drugs in Focus:*** **Drugs Affecting Posterior Pituitary Hormones**

Drug Name	Dosage/Route	Usual Indications
conivaptan (*Vaprisol*)	20 mg IV loading dose over 30 min, then 20–40 mg by continuous IV infusion over 24 h	Treatment of hypervolemic or euvolemic hyponatremia in hospitalized patients
desmopressin (*DDAVP, Stimate*)	*Adult:* 0.1–0.4 mL/d PO, IV, subcutaneously, intranasal for diabetes insipidus; 0.3 mcg/kg IV over 15–30 min for von Willebrand's disease; 20 mcg intranasal at bedtime for nocturnal enuresis *Pediatric:* 0.05–0.3 mL/d intranasal for diabetes insipidus; 0.3 mcg/kg IV over 15–30 min for von Willebrand's disease	Treatment of neurogenic diabetes insipidus, von Willebrand's disease, hemophilia; being studied for the treatment of chronic autonomic failure
tolvaptan (*Samsca*)	Initially 15 mg PO; titrate to a maximum of 60 mg/d PO based on patient response	Treatment of hypervolemic and euvolemic hyponatremia that is resistant to correction with fluid restriction

of the drug. Caution should be used with any known vascular disease *because of its effects on vascular smooth muscle,* epilepsy, asthma, and hyponatremia, *which could be exacerbated by the effects of the drug.* These drugs should not be used during pregnancy *because of the risk of uterine contractions that would harm the fetus* or lactation *because of the potential for adverse effects to the fetus or baby.*

All of these drugs should be stopped during acute illnesses that might lead to fluid and/or electrolyte imbalance, and caution should be used in patients who consume large amounts of fluid *because of the increased risk of electrolyte dilution and hyponatremia.*

Adverse Effects

The adverse effects associated with the use of desmopressin include water intoxication (drowsiness, light-headedness, headache, coma, convulsions) related to the shift to water retention and resulting electrolyte imbalance; tremor, sweating, vertigo, and headache related to water retention (a "hangover" effect); abdominal cramps, flatulence, nausea, and vomiting related to stimulation of GI motility; and local nasal irritation related to nasal administration. Local reaction at injection sites is fairly common. Hypersensitivity reactions have also been reported, ranging from rash to bronchial constriction. The adverse effects associated with conivaptan and tolvaptan are associated with rapid volume shifts (polyuria, blood pressure changes, hyperglycemia, arrhythmias). Constipation, dry mouth, and thirst have also been reported.

Clinically Important Drug–Drug Interactions

There is an increased risk of antidiuretic effects if desmopressin is combined with carbamazepine or chlorpropamide; use caution if these combinations are used. Tolvaptan and conivaptan should be used with care with digoxin, angiotensin-converting enzyme inhibitors, angiotensin receptor blockers, and potassium-sparing diuretics, all of which could cause hyperkalemia. Tolvaptan should not be combined with telithromycin, because of a risk of severe tolvaptan toxicity.

Prototype Summary: Desmopressin

Indications: Treatment of neurogenic diabetes insipidus, hemophilia A.

Actions: Has pressor and antidiuretic effects; increases levels of clotting factor VIII.

Pharmacokinetics:

Route	Onset	Peak	Duration
Oral	1 h	60–90 min	7 h
IV, subcutaneous	30 min	90–120 min	Varies
Nasal	15–60 min	1–5 h	5–21 h

$T_{1/2}$: 7.8 minutes, then 75.5 minutes (IV); 1.5 to 2.5 hours (oral); 3.3 to 3.5 hours (nasal); metabolized in the tissues, excretion is unknown.

Adverse Effects: Headache, facial flushing, nausea, fluid retention, slight increase in blood pressure, local reaction at injection site, water intoxication at high doses.

Nursing Considerations for Patients Receiving Drugs Affecting Posterior Pituitary Hormones

Assessment: History and Examination

- Assess for history of allergy to any antidiuretic hormone preparation or components *to avoid hypersensitivity reactions,* vascular diseases, epilepsy, renal dysfunction, pregnancy, and lactation, *which could be cautions or contraindications to use of the drug.*
- Assess skin for lesions; orientation, affect, and reflexes; blood pressure and pulse; respiration and adventitious sounds; abdominal examination; renal function tests; and serum electrolytes, *to determine baseline status before beginning therapy and for any potential adverse effects.*

Nursing Diagnoses

Nursing diagnoses related to drug therapy might include the following:

- Altered urinary elimination
- Changes in fluid volume related to water retention or excretion
- Deficient knowledge regarding drug therapy

Planning

- The patient will receive the best therapeutic effect from the drug therapy.
- The patient will have limited adverse effects to the drug therapy.
- The patient will have an understanding of the drug therapy, adverse effects to anticipate, and measures to relieve discomfort and improve safety.

Implementation with Rationale

- Monitor patient fluid volume *to watch for signs of water intoxication and fluid excess or excessive fluid loss;* arrange to decrease dose as needed.
- Monitor patients with vascular disease for any sign of exacerbation *to provide for immediate treatment.*
- Monitor condition of nasal passages if given intranasally *to observe for nasal ulceration, which can occur and could affect absorption of the drug.*
- Provide thorough patient teaching, including measures to avoid adverse effects, warning signs of problems, and the need for regular evaluation, including blood tests,

to enhance patient knowledge about drug therapy and promote compliance.

Evaluation

- Monitor patient response to the drug (maintenance of fluid balance).
- Monitor for adverse effects (GI problems, water intoxication, fluid loss, headache, skin rash).
- Evaluate the effectiveness of the teaching plan (patient can name drug, dosage, adverse effects to watch for, and specific measures to avoid them; patient can demonstrate proper administration of nasal preparations).
- Monitor the effectiveness of comfort measures and compliance with the regimen.

KEY POINTS

- Posterior pituitary hormones are produced in the hypothalamus and stored in the posterior pituitary. They include oxytocin and ADH.
- Lack of ADH produces diabetes insipidus, which is characterized by large amounts of dilute urine and excessive thirst.
- ADH replacement uses an analogue of ADH, desmopressin, and can be administered parenterally or intranasally.
- Vasopressin blockers are used to restore sodium balance in patients with severe hyponatremia.
- Fluid balance needs to be monitored when patients are taking drugs that affect ADH.

SUMMARY

- Hypothalamic-releasing factors stimulate the anterior pituitary to release hormones.
- Hypothalamic-releasing factors are used mostly for diagnostic testing and for treating some forms of cancer.
- Anterior pituitary hormones stimulate endocrine glands or cell metabolism.
- GH deficiency can cause dwarfism in children and SDS in adults.
- GH replacement is done with drugs produced by rDNA processes; these agents are more reliable and cause fewer problems than drugs used in the past.
- GH excess causes gigantism in patients whose epiphyseal plates have not closed and acromegaly in patients with closed epiphyseal plates.
- GH antagonists include octreotide and bromocriptine. Blockage of other endocrine activity may occur when these drugs are used.
- Posterior pituitary hormones are produced in the hypothalamus and stored in the posterior pituitary. They include oxytocin and ADH.
- Lack of ADH produces diabetes insipidus, which is characterized by large amounts of dilute urine and excessive thirst.
- ADH replacement uses desmopressin, an analogue of ADH, which can be administered parenterally or intranasally.
- Vasopressin blockers are used to restore sodium balance in patients with severe hyponatremia by preventing ADH from working and greater amounts of urine being produced leading to a concentration of serum.
- Fluid balance needs to be monitored when patients are taking drugs that affect ADH.

CHECK YOUR UNDERSTANDING

Answers to the questions in this chapter can be found in Answers to Check Your Understanding Questions on thePoint®.

MULTIPLE CHOICE

Select the best answer to the following.

1. Hypothalamic hormones are normally present in very small amounts. When used therapeutically, their main indication is
  a. diagnosis of endocrine disorders and treatment of specific cancers.
  b. treatment of multiple endocrine disorders.
  c. treatment of CNS-related abnormalities.
  d. treatment of autoimmune-related problems.

2. Somatropin (*Nutropin* and others) is a genetically engineered GH that is used
  a. to diagnose hypothalamic failure.
  b. to treat precocious puberty.
  c. in the treatment of children with growth failure.
  d. to stimulate pituitary response.

(continues on page 590)

3. GH deficiencies
   a. occur only in children.
   b. always result in dwarfism.
   c. are treated only in children because GH is usually produced only until puberty.
   d. can occur in adults as well as children.

4. Patients who are receiving GH replacement therapy must be monitored very closely. Routine follow-up examinations would include
   a. a bowel program to deal with constipation.
   b. tests of thyroid function and glucose tolerance.
   c. a calorie check to control weight gain.
   d. tests of adrenal hormone levels.

5. Acromegaly and gigantism are both conditions related to excessive secretion of
   a. thyroid hormone.
   b. melanin-stimulating hormone.
   c. GH.
   d. oxytocin.

6. Diabetes insipidus is a relatively rare disease characterized by
   a. excessive secretion of ADH.
   b. renal damage.
   c. the production of large amounts of dilute urine containing no glucose.
   d. insufficient pancreatic activity.

7. Treatment with ADH preparations is associated with adverse effects, including
   a. constipation and paralytic ileus.
   b. cholecystitis and bile obstruction.
   c. nocturia and bed wetting.
   d. "hangover" symptoms, including headache, sweating, and tremors.

8. A patient who is receiving an ADH preparation for diabetes insipidus may need instruction in administering the drug
   a. PO or IM.
   b. PO or intranasally.
   c. PR or PO.
   d. intranasally or by dermal patch.

MULTIPLE RESPONSE

Select all that apply.

1. Octreotide (*Sandostatin*) would be the drug of choice in the treatment of acromegaly in a client with which of the following conditions?
   a. Diabetes
   b. Gallbladder disease
   c. Adrenal insufficiency
   d. Hypothalamic lesions
   e. Intolerance to other therapies
   f. Acromegaly in a client older than the age of 18 years

2. A father brought his 15-year-old son to the endocrine clinic because the boy was only 5 feet tall. He wanted his son to receive GH therapy because short stature would be a detriment to his success as an adult. The boy would be considered for this therapy under which of the following circumstances?
   a. If he were against the use of cadaver parts
   b. If his epiphyses were closed
   c. If his GH levels were very low
   d. If he were also diabetic
   e. If he had chronic renal failure
   f. If he had hypothyroidism

BIBLIOGRAPHY AND REFERENCES

Andrews, M., & Boyle, J. (2012). *Transcultural concepts in nursing care* (6th ed.). Philadelphia, PA: Lippincott Williams & Wilkins.

Brunton, L., Chabner, B., & Knollman, B. (2011). *Goodman and Gilman's the pharmacological basis of therapeutics* (12th ed.). New York: McGraw-Hill.

Facts and Comparisons. (2015). *Drug facts and comparisons*. St. Louis, MO: Author.

Hall, J. (2015). *Guyton and Hall's textbook of medical physiology* (13th ed.). Philadelphia, PA: Saunders

John, C. A., & Day, M. W. (2012). Central neurogenic diabetes insipidus, syndrome of inappropriate secretion of ADH, cerebral salt-wasting syndrome in traumatic brain injury. *Critical Care Nurse, 32*(2), e1–e7.

Karch, A. M. (2014). *Lippincott's nursing drug guide*. Philadelphia, PA: Lippincott Williams & Wilkins.

Lavin, N. (2009). *Manual of endocrinology and metabolism*. Philadelphia, PA: Lippincott Williams & Wilkins.

Melmed, S., Polonsky, K., Reed, P., et al. (2011). *Williams textbook of endocrinology* (12th ed.). Philadelphia, PA: Saunders.

The Medical Letter. (2015). *The medical letter on drugs and therapeutics*. New Rochelle, NY: Author.

Porth, C. (2013). *Pathophysiology: Concepts of altered health states* (9th ed.). Philadelphia, PA: Lippincott Williams & Wilkins.

Reichlin, S. (2012). *The neurohypophysis: Physiological and clinical aspects*. New York: Springer.

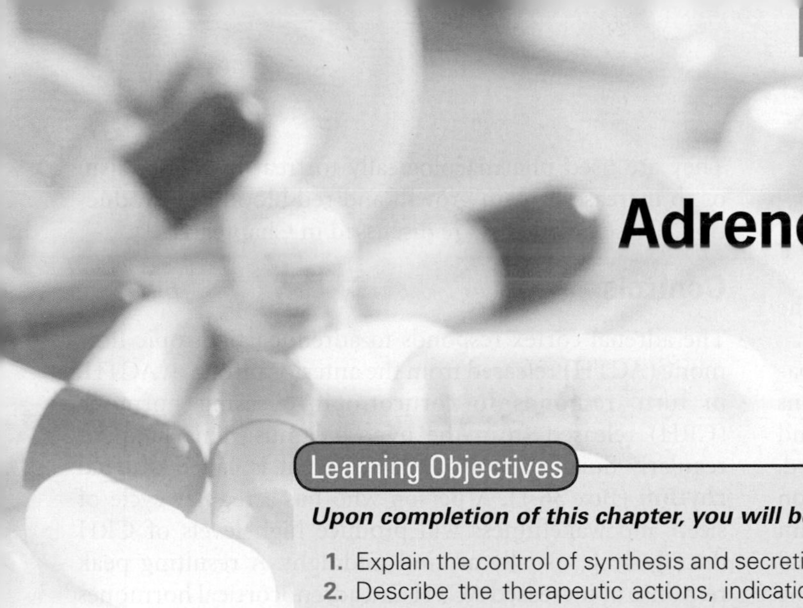

36 Adrenocortical Agents

Learning Objectives

Upon completion of this chapter, you will be able to:

1. Explain the control of synthesis and secretion, and physiological effects of the adrenocortical agents.
2. Describe the therapeutic actions, indications, pharmacokinetics, contraindications, most common adverse reactions, and important drug–drug interactions associated with the adrenocortical agents.
3. Discuss the use of adrenocortical agents across the lifespan.
4. Compare and contrast the prototype drugs prednisone and fludrocortisone with other adrenocortical agents.
5. Outline the nursing considerations, including important teaching points, for patients receiving an adrenocortical agent.

Glossary of Key Terms

adrenal cortex: outer layer of the adrenal gland; produces glucocorticoids and mineralocorticoids in response to adrenocorticotropic hormone (ACTH) stimulation; also responds to sympathetic stimulation

adrenal medulla: inner layer of the adrenal gland; a sympathetic ganglion, it releases norepinephrine and epinephrine into circulation in response to sympathetic stimulation

corticosteroids: steroid hormones produced by the adrenal cortex; include androgens, glucocorticoids, and mineralocorticoids

diurnal rhythm: response of the hypothalamus and then the pituitary and adrenals to wakefulness and sleeping; normally, the hypothalamus begins secretion of corticotropin-releasing factor (CRF) in the evening, peaking at about midnight; adrenocortical peak response is between 6 and 9 AM; levels fall during the day until evening, when the low level is picked up by the hypothalamus and CRF secretion begins again

glucocorticoids: steroid hormones released from the adrenal cortex; they increase blood glucose levels, fat deposits, and protein breakdown for energy

mineralocorticoids: steroid hormones released by the adrenal cortex; they cause sodium and water retention and potassium excretion

Drug List

Adrenocortical Agents

Glucocorticoids
beclomethasone
betamethasone
budesonide
cortisone
dexamethasone
flunisolide
hydrocortisone
methylprednisolone
prednisolone
(P) prednisone
triamcinolone

Mineralocorticoids
cortisone
(P) fludrocortisone
hydrocortisone

Adrenocortical agents are widely used to suppress the immune system and help people to feel better. These drugs do not, however, cure any inflammatory disorders. Once widely used to treat a number of chronic problems, adrenocortical agents are now reserved for short-term use to relieve inflammation during acute stages of illness or for replacement therapy to maintain hormone levels when the adrenal glands are not functioning adequately.

The Adrenal Glands

The two adrenal glands are flattened bodies that sit on top of each kidney. Each gland is made up of an inner core called the adrenal medulla and an outer shell called the adrenal cortex.

The **adrenal medulla** is actually part of the sympathetic nervous system (SNS). It is a ganglion of neurons that releases the neurotransmitters norepinephrine and epinephrine into circulation when the SNS is stimulated. (See Chapter 29 for a review of the SNS.) The secretion of these neurotransmitters directly into the bloodstream allows them to act as hormones, traveling from the adrenal medulla to react with specific receptor sites throughout the body. This is thought to be a backup system for the sympathetic system, adding an extra stimulus to the fight-or-flight response.

The **adrenal cortex** surrounds the medulla and consists of three layers of cells, each of which synthesizes chemically different types of steroid hormones that exert physiological effects throughout the body. The adrenal cortex produces hormones called **corticosteroids**. There are three types of corticosteroids: androgens, glucocorticoids, and mineralocorticoids. Androgens are a form of the male sex hormone testosterone, both men and women produce these hormones. They affect electrolytes, stimulate protein production, and decrease protein breakdown. They are used pharmacologically to treat hypogonadism or to increase protein growth and red blood cell production. These hormones are discussed in Chapter 41.

Controls

The adrenal cortex responds to adrenocorticotropic hormone (ACTH) released from the anterior pituitary. ACTH, in turn, responds to corticotropin-releasing hormone (CRH) released from the hypothalamus. This happens regularly during a normal day in what is called **diurnal rhythm** (Box 36.1). A person who has a regular cycle of sleep and wakefulness will produce high levels of CRH during sleep, usually around midnight. A resulting peak response of increased ACTH and adrenocortical hormones occurs sometime early in the morning, around 6 to 9 AM. This high level of hormones then suppresses any further CRH or ACTH release. The corticosteroids are metabolized and excreted slowly throughout the day and fall to low levels by evening. At this point the hypothalamus and pituitary sense low levels of the hormones and begin the production and release of CRH and ACTH again. This peaks around midnight, and the cycle starts again. It is thought that this diurnal rhythm is partly in response to exposure to light. People who work night shifts and have a different exposure to light cycling do not have the same diurnal schedule as people who are awake in daylight and sleep at night.

BOX 36.1 FOCUS ON The Evidence

Diurnal Rhythm

Research over the years has shown that the adrenocortical hormones are released in a pattern called the diurnal rhythm. The secretion of CRH, ACTH, and cortisol are high in the morning in day-oriented people (those who have a regular cycle of wakefulness during the day and sleep during the night). In such individuals the peak levels of cortisol usually come between 6 and 8 AM. The levels then fall off slowly (with periodic spurts) and reach a low in the late evening, with lowest levels around midnight. Clinically you can see this action. In the morning, most patients will not have a fever because the high levels of corticosteroid block inflammation and immunity, the reactions that cause an increase in body temperature. As the day progresses and the evening shift comes on the fevers rise. This is because the dropping corticosteroids allow the inflammatory and immune systems to get back into action and fevers occur. It is thought that this cycle is related to the effects of sleeping on the hypothalamus and that the hypothalamus is regulating its stimulation of the anterior pituitary in relation to sleep and activity. The cycle may also be connected to the hypothalamic response to light. This is important to keep in mind when treating patients with corticosteroids. In order to mimic the normal diurnal pattern, corticosteroids should be taken immediately on awakening in the morning.

Complications to this pattern arise, however, when patients work shifts or change their sleeping patterns (e.g., college students). In response, the hypothalamus shifts its release of CRH to correspond to the new cycle. For instance, if a person works all night and goes to bed at 8 AM, arising at 3 PM to carry on the day's activities before going to work at 11 PM the hypothalamus will release CRH at about 3 PM in accordance with the new sleep–wake cycle. It usually takes 2 or 3 days for the hypothalamus to readjust. A patient on this schedule who is taking replacement corticosteroids would then need to take them at 3 PM, or on arising. Patients who work several different shifts in a single week may not have time to reregulate their hypothalamus, and the corticosteroid cycle may be thrown off. Patients who have to change their sleep patterns repeatedly often complain about feeling weak, getting sick more easily, or having trouble concentrating. College students frequently develop a pattern of sleeping all day, then staying up all night—a cycle that becomes hard to break as their bodies and endocrine systems try to readjust.

In nursing practice, it is a challenge to help patients understand how the body works and to offer ways to decrease the stress of changing sleep patterns—especially if the nurse is also working several different shifts. Many employers are willing to have employees work several days of the same shift before switching back, mainly because they have noticed an increase in productivity and a decrease in absences when employees have enough time to allow their bodies to adjust to the new shift.

Activation of the stress reaction through the SNS bypasses the usual diurnal rhythm and causes release of ACTH and secretion of the adrenocortical hormones—an important aspect of the stress ("fight-or-flight") response. The stress response is activated with cellular injury or when a person perceives fear or feels anxious. These hormones have many actions, including the following:

- Increasing the blood volume (aldosterone effect)
- Causing the release of glucose for energy
- Slowing the rate of protein production (which preserves energy)
- Blocking the activities of the inflammatory and immune systems (which preserves a great deal of energy)

These actions are important during an acute stress situation, but they can cause adverse reactions in periods of extreme or prolonged stress. For instance, a postoperative patient who is very fearful and stressed may not heal well because protein building is blocked; infections may be hard to treat in such a patient because the inflammatory and immune systems are not functioning adequately.

Aldosterone is also released without ACTH stimulation when the blood surrounding the adrenal gland is high in potassium, a direct stimulus for aldosterone release. Aldosterone causes the kidneys to reabsorb sodium with a resultant excretion of potassium to restore homeostasis.

Adrenal Excess

Excessive adrenocortical excretion results in a disorder called Cushing disease or Cushing syndrome (Box 36.2). This could be the result of an adrenal hyperplasia or tumor, an ACTH secreting tumor, or an early sign of excessive administration of exogenous steroids. The person with this disorder often presents with a moon-like face, central obesity, hypertension, protein breakdown, osteoporosis, and females develop hirsutism (Table 36.1).

Adrenal Insufficiency

Some patients experience a shortage of adrenocortical hormones and develop signs of adrenal insufficiency (Table 36.1). This can occur when a patient does not produce enough ACTH, when the adrenal glands are not able to respond to ACTH, when an adrenal gland is damaged and cannot produce enough hormones (as in Addison's disease), or secondary to surgical removal of the glands.

A more common cause of adrenal insufficiency is prolonged use of corticosteroid hormones. When exogenous corticosteroids are used, they act to negate the regular feedback systems (Figure 36.1). The adrenal glands begin to atrophy because ACTH release is suppressed by the exogenous hormones, so the glands are no longer stimulated to produce or secrete hormones. It takes several weeks to recover from the atrophy caused by this lack of stimulation. To prevent this from happening, patients should receive only short-term steroid therapy and should be weaned slowly from the hormones so that the adrenals have time to recover and start producing hormones again.

BOX 36.2

Cushing Disease Alternative Therapy

In 2015 the U.S. Food and Drug Administration approved pasireotide diaspartate (*Signifor*) for the treatment of adults with Cushing disease for whom pituitary surgery is not an option or for whom pituitary surgery was not curative. This drug is a somatostatin analog. A somatostatin is also known as a growth hormone inhibitor. The drug binds to somatostatin receptors. Corticotroph tumor cells from Cushing disease patients usually overexpress certain somatostatin receptors; activating these leads to inhibition of ACTH secretion and lowering of cortisol secretion within the adrenal gland. The drug is given subcutaneously twice a day with dosing adjusted based on patient response. It is absorbed slowly, metabolized in the liver and kidneys and excreted mainly in the feces. It has a half-life of 12 hours. There is a risk of hypocortisolism, hyperglycemia and diabetes, bradycardia and prolonged QT intervals. Liver function impairment and gall stones have also been reported.

Table 36.1 Signs and Symptoms of Adrenal Dysfunction

Clinical Effects	Hypoadrenal Function (Addison's Syndrome)	Hyperadrenal Function (Cushing Disease)
CNS	Confusion, disorientation	Emotional disturbances
CV system	Hypotension, arrhythmias, CV collapse, loss of extracellular fluid	Cardiac hypertrophy, hypertension
Skin, hair, nails	Hyperpigmentation, sparse axillary and pubic hair; bluish-black oral mucosa	Thin, wrinkled skin; purpura; purple abdominal striae; hirsutism
Metabolic rate	Hyponatremia, hyperkalemia, hypoglycemia; lethargy, fatigue, weakness	Hyperglycemia, hypokalemia; hypernatremia; osteoporosis; renal calculi; amenorrhea
General	Dehydration, fatigue, poor response to stress, limited ability to respond to infection	Moon face; buffalo hump; obesity; immune and inflammatory suppression; risk of gastric ulcers and bleeding

CNS, central nervous system; CV, cardiovascular.

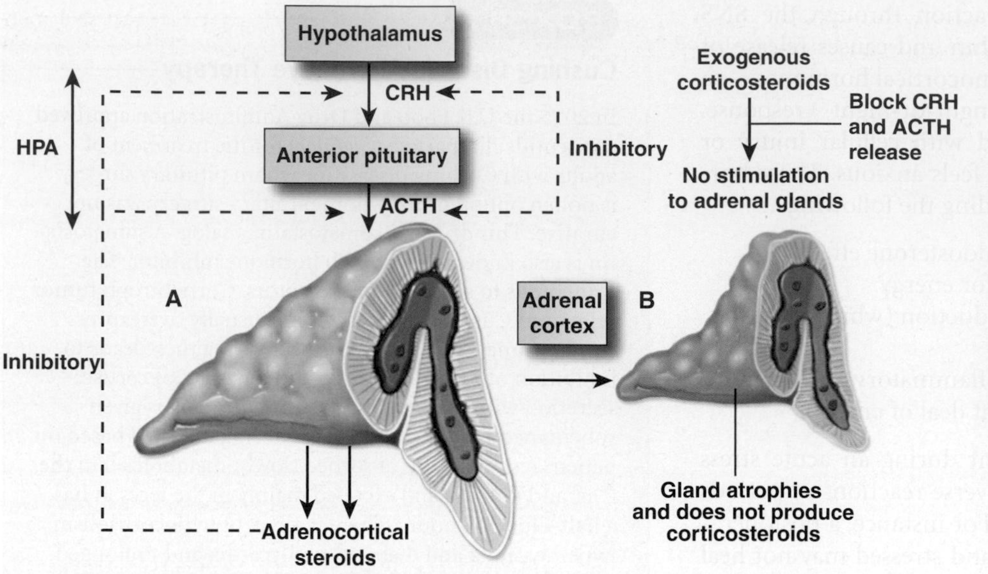

FIGURE 36.1 **A:** Normal controls of adrenal gland. The hypothalamus releases corticotropin-releasing hormone (CRH), which causes release of corticotropin (ACTH) from the anterior pituitary. ACTH stimulates the adrenal cortex to produce and release corticosteroids. Increasing levels of corticosteroids inhibit the release of CRH and ACTH. **B:** Exogenous corticosteroids act to inhibit CRH and ACTH release; the adrenal cortex is no longer stimulated and atrophies. Sudden stopping of steroids results in a crisis of adrenal hypofunction until hypothalamic–pituitary axis controls stimulate the adrenal gland again.

Adrenal Crisis

Patients who have an adrenal insufficiency may do quite well until they experience a period of extreme stress, such as a motor vehicle accident, a surgical procedure, or a massive infection. Because they are not able to supplement the energy-consuming effects of the sympathetic reaction, they enter an adrenal crisis, which can include physiological exhaustion, hypotension, fluid shift, shock, and even death. Patients in adrenal crisis are treated with massive infusion of replacement steroids, constant monitoring, and life support procedures.

KEY POINTS

- There are two adrenal glands, one on top of each kidney.
- Each adrenal gland is composed of the adrenal medulla and the adrenal cortex.
- Corticosteroids help the body to conserve energy for the fight-or-flight response, and help to maintain fluid balance.
- Prolonged use of corticosteroids suppresses the normal hypothalamic–pituitary axis and leads to adrenal atrophy from lack of stimulation.

Adrenocortical Agents

There are three types of corticosteroids: Androgens (discussed in Chapter 41), glucocorticoids, and mineralocorticoids. Not all adrenocortical agents are classified as only glucocorticoids or mineralocorticoids. Hydrocortisone, cortisone, and prednisone have glucocorticoid and some mineralocorticoid activity and affect potassium, sodium, and water levels in the body when present in high levels (Table 36.2). Box 36.3 discusses

Table 36.2 Selected Corticosteroids: Equivalent Strength, Glucocorticoid and Mineralocorticoid Effects, and Duration of Effects

Drug	Equivalent Dose (mg)	Glucocorticoid Effects	Mineralocorticoid Effects	Duration of Effects (h)
Short-Acting Corticosteroids				
cortisone	25	+	++++	8–12
hydrocortisone	20	+	++++	8–12
Intermediate-Acting Corticosteroids				
prednisone	5	++++	++	18–36
prednisolone	5	++++	++	18–36
triamcinolone	4	+++++	—	18–36
methylprednisolone	4	+++++	—	18–36
Long-Acting Corticosteroids				
dexamethasone	0.75	+++++++++	—	36–54
betamethasone	0.75	+++++++++	—	35–54

BOX 36.3 FOCUS ON Drug Therapy Across the Lifespan

Corticosteroids

CHILDREN

Corticosteroids are used in children for the same indications as in adults. The dose for children is determined by the severity of the condition being treated and the response to the drug—not on a weight or age formula.

Children need to be monitored closely for any effects on growth and development, and dose adjustments should be made or drug discontinued if growth is severely retarded.

Topical use of corticosteroids should be limited in children; because their body surface area is comparatively large, the amount of the drug absorbed in relation to weight is greater than in an adult. Apply sparingly and do not use in the presence of open lesions. Do not occlude treated areas with dressings or diapers, which may increase the risk of systemic absorption.

Children need to be supervised when using nasal sprays or respiratory inhalants to ensure that proper technique is being used.

Children receiving long-term therapy should be protected from exposure to infection, and special precautions should be instituted to avoid injury. If injuries or infections do occur the child should be seen by a primary care provider as soon as possible.

ADULTS

Adults should be reminded of the importance of taking these drugs in the morning to approximate diurnal rhythm.

They should also be cautioned about the importance of tapering the drug rather than stopping abruptly.

Several over-the-counter topical preparations contain corticosteroids, and adults should be cautioned to avoid combining these preparations with prescription topical corticosteroids. They also should be cautioned to apply any of these sparingly and to avoid applying them to open lesions or excoriated areas.

With long-term therapy the importance of avoiding exposure to infection—crowded areas, people with colds or the flu, activities associated with injury—should be stressed. If an injury or infection should occur the patient should be encouraged to seek medical care. Monitoring blood glucose levels should be done regularly.

These drugs should not be used during pregnancy because they cross the placenta and could cause adverse effects on the fetus. If the benefit to the mother clearly outweighs the potential risk to the fetus, they should be used with caution. Nursing mothers should find another method of feeding the baby if corticosteroids are needed because of the potential for serious adverse effects on the baby.

OLDER ADULTS

Older adults are more likely to experience the adverse effects associated with these drugs, and the dose should be reduced and the patient monitored very closely. Older adults are more likely to have hepatic and/or renal impairment, which could lead to accumulation of drug and resultant toxic effects. They are also more likely to have medical conditions that could be imbalanced by changes in fluid and electrolytes, metabolism changes, and other drug effects. Such conditions include diabetes, heart failure, osteoporosis, coronary artery disease, and immune suppression. Careful monitoring of drug dose and response to the drug should be done on a regular basis.

their use in different age groups. Figure 36.2 displays the sites of action of the glucocorticoids and the mineralocorticoids.

Glucocorticoids

Glucocorticoids (Table 36.3) are so named because they stimulate an increase in glucose levels for energy. They also increase the rate of protein breakdown and decrease the rate of protein formation from amino acids, another way of preserving energy. Glucocorticoids also cause lipogenesis, or the formation and storage of fat in the body. This stored fat will then be available to be broken down for energy when needed.

Several glucocorticoids are available for pharmacological use. They differ mainly by route of administration and duration of action. Glucocorticoids include beclomethasone (*Beconase AQ*), betamethasone (*Celestone Soluspan*, and others), budesonide (*Rhinocort*, *Entocort EC*), cortisone (generic), dexamethasone (generic), flunisolide (generic), hydrocortisone (*Cortef*, and others), methylprednisolone (*Medrol*), prednisolone (*Omnipred*, *Pred Forte*, and others), prednisone (*Rayos*), and triamcinolone (*Kenalog*, and others).

Therapeutic Actions and Indications

Glucocorticoids enter target cells and bind to cytoplasmic receptors, initiating many complex reactions that are responsible for anti-inflammatory and immunosuppressive effects. Hydrocortisone, cortisone, and prednisone also have some mineralocorticoid activity and affect potassium, sodium, and water levels in the body.

Glucocorticoids are indicated for the short-term treatment of many inflammatory disorders, to relieve discomfort, and to give the body a chance to heal from the effects of inflammation. They block the actions of arachidonic acid, which leads to a decrease in the formation of prostaglandins and leukotrienes. Without these chemicals the normal inflammatory reaction is blocked. They also impair the ability of phagocytes to leave the bloodstream and move to injured tissues, and they inhibit the ability of lymphocytes to act within the immune system, including

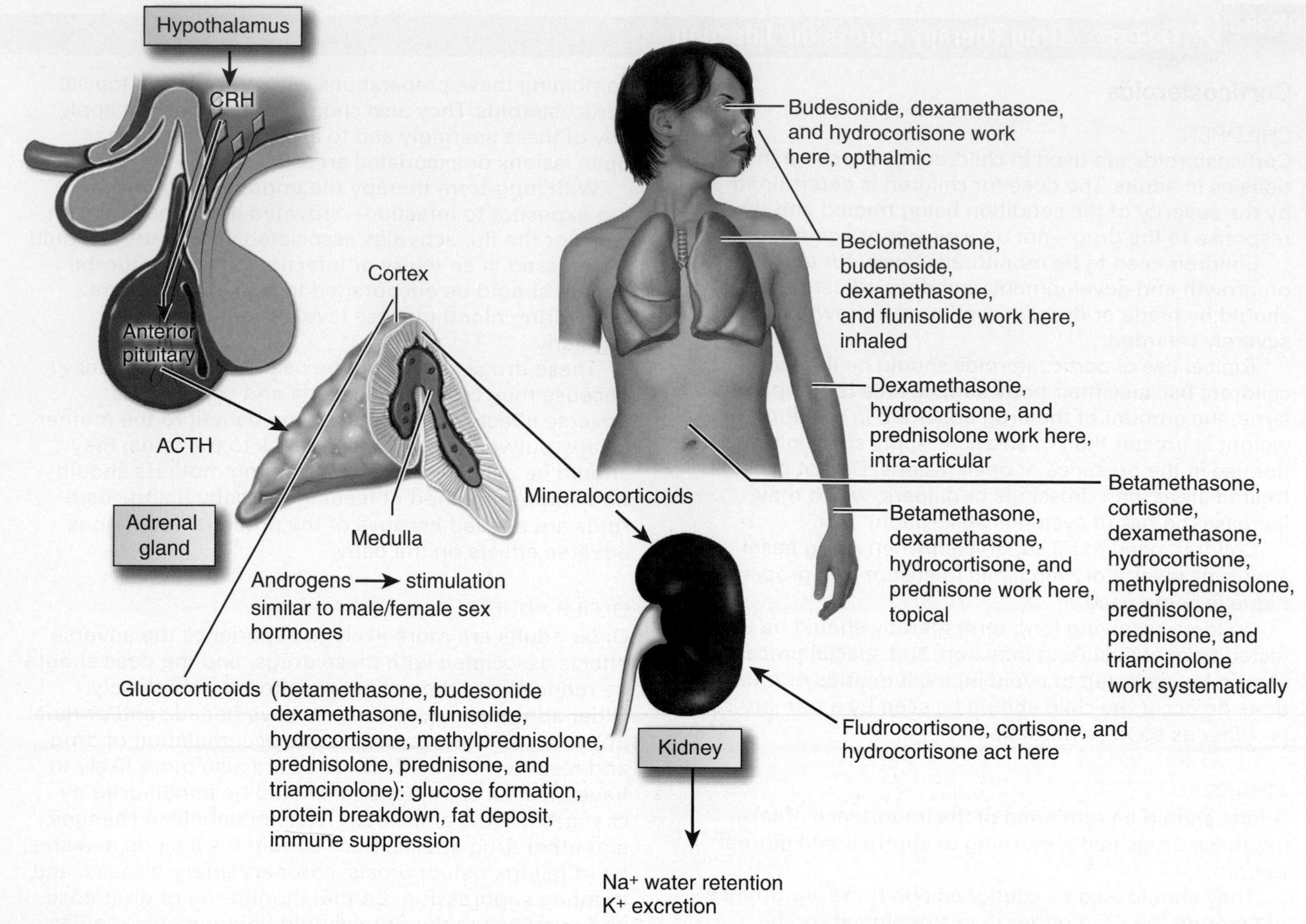

FIGURE 36.2 Sites of action of the adrenocortical agents.

Table 36.3 *Drugs in Focus:* Adrenocortical Agents

Drug Name	Dosage/Route	Usual Indications
Glucocorticoids		
beclomethasone (*Beconase AQ*)	Nasal spray, respiratory inhalant *Adult:* Two inhalations (84–168 mcg) t.i.d. to q.i.d. for respiratory inhalant; one inhalation (42–84 mcg) in each nostril b.i.d. to q.i.d. for nasal spray *Pediatric (6–12 y):* One or two inhalations t.i.d. to q.i.d. for respiratory inhalant *Pediatric (>12 y):* One inhalation in each nostril b.i.d. to q.i.d. for nasal spray	Blocking inflammation in the respiratory tract
betamethasone (*Celestone Soluspan*)	Oral, IM, IV, intra-articular, topical *Adult:* 0.6–7.2 mg/d PO, up to 9 mg/d IV, 0.5–9.0 mg/d IM; apply topical preparation sparingly *Pediatric:* Individualize dose based on severity and response and monitor closely	Management of allergic intra-articular, topical, and inflammatory disorders
budesonide (*Rhinocort, Entocort EC*)	Intranasal *Adult and pediatric (>6 y):* 256 mcg/d given as two sprays in each nostril AM and PM *Pediatric (12 mo–8 y):* 0.5–1 mg once daily in two divided doses using jet nebulizer	Relief of symptoms of seasonal and allergic rhinitis with few side effects, maintenance treatment of asthma, as an oral agent for the treatment of mild-to-moderate active Crohn's disease
cortisone	Oral, IM *Adult:* 25–300 mg/d PO; 20–330 mg IM *Pediatric:* Base dose on response, monitor patient closely	Replacement therapy in adrenal insufficiency, treatment of allergic and inflammatory disorders

Drug Name	Dosage/Route	Usual Indications
Glucocorticoids		
dexamethasone (generic)	Oral, IV, IM, inhalation, intranasal, ophthalmic, topical *Adult and pediatric:* Individualize dose based on response and severity: 0.75–9 mg/d PO, 8–16 mg/d IM, 0.5–9 mg/d IV, two to three inhalations per day for inhalation, one to two sprays in each nostril b.i.d. for nasal spray, 1 drop (gtt) t.i.d. to q.i.d. for ophthalmic solutions; apply topical preparation sparingly	Management of allergic and topical inflammatory disorders, adrenal hypofunction
flunisolide (generic)	Inhalant, intranasal *Adult:* 50–200 mcg intranasal b.i.d. 640 mcg/d via inhalation *Pediatric:* 2 mg/d *AeroBid*; 160 mcg b.i.d. *Aerospan*	Control of bronchial asthma, relief of symptoms of seasonal and allergic rhinitis
hydrocortisone (*Cortef*)	Oral, IV, IM, topical, ophthalmic, rectal, intra-articular *Adult:* 100–500 mg IM or IV q2–6 h, 100 mg half-strength by retention enema for 21 d, one applicator-full daily to b.i.d. intrarectal; apply topical sparingly; 5–20 mg/d PO based on response *Pediatric:* 20–240 mg/d PO, IM, or subcutaneously; 100 mg half-strength by retention enema for 21 d; one applicator-full daily to b.i.d. intrarectal; apply topical sparingly; 5–20 mg/d PO based on response	Replacement therapy, treatment of allergic and inflammatory disorders
methylprednisolone (*Medrol*)	Oral, IV, IM, intra-articular *Adult:* 40–120 mg/d PO or IM, 10–40 mg IV slowly *Pediatric:* Base dose on severity and response	Treatment of allergic and inflammatory disorders
prednisolone (*Omnipred, Pred Forte*)	Oral, IV, IM, ophthalmic, intra-articular *Adult:* 5–60 mg/d PO, 4–60 mg IM or IV, 1–2 gtt in affected eye t.i.d. to q.i.d. *Pediatric:* Base dose on severity and response	Treatment of allergic and inflammatory disorders
prednisone (*Rayos*)	Oral *Adult:* 0.1–0.15 mg/kg/d PO *Pediatric:* Base dose on severity and response	Replacement therapy for adrenal insufficiency, treatment of allergic and inflammatory disorders
triamcinolone (*Kenalog*)	Oral, IM, inhalant, intra-articular, topical *Adult:* 4–60 mg/d PO, 2.5–60 mg/d IM, two inhalations t.i.d. to q.i.d. *Pediatric:* Individualize dose based on severity and response *Pediatric (6–12 y):* One to two inhalations t.i.d. to q.i.d.	Treatment of allergic and inflammatory disorders, management of asthma; treatment of adrenal insufficiency when combined with a mineralocorticoid
(*Triesence*)	4 mg by ocular injection, 1–4 mg intravitreally for visualization	Treatment of sympathetic ophthalmia, temporal arteritis, uveitis; visualization during vitrectomy
Mineralocorticoids		
cortisone (generic)	Oral, IM *Adult:* 25–300 mg/d PO *or* 20–330 mg/d IM *Pediatric:* Base dose on severity and response	Used for replacement therapy in adrenal insufficiency, treatment of allergic and inflammatory disorders
fludrocortisone (generic)	*Adult:* 0.1–0.2 mg/d PO	Used for replacement therapy and treatment of salt-losing adrenogenital syndrome with a glucocorticoid, not recommended for children, being tried for treatment of severe orthostatic hypotension because sodium and water retention effects can lead to increased blood pressure
hydrocortisone (*Cortef*)	Oral, IV, IM, topical, ophthalmic, rectal, intra-articular *Adult:* 20–240 mg/d PO, 100–500 mg IM or IV q2–6 h, 100-mg half-strength by retention enema, one applicator-full rectal foam q.i.d. to b.i.d.; apply topical preparation sparingly *Pediatric:* Base dose on response and severity, 20–240 mg/d PO, 20–240 mg/d IM or subcutaneous, 100-mg half-strength by retention enema, one applicator-full rectal foam q.i.d. to b.i.d.; apply topical preparation sparingly	Used for replacement therapy, treatment of allergic and inflammatory disorders

a blocking of the production of antibodies. They can be used to treat local inflammation as topical agents, intranasal or inhaled agents, intra-articular injections, and ophthalmic agents. Systemic use is indicated for the treatment of some cancers, hypercalcemia associated with cancer, hematological disorders, and some neurological infections. When combined with mineralocorticoids, some of these drugs can be used in replacement therapy for adrenal insufficiency. See Table 36.3 for information on each type of glucocorticoid agent.

Pharmacokinetics

These drugs are absorbed well from many sites. They are metabolized by natural systems, mostly within the liver, and are excreted in the urine. The glucocorticoids are known to cross the placenta and to enter breast milk; they should be used during pregnancy and lactation only if the benefits to the mother clearly outweigh the potential risks to the fetus or neonate.

Beclomethasone and flunisolide are available in the form of a respiratory inhalant and nasal spray.

Betamethasone is a long-acting steroid available for systemic, parenteral use in acute situations, as well as orally and as a topical application.

Budesonide is available for intranasal use.

Cortisone is used orally and parenterally.

Dexamethasone and triamcinolone are available in multiple forms for dermatological, ophthalmological, intra-articular, parenteral, and inhalational uses. They peak quickly, and effects can last for 2 to 3 days.

Hydrocortisone has largely been replaced for other uses (e.g., intra-articular, IV) by other steroid hormones with less mineralocorticoid effect. It may be preferred for use as a topical or ophthalmic agent.

Methylprednisolone is available in multiple forms, including oral, parenteral, intra-articular, and retention enema preparations.

Prednisolone is an intermediate-acting corticosteroid with effects lasting only a day or so. It is used for intralesional and intra-articular injection and is also available in oral and topical forms.

Prednisone is available only as an oral agent.

Contraindications and Cautions

These drugs are contraindicated in the presence of any known allergy to any steroid preparation *to avoid hypersensitivity reactions*; in the presence of an acute infection, *which could become serious or even fatal if the immune and inflammatory responses are blocked*; and with lactation *because the anti-inflammatory and immunosuppressive actions could be passed to the baby.*

Caution should be used in patients with diabetes *because the glucose-elevating effects disrupt glucose control*; with acute peptic ulcers *because steroid use is associated with the development of ulcers*; with other endocrine disorders, *which could be sent into imbalance*; and in pregnancy *because of the potential for adverse effects on the fetus.*

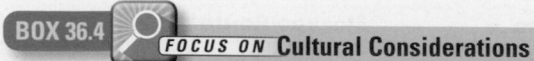

BOX 36.4 FOCUS ON Cultural Considerations

Steroid Toxicity in African Americans

African Americans develop increased toxicity to the corticosteroid methylprednisolone—particularly when it is used for immunosuppression after renal transplantation. This toxicity can include severe steroid-induced diabetes mellitus. African Americans are almost four times as likely as White Americans to develop end-stage renal disease, so this complication is not an unusual problem. If an African American patient is being treated with methylprednisolone, extreme care should be taken to adjust doses appropriately and to treat adverse effects as they arise.

Adverse Effects

Methylprednisolone is associated with increased toxicity in African Americans (Box 36.4). Children are at risk for growth retardation associated with suppression of the hypothalamic–pituitary system. Additional adverse effects associated with the glucocorticoids are related to the route of administration that is used. Local use is associated with local inflammations and infections, as well as burning and stinging sensations.

FOCUS ON Safe Medication Administration

Adverse Effects of Corticosteroid Use Associated with Various Routes of Administration

Systemic: *Systemic effects are most likely to occur when the corticosteroid is given by the oral, IV, IM, or subcutaneous route. Systemic absorption is possible, however, if other routes of administration are not used correctly or if tissue breakdown or injury allows direct absorption.*

Central nervous system (CNS): *Vertigo, headache, paresthesias, insomnia, convulsions, psychosis*

Gastrointestinal: *Peptic or esophageal ulcers, pancreatitis, abdominal distention, nausea, vomiting, increased appetite, weight gain*

Cardiovascular: *Hypotension, shock, heart failure secondary to fluid retention, thromboembolism, thrombophlebitis, fat embolism, arrhythmias secondary to electrolyte disturbances*

Hematological: *Sodium and fluid retention, hypokalemia, hypocalcemia, increased blood sugar, increased serum cholesterol, decreased thyroid hormone levels*

Musculoskeletal: *Muscle weakness, steroid myopathy, loss of muscle mass, osteoporosis, spontaneous fractures*

Eyes, ears, nose, and throat: *Cataracts, glaucoma*

Dermatological: *Frail skin, petechiae, ecchymoses, purpura, striae, subcutaneous fat atrophy*

Endocrine: *Amenorrhea, irregular menses, growth retardation, decreased carbohydrate tolerance, diabetes*

Other: *Immunosuppression, aggravation or masking of infections, impaired wound healing, suppression of hypothalamic–pituitary axis*

Intramuscular repository injections: *Atrophy at the injection site*
Retention enema: *Local pain, burning; rectal bleeding*
Intra-articular injection: *Osteonecrosis, tendon rupture, infection*
Intraspinal: *Meningitis, adhesive arachnoiditis, conus medullaris syndrome*
Intrathecal administration: *Arachnoiditis*
Topical: *Local burning, irritation, acneiform lesions, striae, skin atrophy*
Respiratory inhalant: *Oral, laryngeal, and pharyngeal irritation; fungal infections*
Intranasal: *Headache, nausea, nasal irritation, fungal infections, epistaxis, rebound congestion, perforation of the nasal septum, anosmia, urticaria*
Ophthalmic: *Infections, glaucoma, cataracts*
Intralesional: *Blindness when used on the face and head (rare)*

(P) Prototype Summary: Prednisone

Indications: Replacement therapy in adrenal cortical insufficiency, short-term management of various inflammatory and allergic disorders, hypercalcemia associated with cancer, hematological disorders, ulcerative colitis, acute exacerbations of multiple sclerosis, palliation in some leukemias, trichinosis with systemic involvement.

Actions: Enters target cells and binds to intracellular corticosteroid receptors, initiating many complex reactions responsible for its anti-inflammatory and immunosuppressive effects.

Pharmacokinetics:

Route	Onset	Peak	Duration
PO	Varies	1–2 h	1–1.5 d

$T_{1/2}$: 3.5 hours; metabolized in the liver and excreted in the urine.

Adverse Effects: Vertigo, headache, hypotension, shock, sodium and fluid retention, amenorrhea, increased appetite, weight gain, immunosuppression, aggravation or masking of infections, impaired wound healing.

Clinically Important Drug–Drug Interactions

Therapeutic and toxic effects increase if corticosteroids are given with erythromycin, ketoconazole, or troleandomycin. Serum levels and effectiveness may decrease if corticosteroids are combined with salicylates, barbiturates, phenytoin, or rifampin.

Nursing Considerations for Patients Receiving Glucocorticoids

Assessment: History and Examination

- Assess for history of allergy to any steroid preparations, acute infections, peptic ulcer disease, pregnancy, lactation, endocrine disturbances, and renal dysfunction, *which could be cautions or contraindications to use of the drug.*
- Assess weight; temperature; orientation and affect; grip strength; eye examination; blood pressure, pulse, peripheral perfusion, and vessel evaluation; respiration and adventitious breath sounds; glucose tolerance, renal function, serum electrolytes, and endocrine function tests as appropriate, *to determine baseline status before beginning therapy and for any potential adverse effects.*

Refer to the Critical Thinking Scenario for a full discussion of nursing care for a patient who is receiving glucocorticoids.

Nursing Diagnoses

Nursing diagnoses related to drug therapy might include the following:

- Altered cardiac output related to fluid retention
- Excess fluid volume related to water retention
- Disturbed sensory perception (visual, kinesthetic)
- Risk for infection related to immunosuppression
- Ineffective coping related to body changes caused by the drug
- Deficient knowledge regarding drug therapy
- Imbalanced nutrition: More than body requirements related to metabolic changes

Planning

- The patient will receive the best therapeutic effect from the drug therapy.
- The patient will have limited adverse effects to the drug therapy.
- The patient will have an understanding of the drug therapy, adverse effects to anticipate, and measures to relieve discomfort and improve safety

Implementation with Rationale

- Administer drug daily at 8 to 9 AM *to mimic normal peak diurnal concentration levels and thereby minimize suppression of the hypothalamic–pituitary axis.*
- Space multiple doses evenly throughout the day *to try to achieve homeostasis.*

(continues on page 600)

- Use the minimal dose for the minimal amount of time *to minimize adverse effects.*
- Taper doses when discontinuing from high doses or from long-term therapy *to give the adrenal glands a chance to recover and produce adrenocorticoids.*
- Arrange for increased dose when the patient is under stress *to supply the increased demand for corticosteroids associated with the stress reaction.*
- Use alternate day maintenance therapy with short-acting drugs whenever possible *to decrease the risk of adrenal suppression.*
- Do not give live virus vaccines when the patient is immunosuppressed *because there is an increased risk of infection.*
- Protect the patient from unnecessary exposure to infection and invasive procedures *because the steroids suppress the immune system and the patient is at increased risk for infection.*
- Assess the patient carefully for any potential drug–drug interactions *to avoid adverse effects.*
- Provide thorough patient teaching, including measures to avoid adverse effects, warning signs of problems, and the need for regular evaluation, including blood tests, *to enhance patient knowledge of drug therapy and promote compliance.* Explain the need to protect the patient from exposure to infections *to prevent serious adverse effects.*

Evaluation

- Monitor patient response to the drug (relief of signs and symptoms of inflammation, return of adrenal function to within normal limits).
- Monitor for adverse effects (increased susceptibility to infections, skin changes, endocrine dysfunctions, fatigue, fluid retention, peptic ulcer, psychological changes).
- Evaluate the effectiveness of the teaching plan (patient can name drug, dosage, adverse effects to watch for, and specific measures to avoid them).

CRITICAL THINKING SCENARIO

Adrenocortical Agents

THE SITUATION

M.W., a 48-year-old woman, was diagnosed with severe rheumatoid arthritis 7 years ago. She has been retired, on disability, from her job as an art teacher in the local high school. Her pain is no longer controlled by aspirin, and her physician ordered 5-mg prednisone three times a day. Over the next 4 weeks, M.W.'s symptoms were markedly relieved; she was able to start painting again, and she became much more mobile. She also noted that for the first time in years she felt "really good." Her appetite increased, she was no longer fatigued, and her outlook on life was markedly improved. At her follow-up visit, M.W. had gained 9 pounds; she had slight edema in both ankles, and her blood pressure was 150/92 mm Hg. An inflamed, oozing lesion was found on her right hand, which she stated became infected a few weeks ago after she cut her hand while peeling potatoes. Her range of motion and joints were markedly improved. The physician decided that M.W. was past her crisis and that the prednisone should be tapered to 5 mg/d over a 4-week period.

CRITICAL THINKING

Think about the pathophysiology of rheumatoid arthritis.

What effects did the prednisone have on the process at work in M.W.'s joints?

What effects does the adrenocorticoid steroid have on the rest of M.W.'s body?

What can be expected to occur when a patient is on prednisone for a month?

What precautions should be taken?

What nursing interventions are appropriate for M.W. at this visit?

DISCUSSION

The most urgent problem for M.W. at this time is the infected lesion on her hand.

Because steroids interfere with the normal inflammatory and immune response to infection the lesion could progress to a very serious problem. The lesion should be cultured, cleansed, and dressed. M.W. should be instructed in how to care for her hand and how to protect it from water or further injury. An antibiotic might be prescribed and then evaluated for its appropriateness when the culture report comes back.

The real nursing challenge with M.W. will be helping her to cope with and understand the need to taper her prednisone. The drug-teaching information for prednisone should be thoroughly reviewed with M.W., pointing out the side effects of drug therapy that she is already experiencing and explaining, again, the effect that prednisone has on her body. A calendar

Adrenocortical Agents (continued)

should be prepared for M.W. to help her schedule the tapering of the drug. It usually progresses from 5 mg twice daily for 2 weeks to 5 mg/d. M.W. will need a great deal of encouragement and support to cope with the decrease in therapeutic benefit caused by the need to reduce the prednisone dose. She has felt so good and done so much better while receiving the drug that she may have a real dread of losing those benefits. She should be encouraged to discuss her feelings and to call for support if she needs it. M.W. should be given an appointment for a return visit in 2 weeks to evaluate the lesion on her hand and to check her progress in the tapering of the drug. She should be urged to call if the lesion looks worse to her or if she has any difficulties with her drug therapy.

M.W.'s case is a common example of the clinical problems that are encountered when a patient with a chronic inflammatory condition begins steroid therapy. These patients require strong nursing support and continual teaching.

NURSING CARE GUIDE FOR M.W.: ADRENOCORTICAL AGENTS

Assessment: History and Examination

Assess for allergies to any steroids and for heart failure, pregnancy, hypertension, acute infection, peptic ulcer, vaccination with a live virus, or endocrine disorders.

Also assess for concurrent use of ketoconazole, troleandomycin, estrogens, barbiturates, phenytoin, rifampin, or salicylates.

Focus the physical examination on the following:

Neurological: Orientation, reflexes, affect

General: Temperature, weight, site of hand infection

Cardiovascular: Pulse, cardiac auscultation, blood pressure, edema

Respiratory: Respiratory rate, adventitious sounds

Laboratory tests: Urinalysis, blood glucose level, stool guaiac test, renal function tests, culture and sensitivity of wound specimen

Nursing Diagnoses

Decreased cardiac output related to fluid retention

Disturbed sensory perception related to CNS effects

Risk for infection related to immunosuppression

Ineffective coping related to body changes caused by drug

Excess fluid volume related to water retention

Deficient knowledge regarding drug therapy

Planning

The patient will receive the best therapeutic effect from the drug therapy.

The patient will have limited adverse effects to the drug therapy.

The patient will have an understanding of the drug therapy, adverse effects to anticipate, and measures to relieve discomfort and improve safety.

Implementation

Administer around 9 AM to mimic normal diurnal rhythm.

Use the minimal dose for the minimal period of time that the dose is needed.

Arrange for increased doses during times of stress.

Taper gradually to allow adrenal glands to recover and produce their own steroids.

Protect the patient from unnecessary exposure to infection.

Provide support and reassurance to deal with drug therapy.

Provide patient teaching regarding drug name, dosage, adverse effects, precautions, and warning signs to report.

Evaluation

Evaluate drug effects: Relief of signs and symptoms of inflammation.

Monitor for adverse effects: Infection, peptic ulcer, fluid retention, hypertension, electrolyte imbalance, or endocrine changes.

Monitor for drug–drug interactions as listed.

Evaluate the effectiveness of the patient-teaching program.

Evaluate the effectiveness of comfort and safety measures and support offered.

PATIENT TEACHING FOR M.W.

- The drug that has been prescribed for you is called prednisone. Prednisone is from a class of drugs called corticosteroids, which are similar to steroids produced naturally in your body. They affect a number of bodily functions, including your body's glucose levels, blocking your body's inflammatory and immune responses, and slowing the healing process.
- You should never stop taking your drug suddenly. If your prescription is low or you are unable to take the medication for any reason, notify your health care provider.
- Some of the following adverse effects may occur:
  - *Increased appetite:* This may be a welcome change, but if you notice a continual weight gain, you may want to watch your calories.
  - *Restlessness, trouble sleeping:* Some people experience elation and a feeling of new energy; take frequent rest periods.

(continues on page 602)

Adrenocortical Agents (continued)

- *Increased susceptibility to infection:* Because your body's normal defenses will be decreased, you should avoid crowded places and people with known infections. If you notice any signs of illness or infection, notify your health care provider at once.
- Report any of the following to your health care provider: *Sudden weight gain; fever or sore throat; black, tarry stools; swelling of the hands or feet; any signs of infection; or easy bruising.*
- If you are taking this drug for a prolonged period, limit your intake of salt and salted products and add proteins to your diet.
- Avoid the use of any over-the-counter medication without first checking with your health care provider. Several of these medications can interfere with the effectiveness of this drug.
- Tell any doctor, nurse, or other health care provider involved in your care that you are taking this drug.
- Because this drug affects your body's natural defenses, you will need special care during any stressful situations. You may want to wear or carry medical identification showing that you are taking this medication. This identification alerts any medical personnel taking care of you in an emergency to the fact that you are taking this drug.
- It is important to have regular medical follow-up. If your drug dose is being tapered, notify your health care provider if any of the following occurs: Fatigue, nausea, vomiting, diarrhea, weight loss, weakness, or dizziness.
- Keep this drug out of the reach of children. Do not give this medication to anyone else or take any similar medication that has not been prescribed for you

KEY POINTS

- The glucocorticoids increase glucose production, stimulate fat deposition and protein breakdown, and inhibit protein formation. They are used clinically to block inflammation and the immune response and in conjunction with mineralocorticoids to treat adrenal insufficiency.
- Patients receiving glucocorticoids need to be protected from exposure to infection, have their blood sugar monitored regularly and dietary changes made as needed, and will not heal well because of the blocking protein formation.

Mineralocorticoids

Mineralocorticoids (Table 36.3) affect electrolyte levels and homeostasis. These steroid hormones directly affect the levels of electrolytes in the system. The classic mineralocorticoid is aldosterone. Aldosterone holds sodium—and, with it, water—in the body and causes the excretion of potassium by acting on the renal tubule. Aldosterone is no longer available for pharmacological use. Mineralocorticoids that are available include cortisone, fludrocortisone (generic), and hydrocortisone (*Cortef*).

Therapeutic Actions and Indications

The mineralocorticoids increase sodium reabsorption in renal tubules, leading to sodium and water retention, and increase potassium excretion (see Figure 36.2). Fludrocortisone is a powerful mineralocorticoid and is preferred for replacement therapy over cortisone and hydrocortisone; it is used in combination with a glucocorticoid. Hydrocortisone and cortisone also exert mineralocorticoid effects at high doses; however, this effect usually is not enough to maintain electrolyte balance in adrenal insufficiency. These drugs are indicated (in combination with a glucocorticoid) for replacement therapy in primary and secondary adrenal insufficiency. They are also indicated for the treatment of salt-wasting adrenogenital syndrome when taken with appropriate glucocorticoids. See Table 36.3 for Usual Indications for each mineralocorticoid.

Pharmacokinetics

These drugs are absorbed slowly and distributed throughout the body. They undergo hepatic metabolism to inactive forms. They are known to cross the placenta and to enter breast milk. They should be avoided during pregnancy and lactation *because of the potential for adverse effects in the fetus or baby.*

Contraindications and Cautions

These drugs are contraindicated in the presence of any known allergy to the drug *to avoid hypersensitivity reactions*; with severe hypertension, heart failure, or cardiac disease *because of the resultant increased blood pressure*; and with lactation *due to potential adverse effects on the baby.* Caution should be used in pregnancy *because of the potential for adverse effects to the fetus*; in the presence of any infection, *which will alter adrenal response*; and with high sodium intake *because severe hypernatremia could occur.*

Adverse Effects

Adverse effects commonly associated with the use of mineralocorticoids are related to the increased fluid volume seen with sodium and water retention (e.g., headache, edema, hypertension, heart failure, arrhythmias, weakness) and possible hypokalemia (Figure 36.3). Allergic reactions, ranging from skin rash to anaphylaxis, have also been reported.

Clinically Important Drug–Drug Interactions

Decreased effectiveness of salicylates, barbiturates, hydantoins, rifampin, and anticholinesterases has been reported when these drugs are combined with mineralocorticoids. Such combinations should be avoided if possible, but if they are necessary the patient should be monitored closely and the dose increased as needed.

Ⓟ Prototype Summary: Fludrocortisone

Indications: Partial replacement therapy in cortical insufficiency conditions, treatment of salt-losing adrenogenital syndrome; off-label use: treatment of hypotension.

Actions: Increases sodium reabsorption in the renal tubules and increases potassium and hydrogen excretion, leading to water and sodium retention.

Pharmacokinetics:

Route	Onset	Peak	Duration
PO	Gradual	1.7 h	18–36 h

$T_{1/2}$: 3.5 hours; metabolized in the liver and excreted in the urine.

Adverse Effects: Frontal and occipital headaches, arthralgia, weakness, increased blood volume, edema, hypertension, heart failure, rash, anaphylaxis.

Nursing Considerations for Patients Receiving Mineralocorticoids

Assessment: History and Examination

- Assess for allergy to these drugs *to avoid hypersensitivity reactions*; history of heart failure, hypertension, or infections; high sodium intake; lactation; and pregnancy, *which could be cautions or contraindications to use of the drug.*
- Assess blood pressure, pulse, and adventitious breath sounds; weight and temperature; tissue turgor; reflexes and bilateral grip strength; and serum electrolyte levels, *to determine baseline status before beginning therapy and for any potential adverse effects.*

Nursing Diagnoses

Nursing diagnoses related to drug therapy might include the following:

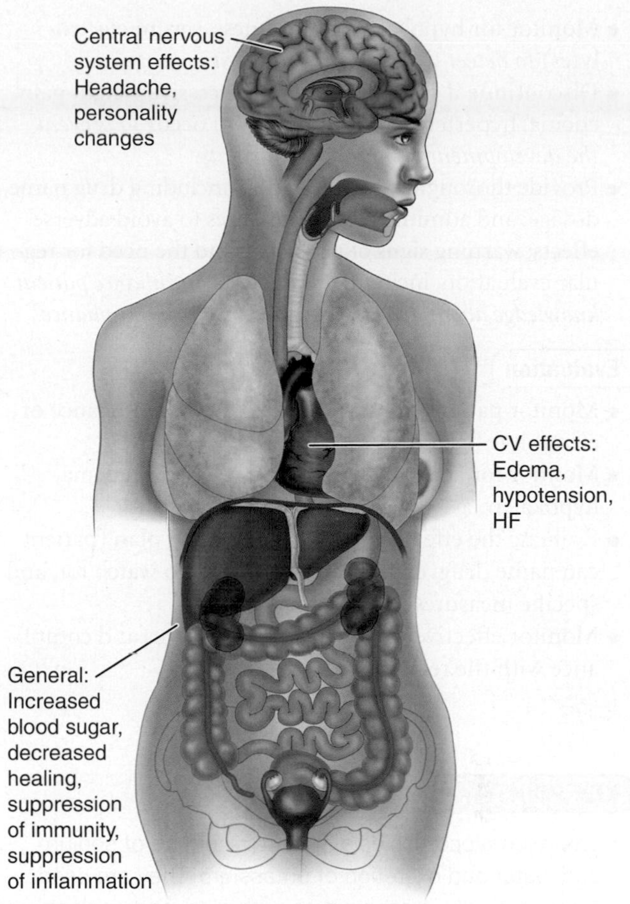

FIGURE 36.3 Variety of adverse effects and toxicities associated with adrenocortical agents.

- Imbalanced nutrition: More than body requirements related to metabolic changes
- Excess fluid volume related to sodium retention
- Impaired urinary elimination related to sodium retention
- Deficient knowledge regarding drug therapy

Planning

- The patient will receive the best therapeutic effect from the drug therapy.
- The patient will have limited adverse effects to the drug therapy.
- The patient will have an understanding of the drug therapy, adverse effects to anticipate, and measures to relieve discomfort and improve safety.

Implementation with Rationale

- Use only in conjunction with appropriate glucocorticoids to maintain control of electrolyte balance.
- Increase dose in times of stress to prevent adrenal insufficiency and to meet increased demands for corticosteroids under stress.

(continues on page 604)

- Monitor for hypokalemia (weakness, serum electrolytes) *to detect the loss early and treat appropriately.*
- Discontinue if signs of overdose (excessive weight gain, edema, hypertension, cardiomegaly) occur *to prevent the development of more severe toxicity.*
- Provide thorough patient teaching, including drug name, dosage, and administration; measures to avoid adverse effects; warning signs of problems; and the need for regular evaluation, including blood tests, *to enhance patient knowledge about drug therapy and promote compliance.*

Evaluation

- Monitor patient response to the drug (maintenance of electrolyte balance).
- Monitor for adverse effects (fluid retention, edema, hypokalemia, headache).
- Evaluate the effectiveness of the teaching plan (patient can name drug, dosage, adverse effects to watch for, and specific measures to avoid them).
- Monitor effectiveness of comfort measures and compliance with the regimen.

KEY POINTS

- The mineralocorticoids stimulate retention of sodium and water and excretion of potassium. They are used therapeutically in conjunction with glucocorticoids to treat adrenal insufficiency.
- Patients receiving mineralocorticoids need to be evaluated for possible hypokalemia and its associated cardiac effects and for fluid retention that could exacerbate heart failure and cause electrolyte abnormalities.

SUMMARY

- The adrenal medulla is basically a sympathetic nerve ganglion that releases norepinephrine and epinephrine into the bloodstream in response to sympathetic stimulation.
- The adrenal cortex produces three types of corticosteroids: Androgens (similar to male sex hormones), glucocorticoids, and mineralocorticoids.
- The corticosteroids are released normally in a diurnal rhythm, with the hypothalamus producing peak levels of CRH around midnight; peak adrenal response occurs around 9 AM. The steroid levels drop slowly during the day to reach low levels in the evening, when the hypothalamus begins CRH secretion, with peak levels again occurring around midnight. Corticosteroids are also released as part of the sympathetic stress reaction to help the body conserve energy for the fight-or-flight response.
- Prolonged use of corticosteroids suppresses the normal hypothalamic–pituitary axis and leads to adrenal atrophy from lack of stimulation. Corticosteroids need to be tapered slowly after prolonged use to allow the adrenals to resume steroid production.
- The glucocorticoids increase glucose production, stimulate fat deposition and protein breakdown, and inhibit protein formation. They are used clinically to block inflammation and the immune response and in conjunction with mineralocorticoids to treat adrenal insufficiency.
- The mineralocorticoids stimulate retention of sodium and water and excretion of potassium. They are used therapeutically in conjunction with glucocorticoids to treat adrenal insufficiency.
- Adverse effects of corticosteroids are related to exaggeration of the physiological effects; they include immunosuppression, peptic ulcer formation, fluid retention, and edema.
- Corticosteroids are used topically and locally to achieve the desired anti-inflammatory effects at a particular site without the systemic adverse effects that limit the usefulness of these drugs.

CHECK YOUR UNDERSTANDING

Answers to the questions in this chapter can be found in Answers to Check Your Understanding Questions on thePoint®.

MULTIPLE CHOICE

Select the best answer to the following.

1. Adrenocortical agents are widely used
   - a. to cure chronic inflammatory disorders.
   - b. for short-term treatment to relieve inflammation.
   - c. for long-term treatment of chronic disorders.
   - d. to relieve minor aches and pains and to make people feel better.

2. If a nurse was asked to explain the adrenal medulla to a patient, it would be appropriate for her to tell that patient that it
   - a. is the outer core of the adrenal gland.
   - b. is the site of production of aldosterone and corticosteroids.
   - c. is actually a neural ganglion of the SNS.
   - d. consists of three layers of cells that produce different hormones.

3. Glucocorticoids are hormones that
   a. are released in response to high glucose levels.
   b. help to regulate electrolyte levels.
   c. help to regulate water balance in the body.
   d. promote the preservation of energy through increased glucose levels, protein breakdown, and fat formation.

4. Diurnal rhythm in a person with a regular sleep cycle would show
   a. high levels of ACTH during the night while sleeping.
   b. rising levels of corticosteroids throughout the day.
   c. peak levels of ACTH and corticosteroids early in the morning.
   d. hypothalamic stimulation to release CRH around noon.

5. Patients who have been receiving corticosteroid therapy for a prolonged period and suddenly stop the drug will experience an adrenal crisis because their adrenal glands will not be producing any adrenal hormones. Your assessment of a patient for the possibility of adrenal crisis may include
   a. physiological exhaustion, shock, and fluid shift.
   b. acne development and hypertension.
   c. water retention and increased speed of healing.
   d. hyperglycemia and water retention.

6. A patient is started on a regimen of prednisone because of a crisis in her ulcerative colitis. Nursing care of this patient would need to include
   a. immunizations to prevent infections.
   b. increased calories to deal with metabolic changes.
   c. fluid restriction to decrease water retention.
   d. administration of the drug around 8 or 9 AM to mimic normal diurnal rhythm.

7. A patient who is taking corticosteroids is at increased risk for infection and should
   a. be protected from exposure to infections and invasive procedures.
   b. take anti-inflammatory agents regularly throughout the day.
   c. receive live virus vaccine to protect him or her from infection.
   d. be at no risk if elective surgery is needed.

8. Mineralocorticoids are used to maintain electrolyte balance in situations of adrenal insufficiency. Mineralocorticoids
   a. are usually given alone.
   b. can be given only IV.
   c. are always given in conjunction with appropriate glucocorticoids.
   d. are separate in their function from the glucocorticoids.

MULTIPLE RESPONSE

Select all that apply.

1. Patients who are taking corticosteroids would be expected to report which of the following?
   a. Weight gain
   b. Round or "moon face" appearance
   c. Feeling of well-being
   d. Weight loss
   e. Excessive hair growth
   f. Fragile skin

2. Corticosteroid hormones are released during a sympathetic stress reaction. They would act to do which of the following?
   a. Increase blood volume
   b. Cause the release of glucose for energy
   c. Increase the rate of protein production
   d. Block the effects of the inflammatory and immune systems
   e. Store glucose to preserve energy
   f. Block protein production to save energy

BIBLIOGRAPHY AND REFERENCES

Andrews, M., & Boyle, J. (2012). *Transcultural concepts in nursing care* (6th ed.). Philadelphia, PA: Lippincott Williams & Wilkins.

Brunton, L., Chabner, B., & Knollman, B. (2011). *Goodman and Gilman's the pharmacological basis of therapeutics* (12th ed.). New York: McGraw-Hill.

Facts and Comparisons. (2015). *Drug facts and comparisons*. St. Louis, MO: Author.

Goulding, N., & Flower, R. (Eds.). (2013). *Glucocorticoids, milestones in drug therapy*. Boston, MA; Birkhauser.

Hall, J. (2015). *Guyton and Hall's textbook of medical physiology* (13th ed.). Philadelphia, PA: Saunders.

Karch, A. M. (2014). *Lippincott's nursing drug guide*. Philadelphia, PA: Lippincott Williams & Wilkins.

Kuehn, B. (2009). Inhaled corticosteroids in patients with COPD. *Journal of the American Medical Association, 301*(14), 1433.

Lavin, N. (2009). *Manual of endocrinology and metabolism*. Philadelphia, PA: Lippincott Williams & Wilkins.

Linos, D. A., & van Heerden, J. A. (2011). *Adrenal glands, diagnostic aspects and surgical therapy*. New York: Springer.

The Medical Letter. (2015). *The medical letter on drugs and therapeutics*. New Rochelle, NY: Author.

Melmed, S., Polonsky, K., Reed, P., et al. (2011). *Williams textbook of endocrinology* (12th ed.). Philadelphia, PA: Saunders.

Porth, C. (2013). *Pathophysiology: Concepts of altered health states* (9th ed.). Philadelphia, PA: Lippincott Williams & Wilkins.

37 Thyroid and Parathyroid Agents

Learning Objectives

Upon completion of this chapter, you will be able to:

1. Explain the control of synthesis and secretion of thyroid hormones and parathyroid hormones, applying this to alterations in the control process (e.g., using thyroid hormones to treat obesity, Paget's disease, etc.).
2. Describe the therapeutic actions, indications, pharmacokinetics, contraindications, most common adverse reactions, and important drug–drug interactions associated with thyroid and parathyroid agents.
3. Discuss the use of thyroid and parathyroid drugs across the lifespan.
4. Compare and contrast thyroid and parathyroid prototype drugs with agents in their class.
5. Outline nursing considerations, including important teaching points, for patients receiving drugs used to affect thyroid or parathyroid function.

Glossary of Key Terms

bisphosphonates: drugs used to block bone resorption and lower serum calcium levels in several conditions

calcitonin: hormone produced by the parafollicular cells of the thyroid; counteracts the effects of parathyroid hormone to maintain calcium levels

cretinism: lack of thyroid hormone in an infant; if untreated, leads to mental retardation

follicles: structural unit of the thyroid gland; cells arranged in a circle

hypercalcemia: excessive calcium levels in the blood

hyperparathyroidism: excessive parathormone

hyperthyroidism: excessive levels of thyroid hormone

hypocalcemia: calcium deficiency

hypoparathyroidism: rare condition of absence of parathormone; may be seen after thyroidectomy

hypothyroidism: lack of sufficient thyroid hormone to maintain metabolism

iodine: important dietary element used by the thyroid gland to produce thyroid hormone

levothyroxine: a synthetic salt of thyroxine (T_4), a thyroid hormone; the most frequently used replacement hormone for treating thyroid disease

liothyronine: the L-isomer of triiodothyronine (T_3), and the most potent thyroid hormone, with a short half-life of 12 hours

metabolism: rate at which the cells burn energy

myxedema: severe lack of thyroid hormone in adults

Paget's disease: a genetically linked disorder of overactive osteoclasts that are eventually replaced by enlarged and softened bony structures

parathormone: hormone produced by the parathyroid glands; responsible for maintaining calcium levels in conjunction with calcitonin

postmenopausal osteoporosis: condition in which dropping levels of estrogen allow calcium to be pulled out of the bone, resulting in a weakened and honeycombed bone structure

thioamides: drugs used to prevent the formation of thyroid hormone in the thyroid cells, lowering thyroid hormone levels

thyroxine: a thyroid hormone that is converted to triiodothyronine in the tissues; it has a half-life of 1 week

Drug List

Thyroid Agents
Thyroid Hormones
- (P) levothyroxine
- liothyronine
- liotrix
- thyroid desiccated

Antithyroid Agents
Thioamides
- methimazole
- (P) propylthiouracil

Iodine Solutions
- sodium iodide I^{131}
- (P) strong iodine solution
- potassium iodide

Parathyroid Agents
Antihypocalcemic Agents
- (P) calcitriol
- parathyroid hormone
- teriparatide

Antihypercalcemic Agents	ibandronate	risedronate	*Calcitonins*
Bisphosphonates	pamidronate	zoledronic acid	(P) calcitonin salmon
(P) alendronate			
etidronate			

This chapter reviews drugs that are used to affect the function of the thyroid and parathyroid glands. These two glands are closely situated in the middle of the neck and they do share a common goal of calcium homeostasis. Serum calcium levels need to be maintained within a narrow range to promote effective blood coagulation, as well as nerve and muscle function. In most respects, however, these glands are very different in structure and function.

The Thyroid Gland

The thyroid gland is located in the middle of the neck, where it surrounds the trachea like a shield (Figure 37.1). Its name comes from the Greek words *thyros* (shield) and *eidos* (gland). It produces two hormones—thyroid hormone and calcitonin.

Structure and Function

The thyroid is a vascular gland with two lobes—one on each side of the trachea—and a small isthmus connecting the lobes. The gland is made up of cells arranged in circular **follicles**. The center of each follicle is composed of colloid tissue in which the thyroid hormones produced by the gland are stored. Cells found around the follicle of the thyroid gland are called parafollicular cells (see Figure 37.1). These cells produce another hormone, **calcitonin**, which affects calcium levels and acts to balance the effects of the parathyroid hormone (PTH), **parathormone**. Calcitonin will be discussed later in connection with the parathyroid glands.

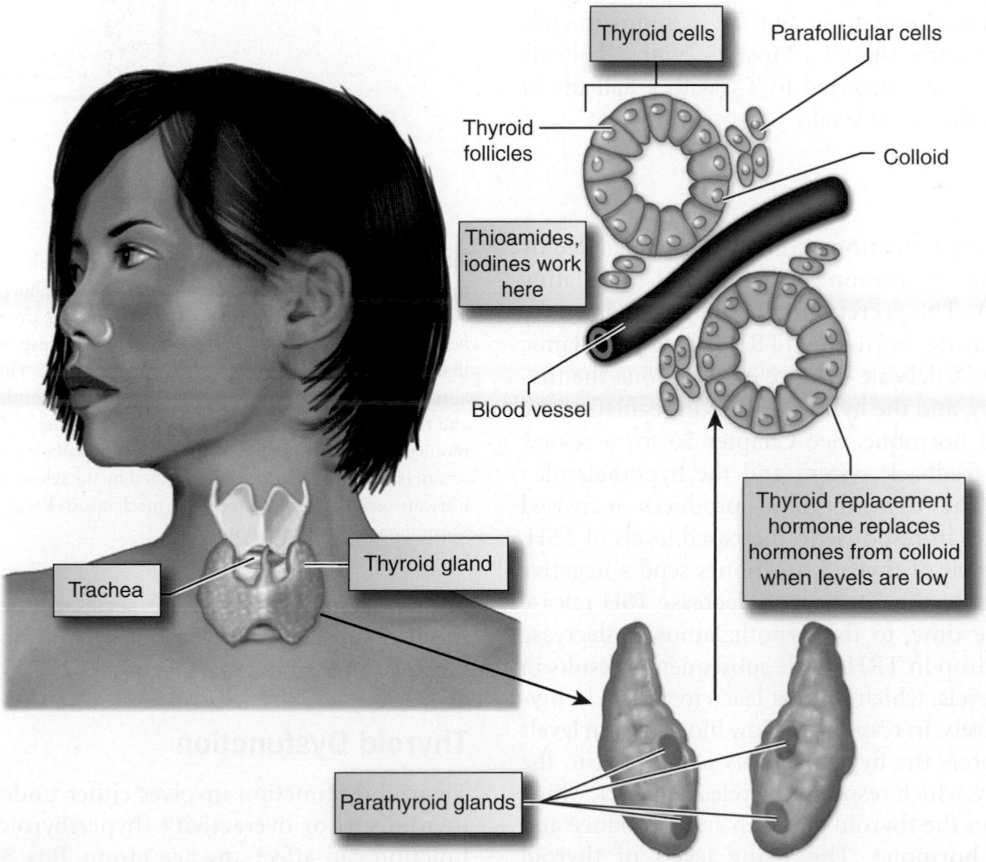

FIGURE 37.1 The thyroid and parathyroid glands. The basic unit of the thyroid gland is the follicle.

The thyroid gland produces two slightly different thyroid hormones, using **iodine** that is found in the diet: Thyroxine, or tetraiodothyronine (T_4), so-named because it contains four iodine atoms, which is given therapeutically in the synthetic form **levothyroxine**, and triiodothyronine (T_3), so-named because it contains three iodine atoms, which is given in the synthetic form **liothyronine**. The thyroid cells remove iodine from the blood, concentrate it, and prepare it for attachment to tyrosine, an amino acid. A person must obtain sufficient amounts of dietary iodine to produce thyroid hormones. The thyroid hormone regulates the rate of **metabolism**—that is, the rate at which energy is burned—in almost all the cells of the body. The thyroid hormones affect heat production and body temperature; oxygen consumption and cardiac output; blood volume; enzyme system activity; and metabolism of carbohydrates, fats, and proteins. Thyroid hormone is also an important regulator of growth and development, especially within the reproductive and nervous systems. Because the thyroid has such widespread effects throughout the body, any dysfunction of the thyroid gland will have numerous systemic effects.

When thyroid hormone is needed in the body the stored thyroid hormone molecule is absorbed into the thyroid cells, where the T_3 and T_4 are broken off and released into circulation. These hormones are carried on plasma proteins, which can be measured as protein-bound iodine levels. The thyroid gland produces more T_4 than T_3. More T_4 is released into circulation, but T_3 is approximately four times more active than T_4. Most T_4 (with a half-life of about 12 hours) is converted to T_3 (with a half-life of about 1 week) at the tissue level.

Control

Thyroid hormone production and release are regulated by the anterior pituitary hormone called thyroid-stimulating hormone (TSH). The secretion of TSH is regulated by thyrotropin-releasing hormone (TRH), a hypothalamic regulating factor. A delicate balance exists among the thyroid, the pituitary, and the hypothalamus in regulating the levels of thyroid hormone. See Chapter 36 for a review of the negative feedback system and the hypothalamic–pituitary axis. The thyroid gland produces increased thyroid hormones in response to increased levels of TSH. The increased levels of thyroid hormones send a negative feedback message to the pituitary to decrease TSH release and, at the same time, to the hypothalamus to decrease TRH release. A drop in TRH levels subsequently results in a drop in TSH levels, which in turn leads to a drop in thyroid hormone levels. In response to low blood serum levels of thyroid hormone the hypothalamus sends TRH to the anterior pituitary, which responds by releasing TSH, which in turn stimulates the thyroid gland to again produce and release thyroid hormone. The rising levels of thyroid hormone are sensed by the hypothalamus, and the cycle begins again. This intricate series of negative feedback mechanisms keeps the level of thyroid hormone within a narrow range of normal (Figure 37.2).

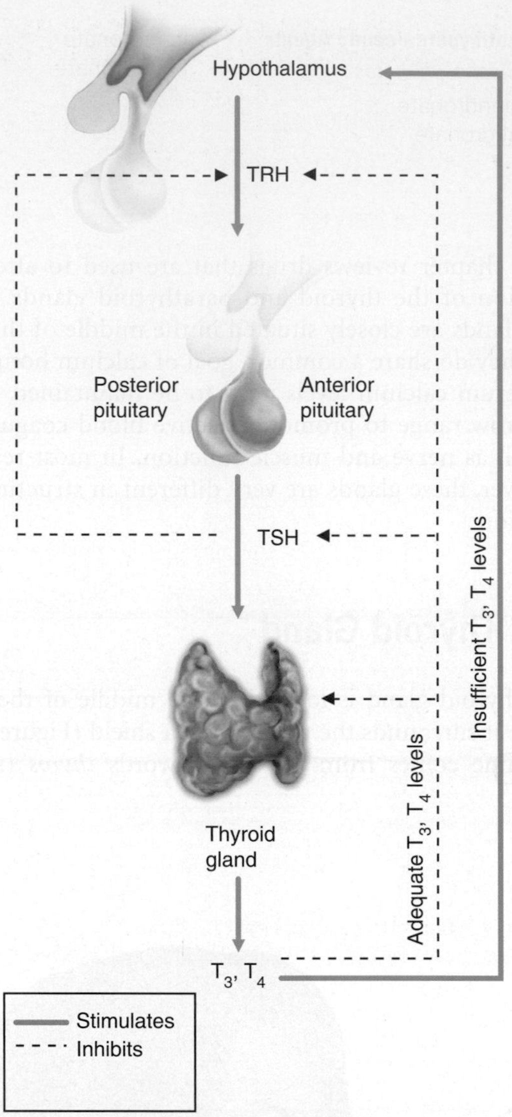

FIGURE 37.2 In response to low blood serum levels of thyroid hormone the hypothalamus sends the thyrotropin-releasing hormone (TRH) to the anterior pituitary, which responds by releasing the thyroid-stimulating hormone (TSH) to the thyroid gland; it, in turn, responds by releasing the thyroid hormone (T_3 and T_4) into the bloodstream. The anterior pituitary is also sensitive to the increase in blood serum levels of the thyroid hormone and responds by decreasing production and release of TSH. As thyroid hormone production and release subside, the hypothalamus senses the lower serum levels, and the process is repeated by the release of TRH again. This intricate series of negative feedback mechanisms keeps the level of thyroid hormone within normal limits.

Thyroid Dysfunction

Thyroid dysfunction involves either underactivity (hypothyroidism) or overactivity (hyperthyroidism). This dysfunction can affect any age group. Box 37.1 explains the use of thyroid agents across the lifespan.

BOX 37.1 FOCUS ON Drug Therapy Across the Lifespan

Thyroid and Parathyroid Agents

CHILDREN

Thyroid replacement therapy is required when a child is hypothyroid. Levothyroxine is the drug of choice in children. Dose is determined based on serum thyroid hormone levels and the response of the child, including growth and development. Dose in children tends to be higher than in adults because of the higher metabolic rate of the growing child. Usually, the starting dose to consider is 10 to 15 mcg/kg/d.

Regular monitoring, including growth records, is necessary to determine the accurate dose as the child grows. Maintenance levels at the adult dose usually occurs after puberty and when active growing stops.

If an antithyroid agent is needed, methimazole is the drug of choice because it is less toxic to the liver. PTU is no longer recommended for children. Unless other agents are ineffective, radioactive agents are not used in children because of the effects of radiation on chromosomes and developing cells.

Hypercalcemia is relatively rare in children, although it may be seen with certain malignancies. If a child develops a malignancy-related hypercalcemia, the bisphosphonates may be used, with dose adjustments based on age and weight. Serum calcium levels should be monitored very closely in the child and dose adjustments made as necessary.

ADULTS

Adults who require thyroid replacement therapy need to understand that this will be a lifelong replacement need. An established routine of taking the tablet first thing in the morning may help the patient to comply with the drug regimen. These drugs should always be taken with a full glass of water to decrease the risk of esophageal atresia. Levothyroxine is the drug of choice for replacement, but in some cases other agents may be needed. Periodic monitoring of thyroid hormone levels is necessary to ensure that dose needs have not changed.

If antithyroid drugs are needed, the patient's underlying problems should be considered. Methimazole is associated with bone marrow suppression and more GI and CNS effects than is PTU. Sodium iodide I^{131} should not be used in adults in their reproductive years unless they are aware of the possibility of adverse effects on fertility.

Alendronate and risedronate are commonly used drugs for osteoporosis and calcium lowering. Serum calcium levels need to be monitored carefully with any of the drugs that affect calcium levels. Patients should be encouraged to take calcium and vitamin D in their diet or as supplements in cases of hypocalcemia, and also for prevention and treatment of osteoporosis.

Thyroid replacement therapy is necessary during pregnancy for women who have been maintained on this regimen. It is not uncommon for hypothyroidism to develop during pregnancy. Levothyroxine is again the drug of choice.

If an antithyroid drug is essential during pregnancy, PTU is the drug of choice because it is less likely to cross the placenta and cause problems for the fetus. Radioactive agents should not be used. Bisphosphonates should be used during pregnancy only if the benefit to the mother clearly outweighs the potential risk to the fetus. Nursing mothers who need thyroid replacement therapy should continue with their prescribed regimen and report any adverse reactions in the baby. Bisphosphonates and antithyroid drugs should not be used during lactation because of the potential for adverse reactions in the baby; another method of feeding the baby should be used.

OLDER ADULTS

Because the signs and symptoms of thyroid disease mimic many other problems that are common to older adults—hair loss, slurred speech, fluid retention, heart failure, and so on—it is important to screen older adults for thyroid disease carefully before beginning any therapy. The dose should be started at a very low level and increased based on the patient response. Levothyroxine is the drug of choice for hypothyroidism. Periodic monitoring of thyroid hormone levels, as well as cardiac and other responses, is essential with this age group.

If antithyroid agents are needed, sodium iodide I^{131} may be the drug of choice because it has fewer adverse effects than the other agents and surgery. The patient should be monitored closely for the development of hypothyroidism, which usually occurs within a year after initiation of antithyroid therapy.

Older adults may have dietary deficiencies related to calcium and vitamin D. They should be encouraged to eat dairy products and foods high in calcium and to supplement their diet if necessary. Postmenopausal women, who are prone to develop osteoporosis, may want to consider hormone replacement therapy and calcium supplements to prevent osteoporosis, though this decision has to be made with full consideration of the risks of using hormone replacement therapy. Many postmenopausal women, and some older men, respond well to the effect of bisphosphonates in moving calcium back into the bone. They need specific instructions on the proper way to take these drugs and may not be able to comply with the restrictions about staying upright and swallowing the tablet with a full glass of water.

Older adults have a greater incidence of renal impairment, and kidney function should be evaluated before starting any of these drugs. Bisphosphonates should be used in lower doses in patients with moderate renal impairment and are not recommended for those who have severe renal impairment. With any of these drugs, regular monitoring of calcium levels is important to ensure that therapeutic effects are achieved with a minimum of adverse effects.

Hypothyroidism

Hypothyroidism is a lack of sufficient levels of thyroid hormones to maintain a normal metabolism. This condition occurs in a number of pathophysiological states:

- Absence of the thyroid gland
- Lack of sufficient iodine in the diet to produce the needed level of thyroid hormone
- Lack of sufficient functioning thyroid tissue due to tumor or autoimmune disorders
- Lack of TSH due to pituitary disease
- Lack of TRH related to a tumor or disorder of the hypothalamus

Hypothyroidism is the most common type of thyroid dysfunction. It is estimated that approximately 5 to 10% of women older than 50 years of age are hypothyroid. Hypothyroidism is also a common finding in elderly men. The symptoms of hypothyroidism can be varied and vague, such as obesity and fatigue (Box 37.2), and are frequently overlooked or mistaken for signs of normal aging (Table 37.1).

Children who are born without a thyroid gland or who have a nonfunctioning gland develop a condition called **cretinisms**. If untreated, these children will have poor growth and development and mental retardation because of the lack of thyroid hormone stimulation. Severe adult hypothyroidism is called myxedema. **Myxedema** usually develops gradually as the thyroid slowly stops functioning. It can develop as a result of autoimmune thyroid disease (Hashimoto disease), viral infection, or overtreatment with antithyroid drugs or because of surgical removal or irradiation of the thyroid gland. Patients with myxedema exhibit many signs and symptoms. Hypothyroidism is treated with replacement thyroid hormone therapy.

Hyperthyroidism

Hyperthyroidism occurs when excessive amounts of thyroid hormones are produced and released into the circulation. Graves' disease, a poorly understood condition that is thought to be an autoimmune problem, is the most common cause of hyperthyroidism. Goiter (enlargement of the thyroid gland) is an effect of hyperthyroidism, which occurs when the thyroid is overstimulated by TSH. This can happen if the thyroid gland does not make sufficient thyroid hormones to turn off the hypothalamus and anterior pituitary; in the body's attempt to produce the needed amount of thyroid hormone the thyroid is continually stimulated by increasing levels of TSH. Additional signs and symptoms of hyperthyroidism can be found in Table 37.1.

Hyperthyroidism may be treated by surgical removal of the gland or portions of the gland, treatment with radiation to destroy parts or all of the gland, or drug treatment to block the production of **thyroxine** in the thyroid gland or to destroy parts or all of the gland. The metabolism of these patients then must be regulated with replacement thyroid hormone therapy.

BOX 37.2 FOCUS ON The Evidence

Thyroid Hormones for Obesity

Treatment trends for obesity have changed over the years. Not long ago, one of the suggested treatments was the use of thyroid hormone. The thinking was that obese people had slower metabolisms and therefore would benefit from a boost in metabolism from extra thyroid hormone.

If an obese patient is truly hypothyroid, this might be a good idea. Unfortunately, many of the patients who received thyroid hormone for weight loss were not tested for thyroid activity and ended up with excessive thyroid hormone in their systems. This situation triggered a cascade of events. The exogenous thyroid hormone disrupted the hypothalamic–pituitary–thyroid control system, resulting in decreased production of TRH and TSH as the hypothalamus and pituitary sensed the rising levels of thyroid hormone. Because the thyroid was no longer stimulated to produce and secrete thyroid hormone, thyroid levels would actually fall. Lacking stimulation by TSH the thyroid gland would start to atrophy. If exogenous thyroid hormone were stopped the atrophied thyroid would not be able to immediately respond to the TSH stimulation and produce thyroid hormone. Ultimately, these patients experienced an endocrine imbalance. What's more, they also did not lose weight—and in the long run may actually have gained weight as the body's compensatory mechanisms tried to deal with the imbalances.

Today, thyroid hormone is no longer considered a good choice for treating obesity. Other drugs have come and gone, and new drugs are released each year to attack other aspects of the problem. Many patients, especially middle-aged people who may recall that thyroid hormone was once used for weight loss, ask for it as an answer to their weight problem. Patients have even been known to "borrow" thyroid replacement hormones from others for a quick weight loss solution or to order the drug over the Internet without supervision or monitoring.

Obese patients need reassurance, understanding, and education about the risks of borrowed thyroid hormone. Insistent patients should undergo thyroid function tests. If the results are normal, patients should receive teaching about the controls and actions of thyroid hormone in the body and an explanation of why taking these hormones can cause problems. Obesity is a chronic and frustrating problem that poses continual challenges for health care providers.

Table 37.1 Signs and Symptoms of Thyroid Dysfunction

Clinical Effects	Hypothyroidism	Hyperthyroidism
CNS	*Depressed:* Hypoactive reflexes, lethargy, sleepiness, slow speech, emotional dullness	*Stimulated:* Hyperactive reflexes, anxiety, nervousness, insomnia, tremors, restlessness, increased basal temperature
CV system	*Depressed:* Bradycardia, hypotension, anemia, oliguria, decreased sensitivity to catecholamines	*Stimulated:* Tachycardia, palpitations, increased pulse pressure, systolic hypertension, increased sensitivity to catecholamines
Skin, hair, and nails	Skin is pale, coarse, dry, thickened; puffy eyes and eyelids; hair is coarse and thin; hair loss; nails are thick and hard	Skin is flushed, warm, thin, moist, sweating; hair is fine and soft; nails are soft and thin
Metabolic rate	*Decreased:* Lower body temperature; intolerance to cold; decreased appetite, higher levels of fat and cholesterol; weight gain; hypercholesterolemia	Increased, overactive cellular metabolism: low-grade fever; intolerance to heat; increased appetite with weight loss; muscle wasting and weakness, thyroid myopathy
Generalized myxedema	Accumulation of mucopolysaccharides in the heart, tongue, and vocal cords; periorbital edema, cardiomyopathy, hoarseness, and thickened speech	Localized with accumulation of mucopolysaccharides in eyeballs, ocular muscles; periorbital edema, lid lag, exophthalmos; pretibial edema
Ovaries	*Decreased function:* Menorrhagia, habitual abortion, sterility, decreased sexual function	Altered; tendency toward oligomenorrhea, amenorrhea
Goiter	Rare; simple nontoxic type may occur	Diffuse, highly vascular; very frequent

CNS, central nervous system; CV, cardiovascular.

KEY POINTS

- The thyroid gland uses iodine to produce the thyroid hormones that regulate body metabolism.
- Control of the thyroid gland involves an intricate balance among TRH, TSH, and circulating levels of thyroid hormone.
- Hypothyroidism is treated with replacement thyroid hormone; hyperthyroidism is treated with thioamides or iodines.

Thyroid Agents

When thyroid function is low, thyroid hormone needs to be replaced to ensure adequate metabolism and homeostasis in the body. When thyroid function is too high the resultant systemic effects can be serious, and the thyroid will need to be removed or destroyed pharmacologically, and then the hormone normally produced by the gland will need to be replaced with thyroid hormone. Thyroid agents include thyroid hormones and antithyroid drugs, which are further classified as thioamides and iodine solutions. Table 37.2 includes a complete list of each type of thyroid agent.

Thyroid Hormones

Several replacement hormone products are available for treating hypothyroidism. These hormones replace the low or absent levels of natural thyroid hormone and suppress the overproduction of TSH by the pituitary. These products can contain both natural and synthetic thyroid hormone. Levothyroxine (*Synthroid, Levoxyl, Levothroid*), a synthetic salt of T_4, is the most frequently used replacement hormone because of its predictable bioavailability and reliability. Desiccated thyroid (*Armour Thyroid*, and others) is prepared from dried animal thyroid glands and contains both T_3 and T_4; although the ratio of the hormones is unpredictable and the required dose and effects vary widely, this drug is inexpensive, making it attractive to some. Additional thyroid hormones include liothyronine (*Cytomel, Triostat*), a synthetic salt of T_3, and liotrix (*Thyrolar*), a synthetic preparation of T_4 and T_3 in a standard 4:1 ratio.

Therapeutic Actions and Indications

The thyroid replacement hormones increase the metabolic rate of body tissues, increasing oxygen consumption, respiration, heart rate, growth and maturation, and the metabolism of fats, carbohydrates, and proteins. They are indicated for replacement therapy in hypothyroid states, treatment of myxedema coma, suppression of TSH in the treatment and prevention of goiters, and management of thyroid cancer. In conjunction with antithyroid drugs, they also are indicated to treat thyroid toxicity, prevent goiter formation during thyroid overstimulation, and treat thyroid overstimulation during pregnancy. These drugs are not approved for weight loss, and carry a warning that they are not to be used for weight loss. See Table 37.2 for Usual Indications for each drug.

Pharmacokinetics

These drugs are well absorbed from the gastrointestinal (GI) tract and bound to serum proteins. Because it contains only T_3, liothyronine has a rapid onset and a long

Table 37.2 *Drugs in Focus:* Thyroid Agents

Drug Name	Dosage/Route	Usual Indications
Thyroid Hormones		
levothyroxine (*Synthroid, Levoxyl, Levothroid,* others)	*Adult:* 0.05–0.2 mg/d PO *Pediatric:* 0.025–0.4 mg/d PO	Replacement therapy in hypothyroidism; suppression of TSH release; treatment of myxedema coma and thyrotoxicosis
liothyronine (*Cytomel, Triostat*)	*Adult:* 25–100 mcg/d PO *Pediatric:* 20–50 mcg/d PO	Replacement therapy in hypothyroidism; suppression of TSH release; treatment of thyrotoxicosis; synthetic hormone used in patients allergic to desiccated thyroid *Special considerations:* Not for use with cardiac or anxiety problems
liotrix (*Thyrolar*)	*Adult:* 60–120 mg/d PO *Pediatric:* 25–150 mcg/d PO based on age and weight	Replacement therapy in hypothyroidism; suppression of TSH release; treatment of thyrotoxicosis *Special considerations:* Not for use with cardiac dysfunction
thyroid desiccated (*Armour Thyroid*)	*Adult:* 60–120 mg/d PO *Pediatric:* 15–90 mg/d PO	Replacement therapy in hypothyroidism; suppression of TSH release; treatment of thyrotoxicosis
Antithyroid Agents ***Thioamides***		
methimazole (*Tapazole*)	*Adult:* 15 mg/d PO initially, up to 30–60 mg/d may be needed; maintenance, 5–15 mg/d PO *Pediatric:* 0.4 mg/kg/d PO initially; maintenance, 15–20 mg/m^2/d PO in three divided doses	Treatment of hyperthyroidism
propylthiouracil (PTU)	*Adult:* 300–900 mg/d PO initially; maintenance, 100–150 mg/d PO	Treatment of hyperthyroidism
Iodine Solutions		
sodium iodide I^{131} (generic, radioactive iodine)	*Adult (>30 y):* 4–10 mCi PO as needed	Treatment of hyperthyroidism; thyroid blocking in radiation emergencies; destruction of thyroid tissue in patients who are not candidates for surgical removal of the gland
strong iodine solution, potassium iodide (*Thyro-Block*)	*Adult:* One tablet, or 2–6 drops (gtt) PO daily to t.i.d. *Pediatric (>1 y):* Adult dose *Pediatric (<1 y):* ½ tablet or 3 gtt PO daily to t.i.d.	Treatment of hyperthyroidism, thyroid blocking in radiation emergencies; presurgical suppression of the thyroid gland, treatment of acute thyrotoxicosis until thioamide levels can take effect

TSH, thyroid-stimulating hormone.

duration of action. Deiodination of the drugs occurs at several sites, including the liver, kidney, and other body tissues. Elimination is primarily in the bile. Thyroid hormone does not cross the placenta and seems to have no effect on the fetus. Thyroid replacement therapy should not be discontinued during pregnancy, and the need for thyroid replacement often becomes apparent or increases during pregnancy. Thyroid hormone does enter breast milk in small amounts. Caution should be used during lactation.

Contraindications and Cautions

These drugs should not be used with any known allergy to the drugs or their binders *to prevent hypersensitivity reactions,* during acute thyrotoxicosis (unless used in conjunction with antithyroid drugs), or during acute myocardial infarction (unless complicated by hypothyroidism), *because the thyroid hormones could exacerbate these conditions.* Caution should be used during lactation *because the drug enters breast milk and could suppress the infant's thyroid production,* and with hypoadrenal conditions such as Addison disease *because the body will not be able to deal with the drug effects.* Liothyronine and liotrix have a greater incidence of cardiac side effects and are not recommended for use in patients with potential cardiac problems or patients who are prone to anxiety reactions.

Adverse Effects

When the correct dose of the replacement therapy is being used, few if any adverse effects are associated with these drugs. Thyroid function tests should be checked annually in long-term therapy to ensure the correct levels are being maintained. Skin reactions and loss of hair are sometimes seen, especially during the first few months of treatment in children. Symptoms of hyperthyroidism may occur as the drug dose is regulated. Some of the less predictable

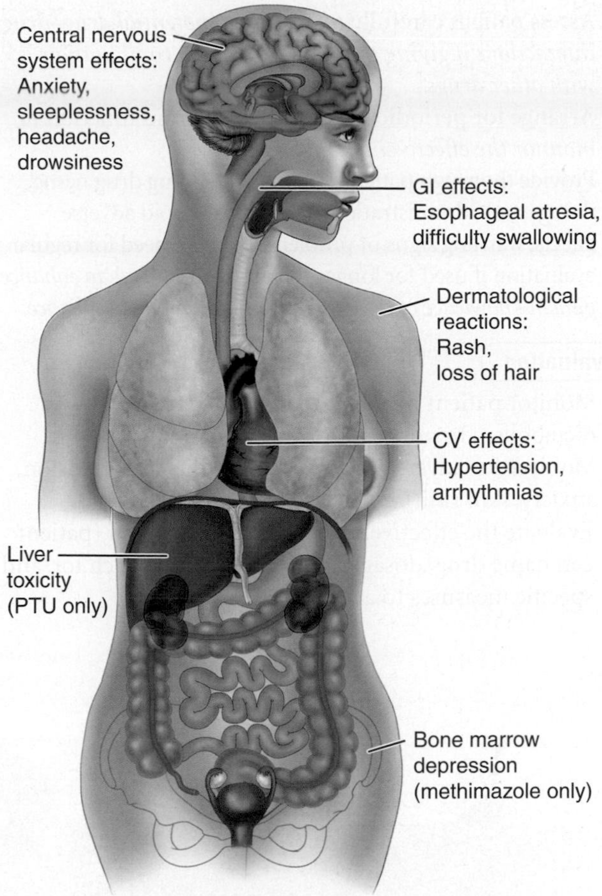

FIGURE 37.3 Variety of adverse effects and toxicities associated with thyroid and parathyroid drugs.

effects are associated with cardiac stimulation (arrhythmias, hypertension), central nervous system (CNS) effects (anxiety, sleeplessness, headache), and difficulty swallowing and esophageal atresia (taking the drug with a full glass of water is strongly recommended to alleviate this effect) (Figure 37.3).

Clinically Important Drug–Drug Interactions

Decreased absorption of the thyroid hormones occurs if they are taken concurrently with cholestyramine. If this combination is needed the drugs should be taken 2 hours apart.

The effectiveness of oral anticoagulants is increased if they are combined with thyroid hormone. Because this may lead to increased bleeding the dose of the oral anticoagulant should be reduced and the bleeding time checked periodically.

Decreased effectiveness of digitalis glycosides can occur when these drugs are combined. Consequently, digitalis levels should be monitored, and increased dose may be required.

Theophylline clearance is decreased in hypothyroid states. As the patient approaches normal thyroid function the theophylline dose may need to be adjusted frequently.

Ⓟ Prototype Summary: Levothyroxine

Indications: Replacement therapy in hypothyroidism; pituitary TSH suppression in the treatment of euthyroid goiters and in the management of thyroid cancer; thyrotoxicosis in conjunction with other therapy; myxedema coma.

Actions: Increases the metabolic rate of body tissues, increasing oxygen consumption, respiration, and heart rate; the rate of fat, protein, and carbohydrate metabolism; and growth and maturation.

Pharmacokinetics:

Route	Onset	Peak	Duration
PO	Slow	1–3 wk	1–3 wk
IV	6–8 h	24–48 h	Unknown

$T_{1/2}$: 6 to 7 days; metabolized in the liver and excreted in the bile.

Adverse Effects: Tremors, headache, nervousness, palpitations, tachycardia, allergic skin reactions, loss of hair in the first few months of therapy in children, diarrhea, nausea, vomiting.

Nursing Considerations for Patients Receiving Thyroid Hormones

Assessment: History and Examination

- Assess for history of allergy to any thyroid hormone or binder, lactation, Addison disease, acute myocardial infarction not complicated by hypothyroidism, and thyrotoxicosis, *which could be contraindications or cautions to use of the drug.*
- Assess for the presence of any skin lesions; orientation and affect; baseline pulse, blood pressure, and electrocardiogram; respiration and adventitious sounds; and thyroid function tests, *to determine baseline status before beginning therapy and for any potential adverse effects.*

Refer to the Critical Thinking Scenario for a full discussion of nursing care for a patient who is receiving a thyroid hormone.

Nursing Diagnoses

Nursing diagnoses related to drug therapy might include the following:

- Decreased cardiac output related to cardiac effects
- Imbalanced nutrition: Less than body requirements related to changes in metabolism
- Ineffective tissue perfusion related to thyroid activity
- Deficient knowledge regarding drug therapy

(continues on page 614)

Planning

- The patient will receive the best therapeutic effect from the drug therapy.
- The patient will have limited adverse effects to the drug therapy.
- The patient will have an understanding of the drug therapy, adverse effects to anticipate, and measures to relieve discomfort and improve safety.

Implementation with Rationale

- Administer a single daily dose before breakfast each day, ensure that the drug is not expired before use *to ensure consistent therapeutic levels.*
- Administer with a full glass of water *to help prevent difficulty swallowing and esophageal atresia.*
- Monitor response carefully when beginning therapy *to adjust dose according to patient response.*
- Monitor cardiac response *to detect cardiac adverse effects.*
- Assess patient carefully *to detect any potential drug–drug interactions if giving thyroid hormone in combination with other drugs.*
- Arrange for periodic blood tests of thyroid function *to monitor the effectiveness of the therapy.*
- Provide thorough patient teaching, including drug name, dosage and administration, measures to avoid adverse effects, warning signs of problems, and the need for regular evaluation if used for longer than recommended, *to enhance patient knowledge of drug therapy and promote compliance.*

Evaluation

- Monitor patient response to the drug (return of metabolism to normal, prevention of goiter).
- Monitor for adverse effects (tachycardia, hypertension, anxiety, skin rash).
- Evaluate the effectiveness of the teaching plan (patient can name drug, dosage, adverse effects to watch for, and specific measures to avoid them).

CRITICAL THINKING SCENARIO

Hypothyroidism

THE SITUATION

H.R., a 38-year-old white woman, complains of "exhaustion, lethargy, and sleepiness." Her past history is sketchy, her speech seems slurred, and her attention span is limited. Mr. R., her husband, reports feeling frustrated with H.R., stating that she has become increasingly lethargic, disorganized, and uninvolved at home. He also notes that she has gained weight and lost interest in her appearance. Physical examination reveals the following remarkable findings: Pulse rate, 52/min; blood pressure, 90/62 mm Hg; temperature, 96.8°F (oral); pale, dry, and thick skin; periorbital edema; thick and asymmetric tongue; height, 5 ft 5 in.; and weight, 165 lb. The immediate impression is that of hypothyroidism. Laboratory tests confirm this, revealing elevated TSH and very low levels of triiodothyronine and thyroxine. *Synthroid*, 0.2 mg daily PO, is prescribed.

CRITICAL THINKING

What teaching plans should be developed for this patient?

What interventions would be appropriate in helping Mr. and Mrs. R. accept the diagnosis and the pathophysiological basis for Mrs. R's complaints and problems?

What body image changes will H.R. experience as her body adjusts to the thyroid therapy?

How can H.R. be helped to adjust to these changes and reestablish her body image and self-concept?

DISCUSSION

Hypothyroidism develops slowly. With it comes fatigue, lethargy, and lack of emotional affect—conditions that result in the patient losing interest in appearance, activities, and responsibilities. In this case, the patient's husband, not knowing that there was a physical reason for the problem, became increasingly frustrated and even angry. Mr. R. should be involved in the teaching program so that his feelings can be taken into consideration. Any teaching content should be written down for later reference. (When H.R. starts to return to normal, her attention span and interest should return; anything that was missed or forgotten can be referred to in the written teaching program.)

H.R. may be encouraged to bring a picture of herself from a year or so ago to help her to understand and appreciate the changes that have occurred. Many patients are totally unaware of changes in their appearance and activity level because the disease progresses so slowly and brings on lethargy and lack of emotional affect.

Hypothyroidism (continued)

The teaching plan should include information about the function of the thyroid gland and the anticipated changes that will be occurring to H.R. over the next week and beyond. The importance of taking the medication daily should be emphasized. The need to return for follow-up to evaluate the effectiveness of the medication and the effects on her body should also be stressed. Both H.R. and her husband will need support and encouragement to deal with past frustrations and the return to normal. Lifelong therapy will probably be needed, so further teaching will be important once things have stabilized.

NURSING CARE GUIDE FOR H.R.: THYROID HORMONE

Assessment: History and Examination

Review the patient's history for allergies to any of these drugs, Addison disease, acute myocardial infarction not complicated by hypothyroidism, lactation, and thyrotoxicosis.

Focus the physical examination on the following:

Neurological: Orientation and affect

Skin: Color and lesions

Cardiovascular (CV): Pulse, cardiac auscultation, blood pressure, and electrocardiogram findings

Respiratory: Respirations, adventitious sounds

Hematological: Thyroid function tests

Nursing Diagnoses

Decreased cardiac output related to cardiac effects

Imbalanced nutrition: Less than body requirements related to effects on metabolism

Ineffective tissue perfusion related to thyroid effects

Deficient knowledge regarding drug therapy

Planning

The patient will receive the best therapeutic effect from the drug therapy.

The patient will have limited adverse effects to the drug therapy.

The patient will have an understanding of the drug therapy, adverse effects to anticipate, and measures to relieve discomfort and improve safety.

Implementation

Administer the drug once a day before breakfast with a full glass of water. Avoid calcium or calcium-containing products at the same time you are taking your thyroid.

Provide comfort, safety measures (e.g., temperature control, rest as needed, safety precautions).

Provide support and reassurance to deal with drug effects and lifetime need.

Provide patient teaching regarding drug name, dosage, adverse effects, precautions, and warning signs to report. Advise the patient to not use a drug past its expiration date.

Evaluation

Evaluate drug effects: Return of metabolism to normal; prevention of goiter.

Monitor for adverse effects: Anxiety, tachycardia, hypertension, skin reaction.

Monitor for drug–drug interactions as indicated for each drug.

Evaluate the effectiveness of the patient-teaching program and comfort and safety measures.

PATIENT TEACHING FOR H.R.

- This hormone is designed to replace the thyroid hormone that your body is not able to produce. The thyroid hormone is responsible for regulating your body's metabolism, or the speed with which your body's cells burn energy. Thyroid hormone actions affect many body systems, so it is very important that you take this medication only as prescribed.
- Never stop taking this drug without consulting with your health care provider. The drug is used to replace a very important hormone and will probably have to be taken for life. Stopping the medication can lead to serious problems.
- Take this drug before breakfast each day with a full glass of water.
- Make sure that you do not use the drug after its expiration date; this drug is known to lose effectiveness over time.
- Thyroid hormone usually causes no adverse effects. You may notice a slight skin rash or hair loss in the first few months of therapy. You should notice the signs and symptoms of your thyroid deficiency subsiding, and you will feel "back to normal."
- Report any of the following to your health care provider: Chest pain, difficulty breathing, sore throat, fever, chills, weight gain, sleeplessness, nervousness, unusual sweating, or intolerance to heat.
- Avoid taking any over-the-counter medication without first checking with your health care provider because several of these medications can interfere with the effectiveness of this drug.
- Tell any doctor, nurse, or other health care provider involved in your care that you are taking this drug. You may also want to wear or carry medical identification showing that you are taking this medication. This would alert any health care personnel taking care of you in an emergency to the fact that you are taking this drug.
- While you are taking this drug, you will need regular medical follow-up, including blood tests to check the activity of your thyroid gland, to evaluate your response to the drug and any possible underlying problems.
- Keep this drug, and all medications, out of the reach of children. Do not give this medication to anyone else or take any similar medication that has not been prescribed for you.

Antithyroid Agents

Drugs used to block the production of thyroid hormone and to treat hyperthyroidism include the thioamides and iodide solutions (Table 37.2). Although these groups of drugs are not chemically related, they both block the formation of thyroid hormones within the thyroid gland (see Therapeutic Actions and Indications).

Therapeutic Actions and Indications

The Thioamides

Thioamides lower thyroid hormone levels by preventing the formation of thyroid hormone in the thyroid cells, which lowers the serum levels of thyroid hormone. They also partially inhibit the conversion of T_4 to T_3 at the cellular level. These drugs are indicated for the treatment of hyperthyroidism. Thioamides include propylthiouracil (PTU) and methimazole (*Tapazole*).

Iodine Solutions

Low doses of iodine are needed in the body for the formation of thyroid hormone. High doses, however, block thyroid function. Therefore, iodine preparations are sometimes used to treat hyperthyroidism but are not used as often as they once were in the clinical setting (see Pharmacokinetics). The iodine solutions cause the thyroid cells to become oversaturated with iodine and stop producing thyroid hormone. In some cases the thyroid cells are actually destroyed. Radioactive iodine (sodium iodide I^{131}) is taken up into the thyroid cells, which are then destroyed by the beta-radiation given off by the radioactive iodine. Except during radiation emergencies the use of sodium iodide is reserved for those patients who are not candidates for surgery, women who cannot become pregnant, and elderly patients with such severe, complicating conditions that immediate thyroid destruction is needed. Iodine solutions include strong iodine solution, potassium iodide (*Iosat, Thyrosafe, Thyroshield*), and sodium iodide I^{131} (generic). See Table 37.2 for Usual Indications for each drug.

Pharmacokinetics

Thioamides

These drugs are well absorbed from the GI tract and are then concentrated in the thyroid gland. The onset and duration of PTU varies with each patient. Methimazole has an onset of action of 30 to 40 minutes and peaks in about 60 minutes. Some excretion can be detected in the urine. Methimazole crosses the placenta and is found in a high ratio in breast milk. PTU has a low potential for crossing the placenta and for entering breast milk (see Contraindications and Cautions).

Iodine Solutions

These drugs are rapidly absorbed from the GI tract and widely distributed throughout the body fluids. Excretion occurs through the urine. Strong iodine products, potassium iodide, and sodium iodide are taken orally and have a rapid onset of action, with effects seen within 24 hours and peak effects seen in 10 to 15 days. The effects are short-lived and may even precipitate further thyroid enlargement and dysfunction (see Adverse Effects). For this reason, and because of the availability of the more predictable thioamides, iodides are not used as often as they once were in the clinical setting. They are used in cases of radiation emergencies.

The strong iodine products cross the placenta and are known to enter breast milk, but the effects on the neonate are not known. Sodium iodide I^{131} enters breast milk and is rated pregnancy category X (see Contraindications and Cautions).

Contraindications and Cautions

Antithyroid agents are contraindicated in the presence of any known allergy to antithyroid drugs *to prevent hypersensitivity reactions* and during pregnancy *because of the risk of adverse effects on the fetus and the development of cretinism.* (If an antithyroid drug is absolutely essential and the mother has been informed about the risk of cretinism in the infant, PTU is the drug of choice, but caution should still be used.) Another method of feeding the baby should be chosen if an antithyroid drug is needed during lactation *because of the risk of antithyroid activity in the infant, including the development of a neonatal goiter.* (Again, if an antithyroid drug is needed, PTU is the drug of choice.) PTU has been associated with severe liver toxicity and is no longer recommended for use in children *because they are more susceptible to the toxic effects on the liver.*

Use of strong iodine products is also contraindicated with pulmonary edema or pulmonary tuberculosis.

> **FOCUS ON Safe Medication Administration**
>
> *Name confusion has been reported between propylthiouracil and* ***Purinethol*** *(mercaptopurine), an antineoplastic agent. Both drugs are often referred to as PTU. Serious adverse effects could occur. Use extreme caution when using these drugs.*

Adverse Effects

Thioamides

The adverse effects most commonly seen with thioamides are the effects of thyroid suppression: Drowsiness, lethargy, bradycardia, nausea, skin rash, and so on. PTU is associated with nausea, vomiting, GI complaints, and severe liver toxicity. GI effects are somewhat less pronounced with methimazole, so it may be the drug of choice for patients who are unable to tolerate PTU or patients with known liver dysfunction. Methimazole is also associated with bone marrow suppression, so the patient using this drug must have frequent blood tests to monitor for this effect.

Iodine Solutions

The most common adverse effect of iodine solutions is hypothyroidism; the patient will need to be started on replacement thyroid hormone to maintain homeostasis. Other adverse effects include iodism (metallic taste and burning in the mouth, sore teeth and gums, diarrhea, cold symptoms, and stomach upset), staining of teeth, skin rash, and the development of goiter.

Sodium iodide (radioactive I^{131}) is usually reserved for use in patients who are older than 30 years of age because of the adverse effects associated with the radioactivity.

Clinically Important Drug–Drug Interactions

Thioamides

An increased risk for bleeding exists when PTU is administered with oral anticoagulants. Changes in serum levels of theophylline, metoprolol, propranolol, and digitalis may lead to changes in the effects of PTU as the patient moves from the hyperthyroid to the euthyroid state.

Iodine Solutions

Because the use of drugs to destroy thyroid function moves the patient from hyperthyroidism to hypothyroidism, patients who are taking drugs that are metabolized differently in hypothyroid and hyperthyroid states or drugs that have a small margin of safety that could be altered by the change in thyroid function should be monitored closely. These drugs include anticoagulants, theophylline, digoxin, metoprolol, and propranolol.

Prototype Summary: Methimazole

Indications: Treatment of hyperthyroidism.

Actions: Inhibits the synthesis of thyroid hormones.

Pharmacokinetics:

Route	Onset	Duration
PO	30–60 min	2–4 h

$T_{1/2}$: 6 to 13 hours; excreted in the urine.

Adverse Effects: Paresthesias, neuritis, vertigo, drowsiness, skin rash, urticaria, skin pigmentation, nausea, vomiting, epigastric distress, nephritis, bone marrow suppression, arthralgia, myalgia, edema.

Prototype Summary: Strong Iodine Products

Indications: Adjunct therapy for hyperthyroidism; thyroid blocking in a radiation emergency.

Actions: Inhibit the synthesis of thyroid hormones and inhibit the release of these hormones into the circulation.

Pharmacokinetics:

Route	Onset	Peak	Duration
PO	24 h	10–15 d	6 wk

$T_{1/2}$: Unknown; metabolized in the liver and excreted in the urine.

Adverse Effects: Rash, hypothyroidism, goiter, swelling of the salivary glands, iodism (metallic taste, burning mouth and throat, sore teeth and gums, head cold symptoms, stomach upset, diarrhea), allergic reactions.

Nursing Considerations for Patients Receiving Antithyroid Agents

Assessment: History and Examination

- Assess for history of allergy to any antithyroid drug; pregnancy and lactation status, liver dysfunction; and pulmonary edema or pulmonary tuberculosis if using strong iodine solutions, *which could be cautions or contraindications to use of the drug.*
- Assess for skin lesions; orientation and affect; baseline pulse, blood pressure, and electrocardiogram; respiration and adventitious sounds; and thyroid function tests, *to determine baseline status before beginning therapy and for any potential adverse effects.*

Nursing Diagnoses

Nursing diagnoses related to drug therapy might include the following:

- Decreased cardiac output related to cardiac effects
- Imbalanced nutrition: More than body requirements related to changes in metabolism
- Risk for injury related to bone marrow suppression
- Deficient knowledge regarding drug therapy

Planning

- The patient will receive the best therapeutic effect from the drug therapy.
- The patient will have limited adverse effects to the drug therapy.
- The patient will have an understanding of the drug therapy, adverse effects to anticipate, and measures to relieve discomfort and improve safety.

(continues on page 618)

Implementation with Rationale

- Administer propylthiouracil three times a day, around the clock, *to ensure consistent therapeutic levels.*
- Give iodine solution through a straw *to decrease staining of teeth*; tablets can be crushed.
- Monitor response carefully and arrange for periodic blood tests *to assess patient response and to monitor for adverse effects.*
- Monitor patients receiving iodine solution for any sign of iodism *so the drug can be stopped immediately if such signs appear.*
- Provide thorough patient teaching, including measures to avoid adverse effects, warning signs of problems, and the need for regular evaluation if used for longer than recommended, *to enhance patient knowledge of drug therapy and promote compliance.*

Evaluation

- Monitor patient response to the drug (lowering of thyroid hormone levels).
- Monitor for adverse effects (bradycardia, anxiety, blood dyscrasias, skin rash).
- Evaluate the effectiveness of the teaching plan (patient can name drug, dosage, adverse effects to watch for, and specific measures to avoid them).
- Monitor the effectiveness of comfort measures and compliance to the regimen.

KEY POINTS

- Hypothyroidism, or lower-than-normal levels of thyroid hormone, is treated with replacement thyroid hormone.
- Hyperthyroidism, or higher-than-normal levels of thyroid hormone, is treated with thioamides, which block the thyroid from producing thyroid hormone, or with iodines, which prevent thyroid hormone production or destroy parts of the gland.

The Parathyroid Glands

The parathyroid glands are four very small groups of glandular tissue located on the back of the thyroid gland (Figure 37.4). The parathyroid glands produce PTH, an important regulator of serum calcium levels.

Structure and Function

As mentioned earlier, the parafollicular cells of the thyroid gland produce the hormone calcitonin. Calcitonin responds to high calcium levels to cause lower serum calcium levels and acts to balance the effects of the PTH, which works to elevate calcium levels. PTH is the most important regulator of serum calcium levels in the body. PTH has many actions, including the following:

- Stimulation of osteoclasts or bone cells to release calcium from the bone
- Increased intestinal absorption of calcium

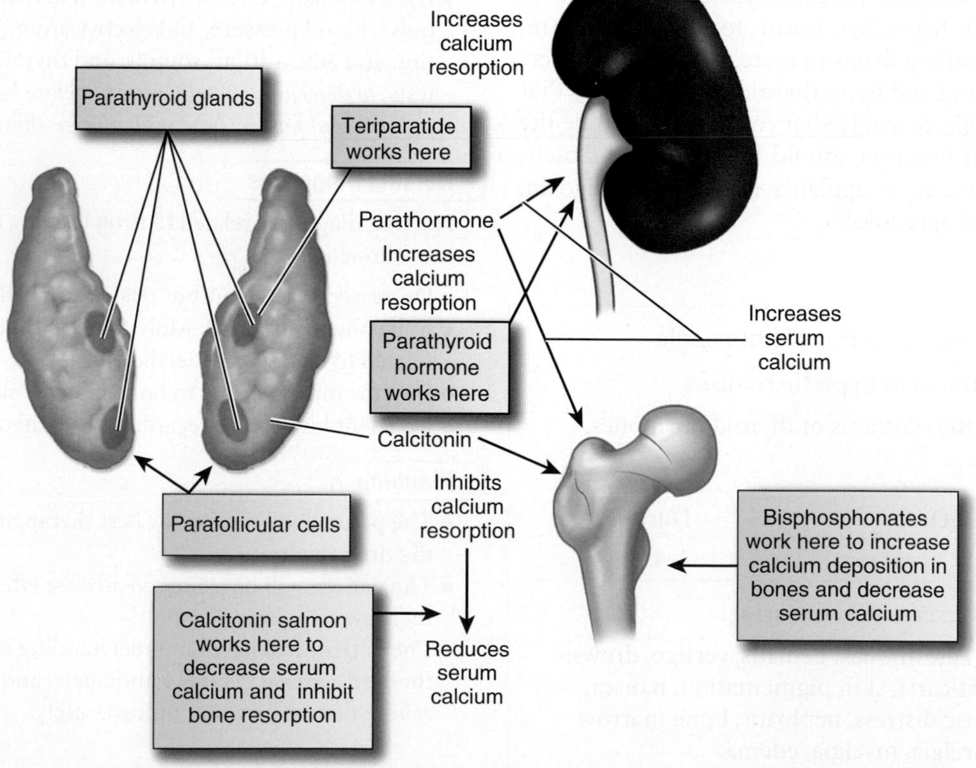

FIGURE 37.4 Calcium control. Parathormone and calcitonin work to maintain calcium homeostasis in the body.

- Increased calcium reabsorption from the kidneys
- Stimulation of cells in the kidney to produce calcitriol, the active form of vitamin D, which stimulates intestinal transport of calcium into the blood

Control

Calcium is an electrolyte that is used in many of the body's metabolic processes. These processes include membrane transport systems, conduction of nerve impulses, muscle contraction, and blood clotting. To achieve all of these effects, the serum levels of calcium must be maintained between 9 and 11 mg/dL. This is achieved through regulation of serum calcium by PTH and calcitonin (Figure 37.5).

The release of calcitonin is not controlled by the hypothalamic–pituitary axis but is regulated locally at the cellular level. Calcitonin is released when serum calcium levels rise. Calcitonin works to reduce calcium levels by blocking bone resorption and enhancing bone formation. This action pulls calcium out of the serum for deposit into the bone. When serum calcium levels are low, PTH release is stimulated. When serum calcium levels are high, PTH release is blocked.

Another electrolyte—magnesium—also affects PTH secretion by mobilizing calcium and inhibiting the release of PTH when concentrations rise above or fall below normal. An increased serum phosphate level indirectly stimulates parathyroid activity. Renal tubular phosphate reabsorption is balanced by calcium secretion into the

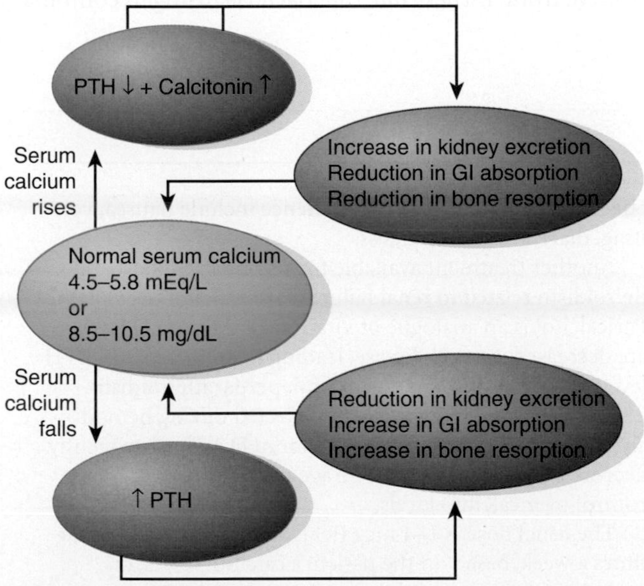

FIGURE 37.5 Regulation of serum calcium. Parathyroid hormone (PTH) and calcitonin regulate normal serum calcium. As serum calcium rises, PTH is inhibited by calcitonin. The kidney then excretes more calcium, the gastrointestinal (GI) system absorbs less, and a reduction in bone resorption occurs. As serum calcium falls, PTH is secreted and raises the calcium level by decreasing the amount of calcium lost in the kidney, increasing the amount absorbed in the GI tract and increasing bone resorption.

urine, which causes a drop in serum calcium, stimulating PTH secretion. The hormones PTH and calcitonin work together to maintain the delicate balance of serum calcium levels in the body and to keep serum calcium levels within the normal range.

Parathyroid Dysfunction and Related Disorders

Parathyroid dysfunction involves either absence of PTH (hypoparathyroidism) or overproduction of PTH (hyperparathyroidism). This dysfunction can affect any age group. Box 37.1 explains the use of parathyroid agents across the lifespan.

Hypoparathyroidism

The absence of PTH results in a low calcium level (**hypocalcemia**) and a relatively rare condition called **hypoparathyroidism.** This is most likely to occur with the accidental removal of the parathyroid glands during thyroid surgery. Treatment consists of calcium and vitamin D therapy to increase serum calcium levels (see Antihypocalcemic Agents).

Hyperparathyroidism

The excessive production of PTH leads to an elevated calcium level (**hypercalcemia**) and a condition called **hyperparathyroidism.** This can occur as a result of parathyroid tumor or certain genetic disorders. The patient presents with signs of high calcium levels (see Table 37.3). Primary hyperparathyroidism occurs more often in women between 60 and 70 years of age. Secondary hyperparathyroidism occurs most frequently in patients with chronic renal failure (see Box 37.3 for more information). When the plasma concentrations of calcium are elevated secondary to high PTH levels, inorganic phosphate levels are usually decreased. Pseudorickets (renal fibrocystic osteosis or renal rickets) may occur as a result of this phosphorus retention (hyperphosphatemia), which results from increased stimulation of the parathyroid glands and increased PTH secretion.

The genetically linked disorder **Paget's disease** is a condition of overactive osteoclasts that are eventually replaced by enlarged and softened bony structures. Patients with this disease complain of deep-bone pain, headaches, and hearing loss and usually have cardiac failure and bone malformation.

Postmenopausal osteoporosis can occur when dropping levels of estrogen allow calcium to be pulled out of the bone, resulting in a weakened and honeycombed bone structure. Estrogen normally causes calcium deposits in the bone; osteoporosis is one of the many complications that accompany the loss of estrogen at menopause (Box 37.4).

Table 37.3 Signs and Symptoms of Calcium Imbalance

System	Hypocalcemia	Hypercalcemia
CNS	Hyperactive reflexes, paresthesias, positive Chvostek and Trousseau signs	Lethargy, personality and behavior changes, polydipsia, stupor, coma
CV	Hypotension, prolonged QT interval, edema, and signs of cardiac insufficiency	Hypertension, shortening of the QT interval, atrioventricular block
GI	Abdominal spasms and cramps	Anorexia, nausea, vomiting, constipation
Muscular	Tetany, skeletal muscle cramps, carpopedal spasm, laryngeal spasm, tetany	Muscle weakness, muscle atrophy, ataxia, loss of muscle tone
Renal		Polyuria, flank pain, kidney stones, acute and/or chronic renal insufficiency
Skeletal	Bone pain, osteomalacia, bone deformities, fractures	Osteopenia, osteoporosis

CNS, central nervous system; CV, cardiovascular; GI, gastrointestinal.

KEY POINTS

- Parathyroid glands produce PTH, which, together with calcitonin, maintains the body's calcium balance.
- A low calcium level (hypocalcemia) is treated with vitamin D and calcium replacement therapy.
- Hypercalcemia and hypercalcemic states are associated with postmenopausal osteoporosis, Paget's disease, and renal failure and malignancies.

Parathyroid Agents

The drugs used to treat disorders associated with parathyroid function are drugs that affect serum calcium levels. There are two parathyroid replacement hormones available and one form of calcitonin; other drugs affect calcium levels in different ways.

Antihypocalcemic Agents

Deficient levels of PTH result in hypocalcemia (calcium deficiency). Vitamin D stimulates calcium absorption from the intestine and restores the serum calcium to a normal level. Hypoparathyroidism is treated primarily with vitamin D and, if necessary, dietary supplements of calcium. However, there are two PTH forms available for therapeutic use, teriparatide (*Forteo*), a PTH genetically engineered from *Escherichia coli* bacteria using recombinant

BOX 37.3

Treatments for Secondary Hyperparathyroidism

A newer class of calcimimetic agents, cinacalcet hydrochloride (*Sensipar*), is available for treatment of secondary hyperparathyroidism in patients undergoing dialysis for chronic kidney disease and for treatment of hypercalcemia in patients with parathyroid carcinoma. Cinacalcet is a calcimimetic drug that increases the sensitivity of the calcium-sensing receptors to activation by extracellular calcium. In increasing the receptors' sensitivity, cinacalcet lowers PTH levels, causing a concomitant decrease in serum calcium levels.

The usual initial adult doses for secondary hyperparathyroidism are 30 mg/d PO, after which PTH, serum calcium, and serum phosphorus levels are monitored to achieve the desired therapeutic effect. The usual dose range is 60–180 mg/d. The drug must be used in combination with vitamin D and/or phosphate binders.

For parathyroid carcinoma the initial dose is 30 mg PO twice a day titrated every 2–4 weeks to maintain serum calcium levels within a normal range; 30–90 mg twice a day up to 90 mg three to four times daily may be needed. Side effects that the patient may experience include nausea, vomiting, diarrhea, and dizziness.

Another treatment available for secondary hyperparathyroidism related to renal failure is paricalcitol (*Zemplar*). Paricalcitol is an analogue of vitamin D. Vitamin D levels are decreased in renal disease, leading to an increase in PTH levels and signs and symptoms of hyperparathyroidism. *Zemplar* is taken orally or can be injected during hemodialysis. The body recognizes the vitamin D and subsequently decreases the synthesis and storage of PTH, allowing a control over calcium levels.

The usual dose is 1–4 mcg PO from once a day to three times a week, based on the patient's calcium levels, or 0.04–0.1 mcg/kg injected during hemodialysis. The drug is rapidly absorbed with peak levels within 3 hours. The drug has a half-life of 12–20 hours. Patients will need regular serum calcium checks, and dose will be adjusted based on individual response. Adverse effects are usually mild, as long as the calcium levels are monitored. Diarrhea, headache, and mild hypertension have been reported.

BOX 37.4 FOCUS ON Gender Considerations

Osteoporosis

Osteoporosis is the most common bone disease found in adults. It results from a lack of bone-building cell (osteoclast) activity and a decrease in bone matrix and mass, with less calcium and phosphorus being deposited in the bone. This can occur with advancing age, when the endocrine system is slowing down and the stimulation to build bone is absent; with menopause, when the calcium-depositing effects of estrogen are lost; with malnutrition states, when vitamin C and proteins essential for bone production are absent from the diet; and with a lack of physical stress on the bones from lack of activity, which promotes calcium removal and does not stimulate osteoclast activity. The inactive, elderly, postmenopausal woman with a poor diet is a prime candidate for osteoporosis. Fractured hips and wrists, shrinking size, and curvature of the spine are all evidence of osteoporosis in this age group. Besides the use of bisphosphonates to encourage calcium deposition in the bone, several other interventions can help prevent severe osteoporosis in this group or in any other people with similar risk factors.

- *Aerobic exercise:* Walking, even 10 minutes a day, has been shown to help increase osteoclast activity. Encourage people to walk around the block or to park their car far from the door and walk. Exercise does not have to involve vigorous gym activity to be beneficial.
- *Proper diet:* Calcium and proteins are essential for bone growth. The person who eats only pasta and avoids milk products could benefit from calcium supplements and encouragement to eat protein at least two or three times a week. Weight loss can also help to improve activity and decrease pressure on bones at rest.
- *Hormone replacement therapy (HRT):* For women, HRT has been very successful in decreasing the progression of osteoporosis. However, results of the Women's Health Study showed an increase in CV events and dementia with long-term HRT, making it a less desirable treatment. The use of HRT has often been linked to increased risk of breast cancer. The use of bisphosphonates might be a better choice of drug therapy for many patients.

The risk of osteoporosis should be taken into consideration as part of the health care regimen for all people as they age. Prevention can save a great deal of pain and debilitation in the long run.

DNA technology, and parathyroid hormone (*Natapara*). Teriparatide is approved to increase bone mass in postmenopausal women and men with primary or hypogonadal osteoporosis who are at high risk for fracture. Parathyroid hormone (*Natapara*) is approved to help control calcium levels in patients with hypoparathyroidism. An additional hypocalcemic agent is calcitriol (*Rocaltrol*), which is the most commonly used form of vitamin D (Table 37.4).

Therapeutic Actions and Indications

Vitamin D compounds regulate the absorption of calcium and phosphate from the small intestine, mineral resorption in bone, and reabsorption of phosphate from the renal tubules. Working along with PTH and calcitonin to regulate calcium homeostasis, vitamin D actually functions as a hormone. With once-daily administration, teriparatide stimulates new bone formation, leading to an increase in skeletal mass. It increases serum calcium and decreases serum phosphorus. Parathyroid hormone acts as a replacement for missing PTH.

Use of these agents is indicated for the management of hypocalcemia in patients undergoing chronic renal dialysis and for the treatment of hypoparathyroidism; teriparatide is also used for the treatment of postmenopausal or hypogonadal osteoporosis and osteoporosis associated with sustained systemic glucocorticoid therapy, which could lead to fractures (see Table 37.4). Parathyroid hormone is only approved for maintenance of calcium levels in patients with hypoparathyroidism.

Pharmacokinetics

Calcitriol is well absorbed from the GI tract and widely distributed throughout the body. It is stored in the liver, fat, muscle, skin, and bones. Calcitriol has a half-life of approximately 5 to 8 hours and a duration of action of 3 to 5 days. After being metabolized in the liver, it is primarily excreted in the bile, with some found in the urine (see Contraindications and Cautions for use of these drugs during pregnancy and lactation).

Teriparatide is given by subcutaneous injection every day. It is rapidly absorbed from the subcutaneous tissues, reaching peak concentration within 3 hours. The half-life of teriparatide is about 1 hour. Serum calcium levels will begin to decline after about 6 hours and return to baseline 16 to 24 hours after dosing. This drug is believed to be metabolized in the liver and excreted through the kidneys.

Parathyroid hormone is given as a daily subcutaneous injection. It reaches peak levels in 5 to 30 minutes and has a half-life of 3 hours. It is thought to be metabolized in the liver and excreted through the kidneys.

Contraindications and Cautions

These drugs should not be used in the presence of any known allergy to any component of the drug *to avoid hypersensitivity reactions*, or hypercalcemia or vitamin D toxicity, *which would be exacerbated by these drugs.* At therapeutic levels, these drugs should be used during pregnancy only if the benefit to the mother clearly outweighs

Table 37.4 *Drugs in Focus:* Parathyroid Agents

Drug Name	Usual Dosage	Usual Indications
Antihypocalcemic Agents		
calcitriol (*Rocaltrol*)	0.5–2 mcg/d PO in the morning	Management of hypocalcemia and reduction of parathormone levels
parathyroid hormone (*Naptara*)	50 mcg/day subcutaneously, adjust dose to maintain serum calcium levels in the lower range of normal	Maintenance of serum calcium levels in adults with hypoparathyroidism
teriparatide (*Forteo*)	20 mg subcutaneously daily	Management of osteoporosis in postmenopausal women and men with primary hypogonadal osteoporosis who do not respond to standard therapy; treatment of patients on sustained systemic glucocorticoid therapy at high risk for fractures
Antihypercalcemic Agents ***Bisphosphonates***		
alendronate (*Fosamax*)	10 mg/d PO; for males and for postmenopausal osteoporosis, 70 mg PO every week *or* 10 mg/d PO for treatment, 35 mg PO every week *or* 5 mg/d PO for prevention	Treatment of Paget's disease, postmenopausal osteoporosis treatment and prevention, treatment of glucocorticoid-induced osteoporosis, osteoporosis in men
etidronate (*Didronel*)	5–10 mg/kg/d PO for 6 mo for Paget's disease; 20 mg/kg/d PO for 2 wk, then 10 mg/kg/d PO for 10 wk for heterotopic ossification	Treatment of Paget's disease, postmenopausal osteoporosis, heterotopic ossification
ibandronate (*Boniva*)	2.5 mg/d PO or 150 mg PO once per month on the same day each month; 3 mg IV given over 15–30 s once every 3 mo	Treatment and prevention of osteoporosis in postmenopausal women
pamidronate (*Aredia*)	30–90 mg IV as an infusion	Treatment of Paget's disease, postmenopausal osteoporosis in women, hypercalcemia of malignancy, osteolytic bone lesions in cancer patients
risedronate (*Actonel*)	30 mg/d PO for 2 mo; reduce dose in renal dysfunction; 5 mg/d PO for osteoporosis *or* 35 mg PO once per week *or* 150 mg PO once per month; 35 mg PO once per week for men to increase bone mass	Treatment of symptomatic Paget's disease in patients who are at risk for complications; treatment and prevention of osteoporosis (postmenopausal, glucocorticoid related and in men)
zoledronic acid (*Zometa, Reclast*)	4 mg IV as a single infusion over not less than 15 min (given once every 2 y for postmenopausal osteoporosis)	Treatment of Paget's disease, postmenopausal osteoporosis in women, hypercalcemia of malignancy, osteolytic bone lesions in certain cancer patients; prevention of new fractures in patients with low-trauma hip fractures
Calcitonins		
calcitonin salmon (*Miacalcin*)	*Paget's disease:* 50–100 IU/d subcutaneous or IM *Postmenopausal osteoporosis:* 100 IU/d subcutaneous or IM with calcium and vitamin D *Hypercalcemia:* 4–8 IU/kg subcutaneous or IM q12 h	Treatment of Paget's disease, postmenopausal osteoporosis in conjunction with vitamin D and calcium supplements; emergency treatment of hypercalcemia
(*Fortical*)	200 IU/d intranasally; alternate nostrils daily	Treatment of postmenopausal osteoporosis in conjunction with calcium supplements and vitamin D

the potential for adverse effects on the fetus. Calcitriol has been associated with hypercalcemia (excessive calcium levels in the blood) in the baby when used by nursing mothers; therefore, another method of feeding the baby should be used if these drugs are needed during lactation. Caution should be used with a history of renal stones or during lactation, *when high calcium levels could cause problems.*

Teriparatide and parathyroid hormone are associated with osteosarcoma—a bone cancer—in animal studies, so its use is limited to postmenopausal women who have osteoporosis, are at high risk for fractures, and are intolerant to standard therapies and to men with primary or hypogonadal osteoporosis or patients on sustained systemic glucocorticoid therapy who are at high risk for fracture and are intolerant to standard therapies. Patients should be informed of the risk of osteosarcoma. These patients should also take supplemental calcium and vitamin D, increase weight-bearing exercise, and decrease risk factors such as smoking and alcohol consumption. Parathyroid hormone is only available through a limited access program.

Adverse Effects

The adverse effects most commonly seen with these drugs are related to GI effects: Metallic taste, nausea, vomiting, dry mouth, constipation, and anorexia. CNS effects such as weakness, headache, somnolence, and irritability may also occur. These are possibly related to the changes in electrolytes that occur with these drugs. Patients with liver or renal dysfunction may experience increased levels of the drugs and/or toxic effects. Severe hypocalcemia and hypercalcemia have occurred with the use of parathyroid hormone.

Clinically Important Drug–Drug Interactions

The risk of hypermagnesemia increases if these drugs are taken with magnesium-containing antacids. This combination should be avoided.

Reduced absorption of these compounds may occur if they are taken with cholestyramine or mineral oil because they are fat-soluble vitamins. If this combination is used the drugs should be separated by at least 2 hours.

Digoxin toxicity can occur with hypercalcemia. If combining these drugs with digoxin, digoxin serum levels and serum calcium levels should be monitored closely.

Ⓟ Prototype Summary: Calcitriol

Indications: Management of hypocalcemia in patients on chronic renal dialysis, management of hypocalcemia associated with hypoparathyroidism.

Actions: A vitamin D compound that regulates the absorption of calcium and phosphate from the small intestine, mineral resorption in bone, and reabsorption of phosphate from the renal tubules, increasing the serum calcium level.

Pharmacokinetics:

Route	Onset	Peak	Duration
PO	Slow	4 h	3–5 d

$T_{1/2}$: 5 to 8 hours; metabolized in the liver and excreted in the bile.

Adverse Effects: Weakness, headache, nausea, vomiting, dry mouth, constipation, muscle pain, bone pain, metallic taste.

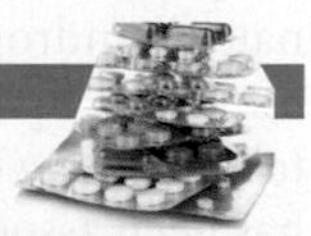

Nursing Considerations for Patients Receiving Antihypocalcemic Agents

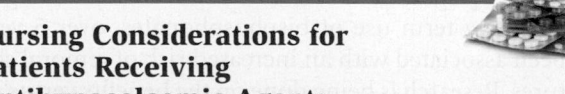

Assessment: History and Examination

- Assess for history of allergy to any component of the drugs, hypercalcemia, vitamin toxicity, renal stone, and pregnancy or lactation, *which could be cautions or contraindications to use of the drug.*
- Assess for the presence of any skin lesions; orientation and affect; liver evaluation; serum calcium, magnesium, and alkaline phosphate levels; and radiographs of bones as appropriate, *to determine baseline status before beginning therapy and any potential adverse effects.*

Nursing Diagnoses

Nursing diagnoses related to drug therapy might include the following:

- Acute pain related to GI or CNS effects
- Imbalanced nutrition: Less than body requirements related to GI effects
- Deficient knowledge regarding drug therapy

Planning

- The patient will receive the best therapeutic effect from the drug therapy.
- The patient will have limited adverse effects to the drug therapy.
- The patient will have an understanding of the drug therapy, adverse effects to anticipate, and measures to relieve discomfort and improve safety

Implementation with Rationale

- Monitor serum calcium concentration before and periodically during treatment *to allow for adjustment of dose to maintain calcium levels within normal limits.*
- Provide supportive measures *to help the patient deal with GI and CNS effects of the drug* (analgesics, small and frequent meals, help with activities of daily living).
- Arrange for a nutritional consultation if GI effects are severe *to ensure nutritional balance.*
- Provide thorough patient teaching, including measures to avoid adverse effects, warning signs of problems, and the need for regular evaluation, *to enhance the patient's knowledge about drug therapy and promote compliance.*

Evaluation

- Monitor patient response to the drug (return of serum calcium levels to normal).
- Monitor for adverse effects (weakness, headache, GI effects).
- Evaluate the effectiveness of the teaching plan (patient can name drug, dosage, adverse effects to watch for, and specific measures to avoid them).
- Monitor the effectiveness of comfort measures and compliance with the regimen.

Antihypercalcemic Agents

Drugs used to treat PTH excess or hypercalcemia include the bisphosphonates and calcitonin salmon. These drugs act on the serum levels of calcium and do not suppress the parathyroid gland or PTH (see Table 37.4).

Therapeutic Actions and Indications

Bisphosphonates

The **bisphosphonates** act to slow or block bone resorption; by doing this, they help to lower serum calcium levels, but they do not inhibit normal bone formation and mineralization. Bisphosphonates include etidronate (*Didronel*), ibandronate (*Boniva*), pamidronate (*Aredia*), risedronate (*Actonel*), alendronate (*Fosamax*), and zoledronic acid (*Zometa*). These drugs are used in the treatment of Paget's disease and of postmenopausal osteoporosis in women, and alendronate is also used to treat osteoporosis in men. Zoledronic acid is also used to prevent new fractures in patients with low-trauma hip fractures and to treat patients with multiple myeloma or documented bone metastases from solid tumors. See Table 37.4 for Usual Indications for each drug.

Calcitonins

The calcitonins are hormones secreted by the thyroid gland to balance the effects of PTH. Currently the only calcitonin readily available is calcitonin salmon (*Fortical*, *Miacalcin*). This hormone inhibits bone resorption, lowers serum calcium levels in children and in patients with Paget's disease, and increases the excretion of phosphate, calcium, and sodium from the kidney. See Table 37.4 for Usual Indications of this drug.

Pharmacokinetics

Bisphosphonates

These drugs are well absorbed from the small intestine and do not undergo metabolism. They are excreted relatively unchanged in the urine. The onset of action is slow, and the duration of action is days to weeks. Patients with renal dysfunction may experience toxic levels of the drug and should be evaluated for a dose reduction. See Contraindications and Cautions for use of these drugs during pregnancy and lactation.

Calcitonins

These drugs are metabolized in the body tissues to inactive fragments, which are excreted by the kidney. Calcitonins cross the placenta and have been associated with adverse effects on the fetus in animal studies. These drugs inhibit lactation in animals; it is not known whether they are excreted in breast milk (see Contraindications and Cautions). Salmon calcitonin can be given by injection or by nasal spray. By either route, peak effects are seen within 40 minutes, and the duration of effect is 8 to 24 hours.

Contraindications and Cautions

Bisphosphonates

These drugs should not be used in the presence of hypocalcemia, *which could be made worse by lowering calcium levels*, or with a history of any allergy to bisphosphonates *to avoid hypersensitivity reactions. Fetal abnormalities have been associated with these drugs in animal trials,* and they should not be used during pregnancy unless the benefit to the mother clearly outweighs the potential risk to the fetus or neonate. Extreme caution should be used when nursing *because of the potential for adverse effects on the baby.* Alendronate should not be used by nursing mothers *because of potential risk for adverse effects on the baby.* Caution should be used in patients with renal dysfunction, *which could interfere with excretion of the drug,* or with upper GI disease, *which could be aggravated by the drug.*

Alendronate, ibandronate, and risedronate need to be taken on arising in the morning, with a full glass of water, fully 30 minutes before any other food or beverage, and the patient must then remain upright for at least 30 minutes; *taking the drug with a full glass of water and remaining upright for at least 30 minutes facilitates delivery of the drug to the stomach.* These drugs should not be given to anyone who is unable to remain upright for 30 minutes after taking the drug *because serious esophageal erosion can occur.*

Zoledronic acid should be used cautiously in aspirin-sensitive asthmatic patients. It may be given as an IV infusion once every 2 years for osteoporosis. Alendronate and risedronate are now available in a once-a-week formulation *to decrease the number of times the patient must take the drug,* which should increase compliance with the drug regimen. Ibandronate is available in a once-a-month formulation and in an IV preparation for use when oral drugs cannot be taken.

Calcitonins

This drug should be used in pregnancy only if the benefit to the mother clearly outweighs the *potential risk to the fetus.* It should not be used during lactation *because the calcium-lowering effects could cause problems for the baby.* Calcitonin salmon should not be used with a known allergy to salmon or fish products. This drug should be used with caution in patients with renal dysfunction or pernicious anemia, *which could be exacerbated by these drugs.*

Adverse Effects

Bisphosphonates

The most common adverse effects seen with bisphosphonates are headache, nausea, and diarrhea. There is also an increase in bone pain in patients with Paget's disease, but this effect usually passes after a few days to a few weeks. Esophageal erosion has been associated with alendronate, ibandronate, and risedronate if the patient has not remained upright for at least 30 minutes after taking the tablets. Long-term use of bisphosphonates, over 5 years, has been associated with an increased risk of femoral shaft fractures. Research is being done on the benefits versus risk of long-term use of these drugs in postmenopausal women and the current guideline is to limit the use to a 3–5 year maximum in patients at low risk for fractures.

Calcitonins

The most common adverse effects seen with this drug is flushing of the face and hands, skin rash, nausea and vomiting, urinary frequency, and local inflammation at the site of injection. Many of these side effects lessen with time, the time varying with each individual patient.

Clinically Important Drug–Drug Interactions

Bisphosphonates

Oral absorption of bisphosphonates is decreased if they are taken concurrently with antacids, calcium products, iron, or multiple vitamins. If these drugs need to be taken, they should be separated by at least 30 minutes.

GI distress may increase if bisphosphonates are combined with aspirin; this combination should be avoided if possible.

Calcitonins

There have been no clinically important drug–drug interactions reported with the use of calcitonin.

Ⓟ Prototype Summary: Alendronate

Indications: Treatment and prevention of osteoporosis in postmenopausal women and in men; treatment of glucocorticoid-induced osteoporosis; treatment of Paget's disease in certain patients.

Actions: Slows normal and abnormal bone resorption without inhibiting bone formation and mineralization.

Pharmacokinetics:

Route	Onset	Duration
PO	Slow	Days

$T_{1/2}$: Greater than 10 days; not metabolized, but excreted in the urine.

Adverse Effects: Headache, nausea, diarrhea, increased or recurrent bone pain, esophageal erosion.

Ⓟ Prototype Summary: Calcitonin Salmon

Indications: Paget's disease, postmenopausal osteoporosis, emergency treatment of hypercalcemia.

Actions: Inhibits bone resorption; lowers elevated serum calcium in children and patients with Paget's disease; increases the excretion of filtered phosphate, calcium, and sodium by the kidney.

Pharmacokinetics:

Route	Onset	Peak	Duration
IM, subcutaneous	15 min	3–4 h	8–24 h
Nasal	Rapid	31–39 min	8–24 h

$T_{1/2}$: 1.43 hours; metabolized in the kidneys and excreted in the urine.

Adverse Effects: Flushing of face and hands, nausea, vomiting, local inflammatory reactions at injection site, nasal irritation if nasal form is used.

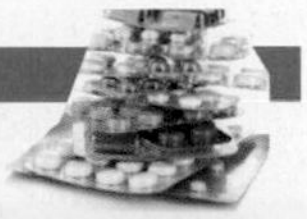

Nursing Considerations for Patients Receiving Antihypercalcemic Agents

Assessment: History and Examination

- Assess for history of allergy to any of these products or to fish products with salmon calcitonin *to avoid hypersensitivity reaction*; pregnancy or lactation; hypocalcemia; and renal dysfunction, *which could be cautions or contraindications to use of the drug.*
- Assess for the presence of any skin lesions; orientation and affect; abdominal examination; serum electrolytes; and renal function tests, *to determine baseline status before beginning therapy and for any potential adverse effects.*

Nursing Diagnoses

Nursing diagnoses related to drug therapy might include the following:

- Acute pain related to GI or skin effects
- Imbalanced nutrition: Less than body requirements related to GI effects
- Anxiety related to the need for parenteral injections (specific drugs)
- Deficient knowledge regarding drug therapy

Planning

- The patient will receive the best therapeutic effect from the drug therapy.
- The patient will have limited adverse effects to the drug therapy.
- The patient will have an understanding of the drug therapy, adverse effects to anticipate, and measures to relieve discomfort and improve safety.

Implementation with Rationale

- Ensure adequate hydration with any of these agents *to reduce the risk of renal complications.*
- Arrange for concomitant vitamin D, calcium supplements, and hormone replacement therapy *if used to treat postmenopausal osteoporosis.*
- Rotate injection sites and monitor for inflammation if using calcitonins *to prevent tissue breakdown and irritation.*
- Monitor serum calcium regularly *to allow for dose adjustment as needed.*
- Assess the patient carefully for any potential drug–drug interactions if giving in combination with other drugs *to prevent serious effects.*
- Arrange for periodic blood tests of renal function if using gallium *to monitor for renal dysfunction.*
- Provide comfort measures and analgesics *to relieve bone pain if it returns as treatment begins.*
- Provide thorough patient teaching, including measures to avoid adverse effects, warning signs of problems, the

(continues on page 626)

need for regular evaluation if used for longer than recommended, and proper administration of nasal spray, *to enhance patient knowledge about drug therapy and promote compliance.*

Evaluation

- Monitor patient response to the drug (return of calcium levels to normal; prevention of complications of osteoporosis; control of Paget's disease).
- Monitor for adverse effects (skin rash; nausea and vomiting; hypocalcemia; renal dysfunction; monitor length of bisphosphonate use).
- Evaluate the effectiveness of the teaching plan (patient can name drug, dosage, adverse effects to watch for, and specific measures to avoid them).
- Monitor the effectiveness of comfort measures and compliance with the regimen.

KEY POINTS

- The parathyroid glands are located behind the thyroid gland and produce PTH, which works with calcitonin, produced by thyroid cells, to maintain the calcium balance in the body.
- Hypocalcemia, or low levels of calcium, is treated with vitamin D products and calcium replacement therapy.
- Hypercalcemia can occur in postmenopausal osteoporosis and Paget's disease, as well as hypercalcemia related to malignancy
- Hypercalcemia is treated with bisphosphonates, which slow or block bone resorption to lower serum calcium levels, or calcitonin, which inhibits bone resorption, lowers serum calcium levels in children and patients with Paget's disease, and increases the excretion of phosphate, calcium, and sodium from the kidney.

SUMMARY

- The thyroid gland uses iodine to produce thyroid hormones. Thyroid hormones control the rate at which most body cells use energy (metabolism).
- Control of the thyroid gland is an intricate process between TRH, released by the hypothalamus; TSH, released by the anterior pituitary; and circulating levels of thyroid hormone.
- Hypothyroidism, or lower-than-normal levels of thyroid hormone, is treated with replacement thyroid hormone.
- Hyperthyroidism, or higher-than-normal levels of thyroid hormone, is treated with thioamides, which block the thyroid from producing thyroid hormone, or with iodines, which prevent thyroid hormone production or destroy parts of the gland.
- The parathyroid glands are located behind the thyroid gland and produce PTH, which works with calcitonin, produced by thyroid cells, to maintain the calcium balance in the body.
- Hypocalcemia, or low levels of calcium, is treated with vitamin D products and calcium replacement therapy.
- Hypercalcemia and hypercalcemic states include postmenopausal osteoporosis and Paget's disease, as well as hypercalcemia related to malignancy.
- Hypercalcemia is treated with bisphosphonates or calcitonin. Bisphosphonates slow or block bone resorption, which lowers serum calcium levels. Calcitonin inhibits bone resorption, lowers serum calcium levels in children and patients with Paget's disease, and increases the excretion of phosphate, calcium, and sodium from the kidney.

CHECK YOUR UNDERSTANDING

Answers to the questions in this chapter can be found in Answers to Check Your Understanding Questions on thePoint®.

MULTIPLE CHOICE

Select the best answer to the following.

1. The thyroid gland produces the thyroid hormones triiodothyronine (T_3) and tetraiodothyronine (T_4), which are dependent on the availability of
   a. iodine produced in the liver.
   b. iodine found in the diet.
   c. iron absorbed from the GI tract.
   d. PTH to promote iodine binding.

2. The thyroid gland is dependent on the hypothalamic–pituitary axis for regulation. Increasing the levels of thyroid hormone (by taking replacement thyroid hormone) would
   a. increase hypothalamic release of TRH.
   b. increase pituitary release of TSH.
   c. suppress hypothalamic release of TRH.
   d. stimulate the thyroid gland to produce more T_3 and T_4.

3. Goiter, or enlargement of the thyroid gland, is usually associated with
   a. hypothyroidism.
   b. iodine deficiency.
   c. hyperthyroidism.
   d. underactive thyroid tissue.

4. Thyroid replacement therapy is indicated for the treatment of
   a. obesity.
   b. myxedema.
   c. Graves' disease.
   d. acute thyrotoxicosis.

5. Assessing a patient's knowledge of his or her thyroid replacement therapy would show good understanding if the patient stated:
   a. "My wife may use some of my drug, since she wants to lose weight."
   b. "I should only need this drug for about 3 months."
   c. "I can stop taking this drug as soon as I feel like my old self."
   d. "I should call if I experience unusual sweating, weight gain, or chills and fever."

6. Administration of propylthiouracil would include giving the drug
   a. once a day in the morning.
   b. around the clock to assure therapeutic levels.
   c. once a day at bedtime to decrease adverse effects.
   d. if the patient is experiencing slow heart rate, skin rash, or excessive bleeding.

7. The parathyroid glands produce PTH, which is important in the body as
   a. a modulator of thyroid hormone.
   b. a regulator of potassium.
   c. a regulator of calcium.
   d. an activator of vitamin D.

8. The drug of choice for the treatment of postmenopausal osteoporosis would be
   a. risedronate.
   b. alendronate.
   c. zoledronic acid
   d. calcitriol.

MULTIPLE RESPONSE

Select all that apply.

1. A patient who is receiving a bisphosphonate for the treatment of postmenopausal osteoporosis should be taught
   a. to also take vitamin D, calcium, and hormone replacement.
   b. to restrict fluids as much as possible.
   c. to take the drug before any food for the day, with a full glass of water.
   d. to stay upright for at least 1/2 hour after taking the drug.
   e. to take the drug with meals to avoid GI upset.
   f. to avoid exercise to prevent bone fractures.

2. Hypothyroidism is a very common and often missed disorder. Signs and symptoms of hypothyroidism include
   a. increased body temperature.
   b. thickening of the tongue.
   c. bradycardia.
   d. loss of hair.
   e. excessive weight loss.
   f. oily skin.

BIBLIOGRAPHY AND REFERENCES

American Medical Association. (2012). *AMA drug evaluations.* Chicago, IL: Author.

Blackwell, J. (2004). Evaluation and treatment of hyperthyroidism and hypothyroidism. *Journal of the American Academy of Nurse Practitioners, 16*(10), 422–425.

Brunton, L., Chabner, B., & Knollman, B. (2011). *Goodman and Gilman's the pharmacological basis of therapeutics* (12th ed.). New York: McGraw-Hill.

Cooper, D. S. (2005). Drug therapy: Antithyroid drugs. *New England Journal of Medicine, 352,* 905–917.

Fact and Comparisons. (2015). *Drug facts and comparisons.* St. Louis, MO: Author.

Karch, A. M. (2014). *Lippincott's nursing drug guide.* Philadelphia, PA: Lippincott Williams & Wilkins.

Khan, A., & Clark, O. (2011). *Parathyroid and calcium disorders.* New York: Humana Press.

Licata, A., & Lerma, E. (Eds.). (2012). *Diseases of the parathyroid glands.* New York. Springer.

Monaco, F. (2012). *Thyroid diseases.* Philadelphia, PA: Taylor & Francis

Park-Willie, L, Mamdani, M., Mamdani, M. M., et al. (2011). Bisphosphonate use and the risk of subtrochanteric or femoral shaft fractures in older women. *Journal of the American Medical Association, 305*(8),783–789.

The Medical Letter. (2015). *The medical letter on drugs and therapeutics.* New Rochelle, NY: Author.

Wondisford, F. E., & Radovick, S. (2009). *Clinical management of thyroid disease.* Philadelphia, PA: Saunders.

38 Agents to Control Blood Glucose Levels

Learning Objectives

Upon completion of this chapter, you will be able to:

1. Describe the pathophysiology of diabetes mellitus, including alterations in metabolic pathways and changes to basement membranes.
2. Describe the therapeutic actions, indications, pharmacokinetics, contraindications, most common adverse reactions, and important drug–drug interactions associated with insulin and other antidiabetic and glucose-elevating agents.
3. Discuss the use of antidiabetic and glucose-elevating agents across the lifespan.
4. Compare and contrast the prototype drugs insulin, chlorpropamide, glyburide, metformin, liraglitude, sitagliptin, and canagliflozin with other antidiabetic agents in their class.
5. Outline the nursing considerations, including important teaching points, for patients receiving an antidiabetic or glucose-elevating agent.

Glossary of Key Terms

adiponectin: hormone produced by adipocytes that acts to increase insulin sensitivity, decrease the release of glucose from liver, and protect the blood vessels from inflammatory changes

diabetes mellitus: a metabolic disorder characterized by high blood glucose levels and altered metabolism of proteins and fats; associated with thickening of the basement membrane, leading to numerous complications

dipeptidyl peptidase-4 (DDP-4): enzyme that quickly metabolizes glucagon-like polypeptide-1

endocannabinoid receptors: receptors found in the adipose tissue, muscles, liver, satiety center, and gastrointestinal (GI) tract that are part of a signaling system within the body to keep the body in a state of energy gain

glucagon-like polypeptide-1 (GLP-1): a peptide produced in the GI tract in response to carbohydrates that increases insulin release, decreases glucagon release, slows GI emptying, and stimulates the satiety center in the brain

glycogen: storage form of glucose; can be broken down for rapid glucose level increases during times of stress

glycosuria: presence of glucose in the urine

glycosylated hemoglobin: a blood glucose marker that provides a 3-month average of blood glucose levels

hyperglycemia: elevated blood glucose levels (>106 mg/dL) leading to multiple signs and symptoms and abnormal metabolic pathways

hypoglycemia: lower-than-normal blood sugar (<40 mg/dL); often results from imbalance between insulin or oral agents and patient's eating, activity, and stress

incretins: peptides that are produced in the GI tract in response to food that help to modulate insulin and glucagon activity

insulin: hormone produced by the beta cells in the pancreas; stimulates insulin receptor sites to move glucose into the cells; promotes storage of fat and glucose in the body

ketosis: breakdown of fats for energy, resulting in an increase in ketones to be excreted from the body

polydipsia: increased thirst; seen in diabetes when loss of fluid and increased tonicity of the blood lead the hypothalamic thirst center to make the patient feel thirsty

polyphagia: increased hunger; sign of diabetes when cells cannot use glucose for energy and feel that they are starving, causing hunger

sulfonylureas: oral antidiabetic agents used to stimulate the pancreas to release more insulin

Drug List

Insulin	Other Antidiabetic Agents	Glucagon-like Polypeptide Receptor Agonists	Sodium–Glucose Cotransporter-2 Inhibitors
(P) insulin	*Alpha-Glucosidase Inhibitors*	abiglutide	(P) canagliflozin
Sulfonylureas and Other Antidiabetic Agents	acarbose	dulaglutide	dapagliflozin
Sulfonylureas	miglitol	liraglutide	empagliflozin
First-Generation Sulfonylureas	*Biguanide*	teduglutide	*Thiazolidinediones*
(P) chlorpropamide	(P) metformin	*Human Amylins*	pioglitazone
tolazamide	*Dipeptidyl Peptidase-4 Inhibitors*	pramlintide	rosiglitazone
tolbutamide	alogliptin	*Incretin Mimetic*	**Glucose-Elevating Agents**
Second-Generation Sulfonylureas	linagliptin	exenatide	diazoxide
glimepiride	saxagliptin	*Meglitinides*	(P) glucagon
glipizide	(P) sitagliptin	nateglinide	
(P) glyburide		repaglinide	

Antidiabetic agents, as the name implies, are used to treat **diabetes mellitus**, the most common of all metabolic disorders. It is estimated that 10 million people in the United States have been diagnosed with diabetes mellitus, and there are many others not yet diagnosed. Diabetes is a complicated disorder that alters the metabolism of glucose, fats, and proteins, affecting many end organs and causing numerous clinical complications. It is part of the metabolic syndrome, a collection of conditions that predispose to cardiovascular (CV) disease (Chapter 46). Treatment of diabetes is aimed at regulating the blood glucose level through the use of insulin or other glucose-lowering drugs. Maintaining the level of serum glucose within a certain range is very important to the nervous system. The nerves in the central nervous system (CNS) receive glucose by diffusion; they do not have insulin receptor sites like all other cells. The presence of too much glucose, which is a large molecule, takes water into the CNS and can cause swelling and nerve instability. The presence of too little glucose results in less energy for the nerves to use to function and loss of cell membrane integrity. Maintaining the appropriate glucose level is a complicated process that involves diet, exercise, and drug management. At times, the blood glucose level is lowered too much, producing a state of hypoglycemia. When this occurs, glucose-elevating agents need to be used to quickly return the serum glucose levels to a normal level. Considerations related to the use of insulin and other antidiabetic agents based on age are highlighted in Box 38.1.

Glucose Regulation

Glucose is the leading energy source for the human body. Glucose is stored in the body for rapid release in times of stress. As a result, blood glucose levels can be readily maintained so that the neurons always receive a constant supply of glucose to function. The body's control of glucose is intricately related to fat and protein metabolism, balancing energy conservation with energy consumption to maintain homeostasis in a variety of situations. Many factors have an impact on this balance and the body's ability to adapt and to maintain metabolism.

The Pancreas

The pancreas is both an endocrine gland, producing hormones, and an exocrine gland, releasing sodium bicarbonate and pancreatic enzymes directly into the common bile duct to be released into the small intestine, where they neutralize the acid chyme from the stomach and aid digestion. The endocrine part of the pancreas produces hormones in collections of tissue called the islets of Langerhans. These islets contain endocrine cells that produce specific hormones. The alpha cells release glucagon in direct response to low blood glucose levels. The beta cells release insulin in direct response to high blood glucose levels and when stimulated by incretins. Delta cells produce somatostatin (growth hormone–inhibiting factor) in response to very low blood glucose levels; somatostatin blocks the secretion of both insulin and glucagon. These hormones work together to maintain the blood glucose level within normal limits.

Insulin

Insulin is the hormone produced by the pancreatic beta cells of the islets of Langerhans. The hormone is released into circulation when the levels of glucose around these cells rise. It is also released in response to **incretins**, peptides that are produced in the gastrointestinal (GI) tract in response to food. One of these incretins, **glucagon-like**

BOX 38.1 FOCUS ON Drug Therapy Across the Lifespan

Antidiabetic Agents

CHILDREN

Treatment of diabetes in children is a difficult challenge of balancing diet, activity, growth, stressors, and insulin requirements. Children need to be carefully monitored for any sign of hypoglycemia or hyperglycemia and treated quickly because their fast metabolism and lack of body reserves can push them into a severe state quickly.

Insulin dose, especially in infants, may be so small that it is difficult to calibrate. Insulin often needs to be diluted to a volume that can be detected on the syringe. A second person should always check the calculations and dose of insulin being given to small children.

Teenagers often present a real challenge for diabetes management. The desire to be "normal" often leads to a resistance to dietary restrictions and insulin injections. The metabolism of the teenager is also in flux, leading to complications in regulating insulin dose. A team approach, including the child, family members, teachers, coaches, and even friends, may be the best way to help the child deal with the disease and the required therapy. New delivery methods for insulin may help this age group cope with the drug therapy in the future.

Metformin is the only oral antidiabetic drug approved for children. It has established dosing for children 10 years of age and older. With the increasing number of children being diagnosed with type 2 diabetes the use of other agents in children is being tested.

ADULTS

Adults need extensive education about the disease, as well as about the drug therapy. Warning signs and symptoms should be stressed repeatedly as the adult learns to juggle insulin needs with exercise, stressors, other drug effects, and diet. Adults maintained on oral agents need to be monitored for changes in response to the drugs. Often additional drugs are added or doses are changed as the disease progresses over time.

Exercise and diet should always be emphasized as the mainstay of dealing with diabetes. Adults need to be cautioned about the use of over-the-counter and herbal or alternative therapies. Many of these products contain agents that alter blood glucose levels and will change insulin or oral agent requirements. Adults should always be asked specifically whether they use any of these agents, and adjustments should be made accordingly.

Insulin therapy is the best choice for diabetics during pregnancy and lactation, which are times of high stress and metabolic demands. Needs may change on a daily basis, and the mother should have ready support and extensive teaching about what to do if hypoglycemia or hyperglycemia occurs. The period of labor and delivery is often a critical time in diabetes management because of the stress and sudden changes in body fluid volume and hormone levels. The obstetrician and the endocrinologist or primary care provider should consult frequently about the best way to support the patient through this period.

OLDER ADULTS

Older adults can have many underlying problems that complicate diabetic therapy. Poor vision and/or coordination may make it difficult to prepare a syringe. A week's supply of syringes can be prepared and refrigerated for the usual dose of insulin.

Dietary deficiencies related to changes in taste, absorption, or attitude may lead to wide fluctuations in blood sugar levels, making it difficult to control diabetes. Many areas have nutritional assistance programs for older adults (e.g., Meals on Wheels) or have places that can refer patients to appropriate agencies that might be able to offer assistance.

Older adults have a greater incidence of renal or hepatic impairment, and kidney and liver function should be evaluated before starting any of these drugs. Combinations of oral agents may not be feasible with severe dysfunction, and the patient may need to use insulin to control blood glucose levels.

Older adults should receive periodic educational reminders about diet, the need for exercise, skin and foot care, and warning signs to report to the health care provider.

The older patient is also more likely to experience end organ damage related to the diabetes—loss of vision, kidney problems, coronary artery disease, and infections—and the drug regimen of these patients can become quite complex. Careful screening for drug interactions is an important aspect of the assessment of these patients.

polypeptide-1 (GLP-1), increases insulin release and decreases glucagon release (in preparation for the nutrients that will soon be absorbed). GLP-1 also slows GI emptying to allow more absorption of nutrients and stimulates the satiety center in the brain to decrease the desire to eat because food is already in the GI tract. GLP-1 has a very short half-life and is metabolized by the enzyme **dipeptidyl peptidase-4 (DDP-4)**.

Insulin circulates through the body and reacts with specific insulin receptor sites to stimulate the transport of glucose into the cells to be used for energy, a process called facilitated diffusion. Insulin also stimulates the synthesis of **glycogen** (glucose stored for immediate release during times of stress or low glucose), the conversion of lipids into fat stored in the form of adipose tissue, and the synthesis of needed proteins from amino acids.

Insulin is released after a meal, in response to incretin release and when the blood glucose levels rise. It circulates and affects metabolism, allowing the body to either store or use the nutrients from the meal effectively. As a result of the insulin release, blood glucose levels fall and insulin release drops off. Sometimes, an insufficient amount of insulin is released. This may occur because the pancreas cannot produce enough insulin, the insulin receptor sites have lost their sensitivity to insulin and they require more insulin to lower glucose effectively, or the person does not have enough receptor sites to support his or her body size, as in obesity.

Glucagon

Glucagon is released from the alpha cells in the islets of Langerhans in response to low blood glucose levels. Glucagon causes an immediate mobilization of glycogen stored in the liver and raises blood glucose levels.

Other Factors Affecting Glucose Control

Other factors in the body have been found to have an impact on glucose, fat, and protein metabolism. These factors play a role in the overall energy balance in the body.

Adipocytes, or fat cells, were once thought to just store fat for energy. However, they have been found to have a major impact on glucose and fat metabolism throughout the body through the secretion of **adiponectin**. This hormone acts to increase insulin sensitivity, decrease the release of glucose from the liver, and protect the blood vessels from inflammatory changes. When adiponectin levels are high, it exerts a protective effect on the body. When adiponectin levels are low, as in cases of intraabdominal fat accumulation, glucose levels rise and blood vessel injury increases.

Endocannabinoid receptors have been identified in adipose tissue, muscles, liver, the satiety center, and the GI tract. These receptors seem to be part of a signaling system within the body to keep the body in a state of energy gain, to prepare for stressful situations. When stimulated, these receptors promote food intake, decrease adiponectin release, increase fat breakdown, decrease insulin sensitivity, increase fat storage, and alter gastric emptying to promote greater nutrient absorption. Patients who are obese have been shown to have increased stimulation of these receptors.

The sympathetic nervous system (SNS), through norepinephrine and epinephrine effects, directly causes a decrease in insulin release, an increase in the release of stored glucose, and an increase in fat breakdown. A person under stress will have increased glucose levels and increased free fatty acid (FFA) levels, which will provide the energy needed for the immediate "fight or flight" associated with a stress reaction. Prolonged stress can alter the control of metabolism that regulates the body's energy balance.

Corticosteroids, which are released diurnally but also during a stress reaction, decrease insulin sensitivity, increase glucose release, and decrease protein building. All of these actions conserve energy and provide immediate glucose for any stressful situation.

Growth hormone causes decreased insulin sensitivity, increase of FFAs, and increase in protein building. Fluctuating levels of growth hormone can upset metabolic homeostasis. Box 38.2 summarizes the effects of various factors on blood glucose levels.

BOX 38.2

Glucose Control Mechanisms

Insulin	Decreases blood glucose; glycogen storage; adipose tissue deposit; synthesis of proteins to form amino acids
Glucagon	Increases blood glucose
Somatostatin	Decreases insulin release; decreases glucagon release; slows GI emptying
Growth hormone	Decreases insulin sensitivity; increases protein building; increases FFA formation
Incretins	Increases insulin release; decreases glucagon release; stimulates satiety center; slows GI emptying
Adiponectin	Increases insulin sensitivity; decreases glucose output from liver; protects vessels from inflammatory reactions
Catecholamines	Decreases insulin release; increases glucose output from liver and muscles; increases breakdown of fat to FFAs
Corticosteroids	Increases glucose output; decreases insulin sensitivity
Endocannabinoid system	Increases food intake by blocking satiety signals; decreases adiponectin release; decreases insulin sensitivity; increases fat synthesis; alters gastric motility

Loss of Blood Glucose Control

When an insufficient amount of insulin is released or insulin receptors are no longer responding, several metabolic changes occur, beginning with hyperglycemia, or increased blood sugar. Hyperglycemia results in **glycosuria**: Sugar is spilled into the urine because the concentration of glucose in the blood is too high for complete reabsorption. Because this sugar-rich urine is an ideal environment for bacteria, cystitis is a common finding. The patient experiences fatigue because the body's cells cannot use the glucose that is there; they need insulin to facilitate transport of the glucose into the cells. **Polyphagia** (increased hunger) occurs because the hypothalamic centers cannot take in glucose; thus the cells sense that they are starving. **Polydipsia** (increased thirst) occurs because the tonicity of the blood is increased owing to the increased glucose and waste products in the blood and the loss of fluid with glucose in the urine. The hypothalamic cells that are sensitive to fluid levels sense a need to increase fluid in the system, which in turn causes the patient to feel thirsty.

Lipolysis, or fat breakdown, occurs as the body breaks down stored fat into FFAs for energy because glucose is not usable. The patient experiences **ketosis** as metabolism shifts to the use of fat for energy. Ketones are produced that cannot be removed effectively. Acidosis also occurs because the liver cannot remove all of the waste products (acid being a primary waste product) that result from the breakdown of glucose, fat, and proteins. Muscles break down because proteins are being broken down for their essential amino acids. The breakdown of proteins results in an increase in nitrogen wastes, which is manifested by an elevated blood urea nitrogen concentration and sometimes by protein in the urine. Patients with hyperglycemia do not heal quickly, because of this protein breakdown, as well as the lack of a stimulus to initiate protein building. All of these actions eventually contribute to development of the complications associated with chronic hyperglycemia or diabetes.

Diabetes Mellitus

Diabetes mellitus (literally, "honey urine") is characterized by complex disturbances in metabolism. Diabetes affects carbohydrate, protein, and fat metabolism. The most frequently recognized clinical signs of diabetes are hyperglycemia (fasting blood sugar level >126 mg/dL) and glycosuria (the presence of sugar in the urine). The alteration in the body's ability to effectively deal with carbohydrate, fat, and protein metabolism over the long-term results in a thickening of the basement membrane (a thin layer of collagen filament that lies just below the endothelial lining of blood vessels) in large and small blood vessels. This thickening leads to changes in oxygenation of the vessel lining; damage to the vessel lining, which leads to narrowing, vessel remodeling, and decreased blood flow through the vessel; and an inability of oxygen to rapidly diffuse across the membrane to the tissues. These changes result in an increased incidence of a number of disorders, including the following:

- *Atherosclerosis:* Heart attacks and strokes related to the development of atherosclerotic plaques in the vessel lining
- *Retinopathy:* Resultant loss of vision as tiny vessels in the eye are narrowed and closed
- *Neuropathies:* Motor and sensory changes in the feet and legs and progressive changes in other nerves as the oxygen supply to these nerves is slowly cut off
- *Nephropathy:* Renal dysfunction related to changes in the basement membrane of the glomerulus

The overall metabolic disturbances associated with diabetes were once thought to be caused by a lack of the hormone insulin. It is now thought that a mosaic of problems, including low insulin and loss of insulin receptor sensitivity, are involved. There is debate over whether prolonged high glucose levels lead to basement membrane changes and complications of diabetes or whether basement membrane thickening is the initial problem that leads to lack of insulin and changes in insulin receptors; whichever comes first, replacement or stimulation of insulin release is the mainstay for treatment of diabetes mellitus.

The diagnosis of diabetes mellitus has involved monitoring of fasting blood glucose levels and sometimes challenging the system with glucose for a glucose tolerance test. However, recent research indicates that the body's response to food may be a more important indicator of impending diabetes. Current thinking is that a fasting blood glucose level may not be as important as a postprandial blood glucose level, which reveals the body's ability to respond to a glucose challenge. The importance of looking at a variety of different glucose markers is being stressed. Box 38.3 highlights some cultural variations in blood glucose levels.

Glycosylated hemoglobin levels, or an HbA1c test, provide a 3-month average of glucose levels. Red blood cells are freely permeable to glucose, and this test gives an average range of glucose exposure over the life of the red blood cell, about 120 days. This test does not require fasting before blood is drawn or the oral intake of glucose before testing. Elevations at or above 6.5% may be an early indicator of a prediabetic state, before changes are noted in the fasting blood sugar level. Once a baseline is established the goal of therapy for a diabetic patient is an HbA1c level <7%. Researchers believe that very early intervention—diet, exercise, and lifestyle changes—may delay the onset of diabetes and the complications, including coronary artery disease, that come with it.

Diabetes mellitus is classified as either type 1, once called insulin-dependent diabetes mellitus, or type 2, once called noninsulin-dependent diabetes mellitus or adult onset diabetes. Type 1 diabetes is usually associated with rapid onset, mostly in younger people, and is connected in many cases to viral destruction of the beta cells of the pancreas. Type 1 diabetes always requires insulin replacement because the beta cells are no longer functioning.

BOX 38.3 FOCUS ON Cultural Considerations

Diabetes and Blood Glucose Variations

Certain ethnic groups tend to have a genetically predetermined variation in blood glucose levels, possibly caused by a variation in metabolism. For example, Native Americans, Hispanic Americans, and Japanese Americans have higher blood glucose levels than White Americans do. The clinical importance of this fact relates to proper screening of patients for hypoglycemia and diabetes mellitus. Patients in these groups who have fasting glucose tolerance tests need to have the standard readjusted before a diagnosis is made. Such patients also require an understanding of potential differences in normal levels on home glucose-monitoring units when they are regulating insulin at home.

Groups that are more likely to develop diabetes mellitus include African Americans, Native Americans, and Hispanic Americans. People in these groups should be screened regularly for diabetes. They also can benefit from teaching about warning signs of diabetes.

Type 2 diabetes was once thought to be a disease of mature adults with a slow and progressive onset. However, studies released in 2001 reported that the incidence of type 2 diabetes in teenagers and young adults is increasing markedly. Patients with type 2 diabetes are able to produce insulin, but perhaps not enough to maintain glucose control, or perhaps their insulin receptors are not sensitive enough to insulin, leading to increased serum glucose levels.

Questions are being raised about the impact of early diet and lack of exercise in contributing to this new increase in type 2 diabetes in young people. The treatment of type 2 diabetes usually begins with changes in diet and exercise. Dieting controls the amount and timing of glucose introduction into the body, and weight loss decreases the number of insulin receptor sites that need to be stimulated, as well as the intraabdominal fat that blocks adiponectin release. Exercise increases the movement of glucose into the cells by SNS activation and by the increased potassium in the blood that occurs directly after exercising. Potassium acts as part of a polarizing system during exercise that pushes glucose into the cells. Clinical studies have shown that controlling serum glucose levels can decrease the risk of complications by up to 40% (ADA, 2015).

When diet and exercise no longer work, other agents (discussed later) are tried to stimulate the production of insulin in the pancreas, increase the sensitivity of the insulin receptor sites, or control the entry of glucose into the system. Injection of insulin may eventually be needed. This concept is often confusing to patients who are learning about diabetes. Type 2 diabetes may evolve over time and the patient eventually require replacement insulin. Timing of the injections of insulin is correlated with food intake and anticipated increases in blood glucose levels, as well as exercise levels and anticipated stress (ADA, 2015). See Box 38.4 for more information about managing glucose levels during stress.

Hyperglycemia

Hyperglycemia, or high blood sugar, results when there is an increase in glucose in the blood. Recent guidelines suggest a fasting glucose level of 130 or above is indicative of hyperglycemia. Clinical signs and symptoms include fatigue, lethargy, irritation, glycosuria, polyphagia, polydipsia, and itchy skin (from accumulation of wastes that the liver cannot clear). If the hyperglycemia goes unchecked the patient will experience ketoacidosis and CNS changes that can progress to coma. Signs of impending dangerous complications of hyperglycemia include the following:

- Fruity breath as the ketones build up in the system and are excreted through the lungs

BOX 38.4 FOCUS ON The Evidence

Managing Glucose Levels during Stress

The body has many compensatory mechanisms for ensuring that blood glucose levels stay within a safe range. The sympathetic stress reaction elevates blood glucose levels to provide ready energy for fight or flight (see Chapter 29). The stress reaction causes the breakdown of glycogen to release glucose and the breakdown of fat and proteins to release other energy.

Stress Reactions

The stress reaction elevates the blood glucose concentration above the normal range. In severe stress situations—such as an acute myocardial infarction or an automobile accident—the blood glucose level can be very high (300–400 mg/dL). The body uses that energy to fight the insult or flee from the stressor.

Nurses in acute care situations need to be aware of this reflex elevation in glucose when caring for patients in acute stress, especially patients in emergency situations whose medical history is unknown. The usual medical response to a blood glucose concentration of 400 mg/dL would be the administration of insulin. In many situations, that is exactly what is done, especially if the patient's history is not known and the effects of such a high glucose level could cause severe systemic reactions. Insulin administration causes a drop in the blood glucose level as glucose enters cells to be either used for energy or converted to glycogen for storage.

However, a problem may arise in the acute care setting, particularly in a nondiabetic patient. Relieving the stress reaction can also drop glucose levels as the stimulus to increase these levels is lost and the glucose that was there is used for energy. A patient in this situation who has been treated with insulin is at risk for development of potentially severe hypoglycemia. The body's response to low glucose levels is a sympathetic stress reaction, which again elevates the blood glucose concentration. If treated, the patient potentially can enter a cycle of high and low glucose levels.

Best Nursing Practice

Nurses are often the ones in closest contact with the highly stressed patient—in the emergency room, the intensive care unit, and the postanesthesia room—and should be constantly aware of the normal and reflex changes in blood glucose that accompany stress. Careful monitoring, with awareness of stress and the relief of stress, can prevent a prolonged treatment program to maintain blood glucose levels within the range of normal, a situation that is not "normal" during a stress reaction.

Diabetic patients who are in severe stress situations require changes in their insulin doses. They should be allowed some elevation of blood glucose, even though their inability to produce sufficient insulin will make it difficult for their cells to make effective use of the increased glucose levels. It is a clinical challenge to balance glucose levels with the needs of the patient because so many factors can affect the glucose level.

Source: American Diabetes Association. (2015). Standards of medical care for patients with diabetes mellitus. *Diabetes Care, 38*(Suppl. 1), S1–S94.

Table 38.1 Signs and Symptoms of Hypoglycemia and Hyperglycemia

Clinical Effects	Hypoglycemia	Hyperglycemia
CNS	Headache, blurred vision, diplopia; drowsiness progressing to coma; ataxia; hyperactive reflexes	Decreased level of consciousness, sluggishness progressing to coma; hypoactive reflexes
Neuromuscular	Paresthesias; weakness; muscle spasms; twitching progressing to seizures	Weakness, lethargy
CV	Tachycardia; palpitations; normal to high blood pressure	Tachycardia; hypotension
Respiratory	Rapid, shallow respirations	Rapid, deep respirations (Kussmaul); acetone-like or fruity breath
GI	Hunger, nausea	Nausea; vomiting; thirst
Other	Diaphoresis; cool and clammy skin; normal eyeballs	Dry, warm, flushed skin; soft eyeballs
Laboratory tests	Urine glucose negative; blood glucose low	Urine glucose strongly positive; urine ketone levels positive; blood glucose levels high
Onset	Sudden; patient appears anxious, drunk; associated with overdose of insulin, missing a meal, increased stress	Gradual; patient is slow and sluggish; associated with lack of insulin, increased stress

CNS, central nervous system; CV, cardiovascular; GI, gastrointestinal.

- Dehydration as fluid and important electrolytes are lost through the kidneys
- Slow, deep respirations (Kussmaul respirations) as the body tries to rid itself of high acid levels
- Loss of orientation and coma

This level of hyperglycemia needs to be treated immediately with insulin.

Hypoglycemia

Hypoglycemia, or a blood glucose concentration lower than 60 mg/dL, occurs in a number of clinical situations, including starvation, and if treatment of hyperglycemia with insulin or oral agents lowers the blood glucose level too far. The body immediately reacts to lowered blood glucose because the cells require glucose to survive, the neurons being among the cells most sensitive to the lack of glucose. The initial reaction to falling blood glucose level is parasympathetic stimulation—increased GI activity to increase digestion and absorption. Rather rapidly, the SNS responds with a "fight-or-flight" reaction that increases blood glucose levels by initiating the breakdown of fat and glycogen to release glucose for rapid energy. The pancreas releases glucagon, a hormone that counters the effects of insulin and works to increase glucose levels and somatostatin, which help the body to conserve energy. In many cases the response to the hypoglycemic state causes a hyperglycemic state. Balancing the body's responses to glucose is sometimes difficult when one is trying to treat and control diabetes. Table 38.1 offers a comparison of the signs and symptoms of hyperglycemia and hypoglycemia. Periodically, the focus of glucose control changes from tight control to less strict control. In 2010, studies were published that showed that patients with very tight control tended to have more CV events and death than patients with less strict control. The incidence of hypoglycemic episodes associated with tight control has been implicated in causing the problems. The new standard, in 2011, is a less rigorous control of blood sugar levels. History shows, however, that this standard may change again in a few years after more studies are conducted.

Insulin

Insulin is the only parenteral antidiabetic agent available for exogenous replacement of low levels of insulin (Table 38.2). It is used to treat type 1 diabetes and to treat type 2 diabetes in adults who have no response to diet, exercise, and other agents. (See Box 38.1 for considerations related to the use of insulin based on age.) The types of insulin that are available include insulin analog or lispro (*Humalog*), insulin aspart (*NovoLog*), insulin glargine (*Lantus, Toujeo*), insulin glulisine (*Apidra*), insulin detemir (*Levemir*), regular insulin (*Novolin R*), NPH (Neutral Protamine Hagedorn) insulin (*Novolin N*), and inhaled insulin (*Afreeza*).

FOCUS ON Safe Medication Administration

In 2009 lente insulin was removed from the market. Name confusion had occurred between ***Lantus*** *insulin and lente insulin. The pharmacokinetics and dose varied greatly. Use caution to make sure you know which insulin was intended for your patient.* ***Lantus*** *and* ***Levemir*** *insulin cannot be mixed in a syringe with any other insulin or any other drug. Use caution when working with these two insulins. Many of the antidiabetic agents need to be administered with specific timing around food intake. If a patient is not able to eat, adjustments need to be made. Use care in teaching patients about timing and eating and in administering insulin in institutions, where timing of food delivery may vary or patients may be NPO for tests or procedures. IV insulin is considered a high-risk drug. The patient is in a precarious situation and rapid swings in blood sugar can occur. Extreme caution needs to be used when giving insulin IV.*

Table 38.2 *Drugs in Focus:* Insulin

Drug Name	Dosage/Route	Usual Indications
Insulin (various types)	Varies based on patient response, diet, and activity level ***Insulin*** *Aspart:* Given within 5–10 min of a meal *Lispro:* Given with 15 min of a meal *Regular insulin:* Given within 30 min of a meal *Glulisine:* Given 15 min before or within 20 min of the start of a meal *Detemir:* Given once daily at bedtime *Glargine:* Given once or twice daily at the same time each day	Treatment of type 1 diabetes mellitus; treatment of type 2 diabetes mellitus in patients whose diabetes cannot be controlled by diet or other agents; treatment of severe ketoacidosis or diabetic coma; treatment of hyperkalemia (in conjunction with a glucose infusion to produce a shift of potassium into the cells [polarizing solution]); also used for short courses of therapy during periods of stress (e.g., surgery, disease) in patients with type 2 diabetes, for newly diagnosed patients being stabilized, for patients with poor control of glucose levels, and for patients with gestational diabetes

Originally, insulin was prepared from pork and beef pancreas. Today, virtually all insulin is prepared by recombinant DNA technology and is human insulin produced by genetically altered bacteria. This purer form of insulin is not associated with the sensitivity problems that many patients developed with the animal products. Animal insulins may still be obtained for patients who are most responsive to them, but they are not generally used. Box 38.5 describes the various forms of insulin delivery that are available or under study for future use.

BOX 38.5

Insulin Delivery: Past, Present, and Future

Past

Subcutaneous Insulin Injection: The delivery of insulin by subcutaneous injection was introduced in the 1920s and changed the way that diabetic patients were managed clinically, giving them a chance for a normal lifestyle. Research is ongoing to find more efficient and acceptable ways to deliver insulin to diabetic patients.

Present

Subcutaneous Insulin Injection: This remains the primary delivery system.

Insulin Jet Injector: This cylindrical device shoots a fine spray of insulin through the skin under very high pressure. Although it is appealing for people who do not like needles or have problems disposing of needles properly, it can be very expensive.

Insulin Pen: This syringe-like device looks like a pen. It has a small needle at the tip and a barrel that holds insulin. The patient "dials" the amount of insulin to be given and injects the insulin subcutaneously by pressing on the top of the pen. This is advantageous for people who need insulin two or three times during the day but cannot easily transport syringes and needles. It is a subtle way to give insulin and is popular with students and business people on the go. It is important to rotate the syringe 15 to 20 times before injecting the insulin to disperse it. Patients often forget this point after using the pens for a while, and as a result may inject far too much or too little insulin when it is needed. Periodic reinforcement of the administration instructions is important.

External Insulin Pump: This pump device can be worn on a belt or hidden in a pocket and is attached to a small tube inserted into the subcutaneous tissue of the abdomen. The device slowly leaks a base rate of insulin into the abdomen all day; the patient can pump or inject booster doses throughout the day to correspond with meals and activity. The device does have several disadvantages. For example, it is awkward, the tubing poses an increased risk of infection and requires frequent changing, and the patient has to frequently check blood glucose levels throughout the day to monitor response.

IV Insulin: In emergency situations or when rapid and continual control of blood glucose is needed, insulin can be given IV. Insulin is considered a high-risk drug when given this way. There is potential for rapid changes in blood glucose and resultant risk to the CNS and heart. IV insulin should be given using a controlled delivery pump and the patient should be constantly monitored and frequent blood glucose levels should be done to adjust the dosage appropriately.

Long-Acting Insulin: The year 2001 brought the release of a subcutaneous insulin that lasts two to three times longer than NPH insulin. This should decrease the need for multiple injections and may increase glucose control, especially for patients with erratic glucose levels during the night. The long-term effects of this type of insulin therapy are not yet known.

Inhaled Insulin: The lung tissue is one of the best sites for insulin absorption. An aerosol delivery system has been developed that delivers a powdered insulin formulation directly into the lung tissue. In early 2006 the FDA approved *Exubera* for the treatment of adult patients with diabetes mellitus for the control of hyperglycemia. In patients with type 1 diabetes, it was designed to be used in combination with longer acting insulins; patients with type 2 diabetes could use it as monotherapy or in combination with other antidiabetic agents. In 2007, however, *Exubera*

(continues on page 636)

BOX 38.5

Insulin Delivery: Past, Present, and Future (continued)

was withdrawn from the market with disappointing sales. Although pulmonary function was shown to decline while using this form of insulin, this was not cited as a cause for the withdrawal; phase III studies showed an increase in insulin antibody formation in patients using inhaled insulin in clinical trials, sending the drug back for further refinement and research. Inhaled insulin was released again in 2014 as *Afreeza*. There are warnings that problems could occur with people who have asthma, COPD, or lung cancer and a baseline and periodic spirometry is suggested. It is a rapid-acting insulin that is inhaled at the beginning of a meal. If used in type 1 diabetes, it must be combined with a long-acting insulin. The most common adverse effects are cough, throat irritation, and hypoglycemia. Because of adverse effects seen in clinical studies it is suggested that patients using this form of insulin may experience more ketoacidosis, hypokalemia, and life-threatening hypoglycemia than patients receiving insulin by injection. Careful monitoring and patient teaching is important.

Future

Implantable Insulin Pump: This pump is surgically implanted into the abdomen and delivers base insulin as well as insulin boluses as needed directly into the abdomen to be absorbed by the liver, just as pancreatic insulin is. The disadvantages are risk of infection, mechanical problems with the pump, and lack of long-term data on its effectiveness. This method is not yet available for general use.

Insulin Patch: The patch is placed on the skin and delivers a constant low dose of insulin. When the patient eats a meal, tabs are pulled on the patch to release more insulin. The problem with this delivery method is that insulin does not readily pass through the skin, so there is tremendous variability in its effects. This route is not yet commercially available.

The most up-to-date information on insulin delivery research is available online at: http://www.niddk.nih.gov

Therapeutic Actions and Indications

Insulin is a hormone that promotes the storage of the body's fuels, facilitates the transport of various metabolites and ions across cell membranes, and stimulates the synthesis of glycogen from glucose, of fats from lipids, and of proteins from amino acids. Insulin does these things by reacting with specific receptor sites on the cell. Figure 38.1 shows the sites of action of replacement insulin and other drugs used to treat diabetic conditions. See Table 38.2 for Usual Indications.

Pharmacokinetics

Various preparations of insulin are available to provide short- and long-term coverage. These preparations are processed within the body like endogenous insulin. However,

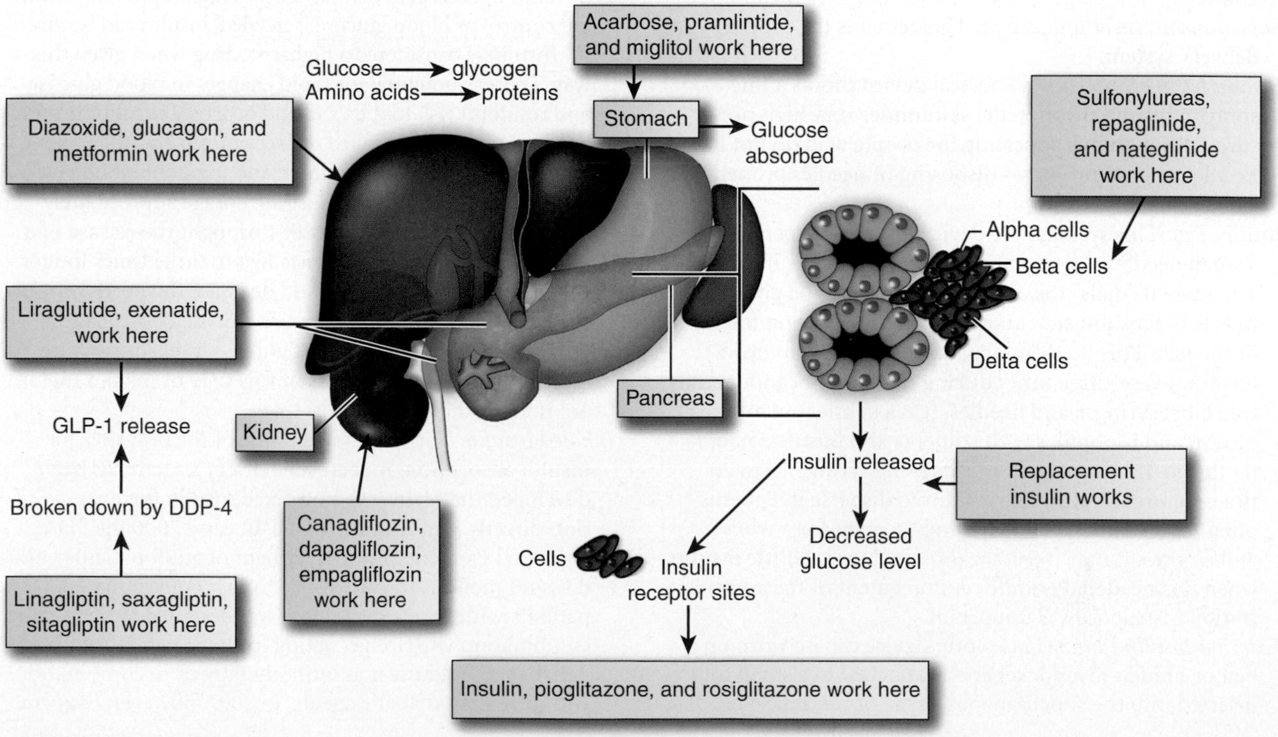

FIGURE 38.1 Sites of action of drugs used to treat diabetic conditions.

the peak, onset, and duration of each vary because of the placement or addition of glycine and/or arginine chains. Maintenance doses are given by the subcutaneous or inhaled routes. Injection sites need to be rotated regularly to avoid damage to muscles and to prevent subcutaneous atrophy. Regular insulin is given IM or IV in emergency situations.

FOCUS ON Safe Medication Administration

Insulin is usually given by subcutaneous injection. Using an insulin syringe, inject the insulin into the loose connective tissue underneath the skin (Figure 38.2). The areas of the body that are best able to be pinched up to access this tissue are the abdomen, the upper thigh, and the upper arm. Insert the needle at a 45-degree angle. Inject the insulin. Remove the needle and syringe and apply gentle pressure at the injection site. Rotate sites regularly to prevent tissue damage.

Insulin is available in various preparations with a wide range of peaks and durations of action. A patient may receive a combination of regular and NPH insulin in the morning to cover the glucose peak from breakfast (regular onset, 30 to 60 minutes) and the lunch and dinner glucose peaks. The patient may then require another injection before bed. The types of insulin used are determined by the anticipated eating and exercise activities of any particular patient. It is very important to make sure that one is using the correct insulin preparation when administering the drug. Insulin glargine (*Lantus, Toujeo*) and insulin detemir (*Levemir*) cannot be mixed in solution with any other drug, including other insulins.

Contraindications and Cautions

Because insulin is used as a replacement hormone, there are no contraindications other than episodes of hypoglycemia, which could be exacerbated. Care should be taken during pregnancy and lactation to monitor glucose levels closely and adjust the insulin dose accordingly. Insulin does not cross the placenta; therefore, it is the drug of choice for managing diabetes during pregnancy. Insulin does enter breast milk, but it is destroyed in the GI tract and does not affect the nursing infant. However, insulin-dependent mothers may have inhibited milk production because of insulin's effects on fat and protein metabolism. The effectiveness of nursing the infant should be evaluated periodically. Patients using inhaled insulin are at risk for impairment of respiratory function; this route is contraindicated in people with asthma or chronic obstructive pulmonary disease (COPD) and in people with lung cancer or a history of lung cancer.

Adverse Effects

The most common adverse effects related to insulin use are hypoglycemia and ketoacidosis, which can be controlled with proper dose adjustments. Local reactions at injection sites, including lipodystrophy, also can occur. This effect is lessened by rotation of injection sites (Figure 38.3). With inhaled insulin, the most common adverse effects also include cough and throat pain or irritation.

Clinically Important Drug–Drug Interactions

Caution should be used when giving a patient stabilized on insulin any drug that decreases glucose levels (e.g., monoamine oxidase inhibitors, beta-blockers, and salicylates,

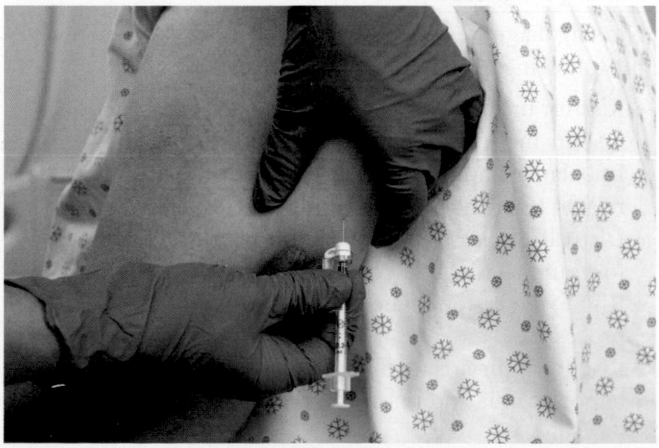

FIGURE 38.2 Insert the needle at a 45-degree angle.

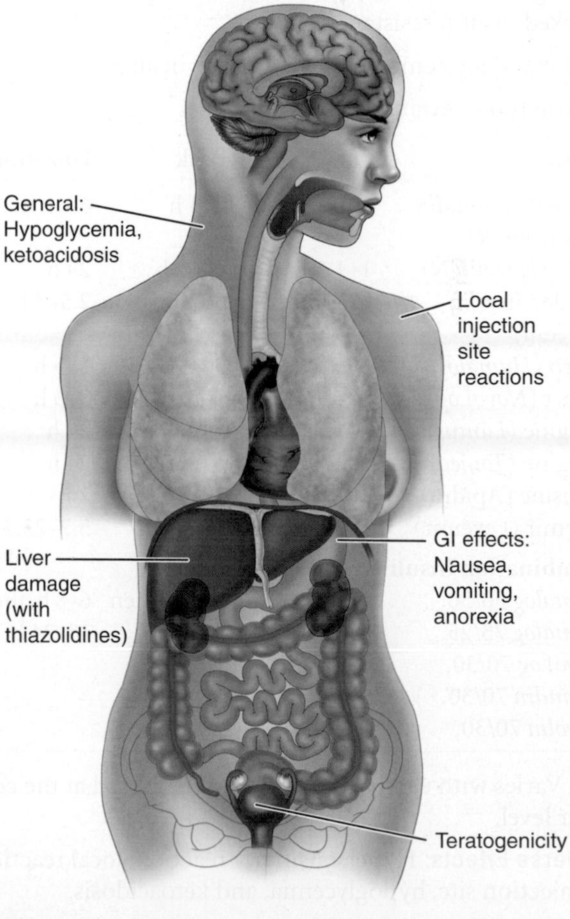

FIGURE 38.3 Variety of adverse effects and toxicities associated with antidiabetic agents.

BOX 38.6 FOCUS ON Herbal and Alternative Therapies

Patients being treated with antidiabetic therapies are at an increased risk of developing hypoglycemia if they use juniper berries, ginseng, garlic, fenugreek, coriander, dandelion root, or celery. If a patient uses these therapies, blood glucose levels should be monitored closely and appropriate dose adjustment made in the prescribed drug.

alcohol). Dose adjustments are needed when any of these drugs is added or removed. Care should also be taken when combining insulin with any beta-blocker. The blocking of the SNS also blocks many of the signs and symptoms of hypoglycemia, hindering the patient's ability to recognize problems. Patients taking beta-blockers need to learn other ways to recognize hypoglycemia. Patients should also be warned about possible interactions with various herbal therapies (Box 38.6).

Prototype Summary: Insulin

Indications: Treatment of type 1 diabetes; treatment of type 2 diabetes when other agents have failed; short-term treatment of type 2 diabetes during periods of stress; management of diabetic ketoacidosis, hyperkalemia, and marked insulin resistance.

Actions: Replacement of endogenous insulin.

Pharmacokinetics:

Route	Onset	Peak	Duration
Regular (*Humulin R, Novolin R*)	30–60 min	2–4 h	6–12 h
NPH (*Novolin N*)	1–1.5 h	4–12 h	24 h
Inhaled insulin (*Afreeza*)	12–15 min	60 min	2.5–3 h
lispro (*Humalog*)	<15 min	30–90 min	2–5 h
aspart (*NovoLog*)	10–20 min	1–3 h	3–5 h
glargine (*Lantus*)	60–70 min	None	24 h
glargine (*Toujeo*)	60–70 min	None	24 h
glulisine (Apidra)	2–5 min	30–90 min	2 h
detemir (Levemir)	1–2 h	3–6 h	5.7–23.3 h
Combination Insulins			
Humalog 50/50, *Humalog* 75/25, *NovoLog* 70/30, *Humulin* 70/30, *Novolin* 70/30	30–60 min, then 1–2 h	2–4 h, then 6–12 h	6–8 h, then 18–24 h

$T_{1/2}$: Varies with each preparation; metabolized at the cellular level.

Adverse Effects: Hypersensitivity reaction, local reactions at injection site, hypoglycemia, and ketoacidosis.

Nursing Considerations for Patients Taking Insulin

Assessment: History and Examination

- Assess for contraindications or cautions: Any known allergy to any insulin and current status of pregnancy or lactation *so that appropriate monitoring and dose adjustments can be completed, including possible need to use animal source insulin.* Assess for history of asthma or COPD if using inhaled insulin *to prevent exacerbation of these conditions and decline in respiratory function.*
- Perform a physical assessment *to establish a baseline before beginning therapy*, and during therapy, *to evaluate the effectiveness of therapy and for any potential adverse effects.*
- Assess for presence of any skin lesions; orientation and reflexes; baseline pulse and blood pressure; respiration or adventitious breath sounds; spirometry if using inhaled form, *which could indicate response to high or low glucose levels and potential risk factors in giving insulin.*
- Assess body systems *for changes suggesting possible complications associated with poor blood glucose control.*
- Investigate nutritional intake, *noting any problems with intake and adherence to prescribed diet that could alter the anticipated response to insulin therapy.*
- Assess activity level, including amount and degree of exercise, *which could alter anticipated response to insulin therapy.*
- Inspect skin areas that will be used for injection of insulin; note any areas that are bruised, thickened, or scarred, *which could interfere with insulin absorption and alter anticipated response to insulin therapy.*
- Obtain blood glucose levels as ordered *to monitor response to insulin and need to adjust dose as needed.*
- Monitor the results of laboratory tests, including urinalysis, *for evidence of glucosuria.*

Refer to the Critical Thinking Scenario for a full discussion of nursing care for a patient with type 1 diabetes mellitus.

Nursing Diagnoses

Nursing diagnoses related to drug therapy might include the following:

- Risk for unstable blood glucose related to the use of insulin and underlying disease processes
- Imbalanced nutrition: Less than body requirements related to metabolic effects of the drug
- Disturbed sensory perception (kinesthetic, visual, auditory, and tactile) related to glucose levels
- Risk for infection related to injections and disease processes
- Risk for Injury related to potential hyperglycemia or hypoglycemia and injection technique

- Ineffective coping related to diagnosis and the need for injection therapy
- Deficient knowledge regarding drug therapy

Planning

- The patient will receive the best therapeutic effect from the drug therapy.
- The patient will have limited adverse effects to the drug therapy.
- The patient will have an understanding of the drug therapy, adverse effects to anticipate, and measures to relieve discomfort and improve safety.

Implementation with Rationale

- Ensure that the patient is following a dietary and exercise regimen and using good hygiene practices *to improve the effectiveness of the insulin and decrease adverse effects of the disease.*
- Gently rotate the vial containing the agent and avoid vigorous shaking *to ensure uniform suspension of insulin.*
- Select a site that is free of bruising and scarring *to ensure good absorption of the insulin.*
- Give maintenance doses by the subcutaneous or inhaled routes only (see Focus on Safe Medication Administration under Pharmacokinetics for insulin), and rotate injection sites regularly *to avoid damage to muscles and to prevent subcutaneous atrophy.* Give regular insulin IM or IV in emergency situations.
- Monitor response carefully *to avoid adverse effects*; blood glucose monitoring is the most effective way to evaluate insulin dose.
- Monitor the patient for signs and symptoms of hypoglycemia, especially during peak insulin times, when these signs and symptoms would be most likely to appear, *to assess the response to insulin and the need for dose adjustment or medical intervention.*
- Always verify the name of the insulin being given *because each insulin has a different peak and duration, and the names can be confused.*
- Use caution when mixing types of insulin; administer mixtures of regular and NPH insulins within 15 minutes after combining them *to ensure appropriate suspension and therapeutic effect.*
- Store insulin in a cool place away from direct sunlight *to ensure effectiveness.* Predrawn syringes are stable for 1 week if refrigerated; *they offer a good way to ensure the proper dose for patients who have limited vision.*
- Monitor the patient during times of trauma or severe stress *for potential dose adjustment needs.*
- Monitor the patient's food intake; ensure that the patient eats when using insulin *to ensure therapeutic effect and avoid hypoglycemia.*
- Monitor the patient's exercise and activities; ensure that the patient considers the effects of exercise in relationship to eating and insulin dose *to ensure therapeutic effect and avoid hypoglycemia.*
- Protect the patient from infection, including good skin care and foot care, *to prevent the development of serious infections and changes in therapeutic insulin doses.*
- Monitor the patient's sensory losses *to incorporate his or her needs into safety issues, as well as potential problems in drawing up and administering insulin.*
- Help the patient to deal with necessary lifestyle changes, including diet and exercise needs, sensory loss, and the impact of a drug regimen that includes giving injections, *to help encourage compliance with the treatment regimen.*
- Instruct patients who are also receiving beta-blockers about ways to monitor glucose levels and signs and symptoms of glucose abnormalities *to prevent hypoglycemic and hyperglycemic episodes when SNS and warning signs are blocked.*
- Provide thorough patient teaching, including diet and exercise needs; measures to avoid adverse effects, including proper food care and screening for injuries; warning signs of problems, including signs and symptoms of hypoglycemia and hyperglycemia; the importance of increased screening when ill or unable to eat properly; proper administration techniques and proper disposal of needles and syringes in the provided sharps bucket and to return this when full to a community take-back center or pharmacy; to never reuse needles or share needles with other people and the need to monitor disease status, *to enhance patient knowledge about drug therapy and promote compliance.*

Evaluation

- Monitor patient response to the drug (stabilization of blood glucose levels).
- Monitor for adverse effects (hypoglycemia, ketoacidosis, lung function decline with inhaled insulin, and injection site irritation).
- Evaluate the effectiveness of the teaching plan (patient can name drug, dosage, adverse effects to watch for, specific measures to avoid them, and proper administration technique).
- Monitor the effectiveness of comfort measures and compliance with the regimen.

CRITICAL THINKING SCENARIO

Type 1 Diabetes Mellitus

THE SITUATION

M.J. is a 22-year-old woman who has newly diagnosed type 1 diabetes mellitus. She was stabilized on insulin while hospitalized for diagnosis and management. One week after discharge, M.J. experienced nausea and anorexia. She was unable to eat, but she took her insulin as usual in the morning. That afternoon, she experienced profuse sweating and was tremulous and apprehensive, so she went to the hospital emergency room. The initial diagnosis was insulin reaction from taking insulin and not eating, combined with the stress of her GI upset. M.J. was treated at the emergency room with intravenous glucose. After she had rested and her glucose levels had returned to normal, she was discharged to home.

CRITICAL THINKING

What instructions should M.J. receive before she leaves? Think about the ways that stress can alter the blood glucose levels. Then consider the stress that a newly diagnosed type 1 diabetic patient undergoes while trying to cope with the diagnosis, learn self-injection, and think about complications of the disease that may arise in the future.

What teaching approaches could help M.J. to decrease her stress and to effectively plan her medical regimen?

What sort of support would be useful for M.J. as she adjusts to her new life?

DISCUSSION

The diagnosis of type 1 diabetes is a life-changing event. M.J. had to learn about the disease and how to test her blood and give herself injections, manage a new diet and exercise program, and cope with the knowledge that the long-term complications of diabetes can be devastating. Many patients who are regulated on insulin in the hospital experience a change in insulin demand after discharge. The SNS is active in the hospital, and one of the effects of SNS activity is increased glucose level—preparing the body for fight or flight. For some patients, returning home eases the stress that activated the SNS, and glucose levels fall. If the patient continues to use the same insulin dose, hypoglycemia can occur. Other patients may feel protected in the hospital and experience stress when they are sent home. They may feel anxious about taking care of themselves while coping with everyday problems and tensions. In addition, it may be overwhelming to learn the proper preparation and administration of a subcutaneous injection. Learning how to properly dispose of needles and syringes may be just one more stressor added to the list. These patients need an increased insulin dose because their stress reaction intensifies when they get home, driving their blood glucose level up.

Patients are taught how to measure their blood glucose levels before they leave the hospital. After they get used to doing this and regulating their insulin based on glucose concentrations, they usually manage well. The first few days to weeks are often the hardest. The nurse should review with M.J. how to test her glucose, draw up her insulin, and regulate the dose. The nurse also should give M.J. written information that she can refer to later.

In addition, the nurse should give M.J. a chance to talk and to vent her feelings about her diagnosis and her future. To help decrease M.J.'s stress and to avoid problems during this adjustment period the nurse can give M.J. a telephone number to call if she has problems or questions. M.J. should return in a few days to review her progress and have any questions answered. In the meantime the nurse should encourage M.J. to write down any questions or problems that arise so that they can be addressed during the follow-up visit. Support and encouragement will be crucial to helping M.J. adjust to her disease and her drug therapy. She can also be referred to the American Diabetic Association, which in many communities offers support services to help diabetics.

NURSING CARE GUIDE FOR M.J.: TYPE 1 DIABETES MELLITUS

Assessment: History and Examination

Review the patient's history for allergies to drug products, pregnancy, breastfeeding, and other drugs in current use. M.J. denies allergies, pregnancy, and lactation. She is taking no other medications.

Focus the physical examination on the following:

Neurological: Orientation, reflexes; M.J. appears shaky, and her pupils are dilated.

Skin: Coloration and/or lesions; M.J.'s appearance (pale and sweaty) is consistent with diaphoresis.

CV: Pulse, 110 beats/min; blood pressure, 155/92 mm Hg.

Respiratory: Respiratory rate, 24/min; lungs clear on auscultation; rapid respiratory rate is indicative of acidosis.

Laboratory tests: Urinalysis—negative for glucose, positive for ketones; blood glucose level, 72 mg/dL.

Nursing Diagnoses

Imbalanced nutrition: Less than body requirements related to metabolic effects

Disturbed sensory perception (kinesthetic, visual, auditory, and tactile) related to effects on glucose levels

Type 1 Diabetes Mellitus (continued)

Risk for infection related to injections and disease process
Ineffective coping related to diagnosis and injections
Deficient knowledge regarding drug therapy

Planning

The patient will receive the best therapeutic effect from the drug therapy.
The patient will have limited adverse effects to the drug therapy.
The patient will have an understanding of the drug therapy, adverse effects to anticipate, and measures to relieve discomfort and improve safety.

Implementation

Provide patient teaching regarding drug name, dosage, adverse effects, precautions, warning signs to report, and proper administration technique.
Assist M.J. to restore blood glucose to normal levels by using insulin and constantly monitoring blood glucose levels during normal times and during times of stress and trauma so that insulin dose can be adjusted to needed amount.
Review proper subcutaneous injection technique and site rotation.
Provide support and reassurance to help M.J. deal with drug injections, this hypoglycemic episode, and her lifetime need for insulin.
Teach M.J. how to store insulin in a cool place away from light and to use caution when mixing insulin types.
Review with M.J. the name and type of insulin, dosage, adverse effects, precautions, warning signs of adverse effects to report, and proper administration technique and proper disposal of needles and syringes.

Evaluation

Evaluate drug effects: Return of glucose levels to normal.
Monitor for adverse effects: Hypoglycemia and/or injection site reaction.
Monitor for drug–drug interactions as indicated for insulin.
Evaluate the effectiveness of patient-teaching program and comfort and safety measures.

PATIENT TEACHING FOR M.J.

- Diet modifications and increased exercise are very important aspects of your diabetes management. You should also practice good skin care and hygiene measures. Check for any injury or sign of infection regularly.
- Insulin is a hormone that is normally produced by your pancreas. It helps to regulate your energy balance by affecting the way the body uses sugar and fats. The lack of insulin produces a disease called diabetes mellitus. By injecting insulin each day, you can help your body use the sugars and fats in your food effectively.
- Check the expiration date on your insulin. Store the insulin at room temperature and avoid extremes of heat and light. Gently rotate the vial between your palms before use to disperse any crystals that may have formed. Do not shake the vial because vigorous shaking can inactivate the drug. Rotate your injection sites on a regular basis.
- A prescription is required to get the syringes that you will need to administer your insulin. Keep the syringes sealed until ready to use, and dispose of them appropriately in the sharps bucket provided; when full return this to a community drug take-back center or a pharmacy. Rotate your injection sites regularly to prevent tissue damage and to ensure that the proper amount of insulin is absorbed. Never reuse needles and never share needles with other people.
- You should be aware of the signs and symptoms of hypoglycemia (too much insulin). If any of these occur, eat or drink something high in sugar, such as candy, orange juice, honey, or sugar. The signs and symptoms to watch for include the following: Nervousness, anxiety, sweating, pale and cool skin, headache, nausea, hunger, and shakiness. These may happen if you skip a meal, exercise too much, or experience extreme stress. If these symptoms happen very often, notify your health care provider. If you cannot eat because of illness or other problems, do not take your usual insulin dose. Contact your health care provider for assistance.
- Avoid the use of any over-the-counter medications or herbal therapies without first checking with your health care provider. Several of these medications and many commonly used herbs can interfere with the effectiveness of insulin. Avoid the use of alcohol because it increases the chances of having hypoglycemic attacks.
- Tell any doctor, nurse, or other health care provider involved in your care that you are taking this drug. You may want to wear or carry a MedicAlert tag showing that you are on this medication. This would alert any medical personnel taking care of you in an emergency to the fact that you are taking this drug.
- Report any of the following to your health care provider: Loss of appetite, blurred vision, fruity odor to your breath, increased urination, increased thirst, nausea, or vomiting.
- While you are taking this drug, it is important to have regular medical follow-up, including blood tests to monitor your blood glucose levels, to evaluate you for any adverse effects of your diabetes.
- Keep this drug and your syringes out of the reach of children. Use proper disposal techniques for your needles and syringes. Do not give this medication to anyone else or take any similar medication that has not been prescribed for you.

KEY POINTS

- Insulin replaces the endogenous hormone when the body does not produce enough insulin or when there are not enough insulin receptor sites to provide adequate glucose control.
- Blood glucose levels vary with food intake, exercise, and stress levels, possibly necessitating a change in insulin dose.
- Patients need to learn to recognize the signs of hypoglycemia and hyperglycemia to effectively manage their drug therapy.

Sulfonylureas and Other Antidiabetic Agents

Other antidiabetic agents may be used in patients who still have a functioning pancreas. These agents include the sulfonylureas and other antidiabetic agents (see Table 38.3). The sulfonylureas were the first oral agents introduced to treat type 2 diabetes. They stimulate the pancreas to release insulin. Other agents discussed in this section have been introduced more recently for use in patients with type 1 and type 2 diabetes. These agents interact with the body's glucose controls in a number of ways, including affecting insulin release, decreasing insulin resistance, or altering

Table 38.3 ***Drugs in Focus:* Other Antidiabetic Agents**

Drug Name	Dosage/Route	Usual Indications
Sulfonylureas		
First-Generation Sulfonylureas		
chlorpropamide (*Diabinese*)	100–250 mg/d PO; lower doses with geriatric patients	Adjunct to diet for the management of type 2 diabetes
tolazamide (generic)	100–250 mg/d PO; lower doses with geriatric patients	Adjunct to diet for the management of type 2 diabetes; adjunct to insulin for management in certain type 2 diabetics, reducing the insulin dose and decreasing the risks of hypoglycemia
tolbutamide (generic)	0.25–3 g/d PO; lower doses with geriatric patients	Adjunct to diet for the management of type 2 diabetes; adjunct to insulin for management in certain type 2 diabetics, reducing the insulin dose and decreasing the risks of hypoglycemia
Second-Generation Sulfonylureas		
glimepiride (*Amaryl*)	1–4 mg/d PO; lower doses with geriatric patients	Adjunct to diet for the management of type 2 diabetes; adjunct to insulin for management in certain type 2 diabetics, reducing the insulin dose and decreasing the risks of hypoglycemia
glipizide (*Glucotrol*)	5 mg PO daily, titrate based on response; do not exceed 15 mg/d; use lower doses with geriatric and hepatic-impaired patients; extended release: 5 mg/d, adjust to a maximum of 20 mg/d	Adjunct to diet for the management of type 2 diabetes; adjunct to insulin for management in certain type 2 diabetics, reducing the insulin dose and decreasing the risks of hypoglycemia
glyburide (*DiaBeta, Micronase, Glynase PresTab*)	1.25–20 mg/d PO (*DiaBeta, Micronase*), 0.75–12 mg/d PO (*Glynase*); lower doses with geriatric patients	Adjunct to diet for the management of type 2 diabetes; adjunct to insulin for management in certain type 2 diabetics, reducing the insulin dose and decreasing the risks of hypoglycemia
Other Antidiabetic Agents		
Alpha-Glucosidase Inhibitors		
acarbose (*Precose*)	100 mg PO t.i.d. at the start of each meal	Adjunct to diet to lower blood glucose in type 2 diabetics; in combination with sulfonylureas to control blood sugar in patients whose diabetes cannot be controlled with either drug alone
miglitol (*Glyset*)	50–100 mg PO t.i.d. with the first bite of each meal	Adjunct to diet to lower blood glucose in type 2 diabetics; in combination with sulfonylureas to control blood sugar in patients whose diabetes cannot be controlled with either drug alone
Biguanide		
metformin (*Glucophage*)	500–850 mg/d PO in divided doses; reduce dose in geriatric and renal-impaired patients; maximum dose: 2,550 mg/d *Pediatric (10–16 y):* 500 mg/d PO with a maximum dose of 2,000 mg/d; do not use extended release form	Adjunct to diet to lower blood glucose in type 2 diabetics

Drug Name	Dosage/Route	Usual Indications
DDP-4 Inhibitors		
alogliptin (*Nesina*)	25 mg/d PO	Adjunct to diet and exercise to improve glucose control in patients with type 2 diabetes
linagliptin (*Tradjenta*)	5 mg/d PO	Adjunct to diet and exercise to improve glucose control in patients with type 2 diabetes
saxagliptin (*Onglyza*)	2.5–5 mg/d PO	Adjunct to diet and exercise to improve glucose control in patients with type 2 diabetes
sitagliptin (*Januvia*)	100 mg/d PO	Adjunct to diet and exercise to improve glucose control in patients with type 2 diabetes, as monotherapy or combined with metformin, pioglitazone, or other agents
Human Amylin		
pramlintide acetate (*Symlin*)	*Type 2 diabetes:*60 mcg by subcutaneous injection immediately before major meals; may be increased to 120 mcg *Type 1 diabetes:* Initially 15 mcg by subcutaneous injection; maintenance 30–60 mcg/dose	Adjunct to treatment of type 2 or type 1 diabetics using meal time insulin but without glycemic control
Incretin Mimetic		
exenatide (*Baraclude, Bydureon*)	5 mcg by subcutaneous injection within 60 min before morning and evening meals; may be increased to 10 mcg b.i.d. after 1 mo; extended release form give 2 mg by subcutaneous injection every 7 d	Adjunct to diet and oral agents to improve glycemic control in patients with type 2 diabetes
GLP-1 Agonists		
abiglutide (*Tanzeum*)	30–50 mg by subcutaneous injection once a week	Adjunct to diet and exercise to improve glucose control in patients with type 2 diabetes; consider risk of thyroid tumor and limit use to patients in whom the benefit outweighs the risk
dulaglutide (*Trulicity*)	0.75–1.5 mg by subcutaneous injection once a week	Adjunct to diet and exercise to improve glucose control in patients with type 2 diabetes; consider risk of thyroid tumor and limit use to patients in whom the benefit outweighs the risk
luraglutide (*Victoza*)	0.6 mg by subcutaneous injection once a day for 1 wk; increase dose based on patient response after 1 wk to a maximum of 1.8 mg/d	Adjunct to diet and exercise to improve glucose control in patients with type 2 diabetes; consider risk of thyroid tumor and limit use to patients in whom the benefit outweighs the risk
Meglitinides		
nateglinide (*Starlix*)	120 mg PO t.i.d. with each meal	Adjunct to diet to lower blood glucose in type 2 diabetics; in combination with metformin to control blood sugar in patients whose diabetes cannot be controlled with either drug alone
repaglinide (*Prandin*)	0.5–4 mg PO before meals, do not exceed 16 mg/d	Adjunct to diet to lower blood glucose in type 2 diabetics; in combination with metformin to control blood sugar in patients whose diabetes cannot be controlled with either drug alone
SGLT-2 Inhibitors		
canagliflozin (*Inkovana*)	100 mg/d PO with the first meal of the day; maximum 300 mg/d	Adjunct to diet to improve glycemic control in type 2 diabetics
dapagliflozin (*Farxiga*)	5 mg/d PO in the morning; maximum 10 mg/d	Adjunct to diet to improve glycemic control in type 2 diabetics
empagliflozin (*Jardiance*)	10mg/d PO in the morning; maximum 25 mg/d	Adjunct to diet to improve glycemic control in type 2 diabetics
Thiazolidinediones		
pioglitazone (*Actos*)	15–30 mg/d PO as a single dose; use caution with hepatic impairment	Adjunct to diet to lower blood glucose in type 2 diabetics; in combination with insulin or sulfonylureas to control blood sugar in patients whose diabetes cannot be controlled with either drug alone
rosiglitazone (*Avandia*)	4–8 mg/d PO as a single dose; use caution with hepatic impairment	Adjunct to diet to lower blood glucose in type 2 diabetics; in combination with insulin or sulfonylureas to control blood sugar in patients whose diabetes cannot be controlled with either drug alone

DDP-4, dipeptidyl peptidase-4; GLP-1, glucagon-like peptide-1; SGLT-2, sodium–glucose cotransporter-2.

glucose absorption from the GI tract and release of glucose by the liver. They often are combined with a sulfonylurea to increase glycemic control.

Sulfonylureas

The **sulfonylureas** bind to potassium channels on pancreatic beta cells. They may improve insulin binding to insulin receptors and increase the number of insulin receptors. They are also known to increase the effect of antidiuretic hormone on renal cells. They are effective only in patients who have functioning beta cells. They are not effective for all diabetics and may lose their effectiveness over time with others. Sulfonylureas are further classified as first-generation or second-generation sulfonylureas. All of the sulfonylureas can cause hypoglycemia.

First-Generation Sulfonylureas

The first-generation sulfonylureas include chlorpropamide (*Diabinese*), tolazamide (generic), and tolbutamide (generic). However, the use of these drugs has been steadily declining as more effective drugs have become available. Some patients may still be treated with these drugs. See Table 38.3 for Usual Indications for first-generation sulfonylureas.

Chlorpropamide has been the most frequently used of the group because it has the most predictable effects and has been proven to be very reliable. Tolbutamide is preferred for patients with renal dysfunction, who may not be able to excrete chlorpropamide, because it is more easily cleared from the body. Tolazamide, which is used even less frequently, is usually tried after the first two drugs have been shown to be ineffective. It is not as predictably effective in many patients, but it can be very effective in some patients who do not respond to chlorpropamide. Tolbutamide and tolazamide are sometimes used in combination with insulin to reduce the insulin dose and decrease the risk of hypoglycemia in certain type 2 diabetics who have begun to use insulin to control their blood glucose level.

The first-generation sulfonylureas were associated with an increased risk of CV disease and death in a somewhat controversial study. They are now thought to possibly cause an increase in CV deaths.

FOCUS ON Safe Medication Administration

*Name confusion has been reported between chlorpropamide (the antidiabetic agent **Diabinese**) and chlorpromazine (the antipsychotic agent **Thorazine**). A mix-up can be deadly. Use caution to make sure you know which drug was ordered for your patient.*

Second-Generation Sulfonylureas

The second-generation drugs include glimepiride (*Amaryl*), glipizide (*Glucotrol*), and glyburide (*DiaBeta*, and others). See Table 38.3 for Usual Indications for each drug. Second-generation sulfonylureas have several advantages over the first-generation drugs, including the following:

- They are excreted in the urine and bile, making them safer for patients with renal dysfunction.
- They do not interact with as many protein-bound drugs as the first-generation drugs.
- They have a longer duration of action, making it possible to take them only once or twice a day, thus increasing compliance.

Glimepiride is a much less expensive drug than most of the other sulfonylureas, which has advantages for some people. Prescribers may try different agents (first- or second-generation drugs) before finding the one that is most effective for a given patient.

Therapeutic Actions and Indications

The sulfonylureas stimulate insulin release from the beta cells in the pancreas (see Figure 38.1). They improve insulin binding to insulin receptors and may actually increase the number of insulin receptors. They are indicated as an adjunct to diet and exercise to lower blood glucose levels in type 2 diabetes mellitus. They have the off-label use of being an adjunct to insulin and metformin to improve glucose control in type 2 diabetics.

Pharmacokinetics

These drugs are rapidly absorbed from the GI tract and undergo hepatic metabolism. They are excreted in the urine. The peak effects and duration of effects differ because of the activity of various metabolites of the different drugs.

Contraindications and Cautions

Sulfonylureas are contraindicated in the presence of known allergy to any sulfonylureas *to avoid hypersensitivity reactions* and in diabetes complicated by fever, severe infection, severe trauma, major surgery, ketoacidosis, severe renal or hepatic disease, pregnancy, or lactation, *which require tighter control of glucose levels using insulin.* These drugs are also contraindicated for use in type 1 diabetics, *who do not have functioning beta cells and would have no benefit from the drug.*

These drugs are not for use during pregnancy. Insulin should be used if an antidiabetic agent is needed during pregnancy. Some of these drugs cross into breast milk, and adequate studies are not available on others. *Because of the risk of hypoglycemic effects in the baby*, these drugs should not be used during lactation. Another method of feeding the baby should be used. The safety and efficacy of these drugs for use in children have not been established.

Adverse Effects

The most common adverse effects related to the sulfonylureas are hypoglycemia (caused by an imbalance in levels of glucose and insulin) and GI distress, including nausea, vomiting, epigastric discomfort, heartburn, and anorexia. (Anorexia should be monitored because affected patients may not eat after taking the sulfonylurea, which could lead to hypoglycemia.) Allergic skin reactions have been reported with some of these drugs, and, as mentioned earlier, there may be an increased risk of CV mortality, particularly with the first-generation agents.

Clinically Important Drug–Drug Interactions

Care should be taken with any drug that acidifies the urine because excretion of the sulfonylurea may be decreased. Caution should also be used with beta-blockers, which may mask the signs of hypoglycemia, and with alcohol, which can lead to altered glucose levels when combined with sulfonylureas. Caution must also be used with many herbal therapies that could alter blood glucose levels.

Prototype Summary: Chlorpropamide

Indications: Adjunct to diet and exercise to lower blood glucose level in type 2 diabetics.

Actions: Stimulates the release of insulin from functioning cells in the pancreas; may improve the binding of insulin-to-insulin receptor sites or increase the number of insulin receptor sites.

Pharmacokinetics:

Route	Onset	Peak	Duration
Oral	1 h	3–4 h	60 h

$T_{1/2}$: 36 hours; metabolized in the liver and excreted in the urine and bile.

Adverse Effects: GI discomfort, anorexia, heartburn, vomiting, nausea, and hypoglycemia.

Prototype Summary: Glyburide

Indications: Adjunct to diet and exercise in the management of type 2 diabetes; with metformin or insulin for stabilization of diabetic patients.

Actions: Stimulates insulin release from functioning beta cells in the pancreas; may improve insulin binding to insulin receptor sites or increase the number of insulin receptor sites.

Pharmacokinetics:

Route	Onset	Duration
Oral	1 h	24 h

$T_{1/2}$: 4 hours; metabolized in the liver and excreted in the bile and urine.

Adverse Effects: GI discomfort, anorexia, nausea, vomiting, heartburn, diarrhea, allergic skin reactions, and hypoglycemia.

Other Antidiabetic Agents

Several other antidiabetic agents are available. Although these drugs are structurally unrelated to the sulfonylureas, they frequently are effective when used in combination with sulfonylureas or insulin. These drugs include the alpha-glucosidase inhibitors acarbose (*Precose*) and miglitol (*Glyset*); the biguanide metformin (*Glucophage*); the meglitinides repaglinide (*Prandin*) and nateglinide (*Starlix*); the thiazolidinediones pioglitazone (*Actos*) and rosiglitazone (*Avandia*); the incretin mimetic exenatide (*Byetta, Bydureon*), the glucagon-like polypeptide receptor agonists abiglutide (*Tanzeum*), dulaglutide (*Trulicity*), and liraglutide (*Victoza*); the human amylin pramlintide (*Symlin*); and the DDP-4 inhibitors alogliptin (*Nesina*), linagliptin (*Tradjenta*), saxagliptin (*Onglyza*), and sitagliptin (*Januvia*); and the newest class, the sodium–glucose cotransporter 2 inhibitors canagliflozin (*Invokana*), dapagliflozin (*Farxiga*), and empagliflozin (*Jardiance*) (see Table 38.3).

Acarbose and miglitol are inhibitors of alpha-glucosidase (an enzyme that breaks down glucose for absorption); they delay the absorption of glucose. They have only a mild effect on glucose levels and have been associated with severe hepatic toxicity. They do not enhance insulin secretion, so their effects are additive to those of the sulfonylureas in controlling blood glucose. These drugs are used in combination with sulfonylureas, metformin, and insulin for patients whose glucose levels cannot be controlled with a single agent or diet and exercise alone.

Metformin decreases the production and increases the uptake of glucose. It is effective in lowering blood glucose levels and does not cause hypoglycemia as the sulfonylureas do. It has been associated with the development of lactic acidosis. Both acarbose and metformin can cause GI distress. Metformin is approved for use in children 10 years of age and older. It is also being used in the treatment of women with polycystic ovary syndrome (see Box 38.7).

The meglitinides include repaglinide and nateglinide and act like the sulfonylureas to increase insulin release. These are rapid-acting drugs with a very short half-life. They are oral drugs used just before meals to lower postprandial glucose levels. These drugs can be used in combination with metformin or a thiazolidinedione for better glycemic control. These drugs are associated with GI upset and diarrhea.

The thiazolidinediones are drugs that decrease insulin resistance; they are used in combination with sulfonylureas, insulin, or metformin to treat patients with insulin resistance. The first drug of this class, troglitazone, was withdrawn from the market after reports of serious hepatotoxicity. The two drugs that are available now—pioglitazone and rosiglitazone—are not associated with the same severe liver toxicity, although in late 2007 reports were published linking these drugs to an increase in CV events. Some European countries have pulled these drugs from the market because of studies showing the increased risk

BOX 38.7

Polycystic Ovary Syndrome and Antidiabetic Drugs

Polycystic ovary syndrome is an ovarian function disorder associated with obesity, infrequent or absent menses, and infertility. Women who have this disorder have elevated insulin levels with normal fasting blood glucose levels, elevated luteinizing hormone (LH) levels, and normal estrogen and follicle-stimulating hormone levels. Because of the alterations in hormone activity, follicles develop on the ovaries, but ovulation does not occur, and the developed follicles turn into cysts. High LH levels tend to cause an increase in androgen production, which is associated with insulin resistance.

Treatment is aimed at altering the metabolic changes to allow ovulation (if pregnancy is desired) or stop the follicle development (if pregnancy is not desired). Weight loss is very important and may correct the alterations in metabolism and allow ovulation to occur without medical treatment. Metformin and pioglitazone have proven effective in increasing insulin sensitivity and decreasing androgen and LH levels to break the cycle and allow ovulation to occur if pregnancy is desired. A fertility drug is often used with the antidiabetic agent. Hormonal contraceptives are used if pregnancy is not desired to halt the development of the follicles and stop the cyst production.

of CV problems. The U.S. Food and Drug Administration (FDA) limited the availability of rosiglitazone due to the links to CV events, putting it in a limited access program that included education about the associated use of the drug. In 2014 further studies seemed to indicate that the drug was not as tightly linked to CV problems and the limited access was lifted. The drug does have a black box warning that CV risk may exist. Pioglitazone has been strongly linked to an increased risk of bladder cancer if it is used for over 1 year. All patients taking either drug should be screened for cardiovascular risk before starting on these drugs and all patients on the drugs should be monitored carefully for CV problems. Patients should also still be monitored for any change in liver function while they are taking these drugs. These drugs are also being studied for use in increasing ovulation frequency in woman who have polycystic ovary syndrome (Box 38.7). Box 38.8 describes some of the new fixed combination oral agents, which provide two different agents in one tablet to make it easier for the patient to be compliant with the drug regimen.

Therapeutic actions and indications, pharmacokinetics, contraindications and cautions, adverse effects, and clinically important drug–drug interactions for these drugs are basically the same as for the sulfonylureas. The safety and efficacy of these drugs for use in children have not been established, except for the use of metformin in children 10 years of age and older.

BOX 38.8

Available Fixed Combination Oral Agents

Several fixed combination oral antidiabetic agents have become available in the last 5 years. These combination products are intended to decrease the number of tablets the patient needs to take each day and thereby increase compliance with the drug regimen. The patient should be stabilized on the individual product first and then switched to the combination product after the correct dose combination for that patient has been established. The patient should be reminded that diet and exercise are still the key parts of the antidiabetic treatment regimen.

- *Glucovance* is a combination of glyburide and metformin and is available in three sizes: 1.25-mg glyburide with 250-mg metformin, 2.5-mg glyburide with 500-mg metformin, and 5-mg glyburide with 500-mg metformin.
- *Avandamet* is a combination of rosiglitazone and metformin and is available in three sizes: 1-, 2-, or 4-mg rosiglitazone with 500-mg metformin.
- *Avandaryl* is a combination of rosiglitazone and glimepiride and is available in three sizes: 1-, 2-, or 4-mg glimepiride with 4-mg rosiglitazone.
- *Duetact* is a combination of pioglitazone and glimepiride, available with 30-mg pioglitazone and 2- or 4-mg glimepiride.
- *Actoplus Met* is a combination of pioglitazone and metformin and is available in two sizes: 500- or 850-mg metformin with 15-mg pioglitazone.
- *Janumet* is a combination of sitagliptin and metformin and is available in two sizes: 50-mg sitagliptin with 500- or 1,000-mg metformin. *Janumet XR* combines 50-mg sitagliptin with 500- or 1,000-mg metformin or 100-mg sitagliptin with 1,000-mg metformin.
- *PrandiMet* is a combination of repaglinide and metformin and is available in two sizes: 500-mg metformin with 1- or 2-mg repaglinide.
- *Kombiglyze XR* is a combination of saxigliptin and extended release metformin available as 5-mg saxigliptin with 500- or 1,000-mg extended release metformin or 2.5-mg saxigliptin with 500-mg extended release metformin.
- *Kazano* is a combination of alogliptin and metformin and is available in two doses, 12.5-mg alogliptin with 500- or 1,000-mg metformin.
- *Oseni* is a combination of alogliptin and pioglitazone and is available in six doses, 12.5-mg alogliptin with 15-, 30-, or 45-mg pioglizazone and 25-mg alogliptin with 15-, 30-, or 45-mg pioglitazone.
- *Invoakamet* is a combination of canagliflozin and metformin, available as 50- or 150-mg canagliflozin with 500- or 1,000-mg metformin.
- *Xigduo XR* is a combination of dapagliflozin and metformin. It is an extended release form with 5- or 10-mg dapagliflozin combined with 500- or 1,000-mg metformin.
- *Glaxambi* is a combination of 10- or 25-mg empagliflozin with 5-mg linagliptin.
- *Jenatdueto* is a combination of 2.5-mg linagliptin with 500-, 850-, or 1,000-mg metformin.
- *Synjardy* is a combination of 5- or 12.5-mg empagliflozin with 500- or 1,000-mg metformin.

Pramlintide is a human amylin that works to modulate gastric emptying after a meal, causes a feeling of fullness or satiety, and prevents the postmeal rise in glucagon that usually elevates glucose levels. It is a synthetic form of human amylin, a hormone produced by the beta cells in the pancreas that is important in regulating postmeal glucose levels. It is injected subcutaneously immediately before a major meal and can be used in combination with insulins and oral agents. It has a rapid onset of action and peaks in 21 minutes. It should be injected before each major meal of the day, at least 2 inches away from any insulin injection site. It cannot be combined in the syringe with insulin. This drug should not be used if the patient is unable to eat.

Exenatide is an incretin that mimics the effects of GLP-1: Enhancement of glucose-dependent insulin secretion by the beta cells in the pancreas, depression of elevated glucagon secretion, and slowed gastric emptying to help moderate and lower blood glucose levels. Exenatide is given by subcutaneous injection twice a day, within 60 minutes before the morning and evening meals. It has a rapid onset of action and peaks within 2 hours; its effects last 8 to 10 hours. It is given in combination with oral agents to improve glycemic control in type 2 diabetes patients who cannot achieve glycemic control on oral agents alone. It should not be given if the patient is unable to eat. An extended release form is now available that is given by subcutaneous injection once every 7 days.

The GLP-1 receptor agonists increase insulin release and decrease glucagon release (in preparation for the nutrients that will soon be absorbed). GLP-1 also slows GI emptying to allow more absorption of nutrients and stimulate the satiety center in the brain to decrease the desire to eat because food is already in the GI tract. See Box 38-9 for a new use for the GLP-1 agonists. GLP-1 has a very short half-life and is metabolized by the enzyme DDP-4. Luraglutide, the first drug in this class has the advantage of once-a-day subcutaneous injection and can be given without consideration of meal time. It is absorbed within 8 to 12 hours and excreted mostly in the urine with a half-life of 13 hours. Abiglutide and dulaglutide are administered subcutaneously once weekly. They are absorbed slowly with a half-life of 5 days. There is a risk of pancreatitis with these drugs. All of the drugs in this class have a black box warning of a risk of thyroid C-cell tumors in animals, and patients need to be made aware of the risk and taught to be aware of the signs and symptoms of thyroid tumors.The drugs should not be used in patients with a history or family history of thyroid cancer of multiple endocrine neoplasia syndrome.

The DDP-4 inhibitors slow the breakdown of GLP-1 in the body, prolonging the effects of increased insulin secretion, decreased glucagon secretion, and slowed GI emptying. There are currently four drugs available in this class, alogliptin, linagliptin, saxagliptin, and sitagliptin. They are oral drugs, taken once a day, often in combination with other agents. They are rapidly absorbed, with peak effects varying from 1 to 5 hours. The half-life varies with each drug and they are excreted unchanged in the urine. Few adverse effects have been reported with these drugs, but they must be used in combination with an appropriate diet and exercise program.

The newest class of drugs developed to control glucose levels is the sodium–glucose cotransporter-2 inhibitors. These drugs work in a unique way to promote the loss of glucose through the urine. Glucose is filtered at the glomerulus, but is such a big molecule it needs to actively be reabsorbed using the sodium–glucose cotransporter. If all of the cotransporter sites are occupied, glucose is spilled in the urine, usually indicating a serum glucose over 200. These drugs block the cotransporter system and glucose is not reabsorbed, but lost in the urine. Glucose is a large molecule and takes water with it (the polyuria described above). The serum glucose levels fall since glucose is not reabsorbed. The patient is at risk for dehydration and hypotension, as well as for urinary tract infections (UTIs) and genital fungal infections because of the large amount of glucose in the urine. Patients taking these drugs are at increased risk for diabetic ketoacidosis and need to be monitored accordingly. Canagliflozin has been linked to loss of bone density and bone fractures; patients receiving this drug need to be screened for risk of bone loss, and bone density should be monitored. Canagliflozin, dapaglifozin, and empagliflozin are the drugs in this class. These drugs are absorbed from the GI tract, reaching peak levels in 1.5 hours, and have a half-life of 12 hours. They must be used cautiously with any renal impairment or history of urinary tract infections.

In 2009, an old drug, bromocriptine, was approved to improve glycemic control in type 2 diabetics, a unique, CNS approach to treating type 2 diabetes. This drug is explained in Box 38.10.

The goal of all of these drugs is to achieve glycemic control as adjunct therapy to diet and exercise. Patients may be on several different drugs, working at different points in the body to achieve that control. Regular medical follow-up and teaching are critical with these patients.

BOX 38.9

GLP-2 Analog

Teduglutide (*Gattex*) is a GLP-2 analog. This GLP is secreted by cells in the distal intestine. Its effects include increasing intestinal and portal blood flow and decreasing gastric acid secretion. Teduglutide binds to the receptors for this glucagon peptide and causes the release of many mediators including insulin-like growth factor, nitric oxide and keratinocyte growth factor. Its actions increase intestinal absorption through increased blood flow and decreased acid secretion. This drug is approved to treat adults with short bowel syndrome who are dependent on parenteral support. It is given by subcutaneous injection once daily. Teduglutide is associated with neoplastic growth, intestinal obstruction, biliary and pancreatic disorders, and fluid overload. It is important to differentiate this drug and its actions from the GLP-1 agonists that are used to maintain glycemic control.

BOX 38.10

New Approach to Treating Type 2 Diabetes

In 2009 the FDA granted approval for a new use of an old drug, bromocriptine (*Cycloset*). Bromocriptine is a dopamine agonist that is used to treat Parkinson's disease (see Chapter 24 for a full discussion of bromocriptine). *Cycloset* is taken orally in the morning, within 2 hours of waking, and with food. It is not clear how *Cycloset* improves glycemic control, but studies in diabetic animals show that boosting dopamine activity in the morning can "reset" the biological clock to improve metabolism problems related to diabetes. In preapproval studies, type 2 diabetics taking *Cycloset* had improved HbA1c levels, showing better glycemic control, and were less likely to have a heart attack or stroke or to die of heart disease.

Prototype Summary: Metformin

Indications: Adjunct to diet and exercise for the treatment of type 2 diabetics older than 10 years of age; extended release form for patients older than 17 years of age; adjunct treatment with polycystic ovary syndrome.

Actions: May increase the peripheral use of glucose, increase production of insulin, decrease hepatic glucose production, and alter intestinal absorption of glucose.

Pharmacokinetics:

Route	Onset	Peak	Duration
Oral	Slow	2–2.5 h	10–16 h

$T_{1/2}$: 6.2 and then 17 hours; metabolized in the liver and excreted in the urine.

Adverse Effects: Hypoglycemia, lactic acidosis, GI upset, nausea, anorexia, diarrhea, heartburn, and allergic skin reaction.

Prototype Summary: Luraglutide

Indications: Adjunct to diet and exercise for the treatment of adults with type 2 diabetes.

Actions: Acts on beta cells to increase insulin release, decrease glucagon release; slows GI absorption and stimulates the satiety center to decrease appetite.

Pharmacokinetics:

Route	Onset	Peak	Duration
Subcutaneous	Slow	8–12 h	24 h

$T_{1/2}$: 13 hours; metabolized in the tissues.

Adverse Effects: Hypoglycemia, headache, nausea, anorexia, diarrhea, allergic skin reaction, pancreatitis, renal impairment, thyroid C-cell tumors.

Prototype Summary: Sitagliptin

Indications: Adjunct to diet and exercise for the treatment of type 2 diabetes.

Actions: DPP-4 inhibitor, slows the breakdown of GLP-1 which leads to increased insulin release, decreased glucagon release and slowed GI absorption.

Pharmacokinetics:

Route	Onset	Peak	Duration
Oral	Rapid	1–4 h	10–16 h

$T_{1/2}$: 12.4 hours; metabolized in the liver and excreted in the urine.

Adverse Effects: Hypoglycemia, headache, vomiting, acute pancreatitis.

Prototype Summary: Canagliflozin

Indications: Adjunct to diet and exercise for the treatment of type 2 diabetes.

Actions: Sodium–glucose cotransporter-2 inhibitor, increases the excretion of glucose from the kidney leading to lowered serum glucose levels.

Pharmacokinetics:

Route	Onset	Peak	Duration
Oral	Rapid	1–2 h	10–16 h

$T_{1/2}$: 10–13 hours; excreted in the urine.

Adverse Effects: Dehydration, hypotension, UTI, genital fungal infections.

Nursing Considerations for Patients Taking Other Antidiabetic Agents

Assessment: History and Examination

- Assess for contraindications or cautions: History of allergy to any of these agents *to avoid hypersensitivity reactions*; severe renal or hepatic dysfunction, *which could interfere with metabolism and excretion of the drugs*; and status of pregnancy or lactation, *which are contraindications to the use of these agents.*
- Perform a complete physical assessment to establish baseline status *before beginning therapy and to evaluate effectiveness and any potential adverse effects during therapy.*
- Assess for the presence of any skin lesions *for indication of possible infection and to establish appropriate*

sites for subcutaneous administration as appropriate; orientation and reflexes; baseline pulse and blood pressure; adventitious breath sounds; abdominal sounds and function, *to monitor effects of altered glucose levels.*

- Assess body systems *for changes suggesting possible complications associated with poor blood glucose control.*
- Investigate nutritional intake, noting any problems with intake and adherence to prescribed diet, *to help prevent adverse reactions to drug therapy.*
- Assess activity level, including amount and degree of exercise, *which can alter serum glucose levels and dosage needs for these drugs.*
- Monitor blood glucose levels as ordered *to evaluate effectiveness of drug and glycemic control.*
- Monitor results of laboratory tests, including urinalysis, for evidence of glucosuria, and renal function tests, especially with the sodium–glucose cotransporter-2 inhibitors; and liver function tests, especially with use of the thiazolidinediones, which can cause liver failure, *to determine the need for possible dose adjustment and evaluate for signs of toxicity.*

Nursing Diagnoses

Nursing diagnoses related to drug therapy might include the following:

- Risk for unstable blood glucose related to ineffective dosing of antidiabetic agents
- Imbalanced nutrition: Less than body requirements related to metabolic effects
- Disturbed sensory perception (kinesthetic, visual, auditory, and tactile) related to glucose levels
- Ineffective coping related to diagnosis and therapy
- Deficient knowledge regarding drug therapy

Planning

- The patient will receive the best therapeutic effect from the drug therapy.
- The patient will have limited adverse effects to the drug therapy.
- The patient will have an understanding of the drug therapy, adverse effects to anticipate, and measures to relieve discomfort and improve safety.

Implementation with Rationale

- Administer the drug as prescribed in an appropriate relationship with meals *to ensure therapeutic effectiveness.*
- Ensure that the patient is following diet and exercise modifications *to improve effectiveness of the drug and decrease adverse effects.*
- Monitor nutritional status *to provide nutritional consultation as needed.*
- Monitor response carefully; blood glucose monitoring is the most effective way *to evaluate dose.* Obtain blood glucose levels as ordered *to monitor drug effectiveness.*
- Monitor liver enzymes of patients receiving pioglitazone or rosiglitazone very carefully *to avoid liver toxicity*; arrange to discontinue the drug *to avert serious liver damage if liver toxicity develops.*
- Monitor patients during times of trauma, pregnancy, or severe stress, *and arrange to switch to insulin coverage as needed.*
- Provide thorough patient teaching, including drug name, dosage, and schedule for administration; administration technique if appropriate; proper disposal of needles and syringes in a sharps bucket with return to a community take-back site or pharmacy; never to reuse needles or share needles with other people; need for food intake within specified time period; signs and symptoms of hypoglycemia and hyperglycemia; skin assessment, including daily inspection of feet; signs and symptoms to report immediately; measures to use when ill or unable to eat; proper diet and exercise program; hygiene measures; recommended schedule for follow-up and disease monitoring; and the need for follow-up lab testing, *to enhance patient knowledge of drug therapy and to promote compliance.*

Evaluation

- Monitor patient response to the drug (stabilization of blood glucose levels).
- Monitor for adverse effects (hypoglycemia, UTI, pancreatitis, and GI distress).
- Evaluate the effectiveness of the teaching plan (patient can name drug, dosage, adverse effects to watch for, and specific measures to avoid them).
- Monitor the effectiveness of comfort measures and compliance with the regimen.

KEY POINTS

- Sulfonylureas work only if the pancreas has functioning beta cells.
- Other antidiabetic agents work to slow GI absorption of glucose, increase release of insulin by beta cells, increase insulin receptor site sensitivity, and/or block liver release of glucose and prevent the reabsorption of glucose in the kidney.
- In times of severe stress, patients regulated on other antidiabetic agents usually need to be switched to insulin to control blood glucose levels.
- Proper diet and exercise are the backbone of antidiabetic therapy; antidiabetic drugs are adjuncts to help control blood glucose levels.

Table 38.4 *Drugs in Focus:* Glucose-Elevating Agents

Drug Name	Dosage/Route	Usual Indications
diazoxide (*Proglycem, Hyperstat*)	*Adult and pediatric:* 3–8 mg/kg/d PO in two to three divided doses q8–12 h	Oral management of hypoglycemia; intravenous use for management of severe hypertension
glucagon (*GlucaGen*)	*Adult and pediatric (>20 kg):* 0.5–1 mg subcutaneous, IM, or IV *Pediatric (<20 kg):* 0.5 mg subcutaneous, IM, or IV	To counteract severe hypoglycemic reactions

Glucose-Elevating Agents

Glucose-elevating agents, as the name implies, raise the blood level of glucose when severe hypoglycemia occurs (<40 mg/dL). Some adverse conditions are associated with hypoglycemia, including pancreatic disorders, kidney disease, certain cancers, disorders of the anterior pituitary, and unbalanced treatment of diabetes mellitus (which can occur if the patient takes the wrong dose of insulin or antidiabetic agents or if something interferes with food intake or changes stress or exercise levels). Two agents are used to elevate glucose in these conditions: Diazoxide (*Proglycem*) and glucagon (*GlucaGen*). Pure glucose can also be given orally or IV to increase glucose levels. Oral glucose tablets or gels (*Glutose, Insta-Glucose*, and *BD Glucose*) are available over the counter for patients to keep on hand for management of moderate hypoglycemic episodes (see Table 38.4).

Therapeutic Actions and Indications

These agents increase the blood glucose level by decreasing insulin release and accelerating the breakdown of glycogen in the liver to release glucose. They are indicated for the treatment of hypoglycemic reactions related to insulin or oral antidiabetic agents, for the treatment of hypoglycemia related to pancreatic or other cancers, and for short-term treatment of acute hypoglycemia related to anterior pituitary dysfunction (Table 38.4).

Pharmacokinetics

Diazoxide is administered orally. Glucagon is given parenterally only and is the preferred agent for emergency situations. Glucagon and diazoxide are rapidly absorbed and widely distributed throughout the body. They are excreted in the urine.

Contraindications and Cautions

Diazoxide is contraindicated with known allergies to sulfonamides or thiazides. Diazoxide has been associated with adverse effects on the fetus including pulmonary hypertension and should not be used during pregnancy. There are no adequate studies on glucagon and pregnancy, so use should be reserved for those situations in which the benefits to the mother outweigh any potential risks to the fetus. Caution should be used during lactation because the drugs may cause hyperglycemic effects in the baby. Caution should be used in patients with renal or hepatic dysfunction or CV disease.

Adverse Effects

Glucagon is associated with GI upset, nausea, and vomiting. Diazoxide has been associated with vascular effects, including hypotension, headache, cerebral ischemia, weakness, heart failure, and arrhythmias; these reactions are associated with diazoxide's ability to relax arteriolar smooth muscle.

Clinically Important Drug–Drug Interactions

Taking diazoxide in combination with thiazide diuretics causes an increased risk of toxicity because diazoxide is structurally similar to these diuretics.

Increased anticoagulation effects have been noted when glucagon is combined with oral anticoagulants. If this combination is needed, the dose should be adjusted.

Prototype Summary: Glucagon

Indications: Counteracts severe hypoglycemic reactions in diabetic patients treated with insulin.

Actions: Accelerates the breakdown of glycogen to glucose in the liver, causing an increase in blood glucose levels.

Pharmacokinetics:

Route	Onset	Peak	Duration
IV	1 min	15 min	9–20 min

$T_{1/2}$: 3 to 10 minutes; metabolized in the liver and excreted in the urine and bile.

Adverse Effects: Hypotension, hypertension, nausea, vomiting, respiratory distress with hypersensitivity reactions, and hypokalemia with overdose.

Nursing Considerations for Patients Taking Glucose-Elevating Agents

Assessment: History and Examination

- Assess for contraindications and cautions: History of allergy to thiazides if using diazoxide *to avoid hypersensitivity reactions*; severe renal or hepatic dysfunction, *which could alter metabolism and excretion of the drug*; CV disease, *which could be exacerbated by the effects of the drug*; and current status of pregnancy or lactation, *which could require caution.*
- Perform a complete physical assessment *to establish a baseline before beginning therapy, monitor effectiveness of therapy, and evaluate for any potential adverse effects during therapy.*
- Assess orientation and reflexes and baseline pulse, blood pressure, and adventitious sounds *to monitor the effects of altered glucose levels*, and abdominal sounds and function, *which could be altered by these drugs.*
- Monitor blood glucose levels as ordered *to assess the effectiveness of the drug and patient response to treatment.*
- Monitor the results of laboratory tests, including urinalysis, *to evaluate for glucosuria*, serum glucose levels *to evaluate response to therapy*, and renal and liver function tests *to determine the need for possible dose adjustment or identify possible toxic effects.*

Nursing Diagnoses

Nursing diagnoses related to drug therapy might include the following:

- Risk for unstable blood glucose related to ineffective dosing of the drug
- Imbalanced nutrition: More than body requirements related to metabolic effects, and less than body requirements related to GI upset
- Disturbed sensory perception (kinesthetic, visual, auditory, and tactile) related to glucose levels
- Deficient knowledge regarding drug therapy

Planning

- The patient will receive the best therapeutic effect from the drug therapy.
- The patient will have limited adverse effects to the drug therapy.
- The patient will have an understanding of the drug therapy, adverse effects to anticipate, and measures to relieve discomfort and improve safety

Implementation with Rationale

- Monitor blood glucose levels *to evaluate the effectiveness of the drug.*
- Have insulin on standby during emergency use *to treat severe hyperglycemia if it occurs as a result of overdose.*
- Monitor nutritional status *to provide nutritional consultation as needed.*
- Monitor patients receiving diazoxide for potential CV effects, including blood pressure, heart rhythm and output, and weight changes, *to avert serious adverse reactions.*
- Provide thorough patient teaching, including drug name, dosage, and schedule for administration; signs and symptoms of hyperglycemia; administration technique if indicated; signs and symptoms of adverse effects; need for follow-up monitoring and laboratory testing if indicated; nutritional measures; and blood glucose monitoring, *to improve patient knowledge and increase compliance to drug regimen.*

Evaluation

- Monitor patient response to the drug (stabilization of blood glucose levels).
- Monitor for adverse effects (hyperglycemia and GI distress).
- Evaluate the effectiveness of the teaching plan (patient can name drug, dosage, adverse effects to watch for, and specific measures to avoid them).
- Monitor the effectiveness of comfort measures and compliance to the regimen.

KEY POINTS

- Glucose-elevating agents are used to increase glucose when levels become dangerously low. Imbalance in glucose levels while taking insulin or oral agents is a common cause of hypoglycemia.
- Patients need to be carefully monitored to determine the effectiveness of therapy with these drugs and to prevent inadvertent overdose, which could lead to hyperglycemia.

SUMMARY

- Diabetes mellitus is the most common metabolic disorder. It is characterized by high blood glucose levels and alterations in the metabolism of fats, proteins, and glucose.
- Glucose control is a complicated process affected by various hormones, enzymes, and receptor sites.
- Diabetes mellitus is complicated by many end organ problems. These are related to thickening of basement membranes and the resultant decrease in blood flow to these areas.
- Treatment of diabetes involves control of blood glucose levels using diet and exercise, a combination of other agents to stimulate insulin release or alter glucose absorption, or the injection of replacement insulin.
- Replacement insulin was once obtained from beef and pork pancreas. Today, replacement insulin is human, derived from genetically altered bacteria.

- The amount and type of insulin given must be regulated daily. Patients taking insulin must learn to inject the drug, to properly dispose of needles and syringes, to test their blood glucose levels, and to recognize the signs of hypoglycemia and hyperglycemia.
- Insulin is used for type 1 diabetes and for type 2 diabetes in times of stress or when other therapies have failed.
- Other antidiabetic agents include first- and second-generation sulfonylureas, which stimulate the pancreas to release insulin, and other agents that alter glucose absorption, decrease insulin resistance, or decrease the formation of glucose. These agents are often used in combination to achieve effectiveness.
- Glucose-elevating agents are used to increase glucose when levels become dangerously low. Imbalance in glucose levels while taking insulin or oral agents is a common cause of hypoglycemia.

CHECK YOUR UNDERSTANDING

Answers to the questions in this chapter can be found in Answers to Check Your Understanding Questions on thePoint®.

MULTIPLE CHOICE

Select the best answer to the following.

1. Currently, the medical management of diabetes mellitus is aimed at
- **a.** controlling caloric intake.
- **b.** increasing exercise levels.
- **c.** regulating blood glucose levels.
- **d.** decreasing fluid loss.

2. The HbA1c blood test is a good measure of overall glucose control because
- **a.** it reflects the level of glucose after a meal.
- **b.** fasting for 8 hours before the test ensures accuracy.
- **c.** it reflects a 3-month average glucose level in the body.
- **d.** the test can be affected by the glucose challenge.

3. A patient with hyperglycemia will present with
- **a.** polyuria, polydipsia, and polyphagia.
- **b.** polycythemia, polyuria, and polyphagia.
- **c.** polyadenitis, polyuria, and polydipsia.
- **d.** polydipsia, polycythemia, and polyarteritis.

4. The long-term alterations in fat, carbohydrate, and protein metabolism associated with diabetes mellitus result in
- **a.** obesity.
- **b.** thickening of the capillary basement membrane.
- **c.** chronic obstructive pulmonary disease.
- **d.** lactose intolerance.

5. Insulin is available in several forms or suspensions, which differ in their
- **a.** effect on the pancreas.
- **b.** onset and duration of action.
- **c.** means of administration.
- **d.** tendency to cause adverse effects.

6. A patient on a fixed income would benefit from a second-generation sulfonylurea to control blood glucose levels. The drug of choice for this patient is
- **a.** glipizide.
- **b.** glyburide.
- **c.** tolbutamide.
- **d.** glimepiride.

7. Miglitol differs from the sulfonylureas in that it
- **a.** greatly stimulates pancreatic insulin release.
- **b.** greatly increases the sensitivity of insulin receptor sites.
- **c.** delays the absorption of glucose, leading to lower glucose levels.
- **d.** cannot be used in combination with other antidiabetic agents.

8. Teaching subjects for the patient with diabetes should include
- **a.** diet and exercise changes that are needed.
- **b.** the importance of avoiding exercise and eating one meal a day.
- **c.** protection from exposure to any infection and avoiding tiring activities.
- **d.** avoiding pregnancy and taking hygiene measures.

MULTIPLE RESPONSE

Select all that apply.

1. Treatment of diabetes may include which of the following?
   a. Replacement therapy with insulin
   b. Control of glucose absorption through the GI tract
   c. Drugs that stimulate insulin release or increase sensitivity of insulin receptor sites
   d. Surgical clearing of the capillary basement membranes
   e. Slowing of gastric emptying
   f. Diet and exercise programs

2. A client is recently diagnosed with diabetes. In reviewing his past history, which of the following would be early indicators of the problem?
   a. Lethargy
   b. Fruity-smelling breath
   c. Boundless energy
   d. Weight loss
   e. Increased sweating
   f. Getting up often at night to go to the bathroom

BIBLIOGRAPHY AND REFERENCES

American Diabetes Association (ADA). (2008). Tests of glycemia in diabetes. *Diabetes Care, 31*, S19–S93.

American Diabetes Association (ADA). (2015). Standards of medical care for patients with diabetes mellitus: 2015. *Diabetes Care, 38*(Suppl. 1), S1–S94.

Anabtawi, A., Hurst, M., Titi, M., et al. (2010). Incidence of hypoglycemia with tight glycemic control protocols: A comparative study. *Diabetes Technology and Therapeutics, 12*(8), 635–639.

Andrews, M., & Boyle, J. (2013). *Transcultural concepts in nursing care* (6th ed.). Philadelphia, PA: Lippincott Williams & Wilkins.

Brunton, L., Chabner, B., & Knollman, B. (2011). *Goodman and Gilman's the pharmacological basis of therapeutics* (12th ed.). New York: McGraw-Hill.

Burant, C. F. (Ed.). (2012). *Medical management of type 2 diabetes.* Alexandria, VA: American Diabetes Association.

Fact and Comparisons. (2015). *Drug facts and comparisons.* St. Louis, MO: Author.

Hall, J. (2015). *Guyton and Hall's textbook of medical physiology* (13th ed.). Philadelphia, PA: Saunders.

Holt, R., Clive, C., Flyvbjerg, A., et al. (Eds.). (2010). *Textbook of diabetes.* Chichester, UK: Wiley-Blackwell.

Karch, A. M. (2014). *Lippincott's nursing drug guide.* Philadelphia, PA: Lippincott Williams & Wilkins.

Moghissi, E. (2010). Reexamining the evidence for inpatient glucose control. *American Journal of Health Promotion, 67*(16), 53–58.

Trikudanathan, S. (2015). Polycystic ovarian syndrome. *Medical Clinics of North America, 99*(1), 221–235.

Wang, M. (2011). *Metabolic syndrome: Underlying mechanisms and drug therapy.* Hoboken, NJ: John Wiley & Sons.

Wilson, Y. (2013). Type 2 diabetes: An epidemic in children. *Nursing Children and Young People, 25*(2), 14–17.

PART 7

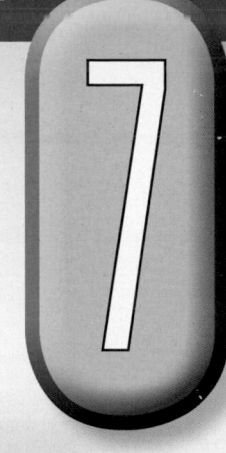

DRUGS ACTING ON THE REPRODUCTIVE SYSTEM

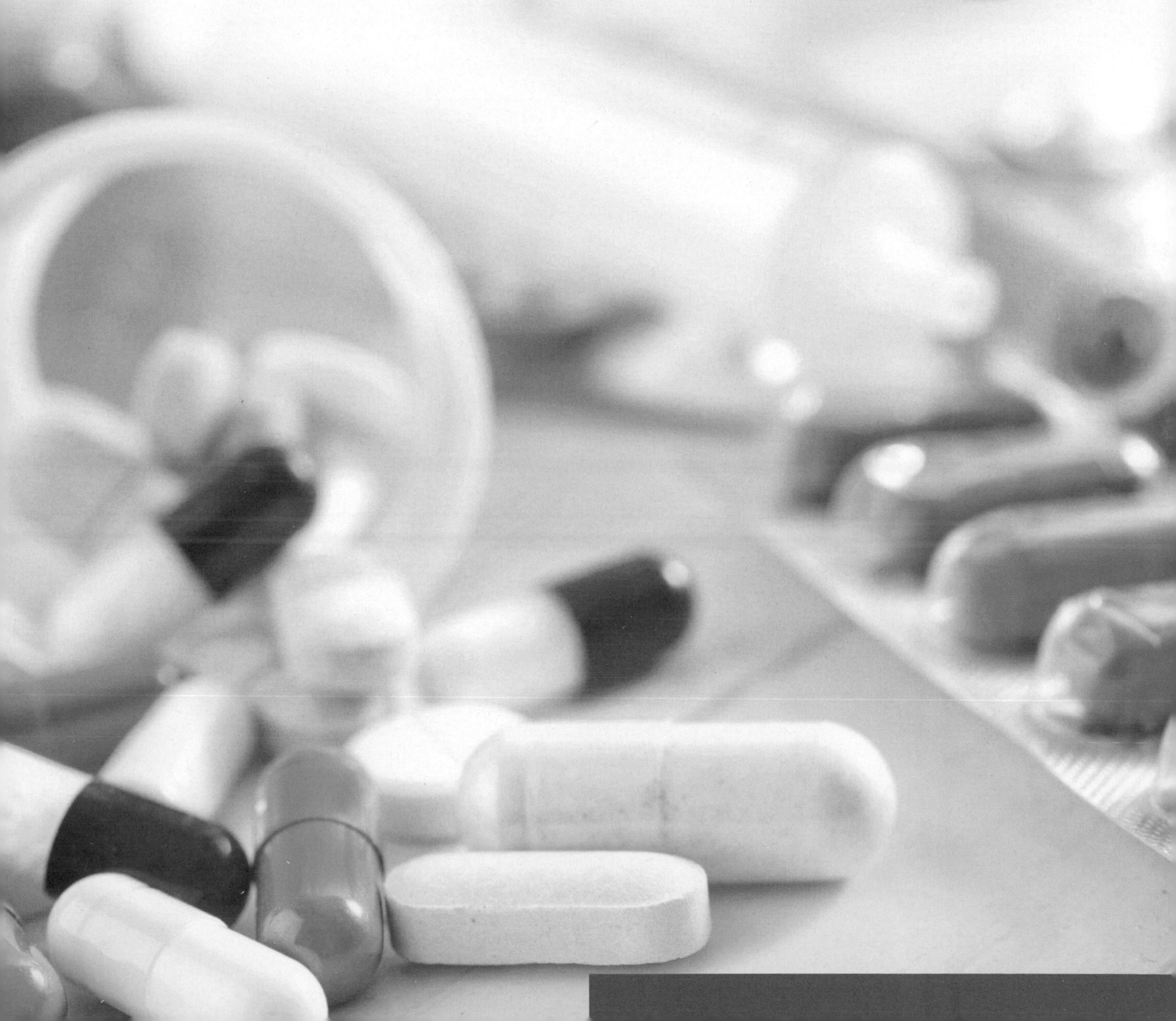

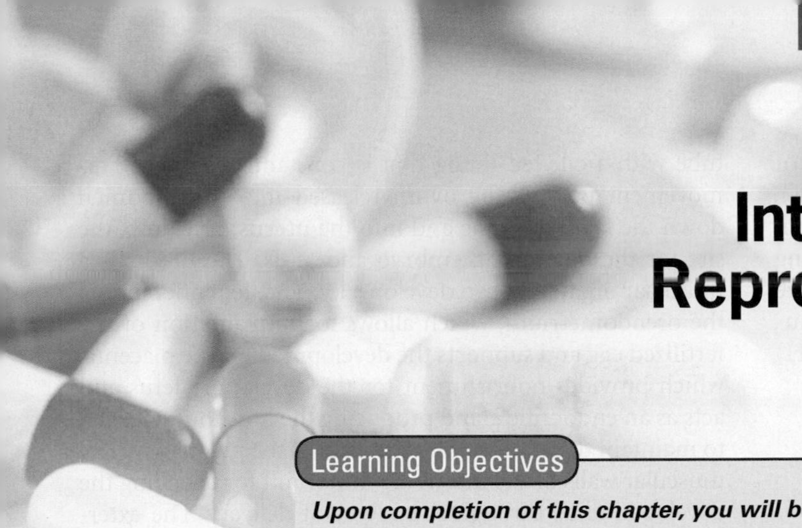

39 Introduction to the Reproductive System

Learning Objectives

Upon completion of this chapter, you will be able to:

1. Label a diagram depicting the structures of the female ovaries and male testes as part of the reproductive systems and explain the function of each structure.
2. Outline the control mechanisms involved with the male and female reproductive systems, using this outline to explain the negative feedback systems involved with each system.
3. List five effects for each of the sex hormones: Estrogen, progesterone, and testosterone.
4. Describe the changes that occur to the female body during pregnancy.
5. Describe the phases of the human sexual response and briefly describe the clinical presentation of each stage.

Glossary of Key Terms

andropause: decrease in gonadal function in males, associated with advancing age, analogous to female menopause

corpus luteum: remains of a follicle that releases mature ovum at ovulation; becomes an endocrine gland producing estrogen and progesterone

estrogen: hormone produced by the ovary, placenta, and adrenal gland; stimulates development of female characteristics and prepares the body for pregnancy

follicle: storage site of each ovum in the ovary; allows the ovum to grow and develop; produces estrogen and progesterone

inhibin: estrogen-like substance produced by seminiferous tubules during sperm production; acts as a negative feedback stimulus to decrease release of follicle-stimulating hormone (FSH)

interstitial or Leydig cells: part of the testes that produce testosterone in response to stimulation by luteinizing hormone (LH)

menarche: the onset of the menstrual cycle

menopause: depletion of the female ova; results in lack of estrogen and progesterone

menstrual cycle: cycling of female sex hormones in interaction with the hypothalamus and anterior pituitary feedback systems

menstruation: expulsion of the uterine lining occurring approximately every 28 to 32 days

ova: eggs, the female gamete, contain half of the information needed in a human nucleus

ovaries: female sexual glands that store ova and produce estrogen and progesterone

ovulation: release of the ovum from the follicle into the abdomen

progesterone: hormone produced by the ovary, placenta, and adrenal gland; promotes maintenance of pregnancy

puberty: point at which the hypothalamus starts releasing gonadotropin-releasing factor (GnRF) to stimulate the release of FSH and LH and begin sexual development

seminiferous tubules: part of the testes that produce sperm in response to stimulation by FSH

sperm: male gamete; contains half of the information needed for a human cell nucleus

testes: male sexual glands that produce sperm and testosterone

testosterone: male sex hormone; produced by the interstitial or Leydig cells of the testes

uterus: the womb; site of growth and development of the embryo and fetus

The reproductive systems in males and females are composed of the structures that support conception and development of a fetus and the endocrine glands that produce the hormones necessary for the regulation and maintenance of these structures and that facilitate reproduction. Though anatomically the two systems appear to be very different, they have many underlying similarities. The same fetal cells in males and females give rise to the glands that produce sexual hormones. In the female, those cells remain in the abdomen and develop into the **ovaries**, the female sexual glands. In the male the cells migrate out of the abdomen to form the **testes** (the male sexual glands), which are suspended from the body in the scrotum. Both male and female glands respond to follicle-stimulating hormone (FSH) and luteinizing hormone (LH), which are released from the anterior pituitary in response to stimulation from gonadotropin-releasing hormone (GnRH) released from the hypothalamus.

Female Reproductive System

The female reproductive system consists of two ovaries, two fallopian tubes, the uterus, and accessory structures, including the vagina, clitoris, labia, and breast tissue. The hormones that stimulate and maintain these structures are estrogen and progesterone. See Figure 39.1.

Structures

The ovaries are almond-shaped organs located on each side of the pelvic cavity. The ovaries store the **ova**, or eggs. Eggs contain half of the genetic material needed to produce a whole cell. At birth, a female's ovaries contain all of the ova that a woman will have; they develop in the fetus. No new ova will ever be produced by the ovaries. The ova are released into the abdomen throughout a woman's life or slowly degenerate over time. Each ovum is contained in a storage site called a **follicle**; the follicles act as endocrine glands producing the hormones **estrogen** and **progesterone**. The primary goal of these hormones is to prepare the body for pregnancy and to maintain the pregnancy until delivery. Very near to each ovary is a fallopian tube. The fallopian tube is a muscular tube with a ciliated lining that is constantly moving. This movement propels the ovum released into the abdomen down the fallopian tube and into the **uterus**, or womb, the site for the developing embryo and fetus. The uterus is a muscular organ that can develop a blood-filled inner lining, the orendometrium, which allows for implantation of the fertilized egg and supports the development of the placenta, which provides nourishment for the developing fetus and acts as an endocrine gland producing the hormones needed to maintain the active metabolic state of the pregnancy. The muscular walls of the uterus are important for expelling the developed fetus through the vagina at delivery. The external genitalia—the clitoris, labia, and vagina—are sites of erogenous stimulation and the entry way for sperm to reach the uterus to allow conception and the exit path for the developed fetus at birth. Development of the breast tissue, also considered a secondary sex characteristic, is controlled by the female sex hormones and is necessary for producing milk for the nourishment of the baby when it has been expelled from the uterus and is no longer able to be dependent on the mother's blood supply for nourishment.

Hormones

The hormones produced in the ovaries are estrogen and progesterone. These two hormones influence many other body systems while preparing the body for pregnancy or maintenance of pregnancy.

Estrogen

The estrogens produced by the ovaries include estradiol, estrone, and estriol. The estrogens enter cells and bind to receptors within the cytoplasm to promote messenger

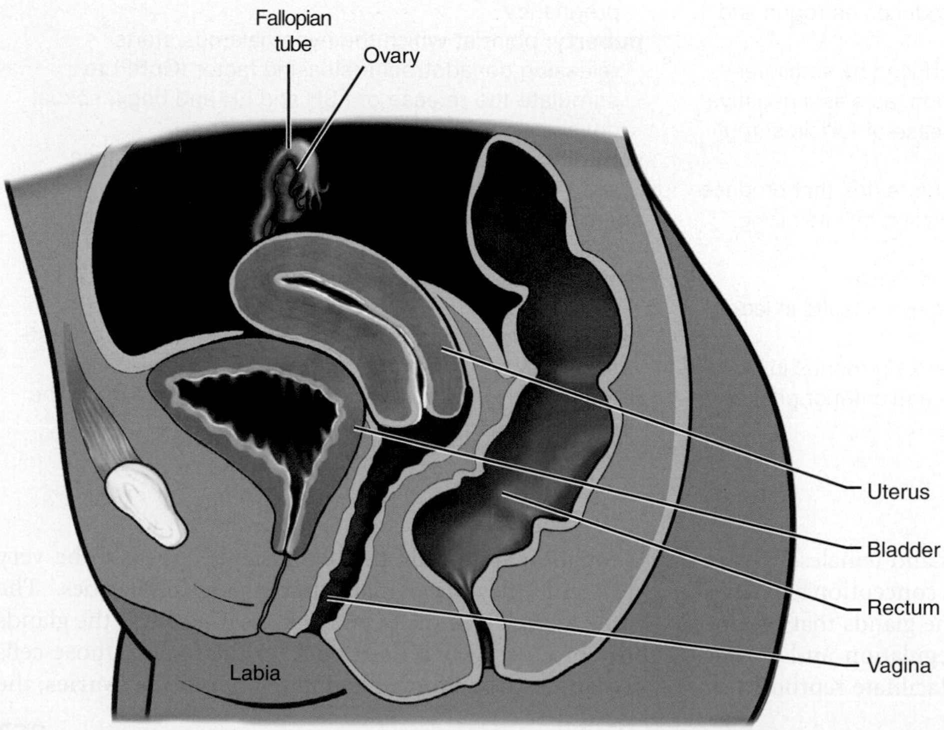

FIGURE 39.1 The female reproductive system.

BOX 39.1

Effects of Estrogen

Growth of genitalia (in preparation for childbirth)
Growth of breast tissue (in preparation for pregnancy and lactation)
Characteristic female pubic hair distribution (a triangle)
Stimulation of protein building (important for the developing fetus)
Increased total blood cholesterol (for energy for the mother as well as the developing fetus) with an increase in high-density lipoprotein levels ("good" cholesterol, which serves to protect the female blood vessels against atherosclerosis)
Retention of sodium and water (to provide cooling for the heat generated by the developing fetus and to increase diffusion of sodium and water to the fetus through the placenta)
Inhibition of calcium resorption from the bones (helps to deposit calcium in the fetal bone structure; when this property is lost at menopause, osteoporosis, or loss of calcium from the bone, is common)
Alteration of pelvic bone structure to a wider and flaring pelvis (to promote easier delivery)
Closure of the epiphyses (to conserve energy for the fetus by halting growth of the mother)
Increased thyroid hormone globulin (metabolism needs to be increased greatly during pregnancy, and the increase in thyroid hormone facilitates this)
Increased elastic tissue of the skin (to allow for the tremendous stretch of the abdominal skin during pregnancy)
Increased vascularity of the skin (to allow for radiation loss of heat generated by the developing fetus)
Increased uterine motility (estrogen is high when the ovum first leaves the ovary, and increased uterine motility helps to move the ovum toward the uterus and to propel the sperm toward the ovum)
Thin, clear cervical mucus (allows easy penetration of the sperm into the uterus as ovulation occurs; used in fertility programs as an indication that ovulation will soon occur)
Proliferative endometrium (to prepare the lining of the uterus for implantation with the fertilized egg)
Anti-insulin effect with increased glucose levels (to allow increased diffusion of glucose to the developing fetus)
T-cell inhibition (to protect the nonself cells of the embryo from the immune surveillance of the mother)

ribonucleic acid (mRNA) activity, which results in specific proteins for cell activity or structure. Many of these effects are first noticed at menarche (the onset of the menstrual cycle), when the hormones begin cycling for the first time. Female characteristics are associated with the effects of estrogen on many of the body's systems—wider hips, soft skin, breast growth, and so on. Box 39.1 summarizes the effects of estrogen on the body.

Progesterone

Progesterone is released into circulation after ovulation. Progesterone has many effects that support the early development of the fetus. Progesterone's effects on body

BOX 39.2

Effects of Progesterone

Decreased uterine motility (to provide increased chance that implantation can occur)
Development of a secretory endometrium (to provide glucose and a rich blood supply for the developing placenta and embryo)
Thickened cervical mucus (to protect the developing embryo and keep out bacteria and other pathogens; this is lost at the beginning of labor as the mucous plug)
Breast growth (to prepare for lactation)
Increased body temperature (a direct hypothalamic response to progesterone, which stimulates metabolism and promotes activities for the developing embryo; this increase in temperature is monitored in the "rhythm method" of birth control to indicate that ovulation has occurred)
Increased appetite (this is a direct effect on the satiety centers of the hypothalamus and results in increased nutrients for the developing embryo)
Depressed T-cell function (again, this protects the nonself cells of the developing embryo from the immune system)
Anti-insulin effect (to generate a higher blood glucose concentration to allow rapid diffusion of glucose to the developing embryo)

temperature are monitored in the "rhythm method" of birth control to indicate that ovulation has just occurred. Box 39.2 summarizes the effects of progesterone on the body.

Control Mechanisms

The developing hypothalamus is sensitive to the androgens released by the adrenal glands and does not release GnRH during childhood. As the hypothalamus matures, it loses its sensitivity to the androgens and starts to release GnRH. This occurs at **puberty**, the beginning of sexual development. The onset of puberty leads to a number of hormonal changes. See Figure 39.2.

GnRH stimulates the anterior pituitary to release FSH and LH. FSH and LH stimulate the follicles on the outer surface of the ovaries to grow and develop. These follicles, called Graafian follicles, produce progesterone, which is retained in the follicle, and estrogen, which is released into circulation. When the circulating estrogen level rises high enough, it stimulates a massive release of LH from the anterior pituitary. This is called the "LH surge." This burst of LH causes one of the developing follicles to burst and release the ovum with its stored hormones into the system. LH also causes the rest of the developing follicles to shrink in on themselves, or involute, and eventually disappear. The release of an ovum from the follicle is called **ovulation.**

The ovum is released into the abdomen near the end of one of the fallopian tubes, and the constant movement of cilia within the tube helps to propel the ovum

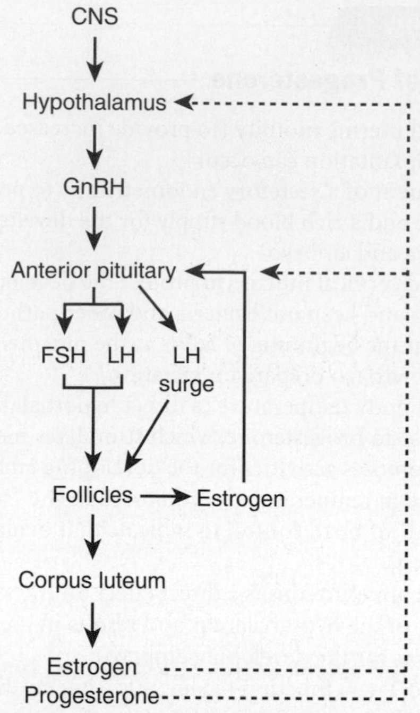

FIGURE 39.2 Interaction of the hypothalamic, pituitary, and ovarian hormones that underlie the menstrual cycle. *Dotted lines* indicate negative feedback surge. CNS, central nervous system; FSH, follicle-stimulating hormone; GnRH, gonadotropin-releasing hormone; LH, luteinizing hormone.

into the fallopian tube and then into the uterus. The ruptured follicle becomes a functioning endocrine gland called the **corpus luteum**. It will continue to produce estrogen and progesterone for 10 to 14 days unless pregnancy occurs

Fertilization of the ovum and implantation in the uterine wall result in the production of human chorionic gonadotropin. This hormone stimulates the corpus luteum to continue to produce estrogen and progesterone until the placenta develops and becomes functional, producing these hormones at a level high enough to sustain the pregnancy.

If pregnancy does not occur the corpus luteum involutes and becomes a white scar on the ovary. This scar is called the corpus albicans. Initially, the rising levels of estrogen and progesterone produced by the corpus luteum act as a negative feedback system to the hypothalamus and the pituitary, stopping the production and secretion of GnRH, FSH, and LH. Later in the cycle, the corpus luteum atrophies, the falling levels of estrogen and progesterone stimulate the hypothalamus to once again release GnRH, and the cycle begins again.

Factors Influencing Control Mechanisms

Because of its position in the brain, the hypothalamus is influenced by many internal and external factors. For example, high levels of stress can interrupt the reproductive cycle. Tremendous amounts of energy are expended in reproduction, and if the body needs energy for fight or flight the hypothalamus shuts down the reproductive activities, stopping the release of GnRH, which results in no FSH or LH release and no stimulation of the follicles. This saves a tremendous amount of energy in the body, energy that the body will use for fight or flight. In addition to stress, starvation, extreme exercise, and emotional problems are all associated with a decrease in reproductive capacity related to the controls of the hypothalamus.

Of interest, light has been found to have an influence on the functioning of the hypothalamus. Increased light levels boost the release of FSH and LH and increase the release of estrogen and progesterone. This is thought to contribute to the early sexual maturation of girls who live near the equator. Longer and earlier exposure to light leads to earlier GnRH release by the hypothalamus and earlier sexual development. Girls living in areas with prolonged periods of darkness (above the Arctic Circle, for example) go through puberty and sexual development at a much later age.

The Menstrual Cycle

The cyclical nature of the female sex hormones on the body produces the **menstrual cycle**. The onset of the menstrual cycle at puberty is called the **menarche**. Each cycle starts with release of FSH and LH and stimulation of the ovarian follicles. For about the next 14 days the developing follicles release estrogen into the body. Thus, the woman may notice the many effects of estrogen, such as breast tenderness and water retention. In addition, estrogen thins cervical mucosa and increases susceptibility to infections.

By about day 14, the estrogen levels have caused the LH surge, and ovulation occurs. The woman experiences increased body temperature, increased appetite, breast tenderness, bloating and abdominal fullness, constipation, among others—the effects associated with progesterone, which is released into the system when the follicle ruptures. The uterus becomes thicker and more vascular as the cycle progresses and develops a proliferative endometrium. After ovulation the lining of the uterus begins to produce glucose and other nutrients that would nurture a growing embryo; this is called a secretory endometrium. If pregnancy does not occur, after about 14 days, the corpus luteum involutes, and the levels of estrogen and progesterone drop off (Figure 39.3).

The dropping levels of estrogen and progesterone trigger the release of GnRH and then FSH and LH again, along with the start of another menstrual cycle. Lowered hormone levels also cause the inner lining of the uterus to slough off because it is no longer stimulated by the hormones. High levels of plasminogen in the uterus prevent clotting of the lining as the vessels shear off. Prostaglandins in the uterus stimulate uterine contraction to clamp off vessels as the lining sheds away. This causes menstrual cramps. This loss of the uterine lining, called **menstruation**, repeats

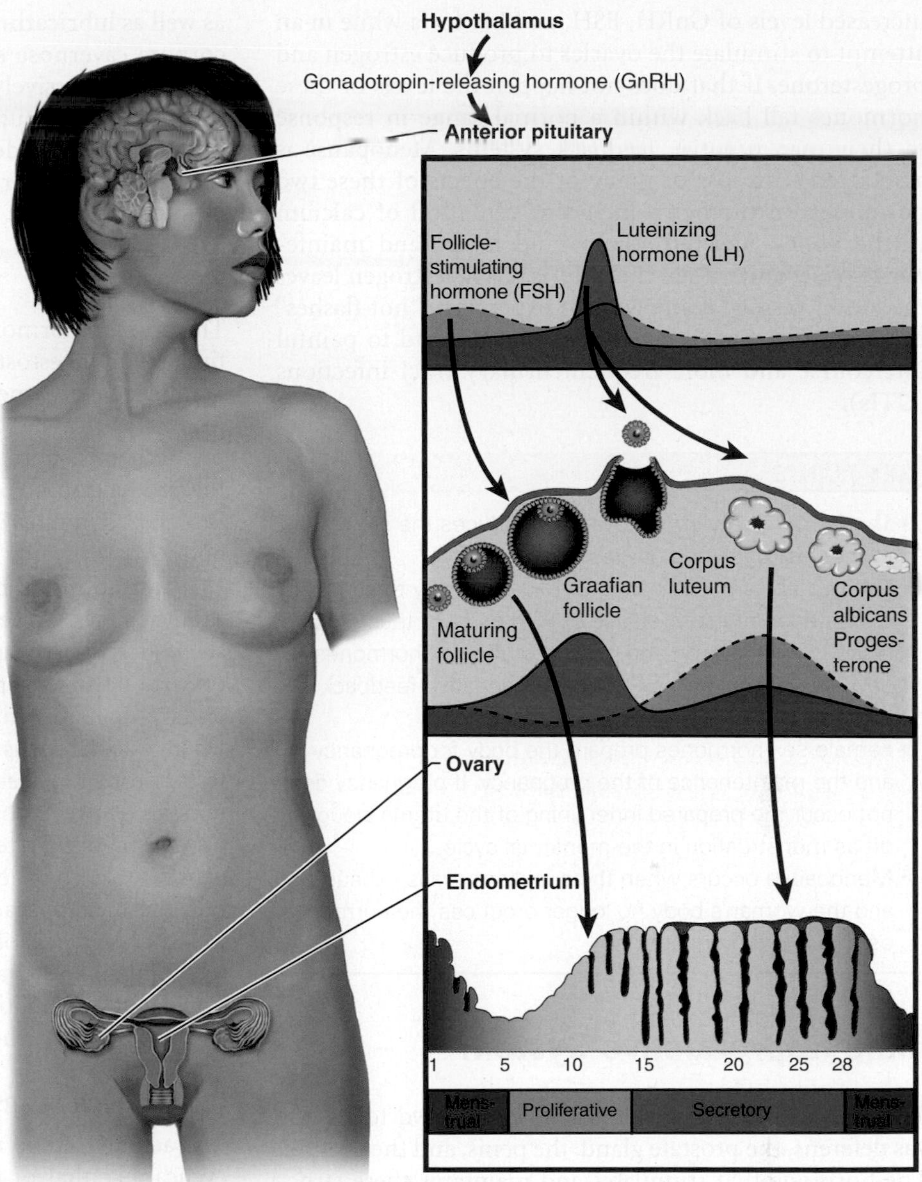

FIGURE 39.3 Relation of pituitary and ovarian hormone levels to the menstrual cycle and to ovarian and endometrial function.

approximately every 28 to 32 days. Figure 39.3 depicts the various phases of the menstrual cycle.

Pregnancy

When the ovum is fertilized by a sperm a new cell is produced that rapidly divides to produce the embryo. The embryo implants in the wall of the uterus, and the interface between the fetal cells and the uterus produces the placenta, a large, vascular organ that serves as a massive endocrine gland and a transfer point for nutrients from the mother to the fetus. The placenta maintains high levels of estrogens and progesterone to support the uterus and the developing fetus. When the placenta ages the levels of progesterone and estrogen fall off.

Eventually, the tendency to block uterine activity (an effect of progesterone) is overcome by the stimulation to increase uterine activity caused by oxytocin (a hypothalamic hormone stored in the posterior pituitary). At this point, local prostaglandins stimulate uterine contraction and the onset of labor. Once the fetus and the placenta have been expelled from the uterus, the hormone levels plummet toward the nonpregnant state. It often takes 6 to 8 weeks to reverse the effects of these hormones because they cause their effects by actually entering the cell, not by reacting with a receptor site on the cell membrane. This postpartum period is a time of tremendous adjustment for the body as it tries to reachieve homeostasis.

Menopause

The follicles contained in the ovary become depleted over time, the ovaries no longer produce estrogen and progesterone, and **menopause**—the cessation of menses—occurs. The hypothalamus and pituitary produce increased levels of GnRH, FSH, and LH for a while in an attempt to stimulate the ovaries to produce estrogen and progesterone. If that does not happen the levels of these hormones fall back within a normal range in response to their own negative feedback systems. Menopause is associated with loss of many of the effects of these two hormones on the body, including retention of calcium in the bones, lowered serum lipid levels, and maintenance of secondary sex characteristics. As estrogen leaves the blood vessels, many women experience "hot flashes" or vasospasm. Drying vaginal tissue can lead to painful intercourse and more frequent urinary tract infections (UTIs).

KEY POINTS

- The female ovary stores ova and produces the sex hormones estrogen and progesterone.
- The hypothalamus releases GnRH at puberty to stimulate the anterior pituitary release of FSH and LH, thus stimulating the production and release of the sex hormones. Levels are controlled by a series of negative feedback systems.
- Female sex hormones prepare the body for pregnancy and the maintenance of the pregnancy. If pregnancy does not occur the prepared inner lining of the uterus sloughs off as menstruation in the menstrual cycle.
- Menopause occurs when the supply of ova is exhausted and the woman's body no longer produces the hormones estrogen and progesterone.

Male Reproductive System

The male reproductive system consists of two testes, the vas deferens, the prostate gland, the penis, and the urethra. The hormone that stimulates and maintains these structures is testosterone.

Structures

The male reproductive system originates from the same fetal cells as in the female. The major male reproductive system structure is the testes, the two endocrine glands that continually produce **sperm**, as well as the hormone **testosterone**. During fetal development the two testes migrate down the abdomen and descend into the scrotum outside the body. There they are protected from the heat of the body to prevent injury to the sperm-producing cells. The testes are made up of two distinct parts: The **seminiferous tubules**, which produce the sperm, and the **interstitial or Leydig cells**, which produce the hormone testosterone. Other components include the vas deferens, which stores produced sperm and carries sperm from the testes to be ejaculated from the body; the prostate gland, which produces enzymes to stimulate sperm maturation, as well as lubricating fluid; the penis, which includes two corpora cavernosa and a corpus spongiosum, structures that allow massively increased blood flow and erection; the urethra, through which urine and the sperm and seminal fluid are delivered; and other glands and ducts that promote sperm and seminal fluid development (Figure 39.4).

Hormones

The primary hormone associated with the male reproductive system is testosterone. Testosterone is responsible for many sexual and metabolic effects in the male. Like estrogen, testosterone enters the cell and reacts with a cytoplasmic receptor site to influence mRNA activity, resulting in the production of proteins for cell structure or function. Box 39.3 summarizes the effects of testosterone on the body.

Castration, or removal of the testes, before puberty results in lack of development of the normal male characteristics, as well as sterility. If the testes are lost before puberty occurs, there will be no development of the secondary male sex characteristics or the other effects seen when testosterone is released. Such a person would require testosterone replacement therapy to develop these characteristics. However, once puberty and the physical changes brought about by testosterone have occurred the androgens released by the adrenal glands are sufficient to sustain the male characteristics. Androgens are very similar in structure to testosterone and are able to influence cells to maintain the changes caused by testosterone. This is important information for adult patients undergoing testicular surgery or chemical castration.

Control Mechanisms

The activity of the male sex glands is not thought to be cyclical like that of the female. The hypothalamus in the male child is also sensitive to circulating levels of adrenal androgens and suppresses GnRH release. After the hypothalamus matures, this sensitivity is lost and the hypothalamus releases GnRH. This in turn stimulates the anterior pituitary to release FSH and LH, or what is sometimes called interstitial cell–stimulating hormone (ICSH) in males. FSH directly stimulates the seminiferous tubules to produce sperm, a process called spermatogenesis. FSH also stimulates the Sertoli cells in the seminiferous tubules to produce estrogens, which provide negative feedback to the pituitary and hypothalamus to cause a decrease in the release of GnRH, FSH, and LH.

The Sertoli cells also produce a substance called **inhibin**, an estrogen-like molecule. Upon the sensing of inhibin by the hypothalamus and anterior pituitary a negative feedback response occurs, decreasing the circulating level of FSH. When the FSH level falls low enough the hypothalamus is stimulated to again release GnRH to stimulate FSH release. This feedback system prevents

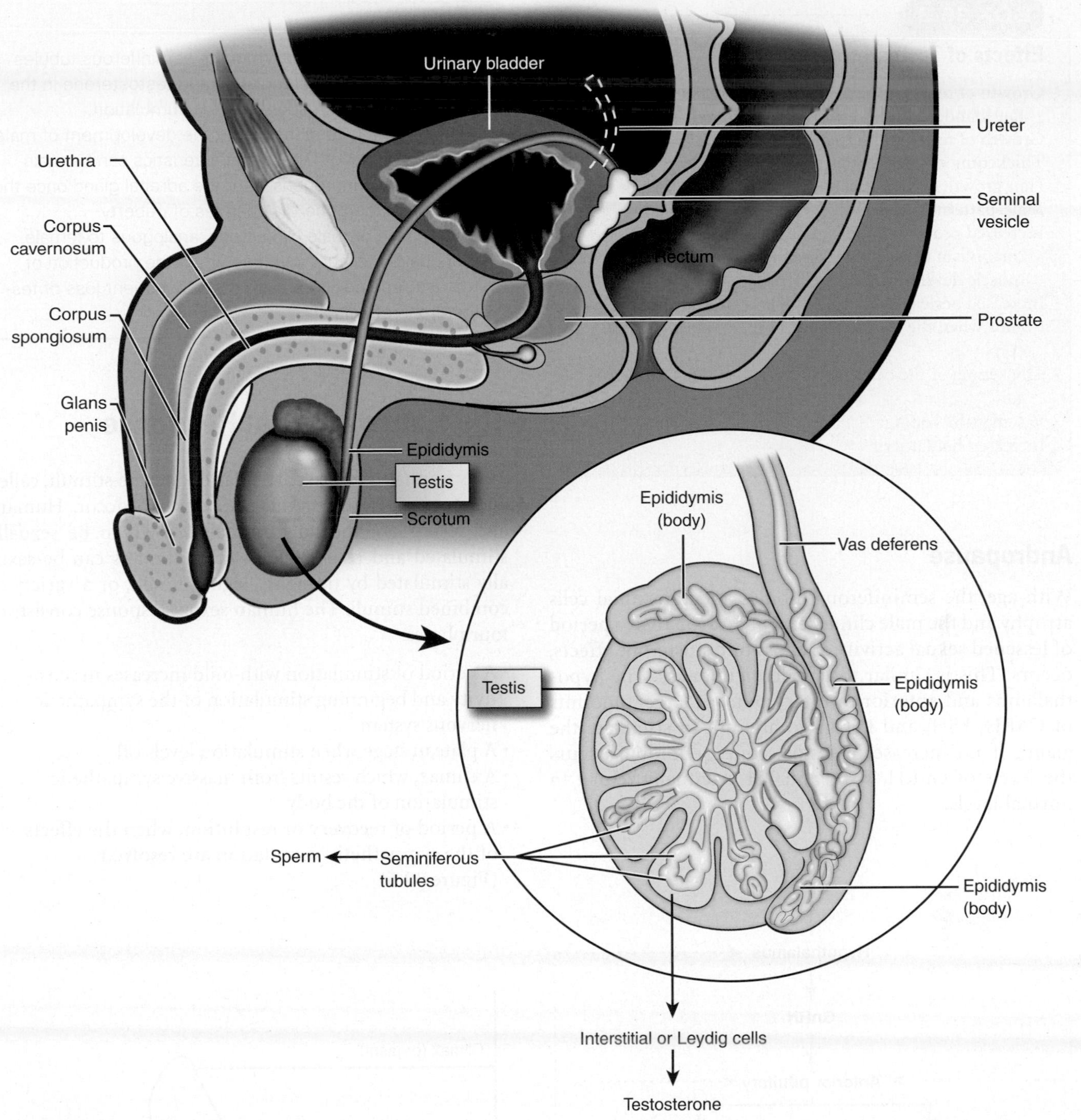

FIGURE 39.4 The male reproductive system.

overproduction of sperm in the testes (Figure 39.5). Inhibin has been investigated for many years as a possible male birth control drug because it is thought to affect only sperm production.

The LH or ICSH stimulates the interstitial (Leydig) cells to produce testosterone. The concentration of testosterone acts in a similar negative feedback system with the hypothalamus. When the concentration is high enough the hypothalamus decreases GnRH release, leading to a subsequent decrease in FSH and LH release. The levels of testosterone are thought to remain within a fairly well-defined range of normal. It has been documented, however, that light affects the male sexual hormones in a similar fashion to its effect on female hormones. "Spring fever," with increased exposure time to sunlight, does increase testosterone levels in men. Other factors that may also have an influence on male hormone levels are likely to be identified in the future.

BOX 39.3

Effects of Testosterone

Growth of male and sexual accessory organs (penis, prostate gland, seminal vesicles, vas deferens)
Growth of testes and scrotal sac
Thickening of vocal cords, producing the deep, male voice
Hair growth on the face, body, arms, legs, and trunk
Male-pattern baldness
Increased protein anabolism and decreased protein catabolism (this causes larger and more powerful muscle development)
Increased bone growth in length and width, which ends when the testosterone stimulates closure of the epiphyses
Thickening of the cartilage and skin, leading to the male gait
Vascular thickening
Increased hematocrit

Andropause

With age, the seminiferous tubules and interstitial cells atrophy and the male climacteric or **andropause**, a period of lessened sexual activity and loss of testosterone effects, occurs. This is similar to female menopause. The hypothalamus and anterior pituitary put out larger amounts of GnRH, FSH, and LH in an attempt to stimulate the gland. If no increase in testosterone or inhibin occurs the levels of GnRH, FSH, and LH eventually return to normal levels.

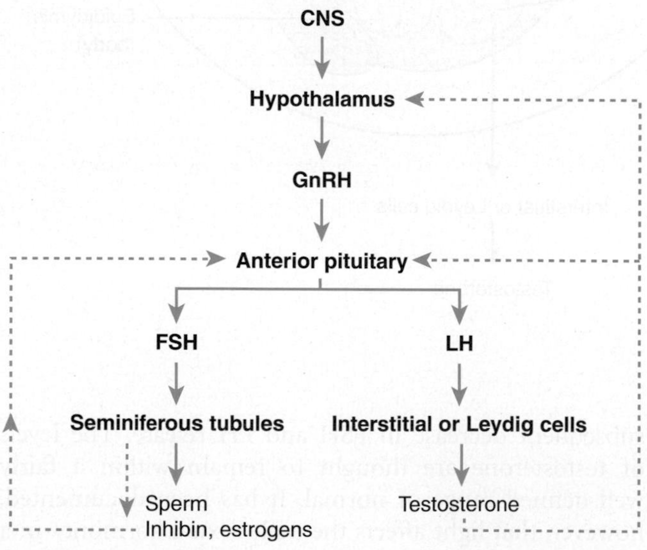

FIGURE 39.5 Interaction of the hypothalamic, pituitary, and testicular hormones that underlie the male sexual hormone system. CNS, central nervous system; FSH, follicle-stimulating hormone; GnRH, gonadotropin-releasing hormone; LH, luteinizing hormone.

KEY POINTS

- The testes produce sperm in the seminiferous tubules in response to FSH stimulation and testosterone in the interstitial cells in response to LH stimulation.
- Testosterone is responsible for the development of male sex characteristics. These characteristics can be maintained by the androgens from the adrenal gland once the body has undergone the changes of puberty.
- Andropause or male climacteric, analogous to female menopause, occurs with age when the production of testosterone declines, with the subsequent loss of testosterone effects.

The Human Sexual Response

Many animals require particular endocrine stimuli, called an estrous cycle, for sexual response to occur. Humans and ferrets are the only animals known to be sexually stimulated and responsive at will. Humans can be sexually stimulated by thoughts, sights, touch, or a variety of combined stimuli. The human sexual response consists of four phases:

- A period of stimulation with mild increases in sensitivity and beginning stimulation of the sympathetic nervous system
- A plateau stage when stimulation levels off
- A climax, which results from massive sympathetic stimulation of the body
- A period of recovery or resolution, when the effects of the sympathetic stimulation are resolved (Figure 39.6)

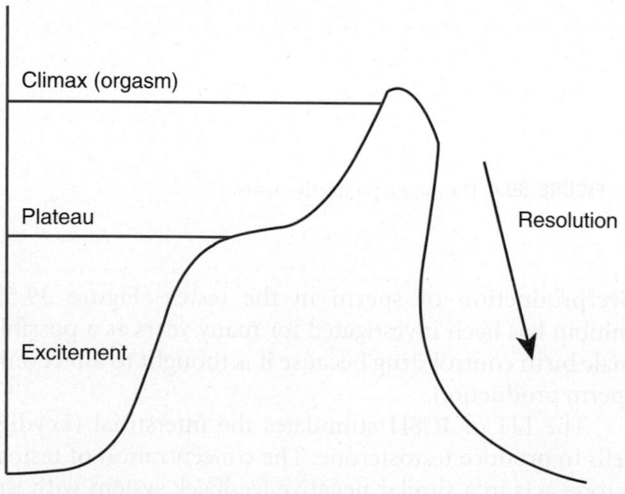

FIGURE 39.6 Human sexual response.

Previously, it was believed that male and female responses were very different. However, it is now thought that the physiology of the responses is quite similar. Sexual stimulation and activity are a normal response and, in healthy individuals, are probably necessary for complete health of the body's systems. The sympathetic stimulation causes increased heart rate, increased blood pressure, sweating, pupil dilation, glycogenolysis (breakdown of stored glycogen to glucose for energy), and other sympathetic responses. This stimulation could be dangerous in some cardiovascular conditions that could be exacerbated by the sympathetic effects. In the male the increased blood flow to the penis causes erection, which is necessary for penetration of the female and deposition of the sperm. Any drug therapy or disease process that interferes with the sympathetic response or the innervation of the sexual organs will change the person's ability to experience the human sexual response. This is important to keep in mind when doing patient teaching and when evaluating the effects of a drug. Beta-blockers, which block the sympathetic nervous system, often cause loss of sexual function. This is important to keep in mind when teaching patients about what effects to expect.

KEY POINTS

- The human sexual response involves activation of the sympathetic nervous system to allow a four-phase response: Stimulation, plateau, climax, and resolution.
- Sexual stimulation and activity are a normal response and, in healthy individuals, are probably necessary for complete health of the body's systems.
- Since activation of the sympathetic response is an integral part of the human sexual response, any disease process or drug therapy that interferes with the sympathetic response will alter the patient's ability to experience a sexual response.

SUMMARY

- Male and female reproductive systems arise from the same fetal cells. The female ovaries store ova and produce the sex hormones estrogen and progesterone; the male testes produce sperm and the sex hormone testosterone.
- The hypothalamus releases GnRH at puberty to stimulate the anterior pituitary release of FSH and LH, thus stimulating the production and release of the sex hormones. Levels are controlled by a series of negative feedback systems.
- Female sex hormones are released in a cyclical fashion. Release of an ovum for possible fertilization is termed ovulation. The female hormones prepare the body for pregnancy, including maintenance of the pregnancy if fertilization occurs.
- If pregnancy does not occur the prepared inner lining of the uterus is sloughed off as menstruation in the menstrual cycle, so that the lining can be prepared again when ovulation reoccurs.
- Menopause in women and the male climacteric in men occur when the body no longer produces sex hormones; the hypothalamus and anterior pituitary respond by releasing increasing levels of GnRH, FSH, and LH in an attempt to achieve higher levels of sex hormones.
- The testes produce sperm in the seminiferous tubules in response to FSH stimulation and testosterone in the interstitial cells in response to LH stimulation.
- Testosterone is responsible for the development of male sex characteristics. These characteristics can be maintained by the androgens from the adrenal gland once the body has undergone the changes of puberty.
- The human sexual response involves activation of the sympathetic nervous system to allow a four-phase response: Stimulation, plateau, climax, and resolution.

CHECK YOUR UNDERSTANDING

Answers to the questions in this chapter can be found in Answers to Check Your Understanding Questions on thePoint®.

MULTIPLE CHOICE

Select the best answer to the following.

1. In a nonpregnant woman the levels of the sex hormones fluctuate in a cyclical fashion until
  a. all of the ova are depleted.
  b. the FSH and LH are depleted.
  c. the hypothalamus no longer senses FSH and LH.
  d. the hypothalamus becomes more sensitive to androgens.

2. A woman develops ova, or eggs,
  a. continually until menopause.
  b. during fetal life.
  c. until menopause.
  d. starting with puberty.

(continues on page 666)

3. Control of the female sex hormones starts with the release of GnRH from the hypothalamus. Because of this, the cycling of these hormones may be influenced by
   a. body temperature.
   b. stress or emotional problems.
   c. age.
   d. androgen release.

4. The rhythm method of birth control depends on the effects of progesterone
   a. to increase uterine motility.
   b. to decrease and thicken cervical secretions.
   c. to elevate body temperature.
   d. to depress appetite.

5. The menstrual cycle
   a. always repeats itself every 28 days.
   b. is associated with changing hormone levels.
   c. is necessary for a human sexual response.
   d. cannot occur if ovulation does not occur.

6. In the male reproductive system,
   a. the seminiferous tubules produce sperm and testosterone.
   b. the interstitial cells produce sperm.
   c. the seminiferous tubules produce sperm and the interstitial cells produce testosterone.
   d. the interstitial cells produce sperm and testosterone.

7. Spring fever occurs as a result of increased light. In males, this increase in light causes an increase in the production of
   a. inhibin.
   b. adrenal androgens.
   c. estrogen.
   d. testosterone.

8. The human sexual response depends on stimulation of
   a. the sympathetic nervous system.
   b. the parasympathetic nervous system.
   c. the hypothalamic sex drive center.
   d. adrenal androgens.

MULTIPLE RESPONSE

Select all that apply.

1. After teaching a group of students about the effects of the various sex hormones the instructor determines that the teaching was successful when the group identifies which of the following as related to estrogen?
   a. Increased levels of high-density lipoproteins
   b. Increased calcium density in the bone
   c. Closing of the epiphyses
   d. Development of a thick cervical plug
   e. Increased body temperature
   f. Triangle-shaped body hair distribution

2. A group of students are reviewing material in preparation for an examination on the sex hormones. Which of the following, if identified by the students as effects of testosterone, demonstrates understanding of the information?
   a. Thickening of skin and vocal cords
   b. Development of a wide and flat pelvis
   c. Development of facial hair
   d. Closure of the epiphyses
   e. Increased hematocrit
   f. Increased aggression

BIBLIOGRAPHY AND REFERENCES

Basson, R. (2007). Women's sexual function and dysfunction. *Journal of the American Medical Association, 297*, 895–897.

Camacho, P. M., Gharib, H., & Sizemore, G. W. (Eds.). (2012). *Evidence-based endocrinology* (3rd ed.). Philadelphia, PA: Lippincott Williams & Wilkins.

Girard, J. (1992). *Endocrinology of puberty*. Farmington, CT: Karger Classic.

Greenspan, F. S., & Gardner, D. G. (Eds.). (2011). *Basic and clinical endocrinology* (9th ed.). New York: Lange Medical Books.

Hall, J. (2015). *Guyton and Hall's textbook of medical physiology* (13th ed.). Philadelphia, PA: Saunders.

Jones, R. (2013). *Human reproductive biology* (4th ed.). St. Louis, MO: Academic Press.

Karch, A. M. (2014). *Lippincott's nursing drug guide*. Philadelphia, PA: Lippincott Williams & Wilkins.

Kronenberg, H. M., Melmed, S., Polonsky, K. S., et al. (Eds.). (2011). *Williams textbook of endocrinology* (12th ed.). Philadelphia, PA: W. B. Saunders.

40 Drugs Affecting the Female Reproductive System

Learning Objectives

Upon completion of this chapter, you will be able to:

1. Integrate knowledge of the effects of sex hormones on the female body to explain the therapeutic and adverse effects of these agents when used clinically.
2. Describe the therapeutic actions, indications, pharmacokinetics, contraindications, most common adverse reactions, and important drug–drug interactions associated with drugs that affect the female reproductive system.
3. Discuss the use of drugs that affect the female reproductive system across the lifespan.
4. Compare and contrast the prototype drugs estradiol, raloxifene, norethindrone, clomiphene, oxytocin, and dinoprostone with other agents in their class.
5. Outline the nursing considerations, including important teaching points to stress, for patients receiving drugs that affect the female reproductive system.

Glossary of Key Terms

abortifacients: drugs used to stimulate uterine contractions and promote evacuation of the uterus to cause abortion or to empty the uterus after fetal death

fertility drugs: drugs used to stimulate ovulation and pregnancy in women with functioning ovaries who are having trouble conceiving

oxytocics: drugs that act like the hypothalamic hormone oxytocin; they stimulate uterine contraction and contraction of the lacteal glands in the breast, promoting milk ejection

progestins: the endogenous female hormone progesterone and its various derivatives, important in maintaining a pregnancy and supporting many secondary sex characteristics

Drug List

Sex Hormones and Estrogen Receptor Modulators

Sex Hormones

Estrogens

- (P) estradiol
- estrogens, conjugated
- estrogens, esterified
- estropipate

Progestins

- desogestrel
- drospirenone
- etonogestrel
- levonorgestrel
- medroxyprogesterone
- (P) norethindrone acetate
- norgestrel
- progesterone
- ulipristal

Estrogen Receptor Modulators

- (P) raloxifene
- toremifene

Fertility Drugs

- cetrorelix
- chorionic gonadotropin
- chorionic gonadotropin alpha
- (P) clomiphene
- follitropin alfa
- follitropin beta
- ganirelix
- menotropins
- urofollitropin

Uterine Motility Drugs

Oxytocics

- methylergonovine
- (P) oxytocin

Abortifacients

- carboprost
- (P) dinoprostone
- mifepristone

The female reproductive system functions in a cyclical fashion, not in the steady-state fashion seen with much of the rest of the endocrine system. Altering any component of this cycle or the system can have a wide variety of effects on the entire body. Drugs that affect the female reproductive system typically include hormones and hormonal-like agents. Figure 40.1 reviews the female reproductive system and sites of action of the drugs used to affect the system. Box 40.1 highlights considerations related to the use of drugs discussed in this chapter as

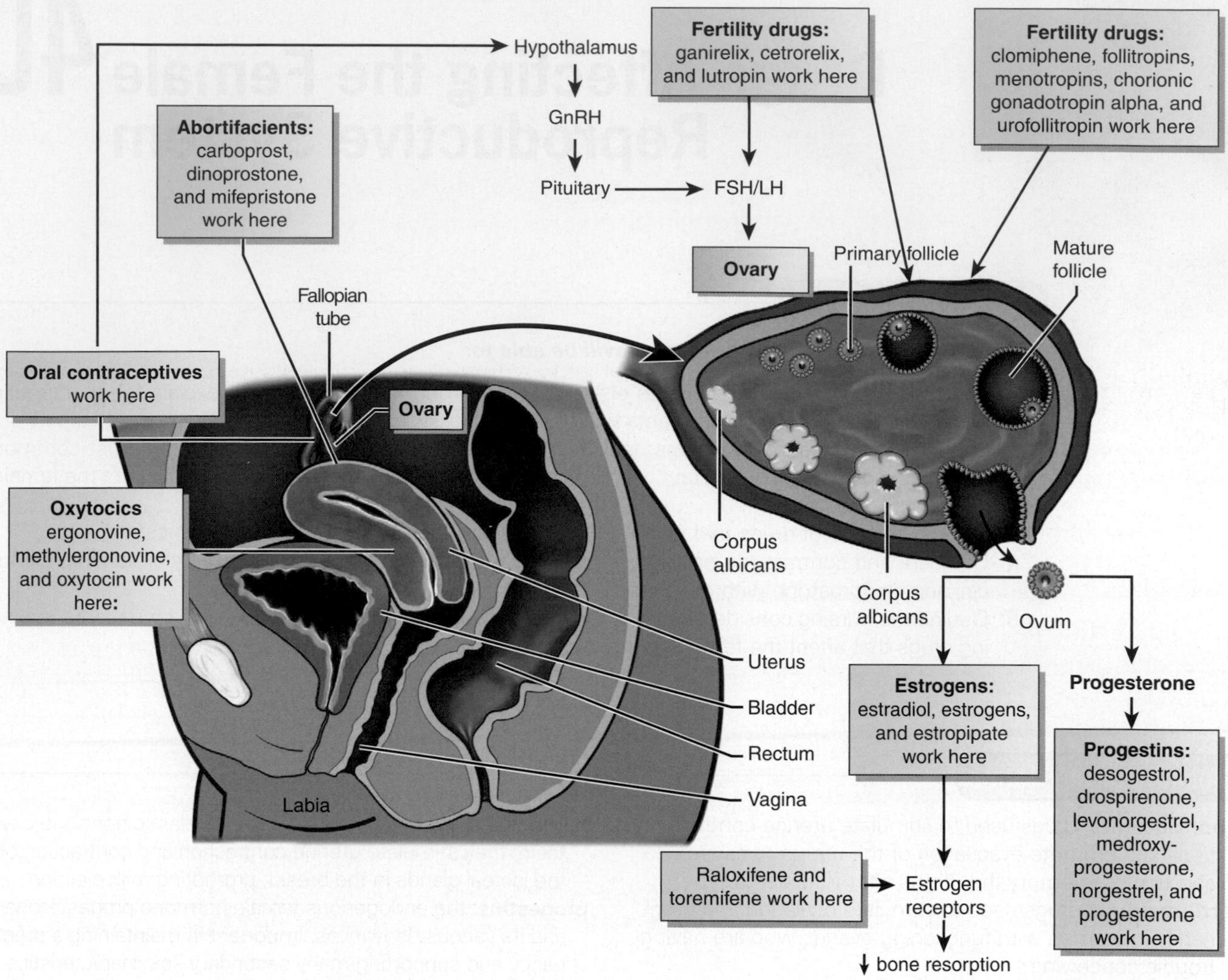

FIGURE 40.1 Sites of action of drugs affecting the female reproductive system.

BOX 40.1 FOCUS ON **Drug Therapy Across the Lifespan**

Drugs Affecting the Female Reproductive System

CHILDREN

The estrogens and progestins have undergone little testing in children. Because of their effects on closure of the epiphyses, they should be used only with great caution in growing children.

If oral contraceptives are prescribed for teenage girls the smallest dose possible should be used and the child should be monitored carefully for metabolic and other effects.

ADULTS

Women who are receiving any of these drugs should receive an annual medical examination, including breast examination and Pap smear, to monitor for adverse effects and underlying medical conditions. The potential for adverse effects should be discussed and comfort measures provided. Women taking estrogen should be advised not to smoke because of the increased risk of thrombotic events.

If any of these drugs is used in males for the treatment of specific cancers the patient should be advised about the possibility of estrogenic effects, and appropriate support should be offered.

When combinations of these hormones are used as part of fertility programs, women need a great deal of psychological support and comfort measures to cope with the many adverse effects associated with these drugs. The risk of multiple births should be explained, as should the need for frequent monitoring.

When abortifacients are used, patients need a great deal of psychological support. Written lists of signs and symptoms to report and what to expect are more effective than just verbal lists in this time of potential stress.

These agents are not for use during pregnancy or lactation because of the potential for adverse effects on the fetus or neonate.

OLDER ADULTS

HRT is no longer commonly used by postmenopausal women. Reports of benefits and risks are frequent and conflicting, and patients need support and reliable information to make informed decisions about the use of these drugs.

If patients are also using alternative therapies, their effects on the HRT and other possible prescription drugs need to be carefully evaluated.

they affect the female reproductive system throughout the lifespan.

Sex Hormones and Estrogen Receptor Modulators

The female sex hormones can be used to replace hormones that are missing or to act on the control mechanisms of the endocrine system to decrease the release of endogenous hormones. Drugs that act like estrogen, particularly at specific estrogen receptors, are also used to stimulate the effects of estrogen in the body with fewer of the adverse effects. See Table 40.1 for information on these agents.

Sex Hormones

Female sex hormones include estrogens and the **progestins** (the endogenous female hormone progesterone and its various derivatives). Estrogens that are available for

Table 40.1 *Drugs in Focus:* Sex Hormones and Estrogen Receptor Modulators

Name	Usual Dosage	Usual Indications
Sex Hormones ***Estrogens***		
estradiol (*Estrace*)	1–2 mg/d PO; 1–5 mg IM every 3–4 wk; 10–20 mg valerate in oil IM q4 wk *or* 1–5 mg cypionate in oil IM every 3–4 wk; 2–4 g intravaginal cream daily; apply vaginal ring once every 90 d	Palliation of signs and symptoms of menopause, prostate cancer, inoperable breast cancer; treatment of female hypogonadism, postpartum breast engorgement
estrogens, conjugated (*C.E.S., Premarin*)	0.3–1.25 mg/d PO	Palliation of signs and symptoms of menopause, prostate cancer, inoperable breast cancer; treatment of female hypogonadism, postpartum breast engorgement; to retard the progress of osteoporosis
estrogens, esterified (*Menest*)	0.3–1.25 mg/d PO	Palliation of signs and symptoms of menopause, prostate cancer, inoperable breast cancer; treatment of female hypogonadism
estropipate (*Ogen*)	0.625–5 mg/d PO	Palliation of signs and symptoms of menopause; treatment of female hypogonadism
Progestins		
desogestrel (*Kariva, Cyclessa*)	0.15 mg with 20 mcg ethinyl estradiol PO 0.1 mg, then 0.125 mg, and then 0.15 mg with 25 mcg ethinyl estradiol PO	Available only in combination form, used as oral contraceptive
drospirenone (*Yasmin*)	3 mg with 30 mcg ethinyl estradiol PO	Used in combination contraceptives; treatment of acne and PMDD; relief of signs and symptoms of menopause
drospirenone (*Yaz*)	3 mg with 0.02 mg estradiol PO	
etonogestrel (*Implanon*)	68 mg implanted subdermally for up to 3 y, may be replaced at that time	Contraceptive for women; being investigated as a male contraceptive agent
etonogestrel (*NuvaRing*)	0.12 mg with 0.015-mg ethinyl estradiol as a vaginal ring	
levonorgestrel (*Mirena, Plan B*)	*Mirena:* 53 mg inserted intrauterine for up to 5 y *Plan B:* 0.75 mg PO taken within 72 h of sexual intercourse and repeated in 12 h	Intrauterine contraceptives; also used as "morning after" pill; component in many combination contraceptives
medroxyprogesterone (*Provera*)	5–10 mg/d PO for 5–10 d for amenorrhea; 400–1,000 mg/wk IM for cancer therapy	Treatment of amenorrhea (orally); palliation of certain cancers (injection)
norethindrone acetate (*Aygestin*)	2.5–10 mg/d PO	Used in combination contraceptives; used alone for treatment of amenorrhea
norgestrel (generic)	0.075–0.35 mg/d PO	Used as contraceptive (most effective when used in combination form)
progesterone (generic)	5–10 mg/d IM for 6–8 d; 90 mg/d intravaginally	Used as contraceptive and in fertility programs; treatment of amenorrhea
ulipristal (*Ella*)	30 mg PO within 72 h of unprotected intercourse	Postcoital contraception

(table continues on page 670)

Table 40.1 *Drugs in Focus:* Sex Hormones and Estrogen Receptor Modulators (continued)

Name	Usual Dosage	Usual Indications
Estrogen Receptor Modulators		
raloxifene (*Evista*)	60 mg/d PO	Used therapeutically to stimulate specific estrogen receptor sites, which results in an increase in bone mineral density without stimulating the endometrium in women; reduces risk of invasive breast cancer in postmenopausal women with osteoporosis who are at high risk for invasive breast cancer
toremifene (*Fareston*)	60 mg/d PO until disease progression occurs	Used as an antineoplastic agent because of its effects on estrogen receptor sites (see Chapter 14) for treatment of advanced breast cancer in postmenopausal women with estrogen receptor–positive and estrogen receptor–unknown tumors

PMDD, premenstrual dysphoric disorder.

use include estradiol (*Estrace*, *Climara*, and others), conjugated estrogens (*Premarin*), esterified estrogen (*Menest*), and estropipate (*Ogen*).

Progestins include drospirenone (*Yasmin*, *Yaz*), etonogestrel (*Implanon*), levonorgestrel (*Mirena*), medroxyprogesterone (*Provera*), norethindrone (*Aygestin*), norgestrel (generic), progesterone (*Prometrium*, and others), desogestrel (found in many contraceptive combinations), and ulipristal (*Ella*) used as a postcoital contraceptive.

Therapeutic Actions and Indications

Estrogens

Estrogens are used in many clinical situations; for example, in small doses, they are used for hormone replacement therapy (HRT) when ovarian activity is blocked or absent. (Box 40.2 lists combination of products used as HRT.) Estrogens are also used as palliation for the discomforts of menopause in the first few years of menopause, when many of the beneficial effects of estrogen are lost, to treat female hypogonadism and ovarian failure, to prevent postpartum breast engorgement, as part of combination contraceptives, to slow bone loss in osteoporosis, and for palliation in certain cancers that have known receptor sensitivity (see Chapter 14). See Table 40.1 for Usual Indications for each type of estrogen.

Estrogens are important for the development of the female reproductive system and secondary sex characteristics. They affect the release of pituitary follicle-stimulating hormone (FSH) and luteinizing hormone (LH); cause capillary dilation, fluid retention, and protein anabolism and thin the cervical mucus; conserve calcium and phosphorus and encourage bone formation; inhibit ovulation; and prevent postpartum breast discomfort. Estrogens also are responsible for the proliferation of the endometrial lining (Figure 40.1). An absence or decrease in estrogen produces the signs and symptoms of menopause in the uterus, vagina, breasts, and cervix. Estrogens are known to compete with androgens for receptor sites; this trait makes them beneficial in certain androgen-dependent prostate cancers. Estrogens produce a wide variety of systemic effects, including protecting the heart from atherosclerosis, retaining calcium in the bones, and maintaining the secondary female sex characteristics (see Box 39.1 for a complete list of estrogen effects). However, the results of a study by the Women's Health Initiative showed some serious negative reactions to exogenous estrogen in postmenopausal women when used in HRT over a period of time (see Boxes 40.3 and 40.4). (See Box 40.5 for information about treating dyspareunia during menopause.)

BOX 40.2

Combination Drugs Used for Menopause

Many fixed combination drugs containing estrogen and a progestin are available specifically for relieving the signs and symptoms associated with menopause in women who have an intact uterus. The benefits include reduction in the risk of osteoporosis and coronary artery disease with short-term use. These drugs are taken as one tablet, once a day. Patients should receive regular medical follow-up and monitoring while taking these drugs.

Estradiol/norethindrone (*Activella*)
Estradiol/norgestimate (*Ortho-Prefest*)
Estradiol/drospirenone (*Yaz*)
Ethinyl estradiol/norethindrone acetate (*Femhrt 1/5*)
Estrogen/medroxyprogesterone (*Premphase*)
Estrogen/medroxyprogesterone/conjugated estrogens (*Prempro*)
Estradiol/drospirenone (*Angeliq*)
Also available is a combination patch (which should be changed twice each week).
Estrogen/norethindrone (*CombiPatch*)
Estradiol/levonorgestrel (*Climara Pro*)

BOX 40.3

Contraceptives: Forms and Dosing

Oral contraceptives are available as monophasic, biphasic, and triphasic preparations. One tablet is taken orally for 21 days, beginning on the day 5 of the cycle (day 1 of the cycle is the first day of menstrual bleeding). Inert tablets or no tablets are taken for the next 7 days, and then a new course of 21 days is started.

Missed doses: If one tablet is missed, take it as soon as possible or take two tablets the next day. If two consecutive tablets are missed, take two tablets daily for the next 2 days and then resume the regular schedule. If three consecutive tablets are missed, begin a new cycle of tablets 7 days after the last tablet was taken, and use an additional method of birth control until the start of the next menstrual period.

Postcoital or emergency contraception ("morning after" regimen): The doses are as follows:

Plan B (levonorgestrel)	Take one tablet within 72 h after intercourse and a second tablet 12 h later
Plan B One-Step (levonorgestrel)	Take one tablet within 72 h after unprotected intercourse, available over the counter for patients 17 y and older
Ella (ulipristal)	Take one tablet within 5 d of unprotected intercourse

Monophasic OCs

Aviane, Lessina Lutera, Orsythia, Sronyx	20-mcg estradiol, 0.10-mg levonorgestrel
Apri, Desogen, Emoquette, Ortho-Cept, Reclipsen, Solia	30-mcg ethinyl estradiol, 0.15-mg desogestrel
Balziva, Femcon FE chewable tablets, Ovcon- 35, Zenchent	35-mcg estradiol, 0.4-mg norethindrone
Beyaz	3-mg drospirenone, 0.2-mg ethinyl estradiol, 0.45-mg levomefolate
Brevicon, Modicon, Necon 0.5/35, Zenchent	35-mcg ethinyl estradiol, 0.5-mg norethindrone
Cryselle, Low-Ogestrel	30-mcg ethinyl estradiol, 0.3-mg norgestrel
Kelnar 1/35, Zovia 1/35E	35-mcg ethinyl estradiol, 1-mg ethynodiol diacetate
Estarylla, MonoNessa, Ortho-Cyclen, Previform, Sprintec	35-mcg ethinyl estradiol, 0.25-mg norgestimate
Gianvi, Loryna, Yaz	30-mg drospirenone, 20-mcg ethinyl estradiol
Junel Fe 1/20, Junel 21 day 1/20, Loestrin 21 1/20, Loestrin Fe 1/20, Loestrin 24 Fe, Microgestin Fe 1/20, Minastrin 24 Fe	20-mcg ethinyl estradiol, 1-mg norethindrone
Junel Fe 1.0/30, Junel 21 day 1.5/30, Loestrin 21 1.5/30, Loestrin Fe 1.5/30, Microgestin Fe 1.5/30	30-mcg ethinyl estradiol, 1.5-mg norethindrone
Necon 1/35, Norinyl 1+35, Ortho-Novum 1/35	35-mcg ethinyl estradiol, 1-mg norethindrone
Necon 1/50, Norinyl 1+50	50-mcg mestranol, 1-mg norethindrone
Ocella, Syeda, Yasmin, Zarah	3-mg drospirenon, 30-mcg ethinyl estradiol
Ogestrel	50-mcg ethinyl estradiol, 0.5-mg norgestrel
Ovcon 50	50-mcg ethinyl estradiol, 1-mg norethindrone
Seasonale, Quasense, Seasonique	0.15-mg levonorgestrel, 0.03-mg ethinyl estradiol for 84 d, 7 d inactive
Sfyral	30-mcg ethinyl estradiol, 3-mg drospirenone
Zovia 1/50E	50-mcg ethinyl estradiol/1-mg ethynodiol diacetate

Biphasic OCs

Necon 10/11	Phase 1, 10 tablets: 0.5-mg norethindrone, 35-mcg ethinyl estradiol; phase 2, 11 tablets: 1-mg norethindrone, 35-mcg ethinyl estradiol
Azurette, Kariva, Mircette	Phase 1, 21 tablets: 0.15-mg desogestrel/20-mcg ethinyl estradiol Phase 2, 5 tablets: 10-mcg ethinyl estradiol
LoLoestrin Fe	Phase 1, 24 tablets: 1-mg norethindrone/10-mcg ethinyl estradiol Phase 2, 2 tablets: 10-mcg ethinyl estradiol
LoSeasonique	Phase 1, 84 tablets: 0.15-mg levonorgestrel/20-mcg ethinyl estradiol Phase 2, 7 tablets: 10-mcg ethinyl estradiol
Seasonique	Phase 1, 84 tablets: 0.15-mg levonorgestrel/30-mcg ethinyl estradiol Phase 2, 7 tablets: 10-mcg ethinyl estradiol

Triphasic OCs

Aranelle, Leena, Tri-Norinyl	Phase 1, 7 tablets: 0.5-mg norethindrone, 35-mcg ethinyl estradiol Phase 2, 9 tablets: 1-mg norethindrone, 35-mcg ethinyl estradiol Phase 3, 5 tablets: 0.5-mg norethindrone, 35-mcg ethinyl estradiol
Caziant, Cesia, Cyclessa, Velivet	Phase 1, 7 tablets: 0.1-mg desogestrel, 25-mcg ethinyl estradiol Phase 2, 7 tablets: 0.125-mg desogestrel, 25-mcg ethinyl estradiol Phase 3, 5 tablets: 0.15-mg desogestrel, 25-mcg ethinyl estradiol

(continues on page 672)

BOX 40.3

Contraceptives: Forms and Dosing (*continued*)

Estrostep Fe, Tilia Fe, Tri-Legest Fe	Phase 1, 5 tablets: 1-mg norethindrone, 20 mcg ethinyl estradiol, 75-mg ferrous fumarate Phase 2, 7 tablets: 1-mg norethindrone, 30-mcg ethinyl estradiol, 75-mg ferrous fumarate Phase 3, 9 tablets: 1-mg norethindrone, 35-mcg ethinyl estradiol, 75-mg ferrous fumarate
Ortho-Novum 7/7/7, Necon 7/7/7	Phase 1, 7 tablets: 0.5-mg norethindrone, 35-mcg ethinyl estradiol Phase 2, 7 tablets: 0.75-mg norethindrone, 35-mcg ethinyl estradiol Phase 3, 7 tablets: 1-mg norethindrone, 35-mcg ethinyl estradiol
Ortho Tri-Cyclen, Tri-Estarylla, TriNessa, Tri-Previfem, Tri-Sprintec	Phase 1, 7 tablets: 0.18-mg norgestimate, 35-mcg ethinyl estradiol Phase 2, 7 tablets: 0.215-mg norgestimate, 35-mcg ethinyl estradiol Phase 3, 7 tablets: 0.25-mg norgestimate, 35-mcg ethinyl estradiol
Ortho Tri-Cyclen LO	Phase 1, 7 tablets: 0.18-mg norgestimate, 25-mcg ethinyl estradiol Phase 2, 7 tablets: 0.215-mg norgestimate, 25-mcg ethinyl estradiol Phase 3, 7 tablets: 0.25-mg norgestimate, 25-mcg ethinyl estradiol
Tri-Legest	Phase 1, 5 tablets: 1-mg norethindrone, 20-mcg ethinyl estradiol Phase 2, 7 tablets: 1-mg norethindrone, 30-mcg ethinyl estradiol Phase 3, 9 tablets: 1-mg norethindrone, 35-mcg ethinyl estradiol
Trivora 28	Phase 1, 6 tablets: 0.5-mg levonorgestrel, 30-mcg ethinyl estradiol Phase 2, 5 tablets: 0.075-mg levonorgestrel, 40-mcg ethinyl estradiol Phase 3, 10 tablets: 0.125-mg levonorgestrel, 30-mcg ethinyl estradiol
Multiphasic Oral Contraceptive	
Natazia	Phase 1, 2 tablets: 3-mg estradiol valerate Phase 2, 5 tablets: 2-mg estradiol valerate, 2-mg dienogest Phase 3, 17 tablets: 2-mg estradiol valerate, 3-mg dienogest Phase 4, 2 tablets: 1-mg estradiol valerate
Quartette	Phase 1, 42 tablets: 0.15-mg levonorgestrel, 0.02-mg ethinyl estradiol Phase 2, 21 tablets: 0.15-mg levonorgestrel, 0.025-mg ethinyl estradiol Phase 3, 21 tablets: 0.15-mg levonorgestrel, 0.03-mg ethinyl estradiol Phase 4, 7 tablets: 0.01-mg ethinyl estradiol
Progestin only contraceptives	
Camila, Errin	0.35-mg norethindrone
Injectables	
Depo-Provera	150-mg medroxyprogesterone, given 1 mL by deep IM injection q3 mo; **black box warning: risk of significant bone loss**
depo-sub Q provera 104	104-mg medroxyprogesterone, give 0.65 mL subcutaneously
Intrauterine System	
Mirena	52-mg levonorgestrel, inserted into the uterus, releases low-dose levonorgestrel over a 5-y period
Skyla	13.5-mg levonorgestrel inserted into uterus for up to 3 y
Transdermal System	
Ortho Evra	6-mg norelgestromin, 0.75-mg ethinyl estradiol; three patches per cycle, each worn for 1 wk; releases estrogen and progestin to prevent ovulation; found to be as safe and effective as oral contraceptives and easier to remember to use for some patients
Vaginal Ring	
NuvaRing	0.12-mg etonogestrel, 0.015-mg ethinyl estradiol ring inserted vaginally once a month and kept in place for 3 wk; after 1-wk rest, a new ring is inserted
Subdermal Implant	
Implanon. Nexplanon	68-mg etonogestrel implanted subdermally, effective up to 3 y, may be replaced at that time if desired

BOX 40.4 FOCUS ON The Evidence

Menopause and Hormone Replacement Therapy—The Women's Health Initiative

Women experience the menarche (onset of the menstrual cycle) in adolescence and menopause (cessation of the menstrual cycle) in midlife. The age at which a woman experiences menopause or "the change" of life varies. The family history of onset of menopause is a good guide for when the effects can be expected. Just as the physical changes associated with puberty can take a few years to be accomplished, so too can the changes associated with menopause. The signs and symptoms of menopause (vaginal dryness, hot flashes, moodiness, loss of bone density, increased risk of CV disease, somnolence) are related to the loss of estrogen and progesterone effects on the body.

Hormone Replacement Therapy or Not?

For centuries, women have proceeded through this time in their lives without pharmacological intervention, although many herbal and alternative therapies may help to ease the transition through menopause (see Box 40.7). Women who rely on these therapies need to be cautioned about potential drug–drug interactions and advised to always report the use of these agents to their health care providers. Today, with more research and safer drugs available to counteract some of the effects of menopause, many women choose to use HRT if the adverse effects of menopause become too uncomfortable or difficult to tolerate. The use of HRT can decrease the discomforts associated with menopause, although various forms of HRT have been associated with increased risks for breast and cervical cancer, heart disease, and stroke. Many women are reluctant to consider HRT because of these effects. The newer drugs used in HRT have been shown to be associated with only a possible increase in risk of breast and cervical cancer, but with long-term use they are associated with an increased risk for CV events. Patients with many risk factors for developing these cancers are at greater risk than patients with no risk factors. Other drugs—the estrogen receptor modulators—have antiestrogen effects on the breast and may remove the cancer risk. However, these drugs may be less reliable in their management of the signs and symptoms of menopause and have not been correlated with a reduction in the risk of coronary artery disease.

Early Research

The Women's Health Initiative was a long-term, multisite study of the effects of hormones on menopausal women. When the initial reports were published, after the third and fourth years of the study, it seemed that the use of HRT was protective in many ways. It seemed that women using HRT had decreased coronary artery disease and CV events, decreased osteoporosis and bone fractures, decreased breast and colon cancer, and improved memory. HRT was then being prescribed to prevent a number of these chronic conditions.

Later Research

In 2002, however, the study was stopped when it was found that women using HRT for 5 or more years had an increased incidence of CV disease and stroke, as well as blood clots, gallstones, and ovarian cancer. The news headlines were confusing at best; many women simply stopped HRT, and women new to menopause would not even consider it.

Applying the Evidence

The woman who is entering menopause should have all of the information available before deciding whether HRT is for her. This can be a very difficult decision for many women, because the risks involved may outweigh the benefits or vice versa. The nurse is often in the best position to provide information, listen to concerns, and help the patient to decide what is best for her.

A complete family and personal history of cancer and coronary artery disease risk factors should be completed to help the patient balance the benefits versus the risks of this therapy. If the decision is made to use HRT the patient may need support in dealing with the effects of the drugs and may have to try several different preparations before the one best suited to her is found. This can be a very frustrating time, so the patient will need a consistent, reliable person to turn to with questions and for support. As researchers continue to study women's health issues, better therapies may be developed to help women through this transition in life. Keeping up with the research as it is reported can be a difficult task, but for anyone who works with women in clinical practice it is a necessity.

The current recommendation of the U.S. Preventative Services Task Force is that women should feel comfortable taking HRT to reduce the symptoms of menopause for short-term therapy (fewer than 5 years). The task force summarized all of the studies and noted that long-term use of HRT provides a decreased risk of osteoporosis and related fractures, possibly a reduced risk of dementia, and a reduction in risk of colon cancer. The negative aspects of this therapy include a definite but small increased risk for heart disease, stroke, and breast cancer. The harms of long-term use outweigh the benefits for most women. The benefits of short-term use, however, must be considered if a woman is having a difficult time getting through menopause (USPSTF, 2012).

Critics of the study also point out that the women in the study were much older than most early postmenopausal groups who could benefit from HRT; they concluded that more research is needed on this. Follow-up research using this study has found no correlation between the use of HRT and the prevention of Alzheimer's disease and no drop in bone fractures in women using HRT.

BOX 40.5

Treating Dyspareunia During Menopause

In 2013 the FDA approved a drug for the treatment of moderate to severe dyspareunia during menopause. This is a condition of painful intercourse associated with the vaginal dryness and changes that occur with menopause. The drug, ospemifene (*Osphena*), is an estrogen agonist/antagonist. It is taken orally, once a day. *Osphena* has a black box warning that its use increases the risk of endometrial cancer and of CV events including stroke, myocardial infarction, and deep-vein thrombosis. Women should be screened for appropriate use. The drug is contraindicated with any undiagnosed genital bleeding, known or suspected estrogen-dependent cancers, active thromboembolic disease, or known or suspected pregnancy. It is advised that a progestin be added to the drug regimen in women with an intact uterus to decrease the endometrial cancer risk. When taking the drug, women may experience hot flashes, vaginal discharge, muscle spasms, and increased sweating. Because of the potential risk associated with the use of the drug, it is recommended that every 3–6 months the use of the drug be reevaluated. This was the first drug approved to help women having problems with intercourse. Erectile dysfunction drugs have been around for many years to help men. Advocates for equality in health care see this as a breakthrough drug in addressing woman-specific needs.

Progestins

Progestins are used as contraceptives, most effectively in combination with estrogens (Box 40.3 lists available contraceptives). They are used to treat primary and secondary amenorrhea and functional uterine bleeding and as part of fertility programs. Like the estrogens, some progestins are useful in treating specific cancers with specific receptor site sensitivity (see Chapter 14). See Table 40.1 for Usual Indications for each type of progestin.

The progestins transform the proliferative endometrium into a secretory endometrium, inhibit the secretion of FSH and LH, prevent follicle maturation and ovulation, inhibit uterine contractions, and may have some anabolic and estrogenic effects. When they are used as contraceptives the exact mechanism of action is not known, but it is thought that circulating progestins and estrogens "trick" the hypothalamus and pituitary and prevent the release of gonadotropin-releasing hormone (GnRH), FSH, and LH, thus preventing follicle development and ovulation. The low levels of these hormones do not produce a thick and vascular endometrium that is receptive to implantation, and if ovulation and fertilization were to occur the chances of implantation would be remote.

Pharmacokinetics

Estrogens

Oral estrogens are well absorbed through the gastrointestinal (GI) tract and undergo extensive hepatic metabolism. They are excreted in the urine. Estrogens cross the placenta and enter breast milk. See Table 40.2 for available forms of estrogen.

Progestins

The progestins are well absorbed, undergo hepatic metabolism, and are excreted in the urine. They are known to cross the placenta and to enter breast milk. Like estrogens,

Table 40.2 Available Forms of Estrogen and Progestin

	Oral	Injection	Vaginal Cream or Gel	Transdermal Patch	Vaginal Ring	Implanted Uterine Device
Estrogens						
estradiol	×	×	×	×	×	—
estrogens, conjugated	×	×	×	—	—	—
estrogens, esterified	×	—	—	—	—	—
estrone	—	×	—	—	—	—
estropipate	×	—	×	—	—	—
Progestins						
desogestrel	×					
drospirenone	×					
etonogestrel	—	—	—	—	×	
hydroxyprogesterone	—	×	—	—	—	
levonorgestrel	×	—	—	—	—	×
medroxyprogesterone	×	×	—	—	—	—
norelgestromin	×	—	—	×	—	—
norethindrone	×	—	—	—	—	—
norgestrel	×	—	—	—	—	—
progesterone	—	×	×	—	—	—

progestins are available in several forms (see Table 40.2). Etonogestrel, in addition to being available as a vaginal ring, *NuvaRing*, is available as a subdermal implant that may be left in place for up to 3 years and then must be removed. Another implant could be placed at that time. Levonorgestrel was once available as an implant system (*Norplant System*) but now is available only in combination-form oral contraceptives or as a uterine insert. It is also used as a "morning after" pill (*Plan B, Plan B OneStep*) (Box 40.6). Ulipristal (*Ella*) is only available as a postcoital or "morning after" contraceptive and is classified as a progesterone agonist/antagonist.

Contraindications and Cautions

Estrogens

Estrogens are contraindicated in the presence of any known allergies to estrogens *to avoid hypersensitivity reactions* and in patients with idiopathic vaginal bleeding, breast cancer, or any estrogen-dependent cancer, *all of which could be exacerbated by the drug*; with a history of thromboembolic disorders, including cerebrovascular accident, or with heavy smokers *because of the increased risk of thrombus and embolus development*; or with hepatic dysfunction, *because of the effects of estrogen on liver function.*

Estrogens are contraindicated during pregnancy *due to the risk of serious fetal defects.* They should be avoided during breastfeeding *because of possible effects on the neonate.* Estrogens should be used cautiously in patients with metabolic bone disease *because of the bone-conserving effect of estrogen, which could exacerbate the disease*; with renal insufficiency, *which could interfere with the renal excretion of the drug and increase the risk for potential adverse effects on fluid and electrolyte balance*; and with hepatic impairment, *which could alter the metabolism of the drug and increase the risk for adverse effects, including those on the liver and GI tract.*

Progestins

Contraindications and cautions for progestins are similar to those for estrogens. Progestins are also contraindicated in the presence of pelvic inflammatory disease (PID), sexually transmitted diseases, endometriosis, or pelvic surgery *because of the effects of progestins on the vasculature of the uterus.* Drospirenone is contraindicated in patients who are at risk for hyperkalemia due to renal disorders, liver disease, adrenal dysfunction, or the use of other drugs that can affect potassium levels *because of its antimineralocorticoid effects and the risk of hyperkalemia.*

Progestins should be used with caution in patients with epilepsy, migraine headaches, asthma, or cardiac or renal dysfunction *because of potential exacerbation of these conditions.*

BOX 40.6 FOCUS ON The Evidence

Over-the-Counter Availability of the "Morning After" Pill

In late 2003 and again in 2005 the FDA was advised to approve OTC use of the morning-after birth control product *Plan B* (levonorgestrel). This drug is used within 72 hours after intercourse and is 89% effective in preventing pregnancy. Critics, however, are concerned that women will not receive appropriate education and follow-up after the use of these products, will not receive appropriate screening, or that the availability will lead to more unprotected sex. Supporters believe that these drugs will decrease the number of unwanted pregnancies and abortions in the population of women who would take advantage of the availability of these drugs. Others proposed that it should only be available to women older than 17 years of age, although it was also argued that this would be too difficult to enforce. In 2013 the FDA approved the sale of *Plan B* OTC to any woman or girl. A generic levonorgestrel is available for sale through a pharmacist. The full report and continuing discussion of the controversy are available online at: http://www.fda.gov

FOCUS ON Safe Medication Administration

By 2104 all estrogen, estrogen-like, and progesterone products carried a black box warning of potential risks. Estrogen-only products are associated with risk of endometrial cancer in women with an intact uterus and no concurrent progesterone therapy; high risk for stroke and thrombotic disorders and possible increased risk for dementia in postmenopausal women; these products are not to be used for the prevention of cardiovascular (CV) disease or dementia, When estrogen and progesterone products are used together there is warning of increased risk of stroke, deep-vein thrombosis, pulmonary embolism, and myocardial infarction; increased risk of invasive breast cancer; increased risk of dementia in postmenopausal women; and these products are also not approved for prevention of CV disease or dementia. Women who take any of these products should be alerted to these possible risks, should have annual pelvic and breast examinations, breast cancer screening, and should be monitored for any signs of thrombotic disorders and alerted to what signs they need to report. Smoking increases the risk of thrombotic events and all women taking these products should be advised not to smoke.

Adverse Effects

Estrogens

Many of the most common adverse effects associated with estrogens involve the genitourinary (GU) tract. They include breakthrough bleeding, menstrual irregularities, dysmenorrhea, amenorrhea, and changes in libido. Other effects can result from the systemic effects of estrogens, including fluid retention, electrolyte disturbances, headache, dizziness, mental changes, weight changes, and edema. GI effects also are fairly common and include nausea, vomiting, abdominal cramps and bloating, and

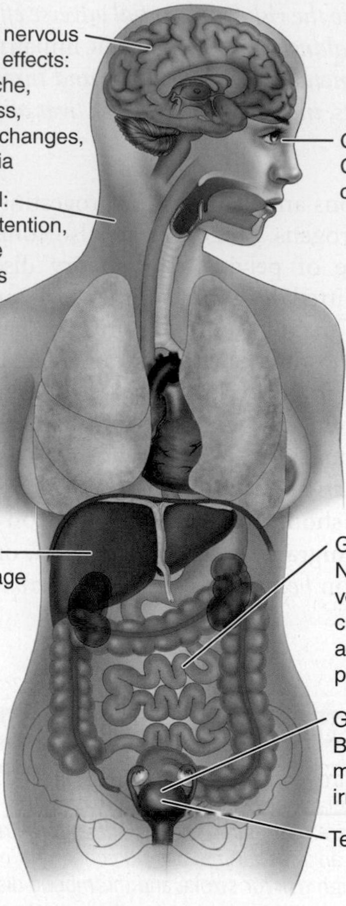

FIGURE 40.2 Variety of adverse effects and toxicities associated with drugs affecting the female reproductive system.

colitis. Potentially serious GI effects, including acute pancreatitis, cholestatic jaundice, and hepatic adenoma, have been reported with the use of estrogens (Figure 40.2).

Progestins

Adverse effects associated with progestins vary with the administration route used. Systemic effects are very similar to the adverse effects of estrogen. Dermal patch contraceptives are associated with the same systemic effects, as well as local skin irritation. Vaginal gel use is associated with headache, nervousness, constipation, breast enlargement, and perineal pain. Intrauterine systems are associated with abdominal pain, endometriosis, abortion, PID, and expulsion of the intrauterine device. Vaginal use is associated with local irritation and swelling. Drospirenone, used in combination contraceptives, has antimineralocorticoid activity and can block aldosterone, leading to increased potassium levels.

Clinically Important Drug–Drug Interactions

Estrogens

If estrogens are given in combination with drugs that enhance their hepatic metabolism (e.g., barbiturates, rifampin, tetracyclines, phenytoin), serum estrogen levels may decrease. Whenever a drug is added to or removed from a drug regimen that contains estrogens the nurse should evaluate that drug for possible interactions and consult with the prescriber for appropriate dose adjustments.

Estrogens have been associated with increased therapeutic and toxic effects of corticosteroids, so patients taking both drugs should be monitored very closely.

Smoking while taking estrogens should be strongly discouraged because the combination with nicotine increases the risk for development of thrombi and emboli.

Grapefruit juice can inhibit the metabolism of estradiols, leading to increased serum levels. Patients should be discouraged from drinking large quantities of grapefruit juice if they are taking estrogens. St. John's wort can affect the metabolism of estrogens and can make estrogen-containing contraceptives less effective. This combination should be discouraged. Other herbal and alternative therapies used for menopausal symptoms may interact with estrogens (Box 40.7).

BOX 40.7 *FOCUS ON* **Herbal and Alternative Therapies**

Black cohosh: 40-mg/d active ingredient, should not be used for longer than 60 days; monitor for dizziness, nausea, vomiting, visual disturbances; contains alcohol—do not combine with disulfiram, metronidazole.

Borage: 90–500 mg/d PO in softgel capsules, not for long-term use; use caution with seizure disorders or liver impairment.

Chaste tree: 150–325 mg PO once or twice daily; may cause increased blood pressure—avoid use with antihypertensives or beta-blockers; may cause rash and itching.

Clary: 8 drops (gtt) in 1 ounce of water daily as an atomizer or dissolved in bath water; may cause sedation—avoid use with alcohol; not for internal use.

Devil's claw: 1.5–6 g/d PO depending on preparation; increases stomach acid and may interfere with many prescription drugs; use with caution.

Dong quai: 500 mg/d PO; causes photosensitivity—avoid exposure to the sun; do not use with warfarin—increased bleeding can occur.

False unicorn root: 1–2 mL PO three times a day; do not use with estrogen or progestins—may alter uterine effects.

Red clover: 4 g PO three times a day as tea; 30–60 gtt PO three times a day of liquid extract; do not use with heparin or warfarin because of increased bleeding effects; do not combine with HRT because of risk for increased estrogenic effects.

Soy: 25 g/d PO; do not use with calcium, iron, or zinc products; may decrease effects of estrogen, raloxifene, tamoxifen—alert the health care provider if combining these drugs.

Wild yam: 1–6 g/d PO; contains progesterone—do not use with HRT; may cause increased blood glucose and other toxic effects; do not combine with disulfiram or metronidazole—severe reaction may occur.

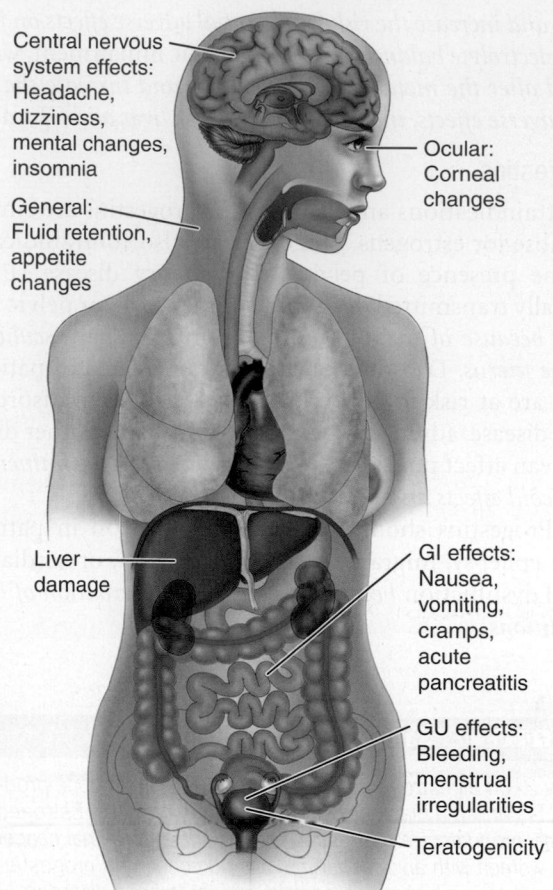

Progestins

Interaction with barbiturates, carbamazepine, phenytoin, griseofulvin, penicillins, tetracyclines, or rifampin may reduce the effectiveness of progestins. Patients using any of these drugs should use another method of contraception if birth control is needed. St. John's wort can affect the metabolism of progestins and can make progestin-containing contraceptives less effective. This combination should be discouraged.

Prototype Summary: Estradiol

Indications: Palliation of moderate to severe vasomotor symptoms associated with menopause; prevention of postmenopausal osteoporosis; treatment of female hypogonadism, female castration, female ovarian failure; palliation of inoperable and progressing breast cancer and inoperable prostatic cancer.

Actions: The most potent endogenous female sex hormone, responsible for estrogen effects on the body.

Pharmacokinetics:

Route	Onset	Peak	Duration
PO	Slow	Days	Unknown

Topical preparations are not generally absorbed systemically.

$T_{1/2}$: Not known; metabolized in the liver and excreted in the urine.

Adverse Effects: Corneal changes, photosensitivity, peripheral edema, chloasma, hepatic adenoma, nausea, vomiting, abdominal cramps, bloating, breakthrough bleeding, change in menstrual flow, dysmenorrhea, premenstrual-like syndrome.

Prototype Summary: Norethindrone Acetate

Indications: Treatment of amenorrhea, abnormal uterine bleeding due to hormonal imbalance; treatment of endometriosis; component of some hormonal contraceptives.

Actions: Progesterone derivative that transforms the proliferative endometrium into a secretory endometrium; inhibits the secretion of pituitary FSH and LH, which prevents ovulation; inhibits uterine contractions.

Pharmacokinetics:

Route	Onset	Peak	Duration
PO	Varies	Unknown	Unknown

$T_{1/2}$: Unknown; metabolized in the liver and excreted in the feces and urine.

Adverse Effects: Venous thromboembolism, loss of vision, diplopia, migraine headache, rash, acne, chloasma, alopecia, breakthrough bleeding, spotting, amenorrhea, fluid retention, edema, increase in weight.

Estrogen Receptor Modulators

Two available estrogen receptor modulators are raloxifene (*Evista*) and toremifene (*Fareston*). The long-term effects of these two drugs are still being studied.

Therapeutic Actions and Indications

Estrogen receptor modulators are not hormones but affect specific estrogen receptor sites, stimulating some and blocking others. They were developed to produce some of the positive effects of estrogen replacement while limiting the adverse effects. See Table 40.1 for Usual Indications for these drugs. Toremifene is discussed in greater detail in Chapter 14, which discusses antineoplastic agents.

Pharmacokinetics

Administered orally, raloxifene is well absorbed from the GI tract and is metabolized in the liver. Excretion occurs through the feces. It is known to cross the placenta and enter into breast milk.

Contraindications and Cautions

Raloxifene is contraindicated in the presence of any known allergy to raloxifene *to avoid hypersensitivity reactions* and during pregnancy and lactation *because of potential effects on the fetus or neonate.* Caution should be used in patients with a history of venous thrombosis or smoking *because of an increased risk of blood clot formation if smoking and estrogen are combined.*

Adverse Effects

Raloxifene has been associated with GI upset, nausea, and vomiting. Changes in fluid balance may also cause headache, dizziness, visual changes, and mental changes. Hot flashes, skin rash, edema, and vaginal bleeding may occur secondary to specific estrogen receptor stimulation. Venous thromboembolism is a potentially dangerous side effect that has been reported.

Clinically Important Drug–Drug Interactions

Cholestyramine reduces the absorption of raloxifene. Highly protein-bound drugs, such as diazepam (*Valium*), ibuprofen (*Motrin*), indomethacin (*Indocin*), and naproxen (*Naprosyn*), may interfere with binding sites. Warfarin taken with raloxifene may decrease the prothrombin time; patients using this combination must be monitored closely.

Ⓟ Prototype Summary: Raloxifene

Indications: Prevention and treatment of osteoporosis in postmenopausal women.

Actions: Increases bone mineral density without stimulating the endometrium; modulates effects of endogenous estrogen at specific receptor sites.

Pharmacokinetics:

Route	Onset	Peak	Duration
PO	Varies	4–7 h	24 h

$T_{1/2}$: 27.7 hours; metabolized in the liver and excreted in the urine.

Adverse Effects: Venous thromboembolism, hot flashes, skin rash, nausea, vomiting, vaginal bleeding, depression, light-headedness.

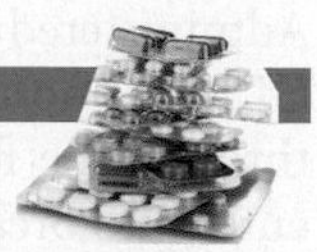

Nursing Considerations for Patients Receiving Sex Hormones or Estrogen Receptor Modulators

Assessment: History and Examination

- Assess for contraindications or cautions: History of allergy to any sex hormone or component of the drug product *to avoid hypersensitivity reactions*; current status related to pregnancy and lactation *due to adverse effects on the fetus and neonate*; hepatic dysfunction *that might interfere with drug metabolism*; CV disease, breast or genital cancer, renal disease, or metabolic bone disease, *which could be exacerbated by estrogen use*; history of thromboembolism or smoking, *which may increase the patient's risk for embolic conditions*; idiopathic vaginal bleeding or pelvic disease, *which could represent an underlying problem that could be exacerbated with the use of these drugs*; and history of asthma or epilepsy, *which could be exacerbated by progestin use.*
- Perform a physical assessment to establish a baseline status before beginning therapy and during therapy *to determine the effectiveness of therapy and evaluate for any potential adverse effects.*
- Assess abdomen, including auscultation of bowel sounds and palpation of the liver, *to identify abnormalities.* Measure abdominal girth as indicated *to evaluate for bloating.*
- Assess skin color, lesions, and texture; affect, orientation, mental status, and reflexes; and blood pressure, pulse, cardiac auscultation, edema, and perfusion, *which will reflect circulatory status and show any changes associated with thromboembolism.*
- Complete or assist with pelvic and breast examinations. Ensure specimen collection for Pap smear; obtain a history of the patient's menstrual cycle *to provide baseline data and to monitor for any adverse effects that could occur.*
- Arrange for ophthalmic examination (particularly if the patient wears contact lenses) *because hormonal changes can alter the fluid in the eye and curvature of the cornea, which can change the fit of contact lenses and alter visual acuity.*
- Monitor the results of laboratory tests, including urinalysis and renal and/or hepatic function tests, *to determine the need for possible dose adjustment and identify early indications of dysfunction.*

See the Critical Thinking Scenario for additional information related to a patient who is taking contraceptives.

Nursing Diagnoses

Nursing diagnoses related to drug therapy might include the following:

- Excess fluid volume related to fluid retention
- Acute pain related to systemic side effects of GI pain and headache
- Ineffective tissue perfusion (cerebral, cardiopulmonary, peripheral) related to changes in the blood vessels concerning drug therapy and risk of thromboemboli
- Unbalanced nutrition: Less than body requirements related to GI distress associated with drug therapy
- Risk for ineffective management of therapeutic regimen related to complexities of drug regimen
- Deficient knowledge regarding drug therapy

Planning

- The patient will receive the best therapeutic effect from the drug therapy.
- The patient will have limited adverse effects to the drug therapy.
- The patient will have an understanding of the drug therapy, adverse effects to anticipate, and measures to relieve discomfort and improve safety.

Implementation with Rationale

- Administer drug as prescribed *to prevent adverse effects*; administer with food if GI upset is severe *to relieve GI distress.*
- Provide analgesics *for relief of headache as appropriate.*
- Strongly urge the patient to stop smoking *to reduce the risk of thromboemboli.*
- Encourage the use of small, frequent meals *to assist with nausea and vomiting.*
- Monitor for swelling and changes in vision or fit of contact lenses *to monitor for fluid retention and fluid changes.*
- Arrange for at least an annual physical examination, including pelvic examination, Pap smear, and breast

examination, *to reduce the risk of adverse effects and to monitor drug effects.*
- Assess the patient periodically for changes in perfusion or signs of vessel occlusion *because of the risk of thromboemboli.*
- Monitor liver function periodically for the patient on long-term therapy *to evaluate liver function and ensure discontinuation of the drug at any sign of hepatic dysfunction.*
- Offer support and reassurance *to deal with the drug and drug effects.*
- Provide thorough patient teaching, including steps to take if a dose is missed or lost, measures to avoid adverse effects, signs and symptoms that may indicate a problem, and the need for regular evaluation, *to enhance patient knowledge about drug therapy and to promote compliance.*

Evaluation

- Monitor patient response to the drug (palliation of signs and symptoms of menopause, prevention of pregnancy, decreased risk factors for coronary artery disease, palliation of certain cancers).
- Monitor for adverse effects (liver changes, GI upset, edema, changes in secondary sex characteristics, headaches, thromboembolic episodes, breakthrough bleeding).
- Monitor for potential drug–drug interactions as indicated.
- Evaluate the effectiveness of the teaching plan (the patient can name the drug, dosage, adverse effects to watch for, specific measures to avoid them, and warning signs and symptoms).
- Monitor the effectiveness of comfort measures and compliance with the regimen.

CRITICAL THINKING SCENARIO

Birth Control

THE SITUATION

J.M. is a 25-year-old woman who is being seen in her gynecologist's office for a routine annual physical examination and Pap test. J.M. reports that she has just become sexually active and would like to start using contraceptives. She has some concerns about stories she has heard about "the pill" and would like to know the safest and most effective birth control to use. She is interested in what other methods are available and what the advantages and disadvantages of each form might be.

CRITICAL THINKING

What teaching and counseling issues will be important for J.M. at this time?

What important issues should be discussed when explaining the benefits and drawbacks of various contraceptive measures?

What teaching information needs to be stressed with J.M. if she elects to use oral contraceptives?

DISCUSSION

This appointment presents a good opportunity for the health care provider to allow J.M. to discuss this new aspect of her life. She may have questions about the experience and about things she should be doing or should be questioning. The risk of sexually transmitted diseases, as well as pregnancy, can be discussed. J.M. needs full information about the various forms of birth control that are available for use. Nonpharmacological measures such as condoms and the rhythm method and their reliability can be discussed.

The use of hormones for birth control should then be explained, including the 96 to 98% reliability of these methods when used correctly. The numerous delivery methods for these hormones should be outlined. A variety of possibilities exist, ranging from the transdermal patch, to injection, to the vaginal ring, to the traditional tablet, and the use of the subdermal implant and intrauterine devices. J.M. elected to go with an oral contraceptive (OC). She stated that she has a good memory, and taking them every day won't be a problem. She swims regularly and thought that the patch might be an issue if it came off, and she was not comfortable with anything being injected or inserted into her body. J.M. will need teaching about drug and herbal interactions with the OC and will need to have written instructions on what to do if a dose is missed. The action that should be taken if a dose is missed can be very complicated and involves knowing on which day in the cycle the dose was missed.

It is also important to stress that the OC will not protect J.M. from sexually transmitted diseases and that precautions will need to be taken to avoid exposure to these diseases. She should also be advised not to smoke because smoking combined with OC

(continues on page 680)

Birth Control (continued)

use increases the risk for emboli. The adverse effects that she might experience should be reviewed, and the importance of an annual pelvic examination and Pap test should be stressed. A trusting nurse–patient relationship is important at this time so that J.M. can feel free to call with questions or problems in the future.

NURSING CARE GUIDE FOR J.M.: ORAL CONTRACEPTIVES

Assessment: History and Examination

Assess the patient's health history for allergies to any estrogens; pregnancy or lactation status; breast or genital cancer; hepatic dysfunction; coronary artery disease; thromboembolic disease; renal disease; idiopathic vaginal bleeding; metabolic bone disease; diabetes; and smoking history.

Focus the physical examination on the following:

Neurological: Orientation, reflexes, affect, mental status

Skin: Color, lesions

CV: Pulse, cardiac auscultation, blood pressure, edema, perfusion

GI: Abdominal examination, liver examination

GU: Pelvic examination, Pap smear, urinalysis

Eye: Ophthalmological examination

Nursing Diagnoses

Excess fluid volume related to fluid retention

Acute pain related to systemic side effects of GI pain or headache

Ineffective tissue perfusion (cerebral, cardiopulmonary, peripheral) related to changes in the blood vessels in connection with drug therapy, and risk of thromboemboli if also smoking

Risk for ineffective management of therapeutic regimen related to complexities of the drug regimen

Deficient knowledge regarding drug therapy

Planning

The patient will receive the best therapeutic effect from the drug therapy.

The patient will have limited adverse effects to the drug therapy.

The patient will have an understanding of the drug therapy, adverse effects to anticipate, and measures to relieve discomfort and improve safety.

Implementation

Administer medication as prescribed.

Administer with meals if upset stomach is a problem.

Provide analgesics for headache if appropriate.

Advise the patient that if she wears contact lenses the shape of her cornea may change and she may need a new prescription or may no longer be able to wear them.

Provide at least an annual physical examination, including Pap smear and breast examination.

Monitor perfusion and complaints of pain, tingling, or numbness.

Provide support and reassurance to deal with drug therapy.

Provide patient teaching regarding drug name, dosage, what to do if a dose is missed, adverse effects, precautions, warnings to report, and safe administration.

Evaluation

Evaluate drug effects: Prevention of pregnancy.

Monitor for adverse effects: Signs of liver dysfunction; GI upset; edema; changes in secondary sex characteristics; headaches; thromboembolic episodes; breakthrough bleeding.

Evaluate the effectiveness of the patient-teaching program and comfort and safety measures.

PATIENT TEACHING FOR J.M.

- An OC, or birth control pill, contains specific amounts of female sex hormones that work to make the body unreceptive to pregnancy and to prevent ovulation (the release of the egg from the ovary). Because these hormones affect many systems in your body, it is important to have regular physical checkups while you are taking this drug.
- Many drugs affect the way that OCs work. To be safe, avoid the use of over-the-counter (OTC) drugs, herbal therapies, and other drugs unless you first check with your health care provider.
- It is important to know that this drug does not protect you against sexually transmitted diseases and appropriate precautions should be taken.
- Some of the following adverse effects may occur:
  - *Headache, nervousness:* Check with your health care provider about the use of an analgesic; this effect usually passes after a few months on the drug.
  - *Nausea, loss of appetite:* This usually passes with time; consult your health care provider if it is a problem.
  - *Swelling, weight gain:* Water retention is a normal effect of these hormones. Limiting salt intake may help. You may have trouble with contact lenses if you wear them because the body often retains fluid, which may change the shape of your eye. This usually adjusts over time.
  - *Blood clots in women who smoke cigarettes:* Cigarette smoking can aggravate serious side effects of OCs, such as the formation of blood clots. When taking OCs, it is advisable to cut down, or preferably to stop, cigarette smoking.

Birth Control (continued)

- Tell any doctor, nurse, or other health care provider that you are taking this drug.
- Report any of the following to your health care provider: Pain in the calves or groin; chest pain or difficulty breathing; lump in the breast; severe headache, dizziness, visual changes; severe abdominal pain; yellowing of the skin; pregnancy.
- Bleeding (a false menstrual period) should occur during the time that the drug is withdrawn. Report bleeding at *any* other time to your health care provider.
- It is important to have regular medical checkups, including Pap tests, while you are taking this drug. If you decide to stop the drug to become pregnant, consult with your health care provider.
- A patient package insert is included with the drug. Read this information and feel free to ask any questions that you might have.
- Keep this drug and all medications out of the reach of children.

KEY POINTS

- Estrogens are hormones associated with the development of the female reproductive system and secondary sex characteristics; pharmacologically, estrogens are used to prevent conception, to stimulate ovulation in women with hypogonadism, and to a lesser extent to replace hormones after menopause.
- Progestins maintain pregnancy and are also involved with development of secondary sex characteristics. Progestins are used as part of combination contraceptives, to treat amenorrhea and functional uterine bleeding, and as part of fertility programs.
- Estrogen receptor modulators are used to stimulate specific estrogen receptors to achieve therapeutic effects of increased bone mass without stimulating the endometrium and causing other, less desirable estrogen effects.

Fertility Drugs

Fertility drugs stimulate the female reproductive system. The following fertility drugs are in use: Cetrorelix (*Cetrotide*), chorionic gonadotropin (*Pregnyl*), chorionic gonadotropin alpha (*Ovidrel*), clomiphene (*Clomid*, and others), follitropin alfa (*Gonal-F*), follitropin beta (*Follistim AQ*), ganirelix (generic), menotropins (*Pergonal*), and urofollitropin (*Bravelle*). Table 40.3 gives more information on these agents.

Therapeutic Actions and Indications

Women without primary ovarian failure who cannot get pregnant after 1 year of trying may be candidates for the use of fertility drugs. Fertility drugs work either directly to stimulate follicles and ovulation or stimulate the hypothalamus to increase FSH and LH levels, leading to ovarian follicular development and maturation of ova. Given in sequence with human chorionic gonadotropin (HCG) to maintain the follicle and hormone production, these drugs are used to treat infertility in women with functioning ovaries whose partners are fertile. Fertility drugs also may be used to stimulate multiple follicle development for the harvesting of ova for in vitro fertilization. Menotropins also stimulate spermatogenesis in men with low sperm counts and otherwise normally functioning testes.

Cetrorelix inhibits premature LH surges in women undergoing controlled ovarian stimulation by acting as a GnRH antagonist. Chorionic gonadotropin is used to stimulate ovulation by acting like GnRH and affecting FSH and LH release. Follitropin alfa and follitropin beta are FSH molecules; they are injected to stimulate follicular development in the treatment of infertility and for harvesting of ova for in vitro fertilization. Menotropins, a purified gonadotropin (similar to FSH and LH), are also used to stimulate spermatogenesis. The urofollitropin now available is a less toxic form of human urofollitropin which used to be prepared from the urine of postmenopausal women and was associated with many immune reactions. Urofollitropin is used to stimulate follicle development and induce ovulation. See Table 40.3 for Usual Indications for each fertility drug.

Pharmacokinetics

These drugs are well absorbed and are treated like endogenous hormones within the body, undergoing hepatic metabolism and renal excretion. Drugs that are available in injectable form include cetrorelix, chorionic gonadotropin, chorionic gonadotropin alpha, follitropin alfa, follitropin beta, menotropins, ganirelix, and urofollitropin. Clomiphene is available as an oral agent.

Table 40.3 *Drugs in Focus:* Fertility Drugs

Drug Name	Dosage/Route	Usual Indications
cetrorelix (*Cetrotide*)	3 mg subcutaneously during early follicular phase *or* 0.25 mg subcutaneously on day 5 or 6 of stimulation and then every day until HCG is administered	Inhibition of premature LH surges in women undergoing controlled ovarian stimulation
chorionic gonadotropin (*Pregnyl*)	500–10,000 IU subcutaneously depending on timing and indication	Stimulation of ovulation, hypogonadism, prepubertal cryptorchidism
chorionic gonadotropin alpha (*Ovidrel*)	250 mcg subcutaneously, timing depending on indication	Induction of final follicular maturation and ovulation induction in infertile women
clomiphene (*Clomid*, and others)	50–100 mg/d PO, with the length of therapy and timing dependent on the particular situation	Treatment of infertility; also found to be effective in the treatment of male infertility
follitropin alfa (*Gonal-F*)	75–150 IU/d subcutaneously, dose increases based on response; do not exceed 300 IU/d	Stimulation of follicular development in the treatment of infertility and for harvesting of ova for in vitro fertilization
follitropin beta (*Follistim AQ*)	75–225 IU/d subcutaneously, dose increases based on response; do not exceed 300 IU/d	Stimulation of follicular development in the treatment of infertility and for harvesting of ova for in vitro fertilization
ganirelix (generic)	250 mcg/d subcutaneously during early follicular phase	Inhibition of premature LH surges in women undergoing controlled ovarian hyperstimulation as part of a fertility program
menotropins (*Pergonal*)	Treatment scheduled with HCG; 150 IU FSH/150 IU LH IM for 9–12 d is often used	Stimulation of ovulation in women and spermatogenesis in men
urofollitropin, (*Bravelle*)	150 IU/d subcutaneously or IM, maximum daily dose of 450 IU	Induction of ovulation in women who have previously received pituitary suppression; stimulation of multiple follicles in ovulatory patients

HCG, human chorionic gonadotropin; LH, luteinizing hormone; FSH, follicle-stimulating hormone.

Contraindications and Cautions

These drugs are contraindicated in the presence of primary ovarian failure (*they only work to stimulate functioning ovaries*); thyroid or adrenal dysfunction *because of the effects on the hypothalamic–pituitary axis*; ovarian cysts, *which could be stimulated and become larger due to the effects of the drugs*; pregnancy *due to the potential for serious fetal effects*; idiopathic uterine bleeding, *which could represent an underlying problem that could be exacerbated by the stimulatory effects of these drugs*; and known allergy to any fertility drug *to avoid hypersensitivity reactions.*

Caution should be used in women who are breastfeeding *because of the risk of adverse effects on the baby* and in those with thromboembolic diseases *because of the risk of increased thrombus formation*, as well as in women with respiratory diseases *because of alterations in fluid volume and blood flow that could overtax the respiratory system.*

Adverse Effects

Adverse effects associated with fertility drugs include a greatly increased risk of multiple births and birth defects; ovarian overstimulation (abdominal pain, distention, ascites, pleural effusion); and headache, fluid retention, nausea, bloating, uterine bleeding, ovarian enlargement, gynecomastia, and febrile reactions (possibly due to stimulation of progesterone release).

Ⓟ Prototype Summary: Clomiphene

Indications: Treatment of ovarian failure in patients with normal liver function and normal endogenous estrogens; off-label use; treatment of male sterility.

Actions: Binds to estrogen receptors, decreasing the number of available estrogen receptors, which gives the hypothalamus the false signal to increase FSH and LH secretion, leading to ovarian stimulation.

Pharmacokinetics:

Route	Onset	Peak	Duration
PO	5–8 d	Unknown	6 wk

$T_{1/2}$: 5 days; metabolized in the liver and excreted in the urine.

Adverse Effects: Vasomotor flushing, visual changes, abdominal discomfort, distention and bloating, nausea, vomiting, ovarian enlargement, breast tenderness, ovarian overstimulation, multiple pregnancies.

Nursing Considerations for Patients Receiving Fertility Drugs

Assessment: History and Examination

Assess for contraindications or cautions: History of allergy to any fertility drug *to avoid hypersensitivity reactions*; current status of pregnancy and lactation, *which are contraindications or cautions to the use of the drug*; primary ovarian failure, *which would not respond to these agents*; thyroid or adrenal dysfunction *due to effects on the hypothalamic–pituitary axis*; ovarian cysts, *which could be stimulated and become larger as a result of the drug's stimulatory effects*; idiopathic uterine bleeding, *which could reflect an underlying medical problem that could be exacerbated by the stimulatory effects of the drug*; thromboembolic diseases, *which could increase the patient's risk for thrombus formation*; and respiratory diseases, *which would be exacerbated by the effects of the drug*.

- Perform a complete physical assessment to establish *baseline status before beginning therapy and during therapy to monitor for any potential adverse effects.*
- Perform a psychological assessment to determine teaching and support needs *as these patients are often very stressed, anxious, and can experience bouts of depression which the nurse will need to be ready to address.*
- Assess skin and lesions; orientation, affect, and reflexes; and blood pressure, pulse, respiration, and adventitious sounds *to determine cardiac function and perfusion and to detect changes in blood flow or thromboemboli.*
- Complete or assist with pelvic and breast examinations and ensure collection of specimen for Pap smear *to establish a baseline of GU health and detect early changes as a result of drug therapy.*
- Monitor the results of laboratory tests, such as renal and hepatic function studies, *to evaluate for possible dysfunction that might interfere with metabolism and excretion of the drug*; and check hormonal levels as indicated *to determine the effectiveness of therapy and reduce the risk of ovarian hyperstimulation.*

Nursing Diagnoses

Nursing diagnoses related to drug therapy might include the following:

- Disturbed body image related to drug treatment and diagnosis
- Acute pain related to headache, fluid retention, or GI upset
- Sexual dysfunction related to alterations in normal hormone control
- Deficient knowledge regarding drug therapy
- Risk for impaired tissue perfusion (cardiopulmonary, peripheral) related to increased risk for thrombus formation
- Situational low self-esteem related to the need for fertility drugs

Planning

- The patient will receive the best therapeutic effect from the drug therapy.
- The patient will have limited adverse effects to the drug therapy.
- The patient will have an understanding of the drug therapy, adverse effects to anticipate, and measures to relieve discomfort and improve safety.

Implementation with Rationale

- Assess the cause of dysfunction before beginning therapy *to ensure appropriate use of the drug.*
- Complete a pelvic examination before each use of the drug *to rule out ovarian enlargement, pregnancy, or uterine problems.*
- Check urine estrogen and estradiol levels before beginning therapy *to verify ovarian function.*
- Administer with an appropriate dose of HCG as indicated *to ensure beneficial effects.*
- Discontinue the drug at any sign of ovarian overstimulation and arrange for hospitalization *to monitor and support the patient* if this occurs.
- Provide women with a calendar of treatment days, explanations of adverse effects to anticipate, and instructions on when intercourse should occur *to increase the therapeutic effectiveness of the drug.*
- Provide warnings about the risk and hazards of multiple births *so the patient can make informed decisions about drug therapy.*
- Offer support and encouragement *to deal with low self-esteem, stress, anxiety, and possible depression issues associated with infertility.*
- Provide patient teaching about proper administration technique, appropriate disposal of needles and syringes, measures to avoid adverse effects, warning signs of problems, and the need for regular evaluation *to enhance patient knowledge about drug therapy and to promote compliance.*

Evaluation

- Monitor patient response to the drug (ovulation).
- Monitor for adverse effects (abdominal bloating, weight gain, ovarian overstimulation, multiple births).
- Evaluate the effectiveness of the teaching plan (the patient can name the drug, dosage, adverse effects to watch for, and specific measures to avoid them).
- Monitor effectiveness of comfort measures and compliance with the regimen.

KEY POINTS

- In women with functioning ovaries, fertility drugs increase follicle development by stimulating FSH and LH to increase the chances for pregnancy.
- Women receiving fertility drugs need to be monitored for ovarian overstimulation, need to be aware of the possibility of multiple births, and need support and encouragement to deal with the self-esteem issues associated with infertility.

Uterine Motility Drugs

Uterine motility drugs stimulate uterine contractions to assist labor (oxytocics) or induce abortion (abortifacients). Tocolytics are drugs used to slow uterine activity. Terbutaline, a $beta_2$-selective adrenergic agonist, was widely used off-label as a tocolytic agent to relax the gravid uterus to prolong pregnancy. In 2011 the U.S. Food and Drug Administration (FDA) required a black box warning on this drug alerting prescribers to significant risks in using the drug for this purpose and stressing that this was not an approved indication for the drug. That same year, hydroxyprogesterone caproate (*Makena*) was approved to reduce the risk of preterm birth in women with a single-fetus pregnancy and a history of singleton spontaneous preterm birth. It is not approved for use in multiple-fetus pregnancies. It is a synthetic progestin and has the effects and adverse effects of the progestins. It is given by IM injection by a health care provider once a week, starting between 16 and 20 weeks of gestation and continuing until the 37th week. Oxytocics and abortifacients are discussed in detail in this section and in Table 40.4.

Oxytocics

Oxytocics stimulate contraction of the uterus, much like the action of the hypothalamic hormone oxytocin, which is stored in the posterior pituitary. These drugs include methylergonovine (*Methergine*), and oxytocin (*Pitocin*)

Therapeutic Actions and Indications

The oxytocics directly affect neuroreceptor sites to stimulate contraction of the uterus. They are especially effective in the gravid uterus. Oxytocin, a synthetic form of the hypothalamic hormone, also stimulates the lacteal glands in the breast to contract, promoting milk ejection in lactating women. Oxytocics are indicated for the prevention and treatment of uterine atony after

Table 40.4 ***Drugs in Focus:* Uterine Motility Drugs**

Drug Name	Dosage/Route	Usual Indications
Oxytocics		
methylergonovine (*Methergine*)	0.2 mg IM or IV, may repeat q2–4 h; 0.2 mg PO t.i.d. during the puerperium for up to 1 wk	Promotion of postpartum uterine involution; stimulation of last stage of labor
oxytocin (*Pitocin*)	1–2 mU/min IV through an infusion pump, increase as needed, do not exceed 20 mU/min; 10 units IM after delivery of the placenta; one spray in each nostril 2–3 min before breastfeeding	Induction of labor; promotion of uterine contractions postpartum; used nasally to stimulate milk "let down" in lactating women; also being evaluated as a diagnostic agent to test abnormal fetal heart rates (oxytocin challenge) and to treat breast engorgement
Abortifacients		
carboprost (*Hemabate*)	250 mcg IM at intervals of 1.5–3.5 h, not to exceed 12-mg total dose; 250 mcg IM to control postpartum bleeding, not to exceed 2-mg total dose	Stimulates uterine muscle contraction (similar to labor contractions) for termination of early pregnancy; evacuation of missed abortion; control of postpartum hemorrhage and uterine atony that does not respond to other therapy
dinoprostone (*Cervidil, Propedil Gel, Prostin E2*)	20-mg vaginal suppository, may repeat q3–5 h as needed for termination of pregnancy; 0.5-mg gel via cervical catheter, repeated in 6 h if needed for cervical ripening, then wait 6–12 h before using oxytocin	A prostaglandin used for evacuation of the uterus; stimulation of cervical ripening before labor
mifepristone (*Mifeprex, RU-486*)	600 mg PO as a single dose; if pregnancy not terminated by day 3, 400-mcg misoprostol PO; if not terminated by day 14, surgical intervention is suggested	Approved for use in terminating early pregnancy during the first 49 d by acting as an antagonist of progesterone to stimulate uterine activity by sites in the endometrium to dislodge or prevent the implantation of any fertilized eggs

delivery. This is important to prevent postpartum hemorrhage. See Table 40.4 for Usual Indications for each of these drugs.

Pharmacokinetics

The oxytocics are rapidly absorbed after parenteral or oral administration, metabolized in the liver, and excreted in the urine and feces. They cross the placenta and enter breast milk.

The oxytocics are administered IM or IV. Methylergonovine is administered as such directly after delivery and then continued in the oral form to promote uterine involution. Oxytocin is also used in a nasal form to stimulate milk "let down" in lactating women.

Contraindications and Cautions

Oxytocics are contraindicated in the presence of any known allergy to oxytocics *to avoid hypersensitivity reactions* and with cephalopelvic disproportion, unfavorable fetal position, complete uterine atony, or early pregnancy, *which could be compromised by uterine stimulation.* Oxytocin is used during lactation because of its effects on milk ejection, but the baby should be evaluated for any adverse effects associated with the hormone. Caution should be used in patients with coronary disease and hypertension *due to the effect of causing arterial contraction, which could raise blood pressure or compromise coronary blood flow,* or in patients who have had previous cesarean births *because of the effects on uterine contraction, which could compromise scars from previous procedures.* Caution should be used in hepatic or renal impairment, *which could alter the metabolism or excretion of the drug.*

Adverse Effects

The adverse effects most often associated with the oxytocics are related to excessive effects (e.g., uterine hypertonicity and spasm, uterine rupture, postpartum hemorrhage, decreased fetal heart rate). GI upset, nausea, headache, and dizziness also are common. Methylergonovine can produce ergotism, manifested by nausea, blood pressure changes, weak pulse, dyspnea, chest pain, numbness and coldness in extremities, confusion, excitement, delirium, convulsions, and even coma. Oxytocin has caused severe water intoxication with coma and even maternal death when used for a prolonged period. This is thought to occur because of related effects of antidiuretic hormone, which is also stored in the posterior pituitary and may be released in response to oxytocin activity, causing water retention by the kidney.

Ⓟ Prototype Summary: Oxytocin

Indications: To initiate or improve uterine contractions for early vaginal delivery; to stimulate or reinforce labor in selected cases of uterine inertia; to manage inevitable or incomplete abortion; for second-trimester abortion; to control postpartum bleeding or hemorrhage; to treat lactation deficiency.

Actions: Synthetic form stimulates the uterus, especially the gravid uterus; causes myoepithelium of the lacteal glands to contract, resulting in milk ejection in lactating women.

Pharmacokinetics:

Route	Onset	Peak	Duration
IV	Immediate	Unknown	60 min
IM	3–5 min	Unknown	2–3 h

$T_{1/2}$: 1 to 6 minutes; metabolized in the tissue and excreted in the urine.

Adverse Effects: Cardiac arrhythmias, hypertension, fetal bradycardia, nausea, vomiting, uterine rupture, pelvic hematoma, uterine hypertonicity, severe water intoxication, anaphylactic reaction.

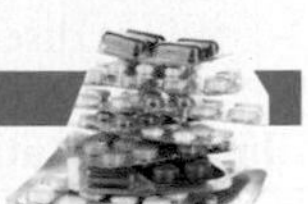

Nursing Considerations for Patients Receiving Oxytocics

Assessment: History and Examination

- Assess for contraindications or cautions: History of allergy to oxytocics *to avoid hypersensitivity reactions;* early status of pregnancy, *which might lead to early onset of labor;* current status of lactation; uterine atony, undesirable fetal position, and cephalopelvic disproportion, *which could be compromised by the stimulatory effects of the drug;* hypertension, *which could be exacerbated due to the drug's effect on arteries;* and history of cesarean birth, *which could lead to uterine rupture or damage to previous surgical sites due to the drug's stimulatory effect on uterine contraction.*
- Perform a complete physical assessment *to establish a baseline before beginning therapy and during therapy to evaluate drug effectiveness and to determine potential adverse effects.*
  - Assess the patient's neurological status, including level of orientation, affect, reflexes, and papillary response.
  - Monitor vital signs, including pulse and blood pressure; auscultate lungs for evidence of adventitious sounds.
  - Assess labor pattern, including uterine contractions, cervical dilation and effacement, and fetal status,

(continues on page 686)

including fetal heart rate, rhythm, and position. Institute electronic fetal monitoring as appropriate.
- Evaluate uterine tone, noting any indications of atony; assess fundal height and uterine involution, and amount and characteristics of vaginal bleeding.
- Monitor the results of laboratory tests, including coagulation studies and complete blood count *to evaluate hematological status.*

Nursing Diagnoses

Nursing diagnoses related to drug therapy might include the following:

- Acute pain related to increased frequency and intensity of uterine contractions or headache
- Excess fluid volume related to ergotism or water intoxication
- Deficient knowledge regarding drug therapy

Planning

- The patient will receive the best therapeutic effect from the drug therapy.
- The patient will have limited adverse effects to the drug therapy.
- The patient will have an understanding of the drug therapy, adverse effects to anticipate, and measures to relieve discomfort and improve safety.

Implementation with Rationale

- Ensure fetal position (if appropriate) and cephalopelvic proportions *to prevent serious complications of delivery.*
- Regulate oxytocin delivery using an infusion pump between contractions if it is being given to stimulate labor *to regulate dose appropriately.*
- Monitor blood pressure and fetal heart rate frequently during and after administration *to monitor for adverse effects.* Discontinue the drug if blood pressure rises dramatically.
- Monitor uterine tone and involution and amount of bleeding *to ensure safe and therapeutic drug use.*
- Discontinue the drug at any sign of uterine hypertonicity *to avoid potentially life-threatening effects*; provide life support as needed.
- Monitor fetal heart rate and rhythm if given during labor *to ensure safety of the fetus.*
- Provide nasal oxytocin at bedside with the bottle sitting upright. Have the patient invert the squeeze bottle and exert gentle pressure to deliver the drug just before nursing *to achieve greatest therapeutic effect to stimulate milk "let down."*
- Provide patient teaching about administration technique for nasal oxytocin if indicated, required monitoring and assessments, danger signs and symptoms to report immediately, possible adverse effects, measures to be instituted to reduce the risk of adverse effects, safety and comfort measures, measures to promote effective breastfeeding as appropriate (for nasal administration of oxytocin), and ongoing need for continued monitoring and evaluation *to enhance patient knowledge of drug therapy and to promote compliance.*

Evaluation

- Monitor patient response to the drug (uterine contraction, prevention of hemorrhage, milk "let down").
- Monitor for adverse effects (blood pressure changes, uterine hypertonicity, water intoxication, ergotism).
- Evaluate the effectiveness of the teaching plan (the patient can name the drug, dosage, adverse effects to watch for, and specific measures to avoid them).
- Monitor the effectiveness of comfort measures and compliance with the regimen.

Abortifacients

Abortifacients are used to evacuate uterine contents via intense uterine contractions. These drugs include carboprost (*Hemabate*), dinoprostone (*Cervidil, Prepidil Gel, Prostin E2*), and mifepristone (RU-486, *Mifeprex*). Some serious name confusion has been reported with dinoprostone and other drugs.

FOCUS ON Safe Medication Administration

Name confusion has been reported among ***Prostin VR Pediatric*** *(alprostadil),* ***Prostin E2*** *(dinoprostone), and* ***Prostin 15*** *(carboprost, available in Europe). Confusion has also been reported between* ***Prepidil*** *(dinoprostone) and bepridil, a calcium-channel blocker. Use extreme caution to make sure that your patient is receiving the correct drug. Serious adverse effects and lack of therapeutic effects can occur if the wrong drug is given to the patient.*

Therapeutic Actions and Indications

The abortifacients stimulate uterine activity, dislodging any implanted trophoblasts and preventing implantation of any fertilized egg. These drugs are approved for use to terminate pregnancy at 12 to 20 weeks from the date of the last menstrual period. See Table 40.4 for Usual Indications for each of these agents.

Pharmacokinetics

These drugs are well absorbed when administered. They are metabolized in the liver and excreted in the urine. Because of their effects on the uterus, they are used during pregnancy only to end the pregnancy. Mifepristone is administered orally and takes 5 to 7 days to produce the desired effect.

Carboprost is available as an IM injection, with an onset of 15 minutes and a duration of 2 hours. Dinoprostone is given by intravaginal suppository, with an onset of effects in 10 minutes and a duration of effects of 2 hours.

Contraindications and Cautions

Abortifacients should not be used with any known allergy to abortifacients or prostaglandins *to avoid hypersensitivity reactions*; after 20 weeks from the last menstrual period, *which would be too late into the pregnancy for an abortion*; or with active PID or acute CV, hepatic, renal, or pulmonary disease, *which could be exacerbated by the effects of these drugs.* They are not recommended for use during lactation *because of the potential for serious effects on the neonate.* If these drugs are to be used by a lactating mother, another method of feeding the baby should be used.

Caution should be used with any history of asthma, hypertension, or adrenal disease, *which could be exacerbated by the drug effects*, and with acute vaginitis (inflammation of the vagina) or scarred uterus, *which could be aggravated by the uterine contractions.*

Adverse Effects

Adverse effects associated with abortifacients include abdominal cramping, heavy uterine bleeding, perforated uterus, and uterine rupture, all of which are related to exaggeration of the desired effects of the drug. Other adverse effects include headache, nausea and vomiting, diarrhea, diaphoresis (sweating), backache, and rash.

Ⓟ Prototype Summary: Dinoprostone

Indications: Termination of pregnancy 12 to 20 weeks from the first day of the last menstrual period; evacuation of the uterus in the management of missed abortion or intrauterine fetal death; management of nonmetastatic gestational trophoblastic disease; initiation of cervical ripening.

Actions: Stimulates the myometrium of the pregnant uterus to contract, evacuating the contents of the uterus.

Pharmacokinetics:

Route	Onset	Peak	Duration
Intravaginal	10 min	15 min	2–3 h

$T_{1/2}$: 5 to 10 hours; metabolized in the tissue and excreted in the urine.

Adverse Effects: Headache, paresthesias, hypotension, vomiting, diarrhea, nausea, uterine rupture, uterine or vaginal pain, chills, diaphoresis, backache, fever.

Nursing Considerations for Patients Receiving Abortifacients

Assessment: History and Examination

- Assess for contraindications or cautions: History of allergy to any abortifacient or prostaglandin preparation *to avoid hypersensitivity reactions*; active pelvic inflammatory disease, *which could be exacerbated by the increased uterine activity*; cardiac, hepatic, pulmonary, or renal disease problems, *which could be exacerbated by the effects of the drug*; history of asthma, *which predisposes the patient to hypersensitivity reactions*; hypotension, hypertension, and epilepsy, *which require cautious use of the drug*; and scarred uterus or acute vaginitis, *which could be exacerbated by the strong uterine contractions.*
- Perform a psychological assessment to determine teaching and support needs *as these patients are often very stressed, anxious, and can experience bouts of depression which the nurse will need to be ready to address.*
- Perform a complete physical assessment before beginning therapy *to establish baseline status and during therapy to determine drug effectiveness and evaluate for any potential adverse effects.*
- Confirm date of last menstrual period and estimated duration of pregnancy *to ensure appropriate use of the drug.*
- Assess vital signs, including skin and lesions; orientation and affect; and blood pressure, pulse, and respiration; and auscultate lung sounds, *to monitor for vascular effects, including bleeding and hypersensitivity reactions.*
- Assist with or complete a pelvic examination, observe for vaginal discharge, and evaluate uterine tone to *monitor effectiveness of the drug and the occurrence of adverse effects.*
- Monitor the results of laboratory tests, including complete blood count (e.g., leukocyte count, hemoglobin, and hematocrit), *to monitor for excess bleeding*, and urinalysis to *monitor for potential infection or reaction to the procedure.*

Nursing Diagnoses

Nursing diagnoses related to drug therapy might include the following:

- Acute pain related to uterine contractions or headache
- Ineffective coping related to abortion or fetal death
- Risk for injury related to increased risk for heavy vaginal bleeding
- Risk for fluid volume deficit related to blood loss, diarrhea, and diaphoresis
- Deficient knowledge regarding drug therapy

(continues on page 688)

Planning

- The patient will receive the best therapeutic effect from the drug therapy.
- The patient will have limited adverse effects to the drug therapy.
- The patient will have an understanding of the drug therapy, adverse effects to anticipate, and measures to relieve discomfort and improve safety.

Implementation with Rationale

- Administer via route indicated, following the manufacturer's directions for storage and preparation, *to ensure safe and therapeutic use of the drug.*
- Confirm the age of the pregnancy before administering the drug *to ensure appropriate use of the drug.*
- Confirm that abortion or uterine evacuation is complete by assessing vaginal bleeding and passing of tissue in the vaginal blood *to avoid potential bleeding problems*; prepare for dilation and curettage if necessary *to stop excessive blood loss.*
- Monitor blood pressure frequently during and after administration *to assess for adverse effects*; discontinue the drug if blood pressure rises dramatically.
- Monitor uterine tone and involution and the amount of bleeding during and for several days after use of the drug *to ensure appropriate response to and recovery from the drug.*
- Provide support and appropriate referrals *to help the patient deal with abortion or fetal death.*
- Provide patient teaching, including monitoring necessary during drug administration, comfort measures, signs and symptoms of adverse effects, measures to minimize or prevent adverse effects, danger signs and symptoms to report immediately, need for follow-up monitoring and evaluation, and sources for support and referrals *to enhance patient knowledge about drug therapy and to promote compliance.*

Evaluation

- Monitor patient response to the drug (evacuation of uterus).
- Monitor for adverse effects (GI upset, nausea, blood pressure changes, hemorrhage, uterine rupture).
- Evaluate the effectiveness of the teaching plan (the patient can name the drug, dosage, adverse effects to watch for, and specific measures to avoid them).
- Monitor the effectiveness of comfort measures and compliance with the regimen.

KEY POINTS

- Oxytocic drugs act like the hypothalamic hormone oxytocin to stimulate uterine contractions and induce or speed up labor and to control bleeding and promote postpartum involution of the uterus.
- Abortifacients are drugs that stimulate uterine activity to cause uterine evacuation. These drugs can be used to induce abortion in early pregnancy or to promote uterine evacuation after intrauterine fetal death.
- Tocolytics are drugs that relax the uterine smooth muscle; they are used to stop premature labor in patients after 20 weeks of gestation. Hydroxyprogesterone caproate is the only drug available for this purpose.

SUMMARY

- Estrogens primarily are used pharmacologically to replace hormones lost at menopause to reduce the signs and symptoms associated with menopause, to stimulate ovulation in woman with hypogonadism, and in combination with progestins for oral contraceptives.
- Progestins, which include progesterone and all of its derivatives, are female sex hormones that are responsible for the maintenance of a pregnancy and for the development of some secondary sex characteristics.
- Progestins are used in combination with estrogens for contraception, to treat uterine bleeding, and for palliation in certain cancers with sensitive receptor sites.
- Fertility drugs stimulate FSH and LH in women with functioning ovaries to increase follicle development and improve the chances for pregnancy.
- A major adverse effect of fertility drugs is multiple births and birth defects.
- Oxytocic drugs act like the hypothalamic hormone oxytocin to stimulate uterine contractions and induce or speed up labor and to control bleeding and promote postpartum involution of the uterus.
- Abortifacients are drugs that stimulate uterine activity to cause uterine evacuation. These drugs can be used to induce abortion in early pregnancy or to promote uterine evacuation after intrauterine fetal death.
- Tocolytics are drugs that relax the uterine smooth muscle; they are used to stop premature labor in patients after 20 weeks of gestation. Hydroxyprogesterone caproate is the only drug approved for this purpose in the United States.

CHECK YOUR UNDERSTANDING

Answers to the questions in this chapter can be found in Answers to Check Your Understanding Questions on thePoint.

MULTIPLE CHOICE

Select the best answer to the following.

1. A postmenopausal woman is to receive short-term HRT to control her menopausal symptoms. Which of the following would the nurse include when teaching the woman about possible adverse effects of this therapy?
a. Constipation
b. Breakthrough bleeding
c. Weight loss
d. Persistently elevated body temperature

2. An estrogen receptor modulator might be the drug of choice in the treatment of postmenopausal osteoporosis in a patient with a family history of breast or uterine cancer. The nurse would instruct the patient that she might experience which of the following?
a. Constipation and dry, itchy skin
b. Flushing and dry vaginal mucosa
c. Hot flashes and vaginal bleeding
d. Diarrhea and weight loss

3. Combination estrogens and progestins are commonly used as OCs. It is thought that this combination has its effect by
a. acting to block the release of FSH and LH, preventing follicle development.
b. directly suppressing the ovaries and preventing ovulation.
c. keeping the endometrium constantly thick and blood filled.
d. preventing menstruation, which prevents pregnancy.

4. Any patient who is taking estrogens, progestins, or combination products should be cautioned to avoid smoking because
a. nicotine increases the metabolism of the hormones, making them less effective.
b. the risk for potentially dangerous thromboembolic episodes increases.
c. nicotine amplifies the adverse effects of the hormones.
d. nicotine blocks hormone receptor sites, and they may no longer be effective.

5. Oxytocin, a synthetic form of the hypothalamic hormone, is used to
a. induce abortion via uterine expulsion.
b. stimulate milk "let down" in the lactating woman.
c. increase fertility and the chance of conception.
d. relax the gravid uterus to prevent preterm labor.

6. The use of an abortifacient drug is contraindicated in a woman
a. who is 15 weeks pregnant.
b. who is older than 50 years of age.
c. who has a history of four previous cesarean births.
d. who is 10 weeks pregnant.

7. A young woman chooses OCs because she feels that it is not the right time for her to get pregnant. You would evaluate her teaching about the drug to be effective if she tells you which of the following?
a. "I shouldn't smoke for the first month to make sure I don't react severely to the pills."
b. "If I forget to take a pill, I'll just start over the next day with a new series of pills."
c. "I may not be able to wear my contact lenses while taking these pills, or I might have to be fitted for a new pair."
d. "If I have to take an antibiotic while I am using these pills, I should take double pills on those days that I am using the antibiotic."

MULTIPLE RESPONSE

Select all that apply.

1. Estrogens produce a wide variety of systemic effects. Effects attributed to estrogen include
a. protecting the heart from atherosclerosis.
b. retaining calcium in the bones.
c. maintaining the secondary female sex characteristics.
d. relaxing the gravid uterus to prolong pregnancy.
e. stimulating the uterus to increase the chances of conception.
f. relaxing blood vessels.

(continues on page 690)

2. A client is taking clomiphene after 6 years of inability to conceive a child. The client will need to be informed about which of the following?
a. The need for a complete physical and pelvic examination before each course of drug therapy
b. The risks and hazards of multiple births
c. The importance of scheduling treatments and intercourse to increase the chance of conception
d. The need to use OCs during drug therapy
e. The need to report blurred vision
f. Common adverse effects include light-headedness, dizziness, and drowsiness

3. A client is receiving an oxytocic drug to stimulate labor. The nursing care of this client would include which of the following?
a. Monitoring of fetal heart rate during labor
b. Regulation of drug delivery between contractions
c. Administration of blood pressure–lowering drugs to balance hypertensive effects
d. Monitoring of maternal blood pressure periodically during and after administration
e. Close monitoring of maternal blood loss following delivery
f. Isolation of the mother and newborn to prevent infection

BIBLIOGRAPHY AND REFERENCES

Aschenbrenner, D. (2004). HRT reconsidered: What should you tell the patient about it now? *American Journal of Nursing, 104*, 51–53.

Bernstein, P., & Pohost, G. (2010). Progesterone, progestins and the heart. *Reviews in Cardiovascular Medicine, 11*(4), 228–236.

Brunton, L., Chabner, B., & Knollman, B. (2011). *Goodman and Gilman's the pharmacological basis of therapeutics* (12th ed.). New York: McGraw-Hill.

Facts and Comparisons. (2015). *Drug facts and comparisons*. St. Louis, MO: Author.

FDA's decision regarding Plan B [*U.S. Food and Drug Administration*]. Available online at: http://www.fda.gov/Drugs/DrugSafety/PostmarketDrugSafetyInformationforPatientsandProviders/ucm109795.htm

Foster, D., Biggs, M., Phillips, K., et al. (2015). Potential public sector cost-savings from OTC access to oral contraceptives. *Contraception, 91*(5), 373–379.

Heiss, G., Wallace, R., Anderson, G. L., et al. (2008). Health risks and benefits 3 years after stopping randomized treatment with estrogen and progestin. *Journal of the American Medical Association, 299*, 1036–1045.

Karch, A. M. (2014). *Lippincott's nursing drug guide*. Philadelphia, PA: Lippincott Williams & Wilkins.

Langer, R. D. (2010). The need to clarify and disseminate contemporary knowledge of hormone therapy initiated near menopause. *Climacteric, 13*(4), 303–306

Lindahl, S. H. (2011). Contraception update. *Advance for Nurse Practitioners and Physician Assistants, 2*(1), 31–34.

Moynihan, R. (2014). Evening the score on sex drugs: Feminist movement or marketing masquerade? *British Medical Journal, 349*, 8246.

Panya, N., Hamoda, H., Arya, R., et al. (2013). The 2013 British Menopause Society and Women's Health Concern recommendations on hormone replacement therapy. *Post Reproductive Health, 19*(2), 59–68.

Potera, C. (2011). Unneeded pelvic exams in women seeking birth control. *American Journal of Nursing, 111*(3), 17–20.

Raymond, E. G., Halpern, V., & Lopez, L. M. (2011). Pericoital oral contraception with levonorgestrol: A systematic review. *Obstetrician Gynecology, 117*(3), 673–681.

Taylor, H. S., & Manson, J. E. (2011). Update on hormone therapy use in menopause. *Journal of Clinical Endocrinology and Metabolism, 96*(2), 255–264.

Toh, S., Hernandez-Diaz, S., Logan, R., et al. (2010). Coronary heart disease in postmenopausal recipients of estrogen and progestin therapy: Does the risk ever disappear? *Annals of Internal Medicine, 152*, 211–217.

USPSTF. (2012). Hormone replacement therapy for the prevention of chronic conditions in postmenopausal women [*U.S. Preventative Services Task Force*]. Available online at: http://www.uspreventiveservicestaskforce.org/uspstf/uspspmho.htm

41 Drugs Affecting the Male Reproductive System

Learning Objectives

Upon completion of this chapter, you will be able to:

1. Discuss the effects of testosterone and androgens on the male body and use this information to explain the therapeutic and adverse effects of these agents when used clinically.
2. Describe the therapeutic actions, indications, pharmacokinetics, contraindications, most common adverse reactions, and important drug–drug interactions associated with drugs affecting the male reproductive system.
3. Discuss the use of drugs that affect the male reproductive system across the lifespan.
4. Compare and contrast the prototype drugs testosterone, oxandrolone, and sildenafil with other agents in their class.
5. Outline the nursing considerations, including important teaching points, for patients receiving drugs used to affect the male reproductive system.

Glossary of Key Terms

anabolic steroids: androgens developed with more anabolic or protein-building effects than androgenic effects

androgenic effects: effects associated with development of male sexual characteristics and secondary characteristics (e.g., deepening of voice, hair distribution, genital development, acne)

androgens: male sex hormones, primarily testosterone; produced in the testes and adrenal glands

hirsutism: hair distribution associated with male secondary sex characteristics (e.g., increased hair on trunk, arms, legs, face)

hypogonadism: underdevelopment of the gonads (testes in the male)

penile erectile dysfunction: condition in which the corpus cavernosum does not fill with blood to allow for penile erection; can be related to aging or to neurological or vascular conditions

phosphodiesterase type 5 inhibitors: drugs used in the treatment of erectile dysfunction that cause smooth muscle relaxation, allowing the flow of blood into the corpus cavernosum.

priapism: a painful and continual erection of the penis

Drug List

Androgens
danazol
fluoxymesterone
methyltestosterone
Ⓟ testosterone

Anabolic Steroids
Ⓟ oxandrolone
oxymetholone

Drugs for Treating Penile Erectile Dysfunction
alprostadil
avanafil
Ⓟ sildenafil
tadalafil
vardenafil

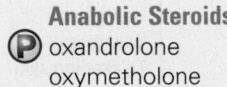

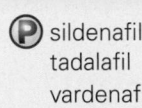

Drugs that are used to affect the male reproductive system include androgens (male steroid hormones), anabolic steroids, and drugs that act to improve penile dysfunction. The male steroids are produced in the testes and affect the entire male reproductive system (Figure 41.1). Box 41.1 describes the effect of these drugs across the lifespan.

Drugs used to treat prostatic hypertrophy are discussed in Chapter 52.

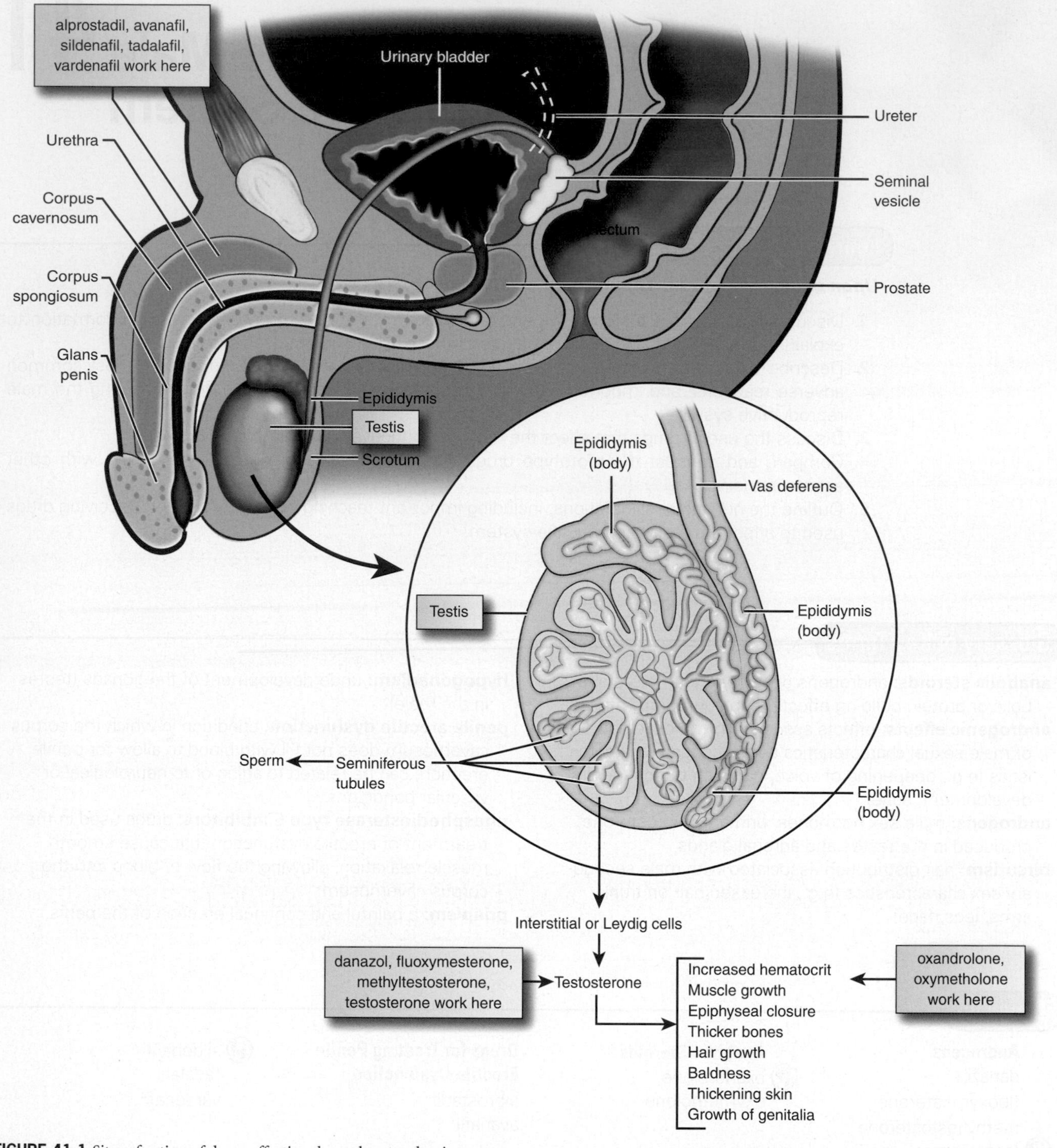

FIGURE 41.1 Sites of action of drugs affecting the male reproductive system.

Androgens

Androgens are male sex hormones and include testosterone, which is produced in the testes, and the androgens, which are produced in the adrenal glands. Testosterone (*Duratest*, *Testoderm*, and others), the primary natural androgen, is the classic androgen in use today. It is used for replacement therapy in cases of **hypogonadism** (underdeveloped testes) and to treat certain breast cancers. Testosterones are all class III controlled substances. Other androgens include danazol (generic), fluoxymesterone (*Android*), and methyltestosterone (*Testred*). See Table 41.1 for more information about these agents.

Therapeutic Actions and Indications

Because the androgens are forms of testosterone, they are responsible for the growth and development of male sex organs and the maintenance of secondary male sex

BOX 41.1 FOCUS ON Drug Therapy Across the Lifespan

Drugs Affecting the Male Reproductive System

CHILDREN

These drugs are used in children as replacement therapy and to increase red blood cell production in renal failure. Because of the effects of these hormones on epiphyseal closure, children should be closely monitored with hand and wrist radiographs pretreatment and every 6 months. If precocious puberty occurs the drug should be stopped.

Adolescents who are prescribed androgens should be alerted to the potential for increased acne and other effects.

Adolescent athletes need constant education about the risks associated with the use of anabolic steroids to improve athletic prowess and the lack of scientific evidence of beneficial effects.

ADULTS

Adults also need reinforcement of the information about anabolic steroid use and athletics.

Women who are prescribed these drugs may experience masculinizing effects and may need support in coping with these body changes. Men who are receiving these drugs for replacement therapy may need to learn self-injection techniques and may benefit from information on depot forms or dermal systems. Periodic liver function tests are important in monitoring the effects of these drugs on the liver.

These drugs are not indicated for use in pregnancy or lactation because of the potential for serious effects on the fetus or neonate.

OLDER ADULTS

Older adults may have problems with androgen therapy because of underlying conditions that are aggravated by the drug effects. Hypertension, heart failure, and coronary artery disease may be aggravated by the fluid retention associated with these drugs. Benign prostatic hypertrophy, a common problem in older men, may be aggravated by androgenic effects that may enlarge the prostate further, leading to urinary difficulties and increased risk of prostate cancer.

Many older adults have hepatic dysfunction, and these drugs can be hepatotoxic. Older patients should be monitored very carefully and dose should be reduced. If signs of liver failure or hepatitis occur the drug should be stopped immediately.

characteristics. They act to increase the retention of nitrogen, sodium, potassium, and phosphorus and to decrease the urinary excretion of calcium. Testosterones increase protein anabolism and decrease protein catabolism (breakdown). They also increase the production of red blood cells. Danazol is used to treat endometriosis, fibrocystic breast disease (in females) and hereditary angioedema. Because it is an androgen, it is able to inhibit the hypothalamic–pituitary–adrenal axis and gonadotropin-releasing hormone, leading to a drop in follicle-stimulating hormone and luteinizing hormone when used in females.

Pharmacokinetics

Testosterone is long acting and is available in several forms, including depot (deep, slow-release) injections,

Table 41.1 ***Drugs in Focus:* Androgens**

Drug Name	Usual Dosage	Usual Indications
danazol (generic)	100–600 mg/d PO, depending on use and response	Blockade of follicle-stimulating hormone and luteinizing hormone release in women to prevent ovulation for treatment of endometriosis, prevention of hereditary angioedema
fluoxymesterone (*Androïd*)	5–20 mg/d PO for replacement therapy, 10–40 mg/d PO for certain breast cancers	Replacement therapy in hypogonadism, treatment of delayed puberty in male patients and certain breast cancers in postmenopausal women
testosterone (*Androderm, Depo-testosterone, Striant, Androgel, Fortesta, Axiron, Natesto, Aveed*)	50–400 mg IM every 2–4 wk, dose varies with preparation; some long-acting depository forms are available; dermatological patch 4–6 mg/d, replace patch daily *Fortesta:* 4 pumps to thighs in the morning *Androgel:* 5 mg applied daily to shoulders, upper arms, or abdomen *Axiron*: 1 pump under each axilla each day *Striant:* 1 system (30 mg) applied to gum region twice a day, 12 h apart *Natesta:* 1 pump in each nostril 3 times each day *Aveed:* 3 mL IM at 0, 4 wk and then every 10 wk	Replacement therapy in hypogonadism, treatment of delayed puberty in male patients and certain breast cancers in postmenopausal women, prevention of postpartum breast engorgement
methyltestosterone (*Testred*)	*Males:* 10–50 mg/d PO *Females:* 50–200 mg/d PO	Replacement therapy in hypogonadism, treatment of delayed puberty in male patients and certain breast cancers in postmenopausal women

buccal systems, topical gels, topical sprays, urethral pellets, and a dermal patch. Danazol, a synthetic androgen, is also long acting but is available only in oral form. Methyltestosterone and fluoxymesterone have long half-lives and are available in the oral form. The androgens are well absorbed and widely distributed throughout the body. They are metabolized in the liver and excreted in the urine. It is not known whether androgens enter breast milk (see Contraindications and Cautions).

Contraindications and Cautions

These drugs are contraindicated with any known allergy to the drug or ingredients in the drug *to prevent hypersensitivity reactions*, during pregnancy and lactation *because of potential adverse effects on the neonate* (another method of feeding the baby should be used if these drugs are needed during lactation), and in the presence of prostate or breast cancer in men, *which could be aggravated by the testosterone effects of the drugs*. They should be used cautiously in the presence of any liver dysfunction or cardiovascular disease *because these disorders could be exacerbated by the effects of the hormones*. The topical forms of testosterone have a black box warning alerting the user to the risk of virilization in children who come in contact with the drug from touching the clothes and skin of the man using the drug. They are advised to cover all application areas if coming in contact with children and wash all clothing that has touched the area before children come in contact with it. Danazol has a black box warning regarding the risk for thromboembolic events, fetal abnormalities, hepatitis, and intracranial hypertension. Health care providers are advised that the drug is not for long-term use and to take appropriate precautions with all patients.

Adverse Effects

Androgenic effects include acne, edema, **hirsutism** (increased hair distribution), deepening of the voice, oily skin and hair, weight gain, decrease in breast size, and testicular atrophy. Antiestrogen effects—flushing, sweating, vaginitis, nervousness, and emotional lability—can be anticipated when these drugs are used with women. Other common effects include headache (possibly related to fluid and electrolyte changes), dizziness, sleep disorders and fatigue, rash, and altered serum electrolytes (Figure 41.2). A potentially life-threatening effect that has been documented is hepatocellular cancer. This may occur because of the effect of testosterone on hepatic cells. Patients on long-term therapy should have hepatic function tests monitored regularly—before beginning therapy and every 6 months during therapy. Inappropriate use of testosterone has led to cardiovascular events including myocardial infarction (MI) and stroke and venous embolic events, including deep-vein thrombosis (DVT) and pulmonary embolism (PE). The U.S. Food and Drug Administration (FDA) has issued warnings for all testosterone products after follow-up studies showed the risk of using these products for unapproved indications. The media pushing treatment for "Low-T syndrome" (see Box 41.2) led to these warnings, and further studies are being conducted. All testosterone products now carry a general warning about the risks of cardiovascular events and the need to evaluate the patient carefully for appropriate use of the drugs.

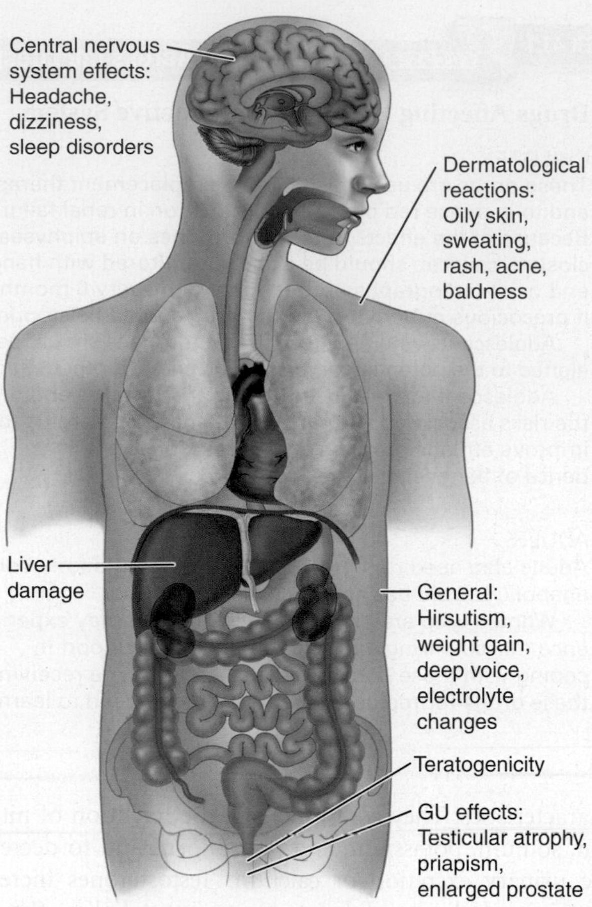

FIGURE 41.2 Variety of adverse effects and toxicities associated with the use of drugs that affect the male reproductive system.

Clinically Significant Drug–Laboratory Test Interferences

While a patient is taking androgens, there may be decreased thyroid function as well as increased creatinine and creatinine clearance, results that are not associated with disease states. These effects can last up to 2 weeks after discontinuation of therapy.

BOX 41.2

Low-Testosterone Syndrome

2013 saw many mass media ads promoting the use of testosterone for treating "Low T syndrome." The signs and symptoms that men were told to look for as they were aging included fatigue, loss of hair, depression, muscle weakness, and decreased energy. Many could report those signs and symptoms without a problem with testosterone. Low testosterone levels can be associated with many chronic diseases, such as chronic obstructive pulmonary disease (COPD), renal failure, or diabetes mellitus. There is little evidence-based research on the effects of a normally falling level of testosterone associated with age. The testosterone replacement drugs that have been tested and approved are for the treatment of hypogonadism or certain cancers. They have not been approved to treat a declining testosterone level associated with age. With many men demanding testosterone replacement for their "Low T syndrome," data started to accumulate of the risks associated with using testosterone replacement for unapproved indications. Reports of cardiovascular events, including MI, strokes, and thromboemboli, led to a general warning on all testosterone products that patients should be cautioned about this risk and the drugs should be avoided with known cardiovascular problems and a reminder that the drugs should only be used for approved indications. In 2015 more problems were reported and a new general warning was issued about the risk of venous clots, including DVT and PE. This warning included another reminder that approved testosterone products are for men with documented low testosterone levels associated with medical conditions. In our electronic age, it is often a challenge to separate evidence from advertising in an attempt to ensure patient safety.

Nursing Considerations for Patients Receiving Androgens

Assessment: History and Examination

- Assess for contraindications or cautions to the use of the drug, including history of allergy to any testosterone or androgen *to avoid hypersensitivity reactions*, pregnancy or lactation *to avoid potential adverse effects on the fetus or baby*, hepatic dysfunction *to avoid the risk of hepatocellular disorders*, and cardiovascular disease and breast or prostate cancer in men, *which could be aggravated by the drug.*
- Perform a physical assessment *to determine baseline status before beginning therapy and for any potential adverse effects.*
- Assess skin color, lesions, texture, and hair distribution *to monitor for drug effects on the body and potential adverse effects.*
- Monitor affect, orientation, and peripheral sensation *to assess CNS effects related to drug use.*
- Perform abdominal examination and serum electrolytes, serum cholesterol, and liver function tests *to monitor for potential effects on liver function.*
- Arrange for radiographs of the long bones in children *to assess for testosterone effects on growth.*

Nursing Diagnoses

Nursing diagnoses related to drug therapy might include the following:

- Disturbed body image related to androgenic effects
- Acute pain related to need for injections
- Sexual dysfunction related to androgenic effects
- Deficient knowledge regarding drug therapy

Planning

- The patient will receive the best therapeutic effect from the drug therapy.
- The patient will have limited adverse effects to the drug therapy.
- The patient will have an understanding of the drug therapy, adverse effects to anticipate, and measures to relieve discomfort and improve safety.

Implementation with Rationale

- Reconstitute the drug according to the manufacturer's directions *to ensure proper reconstitution and to administer as prescribed.*
- Remove an old dermal system before applying a new system to clean, dry, intact skin *to ensure accurate administration and decrease risk of toxic levels.*
- When using any of the topical testosterones or nasal testosterone, follow the manufacturer's guidelines regarding placement, frequency, and protection of the area being used for application *to ensure therapeutic effectiveness and decrease the incidence of adverse effects.*
- Monitor response carefully when beginning therapy *so that the dose can be adjusted accordingly.*
- Monitor liver function periodically with long-term therapy and *arrange to discontinue the drug at any sign of hepatic dysfunction.*

(continues on page 696)

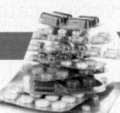

- Provide thorough patient teaching, including measures to avoid adverse effects, warning signs of problems, and the need for regular evaluation, including blood tests. Instruct a family member or caregiver in proper preparation and administration techniques as appropriate *to enhance patient knowledge about drug therapy and to promote compliance with the drug regimen.*

Evaluation

- Monitor patient response to the drug (onset of puberty, maintenance of male sexual characteristics, palliation of breast cancer, blockage of ovulation, prevention of postpartum breast engorgement, relief of angioedema).
- Monitor for adverse effects (androgenic effects, hypoestrogenic effects, serum electrolyte imbalance, headache, sleep disturbances, rash, hepatocellular carcinoma).
- Evaluate the effectiveness of the teaching plan (patient can name drug, dosage, adverse effects to watch for, and specific measures to avoid them; family member or caregiver can demonstrate proper technique for preparation and administration of the drug as appropriate).
- Monitor the effectiveness of comfort measures and compliance with the regimen.

Prototype Summary: Testosterone

Indications: Replacement therapy in hypogonadism, inoperable breast cancer.

Actions: Primary natural androgen, responsible for growth and development of male sex organs and maintenance of secondary sex characteristics; increases the retention of nitrogen, sodium, potassium, and phosphorus; decreases urinary excretion of calcium; increases protein anabolism; stimulates red blood cell production.

Pharmacokinetics:

Route	Onset	Peak
Buccal	Slow	10–12 h
IM	Slow	1–3 d
IM cypionate	Slow	2–4 wk
IM enanthate	Slow	2–4 wk
Dermal	Rapid	24 h
Nasal	Rapid	40 min

$T_{1/2}$: 10 to 100 minutes; metabolized in the liver and excreted in the urine and feces.

Adverse Effects: Dizziness, headache, sleep disorders, fatigue, rash, androgenic effects (acne, deepening voice, oily skin), hypoestrogenic effects (flushing, sweating, vaginitis), polycythemia, nausea, hepatocellular carcinoma.

KEY POINTS

- Androgens are the male sex hormones that are responsible for the development and maintenance of male sex characteristics and secondary sex characteristics or androgenic effects.
- Androgens are used for replacement therapy or to block other hormonal effects.

Anabolic Steroids

The **anabolic steroids** are analogues of testosterone that have been developed to produce the tissue-building effects of testosterone with less androgenic effect. Anabolic steroids include oxandrolone (*Oxandrin*) and oxymetholone (*Anadrol-50*).

Therapeutic Actions and Indications

Anabolic steroids promote body tissue–building processes, reverse catabolic or tissue-destroying processes, and increase hemoglobin and red blood cell mass. Indications for particular anabolic steroids vary with the drug (see Table 41.2). They can be used to treat anemias, certain cancers, and angioedema and to promote weight gain and tissue repair in debilitated patients and protein anabolism in patients who are receiving long-term corticosteroid therapy.

Anabolic steroids are also known to be used illegally for the enhancement of athletic performance by promoting increased muscle mass, increased hematocrit, and theoretically an increase in strength and endurance. They are class III controlled substances. The adverse effects of these drugs can be deadly when they are used in the amounts needed for enhanced athletic performance (see Adverse Effects).

Pharmacokinetics

Oxandrolone and oxymetholone are available orally. Like the androgens, the anabolic steroids are well absorbed and widely distributed throughout the body. They are metabolized in the liver and excreted in the urine. Anabolic steroids are contraindicated for use in pregnancy because of adverse effects on the fetus. It is not known whether anabolic steroids enter breast milk, but because of the potential for adverse effects another method of feeding the baby should be used if these drugs are needed during lactation.

Contraindications and Cautions

These drugs are contraindicated in the presence of any known allergy to anabolic steroids *to prevent hypersensitivity reactions*, during pregnancy and lactation *because of potential masculinization in the neonate*, and in the presence

Table 41.2 Drugs in Focus: Anabolic Steroids

Drug Name	Usual Dosage	Usual Indications
oxandrolone (*Oxandrin*)	*Adult:* 2.5 mg PO two to four times daily, maximum dose 20 mg/d *Pediatric:* <0.1 mg/kg/d PO, monitor closely, may be repeated intermittently	Promotion of weight gain in debilitated patients, treatment of certain cancers, relief of bone pain of osteoporosis, promotion of catabolism with prolonged corticosteroid use
oxymetholone (*Anadrol-50*)	1–5 mg/kg/d PO	Treatment of anemias in adults

of liver dysfunction (*because these drugs are metabolized in the liver and are known to cause liver toxicity*), coronary disease (*because of cholesterol-raising effects through effects on the liver and direct effects on the vascular system*), or prostate or breast cancer in males, *which would be exacerbated by the effects of these drugs.*

Adverse Effects

In prepubertal males, adverse effects include virilization (e.g., phallic enlargement, hirsutism, increased skin pigmentation). Postpubertal males may experience inhibition of testicular function, gynecomastia, testicular atrophy, **priapism** (a painful and continual erection of the penis), baldness, and change in libido (increased or decreased). Women may experience hirsutism, hoarseness, deepening of the voice, clitoral enlargement, baldness, and menstrual irregularities. As with the androgens, serum electrolyte changes, liver dysfunction (including life-threatening hepatitis), insomnia, and weight gain may occur. These drugs all have black box warnings as alerts to the potentially serious effects of liver tumors, hepatitis, and blood lipid level changes that might be associated with increased risk of coronary artery disease. There is an increased risk of prostate problems, especially in geriatric patients.

See the Critical Thinking Scenario for additional information about treating a patient experiencing adverse effects of anabolic steroids.

Cardiomyopathy, hepatic carcinoma, personality changes, and sexual dysfunction are all associated with the excessive and off-label use of anabolic steroids. These drugs are class III controlled substances, which provides monitoring of their use. There is an increased effort to encourage the use of herbal products to improve athletic performance. These products are advertised as "safe" alternatives (Box 41.3).

BOX 41.3 FOCUS ON Herbal and Alternative Therapies

With an increasing awareness of the risks associated with anabolic steroid use and increasing pressures to make it difficult to get these drugs even illegally, there is an increased push in advertising of alternative or "natural" products that are reported to enhance athletic performance.

Bee pollen: Reported to contain amino acids and other minerals and enzymes. There are no scientific studies regarding its effectiveness. Serious allergic reactions have been reported with the use of this product. Random studies have found a wide variety of ingredients in each product, depending on the season, growing conditions, and geographical area.

Creatine: Contains a substance that is found in muscle and naturally occurs in red meats and other dietary sources. No scientific data are available on its actual effects on energy or athletic performance. It interacts with many other drugs, including nonsteroidal anti-inflammatory drugs, cimetidine, probenecid, and trimethoprim, and can cause serious effects on kidney functioning. Users should be advised to drink plenty of fluids while taking this drug and to monitor for swelling, muscle cramps, and dizziness. Suggested only for short-term use.

Damiana: Used to increase muscle strength, as an aphrodisiac, and to boost mental health. It can cause liver toxicity. It interferes with antidiabetic agents and causes elevated blood sugar concentrations. Users should report muscle spasms or hallucinations.

Spirulina: Used to increase energy and boost metabolism. It may contain toxic metals and can cause serious reactions in children and pets. It interferes with vitamin B_{12} absorption. No scientific studies validate the claims of its effectiveness.

Wild yam: Found to have many estrogen-like effects, this herb is used to increase athletic performance because it may contain a constituent of dehydroepiandrosterone used to slow the aging process and to improve energy and stamina. Preparations interact with disulfiram and metronidazole because they contain alcohol. It is known to be toxic to the liver. Users may experience estrogen-like effects, including breast pain. Users should be monitored closely and urged to report any adverse effects.

Patients who are taking a prescribed androgen or anabolic steroid for a medical condition should be advised to avoid taking any of these herbal remedies because of a risk of adverse effects.

CRITICAL THINKING SCENARIO

Adverse Effects of Anabolic Steroids

THE SITUATION

Senior nursing student K.S. recently became engaged. Her fiancé is a college senior who is training as a javelin thrower in hopes of competing in the Olympics. K.S. noticed that her fiancé had been suffering from gastrointestinal (GI) upset for the last 3 weeks and more recently had developed tremors and muscle cramps. K.S. first suspected that he was suffering from a viral infection, but when the symptoms did not resolve, she became concerned. K.S. tried to get her fiancé to see a doctor, but he refused. Eventually, he admitted that he had begun using anabolic steroids to develop his muscles and improve his athletic prowess. He said that the friend who gave him the drugs told him that stomach upset was normal. He refuses to see a physician because he knows that the use of these drugs is illegal. He believes that using the anabolic steroids for a while will put him closer to his goal. K.S. accepts his explanation but is upset about the use of anabolic steroids. She consults with her clinical instructor about the effects of these drugs.

CRITICAL THINKING

What does K.S. need to know? *Think about the systemic effects of anabolic steroids and the possible long-term effects from their abuse.*

What implications do these effects have for the athlete? *Consider the concern that K.S. must be experiencing. Suggest ways for K.S. to share the information about the actual effects of anabolic steroids with her fiancé and still cope with her own feelings and concerns.*

What are the ethical and legal issues involved when a heath care provider knows about illegal drug use and abuse? *Outline a plan for helping K.S. and her fiancé cope with this issue and its implications for their futures.*

DISCUSSION

Use of anabolic steroids is illegal in almost all organized athletic contests. Random drug testing is done to rule out use of these and other drugs. Not surprisingly, K.S. feels insecure about her fiancé's decision. She needs to know that her discussion will be confidential and that she will receive support for her concerns and her fears. K.S. needs to review the effects of anabolic steroids. Although they do promote muscle development, there has never been any evidence that they actually improve athletic performance. The potential adverse effects of these drugs can be deadly, especially if K.S.'s fiancé is receiving the drugs from a friend and has no medical evaluation or dosage guidance to reduce the risk. Personality changes, cardiomyopathy, liver cancer, and impotence are just a few of the possible adverse effects.

K.S. is in a precarious position. She does not want to interfere with her fiancé's dreams or cause problems in their relationship. She should be encouraged to explain the adverse effects of the drugs to her fiancé, pointing out that he is already experiencing some of them. Adverse effects associated with the drugs can ultimately interfere with, not enhance, his athletic performance. She might be encouraged to practice what she will tell her fiancé and to seek other support as needed.

The sale or distribution of anabolic steroids without a prescription is illegal, and this fact further complicates the situation for K.S. Because she is planning to become a health care provider, she may be obligated by state law to report this information to the authorities. K.S. should research these issues and discuss them further with her clinical instructor and other resource people.

NURSING CARE GUIDE FOR K.S.: ANDROGENS, ANABOLIC STEROIDS

A patient receiving an anabolic steroid for a medical condition would have the following care plan.

Assessment: History and Examination

Assess the patient's health history for allergies to any steroids, breast cancer or prostate cancer in men, hepatic dysfunction, coronary artery disease, pregnancy or breastfeeding in women, or concurrent use of insulin or oral anticoagulants.

Focus the physical examination on the following:

Neurological: Orientation, reflexes, affect

Skin: Color, lesions, hair

CV: Pulse, cardiac auscultation, blood pressure, edema

Genitourinary (GI): Abdominal examination, liver examination

Laboratory tests: Serum electrolytes, hepatic function tests, long-bone x-ray studies

Nursing Diagnoses

Disturbed body image related to drug effects
Sexual dysfunction
Acute pain related to injections
Deficient knowledge regarding drug therapy

Planning

The patient will receive the best therapeutic effect from the drug therapy.

The patient will have limited adverse effects to the drug therapy.

The patient will have an understanding of the drug therapy, adverse effects to anticipate, and measures to relieve discomfort and improve safety.

Adverse Effects of Anabolic Steroids (continued)

Implementation

Administer as prescribed.

Monitor liver function before and periodically during therapy.

Monitor patient response and adjust dose as appropriate.

Provide support and reassurance to deal with drug therapy.

Provide patient teaching regarding drug name, dosage, adverse effects, precautions, warnings to report, and safe administration.

Evaluation

Evaluate drug effects: Maintenance of male sex characteristics, suppression of lactation in women.

Monitor for adverse effects: Androgenic effects, hypoestrogenic effects, hepatic dysfunction, electrolyte imbalance, endocrine changes.

Monitor for drug–drug interactions: Decreased need for insulin, increased bleeding with oral anticoagulants.

Evaluate the effectiveness of the patient-teaching program and comfort and safety measures.

PATIENT TEACHING FOR K.S.

If the patient is taking these drugs to increase body mass following severe weight loss due to trauma, you would teach about the following (sharing this information with those considering the unprescribed use of the drugs might be helpful):

- Androgens or anabolic steroids have properties similar to those of the male sex hormones. Because the formulations have widespread effects, there are often many adverse effects associated with their use.
- These drugs are controlled substances because the tendency for people, and athletes in particular, to abuse them can cause serious medical problems. When the drug is used as prescribed, it is safe, but you will need to be monitored.
- Some of the following adverse effects may occur:
    - *GI upset, nausea, vomiting:* Taking the drug with food usually helps to relieve these effects.
    - *Acne:* This is a hormonal effect; washing your face regularly and avoiding oily foods may help.
    - *Increased facial hair, decreased head hair:* These are hormonal effects; if they become bothersome, consult with your health care provider.
    - *Menstrual irregularities (women):* This is a normal effect of the androgens; if you suspect that you might be pregnant, consult with your health care provider immediately.
    - *Weight gain, increased muscle development:* These are common hormonal effects.
    - *Change in sex drive:* This can be distressing and difficult to deal with; consult with your health care provider if this is a serious concern.
- Report any of the following to your health care provider: Swelling in fingers or legs; continual erection; uncontrollable sex drive; yellowing skin; fever, chills, or rash; chest pain or difficulty breathing; hoarseness; loss of hair or growth of facial hair (women).
    - Tell any doctor, nurse, or other health care provider involved in your care that you are taking this drug.
    - Take this medicine only as directed. In addition, schedule regular medical follow-up, including blood tests, to monitor your response to this drug.
    - Keep this drug and all medications out of the reach of children. Do not give this medication to anyone else or take any similar medication that has not been prescribed for you.

Clinically Important Drug–Drug Interactions

Because the anabolic steroids affect the liver, there is a potential for interaction with oral anticoagulants and a potentially decreased need for antidiabetic agents, which may not be metabolized normally. They may alter lipid metabolism and cause a lack of effectiveness for lipid-lowering agents. Patients should be monitored closely and appropriate dose adjustments made.

Prototype Summary: Oxandrolone

Indications: Adjunctive therapy to promote weight gain after weight loss associated with extensive surgery, chronic infections, or trauma; to offset protein catabolism associated with prolonged corticosteroid use; orphan drug uses: short-stature syndrome; HIV-related cachexia and wasting.

Actions: Testosterone analogue with androgenic and anabolic activity, promotes tissue building, reverses catabolic processes, increases red blood cell mass.

Pharmacokinetics:

Route	Onset
PO	Slow

$T_{1/2}$: 9 hours; metabolized in the liver and excreted in the urine.

Adverse Effects: Excitation; insomnia; virilization; hepatitis; liver cell tumors; blood lipid changes; retention of sodium, water, and chloride; acne; masculinization of females; inhibition of testicular function; priapism; baldness; loss of libido in postpubertal males.

Nursing Considerations for Patients Receiving Anabolic Steroids

Assessment: History and Examination

- Assess for the following conditions, *which could be cautions or contraindications to use of the drug*: History of allergy to any androgens or anabolic steroids, pregnancy or lactation *because of masculinization of the neonate*, prostrate or breast cancer, coronary disease, and hepatic dysfunction.
- Perform a physical assessment *to determine baseline status before beginning therapy and for any potential adverse effects*.
- Assess skin color, lesions, texture, and hair distribution *to monitor for drug effects on the body and potential adverse effects*.
- Monitor affect, orientation, and peripheral sensation *to assess CNS effects related to drug use*.
- Perform abdominal examination and serum electrolytes, serum cholesterol, and liver function tests *to monitor for potential effects on liver function*.
- Arrange for radiographs of the long bones in children *to assess for testosterone effects on growth*.

Nursing Diagnoses

Nursing diagnoses related to drug therapy might include the following:

- Disturbed body image related to systemic effects
- Acute pain related to GI or CNS effects
- Risk for impaired liver function related to liver toxic effects
- Deficient knowledge regarding drug therapy

Planning

- The patient will receive the best therapeutic effect from the drug therapy.
- The patient will have limited adverse effects to the drug therapy.
- The patient will have an understanding of the drug therapy, adverse effects to anticipate, and measures to relieve discomfort and improve safety.

Implementation with Rationale

- Administer with food if GI effects are severe *to relieve GI distress*.
- Monitor endocrine function, hepatic function, and serum electrolytes before and periodically during therapy *so that dose can be adjusted appropriately and severe adverse effects can be avoided*.
- Arrange for radiographs of the long bones of children every 3 to 6 months *so that the drug can be discontinued if bone growth reaches the norm for the child's age*.
- Provide thorough patient teaching, including measures to avoid adverse effects and warning signs of problems, as well as the need for regular evaluation, including blood tests, *to enhance patient knowledge about drug therapy and to promote compliance with the drug regimen*.

Evaluation

- Monitor patient response to the drug (increase in hematocrit, protein anabolism).
- Monitor for adverse effects (androgenic effects, serum electrolyte disturbances, epiphyseal closure, hepatic dysfunction, personality changes, cardiac effects).
- Evaluate the effectiveness of the teaching plan (patient can name drug, dosage, adverse effects to watch for, and specific measures to avoid them).
- Monitor the effectiveness of comfort measures and compliance with the regimen.

KEY POINTS

- Anabolic steroids are testosterone analogues with more anabolic or protein-building effects than androgenic effects.
- Deadly effects may result from the abuse of anabolic steroids by athletes trying to build muscle mass and improve performance.

Drugs for Treating Penile Erectile Dysfunction

Penile erectile dysfunction is a condition in which the corpus cavernosum does not fill with blood to allow for penile erection. This can result from the aging process and in vascular and neurological conditions. Two very different types of drugs are approved for the treatment of this condition. These include the prostaglandin alprostadil (*Caverject*, *Muse*) and the **phosphodiesterase type 5 (PDE5)** receptor inhibitors sildenafil (*Viagra*, also available as *Revatio* for the treatment of pulmonary hypertension), tadalafil (*Cialis* also available as *Adcirca*), and vardenafil (*Levitra*). Box 41.4 contains more information about *Viagra*.

Therapeutic Actions and Indications

When injected directly into the cavernosum, alprostadil acts locally to relax the vascular smooth muscle and allow filling of the corpus cavernosum, causing penile erection. The PDE5 inhibitors avanafil, sildenafil, tadalafil, and vardenafil are selective inhibitors of cyclic guanosine monophosphate (cGMP). The PDE5 inhibitors are taken orally and act to increase nitrous oxide levels in the corpus cavernosum. Nitrous oxide activates the

BOX 41.4 FOCUS ON The Evidence

Viagra—Wonder Drug?

The release of the drug Sildenafil (*Viagra*) to treat penile erectile dysfunction caused a tremendous stir in American society. This was the first oral drug developed to treat a disorder that was common in aging men but was seldom mentioned or discussed. *Viagra*, which facilitates penile erection approximately 1 hour after it is taken, returned sexual function to many of these men.

For many months after its release the drug was the center of controversy, news coverage, and debate. Stand-up comedians, television situation comedies, and Internet joke networks were buzzing with the latest *Viagra* jokes. Insurance companies debated covering the cost of this drug. Was it like cosmetic surgery, and not a necessary treatment, or was it a necessary aid to human physiology? Most insurance companies ended up covering the cost of *Viagra*.

Women's rights groups voiced concern that no drug was approved and covered to help facilitate a woman's sexual response. *Viagra* has gone through clinical trials for the treatment of sexual dysfunction in women; repeated reports seem to indicate that it is not effective. However, *Viagra* has proved to be very effective at increasing sexual functioning for many men. Its success has led to the development of three other drugs in the same class of PDE5 inhibitors—avanafil (*Stendra*), tadalafil (*Cialis*), and vardenafil (*Levitra*).

The use of these drugs is not without risks. Deaths have occurred when these drugs were combined with nitrates (e.g., nitroglycerin) or alpha-adrenergic blockers. Headache, flushing, stomach upset, and urinary tract infections often occur. There have been reports of sudden loss of vision and hearing. These drugs do not work without sexual stimulation. Absorption is delayed if they are taken with a high-fat meal, and patients need to plan accordingly. Patients also should be reminded that they need to use protection against sexually transmitted diseases.

When *Viagra* was the hot, new drug, there was tremendous demand for it from the public. This demand continues, and puts health care providers in the position of ensuring that the drug is right for the patient's actual needs. The cause of penile erectile dysfunction should be determined, if at all possible. If this is a problem that the patient has never before discussed with the health care provider, there could be an underlying medical condition that should be addressed. The adverse effects, timing of administration, and drug combinations to avoid should be discussed with the patient before the drug is prescribed.

With pharmaceutical companies advertising in magazines, on television, and over the Internet, health care providers are often asked for specific prescription drugs based on media advertising. This relatively new phenomenon in health care presents new challenges to the health care provider to ensure quality patient teaching to help the patient understand the actual uses, effects, and rationales for a specific drug therapy.

enzyme cGMP, which causes smooth muscle relaxation, allowing the flow of blood into the corpus cavernosum. They prevent the breakdown of cGMP by phosphodiesterase, leading to increased cGMP levels and prolonged smooth muscle relaxation, thus promoting the flow of blood into the corpus cavernosum, resulting in penile erection.

The prostaglandin alprostadil and the PDE5 inhibitors are indicated for the treatment of penile erectile dysfunction. The PDE5 inhibitors have the advantage of being oral drugs that can be timed in coordination with sexual activity, based on the drug's onset. Sildenafil (*Revatio*) and tadalafil (*Adcirca*) are also approved for the treatment of pulmonary arterial hypertension. These drugs are used for both male and female patients with the disease. By relaxing smooth muscle the pulmonary artery relaxes, and there is less resistance and pressure in the pulmonary bed. For this use the drug is available in oral tablet or suspension and in an IV form. Tadalafil is also approved for daily use in men who are very active sexually. A patient might select this drug if the timing of sexual stimulation is not known and may be several hours away. Vardenafil is available in an orally disintegrating tablet, offering an advantage to men who might have trouble swallowing tablets. See Table 41.3 for Usual Indications for all four of these drugs.

Pharmacokinetics

After injection, alprostadil is metabolized to inactive compounds in the lungs and excreted in the urine. The PDE5 inhibitors are well absorbed from the GI tract, undergo metabolism in the liver, and are excreted in the feces. The differences among the three PDE5 inhibitors lie in their onset and duration of action. Sildenafil has a median onset of 27 minutes and a duration of 4 hours. Patients are encouraged to take the drug 1 hour before anticipated sexual stimulation. Vardenafil has a mean onset of action of 26 minutes and a duration of 4 hours; it is also intended to be taken 1 hour before sexual stimulation. Tadalafil has an onset of action of 45 minutes and a duration of 36 hours. Avanafil, the newest drug in this class, has a rapid onset with peak effects in 30–40 minutes and a duration of 2–3 hours. It can be taken 15–30 minutes before sexual stimulation.

Originally none of these drugs was indicated for use in women, so little was known about use during pregnancy and lactation. These drugs are now used to treat pulmonary hypertension in women and men; it is suggested that they be used during pregnancy or lactation only if clearly indicated and benefits outweigh potential risks. Because the effects on pregnancy are not known, if alprostadil is being used, condoms should be used during intercourse with a pregnant woman.

Table 41.3 ***Drugs in Focus:*** **Drugs Used to Treat Penile Erectile Dysfunction**

Drug Name	Dosage/Route	Usual Indications
alprostadil (*Caverject, Muse*)	2.5 mcg injected intracavernously, titrate the dose to one that will allow a satisfactory erection that is maintained no longer than 1 h; mean dose after 6 mo is reported to be 20.7 mcg	Treatment of penile erectile dysfunction
avanafil (*Stendra*)	100 mg PO 15–30 min before sexual stimulation	Treatment of penile erectile dysfunction
sildenafil (*Viagra, Revatio*)	*Viagra:* 25–100 mg PO taken 1 h before sexual stimulation *Revatio:* 20 mg PO t.i.d., at least 4–6 h apart	Treatment of penile erectile dysfunction Treatment of pulmonary arterial hypertension in men and women
tadalafil (*Cialis, Adcirca*)	*Cialis:* 10 mg PO taken before sexual activity, range 5–20 mg PO, limit use to once a day, 2.5–5 mg/d PO for very sexually active males *Adcirca:* 40 mg/d PO	Treatment of penile erectile dysfunction Treatment of pulmonary artery hypertension in men and women
vardenafil (*Levitra, Staxyn*)	5–10 mg PO taken 1 h before sexual stimulation, range 5–20 mg, limit use to once a day; 10 mg/d PO orally disintegrating tablets	Treatment of penile erectile dysfunction

Contraindications and Cautions

These drugs are contraindicated in the presence of any anatomical obstruction or condition that might predispose to priapism *because the risk could be exacerbated by these drugs.*

They cannot be used with penile implants, and they are not indicated for use to improve sexual performance in women (although sildenafil has been studied for the treatment of sexual dysfunction in women, without positive results). However, sildenafil and tadalafil are used in women for the treatment of pulmonary arterial hypertension.

Caution should be used in patients with bleeding disorders. The PDE5 inhibitors should also be used cautiously in patients with coronary artery disease, active peptic ulcer, retinitis pigmentosa, optic neuropathy, hypotension or severe hypertension, congenital prolonged QT interval, or severe hepatic or renal disorders *because of the risk of exacerbating these diseases.*

FOCUS ON Safe Medication Administration

Patients who are using PDE5 inhibitors need to be advised to avoid drinking grapefruit juice while using the drug. Grapefruit juice can cause a decrease in the metabolism of the PDE5 inhibitor, leading to increased serum levels and a risk of toxicity. They need to know that it takes 48 hours for grapefruit juice to be processed by the body, so they need to avoid it for several days around taking the drug. They should also be advised to avoid taking the drug with or just after a high-fat meal. The presence of fat in the GI tract will delay the absorption and onset of action of the drug, which could cause problems for patients who are timing onset of action with their sexual activity. Administration of the drugs should balance these dietary factors.

Adverse Effects

Adverse effects associated with alprostadil are local effects such as pain at the injection site, infection, priapism, fibrosis, and rash. The PDE5 inhibitors are associated with more systemic effects, including headache, flushing (related to relaxation of vascular smooth muscle), dyspepsia, urinary tract infection, diarrhea, dizziness, optic neuropathy, eighth cranial nerve toxicity and loss of hearing, increased risk of melanoma and rash.

Clinically Important Drug–Drug Interactions

The PDE5 inhibitors cannot be taken in combination with any organic nitrates or alpha-adrenergic blockers, drugs which cause a drop in blood pressure; serious cardiovascular effects, including death, have occurred. There is also a possibility of increased vardenafil or tadalafil levels and effects if PDE5 inhibitors are taken with ketoconazole, itraconazole, or erythromycin; monitor the patient and reduce dose as needed.

Vardenafil and tadalafil serum levels can increase if these drugs are combined with indinavir or ritonavir. If these drugs are being used, limit the dose of the PDE5 inhibitor.

Prototype Summary: Sildenafil

Indications: Treatment of erectile dysfunction in the presence of sexual stimulation, treatment of pulmonary arterial hypertension.

Actions: Inhibits PDE5 receptors, leading to a release of nitrous oxide, which activates cyclic guanosine monophosphate to cause a prolonged smooth muscle relaxation, allowing the flow of blood into the corpus cavernosum and facilitating erection.

Pharmacokinetics:

Route	Onset	Peak	Duration
PO	15–30 min	30–120 min	4 h

$T_{1/2}$: 4 hours; metabolized in the liver and excreted in the urine and feces.

Adverse Effects: Headache, abnormal vision, flushing, dyspepsia, urinary tract infection, rash.

Nursing Considerations for Patients Receiving Drugs to Treat Penile Erectile Dysfunction

Assessment: History and Examination

- Assess for the following conditions, *which could be cautions or contraindications to the use of the drug*: History of allergy to any of the preparations, penile structural abnormalities, penile implants, bleeding disorders, active peptic ulcer, coronary artery disease, hypotension or severe hypertension, congenital prolonged QT interval, or severe hepatic or renal disorders.
- Assess baseline status before beginning therapy *to determine any potential adverse effects.*
- Assess skin and lesions *to monitor for adverse reactions to the drug and cardiovascular perfusion.*
- Monitor orientation, affect, and reflexes *to evaluate CNS changes that might be related to changes in blood pressure and blood flow.*
- Assess blood pressure, pulse, respiration, and adventitious sounds *to evaluate blood flow and potential changes in cardiovascular function.*
- When using alprostadil, perform a local inspection of the penis *to assess local reaction to injection and to monitor for potential infection.*
- Evaluate laboratory tests for bleeding time and liver function *to monitor potential adverse effects on the liver.*

Nursing Diagnoses

Nursing diagnoses related to drug therapy might include the following:

- Disturbed body image related to drug effects and indication
- Acute pain related to injection of alprostadil
- Sexual dysfunction
- Deficient knowledge regarding drug therapy

Planning

- The patient will receive the best therapeutic effect from the drug therapy.
- The patient will have limited adverse effects to the drug therapy.
- The patient will have an understanding of the drug therapy, adverse effects to anticipate, and measures to relieve discomfort and improve safety.

Implementation with Rationale

- Assess the cause of dysfunction before beginning therapy *to ensure appropriate use of these drugs.*
- Monitor patients with vascular disease for any sign of exacerbation *so that the drug can be discontinued before severe adverse effects occur.*
- Instruct the patient in the injection of alprostadil, storage of the drug, filling of the syringe, sterile technique, site rotation, and proper disposal of needles *to ensure safe and proper administration of the drug.*
- Monitor patients who are taking PDE5 inhibitors for use of nitrates or alpha-blockers *to avert potentially serious cardiovascular drug–drug interactions.*
- Provide thorough patient teaching, including measures to avoid adverse effects and warning signs of problems, as well as the need for regular evaluation, *to enhance patient knowledge about drug therapy and to promote compliance with the drug regimen.*

Evaluation

- Monitor patient response to the drug (improvement in penile erection).
- Monitor for adverse effects (dizziness, flushing, local inflammation or infection, fibrosis, diarrhea, dyspepsia).
- Evaluate the effectiveness of the teaching plan (patient can name drug, dosage, adverse effects to watch for, and specific measures to avoid them; patient can demonstrate proper administration of injected drug).
- Monitor the effectiveness of comfort measures and compliance with the regimen.

KEY POINTS

- Penile erectile dysfunction can inhibit erection and male sexual function.
- Alprostadil, a prostaglandin, can be injected into the penis to stimulate erection.
- The PDE5 inhibitors are oral agents that act quickly to promote vascular filling of the corpus cavernosum and promote penile erection. They differ in duration and time of onset. They are effective only in the presence of sexual stimulation.

SUMMARY

- Androgens are male sex hormones—specifically testosterone or testosterone-like compounds.
- Androgens are responsible for the development and maintenance of male sex characteristics and secondary sex characteristics or androgenic effects.
- Side effects related to androgen use involve excess of the desired effects as well as potentially deadly hepatocellular carcinoma.
- Androgens can be used for replacement therapy or to block other hormone effects, as is seen with their use in the treatment of specific breast cancers.
- Anabolic steroids are analogues of testosterone that have been developed to have more anabolic or protein-building effects and fewer androgenic effects.

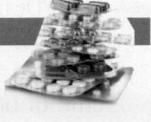

- Anabolic steroids have been abused to enhance muscle development and athletic performance, often with deadly effects.
- Anabolic steroids are used to increase hematocrit and improve protein anabolism in certain depleted states.
- Penile erectile dysfunction can inhibit erection and male sexual function.
- Alprostadil, a prostaglandin, can be injected into the penis to stimulate erection.
- The PDE5 inhibitors are oral agents that act quickly to promote vascular filling of the corpus cavernosum and promote penile erection. They differ in duration and time of onset. They are effective only in the presence of sexual stimulation. They are also used in the treatment of pulmonary arterial hypertension.
- Dangerous cardiovascular effects, including death, have occurred when the PDE5 inhibitors are combined with organic nitrates or alpha-blockers. Careful patient teaching is very important to avoid this drug–drug interaction.

CHECK YOUR UNDERSTANDING

Answers to the questions in this chapter can be found in Answers to Check Your Understanding Questions on thePoint®.

MULTIPLE CHOICE

Select the best answer to the following.

1. Testosterone is approved for use in
  a. treatment of breast cancers.
  b. increasing muscle strength in athletes.
  c. oral contraceptives.
  d. increasing hair distribution in male pattern baldness.

2. Illegal use of large quantities of unprescribed anabolic steroids to enhance athletic performance has been associated with
  a. increased sexual prowess.
  b. muscle rupture from overexpansion.
  c. development of chronic obstructive pulmonary disease.
  d. cardiomyopathy and liver cancers.

3. Anabolic steroids would be indicated for the treatment of
  a. hair loss.
  b. angioedema.
  c. debilitation and severe weight loss.
  d. breast cancers in males.

4. Erectile penile dysfunction is a condition in which
  a. problems with childhood authority figures prevent a male erection.
  b. the corpus cavernosum does not fill with blood to allow for penile erection.
  c. the sympathetic nervous system fails to function.
  d. past exposure to sexually transmitted disease causes physical damage within the penis.

5. A potentially deadly drug–drug interaction can occur if a PDE5 inhibitor (sildenafil, avanafil, tadalafil, or vardenafil) is combined with
  a. corticosteroids.
  b. oral contraceptives.
  c. organic nitrates.
  d. halothane anesthetics.

6. To achieve erection, a patient taking sildenafil (Viagra) would require
  a. sexual stimulation of the penis.
  b. no additional stimulation.
  c. privacy.
  d. 10 to 15 minutes after taking the oral drug.

7. Men taking alprostadil for treatment of erectile dysfunction must
  a. take the drug orally about 1 hour before anticipated intercourse.
  b. arrange for sexual stimulation to promote erection.
  c. learn to inject the drug directly into the penis.
  d. avoid the use of nitrates for cardiovascular disorders.

8. *Viagra* is known to
  a. cause unexpected and enlarged erections.
  b. make a person young and agile.
  c. promote interpersonal relationships between partners.
  d. increase nitrous oxide levels in the corpus cavernosum, causing vascular relaxation and promoting blood flow into the corpus cavernosum.

MULTIPLE RESPONSE

Select all that apply.

1. In assessing a client for androgenic effects, you would expect to find which of the following?
a. Hirsutism
b. Deepening of the voice
c. Testicular enlargement
d. Acne
e. Elevated body temperature
f. Sudden growth

2. A child treated with anabolic steroids because of anemia associated with renal disease will need
a. early sex education classes because of the effects of the drug.
b. x-rays of the long bones every 3 to 6 months so the drug can be stopped when the bone size is appropriate to the child's age.
c. to learn to shave.
d. to learn to cope with an altered body image.
e. regular monitoring of liver function tests.
f. monitoring for the development of edema.

BIBLIOGRAPHY AND REFERENCES

Brunton, L., Chabner, B., & Knollman, B. (2011). *Goodman and Gilman's the pharmacological basis of therapeutics* (12th ed.). New York: McGraw-Hill.

Emmelot-Vork, M., Verhaar, H., Nakhai Pour, H. R., et al. (2008). Effect of testosterone supplementation on function, mobility, cognition and other parameters in older men. *Journal of the American Medical Association, 299*(1), 39–52.

Facts and Comparisons. (2015). *Drug facts and comparisons.* St. Louis, MO: Author.

Fried, R. (2014). *Erectile dysfunction as a cardiovascular impairment.* Philadelphia, PA: Academic Press

Hall, J. (2015). *Guyton and Hall's textbook of medical physiology* (13th ed.). Philadelphia, PA: Saunders.

Karch, A. M. (2014). *Lippincott's nursing drug guide.* Philadelphia, PA: Lippincott Williams & Wilkins.

Nieschlag, E. (2010). *Andrology: Male reproductive health and dysfunction* (3rd ed.). Philadelphia, PA: Springer.

The Medical Letter. (2015). *The medical letter on drugs and therapeutics.* New Rochelle, NY: Author.

Vigen, W., O'Donnell, C., Baron, A., et al. (2013). Association of testosterone therapy with mortality, myocardial infarction and stroke in men with low testosterone levels. *Journal of the American Medical Association, 310*(17), 1829–1836.

Wein, A. J., Kavoussi, L. R., Novick, A. C., et al. (Eds.). (2011). *Campbell–Walsh urology* (10th ed.). Philadelphia, PA: W. B. Saunders.

PART

8

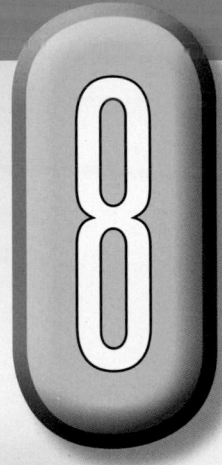

DRUGS ACTING ON THE CARDIOVASCULAR SYSTEM

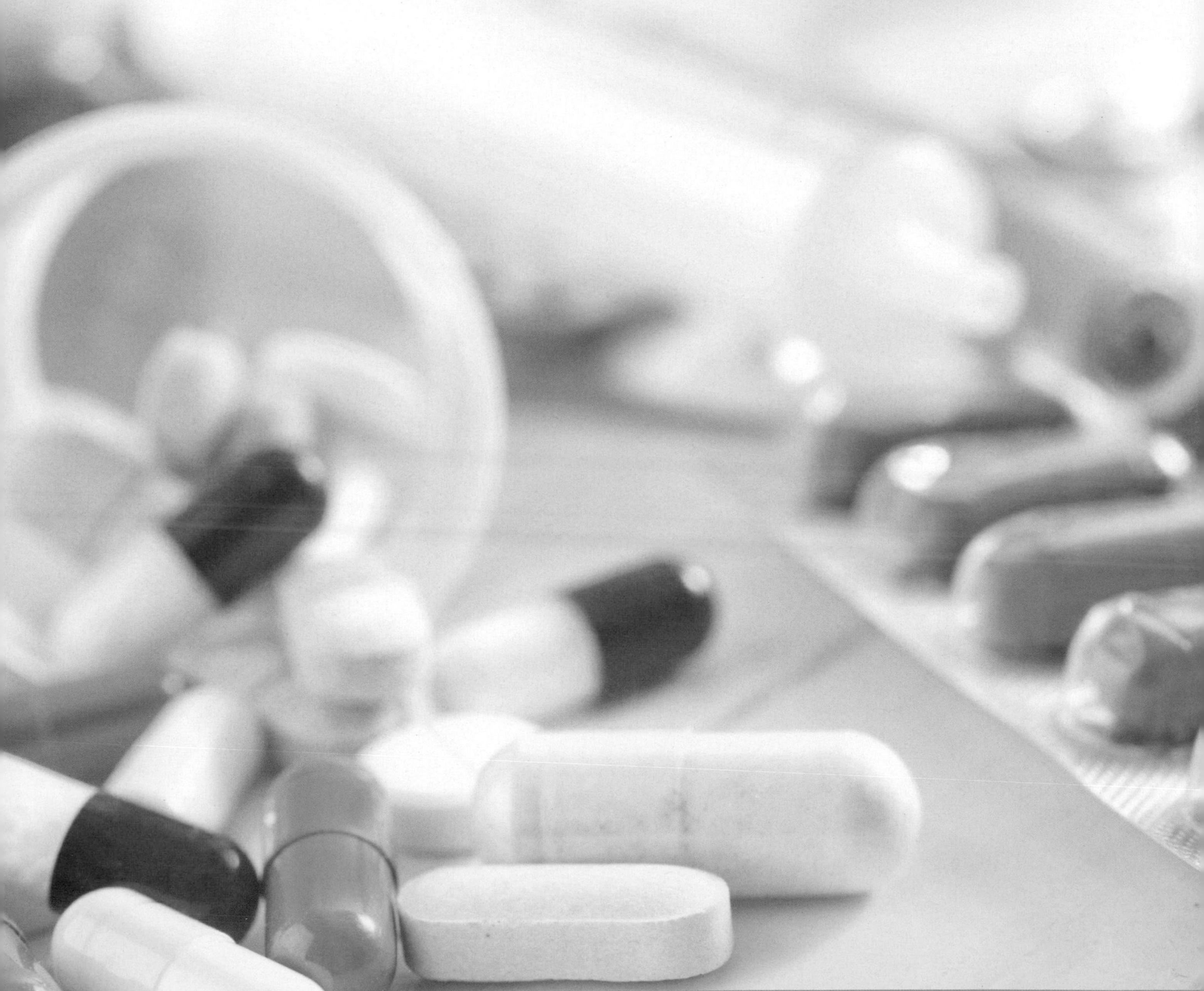

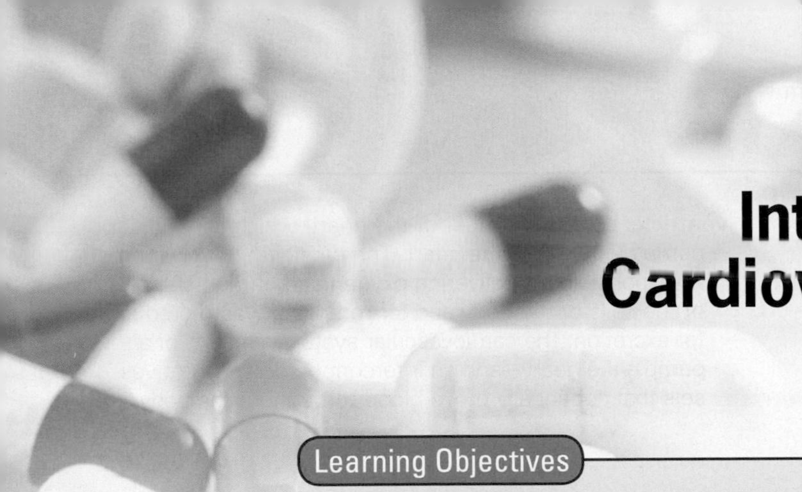

42 Introduction to the Cardiovascular System

Learning Objectives

Upon completion of this chapter, you will be able to:

1. Label a diagram of the heart, including all chambers, valves, great vessels, coronary vessels, and the conduction system.
2. Describe the flow of blood during the cardiac cycle, including flow to the cardiac muscle.
3. Outline the conduction system of the heart, correlating the normal electrocardiogram (ECG) pattern with the underlying electrical activity in the heart.
4. Discuss four normal controls of blood pressure.
5. Describe the capillary fluid shift, including factors that influence the movement of fluid in clinical situations.

Glossary of Key Terms

actin: thin filament, a component of a sarcomere, or muscle unit

ADH: antidiuretic hormone, released from the posterior pituitary, causes retention of water

aldosterone: a hormone released from the adrenal cortex, which causes retention of sodium and water

angiotensin: a peptide hormone that causes vasoconstriction, stimulates aldosterone and ADH release; part of the renin–angiotensin system

arrhythmia: a disruption in cardiac rate or rhythm

arteries: vessels that take blood away from the heart; muscular, resistance vessels

atrium: top chamber of the heart, receives blood from veins

auricle: appendage on the atria of the heart, holds blood to be pumped out with atrial contraction

automaticity: property of heart cells to generate an action potential without an external stimulus

capacitance system: the venous system; distensible, flexible veins that are capable of holding large amounts of blood

capillary: small vessel made up of loosely connected endothelial cells that connect arteries to veins

cardiac cycle: a period of cardiac muscle relaxation (diastole) followed by a period of contraction (systole) in the heart

conductivity: property of heart cells to rapidly conduct an action potential of electrical impulse

diastole: resting phase of the heart; blood is returned to the heart during this phase

dysrhythmia: a disruption in cardiac rate or rhythm, also called an arrhythmia

ectopic focus: a shift in the pacemaker of the heart from the sinoatrial node to some other site

electrocardiogram: an electrical tracing reflecting the conduction of an electrical impulse through the heart muscle; does not reflect mechanical activity

myocardium: the muscle of the heart

myosin: thick filament with projections, a component of a sarcomere, or muscle unit

natriuretic peptide: a peptide produced by the brain, heart, and vasculature which causes natriuresis, excretion of sodium in the urine; degraded by the enzyme neprilysin

oncotic pressure: the pulling pressure of the plasma proteins, responsible for returning fluid to the vascular system at the capillary level

pulse pressure: the systolic blood pressure minus the diastolic blood pressure; reflects the filling pressure of the coronary arteries

resistance system: the arteries; the muscles of the arteries provide resistance to the flow of blood, leading to control of blood pressure

sarcomere: functional unit of a muscle cell, composed of actin and myosin molecules arranged in layers to give the unit a striped or striated appearance

sinoatrial (SA) node: the normal pacemaker of the heart; composed of primitive cells that constantly generate an action potential

Starling's law of the heart: addresses the contractile properties of the heart: the more the muscle is stretched, the stronger it will react, until it is stretched to a point at which it will not react at all

syncytia: intertwining networks of muscle fibers that make up the atria and the ventricles of the heart; allow for a coordinated pumping contraction

systole: contracting phase of the heart, during which blood is pumped out of the heart

(continues on page 710)

Glossary of Key Terms (continued)

troponin: chemical in heart muscle that prevents the reaction between actin and myosin, leading to muscle relaxation; it is inactivated by calcium during muscle stimulation to allow actin and myosin to react, causing muscle contraction

veins: vessels that return blood to the heart; distensible tubes

ventricle: bottom chamber of the heart, which contracts to pump blood out of the heart. The cardiovascular system is responsible for delivering oxygen and nutrients to all of the cells of the body and for removing waste products for excretion. The cardiovascular system consists of a pump—the heart—and an interconnected series of vessels that continually move blood throughout the body.

Structure and Function of the Heart

The heart is a hollow, muscular organ that is divided into four chambers. The heart may actually be viewed as two joined hearts: a right heart and a left heart, each of which is divided into two parts, an upper part called the **atrium** (literally "porch" or entryway) and a lower part called the **ventricle**.

Attached to each atrium is an appendage called the **auricle**, which collects blood that is then pumped into the ventricles by atrial contraction. The right auricle is quite large; the left auricle is very small. The ventricles pump blood out of the heart to the lungs or the body. Between the atria and ventricles are two cardiac valves—thin tissues that are anchored to an annulus, or fibrous ring, which also gives the hollow organ some structure and helps to keep the organ open and divided into distinct chambers.

A partition called a septum separates the right half of the heart from the left half. The right half receives deoxygenated blood from everywhere in the body through the **veins** (vessels that carry blood toward the heart) and directs that blood into the lungs through the pulmonary artery. The left half receives the now-oxygenated blood from the lungs and directs it into the aorta. The aorta delivers blood into the systemic circulation by way of **arteries** (vessels that carry blood away from the heart) (Figure 42.1). The aorta delivers blood into the systemic circulation by way of arteries. The two semilunar valves, the aortic valve and the pulmonic valve, separate these great vessels from the heart and are also anchored onto two fibrous rings or annuli. These valves, like the atrioventricular (AV) valves, keep the blood flowing in one direction. The circulatory system is composed of about 60,000 miles of interconnecting blood vessels that carry the needed oxygen and nutrients to the cells and carry away the metabolic waste products from the tissues.

Cardiac Cycle

The heart, a muscle that contracts thousands of millions of times in a lifetime, possesses structural and functional properties that are different from those of other muscles. The fibers of the cardiac muscle, or **myocardium**, form two intertwining networks called the atrial and ventricular **syncytia**. These interlacing structures enable the atria and then the ventricles to contract synchronously when excited by the same stimulus.

Simultaneous contraction is a necessary property for a muscle that acts as a pump. A hollow pumping mechanism must also pause long enough in the pumping cycle to allow the chambers to fill with fluid. The heart muscle relaxes long enough to ensure adequate filling; the more completely it fills the stronger is the subsequent contraction. This occurs because the muscle fibers of the heart, stretched by the increased volume of blood that has returned to them, spring back to normal size. This is similar to the stretching of a rubber band, which returns to its normal size after it is stretched—the further it is stretched, the stronger is the spring back to normal. This property is defined through **Starling's law of the heart.**

During **diastole**—the period of cardiac muscle relaxation—blood returns to the heart from the systemic

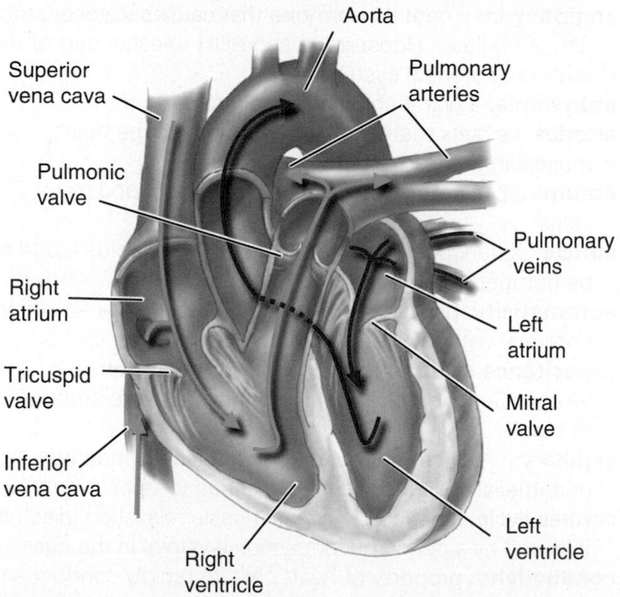

FIGURE 42.1 Blood flow into and out of the heart. Deoxygenated blood enters the right atrium from the great cardiac vein and the superior and inferior venae cavae and flows through the tricuspid valve into the right ventricle, which contracts and sends the blood through the pulmonic valve into the pulmonary artery and to the lungs. Oxygenated blood from the lungs enters the left atrium through the pulmonary veins and passes through the mitral valve into the left ventricle, which contracts and ejects the blood through the aortic valve into the aorta and out to the systemic circulation.

and pulmonary veins, flowing into the right and left atria, respectively. When the pressure generated by the blood volume in the atria is greater than the pressure in the ventricles, blood flows through the AV valves into the ventricles. The valve on the right side of the heart is called the tricuspid valve because it is composed of three leaflets or cusps. The valve on the left side of the heart, called the mitral or bicuspid valve, is composed of two leaflets or cusps (see Figure 42.1). Just before the ventricles are stimulated to contract, the atria contract, pushing about one more tablespoon of blood into each ventricle. The much more powerful ventricles then contract, pumping blood out to the lungs through the pulmonary valve or out to the aorta through the aortic valve and into the systemic circulation. The contraction of the ventricles is referred to as **systole**. Each period of systole followed by a period of diastole is called a **cardiac cycle**. The heart's series of one-way valves keeps the blood flowing in the correct direction:

- *Deoxygenated blood enters* the right atrium, flows through the tricuspid valve to the right ventricle, and flows through the pulmonary valve to the pulmonary arteries and the lungs.
- *Oxygenated blood from the lungs returns* through the pulmonary veins to the left atrium, flows through the mitral valve into the left ventricle, and then flows through the aortic valve to the aorta and the rest of the body.

The AV valves close very tightly when the ventricles contract, preventing blood from flowing backward into the atria, thereby keeping blood moving forward through the system. The pulmonary and aortic valves open with the pressure of ventricular contraction and close tightly during diastole, keeping blood from flowing backward into the ventricles. These valves operate much like one-way automatic doors: You can go through in the intended direction, but if you try to go the wrong way, the doors close and stop your movement. The proper functioning of the cardiac valves is important in maintaining the functioning of the cardiovascular system.

Cardiac Conduction

Each cycle of cardiac contraction and relaxation is controlled by impulses that arise spontaneously in certain pacemaker cells of the **sinoatrial (SA) node** of the heart. These impulses are conducted from the pacemaker cells by a specialized conducting system that activates all of the parts of the heart muscle almost simultaneously. These continuous, rhythmic contractions are controlled by the heart itself; the brain does not stimulate the heart to beat. This safety feature allows the heart to beat as long as it has enough nutrients and oxygen to survive, regardless of the status of the rest of the body. This property protects the vital cardiovascular function in many disease states; it is the same property that allows the heart to continue functioning in a patient who is "brain dead."

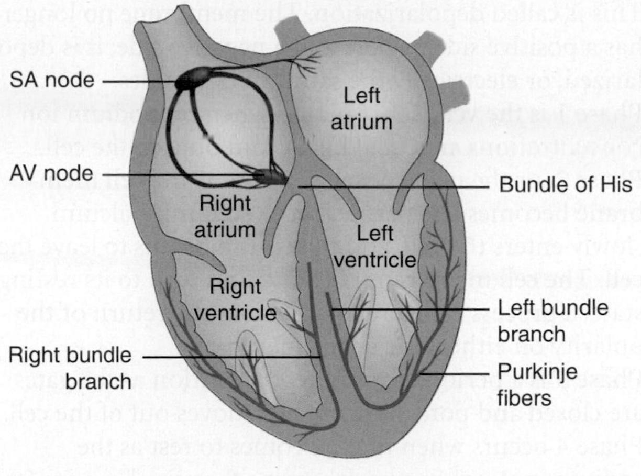

FIGURE 42.2 The conducting system of the heart. Impulses originating in the sinoatrial (SA) node are transmitted through the atrial bundles to the atrioventricular (AV) node and down the bundle of His and the bundle branches by way of the Purkinje fibers through the ventricles.

The conduction system of the heart consists of the SA node, atrial bundles, AV node, bundle of His, bundle branches, and Purkinje fibers (Figure 42.2). The SA node, which is located near the top of the right atrium, acts as the pacemaker of the heart. Atrial bundles conduct the impulse through the atrial muscle. The AV node, which is located near the bottom of the right atrium, slows the impulse and allows the delay needed for ventricular filling. The AV node then sends the impulse from the atria into the ventricles by way of the bundle of His, which enters the septum and then divides into three bundle branches. These bundle branches, which conduct the impulses through the ventricles, break into a fine network of conducting fibers called the Purkinje fibers, which deliver the impulse to the ventricular cells.

Automaticity

The cells of the impulse-forming and conducting system are rather primitive, uncomplicated cells called pale or P cells. Because of their simple cell membrane, these cells possess a special property that differentiates them from other cells: They can generate action potentials or electrical impulses without being excited to do so by external stimuli. This property is called **automaticity**.

All cardiac cells possess some degree of automaticity. During diastole or rest, these cells undergo a spontaneous depolarization because they decrease the flow of potassium ions out of the cell and probably leak sodium into the cell, causing an action potential. This action potential is basically the same as the action potential of the neuron (see Chapter 19). The action potential of the cardiac muscle cell consists of five phases:

- Phase 0 occurs when the cell reaches a point of stimulation. The sodium gates open along the cell membrane, and sodium rushes into the cell, resulting in a positive flow of electrons into the cell—an electrical potential.

This is called depolarization. The membrane no longer has a positive side or pole and a negative side; it is depolarized, or electrically the same on both sides.

- Phase 1 is the very short period when the sodium ion concentrations are equal inside and outside the cell.
- Phase 2, or the plateau stage, occurs as the cell membrane becomes less permeable to sodium. Calcium slowly enters the cell, and potassium begins to leave the cell. The cell membrane is trying to return to its resting state, a process called repolarization, the return of the polarity on either side of the membrane.
- Phase 3 is a period of rapid repolarization as the gates are closed and potassium rapidly moves out of the cell.
- Phase 4 occurs when the cell comes to rest as the sodium–potassium pump returns the membrane to its previous state, with more sodium outside and more potassium inside the cell. Spontaneous depolarization begins again.

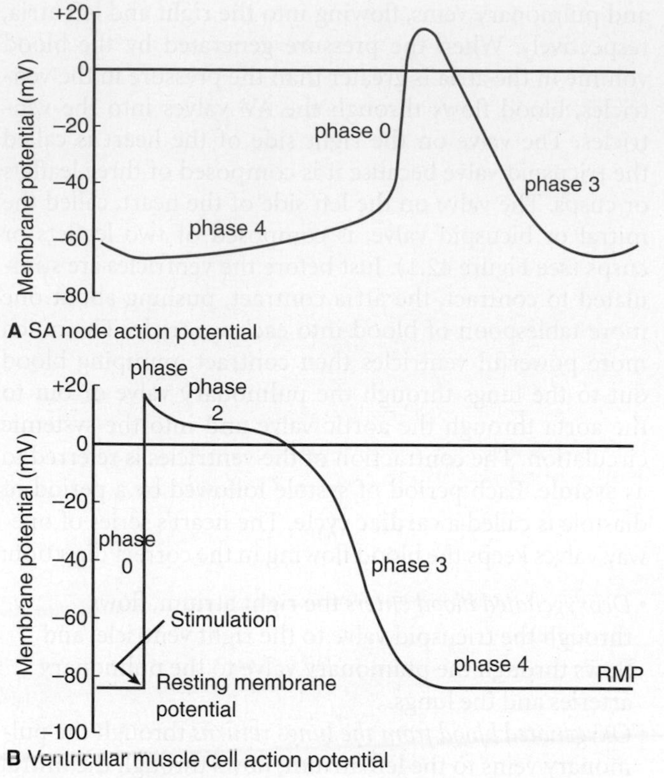

FIGURE 42.3 Action potentials recorded from a cell in the sinoatrial (SA) node (**A**) showing diastolic depolarization in phase 4 and recorded from a ventricular muscle cell (**B**). In phase 0 the cell is stimulated, sodium rushes into the cell, and the cell is depolarized. In phase 1, sodium levels equalize. In phase 2, the plateau phase, calcium enters the cell (the slow current) and potassium and sodium leave. In phase 3 the slow current stops and sodium and potassium leave the cell. In phase 4 the resting membrane potential (RMP) returns and the pacemaker potential begins in the SA node cell.

Each area of the heart has an action potential that appears slightly different from the other action potentials, reflecting the complexity of the cells in that particular area. Because of these differences in the action potential, each area of the heart has a slightly different rate or rhythm. The SA node generates an impulse about 90 to 100 times a minute, the AV node about 40 to 50 times a minute, and the complex ventricular muscle cells only about 10 to 20 times a minute (Figure 42.3).

Conductivity

Normally, the SA node sets the pace for the heart rate because it depolarizes faster than any cell in the heart. However, the other cells in the heart are capable of generating an impulse if anything happens to the SA node, which is another protective feature of the heart. As mentioned earlier, the SA node is said to be the pacemaker of the heart because it acts to stimulate the rest of the cells to depolarize at its rate. When the SA node sets the pace for the heart rate the person is said to be in sinus rhythm.

The specialized cells of the heart can conduct an impulse rapidly through the system so that the muscle cells of the heart are stimulated at approximately the same time. This property of cardiac cells is called **conductivity**. The conduction velocity, or the speed at which the cells can pass on the impulse, is slowest in the AV node and fastest in the Purkinje fibers.

A delay in conduction at the AV node, between the atria and the ventricles, accounts for the fact that the atria contract a fraction of a second before the ventricles contract. This allows extra time for the ventricles to fill completely before they contract. The almost simultaneous spread of the impulse through the Purkinje fibers permits a simultaneous and powerful contraction of the ventricle muscles, making them an effective pump.

After a cell membrane has conducted an action potential, there is a span of time, called the absolute refractory period, in which it is impossible to stimulate that area of membrane. The absolute refractory period is the minimal amount of time that must elapse between two stimuli applied at one site in the heart for each of these stimuli to cause an action potential. This time reflects the responsiveness of the heart cells to stimuli. Cardiac drugs may affect the refractory period of the cells to make the heart more or less responsive.

Autonomic Influences

The heart can generate action potentials on its own and could function without connection to the rest of the body. However, the autonomic nervous system (see Chapter 29) can influence the heart rate and rhythm and the strength of contraction. The parasympathetic nerves—primarily the vagus or tenth cranial nerve—can slow the heart rate and decrease the speed of conduction through the AV node. This allows the heart to rest and conserve its strength. In addition, the parasympathetic influence on the SA node is the dominant influence most of the time, keeping the resting heart rate at 70 to 80 beats/min.

The sympathetic nervous system stimulates the heart to beat faster, speeds conduction through the AV node, and causes the heart muscle to contract harder. This action is important during exercise or stress, when the body's cells need to have more oxygen delivered.

These two branches of the autonomic nervous system work together to help the heart meet the body's demands. Drugs that influence either branch can exert autonomic effects on the heart.

Myocardial Contraction

The end result of the electrical stimulation of the heart cells is the unified contraction of the atria and ventricles, which moves the blood throughout the vascular system. The basic unit of the cardiac muscle is the **sarcomere.** A sarcomere is made up of two contractile proteins: **Actin**, a thin filament, and **myosin**, a thick filament with small projections on it. These proteins are anchored at the Z bands, the outer edges of each sarcomere. These proteins readily react with each other, but at rest they are kept apart by the protein **troponin** (Figure 42.4).

When a cardiac muscle cell is stimulated, calcium enters the cell through channels in the cell membrane and also from storage sites within the cell. This occurs during phase 3 of the action potential, when the cell is starting to repolarize. The calcium reacts with the troponin and inactivates it. This action allows the actin and myosin proteins to react with each other, forming actomyosin bridges. These bridges then break quickly, and the myosin slides along to form new bridges.

As long as calcium is present the actomyosin bridges continue to form. This action slides the proteins together, shortening or contracting the sarcomere. Cardiac muscle cells are linked together: When one cell is stimulated to contract, they are all stimulated to contract.

The shortening of numerous sarcomeres causes the contraction and pumping action of the heart muscle. As the cell reaches its repolarized state, calcium is removed from the cell by a sodium–calcium pump, and calcium released from storage sites within the cell returns to the storage sites. The contraction process requires energy and oxygen for the chemical reaction that allows the formation of the actomyosin bridges and calcium to allow the bridge formation to occur.

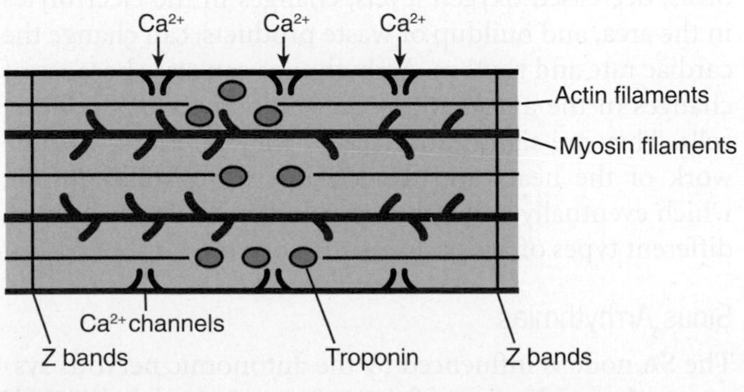

FIGURE 42.4 A sarcomere, the functioning unit of cardiac muscle.

The degree of shortening (the strength of contraction) is determined by the amount of calcium present—the more calcium present the more bridges will be formed—and by the stretch of the sarcomere before contraction begins. The further apart the actin and myosin proteins are before the cell is stimulated the more bridges will be formed and the stronger the contraction will be. This correlates with Starling's law of the heart. The more the cardiac muscle is stretched the greater is the contraction. The more blood that enters the heart the greater is the contraction that is needed to empty the heart, up to a point; however, if the actin and myosin molecules are stretched too far apart, they will not be able to reach each other to form the actomyosin bridges, and no contraction will occur.

KEY POINTS

- The heart, a hollow muscle with four chambers comprising two upper atria and two lower ventricles, pumps oxygenated blood to the body's cells and also collects waste products from the tissues.
- The two-step process known as the cardiac cycle includes diastole (resting period when the veins carry blood back to the heart) and systole (contraction period when the heart pumps blood out to the arteries for distribution to the body).
- Impulses generated in the heart—not the brain—stimulate contraction of the heart muscle.
- The heart's conduction (or stimulatory) system consists of the SA node, the atrial bundles, the AV node, the bundle of His, the bundle branches, and the Purkinje fibers.

Electrocardiography

Electrocardiography is a process of recording the patterns of electrical impulses as they move through the heart. It is an important diagnostic tool in the care of the cardiac patient. The electrocardiography machine detects the patterns of electrical impulse generation and conduction through the heart and translates that information into a recorded pattern, which is displayed as a waveform on a cardiac monitor or printout on calibrated paper. An **electrocardiogram (ECG)** is a measure of electrical activity; it provides no information about the mechanical activity of the heart. The important aspect of cardiac output—the degree to which the heart is doing its job of pumping blood out to all of the tissues—needs to be carefully assessed by looking at and evaluating the patient.

The normal ECG waveform is made up of five main waves: the P wave, which is formed as impulses originating in the SA node or pacemaker pass through the atrial tissues; the QRS complex, which represents depolarization of the bundle of His (Q) and the ventricles (RS); and the T wave, which represents repolarization of the ventricles (Figure 42.5).

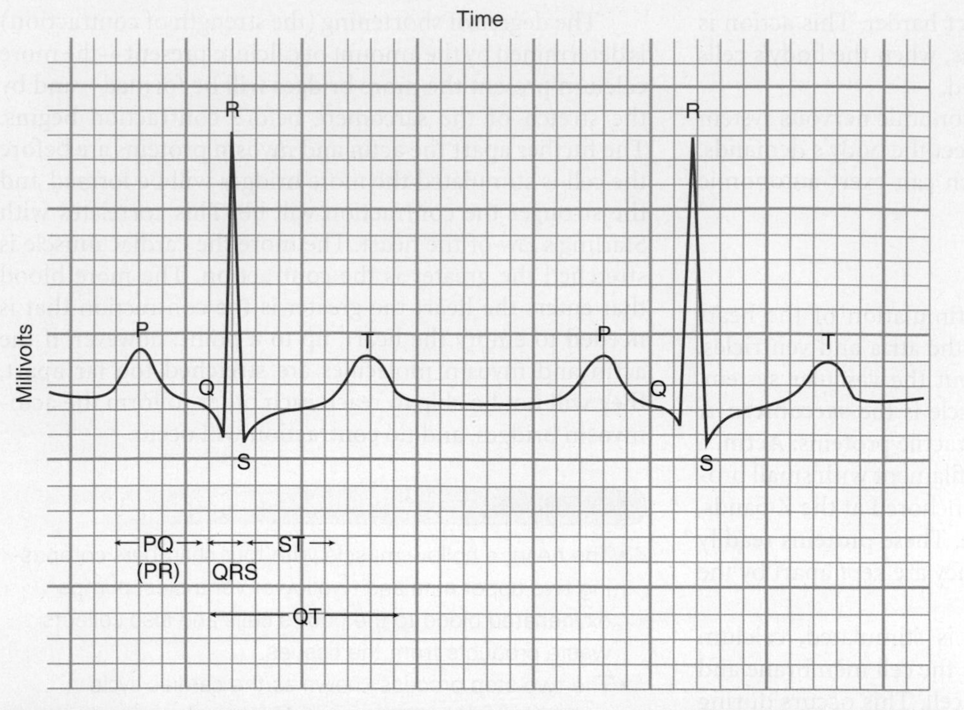

Key:

Each vertical square represents 0.1 mV of electrical charge.

Each horizontal square equals 0.04 s of time.

Approximate values for normal intervals:

PQ (PR) interval—0.16 s
QT interval—0.3 s
QRS interval—0.08 s
P wave—0.08 s
ST interval—0.1 s

P wave = Electrical changes associated with atrial depolarization
QRS complex = Electrical changes associated with ventricular depolarization
T wave = Electrical changes associated with ventricular repolarization
The electrical changes associated with atrial repolarization normally coincide with the QRS complex and are obscured by it.

FIGURE 42.5 The normal electrocardiogram waveform.

The P wave immediately precedes the contraction of the atria. The QRS complex immediately precedes the contraction of the ventricles and then relaxation of the ventricles during the T wave. The repolarization of the atria (the Ta wave) occurs during the QRS complex and usually is not seen on an ECG. In certain conditions of atrial hypertrophy the Ta wave may appear around the QRS complex.

In addition to the five waves, several areas represent critical points on the ECG. These include the following:

P–R interval: Reflects the normal delay of conduction at the AV node

Q–T interval: Reflects the critical timing of repolarization of the ventricles

S–T segment: Reflects important information about the repolarization of the ventricles

A person with a normal ECG pattern and a heart rate within the normal range for that person's age group is said to be in normal sinus rhythm. However, abnormalities in the shape or timing of each part of an ECG tracing help to reveal the presence of particular cardiac disorders.

Arrhythmias

A disruption in cardiac rate or rhythm is called an **arrhythmia**, or **dysrhythmia**. Various factors, such as drugs, acidosis, decreased oxygen levels, changes in the electrolytes in the area, and buildup of waste products, can change the cardiac rate and rhythm. Arrhythmias can arise because of changes in the automaticity or conductivity of the heart cells. They are significant because they interfere with the work of the heart and can disrupt the cardiac output, which eventually will affect every cell in the body. Several different types of arrhythmias may occur.

Sinus Arrhythmias

The SA node is influenced by the autonomic nervous system to change the rate of firing to meet the body's demands for oxygen. A faster-than-normal heart rate—usually anything faster than 100 beats/min in an adult—with a normal-appearing ECG pattern is called sinus tachycardia. If sinus tachycardia becomes too fast, it can lead to decreased time for cardiac filling and a decrease in cardiac output. Many activities or conditions can cause a sinus tachycardia, such as exercise, fear, or stress. The underlying physical condition of the patient will determine whether this fast heart rate is problematic. Sinus bradycardia is a slower-than-normal heart rate (usually less than 60 beats/min) with a normal-appearing ECG pattern. Sinus bradycardia allows increased time for ventricular and an increased cardiac output. This is often seen with athletes who have a slow heart rate. In other people, this rate might be too slow to adequately perfuse all of the tissues.

Supraventricular Arrhythmias

Arrhythmias that originate above the ventricles but not in the SA node are called supraventricular arrhythmias. These arrhythmias feature an abnormally shaped P wave because the site of origin is not the sinus node. However, they show normal QRS complexes because the ventricles are still conducting impulses normally. Supraventricular arrhythmias include the following:

- *Premature atrial contractions*, which reflect an **ectopic focus** (a shift in the pacemaker of the heart from the SA node to some other site) in the atria that is generating an impulse out of the normal rhythm
- *Paroxysmal atrial tachycardia*, sporadically occurring runs of rapid heart rate originating in the atria
- *Atrial flutter*, characterized by sawtooth-shaped P waves reflecting a single ectopic focus that is generating a regular, fast atrial depolarization
- *Atrial fibrillation*, with irregular P waves representing many ectopic foci firing in an uncoordinated manner through the atria

With atrial flutter, often one of every two or one of every three impulses is transmitted to the ventricles. The person may have a 2:1 or 3:1 ratio of P waves to QRS complexes. The ventricles beat faster than normal, losing some efficiency. With atrial fibrillation, so many impulses are bombarding the AV node that an unpredictable number of impulses are transmitted to the ventricles. The ventricles are stimulated to beat in a fast, irregular, and often inefficient manner.

Atrioventricular Block

Atrioventricular block, also called heart block, reflects a slowing or lack of conduction at the AV node. This can occur because of structural damage, hypoxia, or injury to the heart muscle. First-degree heart block, in which all of the impulses from the SA node arrive in the ventricles but after a longer-than-normal period, is characterized by a lengthening of the P–R interval beyond the normal 0.16 to 0.20 seconds. Each P wave is followed by a QRS complex. In second-degree heart block, some of the impulses are lost and do not get through, resulting in a slow rate of ventricular contraction. With this arrhythmia a QRS complex may follow one, two, three, or four P waves. In third-degree heart block, or complete heart block, no impulses from the SA node get through to the ventricles, and the much slower ventricular automaticity takes over. The waveform shows a total dissociation of P waves from QRS complexes and T waves. Because the P waves can come at any time the P–R interval is not constant. The QRS complexes appear at a very slow rate and may not be sufficient to meet the body's needs.

Ventricular Arrhythmias

Impulses that originate below the AV node originate from ectopic foci that do not use the normal conduction pathways. The QRS complexes appear wide and prolonged, and the T waves are inverted, reflecting the slower conduction across cardiac tissue that is not part of the rapid conduction system. Premature ventricular contractions (PVCs) can arise from a single ectopic focus in the ventricles, with all of them having the same shape, or from many ectopic foci, which produces PVCs with different shapes. Runs or bursts of PVCs from many different foci are more ominous because they can reflect extensive damage or hypoxia in the myocardium. Runs of several PVCs at a rapid rate are called ventricular tachycardia. Ventricular fibrillation is seen as a bizarre, irregular, distorted wave. It is potentially fatal because it reflects a lack of any coordinated stimulation of the ventricles. The ventricles' inability to contract in a coordinated fashion results in no blood being pumped to the body or the brain. Thus, there is a total loss of cardiac output.

KEY POINTS

- The normal ECG waveform is made up of five main waves: The P wave, which is formed as impulses originating in the SA node or pacemaker pass through the atrial tissues; the QRS complex, which represents depolarization of the bundle of His (Q) and the ventricles (RS); and the T wave, which represents repolarization of the ventricles.
- A person with a normal ECG pattern and a heart rate within the normal range for that person's age group is said to be in normal sinus rhythm.
- When the generation of impulses is altered the result is known as an arrhythmia (or dysrhythmia) that can upset the normal balance in the cardiovascular system. A decrease in cardiac output, which affects all of the cells of the body, follows.

Circulation

The purpose of the heart's continual pumping action is to keep blood flowing to and from all of the body's tissues and cells. Blood delivers oxygen and much-needed nutrients to the cells for producing energy, and it carries away carbon dioxide and other waste products of metabolism. The steady circulation of blood is essential for the proper functioning of all of the body's organs, including the heart.

The circulation of the blood follows two courses:

- *Heart–lung or pulmonary circulation*: The right side of the heart sends blood to the lungs, where carbon dioxide and some waste products are removed from the blood and oxygen is picked up by the red blood cells.
- *Systemic circulation*: The left side of the heart sends oxygenated blood out to all of the cells in the body.

In addition, the heart muscle, like any other muscle, requires adequate oxygen and nutrients to function. This is accomplished via coronary circulation.

The blood moves from areas of high pressure to areas of lower pressure. The system is a "closed" system; that is, it has no openings or holes that would allow blood to leak out. The closed nature of the system is what keeps the pressure differences in the proper relationship so that blood always flows in the direction in which it is intended to flow (Figure 42.6).

Pulmonary Circulation

The right atrium is a very low-pressure area in the cardiovascular system. All of the deoxygenated blood from the body flows into the right atrium from the inferior and superior venae cavae (see Figure 42.1) and from the great cardiac vein, which returns deoxygenated blood from the heart muscle. As the blood flows into the atrium, the pressure increases. When the pressure becomes greater than the pressure in the right ventricle, most of the blood flows into the right ventricle; this is called the rapid-filling phase. At this point in the cardiac cycle the atrium is stimulated to contract and pushes the remaining blood into the right ventricle. The ventricle is then stimulated to contract; it generates pressure that opens the pulmonic valve (see Figure 42.1) and sends blood into the pulmonary artery, which takes the blood into the lungs, a very low–pressure area. The blood then circulates around the alveoli of the lungs, picking up oxygen and getting rid of carbon dioxide; flows through pulmonary capillaries (the tiny blood vessels that connect arteries and veins) into the pulmonary veins; and then returns to the left atrium.

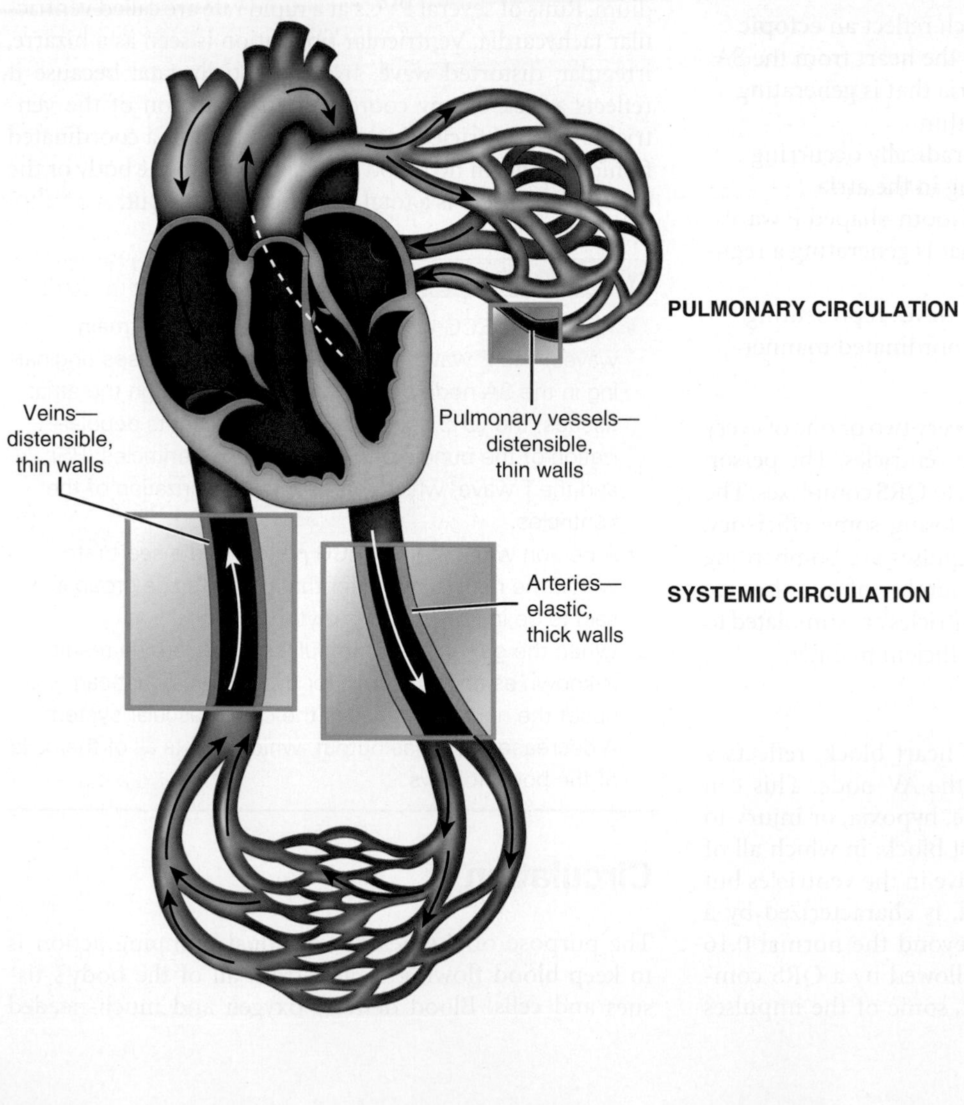

FIGURE 42.6 Blood flow through the systemic and pulmonary vasculature circuits.

Systemic Circulation

When the pressure of blood volume in the left atrium is greater than the pressure in the large left ventricle, this oxygenated blood flows into the left ventricle. The left atrium contracts and pushes any remaining blood into the left ventricle, which is stimulated to contract and generates tremendous pressure to push the blood out the aorta, carrying it throughout the body. The aorta and other large arteries have thick, muscular walls. The entire arterial system contains muscles in the walls of the vessels all the way to the terminal branches or arterioles, which consist of fragments of muscle and endothelial cells. These muscles offer resistance to the blood that is sent pumping into the arterial system by the left ventricle, generating pressure. The arterial system is referred to as a **resistance system**. The vessels can either constrict or dilate, increasing or decreasing resistance, respectively, based on the needs of the body. The arterioles are able to completely shut off blood flow to some areas of the body; that is, they can shunt blood to another area where it is needed more. The arterioles, because of their ability to increase or decrease resistance in the system, are one of the main regulators of blood pressure.

Blood from the tiny arterioles flows into the **capillary** system, which connects the arterial and venous systems. These microscopic vessels are composed of loosely connected endothelial cells. Oxygen, fluid, and nutrients are able to pass through the arterial end of the capillaries and enter the interstitial area between tissue cells. Fluid at the venous end of the capillary, which contains carbon dioxide and other waste products, is drawn back into the vessel. This shifting of fluid in the capillaries, called the capillary fluid shift, is carefully regulated by a balance between hydrostatic (fluid pressure) forces on the arterial end of the capillary and **oncotic pressure** (OP, the pulling pressure of the large, vascular proteins) on the venous end of the capillary. In a normal situation, the higher pressure at the arterial end of a capillary forces fluid out of the vessel and into the tissue, and the now-concentrated proteins (which are too large to leave the capillary) exert a pull on the fluid at the venous end of the capillary to pull it back in. A disruption in the hydrostatic pressure (HP) or in the concentration of proteins in the capillary can lead to fluid being left in the tissue, a condition referred to as edema. The capillaries merge into venules, which merge into veins, the vessels responsible for returning the blood to the heart (Figure 42.7).

The veins are thin-walled, very elastic, low-pressure vessels that can hold large quantities of blood if necessary. The venous system is referred to as a **capacitance system** because the veins have the capacity to hold large quantities of fluid as they distend with fluid volume. These capacitance vessels have a great deal of influence on the venous return to the heart—the amount of blood that is delivered to the right atrium.

Coronary Circulation

The heart muscle requires a constant supply of oxygenated blood to keep contracting. The myocardium receives its blood through two main coronary arteries that branch off the base of the aorta from an area called the sinuses of Valsalva. These arteries encircle the heart in a pattern resembling a crown, which is why they are called "coronary" arteries.

The left coronary artery arises from the left side of the aorta and bifurcates, or divides, into two large vessels

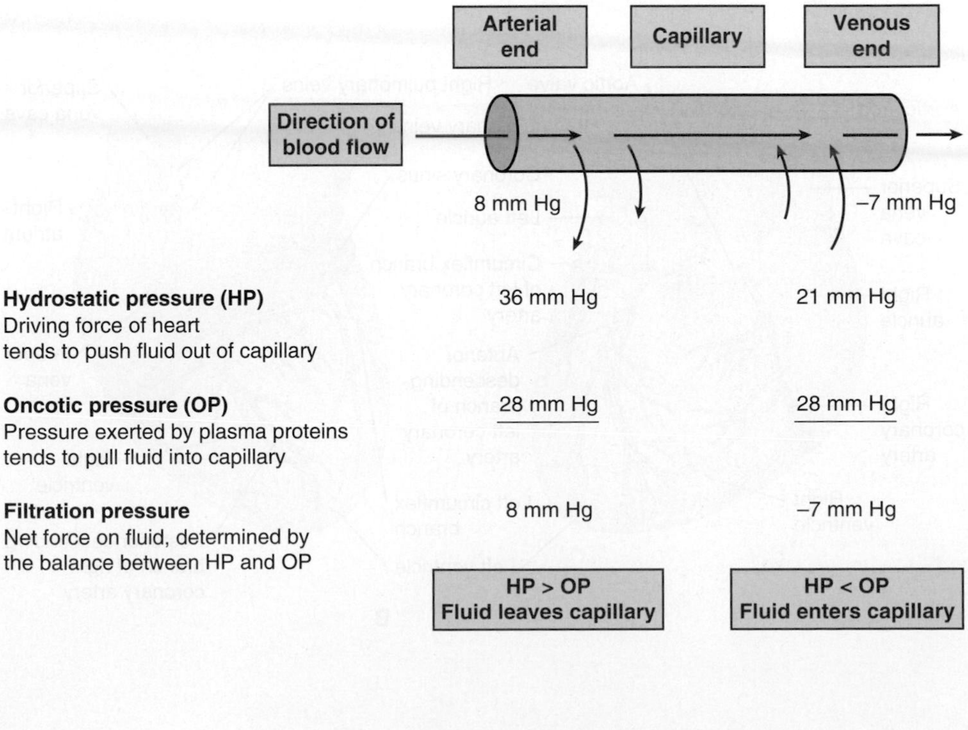

FIGURE 42.7 The net shift of fluid out of and into the capillary is determined by the balance between the hydrostatic pressure (HP) and the oncotic pressure (OP). The HP tends to push fluid out of the capillary, and the OP tends to pull it back into the capillary. At the arterial end of the capillary bed the blood pressure is higher than at the venous end. At the arterial end, HP exceeds OP and fluid filters out. At the venous end, HP has fallen and is less than OP; fluid is pulled back into the capillary from the surrounding tissue. The lymphatic system also returns fluids and substances from the tissues to the circulation.

called the left circumflex artery (which travels down the left side of the heart and feeds most of the left ventricle) and the left anterior descending coronary artery (which travels down the front of the heart and feeds the septum and anterior areas, including much of the conduction system). The artery arising from the right side of the aorta, called the right coronary artery, supplies most of the right side of the heart, including the SA node.

The coronary arteries receive blood during diastole, when the muscle is at rest and relaxed so that blood can flow freely into the muscle. When the ventricle contracts, it forces the aortic valve open, which in turn causes the leaflets of the valve to cover the openings of the coronary arteries. When the ventricles relax the blood is no longer pumped forward and starts to flow back toward the ventricle. The blood flowing down the sides of the aorta closes the aortic valve and fills the coronary arteries. The pressure that fills the coronary arteries is the difference between the systolic (ejection) pressure and the diastolic (resting) pressure. This is called the **pulse pressure** (systolic minus diastolic blood pressure readings). The pulse pressure is monitored clinically to evaluate the filling pressure of the coronary arteries. The oxygenated blood that is fed into the heart by the coronary circulation reaches every cardiac muscle fiber as the vessels divide and subdivide throughout the myocardium (Figure 42.8).

The heart has a pattern of circulation called end artery circulation. The arteries go into the muscle and end without a great deal of backup or collateral circulation. Normally, this is an efficient system and is able to meet the needs of the heart muscle. The heart's supply of and demand for oxygen are met by changes in the delivery of oxygen through the coronary artery system. Problems can arise, however, when an imbalance develops between the supply of oxygen delivered to the heart muscle and the myocardial demand for oxygen.

The main forces that determine the heart's use of oxygen or oxygen consumption include the following:

- *Heart rate*: The more the heart has to pump the more oxygen it requires.
- *Preload (amount of blood that is brought back to the heart to be pumped throughout the body)*: The more blood that is returned to the heart the harder it will have to work to pump the blood around. The volume of blood in the system is a determinant of preload.
- *Afterload (resistance against which the heart has to beat)*: The higher the resistance in the system the harder the heart will have to contract to force open the valves and pump the blood along. Blood pressure is a measure of afterload.
- *Stretch on the ventricles*: If the ventricular muscle is stretched before it is stimulated to contract, more actomyosin bridges will be formed, which will take more energy; alternatively, if the muscle is stimulated to contract harder than usual (which happens with sympathetic stimulation), more bridges will be formed, which also will require more energy.

The muscle can be stretched, as in ventricular hypertrophy related to chronic hypertension or cardiac muscle damage, or in heart failure (HF) when the ventricle does not empty completely and blood backs up in the system.

The supply of blood to the myocardium can be altered if the heart fails to pump effectively and cannot deliver blood to the coronary arteries. This happens in HF and cases of hypotension. The supply is most frequently altered, however, when the coronary vessels become narrowed and unresponsive to stimuli to dilate and deliver more blood. This happens in atherosclerosis or coronary artery disease. The end result of this narrowing can be total blockage of a coronary artery, leading to hypoxia and eventual death of the cells that depend on that vessel for oxygen.

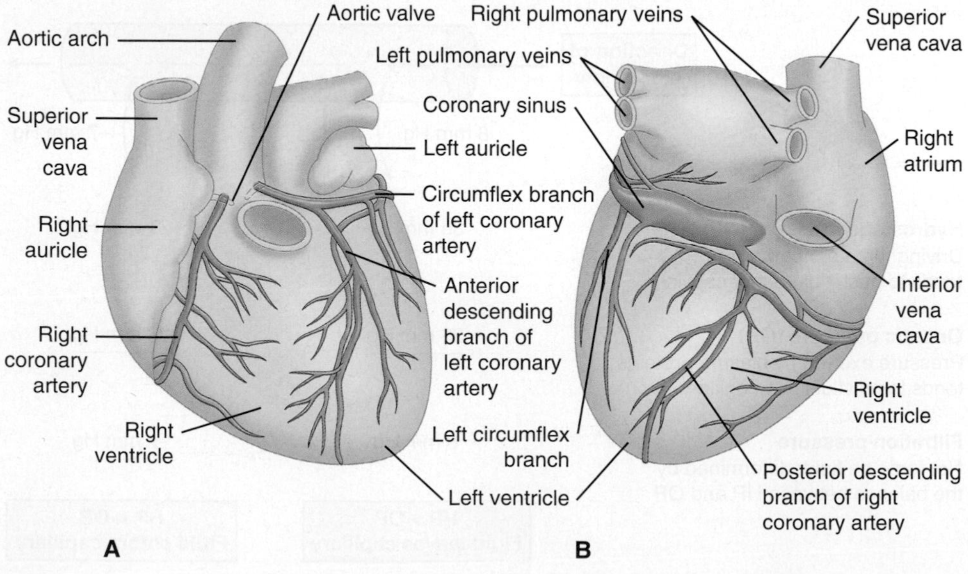

FIGURE 42.8 Coronary arteries and veins. **A.** Anterior view. **B.** Posterior view.

This is called a myocardial infarction, and it is the leading cause of death in the United States.

Systemic Arterial Pressure

The contraction of the left ventricle, which sends blood surging out into the aorta, creates a pressure that continues to force blood into all of the branches of the aorta. This pressure against arterial walls is greatest during systole (cardiac contraction) and falls to its lowest level during diastole. Measurement of both the systolic and the diastolic pressure indicates both the pumping pressure of the ventricle and the generalized pressure in the system, or the pressure the ventricle has to overcome to pump blood out of the heart.

Hypotension

The pressure of the blood in the arteries needs to remain relatively high to ensure that blood is delivered to every cell in the body and to keep the blood flowing from high-pressure to low-pressure areas. The pressure can fall dramatically—termed hypotension—from loss of blood volume or from failure of the heart muscle to pump effectively. Severe hypotension can progress to shock and even death as cells are cut off from their oxygen supply.

Hypertension

Constant, excessive high blood pressure—called hypertension—can damage the fragile inner lining of blood vessels and cause a disruption of blood flow to the tissues. It also puts a tremendous strain on the heart muscle, increasing myocardial oxygen consumption and putting the heart muscle at risk. Hypertension can be caused by neurostimulation of the blood vessels that causes them to constrict, subsequently raising pressure, or by increased volume in the system. In most cases, the cause of hypertension is not known, and drug therapy to correct it is aimed at changing one or more of the normal reflexes that control vascular resistance or the force of cardiac muscle contraction.

Vasomotor Tone

The smooth muscles in the walls of the arteries receive constant input from nerve fibers of the sympathetic nervous system. These impulses work to dilate the vessels if more blood flow is needed in an area, to constrict vessels if increased pressure is needed in the system, and to maintain muscle tone so that the vessel remains patent and responsive.

The coordination of these impulses is regulated through the medulla in an area called the cardiovascular center. If increased pressure is needed, this center increases sympathetic flow to the vessels. If pressure rises too high, this is sensed by baroreceptors or pressure receptors, and the sympathetic flow is decreased. Chapter 43 discusses the drugs that are used to influence the stimulation of vessels to alter blood pressure.

Renin–Angiotensin–Aldosterone System

Another determinant of blood pressure is the renin–angiotensin–aldosterone system. This system is activated when blood flow to the kidneys is decreased. The juxtoglomerular cells, near the afferent arterioles in the kidney, release an enzyme called renin. Renin is transported to the liver, where it converts angiotensinogen (produced in the liver) to **angiotensin** I. Angiotensin I travels to the lungs, where it is converted by angiotensin-converting enzyme to angiotensin II. Angiotensin II travels through the body and reacts with angiotensin II receptor sites on blood vessels to cause a severe vasoconstriction. This increases blood pressure and should increase blood flow to the kidneys to decrease the release of renin. Like angiotensin III, it also causes the release of **aldosterone** from the adrenal cortex, which causes retention of sodium and water and stimulates the release of antidiuretic hormone (**ADH**) from the posterior pituitary to retain water, both of which increase blood volume. Increasing blood volume increases blood flow to the kidney. This system works constantly, whenever a position change alters flow to the kidney or blood volume or pressure changes, to help maintain the blood pressure within a range that ensures perfusion (delivery of blood to all of the tissues) (Figure 42.9).

Natriuretic Peptides

Natriuretic peptides are formed in the atria of the heart, where they are called atrial natriuretic peptides (ANPs), and in the brain, where they are called brain natriuretic peptides (BNPs). There are other natriuretic peptides, labeled CNPs (C-type natriuretic peptides), thought to act in the vasculature, and DNPs (dendroaspis natriuretic peptides), thought to be released from the atria; though not as much research is available on these two peptides. The natriuretic peptides act to inhibit the renin–angiotensin–aldosterone system and cause a diuretic, natriuretic, and blood pressure lowering effect. They are broken down in the body by the enzyme neprilysin. ANP and BNP are released in response to high ventricular filling pressures. This could be related to fluid overload or failure of the heart muscle. The levels of these peptides are linked to HF, and new treatments are aimed at utilizing the effects of these peptides to decrease volume, pressure, and cardiac workload.

Venous Pressure

Blood in the veins also exerts a pressure that may sometimes rise above normal. This can happen if the heart is not pumping effectively and is unable to pump out all of the blood that is trying to return to it. This results in a backup or congestion of blood waiting to enter the heart. Pressure rises in the right atrium and then in the veins that are trying to return blood to the heart as they encounter resistance. The venous system begins to back up or become congested with blood.

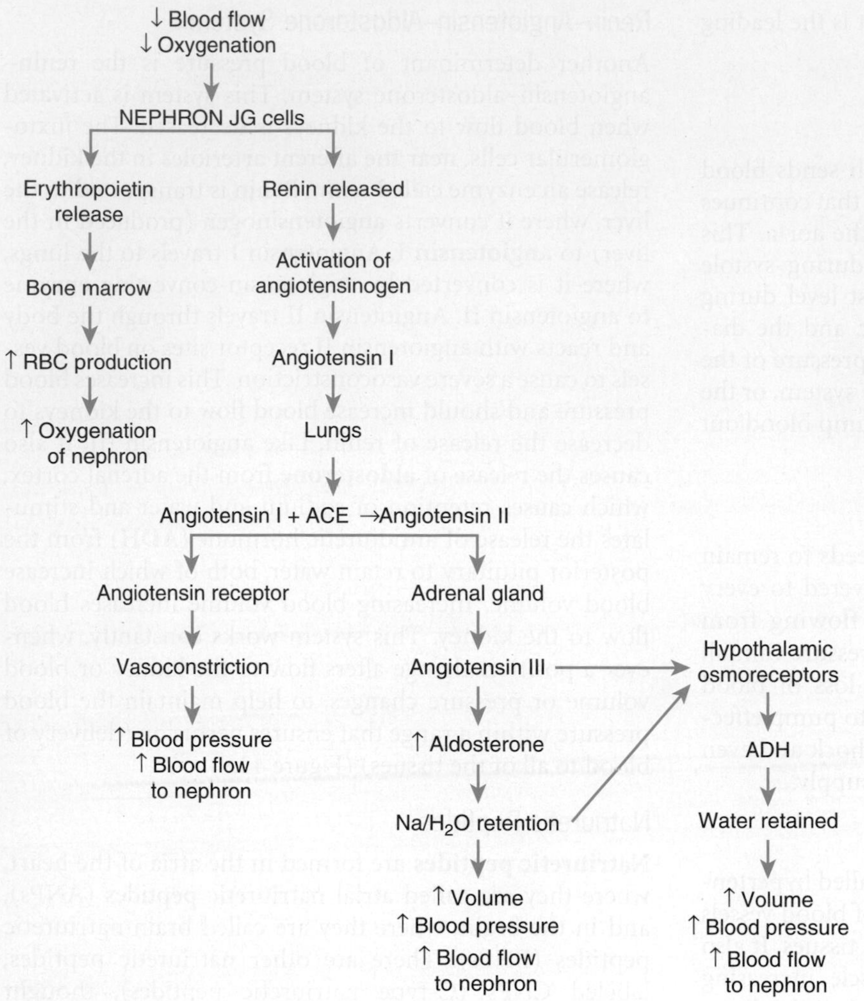

FIGURE 42.9 The renin–angiotensin–aldosterone system for reflex maintenance of blood pressure control.

Heart Failure

If the heart muscle fails to do its job of effectively pumping blood through the system, blood backs up and the system becomes congested. This is called heart failure. The rise in venous pressure that results from this backup of blood increases the HP on the venous end of the capillaries. The HP pushing fluid out of the capillary is soon higher than the OP that is trying to pull the fluid back into the vessel, causing fluid to be lost into the tissues. This shift of fluid accounts for the edema seen with HF. Pulmonary edema results when the left side of the heart fails; peripheral, abdominal, and liver edema occur when the right side of the heart fails.

Other factors can contribute to a loss of fluid in the tissues, including protein loss and fluid retention. Protein loss can lead to a fall in OP and an inability to pull fluid back into the vascular system. Protein levels fall in renal failure, when protein is lost in the urine, and in liver failure, when the liver is no longer able to produce plasma proteins. Fluid retention, which often is stimulated by aldosterone and ADH as described earlier, can increase the HP so much that fluid is pushed out under higher pressure and the balancing pressure to pull it back into the vessel is not sufficient. Drugs that are used to treat HF may affect the vascular system at any of these areas in an attempt to return a balance to the pressures in the system.

KEY POINTS

- Blood pressure is maintained by stimulus from the sympathetic system and reflex control of blood volume and pressure by the renin–angiotensin system and the aldosterone–ADH system. Alterations in blood pressure (hypotension or hypertension) can upset the balance of the cardiovascular system and lead to problems in blood delivery.
- Fluid shifts out of the blood at the arterial ends of capillaries to deliver oxygen and nutrients to the tissues. It moves out due to the hydrostatic or fluid pressure of the arterial side of the system. Fluid returns to the system at the venous end of the capillaries because of the oncotic pull of proteins in the vessels. Disruptions in these pressures can lead to edema or loss of fluid in the tissues.

SUMMARY

- The heart is a hollow muscle that is divided into a right and a left side by a thick septum and into four chambers—the two upper atria and the two lower ventricles. The right side of the heart receives all of the deoxygenated blood from the body through the veins and directs it into the lungs. The left side of the heart receives oxygenated blood from the lungs and pumps it out to every cell in the body through the arteries.
- The heart is responsible for pumping oxygenated blood to every cell in the body and for picking up waste products from the tissues.
- The cardiac cycle consists of a period of rest, or diastole, when blood is returned to the heart by veins, and a period of contraction, or systole, when the blood is pumped out of the heart.
- The heart muscle possesses the properties of automaticity (the ability to generate an action potential in the absence of stimulation) and conductivity (the ability to rapidly transmit an action potential).
- The heart muscle is stimulated to contract by impulses generated in the heart, not by stimuli from the brain. The autonomic nervous system can affect the heart to increase (sympathetic) or decrease (parasympathetic) activity.
- In normal sinus rhythm, cells in the SA node generate an impulse that is transmitted through the atrial bundles and delayed slightly at the AV node before being sent down the bundle of His into the ventricles. When cardiac muscle cells are stimulated, they contract.
- Alterations in the generation of conduction of impulses in the heart cause arrhythmias (dysrhythmias), which can upset the normal balance in the cardiovascular system and lead to a decrease in cardiac output, affecting all of the cells of the body.
- Heart muscle contracts by the sliding of actin and myosin filaments in a functioning unit called a sarcomere. Contraction requires energy and calcium to allow the filaments to react with each other and slide together.
- The heart muscle needs a constant supply of blood, which is furnished by the coronary arteries. Increase in demand for oxygen can occur with changes in heart rate, preload, afterload, or stretch on the muscle.
- The cardiovascular system is a closed pressure system that uses arteries (muscular, pressure, or resistance vessels) to carry blood from the heart, veins (flexible, distensible capacitance vessels) to return blood to the heart, and capillaries (which connect arteries to veins) to keep blood flowing from areas of high pressure to areas of low pressure.
- Blood pressure is maintained by stimulus from the sympathetic system and reflex control of blood volume and pressure by the renin–angiotensin system and the aldosterone–ADH system. Alterations in blood pressure (hypotension or hypertension) can upset the balance of the cardiovascular system and lead to problems in blood delivery.
- Fluid shifts out of the blood at the arterial ends of capillaries to deliver oxygen and nutrients to the tissues. It moves out due to the hydrostatic or fluid pressure of the arterial side of the system. Fluid returns to the system at the venous end of the capillaries because of the oncotic pull of proteins in the vessels. Disruptions in these pressures can lead to edema or loss of fluid in the tissues.

CHECK YOUR UNDERSTANDING

Answers to the questions in this chapter can be found in Answers to Check Your Understanding Questions on thePoint®.

MULTIPLE CHOICE

Select the best answer to the following.

1. When describing heart valves to a group of students, which of the following would the instructor include?
   a. The closing of the AV valves is what is responsible for heart sounds.
   b. Small muscles attached to the AV valves are responsible for opening and closing the valves.
   c. The aortic valve opens when the pressure in the left ventricle becomes greater than the aortic pressure.
   d. The valves leading to the great vessels are called the cuspid valves.
2. In the heart,
   a. the ventricles will not contract unless they are stimulated by action potentials arising from the SA node.
   b. fibrillation of the atria will cause blood pressure to fall to zero.
   c. spontaneous depolarization of the muscle membrane can occur in the absence of nerve stimulation.
   d. the muscle can continue to contract for a long period of time in the absence of oxygen.

(continues on page 722)

3. The activity of the heart depends on both the inherent properties of the cardiac muscle cells and the activity of the autonomic nerves to the heart. Therefore,
   a. cutting all of the autonomic nerves to the heart produces a decrease in heart rate.
   b. blocking the parasympathetic nerves to the heart decreases the heart rate.
   c. stimulating the sympathetic nerves to the heart increases the time available to fill the ventricles during diastole.
   d. the heart rate will increase in cases of dehydration, which lead to low cardiac output.

4. A heart transplantation patient has no nerve connections to the transplanted heart. In such an individual, one would expect to find
   a. a slower-than-normal resting heart rate.
   b. atria that contract at a different rate than ventricles.
   c. an increase in heart rate during emotional stress.
   d. inability to exercise because there is no way to increase heart rate.

5. The baroreceptors in the carotid sinus and aortic arch
   a. are in appropriate positions to protect the brain.
   b. decrease the frequency of impulses sent to the cardiovascular center when arterial blood pressure is increased.
   c. monitor the magnitude of concentration of oxygen in the vessels.
   d. react to high levels of carbon dioxide in the aorta or carotid artery.

6. Cardiac cells differ from skeletal muscle cells in that
   a. they contain actin and myosin.
   b. they possess automaticity and conductivity.
   c. calcium must be present for muscle contraction to occur.
   d. they do not require oxygen to survive.

7. Clinically, dysrhythmias, or arrhythmias, cause
   a. altered cardiac output that could affect all cells.
   b. changes in capillary filling pressures.
   c. alterations in osmotic pressure.
   d. valvular dysfunction.

8. A client is brought to the emergency room with a suspected myocardial infarction. The client is very upset because he had just had an ECG in his doctor's office and it was fine. The explanation of this common phenomenon would include the fact that
   a. the ECG only reflects changes in cardiac output.
   b. the ECG is not a very accurate test.
   c. the ECG only measures the flow of electrical current through the heart.
   d. the ECG is not related to the heart problems.

9. Blood flow to the myocardium differs from blood flow to the rest of the cells of the body in that
   a. blood perfuses the myocardium during systole.
   b. blood flow is determined by many local factors, including buildup of acid.
   c. blood perfuses the myocardium during diastole.
   d. oxygenated blood flows to the myocardium via veins.

MULTIPLE RESPONSE

Select all that apply.

1. During diastole, which of the following would occur?
   a. Opening of the AV valves
   b. Relaxation of the myocardial muscle
   c. Flow of blood from the atria to the ventricles
   d. Contraction of the ventricles
   e. Closing of the semilunar valves
   f. Filling of the coronary arteries

2. The sympathetic nervous system would be expected to have which of the following effects?
   a. Stimulate the heart to beat faster
   b. Speed conduction through the AV node
   c. Cause the heart muscle to contract harder
   d. Slow conduction through the AV node
   e. Decrease overall vascular volume
   f. Increase total peripheral resistance

BIBLIOGRAPHY AND REFERENCES

Barrett, K., Barman, S., Boitano, S., et al. (2015). *Ganong's review of medical physiology* (25th ed.). New York: McGraw-Hill.

Bonow, R. O., Mann, D. L., Libby, P., et al. (2014). *Braunwald's heart disease: A textbook of cardiovascular medicine* (10th ed.). Philadelphia, PA: W. B. Saunders.

Brunton, L., Chabner, B., & Knollman, B. (2011). *Goodman and Gilman's the pharmacological basis of therapeutics* (12th ed.). New York: McGraw-Hill.

Fuster, V., Alexander, R. W., & Rourke, R. A. (Eds.). (2011). *Hurst's the heart* (13th ed.). New York: McGraw-Hill.

Hall, J. (2015). *Guyton and Hall's textbook of medical physiology* (13th ed.). Philadelphia, PA: W. B. Saunders.

Karch, A. M. (2014). *Lippincott's nursing drug guide.* Philadelphia, PA: Lippincott Williams & Wilkins.

Porth, C. M. (2013). *Pathophysiology: Concepts of altered health states* (9th ed.). Philadelphia, PA: Lippincott Williams & Wilkins.

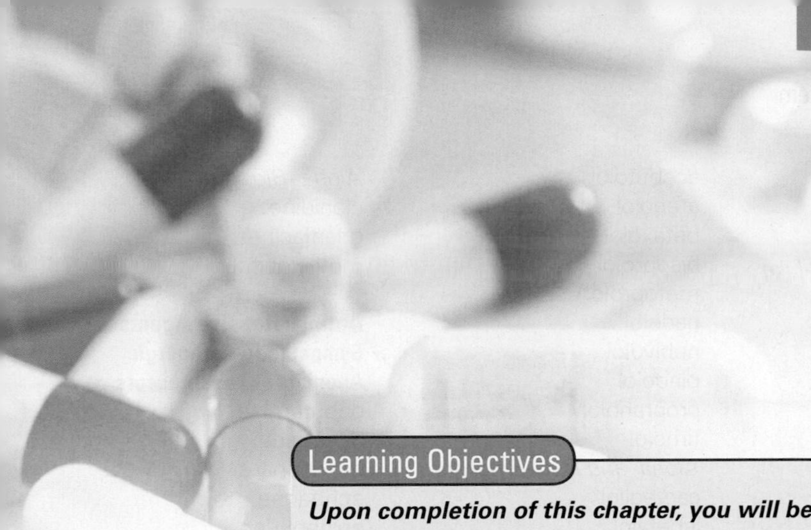

43 Drugs Affecting Blood Pressure

Learning Objectives

Upon completion of this chapter, you will be able to:

1. Outline the normal controls of blood pressure and explain how the various drugs used to treat hypertension or hypotension affect these controls.
2. Describe the therapeutic actions, indications, pharmacokinetics, contraindications, most common adverse reactions, and important drug–drug interactions associated with drugs affecting blood pressure.
3. Discuss the use of drugs that affect blood pressure across the lifespan.
4. Compare and contrast the prototype drugs captopril, losartan, diltiazem, nitroprusside, and droxidopa with other agents in their class and with other agents used to affect blood pressure.
5. Outline the nursing considerations, including important teaching points, for patients receiving drugs used to affect blood pressure.

Glossary of Key Terms

angiotensin-converting enzyme (ACE) inhibitor: drug that blocks ACE, the enzyme responsible for converting angiotensin I to angiotensin II in the lungs; this blocking prevents the vasoconstriction and aldosterone release related to angiotensin II

angiotensin II receptors: specific receptors found in blood vessels and in the adrenal gland that react with angiotensin II to cause vasoconstriction and release of aldosterone

baroreceptor: pressure receptor; located in the arch of the aorta and in the carotid artery; responds to changes in pressure and influences the medulla to stimulate the sympathetic system to increase or decrease blood pressure

cardiovascular center: area of the medulla at which stimulation will activate the sympathetic nervous system to increase blood pressure, heart rate, and so forth

essential hypertension: sustained blood pressure above normal limits with no discernible underlying cause

hypotension: sustained blood pressure that is lower than that required to adequately perfuse all of the body's tissues

peripheral resistance: force that resists the flow of blood through the vessels, mostly determined by the arterioles, which contract to increase resistance; important in determining overall blood pressure

renin–angiotensin–aldosterone system: compensatory process that leads to increased blood pressure and blood volume to ensure perfusion of the kidneys; important in the continual regulation of blood pressure

shock: severe hypotension that can lead to accumulation of waste products and cell death

stroke volume: the amount of blood pumped out of the ventricle with each beat; important in determining blood pressure

Drug List

Antihypertensive Agents

Drugs Affecting the Renin-Angiotensin-Aldosterone System

Angiotensin-Converting Enzyme Inhibitors

benazepril
(P) captopril
enalapril
enalaprilat
fosinopril
lisinopril
moexipril
perindopril
quinapril
ramipril
trandolapril

Angiotensin II Receptor Blockers

azilsartan
candesartan
eprosartan
irbesartan
(P) losartan
olmesartan
telmisartan
valsartan

Renin Inhibitor

aliskiren

Calcium-Channel Blockers

amlodipine
clevidipine
(P) diltiazem
felodipine
isradipine

(continues on page 724)

nicardipine
nifedipine
nisoldipine
verapamil

Vasodilators
hydralazine
minoxidil
nitroprusside

Vasodilators for Pulmonary Artery Hypertension
ambrisentan
bosentan
epoprostenol
iloprost
sildenafil
tadalafil
treprostinil

Other Antihypertensive Agents
Diuretic Agents

Thiazide and Thiazide-Like Diuretics
bendroflumethiazide
chlorothiazide
hydrochlorothiazide
methyclothiazide
chlorthalidone
indapamide
metolazone
Potassium-Sparing Diuretics
amiloride
spironolactone
triamterene

Sympathetic Nervous System Drugs
Beta-Blockers
acebutolol
atenolol
betaxolol
bisoprolol
metoprolol
nadolol
nebivolol
pindolol
propranolol
timolol
Alpha- and Beta-Blockers
carvedilol
labetalol
Alpha-Adrenergic Blockers
phenoxybenzamine
phentolamine
Alpha$_1$-Blockers
doxazosin
prazosin
terazosin
Alpha$_2$-Blockers
clonidine
guanfacine
methyldopa

Antihypotensive Agents
Sympathetic Adrenergic Agonists or Vasopressors
dobutamine
dopamine
droxidopa
ephedrine
epinephrine
isoproterenol
midodrine
norepinephrine
phenylephrine

The cardiovascular (CV) system is a closed system of blood vessels that is responsible for delivering oxygenated blood to the tissues and removing waste products from the tissues. The blood in this system flows from areas of higher pressure to areas of lower pressure. The area of highest pressure in the system is always the left ventricle during systole. The pressure in this area propels the blood out of the aorta and into the system. The lowest pressure is in the right atrium, which collects all of the deoxygenated blood from the body. The maintenance of this pressure system is controlled by specific areas of the brain and various hormones. If the pressure becomes too high the person is said to be hypertensive. If the pressure becomes too low and blood cannot be delivered effectively the person is said to be hypotensive. Severe low blood pressure (BP) is called shock and is a life-threatening situation. Helping the patient to maintain the BP within normal limits is the goal of drug therapy.

Review of Blood Pressure Control

The pressure in the CV system is determined by three elements:

- Heart rate
- **Stroke volume**, or the amount of blood that is pumped out of the ventricle with each heartbeat (primarily determined by the volume of blood in the system)
- Total **peripheral resistance**, or the resistance of the muscular arteries to the blood being pumped through

The small arterioles are thought to be the most important factors in determining peripheral resistance. Because they have the smallest diameter, they are able to almost stop blood flow into capillary beds when they constrict, building up tremendous pressure in the arteries behind them as they prevent the blood from flowing through. The arterioles are very responsive to stimulation from the sympathetic nervous system; they constrict when the sympathetic system is stimulated, increasing total peripheral resistance and BP. The body uses this responsiveness to regulate BP on a constant basis to ensure that there is enough pressure in the system to deliver sufficient blood to the brain.

Baroreceptors

As the blood leaves the left ventricle through the aorta, it influences specialized cells in the arch of the aorta called **baroreceptors** (pressure receptors). Similar cells are located in the carotid arteries, which deliver blood directly to the brain. If there is sufficient pressure in these vessels the baroreceptors are stimulated, sending that information to the brain. If the pressure falls the stimulation of the baroreceptors falls off. That information is also sent to the brain.

The sensory input from the baroreceptors is received in the medulla in an area called the **cardiovascular center**, or vasomotor center. If the pressure is high the medulla stimulates vasodilation and a decrease in cardiac rate and output, causing the pressure in the system to drop. If the pressure is low the medulla directly stimulates an increase in cardiac rate and output and vasoconstriction; this increases total peripheral resistance and raises the BP. The medulla mediates these effects through the autonomic nervous system (see Chapter 29).

The baroreceptor reflex functions continually maintain BP within a predetermined range of normal. For example, if you have been lying down flat and suddenly stand up the blood will rush to your feet (an effect of gravity). You may even feel light-headed or dizzy for a short time. When you stand and the blood flow drops the baroreceptors are not stretched. The medulla senses this drop in stimulation of the baroreceptors and stimulates a rise in heart rate and cardiac output and a generalized vasoconstriction, which increases total peripheral resistance and BP. These increases should raise pressure in the system, which restores blood flow to the brain and stimulates the baroreceptors. The stimulation of the baroreceptors leads to a decrease in stimulatory impulses from the medulla, and the BP falls back within normal limits (Figure 43.1).

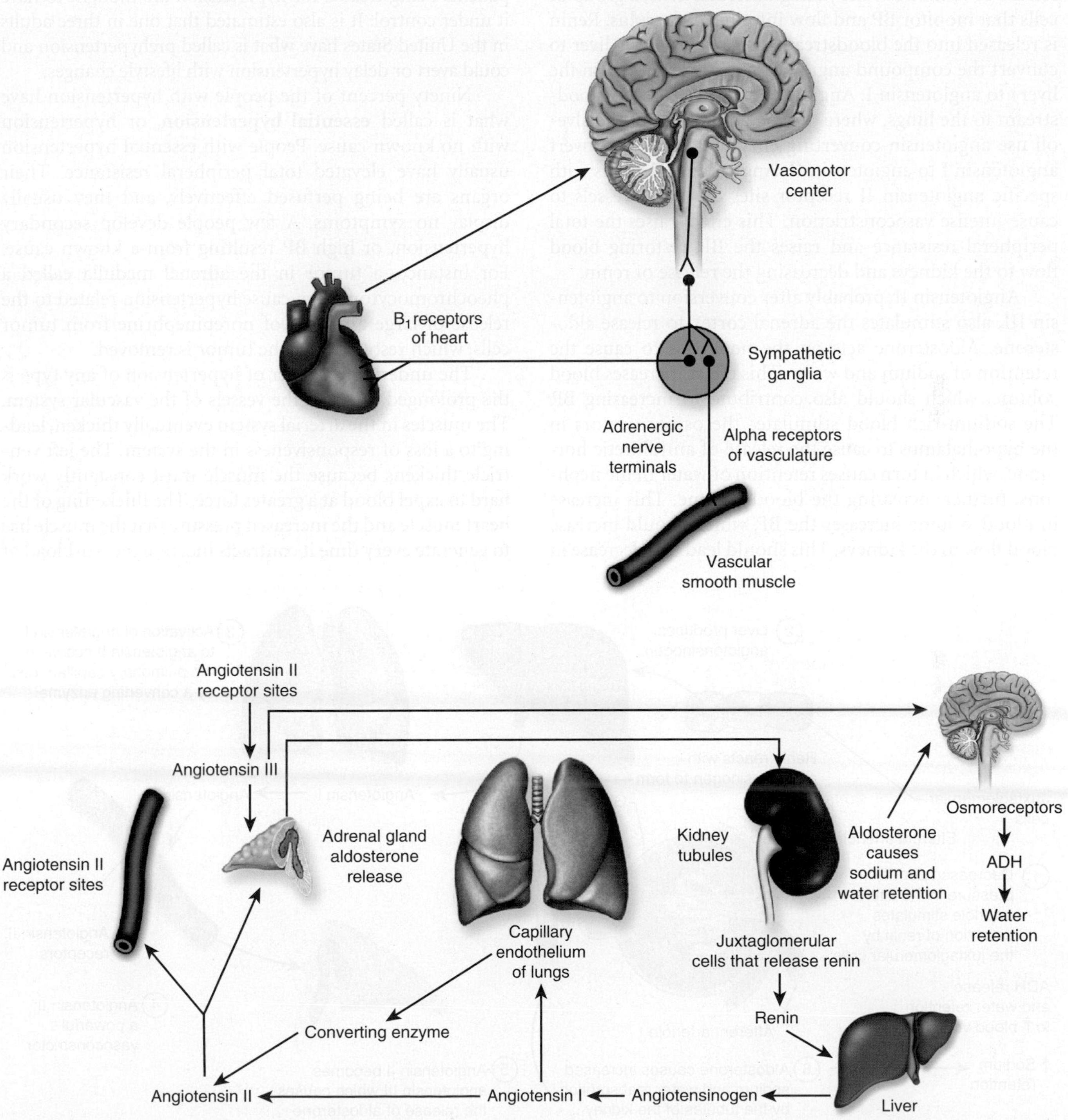

FIGURE 43.1 Control of blood pressure. The vasomotor center in the medulla responds to stimuli from aortic and carotid baroreceptors to cause sympathetic stimulation. The kidneys release renin to activate the renin–angiotensin system, causing vasoconstriction and increased blood volume.

Renin–Angiotensin–Aldosterone System

Another compensatory system is activated when the BP within the kidneys falls. Because the kidneys require constant perfusion to function properly, they have a compensatory mechanism to help ensure that blood flow is maintained. This mechanism is called the **renin–angiotensin–aldosterone system** (RAS).

Low BP or poor oxygenation of a nephron causes the release of renin from the juxtaglomerular cells, a group of cells that monitor BP and flow into the glomerulus. Renin is released into the bloodstream and arrives in the liver to convert the compound angiotensinogen (produced in the liver) to angiotensin I. Angiotensin I travels in the bloodstream to the lungs, where the metabolic cells of the alveoli use angiotensin-converting enzyme (ACE) to convert angiotensin I to angiotensin II. Angiotensin II reacts with specific angiotensin II receptor sites on blood vessels to cause intense vasoconstriction. This effect raises the total peripheral resistance and raises the BP, restoring blood flow to the kidneys and decreasing the release of renin.

Angiotensin II, probably after conversion to angiotensin III, also stimulates the adrenal cortex to release aldosterone. Aldosterone acts on the nephrons to cause the retention of sodium and water. This effect increases blood volume, which should also contribute to increasing BP. The sodium-rich blood stimulates the osmoreceptors in the hypothalamus to cause the release of antidiuretic hormone, which in turn causes retention of water in the nephrons, further increasing the blood volume. This increase in blood volume increases the BP, which should increase blood flow to the kidneys. This should lead to a decrease in the release of renin, thus causing the compensatory mechanisms to stop (Figure 43.2).

Hypertension

When a person's BP is above normal limits for a sustained period a diagnosis of hypertension is made. It is estimated that at least 29% of the people in the United States have hypertension, and many are unaware of it. Only about 52% of the patients being treated for hypertension are thought to have it under control. It is also estimated that one in three adults in the United States have what is called prehypertension and could avert or delay hypertension with lifestyle changes.

Ninety percent of the people with hypertension have what is called **essential hypertension**, or hypertension with no known cause. People with essential hypertension usually have elevated total peripheral resistance. Their organs are being perfused effectively, and they usually display no symptoms. A few people develop secondary hypertension, or high BP resulting from a known cause. For instance, a tumor in the adrenal medulla called a pheochromocytoma can cause hypertension related to the release of large amounts of norepinephrine from tumor cells, which resolves after the tumor is removed.

The underlying danger of hypertension of any type is the prolonged force on the vessels of the vascular system. The muscles in the arterial system eventually thicken, leading to a loss of responsiveness in the system. The left ventricle thickens because the muscle must constantly work hard to expel blood at a greater force. The thickening of the heart muscle and the increased pressure that the muscle has to generate every time it contracts increase the workload of

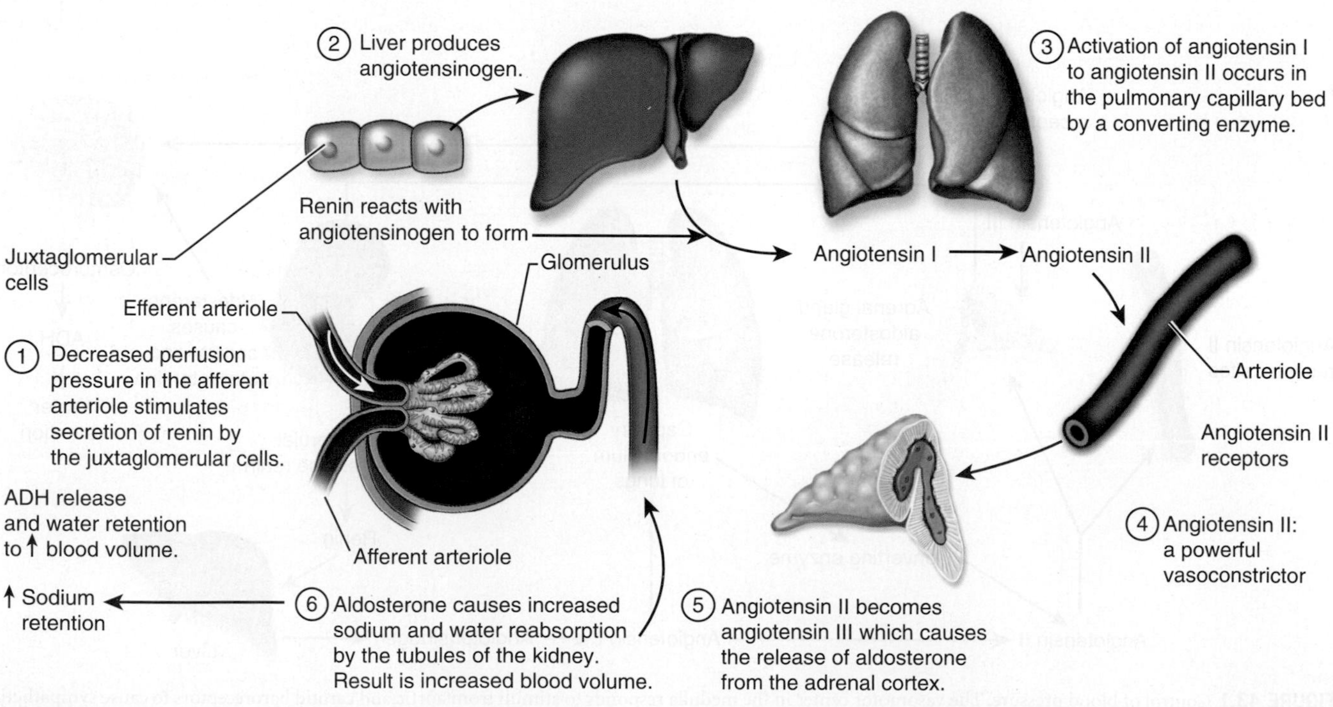

FIGURE 43.2 The renin–angiotensin–aldosterone system.

BOX 43.1

Treatment Recommendations for Hypertension

Treatment Goals

General population 60 years or older: <150/<90
General population under 60 years: <140/<90
Patients 18 years or older with chronic kidney disease: <140/<90
Patients 18 years or older with diabetes: <140/<90

Treatment Guidelines

Nonblack patients, including diabetics: Initiate treatment with a thiazide diuretic, then calcium-channel blocker, ACE inhibitor, ARB.
Black patients, including diabetics: Initiate treatment with thiazide diuretic or calcium-channel blocker.
Patients 18 years or older with chronic kidney disease: Initiate treatment with an ACE inhibitor or ARB.

The main objective of hypertension treatment is to attain and maintain goal BP. If goal BP is not reached within a month of treatment the clinician should increase the dose of the initial drug or add a second drug from one of the classes in recommendation 6 (thiazide-type diuretic, calcium-channel blocker, ACE inhibitor, or ARB). The clinician should continue to assess BP and adjust the treatment regimen until goal BP is reached. If goal BP cannot be reached with two drugs, a third drug from the list provided should be added and titrated. An ACEI and an ARB should not be used together in the same patient. If goal BP cannot be reached using only the drugs recommended or a contraindication or the need to use more than three drugs to reach goal BP, antihypertensive drugs from other classes can be used. Referral to a hypertension specialist may be indicated for patients in whom goal BP cannot be attained using the above strategy or for the management of complicated patients for whom additional clinical consultation is needed.

Adapted from JNC 8 recommendations for managing hypertension.

the heart and the risk of coronary artery disease (CAD) as well. The inner linings of the arteries are damaged by the force of the blood being propelled against them, making these vessels susceptible to atherosclerosis and to narrowing of the lumen of the vessels (see Chapter 46). Tiny vessels can be damaged and destroyed, leading to losses of vision (if the vessels are in the retina), kidney function (if the vessels include the glomeruli in the nephrons), or cerebral function (if the vessels are small and fragile vessels in the brain).

Untreated hypertension increases a person's risk for the following conditions: CAD and cardiac death, stroke, renal failure, and loss of vision. Because hypertension has no symptoms, it is difficult to diagnose and treat, and it is often called the "silent killer." All of the drugs used to treat hypertension have adverse effects, many of which are seen as unacceptable by otherwise healthy people. See Box 43.1 for treatment recommendations for hypertension. Nurses face a difficult challenge trying to convince patients to comply with their drug regimens when they experience adverse effects and do not see any positive effects on their bodies. Research into the cause of hypertension is ongoing. Many theories have been proposed for the cause of the disorder, and it may well be due to a mosaic of factors. Factors that are known to increase BP in some people include high levels of psychological stress, exposure to high-frequency noise, a high-salt diet, lack of rest, and genetic predisposition (see Boxes 43.1, 43.2, and 43.3).

BOX 43.2 FOCUS ON The Evidence

"White Coat" Hypertension

The diagnosis of hypertension is accompanied by the impact of serious ramifications, such as increased risk for numerous diseases and cardiovascular death, the potential need for significant lifestyle changes, and the potential need for drug therapy, which may include many unpleasant adverse effects. Consequently, it is important that a patient be correctly diagnosed before being labeled hypertensive.

Researchers in the 1990s discovered that some patients were hypertensive only when they were in their doctor's office having their BP measured. This was correlated to a sympathetic stress reaction (which elevates systolic blood pressure) and a tendency to tighten the muscles (isometric exercise, which elevates diastolic blood pressure) while waiting to be seen and during BP measurement. The researchers labeled this phenomenon "white coat" hypertension.

The American Heart Association has put forth new guidelines for the diagnosis of hypertension. A patient should have three consecutive BP readings above normal, when taken by a nurse, over a period of 2 to 3 weeks. (It was assumed that nurses were not as threatening or stress provoking as doctors.) These guidelines point out the importance of using the correct technique when taking a patient's BP, especially because the results can have such a tremendous impact on a patient. It is good practice to periodically review the process for performing this routine task. For example, the nurse should:

- Select a cuff that is the correct size for the patient's arm (a cuff that is too small may give a high reading; a cuff that is too large may give a lower reading).
- Try to put the patient at ease; remember that waiting alone in a cold room can be stressful to the body and mind and can increase the blood pressure.

(continues on page 728)

BOX 43.2 FOCUS ON **The Evidence** *(continued)*

- Ensure that the arm that will be used for the cuff is supported.
- Make sure the rest of the patient's muscles are not tensed while the BP is being taken.
- Place both the cuff and the stethoscope directly on the patient instead of on clothing.
- Listen carefully and record the first sound heard, the muffling of sounds, and the absence of sound (the actual diastolic pressure is thought to be between these two sounds).

BP machines found in grocery stores and pharmacies often give higher readings than the actual BP, so patients should not be encouraged to use these machines for follow-up readings. The American Heart Association offers many good guidelines for accurate BP measurement. Nurses are often the health care providers most likely to be taking and recording patient BP, so it is important to always use a proper technique and to make accurate records.

Hypotension

If BP becomes too low the vital centers in the brain, as well as the rest of the tissues of the body, may not receive enough oxygenated blood to continue functioning. **Hypotension** can progress to **shock**, in which the body is in serious jeopardy as waste products accumulate and cells die from lack of oxygen. Hypotensive states can occur in the following situations:

- When the heart muscle is damaged and unable to pump effectively
- With severe blood or fluid loss, when volume drops dramatically
- When there is extreme stress and the body's levels of norepinephrine are depleted, leaving the body unable to respond to stimuli to raise BP

BOX 43.3 FOCUS ON **Cultural Considerations**

Antihypertensive Therapy

In the United States, African Americans are at highest risk for developing hypertension, with men more likely than women to develop the disease. African Americans have documented differences in response to antihypertensive therapy. For example, African Americans are:

- Most responsive to single-drug therapy (as opposed to combination drug regimens).
- More responsive to diuretics, calcium-channel blockers, and alpha-adrenergic blockers.
- Less responsive to ACE inhibitors and beta-blockers.

Increased adverse effects (depression, fatigue, drowsiness) often occur when using thiazide and thiazide-like diuretics, potentially requiring the use of different diuretics or lower doses of the thiazide diuretics.

Screening for hypertension among African Americans is very important to detect hypertension early and to prevent the organ damage that occurs with prolonged hypertension. Because African Americans are more responsive to diuretics the treatment approach should include the first-line use of a diuretic in combination with diet and other lifestyle changes. The use of calcium-channel blockers or alpha-adrenergic blockers should follow.

KEY POINTS

- The CV system depends on pressure changes to circulate blood to the tissues and back to the heart.
- Heart rate, stroke volume, and peripheral vascular resistance are factors that determine BP.
- Constriction and relaxation of the arterioles result in peripheral resistance.
- The baroreceptors stimulate the medulla, which stimulates the sympathetic nervous system to constrict the blood vessels and increase fluid retention if pressure is low in the aorta and the carotid arteries. If pressure is too high, vasodilation and loss of fluid result.
- A decrease in blood flow to the kidneys triggers the RAS, by which the blood vessels constrict and water is retained. This activity increases BP and restores blood flow to the kidney.
- Hypertension is a sustained state of higher-than-normal BP that can lead to blood vessel damage, atherosclerosis, and damage to small vessels in end organs.
- The cause of essential hypertension is unknown; treatment varies among individuals and is aimed at altering the normal reflex responses that control BP.

Antihypertensive Agents

Because an underlying cause of hypertension is usually unknown, altering the body's regulatory mechanisms is the best treatment currently available. Drugs used to treat hypertension work to alter the normal reflexes that control BP. See Figure 43.3 for a review of the sites of action of drugs used to treat hypertension. Treatment for essential hypertension does not cure the disease but is aimed at maintaining the BP within normal limits to prevent the damage that hypertension can cause. Not all patients respond in the same way to antihypertensive drugs because different factors may contribute to each person's hypertension. Patients may have complicating conditions, such as diabetes or acute myocardial infarction (MI) that make it unwise to use certain drugs.

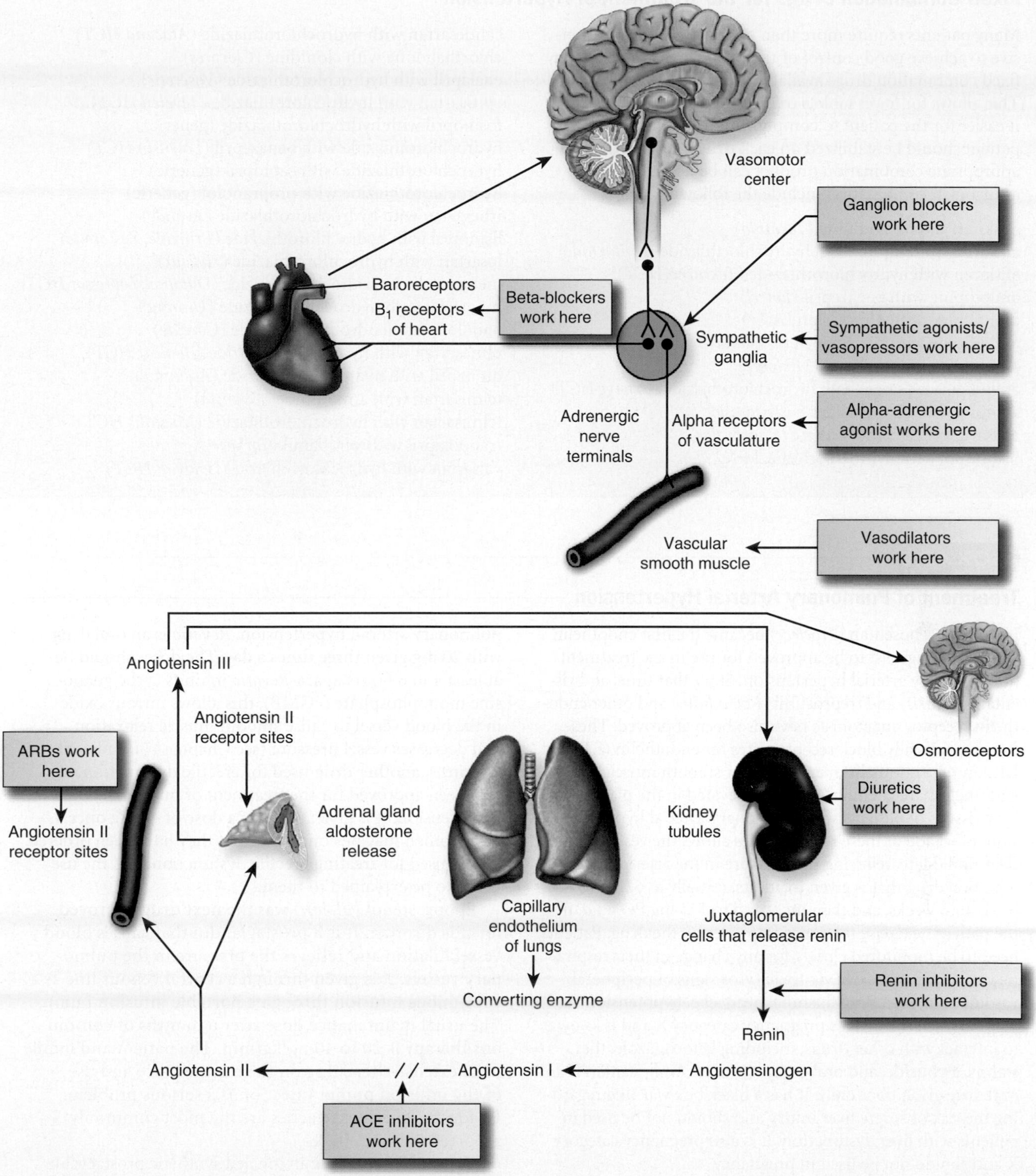

FIGURE 43.3 Sites of action of antihypertensive drugs.

Several different types of drugs that affect different areas of BP control may need to be used in combination to maintain a patient's BP within normal limits. Trials of drugs and combinations of drugs are often needed to develop an individual regimen that is effective without producing adverse effects that are unacceptable to the patient (Box 43.4). Research is ongoing into the treatment of more-specific hypertensions (e.g., pulmonary hypertension). The development of drugs that target specific blood vessel sites and chemicals could lead to a new approach to the treatment of essential hypertension (Box 43.5).

BOX 43.4

Fixed Combination Drugs for the Treatment of Hypertension

Many patients require more than one type of antihypertensive to achieve good control of their BP. There are now many fixed combination drugs available for treating hypertension. This allows for fewer tablets or capsules each day, making it easier for the patient to comply with drug therapy. The patient should be stabilized on each drug first, and then an appropriate combination product can be used. The drugs available in combination include the following:

aliskiren with amlodipine (*Tekamlo*)
aliskiren, amlodipine with hydrochlorthiazide (*Amturnide*)
aliskiren with hydrochlorothiazide (*Tekturna HCT*)
amlodipine with benazepril (*Lotrel*)
amlodipine with olmesartan (*Azor*)
amlodipine with perindopril (*Prestalia*)
amlodipine with valsartan (*Exforge*)
amlodipine, valsartan with hydrochlorothiazide (*Exforge HCT*)
atenolol with chlorthalidone (*Tenoretic*)
azilsartan with chlothalidone (*Edarbyclor*)
bisoprolol with hydrochlorothiazide (*Ziac*)
candesartan with hydrochlorothiazide (*Atacand HCT*)
chlorthalidone with clonidine (*Clorpres*)
enalapril with hydrochlorothiazide (*Vaseretic*)
eprosartan with hydrochlorothiazide (*Teveten HCT*)
fosinopril with hydrochlorothiazide (generic)
hydrochlorothiazide with benazepril (*Lotensin HCT*)
hydrochlorothiazide with captopril (generic)
hydrochlorothiazide with propranolol (generic)
irbesartan with hydrochlorothiazide (*Avalide*)
lisinopril with hydrochlorothiazide (*Prinzide, Zestoretic*)
losartan with hydrochlorothiazide (*Hyzaar*)
metoprolol with hydrochlorothiazide (*Dutoprol, Lopressor HCT*)
moexipril with hydrochlorothiazide (*Uniretic*)
nadolol with bendroflumethiazide (*Corzide*)
olmesartan with hydrochlorothiazide (*Benicar HCT*)
quinapril with hydrochlorothiazide (*Accuretic*)
telmisartan with amlodipine (*Twynsta*)
telmisartan with hydrochlorothiazide (*Micardis HCT*)
trandolapril with verapamil (*Tarka*)
valsartan with hydrochlorothiazide (*Diovan HCT*)

BOX 43.5

Treatment of Pulmonary Arterial Hypertension

In late 2001, bosentan (*Tracleer*) became the first endothelin receptor antagonist to be approved for use in the treatment of pulmonary arterial hypertension. Since that time, ambrisentan (*Letairis*) and treprostinil (*Remodulin*) and other endothelin receptor antagonists have also been approved. These drugs specifically block receptor sites for endothelin (ET_A and ET_B) in the endothelium and vascular smooth muscles; these endothelins are chemicals that are elevated in the plasma and lung tissues of patients with pulmonary arterial hypertension. Blockade of these receptor sites allows the vessels to relax and dilate, relieving the pressure in the arteries. *Tracleer* is an oral drug that is given to adults, initially as 62.5 mg PO b.i.d. for 4 weeks, and then increased to 125 mg PO b.i.d. if the patient's exercise tolerance improves on the drug. Patients need to be monitored closely for any change in their respiratory function, signs of liver toxicity, or signs of peripheral vasodilation, including flushing, headache, hypotension, and palpitations. The drug is pregnancy category X and is known to interact with other drugs, including ketoconazole, the statins, glyburide, and oral contraceptives. Ambrisentan is an oral drug given once daily. It has a black box warning regarding the risk of severe liver injury and should not be used in patients with liver dysfunction. It is also pregnancy category X and should not be used in pregnancy.

Treprostinil (*Remodulin*) is a drug that can be given only by continuous subcutaneous infusion. The patient needs to learn how to care for the infusion port and use the pump. Dosage adjustments are made based on the patient's response and exercise tolerance. Headache and injection site pain are common and may be relieved by the use of analgesics. The drug cannot be discontinued abruptly, but it needs to be tapered to prevent a rebound worsening of the condition.

In 2005, sildenafil, a drug known for the treatment of erectile dysfunction, was approved for the treatment of pulmonary arterial hypertension. *Revatio* is an oral drug, with 20 mg given three times a day. The doses should be at least 4 to 6 hours apart. *Revatio* inhibits cyclic guanosine monophosphate (cGMP); this allows nitrous oxide in the blood vessel to cause smooth muscle relaxation and decreases vessel pressure (see Chapter 41). Tadalafil (*Adcirca*), another drug used for erectile dysfunction, has also been approved for the treatment of pulmonary arterial hypertension. It is given orally at a dose of 40 mg once a day. Women may be concerned that they have been ordered a drug used for treating erectile dysfunction, and the use needs to be explained to them.

Epoprostenol (*Flolan*) was the next drug approved for this disorder. It is a prostaglandin that causes blood vessel dilation and relieves the pressure in the pulmonary vessels. It is given through a central venous line as a continuous infusion through a portable infusion pump. The usual maintenance dose after 6 months of continuous therapy is 20 to 40 ng/kg/min. The patient and family need extensive teaching on the maintenance and use of the infusion pump. Infection is a serious problem. Headache and muscle aches are the most commonly reported adverse effects.

Iloprost (*Ventavis*) is an inhaled synthetic prostacyclin that directly dilates the pulmonary vascular bed, reducing pressure in the pulmonary vascular system, increasing gas exchange, and easing the signs and symptoms of pulmonary arterial hypertension. It is inhaled using a special delivery device six to nine times a day while awake. Patients report dizziness and syncope after using the drug and are encouraged to change position slowly. They should not ingest the drug or get it on their skin. It is a pregnancy category C drug and can be used in pregnancy if the benefit clearly outweighs the potential risk to the fetus.

Antihypertensive agents include ACE inhibitors, angiotensin II receptor blockers (ARBs), calcium-channel blockers, vasodilators, and other antihypertensive agents, including diuretic agents, renin inhibitors, and sympathetic nervous system drugs. See Table 43.1 for a complete list of antihypertensive agents. See Box 43.6 for use of these agents across the lifespan.

Table 43.1 ***Drugs in Focus:* Antihypertensive Agents**

Drug Name	Usual Dosage	Usual Indications
ACE Inhibitors		
benazepril (*Lotensin*)	20–40 mg/d PO, reduce dose with older patients and patients with renal impairment	Approved only for treatment of hypertension in adults
captopril (*Capoten*)	25 mg PO b.i.d. to t.i.d. for hypertension, 50–100 mg PO t.i.d. for HF, 50 mg PO t.i.d. for ventricular dysfunction, 25 mg PO t.i.d. for diabetic nephropathy; reduce dose in patients with renal impairment and in geriatric patients	Treatment of hypertension; adjunct therapy for HF; treatment of left ventricular dysfunction after MI, diabetic nephropathy; for use in adults
enalapril (*Vasotec*)	10–40 mg/d PO; reduce dose in geriatric patients and patients with renal impairment; 2.5 mg PO b.i.d. for HF or left ventricular dysfunction	Treatment of hypertension, HF, left ventricular dysfunction in adults
enalaprilat (generic)	1.25 mg q6 h IV over 5 min	Short-term treatment of acute hypertension when oral therapy is not feasible
fosinopril (generic)	20–40 mg/d PO	Treatment of hypertension, adjunct therapy for HF; for use in adults
lisinopril (*Prinivil*)	20–40 mg/d PO for hypertension, 5–20 mg/d PO for HF, 5–10 mg/d PO after MI; decrease dose in geriatric patients and patients with renal impairment	Treatment of hypertension, HF; treatment of stable patients within 24 h after acute MI to increase survival; for use in adults
moexipril (*Univasc*)	7.5–30 mg/d PO, based on response; reduce dose in patients with renal impairment and in geriatric patients	Treatment of hypertension in adults
perindopril (*Aceon*)	4 mg/d PO; reduce dose in geriatric patients and patients with renal impairment	Treatment of hypertension, may be used alone or as combination drug to control BP; for use in adults
quinapril (*Accupril*)	20–80 mg/d PO, based on response for hypertension; 10–20 mg PO b.i.d. for HF; reduce dose in patients with renal impairment and in geriatric patients	Treatment of hypertension, adjunctive treatment of HF; for use in adults
ramipril (*Altace*)	2.5–20 mg/d PO for hypertension, 5 mg PO b.i.d. for HF; reduce dose in geriatric patients and patients with renal impairment	Treatment of hypertension, adjunctive treatment of HF; for use in adults
trandolapril (*Mavik*)	1–2 mg PO q.i.d. for hypertension; 4 mg/d PO, titrate slowly to that level for HF; reduce dose in patients with renal or hepatic impairment	Treatment of hypertension, HF, and after MI; for use in adults
Angiotensin II Receptor Blockers		
azilsartan (*Edarbi*)	80 mg/d PO	Used alone or as part of combination therapy for treatment of hypertension in adults
candesartan (*Atacand*)	16–32 mg/d PO	Used alone or as part of combination therapy for treatment of hypertension in adults
eprosartan (*Teveten*)	400–800 mg/d PO	Used alone or as part of combination therapy for treatment of hypertension in adults
irbesartan (*Avapro*)	150–300 mg/d PO	Used alone or as part of combination therapy for treatment of hypertension in adults, slowing progression of diabetic nephropathy in patients with hypertension and type 2 diabetes
losartan (*Cozaar*)	25–100 mg/d PO	Used alone or as part of combination therapy for treatment of hypertension in adults, slowing progression of diabetic nephropathy with elevated serum creatinine and proteinuria in patients with hypertension and type 2 diabetes

(table continues on page 732)

Table 43.1 *Drugs in Focus:* Antihypertensive Agents *(continued)*

Drug Name	Usual Dosage	Usual Indications
olmesartan (*Benicar*)	20–40 mg/d PO	Used alone or as part of combination therapy to treat hypertension in adults (newest angiotensin II receptor blocker)
telmisartan (*Micardis*)	40–80 mg/d PO	Used alone or as part of combination therapy for treatment of hypertension in adults
valsartan (*Diovan*)	80–320 mg/d PO based on response	Used alone or as part of combination therapy for treatment of hypertension in adults, treatment of heart failure in patients who are intolerant to ACE inhibitors
Renin Inhibitor		
aliskiren (*Tekurna*)	150-300 mg/d PO based on response	Used alone or as part of combination therapy in treatment of adults with hypertension
Calcium-Channel Blockers		
amlodipine (*Norvasc*)	5–10 mg/d PO, reduce dose in patients with hepatic impairment and in geriatric patients	Used alone or in combination with other agents for treatment of hypertension and angina in adults
clevidipine (*Cleviprex*)	Initially 1–2 mg/h by IV infusion, titrate quickly by doubling the dose every 90 s, usual maintenance dose 4–6 mg/h	Reduction of BP when oral therapy is not possible or desirable
diltiazem (*Cardizem*)	60–120 mg PO b.i.d.	Extended release preparation used to treat hypertension in adults, other preparations are used for angina
felodipine (*Plendil*)	10–15 mg/d PO, do not exceed 10 mg/d in geriatric patients or in patients with hepatic impairment	Used alone or in combination with other agents for treatment of hypertension in adults
isradipine (generic)	2.5–10 mg PO b.i.d., 5–10 mg/d PO—controlled release	Used alone or in combination with thiazide diuretics for treatment of hypertension in adults
nicardipine (*Cardene*)	20–40 mg PO t.i.d.; 0.5–2.2 mg/h IV based on response, switch to oral form as soon as feasible; reduce dose in geriatric patients and in patients with hepatic or renal impairment; 30–60 mg PO b.i.d.—sustained release	Used alone or in combination with other agents for treatment of hypertension and angina, IV form for short-term use when oral route is not feasible; for use in adults
nifedipine (*Procardia XL*)	30–60 mg/d PO	Extended release preparations only for the treatment of hypertension in adults, other preparations are used for angina
nisoldipine (*Sular*)	20–40 mg/d PO; reduce dose in geriatric patients and in patients with hepatic impairment	Extended release tablets used as monotherapy or as part of combination therapy for treatment of hypertension in adults, other preparations are used for angina
verapamil (*Calan SR*)	120–240 mg/d PO, reduce dose in the morning; extended release capsules: 100–300 mg/d PO at bedtime	Extended release formulations for the treatment of essential hypertension, other preparations are used for angina and treating various arrhythmias in adults
Vasodilators		
hydralazine (generic)	*Adult:* 20–40 mg IM or IV repeated as necessary *Pediatric:* 1.7–3.5 mg/kg per 24 h IV or IM in four to six divided doses	Treatment of severe hypertension
minoxidil (generic)	*Adult:* 10–40 mg/d PO in divided doses *Pediatric (<12 y):* 0.25–1 mg/kg/d PO as a single dose	Treatment of severe hypertension unresponsive to other therapy
nitroprusside (*Nitropress*)	*Adult and pediatric:* 3 mcg/kg/min, do not exceed 10 mcg/kg/min	Treatment of hypertensive crisis, also used to maintain controlled hypotension during surgery
Other Antihypertensive Agents ***Diuretic Agents***		
See Chapter 51	See Chapter 51	Treatment of mild hypertension, often first agents used, often used in combination with other agents
Sympathetic Nervous System Blockers		
See Chapter 31	See Chapter 31	

ACE, angiotensin-converting enzyme; HF, heart failure; MI, myocardial infarction; BP, blood pressure.

BOX 43.6 FOCUS ON Drug Therapy Across the Lifespan

Drugs Affecting Blood Pressure

CHILDREN

National standards for determining normal levels of BP in children are quite new. It has been determined that hypertension may start as a childhood disease, and more screening studies are being done to establish normal values for each age group.

Children are thought to be more likely to have secondary hypertension, caused by renal disease or congenital problems such as coarctation of the aorta.

Treatment of childhood hypertension should be done very cautiously because the long-term effects of the antihypertensive agents are not known. Lifestyle changes should be instituted before drug therapy if at all possible. Weight loss and increased activity may bring an elevated BP back to normal in many children.

If drug therapy is used a mild diuretic may be tried first, with monitoring of blood glucose and electrolyte levels on a regular basis. Beta-blockers have been used with success in some children; adverse effects may limit their usefulness in others. The safety and efficacy of the ACE inhibitors and the ARBs have not been established in children. Calcium-channel blockers have been used to treat hypertension in children and may be a first consideration if drug therapy is needed. Careful follow-up of the growing child is essential to monitor for changes in BP, as well as for adverse effects.

ADULTS

Adults receiving any of these drugs need to be instructed about adverse reactions that should be reported immediately. They need to be reminded of safety precautions that may be needed in hot weather or with conditions that cause fluid depletion (e.g., diarrhea, vomiting). If they are taking any other drugs the interacting effects of the various drugs should be evaluated. The importance of other measures to help lower BP—weight loss, smoking cessation, and increased activity—should be stressed.

The safety for the use of these drugs during pregnancy has not been established. ACE inhibitors, ARBs, and renin inhibitors should not be used during pregnancy, and women of childbearing age should be advised to use barrier contraceptives to prevent pregnancy while taking these drugs. Calcium-channel blockers and vasodilators should not be used in pregnancy unless the benefit to the mother clearly outweighs the potential risk to the fetus. The drugs do enter breast milk and can cause serious adverse effects in the baby. Caution should be used or another method of feeding the baby should be used if one of these drugs is needed during lactation.

OLDER ADULTS

Older adults frequently are prescribed one of these drugs. They are more susceptible to the toxic effects of the drugs and are more likely to have underlying conditions that could interfere with drug metabolism and excretion. Renal or hepatic impairment can lead to accumulation of the drugs in the body. If renal or hepatic dysfunction is present the dose should be reduced and the patient monitored very closely.

The total drug regimen of the older patient should be coordinated, with careful attention to interactions among drugs and alternative therapies.

Older adults need to use special caution in any situation that could lead to a fall in BP, such as loss of fluids from diarrhea or vomiting, lack of fluid intake, or excessive heat with decreased sweating that comes with age. Dizziness, falls, or syncope can occur if the BP falls too far in these situations. The BP should always be taken immediately before an antihypertensive is administered to an older adult in an institutional setting to avoid excessive lowering of BP.

Older patients should be especially cautioned about sustained release antihypertensives that cannot be cut, crushed, or chewed to avoid the potential for excessive dosing if these drugs are inappropriately cut.

Stepped Care Approach to Treating Hypertension

The importance of treating hypertension has been proven in numerous research studies. If hypertension is controlled the patient's risk for CV death and disease is reduced. The risk for developing CV complications is directly related to the patient's degree of hypertension. Lowering the degree of hypertension lowers the risk.

The *Seventh Report of the Joint National Committee on Prevention, Detection, Evaluation, and Treatment of Hypertension*, from the National Institutes of Health, established a stepped care approach to treating hypertension that has proved effective in national studies (Box 43.7). It is still the basis for good patient care when it comes to treating hypertension.

Hypertensive treatment is further complicated by the presence of other chronic conditions including diabetes, age, etc. The Joint National Committee published evidence-based recommendations for the treatment of hypertension to help prescribers select an antihypertensive agent in light of complicating conditions (Figure 43.4). A patient's response to a given antihypertensive agent is very individual, so the drug of choice for one patient may have little to no effect on another patient.

Drugs Affecting the Renin–Angiotensin–Aldosterone System

The RAS is one of the body's main reflexes for maintaining BP. In the absence of a known cause for hypertension, one approach to lowering BP is to affect the reflexes that

BOX 43.7

Stepped Care Management of Hypertension

Step 1: Lifestyle Modifications Are Instituted
- Weight reduction
- Smoking cessation
- Moderation of alcohol intake
- Reduction of salt in diet
- Increase in physical activity

Step 2: Inadequate Response
Continue lifestyle modifications. If measures in step 1 are not sufficient to lower BP to an acceptable level, then drug therapy is added:

- Diuretic (decreases serum sodium levels and blood volume)
- ACE inhibitor (blocks the conversion of angiotensin I to angiotensin II)
- Calcium-channel blocker (which relaxes muscle contraction) or other autonomic blockers
- Angiotensin II receptor blocker (blocks the effects of angiotensin on the blood vessel)

Step 3: Inadequate Response
Consider change in drug dose or class, or addition of another drug for combined effect. (Note: Fixed combination drugs should only be used when the patient has been stabilized on each drug separately; see Box 43.4.)

Step 4: Inadequate Response
- All of the above measures are continued.
- A second or third agent or diuretic is added if not already prescribed.

control BP levels. Three classes of drugs have been developed that alter the RAS. The ACE inhibitors, which block the conversion of angiotensin I to angiotensin II, the ARBs, which block the angiotensin receptor site on the blood vessels, and a renin inhibitor, which blocks the reflex at the beginning by inhibiting renin.

Angiotensin-Converting Enzyme Inhibitors

The **angiotensin-converting enzyme inhibitors** include the following agents: benazepril (*Lotensin*), captopril (*Capoten*), enalapril (*Vasotec*), enalaprilat (*generic*),

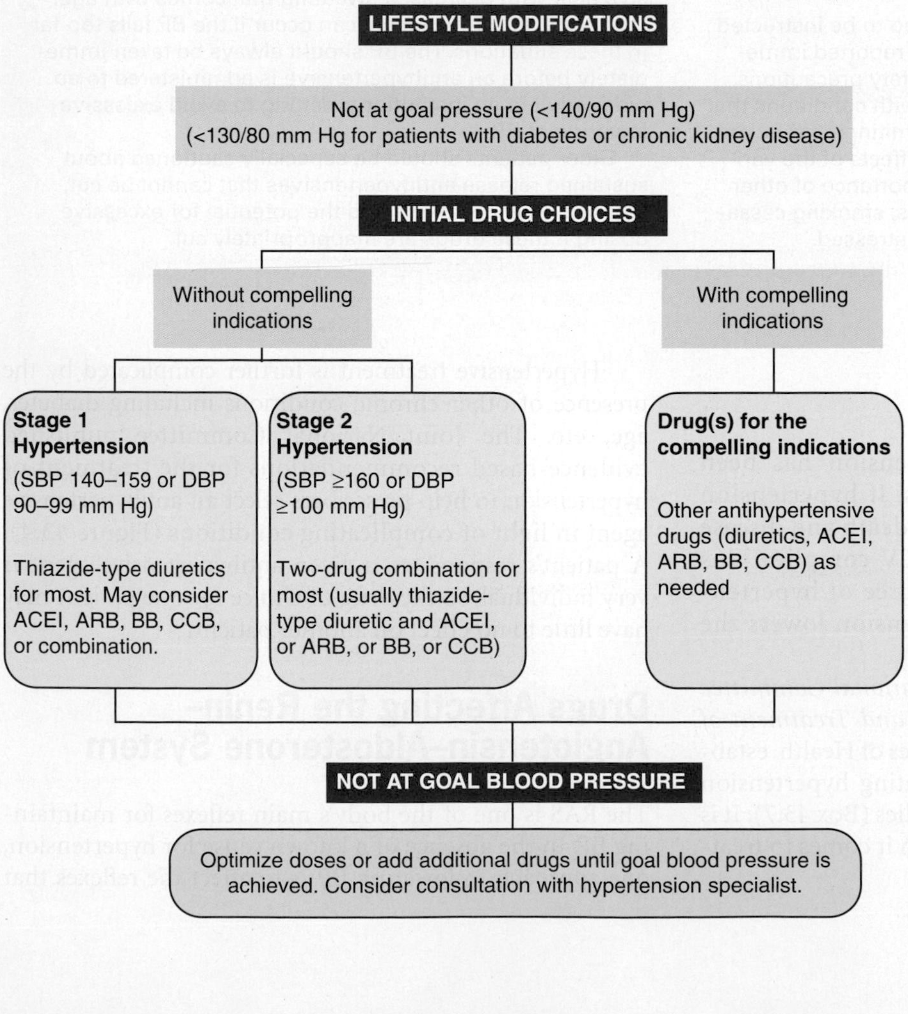
LIFESTYLE MODIFICATIONS
Not at goal pressure (<140/90 mm Hg)
(<130/80 mm Hg for patients with diabetes or chronic kidney disease)
INITIAL DRUG CHOICES
Without compelling indications
With compelling indications
Stage 1 Hypertension
(SBP 140–159 or DBP 90–99 mm Hg)
Thiazide-type diuretics for most. May consider ACEI, ARB, BB, CCB, or combination.
Stage 2 Hypertension
(SBP ≥160 or DBP ≥100 mm Hg)
Two-drug combination for most (usually thiazide-type diuretic and ACEI, or ARB, or BB, or CCB)
Drug(s) for the compelling indications
Other antihypertensive drugs (diuretics, ACEI, ARB, BB, CCB) as needed
NOT AT GOAL BLOOD PRESSURE
Optimize doses or add additional drugs until goal blood pressure is achieved. Consider consultation with hypertension specialist.

FIGURE 43.4 Algorithm for the treatment of hypertension. [From the *Seventh Report of the Joint National Committee on Prevention, Detection, Evaluation, and Treatment of High Blood Pressure* (NIH Publication No. 04-5230) (2004). Bethesda, MD: National Heart, Lung and Blood Institute, National Institutes of Health. Available online at: http://www.nhlbi.nih.gov/guidelines/hypertension/jnc7full.htm]. Though the 8th JNC report on hypertension has been published, this algorithm is still effective.

fosinopril (generic), lisinopril (*Prinivil, Zestril*), moexipril (*Univasc*), perindopril (*Aceon*), quinapril (*Accupril*), ramipril (*Altace*), and trandolapril (*Mavik*).

Therapeutic Actions and Indications

ACE inhibitors act in the lungs to prevent ACE from converting angiotensin I to angiotensin II, a powerful vasoconstrictor and stimulator of aldosterone release (see Figure 43.3). This action leads to a decrease in BP and in aldosterone secretion, with a resultant slight increase in serum potassium and a loss of serum sodium and fluid.

These drugs are indicated for the treatment of hypertension, alone or in combination with other drugs. They are also used in conjunction with digoxin and diuretics for the treatment of heart failure and left ventricular dysfunction. Their therapeutic effect in these cases is thought to be related to a decrease in cardiac workload associated with the decrease in peripheral resistance and blood volume. They are also approved for the treatment of diabetic nephropathy. It is thought that the decrease in stimulation of the angiotensin receptors in the renal artery will slow the damage to the renal artery that occurs in diabetes. See Table 43.1 for Usual Indications for each of these drugs.

Pharmacokinetics

All of the ACE inhibitors are administered orally. Enalapril also has the advantage of parenteral use (enalaprilat) if oral use is not feasible or rapid onset is desirable. These drugs are well absorbed, widely distributed, metabolized in the liver, and excreted in the urine and feces. They have been detected in breast milk, are known to cross the placenta, and have been associated with serious fetal abnormalities, and so they should not be used during pregnancy.

Contraindications and Cautions

ACE inhibitors are contraindicated in the presence of allergy to any of the ACE inhibitors *to prevent hypersensitivity reactions* and with impaired renal function, *which could be exacerbated by the effects of this drug in decreasing renal blood flow.* Caution should be used in patients with heart failure *because the change in hemodynamics could be detrimental in some cases* and in those with salt/volume depletion, *which could be exacerbated by the drug effects.* Women of childbearing age who choose to use one of these drugs should be encouraged to use barrier contraceptives to avoid pregnancy while taking the drug. Use is contraindicated during pregnancy *because of the potential for serious adverse effects on the fetus* and during lactation *because of potential decrease in milk production and effects on the neonate.*

Adverse Effects

The adverse effects most commonly associated with the ACE inhibitors are related to the effects of vasodilation and alterations in blood flow. Such effects include reflex tachycardia, chest pain, angina, heart failure, and cardiac arrhythmias; gastrointestinal (GI) irritation, ulcers, constipation, and liver injury; renal insufficiency, renal failure, and proteinuria; and rash, alopecia, dermatitis, and photosensitivity (Figure 43.5). Quinapril, ramipril, and trandolapril are fairly well tolerated and not associated with as many adverse effects as some of the other agents are. Benazepril, enalapril, and fosinopril are generally well tolerated but cause an unrelenting cough, possibly related to effects in the lungs, where the ACE is inhibited, that may lead patients to discontinue the drug.

Captopril, moexipril, and perindopril are associated with more-serious adverse effects. Captopril has been associated with a sometimes-fatal pancytopenia, cough, and unpleasant GI distress. Moexipril is associated with many unpleasant GI and skin effects, cough, and cardiac arrhythmias; fatal MI and pancytopenia have sometimes been associated with this drug as well. Perindopril and lisinopril are associated with a sometimes-fatal pancytopenia, as well as serious-to-fatal airway obstruction (found to occur more frequently in African American patients).

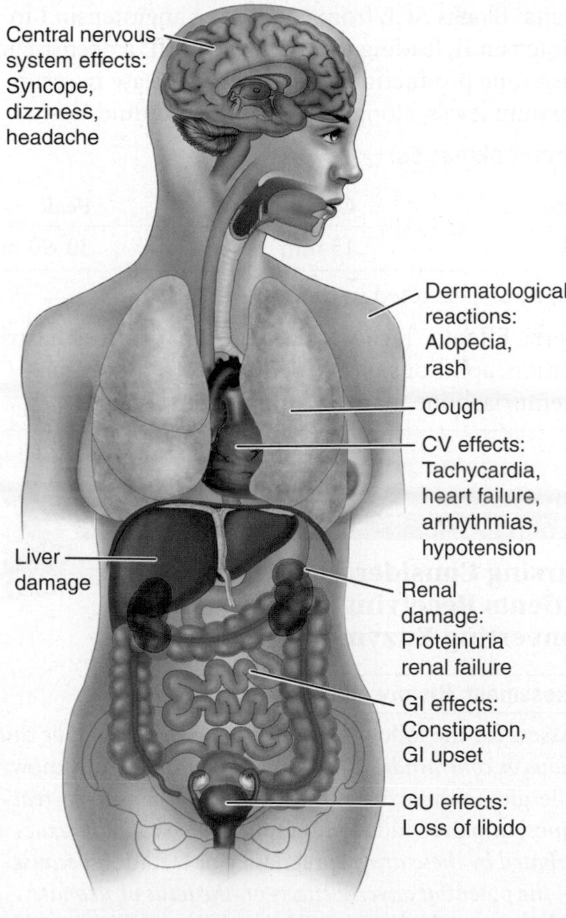

FIGURE 43.5 Variety of adverse effects and toxicities associated with drugs affecting blood pressure.

Clinically Important Drug–Drug Interactions

The risk of hypersensitivity reactions increases if these drugs are taken with allopurinol. There is a risk of decreased antihypertensive effects if taken with nonsteroidal anti-inflammatory drugs; patients should be monitored. The combination of drugs used to alter the RAS is not recommended due to potentially serious adverse effects, and should not be combined with other ACE inhibitors, ARBs, or a renin inhibitor.

Clinically Important Drug–Food Interactions

Absorption of oral ACE inhibitors decreases if they are taken with food. They should be taken on an empty stomach 1 hour before or 2 hours after meals.

Prototype Summary: Captopril

Indications: Treatment of hypertension, heart failure, diabetic nephropathy, and left ventricular dysfunction after an MI.

Actions: Blocks ACE from converting angiotensin I to angiotensin II, leading to a decrease in BP, a decrease in aldosterone production, and a small increase in serum potassium levels, along with sodium and fluid loss.

Pharmacokinetics:

Route	Onset	Peak
Oral	15 min	30–90 min

$T_{1/2}$: 2 hours; excreted in the urine.

Adverse Effects: Tachycardia, MI, rash, pruritus, gastric irritation, aphthous ulcers, peptic ulcers, dysgeusia, proteinuria, bone marrow suppression, cough.

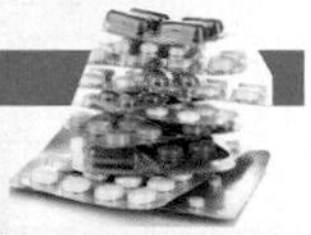

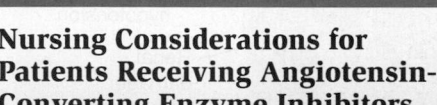

Nursing Considerations for Patients Receiving Angiotensin-Converting Enzyme Inhibitors

Assessment: History and Examination

- Assess for the following conditions, *which could be cautions or contraindications to use of the drug*: Any known allergies to these drugs *to prevent hypersensitivity reactions*; impaired kidney function, *which could be exacerbated by these drugs*; pregnancy or lactation *because of the potential adverse effects on the fetus or neonate*; salt/volume depletion and heart failure, *which could be exacerbated by these drugs.*
- Assess baseline status before beginning therapy *to determine any potential adverse effects.* This includes body temperature and weight; skin color, lesions, and temperature; pulse, BP, baseline electrocardiogram (ECG), and perfusion; respirations and adventitious breath sounds; bowel sounds and abdominal examination; and renal function tests, complete blood count with differential, and serum electrolytes.

Nursing Diagnoses

Nursing diagnoses related to drug therapy might include the following:

- Ineffective tissue perfusion (total body) related to changes in cardiac output
- Impaired skin integrity related to dermatological effects
- Acute pain related to GI distress and cough
- Deficient knowledge regarding drug therapy

Planning

- The patient will receive the best therapeutic effect from the drug therapy.
- The patient will have limited adverse effects to the drug therapy.
- The patient will have an understanding of the drug therapy, adverse effects to anticipate, and measures to relieve discomfort and improve safety.

Implementation with Rationale

- Encourage patient to implement lifestyle changes, including weight loss, smoking cessation, decreased alcohol and salt in the diet, and increased exercise, *to increase the effectiveness of antihypertensive therapy.*
- Administer on an empty stomach 1 hour before or 2 hours after meals *to ensure proper absorption of the drug.*
- Alert the surgeon and mark the patient's chart prominently if the patient is to undergo surgery *to alert medical personnel that the blockage of compensatory angiotensin II could result in hypotension after surgery that would need to be reversed with volume expansion.*
- Give the parenteral form of enalapril only if an oral form is not feasible; transfer to an oral form as soon as possible *to avoid an increased risk for adverse effects.*
- Consult with the prescriber to reduce the dose in patients with renal failure *to account for their decreased production of renin and lower-than-normal levels of angiotensin II.*
- Monitor the patient carefully in any situation that might lead to a drop in fluid volume (e.g., excessive sweating, vomiting, diarrhea, dehydration) *to detect and treat excessive hypotension that may occur.*
- Provide comfort measures *to help the patient tolerate drug effects.* These include small, frequent meals; access to bathroom facilities; bowel program as needed;

environmental controls; safety precautions; and appropriate skin care as needed.
- Provide thorough patient teaching, including the name of the drug, dosage prescribed, measures to avoid adverse effects, warning signs of problems, and the need for periodic monitoring and evaluation, *to enhance patient knowledge about drug therapy and to promote compliance.*
- Offer support and encouragement *to help the patient deal with the diagnosis and the drug regimen.*

Evaluation

- Monitor patient response to the drug (maintenance of BP within normal limits).
- Monitor for adverse effects (hypotension, cardiac arrhythmias, renal dysfunction, skin reactions, cough, pancytopenia, heart failure).
- Evaluate the effectiveness of the teaching plan (patient can name drug, dosage, adverse effects to watch for, specific measures to avoid them, and the importance of continued follow-up).
- Monitor the effectiveness of comfort measures and compliance with the treatment regimen.

Angiotensin II Receptor Blockers

The ARBs include the following drugs: Azilsartan (*Edarbi*), candesartan (*Atacand*), eprosartan (*Teveten*), irbesartan (*Avapro*), losartan (*Cozaar*), olmesartan (*Benicar*), telmisartan (*Micardis*), and valsartan (*Diovan*).

Therapeutic Actions and Indications

The ARBs selectively bind with the **angiotensin II receptors** in vascular smooth muscle and in the adrenal cortex to block vasoconstriction and the release of aldosterone. These actions block the BP-raising effects of the renin–angiotensin system and lower BP. They are indicated to be used alone or in combination therapy for the treatment of hypertension and for the treatment of heart failure in patients who are intolerant to ACE inhibitors. Recently, they were also found to slow the progression of renal disease in patients with hypertension and type 2 diabetes. This action is thought to be related to the effects of blocking angiotensin receptors in the vascular endothelium. See Table 43.1 for Usual Indications for each drug.

Pharmacokinetics

These agents are all given orally. They are well absorbed and undergo metabolism in the liver by the cytochrome P450 system. They are excreted in the feces and urine. The ARBs cross the placenta. It is not known whether they enter breast milk during lactation (see Contraindications and Cautions).

Contraindications and Cautions

The ARBs are contraindicated in the presence of allergy to any of these drugs *to prevent hypersensitivity reactions.* Caution should be used in the presence of hepatic or renal dysfunction, *which could alter the metabolism and excretion of these drugs,* and with hypovolemia *because of the blocking of potentially life-saving compensatory mechanisms.* These drugs are also contraindicated during pregnancy *because of association with serious fetal abnormalities and even death.* Although it is not known whether the ARBs enter breast milk during lactation, these drugs should not be used during lactation *because of the potential for serious adverse effects in the neonate.* Women of childbearing age should be advised to use barrier contraceptives to avoid pregnancy; if a pregnancy does occur the ARB should be discontinued immediately.

Adverse Effects

The adverse effects most commonly associated with ARBs include the following: Headache, dizziness, syncope, and weakness, which could be associated with drops in BP; hypotension; GI complaints, including diarrhea, abdominal pain, and nausea; dry mouth, and tooth pain; symptoms of upper respiratory tract infections and cough; and rash, dry skin, and alopecia. In preclinical trials, these drugs have been associated with the development of various cancers. They have also been associated with renal damage in some patients; it is important to monitor renal function regularly when using these drugs.

Clinically Important Drug–Drug Interactions

The risk of decreased serum levels and loss of effectiveness increases if the ARB is taken in combination with phenobarbital, indomethacin, or rifamycin. If this combination is used the patient should be monitored closely and dose adjustments made. There may be a decrease in anticipated antihypertensive effects if the drug is combined with ketoconazole, fluconazole, or diltiazem. Monitor the patient closely and adjust dose as needed. These drugs should not be used with ACE inhibitors or a renin inhibitor because of the potential for serious adverse effects.

Ⓟ Prototype Summary: Losartan

Indications: Alone or as part of combination therapy for the treatment of hypertension; treatment of diabetic nephropathy with an elevated serum creatinine and proteinuria in patients with type 2 diabetes and hypertension.

Actions: Selectively blocks the binding of angiotensin II to specific tissue receptors found in the vascular smooth muscle and adrenal glands; blocks the vasoconstriction and release of aldosterone associated with the RAS.

Pharmacokinetics:

Route	Onset	Peak	Duration
Oral	Varies	1–3 h	24 h

$T_{1/2}$: 2 hours, then 6 to 9 hours; metabolized in the liver and excreted in urine and feces.

Adverse Effects: Dizziness, headache, diarrhea, abdominal pain, symptoms of upper respiratory tract infection, cough, back pain, fever, muscle weakness, hypotension.

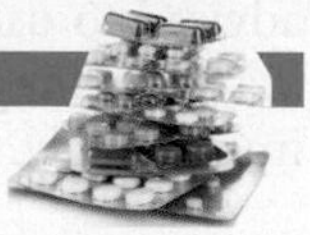

Nursing Considerations for Patients Receiving Angiotensin II Receptor Blockers

Assessment: History and Examination

- Assess for the following conditions, *which could be cautions or contraindications to use of the drug*: Any known allergies to these drugs *to prevent hypersensitivity reactions*; impaired kidney or liver function, *which could be exacerbated by these drugs*; pregnancy and lactation *because of the potential adverse effects on the fetus and neonate*; and hypovolemia, *which could potentiate the BP-lowering effects.*
- Assess baseline status before beginning therapy *to determine any potential adverse effects*; this includes body temperature and weight; skin color, lesions, and temperature; pulse, BP, baseline ECG, and perfusion; respirations and adventitious breath sounds; bowel sounds and abdominal examination; and renal and liver function tests.

Nursing Diagnoses

Nursing diagnoses related to drug therapy might include the following:

- Ineffective tissue perfusion (total body) related to changes in cardiac output
- Impaired skin integrity related to dermatological effects
- Acute pain related to GI distress, cough, skin effects, and headache
- Deficient knowledge regarding drug therapy

Planning

- The patient will receive the best therapeutic effect from the drug therapy.
- The patient will have limited adverse effects to the drug therapy.
- The patient will have an understanding of the drug therapy, adverse effects to anticipate, and measures to relieve discomfort and improve safety.

Implementation with Rationale

- Encourage patient to implement lifestyle changes, including weight loss, smoking cessation, decreased alcohol and salt in the diet, and increased exercise, *to increase the effectiveness of antihypertensive therapy.*
- Administer without regard to meals; give with food *to decrease GI distress if needed.*
- Alert the surgeon and mark the patient's chart prominently if the patient is to undergo surgery *to notify medical personnel that the blockage of compensatory angiotensin II could result in hypotension after surgery that would need to be reversed with volume expansion.*
- Ensure that the female patient is not pregnant before beginning therapy, and suggest the use of barrier contraceptives while she is taking these drugs, *to avert potential fetal abnormalities and fetal death, which have been associated with these drugs.*
- Find an alternative method of feeding the baby if the patient is nursing *to prevent the potentially dangerous blockade of the RAS in the neonate.*
- Monitor the patient carefully in any situation that might lead to a drop in fluid volume (e.g., excessive sweating, vomiting, diarrhea, dehydration) *to detect and treat excessive hypotension that may occur.*
- Provide comfort measures *to help the patient tolerate drug effects*, including small, frequent meals; access to bathroom facilities; safety precautions if central nervous system (CNS) effects occur; environmental controls; appropriate skin care as needed; and analgesics as needed.
- Provide thorough patient teaching, including the name of the drug, dosage prescribed, measures to avoid adverse effects, warning signs of problems, and the need for periodic monitoring and evaluation, *to enhance patient knowledge about drug therapy and to promote compliance.*
- Offer support and encouragement *to help the patient deal with the diagnosis and the drug regimen.*

Evaluation

- Monitor patient response to the drug (maintenance of BP within normal limits).
- Monitor for adverse effects (hypotension, GI distress, skin reactions, cough, headache, dizziness).
- Evaluate the effectiveness of the teaching plan (patient can name drug, dosage, adverse effects to watch for, measures to avoid them, and the importance of continued follow-up).
- Monitor the effectiveness of comfort measures and compliance with the regimen.

Renin Inhibitor

In late 2007 a new class of drugs for treating hypertension was introduced with the approval of aliskiren (*Tekturna*). Aliskiren directly inhibits renin, leading to decreased plasma renin activity and inhibiting the conversion of angiotensinogen to angiotensin I. This inhibition of the RAS leads to decreased BP, decreased aldosterone release, and decreased sodium reabsorption. It is slowly absorbed from the GI tract, with peak levels in 3 hours. It is metabolized in the liver, with a half-life of 24 hours, and is excreted in the urine. Aliskiren crosses the placenta and enters breast milk. It should be avoided in pregnancy because of the potential for serious adverse effects on the fetus. It is suggested that women of childbearing age use contraceptive measures while on this drug. Women who are breastfeeding should find another method of feeding the baby if this drug is needed. Because it blocks the renin–angiotensin system and aldosterone will not be stimulated to be released, there is a risk of hyperkalemia. Patients should have their potassium levels monitored before and periodically during therapy. If aliskiren is combined with furosemide, there may be a loss of diuretic effect. This drug should not be combined with ACE inhibitors or ARBs, because the combined adverse effects can be severe. These patients should be monitored closely. Although it is generally well tolerated, cases of angioedema with respiratory involvement have been reported in patients using this drug. Patients should be advised to report any difficulty in breathing or swelling of the face, lips, or tongue.

Calcium-Channel Blockers

Calcium-channel blockers decrease BP, cardiac workload, and myocardial oxygen consumption. The effects of these drugs on cardiac workload also make them very effective in the treatment of angina (see Chapter 46). The calcium-channel blockers available in immediate release and sustained release forms that are used in treating hypertension include amlodipine (*Norvasc*), felodipine (*Plendil*), isradipine (generic), and nicardipine (*Cardene*). Other calcium-channel blockers are safe and effective for treating hypertension only if they are given as sustained release or extended release preparations. These include diltiazem (*Cardizem CD*), nifedipine (*Procardia XL*), nisoldipine (*Sular*), and verapamil (*Calan SR*). See Contraindications and Cautions for important safety information regarding use of controlled release products. Clevidipine (*Cleviprex*) is only available in IV form for short-term management of hypertension when an oral calcium-channel blocker cannot be used.

Therapeutic Actions and Indications

Calcium-channel blockers inhibit the movement of calcium ions across the membranes of myocardial and arterial muscle cells, altering the action potential and blocking muscle cell contraction. This effect depresses myocardial contractility, slows cardiac impulse formation in the conductive tissues, and relaxes and dilates arteries, causing a fall in BP and a decrease in venous return. See Table 43.1 for Usual Indications for each of these drugs.

Pharmacokinetics

Calcium-channel blockers are given orally and are generally well absorbed, metabolized in the liver, and excreted in the urine. These drugs cross the placenta and enter breast milk (see Contraindications and Cautions). Nicardipine and clevidipine are available in IV form for short-term use when oral administration is not feasible.

Contraindications and Cautions

These drugs are contraindicated in the presence of allergy to any of these drugs *to prevent hypersensitivity reactions*; with heart block or sick sinus syndrome, *which could be exacerbated by the conduction-slowing effects of these drugs*; and with renal or hepatic dysfunction, *which could alter the metabolism and excretion of these drugs*. Although there are no well-defined studies about effects during pregnancy, fetal toxicity has been reported in animal studies; therefore, these drugs should not be used during pregnancy unless the benefit to the mother clearly outweighs any potential risk to the fetus *because of the potential for adverse effects on the fetus or neonate. Because of the potential for serious adverse effects on the baby*, another method of feeding the infant should be used if these drugs are required during lactation.

FOCUS ON Safe Medication Administration

Several drugs that are used to treat hypertension cannot be cut, crushed, or chewed. This is very important information to share with patients. Sometimes patients cut tablets in half to facilitate swallowing or to get twice the number of days for any given prescription. Most drugs formulated for extended release or sustained release are delivered in a matrix system that slowly dispenses the drug into the system. If the coating of the matrix is cut, all of the drug is released at once, leading to the release of too much drug at one time and, consequently, toxic levels of the drug when first taking it. Then the patient receives no drug as the day goes on. Some antihypertensives to be aware of are diltiazem, isradipine, nicardipine, nifedipine, nisoldipine, and verapamil.

Adverse Effects

The adverse effects associated with these drugs relate to their effects on cardiac output and on smooth muscle. CNS effects include dizziness, light-headedness, headache, and fatigue. GI problems include nausea and hepatic injury related to direct toxic effects on hepatic cells. CV effects include hypotension, bradycardia, peripheral edema, and heart block. Skin flushing and rash may also occur.

Clinically Important Drug–Drug Interactions

Drug–drug interactions vary with each of the calcium-channel blockers used to treat hypertension. A potentially serious effect to note is an increase in serum levels and toxicity of cyclosporine if taken with diltiazem.

Clinically Important Drug–Food Interactions

The calcium-channel blockers are a class of drugs that interact with grapefruit juice. When grapefruit juice is present in the body the concentrations of calcium-channel blockers increase, sometimes to toxic levels. Advise patients to avoid the use of grapefruit juice if they are taking a calcium-channel blocker. If a patient on a calcium-channel blocker reports toxic effects, ask whether he or she is drinking grapefruit juice.

Ⓟ Prototype Summary: Diltiazem

Indications: Treatment of essential hypertension in the extended release form.

Actions: Inhibits the movement of calcium ions across the membranes of cardiac and arterial muscle cells, depressing the impulse and leading to slowed conduction, decreased myocardial contractility, and dilation of arterioles, which lowers BP and decreases myocardial oxygen consumption.

Pharmacokinetics:

Route	Onset	Peak	Duration
Oral, extended release	30–60 min	6–11 h	12 h

$T_{1/2}$: 5 to 7 hours; metabolized in the liver and excreted in the urine.

Adverse Effects: Dizziness, light-headedness, headache, peripheral edema, bradycardia, atrioventricular block, flushing, nausea.

Nursing Considerations for Patients Receiving Calcium-Channel Blockers

The main use of calcium-channel blockers is for the treatment of angina. See Chapter 46 for the nursing considerations of calcium channel blockers. See the Critical Thinking Scenario for the initiation of antihypertensive therapy using calcium-channel blockers.

Vasodilators

If other drug therapies do not achieve the desired reduction in BP, it is sometimes necessary to use a direct vasodilator. Most of the vasodilators are reserved for use in severe hypertension, malignant hypertension, or hypertensive emergencies. These include hydralazine (generic), minoxidil (generic), and nitroprusside (*Nitropress*).

Therapeutic Actions and Indications

The vasodilators act directly on vascular smooth muscle to cause muscle relaxation, leading to vasodilation and drop in BP. They do not block the reflex tachycardia that occurs when BP drops. They are indicated for the treatment of severe hypertension that has not responded to other therapy (see Table 43.1).

Pharmacokinetics

Nitroprusside is used IV; hydralazine is available for oral, IV, and IM use; and minoxidil is available as an oral agent only. These drugs are rapidly absorbed and widely distributed. They are metabolized in the liver and primarily excreted in the urine. They cross the placenta and enter breast milk (see Contraindications and Cautions).

CRITICAL THINKING SCENARIO

Initiating Antihypertensive Therapy

THE SITUATION

B.R., a 46-year-old African American male business executive, was seen for a routine insurance physical. His examination was normal except for a BP reading of 164/102 mm Hg. He also was approximately 20 pounds overweight. Urinalysis and blood work results were all within normal limits. He was given a 1,200-calorie-per-day diet to follow and was encouraged to reduce his salt and alcohol intake, start exercising, and stop smoking. He was asked to return in 3 weeks for a follow-up appointment (step 1). Three weeks later, B.R. returned with a 7-pound weight loss and an average BP reading (of three readings) of 145/92 mm Hg. Discussion was held about starting B.R. on a diuretic (step 2) in addition to the lifestyle

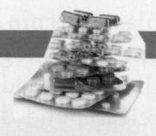

Initiating Antihypertensive Therapy (continued)

changes that B.R. was undertaking. B.R. was reluctant to take a diuretic and, after much discussion, was prescribed a calcium-channel blocker. B.R. asked for a couple more weeks to try to bring his BP down with lifestyle changes before starting the drug.

CRITICAL THINKING

What nursing interventions should be done at this point? *Consider the risk factors that B.R. has for hypertension and the damage that hypertension can cause.*

What are the chances that B.R. can bring his BP within a normal range with lifestyle changes alone?

What additional teaching points should be covered with B.R. before a treatment decision is made?

What implication does the diagnosis of hypertension have for B.R.'s insurance and job security?

What effects could diuretic therapy have on B.R.'s busy business day?

DISCUSSION

B.R. was asked to change many things in his life over the last 3 weeks. These changes themselves can be stressful and can increase a person's BP. B.R.'s reluctance to take a diuretic is understandable for a business executive who might not want his day interrupted by many bathroom stops. African Americans often respond well to diuretic therapy, with a return to normal BP, but they also tend to have more adverse CNS effects with the most commonly used diuretics, the thiazides. This may have an impact on B.R.'s business and home life. The decision to use a calcium-channel blocker may decrease some of the stress B.R. was feeling about the diuretic.

African Americans tend to respond well to monotherapy with calcium-channel blockers, alpha-blockers, or diuretics. B.R. should receive a complete teaching program outlining what is known about hypertension and all of the risk factors involved with the disease. The good effects of weight loss, exercise, and other lifestyle changes should be stressed, and B.R. should be praised for his success over the last 3 weeks.

B.R. may benefit from trying for a couple more weeks to make lifestyle changes that will help bring his BP into normal range. He will then feel that he has some control and input into the situation, and if drug therapy is needed he may be more willing to comply with the prescribed treatment. The diagnosis of hypertension may be delayed for these 2 weeks while B.R. changes his lifestyle. Such a diagnosis should be made only after three consecutive BP readings in the high range are recorded. B.R. may be able to have his BP checked at work in a comfortable environment, which will improve the accuracy of the reading.

In the past, many insurance companies, and some employers, viewed hypertension as a hiring and insurability risk. As a business executive, B.R. may be well aware of this increased risk category—another reason to give him a little more time. He may wish to look into biofeedback for relaxation, a fitness program, smoking cessation programs (if appropriate), and stress reduction. As long as B.R. receives regular follow-up and frequent BP checks, it may be a good idea to allow him to take some control and continue lifestyle changes. If at the end of the 2 weeks no further progress has been made or B.R.'s BP has risen, drug therapy should be considered. Teaching should be aimed at helping B.R. to incorporate the drug effects into his lifestyle, to improve his compliance and tolerance of the therapy.

NURSING CARE GUIDE FOR B.R.: CALCIUM-CHANNEL BLOCKERS

Assessment: History and Examination

Concentrate the health history on allergies to any calcium-channel blocker, renal dysfunction, salt/volume depletion, or heart failure and concurrent use of barbiturates, hydantoins, erythromycin, cimetidine, ranitidine, antifungal agents, and/or grapefruit juice.

Focus the physical examination on the following:

CV: BP, pulse, perfusion, baseline ECG

CNS: Orientation, affect

Skin: Color, lesions, texture, temperature

Respiratory: Respiration, adventitious sounds

GI: Abdominal examination, bowel sounds

Laboratory tests: Renal function tests, complete blood count, electrolyte levels

Nursing Diagnoses

Ineffective tissue perfusion related to changes in cardiac output

Impaired skin integrity related to skin effects

Acute pain related to GI effects of drug

Deficient knowledge regarding drug therapy

Planning

The patient will receive the best therapeutic effect from the drug therapy.

The patient will have limited adverse effects to the drug therapy.

The patient will have an understanding of the drug therapy, adverse effects to anticipate, and measures to relieve discomfort and improve safety.

Implementation

Encourage lifestyle changes to increase drug effectiveness.

(continues on page 742)

Initiating Antihypertensive Therapy (continued)

Do not cut, crush, or chew this tablet. Give with food if GI upset occurs.
Provide comfort and safety measures.
Reduce dosage if patient has renal failure.
Monitor for any situation that might lead to a drop in BP.
Provide support and reassurance to deal with drug effects.
Provide patient teaching regarding drug, dosage, adverse effects, signs and symptoms of problems to report, and safety precautions.

Evaluation

Evaluate drug effects: Maintenance of BP within normal limits.
Monitor for adverse effects: Nausea, dizziness, hypotension, congestive heart failure, skin reactions.
Monitor for drug–drug interactions as listed.
Evaluate effectiveness of patient-teaching program and comfort and safety measures.

PATIENT TEACHING FOR B.R.

- The drug that has been prescribed to treat your hypertension is called a calcium-channel blocker. When used to treat high BP, this drug is called an antihypertensive. High BP is a disorder that may have no symptoms but that can cause serious problems, such as heart attack, stroke, or kidney problems, if left untreated.
- It is very important to take your medication every day, as prescribed, even if you feel perfectly well without the medication. It is possible that you may feel worse because of the adverse effects associated with the medication when you take it. Even if this happens, it is crucial that you take your medication.
- If you find that the adverse effects of this drug are too uncomfortable, discuss the possibility of taking a different antihypertensive medication with your health care provider.
- This drug should be taken on an empty stomach, 1 hour before or 2 hours after meals.
- Common effects of these drugs include:
  - *Dizziness, drowsiness, light-headedness:* These effects often pass after the first few days. Until they do, avoid driving or performing hazardous or delicate tasks that require concentration. If these effects occur, change positions slowly to decrease the light-headedness.
  - *Nausea, vomiting, change in taste perception:* Small, frequent meals may help ease these effects, which may pass with time. If they persist and become too uncomfortable, consult with your health care provider.
  - *Skin rash, mouth sores:* Frequent mouth care may help. Keep the skin dry and use prescribed skin care (lotions, coverings, medication) if needed.
  - Report any of the following to your health care provider: *Difficulty breathing; mouth sores; swelling of the feet, hands, or face; chest pain; palpitations; sore throat; fever or chills.*
- Do not stop taking this drug for any reason. Consult with your health care provider if you have problems taking this medication.
- You should avoid drinking grapefruit juice while you are taking this drug, because the combination of grapefruit juice and a calcium-channel blocker may case toxic effects.
- Tell any doctor, nurse, or others involved in your health care that you are taking this drug.
- Avoid taking over-the-counter medications while you are taking this drug. If you feel that you need one of these, consult with your health care provider for the best choice. Many of these drugs may interfere with the antihypertensive effect that usually occurs with this drug.
- Be extremely careful in any situation that might lead to a drop in BP (e.g., excessive sweating, vomiting, diarrhea, dehydration). If you experience light-headedness or dizziness in any of these situations, consult your health care provider immediately.
- Keep this drug, and all medications, out of the reach of children.

Contraindications and Cautions

The vasodilators are contraindicated in the presence of known allergy to the drug *to prevent hypersensitivity reactions* and with any *condition that could be exacerbated by a sudden fall in BP*, such as cerebral insufficiency. Caution should be used in patients with peripheral vascular disease, CAD, heart failure, or tachycardia, *all of which could be exacerbated by the fall in BP*.

These drugs are also contraindicated with pregnancy unless the benefit to the mother clearly outweighs the potential risk *because of the potential for adverse effects on the fetus or neonate*. If they are needed by a nursing mother, another method of feeding the baby should be selected, *because of the potential for adverse effects on the baby*.

Adverse Effects

The adverse effects most frequently seen with these drugs are related to the changes in BP. These include dizziness, anxiety, and headache; reflex tachycardia, heart failure, chest pain, and edema; skin rash and lesions (abnormal hair growth with minoxidil); and GI upset, nausea, and vomiting. Cyanide toxicity (dyspnea, headache, vomiting, dizziness, ataxia, loss of consciousness, imperceptible pulse, absent reflexes, dilated pupils, pink color, distant heart sounds, and shallow breathing) may occur with nitroprusside, which is metabolized to cyanide and also suppresses iodine uptake and can cause hypothyroidism.

Clinically Important Drug–Drug Interactions

Each of these drugs works differently in the body, so each drug should be checked for potential drug–drug interactions before use.

Prototype Summary: Nitroprusside

Indications: Severe hypertension, maintenance of controlled hypotension during anesthesia, acute heart failure.

Actions: Acts directly on vascular smooth muscle to cause vasodilation and drop of BP; does not inhibit CV reflexes and tachycardia; renin release will occur.

Pharmacokinetics:

Route	Onset	Peak	Duration
IV	1–2 min	Rapid	1–10 min

$T_{1/2}$: 2 minutes; metabolized in the liver and excreted in the urine.

Adverse Effects: Apprehension, headache, retrosternal pressure, palpitations, cyanide toxicity, diaphoresis, nausea, vomiting, abdominal pain, irritation at the injection site.

Nursing Considerations for Patients Receiving Vasodilators

Assessment: History and Examination

- Assess for the following conditions, *which could be cautions or contraindications to use of the drug*: Any known allergies to these drugs, impaired kidney or liver function, pregnancy or lactation *because of the potential adverse effects on the fetus or neonate,* and CV dysfunction, *which could be exacerbated by a fall in BP*.
- Assess baseline status before beginning therapy *to determine any potential adverse effects*; this includes body temperature and weight; skin color, lesions, and temperature; pulse, BP, baseline ECG, and perfusion; respirations and adventitious breath sounds; bowel sounds and abdominal examination; renal and liver function tests; and blood glucose.

Nursing Diagnoses

Nursing diagnoses related to drug therapy might include the following:

- Ineffective tissue perfusion (total body) related to changes in cardiac output
- Impaired skin integrity related to dermatological effects
- Acute pain related to GI distress, skin effects, or headache
- Deficient knowledge regarding drug therapy

Planning

- The patient will receive the best therapeutic effect from the drug therapy.
- The patient will have limited adverse effects to the drug therapy.
- The patient will have an understanding of the drug therapy, adverse effects to anticipate, and measures to relieve discomfort and improve safety.

Implementation with Rationale

- Encourage the patient to implement lifestyle changes, including weight loss, smoking cessation, decreased alcohol and salt in the diet, and increased exercise, *to increase the effectiveness of antihypertensive therapy.*
- Monitor BP closely during administration *to evaluate for effectiveness and to ensure quick response if BP falls rapidly or too much.*
- Monitor blood glucose and serum electrolytes *to avoid potentially serious adverse effects.*
- Monitor the patient carefully in any situation that might lead to a drop in fluid volume (e.g., excessive sweating, vomiting, diarrhea, dehydration) *to detect and treat excessive hypotension that may occur.*
- Provide comfort measures *to help the patient tolerate drug effects,* including small, frequent meals; access to bathroom facilities; safety precautions if CNS effects occur; environmental controls; appropriate skin care as needed; and analgesics as needed.
- Provide thorough patient teaching, including the name of the drug, dosage prescribed, measures to avoid adverse effects, warning signs of problems, and the need for periodic monitoring and evaluation, *to enhance patient knowledge about drug therapy and to promote compliance.*
- Offer support and encouragement *to help the patient deal with the diagnosis and the drug regimen.*

Evaluation

- Monitor patient response to the drug (maintenance of BP within normal limits).
- Monitor for adverse effects (hypotension, GI distress, skin reactions, tachycardia, headache, dizziness).
- Evaluate the effectiveness of the teaching plan (patient can name drug, dosage, adverse effects to watch for, specific measures to avoid them, and the importance of continued follow-up).
- Monitor the effectiveness of comfort measures and compliance with the regimen.

Other Antihypertensive Agents

Diuretic Agents

Diuretics are drugs that increase the excretion of sodium and water from the kidney (Figure 43.3). See Chapter 51 for a detailed discussion of these agents. Diuretics are very important for the treatment of hypertension. These drugs are often the first agents tried in mild hypertension; they affect blood sodium levels and blood volume. A somewhat controversial study, the Antihypertensive and Lipid-Lowering Treatment to Prevent Heart Attack Trial, reported in 2002 and supported with follow-up studies that patients taking the less expensive, less toxic diuretics did better and had better BP control than patients using other antihypertensive agents. Replications of this study have supported its findings, and the use of a thiazide diuretic is currently considered the first drug used in the stepped care management of hypertension. Although these drugs increase urination and can disturb electrolyte and acid–base balances, they are usually tolerated well by most patients. Diuretic agents used to treat hypertension include the following:

- *Thiazide and thiazide-like diuretics:* chlorothiazide (*Diuril*), hydrochlorothiazide (*HydroDIURIL*), methyclothiazide (generic), chlorthalidone (generic), indapamide (generic), and metolazone (*Zaroxolyn*)
- *Potassium-sparing diuretics:* amiloride (*Midamor*), spironolactone (*Aldactone*), and triamterene (*Dyrenium*)

Sympathetic Nervous System Blockers

Drugs that block the effects of the sympathetic nervous system are useful in blocking many of the compensatory effects of the sympathetic nervous system (see Figure 43.3). See Chapters 50 and 31 for a detailed discussion of these drugs.

- Beta-blockers block vasoconstriction, decrease heart rate, decrease cardiac muscle contraction, and tend to increase blood flow to the kidneys, leading to a decrease in the release of renin. These drugs have many adverse effects and are not recommended for all people. They are often used as monotherapy in step 2 treatment, and in some patients they control BP adequately. Beta-blockers used to treat hypertension include the following agents: Acebutolol (*Sectral*), atenolol (*Tenormin*), betaxolol (generic), bisoprolol (*Zebeta*), metoprolol (*Lopressor*), nadolol (*Corgard*), nebivolol (*Bystolic*), pindolol (generic), propranolol (*Inderal*), and timolol (generic).
- Alpha- and beta-blockers are useful in conjunction with other agents and tend to be somewhat more powerful, blocking all of the receptors in the sympathetic system. Patients often complain of fatigue, loss of libido, inability to sleep, and GI and genitourinary disturbances, and they may be unwilling to continue taking these drugs. Alpha- and beta-blockers used to treat hypertension include the following agents: Carvedilol (*Coreg*) and labetalol (*Trandate*).
- Alpha-adrenergic blockers inhibit the postsynaptic alpha$_1$-adrenergic receptors, decreasing sympathetic tone in the vasculature and causing vasodilation, which leads to a lowering of BP. However, these drugs also block presynaptic alpha$_2$-receptors, preventing the feedback control of norepinephrine release. The result is an increase in the reflex tachycardia that occurs when BP decreases. These drugs are used to diagnose and manage episodes of pheochromocytoma, but they have limited usefulness in essential hypertension because of the associated adverse effects. Alpha-adrenergic blockers include the following agents: Phenoxybenzamine (*Dibenzyline*) and phentolamine (*Regitine*).
- Alpha$_1$-blockers are used to treat hypertension because of their ability to block the postsynaptic alpha$_1$-receptor sites. This decreases vascular tone and promotes vasodilation, leading to a fall in BP. These drugs do not block the presynaptic alpha$_2$-receptor sites, and therefore the reflex tachycardia that accompanies a fall in BP does not occur. Alpha$_1$-blockers used to treat hypertension include the following agents: Doxazosin (*Cardura*), prazosin (*Minipress*), and terazosin (generic).
- Alpha$_2$-agonists (see Chapter 30) stimulate the alpha$_2$-receptors in the CNS and inhibit the CV centers, leading to a decrease in sympathetic outflow from the CNS and a resultant drop in BP. These drugs are associated with many adverse CNS and GI effects, as well as cardiac dysrhythmias. Alpha$_2$-blockers used to treat hypertension include the following agents: Clonidine (*Catapres*), guanfacine (*Tenex*), and methyldopa (*generic*).

KEY POINTS

- Hypertension is a sustained state of higher-than-normal BP that can lead to blood vessel damage, atherosclerosis, and damage to small vessels in end organs.
- The cause of essential hypertension is unknown; treatment varies among individuals.
- Drug treatment of hypertension aims to change one or more of the normal reflexes that control BP.
- Sodium levels and fluid volume are decreased by diuretic agents.
- ACE inhibitors prevent the conversion of angiotensin I to angiotensin II, leading to a fall in BP.
- ARBs prevent the body from responding to angiotensin II, causing a loss of effectiveness of the renin–angiotensin system by blocking the angiotensin receptor in blood vessels. Renin inhibitors block the whole system by inhibiting the release of renin.
- Calcium-channel blockers interfere with the ability of muscles to contract, which leads to vasodilation, which in turn reduces BP.

- Other drugs used to treat hypertension include diuretics, which decrease the sodium content in the body, and various sympathetic blockers, which block the BP-raising effects of the sympathetic system.

Antihypotensive Agents

As mentioned earlier, if BP becomes too low (hypotension) the vital centers in the brain and the rest of the tissues of the body may not receive sufficient oxygenated blood to continue functioning. Severe hypotension or shock puts the body in serious jeopardy; it is often an acute emergency situation, with treatment required to save the patient's life. The first-choice drug for treating shock is usually a sympathomimetic drug. See Figure 43.3 for sites of action of drugs used to treat hypotension. Antihypotensive agents are also discussed in Table 43.2.

Sympathetic Adrenergic Agonists or Vasopressors

Sympathomimetic drugs are the first choice for treating severe hypotension or shock. The sympathomimetic drugs are discussed in detail in Chapter 30. Sympathomimetic drugs used to treat shock include the following agents: Dobutamine (generic), dopamine (generic), ephedrine (generic), epinephrine (*Adrenalin*, *AdrenaClick*), isoproterenol (*Isuprel*), norepinephrine (*Levophed*), and phenylephrine (generic).

Therapeutic Actions and Indications

Sympathomimetic drugs react with sympathetic adrenergic receptors to cause the effects of a sympathetic stress response: Increased BP, increased blood volume, and increased strength of cardiac muscle contraction. These actions increase BP and may restore balance to the CV system while the underlying cause of the shock (e.g., volume depletion, blood loss) is treated.

Adverse Effects

The adverse effects related to these drugs are the effects of stimulation of the sympathetic system: Decreased GI activity with nausea and constipation, increased respiratory rate and changes in BP, headache, and changes in peripheral blood flow with numbness, tingling, and even gangrene in extreme cases. These drugs should be used with caution with any disease that limits blood flow, with tachycardia, or with hypertension.

Blood Pressure–Lowering Agents

Midodrine (generic) is an alpha-specific adrenergic agent used to treat orthostatic hypotension—hypotension that occurs with position change—that interferes with a person's ability to function and has not responded to any other therapy (Table 43.2). In 2010 the U.S. Food and Drug Administration (FDA) proposed the withdrawal of this drug from the market. It was a fast-tracked drug that never went through the required testing, and since the required testing of efficacy and safety was never done the FDA felt that the drug should no longer be marketed. It is the only drug available for orthostatic hypotension, and at this time negotiations are still ongoing and the status of the drug's availability is not known.

Therapeutic Actions and Indications

Midodrine activates alpha-receptors in arteries and veins to produce an increase in vascular tone and an increase in BP. It is indicated for the symptomatic treatment of orthostatic hypotension in patients whose lives are impaired by the disorder and who have not had a response to any other therapy.

Pharmacokinetics

Midodrine is rapidly absorbed from the GI tract, reaching peak levels within 1 to 2 hours. It is metabolized in the liver and excreted in the urine with a half-life of 3 to 4 hours. It should be reserved in pregnancy for cases in which the benefit to the mother clearly outweighs the potential risk to the fetus. It is not known whether midodrine enters breast milk, so caution should be used during lactation.

Table 43.2 ***Drugs in Focus:* Antihypotensive Agents**

Drug Name	Usual Dosage	Usual Indications
Drugs for Treating Hypotension		
midodrine (generic)	10 mg PO t.i.d.	Treatment of orthostatic hypotension in adults
droxidopa (*Northera*)	100 mg PO t.i.d.; max 600 mg/d	Treatment of neurogenic hypotension caused by autonomic failure
Sympathetic Adrenergic Agonists or Vasopressors		
See Chapter 30	See Chapter 30	First-choice drugs for treatment of hypotension or shock

Contraindications and Cautions

Midodrine is contraindicated in the presence of supine hypertension, CAD, or pheochromocytoma *because of the risk of precipitating a hypertensive emergency*; with acute renal disease, *which might interfere with excretion of the drug*; with urinary retention *because the stimulation of alpha-receptors can exacerbate this problem*; and with thyrotoxicosis, *which could further increase BP*. Caution should be used with pregnancy and lactation *because of the potential for adverse effects on the fetus or neonate*; with visual problems, *which could be exacerbated by vasoconstriction*; and with renal or hepatic impairment, *which could alter the metabolism and excretion of the drug*.

Adverse Effects

The most common adverse effects associated with this drug are related to the stimulation of alpha-receptors and include piloerection, chills, and rash; hypertension and bradycardia; dizziness, vision changes, vertigo, and headache; and problems with urination.

Clinically Important Drug–Drug Interactions

There is a risk of increased effects and toxicity of cardiac glycosides, beta-blockers, alpha-adrenergic agents, and corticosteroids if they are taken with midodrine. Patients who are receiving any of these combinations should be monitored carefully for the need for a dose adjustment.

Droxidopa (*Northera*) is a newer drug that has gone through the approval process and is indicated for the treatment of orthostatic dizziness, light-headedness, or feeling that "you are about to black out" in adults with symptomatic neurogenic orthostatic hypotension caused by primary autonomic failure, dopamine beta-hydroxylase deficiency, and nondiabetic autonomic neuropathy.

Therapeutic Actions and Indications

Droxidopa is an amino acid analog that is metabolized to norepinephrine by dopadecarboxylase. It is widely distributed throughout the body, and it is thought that its actions on BP are related to the norepinephrine effects causing vasoconstriction.

Pharmacokinetics

This drug is absorbed through the GI tract and reaches peak levels in 1–4 hours. It is widely distributed and metabolized by the normal catecholamine pathways with excretion through the urine. Droxidopa has a half-life of 2.5 hours.

Contraindications and Cautions

There are no contraindications to the use of droxidopa. Caution should be used with any history of CV issues *because the stimulatory effects of norephinephrine can cause exacerbation of these disorders*; with renal impairment *because this could affect the excretion of the drug*. Nursing mothers should select a different method of feeding the baby *because of the potential adverse effects on the baby*.

Adverse Effects

The most common adverse effects associated with this drug are related to the sympathetic effects of the drugs which include supine hypertension, headache, dizziness, nausea, and arrhythmias.

Clinically Important Drug–Drug Interactions

There is a risk of increased effects of droxidopa if combined with any dopadecarboxylase inhibitors.

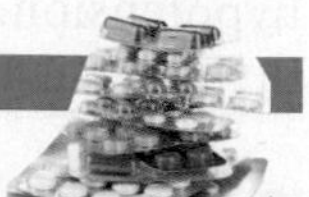

Nursing Considerations for Patients Receiving Antihypotensive Drugs

Assessment: History and Examination

- Assess for the following conditions, *which could be contraindications or cautions*: Any known allergy to the drug *to prevent hypersensitivity reactions*; impaired kidney or liver function, *which could interfere with metabolism and excretion of the drugs*; pregnancy or lactation *because of the potential adverse effects on the fetus or neonate*; CV dysfunction; visual problems; urinary retention; and pheochromocytoma, *which could be exacerbated by the effects of the drugs*.
- Assess baseline status before beginning therapy *to determine any potential adverse effects*; this includes body temperature and weight; skin color, lesions, and temperature; pulse, BP, orthostatic BP, and perfusion; respiration and adventitious sounds; bowel sounds and abdominal examination; and renal and liver function tests.

Nursing Diagnoses

Nursing diagnoses related to drug therapy might include the following:

- Ineffective tissue perfusion (total body) related to changes in cardiac output
- Disturbed sensory perception (visual, kinesthetic, tactile) related to CNS effects
- Acute pain related to GI distress, piloerection, chills, or headache
- Deficient knowledge regarding drug therapy

Planning

- The patient will receive the best therapeutic effect from the drug therapy.

- The patient will have limited adverse effects to the drug therapy.
- The patient will have an understanding of the drug therapy, adverse effects to anticipate, and measures to relieve discomfort and improve safety.

Implementation with Rationale

- Monitor BP carefully *to monitor effectiveness and BP changes.*
- Do not administer the drug to patients who are bedridden, but only to patients who are up and mobile, *to ensure therapeutic effects and decrease the risk of severe supine hypertension.*
- Monitor heart rate regularly when beginning therapy *to monitor for bradycardia*, which commonly occurs at the beginning of therapy; if bradycardia persists, it may indicate a need to discontinue the drug.
- Monitor patient with known visual problems carefully *to ensure that the drug is discontinued if visual fields change.*
- Encourage the patient to void before taking a dose of the drug *to decrease the risk of urinary retention problems.*
- Provide comfort measures *to help the patient tolerate drug effects*, including small, frequent meals; access to bathroom facilities; safety precautions if CNS effects occur; environmental controls; appropriate skin care as needed; and analgesics as needed.
- Provide thorough patient teaching, including the name of the drug, dosage prescribed, measures to avoid adverse effects, warning signs of problems, and the need for periodic monitoring and evaluation, *to enhance patient knowledge about drug therapy and to promote compliance.*
- Offer support and encouragement *to help the patient deal with the diagnosis and the drug regimen.*

Evaluation

- Monitor patient response to the drug (maintenance of BP within normal limits).
- Monitor for adverse effects (hypertension, dizziness, visual changes, headache, chills, urinary problems).
- Evaluate the effectiveness of the teaching plan (patient can name drug, dosage, adverse effects to watch for, specific measures to avoid them, and the importance of continued follow-up).
- Monitor the effectiveness of comfort measures and compliance with the regimen.

KEY POINTS

- Severe hypotension, or shock, is treated with sympathomimetic drugs that stimulate the sympathetic system to increase BP.
- Midodrine and droxidopa are oral drugs used to treat people with orthostatic hypotension whose lives are considerably impaired by the fall in BP when they stand.

SUMMARY

- The CV system is a closed system that depends on pressure differences to ensure the delivery of blood to the tissues and the return of that blood to the heart.
- BP is related to heart rate, stroke volume, and the total peripheral resistance against which the heart has to push the blood.
- Peripheral resistance is primarily controlled by constriction or relaxation of the arterioles. Constricted arterioles raise pressure; dilated arterioles lower pressure.
- Control of BP involves baroreceptor (pressure receptor) stimulation of the medulla to activate the sympathetic nervous system, which causes vasoconstriction and increased fluid retention when pressure is low in the aorta and carotid arteries, and vasodilation and loss of fluid when pressure is too high.
- The kidneys activate the renin–angiotensin–aldosterone system when blood flow to the kidneys is decreased.
- Renin activates the conversion of angiotensinogen to angiotensin I in the liver; angiotensin I is converted by ACE to angiotensin II in the lungs; angiotensin II then reacts with specific receptor sites on blood vessels to cause vasoconstriction to raise BP and in the adrenal gland to cause the release of aldosterone, which leads to the retention of fluid and increased blood volume.
- Hypertension is a sustained state of higher-than-normal BP that can lead to damage to blood vessels, increased risk of atherosclerosis, and damage to small vessels in end organs. Because hypertension often has no signs or symptoms, it is called the silent killer.
- Essential hypertension has no underlying cause, and treatment can vary widely from individual to individual. Treatment approaches include lifestyle changes first, followed by careful addition and adjustment of various antihypertensive drugs.
- Drug treatment of hypertension is aimed at altering one or more of the normal reflexes that control BP: Diuretics decrease sodium levels and volume, sympathetic nervous system drugs alter the sympathetic response and lead to vascular dilation and decreased pumping power of the heart, ACE inhibitors prevent the conversion of angiotensin I to angiotensin II, ARBs prevent the body from responding to angiotensin II, renin inhibitors directly block the effects of renin, calcium-channel blockers interfere with the ability of muscles to contract and lead to vasodilation, and vasodilators directly cause the relaxation of vascular smooth muscle.

- Hypotension is a state of lower-than-normal BP that can result in decreased oxygenation of the tissues, cell death, tissue damage, and even death.
- Hypotension is most often treated with sympathomimetic drugs, which stimulate the sympathetic receptor sites to cause vasoconstriction, fluid retention, and return of normal pressure.

CHECK YOUR UNDERSTANDING

Answers to the questions in this chapter can be found in Answers to Check Your Understanding Questions on thePoint®.

MULTIPLE CHOICE

Select the best answer to the following.

1. The baroreceptors are the most important factor in continual control of BP. The baroreceptors
- **a.** are evenly distributed throughout the body to maintain pressure in the system.
- **b.** sense pressure and immediately send that information to the medulla in the brain.
- **c.** are directly connected to the sympathetic nervous system.
- **d.** are as sensitive to oxygen levels as to pressure changes.

2. Essential hypertension is the most commonly diagnosed form of high BP. Essential hypertension is
- **a.** caused by a tumor in the adrenal gland.
- **b.** associated with no known cause.
- **c.** related to renal disease.
- **d.** caused by liver dysfunction.

3. Hypertension is associated with
- **a.** loss of vision.
- **b.** strokes.
- **c.** atherosclerosis.
- **d.** all of the above.

4. The stepped care approach to the treatment of hypertension includes
- **a.** lifestyle modification, including exercise, diet, and decreased smoking and alcohol intake.
- **b.** use of a diuretic, beta-blocker, or ACE inhibitor to supplement lifestyle changes.
- **c.** a combination of antihypertensive drug classes to achieve desired control.
- **d.** all of the above.

5. ACE inhibitors work on the renin–angiotensin system to prevent the conversion of angiotensin I to angiotensin II. Because this blocking occurs in the cells in the lung, which is usually the site of this conversion, the use of ACE inhibitors often results in
- **a.** spontaneous pneumothorax.
- **b.** pneumonia.
- **c.** unrelenting cough.
- **d.** respiratory depression.

6. A client taking an ACE inhibitor is scheduled for surgery. The nurse should
- **a.** stop the drug.
- **b.** alert the surgeon and mark the client's chart prominently.
- **c.** cancel the surgery and consult with the prescriber.
- **d.** monitor fluid levels and make sure the fluids are restricted before surgery.

7. A patient who is hypertensive becomes pregnant. The drug of choice for this patient is
- **a.** an angiotensin II receptor blocker.
- **b.** an ACE inhibitor.
- **c.** a diuretic.
- **d.** a calcium-channel blocker.

8. Droxidopa, an antihypotensive drug, should be used
- **a.** only with patients who are confined to bed.
- **b.** in the treatment of acute shock.
- **c.** in patients with known pheochromocytoma.
- **d.** to treat orthostatic hypotension in patients whose lives are impaired by the disorder.

MULTIPLE RESPONSE

Select all that apply.

1. Pressure within the vascular system is determined by which of the following?
- **a.** Peripheral resistance
- **b.** Stroke volume
- **c.** Sodium load
- **d.** Heart rate
- **e.** Total intravascular volume
- **f.** Rate of erythropoietin release

2. The renin–angiotensin system is associated with which of the following?
- **a.** Intense vasoconstriction and BP elevation
- **b.** Blood flow through the kidneys
- **c.** Production of surfactant in the lungs
- **d.** Release of aldosterone from the adrenal cortex
- **e.** Retention of sodium and water in the kidneys
- **f.** Liver production of fibrinogen

BIBLIOGRAPHY AND REFERENCES

Andrews, M., & Boyle, J. (2011). *Transcultural concepts in nursing care* (6th ed.). Philadelphia, PA: Lippincott Williams & Wilkins.

Bauchner, H., Fontanorosa, M., & Golub, R. (2014). Updated guidelines for management of high blood pressure; recommendations, review and responsibility. *Journal of the American Medical Association, 311*(5), 377–378.

Bonow, R. O., Mann, D. L., Libby, P., et al. (2014). *Braunwald's heart disease: A textbook of cardiovascular medicine* (10th ed.). Philadelphia, PA: W. B. Saunders.

Brunton, L., Chabner, B., & Knollman, B. (2011). *Goodman and Gilman's the pharmacological basis of therapeutics* (12th ed.). New York: McGraw-Hill.

Eihorn, P. T., Davis, B. R., Wright, J. T., et al. (2010). ALLHAT: Still providing correct answers after seven years. *Hypertension, 53*, 617–623.

Facts and Comparisons. (2015). *Drug facts and comparisons*. St. Louis, MO: Author.

James, P., Oparil, S., Carter, B., et al. (2014). Evidence based guideline for the management of high blood pressure in adults: Report from the panel members appointed to the 8th JNC. *Journal of the American Medical Association, 311*(5), 507–520.

Karch, A. M. (2014). *Lippincott's nursing drug guide*. Philadelphia, PA: Lippincott Williams & Wilkins.

Mozzafarian, D., Benjamin, E. J., Go, A. S., et al. (2015). Heart disease and stroke statistics—2015 update: A report from the American Heart Association. *Circulation, 131*, e29–e322.

Matchar, D. B., McCrory, D. C., Orlando, L. A., et al. (2008). Systematic review: Comparative effectiveness of angiotensin-converting enzyme inhibitors and angiotensin II receptor blockers for treating essential hypertension. *Annals of Internal Medicine, 148*, 16–29.

Porth, C. M. (2014). *Pathophysiology: Concepts of altered health states* (9th ed.). Philadelphia, PA: Lippincott Williams & Wilkins.

The Medical Letter. (2015). *The medical letter on drugs and therapeutics*. New Rochelle, NY: Author.

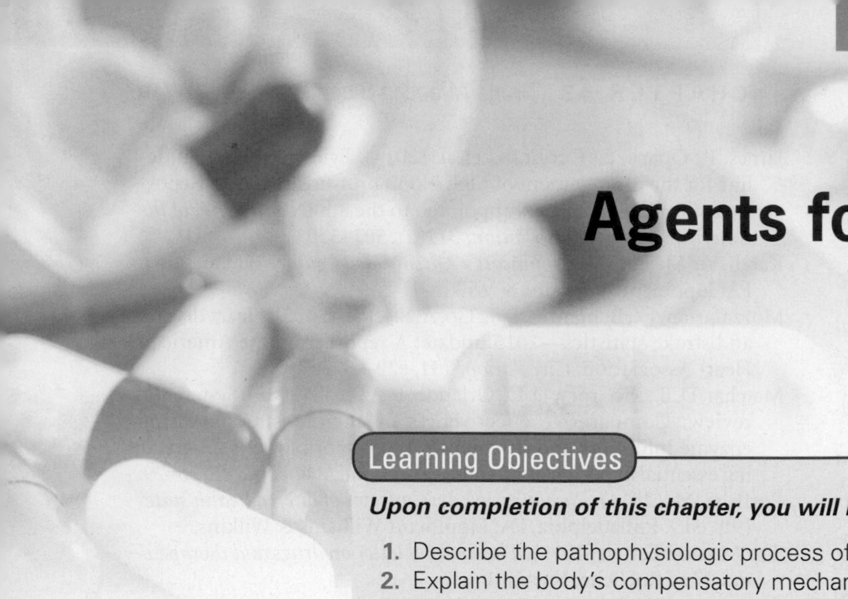

44 Agents for Treating Heart Failure

Learning Objectives

Upon completion of this chapter, you will be able to:

1. Describe the pathophysiologic process of heart failure and the resultant clinical signs.
2. Explain the body's compensatory mechanisms that occur in response to heart failure.
3. Describe the therapeutic actions, indications, pharmacokinetics, contraindications and cautions, most common adverse reactions, and important drug–drug interactions associated with the cardiotonic agents.
4. Discuss the use of cardiotonic agents across the lifespan.
5. Compare and contrast the prototype drugs digoxin, ivabradine, milrinone, and digoxin immune Fab.
6. Outline the nursing considerations, including important teaching points, for patients receiving cardiotonic agents.

Glossary of Key Terms

afterload: resistance against which the heart has to beat

cardiac output: volume of blood being pumped by the heart

cardiomegaly: enlargement of the heart, commonly seen with chronic hypertension, valvular disease, and heart failure

cardiomyopathy: a disease of the heart muscle that leads to an enlarged heart and eventually to complete heart muscle failure and death

dyspnea: discomfort with respirations, often with a feeling of anxiety and inability to breathe, seen with left-sided heart failure

heart failure (HF): a condition in which the heart muscle fails to adequately pump blood around the cardiovascular system, leading to a backup or congestion of blood in the system

hemoptysis: blood-tinged sputum, seen in left-sided heart failure when blood backs up into the lungs and fluid leaks out into the lung tissue

nocturia: getting up to void at night, reflecting increased renal perfusion with fluid shifts in the supine position when a person has gravity-dependent edema related to heart failure; other medical conditions, including urinary tract infection, increase the need to get up and void

orthopnea: difficulty breathing when lying down, often referred to by the number of pillows required to allow a person to breathe comfortably

positive inotropic: effect resulting in an increased force of contraction

preload: amount of blood that is brought back to the heart to be pumped throughout the body

pulmonary edema: severe left-sided heart failure with backup of blood into the lungs, leading to loss of fluid into the lung tissue

tachypnea: rapid and shallow respirations, seen with left-sided heart failure

Drug List

Agents for Heart Failure

Cardiac Glycoside

(P) digoxin

Phosphodiesterase Inhibitor

(P) milrinone

Hyperpolarization-activated Cyclic Nucleotide–Gated Channel Blocker

(P) ivabradine

Two classes of drugs are used primarily for treating heart failure, the cardiotonic agents and a new class, introduced in 2015, the hyperpolarization-activated cyclic nucleotide–gated channel blockers (HCN blockers). Cardiotonic agents are drugs used to increase the contractility of the heart muscle for patients experiencing **heart failure (HF)**. HF is a condition in which the heart fails to pump blood around the body effectively. Because the cardiac cycle normally involves a tight balance between the pumping of the right and left sides of the heart, any failure of the muscle to pump blood out of either side of the heart can result in a backup of blood. If this happens the blood vessels become congested; eventually, the body's cells are deprived of oxygen and nutrients, and waste products build up in the tissues. The primary treatment for HF involves helping the heart muscle to contract more efficiently to restore system balance. The new class of drugs approved for treating heart failure works in the heart's pacemaker affecting the channels responsible for repolarization, leading to a slower heart rate. Slowing the heart rate may help to bring balance back into the cardiac cycle.

Heart Failure

HF, a condition that was once called "dropsy" or decompensation, is a syndrome that usually involves dysfunction of the cardiac muscle, of which the sarcomere is the basic unit. The sarcomere contains two contractile proteins, actin and myosin, which are highly reactive with each other but at rest are kept apart by the chemical troponin. When a cardiac muscle cell is stimulated, calcium enters the cell and inactivates the troponin, allowing the actin and myosin to form actomyosin bridges. The formation of these bridges allows the muscle fibers to slide together or contract (Figure 44.1). The formation of these bridges and subsequent contraction require a constant supply of oxygen, glucose, and calcium. (See Chapter 42 for a review of heart muscle contraction processes.)

HF can occur with any of the disorders that damage or overwork the heart muscle:

- Coronary artery disease (CAD) is the leading cause of HF, accounting for approximately 95% of the cases diagnosed (see Chapter 47 for a discussion of CAD). CAD results in an insufficient supply of blood to meet the oxygen demands of the myocardium. Consequently, the muscles become hypoxic and can no longer function efficiently. When CAD evolves into a myocardial infarction (MI), muscle cells die or are damaged, leading to an inefficient pumping effort.
- **Cardiomyopathy** (a disease of the heart muscle that leads to an enlarged heart, **cardiomegaly**, and eventually to complete muscle failure and death) can occur as a result of a viral infection, alcoholism, anabolic steroid abuse, or a collagen disorder. It causes muscle alterations and ineffective contraction and pumping.
- Hypertension eventually leads to an enlarged cardiac muscle because the heart must work harder than normal to pump against the high pressure in the arteries.

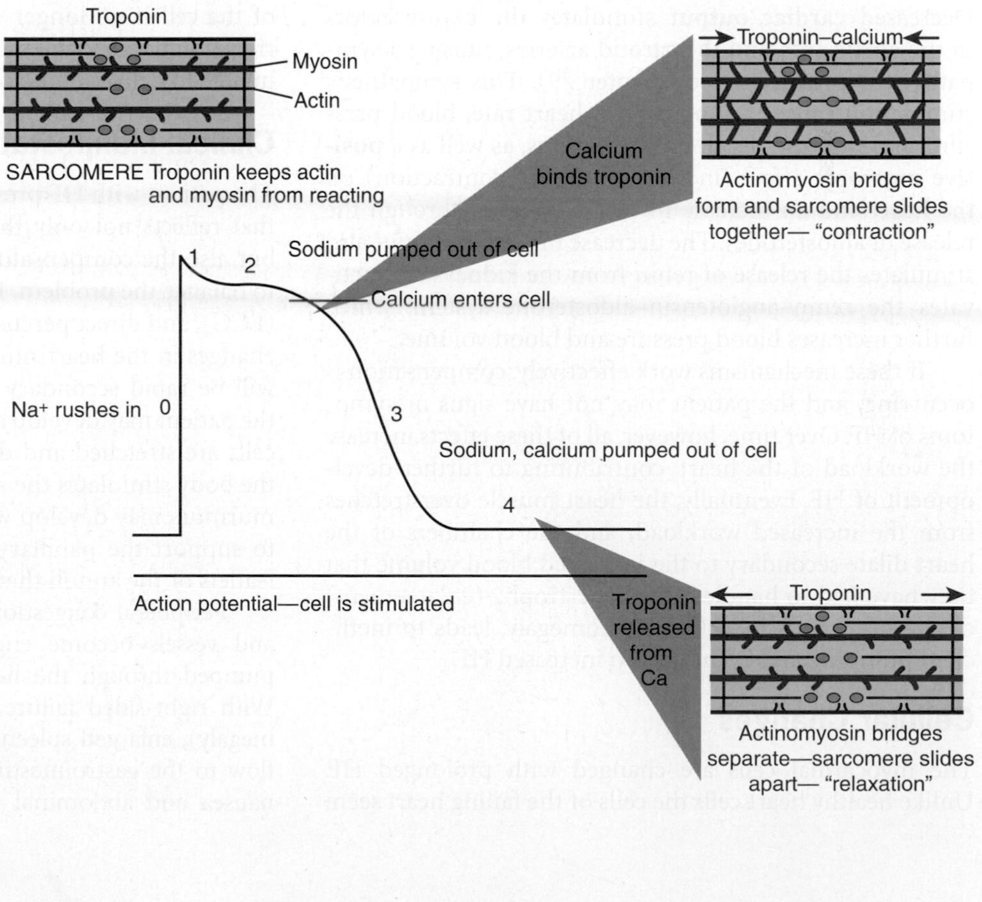

FIGURE 44.1 The sliding filaments of myocardial muscles. Calcium entering the cell deactivates troponin and allows actin and myosin to react, causing contraction. Calcium pumped out of the cell frees troponin to separate actin and myosin; the sarcomere filament slides apart, and the cell relaxes.

Hypertension puts constant increased demands for oxygen on the system because the heart is pumping so forcibly.

- Valvular heart disease leads to an overload of the ventricles because the valves do not close tightly, which allows blood to leak backward into the ventricles. This overloading leads to muscle stretching and increased demand for oxygen and energy as the heart muscle must constantly contract harder. (Valvular heart disease is seen less often today owing to the success of cardiac surgery and effective treatment for rheumatic fever.)

The end result of all of these conditions is that the heart muscle cannot pump blood effectively throughout the vascular system. If the left ventricle pumps inefficiently, blood backs up into the lungs, causing pulmonary vessel congestion and fluid leakage into the alveoli and lung tissue. In severe cases, **pulmonary edema** (manifested by rales, wheezes, blood-tinged sputum, low oxygenation, and development of a third heart sound [S_3]) can occur. If the right side of the heart is the primary problem, blood backs up in the venous system leading to the right side of the heart. Liver congestion and edema of the legs and feet reflect right-sided failure. Because the cardiovascular (CV) system works as a closed system, one-sided failure, if left untreated, eventually leads to failure of both sides, and the signs and symptoms of total HF occur.

Compensatory Mechanisms

Because effective pumping of blood to the cells is essential for life the body has several compensatory mechanisms that function if the heart muscle begins to fail (Figure 44.2). Decreased **cardiac output** stimulates the baroreceptors in the aortic arch and the carotid arteries, causing a sympathetic stimulation (see Chapter 29). This sympathetic stimulation causes an increase in heart rate, blood pressure, and rate and depth of respirations, as well as a **positive inotropic** effect (increased force of contraction) on the heart and an increase in blood volume (through the release of aldosterone). The decrease in cardiac output also stimulates the release of renin from the kidneys and activates the renin–angiotensin–aldosterone system, which further increases blood pressure and blood volume.

If these mechanisms work effectively, compensation is occurring, and the patient may not have signs or symptoms of HF. Over time, however, all of these effects increase the workload of the heart, contributing to further development of HF. Eventually, the heart muscle overstretches from the increased workload, and the chambers of the heart dilate secondary to the increased blood volume that they have had to handle. This hypertrophy (enlargement) of the heart muscle, called cardiomegaly, leads to inefficient pumping and eventually to increased HF.

Cellular Changes

The myocardial cells are changed with prolonged HF. Unlike healthy heart cells the cells of the failing heart seem to lack the ability to produce the energy needed for effective contractions. Movement of calcium ions into and out of the cell is no longer effective, leading to further deterioration because the muscle contracts ineffectively and is unable to deliver blood to the cardiac muscle.

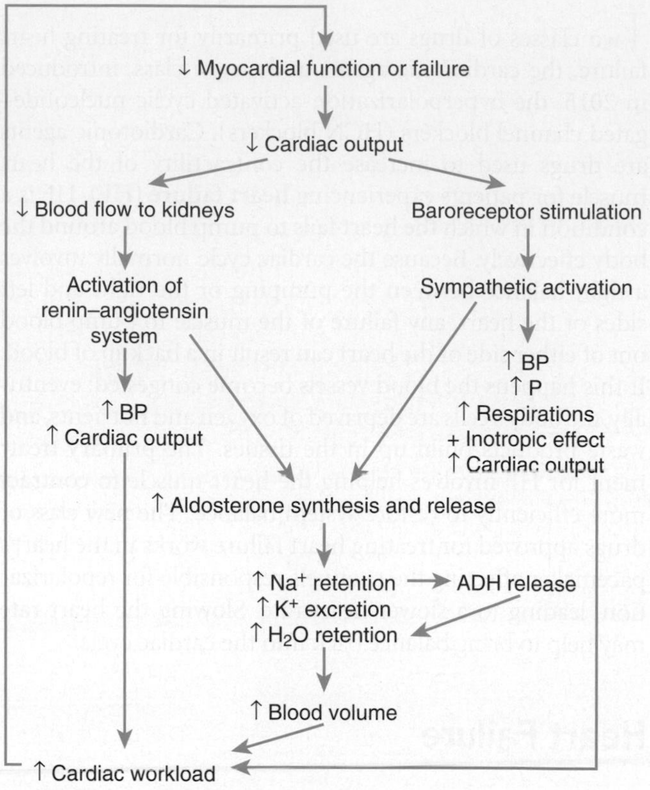

FIGURE 44.2 Compensatory mechanisms in heart failure (HF), which lead to increased cardiac workload and further HF. ADH, antidiuretic hormone; BP, blood pressure; P, pulse.

Clinical Manifestations

The patient with HF presents a predictable clinical picture that reflects not only the problems with heart pumping but also the compensatory mechanisms that are working to balance the problem. Radiography, electrocardiography (ECG), and direct percussion and palpation help to detect changes in the heart muscle and function. The heart rate will be rapid secondary to sympathetic stimulation, and the patient may develop atrial flutter or fibrillation as atrial cells are stretched and damaged. Anxiety often occurs as the body stimulates the sympathetic stress reaction. Heart murmurs may develop when the muscle is no longer able to support the papillary muscles that support the valve leaflets or the annuli that anchor the heart valves.

Peripheral congestion and edema occur as the organs and vessels become engorged waiting for blood to be pumped through the heart as a result of pump failure. With right-sided failure, there is enlarged liver (hepatomegaly), enlarged spleen (splenomegaly), decreased blood flow to the gastrointestinal (GI) tract causing feelings of nausea and abdominal pain, swollen legs and feet, and dependent edema in the coccyx or other dependent areas, with decreased peripheral pulses and hypoxia of those tissues. In addition, with left-sided failure, edema of the lungs reflected in engorged vessels and increased hydrostatic pressure throughout the CV system are also seen (Figure 44.3).

Left-Sided Heart Failure

Left-sided HF reflects engorgement of the pulmonary veins, which eventually leads to difficulty in breathing. Patients complain of **tachypnea** (rapid, shallow respirations), **dyspnea** (discomfort with breathing, often accompanied by a panicked feeling of being unable to breathe), and **orthopnea** (increased difficulty breathing when lying down). Orthopnea occurs in the supine position when the pattern of blood flow changes because of the effects of gravity, which increases pressure and perfusion in the lungs. Orthopnea is usually relieved when the patient sits up, thereby reducing the blood flow through the lungs. The degree of HF is often described by the number of pillows required to get relief (e.g., one-pillow, two-pillow, or three-pillow orthopnea).

The patient with left-sided HF may also experience coughing and **hemoptysis** (coughing up of blood). Rales may be present, signaling the presence of fluid in the lung tissue. In severe cases the patient may develop pulmonary edema; this can be life threatening because, as the spaces in the lungs fill up with fluid, there is no place for gas exchange to occur.

Right-Sided Heart Failure

Right-sided HF usually occurs as a result of chronic obstructive pulmonary disease or other lung diseases that elevate the pulmonary pressure. It often results when the right side of the heart, normally a very low-pressure system, must generate more and more force to move the blood into the lungs. It also commonly occurs with aging, when the venous system fails to deliver blood to the heart effectively and the hydrostatic pressure in the venous end of the capillary

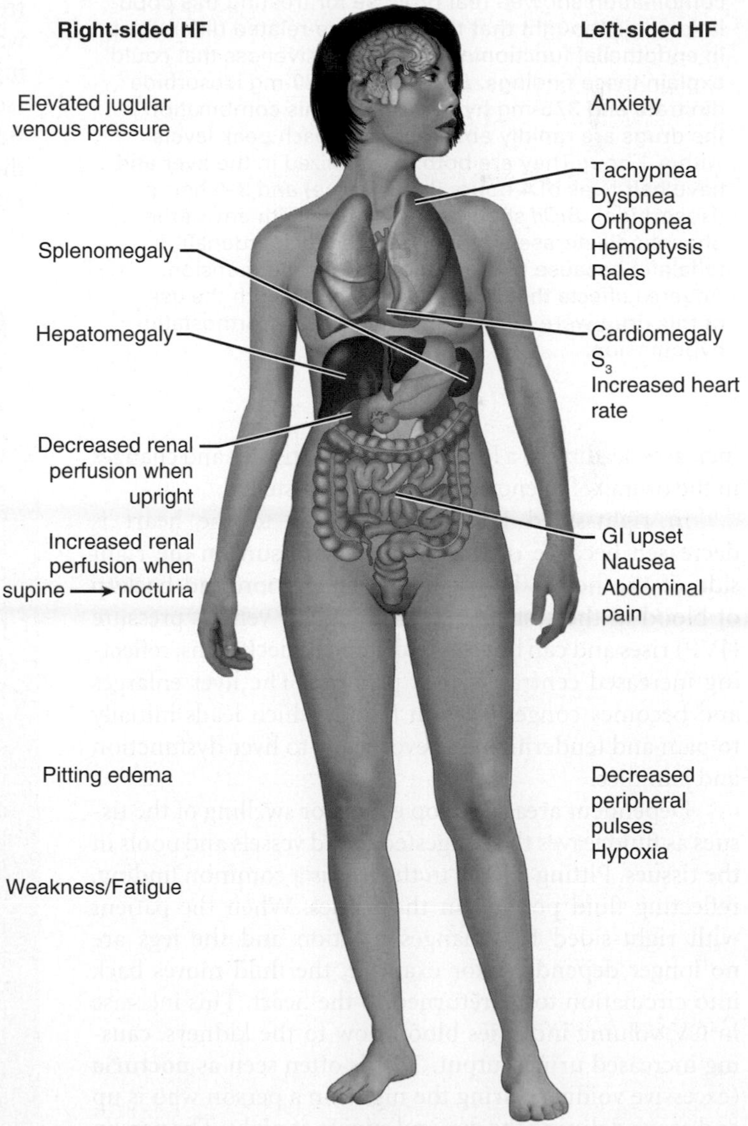

FIGURE 44.3 Signs and symptoms of heart failure (HF).

BOX 44.1 FOCUS ON Cultural Considerations

Drugs for Heart Failure

In 2005, for the first time, the Food and Drug Administration (FDA) approved a drug for use in a specific cultural group. The approval caused a great deal of debate and controversy because of the implications of having a drug approved only for use in African American patients. As a result of much debate the drug was approved for use in self-identified African American patients with severe to moderate HF. The drug, *BiDil*, is a fixed combination drug containing isosorbide dinitrate and hydralazine. This combination of vasodilators was studied in 1999 in the Vasodilator–Heart Failure Study and was found to be only moderately effective in general but was very effective in the subset of African American patients. Further studies were done, and the African American Heart Failure Study (A-HeFT) found that this combination of drugs had a significant impact in decreasing deaths and hospitalizations related to HF in African American patients. African American patients have been found to be less responsive to angiotensin-converting inhibitors, a standard therapy for hypertension and HF; this new combination showed real promise for treating this population. It is thought that there are race-related differences in endothelial functioning and responsiveness that could explain these findings. *BiDil* contains 20-mg isosorbide dinitrate and 37.5-mg hydralazine. In this combination the drugs are rapidly absorbed and reach peak levels within 1 hour. They are both metabolized in the liver and have half-lives of 4 hours (hydralazine) and 3–6 hours (isosorbide). *BiDil* should not be taken with any of the phosphodiesterase inhibitors (sildenafil, vardenafil, tadalafil) because of the risk of serious hypotension. Adverse effects that occurred commonly with the use of this drug were headache, dizziness, and orthostatic hypotension.

increases, leading to a loss of fluid in the tissues and changes in the overall efficiency of the vascular system.

In right-sided HF, venous return to the heart is decreased because of the increased pressure in the right side of the heart. This causes a congestion and backup of blood in the systemic system. Jugular venous pressure (JVP) rises and can be seen in distended neck veins, reflecting increased central venous pressure. The liver enlarges and becomes congested with blood, which leads initially to pain and tenderness and eventually to liver dysfunction and jaundice.

Dependent areas develop edema or swelling of the tissues as fluid leaves the congested blood vessels and pools in the tissues. Pitting edema in the legs is a common finding, reflecting fluid pooling in the tissues. When the patient with right-sided HF changes position and the legs are no longer dependent, for example, the fluid moves back into circulation to be returned to the heart. This increase in CV volume increases blood flow to the kidneys, causing increased urine output. This is often seen as **nocturia** (excessive voiding during the night) in a person who is up and around during the day and supine at night. The person may need to get up during the night to eliminate all of the urine that has been produced as a result of the fluid shift.

Treatments

Several different approaches are used to treat HF. This chapter focuses on the cardiotonic drugs (also called inotropic drugs) that work to directly increase the force of cardiac muscle contraction and the HCN blockers which alter the heart's pacemaker and slow heart rate. Other drug therapies used to treat HF include the following:

- Vasodilators, such as angiotensin-converting enzyme (ACE) inhibitors and nitrates, decrease cardiac workload, relax vascular smooth muscle to decrease **afterload**, and allow pooling in the veins, thereby decreasing **preload** of the heart and helping to improve function (see Chapter 43 for a discussion of ACE inhibitors and Chapter 46 for a discussion of nitrates). In 2005 a combination drug containing a nitrate and vasodilator was approved specifically for treating HF in African American patients (Box 44.1). In 2015, another combination drug was approved for treating HF (Box 44.2). Diuretics decrease blood volume, which decreases venous return and blood pressure, resulting in decreased afterload, preload, and cardiac workload (see Chapter 51 for additional information).
- Beta-adrenergic agonists stimulate the beta receptors in the sympathetic nervous system, increasing calcium flow into the myocardial cells and causing increased contraction, a positive inotropic effect. Other sympathetic

BOX 44.2

New Combination Drug for Treating Heart Failure

In 2015 a new combination drug was approved for reducing hospitalizations and risk for CV death in patients with chronic HF and a reduced ejection fraction. *Entresto* is a combination of valsartan (an ARB) and a new drug sacubitril. Sacubitril is a neprilysin inhibitor. Neprilysin is the enzyme that breaks down the natriuretic peptides in the body. These peptides are responsible for loss of sodium and resultant water in response to ventricular overload. By blocking their breakdown, their effects last longer and more sodium and water are lost. This effect in combination with the blocking of the angiotensin II receptors, which inhibits the effects of the renin–angiotensin–aldosterone system, leads to a decreased cardiac workload, lower vascular volume, lower blood pressure, and improved HF symptoms. The drug is taken orally twice a day. It cannot be used in pregnancy or during breastfeeding (because of the ARB component). It is often used in place of an ACE inhibitor or ARB in combination with other HF drugs. It is contraindicated with ACE inhibitors or aliskiren. Adverse effects include hypotension, hyperkalemia, dizziness, cough, and renal failure. Patients should have regular checks of blood pressure, potassium levels, and renal function.

stimulation effects can cause increased HF because the heart's workload is increased by most sympathetic activity. (See Chapter 30 for additional information.)

- Human B-type natriuretic peptides are normally produced by myocardial cells and brain cells as a compensatory response to increased cardiac workload and increased stimulation by the stress hormones. They bind to endothelial cells, leading to dilation and resulting in decreased venous return, peripheral resistance, and cardiac workload. They also suppress the body's response to the stress hormones, leading to increased fluid loss and further decrease in cardiac workload. Nesiritide (*Natrecor*) is the only drug currently available in a class of drugs called human B-type natriuretic peptides. (See Chapter 50 for more information.)

KEY POINTS

- In HF the heart pumps blood so ineffectively that blood builds up, causing congestion in the CV system.
- HF can result from damage to the heart muscle combined with an increased workload related to CAD, hypertension, cardiomyopathy, valvular disease, or congenital heart abnormalities. As the heart pump fails the muscle cells can no longer work to move calcium into the cell, and cardiac contractions become weak and ineffective.
- Signs and symptoms of HF result from the backup of blood in the vascular system and the loss of fluid in the tissues. Right-sided HF is characterized by edema, liver congestion, elevated JVP, and nocturia, whereas left-sided failure is marked by tachypnea, dyspnea, orthopnea, hemoptysis, anxiety, and poor oxygenation of the blood.
- Treatment agents include vasodilators (to lighten the heart's workload), diuretics (to reduce blood volume and workload), beta-blockers (to decrease the heart's workload by activating sympathetic reaction), human B-type natriuretic peptides (to decrease the heart's workload by vasodilation and suppression of the response to the sympathetic reaction), cardiotonic (inotropic) agents (to stimulate more effective muscle contractions), and HCN blockers (which slow the pacemaker of the heart and decrease heart rate).

Cardiotonic Agents

Cardiotonic (inotropic) drugs affect the intracellular calcium levels in the heart muscle, leading to increased contractility. This increase in contraction strength leads to increased cardiac output, which causes increased renal blood flow and increased urine production. Increased renal blood flow decreases renin release, interfering with the effects of the renin–angiotensin–aldosterone system, and increases urine output, leading to decreased blood volume. The result is a decrease in the heart's workload and relief of HF. Two types of cardiotonic drugs are used: The classic cardiac glycosides, which have been used for hundreds of years, and the newer phosphodiesterase inhibitors. Table 44.1 presents a complete list of these agents. Box 44.3 summarizes the use of cardiotonic drugs in different age groups.

Cardiac Glycosides

The cardiac glycosides were originally derived from the foxglove or digitalis plant. These plants were once ground up to make digitalis leaf. Today, digoxin (*Lanoxin*) is the drug most often used to treat HF.

Table 44.1 ***Drugs in Focus:* Cardiotonic Agents**

Drug Name	Usual Dosage	Usual Indications
Cardiac Glycoside		
digoxin (*Lanoxin*)	*Adult:* Loading dose 0.75–1.25 mg PO *or* 0.125–0.25 mg IV, then maintenance dose of 0.125–0.25 mg/d PO; decrease dose with renal impairment *Pediatric (dose based on age):* 10–60 mcg/kg PO *or* 8–50 mcg/kg IV loading dose; maintenance is 25%–30% of loading dose	Treatment of acute HF, atrial arrhythmias
Phosphodiesterase Inhibitor		
milrinone (generic)	50 mcg/kg IV bolus over 10 min, then 0.375–0.75 mcg/kg/min IV infusion; do not exceed 1.13 mg/kg/d; reduce dose in renal impairment	Short-term management of HF in adults receiving digoxin and diuretics
HCN Blocker		
ivabradine (*Corlanor*)	5 mg PO b.i.d., adjust based on heart rate to maximum 7.5 mg PO b.i.d.	Reduce the risk of hospitalization in stable chronic HF patients with ejection factor of 35% or less and heart rate of 70 or more

HF, heart failure.

BOX 44.3 FOCUS ON Drug Therapy Across the Lifespan

Cardiotonic Agents

CHILDREN

Digoxin is used widely in children with heart defects and related cardiac problems. The margin of safety for the dosage drug is very small with children. The dosage needs to be very carefully calculated and should be double-checked by another nurse before administration.

Children should be monitored closely for any sign of impending digitalis toxicity and should have serum digoxin levels monitored.

The phosphodiesterase inhibitors and HCN blockers are not recommended for use in children.

ADULTS

Adults receiving any of these drugs need to be instructed as to what adverse reactions to report immediately. They should learn to take their own pulse and should be encouraged to keep track of rate and regularity on a calendar. They may be asked to weigh themselves in the same clothing and at the same time of the day to monitor for fluid retention. Any changes in diet, GI activity, or medications should be reported to the health care provider because of the potential for altering serum levels and causing toxic reactions or ineffective dosing.

Patients should also be advised against switching between brands of digoxin because there have been reports of different bioavailabilities, leading to toxic reactions.

The safety for the use of these drugs during pregnancy has not been established. They should not be used in pregnancy unless the benefit to the mother clearly outweighs the potential risk to the fetus. The drugs do enter breast milk, but they have not been associated with any adverse effects in the neonate. Caution should be exercised, however, if one of these drugs is needed during lactation.

OLDER ADULTS

Older adults frequently are prescribed one of these drugs. They, like children at the other end of the life spectrum, are more susceptible to the toxic effects of the drugs and are more likely to have underlying conditions that could interfere with their metabolism and excretion.

Renal impairment can lead to accumulation of digoxin in the body. If renal dysfunction is present the dosage needs to be reduced and the patient monitored very closely for signs of digoxin toxicity.

The total drug regimen of the older patient should be coordinated, with careful attention to interacting drugs or alternative therapies.

For backup in situations of stress or illness a significant other should be instructed in how to take the patient's pulse and the adverse effects to watch for while the patient is taking this drug.

Therapeutic Actions and Indications

Digoxin increases intracellular calcium and allows more calcium to enter myocardial cells during depolarization (Figure 44.4), causing the following effects:

- Increased force of myocardial contraction (a positive inotropic effect)
- Increased cardiac output and renal perfusion (which has a diuretic effect, increasing urine output and decreasing blood volume while decreasing renin release and activation of the renin–angiotensin–aldosterone system)
- Slowed heart rate, owing to slowing of the rate of cellular repolarization (a negative chronotropic effect)
- Decreased conduction velocity through the atrioventricular (AV) node

The overall effect is a decrease in the myocardial workload and relief of HF. Digoxin is indicated for the treatment of HF, atrial flutter, atrial fibrillation, and paroxysmal atrial tachycardia (see Table 44.1). Digoxin has a very narrow margin of safety (meaning that the therapeutic dose is very close to the toxic dose), so extreme care must be taken when using this drug (see Adverse Effects for information on digoxin antidote).

Pharmacokinetics

Digoxin is available for oral and parenteral administration. The drug has a rapid onset of action and rapid absorption (30 to 120 minutes when taken orally, 5 to 30 minutes when given IV). It is widely distributed throughout the body. Digoxin is primarily excreted unchanged in the urine. Because of this, caution should be exercised in the presence of renal impairment because the drug may not be excreted and could accumulate, causing toxicity.

Contraindications and Cautions

Cardiac glycosides are contraindicated in the presence of allergy to any component of the digitalis preparation *to prevent hypersensitivity reactions.* Digoxin is contraindicated in the following conditions: Ventricular tachycardia or fibrillation, *which are potentially fatal arrhythmias and should be treated with other drugs*; heart block or sick sinus syndrome, *which could be made worse by slowing of conduction through the AV node*; idiopathic hypertrophic subaortic stenosis (IHSS) *because the increase in force of contraction could obstruct the outflow tract to the aorta and cause severe problems*; acute MI *because the increase in force of contraction could cause more muscle damage and infarct*; renal insufficiency *because the drug is excreted through the kidneys and toxic levels could develop*; and electrolyte abnormalities (e.g., increased calcium, decreased potassium, decreased magnesium), *which could alter the action potential and change the effects of the drug.*

Digoxin should be used cautiously in patients who are pregnant or lactating *because of the potential for adverse effects on the fetus or neonate.* It is not known whether

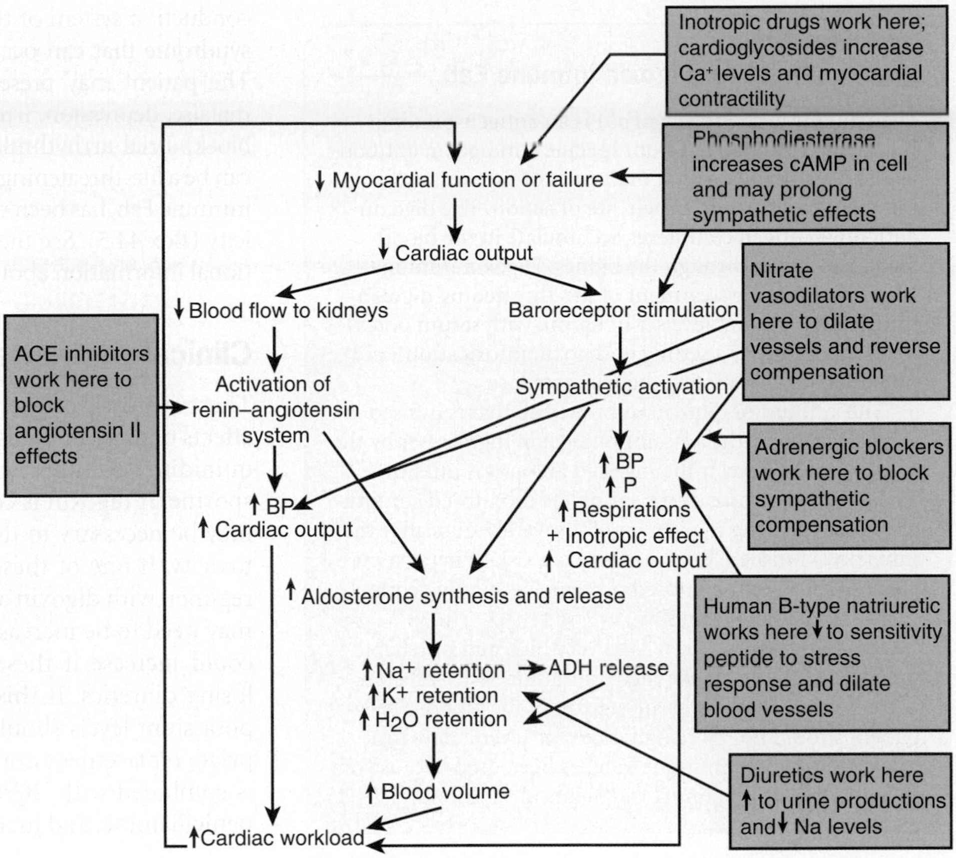

FIGURE 44.4 Sites of action of drugs used to treat heart failure (HF).

digoxin causes fetal toxicity; it should be given during pregnancy only if the benefit to the mother clearly outweighs the risk to the fetus. Digoxin does enter breast milk, but it has not been shown to cause problems for the neonate. Caution should be exercised, however, during lactation. Pediatric and geriatric patients also are at higher risk for adverse effects and should be monitored closely (Box 44.4).

Adverse Effects

The adverse effects most frequently seen with the cardiac glycosides include headache, weakness, drowsiness, and vision changes (a yellow halo around objects is often reported). GI upset and anorexia also commonly occur. Arrhythmias may develop because the glycosides affect the action potential and

BOX 44.4 FOCUS ON **The Evidence**

Preventing Digoxin Toxicity in Children and the Elderly

Pediatric and geriatric patients are at increased risk for digoxin toxicity. Individuals in both of these groups have body masses that are smaller than the average adult body mass, and they may have immature or aging kidneys. Digoxin is excreted unchanged in the kidneys, so any change in kidney function can result in increased serum digoxin levels and subsequent digoxin toxicity. Extreme care should be taken when administering digoxin to patients in either of these age groups.

PEDIATRIC FINDINGS

Many institutions require that pediatric digoxin doses be checked by a second nurse before administration. This practice provides an extra check to help prevent the toxicity of this potentially dangerous drug. The patient should then be assessed before the drug is given, including careful cardiac auscultation and apical pulse measurement to monitor heart rate and rhythm to detect any possible toxic effects.

GERIATRIC FINDINGS

Geriatric patients may not receive the same kind of attention as a policy, but they should be monitored for any factor that might affect digoxin levels when the drug is administered. Such factors may include:

- Renal function (Is the blood urea nitrogen concentration elevated?)
- Low body mass (Is the patient underweight, undernourished, taking laxatives?)
- Current pulse, including quality and rhythm
- Hydration (Is the skin loose? Are the mucous membranes dry? The presence of these conditions could signal potential electrolyte disturbances.)

Many geriatric patients eventually need a decrease in dose, from 0.25 mg once a day to 0.125 mg once a day or 0.25 mg every other day. The nurse administering the drug is often in the best position to detect any changes in the patient's condition that might indicate a need for further evaluation.

BOX 44.5

Digoxin Antidote: Digoxin Immune Fab

Digoxin immune Fab (*DigiFab*) is an antigen-binding fragment (Fab) derived from specific antidigoxin antibodies. These antibodies bind molecules of digoxin, making them unavailable at their site of action. The digoxin antibody–antigen complexes accumulate in the blood and are excreted through the kidney. Digoxin immune Fab is used for the treatment of life-threatening digoxin intoxication (serum levels >10 ng/mL with serum potassium >5 mEq/L in a setting of digoxin intoxication) and potential life-threatening digoxin overdose.

The amount of digoxin immune Fab that is infused IV is determined by the amount of digoxin ingested or by the serum digoxin level if the ingested amount is unknown. The patient's cardiac status should be monitored continually while the drug is given and for several hours after the infusion is finished. Because there is a risk of hypersensitivity reaction to the infused protein, life support equipment should be on standby.

Serum digoxin levels will be very high and unreliable for about 3 days after the digoxin immune Fab infusion because of the high levels of digoxin in the blood. The patient should not be redigitalized for several days to 1 week after digoxin immune Fab has been used because of the potential of remaining fragments in the blood.

conduction system of the heart. Digoxin toxicity is a serious syndrome that can occur when digoxin levels are too high. The patient may present with anorexia, nausea, vomiting, malaise, depression, irregular heart rhythms including heart block, atrial arrhythmias, and ventricular tachycardia. This can be a life-threatening situation. A digoxin antidote, digoxin immune Fab, has been developed to rapidly treat digoxin toxicity (Box 44.5). See the Critical Thinking Scenario for additional information about inadequate digoxin absorption.

Clinically Important Drug–Drug Interactions

There is a risk of increased therapeutic effects and toxic effects of digoxin if it is taken with verapamil, amiodarone, quinidine, quinine, erythromycin, tetracycline, or cyclosporine. If digoxin is combined with any of these drugs, it may be necessary to decrease the digoxin dose to prevent toxicity. If one of these drugs has been part of a medical regimen with digoxin and is discontinued the digoxin dose may need to be increased. The risk of cardiac arrhythmias could increase if these drugs are taken with potassium-losing diuretics. If this combination is used the patient's potassium levels should be checked regularly and appropriate replacement done. Digoxin may be less effective if it is combined with thyroid hormones, metoclopramide, or penicillamine, and increased digoxin dose may be needed.

CRITICAL THINKING SCENARIO

Inadequate Digoxin Absorption

THE SITUATION

G.J. is an 82-year-old white woman with a 50-year history of rheumatic mitral valve disease. She has been stabilized on digoxin for 10 years in a compensated state of HF. G.J. recently moved into an extended care facility because she was having difficulty caring for herself independently. She was examined by the admitting facility physician and was found to be stable. Note was made of an irregular pulse of 76 beats/min with ECG documentation of her chronic atrial fibrillation.

Three weeks after her arrival at the nursing home, G.J. began to develop progressive weakness, dyspnea on exertion, two-pillow orthopnea, and peripheral 2+ pitting edema. These signs and symptoms became progressively worse, and 5 days after the first indication that her HF was returning, G.J. was admitted to the hospital with a diagnosis of HF. Physical examination revealed a heart rate of 96 beats/min with atrial fibrillation, third heart sound, rales, wheezes, 2+ pitting edema bilaterally up to the knees, elevated JVP, cardiomegaly, weak pulses, and poor peripheral perfusion. G.J.'s serum digoxin level was 0.12 ng/mL (therapeutic range, 0.5–2 ng/mL). G.J. was treated with diuretics and was redigitalized in the hospital with close cardiac monitoring.

After her condition stabilized, G.J. reported that she knew she had been taking her digoxin every day because she recognized the pill. The only difference she could identify was that she was given the pill in the afternoon with a dish of ice cream, while at home she always took it on an empty stomach first thing in the morning. The nursing home staff confirmed that G.J. had received the drug daily in the afternoon and that it was the same brand name she had used at home.

CRITICAL THINKING

What nursing interventions should be done at this point? *Think about the signs and symptoms of HF and how they show its progression.*

Inadequate Digoxin Absorption (continued)

How could the change in the timing of drug administration be related to the decreased serum digoxin levels noted on G.J.'s admission?

Consider the factors that affect absorption of a drug. What alterations in dosing could be suggested that would prevent this from happening to G.J. again?

What potential problems with trust could develop for G.J. on her return to the nursing home? Suggest an explanation for what happened to G.J. and possible ways that this problem could have been averted.

DISCUSSION

G.J.'s immediate needs involve trying to alleviate the alteration to her cardiac output that occurred when she lost the therapeutic effects of digoxin. Positioning, cool environment, small and frequent meals, and rest periods can help to decrease the workload on her heart. Digoxin has a small margin of safety and requires an adequate serum level to be therapeutic. G.J. was not absorbing enough digoxin to achieve a therapeutic serum level; consequently, her body began to go through the progression of HF, first right sided and then left sided.

NURSING CARE GUIDE FOR G.J.: DIGOXIN

Assessment: History and Examination

Assess the patient's health history for allergies to any digitalis product, renal dysfunction, IHSS, pregnancy, lactation, arrhythmias, heart block, and electrolyte abnormalities.

Focus the physical examination on the following areas:

CV: Blood pressure, pulse, perfusion, electrocardiography

Central nervous system (CNS): Orientation, affect, reflexes, vision

Skin: Color, lesions, texture, perfusion

Respiratory system: Respiratory rate and character, adventitious sounds

GI: Abdominal examination, bowel sounds

Laboratory tests: Serum electrolytes, body weight

Nursing Diagnoses

Decreased cardiac output related to cardiac effect

Deficient fluid volume related to diuretic effects

Ineffective tissue perfusion related to changes in cardiac output

Impaired gas exchange related to changes in cardiac output

Deficient knowledge regarding drug therapy

Planning

The patient will receive the best therapeutic effect from the drug therapy.

The patient will have limited adverse effects to the drug therapy.

The patient will have an understanding of the drug therapy, adverse effects to anticipate, and measures to relieve discomfort and improve safety.

Implementation

Administer a loading dose to provide rapid therapeutic effects.

Monitor apical pulse for 1 full minute before administering to assess for adverse and therapeutic effects.

Check dose very carefully.

Provide comfort and safety measures: Give small, frequent meals; ensure access to bathroom facilities; avoid intramuscular injection; administer intravenously over 5 minutes; keep emergency equipment on standby.

Provide support and reassurance to deal with drug effects.

Provide patient teaching regarding drug, dosage, adverse effects, what to report, and safety precautions.

Evaluation

Evaluate drug effects: Relief of signs and symptoms of HF, resolution of atrial arrhythmias, serum digoxin levels 0.5–2 ng/mL.

Monitor for adverse effects, including arrhythmias, vision changes (yellow halo), GI upset, headache, and drowsiness.

Monitor for drug–drug interactions as indicated for each drug.

Evaluate the effectiveness of patient-teaching program.

Evaluate the effectiveness of comfort and safety measures.

PATIENT TEACHING FOR G.J.

- Digoxin is a digitalis preparation. Digitalis has many helpful effects on the heart; for example, it helps the heart to beat more slowly and efficiently. These effects promote better circulation and should help to reduce the swelling in your ankles or legs. It also should increase the amount of urine that you produce every day.
- Digoxin is a very powerful drug and must be taken exactly as prescribed. It is important to have regular medical checkups to ensure that the dose of the drug

(continues on page 760)

Inadequate Digoxin Absorption (continued)

is correct for you and that it is having the desired effect on your heart.

- Do not stop taking this drug without consulting your health care provider. Never skip doses and never try to "catch up" any missed doses because serious adverse effects could occur.
- Learn to take your pulse. Take it each morning before engaging in any activity. Write your pulse rate on a calendar so you will be aware of any changes and can notify your health care provider if the rate or rhythm of your pulse shows a consistent change. Your normal pulse rate is _____.
- Try to monitor your weight fairly closely. Weigh yourself every other day, at the same time of the day and in the same amount of clothing. Record your weight on your calendar for easy reference. If you gain or lose 3 pound or more in 1 day, it may indicate a problem with your drug. Consult your health care provider.
- Some of the following adverse effects may occur:
  - *Dizziness, drowsiness, headache:* Avoid driving or performing hazardous tasks or delicate tasks that require concentration if these occur. Consult your health care provider for an appropriate analgesic if the headache is a problem.
  - *Nausea, GI upset, loss of appetite:* Small, frequent meals may help; monitor your weight loss; if it becomes severe, consult your health care provider.
  - *Vision changes, "yellow" halos around objects:* These effects may pass with time. Take extra care in your activities for the first few days. If these reactions do not go away after 3–4 days, consult with your health care provider.
  - Report any of the following to your health care provider: Unusually slow or irregular pulse; rapid weight gain; "yellow vision"; unusual tiredness or weakness; skin rash or hives; swelling of the ankles, legs, or fingers; difficulty breathing.
- Tell any doctor, nurse, dentist, or other health care provider that you are taking this drug.
- Keep this drug, and all medications, out of the reach of children.
- Avoid the use of over-the-counter medications while you are taking this drug. If you think that you need one of these, consult with your health care provider for the best choice. Many of these drugs contain ingredients that could interfere with your digoxin.
- Consider wearing or carrying some form of medical identification to alert any medical personnel who might take care of you in an emergency that you are taking this drug.
- Schedule regular medical checkups to evaluate the actions of the drug and to adjust the dose if necessary.

Absorption of oral digoxin may be decreased if it is taken with cholestyramine, charcoal, colestipol, antacids, bleomycin, cyclophosphamide, or methotrexate. If it is used in combination with any of these agents, the drugs should not be taken at the same time but should be administered 2 to 4 hours apart. Box 44.6 highlights important information about the interactions between digoxin and common herbal remedies.

BOX 44.6 FOCUS ON Herbal and Alternative Therapies

St. John's wort and psyllium have been shown to decrease the effectiveness of digoxin; this combination should be avoided. Increased digoxin toxicity has been reported with ginseng, hawthorn, and licorice. Patients should be advised to avoid these combinations. Licorice acts as a pseudoaldosterone in the body, leading to loss of potassium and retention of sodium and water. This combination can cause serious digoxin toxicity. Patients should be advised to avoid this combination

Ⓟ Prototype Summary: Digoxin

Indications: Treatment of HF, atrial fibrillation.

Actions: Increases intracellular calcium and allows more calcium to enter the myocardial cell during depolarization; this causes a positive inotropic effect (increased force of contraction), increased renal perfusion with a diuretic effect and decrease in renin release, a negative chronotropic effect (slower heart rate), and slowed conduction through the AV node.

Pharmacokinetics:

Route	Onset	Peak	Duration
Oral	30–120 min	2–6 h	6–8 d
IV	5–30 min	1–5 h	4–5 d

$T_{1/2}$: 30 to 40 hours; largely excreted unchanged in the urine.

Adverse Effects: Headache, weakness, drowsiness, visual disturbances, arrhythmias, GI upset.

Nursing Considerations for Patients Receiving Cardiac Glycosides

Assessment: History and Examination

- Assess for contraindications or cautions: Known allergies to any digitalis product *to avoid hypersensitivity reactions*; impaired kidney function, *which could alter the excretion of the drug*; ventricular tachycardia or fibrillation, *which require treatment with other life-saving drugs*; heart block, sick sinus syndrome, or IHSS, *which could be exacerbated by the drug*; acute MI, *which could lead to increased muscle damage and infarction*; electrolyte abnormalities (increased calcium, decreased potassium, or decreased magnesium), *which could alter the action potential and drug effects;* and current status of pregnancy or lactation *to evaluate benefits versus potential risk to the fetus when using the drug.*
- Perform a physical assessment *to establish baseline status before beginning therapy, determine the effectiveness of therapy, and evaluate for any potential adverse effects.*
- Obtain the patient's weight, noting any recent increases or decreases, *to determine the patient's fluid status.*
- Assess cardiac status closely, including pulse and blood pressure, *to identify changes requiring a change in dosage of the drug or the presence of adverse effects,* and auscultate heart sounds, noting any evidence of abnormal sounds, *to identify conduction problems.*
- Inspect the skin and mucous membranes for color, and check nail beds and capillary refill *for evidence of perfusion.*
- Monitor affect, orientation, and reflexes *to evaluate CNS effects of the drug.*
- Assess the patient's respiratory rate and auscultate lungs *for evidence of adventitious breath sounds to monitor for evidence of left-sided HF.*
- Examine the abdomen for distention; auscultate bowel sounds *to evaluate GI motility.*
- Assess voiding patterns and urinary output *to provide a gross indication of renal function.*
- Obtain a baseline ECG *to identify rate and rhythm and evaluate for possible changes.*
- Monitor the results of laboratory tests, including serum electrolyte levels and renal function tests, *to determine the need for possible dose adjustment.*

Nursing Diagnoses

Nursing diagnoses related to drug therapy might include the following:

- Risk for imbalanced fluid volume related to increased renal perfusion secondary to effects of the drug
- Decreased cardiac output related to ineffective cardiac muscle function
- Ineffective tissue perfusion (total body) related to change in cardiac output
- Impaired gas exchange related to changes in cardiac output
- Deficient knowledge related to prescribed drug therapy

Planning

- The patient will receive the best therapeutic effect from the drug therapy.
- The patient will have limited adverse effects to the drug therapy.
- The patient will have an understanding of the drug therapy, adverse effects to anticipate, and measures to relieve discomfort and improve safety.

Implementation with Rationale

- Consult with the prescriber about the need for a loading dose when beginning therapy *to achieve desired results as soon as possible.*
- Monitor apical pulse for 1 full minute before administering the drug *to monitor for adverse effects.* Hold the dose if the pulse is less than 60 beats/min in an adult or less than 90 beats/min in an infant; retake the pulse in 1 hour. If the pulse remains low, document it, withhold the drug, and notify the prescriber *because the pulse rate could indicate digoxin toxicity* (see Table 44.2 for signs and symptoms).
- Monitor the pulse for any change in quality or rhythm *to detect arrhythmias or early signs of toxicity.*
- Check the dose and preparation carefully *because digoxin has a very small margin of safety, and inadvertent drug errors can cause serious problems.*
- Check pediatric dose with extreme care *because children are more apt to develop digoxin toxicity.* Have the dose double-checked by another nurse before administration.
- Follow dilution instructions carefully for IV use; use promptly *to avoid drug degradation.*
- Administer intravenous doses very slowly over at least 5 minutes *to avoid cardiac arrhythmias and adverse effects.*
- Avoid intramuscular administration, *which could be quite painful.*
- Arrange for the patient to be weighed at the same time each day, in the same clothes, *to monitor for fluid retention and HF.* Assess dependent areas for edema; note the amount and degree of pitting *to evaluate the severity of fluid retention.*
- Avoid administering the oral drug with food or antacids *to avoid delays in absorption.*
- Maintain emergency equipment on standby: Potassium salts, lidocaine (*for treatment of arrhythmias*), phenytoin (*for treatment of seizures*), atropine (*to increase heart rate*), and a cardiac monitor, *in case severe toxicity should occur.*

(continues on page 762)

- Obtain digoxin level as ordered; monitor the patient for therapeutic digoxin level (0.5–2 ng/mL) *to evaluate therapeutic dosing and to monitor for the development of toxicity.*
- Provide comfort measures *to help the patient tolerate drug effects.* These include small, frequent meals *to help alleviate GI upset or nausea*; access to bathroom facilities if GI upset is severe and *to accommodate increased urination related to increased cardiac output*; safety precautions *to reduce the risk of injury secondary to weakness and drowsiness*; adequate lighting *to accommodate vision changes if they occur*; positioning for comfort; and frequent rest periods *to balance supply and demand of oxygen.*
- Offer support and encouragement *to help the patient deal with the diagnosis and the drug regimen.*
- Provide thorough patient teaching, including the name of the drug, dosage prescribed, technique for monitoring pulse and acceptable pulse parameters, dietary measures if appropriate, measures to avoid adverse effects, warning signs of possible toxicity and need to notify health care provider, and the need for periodic monitoring and evaluation, including ECGs and laboratory testing, *to enhance patient knowledge about drug therapy and to promote compliance.*

Evaluation

- Monitor patient response to the drug (improvement in signs and symptoms of HF, resolution of atrial arrhythmias, serum digoxin level of 0.5–2 ng/mL).
- Monitor for adverse effects (vision changes, arrhythmias, HF, headache, dizziness, drowsiness, GI upset, nausea).
- Monitor the effectiveness of comfort measures and compliance with the regimen.
- Evaluate the effectiveness of the teaching plan (patient can name drug, dosage, proper administration, adverse effects to watch for, specific measures to avoid them, and the importance of continued follow-up).

Phosphodiesterase Inhibitors

The phosphodiesterase inhibitors (Table 44.1) belong to a second class of drugs that act as cardiotonic (inotropic) agents. The only drug currently available in this class is milrinone (generic).

Therapeutic Actions and Indications

The phosphodiesterase inhibitors block the enzyme phosphodiesterase. This blocking effect leads to an increase in myocardial cell cyclic adenosine monophosphate (cAMP), which increases calcium levels in the cell (Figure 44.4). Increased cellular calcium causes a stronger contraction and prolongs the effects of sympathetic stimulation, which can lead to vasodilation, increased oxygen consumption, and arrhythmias. Milrinone is indicated for the short-term treatment of HF that has not responded to digoxin or diuretics alone or that has had a poor response to digoxin, diuretics, and vasodilators. See Table 44.1 for Usual Indications for each drug. Because this drug has been associated with the development of potentially fatal ventricular arrhythmias, its use is limited to severe situations.

Pharmacokinetics

Milrinone is available only for IV use. It is widely distributed after injection. It is metabolized in the liver and excreted primarily in the urine.

Table 44.2 Congestive HF and Response to Cardiac Glycosides

	Response	
Signs and Symptoms[a]	**During Congestive HF**	**After Full Digitalization**[b]
Heart rate, rhythm, and size	Heart hypertrophied, dilated; rate rapid, irregular; "palpitations"; auscultation—S_3	Dilatation decreased, hypertrophy remains; rate, 70–80 beats/min, may be regular; auscultation—no S_3
Lungs	Dyspnea on exertion; orthopnea; tachypnea; paroxysmal nocturnal dyspnea; wheezing, rales, cough, hemoptysis (pulmonary edema)	Rate of respiration; wheezes, rales gone
Peripheral congestion	Pitting edema of dependent parts, hepatomegaly, JVP, cyanosis, oliguria, nocturia	Cardiac output and renal blood flow leads to urine flow, edema, signs and symptoms of poor perfusion
Other	Weakness, fatigue, anorexia, insomnia, nausea, vomiting, abdominal pain	Appetite: Strength, energy

[a]Because the clinical picture in HF varies with the stage and degree of severity the signs and symptoms may vary considerably in different patients.
[b]Digitalization will not overcome similar symptoms when they are caused by conditions other than HF. Overdosage may actually cause symptoms similar to those of HF (e.g., anorexia, nausea, vomiting, cardiac arrhythmias, peripheral congestion).
HF, heart failure; JVP, jugular venous pressure.

Contraindications and Cautions

Phosphodiesterase inhibitors are contraindicated in the presence of allergy to either of these drugs or to bisulfites *to avoid hypersensitivity reactions*. Milrinone is also contraindicated in the following conditions: Severe aortic or pulmonic valvular disease, *which could be exacerbated by increased contraction*; acute MI, *which could be exacerbated by increased oxygen consumption and increased force of contraction*; fluid volume deficit, *which could be made worse by increased renal perfusion*; and ventricular arrhythmias, *which could be exacerbated by this drug.*

Caution should be exercised in the elderly, *who are more likely to develop adverse effects. There are no adequate studies about the effects of these drugs during pregnancy*, and use should be reserved for situations in which the benefit to the mother clearly outweighs the potential risk to the fetus. *It is not known whether this drug enters breast milk*, so caution should be exercised if the patient is breastfeeding.

Adverse Effects

The adverse effects most frequently seen with this drug is ventricular arrhythmias (which can progress to fatal ventricular fibrillation), hypotension, and chest pain. GI effects include nausea, vomiting, anorexia, and abdominal pain. Thrombocytopenia can occur with milrinone. Hypersensitivity reactions associated with this drug include vasculitis, pericarditis, pleuritis, and ascites. Burning at the IV injection site is also a frequent adverse effect (Figure 44.5).

Clinically Important Drug–Drug Interactions

Precipitates form when milrinone is given in solution with furosemide. Avoid this combination in solution. Use alternate lines if both of these drugs are being given IV.

Ⓟ Prototype Summary: Milrinone

Indications: Short-term treatment of HF in patients who have not responded to digitalis, diuretics, or vasodilators.

Actions: Blocks the enzyme phosphodiesterase, which leads to an increase in myocardial cell cAMP, which increases calcium levels in the cell, causing a stronger contraction and prolonged response to sympathetic stimulation; directly relaxes vascular smooth muscle.

Pharmacokinetics:

Route	Onset	Peak	Duration
IV	Immediate	10 min	8 h

$T_{1/2}$: 2.3–3.5 hours, metabolized in the liver and excreted in the urine and feces.

Adverse effects: Arrhythmias, hypotension, nausea, vomiting, thrombocytopenia, pericarditis, pleuritis, fever, chest pain, burning at injection site.

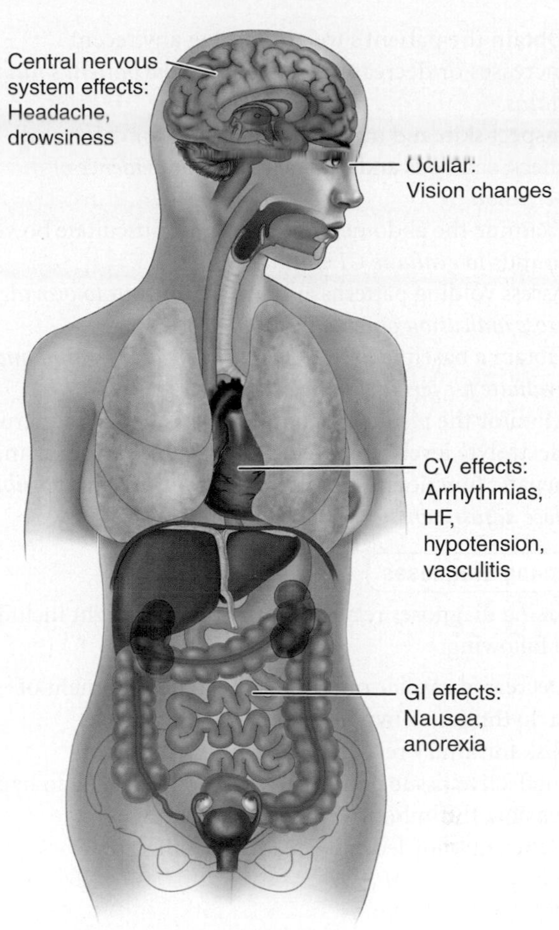

FIGURE 44.5 Variety of adverse effects and toxicities associated with cardiotonic agents.

Nursing Considerations for Patients Receiving a Phosphodiesterase Inhibitor

Assessment: History and Examination

- Assess for contraindications or cautions: Any known allergies to this drug or to bisulfites *to avoid hypersensitivity reactions*; acute aortic or pulmonic valvular disease, acute MI or fluid volume deficit, and ventricular arrhythmias, *which could be exacerbated by these drugs*; and current status of pregnancy and lactation *to prevent potential adverse effects to the fetus or baby*.
- Perform a physical assessment *to establish baseline status before beginning therapy, determine the effectiveness of therapy, and evaluate for any potential adverse effects.*
- Assess cardiac status closely, including pulse and blood pressure, *to identify changes or the presence of adverse effects*; auscultate heart sounds, noting any evidence of abnormal sounds.

(continues on page 764)

- Obtain the patient's weight, noting any recent increases or decreases, *to determine the patient's fluid status.*
- Inspect skin and mucous membranes for color, and check nail beds and capillary refill *for evidence of perfusion.*
- Examine the abdomen for distention; auscultate bowel sounds *to evaluate GI motility.*
- Assess voiding patterns and urinary output *to provide a gross indication of renal function.*
- Obtain a baseline ECG *to identify rate and rhythm and evaluate for possible changes.*
- Monitor the results of laboratory tests, including serum electrolyte levels, complete blood count, and renal and hepatic function tests, *to determine the need for possible dose adjustment.*

Nursing Diagnoses

Nursing diagnoses related to drug therapy might include the following:

- Decreased cardiac output related to development of arrhythmias or hypotension
- Risk for injury related to CNS or CV effects
- Ineffective tissue perfusion (total body) related to hypotension, thrombocytopenia, or arrhythmias
- Deficient knowledge related to drug therapy

Planning

- The patient will receive the best therapeutic effect from the drug therapy.
- The patient will have limited adverse effects to the drug therapy.
- The patient will have an understanding of the drug therapy, adverse effects to anticipate, and measures to relieve discomfort and improve safety.

Implementation with Rationale

- Protect the drug from light *to prevent drug degradation.*
- Ensure that patient has a patent IV access site available *to allow for IV administration of the drug.*
- Monitor pulse and blood pressure frequently during administration *to monitor for adverse effects so that the dose can be altered if needed to avoid toxicity.*
- Monitor input and output and record daily weight *to evaluate the resolution of HF.*
- Monitor platelet counts before and regularly during therapy *to ensure that the dose is appropriate*, inspect the skin for bruising or petechiae *to detect early signs of thrombocytopenia*, and consult with the prescriber about the need *to decrease the dose at the first sign of thrombocytopenia.*
- Monitor IV injection sites and provide comfort measures *if infusion is causing irritation.*
- Provide life support equipment on standby *in case of severe reaction to the drug or development of ventricular arrhythmias.*
- Provide comfort measures *to help the patient tolerate drug effects.* These include small, frequent meals *to alleviate GI upset and anorexia*; access to bathroom facilities to provide needed facilities if GI upset is severe and when increased urination occurs secondary to increased cardiac output; safety precautions *to protect the patient if visual changes, dizziness, or weakness occurs*; and orientation to surroundings *to support the patient if CNS changes occur.*
- Offer support and encouragement *to help the patient deal with the diagnosis and the drug regimen.*
- Provide thorough patient teaching, including the name of the drug, dosage prescribed, measures to avoid adverse effects, warning signs of problems, and the need for periodic monitoring and evaluation, *to enhance patient knowledge about drug therapy and to promote compliance.*

Evaluation

- Monitor patient response to the drug (alleviation of signs and symptoms of HF).
- Monitor for adverse effects (hypotension, cardiac arrhythmias, GI upset, thrombocytopenia).
- Monitor the effectiveness of comfort measures and compliance with the regimen.
- Evaluate the effectiveness of the teaching plan (patient can name drug, dosage, adverse effects to watch for, specific measures to avoid them, and the importance of continued follow-up).

Hyperpolarization-Activated Cyclic Nucleotide–Gated Channel Blockers

In 2015 a new class of drugs was approved for the treatment of patients with chronic HF. The HCN blocker introduced, ivabradine (*Corlanor*), does not affect muscle contraction but does affect the pacemaker of the heart to reduce heart rate.

Therapeutic Actions and Indications

Blocking the HCNs slows the heart's pacemaker, the sinus node, in the repolarizing phase of the action potential. This leads to a reduction in heart rate. Slowing the heart rate allows more time for ventricular filling and improves cardiac output. The systemic effects seen with beta-blockers are not seen with this class of drug. There are no effects on ventricular repolarization or on ventricular contractility. This action also affects channels in the retina, which may alter the retinal response to bright light and explain some of the adverse effects seen with this drug. Ivabradine is indicated to reduce the risk of hospitalization for worsening HF in patients with stable, symptomatic, chronic heart failure with a left ventricular ejection fraction of 35% or less, who are in sinus rhythm with a rate of 70 or more and who are on the maximally tolerated dose of beta-blockers or who have a contraindication to the use of beta blockers. See Table 44.1.

Pharmacokinetics

Ivabradine is rapidly absorbed through the GI tract, reaching peak levels in 1 hour. It is metabolized in the liver and intestines and excreted in the feces and bile with a half-life of 2 hours and effective duration of 6 hours.

Contraindications and Cautions

Ivabradine is contraindicated in the presence of allergy to either of these drugs or to bisulfites *to avoid hypersensitivity reactions.* It is also contraindicated in the following conditions: Active, decompensated HF; hypotension; sick sinus syndrome of AV block; resting heart rate under 60 beats/min; patients completely dependent on a pacemaker, *which could be exacerbated by the drug leading to serious adverse effects*; severe hepatic impairment, *which could lead to drug accumulation;* concurrent use of strong CYP3A4 inhibitors, *which could lead to drug accumulation and toxic effects.*

Caution should be exercised with atrial fibrillation or moderate heart block *because the drug effects may be unpredictable and not therapeutic. Fetal toxicity has been reported* so use should be discouraged in pregnancy and use should be reserved for situations in which the benefit to the mother clearly outweighs the potential risk to the fetus. Women of childbearing age should be encouraged to use contraceptive measures. *It is not known whether this drug enters breast milk,* so it is not recommended to use this drug if breastfeeding.

Adverse Effects

The adverse effects most frequently seen with this drug are bradycardia, hypertension, atrial fibrillation, and luminous phenomena (sudden changes in brightness in parts of the visual field, colored bright lights, image decompensation, multiple images). Safety precautions need to be taken with the visual changes.

Clinically Important Drug–Drug Interactions

Altered plasma concentrations occur with strong CYP3A4 inhibitors or inducers; this combination should be avoided. Severe bradycardia can occur if combined with other negatively chronotropic drugs.

Ⓟ Prototype Summary: Ivabradine

Indications: Treatment of chronic heart failure in stable patients at maximum beta-blocker doses, to prevent rehospitalizations

Actions: Blocks HCNs to slow the heart's pacemaker and reduce heart rate with no effect on muscle contraction

Pharmacokinetics:

Route	Onset	Peak	Duration
PO	Rapid	1 hour	6 h

$T_{1/2}$: 2.5 hours; metabolized in the liver and intestines; excreted in the urine and feces

Adverse Effects: Bradycardia, atrial fibrillation, hypertension, luminous phenomena (visual changes)

Nursing Considerations for Patients Receiving Ivabradine

Assessment: History and Examination

- Assess for contraindications or cautions: Any known allergies to this drug *to avoid hypersensitivity reactions*; AV block, decompensated HF, dependence on a pacemaker, resting heart rate under 60 beats/min, hypotension, *which could be exacerbated by these drugs*; severe hepatic impairment or concurrent use of CYP3A4 inhibitors, *which could lead to accumulation of the drug*; and current status of pregnancy and lactation *to prevent potential adverse effects to the fetus or baby.*
- Perform a physical assessment *to establish baseline status before beginning therapy, determine the effectiveness of therapy, and evaluate for any potential adverse effects.*
- Assess cardiac status closely, including pulse and blood pressure, *to identify changes or the presence of adverse effects*; auscultate heart sounds, noting any evidence of abnormal sounds.
- Obtain the patient's weight, noting any recent increases or decreases, *to determine the patient's fluid status.*
- Inspect skin and mucous membranes for color, and check nail beds and capillary refill *for evidence of perfusion.*
- Assess voiding patterns and urinary output *to provide a gross indication of renal function.*
- Obtain a baseline ECG *to identify rate and rhythm and evaluate for possible changes.*
- Monitor the results of laboratory tests, including serum electrolyte levels, complete blood count, and renal and

(continues on page 766)

hepatic function tests, *to determine the need for possible dose adjustment.*

Nursing Diagnoses

Nursing diagnoses related to drug therapy might include the following:

- Decreased cardiac output related to development of arrhythmias or hypotension
- Risk for injury related to visual or CV effects
- Ineffective tissue perfusion (total body) related to hypotension or bradycardia
- Deficient knowledge related to drug therapy

Planning

- The patient will receive the best therapeutic effect from the drug therapy.
- The patient will have limited adverse effects to the drug therapy.
- The patient will have an understanding of the drug therapy, adverse effects to anticipate, and measures to relieve discomfort and improve safety.

Implementation with Rationale

- Ensure appropriate use of drug *to avoid serious adverse effects.*
- Monitor heart rate and blood pressure regularly *to evaluate drug effects and intervene as needed.*
- Monitor input and output and record daily weight *to evaluate the resolution of HF.*
- Provide safety measures if visual disturbances occur, including limiting driving and operation of hazardous machinery *to ensure patient safety.*
- Provide comfort measures *to help the patient tolerate drug effects.*
- Offer support and encouragement *to help the patient deal with the diagnosis and the drug regimen.*
- Provide thorough patient teaching, including the name of the drug, dosage prescribed, measures to avoid adverse effects, warning signs of problems, and the need for periodic monitoring and evaluation, *to enhance patient knowledge about drug therapy and to promote compliance.*

Evaluation

- Monitor patient response to the drug (alleviation of signs and symptoms of HF).
- Monitor for adverse effects (hypotension, cardiac arrhythmias, visual disturbances).
- Monitor the effectiveness of comfort and safety measures and compliance with the regimen.
- Evaluate the effectiveness of the teaching plan (patient can name drug, dosage, adverse effects to watch for, specific measures to avoid them, and the importance of continued follow-up).

KEY POINTS

- The cardiac glycoside digoxin increases the movement of calcium into the heart muscle. This results in increased force of contraction, which increases blood flow to the kidneys (causing a diuretic effect), slows the heart rate, and slows conduction through the AV node. All of these effects decrease the heart's workload.
- Phosphodiesterase inhibitors block the breakdown of cAMP in the cardiac muscle. This allows more calcium to enter the cell (leading to more intense contraction) and increases the effects of sympathetic stimulation (which can lead to vasodilation but also can increase pulse, blood pressure, and workload on the heart).
- Milrinone, the only phosphodiesterase inhibitor available, is associated with severe effects. It is reserved for use in extreme situations. It is only available for IV use.
- Ivabradine is the first HCN blocker which is used with stable, chronic HF to slow the pacemaker of the heart, reducing heart rate without the systemic effects that occur with beta-blockers. Slowing the heart rate allows more time for ventricular filling and improves cardiac output without the systemic effects seen with beta-blockers.

SUMMARY

- HF, a condition in which the heart muscle fails to effectively pump blood through the CV system, can be the result of a damaged heart muscle and increased demand to work harder.
- The sarcomere—the functioning unit of the heart muscle—is made up of protein fibers: Thin actin fibers and thick myosin fibers, which react with each other when calcium is present to inactivate troponin. The fibers slide together, resulting in contraction. Failing cardiac muscle cells lose the ability to effectively use energy to move calcium into the cell, and contractions become weak and ineffective.
- Cardiotonic (inotropic) agents are one class of drugs used in the treatment of HF. These agents directly stimulate the muscle to contract more effectively.
- Cardiac glycosides increase the movement of calcium into the heart muscle. This results in increased force of contraction, which increases blood flow to the kidneys (causing a diuretic effect), slows the heart rate, and slows conduction through the AV node. All of these effects decrease the heart's workload. Digoxin is the cardiac glycoside most commonly used to treat HF.
- Phosphodiesterase inhibitors block the breakdown of cAMP in the cardiac muscle. This allows more calcium to enter the cell (leading to more intense contraction) and increases the effects of sympathetic stimulation (which can lead to vasodilation but also can increase pulse, blood pressure, and workload on the heart). Because these drugs are associated with severe effects, they are reserved for use in extreme situations.

- HCN blockers slow the repolarization of the heart's pacemaker, leading to a slower heart rate. Slowing the heart rate allows more time for filling and improves cardiac output. This class of drugs does not affect ventricular cell activity. The systemic effects seen with the use of beta-blockers do not occur with this class of drugs.

CHECK YOUR UNDERSTANDING

Answers to the questions in this chapter can be found in Answers to Check Your Understanding Questions on thePoint®.

MULTIPLE CHOICE

Select the best answer to the following.

1. A nurse assessing a patient with HF would expect to find which of the following:
a. Cardiac arrest
b. Congestion of blood vessels
c. An MI
d. A pulmonary embolism

2. Calcium is needed in the cardiac muscle
a. to break apart actin–myosin bridges.
b. to activate troponin.
c. to promote contraction via sliding.
d. to maintain the electrical rhythm.

3. When assessing a patient with right-sided HF the nurse would expect to find edema
a. in gravity-dependent areas.
b. in the hands and fingers.
c. around the eyes.
d. when the patient is lying down.

4. ACE inhibitors and other vasodilators are used in the early treatment of HF. They act to
a. cause loss of volume.
b. increase arterial pressure and perfusion.
c. cause pooling of the blood and decreased venous return to the heart.
d. increase the release of aldosterone and improve fluid balance.

5. A nurse is preparing to administer a prescribed cardiotonic drug to a patient based on the understanding that this group of drugs act in which way?
a. They block the sympathetic nervous system.
b. They block the renin–angiotensin system.
c. They block the parasympathetic influence on the heart muscle.
d. They affect intracellular calcium levels in the heart muscle.

6. A nurse would instruct a patient taking *Lanoxin* (digoxin) for the treatment of HF to do which of the following?
a. Make up any missed doses the next day.
b. Report changes in heart rate.
c. Avoid exposure to the sun.
d. Switch to generic tablets if less expensive.

7. A nurse is about to administer *Lanoxin* to a patient whose apical pulse is 48 beats/min. She should
a. give the drug and notify the prescriber that the heart rate is low.
b. retake the pulse in 15 minutes and give the drug if the pulse has not changed.
c. retake the pulse in 1 hour and withhold the drug if the pulse is still less than 60 beats/min.
d. withhold the drug and notify the prescriber that the heart rate is below 60 beats/min.

8. Before giving digoxin to an infant, the nurse should
a. notify the prescriber that the dose is about to be given and recheck the ordered dose.
b. check the apical pulse and have another nurse double-check the dose.
c. make sure that the infant has eaten, has a full stomach, and has been given an antacid.
d. check the apical pulse and give the drug very slowly.

MULTIPLE RESPONSE

Select all that apply.

1. HF occurs when the heart fails to pump effectively. Which of the following could cause HF?
a. Coronary artery disease
b. Chronic hypertension
c. Cardiomyopathy
d. Fluid overload
e. Pneumonia
f. Cirrhosis

2. A client develops left-sided HF after an MI. Which of the following would the nurse expect to find during the client assessment?
a. Orthopnea
b. Polyuria
c. Tachypnea
d. Dyspnea
e. Blood-tinged sputum
f. Swollen ankles

BIBLIOGRAPHY AND REFERENCES

Bonow, R. O., Mann, D. L., Libby, P., et al. (2014). *Braunwald's heart disease: A textbook of cardiovascular medicine* (10th ed.). Philadelphia, PA: W. B. Saunders.

Brunton, L., Chabner, B., & Knollman, B. (2011). *Goodman and Gilman's the pharmacological basis of therapeutics* (12th ed.). New York: McGraw-Hill.

Carson, P., Ziesche, R., Johnson, G., Cohn, J. N. (1999). Racial differences in response therapy for heart failure: analysis of the vasodilator-heart failure trials. *Journal of Cardiac Failure*, 5(3):178–187.

Facts and Comparisons. (2015). *Drug facts and comparisons*. St. Louis, MO: Author.

Hall, J. (2015). *Guyton and Hall's textbook of medical physiology* (13th ed.). Philadelphia, PA: W. B. Saunders

Harkness, K., Spalling, M., Currie, K., et al. (2015). A systematic review of patient heart failure self-care strategies. *Journal of Cardiovascular Nursing, 30*(2), 121–135.

Karch, A. M. (2014). *Lippincott's nursing drug guide*. Philadelphia, PA: Lippincott Williams & Wilkins.

Mann, D. (2015). *Heart failure: A companion to Braunwald's heart disease*. Philadelphia, PA: W. B. Saunders.

Paul, S. (2008). Hospital discharge education for patients with heart failure: What really works and what is the evidence. *Critical Care Nurse, 28*, 66–82.

Porth, C. M. (2013). *Pathophysiology: Concepts of altered health states* (9th ed.). Philadelphia, PA: Lippincott Williams & Wilkins.

Roubille, F., & Tardif, J.-C. (2013). New therapeutic targets in cardiology: Heart failure and arrhythmia: HCN channels. *Circulation, 127*, 1986–1996.

Taylor, A.. Ziesche, R., Yancy, C., et al. (2004). Combination of isosborbide dinitrate and hydralazine in blacks with heart failure. *The New England Journal of Medicine*, 2004, 351: 2049–2057.

The Medical Letter. (2015). *The medical letter on drugs and therapeutics*. New Rochelle, NY: Author.

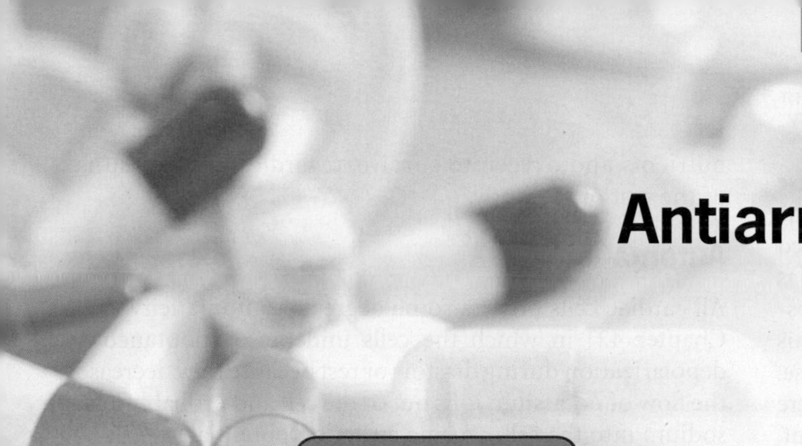

Antiarrhythmic Agents 45

Learning Objectives

Upon completion of this chapter, you will be able to:

1. Describe the cardiac action potential and its phases to explain the changes made by each class of antiarrhythmic agents.
2. Describe the therapeutic actions, indications, pharmacokinetics, contraindications and cautions, most common adverse reactions, and important drug–drug interactions associated with antiarrhythmic agents.
3. Discuss the use of antiarrhythmic agents across the lifespan.
4. Compare and contrast the prototype antiarrhythmic drugs lidocaine, propranolol, sotalol, and diltiazem with other agents in their class and with other classes of antiarrhythmics.
5. Outline the nursing considerations, including important teaching points, for patients receiving antiarrhythmic agents.

Glossary of Key Terms

antiarrhythmics: drugs that affect the action potential of cardiac cells and are used to treat arrhythmias and restore normal rate and rhythm

bradycardia: slower-than-normal heart rate (usually less than 60 beats/min)

cardiac output: the amount of blood the heart can pump per beat; influenced by the coordination of cardiac muscle contraction, heart rate, and blood return to the heart

Cardiac Arrhythmia Suppression Trial (CAST): a large research study run by the National Heart and Lung Institute that found that long-term treatment of arrhythmias may have a questionable effect on mortality and in some cases actually lead to increased cardiac death; basis for the current indication for antiarrhythmics (short-term use to treat life-threatening ventricular arrhythmias)

heart blocks: blocks to conduction of an impulse through the cardiac conduction system; can occur at the atrioventricular node, interrupting conduction from the atria into the ventricles, or in the bundle branches within the ventricles, preventing the normal conduction of the impulse

hemodynamics: the study of the forces moving blood throughout the cardiovascular system

premature atrial contraction (PAC): caused by an ectopic focus in the atria that stimulates an atrial response

premature ventricular contraction (PVC): caused by an ectopic focus in the ventricles that stimulates the cells and causes an early contraction

proarrhythmic: tending to cause arrhythmias; many of the drugs used to treat arrhythmias have been found to generate them

tachycardia: faster-than-normal heart rate (usually greater than 100 beats/min)

Drug List

Antiarrhythmic Agents

Class I Antiarrhythmics

Class Ia
- disopyramide
- procainamide
- quinidine

Class Ib
- (P) lidocaine
- mexiletine

Class Ic
- flecainide
- propafenone

Class II Antiarrhythmics
- acebutolol
- esmolol
- (P) propranolol

Class III Antiarrhythmics
- (P) amiodarone
- dofetilide
- ibutilide
- sotalol

Class IV Antiarrhythmics
- (P) diltiazem
- verapamil

Other Antiarrhythmics
- adenosine
- digoxin
- dronedarone

As discussed in earlier chapters, disruptions in impulse formation and in the conduction of impulses through the myocardium are called arrhythmias. (They also are called dysrhythmias by some health care providers.) Arrhythmias occur in the heart because all of the cells of the heart possess the property of automaticity (discussed later in this chapter) and therefore can generate an excitatory impulse. Disruptions in the normal rhythm of the heart can interfere with myocardial contractions and affect the **cardiac output**, the amount of blood pumped with each beat. Arrhythmias that seriously disrupt cardiac output can be fatal. Drugs used to treat arrhythmias, called antiarrhythmics, suppress automaticity or alter the conductivity of the heart.

Arrhythmias

Arrhythmias involve changes to the automaticity or conductivity of the heart cells. These changes can result from several factors, including electrolyte imbalances that alter the action potential, decreased oxygen delivery to cells that changes their action potential, structural damage that changes the conduction pathway, or acidosis or waste product accumulation that alters the action potential. In some cases, changes to the heart's automaticity or conductivity may result from drugs that alter the action potential or cardiac conduction.

Conductivity

With normal heart function, each cycle of cardiac contraction and relaxation is controlled by impulses arising spontaneously in the sinoatrial (SA) node and transmitted via a specialized conducting system to activate all parts of the heart muscle almost simultaneously (see Chapter 42) (Figure 45.1). These continuous, rhythmic contractions are controlled by the heart itself. This property allows the heart to beat as long as it has enough nutrients and oxygen to survive, regardless of the status of the rest of the body.

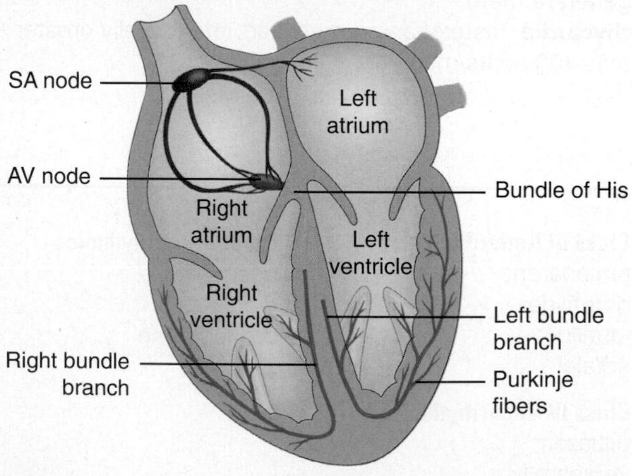

FIGURE 45.1 The conducting system of the heart. Impulses originating in the sinoatrial (SA) node are transmitted through the atrial bundles to the atrioventricular (AV) node and down the bundle of His and the bundle branches by way of the Purkinje fibers through the ventricles.

Automaticity

All cardiac cells possess some degree of automaticity (see Chapter 42) in which the cells undergo a spontaneous depolarization during diastole or rest because they decrease the flow of potassium ions out of the cell and probably leak sodium into the cell, causing an action potential.

The action potential of the cardiac muscle cell consists of five phases:

- *Phase 0* occurs when the cell reaches a point of stimulation. The sodium gates open along the cell membrane, and sodium rushes into the cell; this positive flow of electrons into the cell results in an electrical potential. This is called depolarization as the membrane no longer has a charge difference between the inside and outside of the membrane.
- *Phase 1* is a very short period during which the sodium ion concentration equalizes inside and outside the cell.
- *Phase 2*, or the plateau stage, occurs as the cell membrane becomes less permeable to sodium, calcium slowly enters the cell, and potassium begins to leave the cell. The cell membrane is trying to return to its resting state, a process called repolarization or returning of the charge differences to the membrane.
- *Phase 3* is a time of rapid repolarization as the sodium gates are closed and potassium flows out of the cell.
- *Phase 4* occurs when the cell comes to rest; the sodium–potassium pump returns the membrane to its resting membrane potential, and spontaneous depolarization begins again.

Each area of the heart has a slightly different-appearing action potential that reflects the complexity of the cells in that area. Because of these differences in the action potential, each area of the heart has a slightly different rate of rhythmicity. The SA node generates an impulse about 60 to 100 times per minute, the atrioventricular (AV) node about 40 to 50 times per minute, and the complex ventricular muscle cells about 10 to 20 times per minute.

Hemodynamics

The study of the forces that move blood throughout the cardiovascular system is called **hemodynamics**. The ability of the heart to effectively pump blood depends on the coordinated contraction of the atrial and ventricular muscles, which are stimulated to contract via the conduction system. The conduction system is designed so that atrial stimulation is followed by total atrial contraction and ventricular stimulation is followed by total ventricular contraction.

To pump effectively, these muscles need to contract together. If this orderly initiation and conduction of impulses is altered the result can be a poorly coordinated contraction of the ventricles that is unable to deliver an adequate supply of oxygenated blood to the brain and other organs, including the heart muscle. If these hemodynamic alterations are severe, serious complications can occur. For example, lack of sufficient blood flow to the brain can cause syncope or precipitate stroke; lack of sufficient blood flow to the myocardium can exacerbate atherosclerosis and cause angina or myocardial infarction (MI).

Types of Arrhythmias

Various factors can change the cardiac rate and rhythm, resulting in an arrhythmia. Arrhythmias can be caused by changes in rate (**tachycardia**, which is a faster-than-normal heart rate, or **bradycardia**, which is a slower-than-normal heart rate); by stimulation from an ectopic focus, such as **premature atrial contractions (PACs)** or **premature ventricular contractions (PVCs)**, atrial flutter, atrial fibrillation (AF) (Box 45.1), or ventricular fibrillation; or

BOX 45.1

Understanding Atrial Fibrillation

AF is a relatively common arrhythmia of the atria. It has been associated with coronary artery disease, myocardial inflammation, valvular disease, cardiomegaly, and rheumatic heart disease. The cells of the atria are connected side to side and top to bottom and are relatively simple cells. In contrast, the cells of the ventricles are connected only from top to bottom, with one cell connected only to one or two other cells. It is much easier, therefore, for an ectopic focus in the atria to spread that impulse throughout the entire atria, setting up a cycle of chaotic depolarization and repolarization. It is more difficult to stimulate fibrillation in the ventricles, because one ectopic site cannot rapidly spread impulses to many other cells, only to the cells connected in its two- or three-cell set.

Fibrillation results in lack of any coordinated pumping action, because the muscles are not stimulated to contract and pump out blood. In the ventricles, this is a life-threatening situation. If the ventricles do not pump blood, no blood is delivered to the brain, the tissues of the body, or the heart muscle itself. However, loss of pumping action in the atria per se does not usually cause much of a problem. The atrial contraction is like an extra kick of blood into the ventricles; it provides a nice backup to the system, but the blood will still flow normally without that kick.

Danger of Blood Clots

One of the problems with AF occurs when it exists for longer than 1 week. The auricles (those appendages hanging on the atria to collect blood; see Chapter 42) fill with blood that is not effectively pumped into the ventricles. Over time, this somewhat stagnant blood tends to clot. Because the auricles are sacks of striated muscle fibers, blood clots form around these fibers. In this situation, if the atria were to contract in a coordinated manner, there is a substantial risk that those clots or emboli would be pumped into the ventricles and then into the lungs (from the right auricle), which could lead to pulmonary emboli, or to the brain or periphery (from the left auricle), which could cause a stroke or occlusion of peripheral vessels.

Treatment Choices

Treatment of AF can be complicated if the length of time the patient has been in AF is not known. If a patient goes into AF acutely, drug therapy is available for rapid conversion. For example, ibutilide is often very effective when given IV for rapid conversion of the AF. IM quinidine also may convert AF effectively. In some situations, digoxin has been effective in converting AF. Electrocardioversion, a DC current shock to the chest, may break the cycle of fibrillation and convert a patient to sinus rhythm, after which the rhythm will need to be stabilized with drug therapy. Quinidine is often the drug of choice for long-term stabilization.

If the onset of AF is not known and it is suspected that the atria may have been fibrillating for longer than 1 week the patient is better off staying in AF without drug therapy or electrocardioversion. Prophylactic oral anticoagulants are given to decrease the risk of clot formation and emboli being pumped into the system. There are now several oral anticoagulants available for prophylaxis in atrial fibriallation including warfarin (*Coumadin*), dabigatran (*Pradaxa*), apixiban (*Eliquis*), rivaroxaban (*Xarelto*), and edoxaban (*Savaysa*). Each of these drugs has good points and bad points. They are discussed in Chapter 48. Conversion in this case could result in potentially life-threatening embolization of the lungs, brain, or other tissues.

Supraventricular Tachycardia: Another Danger

The other danger of AF is rapid ventricular response to the atrial stimuli, a condition called supraventricular tachycardia (SVT). With the atria firing impulses, possibly 200 to 300 a minute, the number of stimuli conducted into the ventricles is erratic and irregular. If the ventricle is responding too rapidly—more than 120 times a minute—the filling time of the ventricles is greatly reduced, causing cardiac output to fall dramatically. In these situations, and when AF is anticipated (such as with AF or paroxysmal atrial tachycardia), drugs may be given to slow conduction and protect the ventricles from rapid rates. Flecainide, propafenone, and propranolol are often used to convert rapid SVT. Esmolol, diltiazem, and verapamil are used IV to convert SVT with rapid ventricular response, which could progress to AF.

Implications for Nurses

Careful patient assessment is essential before beginning treatment for AF. If a history cannot be established from patient information and medical records are not available, it is usually recommended that AF be left untreated and anticoagulant therapy be started. This can pose a challenge for the nurse in trying to teach patients about why their rapid and irregular heart rate will not be treated and explaining all of the factors involved in the long-term use of oral anticoagulants.

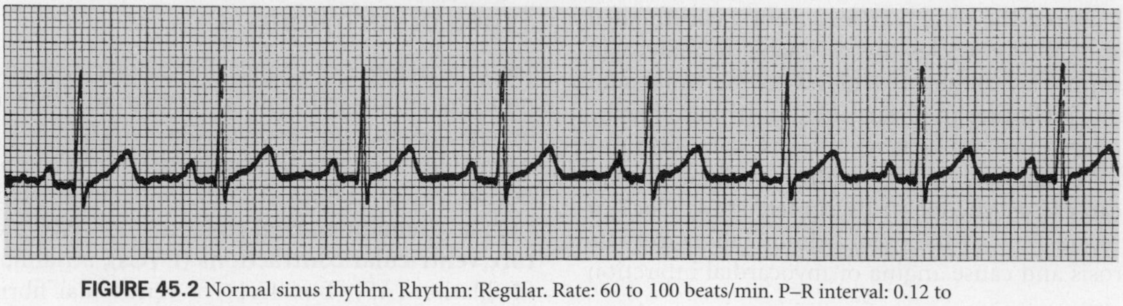

FIGURE 45.2 Normal sinus rhythm. Rhythm: Regular. Rate: 60 to 100 beats/min. P–R interval: 0.12 to 0.20 seconds. QRS: 0.06 to 0.10 seconds.

by alterations in conduction through the muscle, such as **heart blocks** and bundle branch blocks. Figure 45.2 displays an electrocardiogram (ECG) strip showing normal sinus rhythm; Figures 45.3, 45.4, and 45.5 depict various arrhythmias.

KEY POINTS

- Arrhythmias (also called dysrhythmias) are disruptions in the normal rate or rhythm of the heart.
- The cardiac conduction system determines the heart's rate and rhythm. The property by which the cardiac cells generate an action potential internally to stimulate the cardiac muscle without other stimulation is known as automaticity.
- Electrolyte disturbances, decreases in the oxygen delivered to the cells, structural damage in the conduction pathway, drug effects, acidosis, or the accumulation of waste products can trigger arrhythmias.
- Changes in the heart rate, uncoordinated heart muscle contractions, or blocks that alter the movement of impulses through the system can disrupt heart rhythm.
- Arrhythmias change the mechanics of blood circulation (hemodynamics), which can interrupt delivery of blood to the brain, other tissues, and the heart.

Antiarrhythmic Agents

Antiarrhythmics affect the action potential of the cardiac cells by altering their automaticity, conductivity, or both. Because of this effect, antiarrhythmic drugs can also produce new arrhythmias—that is, they are **proarrhythmic.** Antiarrhythmics are used in emergency situations when the hemodynamics arising from the patient's arrhythmia are severe and could potentially be fatal. Box 45.2 contains information regarding use of antiarrhythmic agents across the lifespan.

Antiarrhythmics were widely used on a long-term basis to suppress any abnormal arrhythmia, until the publication of the **Cardiac Arrhythmia Suppression Trial (CAST)** in the early 1990s. This multicenter, randomized, long-term study conducted by the National Heart, Lung, and Blood Institute looked at the mortality rate of patients

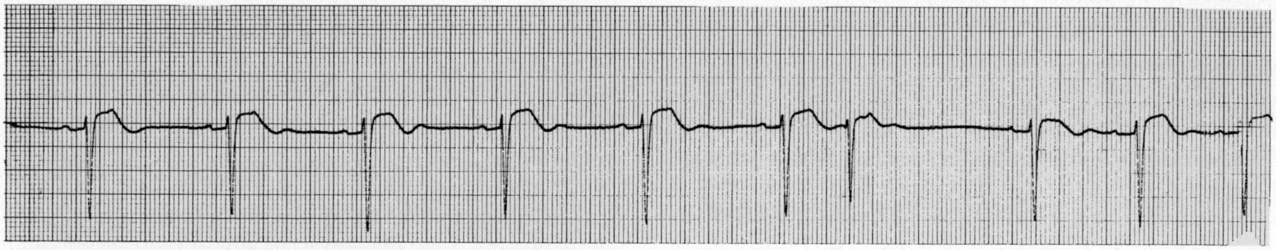

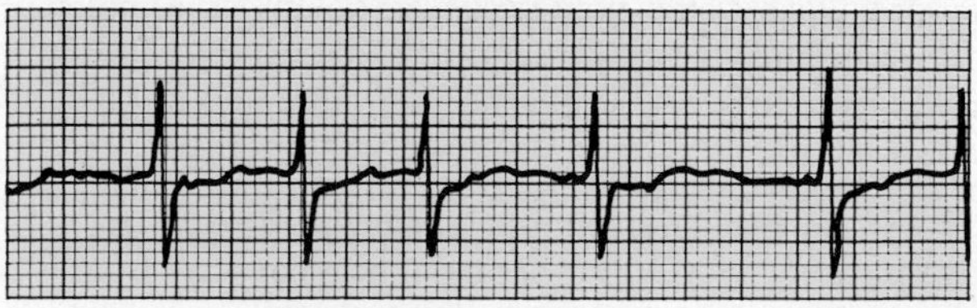

FIGURE 45.3 Atrial arrhythmias: Premature atrial contractions (PACs). Rhythm: Irregular due to the origination of a beat outside the normal conduction system (ectopic). Rate: Normal sinus rate, except for PACs. P–R interval: P wave is abnormal, and interval may be slightly shortened in ectopic beat. QRS: Normal. Atrial fibrillation. Rhythm: Irregularly irregular. Rate: Variable; usually rapid on initiation of rhythm; decreases when controlled by medication. P–R interval: No P waves are seen, replaced by an irregular wavy baseline. The atria are fibrillating because impulses are arising at a rate greater than 350 per minute. The ventricles respond when the atrioventricular (AV) node is stimulated to threshold and can receive the impulse. QRS: Normal.

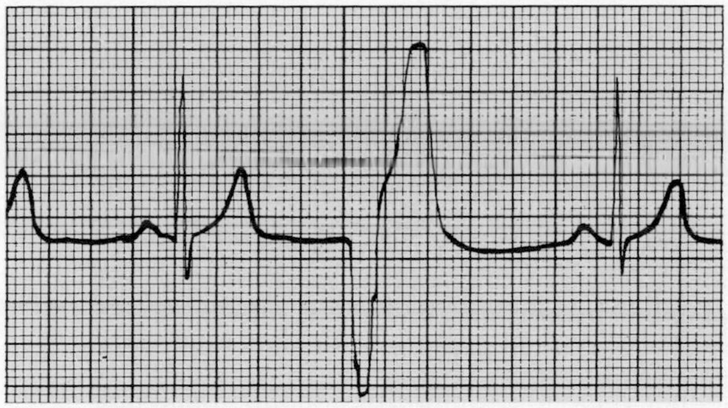

A
Premature ventricular contraction (PVC).

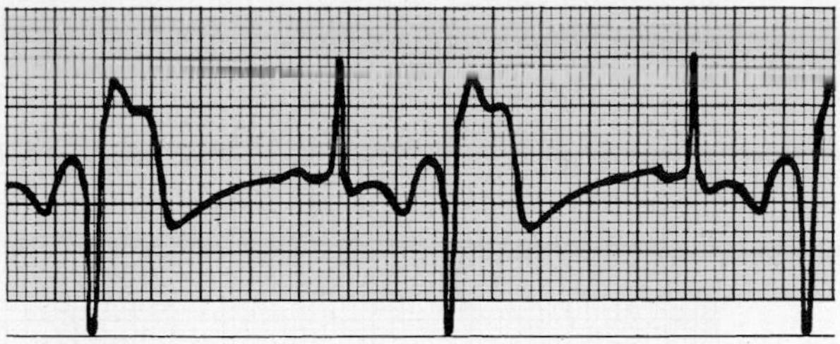

B
Ventricular bigeminy. (Every other beat is a PVC.)

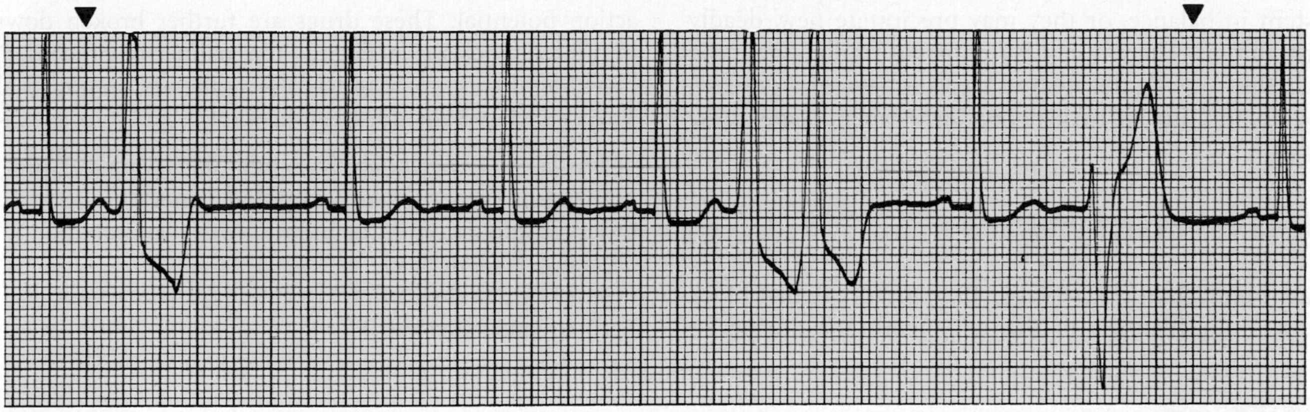

C
Multiformed PVCs.

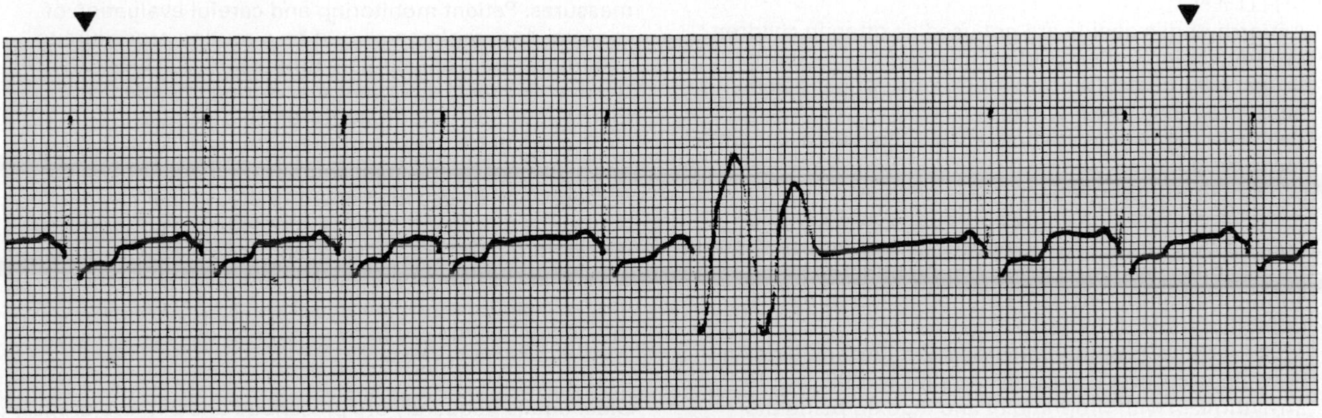

D
Heart block with PVCs.

FIGURE 45.4 Premature ventricular contractions (PVCs) or ventricular premature beats (VPBs). Rhythm: Irregular. Rate: Variable; only interrupts the cycle of the ectopic, ventricular contraction. P–R interval: Normal in sinus beats, not measurable in PVCs. QRS: Wide, bizarre, greater than 0.12 seconds.

with asymptomatic, non–life-threatening arrhythmias being treated with antiarrhythmics. The results showed that long-term use of some antiarrhythmics was associated with an increased risk of death. In fact, the risk of death for some patients was two to three times greater than that for untreated patients. These results prompted more clinical trials to look at the effectiveness of long-term use of antiarrhythmics.

It was found that antiarrhythmics may block some reflex arrhythmias that help to keep the cardiovascular

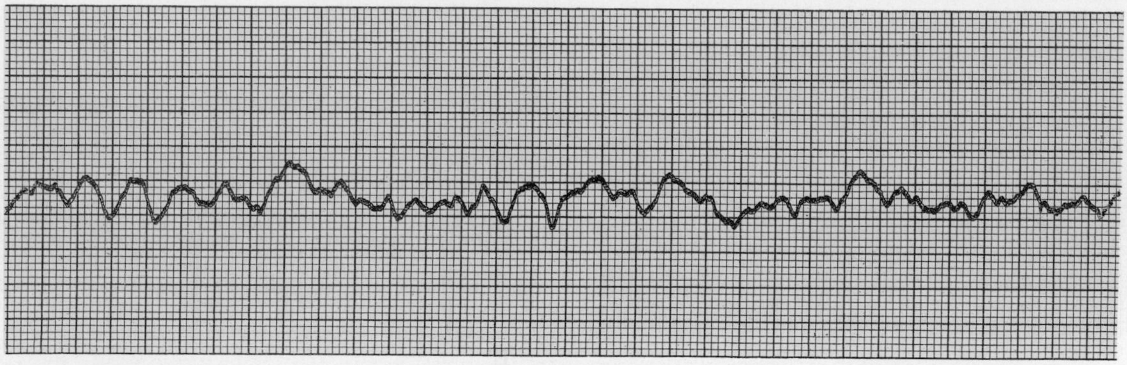

FIGURE 45.5 Ventricular fibrillation. Rhythm: Irregular. Rate: Not measurable. P–R interval: Not measurable. QRS: Not measurable, replaced by an irregular wavy baseline. No coordinated electrical or mechanical activity in the ventricle, no cardiac output.

system in balance, or they may precipitate new, deadly arrhythmias. Therefore, it is important to document the arrhythmia being treated and the rationale for treatment and to monitor a patient regularly when using these drugs.

Class I Antiarrhythmics

Class I antiarrhythmics (Table 45.1) are drugs that block the sodium channels in the cell membrane during an action potential. These drugs are further broken down into three subclasses, reflecting the manner in which their blockage of sodium channels affects the action potential. These subclasses include the following:

- Class Ia antiarrhythmics: Disopyramide (*Norpace*), procainamide (generic), and quinidine (generic)
- Class Ib antiarrhythmics: Lidocaine (*Xylocaine*) and mexiletine (generic)
- Class Ic antiarrhythmics: Flecainide (generic) and propafenone (*Rythmol*)

BOX 45.2 FOCUS ON **Drug Therapy Across the Lifespan**

Antiarrhythmic Agents

CHILDREN

Antiarrhythmic agents are not used as often in children as they are in adults. Children who do require these drugs, after cardiac surgery or because of congenital heart problems, need to be monitored very closely to deal with the related adverse effects that can occur with these drugs.

Digoxin is approved for use in children to treat arrhythmias and has an established recommended dose. If other antiarrhythmics are used the dose should be carefully calculated using weight and age and should be double-checked by another nurse before administration.

Adenosine, propranolol, procainamide, and digoxin have been successfully used to treat supraventricular arrhythmias, with propranolol and digoxin being the drugs of choice for long-term management. Verapamil should be avoided in children.

Many arrhythmias in children are now treated by ablation techniques to destroy the arrhythmia-producing cells. This has been very successful in treating Wolff–Parkinson–White and related syndromes in children. If lidocaine is used for ventricular arrhythmias related to cardiac surgery or digoxin toxicity, serum levels should be monitored regularly to determine the appropriate dose and to avoid the potential for serious proarrhythmias and other adverse effects. The child should receive continuous cardiac monitoring.

ADULTS

Adults receive these drugs most often as emergency measures. Patient monitoring and careful evaluation of the total drug regimen should be a routine procedure to ensure the most effective treatment with the least chance of adverse effects. Frequent monitoring and medical follow-up is very important for these patients.

The safety for the use of these drugs during pregnancy has not been established. They should not be used in pregnancy unless the benefit to the mother clearly outweighs the potential risk to the fetus. The drugs enter breast milk, and some have been associated with adverse effects on the neonate. Class I, III, and IV agents should not be used during lactation; if they are needed, another method of feeding the baby should be used.

OLDER ADULTS

Older adults frequently are prescribed one of these drugs. Older adults are more likely to develop adverse effects associated with the use of these drugs, including arrhythmias, hypotension, and congestive heart failure. They are also more likely to have renal and/or hepatic impairment related to underlying medical conditions, which could interfere with the metabolism and excretion of these drugs.

The dose for older adults should be started at a lower level than that recommended for other adults. The patient should be monitored very closely and the dose adjusted based on patient response. If other drugs are added to or removed from the drug regimen, appropriate dose adjustments may need to be made.

Table 45.1 *Drugs in Focus:* Antiarrhythmic Agents

Drug Name	Usual Dosage	Usual Indications
Class I Antiarrhythmics ***Class Ia***		
disopyramide (*Norpace*)	*Adult:* 400–800 mg/d PO in divided doses q6–12 h; use lower doses with older patients *Pediatric:* 6–30 mg/kg/d PO in divided doses q6 h, base dose on age	Treatment of life-threatening ventricular arrhythmias
procainamide (generic)	*Adult:* 0.5–1 g IM q4–8 h; 500–600 mg IV over 25–30 min, then 2–6 mg/min IV *Pediatric:* 20–30 mg/kg/d IM in divided doses q4–6 h; 3–6 mg/kg IV over 5 min, then 20–80 mcg/kg/min IV	Treatment of life-threatening ventricular arrhythmias; favorable drug with which to start treatment because it is available in IM, IV, and oral forms (can be switched to oral form)
quinidine (generic)	400–600 mg PO q2–3 h; 600 mg IM, then 400 mg IM q2h as needed; 330 mg IV at a rate of 1 mL/min	Treatment of atrial arrhythmias in adults
Class Ib		
lidocaine (*Xylocaine*)	*Adult:* 300 mg of 10% solution IM, 50–100-mg IV bolus at the rate of 20–50 mg/min, 1-4-mg/min IV infusion *Pediatric:* Safety and efficacy not established; 1 mg/kg IV followed by IV infusion 30 mcg/kg/min has been recommended	Treatment of life-threatening ventricular arrhythmias during MI or cardiac surgery; also used as bolus injection in emergencies when monitoring is not available to document exact arrhythmia
mexiletine (generic)	200 mg PO q8 h up to 1,200 mg/d PO may be needed	Approved only for use in life-threatening ventricular arrhythmias in adults
Class Ic		
flecainide (generic)	50–100 mg PO q12 h; reduce dose as needed with older patients or patients with renal impairment	Treatment of life-threatening ventricular arrhythmias in adults; prevention of PAT in symptomatic patients with no structural heart defect
propafenone (*Rythmol*)	150–300 mg PO based on patient response; start with lower dose and increase slowly with older patients	Treatment of life-threatening ventricular arrhythmias in adults; prevention of PAT in symptomatic patients with no structural heart defect
Class II Antiarrhythmics		
acebutolol (*Sectral*)	200–600 mg PO b.i.d., based on patient response; use lower doses with older patients; decrease dose by 50% in patients with renal or hepatic impairment	Management of premature ventricular contractions in adults; intraoperative and postoperative tachycardia; also used as an antihypertensive
esmolol (*Brevibloc*)	Loading dose of 500 mcg/kg/min IV, then 50 mcg/kg/min for 4 min, maintain with IV infusion 100 mcg/kg/min	Short-term management of SVT in adults and tachycardia that is not responding to other measures
propranolol (*Inderal*)	10–30 mg PO t.i.d. to q.i.d.; 1–3 mg IV for life-threatening arrhythmias, may repeat in 2 min, then do not repeat for 4 h	Treatment of SVT caused by digoxin or catecholamines in adults; also used as an antihypertensive, antianginal, and antimigraine headache drug
Class III Antiarrhythmics		
amiodarone (*Cordarone*)	800–1,600 mg/d PO in divided doses for 1–3 wk, then 600–800 mg/d PO for 1 mo; reduce to 400 mg/d PO if rhythm is stable, 1,000 mg IV over 24 h, then 540 mg IV at 0.5 mg/min for 18–96 h	Treatment of adults with life-threatening ventricular arrhythmias not responding to any other drug; preferred antiarrhythmic in the Advanced Cardiac Life Support protocol
dofetilide (*Tikosyn*)	125–500 mcg PO b.i.d. based on creatinine clearance	Conversion of AF/flutter to normal sinus rhythm; maintenance of normal sinus rhythm after conversion for adults
ibutilide (*Corvert*)	1 mg infused IV over 1 min, may be repeated in 10 min if needed	Conversion of recent onset AF/flutter in adults (most effective if the duration of AF/flutter is <90 d)
sotalol (*Betapace*)	80 mg/d PO, may be titrated to 240–320 mg/d PO; reduce dose in patients with renal impairment	Treatment of adults with life-threatening ventricular arrhythmias not responding to any other drug
sotalol (*Betapace AF*)	80–120 mg PO daily to b.i.d. based on patient response	Maintenance of normal sinus rhythm after conversion of atrial arrhythmias in adults

(table continues on page 776)

Table 45.1 *Drugs in Focus:* Antiarrhythmic Agents (*continued*)

Drug Name	Usual Dosage	Usual Indications
Class IV Antiarrhythmics		
diltiazem (generic)	0.25 mg/kg IV bolus, then a second bolus of 0.35 mg/kg IV if needed; maintain with continuous infusion of 5–10 mg/h for up to 24 h	IV to treat paroxysmal SVT in adults
verapamil (generic)	*Adult:* 5–10 mg IV over 2 min, may repeat with 10 mg in 30 min if needed *Pediatric:* 0.1–0.3 mg/kg IV over 2 min; do not exceed 5 mg per dose, may repeat in 30 min if needed	IV to treat paroxysmal SVT; temporarily controls the ventricular response to rapid atrial rates
Other Antiarrhythmics		
adenosine (*Adenocard*)	6 mg IV as a rapid bolus over 1–2 s, may repeat with 12-mg IV bolus after 1–2 min if needed, may be repeated a second time if needed	Treatment of SVTs, including those caused by the use of alternate conduction pathways in adults
digoxin (*Lanoxin*)	*Adult:* 0.75–1.25-mg PO loading dose, then 0.125–0.25 mg/d PO *or* 0.125–0.25-mg IV loading dose, and then 0.125–0.25 mg/d PO *Pediatric:* 10–50-mcg/kg loading dose PO *or* 8–50-mcg/kg loading dose IV, based on age, then maintenance dose of 25–35% of loading dose	Treatment of atrial flutter, AF, PAT
dronedarone (*Multaq*)	400 mg PO b.i.d. with the morning and evening meals	Treatment of paroxysmal or persistent AF or atrial flutter in patients with multiple risk factors for CAD who are currently in sinus rhythm or scheduled for conversion

MI, myocardial infarction; PAT, paroxysmal atrial tachycardia; SVT, supraventricular tachycardia; AF, atrial fibrillation; CAD, coronary artery disease.

Therapeutic Actions and Indications

The class I antiarrhythmics stabilize the cell membrane by binding to sodium channels, depressing phase 0 of the action potential, and changing the duration of the action potential (Figure 45.6). *Class Ia drugs* depress phase 0 of the action potential and prolong the duration of the action potential. *Class Ib drugs* depress phase 0 somewhat and actually shorten the duration of the action potential. *Class Ic drugs* markedly depress phase 0, with a resultant extreme slowing of conduction, but have little effect on the duration of the action potential.

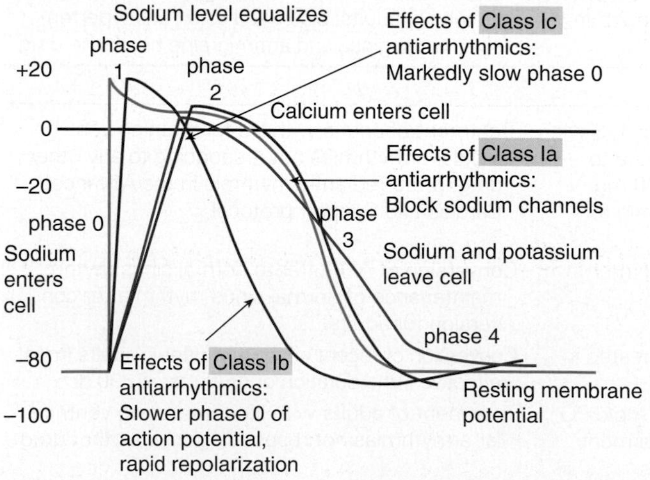

FIGURE 45.6 The cardiac action potentials, showing the effects of class Ia, Ib, and Ic antiarrhythmics.

These drugs are local anesthetics or membrane-stabilizing agents. They bind more quickly to sodium channels that are open or inactive—ones that have been stimulated and are not yet repolarized. This characteristic makes these drugs preferable in conditions such as tachycardia, in which the sodium gates are open frequently. These drugs are indicated for the treatment of potentially life-threatening ventricular arrhythmias and should not be used to treat other arrhythmias because of the risk of a proarrhythmic effect. See Table 45.1 for Usual Indications for each class I antiarrhythmic agent.

Pharmacokinetics

These drugs are widely distributed after injection or after rapid absorption through the gastrointestinal (GI) tract. They undergo extensive hepatic metabolism and are excreted in the urine. These drugs cross the placenta and are found in breast milk (see Contraindications and Cautions).

Disopyramide is available in oral form. Procainamide is available in IM and IV forms. Quinidine is also available for oral, IM, or IV administration and is administered to adults only.

Lidocaine is administered by the IM or IV route and can also be given as a bolus injection in emergencies when monitoring is not available to document the exact arrhythmia. Mexiletine is an oral drug administered to adults only.

Flecainide and propafenone are available in oral form.

Contraindications and Cautions

Class I antiarrhythmics are contraindicated in the presence of allergy to any of these drugs *to prevent hypersensitivity reactions*; with bradycardia or heart block unless an artificial pacemaker is in place *because changes in conduction could lead to complete heart block*; with heart failure (HF), hypotension, or shock, *which could be exacerbated by effects on the action potential*; and with electrolyte disturbances, *which could alter the effectiveness of these drugs*. Caution should be used in patients with renal or hepatic dysfunction, *which could interfere with the biotransformation and excretion of these drugs*.

These drugs cross the placenta, and although no specific adverse effects have been associated with their use, it is suggested that they be used in pregnancy only if the benefits to the mother clearly outweigh the potential risks to the fetus. Class I antiarrhythmics enter breast milk, and *because of the potential for adverse effects on the neonate* they should not be used during lactation. Another method of feeding the baby should be chosen.

Adverse Effects

The adverse effects of the class I antiarrhythmics are associated with their membrane-stabilizing effects and effects on action potentials. Central nervous system (CNS) effects can include dizziness, drowsiness, fatigue, twitching, mouth numbness, slurred speech, vision changes, and tremors that can progress to convulsions. GI symptoms include changes in taste, nausea, and vomiting. Cardiovascular effects include the proarrhythmic effects that lead to the development of arrhythmias (including heart blocks), hypotension, vasodilation, and the potential for cardiac arrest. Respiratory depression progressing to respiratory arrest can also occur (Figure 45.7) Other adverse effects include rash, hypersensitivity reactions, loss of hair, and potential bone marrow depression.

Moricizine, a class Ia drug, is found to increase cardiac deaths because of its proarrhythmic effects. Flecainide is a class Ic drug that was found to increase the risk of death in the CAST study.

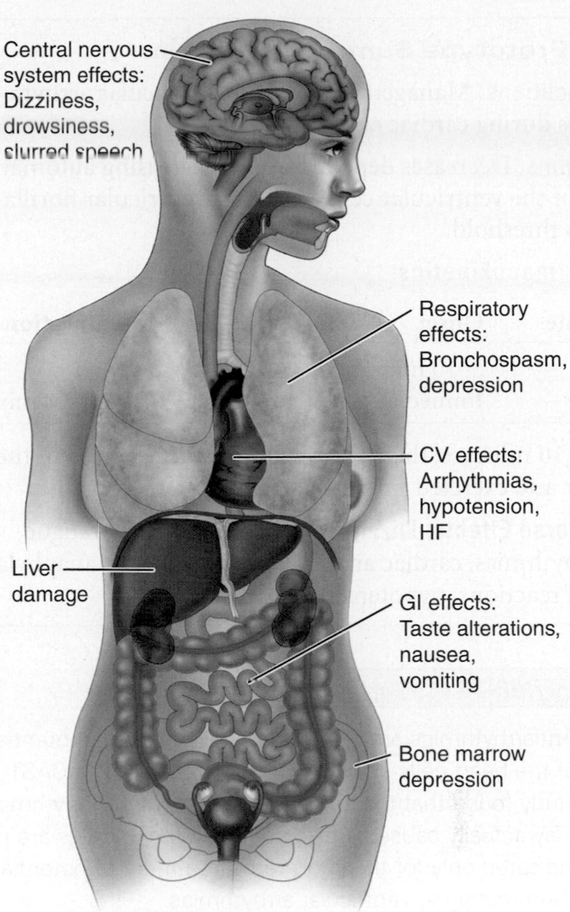

FIGURE 45.7 Variety of adverse effects and toxicities associated with antiarrhythmics.

Clinically Important Drug–Drug Interactions

Several drug–drug interactions have been reported with these agents, so the possibility of an interaction should always be considered before any drug is added to a regimen containing an antiarrhythmic. The risk for arrhythmia increases if these agents are combined with other drugs that are known to cause arrhythmias, such as digoxin and the beta-blockers.

Because quinidine competes for renal transport sites with digoxin the combination of these two drugs can lead to increased digoxin levels and digoxin toxicity. If these drugs are used in combination the patient's digoxin level should be monitored and appropriate dose adjustment made. Serum levels and toxicity of the class Ia antiarrhythmics increase if they are combined with cimetidine; extreme caution should be used if patients are receiving this combination.

The risk of bleeding effects of these drugs increases if they are combined with oral anticoagulants; patients receiving this combination should be monitored closely and have their anticoagulant dose reduced as needed. Check individual drug monographs for specific interactions associated with each drug.

Clinically Important Drug–Food Interactions

Quinidine requires a slightly acidic urine (normal state) for excretion. Patients receiving quinidine should avoid foods that alkalinize the urine (e.g., citrus juices, vegetables, antacids, milk products), which could lead to increased quinidine levels and toxicity. Grapefruit juice has been shown to interfere with the metabolism of quinidine, leading to increased serum levels and toxic effects; this combination should be avoided.

Prototype Summary: Lidocaine

Indications: Management of acute ventricular arrhythmias during cardiac surgery or MI.

Actions: Decreases depolarization, decreasing automaticity of the ventricular cells; increases ventricular fibrillation threshold.

Pharmacokinetics:

Route	Onset	Peak	Duration
IM	5–10 min	5–15 min	2 h
IV	Immediate	Immediate	10–20 min

$T_{1/2}$: 10 minutes, then 1.5 to 3 hours; metabolized in the liver and excreted in the urine.

Adverse Effects: Dizziness, light-headedness, fatigue, arrhythmias, cardiac arrest, nausea, vomiting, anaphylactoid reactions, hypotension, vasodilation.

KEY POINTS

- Antiarrhythmics are drugs that alter the action potential of the heart cells and interrupt arrhythmias. The CAST study found that the long-term treatment of arrhythmias may actually cause cardiac death, so these drugs are now indicated only for the short-term treatment of potentially life-threatening ventricular arrhythmias.
- Class I antiarrhythmics block sodium channels, depress phase 0 of the action potential, and generally prolong the action potential, leading to a slowing of conduction and automaticity.
- Class I antiarrhythmics are membrane stabilizers; the adverse effects seen are related to the stabilization of cell membranes, including those in the CNS and the GI tract.

Class II Antiarrhythmics

The class II antiarrhythmics are beta-adrenergic blockers that block beta-receptors, causing a depression of phase 4 of the action potential (Figure 45.8). Several beta-adrenergic blockers, such as acebutolol (*Sectral*), esmolol (*Brevibloc*), and propranolol (*Inderal*), are used as antiarrhythmics.

Therapeutic Actions and Indications

The class II antiarrhythmics competitively block beta-receptor sites in the heart and kidneys. The result is a decrease in heart rate, cardiac excitability, and cardiac output, a slowing of conduction through the AV node, and a decrease in the release of renin. These effects stabilize excitable cardiac tissue and decrease blood pressure, which decreases the heart's workload and may further stabilize hypoxic cardiac tissue. These drugs are indicated for the treatment of supraventricular tachycardias and PVCs. See Table 45.1 for Usual Indications for each drug.

Pharmacokinetics

Acebutolol is an oral drug. Esmolol is administered IV. Propranolol may be administered orally or IV. These drugs are absorbed from the GI tract or have an immediate effect when given IV and undergo hepatic metabolism. They are excreted in the urine. Food has been found to increase the bioavailability of propranolol, although this effect has not been found with other beta-adrenergic blocking agents.

Contraindications and Cautions

The use of these drugs is contraindicated in the presence of sinus bradycardia (rate less than 45 beats/min) and AV block, *which could be exacerbated by the effects of these drugs*; with cardiogenic shock, HF, asthma, or respiratory depression, *which could worsen due to blockage of beta-receptors*; and with pregnancy and lactation *because of the potential for adverse effects on the fetus or neonate.*

Caution should be used in patients with diabetes and thyroid dysfunction, *which could be altered by the blockade of the beta-receptors*, and in patients with renal and hepatic dysfunction, *which could alter the metabolism and excretion of these drugs.*

Adverse Effects

The adverse effects associated with class II antiarrhythmics are related to the effects of blocking beta-receptors in the sympathetic nervous system. CNS effects include dizziness, insomnia, dreams, and fatigue. Cardiovascular symptoms can include hypotension, bradycardia, AV block, arrhythmias, and alterations in peripheral perfusion. Respiratory effects can include bronchospasm and dyspnea. GI problems frequently include nausea, vomiting, anorexia, constipation, and diarrhea. Other effects to anticipate include a loss of libido, decreased exercise tolerance, and alterations in blood glucose levels.

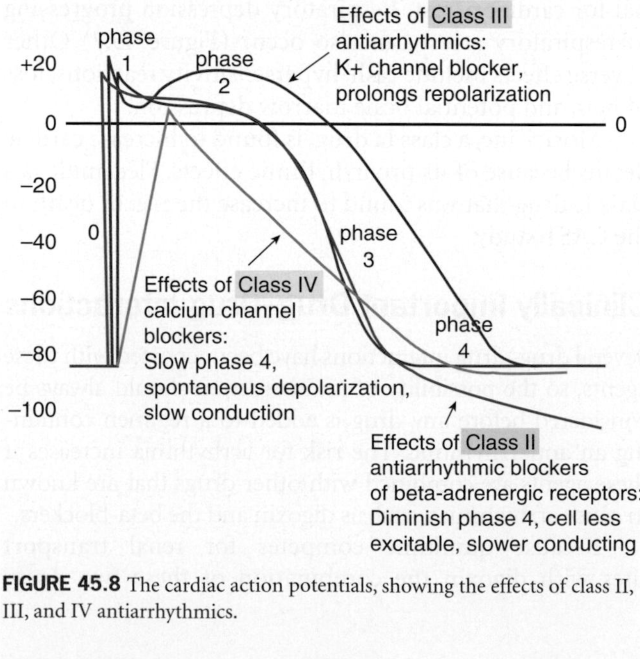

FIGURE 45.8 The cardiac action potentials, showing the effects of class II, III, and IV antiarrhythmics.

Clinically Important Drug–Drug Interactions

The risk of adverse effects increases if these drugs are taken with verapamil; if this combination is used, dose adjustment will be needed.

There is a possibility of increased hypoglycemia if these drugs are combined with insulin; patients should be monitored closely.

Other specific drug interactions may occur with each drug; check a drug reference before combining these drugs with any others.

Prototype Summary: Propranolol

Indications: Treatment of cardiac arrhythmias, especially supraventricular tachycardia; treatment of ventricular tachycardia induced by digitalis or catecholamines.

Actions: Competitively blocks beta-adrenergic receptors in the heart and kidney, has a membrane-stabilizing effect, and decreases the influence of the sympathetic nervous system.

Pharmacokinetics:

Route	Onset	Peak	Duration
Oral	20–30 min	60–90 min	6–12 h
IV	Immediate	1 min	4–6 h

$T_{1/2}$: 3 to 5 hours; metabolized in the liver and excreted in the urine.

Adverse Effects: Bradycardia, heart failure, cardiac arrhythmias, heart blocks, cerebrovascular accident, pulmonary edema, gastric pain, flatulence, nausea, vomiting, diarrhea, impotence, decreased exercise tolerance, antinuclear antibody development.

KEY POINTS

- Class II antiarrhythmics are beta-adrenergic receptor blockers that prevent sympathetic stimulation.
- Adverse effects related to class II antiarrhythmics are associated with blocking of the sympathetic response.

Class III Antiarrhythmics

The class III antiarrhythmics include amiodarone (*Cordarone*), dofetilide (*Tikosyn*), ibutilide (*Corvert*), and sotalol (*Betapace, Betapace AF*).

Therapeutic Actions and Indications

The class III antiarrhythmics block potassium channels and slow the outward movement of potassium during phase 3 of the action potential, prolonging it (Figure 45.7). All of these drugs are proarrhythmic and have the potential of inducing arrhythmias. Although amiodarone has been associated with such serious and even fatal toxic reactions, in 2005 the American Heart Association issued new guidelines for Advanced Cardiac Life Support that named amiodarone the drug of choice for treating ventricular fibrillation or pulseless ventricular tachycardia in cardiac arrest situations. See Table 45.1 for Usual Indications for each drug.

Pharmacokinetics

Amiodarone is available in an oral or IV form. Dofetilide and sotalol are administered only in oral form. Ibutilide is given IV. These drugs are well absorbed after oral administration and are immediately available after IV administration and widely distributed. Absorption of sotalol is decreased by the presence of food. They are metabolized in the liver and excreted in the urine.

Contraindications and Cautions

When these drugs are used to treat life-threatening arrhythmias for which no other drug has been effective, there are no contraindications. Ibutilide and dofetilide should not be used in the presence of AV block, *which could be exacerbated by the drug. Because sotalol is known to be proarrhythmic,* patients should be monitored very closely at the initiation of therapy and periodically during therapy. Caution should be used with all of these drugs in the presence of shock, hypotension, or respiratory depression; with a prolonged QTc (corrected) interval, *which could worsen due to the depressive effects on action potentials*; and with renal or hepatic disease, *which could alter the biotransformation and excretion of these drugs.*

Adverse Effects

The adverse effects associated with these drugs are related to the changes they cause in action potentials. Nausea, vomiting, and GI distress; weakness and dizziness; and hypotension, HF, and arrhythmia are common. Amiodarone has been associated with a potentially fatal liver toxicity, ocular abnormalities, and the development of very serious cardiac arrhythmias.

Clinically Important Drug–Drug Interactions

These drugs can cause serious toxic effects if they are combined with digoxin or quinidine. There is an increased risk of proarrhythmias if they are combined with antihistamines, phenothiazines, or tricyclic antidepressants. There is an increased risk of serious adverse effects if dofetilide is combined with ketoconazole, cimetidine, or verapamil, and so these combinations should be avoided. Sotalol may have a loss of effectiveness if it is combined with nonsteroidal anti-inflammatory drugs, aspirin, or antacids.

Other specific drug–drug interactions have been reported with individual drugs; a drug reference should always be consulted when adding a new drug to a regimen containing any of these agents.

Prototype Summary: Amiodarone

Indications: Treatment of life-threatening ventricular arrhythmias.

Actions: Acts directly on heart muscle cells to prolong repolarization and the refractory period, increasing the threshold for ventricular fibrillation; also acts on peripheral smooth muscle to decrease peripheral resistance.

Pharmacokinetics:

Route	Onset	Peak	Duration
Oral	2–3 d	3–7 h	6–8 h
IV	Immediate	20 min	Infusion

$T_{1/2}$: 10 days; metabolized in the liver and excreted in the urine.

Adverse Effects: Malaise, fatigue, dizziness, heart failure, cardiac arrhythmias, cardiac arrest, constipation, nausea, vomiting, hepatotoxicity, pulmonary toxicity, corneal microdeposits, and vision changes.

KEY POINTS

- Class III antiarrhythmics block potassium channels and prolong phase 3 of the action potential.
- Amiodarone is the drug recommended for use during life support measures. It is associated with serious to potentially fatal hepatotoxicity.

Class IV Antiarrhythmics

Class IV antiarrhythmics include two calcium-channel blockers: Diltiazem (generic) and verapamil (generic).

Therapeutic Actions and Indications

The class IV antiarrhythmics block the movement of calcium ions across the cell membrane, depressing the generation of action potentials and delaying phases 1 and 2 of repolarization, which slows automaticity and conduction (see Figure 45.7). Both diltiazem and verapamil are used as antihypertensives (see Chapter 43) and to treat angina (see Chapter 46). Table 45.1 describes Usual Indications for each drug.

Pharmacokinetics

Diltiazem is administered IV. When used as an antiarrhythmic, verapamil is used IV. These drugs are well absorbed after IV administration. They are highly protein bound, metabolized in the liver, and excreted in the urine. They cross the placenta and enter breast milk.

Contraindications and Cautions

These drugs are contraindicated with known allergy to any calcium channel blocker *to avoid hypersensitivity reactions*, with sick sinus syndrome or heart block (unless an artificial pacemaker is in place) *because the block could be exacerbated by these drugs*, with pregnancy or lactation *because of the potential for adverse effects on the fetus or neonate*, and with HF or hypotension *because of the hypotensive effects of these drugs*. Caution should be used in cases of idiopathic hypertrophic subaortic stenosis, *which could be exacerbated*, or impaired renal or liver function, *which could affect the metabolism or excretion of these drugs*.

Adverse Effects

The adverse effects associated with these drugs are related to their vasodilation of blood vessels throughout the body. CNS effects include dizziness, weakness, fatigue, depression, and headache. GI upset, nausea, and vomiting can occur. Hypotension, HF, shock, arrhythmias, and edema have also been reported.

Clinically Important Drug–Drug Interactions

Verapamil has been associated with many drug–drug interactions, including increased risk of cardiac depression with beta-blockers; additive AV slowing with digoxin; increased serum levels and toxicity of digoxin, carbamazepine, prazosin, and quinidine; increased respiratory depression with atracurium, pancuronium, and vecuronium; and decreased effects if combined with calcium products or rifampin.

There is a risk of severe cardiac effects if these drugs are given IV within 48 hours of IV beta-adrenergic drugs. The combination should be avoided.

Diltiazem can increase the serum levels and toxicity of cyclosporine if the drugs are taken concurrently.

Prototype Summary: Diltiazem

Indications: Treatment of paroxysmal supraventricular tachycardia, atrial fibrillation, and atrial flutter.

Actions: Blocks the movement of calcium ions across the cell membrane, depressing the generation of action potentials, delaying phases 1 and 2 of repolarization, and slowing conduction through the AV node.

Pharmacokinetics:

Route	Onset	Peak	Duration
Oral	30–60 min	2–3 h	6–8 h
IV	Immediate	2–3 min	Unknown

$T_{1/2}$: 3.5 to 6 hours; metabolized in the liver and excreted in the urine.

Adverse Effects: Dizziness, light-headedness, headache, asthenia, peripheral edema, bradycardia, AV block, flushing, nausea, hepatic injury.

KEY POINTS

- Class IV antiarrhythmics are calcium-channel blockers that shorten the action potential, disrupting ineffective rhythms and rates.
- Whichever type of antiarrhythmic is used the patient receiving an antiarrhythmic drug needs to be constantly monitored while being stabilized and throughout the course of therapy to detect the development of arrhythmias or other adverse effects associated with alteration of the action potentials of other muscles or nerves.

Other Antiarrhythmics

Drugs other than those classified as class I, II, III, or IV may be used to treat arrhythmias. Table 45.2 provides a summary of types of arrhythmias and the specific drugs used to treat each type. Additional antiarrhythmics include adenosine (*Adenocard*), digoxin, and dronedarone (*Multaq*).

Adenosine is another antiarrhythmic agent that is used to convert supraventricular tachycardia to sinus rhythm if vagal maneuvers have been ineffective. It is often the drug of choice for terminating supraventricular tachycardias, including those associated with the use of alternative conduction pathways around the AV node (e.g., Wolff–Parkinson–White syndrome), for two reasons: (1) It has a very short duration of action (about 15 seconds), after which it is picked up by circulating red blood cells and cleared through the liver, and (2) it is associated with very few adverse effects (headache, flushing, and dyspnea of short duration). This drug slows conduction through the AV node, prolongs the refractory period, and decreases automaticity in the AV node. It is given IV with continuous monitoring of the patient.

Digoxin (see Chapter 44) is also used at times to treat arrhythmias. This drug slows calcium leaving the cell, prolonging the action potential and slowing conduction and heart rate. Digoxin is effective in the treatment of atrial arrhythmias. The drug exerts a positive inotropic effect, leading to increased cardiac output, which increases perfusion of the coronary arteries and may eliminate the cause of some arrhythmias as hypoxia is resolved and waste products are removed more effectively.

Dronedarone has properties of all four classes of antiarrhythmics, and the mechanism by which it helps suppress atrial arrhythmias is not fully understood. It is used to reduce the risk of hospitalization in patients with paroxysmal or persistent AF of flutter who have risks factors for cardiovascular disease and who are in sinus rhythm or are scheduled to be converted to sinus rhythm. It is an oral drug that is taken twice a day. Many drug–drug interactions have been associated with the drug, and this should always be reviewed before starting or stopping any drugs while on this drug. Grapefruit juice should be avoided while taking this drug. The most common adverse effects seen with dronedarone are HF, prolonged QT interval, nausea, diarrhea, and rash. It should never be used during pregnancy because it has been associated with fetal abnormalities.

Table 45.2 Types of Arrhythmias and Drugs of Choice for Treatment

Arrhythmia	Antiarrhythmic Drugs
Atrial	
Flutter or fibrillation	Class Ia: Quinidine[a] (long term) Class III: Ibutilide[a] (conversion of recent onset), dofetilide (conversion and maintenance), sotalol (maintenance) Other: Dronedarone (maintenance)
Paroxysmal atrial tachycardia	Other: Digoxin
SVT	Class Ic: Flecainide, propafenone[a] Class II: Esmolol[a] (short term), propranolol Class IV: Diltiazem (IV), verapamil (IV) Other: Adenosine[a] (SVT, including those caused by using alternate conduction pathways)
Ventricular	
PVCs	Class Ib: Lidocaine[a] Class II: Acebutolol
Tachycardia or fibrillation Life-threatening ventricular arrhythmias	Class Ib: Lidocaine[a] Class Ia: Disopyramide, procainamide Class Ib: Mexiletine Class Ic: Flecainide[b], propafenone Class III: Amiodarone[a], sotalol[b]

[a]Drug of choice.
[b]Not drug of choice; proarrhythmic.
SVT, supraventricular tachycardia; PVC, premature ventricular contraction.

Nursing Considerations for Patients Receiving Antiarrhythmic Agents

Assessment: History and Examination

- Assess for contraindications or cautions: Any known allergies to these drugs *to avoid hypersensitivity reactions*; impaired liver or kidney function, *which could alter the metabolism and excretion of the drug*; any condition that could be exacerbated by the depressive effects of the drugs (e.g., heart block, HF, hypotension, shock, respiratory dysfunction, electrolyte disturbances) *to avoid exacerbation of these conditions*; and current status of pregnancy and lactation *to prevent potential adverse effects on the fetus or baby*.
- Perform a physical assessment *to establish a baseline before beginning therapy and during therapy to determine the effectiveness of therapy and evaluate for any potential adverse effects*.
- Assess the patient's neurological status, including level of alertness, speech and vision, and reflexes, *to identify possible CNS effects*.
- Assess cardiac status closely, including pulse, blood pressure, heart rate, and rhythm, *to identify changes requiring a change in the dosage of the drug or the presence of adverse effects*; auscultate heart sounds, noting any evidence of abnormal sounds, *for early detection of HF*; and anticipate cardiac monitoring *to evaluate heart rate and rhythm and aid in identifying arrhythmia*.
- Monitor respiratory rate and depth and auscultate lungs, for evidence of adventitious sounds *to identify respiratory depression and detect changes associated with HF*.
- Inspect abdomen *for evidence of distention*; auscultate bowel sounds *to evaluate GI motility*.
- Evaluate skin for color, lesions, and temperature *to detect adverse reactions and to assess cardiac output*.
- Obtain a baseline ECG *to evaluate heart rate and rhythm*; monitor the results of laboratory tests, including complete blood count, *to identify possible bone marrow suppression*, and renal and liver function tests *to determine the need for possible changes in dose and identify toxic effects*.

Nursing Diagnoses

Nursing diagnoses related to drug therapy might include the following:

- Decreased cardiac output related to cardiac effects
- Disturbed sensory perception (visual, auditory, kinesthetic, gustatory, tactile) related to CNS effects
- Risk for injury related to adverse drug effects
- Deficient knowledge regarding drug therapy

Planning

- The patient will receive the best therapeutic effect from the drug therapy.
- The patient will have limited adverse effects to the drug therapy.
- The patient will have an understanding of the drug therapy, adverse effects to anticipate, and measures to relieve discomfort and improve safety.

Implementation with Rationale

- Titrate the dose to the smallest amount needed to achieve control of the arrhythmia *to decrease the risk of severe adverse effects*.
- Continually monitor cardiac rhythm when initiating or changing dose *to detect potentially serious adverse effects and to evaluate drug effectiveness*.
- Ensure that emergency life support equipment is readily available *to treat severe adverse reactions that might occur*.
- Administer parenteral forms as ordered only if the oral form is not feasible; expect to switch to the oral form as soon as possible *to decrease the potential for severe adverse effects*.
- Consult with the prescriber to reduce the dose in patients with renal or hepatic dysfunction; reduced dose may be needed *to ensure therapeutic effects without increased risk of toxic effects*.
- Establish safety precautions, including side rails, lighting, and noise control, if CNS effects occur *to ensure patient safety*.
- Arrange for periodic monitoring of cardiac rhythm when the patient is receiving long-term therapy *to evaluate effects on cardiac status*.
- Provide comfort measures *to help the patient tolerate drug effects*. These include small, frequent meals to minimize nausea and vomiting; access to bathroom facilities; bowel program as needed *to deal with nausea, vomiting, and constipation*; administration of food with drug if GI upset is severe *to alleviate the discomfort*; environmental controls, such as temperature regulation, light control, and decreased noise, *to alleviate overstimulation if CNS effects occur*; and reorientation as needed.
- Offer support and encouragement *to help the patient deal with the diagnosis and the drug regimen*.
- Provide thorough patient teaching, including the name of the drug, dosage prescribed, measures to avoid adverse effects, warning signs of problems, and the need for periodic monitoring and evaluation, *to enhance patient knowledge about drug therapy and to promote compliance*.

Evaluation

- Monitor patient response to the drug (stabilization of cardiac rhythm and output).
- Monitor for adverse effects (sedation, hypotension, cardiac arrhythmias, respiratory depression, CNS effects).
- Evaluate the effectiveness of the teaching plan (patient can name drug, dosage, adverse effects to watch for, specific measures to avoid them, and the importance of continued follow-up).
- Monitor the effectiveness of comfort measures and compliance with the regimen.

See the Critical Thinking Scenario for information on managing the patient on chronic antiarrhythmic therapy.

CRITICAL THINKING SCENARIO

Managing the Patient on Chronic Antiarrhythmic Therapy

THE SITUATION

R.A., a 63-year-old man, developed AF 2 years ago, with a rapid drop in blood pressure and a rapid pulse of 160 beats/min, irregularly irregular. He was cardioverted within a few hours of onset to normal sinus rhythm with a heart rate of 74 beats/min. He was started on dofetilide (*Tikosyn*) and remained stable for more than a year. It was decided to stop the drug and monitor the patient. He did well, but on a long-awaited trip to Italy, he again developed AF, with rapid pulse and drop in blood pressure. He was treated at an Italian clinic with cardioversion and seen by his cardiologist on his return to the United States. He was again placed on *Tikosyn* to maintain his conversion to sinus rhythm. He called the clinic with complaints of palpitations and a severe headache and was told to immediately come in to be evaluated. He was found to be in sinus rhythm with PVCs. He stated that he felt that the headache was related to a cold he had been fighting, and he has been self-medicating with antihistamines.

CRITICAL THINKING

Based on your knowledge of the drug dofetilide and the symptoms reported by R.A., what do you think happened?

What actions should be taken at this time to make sure that R.A.'s heart rhythm remains stable?

What teaching points will be essential to convey to R.A. before he goes home?

What other screening should be done at this time to prevent problems in the future?

DISCUSSION

R.A. has the signs and symptoms of increased dofetilide levels—headache and ventricular arrhythmias. Initially, R.A. should be placed on a cardiac monitor, and he should be supported to ensure that the ventricular arrhythmias do not progress. His dofetilide should be stopped until the situation is stabilized. Emergency life support equipment should be readily available in case the situation deteriorates.

R.A. stabilized rapidly, and he was given IV fluids to dilute the drug effects and encourage excretion. His PVCs became less and less frequent, and he remained in normal sinus rhythm. R.A. was questioned about how and when he takes his drug and any other drugs he might be taking. He was reminded that antihistamines should be avoided while on dofetilide. Because he was self-medicating with antihistamines, it is possible that the toxicity that developed was a drug–drug interaction. He was encouraged to try increased fluid intake, use a room humidifier, and possibly use a nonsteroidal anti-inflammatory drug for pain relief to get through the cold that he was experiencing. Before leaving, he should have drug information reviewed to increase its safe use. He should take the drug twice a day and not skip any doses. If he does miss a dose, he should not catch up doses but should just resume the regular schedule. He should avoid antihistamines, as well as other antiarrhythmics, while on this drug. It is a good idea to keep a complete list of drugs being taken—including over-the-counter drugs and herbal remedies—so the health care provider can check and make sure that there is no potential reaction to be concerned about. He should also be reminded about the importance of regular medical follow-up, which will include an ECG and blood tests, to evaluate the effects of the drug on his body.

While R.A. is within the health care system, it would be a good idea to do a full ECG and to get blood tests to measure his creatinine levels, as well as serum electrolytes, which have an effect on cardiac conduction.

NURSING CARE GUIDE FOR R.A.: DOFETILIDE (ANTIARRHYTHMIC AGENTS)

Assessment: History and Examination

Assess the patient's health history for allergies to dofetilide or ibutilide; for any heart block or prolonged QT intervals; history of AF, including onset of last episode; and drug history for use of antihistamines, drugs that could prolong the QT interval, other antiarrhythmics, or tricyclic antidepressants.

Focus the physical examination on the following areas:

CV: Blood pressure, pulse, heart rhythm, perfusion

CNS: Orientation, affect, reflexes

Respiratory system: Respiratory rate and character, adventitious sounds

Laboratory tests: Renal function tests, serum electrolytes, ECG

Nursing Diagnoses

Decreased cardiac output related to cardiac effects

Disturbed sensory perception (visual, auditory, kinesthetic, gustatory, tactile) related to CNS effects

Risk for injury related to adverse drug effects

Deficient knowledge regarding drug therapy

Planning

The patient will receive the best therapeutic effect from the drug therapy.

The patient will have limited adverse effects to the drug therapy.

(continues on page 784)

Managing the Patient on Chronic Antiarrhythmic Therapy (continued)

The patient will have an understanding of the drug therapy, adverse effects to anticipate, and measures to relieve discomfort and improve safety.

Implementation

Continually monitor cardiac rhythm when initiating or changing dose.

Ensure that emergency life support equipment is readily available.

Establish safety precautions, including side rails, lighting, and noise control, if CNS effects occur.

Arrange for periodic monitoring of cardiac rhythm when the patient is receiving long-term therapy.

Provide comfort measures, including small, frequent meals to minimize nausea and vomiting; access to bathroom facilities; and environmental controls, such as temperature regulation, light control, and decreased noise.

Offer support and encouragement to help the patient deal with the diagnosis and the drug regimen.

Provide patient teaching regarding drug name, dosage, schedule of administration, measures to reduce adverse effects, other drugs to avoid, what to report, and the need for regular, periodic monitoring.

Evaluation

Monitor patient response to the drug (stabilization of cardiac rhythm and output).

Monitor for adverse effects (sedation, hypotension, cardiac arrhythmias, respiratory depression, CNS effects).

Monitor for drug–drug interactions.

Evaluate the effectiveness of the teaching plan (patient can name drug, dosage, adverse effects to watch for, specific measures to avoid them, and the importance of continued follow-up).

Monitor the effectiveness of comfort measures and compliance with the regimen.

PATIENT TEACHING FOR R.A.

- An antiarrhythmic drug, such as dofetilide, acts to stop the irregular rhythm in your heart, helping it to beat more regularly and therefore more efficiently.
- When taking dofetilide, you should remember to take it twice a day. If you miss a dose, do not make up the dose, just return to your regular schedule. Never take more than two doses in a day.
- Do not take antihistamines while you are on this drug; this combination can increase the adverse effects and can be quite serious. There are other drugs that should be avoided; make sure you give your health care provider a complete list of the drugs that you are taking, including over-the-counter drugs and herbal remedies, so the safety of any combinations can be checked.
- Some adverse effects that might occur include the following:
  - *Headache*: Medication may be available to help if this is a problem.
  - *Dizziness, light-headedness*: Avoid driving a car or operating dangerous machinery until you know how this drug will affect you.
  - *Nausea, diarrhea, flatulence*: Small, frequent meals may help to alleviate these problems.
  - Report any of the following to your health care provider: Chest pain, difficulty breathing, palpitations, numbness, or tingling.
- Tell any doctor, nurse, or other health care provider involved in your care that you are taking this drug.
- Keep this drug, and all medications, out of the reach of children.
- Schedule regular medical appointments while you are on this drug to evaluate your heart rhythm and your response to the drug and to monitor your blood levels of important electrolytes that affect heart function.
- Do not stop taking this medication. If you have to stop the medication, contact your health care provider immediately.

SUMMARY

- Disruptions in the normal rate or rhythm of the heart are called arrhythmias (also known as dysrhythmias).
- Electrolyte disturbances, decreases in the oxygen delivered to the cells leading to hypoxia or anoxia, structural damage that changes the conduction pathway, acidosis or the accumulation of waste products, or drug effects can lead to disruptions in the automaticity of the cells or in the conduction of the impulse that result in arrhythmias. The result can be changes in heart rate (tachycardias or bradycardias), stimulation from ectopic foci in the atria or ventricles that cause an uncoordinated muscle contraction, or blocks in the conduction system (e.g., AV heart block, bundle branch blocks) that alter the normal movement of the impulse through the system.
- Arrhythmias cause problems because they alter the hemodynamics of the cardiovascular system. They can cause a decrease in cardiac output related to the uncoordinated pumping action of the irregular rhythm, leading to lack of filling time for the ventricles. Any of these effects can interfere with the delivery of blood to the brain, to other tissues, or to the heart muscle.

- Antiarrhythmics are drugs that alter the action potential of the heart cells and interrupt arrhythmias. The CAST study found that the long-term treatment of arrhythmias may actually cause cardiac death, so these drugs are now indicated only for the short-term treatment of potentially life-threatening ventricular arrhythmias.
- Class I antiarrhythmics block sodium channels, depress phase 0 of the action potential, and generally prolong the action potential, leading to a slowing of conduction and automaticity.
- Class II antiarrhythmics are beta-adrenergic receptor blockers that prevent sympathetic stimulation.
- Class III antiarrhythmics block potassium channels and prolong phase 3 of the action potential.
- Class IV antiarrhythmics are calcium-channel blockers that shorten the action potential, disrupting ineffective rhythms and rates.
- A patient receiving an antiarrhythmic drug needs to be constantly monitored while being stabilized and throughout the course of therapy to detect the development of arrhythmias or other adverse effects associated with alteration of the action potentials of other muscles or nerves.

CHECK YOUR UNDERSTANDING

Answers to the questions in this chapter can be found in Answers to Check Your Understanding Questions on thePoint®.

MULTIPLE CHOICE

Select the best response to the following.

1. Cardiac contraction and relaxation are controlled by
- **a.** a specific area in the brain.
- **b.** the sympathetic nervous system.
- **c.** the autonomic nervous system.
- **d.** spontaneous impulses arising within the heart.

2. Antiarrhythmic drugs alter the action potential of the cardiac cells. Because they alter the action potential, antiarrhythmic drugs often
- **a.** cause HF.
- **b.** alter blood flow to the kidney.
- **c.** cause new arrhythmias.
- **d.** cause electrolyte disturbances.

3. Because of the results of the CAST study,
- **a.** antiarrhythmics are now more widely used.
- **b.** antiarrhythmics are used as prophylactic measures in situations that might lead to an arrhythmia.
- **c.** antiarrhythmics are no longer used in the United States.
- **d.** antiarrhythmics are reserved for use in cases of life-threatening arrhythmias.

4. Ibutilide (*Corvert*) is a class III antiarrhythmic drug that is used for
- **a.** sedation during electrocardioversion.
- **b.** conversion of recent onset AF and flutter.
- **c.** treatment of life-threatening ventricular arrhythmias.
- **d.** treatment of arrhythmias complicated by HF.

5. The drug of choice for the treatment of a supraventricular tachycardia associated with Wolff–Parkinson–White syndrome is
- **a.** digoxin.
- **b.** verapamil.
- **c.** lidocaine.
- **d.** adenosine.

6. A patient who is receiving an antiarrhythmic drug needs
- **a.** constant cardiac monitoring until stabilized.
- **b.** frequent blood tests, including drug levels.
- **c.** an antidepressant to deal with psychological depression.
- **d.** dietary changes to prevent irritation of the heart muscle.

7. A patient is brought into the emergency room with a potentially life-threatening ventricular arrhythmia. Immediate treatment might include
- **a.** a loading dose of digoxin.
- **b.** injection of quinidine.
- **c.** bolus and titrated doses of lidocaine.
- **d.** loading dose of propafenone.

8. A client stabilized on quinidine for the regulation of AF would be cautioned to avoid which of the following?
- **a.** Potassium-rich foods
- **b.** Foods containing tyrosine
- **c.** High-sodium-containing foods
- **d.** Foods that alkalinize the urine

MULTIPLE RESPONSE

Select all that apply.

1. The conduction system of the heart includes which of the following?
  a. The SA node
  b. The sinuses of Valsalva
  c. The atrial bundles
  d. The Purkinje fibers
  e. The coronary sinus
  f. The bundle of His

2. Arrhythmias or dysrhythmias can be caused by which of the following?
  a. Lack of oxygen to the heart muscle cells
  b. Acidosis near a cell
  c. Structural damage in the conduction pathway through the heart
  d. Vasodilation in the myocardial vascular bed
  e. Thyroid hormone imbalance
  f. Electrolyte imbalances

BIBLIOGRAPHY AND REFERENCES

Abhishek, M., Mansour, M., McManus, D., et al. (2014). Novel therapeutic targets in the management of atrial fibrillation. *American Journal of Cardiovascular Drugs, 14*(6), 403–421.

Bonow, R. O., Mann, D. L., Libby, P., et al. (2014). *Braunwald's heart disease: A textbook of cardiovascular medicine* (10th ed.). Philadelphia, PA: W. B. Saunders.

Brunton, L., Chabner, B., & Knollman, B. (2011). *Goodman and Gilman's the pharmacological basis of therapeutics* (12th ed.). New York: McGraw-Hill.

Epstein, A. E., Hallstrom, A. P., Rogers, W. J., et al. (1993). Mortality following ventricular arrhythmia suppression by encainide, flecainide, and moricizine after myocardial infarction. The original design concept of the Cardiac Arrhythmia Suppression Trial (CAST). *Journal of the American Medical Association, 270*, 2451–2455.

Facts and Comparisons. (2015). *Drug facts and comparisons*. St. Louis, MO: Author.

Fuster, V., Alexander, R. W., & Rourke, R. A. (Eds.). (2011). *Hurst's the heart* (13th ed.). New York: McGraw-Hill.

Gross, A., & Stern, T. (2013). Cognitive impact of atrial fibrillation. *Primary Care Companion for CNS Disorders, 15*(1), PCC.12f01471.

Hazinski, M., Nadkarni, V., Hickey, R. et al. (2005). Major changes in the 2005 AHA Guidelines for CPR and ECC. *Circulation*, 112, IV-206-IV-211.

Karch, A. M. (2014). *Lippincott's nursing drug guide*. Philadelphia, PA: Lippincott Williams & Wilkins.

McCabe, P. (2010). Psychological distress in patients diagnosed with atrial fibrillation: The state of the science. *Journal of Cardiovascular Nursing, 25*(1), 40–51.

Porth, C. M. (2013). *Pathophysiology: Concepts of altered health states* (9th ed.). Philadelphia, PA: Lippincott Williams & Wilkins.

Schnabel, R., Aspelund, T., Li, G., et al. (2010). Validation of atrial fibrillation risk algorithm in Whites and African Americans. *Archives of Internal Medicine, 170*, 1909–1917.

The Medical Letter. (2015). *The medical letter on drugs and therapeutics*. New Rochelle, NY: Author.

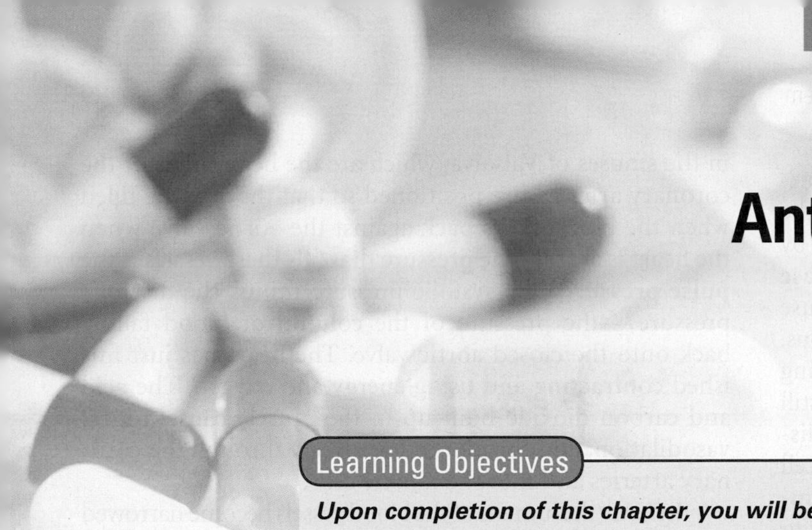

Antianginal Agents 46

Learning Objectives

Upon completion of this chapter, you will be able to:

1. Describe coronary artery disease, including identified risk factors and clinical presentation.
2. Describe the therapeutic actions, indications, pharmacokinetics, contraindications and cautions, most common adverse reactions, and important drug–drug interactions associated with the nitrates, beta-blockers, and calcium channel blockers used to treat angina.
3. Discuss the use of antianginal agents across the lifespan.
4. Compare and contrast the prototype drugs nitroglycerin, metoprolol, and diltiazem with other agents used to treat angina.
5. Outline the nursing considerations, including important teaching points, for patients receiving drugs used to treat angina.

Glossary of Key Terms

angina pectoris: "suffocation of the chest"; pain caused by the imbalance between oxygen being supplied to the heart muscle and demand for oxygen by the heart muscle

atheroma: plaque in the endothelial lining of arteries; contains fats, blood cells, lipids, inflammatory agents, and platelets; leads to narrowing of the lumen of the artery, stiffening of the artery, and loss of distensibility and responsiveness

atherosclerosis: narrowing of the arteries caused by buildup of atheromas, swelling, and accumulation of platelets; leads to a loss of elasticity and responsiveness to normal stimuli

coronary artery disease (CAD): characterized by progressive narrowing of coronary arteries, leading to a decreased delivery of oxygen to cardiac muscle cells; leading killer of adults in the Western world

myocardial infarction: end result of vessel blockage in the heart; leads to ischemia and then necrosis of the area cut off from the blood supply; it can heal, with the dead cells replaced by scar tissue

nitrates: drugs used to cause direct relaxation of smooth muscle, leading to vasodilation and decreased venous return to the heart with decreased resistance to blood flow; this rapidly decreases oxygen demand in the heart and can restore the balance between blood delivered and blood needed in the heart muscle of patients with angina

Prinzmetal angina: drop in blood flow through the coronary arteries caused by a vasospasm in the artery, not by atherosclerosis

pulse pressure: the systolic blood pressure minus the diastolic blood pressure; reflects the filling pressure of the coronary arteries

stable angina: pain due to the imbalance of myocardial oxygen supply and demand; the pain is relieved by rest or stoppage of activity

unstable angina: episode of myocardial ischemia with pain due to the imbalance of myocardial oxygen supply and demand when the person is at rest

Drug List

Antianginal Agents
Nitrates
amyl nitrate
isosorbide dinitrate
isosorbide mononitrate
Ⓟ nitroglycerin

Beta-Blockers
atenolol
Ⓟ metoprolol
nadolol
propranolol

Calcium-Channel Blockers
amlodipine
Ⓟ diltiazem
nicardipine
nifedipine
verapamil

Piperazine acetamide
ranolazine

Antianginal agents are used to help restore the appropriate supply-and-demand ratio in oxygen delivery to the myocardium. An imbalance in this ratio, manifested by pain, is most commonly due to **coronary artery disease (CAD)**. CAD has, for many years, been the leading cause of death in the United States and most Western nations. Despite great strides in understanding the contributing causes of this disease and ways to prevent it, CAD still claims more lives than any other disease. The drugs discussed in this chapter are used to prevent myocardial cell death when the coronary vessels are already seriously damaged and are having trouble maintaining the blood flow to the heart muscle. Chapters 47 and 48 discuss drugs that are used to prevent the blocking of the coronary arteries before they become narrowed and damaged or to restore blood flow through narrowed vessels.

Coronary Artery Disease

The myocardium must receive a constant supply of blood to have the oxygen and nutrients needed to maintain a constant pumping action. The myocardium receives all of its blood from two coronary arteries that exit the sinuses of Valsalva at the base of the aorta. These vessels divide and subdivide to form the capillaries that deliver oxygen to heart muscle fibers.

Unlike other tissues in the body the heart muscle receives its blood supply during diastole, while it is at rest. This is important because when the heart muscle contracts, it becomes tight and clamps the blood vessels closed, rendering them unable to receive blood during systole, which is when all other tissues receive fresh blood. The openings in the sinuses of Valsalva, which are the beginnings of the coronary arteries, are positioned so that they can be filled when the blood flows back against the aortic valve when the heart is at rest. The pressure that fills these vessels is the **pulse pressure** (the systolic pressure minus the diastolic pressure)—the pressure of the column of blood falling back onto the closed aortic valve. The heart has just finished contracting and using energy and oxygen. The acid and carbon dioxide built up in the muscle cause a local vasodilation, and the blood flows freely through the coronary arteries and into the muscle cells.

In CAD the lumens of the blood vessels become narrowed so that blood is no longer able to flow freely to the muscle cells. The narrowing of the vessels is caused by the development of **atheromas**, or fatty tumors in the intima of the vessels, in a process called **atherosclerosis** (Figure 46.1A). These deposits cause damage to the intimal lining of the vessels, attracting platelets and immune factors and causing swelling and the development of a larger deposit. Over time, these deposits severely decrease the size of the vessel. While the vessel is being narrowed by the deposits in the intima, it is also losing its natural elasticity and becoming unable to respond to the normal stimuli to dilate or constrict to meet the needs of the tissues.

The person with atherosclerosis has a classic supply-and-demand problem. The heart may function without problem until increases in activity or other stresses place a demand on it to beat faster or harder. Normally, the heart would stimulate the vessels to deliver more blood when this occurs, but the narrowed vessels are not able to respond and cannot supply the blood needed by the working heart (Figure 46.1B). The heart muscle then becomes hypoxic. This imbalance between oxygen supply and demand is manifested as pain, or **angina pectoris**, which literally means "suffocation of the chest."

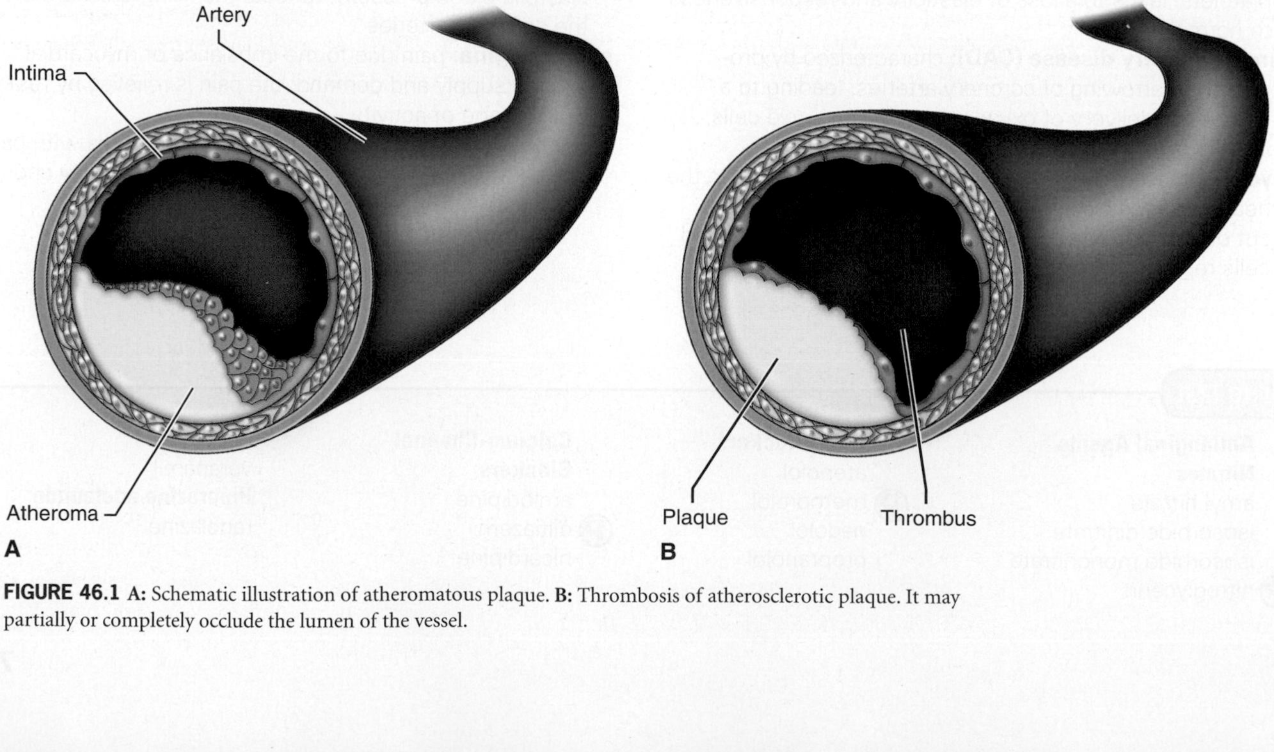

FIGURE 46.1 **A:** Schematic illustration of atheromatous plaque. **B:** Thrombosis of atherosclerotic plaque. It may partially or completely occlude the lumen of the vessel.

Angina

The body's response to a lack of oxygen in the heart muscle is pain, called angina. Although the heart muscle does not have any pain fibers a substance called substance P is released from ischemic myocardial cells, and pain is felt wherever substance P reacts with a pain receptor. For many people this is the chest, and for others it is the left arm; still others have pain in the jaw and teeth. The basic response to this type of pain is to stop whatever one is doing and to wait for the pain to go away. In cases of minor limitations to the blood flow through vessels, stopping activity may bring the supply and demand for blood back into balance. This condition is called **stable angina**. There is no damage to heart muscle, and the basic reflexes surrounding the pain restore blood flow to the heart muscle. This process can go on for a long time with no resultant myocardial infarction (MI). This is called chronic angina, and this condition can severely limit a person's activities and quality of life.

If the narrowing of the coronary arteries becomes more pronounced the heart may experience episodes of ischemia even when the patient is at rest. This condition is called **unstable angina** or preinfarction angina. Although no damage to heart muscle occurs the person is at increased risk of a complete blockage of blood supply to the heart muscle if the heart needs to work harder or the oxygen demand increases.

Prinzmetal angina is an unusual form of angina because it seems to be caused by spasm of the blood vessels and not just by vessel narrowing. The person with this type of angina has angina at rest, often at the same time each day, and usually with an associated electrocardiogram (ECG) pattern change.

Acute Myocardial Infarction

If a coronary vessel becomes completely occluded and is unable to deliver blood to the cardiac muscle the area of muscle that depends on that vessel for oxygen becomes ischemic and then necrotic. This is called a **myocardial infarction**. The pain associated with this event can be excruciating. Nausea and a severe sympathetic stress reaction may also be present. A serious danger of an MI is that arrhythmias can develop in nearby tissue that is ischemic and very irritable. Most of the deaths caused by MI occur as a result of fatal arrhythmias. If the heart muscle has a chance to heal, within 6 to 10 weeks, scar tissue will form in the necrotic area and the muscle will compensate for the injury. If the area of the muscle that is damaged is very large, however, the muscle may not be able to compensate for the loss, and heart failure (HF) and even cardiogenic shock may occur. These conditions can be fatal or can leave a person severely limited by the weakened heart muscle.

KEY POINTS

- CAD involves changes in the coronary vessels that promote atheromas (tumors), which narrow the coronary arteries and decrease their elasticity and responsiveness to normal stimuli.
- Angina pectoris occurs when the narrowed vessels cannot accommodate the myocardial demand for oxygen.
- Stable angina occurs when the heart muscle is perfused adequately except during exertion or increased demand. Unstable or preinfarction angina occurs when the vessels are so narrow that the myocardial cells are deprived of sufficient oxygen even at rest. Prinzmetal angina is a spasm of a coronary vessel that decreases the flow of blood through the narrowed lumen.
- When a coronary vessel is completely occluded the cells that depend on that vessel for oxygen become ischemic, then necrotic, and die. The result is known as an MI.

Antianginal Agents

Antianginal drugs (Table 46.1) are used to help restore the appropriate supply-and-demand ratio in oxygen delivery to the myocardium when rest is not enough. These drugs can work to improve blood delivery to the heart muscle in one of two ways: (1) By dilating blood vessels (i.e., increasing the supply of oxygen) or (2) by decreasing the work of the heart (i.e., decreasing the demand for oxygen). The demand for oxygen by the heart muscle is influenced by heart rate (a faster heart rate requires more energy), the preload (the more blood returned to the heart the more pumping will be done to empty it, which requires more energy), the afterload (the more pressure the heart has to pump against the more energy is required), and stretch on the ventricle (the further apart the actin and myosin fibers the more energy is used as they react and slide or contract). Nitrates, beta-adrenergic blockers, and calcium-channel blockers are used to treat angina (Figure 46.2). A newer class of drugs, the piperazine acetamides, is now available to treat chronic angina. The mechanism of action of this type of drug is not understood, but it decreases myocardial workload without decreasing heart rate or blood pressure.

All antianginal agents are effective and may be used in combination to achieve good pain control. The type of drug that is best for a patient is determined by tolerance of adverse effects and response to the drug. The use of antianginal agents with different age groups is discussed in Box 46.1.

Nitrates

Nitrates are drugs that act directly on smooth muscle to cause relaxation and to depress muscle tone. Because the action is direct, these drugs do not influence any nerve or other activity, and the response is usually quite fast. Nitrates include amyl nitrate (generic), isosorbide dinitrate (*Isordil*), isosorbide mononitrate (*Monoket*), and nitroglycerin (*Nitro-Bid*, *Nitrostat*, and others).

Table 46.1 *Drugs in Focus:* Antianginal Agents

Drug Name	Usual Dosage	Usual Indications
Nitrates		
amyl nitrate (generic)	0.3 mL by inhalation of vapor, may be repeated in 3–5 min	Relief of acute anginal pain in adults
isosorbide dinitrate (*Isordil*)	2.5–5 mg SL; 5-mg chewable tablet; 5–20 mg PO; maintenance 10–40 mg PO q6 h or 40–80 mg PO SR q8–12 h *Acute prophylaxis:* 5–10 mg SL or chewable tablets q2–3 h	Taken before chest pain begins in situations in which exertion or stress can be anticipated for prevention of angina in adults; taken daily for management of chronic angina
isosorbide mononitrate (*Monoket*)	2.5–5 mg SL; 5-mg chewable tablet; 5–20 mg PO; maintenance 10–40 mg PO q6 h or 40–80 mg PO SR q8–12 h *Acute prophylaxis:* 5–10 mg SL or chewable tablets q2–3 h	Taken before chest pain begins in situations in which exertion or stress can be anticipated for prevention of angina in adults; taken daily for management of angina
nitroglycerin (*Nitro-Bid*, *Nitrostat*, and others)	5 mcg/min via IV infusion pump every 3–5 min; one tablet SL every 5 min for acute attack, up to three tablets in 15 min; 0.4-mg metered dose translingual, up to three doses in 15 min for acute attacks *Prevention:* One tablet (0.3–0.6 mg) sublingually 5–10 min before activities that might precipitate an attack: 2.5–9 mg PO of SR tablet q8–12h; doses as high as 26 mg PO q.i.d. have been used; 0.5 in. q8 h for topical application, up to 4–5 in. (1 in. = 15 mg) have been used; one pad (60–75 mg) has been used; one pad transdermal system per day; 1 mg q3–5 h while awake for transmucosal system	Nitrate of choice for treatment of acute angina attack; prevention of anginal attacks
Beta-Blockers		
metoprolol (*Toprol XL*)	100 mg/d PO as single dose, ER tablet; 100–400 mg/d PO in two divided doses regular release	Treatment of angina in adults; prevention of reinfarction within 3–10 d after MI
nadolol (*Corgard*)	40–80 mg/d PO	Long-term management of angina in adults
propranolol (*Inderal*)	10–20 mg PO t.i.d. to q.i.d., titrate based on patient response; 160 mg/d is often needed for maintenance	Long-term management of angina and prevention of reinfarction in patients 1–4 wk after MI in adults
Calcium-Channel Blockers		
amlodipine (*Norvasc*)	5 mg/d PO; reduce dose with hepatic impairment or in geriatric patients	Treatment of chronic, stable angina and of Prinzmetal angina in adults
diltiazem (*Cardizem*, *Cardizem LA*)	180–360 mg/d PO in three or four divided doses; 120–180 mg PO b.i.d. SR	Treatment of angina in adults
nicardipine (*Cardene*)	20–40 mg PO t.i.d.; use immediate release only	Treatment of angina in adults
nifedipine (*Adalat CC*, *Procardia*)	10–20 mg PO t.i.d.	Treatment of angina in adults
verapamil (*Calan*)	320–480 mg/d PO	Treatment of angina in adults; treatment of tachyarrhythmias
Piperazine Acetamide		
ranolazine (*Ranexa*)	500 mg PO b.i.d., to a maximum 1,000 mg PO b.i.d.	Treatment of chronic angina in adults, as primary therapy or in combination with nitrates, amlodipine, or beta-blockers

SL, sublingual; SR, standard release; ER, extended release; MI, myocardial infarction.

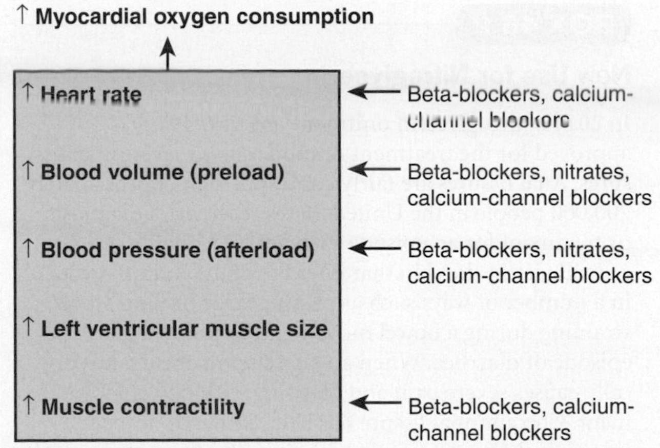

FIGURE 46.2 Interaction of antianginal agents with factors affecting myocardial oxygen demand.

Therapeutic Actions and Indications

The nitrates relax and dilate veins, arteries, and capillaries, allowing increased blood flow through the vessels and lowering systemic blood pressure because of a drop in resistance. Because CAD causes a stiffening and lack of responsiveness in the coronary arteries the nitrates probably have very little effect on increasing blood flow through these arteries. However, they do increase blood flow through healthy coronary arteries. Therefore, the blood supply through any healthy vessels in the heart increases, possibly helping the heart to compensate somewhat.

The main effect of nitrates, however, seems to be related to the drop in blood pressure that occurs. The vasodilation causes blood to pool in veins and capillaries, decreasing preload, while the relaxation of the vessels decreases afterload. The combination of these effects greatly reduces the cardiac workload and the demand for oxygen, thus bringing the supply-and-demand ratio back into balance. Nitrates are indicated for the prevention and treatment of attacks of angina pectoris. See Table 46.1 for Usual Indications for each of these drugs.

Pharmacokinetics

Nitroglycerin is available as a sublingual tablet, a translingual spray, an IV solution (for bolus injection or infusion), a transdermal patch, a topical ointment or paste, or a transmucosal agent. It can be carried with the patient, who then can use it when the need arises. Slow-release forms also are available for use in preventing anginal attacks (Box 46.2).

Amyl nitrate is supplied as a capsule that is broken and waved under the patient's nose for inhalation. The

BOX 46.1 FOCUS ON Drug Therapy Across the Lifespan

Antianginal Agents

CHILDREN

The antianginals are not indicated for any condition commonly found in children. In some situations, particularly congenital heart defects or cardiac surgery, nitroglycerin may be used. The dose of the drug should be determined by considering age and weight. The child should be very carefully monitored for adverse reactions, including potentially dangerous changes in blood pressure.

ADULTS

Adults who receive these drugs should be instructed in their proper administration, particularly if varying forms of nitroglycerin are used. Patients should also be encouraged to determine what activities or situations tend to precipitate an anginal attack so that they can take measures to avoid those circumstances or take an antianginal agent before the event occurs.

With nitroglycerin use, it is important that the patient knows how to use the drug, how to store the drug, how to determine whether it is still effective, and how much to take before seeking emergency medical care.

Patients should know that regular medical follow-up is important and should be instructed in nonpharmacological measures—weight loss, smoking cessation, activity changes, diet changes—that could decrease their risk of CAD and improve the effectiveness of the antianginal therapy.

The safety for the use of these drugs during pregnancy has not been established. There is a significant potential for adverse effects on the fetus related to blood flow changes and direct drug effects when the drugs cross the placenta. The drugs do enter breast milk, and it is advised that another method of feeding the baby be used if one of these drugs is prescribed during lactation.

OLDER ADULTS

Older adults frequently are prescribed one of these drugs. Older adults are more likely to develop adverse effects associated with the use of these drugs—arrhythmias, hypotension, and heart disease. Safety measures may be needed if these effects occur and interfere with the patient's mobility and balance.

Older adults are also more likely to have renal and/or hepatic impairment related to underlying medical conditions, which could interfere with the metabolism and excretion of these drugs. The dose for older adults should be started at a lower level than that recommended for younger adults. The patient should be monitored very closely and dose adjusted based on patient response.

If other drugs are added to or removed from the drug regimen, appropriate dose adjustments may need to be made. If the patient is using a different form of nitroglycerin, special care should be taken to make sure that the proper administration, storage, and timing of use are understood.

FOCUS ON Safe Medication Administration

Sublingual, Transbuccal, and Transdermal Administration of Nitroglycerin

Sublingual administration. *Patients often prefer this route of administration, opting to administer the drug themselves even in the institutional setting. Make sure that the drug is given correctly:*

- *Check under the tongue to make sure there are no lesions or abrasions that could interfere with the absorption of the drug. Have the patient take a sip of water to moisten the mucous membranes so the tablet will dissolve quickly. Then instruct the patient to place the tablet under the tongue, close the mouth, and wait until the tablet has dissolved.*
- *Caution the patient not to swallow the tablet; its effectiveness would be lost if the tablet entered the stomach. If the patient uses translingual drugs often, encourage the patient to alternate sides of the tongue—placing it under the left side for one dose and under the right side for the other dose.*
- *Here's a tip to help in administering sublingual medications to patients who cannot do it themselves or who cannot open their mouths: Use a tongue depressor to move the tongue aside and place the tablet, or slide the tablet down through a straw to the underside of the tongue.*

Transbuccal administration. *Make sure that the tablet the patient is going to use is designed for buccal administration:*

- *Check the inside of the cheeks to be sure there are no ulcerations or abrasions that could interfere with the absorption of the drug. Have the patient place the tablet between his or her gums and cheek pocket and then hold it in place until the tablet dissolves.*
- *Again, caution the patient not to swallow the tablet, and instruct the patient to rotate the site of placement from side to side with each dose.*

Transdermal administration. *Errors have been reported with inappropriate use of nitroglycerin patches and nitroglycerin paste. Make sure to discuss safe administration with the patient:*

- *It is very important, even if it seems like common sense, to teach patients to remove the old transdermal system and to wash the area before placing a new system to prevent adverse effects such as severe hypotension.*
- *Urge patients who are given tubes of nitroglycerin paste to label tubes clearly in large letters and to store them safely away from other people in a secure place. This prevents accidental misuse of nitroglycerin paste for hand cream, which can result in a toxic dose of the drug.*

administration is somewhat awkward for the patient to use by himself or herself. It usually requires another person to administer it properly. It is not used very often because this drug has been abused and sold on the streets as "poppers". It was once available over the counter but is now available only by prescription. Isosorbide dinitrate and isosorbide mononitrate are available in oral form.

BOX 46.2

New Use for Nitroglycerin

In 2011 a nitroglycerin ointment, *Rectiv* 0.4%, was approved for the treatment of moderate to severe anal fissures. Anal fissures are fairly common, with approximately 700,000 people in the United States receiving a diagnosis or treatment for an episode each year. An anal fissure is a small tear in the skin that lines the anus, and can occur in a number of ways such as passing large or hard stools, straining during a bowel movement, or following an episode of diarrhea. When an anal fissure occurs, it typically causes severe pain and bleeding with bowel movement. Chronic anal fissure has been shown to impact significantly on a patient's quality of life. An episode can take 6 to 8 weeks to heal; and if healing does not occur, then surgery may be required. This ointment is applied to the mucosa of the anus every 12 hours for up to 3 weeks. It causes vasodilation and relaxation of smooth muscle, which will decrease sphincter tone and pressure. Patients must be cautioned that this product is not for relief of angina pain and is only for intraanal use.

Nitrates are very rapidly absorbed, metabolized in the liver and excreted in the urine. They cross the placenta and enter breast milk. Nitroglycerin is available in many forms, and absorption, onset of action, and duration vary with the form used (see Prototype Summary). Amyl nitrate, upon inhalation, has an onset of action of about 30 seconds. Isosorbide dinitrate and isosorbide mononitrate, when given orally, have onset of action in 14 to 45 minutes, or up to 4 hours if the sustained release (SR) form is used. The drug may have a duration of action of 4 to 6 hours, or 6 to 8 hours if the SR form is used.

Contraindications and Cautions

Nitrates are contraindicated in the presence of any allergy to nitrates *to prevent hypersensitivity reactions.* These drugs also are contraindicated in the following conditions: Severe anemia *because the decrease in cardiac output could be detrimental in a patient who already has a decreased ability to deliver oxygen because of a low red blood cell count*; head trauma or cerebral hemorrhage *because the relaxation of cerebral vessels could cause intracranial bleeding*; and pregnancy or lactation *because of potential adverse effects on the neonate and ineffective blood flow to the fetus.*

Caution should be used in patients with hepatic or renal disease, *which could alter the metabolism and excretion of these drugs.* Caution also is required for patients with hypotension, hypovolemia, and conditions that limit cardiac output (e.g., tamponade, low ventricular filling pressure, low pulmonary capillary wedge pressure) *because these conditions could be exacerbated, resulting in serious adverse effects.*

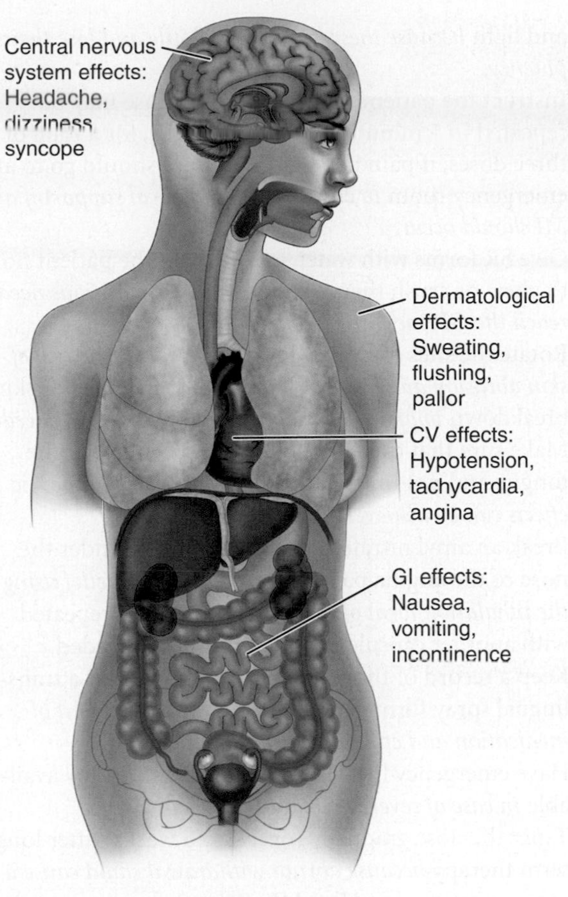

FIGURE 46.3 Variety of adverse effects and toxicities associated with antianginals.

Adverse Effects

The adverse effects associated with these drugs are related to vasodilation and the decrease in blood flow that occurs. Central nervous system (CNS) effects include headache, dizziness, and weakness. Gastrointestinal (GI) symptoms can include nausea, vomiting, and incontinence. Cardiovascular (CV) problems include hypotension, which can be severe and must be monitored; reflex tachycardia that occurs when blood pressure falls; syncope; and angina, which could be exacerbated by the hypotension and changes in cardiac output (Figure 46.3). Skin-related effects include flushing, pallor, and increased perspiration. With the transdermal preparation, there is a risk of contact dermatitis and local hypersensitivity reactions.

Clinically Important Drug–Drug Interactions

There is a risk of hypertension and decreased antianginal effects if these drugs are given with ergot derivatives. There is also a risk of decreased therapeutic effects of heparin if these drugs are given together with heparin; if this combination is used the patient should be monitored and appropriate dose adjustments made. Patients should not combine nitrates with sildenafil, tadalafil, or vardenafil, drugs used to treat erectile dysfunction, because serious hypotension and CV events could occur.

Ⓟ Prototype Summary: Nitroglycerin

Indications: Treatment of acute angina, prophylaxis of angina, IV treatment of angina unresponsive to beta-blockers or organic nitrates, perioperative hypertension, and heart failure associated with acute MI; to produce controlled hypotension during surgery.

Actions: Relaxes vascular smooth muscle with a resultant decrease in venous return and decrease in arterial blood pressure, reducing the left ventricular workload and decreasing myocardial oxygen consumption.

Pharmacokinetics:

Route	Onset	Duration
IV	1–2 min	3–5 min
Sublingual tablet	1–3 min	30–60 min
Translingual spray	2 min	30–60 min
Transmucosal tablet	1–2 min	3–5 min
Oral, SR tablet	20–45 min	8–12 h
Topical ointment	30–60 min	4–8 h
Transdermal	30–60 min	24 h

$T_{1/2}$: 1 to 4 minutes; metabolized in the liver and excreted in the urine.

Adverse Effects: Hypotension, headache, dizziness, tachycardia, rash, flushing, nausea, vomiting, sweating, and chest pain.

Nursing Considerations for Patients Receiving Nitrates

Assessment: History and Examination

- Assess for contraindications or cautions: Any known allergies to nitrates *to avoid hypersensitivity reactions;* impaired liver or kidney function, *which could alter the metabolism and excretion of the drug; any condition that could be exacerbated by the hypotension and change in blood flow caused by these drugs,* such as early MI, head trauma, cerebral hemorrhage, hypotension, hypovolemia, anemia, or low-cardiac-output states; and current status of pregnancy or lactation *because of the potential for adverse effects on the fetus or nursing baby.*
- Perform a physical assessment *to establish baseline status before beginning therapy* and *during therapy to determine effectiveness and to evaluate for any potential adverse effects.*
- Inspect the skin for color, intactness, and any signs of redness, irritation, or breakdown, especially if the patient is using the transdermal or topical form of the drug, *to prevent possible skin reaction and ensure adequate surface for application and absorption of trans-*

(continues on page 794)

dermal or topical drug. Also check the patient's oral or buccal mucosa (including the area under the tongue) if sublingual or buccal forms are ordered *to reduce the risk of irritation and ensure adequate surface for absorption*.

- Assess the patient's complaint of pain, including onset, duration, intensity, location, and measures used to relieve it. Investigate activity level prior to and after the onset of pain *to aid in identifying possible contributing factors to the pain and its progression*.
- Assess the patient's neurological status, including level of alertness, affect, and reflexes, *to evaluate for CNS effects*.
- Monitor respirations and auscultate lungs *to evaluate changes in cardiac output*.
- Assess cardiopulmonary status closely, including pulse rate, blood pressure, heart rate, and rhythm, *to determine the effects of therapy and identify any adverse effects*.
- Obtain an ECG as ordered *to evaluate heart rate and rhythm, which could indicate changes in cardiac perfusion*.
- Monitor laboratory test results, including liver and renal function tests, complete blood count, and hemoglobin level, *to determine the need for possible dose adjustment*.

Nursing Diagnoses

Nursing diagnoses related to drug therapy might include the following:

- Decreased cardiac output related to vasodilation and hypotensive effects
- Risk for injury related to CNS or CV effects
- Ineffective tissue perfusion (total body) related to hypotension or change in cardiac output
- Deficient knowledge regarding drug therapy

Planning

- The patient will receive the best therapeutic effect from the drug therapy.
- The patient will have limited adverse effects to the drug therapy.
- The patient will have an understanding of the drug therapy, adverse effects to anticipate, and measures to relieve discomfort and improve safety

Implementation with Rationale

- Give sublingual preparations under the tongue or in the buccal pouch, and encourage the patient not to swallow, *to ensure that therapeutic effectiveness is achieved* (see Pharmacokinetics for discussion of safe medication administration).
- Ask the patient if the tablet "fizzles" or burns, which indicates potency. Always check the expiration date on the bottle and protect the medication from heat and light *because these drugs are volatile and lose their potency*.
- Instruct the patient that a sublingual dose may be repeated in 5 minutes if relief is not felt, for a total of three doses; if pain persists the patient should go to an emergency room *to ensure proper medical support if an MI should occur*.
- Give SR forms with water, and caution the patient not to chew or crush them *because these preparations need to reach the GI tract intact*.
- Rotate the sites of topical forms *to decrease the risk of skin abrasion and breakdown*; monitor for signs of skin breakdown *to arrange for appropriate skin care as needed*.
- Make sure that translingual spray is used under the tongue and not inhaled *to ensure that the therapeutic effects can be achieved*.
- Break an amyl nitrate capsule and wave it under the nose of the angina patient *to provide rapid relief using the inhalation form of the drug*; this may be repeated with another capsule in 3 to 5 minutes if needed.
- Keep a record of the number of sprays used if a translingual spray form is used *to prevent running out of medication and episodes of untreated angina*.
- Have emergency life support equipment readily available *in case of severe reaction to the drug or MI*.
- Taper the dose gradually (over 4 to 6 weeks) after long-term therapy *because abrupt withdrawal could cause a severe reaction, including MI*.
- Provide comfort measures *to help the patient tolerate drug effects*. These include small, frequent meals *to alleviate GI upset*; access to bathroom facilities if GI upset is severe or the patient experiences incontinence; environmental controls such as temperature, controlled lighting, and noise reduction *to decrease stresses that could aggravate cardiac workload*; safety precautions such as lying or sitting down after taking the drug and assistance with ambulation *to reduce the risk of injury*; reorientation; and appropriate skin care as needed.
- Offer support and encouragement *to help the patient deal with the diagnosis and the drug regimen*.
- Provide thorough patient teaching, including the name of the drug; dosage prescribed; proper technique for administration (oral, sublingual, transbuccal, transdermal, inhalation spray, or topical); need for removal of transdermal or topical drug before application of the next dose; the importance of having an adequate supply of drug (e.g., teaching the patient to count the number of sprays used for a translingual spray so as not to run short); measures to prevent anginal attacks, and actions to take when an attack occurs; use of medication during an attack (such as the number of tablets and time span that the patient can take sublingual tablets); measures to avoid adverse effects, warning signs of problems, and

signs and symptoms to report immediately; and the need for periodic monitoring and evaluation *to enhance patient knowledge about drug therapy and to promote compliance.*

Evaluation

- Monitor patient response to the drug (alleviation of signs and symptoms of angina, prevention of angina).
- Monitor for adverse effects (hypotension, cardiac arrhythmias, GI upset, skin reactions, headache).
- Evaluate the effectiveness of the teaching plan (patient can name drug, dosage, proper administration, adverse effects to watch for, specific measures to avoid them, and the importance of continued follow-up).
- Monitor the effectiveness of comfort measures and compliance with the regimen.

See the Critical Thinking Scenario for measures for handling an angina attack.

KEY POINTS

- Nitrates cause blood vessels to relax and dilate. This results in a drop in peripheral resistance and blood pressure and a decrease in venous return to the heart. These actions will decrease myocardial workload and can restore the appropriate balance in the supply–demand ratio in the heart.
- Nitrates are available in many forms that vary in time of onset and duration of action. Fast-acting nitrates are used to treat acute anginal attacks. Slower-acting nitrates are used to prevent anginal attacks from occurring.

Beta-Adrenergic Blockers

As discussed in Chapter 31, beta-adrenergic blockers are used to block the stimulatory effects of the sympathetic nervous system. The beta-blockers recommended for use

CRITICAL THINKING SCENARIO

Handling an Angina Attack

THE SITUATION

S.W. is a 48-year-old white woman with a 2-year history of angina pectoris. She was given sublingual nitroglycerin to use when she had chest pain. For the past 6 months, she has been stable, experiencing little chest pain. This morning after her exercise class, S.W. had an argument with her daughter and experienced severe chest pain that was unrelieved by four nitroglycerin tablets taken over a 20-minute period. S.W.'s daughter rushed her to the hospital, where she was given oxygen through nasal cannula and placed on a cardiac monitor, which showed a sinus tachycardia of 110 beats/min. A 12-lead ECG showed no changes from her previous ECG of 7 months ago.

S.W. did not have elevated troponin levels. The chest pain subsided within 3 minutes after she received another sublingual nitroglycerin. It was decided that S.W. should stay in the emergency department (ED) for a few hours for observation. The diagnosis of an acute angina attack was made.

CRITICAL THINKING

What nursing interventions are appropriate for S.W. while she is still in the ED? *Consider the progression of CAD and the ways in which that progression can be delayed and chest pain avoided.*

What teaching points should be stressed with this patient?

What type of guilt may the daughter experience after the disagreement with S.W.?

What interventions would be useful in dealing with mother and daughter during this crisis?

Should any further tests or treatments be addressed with S.W. when discussing her heart disease?

DISCUSSION

S.W.'s vital signs should be monitored closely while she is in the ED. If her attack subsides, she will be discharged, and teaching points about CAD will be reviewed with her. It would be a good time to discuss angina with S.W. and her daughter, explaining the pathophysiology of the disease and ways to avoid disrupting the supply-and-demand ratio in the heart muscle.

Because S.W. took four nitroglycerin tablets with no effect before coming to the ED, it would be important to find out the age and potency of her drug. Review the storage requirements for the drug, ways to tell whether it is potent, and the importance of replacing the pills at least every 6 months.

S.W. and her daughter should be encouraged to air their feelings about this episode; for example, guilt or anger may be precipitated by this scare. They should have the opportunity to explore other ways of handling their problems, try to pace activities to avoid excessive demand for oxygen, and plan what to do if this happens again. They should both receive support and encouragement to cope with the angina and its implications.

Written information, including drug information, should be given to S.W. Once her condition is stabilized, further studies may be indicated to monitor the progress of her disease. The use of dietary interventions, avoidance of smoking as appropriate, blood pressure control, and monitoring of activity should be considered.

(continues on page 796)

Handling an Angina Attack (continued)

NURSING CARE GUIDE FOR S.W.: ANTIANGINAL NITRATES

Assessment: History and Examination

Assess S.W. for allergies to any nitrates, renal or hepatic dysfunction, pregnancy and lactation (if appropriate), early MI, head trauma, hypotension, and hypovolemia.

Focus the physical examination on the following areas:

CV: Blood pressure, pulse, perfusion, ECG

CNS: Orientation, affect, reflexes, vision

Skin: Color, lesions, texture

Respiratory system: Respiratory rate and character, adventitious sounds

GI: Abdominal examination, bowel sounds

Laboratory tests: Liver and renal function tests, complete blood count, hemoglobin

Nursing Diagnoses

Decreased cardiac output related to hypotension

Risk for injury related to CNS and CV effects

Ineffective tissue perfusion (total body) related to CV effects

Fear and anxiety related to disease

Deficient knowledge regarding drug therapy

Planning

The patient will receive the best therapeutic effect from the drug therapy.

The patient will have limited adverse effects to the drug therapy.

The patient will have an understanding of the drug therapy, adverse effects to anticipate, and measures to relieve discomfort and improve safety.

Implementation

Ensure proper administration of drug, and protect the drug from heat and light.

Provide comfort and safety measures.

- Offer environmental control for headaches.
- Give drug with food if GI upset occurs.
- Provide skin care as needed.
- Taper dose after long-term use.

Provide support and reassurance to deal with drug effects.

Provide patient teaching regarding drug, dosage, adverse effects, what to report, and safety precautions.

Evaluation

Evaluate drug effects: Relief of signs and symptoms of angina, prevention of angina.

Monitor for adverse effects: Headache, dizziness; arrhythmias; GI upset; skin reactions; hypotension; and CV effects.

Monitor for drug–drug interactions as indicated for each drug.

Evaluate the effectiveness of the patient-teaching program and comfort and safety measures.

PATIENT TEACHING FOR S.W.

- A nitrate is given to patients with chest pain that occurs because the heart muscle is not receiving enough oxygen. The nitrates act by decreasing the heart's workload, and thus its need for oxygen, which it uses for energy. This relieves the pain of angina.
- Besides taking the drug as prescribed, you can also help your heart by decreasing the work that it must do. For example, you can do the following:
  - Reduce weight, if necessary.
  - Decrease or avoid the use of coffee, cigarettes, or alcoholic beverages.
  - Avoid going outside in very cold weather; if this cannot be avoided, dress warmly and avoid exertion while outside.
  - Avoid stressful activities, especially in combination. For example, if you eat a big meal, do not drink coffee or alcoholic beverages with that meal. If you have just eaten a big meal, do not climb stairs; rest for a while.
  - Determine which social interactions are stressful or anxiety producing; then find ways to limit or avoid these situations.
  - Determine ways to vent your feelings (e.g., throwing things, screaming, diversions).
  - Learn to slow down, rest periodically, and schedule your activities to allow your heart to pace its use of energy throughout the day and to help you to maintain your activities without pain.
- Nitroglycerin tablets are taken sublingually. Place one tablet under your tongue. Do not swallow until the tablet has dissolved. The tablet should burn slightly or "fizzle" under your tongue; if this does not occur the tablet is not effective and you should get a fresh supply of tablets.
- Ideally, take the nitroglycerin before your chest pain begins. If you know that a certain activity usually causes chest pain (e.g., eating a big meal, attending a business meeting, engaging in sexual intercourse), take the tablet before undertaking that activity.
- Sublingual nitroglycerin is a very unstable compound. Do not buy large quantities at a time because it does not store well. Keep the drug in a dark, dry place and in a dark-colored glass container, not a plastic bottle, with a tight lid. Leave it in its own bottle. Do not combine it with other drugs.
- Some of the following adverse effects may occur:
  - *Dizziness, light-headedness:* This often passes as you adjust to the drug. Use great care if you are taking sublingual or transmucosal forms of the drug. Sit or lie down to avoid dizziness or falls. Change position slowly to help decrease the dizziness.

Handling an Angina Attack (continued)

- *Headache:* This is a common problem. Over-the-counter headache remedies often provide no relief for the pain. Lying down in a cool environment and resting may help alleviate some of the discomfort.
- *Flushing of the face and neck:* This is usually a very minor problem that passes as the drug's effects pass.
- Report any of the following to your health care provider: *blurred vision, persistent or severe headache, skin rash, more frequent or more severe angina attacks, or fainting.*
- Sublingual nitroglycerin usually relieves chest pain within 3 to 5 minutes. If pain is not relieved within 5 minutes, take another tablet. If pain continues, take another tablet in 5 minutes. A total of ____ tablets may be used, spaced every 5 minutes. If the pain is not relieved after that time, call your health care provider or go to a hospital emergency room as soon as possible.
- Tell any doctor, nurse, or other health care provider involved in your care that you are taking this drug.
- Keep this drug, and all medications, out of the reach of children.
- Avoid taking over-the-counter medications while you are taking this drug. If you feel that you need one of these, consult with your health care provider for the best choice. Many of these drugs can change the effects of this drug and cause problems.
- Avoid alcohol while you are taking this drug because the combination can cause serious problems.
- If you are taking this drug for a prolonged period of time, do not stop taking it suddenly. Your body will need time to adjust to the loss of the drug. The dose must be gradually reduced to prevent serious problems.

in angina include atenolol (*Tenormin*), metoprolol (*Toprol XL*), propranolol (*Inderal*), and nadolol (*Corgard*).

Therapeutic Actions and Indications

The beta-blockers competitively block beta-adrenergic receptors in the heart and juxtaglomerular apparatus, decreasing the influence of the sympathetic nervous system on these tissues. The result is a decrease in the excitability of the heart, a decrease in cardiac output, a decrease in cardiac oxygen consumption, and a lowering of blood pressure. They are indicated for the long-term management of angina pectoris caused by atherosclerosis. These drugs are sometimes used in combination with nitrates to increase exercise tolerance. See Table 46.1 for Usual Indications for each of these drugs.

Beta-blockers are not indicated for the treatment of Prinzmetal angina because they could cause vasospasm due to blocking of beta-receptor sites. Propranolol and metoprolol can also be used to prevent reinfarction in stable patients 1 to 4 weeks after an MI. This effect is thought to be caused by the suppression of myocardial oxygen demand for a prolonged period.

Pharmacokinetics

These drugs are absorbed from the GI tract after oral administration and undergo hepatic metabolism. They reach peak levels in 60 to 90 minutes and have varying duration of effects, ranging from 6 to 19 hours. Food has been found to increase the bioavailability of propranolol, but this effect has not been found with other beta-adrenergic blocking agents.

Contraindications and Cautions

The beta-blockers are contraindicated in patients with bradycardia, heart block, and cardiogenic shock *because blocking of the sympathetic response could exacerbate these diseases.* They also are contraindicated with pregnancy and lactation *because of the potential for adverse effects on the fetus or neonate.*

Caution should be used in patients with diabetes, peripheral vascular disease, asthma, chronic obstructive pulmonary disease, or thyrotoxicosis *because the blockade of the sympathetic response blocks normal reflexes that are necessary for maintaining homeostasis in patients with these diseases.* Many patients with these complicating disorders receive beta-blockers, and these patients need to be monitored carefully to avoid serious adverse effects.

Adverse Effects

Beta-blockers have many adverse effects associated with the blockade of the sympathetic nervous system. However, the dose used to prevent angina is lower than doses used to treat hypertension. Therefore, there is a decreased incidence of adverse effects associated with this specific use of beta-blockers.

Adverse effects do occur. CNS effects include dizziness, fatigue, emotional depression, and sleep disturbances. GI problems include gastric pain, nausea, vomiting, colitis, and diarrhea. CV effects can include HF, reduced cardiac output, and arrhythmias. Respiratory effects can include bronchospasm, dyspnea, and cough. Decreased exercise tolerance and malaise are also common complaints.

Clinically Important Drug–Drug Interactions

A paradoxical hypertension occurs when clonidine is given with beta-blockers, and an increased rebound hypertension with clonidine withdrawal may also occur; it is best to avoid this combination.

A decreased antihypertensive effect occurs when beta-blockers are given with nonsteroidal anti-inflammatory drugs; if this combination is used the patient should be monitored closely and a dose adjustment made.

An initial hypertensive episode followed by bradycardia occurs if these drugs are given with epinephrine, and a possibility of peripheral ischemia exists if beta-blockers are taken in combination with ergot alkaloids.

There also is a potential for a change in blood glucose levels if these drugs are given with insulin or antidiabetic agents, and the patient will not have the usual signs and symptoms of hypoglycemia or hyperglycemia to alert him or her to potential problems. If this combination is used the patient should monitor blood glucose frequently throughout the day and should be alert to new warnings about glucose imbalance.

Ⓟ Prototype Summary: Metoprolol

Indications: Treatment of stable angina pectoris; also used for treatment of hypertension, prevention of reinfarction in MI patients, and treatment of stable, symptomatic HF.

Actions: Competitively blocks beta-adrenergic receptors in the heart and kidneys, decreasing the influence of the sympathetic nervous system on these tissues and the excitability of the heart; decreases cardiac output, which results in a lowered blood pressure and decreased cardiac workload.

Pharmacokinetics:

Route	Onset	Peak	Duration
Oral	15 min	90 min	15–19 h
IV	Immediate	60–90 min	15–19 h

$T_{1/2}$: 3 to 4 hours; metabolized in the liver and excreted in the urine.

Adverse Effects: Dizziness, vertigo, HF, arrhythmias, gastric pain, flatulence, diarrhea, vomiting, impotence, decreased exercise tolerance.

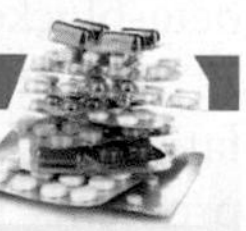

Nursing Considerations for Patients Receiving Beta-Blockers

See Chapter 31 for the nursing considerations associated with beta-blockers.

KEY POINTS

- Beta-blockers are used in the treatment of angina to help restore the balance between supply of oxygen and demand for oxygen.
- Beta-blockers prevent the activation of sympathetic receptors, which normally would increase heart rate, increase blood pressure, and increase cardiac contraction. All of these actions would increase the demand for oxygen; blocking these actions decreases the demand for oxygen.

Calcium-Channel Blockers

Calcium-channel blockers include amlodipine (*Norvasc*), diltiazem (*Cardizem*), nicardipine (*Cardene*), nifedipine (*Adalat CC, Procardia*), and verapamil (*Calan*).

Therapeutic Actions and Indications

Calcium-channel blockers inhibit the movement of calcium ions across the membranes of myocardial and arterial muscle cells, altering the action potential and blocking muscle cell contraction. A loss of smooth muscle tone, vasodilation, and decreased peripheral resistance occur. Subsequently, preload and afterload are decreased, which in turn decreases cardiac workload and oxygen consumption.

Calcium-channel blockers are indicated for the treatment of Prinzmetal angina, chronic angina, effort-associated angina, and hypertension. In Prinzmetal angina, these agents relieve coronary artery vasospasm, increasing blood flow to the muscle cells. Research also indicates that these drugs block the proliferation of cells in the endothelial layer of the blood vessel, slowing the progress of atherosclerosis. Verapamil is also used to treat cardiac tachyarrhythmias because it slows conduction more than the other calcium-channel blockers do. The drug of choice depends on the patient's diagnosis and ability to tolerate adverse drug effects. See Table 46.1 for Usual Indications for each of these drugs.

Pharmacokinetics

These drugs are generally well absorbed after oral administration, metabolized in the liver, and excreted in the urine. They have an onset of action of 20 minutes and a duration of action of 2 to 4 hours. These drugs cross the placenta and enter breast milk.

Contraindications and Cautions

Calcium-channel blockers are contraindicated in the presence of allergy to any of these drugs *to avoid hypersensitivity reactions* and with pregnancy or lactation *because of the potential for adverse effects on the fetus or neonate.*

Caution should be used with heart block or sick sinus syndrome, *which could be exacerbated by the conduction-slowing effects of these drugs*; with renal or hepatic dysfunction, *which could alter the metabolism and excretion of these drugs*; and with HF, *which could be exacerbated by the decrease in cardiac output that could occur.*

Adverse Effects

The adverse effects associated with these drugs are related to their effects on cardiac output and on smooth muscle. CNS effects include dizziness, light-headedness, headache, and fatigue. GI effects can include nausea and hepatic injury related to direct toxic effects on hepatic cells. CV effects include hypotension, bradycardia, peripheral edema, and heart block. Skin effects include flushing and rash.

Clinically Important Drug–Drug Interactions

Drug–drug interactions vary with each of the calcium-channel blockers. Potentially serious effects to keep in mind include increased serum levels and toxicity of cyclosporine if they are taken with diltiazem, and increased risk of heart block and digoxin toxicity if they are combined with verapamil (because verapamil increases digoxin serum levels). Both verapamil and digoxin depress myocardial conduction. If any combinations of these drugs must be used the patient should be monitored very closely and appropriate dose adjustments made. Verapamil has also been associated with serious respiratory depression when given with general anesthetics or as an adjunct to anesthesia.

Ⓟ Prototype Summary: Diltiazem

Indications: Treatment of Prinzmetal angina, effort-associated angina, and chronic stable angina; also used to treat essential hypertension and paroxysmal supraventricular tachycardia.

Actions: Inhibits the movement of calcium ions across the membranes of myocardial and arterial muscle cells, altering the action potential and blocking muscle cell contraction, which depresses myocardial contractility; slows cardiac impulse formation in the conductive tissues, and relaxes and dilates arteries, causing a fall in blood pressure and a decrease in venous return; decreases the workload of the heart and myocardial oxygen consumption; relieves the vasospasm of the coronary artery, increasing blood flow to the muscle cells (Prinzmetal angina).

Pharmacokinetics:

Route	Onset	Peak
Oral	30–60 min	2–3 h
SR, extended release (ER)	30–60 min	6–11 h
IV	Immediate	2–3 min

$T_{1/2}$: 3.5 to 6 hours SR, 5 to 7 hours ER; metabolized in the liver and excreted in the urine.

Adverse Effects: Dizziness, light-headedness, headache, asthenia, peripheral edema, bradycardia, atrioventricular block, flushing, rash, nausea.

Nursing Considerations for Patients Receiving Calcium-Channel Blockers

Assessment: History and Examination

- Assess for contraindications or cautions: Known allergies to any of these drugs *to avoid hypersensitivity reactions*; impaired liver or kidney function, *which could alter the metabolism and excretion of the drug*; heart block, *which could be exacerbated by the conduction depression of these drugs*; and current status of pregnancy or lactation *because of the risk of adverse effects to the fetus or nursing baby.*
- Perform a physical assessment to establish *baseline status before beginning therapy and during therapy to determine the effectiveness and evaluate for any potential adverse effects.*
- Inspect skin for color and integrity *to identify possible adverse skin reactions.*
- Assess the patient's complaint of pain, including onset, duration, intensity, and location, and measures used to relieve the pain. Investigate activity level prior to and after the onset of pain *to aid in identifying possible contributing factors to the pain and its progression.*
- Assess cardiopulmonary status closely, including pulse rate, blood pressure, heart rate, and rhythm, *to determine the effects of therapy and identify any adverse effects.*
- Obtain an ECG as ordered *to evaluate heart rate and rhythm.*
- Monitor respirations and auscultate lungs *to evaluate changes in cardiac output.*
- Monitor laboratory test results, including liver and renal function tests, *to determine the need for possible dose adjustment.*

Nursing Diagnoses

Nursing diagnoses related to drug therapy might include the following:

- Decreased cardiac output related to hypotension and vasodilation
- Risk for injury related to CNS or CV effects
- Ineffective tissue perfusion (total body) related to hypotension or change in cardiac output
- Deficient knowledge regarding drug therapy

Planning

- The patient will receive the best therapeutic effect from the drug therapy.
- The patient will have limited adverse effects to the drug therapy.
- The patient will have an understanding of the drug therapy, adverse effects to anticipate, and measures to relieve discomfort and improve safety.

(continues on page 800)

Implementation with Rationale

- Monitor the patient's blood pressure, cardiac rhythm, and cardiac output closely while the drug is being titrated or dose is being changed *to ensure early detection of potentially serious adverse effects.*
- Monitor blood pressure very carefully if the patient is also taking nitrates *because there is an increased risk of hypotensive episodes.*
- If a patient is on long-term therapy, periodically monitor blood pressure and cardiac rhythm while the patient is using these drugs *because of the potential for adverse CV effects.*
- Provide comfort measures *to help the patient tolerate drug effects.* These include small, frequent meals *to alleviate GI upset*; environmental controls, such as limiting light, maintaining temperature, and avoiding excessive noise and interruptions, *which could aggravate stress and increase myocardial demand*; and taking safety precautions, such as providing periodic rests and assisting with ambulation if dizziness occurs, *to prevent injury.*
- Offer support and encouragement *to help the patient deal with the diagnosis and the drug regimen.*
- Provide thorough patient teaching, including the name of the drug and dosage prescribed; measures to avoid adverse effects and prevent anginal attacks; actions to take when an attack occurs; warning signs of problems, and signs and symptoms to report immediately; and the need for periodic monitoring and evaluation *to enhance patient knowledge about drug therapy and to promote compliance.*

Evaluation

- Monitor patient response to the drug (alleviation of signs and symptoms of angina, prevention of angina).
- Monitor for adverse effects (hypotension, cardiac arrhythmias, GI upset, skin reactions, headache).
- Monitor the effectiveness of comfort measures and compliance with the regimen.
- Evaluate the effectiveness of the teaching plan (patient can name drug, dosage, proper administration, adverse effects to watch for, specific measures to avoid them, and the importance of continued follow-up).

KEY POINTS

- Calcium-channel blockers block muscle contraction in smooth muscle and decrease the heart's workload, relax vasospasm in Prinzmetal angina, and possibly block proliferation of the damaged endothelium in coronary vessels.
- Patients on calcium-channel blockers need to be monitored for signs of decreased cardiac output and response, including slow heart rate, hypotension, dizziness, and headache.

Piperazine Acetamide Agent

In late 2006 the U.S. Food and Drug Administration approved the first new drug in more than 10 years for the treatment of chronic angina. Since its approval, postmarketing studies have shown that the drug is very effective in treating angina and has the added benefits of decreasing blood glucose levels when used in diabetic patients and decreasing the incidence of ventricular fibrillation, atrial fibrillation, and bradycardia in chronic angina patients. Ranolazine (*Ranexa*) is available in an ER tablet form for oral use. The mechanism of action of the drug is not understood. It does prolong the QT interval, it does not decrease heart rate or blood pressure, but it does decrease myocardial workload, bringing the supply and demand for oxygen back into balance. Ranolazine is approved as a first-line treatment for angina or for use in combination with nitrates, beta-blockers, or amlodipine. It is rapidly absorbed, reaching peak levels in 2 to 5 hours. It is metabolized in the liver with a half-life of 7 hours and is excreted in the urine and feces. Ranolazine is contraindicated for use with any known sensitivity to the drug; with preexisting prolonged QT interval or in combination with drugs that would prolong QT intervals; and with hepatic impairment and lactation. Caution should be used with pregnancy or renal impairment. Drug–drug interactions can occur with ketoconazole, diltiazem, verapamil, macrolide antibiotics, and HIV protease inhibitors; these combinations should be avoided because ranolazine levels may become extremely high. Digoxin levels may become high if the two drugs are combined; if this combination is needed the digoxin dose will need to be decreased. Tricyclic antidepressants and antipsychotic drug levels may increase if these agents are combined with ranolazine; if they are combined the dose of these drugs may need to be decreased. Grapefruit juice should be avoided while taking this drug. Dizziness, headache, nausea, and constipation are the most commonly experienced adverse effects. Patients must be cautioned not to cut, crush, or chew the tablets, which need to be swallowed whole. Safety precautions may be needed if dizziness is an issue.

SUMMARY

- CAD, the leading cause of death in the United States and most Western nations, develops when changes in the intima of coronary vessels lead to the development of atheromas or fatty tumors, accumulation of platelets and debris, and a thickening of arterial muscles, resulting in a loss of elasticity and responsiveness to normal stimuli.
- Narrowing of the coronary arteries secondary to atheroma buildup is called atherosclerosis.

- Narrowed coronary arteries eventually become unable to deliver all the blood that is needed by the myocardial cells, causing a problem of supply and demand.
- Angina pectoris, or "suffocation of the chest," occurs when the myocardial demand for oxygen cannot be met by the narrowed vessels. Pain, anxiety, and fatigue develop when the supply-and-demand ratio is upset. Types of angina include stable, unstable, and Prinzmetal angina.
- MI occurs when a coronary vessel is completely occluded and the cells that depend on that vessel for oxygen become ischemic, then necrotic, and die.
- Angina can be treated by drugs that either increase the supply of oxygen or decrease the heart's workload, which decreases the demand for oxygen.
- Nitrates and beta-blockers are used to cause vasodilation and to decrease venous return and arterial resistance—effects that decrease cardiac workload and oxygen consumption.
- Nitroglycerin is the drug of choice for treating an acute anginal attack. It is available in various forms.
- Beta-blockers prevent the activation of sympathetic receptors, which normally would increase heart rate, increase blood pressure, and increase cardiac contraction. All of these actions would increase the demand for oxygen; blocking these actions decreases the demand for oxygen.
- Calcium-channel blockers block muscle contraction in smooth muscle and decrease the heart's workload, relax vasospasm in Prinzmetal angina, and possibly block the proliferation of the damaged endothelium in coronary vessels.
- The newest drug approved for the treatment of angina is the piperazine acetamide agent ranolazine. The mechanism of action of this drug is not understood. It prolongs QT intervals, does not slow heart rate or blood pressure, but decreases myocardial oxygen demand.

CHECK YOUR UNDERSTANDING

Answers to the questions in this chapter can be found in Answers to Check Your Understanding Questions on thePoint®.

MULTIPLE CHOICE

Select the best answer to the following.

1. Coronary artery disease results in
- **a.** an imbalance in cardiac muscle oxygen supply and demand.
- **b.** delivery of blood to the heart muscle during systole.
- **c.** increased pulse pressure.
- **d.** a decreased workload on the heart.

2. Angina
- **a.** causes death of heart muscle cells.
- **b.** is pain due to lack of oxygen to myocardial cells.
- **c.** cannot occur at rest.
- **d.** is not treatable.

3. Nitrates are commonly used antianginal drugs that act to
- **a.** increase the preload on the heart.
- **b.** increase the afterload on the heart.
- **c.** dilate coronary vessels to increase the delivery of oxygen through those vessels.
- **d.** decrease venous return to the heart, decreasing the myocardial workload.

4. Calcium-channel blockers are effective in treating angina because they
- **a.** prevent any CV exercise, preventing strain on the heart.
- **b.** block strong muscle contractions, causing vasodilation.
- **c.** alter the electrolyte balance of the heart, preventing arrhythmias.
- **d.** increase the heart rate, making it more efficient.

5. A nurse would question an order for which of the following if the patient was also receiving verapamil?
- **a.** Oral contraceptives
- **b.** Cyclosporine
- **c.** Digoxin
- **d.** Barbiturate anesthetics

6. Prinzmetal angina occurs as a result of
- **a.** electrolyte imbalance.
- **b.** a spasm of a coronary vessel.
- **c.** decreased venous return to the heart.
- **d.** a ventricular arrhythmia

(continues on page 802)

MULTIPLE RESPONSE

Select all that apply.

1. Treating angina involves modifying factors that could decrease myocardial oxygen consumption. It could be expected that this might include
a. weight loss.
b. use of nitrates.
c. use of angiotensin-converting enzyme inhibitors.
d. activity modification.
e. use of a piperazine acetamide agent.
f. use of a calcium-channel blocker.

2. An acute myocardial infarction is usually associated with which of the following?
a. Permanent injury to the heart muscle
b. Potentially serious arrhythmias
c. Pain
d. The development of hypertension
e. Loss of consciousness
f. A feeling of anxiety

3. When describing the action of antianginal drugs to a patient, which of the following would the nurse include?
a. Decrease the workload on the heart
b. Increase the supply of oxygen to the heart
c. Change the metabolic pathway in the heart muscle to remove the need for oxygen
d. Restore the supply-and-demand balance of oxygen in the heart
e. Decrease venous return to the heart
f. Alter the coronary artery-filling pathway

4. A client who has nitroglycerin to avert an acute anginal attack would need to be taught
a. to take five or six tablets and then seek medical help if no relief occurs.
b. to buy the tablets in bulk to decrease the cost.
c. to protect tablets from light and humidity.
d. to store the tablets in a clearly marked, clear container in open view.
e. to use the nitroglycerin before an event or activity that will most likely precipitate an anginal attack.
f. to discard them if they do not fizzle when placed under the tongue.

BIBLIOGRAPHY AND REFERENCES

AHA/ACC. (2014). 2014 AHA/ACC guideline for the management of patients with Non–ST-elevation acute coronary syndromes [*American Heart Association/American College of Cardiology*]. Available online at: http://circ.ahajournals.org/content/early/2014/09/22/CIR.0000000000000134.full.pdf

Brunton, L., Chabner, B., & Knollman, B. (2011). *Goodman and Gilman's the pharmacological basis of therapeutics* (12th ed.). New York: McGraw-Hill.

DeVon, H., Hogan, N., Ochs, A., et al. (2010). Time to treatment of acute coronary syndromes: The cost of indecision. *Journal of Cardiovascular Nursing, 25*(2), 106–114.

Facts and Comparisons. (2015). *Drug facts and comparisons*. St. Louis, MO: Author.

Fuster, V., Alexander, R. W., & Rourke, R. A. (Eds.). (2011). *Hurst's the heart* (13th ed.). New York: McGraw-Hill.

Jneid, H., Anderson, J. L., Wright, R. S., et al. (2012). 2012 Update guidelines for the management of patients with unstable angina/non-ST-elevation myocardial infarction: A report of the American College of Cardiology/American Heart Association Task Force on Practice Guidelines. *Journal of the American College of Cardiology, 60*(7), 645–681.

Karch, A. M. (2014). *Lippincott's nursing drug guide*. Philadelphia, PA: Lippincott Williams & Wilkins.

Ogle, K. (2010). Heart matters: Analyzing angina. *Nursing Made Incredibly Easy, 8*(6), 9–12.

Porth, C. M. (2013). *Pathophysiology: Concepts of altered health states* (9th ed.). Philadelphia, PA: Lippincott Williams & Wilkins.

The Medical Letter. (2015). *The medical letter on drugs and therapeutics*. New Rochelle, NY: Author.

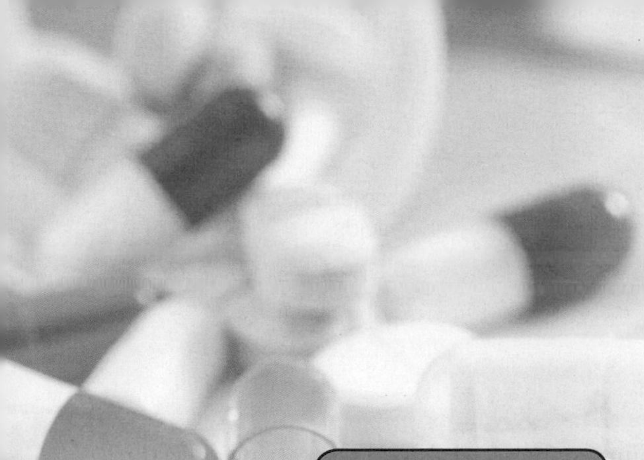

Lipid-Lowering Agents 47

Learning Objectives

Upon completion of this chapter, you will be able to:

1. Outline the mechanisms of fat metabolism in the body and discuss the role of hyperlipidemia as a risk factor for coronary artery disease.
2. Describe the therapeutic actions, indications, pharmacokinetics, contraindications and cautions, most common adverse reactions, and important drug–drug interactions associated with bile acid sequestrants, HMG–CoA inhibitors, cholesterol absorption inhibitors, and other agents used to lower lipid levels.
3. Discuss the use of drugs that lower lipid levels across the lifespan.
4. Compare and contrast the various drugs used to lower lipid levels.
5. Outline the nursing considerations, including important teaching points, for patients receiving drugs used to lower lipid levels.

Glossary of Key Terms

antihyperlipidemic agents: general term used for drugs used to lower lipid levels in the blood

bile acids: cholesterol-containing acids found in the bile that act like detergents to break up fats in the small intestine

cholesterol: necessary component of human cells that is produced and processed in the liver, then stored in the bile until stimulus causes the gallbladder to contract and send the bile into the duodenum via the common bile duct; a fat that is essential for the formation of steroid hormones and cell membranes; it is produced in cells and taken in by dietary sources

chylomicron: carrier for lipids in the bloodstream, consisting of proteins, lipids, cholesterol, and so forth

endocannabinoids: endogenous substances that activate nervous system receptors that are important in the regulation of appetite, food intake, and metabolism

high-density lipoprotein (HDL): loosely packed chylomicron-containing fats, able to absorb fats and fat remnants in the periphery; thought to have a protective effect, decreasing the development of coronary artery disease

hydroxymethylglutaryl–coenzyme A (HMG–CoA) reductase: enzyme that regulates the last step in cellular cholesterol synthesis

hyperlipidemia: increased levels of lipids in the serum, associated with increased risk of coronary artery disease development

low-density lipoprotein (LDL): tightly packed fats that are thought to contribute to the development of coronary artery disease when remnants left over from the LDL are processed in the arterial lining

metabolic syndrome: a collection of factors, including insulin resistance, abdominal obesity, low high-density lipoprotein and high triglyceride levels, hypertension, and proinflammatory and prothrombotic states, that increase the incidence of coronary artery disease

risk factors: factors that have been identified as increasing the risk of the development of a disease; for coronary artery disease, risk factors include genetic predisposition, gender, age, high-fat diet, sedentary lifestyle, gout, hypertension, diabetes, and estrogen deficiency

Drug List

Lipid-Lowering Agents

Bile Acid Sequestrants
- (P) cholestyramine
- colesevelam
- colestipol

HMG–CoA Reductase Inhibitors
- (P) atorvastatin
- fluvastatin
- lovastatin
- pitavastatin
- pravastatin
- rosuvastatin
- simvastatin

Cholesterol Absorption Inhibitor
- (P) ezetimibe

(continues on page 804)

Other Lipid-Lowering Agents **Fibrates** fenofibrate fenofibric acid gemfibrozil	**Vitamin B** niacin	**Omega-3 fatty acids** omega-3-acid ethyl esters	omega-3-carboxylic acids

The drugs discussed in this chapter lower the serum levels of cholesterol and various lipids. These drugs are sometimes called **antihyperlipidemic agents** and are used to treat **hyperlipidemia**—an increase in the level of lipids in the blood. There is mounting evidence that the incidence of coronary artery disease (CAD), the leading killer of adults in the Western world, is higher among people with high serum lipid levels. The cause of CAD is poorly understood, but some evidence indicates that cholesterol and fat may play a major role in disease development. Lipid and triglyceride levels play a role in **metabolic syndrome**, a collection of factors—including insulin resistance, abdominal obesity, low high-density lipoprotein, high triglyceride levels, hypertension, and proinflammatory and prothrombotic states—that has been shown to increase the incidence of CAD. See Table 47.1.

Coronary Artery Disease

As explained in Chapter 46, CAD is characterized by the progressive growth of atheromatous plaques, or atheromas, in the coronary arteries. These plaques, which begin as fatty streaks in the endothelium, eventually injure the endothelial lining of the artery, causing an inflammatory reaction. This inflammatory process triggers the development of characteristic foam cells, containing fats and white blood cells that further injure the endothelial lining. Over time, platelets, fibrin, other fats, and remnants collect on the injured vessel lining and cause the atheroma to grow, further narrowing the interior of the blood vessel and limiting blood flow.

Table 47.1 Clinical Aspects of the Metabolic Syndrome

Parameter	Significant Values
Insulin resistance	Fasting blood sugar >110 mg/dL
Abdominal obesity	Waist measurement >40 inches in men; >35 inches in women
Lipid abnormalities	HDL <40 mg/dL in men or <50 mg/dL in women; any triglyceride levels ≥150 mg/dL
Hypertension	Blood pressure >130/85 mm Hg
Proinflammatory state	Increased macrophages, increased levels of interleukin-6 and tumor necrosis factor
Prothrombotic state	Increased plasminogen activator levels

HDL, high-density lipoproteins.

The injury to the vessel also causes scarring and a thickening of the vessel wall. As the vessel thickens, it becomes less distensible and less reactive to many neurological and chemical stimuli that would ordinarily dilate or constrict it. As a result the coronary vessels no longer are able to balance the myocardial demand for oxygen with increased blood supply. More recent evidence indicates that the makeup of the core of the atheroma may be a primary determinant of which atheromas might rupture and cause acute blockage of a vessel. The softer, more lipid-filled atheromas appear to be more likely to rupture than the stable, harder cores.

Risk Factors

Evidence exists that atheroma development occurs more quickly in patients with elevated cholesterol and lipid levels. Patients who consume high-fat diets are more likely to develop high lipid levels. However, patients without increased lipid levels can also develop atheromas leading to CAD, so other factors evidently contribute to this process. Although the exact mechanism of atherogenesis (atheroma development) is not understood, certain **risk factors** increase the likelihood that a person will develop CAD. Metabolic syndrome occurs when a patient has several risk factors: Increased insulin resistance, high blood pressure, altered lipid levels, and a proinflammatory and prothrombotic state, which seem to increase the risk of CAD development dramatically. Unmodifiable and modifiable risk factors are presented in Box 47.1. Different ethnic groups also have different risk factors, as discussed in Box 47.2, as do different genders, as discussed in Box 47.3.

Treatment

Because an exact cause of CAD is not known, successful treatment involves manipulating a number of these risk factors (Table 47.2). Overall treatment and prevention of CAD should include the following measures: Decreasing dietary fats (decreasing total fat intake and limiting saturated fats seems to have the most impact on serum lipid levels); losing weight, which helps to decrease insulin resistance and the development of type 2 diabetes; eliminating smoking; increasing exercise levels; decreasing stress; and treating hypertension, diabetes, and gout.

KEY POINTS

- CAD is the leading cause of death in the Western world. It is associated with the development of atheromas or plaques in arterial linings that lead to narrowing of the lumen of the

BOX 47.1

Risk Factors for Coronary Artery Disease

Unmodifiable Risk Factors

- *Genetic predispositions*: Coronary artery disease (CAD) is more likely to occur in people who have a family history of the disease, particularly if the disease occurs in relatives younger than the age of 55 years
- *Age*: The incidence of CAD increases with age.
- *Gender*: Men are more likely than premenopausal women to have CAD; however, the incidence is almost equal in men and postmenopausal women, possibly because of a protective effect of estrogens (see Box 47.3).

Modifiable Risk Factors

- *Gout*: Increased uric acid levels seem to injure vessel walls.
- *Cigarette smoking*: Nicotine causes vasoconstriction and may have an effect on the endothelium of blood vessels; over time, smoking can lower oxygen levels in the blood.
- *Sedentary lifestyle*: Exercise increases the levels of chemicals that seem to protect the coronary arteries.
- *High stress levels*: Constant sympathetic reactions increase the myocardial oxygen demand while causing vasoconstriction and may contribute to a remodeling of the blood vessel endothelium, leading to an increased susceptibility to atheroma development.
- *Hypertension*: High pressure in the arteries causes endothelial injury and increases afterload and myocardial oxygen demand.
- *Obesity*: This may reflect altered fat metabolism, and will increases the heart's workload.
- *Diabetes*: Diabetics have a capillary membrane thickening, which accelerates the effects of atherosclerosis, and abnormal fat metabolism, which increases lipid levels.
- *Other factors that, if untreated, may contribute to CAD* include bacterial infections (*Chlamydia* infections have been correlated with onset of CAD, and treatment with tetracycline and fluororoentgenography has been associated with decreased incidence of CAD, indicating a possible bacterial link) and autoimmune processes (some plaques contain antibodies and other products of immune reactions, making autoimmune reactions a possibility).

artery and hardening of the artery wall, with loss of distensibility and responsiveness to stimuli for contraction or dilation.

- The cause of CAD is not understood, but many contributing risk factors have been identified, including increasing age, male gender, genetic predisposition, high-fat diet, sedentary lifestyle, smoking, obesity, high stress levels, bacterial infections, diabetes, hypertension, gout, and menopause. The presence of many of these factors constitutes metabolic syndrome.
- Treatment and prevention of CAD are aimed at manipulating the known risk factors to decrease CAD development and progression.

BOX 47.2 FOCUS ON Cultural Considerations

Variations in Lipoprotein Levels

Despite the fact that White Americans have the highest incidence of CAD, certain known risk factors may place other ethnic groups at greater risk. For example, hypertension and diabetes occur more frequently among African Americans and Native Americans than among Whites. There are identified cultural variations in lipid levels as well.

Cultural variations in key lipid parameters include the following:

- *Serum cholesterol levels:* Whites > African Americans, Native Americans
- *HDL levels:* African Americans, Asian Americans > Whites; Mexican Americans > Whites
- *LDL levels:* African Americans < Whites
- *HDL cholesterol ratio:* African Americans < Whites

BOX 47.3 FOCUS ON Gender Considerations

Women and Heart Disease

Until the late 1990s, heart disease was considered to be a condition that primarily affected men. Because of that belief, women were seldom screened for heart disease, and when they did experience acute cardiac events, they were not treated promptly or adequately. However, recent research has shown that heart disease is the leading cause of death among women, surpassing such diseases as breast and colon cancers. This finding has led to further research, still ongoing, about women and heart disease.

Women enjoy a protective hormone effect against the development of CAD until menopause, when estrogen loss seems to rapidly increase the production of atheromas and the development of CAD. In several studies, women who received hormone replacement therapy (HRT) at menopause had a significantly reduced risk of CAD and MI in the first few years after the onset of menopause. Research showed, however, that after 5 years of HRT the incidence of MI and stroke rose sharply, leading to an early closure of the study. Studies have found that women experience different symptoms of heart disease—jaw and neck pain, fatigue, and insomnia—and sometimes these are overlooked.

HRT is not recommended as a means of reducing the risk of heart disease or stroke, although it is still recommended for the treatment of severe menopausal symptoms in the first few years after menopause. Women should be advised to reduce other cardiac risk factors by eating a diet low in saturated fats, exercising regularly, not smoking, controlling weight, managing stress, and seeking treatment for gout, hypertension, and diabetes.

Clearly, heart disease is not just a disease of men. Research will continue to offer health care professionals new information on preventing and treating heart disease in women.

Table 47.2 Risk Factors for Coronary Artery Disease

Unmodifiable Risks	Modifiable Risks	Suggested Modifications
Family history	Sedentary lifestyle	Exercise
Age	High-fat diet	Low-fat diet (polyunsaturated and monounsaturated fats)
Gender	Smoking	Smoking cessation
	Obesity	Weight loss
	High stress levels	Stress management
	Bacterial infections	Antibiotic treatment
	Diabetes	Control of blood glucose levels
	Hypertension	Control of blood pressure
	Gout	Control of uric acid levels
	Menopause	HRT (first few years of menopause only)

HRT, hormone replacement therapy.

Fats and Biotransformation (Metabolism)

Fats are taken into the body as dietary fats, then broken down in the stomach to fatty acids, lipids, and cholesterol (Figure 47.1). The presence of these products in the duodenum stimulates contraction of the gallbladder and the release of bile. **Bile acids**, which contain high levels of **cholesterol** (a fat), act like a detergent in the small intestine and break up the fats into small units, called micelles, which can be absorbed into the wall of the small intestine. (Imagine ads for dishwashing detergents that break up the grease and fats in the dishwashing water; bile acids do much the same thing.) The bile acids are then reabsorbed and recycled to the gallbladder, where they remain until the gallbladder is again stimulated to release them to facilitate fat absorption.

Fats and water do not mix and cannot be absorbed directly into the plasma. To allow absorption, micelles are carried in a **chylomicron**, a package of fats and proteins. This packaging is done by brush enzymes in the wall of the small intestine. The chylomicrons pass through the wall of the small intestine, are picked up by the surrounding intestinal lymphatic system, travel through the system to the heart, and then are sent out into circulation. The proteins that are exposed on the chylomicron, called apoproteins, determine the fate of the lipids or fats being carried. For example, some of these packages are broken down in the tissues to be used for energy, some are stored in fat deposits for future use as energy, and some continue to the liver, where they are further processed into lipoproteins.

Lipoproteins

The lipoproteins produced in the liver that might have clinical implications are the **low-density lipoproteins (LDLs)** and the **high-density lipoproteins (HDLs)**. LDLs enter circulation as tightly packed cholesterol, triglycerides, and lipids—all of which are carried by proteins that enter circulation to be broken down for energy or stored for future use as energy. When an LDL package is broken down, many remnants or leftovers need to be returned to the liver for recycling. If a person has many of these remnants in the blood vessels, it is thought that the inflammatory process is initiated to help remove this debris. Some experts believe that this may be the underlying process involved in atherogenesis or the development of the atheroma. When considering risk factors for metabolic syndrome, however, LDL levels are not included.

HDLs enter circulation as loosely packed lipids that are used for energy and to pick up remnants of fats and cholesterol that are left in the periphery by LDL breakdown. HDLs serve a protective role in cleaning up remnants in blood vessels. It is known that HDL levels increase during exercise, which could explain why people who exercise regularly lower their risk of CAD. HDL levels also increase in response to estrogen, which could explain some of the protective effect of estrogen before menopause. In metabolic syndrome risk factors, low HDL levels are considered a risk.

Cholesterol

The body needs fats, particularly cholesterol, to maintain normal function. Cholesterol is the base unit for the formation of the steroid hormones (the sex hormones, as well as the adrenal cortical hormones). It is also a basic unit in the formation and maintenance of cell membranes. Cholesterol is usually provided through the diet and the fat metabolism process just described. If dietary cholesterol falls off the body is prepared to produce cholesterol to ensure that the cell membranes and the endocrine system are intact.

Every cell in the body has the metabolic capability of producing cholesterol. The enzyme **hydroxymethylglutaryl–coenzyme A (HMG–CoA) reductase** regulates the early, rate-limiting step in the cellular synthesis of cholesterol. If dietary cholesterol is severely limited the cellular synthesis of cholesterol will increase.

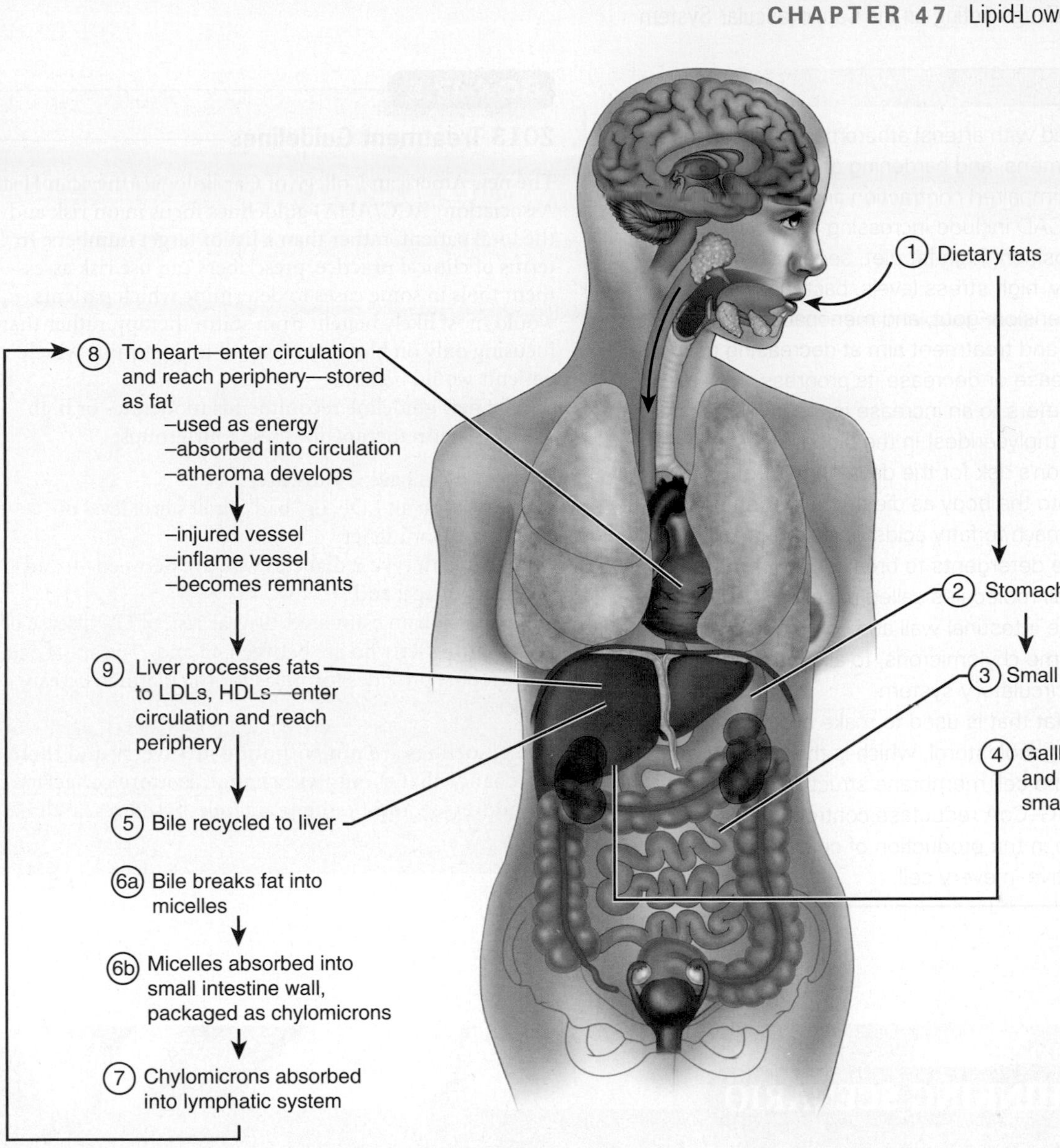

FIGURE 47.1 Metabolism of fats in the body.

Hyperlipidemias

When the levels of lipids in the blood increase, hyperlipidemia occurs. This can result from excessive dietary intake of fats or from genetic alterations in fat metabolism leading to a variety of elevated fats in the blood (e.g., hypercholesterolemia, hypertriglyceridemia, alterations in LDL and HDL concentrations). Cultural variations related to lipid levels also have been identified (Box 47.4).

Dietary modifications are often successful in treating hyperlipidemia that is caused by excessive dietary intake of fats. Drug therapy is needed if the cause is genetically linked alterations in lipid levels or if dietary limits do not decrease the serum lipid levels to an acceptable range. Box 47.5 gives the current standard guidelines for lipid levels. Antihyperlipidemic agents such as bile acid sequestrants, HMG–CoA inhibitors, fibrates, niacin, or cholesterol absorption inhibitors may be used. These drugs are often used in combination and should be part of an overall health care regimen that includes exercise, dietary restrictions, and lifestyle changes.

See the Critical Thinking Scenario for additional information on treating hyperlipidemia.

BOX 47.4 FOCUS ON **Cultural Considerations**

Rosuvastatin and Asian Americans

Rosuvastatin reaches higher serum levels in Asian Americans than in other populations. Higher serum levels are associated with an increased risk for rhabdomyolysis. It is recommended that this drug be reserved for use in non-Asian patients.

KEY POINTS

- CAD is associated with arterial atheromas or plaques, narrowed arterial lumens, and hardening of the artery wall, all of which lead to impaired contraction and vascular dilation.
- Risk factors for CAD include increasing age, male gender, genetic predisposition, high-fat diet, sedentary lifestyle, smoking, obesity, high stress levels, bacterial infections, diabetes, hypertension, gout, and menopause.
- CAD prevention and treatment aim at decreasing risk factors to delay disease or decrease its progress.
- Hyperlipidemia refers to an increase in the level of lipids (cholesterol and triglycerides) in the blood. Hyperlipidemia increases a person's risk for the development of CAD.
- Fats are taken into the body as dietary fats, then broken down in the stomach to fatty acids, lipids, and cholesterol.
- Bile acids act like detergents to break down or metabolize fats into small molecules called micelles, which are absorbed into the intestinal wall and combined with proteins to become chylomicrons, to allow transport throughout the circulatory system.
- Cholesterol is a fat that is used to make bile acids; all cells can produce cholesterol, which is the base for steroid hormones and cell membrane structure.
- The enzyme HMG–CoA reductase controls the early rate-limiting step in the production of cellular cholesterol; HMG–CoA is active in every cell.

BOX 47.5

2013 Treatment Guidelines

The new American College of Cardiology/American Heart Association (ACC/AHA) guidelines focus in on risk and the total patient, rather than a list of target numbers. In terms of clinical practice, prescribers can use risk assessment tools in some cases to determine which patients would most likely benefit from statin therapy, rather than focusing only on blood cholesterol to determine which patients would benefit.

The new guideline recommends moderate- or high-intensity statin therapy for these four groups:

- Patients who have CV disease;
- Patients with an LDL, or "bad" cholesterol level of 190 mg/dL or higher;
- Patients with type 2 diabetes who are between 40 and 75 years of age; and
- Patients with an estimated 10-year risk of CV disease of 7.5% or higher who are between 40 and 75 years of age (the report provides formulas for calculating 10-year risk).

The guidelines are not without controversy and there is a chance that things will change as more concerns are addressed and further evidence-based research is done.

CRITICAL THINKING SCENARIO

Treating Hyperlipidemia

THE SITUATION

M.M., a 55-year-old white businessman, was seen for a routine insurance physical examination. He was found to be obese and borderline hypertensive, with a nonfasting LDL level of 325 mg/dL (very high). M.M. reported smoking two packs of cigarettes a day and noted in his family history that both of his parents died of heart attacks before age 50 years. He described himself as a "workaholic" with no time to exercise and a tendency to eat most of his meals in restaurants. The primary medical regimen suggested for M.M. included ceasing or decreasing smoking, weight loss, dietary changes to eliminate saturated fats, and decreased stress. On a return visit after 4 weeks, M.M. had lost 7 pounds and reported a decrease in smoking, but his LDL levels were unchanged. The use of an antihyperlipidemic drug was discussed. He was started on atorvastatin and advised to continue the diet and exercise program and to return in 3 months for follow-up.

CRITICAL THINKING

What nursing interventions are appropriate at this point? *Consider all of the known risk factors for CAD; then rank M.M.'s risk based on those factors.*

What lifestyle changes can help M.M. to reduce his risk of heart disease?

What support services should be consulted to help M.M.?

Should other tests be done before considering any drug therapy for M.M.? *Think about the kind of patient teaching that would help M.M. to cope with the overwhelming lifestyle changes that have been suggested, yet remain compliant with his medical regimen.*

Treating Hyperlipidemia (continued)

DISCUSSION

M.M.'s description of himself as a workaholic should alert the nurse to the possibility that he will have trouble adapting to any prescribed lifestyle changes. (Workaholics tend to be very organized, goal-driven, and somewhat controlling individuals.) M.M. should first receive extensive teaching about CAD, his risk factors, and his options. The benefits of decreasing or eliminating risk factors should be discussed. Drug therapy is intended as an adjunct to diet and exercise, and the effectiveness of drug therapy improves remarkably when diet and exercise changes are made. M.M. may be more compliant if he exercises some control over his situation, so he should be invited to suggest possible lifestyle changes or adaptations. M.M. also should be encouraged to set short-range goals that are achievable, to help him feel successful. He needs to understand that beginning drug therapy does not mean that exercise and diet are no longer important.

M.M. also needs to understand that antihyperlipidemic drugs can cause dizziness, headaches, gastrointestinal (GI) upset, and constipation. Because of his busy lifestyle, M.M. may have trouble coping with these adverse effects. M.M.'s health care provider may need to try a variety of different drugs or combinations of drugs to find ones that are effective but do not cause unacceptable adverse effects.

The American Heart Association (AHA) has numerous booklets, diets, support groups, and counselors who can help M.M. as he tries to adapt to his medical regimen. He can contact the AHA online at http://www.americanheart.org for a quick reference and referrals to other sources. M.M. will benefit from having a consistent health care provider who can offer him encouragement, answer any questions, and allow him to vent his feelings. Often, lifestyle changes are the most difficult part of this medical regimen, so M.M. will need constant support.

NURSING CARE GUIDE FOR M.M.: HMG–CoA REDUCTASE INHIBITORS

Assessment: History and Examination

Assess M.M.'s health history for allergies to any HMG–CoA reductase inhibitor or fungal byproducts; hepatic dysfunction; or endocrine disorders.

Focus the physical examination on the following areas:

Cardiovascular (CV): Blood pressure, pulse, perfusion
Central nervous system (CNS): Orientation, affect, reflexes, vision
Skin: Color, lesions, texture
Respiratory system: Rate, adventitious sounds
GI: Abdominal examination, bowel sounds
Laboratory tests: Liver and renal function tests, serum lipids

Nursing Diagnoses

Disturbed sensory perception related to CNS effects
Risk for injury related to CNS, liver, and renal effects
Acute pain related to headache, myalgia, and GI effects
Deficient knowledge regarding drug therapy

Planning

The patient will receive the best therapeutic effect from the drug therapy.

The patient will have limited adverse effects to the drug therapy.

The patient will have an understanding of the drug therapy, adverse effects to anticipate, and measures to relieve discomfort and improve safety.

Implementation

Administer the drug at bedtime.
Monitor serum lipids prior to therapy and periodically during therapy.
Provide comfort and safety measures: Give small meals.
Arrange for periodic ophthalmic exams to screen for cataracts.
Give the drug with food if GI upset occurs.
Institute bowel program as needed.
Provide safety measures if needed.
Monitor liver function, and arrange to stop the drug if liver impairment occurs.
Provide support and reassurance to deal with drug effects and the need to make lifestyle, diet, and exercise changes.
Provide patient teaching regarding drug, dosage, adverse effects, what to report, and safety precautions.

Evaluation

Evaluate drug effects: Lowering of serum cholesterol and lipid levels, prevention of first myocardial infarction (MI), slowed progression of CAD.
Monitor for adverse effects: Sedation, dizziness, headache, cataracts, GI upset; hepatic or renal dysfunction; rhabdomyolysis.
Monitor for drug–drug interactions as indicated for each drug.
Evaluate the effectiveness of the patient-teaching program.
Evaluate the effectiveness of comfort and safety measures.

(continues on page 810)

Treating Hyperlipidemia (continued)

PATIENT TEACHING FOR M.M.

- An HMG–CoA reductase inhibitor, or "statin," is an antihyperlipidemic agent, which means that it works to decrease the levels of certain lipids, or fats, in your blood. An increase in serum lipid levels has been associated with the development of many blood vessel disorders, including CAD, which can lead to a heart attack. This drug must be used in conjunction with a low-calorie, low-saturated-fat diet and an exercise program.
- Some of the following adverse effects may occur:
  - *Headache, blurred vision, nervousness, insomnia*: Avoid driving or performing hazardous or delicate tasks that require concentration; these effects may pass with time.
  - *Nausea, vomiting, flatulence, constipation*: Small, frequent meals may help. If constipation becomes a problem, consult with your health care provider for appropriate interventions.
- Report any of the following to your health care provider: *Severe GI upset, vision changes, unusual bleeding, dark urine or light-colored stools, or sudden muscle pain accompanied by fever.*
- You will need to have regular medical examinations to monitor the effectiveness of this drug on your lipid levels and to detect any adverse effects. These examinations will include blood tests and eye examinations.
- Avoid grapefruit juice while you are taking this drug.
- Tell any doctor, nurse, or other health care provider that you are taking this drug.
- Keep this drug, and all medications, out of the reach of children.
- To help to decrease your risk of heart disease, follow these guidelines: Adhere to a diet that is low in calories and saturated fat, exercise regularly, stop smoking, and reduce stress.

Lipid-Lowering Agents

Lipid-lowering agents lower the serum levels of cholesterol and various lipids. These include bile acid sequestrants, HMG–CoA reductase inhibitors, and a cholesterol absorption inhibitor. Other drugs that are used to affect lipid levels do not fall into any of the classes but are also approved for use in combination to lower lipid levels with changes in diet and exercise (see Other Lipid-Lowering Agents). Box 47.6 summarizes the use of lipid-lowering agents in different age groups.

Bile Acid Sequestrants

Bile acid sequestrants are used to decrease plasma cholesterol levels. Three bile acid sequestrants currently in use are cholestyramine (generic), colestipol (*Colestid*), and colesevelam (*WelChol*).

BOX 47.6 FOCUS ON Drug Therapy Across the Lifespan

Lipid-Lowering Agents

CHILDREN

Familial hypercholesterolemia may be seen in children. Because of the importance of lipids in the developing nervous system, treatment is usually restricted to tight dietary restrictions to limit fats and calories.

Clofibrate has been used to treat genetic hypercholesterolemia that is unresponsive to dietary restrictions. The HMG–CoA inhibitors lovastatin, simvastatin, and atorvastatin can be used in postmenarchal girls and boys 10 to 17 years of age for treating familial hypercholesterolemia. Pravastatin has been approved for use in children older than 8 years of age, but these children should be monitored very closely.

ADULTS

Lifestyle changes, including dietary restrictions, exercise, smoking cessation, and stress reduction, should be tried before any antihyperlipidemic drug is used.

HMG–CoA reductase inhibitors are the first drug of choice in the treatment of hypercholesterolemia in patients who are at risk for, or who have already developed, CAD. The drugs are well tolerated and less expensive than some of the other antihyperlipidemic drugs. Combination therapy with a bile acid sequestrant, a fibrate, or niacin may be necessary if lipid levels still cannot be reduced.

Women of childbearing age should not take HMG–CoA reductase inhibitors (pregnancy category X). Bile acid sequestrants are the drug of choice for these women if a lipid-lowering agent is needed.

OLDER ADULTS

No outcome data are available to prove the impact of lipid-lowering agents in decreasing the incidence of MI or cardiac death in the older population.

Lifestyle changes, including dietary restrictions, exercise, smoking cessation, and stress reduction, should be tried before any antihyperlipidemic drug is used.

Lower doses of HMG–CoA reductase inhibitors should be used in elderly patients and in any patient with renal dysfunction. Care must be taken with those drugs that cannot be cut, crushed, or chewed. Patients should be alerted about these restrictions.

Therapeutic Actions and Indications

Bile acid sequestrants bind with bile acids in the intestine to form an insoluble complex that is then excreted in the feces (Figure 47.2). Bile acids contain high levels of cholesterol. As a result the liver must use cholesterol to make more bile acids. The hepatic intracellular cholesterol level falls, leading to an increased absorption of cholesterol-containing LDL segments from circulation to replenish the cell's cholesterol. The serum levels of cholesterol and LDL decrease as the circulating cholesterol is used to provide the cholesterol that the liver needs to make bile acids. These drugs are used to reduce serum cholesterol in patients with primary hypercholesterolemia (manifested by high cholesterol and high LDLs) as an adjunct to diet and exercise. Cholestyramine is also used to treat pruritus associated with partial biliary obstruction. See Table 47.3 for Usual Indications for each of these drugs.

Pharmacokinetics

Bile acid sequestrants are not absorbed systemically. They act while in the intestine and are excreted directly in the feces. Their action is limited to their effects while they are present in the intestine. Cholestyramine is a powder that must be mixed with liquids and taken up to six times a day. Colestipol is available in both powder and tablet form and is taken only four times a day. Colesevelam is available in tablet form and is taken once or twice a day.

Contraindications and Cautions

Bile acid sequestrants are contraindicated in the presence of allergy to any bile acid sequestrant *to prevent*

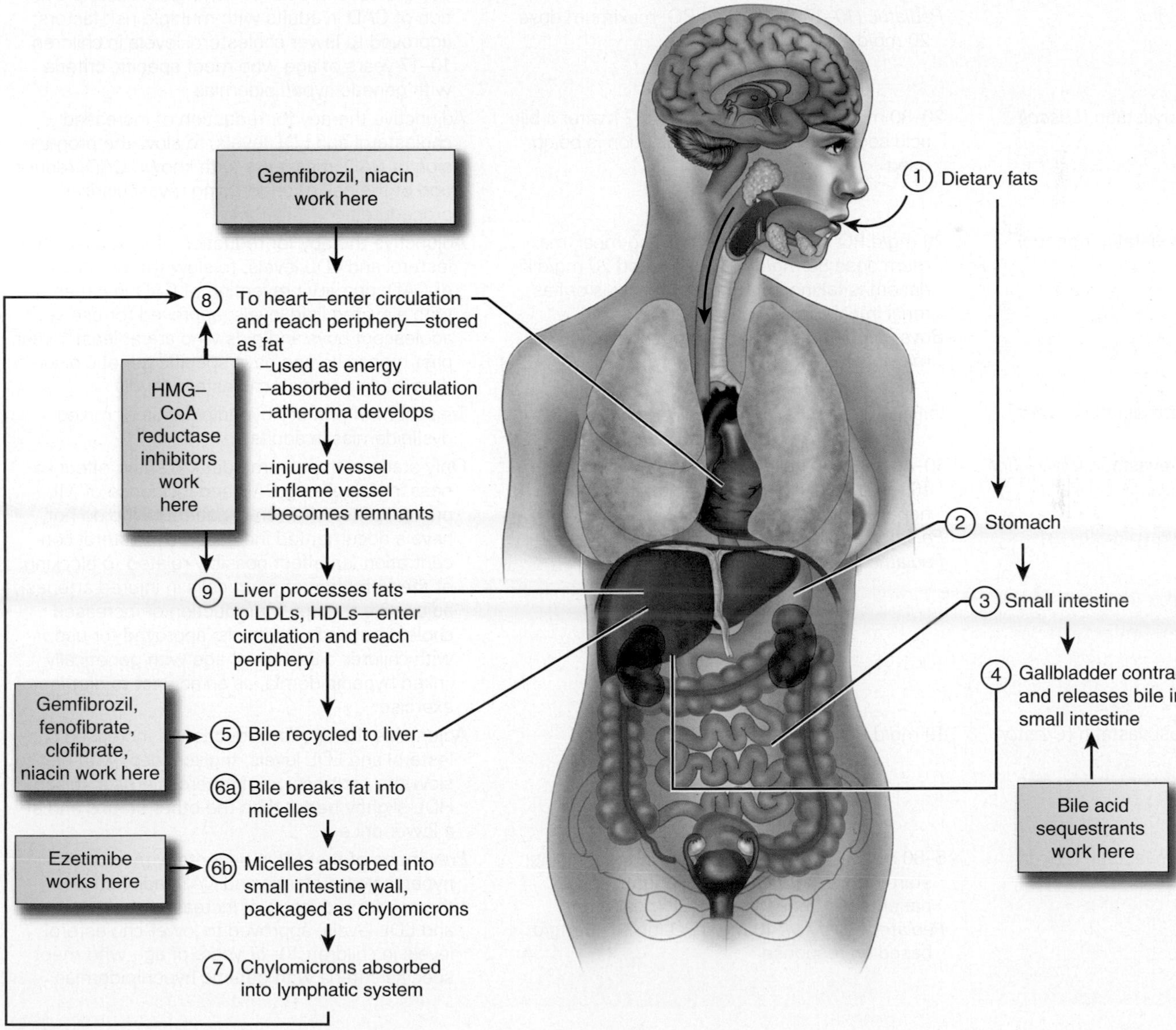

FIGURE 47.2 Sites of action of lipid-lowering agents.

Table 47.3 *Drugs in Focus:* Lipid-Lowering Drugs

Drug Name	Usual Dosage	Usual Indications
Bile Acid Sequestrants		
cholestyramine (generic)	4 g PO one to two times per day, maximum dose 24 g/d; must be mixed with water or other noncarbonated fluids	Adjunctive treatment of primary hypercholesterolemia; treatment of pruritus associated with partial biliary obstruction
colesevelam (*Welchol*)	Three 625-mg tablets taken twice a day with meals, or six tablets taken once daily with a meal	Adjunctive treatment with diet and exercise to reduce LDLs in patients with familial hypercholesterolemia; may be combined with an HMG–CoA reductase inhibitor
colestipol (*Colestid*)	*Granule form:* 5–30 g/d PO; may be taken in divided doses; must be mixed in water or other liquid *Tablet form:* 2–16 g/d PO taken once or in divided doses; tablets must not be cut, crushed, or chewed	Adjunctive treatment of primary hypercholesterolemia
HMG–CoA Reductase Inhibitors		
atorvastatin (*Lipitor*)	10 mg/d PO with a possible dose range of 10–80 mg/d; may be taken at any time of day *Pediatric (10–17 y):* 10 mg/d PO, maximum dose 20 mg/d	Adjunctive therapy for reduction of increased cholesterol and LDL levels, triglycerides; prevention of CAD in adults with multiple risk factors; approved to lower cholesterol levels in children 10–17 years of age who meet specific criteria with genetic hyperlipidemias
fluvastatin (*Lescol*)	20–80 mg PO, taken at bedtime; >2 h after a bile acid sequestrant, if this combination is being used	Adjunctive therapy for reduction of increased cholesterol and LDL levels; to slow the progression of CAD in patients with known CAD; reduction of the risk of undergoing revascularization procedures
lovastatin (generic)	20 mg/d PO taken with the evening meal; maximum dose 80 mg/d; do not exceed 20 mg/d if patient is taking immunosuppressives or has renal impairment *Boys and girls 1 y postmenarche:* 20 mg/d PO, may increase to 80 mg/d	Adjunctive therapy for reduction of increased cholesterol and LDL levels; to slow the progression of CAD; primary prevention of CAD in patients with elevated lipid levels; approved for use with adolescent boys and girls who are at least 1 year past menarche and have specific genetic disorders leading to high cholesterol levels
pitavastatin (*Livalo*)	Initially, 2 mg/d PO, range 1–4 mg/d PO	Treatment of primary hyperlipidemia or mixed dyslipidemias in adults
pravastatin (*Pravachol*)	10–40 mg/d PO taken at bedtime; start with 10 mg/d in elderly patients and patients with hepatic or renal impairment *Pediatric (8–13 y):* 20 mg/d PO *Pediatric (14–18 y):* 40 mg/d PO	Only statin with outcome data to show effectiveness in decreasing CAD and incidence of MI; prevents first MI even in patients who do not have a documented increased cholesterol concentration (an effect possibly related to blocking of the formation of foam cells in injured arteries); adjunctive therapy for reduction of increased cholesterol and LDL levels; approved for use with children >8 years of age with genetically linked hyperlipidemia, as an adjunct to diet in exercise
rosuvastatin (*Crestor*)	10 mg/d PO initial dose range; 5–40 mg/d	Adjunctive therapy for reduction of increased cholesterol and LDL levels, triglycerides; with diet to slow the progression of atherosclerosis; raises HDL slightly better than the other statins and at a lower price
simvastatin (*Zocor*)	5–80 mg/d PO taken once a day in the evening; start with 5 mg/d in elderly patients and in patients with hepatic or renal impairment *Pediatric (10–17 y):* 10 mg/d PO, up to 40 mg/d based on response	Prevention of first MI in patients with known hypercholesterolemia and CAD; adjunctive therapy for reduction of increased cholesterol and LDL levels; approved to lower cholesterol levels in children 10–17 years of age who meet specific criteria with genetic hyperlipidemias

Drug Name	Usual Dosage	Usual Indications
Cholesterol Absorption Inhibitor		
ezetimibe (*Zetia*)	10 mg/d PO	Adjunct to diet and exercise to reduce cholesterol as monotherapy or combined with an HMG–CoA inhibitor or a bile acid sequestrant; adjunct to diet to reduce elevated sitosterol and campesterol levels in homozygous sitosterolemia (to reduce elevated sitosterol and campesterol levels, the enzymes that are elevated when patients have this rare disorder); used in combination with atorvastatin or simvastatin as treatment for homozygous familial hypercholesterolemia
Other Lipid-Lowering Agents ***Fibrates***		
fenofibrate (*TriCor*)	67 mg/d PO given with a meal; may be increased up to 67 mg PO t.i.d. as needed; monitor patients with impaired renal function and the elderly very carefully	Treatment of very high triglyceride levels in adults who are at risk for pancreatitis if not responsive to dietary measures
fenofibric acid (*Trilipix*)	45–135 mg/d PO	Treatment of hypertriglyceridemia or to reduce lipid levels in mixed hyperlipidemia not responsive to other therapies: with a statin to reduce triglyceride levels and raise HDL levels in mixed hyperlipidemias with high risk for CAD
gemfibrozil (*Lopid*)	1,200 mg/d PO divided into two doses and taken before the morning and evening meals	Treatment of very high triglyceride levels with abdominal pain and potential pancreatitis in adults
Vitamin B		
niacin (*Niacor*, *Niaspan*)	1.5–2 g/d PO in divided doses for tablets; 500–2,000 mg/d PO for ER tablets taken at bedtime	Treatment of hyperlipidemia not responding to diet and weight loss; to slow progression of CAD when combined with a bile acid sequestrant
Omega-3 Fatty Acids		
omega-3-acid ethyl esters (*Lovaza*)	4 g/d PO	Adjunct to diet to reduce very high triglycerides
omega-3-carboxylic acids (*Epanova*)	2–4 g/d PO	Adjunct to diet to reduce very high triglycerides

LDL, low-density lipoproteins; HMG–CoA, hydroxymethylglutaryl–coenzyme A; CAD, coronary artery disease; MI, myocardial infarction; HDL, high-density lipoproteins; ER, extended release.

hypersensitivity reactions. These drugs also are contraindicated in the following conditions: Complete biliary obstruction, *which would prevent bile from being secreted into the intestine*; abnormal intestinal function, *which could be aggravated by the presence of these drugs*; and pregnancy or lactation *because the potential decrease in the absorption of fat and fat-soluble vitamins could have a detrimental effect on the fetus or neonate*. If a lipid-lowering drug is needed, however, a bile acid sequestrant is the drug of choice.

Adverse Effects

Adverse effects associated with the use of these drugs include headache, anxiety, fatigue, and drowsiness, which could be related to changes in serum cholesterol levels. Direct GI irritation, including nausea, constipation that may progress to fecal impaction, and aggravation of hemorrhoids, may occur. Other effects include increased bleeding times related to a decreased absorption of vitamin K and consequent decreased production of clotting factors; vitamin A and D deficiencies related to decreased absorption of fat-soluble vitamins; rash; and muscle aches and pains.

Clinically Important Drug–Drug Interactions

Malabsorption of fat-soluble vitamins occurs when they are combined with these drugs. These drugs decrease or delay the absorption of thiazide diuretics, digoxin, warfarin, thyroid hormones, and corticosteroids. Consequently, any of these drugs should be taken 1 hour before or 4 to 6 hours after the bile acid sequestrant.

Ⓟ Prototype Summary: Cholestyramine

Indications: Reduction of elevated serum cholesterol in patients with primary hypercholesterolemia; pruritus associated with partial biliary obstruction.

Actions: Binds with bile acids in the intestine, allowing excretion in the feces instead of reabsorption, causing cholesterol to be oxidized in the liver and serum cholesterol levels to fall.

Pharmacokinetics: Not absorbed systemically.

$T_{1/2}$: Not absorbed systemically; excreted in the feces.

Adverse Effects: Rash, headache, anxiety, vertigo, dizziness, constipation due to fecal impaction, exacerbation of hemorrhoids, cramps, flatulence, nausea, increased bleeding tendencies, vitamin A and D deficiencies, muscle and joint pain.

Nursing Considerations for Patients Receiving Bile Acid Sequestrants

Assessment: History and Examination

- Assess for contraindications or cautions: Known allergies to these drugs *to avoid hypersensitivity reactions*; impaired intestinal function, *which could be exacerbated by these drugs*; biliary obstruction, *which could block the effectiveness of these drugs*; and current status related to pregnancy and lactation *because of the potential for adverse effects on the fetus or nursing baby*.
- Perform a physical assessment *to establish a baseline before beginning therapy and during therapy to determine the effectiveness of therapy and evaluate for any potential adverse effects*.
- Weigh the patient *to establish a baseline and evaluate for changes reflecting lifestyle changes that accompany drug therapy*.
- Inspect the patient's skin for color, bruising, and rash *to evaluate for possible adverse effects*.
- Assess neurological status, including level of orientation and alertness, *to determine any CNS effects*.
- Monitor pulse and blood pressure *for changes related to changes in CAD risk factors*.
- Inspect the abdomen for distention and auscultate bowel sounds *for changes in GI motility*.
- Assess bowel elimination patterns, including frequency of stool passage and stool characteristics, *to identify possible constipation and fecal impaction*.
- Monitor the results of laboratory tests, including serum cholesterol and lipid levels, *to evaluate the effectiveness of drug therapy*.

Nursing Diagnoses

Nursing diagnoses related to drug therapy might include the following:

- Acute pain related to headache and GI effects
- Constipation related to GI effects
- Risk for injury related to CNS changes and potential for bleeding
- Deficient knowledge regarding drug therapy

Planning

- The patient will receive the best therapeutic effect from the drug therapy.
- The patient will have limited adverse effects to the drug therapy.
- The patient will have an understanding of the drug therapy, adverse effects to anticipate, and measures to relieve discomfort and improve safety

Implementation with Rationale

- Do not administer powdered agents in dry form; *these drugs must be mixed in fluids to be effective*. Mix with fruit juices, soups, liquids, cereals, or pulpy fruits. Mix colestipol, but not cholestyramine, with carbonated beverages. Stir, and encourage the patient to swallow all of the dose.
- If the patient is taking tablets, ensure that tablets are not cut, chewed, or crushed *because they are designed to be broken down in the GI tract; if they are crushed, the active ingredients will not be effective*. Urge the patient to swallow tablets whole with plenty of fluid.
- Give the drug before meals *to ensure that the drug is in the GI tract with food*.
- Administer other oral medications 1 hour before or 4 to 6 hours after the bile sequestrant *to avoid drug–drug interactions*.
- Arrange for a bowel program as appropriate *to effectively deal with constipation if it occurs*.
- Provide comfort measures *to help the patient tolerate the drug effects*. These include small, frequent meals to reduce the risk of nausea; ready access to bathroom facilities to prevent constipation; safety precautions to prevent injury if dizziness, CNS changes, or bleeding is a problem; replacement of fat-soluble vitamins; skin care as needed; and analgesics for headache.
- Offer support and encouragement *to help the patient deal with the diagnosis and the drug regimen and lifestyle changes that may be necessary*; refer the patient to services that might help with the high cost of these drugs.
- Provide thorough patient teaching, including the name of the drug, dosage prescribed, and schedule for administration; method to administer the drug, such as mixing the powder form in fluids or taking tablets whole (without crushing, chewing, or cutting); appropriate fluids for mixing drug; measures to avoid adverse

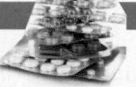

effects, warning signs of problems, and the need for follow-up laboratory testing to monitor cholesterol and lipid levels; dietary and lifestyle changes for risk reduction; and monitoring and evaluation *to enhance patient knowledge about drug therapy and to promote compliance.*

Evaluation

- Monitor patient response to the drug as appropriate (reduction in serum cholesterol levels).
- Monitor for adverse effects (headache, vitamin deficiency, increased bleeding times, constipation, nausea, rash).
- Evaluate the effectiveness of the teaching plan (patient can name drug, dosage, adverse effects to watch for, and specific measures to avoid them; patient understands the importance of continued follow-up).
- Monitor the effectiveness of comfort measures and compliance with the regimen.

KEY POINTS

- Bile acid sequestrants prevent the reabsorption of bile salts, which are very high in cholesterol. Consequently, the liver will pull cholesterol from the blood to make new bile acids, lowering the serum cholesterol level.
- Patients receiving bile acid sequestrants need to learn how to mix the powders, or, if taking the tablet form, the importance of swallowing the tablet whole and not cutting, crushing, or chewing it. Doses should not be taken with other drugs to avoid problems with absorption.
- GI problems are often reported when using bile acid sequestrants, including nausea, bloating, and constipation.

HMG–CoA Reductase Inhibitors

The HMG–CoA reductase inhibitors include atorvastatin (*Lipitor*), fluvastatin (*Lescol*), lovastatin (generic), pitavastatin (*Livalo*), pravastatin (*Pravachol*), rosuvastatin (*Crestor*), and simvastatin (*Zocor*).

Therapeutic Actions and Indications

The early rate-limiting step in the synthesis of cellular cholesterol involves the enzyme HMG–CoA reductase. If this enzyme is blocked, serum cholesterol and LDL levels decrease because more LDLs are absorbed by the cells for processing into cholesterol. In contrast, HDL levels increase slightly with this alteration in fat metabolism. HMG–CoA reductase inhibitors block HMG–CoA reductase from completing the synthesis of cholesterol (see Figure 47.2). Most of these drugs are chemical modifications of compounds produced by fungi. As a group, they are frequently referred to as "statins." Because these drugs undergo a marked first-pass effect in the liver, most of their effects are seen in the liver (see Adverse Effects). These drugs may also have some effects on the process that generates atheromas in vessel walls. That exact mechanism of action is not understood. These drugs are indicated as adjuncts with diet and exercise for the treatment of increased cholesterol and LDL levels that are unresponsive to dietary restrictions alone.

Pravastatin, lovastatin (one of the oldest HMG–CoA drugs available), and simvastatin are indicated for patients with documented CAD to slow progression of the disease. These three agents and atorvastatin are used to prevent a first MI in patients who have multiple risk factors for developing CAD. Table 47.3 discusses Usual Indications for each of the HMG–CoA reductase inhibitors. Several of the statin drugs have been formulated as combination therapy. Examples of combination therapy are highlighted in Box 47.7.

Pharmacokinetics

The statins are all absorbed from the GI tract and undergo first-pass metabolism in the liver. They are excreted through the feces and urine. The peak effect of these drugs is usually seen within 2 to 4 weeks. These drugs are most effective when taken at night when the liver is processing the most lipids. These drugs cross the placenta, and most have been found in breast milk.

Contraindications and Cautions

These drugs are contraindicated in the presence of allergy to any of the statins or to fungal byproducts or compounds *to avoid hypersensitivity reactions.* Statins also are contraindicated in patients with active liver disease or a history of alcoholic liver disease, *which could be exacerbated, leading to severe liver failure*, and with pregnancy or lactation, *because of the potential for adverse effects on the fetus or neonate.* These drugs are labeled as pregnancy category X.

Atorvastatin levels are not affected by renal disease, but patients with renal impairment who are taking other statins require close monitoring *since rhabdomyolysis, a potential adverse effect associated with these drugs, can be very harmful to the kidneys.* Caution should be used in patients with impaired endocrine function *because of the potential alteration in the formation of steroid hormones.*

Adverse Effects

The most common adverse effects associated with these drugs reflect their effects on the GI system: Flatulence, abdominal pain, cramps, nausea, vomiting, and constipation. CNS effects can include headache, dizziness, blurred vision, insomnia, fatigue, and cataract development and may reflect changes in the cell membrane and synthesis of cholesterol. Increased concentrations of liver enzymes commonly occur, and acute liver failure has been reported with the use of atorvastatin and fluvastatin (Figure 47.3). Lovastatin, pravastatin, and simvastatin are not associated

BOX 47.7

Combination and Other Therapies for Treating Coronary Artery Disease

In 2002 the FDA approved *Advicor*, a fixed combination of extended release niacin and lovastatin, for reducing the risk of atherosclerosis in patients with multiple risk factors. It was thought that the convenience of taking one tablet each day in the evening would improve patient compliance with the lipid-lowering therapy.

The drug is not intended as initial therapy. It should be used only after the patient has been stabilized on lovastatin and extended-release niacin and found to tolerate the combination and to have acceptable lower cholesterol levels.

The drug is available in three strengths: 500-mg niacin/20-mg lovastatin, 750-mg niacin/20-mg lovastatin, and 1,000-mg niacin/20-mg lovastatin. The contraindications and cautions for both niacin and lovastatin apply to this drug, and patient teaching should incorporate the same warnings about adverse effects that are used with both agents.

Combination Drugs for Treating CAD

- *Caduet* is a combination of 5- or 10-mg amlodipine and 10-, 20-, 40-, or 80-mg atorvastatin. The patient should first be stabilized on the individual drugs before the correct combination is selected. The combination provides the blood pressure–lowering and antianginal effect of the amlodipine with the lipid-lowering effects of the atorvastatin. The usual adult dose is 5- to 10-mg amlodipine with 10- to 80-mg atorvastatin, based on patient response. The recommended dose in children 10 to 17 years of age is 2.5- to 5-mg amlodipine with 10- to 20-mg atorvastatin.
- *Vytorin*, introduced in 2005, is a combination of ezetimibe and simvastatin, and was approved to help lower lipid levels in patients who did not have good results with single-drug therapy. Ezetimibe decreases the absorption of cholesterol, and simvastatin decreases the body's production of cholesterol. The drug is available in tablets that contain 10-mg ezetimibe and 10-, 20-, 40-, or 80-mg simvastatin. Dose should be determined based on lipid levels. The ENHANCE study reported disappointing effectiveness of this combination.
- *Simcor* is a combination of simvastatin and niacin. The tablets are available as 500- or 750-mg niacin with 20-mg simvastatin. The usual adult dose is a maximum of 2,000-mg niacin with 40-mg simvastatin if needed.
- *Liptruzet* is a combination of ezetimibe (10 mg) with atorvastatin (10, 20, 40, or 80 mg). The usual oral dose is one tablet in the evening. If the patient is also on a bile acid sequestrant, this drug should be given 2 hours before or 4 hours after the bile acid sequestrant.

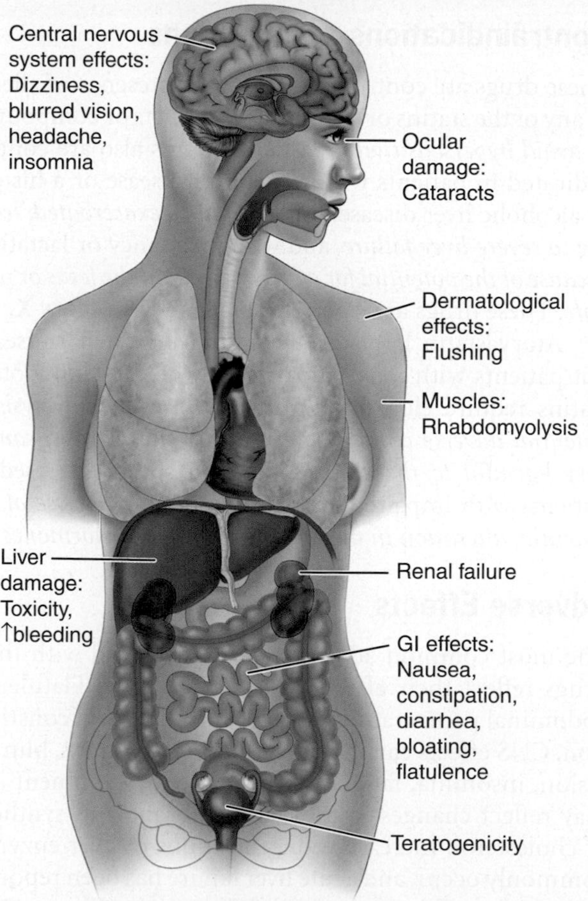

FIGURE 47.3 Variety of adverse effects and toxicities associated with lipid-lowering drugs.

with some of the severe liver toxicity that is seen with the other agents. Rhabdomyolysis, a breakdown of muscles whose waste products can injure the glomerulus and cause acute renal failure, has also occurred with the use of all of these drugs. Rosuvastatin is associated with increased occurrence of rhabdomyolysis in Asian American patients and that should be taken into consideration when picking a statin for those patients. In 2011, studies showed that patients using the highest dose of simvastatin, 80 mg, had increased incidence of CV events and the U.S. Food and Drug Administration (FDA) sent out warnings that the 80-mg dose of simvastatin should not be started on any new patients and only continued if patients taking it had been doing so without adverse effects.

Clinically Important Drug–Drug Interactions

The risk for rhabdomyolysis increases if any of these drugs is combined with erythromycin, cyclosporine, gemfibrozil, niacin, or antifungal drugs; such combinations should be avoided.

Increased serum levels and resultant toxicity can occur if these drugs are combined with digoxin or warfarin; if this combination is used, serum digoxin levels and/or clotting times should be monitored carefully and the prescriber consulted for appropriate dose changes.

Increased estrogen levels can occur if these drugs are taken with oral contraceptives; the patient should be monitored carefully if this combination is used.

Serum levels and the risk of toxicity increase if these drugs are combined with grapefruit juice.

FOCUS ON Safe Medication Administration

Patients who are taking HMG–CoA inhibitors need to be cautioned to avoid drinking grapefruit juice while taking these drugs. Grapefruit juice alters the metabolism of the drugs, leading to an increased serum level of drug and increased risk for adverse effects, such as the potentially fatal rhabdomyolysis with renal failure. The metabolism of the components of grapefruit juice takes about 48 hours. Since the effects may last for several days, just drinking the grapefruit juice at a different time of day does not protect the patient from risk.

Prototype Summary: Atorvastatin

Indications: Adjunct to diet in the treatment of elevated levels of cholesterol, triglycerides, and LDL; to increase HDL cholesterol in patients with primary hypercholesterolemia; treatment of boys and postmenarchal girls aged 10 to 17 years with familial hypercholesterolemia and two or more risk factors for CAD; prevention of CAD in adults without clinically evident heart disease but with multiple risk factors to reduce the risk for CV events.

Actions: Inhibits HMG–CoA, causing a decrease in serum cholesterol levels, LDLs, and triglycerides and an increase in HDL levels.

Pharmacokinetics:

Route	Onset	Peak	Duration
Oral	Slow	1–2 h	20–30 h

$T_{1/2}$: 14 hours; metabolized in the liver and cells and excreted in the bile.

Adverse Effects: Headache, flatulence, abdominal pain, cramps, constipation, rhabdomyolysis with acute renal failure.

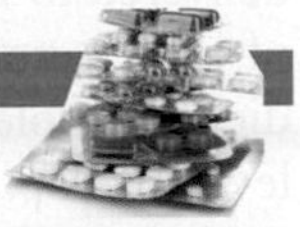

Nursing Considerations for Patients Receiving HMG–CoA Reductase Inhibitors

Assessment: History and Examination

- Assess for contraindications and cautions: Any known allergies to these drugs or to fungal byproducts *to avoid hypersensitivity reactions*; active liver disease or history of alcoholic liver disease, *which could be exacerbated by the effects of these drugs*; current status of pregnancy or lactation *because of potential adverse effects on the fetus or neonate*; and impaired endocrine function, *which could be exacerbated by effects on steroid hormones.*
- Perform a physical assessment *to establish a baseline before beginning therapy and during therapy to determine its effectiveness and evaluate for any potential adverse effects.*
- Weigh the patient *to establish a baseline and evaluate for changes reflecting lifestyle changes that accompany drug therapy.*
- Assess the patient's neurological status, including level of orientation, affect, and reflexes, which show early changes related to CNS function, *to evaluate for possible CNS effects of the drug.*
- Obtain vital signs, including pulse and blood pressure, *to identify changes.*
- Inspect the abdomen for distention and auscultate bowel sounds *for changes in GI motility.*
- Assess bowel elimination patterns, including frequency of stool passage and stool characteristics, *to identify possible constipation.*
- Monitor the results of laboratory tests, including renal and liver function tests, *to identify possible toxicity and serum lipid levels to evaluate the drug's effectiveness.*

Nursing Diagnoses

Nursing diagnoses related to drug therapy might include the following:

- Disturbed sensory perception (visual, kinesthetic, gustatory) related to CNS effects
- Risk for injury related to CNS, liver, and renal effects
- Acute pain related to headache, myalgia, and GI effects
- Deficient knowledge regarding drug therapy

Planning

- The patient will receive the best therapeutic effect from the drug therapy.
- The patient will have limited adverse effects to the drug therapy.
- The patient will have an understanding of the drug therapy, adverse effects to anticipate, and measures to relieve discomfort and improve safety.

Implementation with Rationale

- Administer the drug at bedtime *because the highest rates of cholesterol synthesis occur between midnight and 5 AM, and the drug should be taken when it will be most effective*; give atorvastatin at any time during the day.
- Monitor serum cholesterol and LDL levels before and periodically during therapy *to evaluate the effectiveness of this drug.*
- Arrange for periodic ophthalmic examinations *to monitor for cataract development.*
- Monitor liver function tests before and periodically during therapy *to monitor for liver damage*; consult with the prescriber to discontinue the drug if the aspartate aminotransferase (AST) or alanine aminotransferase (ALT) level increases to three times normal.
- Ensure that the patient has attempted a cholesterol-lowering diet and exercise program for at least 3 to 6 months before beginning therapy *to ensure the need for drug therapy.*

(continues on page 818)

- Encourage the patient to make the lifestyle changes necessary *to decrease the risk for CAD and to increase the effectiveness of drug therapy.*
- Withhold lovastatin, atorvastatin, or fluvastatin in any acute, serious medical condition (e.g., infection, hypotension, major surgery or trauma, metabolic endocrine disorders, seizures) *that might suggest myopathy or serve as a risk factor for the development of renal failure.*
- Suggest the use of barrier contraceptives for women of childbearing age *because there is a risk of severe fetal abnormalities if these drugs are taken during pregnancy.*
- Provide comfort measures *to help the patient tolerate drug effects.* These include small, frequent meals *to minimize nausea and vomiting*; access to bathroom facilities *to ensure adequate bowel evacuation*; bowel program as needed *to address constipation*; use of food with the drug if GI upset is severe *to decrease direct irritating effects*; environmental controls, such as temperature and lighting controls, *to help deal with headaches*; and safety precautions, such as lighting control and activity restrictions, to *protect the patient if vision changes and muscle effects occur.*
- Offer support and encouragement *to help the patient deal with the diagnosis, needed lifestyle changes, and the drug regimen.*
- Provide thorough patient teaching, including the name of the drug, dosage prescribed, and administration at bedtime for best effectiveness; measures to avoid adverse effects, warning signs of problems, and the need for follow-up laboratory testing to monitor cholesterol and lipid levels; importance of follow-up renal and liver function testing; dietary and lifestyle changes for risk reduction; and monitoring and evaluation, *to enhance patient knowledge about drug therapy and to promote compliance.*

See the Critical Thinking Scenario for discussion of a patient receiving an HMG–CoA inhibitor.

Evaluation

- Monitor patient response to the drug (lowering of serum cholesterol and LDL levels, prevention of first MI, slowing of progression of CAD).
- Monitor for adverse effects (headache, dizziness, blurred vision, cataracts, GI upset, liver failure, rhabdomyolysis).
- Monitor the effectiveness of comfort measures and compliance with the regimen.
- Evaluate the effectiveness of the teaching plan (patient can name drug, dosage, adverse effects to watch for, and specific measures to avoid them; patient understands the importance of continued follow-up).

KEY POINTS

- HMG–CoA reductase inhibitors, or statins, block the enzyme HMG–CoA reductase, resulting in lower serum cholesterol levels, a resultant breakdown of LDLs, and a slight increase in HDLs.
- Patients receiving HMG–CoA reductase inhibitors should avoid pregnancy because of serious fetal adverse effects; should take the drug in the evening to mimic the normal patterns of lipid formation; should have liver function monitored regularly; and should be instructed to report any sudden muscle pain, especially if accompanied by fever.

Cholesterol Absorption Inhibitors

The first of a new class of drugs to lower cholesterol levels was approved in 2003—ezetimibe (*Zetia*). Currently there is controversy about this class of cholesterol-lowering drugs because of a trial entitled "Effect of combination ezetimibe and high-dose simvastatin versus simvastatin alone on the atherosclerotic process in subjects with heterozygous familial hypercholesterolemia" (ENHANCE). This study, released in January 2008, looked at the actual postmarketing benefits of antihyperlipidemic therapy. The study failed to find any positive benefit from the addition of ezetimibe to a statin. This finding called into question the whole class of cholesterol-lowering drugs and the benefits or lack of benefits associated with this therapy (Box 47.8). Further studies are still in progress.

Therapeutic Actions and Indications

Ezetimibe works in the brush border of the small intestine to decrease the absorption of dietary cholesterol from the small intestine. As a result, less dietary cholesterol is delivered to the liver, and the liver increases the clearance of cholesterol from the serum to make up for the drop in dietary cholesterol, causing the total serum cholesterol level to drop. See Table 47.3 for Usual Indications.

Pharmacokinetics

Ezetimibe is absorbed well after oral administration, reaching peak levels in 4 to 6 hours. It is metabolized in the liver and the small intestine, with a half-life of 22 hours. Excretion is through the feces and urine. It is not known whether the drug crosses the placenta or enters breast milk.

Contraindications and Cautions

Ezetimibe is contraindicated in patients with an allergy to any component of the drug *to avoid hypersensitivity*

BOX 47.8 FOCUS ON The Evidence

The ENHANCE Study

Modifying the risk factors established through the Framingham study combined with those found in metabolic syndrome remains the key to the prevention of CAD. If, statistically, risk factors can be reduced the chances of a CV event will be smaller. The actual process of atheroma development and vessel occlusion remains elusive, and the role of cholesterol and lipids in the actual process is not clearly understood. Lowering the cholesterol and lipid levels, although putting the patient into a statistically lower risk group, does not seem to really offer much protection against CV events in patients who have not already experienced an event. Watching the television ads or reading magazine ads for the lipid-lowering drugs, you will notice a disclaimer that states that "these drugs have not been proven to reduce your risk of heart disease or heart attack."

When the ENHANCE study was published in 2008, showing that the use of ezetimibe and simvastatin did not slow the progression of atheromas, the action of other lipid-reducing drugs was called into question. The data on the effectiveness of atorvastatin claims a 36% reduction in cardiac events. Based on these data, this means that in a large study, 3% of the patients receiving no drugs suffered a cardiac event, whereas only 2% of the patients taking atorvastatin suffered a CV event. This translates into 1 less heart attack in every 100 people over a 3-year period. The other 99 people taking the drug had no measurable benefit from the drug. The number needed to treat to show effectiveness is very high. Other lipid-lowering drugs show similar or even worse statistics. Should our heath care focus so heavily, then, on lowering cholesterol and lipid levels? The publication of the JUPITER study in 2010 caused a great deal of controversy when it was ended early because of what seemed to be amazing results in preventing CV disease, but on further review, showed no effect. Those who feel health care should focus heavily on lowering lipid levels argue that, with large numbers of people using these drugs, the number of people who are saved from a CV event is actually higher. Those who are now questioning the heavy focus on lipids lowering it wonder whether the cost and adverse effects associated with the drugs are justified for benefiting such a small percentage of patients. At the moment, this seems to be the best we have to offer patients, but as more research is done on the process of CAD, standards may change.

reactions. If it is used in combination with a statin, it should not be used during pregnancy or lactation or with severe liver disease *because of the known effects of statins, including possible liver problems and renal failure.*

The drug should be used with caution as monotherapy during pregnancy or lactation *because the effects on the fetus or neonate are not known* and with elderly patients or patients with liver disease *because of the potential for adverse reactions.*

Adverse Effects

The most common adverse effects associated with ezetimibe are mild abdominal pain and diarrhea. It is not associated with the bloating and flatulence that occurs with the bile acid sequestrants and another class of lipid-lowering drugs called fibrates. Other adverse effects that have been reported include headache, dizziness, fatigue, upper respiratory tract infection (URI), back pain, and muscle aches and pains.

Clinically Important Drug–Drug Interactions

The risk of elevated serum levels of ezetimibe increases if it is given with cholestyramine, fenofibrate, gemfibrozil, or antacids. If these drugs are used in combination, ezetimibe should be taken at least 2 hours before or 4 hours after the other drugs.

The risk for toxicity also increases if ezetimibe is combined with cyclosporine. If this combination cannot be avoided the patient should be monitored very closely.

If ezetimibe is combined with any fibrate the risk of cholethiasis increases. The patient should be monitored closely.

Warfarin levels increase in a patient who is also taking ezetimibe; if this combination is used the patient should be monitored very closely.

Prototype Summary: Ezetimibe

Indications: Adjunct to diet and exercise to lower serum cholesterol levels; in combination with atorvastatin or simvastatin for the treatment of homozygous familial hypercholesterolemia; with diet for the treatment of homozygous sitosterolemia to lower sitosterol and campesterol levels.

Actions: Works in the brush border of the small intestine to inhibit the absorption of cholesterol.

Pharmacokinetics:

Route	Onset	Peak
Oral	Moderate	4–12 h

$T_{1/2}$: 22 hours; metabolized in the liver and small intestine and excreted in the feces and urine.

Adverse Effects: Headache, dizziness, abdominal pain, diarrhea, URI, back pain, myalgia, arthralgia.

Nursing Considerations for Patients Receiving Cholesterol Absorption Inhibitors

Assessment: History and Examination

- Assess for contraindications or cautions: Any known allergies to any component of the drug *to avoid hypersensitivity reactions*; liver dysfunction or advanced age *because the processing of the drug may differ from the norm*; current status of pregnancy or lactation *because the possible effects on the fetus or neonate are not known.*
- Perform a physical assessment to establish a baseline *before beginning therapy and during therapy to determine its effectiveness and evaluate for any potential adverse effects.*
- Monitor orientation and reflexes *to detect changes in CNS function, such as dizziness, that could require safety measures.*
- Monitor respirations and auscultate lungs for *evidence of adventitious sounds to monitor changes in cardiac output.*
- Inspect the abdomen for distention and auscultate bowel sounds for *changes in GI motility.*
- Assess bowel elimination patterns, including frequency of stool passage and stool characteristics, *to identify possible changes that could require intervention.*
- Monitor the results of laboratory tests, including serum cholesterol and lipid levels, *to evaluate the effectiveness of drug therapy*, and liver function studies *to monitor for toxic effects.*

Nursing Diagnoses

Nursing diagnoses related to drug therapy may include the following:

- Disturbed sensory perception (visual, kinesthetic, gustatory) related to CNS effects
- Acute pain related to headache, myalgia, and GI effects
- Deficient knowledge regarding drug therapy

Planning

- The patient will receive the best therapeutic effect from the drug therapy.
- The patient will have limited adverse effects to the drug therapy.
- The patient will have an understanding of the drug therapy, adverse effects to anticipate, and measures to relieve discomfort and improve safety.

Implementation with Rationale

- Monitor serum cholesterol, triglyceride, and LDL levels before and periodically during therapy *to evaluate the effectiveness of this drug.*
- Monitor liver function tests before and periodically during therapy *to detect possible liver damage.*
- Ensure that the patient has attempted a cholesterol-lowering diet and exercise program for at least several months before beginning therapy *to ensure the need for drug therapy.*
- Encourage the patient to make the lifestyle changes necessary *to decrease the risk of CAD and to increase the effectiveness of drug therapy.*
- Suggest the use of barrier contraceptives for women of childbearing age if the drug is being used in combination with a statin *because there is a risk of severe fetal abnormalities if these drugs are taken during pregnancy.*
- Provide comfort measures *to help the patient tolerate drug effects.* These include readily available access to bathroom facilities *to help with episodes of diarrhea*; safety precautions *to protect the patient if dizziness is an issue*; and analgesics for headache and muscle aches if appropriate.
- Offer support and encouragement *to help the patient deal with the diagnosis, needed lifestyle changes, and the drug regimen.*
- Provide thorough patient teaching, including the name of the drug, dosage prescribed, and schedule for administration; measures to avoid adverse effects, warning signs of problems, and the need for follow-up laboratory testing to monitor cholesterol and lipid levels; dietary and lifestyle changes for reducing the risk of CAD and increasing the effectiveness of drug therapy; and monitoring and evaluation *to enhance patient knowledge about drug therapy and to promote compliance.*

Evaluation

- Monitor patient response to the drug (lowering of serum cholesterol and LDL levels, lowering of sitosterol and campesterol levels).
- Monitor for adverse effects (headache, dizziness, GI pain, muscle aches and pains, upper respiratory tract infection).
- Monitor the effectiveness of comfort measures and compliance with the regimen.
- Evaluate the effectiveness of the teaching plan (patient can name drug, dosage, adverse effects to watch for, and specific measures to avoid them; patient understands the importance of continued follow-up).

KEY POINTS

- The cholesterol absorption inhibitor ezetimibe works in the brush border of the small intestine to prevent the absorption of dietary cholesterol, which leads to increased clearance of cholesterol by the liver and a resultant fall in serum cholesterol.
- Change in diet and increased exercise are very important parts of the overall treatment of a patient receiving a cholesterol absorption inhibitor.

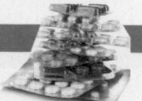

Other Lipid-Lowering Agents

Other drugs that are used to affect lipid levels do not fall into any of the classes discussed previously. They are approved for use in combination with changes in diet and exercise. They include the fibrates (derivatives of fibric acid), omega-3 fatty acids and the vitamin niacin (see Table 47.3). Other drugs have been approved only for treating familial lipid disorders.

Fibrates

The fibrates stimulate the breakdown of lipoproteins from the tissues and their removal from the plasma. They lead to a decrease in lipoprotein and triglyceride synthesis and secretion. The fibrates are absorbed from the GI tract and are metabolized in the liver and excreted in urine. Fibrates in use today include the following agents:

- Fenofibrate (*TriCor*, and others) inhibits triglyceride synthesis in the liver, resulting in reduction of LDL levels; increases uric acid secretion; and may stimulate triglyceride breakdown. It is used for adults with very high triglyceride levels who are not responsive to strict dietary measures and who are at risk for pancreatitis. Peak effects are usually seen within 4 weeks, and the patient's serum lipid levels should be reevaluated at that time.
- Gemfibrozil (*Lopid*) inhibits peripheral breakdown of lipids, reduces production of triglycerides and LDLs, and increases HDL concentrations. It is associated with GI and muscle discomfort. This drug should not be combined with statins. There is an increased risk of rhabdomyolysis from 3 weeks to several months after therapy if this combination is used. If this combination cannot be avoided the patient should be monitored very closely.
- In 2009 the FDA approved a new type of fibrate, a peroxisome proliferator receptor alpha activator. Fenofibric acid (*Trilipix*) is the first drug in this type. This drug works to activate a specific hepatic receptor that results in increased breakdown of lipids, elimination of triglyceride-rich particles from the plasma, and reduction in the production of an enzyme that naturally inhibits lipid breakdown. The result is seen as a decrease in triglyceride levels, changes in LDL production that makes them more easily broken down in the body, and an increase in HDL levels. Fenofibric acid is approved to be used in combination with a statin to reduce triglyceride levels and increase HDL levels in patients with mixed lipid disorders; as monotherapy to decrease triglyceride levels in patients with severe hypertriglyceridemia; and as monotherapy to reduce LDL, total cholesterol, and triglycerides and to increase HDL levels in patients with primary hyperlipidemia or mixed lipid disorders. Fenofibric acid is slowly absorbed from the GI tract, with peak levels occurring in 4 to 5 hours; metabolized in the liver, it has a half-life of 20 hours and is excreted in the urine. Caution should be used in patients with renal impairment, and the drug should be avoided in patients with severe renal impairment. The most common adverse effects that have been reported are headache, back pain, nausea, diarrhea, muscle pain, runny nose, and respiratory infections. Gallstones have also been reported with this drug. Patients complaining of gallstone-type pain should be screened carefully. There is an increased risk of muscle breakdown and rhabdomyolysis if taken with a statin, and patients using this combination need to be monitored closely. Caution must be used with warfarin anticoagulants; increased bleeding can occur. The patient should be monitored closely and the dose of the anticoagulant regulated to achieve therapeutic anticoagulation.

Vitamin B

Vitamin B_3, known as niacin (*Niacor, Niaspan*) or nicotinic acid, inhibits the release of free fatty acids from adipose tissue, increases the rate of triglyceride removal from plasma, and generally reduces LDL and triglyceride levels and increases HDL levels. It may also decrease the levels of apoproteins needed to form chylomicrons. The initial effect on lipid levels is usually seen within 5 to 7 days, with the maximum effect occurring in 3 to 5 weeks. Niacin is associated with intense cutaneous flushing, nausea, and abdominal pain, making its use somewhat limited. It also increases the serum levels of uric acid and may predispose patients to the development of gout. Niacin is often combined with bile acid sequestrants for increased effect. It is given at bedtime to make maximum use of nighttime cholesterol synthesis, and it must be given 4 to 6 hours after the bile sequestrant to ensure absorption.

Omega-3 Fatty Acids

- Omega-3-acid ethyl esters (*Lovaza*) is a combination of omega-3 fatty acids and an activator that inhibits liver enzyme systems to decrease the synthesis of triglycerides, a risk factor in metabolic syndrome, lowering serum triglyceride levels. It is approved to lower triglycerides in adults with very high triglyceride levels. It should be combined with appropriate diet and exercise to help keep overall lipid levels lower. It is not recommended in pregnancy or lactation. There is substantial research evidence to support the effects of this drug, unlike research on the over-the-counter fish oil products, which does not support effectiveness in lowering lipid levels. This drug may prolong bleeding time so caution must be used with any other drugs that affect bleeding. Diarrhea, nausea, abdominal pain, and discomfort are the most common adverse effects.
- Omega-3-carboxylic acids (*Epanova*) is a fish oil mixture of free fatty acids approved as an adjunct to diet to reduce triglyceride levels in adults with severe hypertriglyceridemia (500 mg/dL or over). In some patients

this drug increases LDL levels, which need to be closely monitored. Caution needs to be used in patients with hepatic impairment or allergy to fish or shellfish. These capsules have to be swallowed whole, not cut, crushed, or chewed. This drug may prolong bleeding time so caution must be used with any other drugs that affect bleeding. Diarrhea, nausea, abdominal pain, and discomfort are the most common adverse effects.

Other Therapies

In 2014, two new drugs were approved specifically for the treatment of homozygous familial hypercholesterolemia. Mipomersen (*Kynamro*) and lomitapide (*Juxtapid*) are both oral agents approved as adjuncts to diet, exercise, and other lipid-lowering therapies. Both have black box warnings regarding the potential for serious hepatotoxicity and because of this risk both are available only through a limited access program. Mipomersen inhibits apoprotein B synthesis and lomitapide inhibits the triglyceride transfer protein. Both drugs are indicated only for use with familial hypercholesterolemia and neither drug has any evidence of any effect on CV morbidity or mortality.

Combination Therapy

Frequently, if the patient shows no response to strict dietary modification, exercise, and lifestyle changes, and the use of one lipid-lowering agent, combination therapy may be initiated to achieve desirable serum LDL and cholesterol levels. For example, a bile acid sequestrant might be combined with niacin; the combination would decrease the synthesis of LDLs while lowering the serum levels of LDLs. This combination is thought to help slow the progression of CAD. Numerous fixed combination therapies are available (see Box 47.7). However, care must be taken not to combine agents that increase the risk of rhabdomyolysis. For example, HMG–CoA reductase inhibitors are not usually combined with niacin or gemfibrozil.

Future Therapies

Despite advances in treatment, CAD remains the number one killer of adults in the United States. New drugs are being investigated that would address multiple risk factors simultaneously with hopes of cutting risk successfully. The **endocannabinoids** are substances present in the body that activate various neurological receptors that seem to be very important in the body's regulation of appetite, satiety, and lipid metabolism. With blocking of the endocannabinoid system a series of changes occur that would seem to have a very profound effect on many components of the metabolic syndrome. Blocking the endocannabinoid system results in feelings of satiety and decreased appetite, leading to weight loss; decreased release of growth hormone, increased oxygen and glucose use in the muscle, decreased fat synthesis in the liver, decreased levels of triglycerides and LDLs, and increased levels of HDLs, improving the lipid profile; increased sensitivity of insulin receptor sites, leading to decreased blood glucose levels; decreased fat production and storage; increased levels of adiponectin; and decreased activity of tumor necrosis factor, a proinflammatory agent, and decreased activity of C-reactive protein, which is associated with proinflammatory and prothrombotic states.

Rimonabant is an endocannabinoid blocker that has been used in Europe as a weight loss agent. In early studies in the United States, it has been shown to significantly reduce weight and abdominal adiposity and improve lipid profiles while increasing insulin sensitivity and reducing the proinflammatory and prothrombotic markers. Approval of the drug was denied at one point because of some significant CNS changes that occur, leading to questions of safety. In April 2008, preliminary studies of the drug were published that reported no change in atherosclerosis and disease progression, despite improvement in metabolic syndrome markers, thus showing again that there is no real understanding of the process of CAD and risk modification. Further studies are being conducted with ongoing research into the endothelial lining of the blood vessels and the metabolism of the body.

KEY POINTS

- Other agents used to lower cholesterol include fibrates and niacin. Often lipid-lowering agents are used in combination to lower the cholesterol at different sites.
- Research is being done on the effects of blocking the endocannabinoid system, resulting in weight loss, improved lipid profiles, and decreased proinflammatory and prothrombotic states. Questions have not been answered about the safety or effectiveness of drugs that block this system.

SUMMARY

- CAD is the leading cause of death in the Western world. It is associated with the development of atheromas or plaques in arterial linings that lead to narrowing of the lumen of the artery and hardening of the artery wall, with loss of distensibility and responsiveness to stimuli for contraction or dilation.
- The cause of CAD is not understood, but many contributing risk factors have been identified, including increasing age, male gender, genetic predisposition, high-fat diet, sedentary lifestyle, smoking, obesity, high stress levels, bacterial infections, diabetes, hypertension, gout, and menopause. The presence of many of these factors constitutes metabolic syndrome.
- Treatment and prevention of CAD is aimed at manipulating the known risk factors to decrease CAD development and progression.

- Fats are metabolized with the aid of bile acids, which act as a detergent to break fats into small molecules called micelles. Micelles are absorbed into the intestinal wall and combined with proteins to become chylomicrons, which can be transported throughout the circulatory system.
- Some fats are used immediately for energy or are stored in adipose tissue; others are processed in the liver to LDLs, which are associated with the development of CAD. LDLs are broken down in the periphery and leave many remnants (e.g., fats) that must be removed from blood vessels. This process involves the inflammatory reaction and may initiate or contribute to atheroma production.
- Some fats are processed into HDLs, which are able to absorb fats and remnants from the periphery and offer a protective effect against the development of CAD.
- Cholesterol is an important fat that is used to make bile acids. It is the base for steroid hormones and provides the necessary structure for cell membranes. All cells can produce cholesterol.
- HMG–CoA reductase is an enzyme that controls the final step in the production of cellular cholesterol.
- Patients taking lipid-lowering drugs need to include diet, exercise, and lifestyle changes to reduce the risk of CAD.
- Bile acid sequestrants bind with bile acids in the intestine and lead to their excretion in feces. This results in lower bile acid levels as the liver uses cholesterol to produce more bile acids. The end result is a decrease in serum cholesterol and LDL levels as the liver changes its metabolism of these fats to meet the need for more bile acids.
- HMG–CoA reductase inhibitors, or statins, block the enzyme HMG–CoA reductase, resulting in lower serum cholesterol levels, a resultant breakdown of LDLs, and a slight increase in HDLs.
- The cholesterol absorption inhibitor ezetimibe works in the brush border of the small intestine to prevent the absorption of dietary cholesterol, which leads to increased clearance of cholesterol by the liver and a resultant fall in serum cholesterol.
- Other agents used to lower cholesterol include fibrates, niacin, and omega-3 fatty acids. Often lipid-lowering agents are used in combination to lower the cholesterol at different sites.
- Research is being done on the effects of blocking the endocannabinoid system, resulting in weight loss, improved lipid profiles, and decreased proinflammatory and prothrombotic states. Questions have not been answered about the safety or effectiveness of drugs that block this system.

CHECK YOUR UNDERSTANDING

Answers to the questions in this chapter can be found in Answers to Check Your Understanding Questions on thePoint®.

MULTIPLE CHOICE

Select the best answer to the following.

1. After describing to a community group the ways in which the body uses cholesterol, which of the following, if stated by the group as such as a way, indicates successful teaching?
- **a.** The production of water-soluble vitamins
- **b.** The formation of steroid hormones
- **c.** The mineralization of bones
- **d.** The development of dental plaques

2. The formation of atheromas in blood vessels precedes the signs and symptoms of
- **a.** hepatitis.
- **b.** CAD.
- **c.** diabetes mellitus.
- **d.** chronic obstructive pulmonary disease (COPD).

3. Hyperlipidemia is considered to be
- **a.** a normal finding in adult males.
- **b.** related to stress levels.
- **c.** a treatable CAD risk factor.
- **d.** a side effect of cigarette smoking.

4. The bile acid sequestrants
- **a.** are absorbed into the liver.
- **b.** take several weeks to show an effect.
- **c.** have no associated adverse effects.
- **d.** prevent bile salts from being reabsorbed.

5. HMG–CoA reductase inhibitors work in the
- **a.** process of bile secretion.
- **b.** process of cholesterol formation in the cell.
- **c.** intestinal wall to block fat absorption.
- **d.** kidney to block fat excretion.

(continues on page 824)

6. Which of the following would the nurse include when teaching a patient about HMG–CoA reductase inhibitors?
   a. The patient will not have a heart attack.
   b. The patient will not develop CAD.
   c. The patient might develop cataracts as a result.
   d. The patient might stop absorbing fat-soluble vitamins.

7. Which of the following would the nurse expect the health care provider to prescribe for a patient who has high lipid levels and cannot take fibrates or HMG–CoA reductase inhibitors?
   a. Nicotine
   b. Vitamin C
   c. Niacin
   d. Nitrates

8. Which of the following would alert the nurse to suspect that a patient receiving HMG–CoA reductase inhibitors is developing rhabdomyolysis?
   a. Flatulence and abdominal bloating
   b. Increased bleeding and bruising
   c. The development of cataracts and blurred vision
   d. Muscle pain and weakness

MULTIPLE RESPONSE

Select all that apply.

1. A bile acid sequestrant is the drug of choice for a client who has which of the following?
   a. A high LDL concentration
   b. A high triglyceride concentration
   c. Biliary obstruction
   d. Vitamin K deficiency
   e. A high HDL concentration
   f. Intolerance to statins

2. Teaching a client who is prescribed an HMG–CoA reductase inhibitor to treat high cholesterol and high lipid levels should include which of the following?
   a. The importance of exercise
   b. The need for dietary changes to alter cholesterol levels
   c. That taking a statin will allow a full, unrestricted diet
   d. That drug therapy is always needed when these levels are elevated
   e. The importance of controlling blood pressure and blood glucose levels
   f. That stopping smoking may also help to lower lipid levels

BIBLIOGRAPHY AND REFERENCES

Aronne, L. J. (2007). Therapeutic options for modifying cardiometabolic risk factors. *American Journal of Medicine, 120*(Suppl.), S26–S34.

Bray, G. (2008). *Metabolic syndrome and obesity.* Totowa, NJ: Humana Press.

Brunton, L., Chabner, B., & Knollman, B. (2011). *Goodman and Gilman's the pharmacological basis of therapeutics* (12th ed.). New York: McGraw-Hill

Facts and Comparisons. (2015). *Drug facts and comparisons.* St. Louis, MO: Author.

Gagne, J., & Choudhry, N. (2011). How many "me-too" drugs is too many? *Journal of the American Medical Association, 305*(7), 711–712.

Glynn, R., Koenig, W., Nordestgaard, B., et al. (2010). Rosuvastatin for primary prevention in older persons with elevated C-reactive protein and low to average low-density lipoprotein cholesterol levels: Exploratory analysis of a randomized trial; secondary analysis of the JUPITER study. *Annals of Internal Medicine, 152,* 488–496.

Kakafika, A. I., Mikahilidis, D. P., & Karagiannis, A. (2007). The role of the endocannabinoid system blockade in the treatment of the metabolic syndrome. *Journal of Clinical Pharmacology, 47,* 642–652.

Karch, A. M. (2014). *Lippincott's nursing drug guide.* Philadelphia, PA: Lippincott Williams & Wilkins.

Kastelen, J. J., Adkim, F., Stroes, E. S., et al. (2008). ENHANCE: Simvastatin with or without ezetimibe in familial cholesterolemia. *New England Journal of Medicine, 358,* 1431–1443.

Keany, J., Curfman, G., & Jarcho, J. (2014). A pragmatic view of the new cholesterol treatment guidelines. *New England Journal of Medicine, 370,* 275–278.

Nissen, S. E., Nicholls, S. J., Wolski, K., et al. (2008). Effect of rimonabant on progression of atherosclerosis in patients with abdominal obesity and coronary artery disease. *Journal of the American Medical Association, 229,* 1547–1560.

O'Donnell, C., Elosua, R. (2008). Cardiovascular risk factors. Insight from the Framingham Study. *Revista Española de Cardiología, 61*(3), 299–310.

Porth, C. M. (2013). *Pathophysiology: Concepts of altered health states* (9th ed.). Philadelphia, PA: Lippincott Williams & Wilkins.

Spinler, S. A. (2006). Challenges associated with metabolic syndrome. *Pharmacotherapy, 26,* 209S–217S.

Stone, N., Robinson, J., Lichtenstein, A., et al. (2014). 2013 ACC/AHA guideline on the treatment of blood cholesterol to reduce atherosclerotic cardiovascular risk in adults. *Circulation, 129,* S1–S45.

Woods, S. C. (2007). Role of the endocannabinoid system in regulating cardiovascular and metabolic risk factors. *American Journal of Medicine, 120*(Suppl.), S19–S25.

The Medical Letter. (2015). *The medical letter on drugs and therapeutics.* New Rochelle, NY: Author.

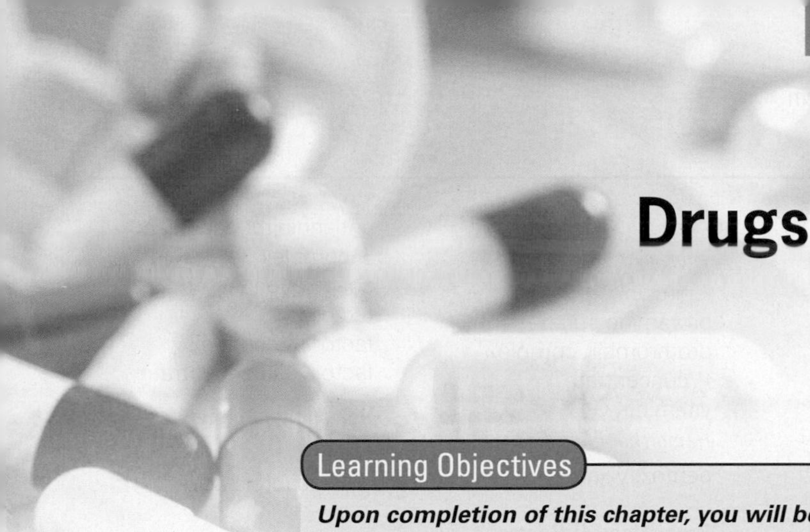

48 Drugs Affecting Blood Coagulation

Learning Objectives

Upon completion of this chapter, you will be able to:

1. Outline the mechanisms by which blood clots dissolve in the body, correlating this information with the actions of drugs used to affect blood clotting.
2. Describe the therapeutic actions, indications, pharmacokinetics, contraindications, most common adverse reactions, and important drug–drug interactions associated with drugs affecting blood coagulation.
3. Discuss the use of drugs that affect blood coagulation across the lifespan.
4. Compare and contrast the prototype drugs aspirin, heparin, urokinase, antihemophilic factor, and aminocaproic acid with other agents used to affect blood coagulation.
5. Outline the nursing considerations, including important teaching points, for patients receiving drugs used to affect blood coagulation.

Glossary of Key Terms

anticoagulants: drugs that block or inhibit any step of the coagulation process, preventing or slowing clot formation

antiplatelet agents: drugs that interfere with the aggregation or clumping of platelets to form the platelet plug

clotting factors: substances formed in the liver—many requiring vitamin K—that react in a cascading sequence to cause the formation of thrombin from prothrombin; thrombin then breaks down fibrin threads from fibrinogen to form a clot

coagulation: the process of blood changing from a fluid state to a solid state to plug injuries to the vascular system

extrinsic pathway: cascade of clotting factors in blood that has escaped the vascular system to form a clot on the outside of the injured vessel

Hageman factor: first factor activated when a blood vessel or cell is injured; starts the cascading reaction of the clotting factors, activates the conversion of plasminogen to plasmin to dissolve clots, and activates the kinin system responsible for activation of the inflammatory response

hemorrhagic disorders: disorders characterized by a lack of clot-forming substances, leading to states of excessive bleeding

hemostatic agents: drugs that stop blood loss, usually by blocking the plasminogen mechanism and preventing clot dissolution

intrinsic pathway: cascade of clotting factors leading to the formation of a clot within an injured vessel

plasminogen: natural clot-dissolving system; converted to plasmin (also called fibrinolysin) by many substances to dissolve clots that have formed and to maintain the patency of injured vessels

platelet aggregation: property of platelets to adhere to an injured surface and then attract other platelets, which clump together or aggregate at the area, plugging up an injury to the vascular system

thromboembolic disorders: disorders characterized by the formation of clots or thrombi on injured blood vessels with potential breaking of the clot to form emboli that can travel to smaller vessels, where they become lodged and occlude the vessel

thrombolytic agents: drugs that lyse, or break down, a clot that has formed; these drugs activate the plasminogen mechanism to dissolve fibrin threads

Drug List

Drugs Affecting Clot Formation and Resolution

Antiplatelet Agents
abciximab
anagrelide
(P) aspirin
cilostazol
clopidogrel
dipyridamole
eptifibatide
ticagrelor
ticlopidine
tirofiban
vorapaxar

Anticoagulants
antithrombin
apixaban
argatroban
bivalirudin
dabigatran
desirudin
edoxaban
fondaparinux
(P) heparin
protein C concentrate
rivaroxaban
warfarin

Thrombolytic Agents
alteplase
reteplase
tenecteplase
(P) urokinase

Other Drugs Affecting Clot Formation
Low-Molecular-Weight Heparins
dalteparin
enoxaparin
fondaparinux
Anticoagulant Adjunctive Therapy
lepirudin
protamine sulfate
prothrombin complex concentrate
vitamin K
Hemorrheologic Agent
pentoxifylline

Drugs Used to Control Bleeding

Antihemophilic Agents
(P) antihemophilic factor
antihemophilic factor Fc fusion protein
antihemophilic factor porcine sequence
anti-inhibitor coagulant complex
coagulation factor VIIa
factor IX
factor IX complex
factor XIII concentrate

Hemostatic Agents
Systemic
(P) aminocaproic acid
Topical
absorbable gelatin
human fibrin sealant
microfibrillar collagen
thrombin
thrombin, recombinant

The cardiovascular (CV) system is a closed system, and blood remains in a fluid state while in it. Because blood is trapped in a closed space, it maintains the difference in pressures required to keep the system moving along. Everything in the CV system moves from higher pressure to lower pressure. If the vascular system is injured—from a cut, a puncture, or capillary destruction—the fluid blood could leak out, causing the system in that area to lose pressure and changing the flow in the system, potentially shutting it down entirely. To deal with the problem of blood leaking and potentially shutting down the system, blood that is exposed to an injury in a vessel almost immediately forms into a solid state, or clot, which plugs the hole in the system and keeps the required pressure differences intact.

Blood Coagulation

People injure blood vessels all the time (e.g., by coughing too hard, by knocking into the corner of the desk when sitting down). Consequently, the vascular system must maintain an intricate balance between the tendency to clot or form a solid state, called **coagulation**, and the need to "unclot," or reverse coagulation, to keep the vessels open and the blood flowing. If a great deal of vascular damage occurs, such as with a major cut or incision, the balance in the area shifts to a procoagulation mode and a large clot is formed. At the same time, the enzymes in the plasma work to dissolve this clot before blood flow to tissues is lost, which otherwise would lead to hypoxia and potential cell death.

Drugs that affect blood coagulation work at various steps in the blood-clotting and clot-dissolving processes to restore the balance that is needed to maintain the CV system. Box 48.1 discusses the uses of these drugs in various age groups.

Clotting Process

Blood coagulation is a complex process that involves vasoconstriction, platelet clumping or aggregation, and a cascade of **clotting factors** produced in the liver that eventually react to break down fibrinogen (a protein also produced in the liver) into insoluble fibrin threads. When a clot is formed, plasmin (another blood protein) acts to break it down. Blood coagulation can be affected at any step in this complicated process to alter the way that blood clotting occurs.

Vasoconstriction

The first reaction to a blood vessel injury is local vasoconstriction (Figure 48.1). If the injury to the blood vessel is very small, this vasoconstriction can seal off any break and allow the area to heal.

Platelet Aggregation

Injury to a blood vessel exposes blood to the collagen and other substances under the endothelial lining of the vessel. This exposure causes platelets in the circulating blood to stick or adhere to the site of the injury. Once they stick the platelets release adenosine diphosphate (ADP), serotonin, and other chemicals that attract other platelets, causing them to gather or aggregate and to stick as well. ADP is also a precursor of the prostaglandins, from which thromboxane A_2 is formed. Thromboxane A_2 causes local vasoconstriction and further **platelet aggregation** and adhesion. This series of events forms a platelet plug at the site of the

BOX 48.1 FOCUS ON Drug Therapy Across the Lifespan

Drugs Affecting Blood Coagulation

CHILDREN

Little research is available on the use of anticoagulants in children. If they are used the child needs to be monitored very carefully to avoid excessive bleeding related to drug interactions or alterations in GI or liver function. People who interact with the child need to understand the importance of preventing injuries and providing safety precautions and should be aware of what to do if the child is injured and begins to bleed.

If heparin is used the dose should be carefully calculated based on weight and age and checked by another person before the drug is administered.

Warfarin is used with children who are to undergo cardiac surgery. Again, the dose must be determined based on weight and age, and the child should be monitored closely. Dabigatran, apixaban, edoxaban, and rivaroxaban are not approved for use in children.

The safety of low-molecular-weight heparins has not been established in children.

At this time, there are no indications for the use of antiplatelet or thrombolytic drugs with children.

ADULTS

Adults receiving these drugs need to be instructed in ways to prevent injury—such as using an electric razor instead of a straight razor, using a soft-bristled toothbrush to protect the gums, and avoiding contact sports—and instructed in what to do if bleeding does occur (apply constant, firm pressure and contact a health care provider). They should receive a written list of signs of bleeding to watch for and to report to their health care provider.

Because so many drugs and alternative therapies are known to interact with these agents, it is very important that these patients be urged to report the use of this drug to any other health care provider and to consult with one before using any over-the-counter drugs or alternative therapies.

It is prudent to advise any patient using one of these drugs in the home setting to carry or wear a MedicAlert notification in case of emergency.

The patient also needs to understand the importance of regular, periodic blood tests to evaluate the effects of the drug.

Because of the many risks associated with increased bleeding or increased blood clotting during pregnancy, these drugs should not be used during pregnancy unless the benefit to the mother clearly outweighs the potential risk to the fetus and to the mother at delivery. Risks of altered blood clotting in the neonate make these drugs generally inadvisable for use during lactation.

OLDER ADULTS

Older adults may have many underlying medical conditions that require the need for drugs that alter blood clotting (e.g., CAD, CVA, peripheral vascular disease, TIAs). Statistically, older adults also take more medications, making them more likely to encounter drug–drug interactions associated with these drugs. The older adult is also more likely to have impaired liver and kidney function, conditions that can alter the metabolism and excretion of these drugs.

The older adult should be carefully evaluated for liver and kidney function, use of other medications, and ability to follow through with regular blood testing and medical evaluation before therapy begins. Therapy should be started at the lowest possible level and adjusted accordingly after the patient response has been noted.

Careful attention needs to be given to the patient's total drug regimen. Starting, stopping, or changing the dose of another drug may alter the body's metabolism of the drug that is being used to affect coagulation, leading to increased risk of bleeding or ineffective anticoagulation.

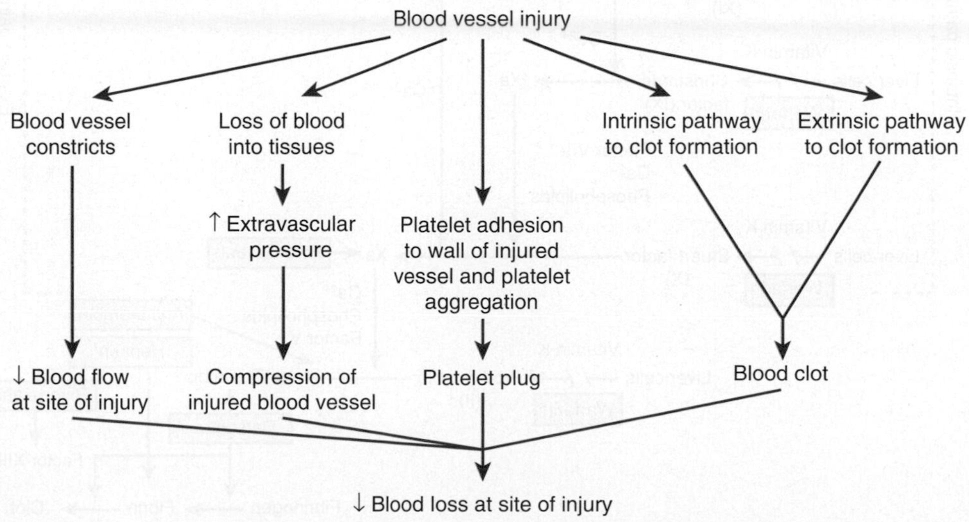

FIGURE 48.1 Process of blood coagulation.

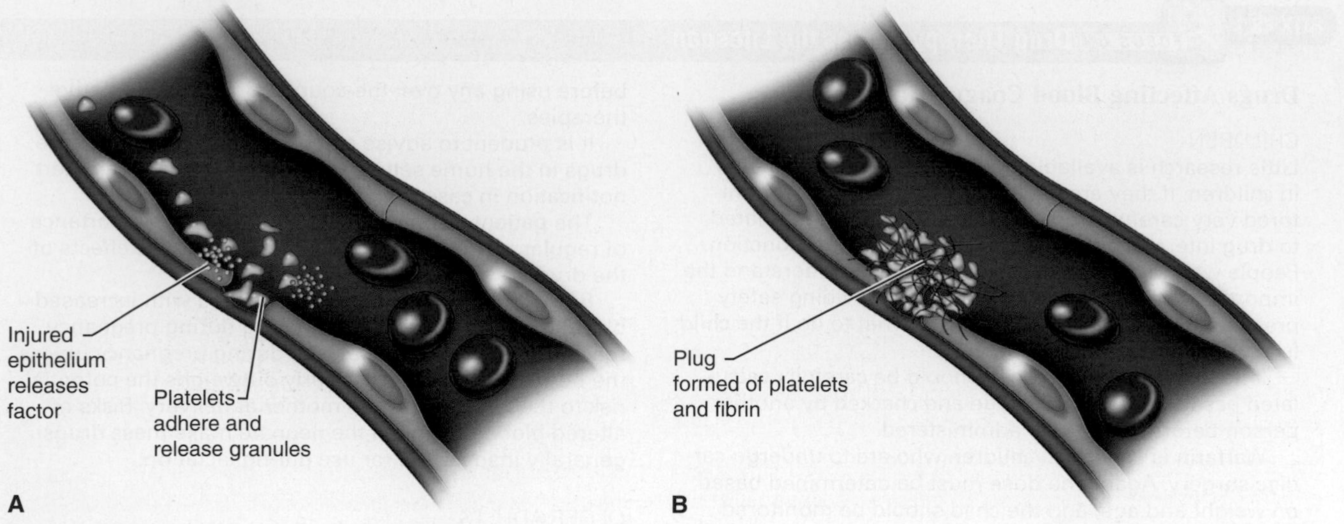

FIGURE 48.2 **A.** Damaged vessel endothelium is a stimulus to circulating platelets, causing platelet adhesion. **B.** Platelets release mediators, and platelet aggregation results.

vessel injury. In many injuries the combination of vasoconstriction and platelet aggregation is enough to seal off the injury and keep the CV system intact (Figure 48.2).

Intrinsic Pathway

As blood comes in contact with the exposed collagen of the injured blood vessel, one of the clotting factors, **Hageman factor** (also called factor XII), a chemical substance that is found circulating in the blood, is activated. (Clotting factors are often known by a name and by a Roman numeral. When one of these factors becomes activated the lowercase letter "a" is added; e.g., activated Hageman factor is also called factor XIIa.) The activation of Hageman factor starts a number of reactions in the area: The clot formation process is activated, the clot-dissolving process is activated, and the inflammatory response is started (see Chapter 15). The activation of Hageman factor first activates clotting factor XI (plasma thromboplastin antecedent) and then activates a cascading series of coagulant substances called the **intrinsic pathway** (Figure 48.3) that ends with the

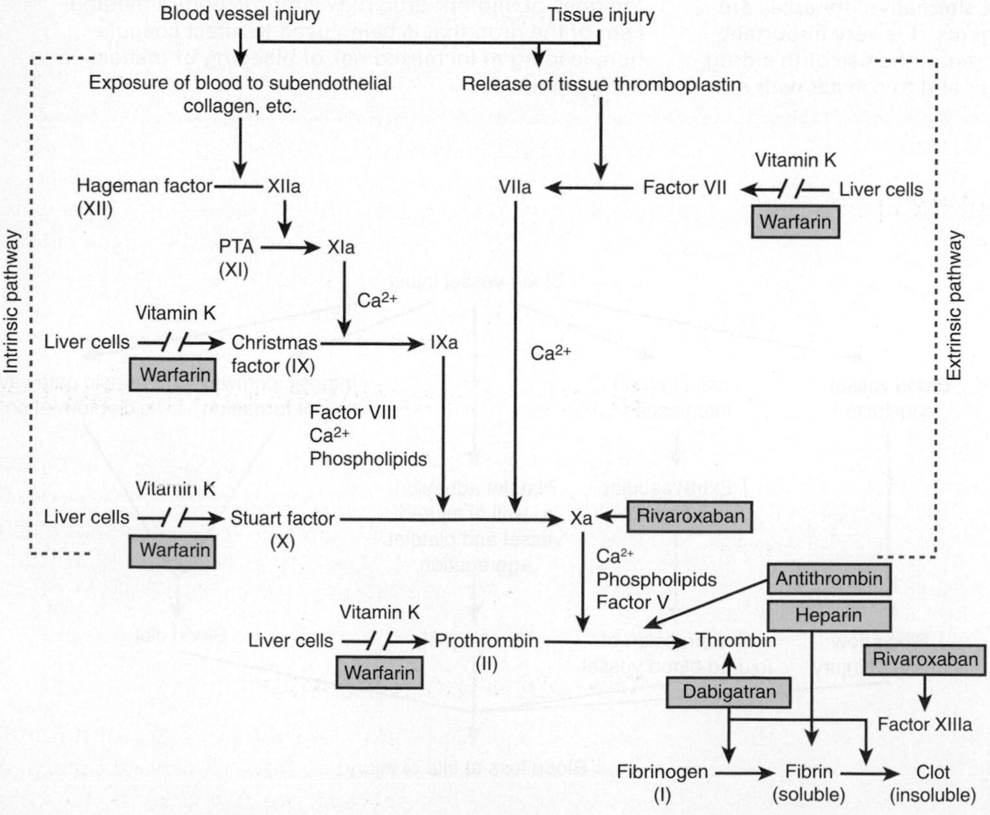

FIGURE 48.3 Details of the intrinsic and extrinsic clotting pathways. The sites of action of some of the drugs that can influence these processes are shown in *red*.

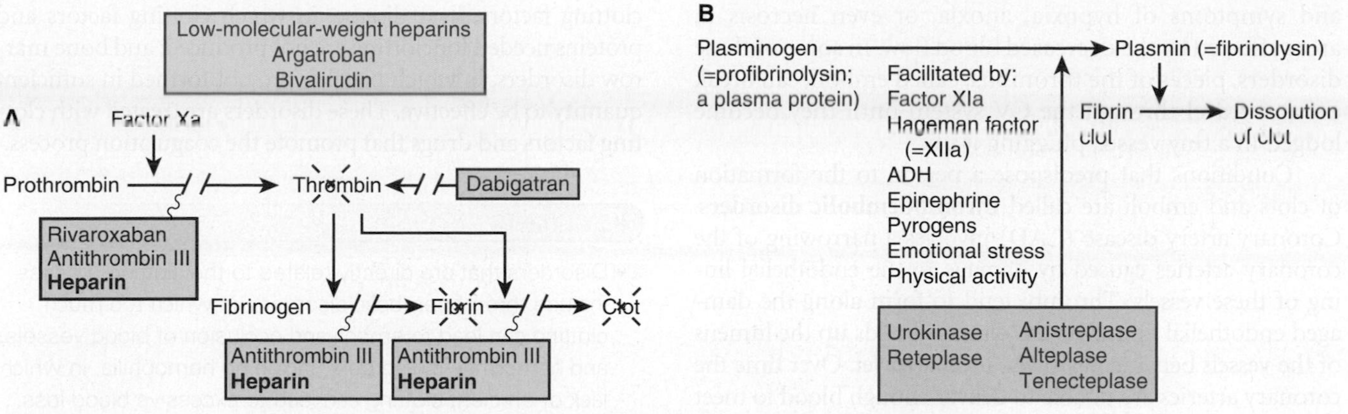

FIGURE 48.4 **A.** Anticlotting process. Antithrombin III (in plasma) and rivaroxaban inhibit the activity of Stuart factor (factor Xa) and thrombin; the drug heparin enhances the activity of antithrombin III. Steps in clot formation that are inhibited by heparin are shown in *red.* Dabigatran directly inhibits thrombin. **B.** Fibrinolytic process: Clots are dissolved. The step that is facilitated by the clot-dissolving drugs and by other agents is shown in *blue.*

conversion of prothrombin to thrombin. Calcium is the catalyst that facilitates this cascade. Activated thrombin breaks down fibrinogen to form insoluble fibrin threads, which form a clot inside the blood vessel. The clot, called a thrombus, acts to plug the injury and seal the system.

Extrinsic Pathway

While the coagulation process is going on inside the blood vessel via the intrinsic pathway the blood that has leaked out of the vascular system and into the surrounding tissues is caused to clot by the **extrinsic pathway.** Injured cells release a substance called tissue thromboplastin, which activates clotting factors in the blood and starts the clotting cascade to form a clot on the outside of the blood vessel. The injured vessel is now vasoconstricted and has a platelet plug, as well as a clot on both the inside and the outside of the blood vessel in the area of the injury. These actions maintain the closed nature of the CV system (see Figure 48.3).

Clot Resolution and Anticlotting Process

Blood plasma also contains anticlotting substances that inhibit clotting reactions that might otherwise lead to an obstruction of blood vessels by blood clots. For example, antithrombin III prevents the formation of thrombin, thus stopping the breakdown of the fibrin threads.

Another substance in the plasma, called plasmin or fibrinolysin, dissolves clots to ensure free movement of blood through the system. Plasmin is a protein-dissolving substance that breaks down the fibrin framework of blood clots and opens up vessels. Its precursor, called **plasminogen,** is made in the liver and is found in the plasma. The conversion of plasminogen to plasmin begins with the activation of Hageman factor and is facilitated by a number of other factors, including antidiuretic hormone, epinephrine, pyrogens, emotional stress, physical activity, and the chemical urokinase. Plasmin helps to keep blood vessels open and functional. Very high levels of plasmin are found in the lungs (which contain millions of tiny, easily injured capillaries) and in the uterus (which in pregnancy must maintain a constant blood flow for the developing fetus). The action of plasmin is evident in the female menstrual flow, in that clots do not form rapidly when the lining of the uterus is shed; the blood oozes slowly over a period of days (Figure 48.4).

KEY POINTS

- The transformation of fluid blood into a solid state to seal breaks in the vascular system is known as coagulation.
- The coagulation process involves vasoconstriction, platelet aggregation to form a plug, and intrinsic and extrinsic clot formation initiated by Hageman factor to plug any breaks in the system.
- The conversion of prothrombin to thrombin, which results in insoluble fibrin threads, is the final step of clot formation.
- To prevent the occlusion of blood vessels and the denying of blood to the tissues a formed clot must be dissolved.
- The base of the clot-dissolving system is the conversion of plasminogen to plasmin (fibrinolysin) by several factors, including Hageman factor. Plasmin dissolves fibrin threads and resolves the clot.

Disorders Affecting Blood Coagulation

Disorders that directly affect the coagulation process fall into two main categories: (1) conditions that involve overproduction of clots, or thromboembolic disorders; and (2) conditions in which the clotting process is not working effectively, resulting in risk for excess bleeding or hemorrhagic disorders.

Thromboembolic Disorders

Medical conditions that involve the formation of thrombi result in decreased blood flow through or total occlusion of a blood vessel. These conditions are marked by the signs and symptoms of hypoxia, anoxia, or even necrosis in areas affected by the decreased blood flow. In some of these disorders, pieces of the thrombus, called emboli, can break off and travel through the CV system until they become lodged in a tiny vessel, plugging it up.

Conditions that predispose a person to the formation of clots and emboli are called **thromboembolic disorders**. Coronary artery disease (CAD) involves a narrowing of the coronary arteries caused by damage to the endothelial lining of these vessels. Thrombi tend to form along the damaged endothelial lining. As the damage builds up the lumens of the vessels become narrower and narrower. Over time the coronary arteries are unable to deliver enough blood to meet the needs of the heart muscle, and hypoxia develops. If a vessel becomes so narrow that a tiny clot occludes it completely the blood supply to that area is cut off and anoxia occurs, followed by infarction and necrosis. With age, many of the vessels in the body can be damaged and develop similar problems with narrowing and blood delivery. These disorders are treated with drugs that interfere with the normal coagulation process to prevent the formation of clots in the system.

Hemorrhagic Disorders

Hemorrhagic disorders, in which excess bleeding occurs, are less common than thromboembolic disorders. These disorders include hemophilia, in which there is a genetic lack of clotting factors; liver disease, in which clotting factors and proteins needed for clotting are not produced; and bone marrow disorders, in which platelets are not formed in sufficient quantity to be effective. These disorders are treated with clotting factors and drugs that promote the coagulation process.

KEY POINTS

- Disorders that are directly related to the clotting process include thromboembolic disorders, in which too much clotting can lead to emboli and occlusion of blood vessels, and hemorrhagic disorders, including hemophilia, in which lack of efficient clotting can lead to excessive blood loss.

Drugs Affecting Clot Formation and Resolution

Drugs that affect clot formation include antiplatelet drugs, which alter platelet aggregation and the formation of the platelet plug; anticoagulants, which interfere with the clotting cascade and thrombin formation; and thrombolytic agents, which break down the thrombus or clot that has been formed by stimulating the plasmin system (see Table 48.1). Box 48.2 discusses the interaction of herbal remedies with these agents.

Table 48.1 ***Drugs in Focus:*** **Drugs Affecting Clot Formation and Resolution**

Drug Name	Usual Dosage	Usual Indications
Antiplatelet Agents		
abciximab (*ReoPro*)	0.25-mg/kg IV bolus 10–60 min before procedure, then continuous infusion of 10 mcg/kg/min for 12 h *Angina:* 0.25 mg/kg by IV bolus, then 10 mcg/kg/min IV for 18–24 h	Prevention of acute cardiac events during transluminal coronary angioplasty when used in conjunction with heparin and aspirin; early treatment of unstable angina and non–Q-wave MI
anagrelide (*Agrylin*)	0.5 mg PO q.i.d. or 1 mg PO b.i.d., may increase by 0.5 mg/d each week; maximum dose 10 mg/d or 2.5 mg as a single dose	Treatment of essential thrombocythemia to reduce elevated platelet count and decrease the risk of thrombosis
aspirin (generic)	1,300 mg/d PO to decrease TIAs; 300–325 mg/d PO to reduce MI risk	Reduction of the incidence of TIAs and strokes in men; reduction of the risk of death or nonfatal MI in patients with a past history of MI or with angina
cilostazol (*Pletal*)	100 mg PO b.i.d.	Reduction of symptoms of intermittent claudication, allowing increased walking distance in adults
clopidogrel (*Plavix*)	75 mg/d PO	Treatment of patients who are at risk for ischemic events; patients with a history of MI, peripheral artery disease, or ischemic stroke; and patients with acute coronary syndrome
dipyridamole (*Persantine*)	50 mg PO t.i.d. for angina; 75–100 mg PO q.i.d. for heart valve patients; 0.142 mg/kg/min IV over 4 min for diagnosis	Prevention of thromboembolism in patients with artificial heart valves when used in combination with warfarin; aids diagnosis of CAD in patients who cannot exercise; may be used in treatment of angina (found to be only "possibly effective" by the FDA)
eptifibatide (*Integrilin*)	180 mcg/kg IV over 1–2 min, then 2 mcg/kg/min IV for up to 72 h for acute coronary syndrome; 135-mcg/kg IV bolus before procedure, then 0.5 mcg/kg/min IV for 20–24 h	Treatment of acute coronary syndrome; prevention of ischemic episodes in patients undergoing percutaneous coronary interventions
ticagrelor (*Brilinta*)	180-mg PO loading dose then 90 mg PO b.i.d. with daily aspirin 0.325-mg loading dose, then 75–100 mg/d	To reduce the rate of thrombotic coronary collateral vessel events in patients with acute coronary syndrome

Table 48.1 ***Drugs in Focus:* Drugs Affecting Clot Formation and Resolution** *(continued)*

Drug Name	Usual Dosage	Usual Indications
ticlopidine (generic)	250 mg PO b.i.d.	Reduction of the risk of thrombotic stroke in patients with TIAs or history of stroke who are intolerant to aspirin therapy
tirofiban (*Aggrastat*)	0.4 mcg/kg/min IV over 30 min, then continuous infusion of 0.1 mcg/kg/min	Treatment of acute coronary syndrome and prevention of cardiac ischemic events during percutaneous coronary intervention; used in combination with heparin
vorapaxar (*Zontivity*)	2.5 mg/d PO	Reduction of thrombolic CV events in patients with a history of MI or peripheral arterial disease
Anticoagulants		
antithrombin (*Thrombate III*)	Dose must be calculated using body weight and baseline levels, given every 2–8 d	Replacement in hereditary antithrombin III deficiency; treatment of patients with this deficiency who are to undergo surgery or obstetrical procedures that might put them at risk for thromboembolism
apixaban (*Eliquis*)	2.5–5 mg PO b.i.d.	Reduction in the risk of stroke and systemic embolism in patients with nonvalvular AF; prevention and treatment of DVT and PE
argatroban (*Acova*)	2 mcg/kg/min IV until the desired effect is seen; then dose is adjusted	Treatment of thrombosis in heparin-induced thrombocythemia
bivalirudin (*Angiomax*)	1-mg/kg IV bolus, then 2.5 mg/kg/h IV for 4 h and 0.2 mg/kg/h IV as a low-dose infusion	Prevention of ischemic events in patients undergoing transluminal coronary angioplasty when used in combination with aspirin
dabigatran (*Pradaxa*)	150 mg PO b.i.d.	Reduction in the risk for stroke and systemic embolism in patients with nonvalvular AF; prevention and treatment of DVT and PE
desirudin (*Iprivask*)	15 mg by subcutaneous injection q12 h beginning 5–15 min before surgery and continuing for 9–12 d	Prevention of DVT in patients undergoing elective hip replacement
edoxaban (*Savaysa*)	60 mg/d PO; 30 mg/d PO with renal impairment	Reduction in the risk of stroke and systemic embolism in patients with nonvalvular AF; treatment of DVT and PE
fondaparinux (*Arixtra*)	*Prevention:* 2.5 mg/d by subcutaneous injection starting 6–8 h after surgical closure and continuing for 5–9 d *Treatment:* 5–10 mg/d by subcutaneous injections for 5–9 d	Prevention and treatment of venous thromboembolic events following surgery for hip fracture, hip replacement, or knee replacement; used with warfarin when appropriate
heparin (generic)	10,000–20,000 units subcutaneous, then 8,000–10,000 units q8 h; 5,000–10,000 units IV q4–6 h *Pediatric:* 50 units/kg IV bolus, then 100 units/kg IV q4 h	Prevention and treatment of venous thrombosis, PE, AF with embolization; prevention of clotting in blood samples, dialysis, and venous tubing; diagnosis and treatment of DIC (Box 48.3); also used as an adjunct in the treatment of MI and stroke
protein C concentrate (*Ceprotin*)	100–120 IU/kg IV injection; then 60–80 IU/kg IV q6 h for three doses *Maintenance:* 45–60 IU/kg IV q6–12 h	Replacement therapy for congenital protein C deficiency
rivaroxaban (*Xarelto*)	10 mg/d PO starting within 6–10 h after surgery, continuing for 35 d after hip replacement or 12 d after knee replacement	Prevention of DVTs that may lead to PE in patients undergoing knee or hip replacement surgery
warfarin (*Coumadin*)	10–15 mg/d PO, then 2–10 mg/d PO based on PT ratio or INR; use lower doses with geriatric patients	Treatment of patients with AF, artificial heart valves, or valvular damage that makes patient susceptible to thrombus and embolus formation; prevention and treatment of venous thrombosis, PE, embolus with AF, systemic emboli after MI
Thrombolytic Agents		
alteplase (*Activase*)	100 mg IV given over 2 h	Treatment of MI, acute PE, and acute ischemic stroke; restoration of function in occluded central venous access devices
reteplase (*Retavase*)	10 IU + 10 IU double-bolus IV, each over 2 min, 30 min apart	Treatment of coronary artery thrombosis associated with an acute MI

(continues on page 832)

Table 48.1 *Drugs in Focus:* Drugs Affecting Clot Formation and Resolution (*continued*)

Drug Name	Usual Dosage	Usual Indications
tenecteplase (*TNKase*)	30–50 mg IV over 5 sec	Reduction of mortality associated with acute MI
urokinase (*Abbokinase*)	4,400–10,000 units/min for up to 2 h, based on clinical response	Lysis of PE; treatment of coronary thrombosis; for clearing occluded intravenous catheters
Other Drugs Affecting Clot Formation ***Low-Molecular-Weight Heparins***		
dalteparin (*Fragmin*)	*DVT:* 2,500–5,000 IU/d subcutaneous starting 1–2 h before surgery and then for 5–10 d *Angina:* 120 IU/kg subcutaneous q12 h with aspirin therapy for 5–8 d	Prevention of DVT that may lead to PE after abdominal surgery or hip replacement; treatment of unstable angina and non–Q-wave MI
enoxaparin (*Lovenox*)	*Hip surgery:* 30 mg subcutaneous q12 h for 7–10 d *Abdominal surgery:* 40 mg/d subcutaneous for 7–10 d *DVT or PE:* 1 mg/kg subcutaneous q12 h *Angina:* 1 mg/kg subcutaneous q12 h *Prevention of DVT in high-risk patients:* 40 mg/d subcutaneous for 6–14 d	Prevention of DVT that may lead to PE after hip replacement or abdominal surgery; with warfarin to treat acute DVT or PE; prevention of ischemic complications of unstable angina or non–Q-wave MI; prevention of DVT in patients with severely restricted mobility due to illness
Anticoagulant Adjunctive Therapy		
lepirudin (*Refludan*)	0.4 mg/kg as an IV bolus followed by continuous IV infusion of 0.15 mg/kg for 2–10 d	Treatment of heparin-induced thrombocytopenia associated with thromboembolic disease (rare allergic reaction to heparin)
protamine sulfate (generic)	1 mg IV neutralized 90–115 USP units of heparin; dose based on specific overdose	Treatment of heparin overdose
prothromin complex concentrate (*Kcentra, Octaplex*)	25–50 units/kg IV based on INR	Treatment of warfarin-related bleeding
vitamin K (generic)	2.5–10 mg IM or by subcutaneous injection; may be repeated in 6–8 h based on PT time	Treatment of anticoagulant-induced prothrombin deficiency
Hemorrheologic Agent		
pentoxifylline (generic)	400 mg PO t.i.d. with meals	Treatment of intermittent claudication to improve function and reduce symptoms; improve blood flow in vascular diseases

MI, myocardial infarction; TIA, transient ischemic attack; CAD, coronary artery disease; FDA, U.S. Food and Drug Administration; AF, atrial fibrillation; DVT, deep-vein thrombosis; PE, pulmonary embolism; DIC, disseminated intravascular coagulation; PT, prothrombin time; INR, international normalized ratio.

Antiplatelet Agents

Antiplatelet agents decrease the formation of the platelet plug by decreasing the responsiveness of the platelets to stimuli that would cause them to stick and aggregate on a vessel wall. Antiplatelet agents available for use include abciximab (*ReoPro*), anagrelide (*Agrylin*), aspirin (generic), cilostazol (*Pletal*), clopidogrel (*Plavix*), dipyridamole (*Persantine*), eptifibatide (*Integrilin*), ticagrelor (*Brilinta*), ticlopidine (generic), tirofiban (*Aggrastat*), and vorapaxar (*Zontivity*).

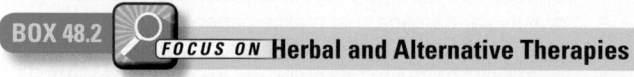

BOX 48.2 FOCUS ON Herbal and Alternative Therapies

Many herbal therapies can cause problems when used with drugs that affect blood coagulation. Patients taking these drugs should be cautioned to avoid angelica, cat's claw, chamomile, chondroitin, feverfew, garlic, ginkgo, goldenseal, grape seed extract, green leaf tea, horse chestnut seed, psyllium, and turmeric. If a patient who is taking an anticoagulant presents with increased bleeding and no other interaction or cause is found, question the patient about the possibility of use of herbal therapies.

Therapeutic Actions and Indications

The antiplatelet agents inhibit platelet adhesion and aggregation by blocking receptor sites on the platelet membrane, preventing platelet–platelet interaction or the interaction of platelets with other clotting chemicals. One drug, anagrelide, blocks the production of platelets in the bone marrow. These agents are used effectively to treat CV diseases that are prone to produce occluded vessels; for the maintenance of venous and arterial grafts; to prevent cerebrovascular occlusion; and as adjuncts to thrombolytic therapy in the treatment of myocardial infarction (MI) and the prevention of reinfarction after MI. The prescriber's choice of drug depends on the intended use and the patient's tolerance of the associated adverse effects. See Table 48.1 for Usual Indications for each of these agents.

Pharmacokinetics

Abciximab, eptifibatide, and tirofiban are administered IV. Antiplatelet agents that are administered orally include anagrelide, aspirin, cilostazol, clopidogrel, ticagrelor, ticlopidine, and vorapaxar. Dipyridamole is used orally or as an IV agent.

These drugs are generally well absorbed and highly bound to plasma proteins. They are metabolized in the liver and excreted in the urine, and they tend to enter breast milk (see Contraindications and Cautions).

Contraindications and Cautions

Antiplatelet agents are contraindicated in the presence of allergy to the specific drug *to avoid hypersensitivity reactions*. Caution should be used in the following conditions: The presence of any known bleeding disorder or active bleeding *because of the risk of excessive blood loss*; recent surgery *because of the risk of increased bleeding in unhealed vessels*; and closed head injuries, history of stroke or transient ischemic attack (TIA) *because of the risk of bleeding in the brain*.

Although there are no adequate studies of these drugs in pregnancy, they are contraindicated with pregnancy *because of the potential for increased bleeding* (see Adverse Effects); they should be used during pregnancy only if the benefits to the mother clearly outweigh the potential risks to the fetus. These drugs are also contraindicated during lactation *because of the potential adverse effects on the fetus or neonate*; if they are needed by a breastfeeding mother, she should find another method of feeding the baby.

Anagrelide should be used with caution with any history of thrombocytopenia *because it decreases the production of platelets in the bone marrow*. Platelet levels should be checked regularly to monitor for thrombocytopenia if a patient is on this drug.

Adverse Effects

The most common adverse effect seen with these drugs is bleeding, which often occurs as increased bruising and bleeding while brushing the teeth. Vorapaxar has a black box warning related to the possibility of serious to fatal bleeding episodes. Other common problems include headache, dizziness, and weakness; the cause of these reactions is not understood (Figure 48.5). Nausea and gastrointestinal (GI) distress may occur because of the direct irritating effects of the oral drug on the GI tract. Skin rash, another common effect, may be related to direct drug effects on the dermis.

Clinically Important Drug–Drug Interactions

The risk of excessive bleeding increases if any of these drugs is combined with another drug that affects blood clotting. Do not use vorapaxar with any CYP3A inhibitors or inducers.

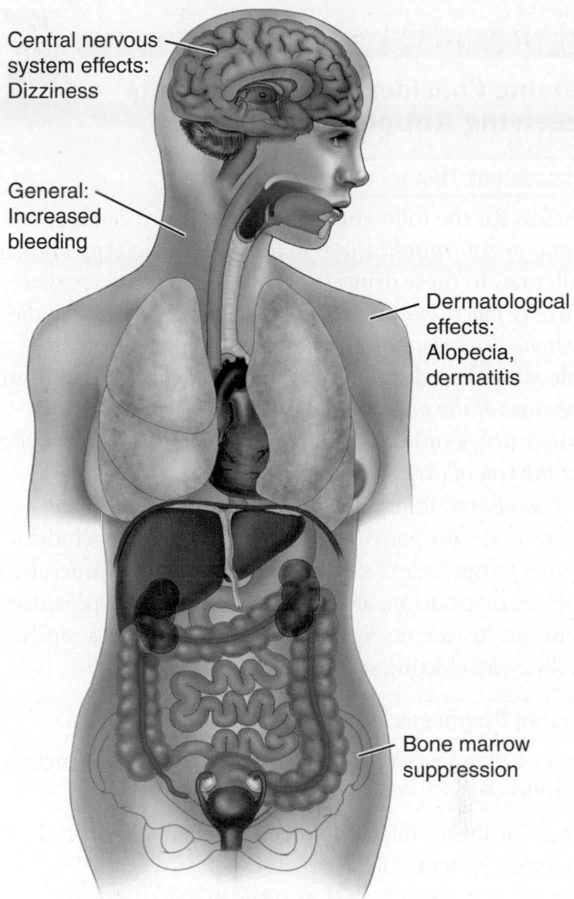

FIGURE 48.5 Variety of adverse effects and toxicities associated with drugs affecting blood coagulation.

Prototype Summary: Aspirin

Indications: Reduction of risk of recurrent TIAs or strokes in men with a history of TIA due to fibrin or platelet emboli; reduction of death or nonfatal MI in patients with a history of infarction or unstable angina; MI prophylaxis; also used for its anti-inflammatory, analgesic, and antipyretic effects.

Actions: Inhibits platelet aggregation by inhibiting platelet synthesis of thromboxane A2.

Pharmacokinetics:

Route	Onset	Peak	Duration
Oral	5–30 min	0.25–2 h	3–6 h

$T_{1/2}$: 15 minutes to 12 hours; metabolized in the liver and excreted in the urine.

Adverse Effects: Acute aspirin toxicity with hyperpnea, possibly leading to fever, coma, and CV collapse; nausea, dyspepsia, heartburn, epigastric discomfort, GI bleeding, occult blood loss, dizziness, tinnitus, difficulty hearing, anaphylactoid reaction.

Nursing Considerations for Patients Receiving Antiplatelet Agents

Assessment: History and Examination

- Assess for the following conditions, *which could be cautions or contraindications to use of the drug*: Any known allergies to these drugs *because of the risk of hypersensitivity reactions*; pregnancy or lactation *because of the potential adverse effects on the fetus or neonate*; and bleeding disorders, recent surgery, or closed head injury *because of the potential for excessive bleeding*; use of other drugs or herbs that could affect bleeding *because of the risk of excessive bleeding.*
- Assess baseline status before beginning therapy *to determine any potential adverse effects.* This includes body temperature; skin color, lesions, and temperature; affect, orientation, and reflexes; pulse, blood pressure, and perfusion; respirations and adventitious sounds; CBC; and clotting studies (see Table 48.2).

Nursing Diagnoses

Nursing diagnoses related to drug therapy might include the following:

- Risk for injury related to bleeding effects or central nervous system (CNS) effects
- Acute pain related to GI or CNS effects
- Deficient knowledge regarding drug therapy

Planning

- The patient will receive the best therapeutic effect from the drug therapy.
- The patient will have limited adverse effects to the drug therapy.
- The patient will have an understanding of the drug therapy, adverse effects to anticipate, and measures to relieve discomfort and improve safety.

Implementation with Rationale

- Provide small, frequent meals *to relieve GI discomfort* if GI upset is a problem.
- Provide comfort measures and analgesia for headache *to relieve pain and improve patient compliance with the drug regimen.*
- Suggest safety measures, including the use of an electric razor and avoidance of contact sports, *to decrease the risk of bleeding.*
- Monitor platelet count if the patient is using anagrelide *to detect thrombocytopenia and increased risk of bleeding.*
- Provide increased precautions against bleeding during invasive procedures; use pressure dressings and ice *to decrease excessive blood loss caused by anticoagulation.*
- Mark the chart of any patient receiving this drug *to alert medical staff that there is a potential for increased bleeding.*
- Provide thorough patient teaching, including the name of the drug, dosage prescribed, measures to avoid adverse effects, warning signs of problems, the need for periodic monitoring and evaluation, and the need to wear or carry a MedicAlert notification, *to enhance patient knowledge about drug therapy and to promote compliance with the drug regimen.*
- Offer support and encouragement *to help the patient deal with the diagnosis and the drug regimen.*

Evaluation

- Monitor patient response to the drug (increased bleeding time, prevention of occlusive events).
- Monitor for adverse effects (bleeding, GI upset, dizziness, headache).
- Evaluate the effectiveness of the teaching plan (patient can name drug, dosage, adverse effects to watch for, and specific measures to avoid them; patient understands the importance of continued follow-up).
- Monitor the effectiveness of comfort measures and compliance with the regimen.

Anticoagulants

Anticoagulants are drugs that interfere with the normal coagulation process by interfering with the clotting cascade and thrombin formation. Drugs in this class include antithrombin III (*Thrombate III*), argatroban (*Acova*), bivalirudin (*Angiomax*), desirudin (*Iprivask*), fondaparinux (Arixtra), heparin (generic), warfarin (*Coumadin*) and the newest oral anticoagulants dabigatran (*Pradaxa*), rivaroxaban (*Xarelto*), apixaban (*Eliquis*), and edoxaban (*Savaysa*); and protein C concentrate (*Ceprotin*).

Therapeutic Actions and Indications

As noted previously, the anticoagulants interfere with the normal cascade of events involved in the clotting process. Warfarin, an oral drug in this class, causes a decrease in the production of vitamin K–dependent clotting factors in the liver. The eventual effect is a depletion of these clotting factors and a prolongation of clotting times. It is used to maintain a state of anticoagulation in situations in which the patient is susceptible to potentially dangerous clot formation (see Table 48.1 for Usual Indications for warfarin). See the Critical Thinking Scenario for additional nursing care for the patient taking warfarin. Newer oral drugs include dabigatran, rivaroxaban, apixaban, and edoxaban. Dabigatran (*Pradaxa*) directly inhibits thrombin, which blocks the last step to

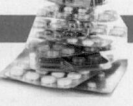

Table 48.2 Review of Clotting Studies

Test	Measure	Therapeutic Range	Uses
aPPT PTT	Activity of intrinsic pathway of coagulation	1.5–2.5 times baseline	Dose adjustment for heparin, low-molecular-weight heparins, desirudin, argatroban, bivalirudin, dabigatran, rivaroxaban
INR	Standardized measure of prothrombin levels	2–3.5	Warfarin dose adjustment, fondaparinux dose adjustment
PT	Time required for clotting to occur; extrinsic pathway activity	1.3–1.5	Warfarin dose adjustment

aPPT, activated partial thromboplastin time; PPT, partial thromboplastin time; INR, international normalized ratio; PT, prothrombin time.

clot formation. It is approved to reduce the risk of stroke and systemic embolism in patients with nonvalvular atrial fibrillation (AF) and for the treatment of deep-vein thrombosis (DVT) and pulmonary embolism (PE) in patients treated with a parenteral anticoagulant for 5 to 10 days and prevention of recurrence of DVT and PE. The high cost of the drug and lack of a quick antidote for overdose have resulted in many health care providers being very cautious about switching to this therapy. Rivaroxaban (*Xarelto*) and edoxaban (*Eliquis*) are factor Xa inhibitors that stop the coagulation cascade at this early step. They are approved to prevent DVT, which might lead to PE, in patients undergoing knee or hip replacement surgery; prevention of stroke in patients with nonvalvular AF and for the prevention and treatment of DVT and PE. The newest of these agents, apixaban (*Savaysa*), is a factor Xa inhibitor that comes with cautions if used in patients with renal impairment. It is also approved for the treatment on nonvalvular AF and the treatment of DVT and PE.

Heparin, argatroban, and bivalirudin block the formation of thrombin from prothrombin. The usual indications for heparin include acute treatment and prevention of venous thrombosis and pulmonary embolism; treatment of AF with embolization; prevention of clotting in blood samples and in dialysis and venous tubing; and diagnosis and treatment of disseminated intravascular coagulation (DIC) (Box 48.3). Because heparin must be injected, it is often not the drug of choice for outpatients, who would be responsible for injecting the drug several times during the day. Patients may be started on heparin in the acute situation and then switched to an oral anticoagulant. Antithrombin and protein C concentrate are blood products that are used for replacement in specific genetic deficiencies.

BOX 48.3

Understanding Disseminated Intravascular Coagulation

DIC is a syndrome in which bleeding and thrombosis are found together. It can occur as a complication of many problems, including severe infection with septic shock, traumatic childbirth or missed abortion, and massive injuries. In these disorders, local tissue damage causes the release of coagulation-stimulating substances into the circulation. These substances then stimulate the coagulation process, causing fibrin clot formation in small vessels in the lungs, kidneys, brain, and other organs. This continuing reaction consumes excessive amounts of fibrinogen, other clotting factors, and platelets. The end result is increased bleeding. In essence the patient clots too much, resulting in the possibility of bleeding to death.

The first step in treating this disorder is to control the problem that initially precipitated it. For example, treating the infection, performing dilation and curettage to clear the uterus, or stabilizing injuries can help stop this continuing process. Whole-blood infusions or the infusion of fibrinogen may be used to buy some time until the patient is stable and can form clotting factors again. There are associated problems with giving whole blood (e.g., development of hepatitis or AIDS), and there is a risk that fibrinogen may set off further intravascular clotting. Paradoxically, the treatment of choice for DIC is the anticoagulant heparin. Heparin prevents the clotting phase from being completed, thus inhibiting the breakdown of fibrinogen. It may also help avoid hemorrhage by preventing the body from depleting its entire store of coagulation factors.

Because heparin is usually administered to prevent blood clotting, and the adverse effects that are monitored with heparin therapy include signs of bleeding, it can be a real challenge for the nursing staff to feel comfortable administering heparin to a patient who is bleeding to death. Understanding the disease process can help alleviate any doubts about the treatment.

CRITICAL THINKING SCENARIO

Oral Anticoagulant Therapy

THE SITUATION

G.R. is a 68-year-old woman with a history of severe mitral valve disease. For the last several years, she has been able to manage her condition with digoxin, a diuretic, and a potassium supplement. However, on a recent visit to her physician she disclosed that she had been experiencing periods of breathlessness, palpitations, and dizziness. Tests showed that she was having frequent periods of AF, with a heart rate of up to 140 beats/min. Because of the danger of emboli as a result of her valve disease and the bouts of AF, warfarin therapy was begun.

CRITICAL THINKING

What nursing interventions should be done at this point?

Why do people with mitral valve disease frequently develop AF? *Think about why emboli form when the atria fibrillate. Stabilizing G.R. on warfarin may take several weeks of blood tests and dose adjustments.*

How can this process be made easier?

What patient teaching points should be covered with G.R. to ensure that she is protected from emboli and does not experience excessive bleeding?

DISCUSSION

G.R.'s situation is complex. She has a progressive degenerative valve disease that usually leads to heart failure (HF) and frequently to other complications, such as AF and emboli formation. Her digoxin and potassium levels should be checked to determine whether her HF is stabilized or the digoxin is causing the AF because of excessive doses or potassium imbalance. If these tests are within normal limits, G.R. may be experiencing AF because of irritation to the atrial cells caused by the damaged mitral valve and associated swelling and scarring. If this is the case an anticoagulant will help protect G.R. against emboli, which form in the auricles when blood pools there while the atria are fibrillating. There is less chance of emboli formation if clotting is slowed.

G.R. will need extensive teaching about warfarin, including the need for frequent blood tests, the list of potential drug–drug interactions, the importance of being alert to the many factors that can affect dose needs (including illness and diet), and how to monitor for subtle blood loss. The patient may need teaching about the reason that this oral anticoagulant was selected for her. Media campaigns and advertising widely urge the use of the other oral agents. This can also be a good opportunity to review teaching about valvular disease and HF and to answer any questions that she might have about how all of these things interrelate. If possible, it would be useful to teach G.R. or a responsible caregiver how to take a pulse so that G.R. can be alerted to potential arrhythmias and avert problems before they begin. It also would be a good idea to check on support services for G.R. to ensure that her blood tests can be done and that her response to the drug is monitored carefully.

NURSING CARE GUIDE FOR G.R.: WARFARIN

Assessment: History and Examination

Assess G.R.'s health history for allergies to warfarin, subacute bacterial endocarditis, hemorrhagic disorders, tuberculosis, renal or hepatic dysfunction, gastric ulcers, thyroid disease, uncontrolled hypertension, severe trauma, or a long-term indwelling catheter (which increases the risk of bleeding). Also assess concurrent use of numerous drugs and herbal therapies.

Focus the physical examination on the following areas:

CV: Blood pressure, pulse, perfusion, baseline electrocardiogram (ECG)

CNS: Orientation, affect, reflexes, vision

Skin: Color, lesions, texture

Respiratory system: Respiratory rate and character, adventitious sounds

GI: Abdominal examination, guaiac stool test results (for occult blood)

Laboratory tests: Liver and renal function tests, prothrombin time (PT), international normalized ratio (INR)

Nursing Diagnoses

Ineffective tissue perfusion (total body) related to alteration in clotting effects

Risk for injury related to anticoagulant effects

Disturbed body image related to alopecia, skin rash

Deficient knowledge regarding drug therapy

Planning

The patient will receive the best therapeutic effect from the drug therapy.

The patient will have limited adverse effects to the drug therapy.

Oral Anticoagulant Therapy (continued)

The patient will have an understanding of the drug therapy, adverse effects to anticipate, and measures to relieve discomfort and improve safety.

Implementation

Ensure proper administration of the drug.

Provide comfort and safety measures, such as small meals, protection from injury during invasive and other procedures, bowel program as needed, standby antidotes (e.g., vitamin K), and careful skin care.

Provide support and reassurance to deal with drug effects.

Provide patient teaching regarding drug, dosage, adverse effects, what to report, and safety precautions.

Evaluation

Evaluate drug effects: Increased bleeding times, PT 1.5–2.5 times control or PT/INR ratio of 2:3.

Monitor for adverse effects: Bleeding, alopecia, rash, GI upset, excessive bleeding.

Monitor for drug–drug interactions (numerous).

Evaluate the effectiveness of the patient-teaching program and comfort and safety measures.

PATIENT TEACHING FOR G.R.

- An anticoagulant slows the body's normal blood-clotting processes to prevent harmful blood clots from forming. This type of drug is often called a "blood thinner"; however, it cannot dissolve any clots that have already formed and does not make your blood thin.
- *Never* change any medication that you are taking—such as adding or stopping another drug, taking a new over-the-counter medication or herbal agent, or stopping one that you have been taking regularly—without consulting with your health care provider. Many other drugs and herbs affect the way that your anticoagulant works; starting or stopping another drug can cause excessive bleeding or interfere with the desired effects of the drug.
- Some of the following adverse effects may occur:
  - *Stomach bloating, cramps:* These problems often pass with time; consult your health care provider if they persist or become too uncomfortable.
  - *Loss of hair, skin rash:* These problems can be very frustrating; you may wish to discuss these with your health care provider.
  - *Orange–yellow discoloration of the urine:* This can be frightening, but it may just be an effect of the drug. If you are concerned that this might be blood, simply add vinegar to your urine; the color should disappear. If the color does not disappear, it may be caused by blood, and you should contact your health care provider.
- Report any of the following to your health care provider: *Unusual bleeding (when brushing your teeth, excessive bleeding from an injury, excessive bruising); black or tarry stools; cloudy or dark urine; sore throat, fever, or chills; severe headache or dizziness.*
- Tell any doctor, nurse, or other health care provider involved in your care that you are taking this drug. You should carry or wear medical identification stating that you are taking this drug to alert emergency medical personnel that you are at increased risk for bleeding.
- Avoid situations in which you could be easily injured—for example, engaging in contact sports or games with children or using a straight razor.
- Keep this drug, and all medications, out of the reach of children.
- Avoid the use of over-the-counter medications and herbal agents while you are taking this drug. If you feel that you need one of these, consult with your health care provider for the best choice. Many of these drugs and herbs can interfere with your anticoagulant.
- Schedule regular, periodic blood tests while you are taking this drug to monitor the effects of the drug on your body and adjust your dose as needed.

Antithrombin interferes with the formation of thrombin from prothrombin; it is a naturally occurring anticoagulant, as mentioned earlier, and a natural safety feature in the clotting system. Fondaparinux inhibits factor Xa and blocks the clotting cascade to prevent clot formation. It is supplied in prefilled syringes, making it convenient for patients who self-administer the drug at home.

Pharmacokinetics

Heparin is injected IV or subcutaneously and has an almost immediate onset of action. It is excreted in the urine. Warfarin, dabigatran, appixaban, edoxaban, and rivaroxaban are used orally. All other drugs in this class (heparin, antithrombin, argatroban, desirudin, fondaparinux, protein C complex, and bivalirudin) are given parenterally. Warfarin is readily absorbed through the GI tract, metabolized in the liver, and excreted in the urine and feces. Warfarin's onset of action is about 3 days; its effects last for 4 to 5 days. Because of the time delay, warfarin is not the drug of choice in an acute situation, but it is convenient and useful for prolonged effects. Dabigatran has a rapid onset of action, peaking in 1 to 2 hours. It has a half-life of 12 to 17 hours and is excreted in the urine after being metabolized in the liver. Rivaroxaban is also absorbed rapidly with peak effects in 2 to 4 hours. It has a slightly shorter half-life of 5 to 9 hours and is excreted in the urine and feces after being metabolized in the liver. Patients must use care in storing dabigatran (in a dark, nonhumid environment) and in the original bottle and it is only stable for 60 days from the time the bottle is opened. Edoxaban reaches peak levels in 1 to 2 hours, is minimally metabolized, and mostly excreted unchanged in the urine with a half-life of 10 to 14 hours. Apixaban reaches peak levels after oral administration in 3 to 4 hours, is metabolized in the liver, and excreted in the feces and urine with a half-life of 12 hours.

Because antithrombin and protein C concentrate are exogenous forms of naturally occurring anticoagulants the body handles them in the same way that it handles the naturally occurring products.. Argatroban is given as a continuous IV infusion. Desirudin and fondaparinux are absorbed quickly from subcutaneous sites and metabolized and excreted by the kidneys. Bivalirudin is given IV and is excreted through the kidneys.

Contraindications and Cautions

The anticoagulants are contraindicated in the presence of known allergy to the drugs *to avoid hypersensitivity reactions*. They also should not be used with any conditions *that could be compromised by increased bleeding tendencies*, including hemorrhagic disorders, recent trauma, spinal puncture (the oral anticoagulants come with black box warnings of the risk of hemorrhage with spinal puncture or anesthesia), GI ulcers, recent surgery, intrauterine device placement, tuberculosis, presence of indwelling catheters, and threatened abortion. The oral anticoagulants are contraindicated in pregnancy *because fetal injury and death have occurred;* in lactation *because of the potential risk to the baby;* and in renal or hepatic disease, *which could interfere with the metabolism and effectiveness of these drugs*. Although some adverse fetal effects have been reported with its use during pregnancy, heparin does not enter breast milk, and so it is the anticoagulant of choice if one is needed during lactation.

Caution should be used in patients with heart failure, thyrotoxicosis, senility, or psychosis *because of the potential for unexpected effects* and in patients with diarrhea or fever, *which could alter the normal clotting process by, respectively, loss of vitamin K from the intestine or activation of plasminogen*. Caution should be used in pregnancy and lactation with anticoagulants other than warfarin *because of the potential for adverse effects*; benefits should outweigh potential risks. Caution must be used in patients with renal failure if using apixaban *because the drug is eliminated unchanged in the urine and toxic levels could occur.*

FOCUS ON Safe Medication Administration

*Injectable vitamin K is used to reverse the effects of warfarin. Vitamin K promotes the liver synthesis of several clotting factors. When these pathways have been inhibited by warfarin, clotting time is increased. If an increased level of vitamin K is provided, more of these factors are produced, and the clotting time can be brought back within a normal range. Because of the way in which vitamin K exerts its effects on clotting, there is a delay of at least 24 hours from the time the drug is given until some change can be seen. This occurs because there is no direct effect on the warfarin, but rather an increased stimulation of the liver, which must then produce the clotting factors. The usual dose for the treatment of anticoagulant-induced prothrombin deficiency is 2.5 to 10 mg IM or subcutaneously or, rarely, 25 mg IM or subcutaneously. Oral doses can be used if injection is not feasible. A prothrombin time response within 6 to 8 hours after parenteral doses or 12 to 48 hours after oral doses will determine the need for a repeat dose. If a response is not seen and the patient is bleeding excessively, fresh-frozen plasma or an infusion of whole blood may be needed. In 2014 a quick reversal agent was approved for warfarin overdose. Prothrombin complex concentrate (**KCentra, Ocaplex**), a blood product, is infused IV to supply the clotting factors needed to restore hemostatic balance. The IV dosing is based on the patient's INR.*

Adverse Effects

The most commonly encountered adverse effect of the anticoagulants is bleeding, ranging from bleeding gums with tooth brushing to severe internal hemorrhage. Patients need teaching about administration, disposal of the syringes, and signs of bleeding to watch for. Periodic blood tests will be needed to assess the effects of the drug on the body. Clotting times should be monitored closely to avoid these problems. Table 48.2 reviews clotting studies that should be monitored. The patient should also be monitored for warfarin overdose. The newer oral anticoagulants cannot be used with artificial heart valves, which can become obstructed. These drugs also have a black box warning of the risk for rebound thromboembolic events when the drugs are suddenly stopped. This is a concern if a patient forgets to get a refill of the drug or is traveling and runs out of the drug. Patient selection must be done carefully and teaching needs to be explicit. These drugs also have a black box warning about the risk for spinal and epidural hematoma if used during spinal anesthesia or spinal puncture; permanent paralysis has occurred.

Serious adverse effects may occur when adding or taking away a drug from the regimen of a patient receiving warfarin without careful patient monitoring and adjustment of the warfarin dose (see Clinically Important Drug–Drug Interactions). Warfarin has been associated with alopecia and dermatitis, as well as bone marrow depression and, less frequently, prolonged and painful erections. The following Focus on Safe Medication Administration discusses the treatment of heparin overdose. Nausea, GI upset, diarrhea, and hepatic dysfunction also may occur secondary to direct drug toxicity.

FOCUS ON Safe Medication Administration

In cases of a heparin overdose the antidote is protamine sulfate (generic). This strongly basic protein drug forms stable salts with heparin as soon as the two drugs come in contact, immediately reversing heparin's anticoagulant effects. Paradoxically, if protamine is given to a patient who has not received heparin, it has anticoagulant effects. The dose is determined by the amount of heparin that was given and the time that elapsed since then. A dose of 1 mg IV protamine neutralizes 90 units of heparin derived from lung tissue or 110 USP of heparin derived from intestinal mucosa. The drug must be administered very slowly—not to exceed 50 mg IV in any 10-minute period. Care must be taken to calculate the amount of heparin that has been given to the patient. Potentially fatal anaphylactic reactions have been reported with the use of protamine sulfate, and so life support equipment should be readily available when it is used.

Clinically Important Drug–Drug Interactions

Increased bleeding can occur if heparin is combined with oral anticoagulants, salicylates, penicillins, or cephalosporins. Decreased anticoagulation can occur if heparin is combined with nitroglycerin.

Warfarin has documented drug–drug interactions with a vast number of other drugs (Table 48.3). It is a wise practice never to add or take away a drug from the regimen of a patient receiving warfarin without careful patient monitoring and adjustment of the warfarin dose to prevent serious adverse effects. Because of the many factors that can affect the therapeutic levels of warfarin, it is often very difficult to reach a stable level and maintain that level. In 2007 the U.S. Food and Drug Administration (FDA) approved a genetic marker to offer some help with that challenge (Box 48.4).

Dabigatran, edoxaban, apixaban, and rivaroxaban must be used with caution with antifungals, erythromycin, ritonavir, phenytoin, and rifampin because of alterations in metabolism. All of these drugs should be used with caution if combined with any other drugs or herbs known to increase bleeding effects.

Prototype Summary: Heparin

Indications: Prevention and treatment of venous thrombosis and PE; treatment of AF with embolization; diagnosis and treatment of DIC; prevention of clotting in blood samples and heparin lock sets.

Actions: Inhibits thrombus and clot production by blocking the conversion of prothrombin to thrombin and fibrinogen to fibrin.

Pharmacokinetics:

Route	Onset	Peak	Duration
IV	Immediate	Minutes	2–6 h
Subcutaneous	20–60 min	2–4 h	8–12 h

$T_{1/2}$: 30 to 180 minutes; metabolized in the cells and excreted in the urine.

Adverse Effects: Loss of hair, bruising, chills, fever, osteoporosis, suppression of renal function (with long-term use). See Anticoagulant Adjunctive Therapy for information on lepirudin (Refludan), a drug developed for the treatment of rare allergic reaction to heparin.

Table 48.3 Clinically Important Drug–Drug Interactions with Warfarin

↑Bleeding Effects	↓Anticoagulation	↑Activity and Effects of Other Drug
salicylates	barbiturates	phenytoin
chloral hydrate	griseofulvin	
phenylbutazone	rifampin	
clofibrate	phenytoin	
disulfiram	glutethimide	
chloramphenicol	carbamazepine	
metronidazole	vitamin K	
cimetidine	vitamin E	
ranitidine	cholestyramine	
cotrimoxazole	aminoglutethimide	
quinidine	ethchlorvynol	
quinine		
oxyphenbutazone		
thyroid drugs		
glucagon		
danazol		
erythromycin		
androgens		
amiodarone		
cefamandole		
cefoperazone		
cefotetan		
moxalactam		
cefazolin		
cefoxitin		
ceftriaxone		
meclofenamate		
mefenamic acid		
famotidine		
nizatidine		
nalidixic acid		

BOX 48.4

Genetic Marker Test for Warfarin

In September 2007 the FDA approved a new genetic test that shows patient sensitivity to warfarin, which will make prescribing and setting doses much easier. It is estimated that at least one-third of patients metabolize the drug differently, which could account for the huge number of adverse events associated with the drug. The new test, the Nanosphere Verigene Warfarin Metabolism Nucleic Acid Test, picks up gene variants that contribute to the abnormal metabolism and alerts the prescriber to related dose requirements. Preliminary postmarketing studies were not as positive as anticipated. Further use may refine use guidelines.

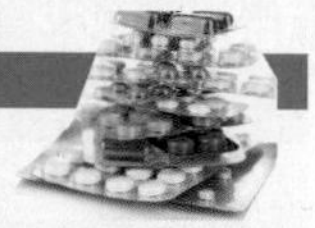

Nursing Considerations for Patients Receiving Anticoagulants

Assessment: History and Examination

- Assess for any known allergies to these drugs *to avoid potential hypersensitivity reactions.* Also screen for conditions *that could be exacerbated by increased bleeding tendencies*, including hemorrhagic disorders, recent trauma, spinal puncture, GI ulcers, recent surgery, intrauterine device placement, tuberculosis, presence of indwelling catheters, and threatened abortion. Also screen for pregnancy *to ensure that benefits outweigh any potential risks* (*contraindicated with warfarin*); lactation *because of the potential for risks to the baby* (use of heparin is suggested if an anticoagulant is needed during lactation); renal or hepatic disease, *which could interfere with the metabolism, excretion, and effectiveness of these drugs*; heart failure; thyrotoxicosis; senility or psychosis *because of the potential for unexpected effects*; and diarrhea or fever, *which could alter the normal clotting process.*
- Assess baseline status before beginning therapy *to determine any potential adverse effects.* This includes body temperature; skin color, lesions, and temperature; affect, orientation, and reflexes; pulse, blood pressure, and perfusion; respirations and adventitious sounds; clotting studies, renal and hepatic function tests, CBC, and stool guaiac; and ECG, if appropriate.

Nursing Diagnoses

Nursing diagnoses related to drug therapy might include the following:

- Risk for injury related to bleeding effects and bone marrow depression
- Disturbed body image related to alopecia and skin rash
- Ineffective tissue perfusion (total body) related to blood loss
- Deficient knowledge regarding drug therapy

Planning

- The patient will receive the best therapeutic effect from the drug therapy.
- The patient will have limited adverse effects to the drug therapy.
- The patient will have an understanding of the drug therapy, adverse effects to anticipate, and measures to relieve discomfort and improve safety.

Implementation with Rationale

- Evaluate for therapeutic effects of warfarin—PT 1.5 to 2.5 times the control value or ratio of PT to INR of 2 to 3—*to evaluate the effectiveness of the drug dose.*
- Evaluate for therapeutic effects of heparin—whole blood clotting time (WBCT) 2.5 to 3 times control or activated partial thromboplastin time (APTT) 1.5 to 3 times the control value—*to evaluate the effectiveness of the drug dose.*
- Evaluate the patient regularly for any sign of blood loss (petechiae, bleeding gums, bruises, dark-colored stools, dark-colored urine) *to evaluate the effectiveness of the drug dose and to determine the need to consult with the prescriber if bleeding becomes apparent.*
- Establish safety precautions *to protect the patient from injury.*
- Provide safety measures, such as use of an electric razor and avoidance of contact sports, *to decrease the risk of bleeding.*
- Provide increased precautions against bleeding during invasive procedures; use pressure dressings; avoid IM injections; and do not rub subcutaneous injection sites *because the state of anticoagulation increases the risk of blood loss.*
- Mark the chart of any patient receiving this drug *to alert the medical staff that there is a potential for increased bleeding.*
- Maintain antidotes on standby (protamine sulfate for heparin, vitamin K or prothrombin complex concentrate for warfarin) *in case of overdose.*
- Ensure a switch to another anticoagulant if apixaban, edoxaban, dabigatran, or rivaroxaban are stopped suddenly for any reason other than pathological bleeding *because of the risk of thromboembolic events.*
- Monitor the patient carefully when any drug or herb is added to or withdrawn from the drug regimen of a patient taking warfarin *because of the risk of drug–drug interactions that would change the effectiveness of the anticoagulant.*
- Make sure that the patient receives regular follow-up and monitoring, including measurement of clotting times, *to ensure maximum therapeutic effects.*

- Provide thorough patient teaching, including the name of the drug, dosage prescribed, measures to avoid adverse effects, warning signs of problems, the need for periodic monitoring and evaluation, and the need to wear or carry a MedicAlert notification, *to enhance patient knowledge about drug therapy and to promote compliance with the drug regimen.*
- Offer support and encouragement *to help the patient deal with the diagnosis and the drug regimen.*

Evaluation

- Monitor patient response to the drug: Increased bleeding time (warfarin PT 1.5 to 2.5 times the control value or warfarin PT/INR ratio of 2 to 3; heparin WBCT of 2.5 to 3 times the control value or APTT of 1.5 to 3 times the control value).
- Monitor for adverse effects (bleeding, bone marrow depression, alopecia, GI upset, rash).
- Evaluate the effectiveness of the teaching plan (patient can name drug, dosage, adverse effects to watch for, and specific measures to avoid them; the patient understands the importance of continued follow-up).
- Monitor the effectiveness of comfort measures and compliance with the regimen.

Thrombolytic Agents

Thrombolytic agents break down the thrombus that has been formed by stimulating the plasmin system. This process is called clot resolution. Thrombolytic agents include alteplase (*Activase*), reteplase (*Retavase*), tenecteplase (*TNKase*), and urokinase (*Abbokinase*).

Therapeutic Actions and Indications

If a thrombus has already formed in a vessel (e.g., during an acute MI), it may be necessary to dissolve that clot to open the vessel and restore blood flow to the dependent tissue. All of the drugs that are available for this purpose work to activate the natural anticlotting system—conversion of plasminogen to plasmin. The activation of this system breaks down fibrin threads and dissolves any formed clot. The thrombolytics are effective only if the patient has plasminogen in the plasma. See Table 48.1 for Usual Indications for each of these agents.

Pharmacokinetics

These drugs are given IV and are cleared from the body after liver metabolism. They cross the placenta, but it is not known whether they enter breast milk (see Contraindications and Cautions).

Contraindications and Cautions

The use of thrombolytic agents is contraindicated in the presence of allergy to any of these drugs *to prevent hypersensitivity reactions*. They also should not be used with any condition *that could be worsened by the dissolution of clots*, including recent surgery, active internal bleeding, cerebrovascular accident (CVA) within the last 2 months, aneurysm, obstetrical delivery, organ biopsy, recent serious GI bleeding, rupture of a noncompressible blood vessel, recent major trauma (including cardiopulmonary resuscitation), known blood-clotting defects, cerebrovascular disease, uncontrolled hypertension, and liver disease, *which could affect normal clotting factors and the production of plasminogen.*

These drugs are also contraindicated in pregnancy *because of the possible adverse effects on the fetus or neonate.* These drugs should not be used during pregnancy unless the benefits to the mother clearly outweigh the potential risks to the fetus. Caution should be used during lactation *because of the potential risk for bleeding effects in the nursing baby.*

Adverse Effects

The most common adverse effect associated with the use of thrombolytic agents is bleeding. Patients should be monitored closely for the occurrence of cardiac arrhythmias (with coronary reperfusion) and hypotension. Hypersensitivity reactions are not uncommon; they range from rash and flushing to bronchospasm and anaphylactic reaction.

Clinically Important Drug–Drug Interactions

The risk of hemorrhage increases if thrombolytic agents are used with any anticoagulant or antiplatelet drug.

Prototype Summary: Urokinase

Indications: Lysis of PE or PE with unstable hemodynamics in adults.

Actions: Converts endogenous plasminogen to plasmin, which breaks down fibrin clots, fibrinogen, and other plasma proteins; lyses thrombi and emboli.

Pharmacokinetics:

Route	Onset	Peak	Duration
IV	Immediate	End of injection	Unknown

$T_{1/2}$: Unknown; metabolized in the plasma; excretion method unknown.

Adverse Effects: Headache, angioneurotic edema, hypotension, skin rash, bleeding, breathing difficulties, bronchospasm, pain, fever, anaphylactic shock.

Nursing Considerations for Patients Receiving Thrombolytic Agents

Assessment: History and Examination

- Assess for any known allergies to these drugs *to prevent hypersensitivity reactions.* Also screen for any conditions *that could be worsened by the dissolution of clots,* including recent surgery, active internal bleeding, CVA within the last 2 months, aneurysm, obstetrical delivery, organ biopsy, recent serious GI bleeding, rupture of a noncompressible blood vessel, recent major trauma (including cardiopulmonary resuscitation), known blood-clotting defects, cerebrovascular disease, uncontrolled hypertension, liver disease, *which could affect normal clotting factors and the production of plasminogen,* and pregnancy or lactation *because of the possible adverse effects on the neonate.*
- Assess baseline status before beginning therapy *to determine any potential adverse effects.* Assess the following: Body temperature; skin color, lesions, and temperature; affect, orientation, and reflexes; pulse, blood pressure, and perfusion; respirations and adventitious sounds; and clotting studies, renal and hepatic function tests, CBC, guaiac test for occult blood in stool, and ECG.

Nursing Diagnoses

Nursing diagnoses related to drug therapy might include the following:

- Risk for injury related to clot-dissolving effects
- Ineffective tissue perfusion (total body) related to possible blood loss
- Decreased cardiac output related to bleeding and arrhythmias
- Deficient knowledge regarding drug therapy

Planning

- The patient will receive the best therapeutic effect from the drug therapy.
- The patient will have limited adverse effects to the drug therapy.
- The patient will have an understanding of the drug therapy, adverse effects to anticipate, and measures to relieve discomfort and improve safety

Implementation with Rationale

- Arrange to administer tenecteplase to reduce mortality associated with acute MI as soon as possible after the onset of symptoms *because the timing for the administration of tenecteplase is critical to resolve the clot before permanent damage occurs to the myocardial cells.*
- Discontinue heparin if it is being given before administration of a thrombolytic agent, unless specifically ordered for coronary artery infusion, *to prevent excessive loss of blood.*
- Evaluate the patient regularly for any sign of blood loss (petechiae, bleeding gums, bruises, dark-colored stools, dark-colored urine) *to evaluate drug effectiveness and for the need to consult with the prescriber if blood loss becomes apparent.*
- Monitor coagulation studies regularly; consult with the prescriber *to adjust the drug dose appropriately.*
- Institute treatment within 6 hours after the onset of symptoms of acute MI *to achieve optimum therapeutic effectiveness.*
- Arrange to type and crossmatch blood *in case of serious blood loss that requires whole-blood transfusion.*
- Monitor cardiac rhythm continuously if the drug is being given for acute MI *because of the risk of alteration in cardiac function;* have life support equipment on standby as needed.
- Provide increased precautions against bleeding during invasive procedures, use pressure dressings and ice, avoid IM injections, and do not rub subcutaneous injection sites *because of the risk of increased blood loss in the anticoagulated state.*
- Mark the chart of any patient receiving this drug *to alert medical staff that there is a potential for increased bleeding.*
- Provide thorough patient teaching, including the name of the drug, dosage prescribed, measures to avoid adverse effects, warning signs of problems, and the need for periodic monitoring and evaluation, *to enhance patient knowledge about drug therapy and to promote compliance with the drug regimen.*
- Offer support and encouragement *to help the patient deal with the diagnosis and the drug regimen.*

Evaluation

- Monitor patient response to the drug (dissolution of the clot and return of blood flow to the area).
- Monitor for adverse effects (bleeding, arrhythmias, hypotension, hypersensitivity reaction).
- Evaluate the effectiveness of the teaching plan (patient can name drug, adverse effects to watch for, and specific measures to avoid them).
- Monitor the effectiveness of comfort measures and compliance with the regimen.

Other Drugs Affecting Clot Formation

Other drugs that affect clot formation are also effective in preventing thromboembolic episodes. These drugs include the low-molecular-weight heparins, adjunctive agents used to help alleviate adverse reactions to these drugs, and one hemorrheologic agent.

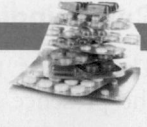

Low-Molecular-Weight Heparins

In the late 1990s a series of low-molecular-weight heparins were developed. These drugs inhibit thrombus and clot formation by blocking factors Xa and IIa. Because of the size and nature of the molecules, these drugs do not greatly affect thrombin, clotting, or the PT; therefore, they cause fewer systemic adverse effects. They also have been found to block angiogenesis, the process that allows cancer cells to develop new blood vessels. They are being studied as possible adjuncts to cancer chemotherapy. These drugs are indicated for very specific uses in the prevention of clots and emboli formation after certain surgeries or prolonged bed rest. The nursing care of a patient receiving one of these drugs is similar to that of a patient receiving heparin. The drug is given just before (or just after) the surgery and then is continued for 7 to 14 days during the postoperative recovery process. Caution must be used to avoid combining these drugs with standard heparin therapy; serious bleeding episodes and deaths have been reported when this combination was inadvertently used. Low-molecular-weight heparins include dalteparin and enoxaparin. See Table 48.1 for additional information about these agents.

Anticoagulant Adjunctive Therapy

Agents used in anticoagulant adjunctive therapy include lepirudin, protamine sulfate, prothrombin complex concentrate, and vitamin K. See Focus on Safe Medication Administration under Adverse Effects for anticoagulants for additional information about vitamin K and protamine sulfate. See also Table 48.1 for additional information for each of these agents.

Lepirudin (*Refludan*) is an IV drug that was developed to treat a rare allergic reaction to heparin. In some patients an allergy to heparin precipitates a heparin-induced thrombocythemia with associated thromboembolic disease. Lepirudin directly inhibits thrombin, blocking the thromboembolic effects of this reaction. A 0.4-mg/kg initial IV bolus followed by a continuous infusion of 0.15 mg/kg for 2 to 10 days is the usual treatment. The patient needs to be monitored for bleeding from any site and for the development of direct hepatic injury.

Hemorrheologic Agent

Pentoxifylline (generic) is known as a hemorrheologic agent, or a drug that can induce hemorrhage. It is a xanthine that, like caffeine and theophylline, decreases platelet aggregation and decreases the fibrinogen concentration in the blood. These effects can decrease blood clot formation and increase blood flow through narrowed or damaged vessels. The mechanism of action by which pentoxifylline does these things is not known. It is one of the very few drugs found to be effective in treating intermittent claudication, a painful vascular problem of the legs.

Because pentoxifylline is a xanthine, it is associated with many CV stimulatory effects; patients with underlying CV problems need to be monitored carefully when taking this drug. Pentoxifylline can also cause headache, dizziness, nausea, and upset stomach. It is taken orally three times a day for at least 8 weeks to evaluate its effectiveness. See Table 48.1 for additional information about this drug.

KEY POINTS

- To keep blood from coagulating, anticoagulants block blood aggregates or interfere with the mechanisms that cause blood to clot.
- Thrombolytic drugs activate the plasminogen system to dissolve clots naturally.

Drugs Used to Control Bleeding

On the other end of the spectrum of coagulation problems are various bleeding disorders. These include the following:

- *Hemophilia*, in which there is a genetic lack of clotting factors that leaves the patient vulnerable to excessive bleeding with any injury.
- *Liver disease*, in which clotting factors and proteins needed for clotting are not produced.
- *Bone marrow disorders*, in which platelets are not formed in sufficient quantity to be effective.

Bleeding disorders are treated with clotting factors and drugs that promote the coagulation process. These include antihemophilic agents and hemostatic agents (systemic and topical) (see Table 48.4).

Antihemophilic Agents

The drugs used to treat hemophilia are replacement factors for the specific clotting factors that are genetically missing in that particular type of hemophilia. These drugs include antihemophilic factor (*Bioclate*, *ReFacto*, and others), coagulation factor VIIa (*NovoSeven*), and factor IX (*BeneFix*, *Profilnine SD*, and others), factor IX complex (*Bebulin VH*, *Profilnine* SD), anti-inhibitor coagulant complex (*Feiba NA*), factor XIII (*Corifact*) and the newest drugs in this group, antihemophilic factor Fc fusion protein (*Eloctate*), and antihemophilic factor porcine sequence (*Obizur*).

Therapeutic Actions and Indications

The antihemophilic drugs replace clotting factors that are either genetically missing or low in a particular type

Table 48.4 *Drugs in Focus:* Drugs Used to Control Bleeding

Drug Name	Usual Dosage	Usual Indications
Antihemophilic Agents		
antihemophilic factor (*Bioclate*, and others)	IV dose based on level of antihemophilic factor, weight, and patient response	Treatment of hemophilia A; to correct or prevent bleeding episodes or to allow necessary surgery
antihemophilic factor Fc fusion protein (*Eloctate*)	IV dose based on factor VIII levels. patient weight, response	Treatment of congenital hemophilia A; to correct or prevent bleeding episodes or to allow necessary surgery
antihemophilic factor porcine sequence (*Obizur*)	200 units/kg IV, dose then titrated based on factor VIII levels	Treatment of bleeding episodes related to acquired hemophilia A in adults
anti-inhibitor coagulant complex (*Feiba NA*)	50–100 units/kg IV at 12-h intervals until bleeding is controlled	Control of spontaneous bleeding episodes or to cover surgical interventions in hemophilia A and B patients with inhibitors
coagulation factor VIIa (*NovoSeven*)	90 mcg/kg IV q2 h until hemostasis is achieved	Treatment of bleeding episodes in patients with hemophilia A or B
factor IX (*Bebulin VH*, *Profilnine SD*)	IV dose based on weight and levels of factor IX	Prevention and control of bleeding in patients with factor IX deficiencies
factor IX complex (*BeneFix*, and others)	IV dose based on factor levels, weight, and desired response	Treatment or prevention of hemophilia B (Christmas disease, a deficiency of factor IX); treatment of bleeding episodes in patients with factor VII and factor VIII deficiencies; controls bleeding episodes in patients with hemophilia A
factor XIII (*Corifact*)	40 units/kg IV, subsequent dosing based on patient response	Prevention of bleeding in patients with congenital factor XIII deficiencies
Hemostatic Agents ***Systemic***		
aminocaproic acid (*Amicar*)	5 mg PO or IV, then 1–1.25 g/h; not to exceed 30 g in 24 h	Treatment of excessive bleeding in hyperfibrinolytic states; prevention of recurrence of bleeding with subarachnoid hemorrhage; sometimes used for treatment of attacks of hereditary angioedema
Topical		
absorbable gelatin (*Gelfoam*)	Smear or press onto surface; do not remove, will be absorbed	Controls bleeding from surface cuts or injury
human fibrin sealant (*Artiss*)	Spray a thin layer on prepared graft bed	Adheres autologous skin grafts to surgically prepared wound beds resulting from burns in adults and children
human fibrin sealant (*Evicel*)	Spray or drip solution onto site to produce a thin, even layer	Adjunct to hemostasis in liver or vascular surgery when control of bleeding by standard surgical techniques is ineffective
microfibrillar collagen (*Avitene*)	Use dry; apply to area and apply pressure for 3–5 min	Controls bleeding from surface cuts or injury
thrombin (*Evithrom*, *Thrombinar*)	100–1,000 units/mL freely mixed with blood	Controls bleeding from surface cuts or injury
thrombin, recombinant (*Recothrom*)	Apply solution directly to bleeding site in conjunction with absorbable gelatin sponge	Adjunct to hemostasis whenever oozing blood and minor bleeding from capillaries and small venules is accessible and control of bleeding by standard surgical techniques is ineffective or impractical; decreases possibility for allergic reactions associated with bovine thrombin

of hemophilia. The drug of choice depends on the particular hemophilia that is being treated. Antihemophilic factor is factor VIII, the clotting factor that is missing in classic hemophilia (hemophilia A). This agent is used to correct or prevent bleeding episodes or to allow necessary surgery.

Coagulation factor VIIa and factor IX complex are used for patients with hemophilia A or B (see Table 48.4 for

Usual Indications for each of these agents). Coagulation factor VIIa is a preparation made from mouse, hamster, and bovine proteins that contains variable amounts of preformed clotting factors (see Contraindications and Cautions). Factor IX complex contains plasma fractions of many of the clotting factors and increases blood levels of factors II, VII, IX, and X. Factor XIII replaces factor XIII in patients with a congenital deficiency. Anti-inhibitor coagulant complex is used to control spontaneous bleeding or to cover surgical procedures in patients with hemophilia A and B with inhibitors. Antihemophilic factor Fc fusion protein is used to prevent and control bleeding episodes in adults and children with hemophilia A (factor VIII deficiency) and antihemophilic factor porcine sequence is used for treating bleeding episodes in adults with acquired hemophilia A. The drug of choice for any given patient is determined by his or her particular coagulation abnormalities.

Pharmacokinetics

These agents replace normal clotting factors and are processed as such by the body. They must be given IV and are processed by the body in the same way that naturally occurring clotting factors are processed in the plasma, usually with a half-life of 24 to 36 hours.

Contraindications and Cautions

Antihemophilic factor is contraindicated in the presence of known allergy to mouse proteins *to prevent hypersensitivity reactions.* Factor IX is contraindicated in the presence of liver disease with signs of intravascular coagulation or fibrinolysis *to prevent serious aggravation of these disorders.* Coagulation factor VIIa is contraindicated with known allergies to mouse, hamster, or bovine products *to prevent hypersensitivity reactions.* These drugs are not recommended for use during lactation, and caution should be used during pregnancy *because of the potential for adverse effects on the baby or fetus.* They should be used during pregnancy only if the benefit to the mother clearly outweighs the potential risk to the fetus. It is recommended that another method of feeding the baby be used if these drugs are needed during lactation. Because these drugs are used to prevent serious bleeding problems or to treat bleeding episodes, there are few contraindications to their use.

Adverse Effects

The most common adverse effects associated with antihemophilic agents involve risks associated with the use of blood products (e.g., hepatitis, AIDS). Headache, flushing, chills, fever, and lethargy may occur as a reaction to the injection of a foreign protein. Nausea and vomiting may also occur, as may stinging, itching, and burning at the site of the injection.

Ⓟ Prototype Summary: Antihemophilic Factor

Indications: Treatment of classic hemophilia to provide temporary replacement of clotting factors to correct or prevent bleeding episodes or to allow necessary surgery.

Actions: Normal plasma protein that is needed for the transformation of prothrombin to thrombin, the final step in the clotting pathway.

Pharmacokinetics:

Route	Onset	Peak	Duration
IV	Immediate	Unknown	Unknown

$T_{1/2}$: 12 hours; cleared from the body by normal protein metabolism.

Adverse Effects: Allergic reaction, stinging at injection site, headache, rash, chills, nausea, hepatitis, AIDS (risks associated with the use of blood products).

Nursing Considerations for Patients Receiving Antihemophilic Agents

Assessment: History and Examination

- Assess for the following conditions, *which could be cautions or contraindications to use of the drug*: Any known allergies to these drugs or to mouse proteins with antihemophilic factor; liver disease.
- Assess for baseline status before beginning therapy *to determine any potential adverse effects.* Assess the following: Body temperature; skin color, lesions, and temperature; affect, orientation, and reflexes; pulse, blood pressure, and perfusion; respirations and adventitious sounds; clotting studies; and hepatic function tests.

Nursing Diagnoses

Nursing diagnoses related to drug therapy might include the following:

- Ineffective tissue perfusion (total body) related to changes in coagulation
- Acute pain related to GI, CNS, or skin effects
- Anxiety or fear related to the diagnosis and use of blood-related products
- Deficient knowledge regarding drug therapy

Planning

- The patient will receive the best therapeutic effect from the drug therapy.
- The patient will have limited adverse effects to the drug therapy.

(continues on page 846)

- The patient will have an understanding of the drug therapy, adverse effects to anticipate, and measures to relieve discomfort and improve safety

Implementation with Rationale

- Ensure that appropriate clotting factor is being used for the patient *to ensure therapeutic effectiveness and prevent inappropriate increase in other clotting factors.*
- Administer by the IV route only *to ensure therapeutic effectiveness.*
- Monitor clinical response and clotting factor levels regularly *to arrange to adjust dose as needed.*
- Monitor the patient for any sign of thrombosis *to arrange to use comfort and support measures as needed* (e.g., support hose, positioning, ambulation, exercise).
- Decrease the rate of infusion if headache, chills, fever, or tingling occurs *to prevent severe drug reaction*; in some individuals the drug will need to be discontinued.
- Arrange to type and crossmatch blood *in case of serious blood loss that will require whole-blood transfusion.*
- Mark the chart of any patient receiving this drug *to alert medical staff that there is a potential for increased bleeding.*
- Provide thorough patient teaching, including the name of the drug, dosage prescribed, measures to avoid adverse effects, warning signs of problems, and the need for periodic monitoring and evaluation, *to enhance patient knowledge about drug therapy and to promote compliance with the drug regimen.*
- Offer support and encouragement *to help the patient deal with the diagnosis and the drug regimen.*

Evaluation

- Monitor patient response to the drug (control of bleeding episodes, prevention of bleeding episodes).
- Monitor for adverse effects (thrombosis, CNS effects, nausea, hypersensitivity reaction, hepatitis, AIDS).
- Evaluate the effectiveness of the teaching plan (patient can name drug, dosage of drug, adverse effects to watch for, specific measures to avoid them, and warning signs to report).
- Monitor the effectiveness of comfort measures and compliance with the regimen.

Hemostatic Agents

Some situations result in a fibrinolytic state with excessive plasminogen activity and risk of bleeding from clot dissolution. For example, patients undergoing repeat coronary artery bypass graft (CABG) surgery are especially prone to excessive bleeding and may require blood transfusion. **Hemostatic agents** are used to stop bleeding. Hemostatic drugs may be either systemic or topical.

The hemostatic drug that is used systemically is aminocaproic acid (*Amicar*). Topical hemostatic agents include absorbable gelatin (*Gelfoam*), human fibrin sealant (*Artiss, Evicel*), microfibrillar collagen (*Avitene*), thrombin (*Evithrom, Thrombostat*), and thrombin recombinant (*Recothrom*).

Therapeutic Actions and Indications

Systemic Hemostatic Agents

The systemic hemostatic agents are used to prevent body-wide or systemic clot breakdown, thus preventing blood loss in situations in which serious systemic bleeding could occur, or hyperfibrinolysis. There is only one systemic hemostatic agent available for use in the United States.

Aminocaproic acid inhibits plasminogen-activating substances and has some antiplasmin activity. When taking the oral form of aminocaproic acid the patient may need to take 10 tablets in the first hour and then continue taking the drug around the clock. Aprotinin, another systemic hemostatic agent used to reduce blood loss and need for transfusions associated with CABG surgery, was pulled from the market in 2008 after reports of increased risk of CV events in patients who had been treated with this drug. See Table 48.4 for Usual Indications for aminocaproic acid.

Topical Hemostatic Agents

Some surface injuries involve so much damage to the small vessels in the area that clotting does not occur and blood is slowly and continually lost. For these situations, topical or local hemostatic agents are often used. The use of these drugs is also incorporated into the care of wounds or decubitus ulcers as adjunctive therapy. The drug of choice depends on the nature of the injury and the prescriber's preference. The newest topical hemostatic agent is human fibrin sealant. Thrombin recombinant is the first topical hemostatic agent approved to be made using recombinant DNA technology (this will decrease many of the potential allergic reactions associated with bovine thrombin; see Contraindications and Cautions). See Table 48.4 for additional information about these agents.

Pharmacokinetics

Systemic Hemostatic Agents

Aminocaproic acid is available in oral and IV forms. It is rapidly absorbed and widely distributed throughout the body. It is excreted largely unchanged in urine, with a half-life of 2 hours.

Topical Hemostatic Agents

Absorbable gelatin and microfibrillar collagen are available in sponge form and are applied directly to the injured area until the bleeding stops.

Human fibrin sealant (*Artiss*) is available in spray form and applied in a thin layer onto the graft bed. *Evicel* is sprayed directly onto any active bleeding site.

Thrombin, which is derived from bovine sources, is a solution that is applied topically and mixed in with the blood. Thrombin recombinant is also a solution and is applied directly to the bleeding site surface in conjunction with absorbable gelatin sponge; the amount needed varies with the area of tissue to be treated.

Contraindications and Cautions

Systemic Hemostatic Agents

Aminocaproic acid is contraindicated in the presence of allergy to the drug *to prevent hypersensitivity reactions* and with acute DIC *because of the risk of tissue necrosis.* Caution should be used in cardiac disease *because of the risk of arrhythmias* and in renal and hepatic dysfunction, *which could alter the excretion of these drug and the normal clotting processes.* Although the safety for use of this drug during pregnancy has not been established, it should be used only if the benefits to the mother clearly outweigh the potential risks to the neonate *because of the potential for adverse effects on the fetus.* It is recommended that nursing mothers use a different method for feeding the baby if this drug is used *because of the potential for adverse effects on the baby.*

Topical Hemostatic Agents

Use thrombin with caution for those patients with an allergy to bovine products. *Because thrombin comes from animal sources, it may precipitate an allergic response; the patient needs to be carefully monitored for such a reaction.* Many of the potential allergic reactions associated with bovine thrombin will be decreased as a result of approval for thrombin recombinant to be made using recombinant DNA technology. Safety for use of thrombin recombinant in children has not been established.

Adverse Effects

Systemic Hemostatic Agents

The most common adverse effect associated with systemic hemostatic agents is excessive clotting. In 2007, there were many reports of increased CV events, including fatalities in patients who received the hemostatic drug aprotinin. Some of the events occurred months after the drug was used. The drug was removed from the market in 2008. CNS effects of aminocaproic acid can include hallucinations, drowsiness, dizziness, headache, and psychotic states, all of which could be related to changes in cerebral blood flow associated with changes in clot dissolution. GI effects, including nausea, cramps, and diarrhea, may be related to excessive clotting in the GI tract, causing reflex GI stimulation. Weakness, fatigue, malaise, and muscle pain can occur as small clots build up in muscles. Intrarenal obstruction and renal dysfunction have also been reported.

Topical Hemostatic Agents

Use of absorbable gelatin and microfibrillar collagen can pose a risk of infection *because bacteria can become trapped in the vascular area when the sponge is applied.* Immediate removal of the sponge and cleaning of the area can help to decrease this risk.

Clinically Important Drug–Drug Interactions

Systemic Hemostatic Agents

Aminocaproic acid is associated with the development of hypercoagulation states if it is combined with oral contraceptives or estrogens. The risk of bleeding increases if it is given with heparin.

Topical Hemostatic Agents

There are no reported drug–drug interactions with the topically applied hemostatic agents.

Prototype Summary: Aminocaproic Acid

Indications: Treatment of excessive bleeding resulting from hyperfibrinolysis; also used to prevent the recurrence of subarachnoid hemorrhage, for management of megakaryocytic thrombocytopenia, to decrease the need for platelet administration, and to abort and treat attacks of hereditary angioneurotic edema.

Actions: Inhibits plasminogen activator substances and has antiplasmin activity that inhibits fibrinolysis and prevents the breakdown of clots.

Pharmacokinetics:

Route	Onset	Peak	Duration
Oral	Rapid	2 h	Unknown
IV	Immediate	Minutes	2–3 h

$T_{1/2}$: 2 hours; excreted unchanged in the urine.

Adverse Effects: Dizziness, tinnitus, headache, weakness, hypotension, nausea, cramps, diarrhea, fertility problems, malaise, elevated serum creatine phosphokinase.

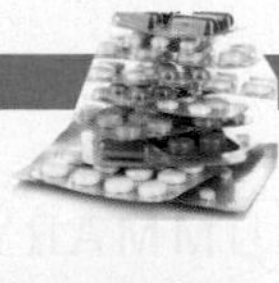

Nursing Considerations for Patients Receiving Systemic Hemostatic Agents

Nursing considerations for a patient receiving topical hemostatic agents are similar to those with the use of any topical drug (see Appendix B).

Assessment: History and Examination

- Assess for the following conditions, *which could be cautions or contraindications to the use of systemic*

(continues on page 848)

hemostatic agents: Any known allergies to any component of the drug *to prevent hypersensitivity reactions*; acute disseminated intravascular coagulation *because of the risk of tissue necrosis*; renal and hepatic dysfunction, *which could alter the excretion of these drugs and the normal clotting processes*; and lactation *because of the potential for adverse effects on the neonate.*

- Assess baseline status before beginning therapy *to determine any potential adverse effects*. Assess the following: Body temperature; skin color, lesions, and temperature; affect, orientation, and reflexes; pulse, blood pressure, and perfusion; respirations and adventitious sounds; bowel sounds and normal output; urinalysis and clotting studies; and renal and hepatic function tests.

Nursing Diagnoses

Nursing diagnoses related to drug therapy might include the following:

- Disturbed sensory perception related to CNS effects
- Acute pain related to GI, CNS, or muscle effects
- Risk for injury related to CNS or blood-clotting effects
- Deficient knowledge regarding drug therapy

Planning

- The patient will receive the best therapeutic effect from the drug therapy.
- The patient will have limited adverse effects to the drug therapy.
- The patient will have an understanding of the drug therapy, adverse effects to anticipate, and measures to relieve discomfort and improve safety.

Implementation with Rationale

- Monitor clinical response and clotting factor levels regularly *to arrange to adjust dose as needed.*
- Monitor the patient for any sign of thrombosis *to arrange to use comfort and support measures as needed* (e.g., support hose, positioning, ambulation, exercise).
- Orient the patient and offer support and safety measures if hallucinations or psychoses occur *to prevent patient injury.*
- Offer comfort measures *to help the patient deal with the effects of the drug*. These include small, frequent meals; mouth care; environmental controls; and safety measures.
- Provide thorough patient teaching, including the name of the drug, dosage prescribed, measures to avoid adverse effects, warning signs of problems, and the need for periodic monitoring and evaluation, *to enhance patient knowledge about drug therapy and to promote compliance with the drug regimen.*
- Offer support and encouragement *to help the patient deal with the diagnosis and the drug regimen.*

Evaluation

- Monitor patient response to the drug (control of bleeding episodes).
- Monitor for adverse effects (thrombosis, CNS effects, nausea, hypersensitivity reaction).
- Evaluate the effectiveness of the teaching plan (patient can name drug, dosage of drug, adverse effects to watch for, specific measures to avoid them, and warning signs to report).
- Monitor the effectiveness of comfort measures and compliance with the regimen.

KEY POINTS

- Hemostatic agents are used to stop bleeding from occurring. They are used in situations that result in a fibrinolytic state with excessive plasminogen activity and the risk of bleeding from clot dissolution. For example, patients undergoing repeat CABG surgery are especially prone to excessive bleeding and may require blood transfusion.
- Aminocaproic acid is a systemic hemostatic agent used to treat conditions resulting from systemic hyperfibrinolysis. Several topical agents are also available for local use on active bleeding sites, often during surgery or with severe injury.

SUMMARY

- Coagulation is the transformation of fluid blood into a solid state to plug up breaks in the vascular system.
- Coagulation involves several processes, including vasoconstriction, platelet aggregation to form a plug, and intrinsic and extrinsic clot formation initiated by Hageman factor to plug any breaks in the system.
- The final step of clot formation is the conversion of prothrombin to thrombin, which breaks down fibrinogen to form insoluble fibrin threads.
- Once a clot is formed, it must be dissolved to prevent the occlusion of blood vessels and loss of blood supply to tissues.
- Plasminogen is the basis of the clot-dissolving system. It is converted to plasmin (fibrinolysin) by several factors, including Hageman factor. Plasmin dissolves fibrin threads and resolves the clot.

- Anticoagulants block blood coagulation by interfering with one or more of the steps involved, such as blocking platelet aggregation or inhibiting the intrinsic or extrinsic pathways to clot formation.
- Thrombolytic drugs dissolve clots or thrombi that have formed. They activate the plasminogen system to stimulate natural clot dissolution.
- Hemostatic drugs are used to stop bleeding. They may replace missing clotting factors or prevent the plasminogen system from dissolving formed clots.
- Hemophilia, a genetic lack of essential clotting factors, results in excessive bleeding. It is treated by replacing missing clotting factors.

CHECK YOUR UNDERSTANDING

Answers to the questions in this chapter can be found in Answers to Check Your Understanding Questions on thePoint®.

MULTIPLE CHOICE

Select the best answer to the following.

1. Blood coagulation is a complex reaction that involves
a. vasoconstriction, platelet aggregation, and plasminogen action.
b. vasodilation, platelet aggregation, and activation of the clotting cascade.
c. vasoconstriction, platelet aggregation, and conversion of prothrombin to thrombin.
d. vasodilation, platelet inhibition, and action of the intrinsic and extrinsic clotting cascades.

2. Warfarin, an oral anticoagulant, acts
a. to directly prevent the conversion of prothrombin to thrombin.
b. to decrease the production of vitamin K clotting factors in the liver.
c. as a catalyst in the conversion of plasminogen to plasmin.
d. immediately, so it is the drug of choice in emergency situations.

3. Heparin reacts to prevent the conversion of prothrombin to thrombin. Heparin
a. is available in oral and parenteral forms.
b. takes about 72 hours to have a therapeutic effect.
c. has its effects reversed with the administration of protamine sulfate.
d. has its effects reversed with the injection of vitamin K.

4. The low-molecular-weight heparin of choice for preventing DVT after hip replacement therapy is
a. heparin.
b. dalteparin.
c. fondaparinux.
d. enoxaparin.

5. A thrombolytic agent could be safely used in
a. CVA within the last 2 months.
b. acute MI within the last 3 hours.
c. recent, serious GI bleeding.
d. obstetrical delivery.

6. Antihemophilic agents are used to replace missing clotting factors to prevent severe blood loss. The most common side effect or side effects associated with the use of these drugs are
a. bleeding.
b. dark stools and urine.
c. hepatitis and AIDS.
d. constipation.

MULTIPLE RESPONSE

Select all that apply.

1. Hageman factor is known to activate which of the following?
a. The clotting cascade
b. The anticlotting process
c. The inflammatory response
d. Platelet aggregation
e. Thromboxane A_2
f. Troponin coupling

2. Plasminogen is converted to plasmin, a clot-dissolving substance, by which of the following?
a. Nicotine
b. Hageman factor
c. Tenecteplase
d. Pyrogens
e. Thrombin
f. Christmas factor

(continues on page 850)

3. Antiplatelet drugs block the aggregation of platelets and keep vessels open. These drugs would be useful in which of the following?
a. Maintaining the patency of grafts
b. Decreasing the risk of fatal MI
c. Preventing reinfarction after MI
d. Dissolving a PE and improving oxygenation
e. Decreasing damage in a subarachnoid bleed
f. Preventing thromboembolic strokes

4. Evaluating a client who is taking an anticoagulant for blood loss would usually include assessing for which of the following?
a. The presence of petechiae
b. Bleeding gums while brushing the teeth
c. Dark-colored urine
d. Yellow color to the sclera or skin
e. The presence of ecchymotic areas
f. Loss of hair

BIBLIOGRAPHY AND REFERENCES

Adam, S. S., McDuffie, J. R., Ortel, T. L., et al. (2012). Comparative Effectiveness of Warfarin and New Oral Anticoagulants for the Management of Atrial Fibrillation and Venous Thromboembolism: A Systematic Review. *Annals of Internal Medicine, 157*(11), 796–807. Available online at: http://annals.org/article.aspx?articleid=1355171

Brunton, L., Chabner, B., & Knollman, B. (2011). *Goodman and Gilman's the pharmacological basis of therapeutics* (12th ed.). New York: McGraw-Hill.

Facts and Comparisons. (2015). *Drug facts and comparisons.* St. Louis, MO: Author.

Karch, A. M. (2014). *Lippincott's nursing drug guide.* Philadelphia, PA: Lippincott Williams & Wilkins.

Mannucci, P. M. (2004). Treatment of von Willebrand's disease. *New England Journal of Medicine, 351*, 683–694.

Porth, C. M. (2013). *Pathophysiology: Concepts of altered health states* (9th ed.). Philadelphia, PA: Lippincott Williams & Wilkins.

Shimol, V., & Gage, B. (2011). Cost-effectiveness of dabigatran for stroke prophylaxis in atrial fibrillation. *Circulation, 123*, 2562–2570.

Streiff, M., & Haut, E. (2009). The CMS ruling on venous thromboembolism after total knee or hip arthroplasty: Weighing risks and benefits. *Journal of the American Medical Association, 301*(10), 1063–1065.

The Medical Letter. (2014). *New oral anticoagulants for acute venous thromboembolism.* New Rochelle, NY: Author.

The Medical Letter. (2015). *The medical letter on edoxaban: The fourth new oral anticoagulant.* New Rochelle, NY: Author.

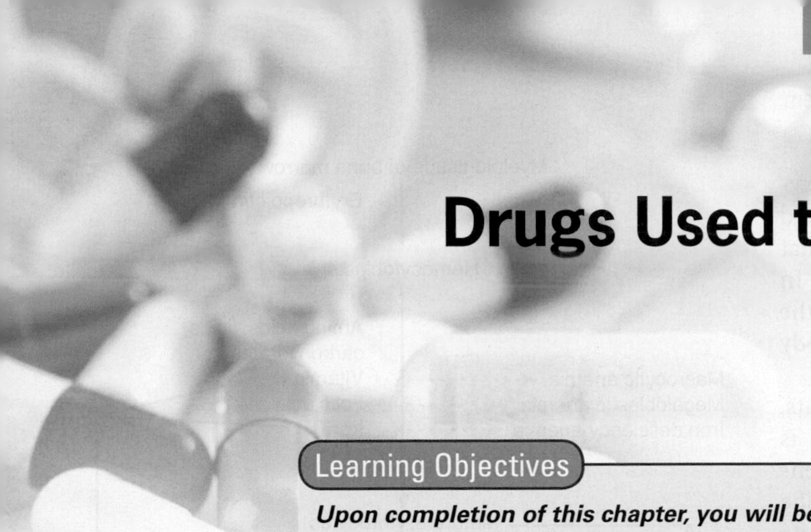

Drugs Used to Treat Anemias 49

Learning Objectives

Upon completion of this chapter, you will be able to:

1. Explain the process of erythropoiesis and its correlation with the development of three types of anemias.
2. Describe the therapeutic actions, indications, pharmacokinetics, contraindications and cautions, most common adverse reactions, and important drug–drug interactions associated with drugs used to treat anemias.
3. Discuss the use of drugs used to treat anemias across the lifespan.
4. Compare and contrast the prototype drugs epoetin alfa, ferrous sulfate, folic acid, and hydroxocobalamin with other agents in their class.
5. Outline the nursing considerations, including important teaching points, for patients receiving drugs used to treat anemias.

Glossary of Key Terms

anemia: disorder involving too few red blood cells (RBCs) or ineffective RBCs that can alter the blood's ability to carry oxygen

erythrocytes: RBCs, responsible for carrying oxygen to the tissues and removing carbon dioxide; they have no nucleus and live approximately 120 days

erythropoiesis: process of RBC production and life cycle; formed by megaloblastic cells in the bone marrow, using iron, folic acid, carbohydrates, vitamin B_{12}, and amino acids; they circulate in the vascular system for about 120 days and then are lysed and recycled

erythropoietin: glycoprotein produced by the kidneys, released in response to decreased blood flow or low oxygen tension in the kidney; stimulates RBC production in the bone marrow

iron deficiency anemia: low RBC count with low iron available because of high demand, poor diet, or poor absorption; treated with iron replacement

megaloblastic anemia: anemia caused by lack of vitamin B_{12} and/or folic acid, in which RBCs are fewer in number and have a weak stroma and a short lifespan; treated by replacement of folic acid and vitamin B_{12}

pernicious anemia: type of megaloblastic anemia characterized by lack of vitamin B_{12} secondary to low production of intrinsic factor by gastric cells; vitamin B_{12} must be replaced by IM injection or nasal spray because it cannot be absorbed through the gastrointestinal tract

plasma: the liquid part of the blood; consists mostly of water and plasma proteins, glucose, and electrolytes

reticulocyte: RBC that has lost its nucleus and entered circulation just recently, not yet fully matured

Drug List

Erythropoiesis-Stimulating Agents
darbepoetin alfa
(P) epoetin alfa

Agents Used for Iron Deficiency Anemia
ferrous aspartate
ferrous fumarate
ferrous gluconate
(P) ferrous sulfate
ferrous sulfate exsiccated
ferumoxytol
iron dextran
iron sucrose
sodium ferric gluconate complex

Agents Used for Other Anemias

Agents for Megaloblastic Anemias
Folic Acid Derivatives
(P) folic acid
leucovorin
levoleucovorin
Vitamin B_{12}
cyanocobalamin
(P) hydroxocobalamin

Agent for Sickle Cell Anemia
(P) hydroxyurea

Blood is essential for cell survival because it carries oxygen and nutrients and removes waste products that could be toxic to the tissues. It also contains clotting factors that help to maintain the vascular system and keep it sealed. In addition, blood contains the important components of the immune and inflammatory systems that protect the body from infection.

Blood is composed of liquid and formed elements. The liquid part of blood is called plasma. **Plasma** is mostly water, but it also contains proteins that are essential for the immune response and for blood clotting. The formed elements of the blood include leukocytes (white blood cells), which are an important part of the immune system (see Chapter 15); **erythrocytes** (red blood cells [RBCs]), which carry oxygen to the tissues and remove carbon dioxide for delivery to the lungs; and platelets, which play an important role in coagulation (see Chapter 48). This chapter discusses drugs that are used to treat **anemias**, which are disorders that involve too few RBCs or ineffective RBCs that can alter the blood's ability to carry oxygen.

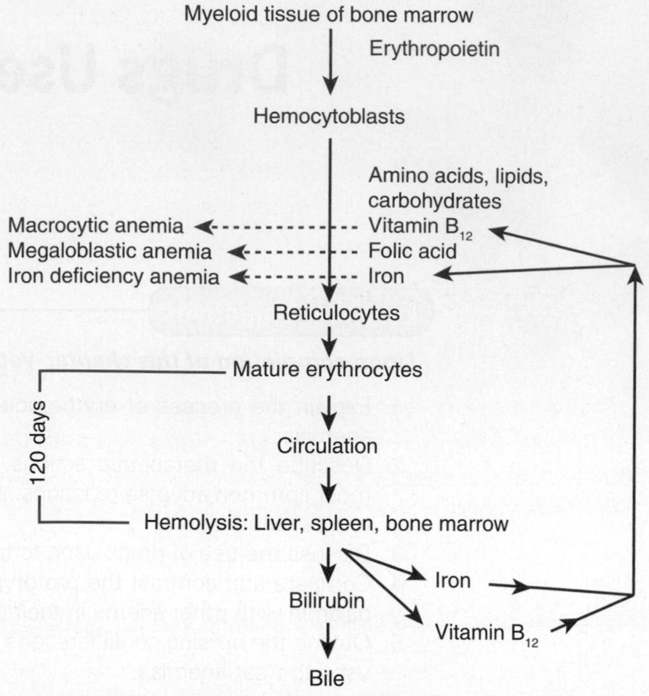

FIGURE 49.1 Erythropoiesis. Red blood cells are produced in the myeloid tissue of the bone marrow in response to the hormone erythropoietin. The hemocytoblasts require various essential factors to produce mature erythrocytes. A lack of any one of these can result in an anemia of the type indicated opposite each factor. Mature erythrocytes survive for about 120 days and are then lysed in the liver, spleen, or bone marrow.

Anemia

Anemia results from some alteration in **erythropoiesis**, the process of RBC production, which occurs in the myeloid tissue of the bone marrow. The rate of RBC production is controlled by the glycoprotein **erythropoietin**, which is released from the kidneys in response to decreased blood flow or decreased oxygen tension in the kidneys. Under the influence of erythropoietin an undifferentiated cell in the bone marrow becomes a hemocytoblast. This cell uses certain amino acids, lipids, carbohydrates, vitamin B_{12}, folic acid, and iron to become an immature RBC. In the last phase of RBC production the cell loses its nucleus and enters circulation. This cell, called a **reticulocyte**, finishes its maturing process in circulation (Figure 49.1).

Although the mature RBC has no nucleus, it does have a vast surface area to improve its ability to transport oxygen and carbon dioxide. Because it lacks a nucleus the RBC cannot reproduce or maintain itself, and so it will eventually wear out. The average lifespan of an RBC is about 120 days. At that time the elderly RBC is lysed in the liver, spleen, or bone marrow. The building blocks of the RBC (e.g., iron, vitamin B_{12}) are then recycled and returned to the bone marrow for the production of new RBCs. The only part of the RBC that cannot be recycled is the toxic pigment bilirubin, which is conjugated in the liver, passed into the bile, and excreted from the body in the feces or the urine. Bilirubin is what gives color to both of these excretions. Erythropoiesis is a constant process by which about 1% of the body's RBCs are destroyed and replaced each day.

Etiology of Anemia

Anemia can occur if erythropoietin levels are low. This is seen in renal failure, when the kidneys are no longer able to produce erythropoietin. It can also occur if the body does not have enough of the building blocks necessary to form RBCs or if a person has genetic predisposition to forming abnormal RBCs, as in sickle cell anemia. To produce healthy RBCs the bone marrow must have the following:

- Adequate amounts of iron, which is used in forming hemoglobin rings to carry the oxygen.
- Minute amounts of vitamin B_{12} and folic acid, to form a strong supporting structure that can survive being battered through blood vessels for 120 days.
- Essential amino acids and carbohydrates to complete the hemoglobin rings, cell membrane, and basic structure.

Normally, an individual's diet supplies adequate amounts of all of these substances, which are absorbed from the gastrointestinal (GI) tract and transported to the bone marrow. However, when the diet cannot supply enough of a nutrient, or enough of the nutrient cannot be absorbed, the person can develop a deficiency anemia. Fewer RBCs are produced, and the ones that are produced are immature and inefficient iron carriers. This type of anemia is called a deficiency anemia.

Another type of anemia is megaloblastic anemia, which involves decreased production of RBCs and ineffectiveness of those RBCs that are produced (they do not usually survive for the 120 days that is normal for the life of an RBC). Patients with megaloblastic anemia usually have a lack of vitamin B_{12} or folic acid.

A third type of anemia is hemolytic anemia, which involves a lysing of RBCs because of genetic factors or from exposure to toxins. Sickle cell anemia is a type of hemolytic anemia.

Iron Deficiency Anemia

All cells in the body require some amount of iron, but iron can be very toxic to cells, especially neurons. To maintain the needed iron levels and avoid toxic levels the body has developed a system for controlling the amount of iron that can enter the body through intestinal absorption. Only enough iron is absorbed to replace the amount of iron that is lost each day. Once iron is absorbed, it is carried by a plasma protein called transferrin, a beta-globulin. This protein carries iron to various tissues to be stored and transports iron from RBC lysis back to the bone marrow for recycling.

Only about 1 mg of iron is actually lost each day in sweat, in sloughed skin, and from GI and urinary tract linings. Because of the body's efficient iron recycling, very little iron is usually needed in the diet, and most diets adequately replace the iron that is lost. However, in situations in which blood is being lost a negative iron balance might occur, and the patient could develop iron deficiency anemia. This can occur in certain rare GI diseases in which the patient is unable to absorb iron from the GI tract, but **iron deficiency anemia** is also a relatively common problem in certain groups, including the following:

- Menstruating women, who lose RBCs monthly
- Pregnant and lactating women, who have increased demands for iron
- Rapidly growing adolescents, especially those who do not have a nutritious diet
- Persons with GI bleeding, including individuals with slow bleeding associated with use of nonsteroidal anti-inflammatory drugs

The person with this type of anemia may complain of being tired because there is insufficient oxygen delivery to the tissues. These conditions are usually treated with iron replacement therapy (see Agents used for Iron Deficiency Anemia).

Megaloblastic Anemias

Megaloblastic anemias result from insufficient amounts of folic acid or vitamin B_{12} to adequately create the stromal structure needed in a healthy RBC, causing a slowing of nuclear DNA synthesis. This effect occurs in rapidly dividing cells such as the bone marrow. The bone marrow contains a large number of megaloblasts, or large, immature RBCs, and because these RBCs are so large, they become crowded in the bone marrow and fewer RBCs are produced, increasing the amount of immature cells in circulation. Cells in the GI tract are additional examples of cells that are often affected. When the GI tract is involved, this can result in the appearance of a characteristic red and glossy tongue and diarrhea.

Folic Acid Deficiency

Folic acid is essential for cell division in all types of tissue. Deficiencies in folic acid are noticed first in rapidly growing cells, such as those in cancerous tissues, in the GI tract, and in the bone marrow. Folic acid is very important for the developing fetus, a site of very rapidly growing cells. Pregnant women are urged to take folic acid supplements to help prevent fetal abnormalities, particularly neural tube defects. Most people can get all the folic acid they need from their diet. For example, folic acid is found in green leafy vegetables, milk, eggs, and liver. Deficiency in folic acid may occur in certain malabsorption states, such as sprue and celiac diseases. Malnutrition that accompanies alcoholism is also a common cause of folic acid deficiency. Repeated pregnancies and extended treatment with certain antiepileptic medications can also contribute to folic acid deficiency. Folic acid deficiency is treated by the administration of folic acid or folate.

Vitamin B_{12} Deficiency

Vitamin B_{12} is used in minute amounts by the body and is stored for use if dietary intake falls. It is necessary not only for the health of the RBCs, but also for the formation and maintenance of the myelin sheath in the central nervous system (CNS). It is found in the diet in meats, seafood, eggs, and cheese. Strict vegetarians who eat nothing but vegetables may develop a vitamin B_{12} deficiency. Such individuals with a dietary insufficiency of vitamin B_{12} typically respond to vitamin B_{12} replacement therapy to reverse their anemia.

The most common cause of this deficiency, however, is inability of the GI tract to absorb the needed amounts of the vitamin. Gastric mucosal cells produce a substance called intrinsic factor, which is necessary for the absorption of vitamin B_{12} by the upper intestine.

Pernicious anemia occurs when the gastric mucosa cannot produce intrinsic factor and vitamin B_{12} cannot be absorbed. The person with pernicious anemia will complain of fatigue and lethargy and will also have CNS effects because of damage to the myelin sheath. Patients will also complain of numbness, tingling, and eventually lack of coordination and motor activity. Pernicious anemia was once a fatal disease, but it is now treated with parenteral or nasal vitamin B_{12} to replace the amount that can no longer be absorbed.

Sickle Cell Anemia

Sickle cell anemia is a chronic hemolytic anemia that occurs almost exclusively in African Americans ("hemolytic" means that the anemia involves a lysing or destruction of RBCs). It is characterized by a genetically inherited hemoglobin S, which gives the RBCs a sickle-shaped appearance. The patient with sickle cell anemia produces fewer than normal RBCs, and the RBCs that are produced are unable to carry oxygen efficiently. The sickle-shaped RBCs can become lodged in tiny blood vessels, where they stack up on one another and occlude the vessel. This occlusion leads to anoxia and infarction of the tissue in that area, which is characterized by severe pain and an acute inflammatory reaction—a condition often called a sickle cell crisis (the patient may even have ulcers on the extremities as a result of such occlusions). Severe, acute episodes of sickling with vessel occlusion may be associated with acute infections and the body's reactions to the immune and inflammatory responses. In the past, sickle cell anemia was treated only with pain medication and support for the patient. Now hydroxyurea has been found to be effective in treating this disease in adults.

KEY POINTS

- RBCs are produced in the bone marrow in a process called erythropoiesis, which is controlled by the glycoprotein erythropoietin, produced in the kidneys. The bone marrow uses iron, amino acids, carbohydrates, folic acid, and vitamin B_{12} to produce healthy, efficient RBCs.
- Anemia is a state of too few RBCs or ineffective RBCs. Anemia can be caused by a lack of erythropoietin or a lack of the components needed to produce RBCs.
- Anemia can be categorized as deficiency (iron deficiency anemia), megaloblastic (folic acid or vitamin B_{12} deficiency), or hemolytic (sickle cell).

Erythropoiesis-Stimulating Agents

Patients who are no longer able to produce enough erythropoietin in the kidneys may benefit from treatment with exogenous erythropoietin, which is available as the drugs epoetin alfa (*Epogen*, *Procrit*) and darbepoetin alfa (*Aranesp*). When agents are used to stimulate the bone marrow to make more RBCs, it is important to ensure that the patient has adequate levels of the components required to make RBCs, including adequate iron. See Table 49.1 for additional information about each of these agents. Box 49.1 highlights important considerations for different age groups when this group of drugs and other drugs used to treat anemia are administered.

Therapeutic Actions and Indications

Epoetin alfa acts like the natural glycoprotein erythropoietin to stimulate the production of RBCs in the bone marrow (Figure 49.2). This drug is indicated in the treatment of anemia associated with renal failure and for patients on dialysis; for anemia associated with AIDS therapy; and for anemia associated with cancer chemotherapy when the bone marrow is depressed and the kidneys may be affected by toxic drugs (*Procrit* only). It is not approved to treat other anemias and is not a replacement for whole blood in the emergency treatment of anemia. See Table 49.1 for additional indications.

Darbepoetin alfa is an erythropoietin-like protein produced in Chinese hamster ovary cells with the use of recombinant DNA technology. This drug gained negative publicity after it was used by athletes to increase their RBC count in the hope that it would give them more endurance and strength. Many athletic governing bodies now screen for the presence of darbepoetin among other banned drugs. This drug has the advantage of once-weekly administration, compared with two to three times a week administration for epoetin. Darbepoetin alfa is approved to treat anemias associated with chronic renal failure, including patients receiving dialysis. Darbepoetin alfa is also used for treatment of anemia induced by cancer chemotherapy. (See also Table 49.1.)

FOCUS ON Safe Medication Administration

With any of these drugs, there is a risk of decreasing the normal levels of erythropoietin if this drug is given to patients who have normal renal functioning and adequate levels of erythropoietin (see Adverse Effects for important safety information related to medication administration). Negative feedback occurs with the renal cells, and less endogenous erythropoietin is produced if exogenous erythropoietin is given. Administration of this drug to an anemic patient with normal renal function can actually cause a more severe anemia if the endogenous levels fall and no longer stimulate RBC production.

Table 49.1 ***Drugs in Focus:* Erythropoiesis-Stimulating Agents**

Drug Name	Usual Dosage	Usual Indications
darbepoetin alfa (*Aranesp*)	0.45 mcg/kg IV or subcutaneously once per week; 2.25 mcg/kg/wk subcutaneously (with chemotherapy)	Treatment of anemia associated with chronic renal failure, including in dialysis patients; treatment of chemotherapy-induced anemia
epoetin alfa (*Epogen*)	50–100 units/kg IV or subcutaneously three times per week; 300 units/kg/d subcutaneously for 15 d (reduction of need for blood transfusions)	Treatment of anemia associated with renal failure and patients on dialysis; reduction in need for transfusions in surgical patients; treatment of anemia associated with AIDS therapy; treatment of anemia associated with cancer chemotherapy
epoetin alfa (*Procrit*)	150 units/kg subcutaneously three times per week	Treatment of anemia associated with cancer chemotherapy

BOX 49.1 FOCUS ON **Drug Therapy Across the Lifespan**

Drugs Used to Treat Anemias

CHILDREN

Proper nutrition should be established for children to provide the essential elements needed for the formation of RBCs. The cause of the anemia should be determined to avoid prolonged problems.

The safety and efficacy of epoetin alfa use have not been established for children. If the drug is used, careful dose calculation should be done based on weight and age, and the child should be monitored very closely for response, iron levels, and nutrition.

Iron doses for replacement therapy are determined by age. If a liquid solution is being used the child should drink it through a straw to avoid staining of the teeth. Periodic blood counts should be performed; it may take 4 to 6 months of oral therapy to reverse an iron deficiency. Remember that iron can be toxic to children, and iron supplements should be kept out of their reach and administration monitored.

Maintenance doses for folic acid have been established for children, based on age. Nutritional means should be used to establish folic acid levels whenever possible.

Children with pernicious anemia require a monthly injection of vitamin B_{12}; the nasal form has not been approved for use with children.

ADULTS

The underlying cause of the anemia should be established and appropriate steps taken to reverse the cause if possible. Adults receiving epoetin alfa or darbepoetin alfa should be monitored closely for response, for the need for iron or other RBC building blocks, and for the possibility of development of pure red cell aplasia.

Advertised heavily in the mass media, epoetin is often requested by adults to help restore energy. Careful patient teaching about the drug and how and why it is administered may be needed.

Adults receiving iron replacement may experience GI upset and frequently experience constipation. Appropriate measures to maintain bowel function may be needed.

Adults also need to know that periodic blood tests will be needed to evaluate response.

Adults being treated for pernicious anemia may opt for nasal vitamin B_{12}. These patients need to receive careful instructions about the proper administration of the drug and should have nasal mucous membranes evaluated periodically.

Proper nutrition during pregnancy and lactation is often still not an adequate way to meet the increased demands of those states. Prenatal vitamins contain iron and folic acid and are usually prescribed for pregnant women. Folic acid is known to be very important for the development of the neural tube, and often women who are considering becoming pregnant are encouraged to take folic acid to build up levels for the planned pregnancy. Use of epoetin alfa or darbepoetin alfa is not recommended during pregnancy or lactation because of the potential for adverse effects on the fetus or baby. Iron replacement is frequently needed postpartum to provide the iron lost during delivery. The new mother should be reminded to keep the drug out of the reach of children and not to combine prescribed iron with an OTC preparation containing high levels of iron.

Women maintained on vitamin B_{12} before pregnancy should continue the treatment during pregnancy. Increased doses may be needed due to changes associated with the pregnancy.

OLDER ADULTS

Older adults may have nutritional problems related to age and may lose more iron through cellular sloughing. Older adults should be assessed for anemia, and possible causes should be evaluated.

Replacement therapy in the older adult can cause the same adverse effects as are seen in the younger person. Bowel-training programs may be needed to prevent severe constipation.

Use of nasal vitamin B_{12} may not be practical. If the patient desires to use this administration technique, nasal mucous membranes should be evaluated before and periodically during treatment.

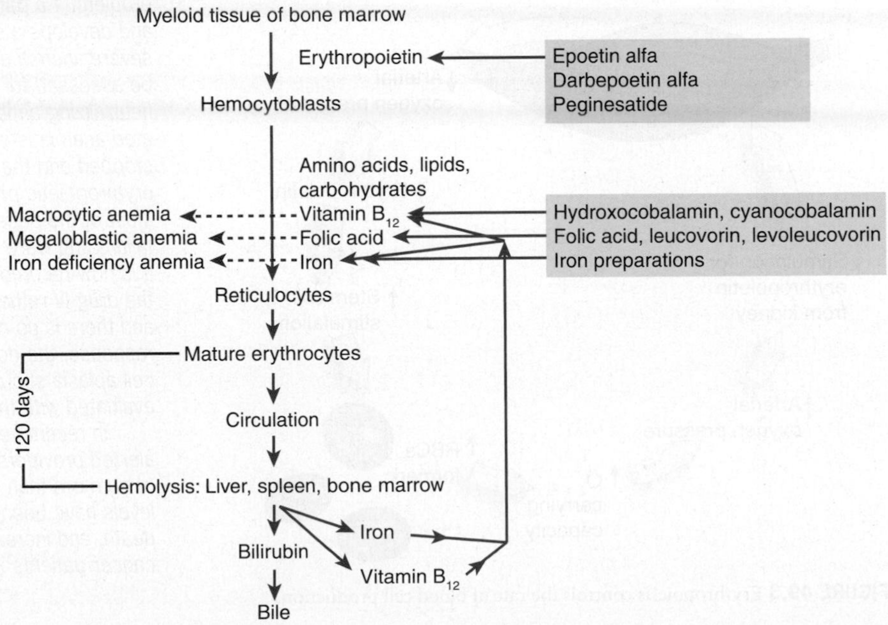

FIGURE 49.2 Sites of action of drugs used to treat anemia.

Pharmacokinetics

Both of these drugs can be given IV or by subcutaneous injection. Epoetin alfa, which is like endogenous erythropoietin, is metabolized in the serum through the normal process that the body uses to clear erythropoietin. It has a slow onset and peaks in 5 to 24 hours, and its duration of effect is usually 24 hours. It has a half-life of 4 to 13 hours and is excreted in the urine. Darbepoetin alfa has a half-life of 21 hours after IV administration or 49 hours after subcutaneous administration. It reaches peak effects in 14 hours (if given IV) or 34 hours (subcutaneously). Duration of effects is 24 to 72 hours, and excretion is through the urine. It is not known whether epoetin alfa enters breast milk.

Contraindications and Cautions

Both of these drugs are contraindicated in the presence of uncontrolled hypertension *because of the risk of even further hypertension when RBC numbers increase and the pressure within the vascular system increases*; with known hypersensitivity to any component of the drug *to avoid hypersensitivity reactions*; and with lactation *because of the potential for allergic-type reactions with the neonate.* There are no adequate studies in pregnancy, and so use should be limited to those situations in which the benefit to the mother clearly outweighs the potential risk to the fetus.

Use caution when administering any of these drugs to patients with normal renal functioning and adequate levels of erythropoietin *because of the rebound decrease in erythropoietin that will occur* and when administering them to a patient with anemia and normal renal function *because this can cause more severe anemia* (Figure 49.3).

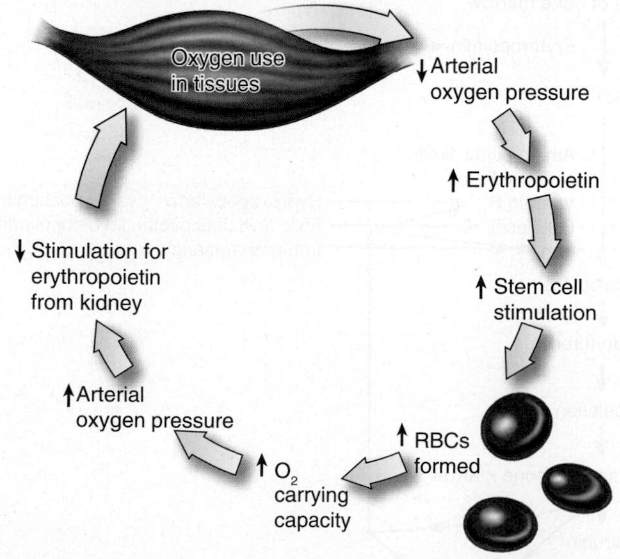

FIGURE 49.3 Erythropoiesis controls the rate of blood cell production.

Adverse Effects

The adverse effects most commonly associated with these drugs include the CNS effects of headache, fatigue, asthenia, and dizziness and the potential for serious seizures. These effects may be the result of a cellular response to the glycoprotein. Nausea, vomiting, and diarrhea also are common effects. Cardiovascular (CV) symptoms can include hypertension, edema, and possible chest pain, all of which may be related to the increase in RBC numbers changing the balance within the CV system. Serious CV effects and increased risk for deep-vein thrombosis (DVT) have been seen when the hemoglobin becomes higher than 11 g/dL. Patients receiving IV administration must also be monitored for possible clotting of the access line related to direct cellular effects of the drug. Rapid growth of cancer is seen when hemoglobin becomes higher than 11 g/dL. Postmarketing studies showed that pure red cell aplasia associated with erythropoietin-neutralizing antibodies could occur with all of these products. In 2008, after analyses of several postmarketing studies, these drugs were required to add black box warnings to their prescribing information as reported in the Focus on Safe Medication Administration below.

FOCUS ON Safe Medication Administration

*In late 2005 the makers of epoetin and darbepoetin sent out warning letters to health care professionals to bring attention to serious adverse effects that had been noted in postmarketing studies. Cases of pure red cell aplasia (defective or insufficient production) and severe anemias, with or without cytopenias (decreased levels of other blood cells), had been reported. These cases were associated with the development of neutralizing antibodies to erythropoietin. Use of any therapeutic protein brings with it the risk of antibody production. All of the erythropoietic proteins (**Aranesp**, **Epogen**, **Procrit**) now carry a warning about the potential for this problem. If a patient is being treated with one of these drugs and develops a sudden loss of response, accompanied by severe anemia and low reticulocyte count, the patient should be assessed for the possible causes. Assays for binding and neutralizing antibodies should be done. If an antibody-mediated anemia is confirmed the drug should be permanently stopped and the patient should **not** be switched to another erythropoietic protein because cross-reaction could occur. Most of the patients in the reported cases had chronic renal failure and were being treated with subcutaneous injections. It is now recommended that patients on hemodialysis receive the drug IV rather than subcutaneously. If the drug is started and there is no response, or if a patient fails to maintain a response, the dose should not be increased, and red blood cell aplasia should be suspected. The patient should be evaluated with the appropriate tests and supported.*

In recent years the U.S. Food and Drug Administration alerted providers to the importance of a target hemoglobin of no more than 11 g/dL when using these drugs. Higher levels have been associated with CV events, including death, and increased rates of tumor progression death in cancer patients in whom the drug was being used to treat anemia associated with toxic drug therapy. Monitoring the hemoglobin levels is critical for safe and therapeutic use of the erythropoiesis-stimulating agents. An increase in tumor growth was also found in cancer patients treated with these drugs when hemoglobin levels were not kept within the guidelines of no more than 11 g/dL. This has been added to the black box warnings for these drugs to alert caregivers to carefully monitor hemoglobin levels to assure patient safety.

Clinically Important Drug–Drug Interactions

These drugs should never be mixed in solution with any other drugs because of a risk of interactions in the solution.

Ⓟ Prototype Summary: Epoetin Alfa

Indications: Treatment of anemia associated with chronic renal failure, related to treatment of HIV infection or to chemotherapy in cancer patients; to reduce the need for allogenic blood transfusions in surgical patients.

Actions: Natural glycoprotein that stimulates RBC production in the bone marrow.

Pharmacokinetics:

Route	Onset	Peak	Duration
Subcutaneous	7–14 d	5–24 h	24 h

$T_{1/2}$: 4 to 13 hours; metabolized in the serum and excreted in the urine.

Adverse Effects: Headache, arthralgias, fatigue, asthenia, dizziness, hypertension, edema, chest pain, nausea, vomiting, diarrhea.

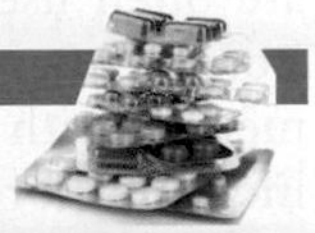

Nursing Considerations for Patients Receiving Erythropoiesis-Stimulating Agents

Assessment: History and Examination

- Assess for contraindications or cautions: Any known allergies to any component of the drug *to avoid hypersensitivity reactions*; severe hypertension, *which could be exacerbated*; and lactation *because of potential adverse effects on the neonate*. These drugs should be used with caution in patients with anemia and normal renal function *to prevent rebound decrease in normal erythropoietin production* and in patients with cancer receiving the drugs to increase hematocrit after antineoplastic chemotherapy *because of the risk of rapid tumor progression if hemoglobin levels exceed guidelines.*
- Perform a physical assessment to establish a *baseline before beginning therapy and during therapy to determine drug effectiveness and evaluate any potential adverse effects.*
- Assess neurological status, including affect, orientation, and muscle strength, *to identify possible adverse CNS effects.*
- Monitor vital signs, including pulse and blood pressure, for changes, and assess CV status *to identify possible CV effects*; and inspect lower extremities *for evidence of edema, which could indicate a change in CV function.*
- Assess respirations and auscultate lung sounds for adventitious breath sounds *for early detection of changes in CV function.*
- Monitor the results of laboratory tests, including renal function tests, complete blood count, hematocrit, iron concentration, transferrin, and electrolyte levels, *to evaluate the effectiveness of therapy and to ensure that the hemoglobin level does not exceed 11 g/dL.* Be aware of variations in hematological test results due to race (Box 49.2).

Nursing Diagnoses

Nursing diagnoses related to drug therapy might include the following:

- Nausea related to adverse GI effects
- Diarrhea related to GI effects
- Risk for injury related to CNS effects
- Risk for imbalanced fluid volume related to CV effects
- Deficient knowledge regarding drug therapy

Planning

- The patient will receive the best therapeutic effect from the drug therapy.
- The patient will have limited adverse effects to the drug therapy.
- The patient will have an understanding of the drug therapy, adverse effects to anticipate, and measures to relieve discomfort and improve safety.

Implementation with Rationale

- Confirm the chronic, renal nature of the patient's anemia before administering the drug to treat renal failure anemia *to ensure proper use of the drug.*
- Give epoetin alfa three times per week, either IV or subcutaneously, *to achieve appropriate therapeutic drug levels.* Administer darbepoetin alfa once per week, subcutaneously or IV.
- Provide the patient with a calendar of marked days *to aid in remembering dates for injection and promote increased compliance with the drug regimen.*
- Do not mix with any other drug solution *to avoid potential incompatibilities.*

(continues on page 858)

- Monitor access lines for clotting and *arrange to clear line as needed.*
- Ensure that prescribed laboratory testing, such as hematocrit levels, is completed before drug administration *to determine correct dose.* If the patient does not respond within 8 weeks, reevaluate the cause of anemia. Anticipate a target hemoglobin of 11 g/dL.
- Evaluate iron stores before and periodically during therapy *because supplemental iron may be needed as the patient makes more RBCs.*
- Maintain seizure precautions on standby *in case seizures occur as a reaction to the drug.*
- Provide comfort measures *to help the patient tolerate the drug effects.* These include small, frequent meals to help minimize nausea and vomiting; readily available access to bathroom facilities should diarrhea occur; and analgesia for headache or arthralgia.
- Offer support and encouragement *to help the patient deal with the diagnosis and the drug regimen.*
- Provide thorough patient teaching, including the name of the drug, dosage prescribed, administration technique and frequency of administration, measures to avoid adverse effects, warning signs of problems and need to notify health care provider, and the need for follow-up laboratory testing, *to enhance patient knowledge about drug therapy and to promote compliance.*

Evaluation

- Monitor patient response to the drug (alleviation of anemia, target hemoglobin level a maximum of 11 g/dL).
- Monitor for adverse effects (headache, hypertension, nausea, vomiting, seizures, dizziness).
- Monitor the effectiveness of comfort measures and compliance with the regimen.
- Evaluate the effectiveness of the teaching plan (patient can name drug, dosage, adverse effects to watch for, and specific measures to avoid them; patient understands the importance of continued follow-up).

BOX 49.2 FOCUS ON **Cultural Considerations**

Hematological Laboratory Test Variations

There are racial variations in hematological laboratory test results:

Hemoglobin/Hematocrit: Levels in African Americans are generally 1 g lower than in other groups.

Serum transferrin levels (children aged 1–3.5 y): The mean value for African American children is 22 mg/100 mL higher than that for white children. (This may be because African Americans have lower hematocrit and hemoglobin; transferrin levels increase normally in the presence of anemia.)

Because of these variations, the diagnosis and treatment of anemia in African Americans should be based on a different norm than with other groups of patients.

KEY POINTS

- Erythropoiesis-stimulating drugs are used to act like erythropoietin and stimulate the bone marrow to produce more RBCs.
- These drugs must be given IV or by subcutaneous injection. Patients must have an adequate supply of the other components of RBCs, including iron, for these drugs to be effective.
- Erythropoiesis-stimulating drugs should be used with a target hemoglobin level of no more than 11 g/dL. Higher levels are associated with an increased risk for CV events and increased tumor growth in cancer patients.

Agents Used for Iron Deficiency Anemia

Although most people get all of the iron they need through diet, in some situations diet alone may not be adequate. The iron preparations that are available include ferrous aspartate (*FE Aspartate*), ferrous fumarate (*Feostat*), ferrous gluconate (*Fergon*), ferrous sulfate (*Feosol*), ferrous sulfate exsiccated (*Feratab, Slow FE*), ferumoxytol (*Feraheme*), iron dextran (*InFeD*), iron sucrose (*Venofer*), and sodium ferric gluconate complex (*Ferrlecit*). See also Table 49.2.

Therapeutic Actions and Indications

Iron preparations elevate the serum iron concentration (see Figure 49.2). They are then either converted to hemoglobin or trapped in reticuloendothelial cells for storage and eventual release and conversion into a usable form of iron for RBC production. Oral iron preparations are often used to help these patients regain a positive iron balance; these preparations need to be supplemented with adequate dietary intake of iron. They are indicated for the treatment of iron deficiency anemias and may also be used as adjunctive therapy in patients receiving an erythropoiesis-stimulating drug. The drug of choice depends on the prescriber's personal preference and experience and often on what kinds of samples are available to give the patient. See Table 49.2 for Usual Indications.

Pharmacokinetics

Ferrous aspartate, ferrous fumarate, ferrous gluconate, ferrous sulfate, and ferrous sulfate exsiccated are available for oral administration. Iron dextran is a parenteral form of iron given by the Z-track method, which may be used if an oral form cannot be given or cannot be tolerated. Patients with severe GI absorption problems may require this form of iron.

Table 49.2 *Drugs in Focus:* Agents Used for Iron Deficiency Anemia

Drug Name	Dosage/Route	Usual Indications
ferrous aspartate (*FE Aspartate*)	*Adult:* 112 mg/d PO	Dietary supplement as iron
ferrous fumarate (*Feostat*)	100–200 mg/d PO *Pediatric 2–12 y:* 50–100 mg/d PO *Pediatric 6 mo–2 y:* 6 mg/kg/d PO *Infants:* 10–25 mg/d PO	Treatment of iron deficiency anemia
ferrous gluconate (*Fergon*)	100–200 mg/d PO *Pediatric 2–12 y:* 50–100 mg/d PO *Pediatric 6 mo–2 y:* 6 mg/kg/d PO *Infants:* 10–25 mg/d PO	Treatment of iron deficiency anemia
ferrous sulfate (*Feosol*)	100–200 mg/d PO *Pediatric 2–12 y:* 50–100 mg/d PO *Pediatric 6 mo–2 y:* 6 mg/kg/d PO *Infants:* 10–25 mg/d PO	Treatment of iron deficiency anemia
ferrous sulfate exsiccated (*Ferralyn Lanacaps, Slow FE*)	100–200 mg/d PO *Pediatric 2–12 y:* 50–100 mg/d PO *Pediatric 6 mo–2 y:* 6 mg/kg/d PO *Infants:* 10–25 mg/d PO	Treatment of iron deficiency anemia
ferumoxytol (*Feraheme*)	500 mg IV followed 3–8 d later with 500 mg IV, depending on patient response	Treatment of iron deficiency anemia in adults with chronic renal failure
iron dextran (*InFeD*)	mg iron = 0.3 × (weight in pound) × {[100 – (hemoglobin in g/dL) × 100]/14.8} given IM, using Z-track technique	Treatment of iron deficiency anemia (parenteral)
iron sucrose (*Venofer*)	100 mg one to three times per week given IV during dialysis sessions, slowly over 1 min	Treatment of iron deficiency in patients undergoing chronic hemodialysis or nondialysis patients with renal failure who are also receiving supplemental erythropoietin therapy
sodium ferric gluconate complex (*Ferrlecit*)	10 mL diluted in 100 mL of 0.9% sodium chloride for injection over 60 min; initially eight doses given at separate dialysis sessions, then give periodically to maintain hematocrit	Treatment of iron deficiency in patients undergoing chronic hemodialysis who are also receiving supplemental erythropoietin therapy

FOCUS ON Safe Medication Administration

Z-Track Injections

The Z-track method is used when injecting iron to reduce the risk of subcutaneous staining and irritation. It is a good idea to review the method of giving Z-track injections before giving one. The area to be injected is prepped for the injection. Place your gloved finger on the skin surface and pull the skin and the subcutaneous layers out of alignment with the muscle lying beneath. Try to move the skin about 1 cm, or 1/2 in. Insert the needle at a 90-degree angle at the point where you originally placed your finger. Inject the drug and then withdraw the needle. Remove your finger from the skin, which will allow the layers to slide back into their normal position. The track that the needle made when inserting into the muscle is now broken by the layers, and the drug is trapped in the muscle (Figure 49.4).

Patients should be switched to the oral form if at all possible because of the pain associated with IM administration of iron. Iron sucrose, ferumoxytol, and sodium ferric gluconate complex are given IV specifically for patients who are undergoing chronic hemodialysis or who are in renal failure and not on dialysis but are receiving supplemental erythropoietin therapy.

Iron is primarily absorbed from the small intestine by an active transport system. It is transported in the blood, bound to transferrin. Small amounts are lost daily in the sweat, urine, sloughing of skin and mucosal cells, and sloughing of intestinal cells, as well as in the menstrual flow of women. Most of the oral drug that is taken is lost in the feces, but slowly some of the metal is absorbed into the intestine and transported to the bone marrow. It can take 2 to 3 weeks to see improvement and up to 6 to 10 months for a return to a stable iron level once a deficiency exists. It is used during pregnancy and lactation to help the mother meet the increased demands for iron that occur at those times.

Contraindications and Cautions

These drugs are contraindicated for patients with known allergy to any of these preparations *because severe hypersensitivity reactions have been associated with the parenteral form of iron*. They also are contraindicated in the following conditions: Hemochromatosis (excessive iron); hemolytic anemias, *which may increase*

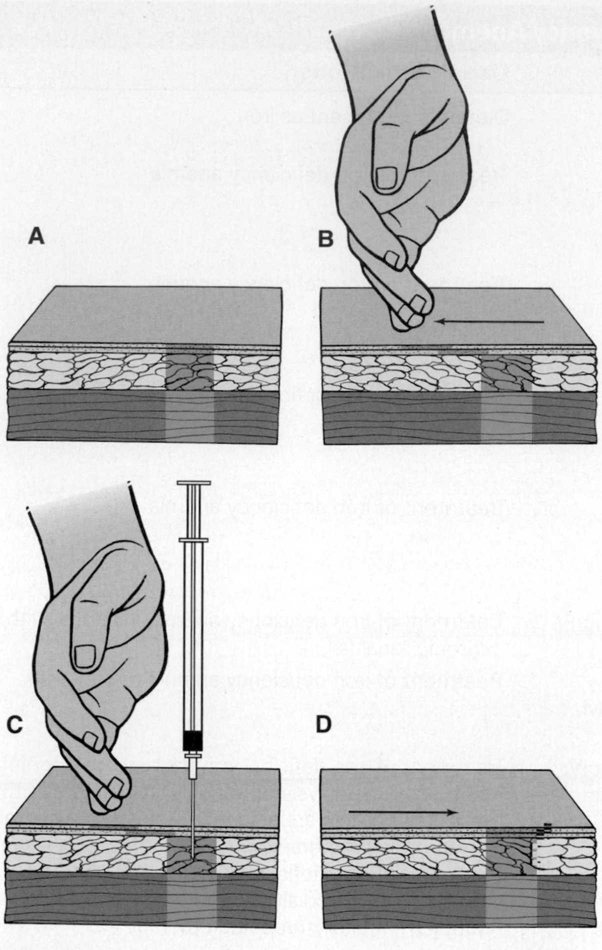

FIGURE 49.4 Use of the Z-track, or zigzag, technique for injections. **A:** Normal skin and tissues. **B:** Move the skin to one side. **C:** Insert the needle at a 90-degree angle and aspirate for blood. **D:** Withdraw the needle, and allow the displaced tissue to return to normal position, thereby keeping the solution from leaving the muscle tissue.

serum iron levels and cause toxicity; normal iron balance *because the drug will not be absorbed and will just pass through the body*; and peptic ulcer, colitis, or regional enteritis *because the drug can be directly irritating to these tissues and can cause exacerbation of diseases*.

Adverse Effects

The most common adverse effects associated with oral iron are related to direct GI irritation; these include GI upset, anorexia, nausea, vomiting, diarrhea, dark stools, and constipation. With increasing serum levels, iron can be directly toxic to the CNS, causing coma and even death. Box 49.3 discusses iron toxicity and drugs that are used to counteract this effect (Figure 49.5). Parenteral iron is associated with severe anaphylactic reactions, local irritation, staining of the tissues, and phlebitis. Ferumoxytol is a supermagnetic iron oxide that can alter magnetic resonance imaging (MRI) images and interpretation for up to 3 months after administration; patients should be aware that they have been given this drug and cautioned to report it before undergoing any

BOX 49.3

Chelating Agents

Heavy metals, including iron, lead, arsenic, mercury, copper, and gold, can cause toxicity in the body by their ability to tie up chemicals in living tissues that need to be free in order for the cell to function normally. When these vital substances (thiols, sulfurs, carboxyls, and phosphoryls) are bound to the metal, certain cellular enzyme systems become deactivated, resulting in failure of cellular function and eventual cell death. Drugs that have been developed to counteract metal toxicity are called chelating agents (from the Greek word for "claw").

Chelating agents grasp and hold a toxic metal so that it can be carried out of the body before it has time to harm the tissues. The chelating agent binds the molecules of the metal, preventing it from damaging the cells within the body. The complex that is formed by the chelating agent and the metal is nontoxic and is excreted by the kidneys.

Chelating Agent	Toxic Metal	Notes
calcium disodium edetate	Lead	Given IM or IV; monitor renal and hepatic function because serious and even fatal toxicity can occur
deferasirox (*Exjade*)	Iron	Oral agent for chronic iron overload in patients over 2 y
deferiprone (*Ferriprox*)	Iron	Oral agent for treatment of transfusional iron overload due to thalassemia syndrome
deferoxamine mesylate (*Desferal*)	Iron	Given IM, subcutaneous, or IV; rash and vision changes are common
dimercaprol (*BAL*)	Arsenic, gold, mercury	Given IM only for 7–10 d; CV toxicity may occur; push fluids and alkalinize urine to increase excretion
succimer (*Chemet*)	Lead	*Children with lead poisoning:* 10 mg/kg *or* 350 mg/m^2 q8 h PO for 5 d; reduce to 10 mg/kg *or* 350 mg/m^2 q12 h PO for 2 wk; make sure patient is well hydrated

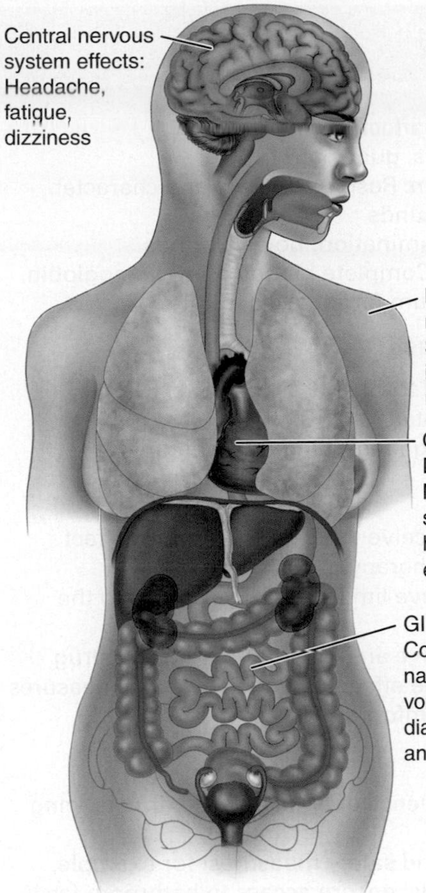

FIGURE 49.5 Variety of adverse effects and toxicities associated with drugs used to treat anemias.

medical testing. See the Critical Thinking Scenario for additional information about iron preparations and toxicity.

Clinically Important Drug–Drug Interactions

Iron absorption decreases if iron preparations are taken with antacids, tetracyclines, or cimetidine; if these drugs must be used, they should be spaced at least 2 hours apart.

Anti-infective response to ciprofloxacin or ofloxacin can decrease if these drugs are taken with iron because of a decrease in absorption; they also should be administered at least 2 hours apart.

Increased iron levels occur if iron preparations are taken with chloramphenicol; patients receiving this combination should be monitored closely for any sign of iron toxicity. The effects of levodopa may decrease if it is taken with iron preparations; patients receiving both of these drugs should take them at least 2 hours apart.

Clinically Important Drug–Food Interactions

Iron is not absorbed if taken with antacids, eggs, milk, coffee, or tea. These substances should not be administered concurrently. Acidic liquids may enhance the absorption of iron and should be not be given concurrently.

CRITICAL THINKING SCENARIO

Iron Preparations and Toxicity

THE SITUATION

L.L., a 28-year-old woman, suffered a miscarriage 6 weeks ago. She lost a great deal of blood during the miscarriage and underwent a dilation and curettage to control the bleeding. On her 6-week routine follow-up visit, she was found to have recovered physically from the event but was still depressed over her loss. Her hematocrit was 31%, and she admitted feeling tired and weak. She was offered emotional support and given a supply of ferrous sulfate tablets, with instructions to take one tablet three times a day.

At home, L.L. transferred the pills to a decorative bottle that had once held vitamins and left it on her table as a reminder to take the tablets. The next day, she discovered her 2-year-old daughter eating the tablets and punished her for getting into them. About 1 hour later the toddler complained of a really bad "tummy ache" and started vomiting. She then became lethargic, and L.L. called the pediatrician, who told them to go immediately to the emergency department and bring the remaining tablets with them. The toddler was found to have a weak, rapid pulse (156 beats/min), rapid, shallow respirations (32/min), and a low blood pressure (60/42 mm Hg). When a diagnosis of acute iron toxicity was made, L.L. became distraught. She said she had no idea that iron could be dangerous because it can be bought over the counter (OTC) in so many preparations. She had not read the written information given to her because it was "just iron."

CRITICAL THINKING

What nursing interventions should be done at this point?
What sort of crisis intervention would be most appropriate for L.L.? *Think about the combined depression from the miscarriage, fear and anxiety related to this crisis, and L.L.'s iron-depleted state.*

(continues on page 862)

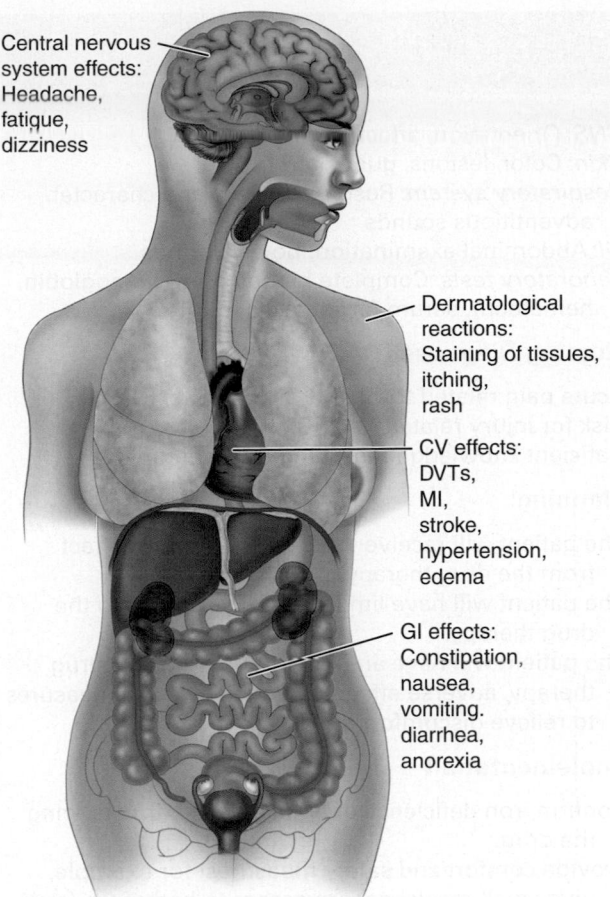

Iron Preparations and Toxicity (continued)

What kind of reserve does she have for dealing with this crisis? Which measures would be appropriate for helping the mother cope with this crisis and for treating the toddler?

DISCUSSION

The first priority is to support and detoxify the child suffering from iron toxicity. In cases of acute iron, eggs and milk are given to bind the iron and prevent absorption. Gastric lavage, using a 1% sodium bicarbonate solution, can be done in a medical facility. This procedure is safe for about the first hour after ingestion. After that time, there is an increased risk of gastric erosion caused by the corrosive iron, making lavage very dangerous. Because this toddler is well beyond the first hour, other measures will be needed. Supportive measures to deal with shock, dehydration, and GI damage will be necessary. In addition, an iron-chelating agent such as deferoxamine mesylate may be tried.

During this crisis, L.L. will need a great deal of support, including a responsible relative or friend or other person who can stay with her. She also will need reassurance and a place to rest. After the situation is stabilized, L.L. will need teaching and additional support. For example, she should be reassured that most people do not take OTC drugs seriously, and many do not even read the labels. However, the nurse can use this opportunity to stress the importance of reading all of the labels and following the directions that come with OTC drugs. L.L. also should be commended for calling the pediatrician and getting medical care for the toddler quickly. Finally, she should receive a review of the iron-teaching information and be encouraged to ask questions.

This case is a good example for a staff in-service program, stressing not only the dangers of iron toxicity, but also the vital importance of providing good patient education before sending a patient home with a new drug. Simply giving a patient written information is often not enough. The nursing care guide and teaching guidelines for L.L. when she was given the iron supplement should have included the following.

NURSING CARE GUIDE FOR L.L.: IRON PREPARATIONS

Assessment: History and Examination

Assess L.L.'s health history for allergies to any iron preparation, colitis, enteritis, hepatic dysfunction, or peptic ulcer.

Then focus the physical examination on the following areas:

CV: Blood pressure, pulse, perfusion

CNS: Orientation, affect, reflexes, vision

Skin: Color, lesions, gums, teeth

Respiratory system: Respiratory rate and character, adventitious sounds

GI: Abdominal examination, bowel sounds

Laboratory tests: Complete blood count, hemoglobin, hematocrit, serum ferritin assays

Nursing Diagnoses

Acute pain related to GI and CNS effects

Risk for injury related to CNS effects

Deficient knowledge regarding drug therapy

Planning

The patient will receive the best therapeutic effect from the drug therapy.

The patient will have limited adverse effects to the drug therapy.

The patient will have an understanding of the drug therapy, adverse effects to anticipate, and measures to relieve discomfort and improve safety.

Implementation

Confirm iron deficiency anemia before administering the drug.

Provide comfort and safety measures; for example, give small meals; ensure access to bathroom facilities; give the drug with food if GI upset occurs; and institute a bowel program as needed.

Arrange for the treatment of the underlying cause of anemia.

Provide support and reassurance to deal with drug effects.

Provide patient teaching regarding drug, dosage, adverse effects, what to report, and safety precautions.

Evaluation

Evaluate drug effects (relief of signs and symptoms of anemia, hematocrit within normal limits).

Monitor for adverse effects: GI upset, CNS toxicity, coma.

Monitor hematocrit and hemoglobin periodically.

Monitor for drug–drug interactions as indicated for each drug.

Evaluate the effectiveness of the patient-teaching program and comfort and safety measures.

PATIENT TEACHING FOR L.L.

- Iron is a naturally occurring mineral found in many foods. It is used by the body to make RBCs, which carry oxygen to all parts of the body. Supplemental iron needs to be taken when the body does not have enough iron available to make healthy RBCs, a condition called anemia.

Iron Preparations and Toxicity (continued)

- Iron is a toxic substance if too much is taken. You must avoid self-medicating with OTC preparations containing iron while you are taking this drug.
- You will need to return for regular medical checkups while taking this drug to determine its effectiveness.
- Take your medication as follows, depending on the specific iron preparation that has been prescribed:
  - Dissolve *ferrous salts* in orange juice to improve the taste.
  - Take *liquid iron preparations* with a straw to prevent the iron from staining teeth.
  - Place iron drops on the back of the tongue to prevent staining of the teeth.
- Some of the following adverse effects may occur:
  - *Dark, tarry, or green stools*: The iron preparations stain the stools; the color remains as long as you are taking the drug and should not cause concern.
  - *Constipation:* This is a common problem; if it becomes too uncomfortable, consult with your health care provider for an appropriate remedy.
  - *Nausea, indigestion, vomiting:* These problems can often be solved by taking the drug with food, making sure to avoid eggs, milk, coffee, and tea.
  - Report any of the following to your health care provider: *Severe diarrhea, severe abdominal pain or cramping, unusual tiredness or weakness, or bluish tint to the lips or fingernail beds.*
- Tell any doctor, nurse, or other health care provider that you are taking this drug.
- Keep this drug, and all medications, out of the reach of children. Because iron can be very toxic, seek emergency medical help immediately if you suspect that a child has taken this preparation unsupervised.
- Because iron can interfere with the absorption of some drugs, do not take iron at the same time as *tetracycline* or *antacids*. These drugs must be taken during intervals when iron is not in the stomach.

P Prototype Summary: Ferrous Sulfate

Indications: Prevention and treatment of iron deficiency anemia; dietary supplement for iron.

Actions: Elevates the serum iron concentration and is then converted into hemoglobin or stored for eventual conversion to a usable form of iron.

Pharmacokinetics:

Route	Onset	Peak	Duration
Oral	4 d	7–10 d	2–4 mo

$T_{1/2}$: Not known; recycled for use, not excreted.

Adverse Effects: GI upset, anorexia, nausea, vomiting, constipation, diarrhea, CNS toxicity progressing to coma and death with overdose.

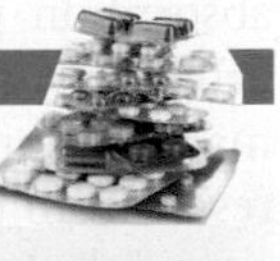

Nursing Considerations for Patients Receiving Iron Preparations

Assessment: History and Examination

- Assess for contraindications or cautions: Any known allergies to this drug *to avoid hypersensitivity reactions*; hyperchromatosis *to avoid increasing already increased iron levels*; colitis, enteritis, or peptic ulcer, *which could lead to increased GI irritation from the drug and exacerbation of the disorder*; and hemolytic anemias, *which could increase serum iron levels and lead to toxicity*.
- Perform a physical assessment to establish a *baseline before beginning therapy and during therapy to determine drug effectiveness and to evaluate for any potential adverse effects.*
- Inspect the color and integrity of the skin and mucous membranes *to identify potential signs and symptoms associated with anemia and evaluate for possible adverse effects of the parenteral form.*
- Assess patient's neurological status, including level of orientation, affect, and reflexes, *to identify possible CNS effects and early signs of possible toxicity.*
- Monitor pulse, blood pressure, perfusion, respirations, and adventitious sounds *to check CV function and detect early signs of toxicity*.
- Inspect abdomen for distention and auscultate bowel sounds *to evaluate GI motility*.
- Inspect the skin integrity of the intended parenteral administration site *to ensure intactness and evaluate for possible staining.*
- Monitor the results of laboratory tests, including complete blood count, hematocrit, hemoglobin, and serum ferritin assays, *to determine drug effectiveness and identify toxic levels.*

Nursing Diagnoses

Nursing diagnoses related to drug therapy might include the following:

- Acute pain related to CNS or GI effects or parenteral administration

(continues on page 864)

- Nausea related to adverse GI effects
- Constipation related to adverse GI effects
- Disturbed body image related to drug staining of the skin from parenteral injection
- Risk for injury related to CNS effects
- Deficient knowledge regarding drug therapy

Planning

- The patient will receive the best therapeutic effect from the drug therapy.
- The patient will have limited adverse effects to the drug therapy.
- The patient will have an understanding of the drug therapy, adverse effects to anticipate, and measures to relieve discomfort and improve safety.

Implementation with Rationale

- Ensure that iron deficiency anemia is confirmed before administering drugs *to ensure proper use of the drug.*
- Consult with the physician to arrange for the treatment of the underlying cause of anemia if possible *because iron replacement will not correct the cause of the iron loss.*
- Administer the oral form with meals that do not include eggs, milk, coffee, and tea *to relieve GI irritation and nausea if GI upset is severe and to prevent drug–food interactions*; have the patient drink oral solutions through a straw *to prevent staining of teeth.*
- Caution the patient that stools may be dark or green *to prevent undue alarm if this occurs.*
- Take measures to help alleviate constipation *to prevent discomfort and the adverse effects of severe constipation.*
- Administer IM only by the Z-track technique *to ensure proper administration and to avoid staining of the tissues brown.* Warn the patient that the injection can be painful.
- Arrange for hematocrit and hemoglobin measurements before administration and periodically during therapy *to monitor drug effectiveness.*
- Provide comfort measures *to help the patient tolerate drug effects.* These include small, frequent meals to minimize nausea and readily available access to bathroom facilities should constipation occur, and increased fiber and fluid intake and increased exercise *to help alleviate constipation.*
- Offer support and encouragement *to help the patient deal with the diagnosis and the drug regimen.*
- Provide thorough patient teaching, including the drug name, dosage, and route of administration; administration technique, such as parenteral Z-track injection or oral solution through a straw, and frequency of administration; foods and fluids to avoid and to include to ensure proper absorption; need for increased fluids and fiber foods in diet and exercise to prevent constipation; notification of change in stool color and consistency; potential for pain at site and staining of skin with parenteral administration; measures to avoid adverse effects; warning signs of problems and need to notify health care provider; and the need for follow-up laboratory testing, *to enhance patient knowledge about drug therapy and to promote compliance.*

Evaluation

- Monitor patient response to the drug (alleviation of anemia).
- Monitor for adverse effects (GI upset and reaction, CNS toxicity, coma).
- Monitor the effectiveness of comfort measures and compliance with the regimen.
- Evaluate the effectiveness of the teaching plan (patient can name drug, dosage, adverse effects to watch for, and specific measures to avoid them; patient understands the importance of continued follow-up).

KEY POINTS

- Iron products are used to replace iron in cases of iron deficiency anemia, which can occur because of deficient iron intake or because of blood loss leading to lower iron levels.
- Iron products commonly cause constipation, nausea, green stools, and GI upset.
- Iron toxicity can cause severe CNS toxicity, coma, and even death because high iron levels are very toxic to nerve cell membranes.

Agents Used for Other Anemias

This section discusses treatment for megaloblastic anemias and sickle cell anemia. Table 49.3 gives a complete list of agents.

Agents for Megaloblastic Anemias

Megaloblastic anemia is treated with folic acid and vitamin B_{12}. Folate deficiencies usually occur secondary to increased demand (as in pregnancy or growth spurts); as a result of absorption problems in the small intestine; because of drugs that cause folate deficiencies; or secondary to the malnutrition of alcoholism. Vitamin B_{12} deficiencies can result from poor diet or increased demand, but the usual cause is lack of intrinsic factor in the stomach, which is necessary for absorption. The drugs are usually given together to ensure that the problem is addressed and the blood cells can be formed properly (Table 49.3). Folic acid derivatives include folic acid (generic), leucovorin (generic), and levoleucovorin (*Fusilev*), which is available only in an IV form. Vitamin B_{12} includes hydroxocobalamin (generic), an injectable drug, and cyanocobalamin (*Nascobal*), a nasal spray.

Table 49.3 ***Drugs in Focus:* Agents Used for Other Anemias**

Drug Name	Dosage/Route	Usual Indications
Agents for Megaloblastic Anemias		
Folic Acid Derivatives		
folic acid (generic)	1 mg/d PO, IM, subcutaneously, or IV	Replacement therapy and treatment of megaloblastic anemia
leucovorin (generic)	1 mg/d IM for replacement; 12–15 g/m² PO, then 10 g/m² PO q6 h for 72 h for rescue	Replacement therapy and treatment of megaloblastic anemia; used as "leucovorin rescue" after chemotherapy, allowing noncancerous cells to survive the chemotherapy; used with fluorouracil for palliative treatment of colorectal cancer (see Chapter 14)
levoleucovorin (*Fusilev*)	7.5 mg IV q6 h; length of treatment determined by patient response and methotrexate levels	To diminish the toxicity and counteract the effects of impaired methotrexate elimination and of inadvertent overdose of folic acid antagonists after high-dose methotrexate therapy in osteosarcoma
Vitamin B_{12}		
cyanocobalamin (*Nascobal*)	One spray (500 mcg) in one nostril once a week	Replacement therapy; treatment of megaloblastic anemia
hydroxocobalamin (generic)	30 mcg/d IM for 5–10 d, then 100–200 mcg/mo IM	
	Pediatric: 1–5 mg IM over ≥2 wk, then 30–50 mcg IM every 4 wk	Replacement therapy; treatment of megaloblastic anemia, pernicious anemia
Agent for Sickle Cell Anemia		
hydroxyurea (*Droxia*)	Initially 15 mg/kg/d PO as a single dose; increase by 5 mg/kg/d every 12 wk to a maximum dose of 35 mg/kg/day PO	Reduction of frequency of painful crises and to decrease the need for blood transfusions in adults with sickle cell anemia

Therapeutic Actions and Indications

Folic acid and vitamin B_{12} are essential for cell growth and division and for the production of a strong stroma in RBCs (see Figure 49.3). Vitamin B_{12} is also necessary for maintenance of the myelin sheath in nerve tissue. Both are given as replacement therapy for dietary deficiencies, as replacement in high-demand states such as pregnancy and lactation, and to treat megaloblastic anemia. Folic acid is used as a rescue drug for cells exposed to some toxic chemotherapeutic agents. Leucovorin is used as a rescue drug following methotrexate therapy to decrease the toxicity of methotrexate caused by decreased elimination or overdose of folic acid antagonists such as trimethoprim and for the treatment of various megaloblastic anemias. Levoleucovorin is the newest drug in this class and is only approved to decrease the toxicity of methotrexate caused by decreased elimination or overdose of folic acid antagonists in the treatment of osteosarcomas. See Table 49.3 for Usual Indications for each of these agents.

Pharmacokinetics

Folic acid can be given in oral, IM, IV, and subcutaneous forms. Parenteral drugs are preferred for patients with potential absorption problems; all other patients should be given the oral form if at all possible. Leucovorin is a reduced form of folic acid that is available for oral, IM, and IV use. Levoleucovorin is only available in an IV form.

Hydroxocobalamin must be given IM every day for 5 to 10 days to build up levels, then once a month for life. It cannot be taken orally because the problem with pernicious anemia is the inability to absorb vitamin B_{12} secondary to low levels of intrinsic factor. It can be used in states of increased demand (e.g., pregnancy, growth spurts) or dietary deficiency, but oral vitamins are preferred in most of those cases. Cyanocobalamin is not as tightly bound to proteins and does not last in the body as long as hydroxocobalamin. This drug is primarily stored in the liver and slowly released as needed for metabolic functions. It is available as an intranasal gel that allows vitamin B_{12} absorption directly through the nasal mucosa. *Nascobal* is used once a week as an intranasal spray in one nostril.

Folic acid and vitamin B_{12} are well absorbed after injection, metabolized mainly in the liver, and excreted in the urine. These vitamins are considered essential during pregnancy and lactation because of the increased demands of the mother's metabolism.

Contraindications and Cautions

These drugs are contraindicated in the presence of known allergies to these drugs or to their components *to avoid hypersensitivity reactions*. They should be used cautiously in patients who are pregnant or lactating or who have other anemias *to ensure that the correct doses of the drug are used to provide the best therapeutic effect and decrease the risk of toxic effects*. Nasal cyanocobalamin should be used with caution in the presence of nasal erosion or ulcers, *which could alter absorption of the drug*.

Adverse Effects

These drugs have relatively few adverse effects because they are used as replacements for required chemicals. Hydroxocobalamin has been associated with itching, rash, and signs of excessive vitamin B levels, which can also include peripheral edema and heart failure. Mild diarrhea has been reported with these drugs. Pain and discomfort can occur at injection sites. Nasal irritation can occur with the use of intranasal spray.

Ⓟ Prototype Summary: Folic Acid

Indications: Treatment of megaloblastic anemia due to sprue, nutritional deficiency.

Actions: Reduced form of folic acid, required for nucleoprotein synthesis and maintenance of normal erythropoiesis.

Pharmacokinetics:

Route	Onset	Peak
Oral, IM, subcutaneous, IV	Varies	30–60 min

$T_{1/2}$: Unknown; metabolized in the liver and excreted in the urine.

Adverse Effects: Allergic reactions, pain and discomfort at injection site.

Ⓟ Prototype Summary: Hydroxocobalamin

Indications: Treatment of vitamin B12 deficiency; to meet increased vitamin B12 requirements related to disease, pregnancy, or blood loss.

Actions: Essential for nucleic acid and protein synthesis; used for growth, cell reproduction, hematopoiesis, and nucleoprotein and myelin synthesis.

Pharmacokinetics:

Route	Onset	Peak
IM	Intermediate	60 min

$T_{1/2}$: 24 to 36 hours; metabolized in the liver and excreted in the urine.

Adverse Effects: Itching, transitory exanthema, mild diarrhea, anaphylactic reaction, heart failure, pulmonary edema, hypokalemia, pain at injection site.

Nursing Considerations for Patients Receiving Folic Acid Derivatives or Vitamin B_{12}

Assessment: History and Examination

- Assess *for contraindications or cautions*: Any known allergies to these drugs or drug components, other anemias, pregnancy, lactation, and nasal erosion.
- Assess baseline status before beginning therapy *to determine any potential adverse effects*. This includes affect, orientation, and reflexes; pulse, blood pressure, and perfusion; respirations and adventitious sounds; and complete blood count, hematocrit, and iron levels, *to determine the effectiveness of drug therapy*.

Nursing Diagnoses

Nursing diagnoses related to drug therapy might include the following:

- Acute pain related to injection or nasal irritation
- Risk for fluid volume imbalance related to CV effects
- Deficient knowledge regarding drug therapy

Planning

- The patient will receive the best therapeutic effect from the drug therapy.
- The patient will have limited adverse effects to the drug therapy.
- The patient will have an understanding of the drug therapy, adverse effects to anticipate, and measures to relieve discomfort and improve safety.

Implementation with Rationale

- Confirm the nature of the megaloblastic anemia *to ensure that the proper drug regimen is being used*.
- Give both types of drugs in cases of pernicious anemia *to ensure therapeutic effectiveness*.
- Parenteral vitamin B_{12} must be given IM each day for 5 to 10 days and then once a month for life *if used to treat pernicious anemia*.
- Arrange for nutritional consultation *to ensure a well-balanced diet*.
- Monitor for the possibility of hypersensitivity reactions; *have life support equipment on standby in case reactions occur*.
- Arrange for hematocrit readings before and periodically during therapy *to monitor drug effectiveness*.
- Provide comfort measures *to help the patient tolerate drug effects*. These include small, frequent meals, access to bathroom facilities, and analgesia for muscle or nasal pain.
- Provide thorough patient teaching, including the name of the drug, dosage prescribed, measures to avoid adverse effects, warning signs of problems, and the need

for periodic monitoring and evaluation, *to enhance patient knowledge about drug therapy and to promote compliance with the drug regimen.*
- Offer support and encouragement *to help the patient deal with the diagnosis and the drug regimen.*

Evaluation

- Monitor patient response to the drug (alleviation of anemia).
- Monitor for adverse effects (nasal irritation, pain at injection site, nausea).
- Evaluate the effectiveness of the teaching plan (patient can name drug, dosage, adverse effects to watch for, and specific measures to avoid them; patient understands the importance of continued follow-up).
- Monitor the effectiveness of comfort measures and compliance with the regimen.

Agent for Sickle Cell Anemia

Patients with sickle cell anemia are treated with antibiotics to help fight the infections that can occur when blood flow is decreased to any area; with pain-relieving activities to help alleviate the pain associated with the anoxia to tissues, which can range from heat applied to the area to OTC pain medications to prescription opioids; and now, for adults, with hydroxyurea (*Droxia*). Hydroxyurea is a cytotoxic antineoplastic drug that is also used to treat leukemia, ovarian cancer, and melanoma.

Therapeutic Actions and Indications

Hydroxyurea, taken for several months, increases the amount of fetal hemoglobin produced in the bone marrow and dilutes the formation of the abnormal hemoglobin S in adults who have sickle cell anemia. This results in less clogging of small vessels and the painful, anoxic effects associated with RBC sickling or stacking. See Table 49.3 for Usual Indications.

Pharmacokinetics

Given orally, hydroxyurea is absorbed well from the GI tract, reaching peak levels in 1 to 4 hours. It is metabolized in the liver and excreted in the urine with a half-life of 3 to 4 hours. It is known to cross the placenta and to enter breast milk.

Contraindications and Cautions

Hydroxyurea is contraindicated with known allergy to any component of the drug *to prevent hypersensitivity reactions* and with severe anemia or leucopenia *because it can cause further bone marrow suppression.* It should be used with caution in the presence of impaired liver or renal function, *which could interfere with metabolism and excretion of the drug,* and it should only be used in pregnancy and lactation if the benefit to the mother clearly outweighs the potential risk to the fetus or baby *because this drug crosses the placenta and enters breast milk and could cause serious effects in the fetus or baby.*

Adverse Effects

Hydroxyurea is cytotoxic and is associated with adverse effects associated with the death of cells, especially in cells that are rapidly turning over. GI effects include anorexia, nausea, vomiting, stomatitis, diarrhea, or constipation; dermatological effects include rash or erythema; and bone marrow suppression usually occurs. Headache, dizziness, disorientation, fever, chills, and malaise have been reported, possibly related to the effects of cell death in the body. As with other cytotoxic drugs, there is an increased risk of cancer development.

Clinically Important Drug–Drug Interactions

There is an increased risk of uric acid levels if this drug is combined with any uricosuric agents; if this combination must be used, dose adjustments will be needed for the uricosuric agent.

P Prototype Summary: Hydroxyurea

Indications: Reduction of frequency of painful crisis and need for blood transfusions in adult patients with sickle cell anemia.

Actions: Increases fetal hemoglobin production in the bone marrow and dilutes the formation of abnormal hemoglobin S.

Pharmacokinetics:

Route	Onset	Peak	Duration
Oral	Varied	1–4 h	18–20 h

$T_{1/2}$: 3 to 4 hours; metabolized in the liver and excreted in the urine.

Adverse Effects: Dizziness, headache, rash, erythema, anorexia, nausea, vomiting, stomatitis, bone marrow depression, cancer.

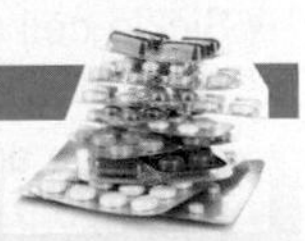

Nursing Considerations for a Patient Receiving Hydroxyurea

See Chapter 14, Antineoplastic Agents, for the nursing considerations for a patient receiving hydroxyurea.

Box 49.4 provides information about eltrombopag (*Promacta*), an oral drug that is now approved for use in treating aplastic anemia and idiopathic thrombocytopenia (ITP).

BOX 49.4

Aplastic Anemia

Aplastic anemia is a disease caused by damage to the bone marrow and the bone marrow stem cells. The damage can be caused by drugs, radiation exposure, infections, immune pancytopenia disorders, and sometimes by genetics. There are deficiencies in all of the blood components formed in the bone marrow, which is called pancytopenia. Low RBC count (anemia), low white blood cell count (leukopenia), and low platelet count (thrombocytopenia) are characteristic of pancytopenia, and, in addition, the stem cell count in the bone marrow becomes very low and that area of the bone marrow is often replaced by fat deposits. The patient with this situation is at high risk for bleeding (loss of platelets), high risk for infection (loss of white cells), and often very tired and pale (loss of red cells). Treatment may involve use of immunosuppressant drugs, corticosteroids, or replacement elements in critical situations; bone marrow transplant is often an option. Eltrombopag (*Promacta*) is an oral drug that is now approved for use in treating aplastic anemia and ITP. It is a thrombopoietin receptor agonist that initiates signaling cascades in the bone marrow leading to proliferation and differentiation of the bone marrow progenitor cells, leading to increased production of blood components. Eltromobopag is absorbed from the GI tract reaching peak levels in 2 to 6 hours; after hepatic metabolism it is excreted primarily in the feces with a half-life of 21 to 32 hours. It has a black box warning about the risk of severe hepatic impairment if used in patients with chronic hepatitis C, though it is also approved for the treatment of thrombocytopenia in patients with chronic hepatitis C to allow for interferon treatment. These patients must be monitored closely. It also has warnings that doses need to be reduced when used in patients of eastern Asian heritage because the drug levels will be higher.

KEY POINTS

- Megaloblastic anemia is treated with folic acid and vitamin B_{12}.
- Levoleucovorin and leucovorin are used as rescue drugs for methotrexate therapy when folate inhibition is high.
- Patients receiving these drugs require periodic blood tests to ensure therapeutic effects and avoid the toxicity associated with high serum levels.
- Sickle cell anemia is a genetic disorder in hemoglobin formation that can lead to clogging of blood vessels, with resulting anoxia and severe pain.
- Hydroxyurea, an antineoplastic drug, is useful in reducing the painful crises and need for blood transfusions in adults with sickle cell anemia. It is associated with many adverse effects because it is a cytotoxic drug.

SUMMARY

- Blood is composed of liquid plasma and formed elements (white blood cells, RBCs, and platelets) and contains oxygen and nutrients that are essential for cell survival; it delivers these to the cells and removes waste products from the tissues.
- RBCs are produced in the bone marrow in a process called erythropoiesis, which is controlled by the glycoprotein erythropoietin, produced by the kidneys.
- RBCs do not have a nucleus, and their lifespan is about 120 days, at which time they are lysed and their building blocks are recycled to make new RBCs.
- The bone marrow uses iron, amino acids, carbohydrates, folic acid, and vitamin B_{12} to produce healthy, efficient RBCs.
- An insufficient number or immaturity of RBCs results in low oxygen levels in the tissues, with tiredness, fatigue, and loss of reserve.
- Anemia is a state of too few RBCs or ineffective RBCs. Anemia can be caused by a lack of erythropoietin or by a lack of the components needed to produce RBCs.
- Iron deficiency anemia occurs when there is inadequate iron intake in the diet or an inability to absorb iron from the GI tract. Iron is needed to produce hemoglobin, which carries oxygen. Iron deficiency anemia is treated with iron replacement.
- Iron is a very toxic mineral at high levels. The body controls the absorption of iron and carefully regulates its storage and movement in the body.
- Folic acid and vitamin B_{12} are needed to produce a strong supporting structure in the RBC so that it can survive 120 days of being propelled through the vascular system. These are usually found in adequate amounts in the diet. Deficiencies are treated with folic acid and vitamin B_{12} replacement.
- A dietary lack of or inability to absorb folic acid, vitamin B_{12}, or both will produce a megaloblastic anemia, in which the RBCs are large and immature and have a short lifespan.
- Pernicious anemia is a lack of vitamin B_{12}, which is also used by the body to maintain the myelin sheath on nerve axons. If vitamin B_{12} is lacking, these neurons will degenerate and cause many CNS effects.
- Pernicious anemia is caused by the deficient production of intrinsic factor by gastric cells.
- Intrinsic factor is needed to allow the body to absorb vitamin B_{12}. If intrinsic factor is lacking, vitamin B_{12} must be given parenterally or intranasally for life to ensure absorption.
- Sickle cell anemia is a genetic disorder characterized by the production of hemoglobin S. The RBCs have a sickle shape and can stack up in blood vessels and cause anoxia, pain, and even cell death.
- Sickle cell anemia is treated with antibiotics, pain-relieving measures, and the cytotoxic drug hydroxyurea, which causes increased fetal hemoglobin production in the bone marrow and dilution of hemoglobin S with a resultant reduction in RBC stacking and clogging of blood vessels.

CHECK YOUR UNDERSTANDING

Answers to the questions in this chapter can be found in Answers to Check Your Understanding Questions on thePoint®.

MULTIPLE CHOICE

Select the best answer to the following.

1. After teaching a group of students about RBC production the instructor determines that the teaching was effective when the group states that the rate of RBC production is controlled by
   a. iron.
   b. folic acid.
   c. erythropoietin.
   d. vitamin B_{12}.

2. RBCs must be continually produced by the body because
   a. the iron within the RBC wears out and must be replaced.
   b. RBCs cannot maintain themselves and wear out.
   c. RBCs are continuously entering and being lost from the GI tract.
   d. RBCs are processed into bile salts and must be replaced.

3. Which of the following would the nurse include in the teaching plan when describing anemia to a patient?
   a. A decreased number of or abnormal RBCs
   b. A lack of iron in the body
   c. A lack of vitamin B_{12} in the body
   d. An excessive number of platelets

4. Megaloblastic anemia is a result of insufficient folic acid or vitamin B_{12}, affecting which of the following?
   a. White blood cell production
   b. Vegetarians
   c. Rapidly turning over cells
   d. Slow-growing cells

5. The nurse would expect the physician to prescribe epoetin alfa (*Epogen*) as the drug of choice
   a. for acute blood loss during surgery.
   b. to replace blood loss from traumatic injury.
   c. for treatment of anemia during lactation.
   d. for treatment of anemia associated with renal failure.

6. A patient with anemia who is given iron salts could expect to show a therapeutic increase in hematocrit
   a. within 72 hours.
   b. within 2 to 3 weeks.
   c. within 6 to 10 months.
   d. within 1 to 2 weeks.

7. To ensure maximum absorption a nurse instructs a patient receiving oral iron therapy to avoid taking the iron with
   a. protein.
   b. antibiotics.
   c. dairy products.
   d. any other drugs.

8. After teaching a patient with pernicious anemia about vitamin B_{12} therapy, which patient statement would indicate that the teaching was successful?
   a. I can take this pill with breakfast.
   b. I should take this pill at bedtime.
   c. I need to inject this drug subcutaneously every day.
   d. I need to inject this drug IM every 5 to 10 days.

MULTIPLE RESPONSE

Select all that apply.

1. Clients are often given iron pills by their clinic. Instructions in giving these pills should include
   a. taking the drug with milk to avoid GI problems.
   b. the potential for constipation.
   c. keeping these potentially toxic pills away from children.
   d. taking the drug with antacids to alleviate GI upset.
   e. having periodic blood tests to evaluate the drug effect.
   f. being aware that stools may be colored green.

2. In a healthy person, very little iron is needed on a daily basis. Loss of iron is associated with which of the following?
   a. Heavy menstrual flow
   b. Bile duct obstruction
   c. Internal bleeding
   d. Penetrating traumatic injury
   e. Bone marrow suppression
   f. Alcoholic cirrhosis

BIBLIOGRAPHY AND REFERENCES

Balducci, L., Ershlor, W., & Bennett, J. (2007). *Anemia in the elderly.* New York: Springer Science.

Bennett, C. L., Silver, S. M., Djulbegovic, B., et al. (2008). Venous thromboembolism and mortality associated with recombinant erythropoietin and darbepoetin administration for the treatment of cancer-associated anemia. *Journal of the American Medical Association, 299*, 914–924.

Brookhurt, M., Schneeweiss, S., Ahorn, J., et al. (2010). Comparative mortality risk of anemia management practices in incident hemodialysis patients. *Journal of the American Medical Association, 303*(9), 857–864.

Brunton, L., Chabner, B., & Knollman, B. (2011). *Goodman and Gilman's the pharmacological basis of therapeutics* (12th ed.). New York: McGraw-Hill.

Facts and Comparisons. (2015). *Drug facts and comparisons.* St. Louis, MO: Author.

Karch, A. M. (2014). *Lippincott's nursing drug guide.* Philadelphia, PA: Lippincott Williams & Wilkins.

Porth, C. M. (2013). *Pathophysiology: Concepts of altered health states* (9th ed.). Philadelphia, PA: Lippincott Williams & Wilkins.

The Medical Letter. (2015). *The medical letter on drugs and therapeutics.* New Rochelle, NY: Author.

Yawn, B., Buchanan, G., Afenyiannan, A., et al. (2014). Management of sickle cell disease: Summary of the 2014 evidence-based report by expert panel members. *Journal of the American Medical Association, 312*(10), 1033–1048.

PART

9

DRUGS ACTING ON THE RENAL SYSTEM

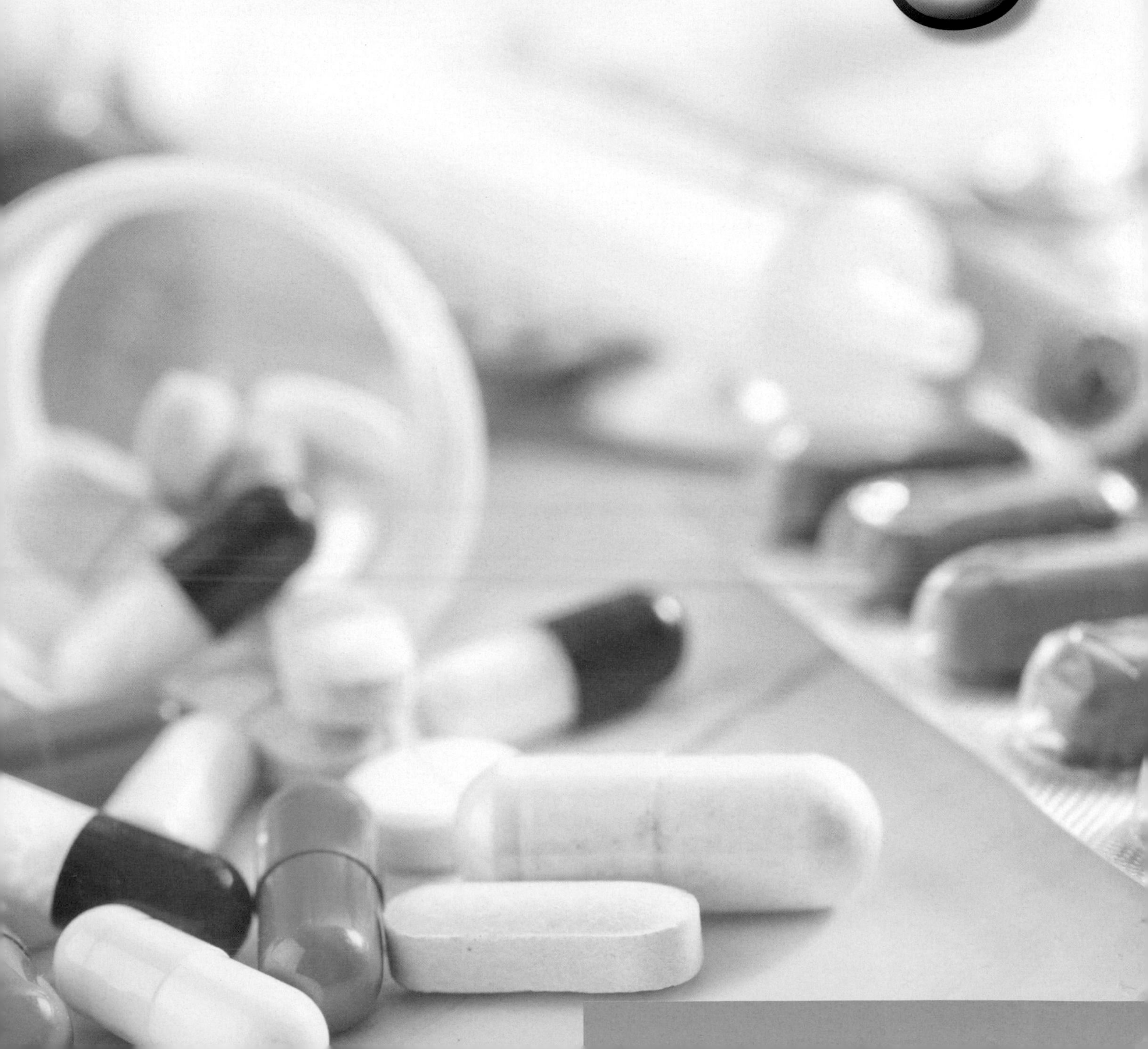

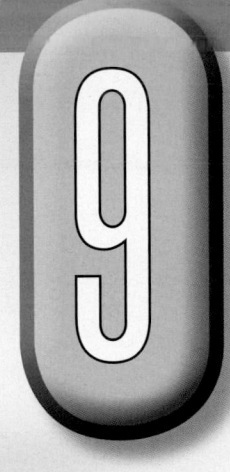

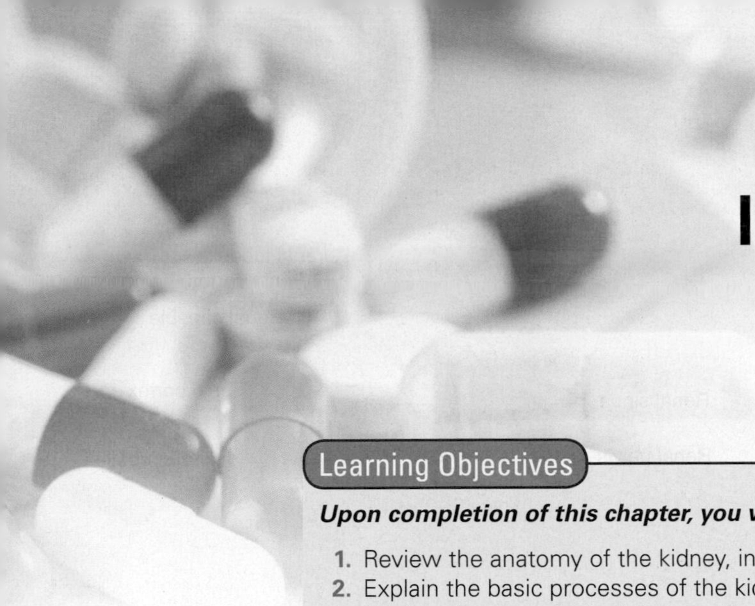

50 Introduction to the Renal System

Learning Objectives

Upon completion of this chapter, you will be able to:

1. Review the anatomy of the kidney, including the structure of the nephron.
2. Explain the basic processes of the kidney and where these processes occur.
3. Explain the control of calcium, sodium, potassium, and chloride in the nephron.
4. Discuss the countercurrent mechanism and the control of urine concentration and dilution, applying these effects to various clinical scenarios.
5. Describe the renin–angiotensin–aldosterone system, including controls and clinical situations where this system is active.
6. Discuss the roles of the kidney in acid–base balance, calcium regulation, and red blood cell production, integrating this information to explain the clinical manifestations of renal failure.

Glossary of Key Terms

aldosterone: hormone produced by the adrenal gland that causes the distal tubule to retain sodium, and therefore water, while losing potassium into the urine

antidiuretic hormone (ADH): hormone produced by the hypothalamus and stored in the posterior pituitary gland; important in maintaining fluid balance; causes the distal tubules and collecting ducts of the kidney to become permeable to water, leading to an antidiuretic effect and fluid retention

carbonic anhydrase: a catalyst that speeds up the chemical reaction combining water and carbon dioxide, which react to form carbonic acid and immediately dissociate to form sodium bicarbonate

countercurrent mechanism: process used by medullary nephrons to concentrate or dilute the urine in response to body stimuli to maintain fluid and electrolyte balance

filtration: passage of fluid and small components of the blood through the glomerulus into the nephron tubule

glomerulus: the tuft of blood vessel between the afferent and efferent arterioles in the nephron; the fenestrated membrane of the glomerulus allows filtration of fluid from the blood into the nephron tubule

nephron: functional unit of the kidney, composed of Bowman's capsule, the proximal and distal convoluted tubules, and the collecting duct

prostate gland: gland located around the male urethra; responsible for producing an acidic fluid that maintains sperm and lubricates the urinary tract

reabsorption: the movement of substances from the renal tubule back into the vascular system

renin–angiotensin–aldosterone system: compensatory process that leads to increased blood pressure and blood volume to ensure perfusion of the kidneys; important in the continual regulation of blood pressure

secretion: the active movement of substances from the blood into the renal tubule for excretion

The renal system is composed of the kidneys and the structures of the urinary tract: The ureters, the urinary bladder, and the urethra. This system has four major functions in the body:

- Maintaining the volume and composition of body fluids within normal ranges, including the following functions:
  - clearing nitrogenous wastes from protein metabolism
  - maintaining acid–base balance and electrolyte levels
  - excreting various drugs and drug metabolites
- Regulating vitamin D activation, which helps to maintain and regulate calcium levels
- Regulating blood pressure through the renin–angiotensin–aldosterone system
- Regulating red blood cell production through the production and secretion of erythropoietin

The Kidneys

The kidneys are two small organs that make up about 0.5% of total body weight but receive about 25% of the cardiac output. Approximately 1,600 L of blood flows through these two small organs each day for cleansing. Most of the fluid that is filtered out by the kidneys is returned to the body, and the waste products that remain are excreted in a relatively small amount of water as urine.

Structure

The kidneys are located under the ribs, for protection from injury. They have three protective layers that make up the renal capsule: A fiber layer, a perirenal or brown fat layer, and the renal parietal layer. The capsule contains pain fibers, which are stimulated if the capsule is stretched secondary to an inflammatory process.

The kidneys have three identifiable regions: The outer cortex, the inner medulla, and the renal pelvises. The renal pelvises drain the urine into the ureters. The ureters are muscular tubes that lead into the urinary bladder, where urine is stored until it is excreted (Figure 50.1).

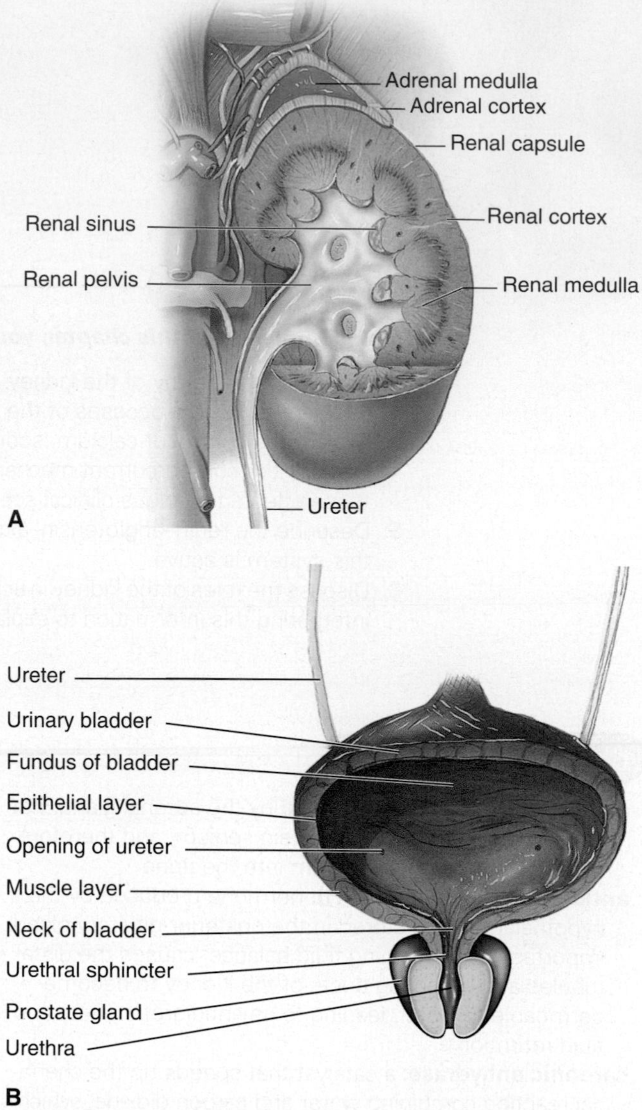

FIGURE 50.1 The kidney (**A**) and organs of the urinary tract (**B**).

Nephron

The functional unit of the kidneys is called the **nephron**. There are approximately 2.4 million nephrons in an adult. All of the nephrons filter fluid and make urine, but only the medullary nephrons can concentrate or dilute urine. It is estimated that only about 25% of the total number of nephrons are necessary to maintain healthy renal function. That means that the renal system is well protected from failure with a large backup system. However, it also means that by the time a patient manifests signs and symptoms suggesting failure of the kidneys, extensive kidney damage has already occurred.

The nephron is basically a tube that begins at Bowman's capsule and becomes the proximal and then distal convoluted tubule (Figure 50.2). Bowman's capsule has a fenestrated or "window-like" epithelium that works like a sieve or a strainer to allow fluid to flow through but keep large components (e.g., proteins) from entering. The tube exits the capsule curling around in a section called the proximal convoluted tubule. From there, it narrows to form the descending and ascending loop of Henle. It widens as the distal convoluted tubule and then flows into the collecting ducts, which meet at the renal pelvises. Each section of the tubule functions in a slightly different manner to maintain fluid and electrolyte balance in the body.

Blood Supply

The blood flow to the nephron is unique. The renal arteries come directly off the aorta and enter each kidney. As a renal artery enters each of the kidneys, it divides to form interlobar arteries, which become smaller arcuate (bowed) arteries and then afferent arterioles. The afferent arterioles branch to form the glomerulus inside Bowman's capsule. The **glomerulus** is like a tuft of blood vessels with a capillary-like endothelium that allows easy passage of fluid and waste products. The efferent arteriole exits from the glomerulus and branches into the peritubular capillary system, which contains very concentrated blood and returns fluid and electrolytes that have been reabsorbed from the tubules to the bloodstream. These capillaries flow into the vasa recta, which flows into intralobar veins, which in turn drain into the inferior vena cava. The two arterioles around the glomerulus work together to closely regulate the flow of fluid into the glomerulus, increasing or decreasing pressure on either side of the glomerulus as needed.

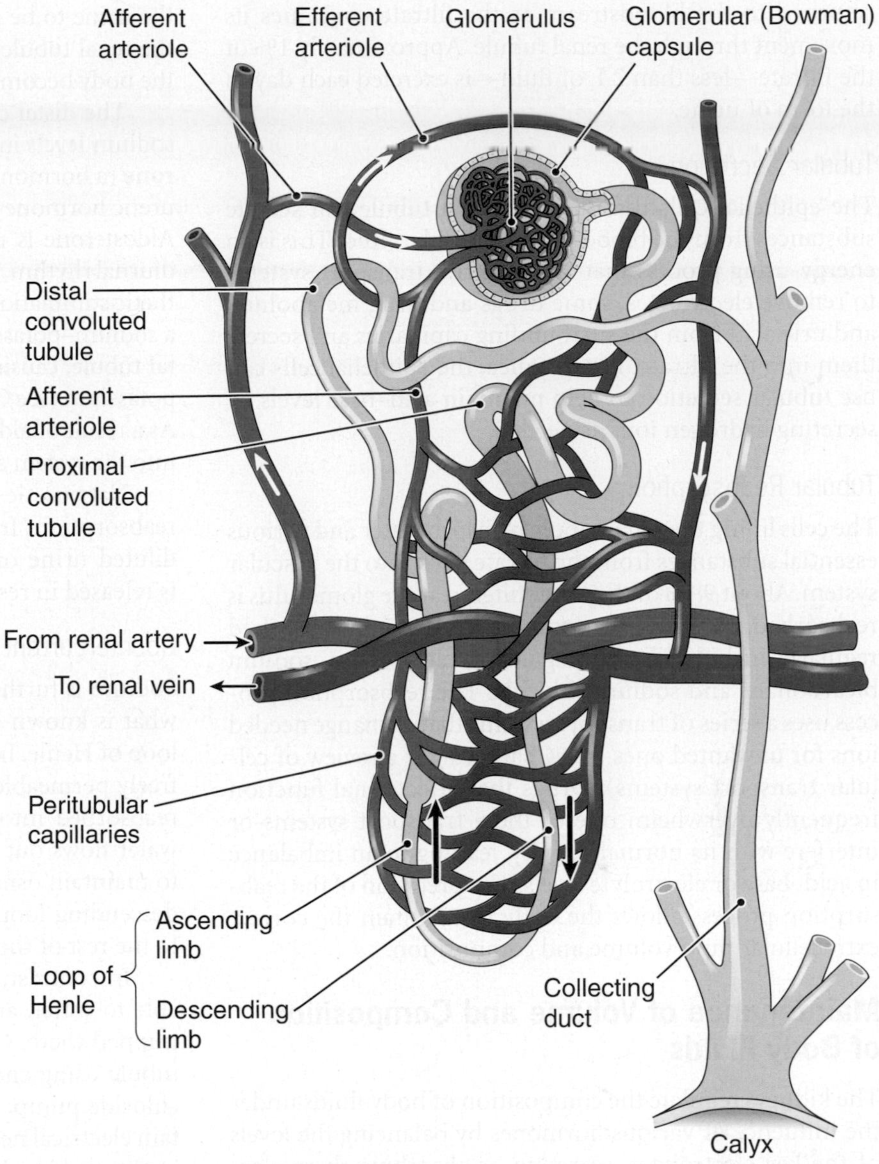

FIGURE 50.2 The nephron—the functional unit of the kidneys. Secretion and reabsorption of water, electrolytes, and other solutes in the various segments of the renal tubule, the loop of Henle, and the collecting duct can be influenced by diuretics, other drugs, and endogenous substances, including certain hormones. In the kidneys the distal convoluted tubule wraps around and is actually next to the afferent arteriole.

Other Structures

A small group of cells, called the juxtaglomerular apparatus, connects the afferent arteriole to the distal convoluted tubule. This is where erythropoietin and renin are produced. Because of their proximity to the afferent arteriole, these cells are especially sensitive to the volume and quality of blood flow into the glomerulus. Surrounding the nephrons is an area called the macula densa, which consists of immune system cells and chemicals that can respond quickly to any cellular damage or injury.

Nephron Function

The nephrons function by using three basic processes: Glomerular **filtration** (passage of fluid and small components of the blood through the glomerulus into the nephron tubule), tubular **secretion** (active movement of substances from the blood into the renal tubule), and tubular **reabsorption** (movement of substances from the renal tubule back into the vascular system).

Glomerular Filtration

The glomerulus acts as an ultrafine filter for all of the blood that flows into it. The semipermeable membrane keeps blood cells, proteins, and lipids inside the vessel, whereas hydrostatic pressure from the blood pushes water and smaller components of the plasma into the tubule. The resulting fluid is called the filtrate. Scarring or swelling of or damage to the semipermeable membrane leads to the escape of larger plasma components, such as blood cells or protein, into the filtrate. The large size of these components prevents them from being reabsorbed by the tubule, and they are lost in the urine. Thus, a clinical sign of renal damage is the presence of blood cells or protein in the urine.

Approximately 125 mL of fluid is filtered out each minute, or 180 L/d. About 99% of the filtered fluid is returned to the bloodstream as the filtrate continues its movement through the renal tubule. Approximately 1% of the filtrate—less than 2 L of fluid—is excreted each day in the form of urine.

Tubular Secretion

The epithelial cells that line the renal tubule can secrete substances from the blood into the tubular fluid. This is an energy-using process that allows active transport systems to remove electrolytes, some drugs and drug metabolites, and uric acid from the surrounding capillaries and secrete them into the filtrate. For instance, the epithelial cells can use tubular secretion to help maintain acid–base levels by secreting hydrogen ions as needed.

Tubular Reabsorption

The cells lining the renal tubule reabsorb water and various essential substances from the filtrate back into the vascular system. About 99% of the water filtered at the glomerulus is reabsorbed. Other filtrate components that are reabsorbed regularly include vitamins, glucose, electrolytes, sodium bicarbonate, and sodium chloride. The reabsorption process uses a series of transport systems that exchange needed ions for unwanted ones (see Chapter 7 for a review of cellular transport systems). Drugs that affect renal function frequently overwhelm one of these transport systems or interfere with its normal activity, leading to an imbalance in acid–base or electrolyte levels. The precision of the reabsorption process allows the body to maintain the correct extracellular fluid volume and composition.

Maintenance of Volume and Composition of Body Fluids

The kidneys regulate the composition of body fluids under the influence of various hormones by balancing the levels of the key electrolytes, secreting or absorbing these electrolytes to maintain the desired levels. The volume of body fluids is controlled by diluting or concentrating the urine.

Sodium Regulation

Sodium is one of the body's major cations (positively charged ions). It filters through the glomerulus and enters the renal tubule; then it is actively reabsorbed in the proximal convoluted tubule to the peritubular capillaries. As sodium is actively moved out of the filtrate, it takes chloride ions and water with it. This occurs by passive diffusion as the body maintains the osmotic and electrical balances on both sides of the tubule.

Sodium ions are also reabsorbed via a transport system that functions under the influence of the catalyst **carbonic anhydrase**. This enzyme speeds the combining of carbon dioxide and water to form carbonic acid. The carbonic acid immediately dissociates to form sodium bicarbonate, using a sodium ion from the renal tubule and a free hydrogen ion (an acid). The hydrogen ion remains in the filtrate, causing the urine to be slightly acidic. The bicarbonate is stored in the renal tubule as the body's alkaline reserve for use when the body becomes too acidic and a buffer is needed.

The distal convoluted tubule acts to further adjust the sodium levels in the filtrate under the influence of **aldosterone** (a hormone produced by the adrenal gland) and natriuretic hormone (probably produced by the hypothalamus). Aldosterone is released into the circulation as part of the diurnal rhythm, in response to high potassium levels, sympathetic stimulation, or angiotensin III. Aldosterone stimulates a sodium–potassium exchange pump in the cells of the distal tubule, causing reabsorption of sodium in exchange for potassium (see Chapter 7 for a review of the sodium pump). As a result of aldosterone stimulation, sodium is reabsorbed into the system and potassium is lost in the filtrate.

Natriuretic hormone causes a decrease in sodium reabsorption from the distal tubules with a resultant diluted urine or increased volume. Natriuretic hormone is released in response to fluid overload or hemodilution.

Countercurrent Mechanism

Sodium is further regulated in the medullary nephrons in what is known as the **countercurrent mechanism** in the loop of Henle. In the descending loop of Henle the cells are freely permeable to water and sodium. Sodium is actively reabsorbed into the surrounding peritubular tissue, and water flows out of the tubule into this sodium-rich tissue to maintain osmotic balance. The filtrate at the end of the descending loop of Henle is concentrated in comparison to the rest of the filtrate.

In contrast, the ascending loop of Henle is impermeable to water, and so water that remains in the tubule is trapped there. Chloride is actively transported out of the tubule using energy in a process that is referred to as the chloride pump; sodium leaves with the chloride to maintain electrical neutrality. As a result, the fluid in the ascending loop of Henle becomes hypotonic in comparison to the hypertonic situation in the peritubular tissue.

Antidiuretic hormone (ADH), which is produced by the hypothalamus and stored in the posterior pituitary gland, is important in maintaining fluid balance. ADH is released in response to falling blood volume, sympathetic stimulation, or rising sodium levels (a concentration that is sensed by the osmotic cells of the hypothalamus).

If ADH is present at the distal convoluted tubule and the collecting duct the permeability of the membrane to water is increased. Consequently, the water remaining in the tubule rapidly flows into the hypertonic tissue surrounding the loop of Henle, where it either is absorbed by the peritubular capillaries or reenters the descending loop of Henle in a countercurrent style. The resulting urine is hypertonic and of small volume. If ADH is not present the tubule remains impermeable to water. The water that has been trapped in the ascending loop of Henle passes into the collection duct, resulting in hypotonic urine of greater volume. This countercurrent mechanism and the influence of the hypothalamus and ADH release allows the body to finely regulate fluid volume by regulating the control of sodium and water (Figure 50.3).

Chloride Regulation

Chloride is an important negatively charged ion that helps to maintain electrical neutrality with the movement of cations across the cell membrane. Chloride is primarily reabsorbed in the loop of Henle, where it promotes the movement of sodium out of the cell.

Potassium Regulation

Potassium is another cation that is vital to proper functioning of the nervous system, muscles, and cell membranes. About 65% of the potassium that is filtered at the glomerulus is reabsorbed at Bowman's capsule and the proximal convoluted tubule. Another 25% to 30% is reabsorbed in the ascending loop of Henle. The fine-tuning of potassium levels occurs in the distal convoluted tubule, where aldosterone activates sodium–potassium exchange, leading to a loss of potassium. If potassium levels are very high the retention of sodium in exchange for potassium also leads to a retention of water and a dilution of blood volume, which further decreases the potassium concentration (see Figure 50.3).

Calcium Regulation

Calcium is important in muscle function, blood clotting, bone formation, contraction of cell membranes, and muscle movement and is another important cation that is regulated by the kidneys. The absorption of calcium from the gastrointestinal (GI) tract is regulated by vitamin D ingested as part of the diet. The vitamin then must be activated in the kidneys to a form that will promote calcium absorption. Once absorbed from the GI tract, calcium levels are maintained within a very tight range by the activity of parathyroid hormone (PTH) and calcitonin.

Calcium is filtered at the glomerulus and mostly reabsorbed in the proximal convoluted tubule and ascending loop of Henle. Fine-tuning of calcium reabsorption occurs in the distal convoluted tubule, where the presence of PTH stimulates reabsorption of calcium to increase serum calcium levels when they are low (see Figure 50.3 and Chapter 37).

Blood Pressure Control

The fragile nephrons require a constant supply of blood and are equipped with a system to ensure that they are perfused. This mechanism, called the **renin–angiotensin–aldosterone system**, involves a total body reaction to decreased blood flow to the nephrons.

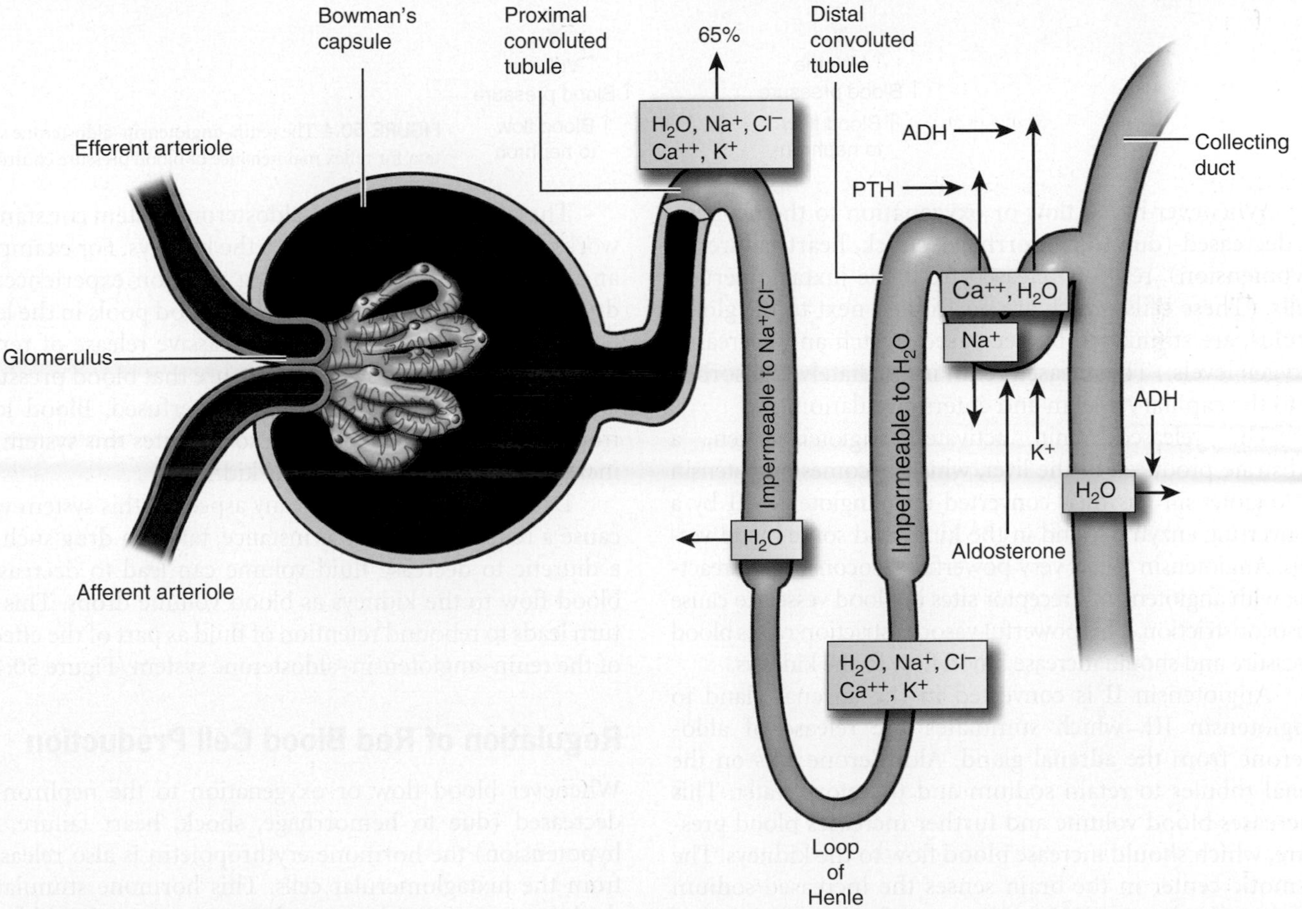

FIGURE 50.3 Nephron and points of regulation of sodium, chloride, potassium, calcium, and water. ADH, antidiuretic hormone; PTH, parathyroid hormone.

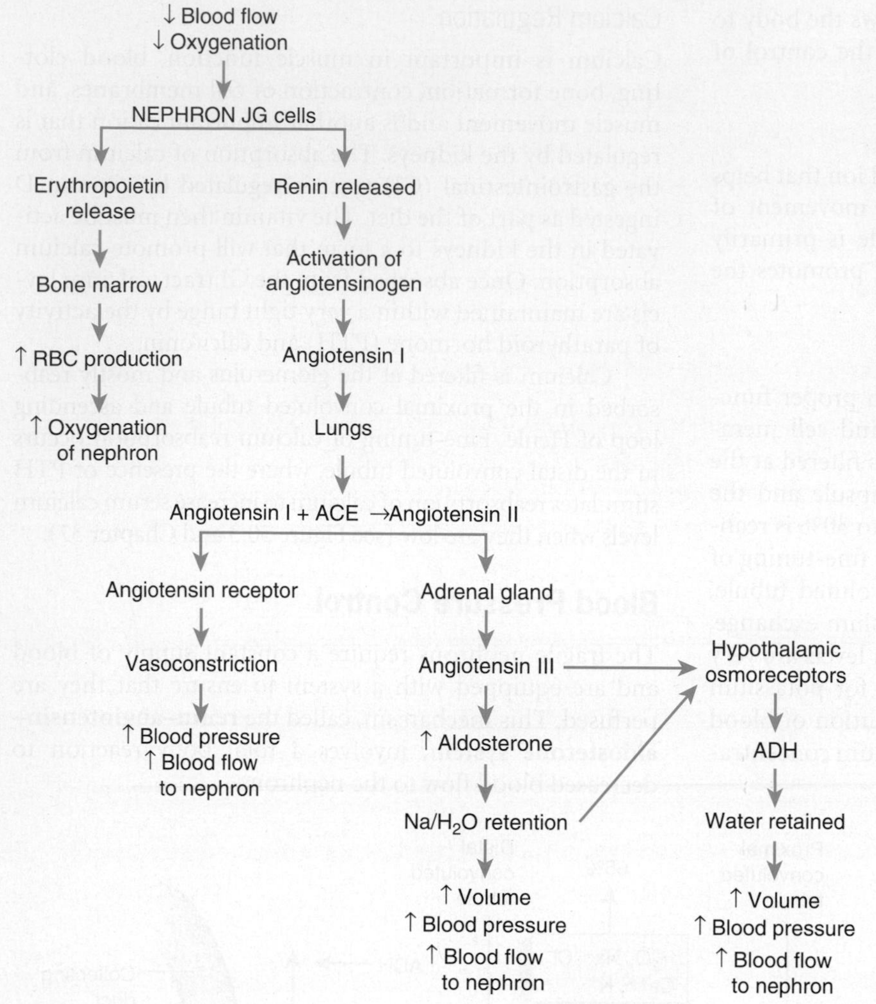

FIGURE 50.4 The renin–angiotensin–aldosterone system for reflex maintenance of blood pressure control.

Whenever blood flow or oxygenation to the nephron is decreased (due to hemorrhage, shock, heart failure, or hypotension), renin is released from the juxtaglomerular cells. (These cells, which are positioned next to the glomerulus, are stimulated by decreased stretch and decreased oxygen levels.) The released renin immediately is absorbed into the capillary system and enters circulation.

The released renin activates angiotensinogen, a substrate produced in the liver, which becomes angiotensin I. Angiotensin I is then converted into angiotensin II by a converting enzyme found in the lungs and some blood vessels. Angiotensin II is a very powerful vasoconstrictor, reacting with angiotensin II receptor sites in blood vessels to cause vasoconstriction. This powerful vasoconstriction raises blood pressure and should increase blood flow to the kidneys.

Angiotensin II is converted in the adrenal gland to angiotensin III, which stimulates the release of aldosterone from the adrenal gland. Aldosterone acts on the renal tubules to retain sodium and therefore water. This increases blood volume and further increases blood pressure, which should increase blood flow to the kidneys. The osmotic center in the brain senses the increased sodium levels and releases ADH, leading to a further retention of water and a further increase in blood volume and pressure, which should again increase blood flow to the kidneys.

The renin–angiotensin–aldosterone system constantly works to maintain blood flow to the kidneys. For example, an individual rising from a lying position experiences a drop in blood flow to the kidneys as blood pools in the legs because of gravity. This causes a massive release of renin and activation of this system to ensure that blood pressure is maintained and the kidneys are perfused. Blood loss from injury or during surgery also activates this system to increase blood flow through the kidneys.

Drugs that interfere with any aspect of this system will cause a reflex response. For instance, taking a drug such as a diuretic to decrease fluid volume can lead to decreased blood flow to the kidneys as blood volume drops. This in turn leads to rebound retention of fluid as part of the effects of the renin–angiotensin–aldosterone system (Figure 50.4).

Regulation of Red Blood Cell Production

Whenever blood flow or oxygenation to the nephron is decreased (due to hemorrhage, shock, heart failure, or hypotension) the hormone erythropoietin is also released from the juxtaglomerular cells. This hormone stimulates the bone marrow to increase the production of red blood cells, which bring oxygen to the kidneys. Erythropoietin is the only known factor that can regulate the rate of red blood cell production. When a patient develops renal failure and the production of erythropoietin drops the production of red blood cells falls and the patient becomes anemic.

KEY POINTS

- The kidneys are two small, bean-shaped organs that receive about 25% of the cardiac output.
- The nephron is the functional unit of the kidneys and is involved in three processes: Glomerular filtration, tubular secretion, and tubular reabsorption.
- The kidney plays a key role in regulating body fluid volume and maintaining blood pressure, red blood cell production, acid–base balance, and electrolyte stability.
- The renin–angiotensin–aldosterone system is activated when blood flow to the nephron is decreased and renin is released. The end result is increased vasoconstriction and increased blood pressure and sodium and water retention, which increase blood volume and pressure.
- Red blood cell production is controlled by erythropoietin released from the juxtaglomerular apparatus when oxygen delivery to the nephron is decreased. Erythropoietin stimulates the bone marrow to produce red blood cells to increase oxygen delivery to the nephrons.

The Urinary Tract

As noted previously, the urinary tract is composed of the ureters, urinary bladder, and urethra (see Figure 50.1).

Ureters

One ureter exits each kidney, draining the filtrate from the collecting ducts. The ureters have a smooth endothelial lining and circular muscular layers. Urine entering the ureter stimulates a peristaltic wave that pushes the urine down toward the urinary bladder.

Urinary Bladder

The urinary bladder is a muscular pouch that stretches and holds the urine until it is excreted from the body. Urine is usually a slightly acidic fluid; this acidity helps to maintain the normal transport systems and to destroy bacteria that may enter the bladder. Control of bladder emptying is learned control over the urethral sphincter; once it is established a functioning nervous system is necessary to maintain control.

Urethra

In the female the urethra is a very short tube that leads from the bladder to an area populated by normal flora, including *Escherichia coli*, which can cause frequent bladder infections or cystitis. In the male the urethra is much longer and passes through the **prostate gland**, a small gland that produces an alkaline fluid that is important in maintaining the sperm and lubricating the tract. Enlargement and infection in the prostate gland are often problems in older men.

KEY POINTS

- The ureters, urinary bladder, and urethra make up the rest of the urinary tract.
- The shorter female urethra leads from the urinary bladder to the outer body into an area rich in gram-negative bacteria. Cystitis, or infection of the urinary bladder, is a common problem for women.
- The longer male urethra passes through the prostate gland, which may enlarge or become infected, a problem often associated with advancing age.

SUMMARY

- The functional unit of the kidneys is called the nephron; it is composed of Bowman's capsule, the proximal convoluted tubule, the loop of Henle, the distal convoluted tubule, and the collecting duct.
- The blood flow to the nephron is unique, allowing autoregulation of blood flow through the glomerulus.
- Sodium levels are regulated throughout the tubule by active and passive movement and are fine-tuned by the presence of aldosterone in the distal tubule.
- The countercurrent mechanism in the medullary nephrons allows for the concentration or dilution of urine under the influence of ADH secreted by the hypothalamus.
- Potassium concentration is regulated throughout the tubule, with aldosterone being the strongest influence for potassium loss.
- The kidneys play a key role in the regulation of calcium by activating vitamin D to allow GI calcium reabsorption and by reabsorbing or excreting calcium from the tubule under the influence of PTH.
- The kidneys influence blood pressure control, releasing renin to activate the renin–angiotensin system, which leads to increased blood pressure and volume and a resultant increased blood flow to the kidney. The balance of this reflex system can lead to water retention or excretion and has an impact on drug therapy that promotes water or sodium loss.
- The ureters, urinary bladder, and urethra make up the rest of the urinary tract. The longer male urethra passes through the prostate gland, which may enlarge or become infected, a problem often associated with advancing age.

CHECK YOUR UNDERSTANDING

Answers to the questions in this chapter can be found in Answers to Check Your Understanding Questions on thePoint®.

MULTIPLE CHOICE

Select the best answer to the following.

1. During severe exertion a man may lose up to 4 L of hypotonic sweat per hour. This loss would result in
   a. decreased plasma volume.
   b. decreased plasma osmolarity.
   c. decreased circulating levels of ADH.
   d. return of body fluid balance to normal after ingestion of 100 mL of water.

2. Urine passes through the ureter by
   a. osmosis.
   b. air pressure.
   c. filtration.
   d. Peristalsis.

3. When describing renal reabsorption to a group of students the instructor would identify it as the movement of which of the following?
   a. Substances from the renal tubule into the blood
   b. Substances from the blood into the renal tubule
   c. Water that is increased in the absence of ADH
   d. Sodium occurring only in the proximal tubule

4. Considering the functions of the kidney, if a patient lost kidney function a nurse would expect to see
   a. increased red blood cell count.
   b. decreased fluid volume.
   c. electrolyte disturbances.
   d. decreased blood pressure.

5. Blood flow to the nephron differs from blood flow to other tissues in that
   a. the venous system is not involved in blood flow around the nephron.
   b. there are no capillaries in the nephron allowing direct flow from artery to vein.
   c. efferent and afferent arterioles allow for autoregulation of blood flow.
   d. the capillary bed has a fenestrated membrane to allow passage of fluid and small particles.

6. Concentration and dilution of urine is controlled by
   a. afferent arterioles.
   b. the renin–angiotensin system.
   c. aldosterone release.
   d. the countercurrent mechanism.

7. Women tend to have more problems with bladder infections than men because
   a. women have *Escherichia coli* in the urinary tract.
   b. women have a short urethra, making access to the bladder easier for bacteria.
   c. the prostate gland secretes a substance that protects men from bladder infections.
   d. women's urine is more acidotic, encouraging the growth of bladder bacteria.

MULTIPLE RESPONSE

Select all that apply.

1. Considering the metabolic functions of the kidneys, renal failure would be expected to cause which of the following?
   a. Anemia
   b. Loss of calcium regulation
   c. Urea buildup on the skin
   d. Respiratory alkalosis
   e. Metabolic acidosis
   f. Changes in the function of blood cells

2. During severe diarrhea, there is a loss of water, bicarbonate, and sodium from the GI tract. Physiological compensation for this would probably include which of the following?
   a. Increased alveolar ventilation
   b. Decreased hydrogen ion secretion by the renal tubules
   c. Decreased urinary excretion of sodium and water
   d. Increased renin secretion
   e. Increased hydrogen ion secretion by the renal tubules
   f. Increased ADH levels

3. Maintenance of blood pressure is important in maintaining the fragile nephrons. Reflex systems that work to ensure blood flow to the kidneys include
   a. the renin–angiotensin system causing vasoconstriction.
   b. baroreceptor monitoring of the renal artery.
   c. aldosterone release secondary to angiotensin stimulation.
   d. ADH release in response to decreased blood volume with increased osmolarity.
   e. release of erythropoietin.
   f. local response of the afferent arterioles.

BIBLIOGRAPHY AND REFERENCES

Barrett, K., Barman, S., Boitano, S., et al. (2015). *Ganong's review of medical physiology* (25th ed.). New York: McGraw-Hill.

Brunton, L., Chabner, B., & Knollman, B. (2011). *Goodman and Gilman's the pharmacological basis of therapeutics* (12th ed.). New York: McGraw-Hill.

Eaton, D. C., & Pooler, J. P. (2013). *Vander's renal physiology* (8th ed.). New York: McGraw-Hill.

Hall, J. (2015). *Guyton and Hall's textbook of medical physiology* (13th ed.). Philadelphia, PA: W. B. Saunders.

Rennke, H. G., & Denker, B. M. (2013). *Renal pathophysiology: The essentials* (4th ed.). Philadelphia, PA: Lippincott Williams & Wilkins.

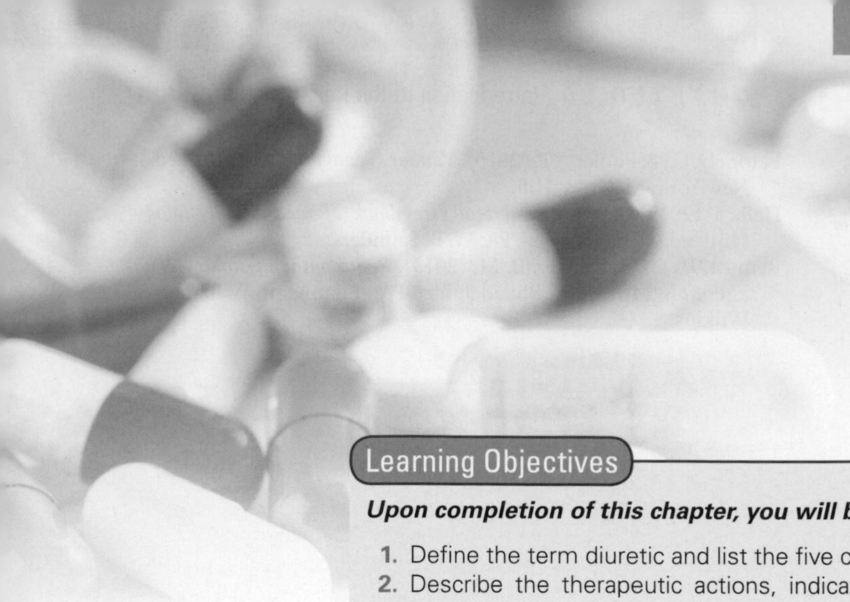

51 Diuretic Agents

Learning Objectives

Upon completion of this chapter, you will be able to:

1. Define the term diuretic and list the five classes of diuretics.
2. Describe the therapeutic actions, indications, pharmacokinetics, contraindications and cautions, most common adverse reactions, and important drug–drug interactions associated with the various classes of diuretic drugs.
3. Discuss the use of diuretic agents across the lifespan.
4. Compare and contrast the prototype drugs of each class of diuretic drugs with other agents in their class.
5. Outline the nursing considerations, including important teaching points, for patients receiving diuretic agents.

Glossary of Key Terms

alkalosis: state of not having enough acid to maintain normal homeostatic processes; seen with loop diuretics, which cause loss of bicarbonate in the urine

edema: movement of fluid into the interstitial spaces; occurs when the balance between osmotic pull (from plasma proteins) and hydrostatic push (from blood pressure) is upset

fluid rebound: reflex reaction of the body to the loss of fluid or sodium; the hypothalamus causes the release of antidiuretic hormone, which promotes water retention, and stress related to fluid loss combines with decreased blood flow to the kidneys to activate the renin–angiotensin–aldosterone system, leading to further water and sodium retention

high-ceiling diuretics: powerful diuretics that work in the loop of Henle to inhibit the reabsorption of sodium and chloride, leading to a sodium-rich diuresis

hyperaldosteronism: excessive output of aldosterone from the adrenal gland, leading to increased sodium and water retention and loss of potassium

hypokalemia: low potassium in the blood, which often occurs after diuretic use; characterized by weakness, muscle cramps, trembling, nausea, vomiting, diarrhea, and cardiac arrhythmias

osmotic pull: drawing force of large molecules on water, pulling it into a tubule or capillary essential for maintaining normal fluid balance within the body; used to draw out excess fluid into the vascular system or the renal tubule

Drug List

Diuretics

Thiazide Diuretics and Thiazide-like Diuretics

Thiazide Diuretics

chlorothiazide
(P) hydrochlorothiazide
hydroflumethiazide
methyclothiazide

Thiazide-like Diuretics

chlorthalidone
indapamide
metolazone

Loop Diuretics

bumetanide
ethacrynic acid
(P) furosemide
torsemide

Carbonic Anhydrase Inhibitors

(P) acetazolamide
methazolamide

Potassium-Sparing Diuretics

amiloride
(P) spironolactone
triamterene

Osmotic Diuretics

(P) Mannitol

Diuretic agents are commonly thought of simply as drugs that increase the amount of urine produced by the kidneys. Most diuretics do increase the volume of urine produced to some extent, but the greater clinical significance of diuretics is their ability to increase sodium excretion.

Most diuretics prevent the cells lining the renal tubules from reabsorbing an excessive proportion of the sodium ions in the glomerular filtrate. As a result, sodium and other ions (and the water in which they are dissolved) are lost in the urine instead of being returned to the blood, where they would cause increased intravascular volume and therefore increased hydrostatic pressure, which could result in leaking of fluids at the capillary level.

Diuretics are indicated for the treatment of edema associated with heart failure (HF), acute pulmonary **edema**, liver disease (including cirrhosis), and renal disease and for the treatment of hypertension. They are also used to decrease fluid pressure in the eye (intraocular pressure [IOP]), which is useful in treating glaucoma. Diuretics that decrease potassium levels may also be indicated in the treatment of conditions that cause hyperkalemia.

HF can cause edema as a result of several factors. The failing heart muscle does not pump sufficient blood to the kidneys, causing activation of the renin–angiotensin system and resulting in increases in blood volume and sodium retention. Because the failing heart muscle cannot respond to the usual reflex stimulation the increased volume is slowly pushed out into the capillary level as venous pressure increases because the blood is not being pumped effectively (see Chapter 44).

Pulmonary edema, or left-sided HF, develops when the increased volume of fluids backs up into the lungs. The fluid pushed out into the capillaries in the lungs interferes with gas exchange. If this condition develops rapidly, it can be life threatening.

Patients with liver failure and cirrhosis often present with edema and ascites. This is caused by (1) reduced plasma protein production, which results in less oncotic pull in the vascular system and fluid loss at the capillary level and (2) obstructed blood flow through the portal system, which is caused by increased pressure from congested hepatic vessels.

Renal disease produces edema because of the loss of plasma proteins into the urine when there is damage to the glomerular basement membrane. Other types of renal disease produce edema because of activation of the renin–angiotensin system as a result of decreasing volume (associated with the loss of fluid into the urine), which causes a drop in blood pressure, or because of failure of the renal tubules to regulate electrolytes effectively.

Hypertension is predominantly an idiopathic disorder; in other words, the underlying pathology is not known. Treatment of hypertension is aimed at reducing the higher-than-normal blood pressure, which can damage end organs and lead to serious cardiovascular (CV) disorders. Diuretics were once the key element in antihypertensive therapy, the goal of which was to decrease volume and sodium, which would then decrease pressure in the system. Then several other classes of drugs, including angiotensin-converting enzyme inhibitors, angiotensin receptor blockers, beta-blockers, and calcium-channel blockers, became available for the initial treatment of hypertension. However, recent studies have repeatedly found that the use of thiazide diuretics is still the most effective way of treating initial hypertension. Diuretics are also often used as an adjunct to improve the effectiveness of these other drugs.

Glaucoma is an eye disease characterized by increased pressure in the eye—known as IOP—which can cause optic nerve atrophy and blindness. Diuretics are used to provide osmotic pull to remove some of the fluid from the eye, which decreases the IOP, or as adjunctive therapy to reduce fluid volume and pressure in the CV system, which also decreases pressure in the eye somewhat.

Diuretics

There are five classes of diuretics, each working at a slightly different site in the nephron or using a different mechanism. Diuretic classes include the thiazide and thiazide-like diuretics, loop diuretics, carbonic anhydrase inhibitors, potassium-sparing diuretics, and osmotic diuretics (Table 51.1). For the most part, the overall nursing care of a patient receiving any diuretic is similar, although there are specific differences. Adverse effects associated with diuretics are also specific to the particular class used. For details, see Adverse Effects for each class of diuretics discussed in this chapter, and refer to Table 51.1. The most common adverse effects seen with diuretics include gastrointestinal (GI) upset, fluid and electrolyte imbalances, hypotension, and electrolyte disturbances.

This chapter presents each class in the order of frequency of use, beginning with the most frequent. Box 51.1 highlights important considerations related to diuretic use based on the patient's age.

FOCUS ON Safe Medication Administration

Explaining Fluid Rebound

Care must be taken when using diuretics to avoid fluid rebound, which is associated with fluid loss. If a patient stops taking in water and takes the diuretic the result will be a concentrated plasma of smaller volume. The decreased volume is sensed by the nephrons, which activate the renin–angiotensin cycle. When the concentrated blood is sensed by the osmotic center in the brain, antidiuretic hormone (ADH) is released to hold water and dilute the blood. The result can be a "rebound" edema as fluid is retained.

Many patients who are taking a diuretic markedly decrease their fluid intake in order to decrease the number of trips to the bathroom. The result is a rebound of water retention after the diuretic effect. This effect can also be seen in many diets that promise "immediate results"; they frequently contain a key provision to increase fluid intake to 8 to 10 full glasses of water daily. The reflex result of diluting the system with so much water is a drop in ADH release and fluid loss.

Some people can lose 5 pounds in a few days by doing this. However, the body's reflexes soon kick in, causing rebound retention of fluid to reestablish fluid and electrolyte balance. Most people get frustrated at this point and give up the fad diet. It is important to be able to explain this effect. Teaching patients about balancing the desired diuretic effect with the actions of the normal reflexes is a clinical skill.

KEY POINTS

- Diuretics increase sodium excretion, and therefore water excretion, from the kidneys.
- Diuretics help to relieve edema associated with HF and pulmonary edema, liver failure and cirrhosis, and various types of renal disease. They are also used in treating hypertension.

Table 51.1 ***Drugs in Focus:* Diuretics**

Drug Name	Usual Dosage	Usual Indications
Thiazide Diuretics *Thiazide Diuretics*		
chlorothiazide (*Diuril*)	*Adult:* 0.5–2 g PO or IV, daily to b.i.d. for edema; 0.5–2 g/d PO for hypertension *Pediatric (<6 mo):* Up to 33 mg/kg/d PO *Pediatric (>6 mo):* 22 mg/kg/d PO in two divided doses	Treatment of edema caused by HF liver disease, or renal disease; monotherapy or as adjunctive treatment of hypertension
hydrochlorothiazide (generic)	*Adult:* 25–100 mg/d PO or intermittently, up to 200 mg/d maximum for edema; 25–100 mg/d PO for hypertension *Pediatric (<6 mo):* Up to 3.3 mg/kg/d PO in two divided doses *Pediatric (6 mo–2 y):* 12.5–37.5 mg/d PO in two divided doses *Pediatric (2–12 y):* 37.6–100 mg/d PO in two divided doses	Treatment of edema caused by HF, liver disease, or renal disease; monotherapy or as adjunctive treatment of hypertension
hydroflumethiazide (*Saluron*)	25–200 mg PO b.i.d. for edema; 50–100 mg/d PO for hypertension	Treatment of edema caused by HF, liver disease, or renal disease; monotherapy or as adjunctive treatment of hypertension
methyclothiazide (generic)	2.5–10 mg/d PO for edema; 2.5–5 mg/d PO for hypertension	Treatment of edema caused by HF, liver disease, or renal disease; monotherapy or as adjunctive treatment of hypertension
Thiazide-like Diuretics		
chlorthalidone (generic)	50–100 mg/d PO for edema; 25–100 mg/d PO for hypertension	Treatment of edema caused by HF or by liver or renal disease; adjunctive treatment of hypertension
indapamide (generic)	2.5–5 mg/d PO for edema or hypertension, based on patient response	Treatment of edema caused by HF or by liver or renal disease; adjunctive treatment of hypertension
metolazone (*Zaroxolyn*)	2.5–5 mg/d PO for hypertension; 5–20 mg/d PO for edema, based on patient response	Treatment of edema caused by HF or by liver or renal disease; adjunctive treatment of hypertension
Loop Diuretics		
bumetanide (generic)	0.5–2 mg/d PO as a single dose repeated to a maximum of 10 mg; 0.5–1 mg IM or IV given over 1–2 min, may be repeated in 2–3 h, not to exceed 10 mg/d *Geriatric or renal-impaired patient:* 12 mg by continuous IV infusion over 12 h may be most effective and least toxic	Treatment of acute HF; acute pulmonary edema; hypertension; and edema of HF, renal disease, or liver disease

Drug Name	Usual Dosage	Usual Indications
ethacrynic acid (*Edecrin*)	50–200 mg/d PO based on patient response; 0.5–1 mg/kg IV slowly *Pediatric:* 25 mg PO with slow titration up as needed; not to be used with infants	Treatment of acute HF; acute pulmonary edema; hypertension; and edema of HF, renal disease, or liver disease
furosemide (*Lasix*)	20–80 mg/d PO, up to 600 mg/d may be given; 20–40 mg IM or IV given slowly; 40 mg IV over 1–2 min for acute pulmonary edema, increase to 80 mg after 1 h if response is not adequate; 40 mg PO b.i.d. for hypertension *Geriatric or renal-impaired patient:* 2–2.5 g/d PO *Pediatric:* 2 mg/kg/d PO for hypertension, not to exceed 6 mg/kg/d; 1 mg/kg IV or IM for edema, increased by 1 mg/kg as needed; not to exceed 6 mg/kg	Treatment of acute HF; acute pulmonary edema; hypertension; and edema of HF, renal disease, or liver disease
torsemide (*Demadex*)	10–20 mg/d PO for IV for HF or chronic renal failure; 5–10 mg/d PO for hypertension	Treatment of acute HF; acute pulmonary edema; hypertension; and edema of HF, renal disease, or liver disease
Carbonic Anhydrase Inhibitors		
acetazolamide (*Diamox*)	500 mg IV repeated in 2–4 h, then 250 mg–1 g/d in divided doses q6 8 h for glaucoma; 8–30 mg/kg/d in divided doses for epilepsy; 250 mg–1 g/d PO given in divided doses four times per day or once or twice a day if using sustained release formulation	Treatment of glaucoma; adjunctive treatment of epilepsy, mountain sickness
methazolamide (generic)	50–100 mg PO b.i.d. to t.i.d.	Treatment of glaucoma
Potassium-Sparing Diuretics		
amiloride (*Midamor*)	15–20 mg/d PO with monitoring of electrolytes	Adjunctive treatment of edema caused by HF, liver disease, or renal disease; hypertension; hyperkalemia; and hyperaldosteronism *Special consideration:* Not for use in children
spironolactone (*Aldactone*)	100–200 mg/d PO for edema; 100–400 mg/d PO for hyperaldosteronism; 50–100 mg/d PO for hypertension *Pediatric:* 3.3 mg/kg/d PO	Adjunctive treatment of edema caused by HF, liver disease, or renal disease; hypertension; hyperkalemia; and hyperaldosteronism *Special consideration:* Can be used in children with careful monitoring of electrolytes
triamterene (*Dyrenium*)	100 mg/d PO b.i.d.	Adjunctive treatment of edema caused by HF, liver disease, or renal disease; hypertension; hyperkalemia; and hyperaldosteronism *Special consideration:* Not for use in children
Osmotic Diuretics		
mannitol (*Osmitrol*)	50–100 g IV for oliguria; 1.5–2 g/kg IV to reduce intracranial pressure; dose not established for children <12 y	Treatment of elevated intracranial pressure, acute renal failure, acute glaucoma; also used to decrease intracranial pressure, prevent oliguric phase of renal failure, and to promote movement of toxic substances through the kidneys

HF, heart failure.

BOX 51.1 FOCUS ON Drug Therapy Across the Lifespan

Diuretic Agents

CHILDREN

Diuretics are often used in children to treat edema associated with heart defects, to control hypertension, and to treat edema associated with renal and pulmonary disorders.

Hydrochlorothiazide and chlorothiazide have established pediatric dosing guidelines. Furosemide is often used when a stronger diuretic is needed; care should be taken not to exceed 6 mg/kg/d when using this drug. Ethacrynic acid may be used orally in some situations but should not be used in infants. Bumetanide, although not recommended for use in children, may be used for children who are taking other ototoxic drugs, including antibiotics, and may cause less hypokalemia, making it preferable to furosemide for children also taking digoxin. Spironolactone is the only potassium-sparing diuretic that is recommended for use in children, but, as with adults, it should not be used in the presence of severe renal impairment.

Because of the size and rapid metabolism of children the effects of diuretics may be rapid and adverse effects may occur suddenly. The child receiving a diuretic should be monitored for serum electrolyte changes; for evidence of fluid volume changes; for rapid weight gain or loss, which could reflect fluid volume; and for signs of ototoxicity.

ADULTS

Adults may be taking diuretics for prolonged periods and need to be aware of the signs and symptoms of fluid imbalance to report to their health care provider. Adults receiving chronic diuretic therapy should weigh themselves on the same scale, in the same clothes, and at the same time each day to monitor for fluid retention or sudden fluid loss. They should be alerted to situations that could aggravate fluid loss, such as diarrhea, vomiting, or excessive heat and sweating, which could change their need for the diuretic. They should also be urged to maintain their fluid intake to help balance their bodies' compensatory mechanisms and to prevent fluid rebound.

Patients taking potassium-losing diuretics should be encouraged to eat foods that are high in potassium and to have their serum potassium levels checked periodically. Patients taking potassium-sparing diuretics should be cautioned to avoid those same foods.

The use of diuretics to change the fluid shifts associated with pregnancy is not appropriate. Women maintained on these drugs for underlying medical reasons should not stop taking them, but they need to be aware of the potential for adverse effects on the fetus. Women who are nursing and need a diuretic should find another method of feeding the baby because of the potential for adverse effects on the baby as well as the lactating mother.

OLDER ADULTS

Older adults often have conditions that are treated with diuretics. They are also more likely to have renal or hepatic impairment, which requires cautious use of these drugs.

Older adults should be started on the lowest possible dose of the drug, and the dose should be titrated slowly based on patient response. Frequent serum electrolyte measurements should be done to monitor for adverse reactions.

The intake and activity level of the patient can alter the effectiveness and need for the diuretic. High-salt diets and inactivity can aggravate conditions that lead to edema, and patients should be encouraged to follow activity and dietary guidelines if possible.

Thiazide and Thiazide-like Diuretics

The thiazide diuretics belong to a chemical class of drugs called the sulfonamides. Thiazide-like diuretics have a slightly different chemical structure but work in the same way as thiazide diuretics.

Thiazide diuretics include chlorothiazide (*Diuril*), hydrochlorothiazide (generic), hydroflumethiazide (*Saluron*), and methyclothiazide (generic). Thiazide-like diuretics include chlorthalidone (generic), indapamide (generic), and metolazone (*Zaroxolyn*). Thiazide and thiazide-like diuretics are among the most frequently used diuretics.

Therapeutic Actions and Indications

Thiazide and thiazide-like diuretics act to block the chloride pump. Chloride is actively pumped out of the tubule by cells lining the ascending limb of the loop of Henle and the distal tubule. Sodium passively moves with the chloride to maintain electrical neutrality. (Chloride is a negative ion, and sodium is a positive ion.) Blocking of the chloride pump keeps the chloride and the sodium in the tubule to be excreted in the urine, thus preventing the reabsorption of both chloride and sodium in the vascular system (Figure 51.1). Because these segments of the tubule are impermeable to water, there is little increase in the volume of urine produced, but it will be sodium rich, a saluretic effect. Thiazides are considered to be mild diuretics compared with the more potent loop diuretics. These drugs are the first-line drugs used to manage essential hypertension when drug therapy is needed. See Table 51.2 for Usual Indications for these agents.

Pharmacokinetics

These drugs are well absorbed from the GI tract after oral administration, with onset of action ranging from 1 to 3 hours. They have peak effects within 4 to

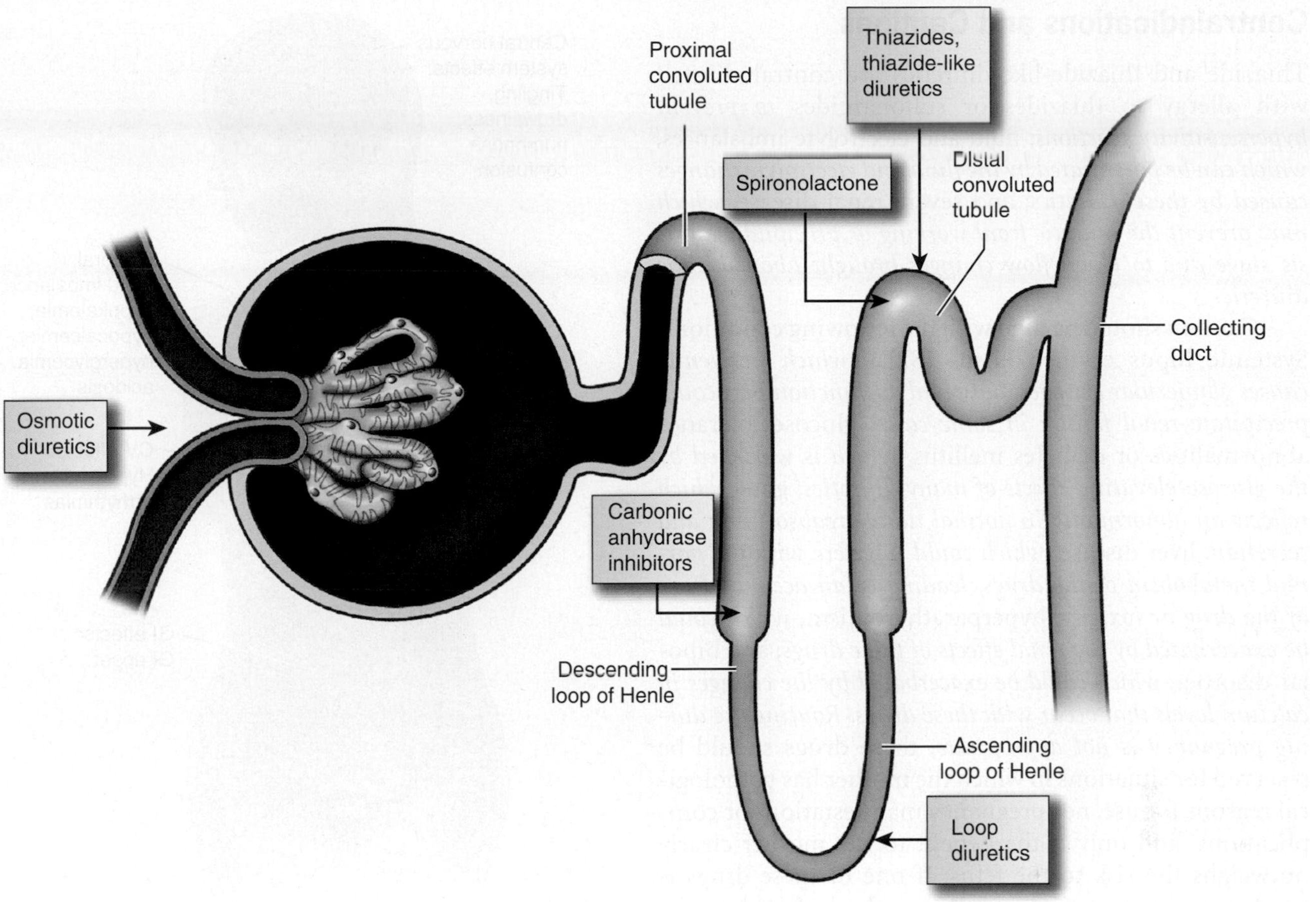

FIGURE 51.1 Sites of action of diuretics in the nephron.

6 hours and duration of effects of 6 to 12 hours. They are metabolized in the liver and excreted in the urine. These diuretics cross the placenta and enter breast milk. Hydrochlorothiazide, the most frequently used of the thiazide diuretics and the prototype of this class, can be used in small doses because it is more potent than chlorothiazide, the oldest drug of this class. Chlorothiazide is also available for IV infusion.

Table 51.2 Comparison of Diuretics

Diuretic Class	Major Site of Action	Usual Indications	Major Adverse Effects
Thiazide, thiazide like	Distal convoluted tubule	Edema of HF, renal and liver disease	GI upset, CNS complications, hypovolemia
Loop	Loop of Henle	Acute HF; acute pulmonary edema; hypertension; edema of HF, liver, and renal disease	Hypokalemia, volume depletion, hypotension, CNS effects, GI upset, hyperglycemia
Carbonic anhydrase inhibitors	Proximal tubule	Glaucoma; diuresis in HF; mountain sickness; epilepsy	GI upset, urinary frequency
Potassium sparing	Distal tubule and collecting duct	Adjunct for edema of HF, liver and renal disease; treatment of hypokalemia; adjunct for hypertension; adjunct for hypertension; hyperaldosteronism	Hyperkalemia, CNS effects, diarrhea
Osmotic	Glomerulus, tubule	Reduction of intracranial pressure; prevention of oliguric phase of renal failure; reduction of IOP; renal clearance of toxic substances	Hypotension, GI upset, fluid and electrolyte imbalances

GI, gastrointestinal; CNS, central nervous system; HF, heart failure; IOP, intraocular pressure.

Contraindications and Cautions

Thiazide and thiazide-like diuretics are contraindicated with allergy to thiazides or sulfonamides *to prevent hypersensitivity reactions*; fluid and electrolyte imbalances, *which can be potentiated by the fluid and electrolyte changes caused by these diuretics*; and severe renal disease, *which may prevent the diuretic from working or precipitate a crisis stage due to blood flow changes brought about by the diuretic.*

Caution should be used with the following conditions: Systemic lupus erythematosus (SLE), *which frequently causes glomerular changes and renal dysfunction that could precipitate renal failure in some cases*; glucose tolerance abnormalities or diabetes mellitus, *which is worsened by the glucose-elevating effects of many diuretics*; gout, *which reflects an abnormality in normal tubule reabsorption and secretion*; liver disease, *which could interfere with the normal metabolism of the drugs, leading to an accumulation of the drug or toxicity*; hyperparathyroidism, *which could be exacerbated by the renal effects of these drugs*; and bipolar disorder, *which could be exacerbated by the changes in calcium levels that occur with these drugs. Routine use during pregnancy is not appropriate*; these drugs should be reserved for situations in which the mother has pathological reasons for use, not pregnancy manifestations or complications, and only if the benefit to the mother clearly outweighs the risk to the fetus. If one of these drugs is needed during lactation, another method of feeding the baby should be used *because of the potential for adverse effects on fluid and electrolyte changes in the fetus and the baby.*

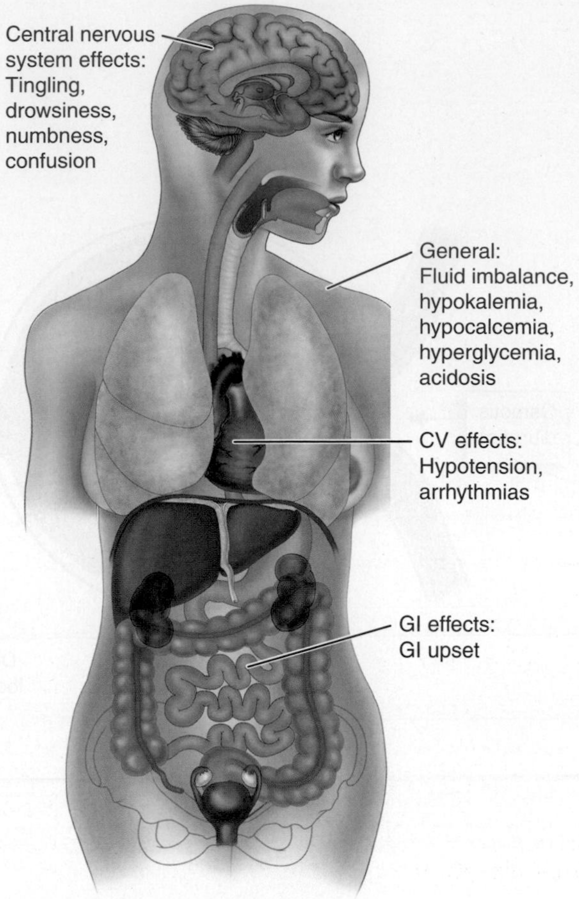

FIGURE 51.2 Variety of adverse effects and toxicities associated with diuretics.

Adverse Effects

The most common adverse effects associated with diuretic agents include GI upset, fluid and electrolyte imbalances, hypotension, and electrolyte disturbances. Adverse effects associated with the use of thiazide and thiazide-like diuretics are related to interference with the normal regulatory mechanisms of the nephron. Potassium is lost at the distal tubule because of the actions on the pumping mechanism, and **hypokalemia** (low blood levels of potassium) may result. Signs and symptoms of hypokalemia include weakness, muscle cramps, and arrhythmias (Figure 51.2). Another adverse effect is decreased calcium excretion, which leads to increased calcium levels in the blood. Uric acid excretion also is decreased because the thiazides interfere with its secretory mechanism. High levels of uric acid can result in gout.

If these drugs are used over a prolonged period, blood glucose levels may increase. This may result from the change in potassium levels (which keeps glucose out of the cells), or it may relate to some other mechanism of glucose control.

Urine is slightly alkalinized when the thiazides or thiazide-like diuretics are used because they block the reabsorption of bicarbonate. This effect can cause problems for patients who are susceptible to bladder infections.

Clinically Important Drug–Drug Interactions

Decreased absorption of these drugs may occur if they are combined with cholestyramine or colestipol. If this combination is used the drugs should be taken separated by at least 2 hours.

The risk of digoxin toxicity increases due to potential changes in potassium levels; serum potassium should be monitored if this combination is used. Risk of quinidine toxicity increases due to decreased quinidine excretion with an alkaline urine, leading to increased serum levels of quinidine. If this combination is used the patient must be monitored closely and quinidine dose decreased as appropriate.

Decreased effectiveness of antidiabetic agents may occur related to the changes in glucose metabolism; dose adjustment of those agents may be needed.

The risk of lithium toxicity may increase if these drugs are combined. Serum lithium levels should be monitored and appropriate dose adjustment made as needed.

Prototype Summary: Hydrochlorothiazide

Indications: Adjunctive therapy for edema associated with HF, cirrhosis, corticosteroid or estrogen therapy, and renal dysfunction; treatment of hypertension as monotherapy or in combination with other antihypertensives.

Actions: Inhibits reabsorption of sodium and chloride in distal renal tubules, increasing the excretion of sodium, chloride, and water by the kidneys.

Pharmacokinetics:

Route	Onset	Peak	Duration
Oral	2 h	4–6 h	6–12 h

$T_{1/2}$: 5.6 to 14 hours; metabolized in the liver and excreted in the urine.

Adverse Effects: Dizziness, vertigo, orthostatic hypotension, nausea, anorexia, vomiting, dry mouth, diarrhea, polyuria, nocturia, muscle cramps, or spasms.

Loop Diuretics

Loop diuretics are so named because they work in the loop of Henle. Loop diuretics are also referred to as **high-ceiling diuretics** because they cause a greater degree of diuresis than other diuretics. Four loop diuretics are available: Ethacrynic acid (*Edecrin*), the first loop diuretic introduced; bumetanide (generic); furosemide (*Lasix*), the most commonly used loop diuretic; and torsemide (*Demadex*).

FOCUS ON Safe Medication Administration

Name confusion has been reported between furosemide and torsemide; the dose and strength of effect of these two drugs are very different. Use extreme caution to make sure you are using the prescribed drug and dose.

Therapeutic Actions and Indications

Loop diuretics block the chloride pump in the ascending loop of Henle, where normally 30% of all filtered sodium is reabsorbed. This action decreases the reabsorption of sodium and chloride. The loop diuretics have a similar effect in the descending loop of Henle and in the distal convoluted tubule, resulting in the production of a copious amount of sodium-rich urine. These drugs work even in the presence of acid–base disturbances, renal failure, electrolyte imbalances, or nitrogen retention.

Because they can produce a loss of fluid of up to 20 pounds/day, loop diuretics are the drugs of choice when a rapid and extensive diuresis is needed. In cases of severe edema or acute pulmonary edema, it is important to remember that these drugs can have an effect only on the blood that reaches the nephrons. If a person is not able to perfuse the kidney because of HF or vascular disease, these drugs will not have an effect. A rapid diuresis occurs, producing a more hypertonic intravascular fluid. In pulmonary edema, this fluid then circulates back to the lungs, pulls fluid out of the interstitial spaces by its oncotic pull, and delivers this fluid to the kidneys, where the water is pulled out, completing the cycle. In the treatment of pulmonary edema, it can sometimes take hours to move all of the fluid out of the lungs because the fluid must be pulled out of the interstitial spaces in the lungs before it can be circulated to the kidneys for removal. Remembering how the drugs work and the way in which fluid moves in the vascular system will make it easier to understand the effects to anticipate.

Loop diuretics are commonly indicated for the treatment of acute HF, acute pulmonary edema, edema associated with HF or with renal or liver disease, and hypertension. See Table 51.1 for Usual Indications for each of these agents. Furosemide is less powerful than bumetanide and torsemide, and therefore has a larger margin of safety for home use.

See the Critical Thinking Scenario for additional information about using furosemide in HF.

Ethacrynic acid is used less frequently in the clinical setting because of the improved potency and reliability of the newer drugs.

Box 51.2 describes nesiritide, a recombinant form of natriuretic peptide, a natural diuretic agent that can cause diuresis, which was approved in 2001 for the treatment of HF.

BOX 51.2

Hormone-like Treatment for Heart Failure

The U.S. Food and Drug Administration has approved nesiritide (*Natrecor*), a recombinant form of natriuretic peptide. This drug acts like natriuretic hormone, a natural substance probably produced by the hypothalamus, which causes a decrease in sodium reabsorption from the distal renal tubules with a resultant dilute urine or increased volume. Natriuretic hormone is normally released in response to fluid overload or hemodilution. In studies, this drug was effective in the treatment of HF, reducing volume and cardiac workload.

Nesiritide is given as an IV bolus of 2 mcg/kg followed by a continuous infusion of 0.01 mcg/kg/min for up to 48 hours. It is approved for the treatment of patients with acutely decompensated HF who have dyspnea at rest or with minimal activity. After therapy with nesiritide, patients reported increased activity tolerance and easier breathing at rest.

Pharmacokinetics

Loop diuretics are available for oral or IV use. Furosemide may also be given IM. They reach peak levels in 60 to 120 minutes (orally) or 30 minutes (parenterally) and are metabolized with a half-life of 30 to 60 minutes and excreted primarily through urine.

Contraindications and Cautions

Among the contraindications to these drugs are allergy to a loop diuretic *to prevent hypersensitivity reactions*; electrolyte depletion, *which could be aggravated by the electrolyte effects of these drugs*; anuria—severe renal failure, *which may prevent the diuretic from working or precipitate a crisis stage due to the blood flow changes brought about by the diuretic*; and hepatic coma, *which could be exacerbated by the fluid shifts associated with drug use. Routine use during pregnancy is not appropriate*; these drugs should be reserved for situations in which the mother has pathological reasons for use, not pregnancy manifestations or complications, and only if the benefit to the mother clearly outweighs the risk to the fetus.

CRITICAL THINKING SCENARIO

Using Furosemide (*Lasix*) in Heart Failure

THE SITUATION

M.R. is a 68-year-old woman with rheumatic mitral valve heart disease. She has refused any surgical intervention and has developed progressively worsening HF. Recently furosemide (*Lasix*), 40 mg/d PO, was prescribed for her along with digoxin. After 10 d with the new prescription, M.R. calls to tell you that she is allergic to the new medicine and cannot take it anymore. She reports extensive ankle swelling and difficulty breathing. You refer her to a cardiologist for immediate review.

CRITICAL THINKING

Think about the physiology of mitral valve disease and the progression of HF in this patient. How does furosemide work in the body?

What additional activities will be important to help maintain some balance in this patient's cardiac status?

What is the nature of M.R.'s reported allergy, and what other options could be tried?

DISCUSSION

Over time, an incompetent mitral valve leads to an enlarged and overworked left ventricle as the backup of blood "waiting to be pumped" continues to progress. Drug therapy for a patient with this disorder is usually aimed at decreasing the workload of the heart as much as possible to maintain cardiac output. Digoxin increases the contractility of the heart muscle, which should lead to better perfusion of the kidneys. Furosemide—a loop diuretic—acts on the loop of Henle to block the reabsorption of sodium and water and lead to a diuresis, which decreases the volume of blood the heart needs to pump and makes the blood that is pumped more efficient. This blood then has an oncotic pull to move fluid from the tissue into circulation, where it can be acted on by the kidneys, leading to further diuresis.

M.R. should be encouraged to maintain fluid intake and to engage in activity as much as possible but to take frequent rest periods. Her potassium level should be monitored regularly (this is especially important because she is also taking digoxin, which is very sensitive to potassium levels), her edematous limbs should be elevated periodically during the day, and she should monitor her sodium intake.

When M.R. was questioned about her reported allergy, it was discovered that her "allergic reaction" was actually increased urination (a therapeutic effect). M.R. needs to learn about the actions of the drug. She also needs information about the timing of administration so that the resultant diuresis will not interfere with rest or with her daily activities. HF is a progressive, incurable disease, so patient education is a very important part of the overall management regimen.

NURSING CARE GUIDE FOR M.R.: DIURETIC AGENTS

Assessment: History and Examination

Assess M.R.'s health history, including allergies to diuretics, fluid or electrolyte disturbances, gout, glucose tolerance abnormalities, liver disease, systemic lupus erythematosus, pregnancy, and breastfeeding.

Focus the physical examination on the following areas:

Neurological: Orientation, reflexes, strength
Skin: color, texture, edema
CV: Blood pressure, pulse, cardiac auscultation
GI: Liver evaluation
Genitourinary (GU): Urinary output

Using Furosemide (*Lasix*) in Heart Failure (continued)

Laboratory tests: Hematology; serum electrolytes, glucose, uric acid; liver function tests

Nursing Diagnoses

Risk for deficient fluid volume related to diuretic effect
Impaired urinary elimination
Imbalanced nutrition: Less than body requirements related to GI upset and metabolic changes
Deficient knowledge regarding drug therapy

Planning

The patient will receive the best therapeutic effect from the drug therapy.
The patient will have limited adverse effects to the drug therapy.
The patient will have an understanding of the drug therapy, adverse effects to anticipate, and measures to relieve discomfort and improve safety.

Implementation

Obtain daily weight, and monitor urine output.
Provide comfort and safety measures: Sugarless lozenges, mouth care, safety precautions, skin care, nutrition.
Administer the drug with food early in the day.
Provide support and reassurance to deal with drug effects and lifestyle changes.
Provide patient teaching regarding drug name, dosage, side effects, precautions, warnings to report, daily weighing, and recording dietary changes as needed.

Evaluation

Evaluate drug effects: Urinary output, weight changes, status of edema, blood pressure changes.
Monitor for adverse effects: Hypotension, hypokalemia, hyperkalemia, hypocalcemia, hypercalcemia, hyperglycemia, increased uric acid levels.
Monitor for drug–drug interactions as indicated.
Evaluate the effectiveness of the patient-teaching program and comfort and safety measures.

PATIENT TEACHING FOR M.R.

- A diuretic, or "water pill," such as furosemide (*Lasix*), will help to reduce the amount of fluid that is in your body by causing the kidneys to pass larger amounts of water and salt into your urine. By removing this fluid the diuretic helps to decrease the work of the heart, lower blood pressure, and get rid of edema, or swelling in your tissues.
- This drug can be taken with food, which may eliminate possible stomach upset. When taking a diuretic, you should maintain your usual fluid intake and try to avoid excessive intake of salt.
- Furosemide is a diuretic that causes potassium loss, so you should eat foods that are high in potassium (e.g., orange juice, raisins, bananas).
- Weigh yourself each day, at the same time of day and in the same clothing. Record these weights on a calendar. Report any loss or gain of 3 pounds or more in 1 day.
- Common effects of this drug include the following:
  - *Increased volume and frequency of urination:* Have ready access to bathroom facilities. Once you are used to the drug, you will know how long the effects last for you.
  - *Dizziness, feeling faint on arising, drowsiness:* Loss of fluid can lower blood pressure and cause these feelings. Change positions slowly; if you feel drowsy, avoid driving or other dangerous activities. These feelings are often increased if alcohol is consumed; avoid this combination or take special precautions if you combine them.
  - *Increased thirst:* As fluid is lost, you may experience a feeling of thirst. Sucking on sugarless lozenges and frequent mouth care might help to alleviate this feeling. Do not drink an excessive amount of fluid while taking a diuretic. Try to maintain your usual fluid intake.
  - Report any of the following to your health care provider: Muscle cramps or pain, loss or gain of more than 3 pounds in 1 day, swelling in your fingers or ankles, nausea or vomiting, unusual bleeding or bruising, trembling or weakness.
- Avoid the use of any over-the-counter (OTC) medication without first checking with your health care provider. Several OTC medications can interfere with the effectiveness of this drug.
- Tell any doctor, nurse, or other health care provider involved in your care that you are taking this drug.
- Keep this drug, and all medications, out of the reach of children.

Caution should be used with the following conditions: SLE, *which frequently causes glomerular changes and renal dysfunction that could precipitate renal failure in some cases*; glucose tolerance abnormalities or diabetes mellitus, *which is worsened by the glucose-elevating effects of many diuretics*; and gout, *which reflects an abnormality in normal tubule reabsorption and secretion.*

Safety for use in children younger than 18 years of age has not been established. If one of these drugs is used for a child, careful monitoring of the child's fluid and electrolyte balance is needed, and emergency support measures should be on standby.

Adverse Effects

Adverse effects are related to the imbalance in electrolytes and fluid that these drugs cause. Hypokalemia is a very common adverse effect because potassium is lost when the transport systems in the tubule try to save some of the sodium being lost. **Alkalosis**, or a rise in serum pH to an alkaline state, may occur as bicarbonate is lost in the urine. Calcium is also lost in the tubules along with the bicarbonate, which may result in hypocalcemia and tetany. The rapid loss of fluid can result in hypotension and dizziness if it causes a rapid imbalance in fluid levels. Long-term use of these drugs may also result in hyperglycemia because of the diuretic effect on blood glucose levels, so susceptible patients need to be monitored for this effect. Ototoxicity and even deafness have been reported with these drugs, but the loss of hearing is usually reversible after the drug is stopped. This may be an effect of electrolyte changes on the conduction of fragile nerves in the central nervous system.

Clinically Important Drug–Drug Interactions

The risk of ototoxicity increases if loop diuretics are combined with aminoglycosides or cisplatin. Anticoagulation effects may increase if these drugs are given with anticoagulants. There may also be a decreased loss of sodium and decreased antihypertensive effects if these drugs are combined with indomethacin, ibuprofen, salicylates, or other nonsteroidal anti-inflammatory agents; a patient receiving this combination should be monitored closely, and appropriate dose adjustments should be made.

Prototype Summary: Furosemide

Indications: Treatment of edema associated with HF, acute pulmonary edema, hypertension.

Actions: Inhibits the reabsorption of sodium and chloride from the distal renal tubules and the loop of Henle, leading to a sodium-rich diuresis.

Pharmacokinetics:

Route	Onset	Peak	Duration
Oral	60 min	60–120 min	6–8 h
IV, IM	5 min	30 min	2 h

$T_{1/2}$: 120 minutes; metabolized in the liver and excreted in the urine.

Adverse Effects: Dizziness, vertigo, paresthesias, orthostatic hypotension, rash, urticaria, nausea, anorexia, vomiting, glycosuria, urinary bladder spasm.

Carbonic Anhydrase Inhibitors

The carbonic anhydrase inhibitors are relatively mild diuretics. Available agents include acetazolamide (*Diamox*) and methazolamide (generic).

FOCUS ON Safe Medication Administration

Name confusion has occurred between acetazolamide and acetohexamide—an antidiabetic agent. Use caution if either of these drugs is prescribed for your patient; make sure that the diagnosis and the treatment are appropriate.

Therapeutic Actions and Indications

The enzyme carbonic anhydrase is a catalyst for the formation of sodium bicarbonate, which is stored as the alkaline reserve in the renal tubule, and for the excretion of hydrogen, which results in a slightly acidic urine. Diuretics that block the effects of carbonic anhydrase slow down the movement of hydrogen ions; as a result, more sodium and bicarbonate are lost in the urine. These drugs are used as adjuncts to other diuretics when a more intense diuresis is needed. Most often, carbonic anhydrase inhibitors are used to treat glaucoma because the inhibition of carbonic anhydrase results in decreased secretion of aqueous humor of the eye. See Table 51.2 for Usual Indications for each of these agents.

Pharmacokinetics

These drugs are rapidly absorbed and widely distributed. Acetazolamide is available orally and for IV use. These drugs peak in 2 to 4 hours (15 minutes if given IV) and have a 6- to 12-hour duration. They are excreted in urine. Some of these agents have been associated with fetal abnormalities, and they should not be used during pregnancy. Because of the potential for adverse effects on the baby, another method of feeding the infant should be used if one of these drugs is needed during lactation.

Contraindications and Cautions

Carbonic anhydrase inhibitors are contraindicated in patients with allergy to the drug or to antibacterial sulfonamides or thiazides *to prevent hypersensitivity reactions*, or in patients with chronic noncongestive angle-closure glaucoma, *which would not be effectively treated by these drugs*. Routine use during pregnancy is not appropriate; these drugs should be reserved for situations in which the mother has pathological reasons for use, not pregnancy manifestations or complications, and only if the benefit to the mother clearly outweighs the risk to the fetus.

Cautious use is recommended in patients who have fluid or electrolyte imbalances, renal or hepatic disease, adrenocortical insufficiency, respiratory acidosis, or chronic obstructive pulmonary disease, *which could be exacerbated by the fluid and electrolyte changes caused by these drugs.*

Adverse Effects

Adverse effects of carbonic anhydrase inhibitors are related to the disturbances in acid–base and electrolyte balances. Metabolic acidosis is a relatively common and potentially dangerous effect that occurs when bicarbonate is lost. Hypokalemia is also common because potassium excretion is increased as the tubule loses potassium in an attempt to retain some of the sodium that is being excreted. Patients also complain of paresthesias (tingling) of the extremities, confusion, and drowsiness, all of which are probably related to the neural effect of the electrolyte changes.

Clinically Important Drug–Drug Interactions

There may be an increased excretion of salicylates and lithium if they are combined with these drugs. Caution should be used to monitor serum levels of patients taking lithium.

Ⓟ Prototype Summary: Acetazolamide

Indications: Adjunctive treatment of open-angle glaucoma, secondary glaucoma; preoperative use in acute angle-closure glaucoma when delay of surgery is indicated; edema caused by heart failure; and drug-induced edema.

Actions: Inhibits carbonic anhydrase, which decreases aqueous humor formation in the eye, IOP, and hydrogen secretion by the renal tubules.

Pharmacokinetics:

Route	Onset	Peak	Duration
Oral	1 h	2–4 h	6–12 h
Sustained release oral	2 h	8–12 h	18–24 h
IV	1–2 min	15–18 min	4–5 h

$T_{1/2}$: 5 to 6 hours; excreted unchanged in the urine.

Adverse Effects: Weakness, fatigue, rash, anorexia, nausea, urinary frequency, renal calculi, bone marrow suppression, weight loss.

Potassium-Sparing Diuretics

The potassium-sparing diuretics are not as powerful as the loop diuretics, but they retain potassium instead of wasting it. Drugs include amiloride (*Midamor*), spironolactone (*Aldactone*), and triamterene (*Dyrenium*). These diuretics are used for patients who are at high risk for hypokalemia associated with diuretic use (e.g., patients receiving digitalis or patients with cardiac arrhythmias).

Therapeutic Actions and Indications

Potassium-sparing diuretics cause a loss of sodium while promoting the retention of potassium. Spironolactone acts as an aldosterone antagonist, blocking the actions of aldosterone in the distal tubule. Amiloride and triamterene block potassium secretion through the tubule. The diuretic effect of these drugs comes from the balance achieved in losing sodium to offset the potassium retained.

Potassium-sparing diuretics are often used as adjuncts with thiazide or loop diuretics or in patients who are especially at risk if hypokalemia develops, such as patients taking certain antiarrhythmics or digoxin and those who have particular neurological conditions. Spironolactone, the most frequently prescribed of these drugs, is the drug of choice for treating **hyperaldosteronism**, a condition seen in cirrhosis of the liver and nephrotic syndrome (see Table 51.2).

Pharmacokinetics

These drugs are well absorbed after oral administration, are protein bound, and are widely distributed. They are metabolized in the liver and primarily excreted in the urine. These diuretics cross the placenta and enter breast milk. Spironolactone has a slow onset of action, 24 to 48 hours, reaches peak effects in 48 to 72 hours, and has a duration of effect of 72 hours. Amiloride and triamterene reach peak effects in 6 to 10 hours and have a duration of effect of 16 to 24 hours.

Contraindications and Cautions

These drugs are contraindicated for use in patients with allergy to the drug *to prevent hypersensitivity reactions*, and hyperkalemia, renal disease, or anuria, *which could be exacerbated by the effects of these drugs. Routine use during pregnancy is not appropriate*; these drugs should be reserved for situations in which the mother has pathological reasons for use, not pregnancy manifestations or complications, and only if the benefit to the mother clearly outweighs the risk to the fetus.

Adverse Effects

The most common adverse effect of potassium-sparing diuretics is hyperkalemia, which can cause lethargy, confusion, ataxia, muscle cramps, and cardiac arrhythmias. Patients taking these drugs need to be evaluated regularly for signs of increased potassium and informed about the signs and symptoms to watch for. They also should be advised to avoid foods that are high in potassium (Box 51.3). Because these drugs work much like aldosterone, they are associated with various androgen (another similar hormone) effects such as hirsutism, gynecomastia, deepening of the voice, and irregular menses.

BOX 51.3

Potassium-Rich Foods

Avocados	Bananas	Broccoli	Cantaloupe	Dried fruits
Grapefruit	Lima beans	Nuts	Navy beans	Oranges
Peaches	Potatoes	Prunes	Rhubarb	*Sanka* coffee
Sunflower seeds	Spinach	Tomatoes	Watermelon	

Clinically Important Drug–Drug Interactions

The diuretic effect decreases if potassium-sparing diuretics are combined with salicylates. Dose adjustment may be necessary to achieve therapeutic effects.

Prototype Summary: Spironolactone

Indications: Primary hyperaldosteronism, adjunctive therapy in the treatment of edema associated with HF, nephrotic syndrome, hepatic cirrhosis; treatment of hypokalemia or prevention of hypokalemia in patients at high risk if hypokalemia occurs; essential hypertension.

Actions: Competitively blocks the effects of aldosterone in the renal tubule, causing loss of sodium and water and retention of potassium.

Pharmacokinetics:

Route	Onset	Peak	Duration
Oral	24–48 h	48–72 h	48–72 h

$T_{1/2}$: 20 hours; metabolized in the liver and excreted in the urine.

Adverse Effects: Dizziness, headache, drowsiness, rash, cramping, diarrhea, hyperkalemia, hirsutism, gynecomastia, deepening of the voice, irregular menses.

Osmotic Diuretics

Osmotic diuretics pull water into the renal tubule without sodium loss. Currently, only one osmotic diuretic is available, mannitol (*Osmitrol*).

Therapeutic Actions and Indications

Some nonelectrolytes are used IV to increase the volume of fluid produced by the kidneys. Mannitol is a sugar that is not well reabsorbed by the tubules; it acts to pull large amounts of fluid into the urine due to the **osmotic pull** exerted by the large sugar molecule. Because the tubule is not able to reabsorb all of the sugar pulled into it, large amounts of fluid are lost in the urine. The effects of this osmotic drug are not limited to the kidneys because the injected substance pulls fluid into the vascular system from extravascular spaces, including the aqueous humor. Therefore, mannitol is often used in acute situations when it is necessary to decrease IOP before eye surgery or during acute attacks of glaucoma. It is also the diuretic of choice in cases of increased cranial pressure or acute renal failure due to shock, drug overdose, or trauma. See Table 51.2 for Usual Indications for mannitol.

Pharmacokinetics

Mannitol is only available for IV use. It is freely filtered at the renal glomerulus, poorly reabsorbed by the renal tubule, not secreted by the tubule, and resistant to metabolism. Action depends on the concentration of osmotic activity in the solution. It is not known whether this drug can cause fetal harm. In addition, the effects during lactation are not well understood.

Contraindications and Cautions

Mannitol is contraindicated in patients with renal disease and anuria from severe renal disease, pulmonary congestion, intracranial bleeding, dehydration, and HF, *which could be exacerbated by the large shifts in fluid related to use of these drugs. Routine use during pregnancy is not appropriate*; it should be reserved for situations in which the mother has pathological reasons for use, not pregnancy manifestations or complications, and only if the benefit to the mother clearly outweighs the risk to the fetus.

Adverse Effects

The most common and potentially dangerous adverse effect related to an osmotic diuretic is the sudden drop in fluid levels. Nausea, vomiting, hypotension, light-headedness, confusion, and headache can be accompanied by cardiac decompensation and even shock. Patients receiving mannitol should be closely monitored for fluid and electrolyte imbalance.

Prototype Summary: Mannitol

Indications: Prevention and treatment of the oliguric phase of renal failure; reduction of intracranial pressure and treatment of cerebral edema; reduction of elevated IOP; promotion of urinary excretion of toxic substances; diagnostic use for measurement of glomerular filtration rate; also available as an irrigant in transurethral prostatic resection and other transurethral procedures.

Actions: Elevates the osmolarity of the glomerular filtrate, leading to a loss of water, sodium, and chloride; creates an osmotic gradient in the eye, reducing IOP; creates an osmotic effect that decreases swelling after transurethral surgery.

Pharmacokinetics:

Route	Onset	Peak	Duration
IV	30–60 min	1 h	6–8 h
Irrigant	Rapid	Rapid	Short

$T_{1/2}$: 15 to 100 minutes; excreted unchanged in the urine.

Adverse Effects: Dizziness, headache, hypotension, rash, nausea, anorexia, dry mouth, thirst, diuresis, fluid and electrolyte imbalances.

Nursing Considerations for Patients Receiving Diuretics

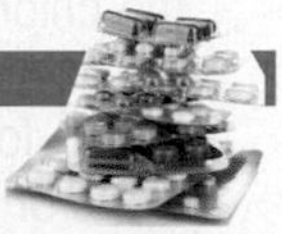

Assessment: History and Examination

- Assess for contraindication or cautions: Any known allergies to thiazides or sulfonamides *to prevent hypersensitivity reactions*; fluid or electrolyte disturbances, *which could be exacerbated by the diuretic or render the diuretic ineffective*; gout, *which reflects an abnormal tubule function and could be worsened by the diuretic or reflect a condition that would render the diuretic ineffective*; glucose tolerance abnormalities, *which may be exacerbated by the glucose-elevating effects*; liver disease, *which could alter the metabolism of the drug, leading to toxic levels*; systemic lupus erythematosus, *which frequently affects the glomerulus and could be exacerbated by the use of a thiazide or thiazide-like diuretic*; hyperparathyroidism and bipolar disorder, *which could be exacerbated due to increased serum concentrations of calcium*; and current status of pregnancy or lactation *because of the potential for adverse effects on the fetus or baby*.
- Perform a physical assessment *to establish baseline data before beginning therapy, to determine the effectiveness of therapy, and to evaluate for occurrence of any adverse effects associated with drug therapy*.
- Inspect the skin carefully for signs and symptoms of edema; note the extent and degree of edema, including evidence of pitting, *to provide a baseline as a reference for drug effectiveness*; check skin turgor *to determine hydration status*.
- Assess cardiopulmonary status, including blood pressure and pulse, and auscultate heart and lung sounds for abnormalities *to evaluate fluid movement and state of hydration and monitor the effects on the heart and lungs*.
- Obtain an accurate body weight *to provide a baseline to monitor fluid balance*.
- Monitor intake and output and assess voiding patterns *to evaluate fluid balance and renal function*.
- Evaluate liver status *to determine potential problems in drug metabolism*.
- Monitor the results of laboratory tests, including serum electrolyte levels, especially potassium and calcium, uric acid, and glucose levels, *to determine the drug's effect*, and renal and liver function tests *to identify the need for possible dose adjustment and toxic effects*.

Nursing Diagnoses

Nursing diagnoses related to drug therapy may include the following:

- Risk for deficient fluid volume related to drug effect
- Impaired urinary elimination related to drug effect
- Imbalanced nutrition: Less than body requirements related to GI upset and metabolic changes
- Risk for injury related to changes in fluid volume and electrolyte balance secondary to drug effects
- Deficient knowledge regarding drug therapy

Planning

- The patient will receive the best therapeutic effect from the drug therapy.
- The patient will have limited adverse effects to the drug therapy.
- The patient will have an understanding of the drug therapy, adverse effects to anticipate, and measures to relieve discomfort and improve safety

Implementation with Rationale

- Administer oral drug with food or milk *to buffer the drug effect on the stomach lining if GI upset is a problem*.
- Administer IV diuretics slowly *to prevent severe changes in fluid and electrolytes*.
- Continuously monitor urinary output, cardiac response, and heart rhythm of patients receiving IV diuretics *to monitor for rapid fluid switch and potential electrolyte disturbances leading to cardiac arrhythmia*. Switch to the oral form, *which is less potent and easier to monitor*, as soon as possible, as appropriate.
- Administer oral form early in the day *so that increased urination will not interfere with sleep*.
- Monitor the dose carefully and reduce the dose of one or both drugs if given with antihypertensive agents; *loss of fluid volume can precipitate hypotension*.
- Monitor the patient response to the drug (e.g., blood pressure, urinary output, weight, serum electrolytes, hydration, periodic blood glucose monitoring) *to evaluate the effectiveness of the drug and monitor for adverse effects*.
- Assess weight daily *to evaluate fluid balance*.
- Check skin turgor *to evaluate for possible fluid volume deficit*, and assess edematous areas for changes, including a decrease in amount or degree of pitting.

(continues on page 896)

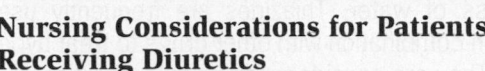

- Provide comfort measures, including skin care and nutrition consultation, *to increase compliance with drug therapy and decrease the severity of adverse effects*; provide safety measures if dizziness and weakness are a problem *to prevent injury.*
- Provide a potassium-rich or low-potassium diet as appropriate *to maintain electrolyte balance and replace lost potassium or prevent hyperkalemia.*
- Provide thorough patient teaching, including the name of the drug and dosage prescribed, *to enhance patient knowledge about drug therapy and to promote compliance.* Additional patient teaching includes the following:
  - Importance of taking the diuretic early in the day to avoid interference with sleep.
  - Administration of the drug with food or meals if GI upset occurs.
  - Need to weigh oneself daily and report any increase in weight of 3 pounds or more in 1 day.
  - Importance of maintaining an adequate fluid intake to prevent **fluid rebound** (see Focus on Safe Medication Administration in this chapter's introduction to diuretic agents).
  - Need to have readily available access to bathroom facilities after taking the prescribed dose.
  - Signs and symptoms of adverse effects, including hypokalemia, hyperkalemia, and hypercalcemia, and the need to notify the health care provider should any occur.
  - Danger signs and symptoms to report immediately.
  - Safety measures, such as moving slowly if dizziness is an issue and avoiding very hot environments and other situations potentially leading to extra loss of fluid.
  - Dietary sources of foods high in potassium, with an emphasis on the need for intake of these foods or the need to avoid these foods if using a potassium-sparing diuretic.
  - Need for compliance with therapy to achieve intended results.
  - Importance of continued follow-up and monitoring, including laboratory testing to determine the effectiveness of therapy.

Evaluation

- Monitor patient response to the drug (weight, urinary output, edema changes, blood pressure).
- Monitor for adverse effects (electrolyte imbalance, orthostatic hypotension, rebound edema, hyperglycemia, increased uric acid levels, acid–base disturbances, dizziness).
- Monitor the effectiveness of comfort measures and compliance with the regimen.
- Evaluate the effectiveness of the teaching plan (patient can name drug, dosage, adverse effects to watch for, and specific measures to avoid them).

SUMMARY

- Diuretics—drugs that increase the excretion of sodium, and therefore water, from the kidneys—are used in the treatment of edema associated with HF and pulmonary edema, liver failure and cirrhosis, and various types of renal disease, and as adjuncts in the treatment of hypertension.
- Classes of diuretics differ in their site of action and intensity of effects. Thiazide diuretics work to block the chloride pump in the distal convoluted tubule. This effect leads to a loss of sodium and potassium and a minor loss of water. Thiazides are frequently used alone or in combination with other drugs to treat hypertension. They are considered to be mild diuretics.
- Loop diuretics work in the loop of Henle and have a powerful diuretic effect, leading to the loss of water, sodium, and potassium. These drugs are the most potent diuretics and are used in acute situations, as well as in chronic conditions not responsive to milder diuretics.
- Carbonic anhydrase inhibitors work to block the formation of carbonic acid and bicarbonate in the renal tubule. These drugs can cause an alkaline urine and loss of the bicarbonate buffer. Carbonic anhydrase inhibitors are used in combination with other diuretics when a stronger diuresis is needed, and they are frequently used to treat glaucoma because they decrease the amount of aqueous humor produced in the eye.
- Potassium-sparing diuretics are mild diuretics that act to spare potassium in exchange for the loss of sodium and water in the urine. These diuretics are preferable if potassium loss could be detrimental to a patient's cardiac or neuromuscular condition. Patients must be careful not to become hyperkalemic while taking these drugs.
- The osmotic diuretic mannitol uses hypertonic pull to remove fluid from the intravascular spaces and to deliver large amounts of water into the renal tubule. There is a danger of sudden change of fluid volume and massive fluid loss with this drug. This drug is used to decrease intracranial pressure, to treat glaucoma, and to help push toxic substances through the kidneys.

CHECK YOUR UNDERSTANDING

Answers to the questions in this chapter can be found in Answers to Check Your Understanding Questions on thePoint®.

MULTIPLE CHOICE

Select the best answer to the following.

1. Most diuretics act in the body to cause
   a. loss of calcium.
   b. loss of sodium.
   c. retention of potassium.
   d. retention of chloride.

2. Diuretics cause a loss of fluid volume in the body. The drop in volume activates compensatory mechanisms to restore the volume, including
   a. suppression of ADH release and stimulation of the countercurrent mechanism.
   b. suppression of aldosterone release and increased ADH release.
   c. activation of the renin–angiotensin–aldosterone system with increased ADH and aldosterone.
   d. stimulation of the countercurrent mechanism with reflex drop in renin release.

3. Thiazide diuretics are considered mild diuretics because
   a. they block the sodium pump in the loop of Henle.
   b. they cause loss of sodium and chloride but little water.
   c. they do not cause fluid rebound when they work in the kidneys.
   d. they have little or no effect on electrolyte levels.

4. The nurse would anticipate an order for a loop diuretic as the drug of choice for a patient with
   a. hypertension.
   b. shock.
   c. pulmonary edema.
   d. fluid retention of pregnancy.

5. When providing care to a patient who is receiving a loop diuretic the nurse would determine the need to regularly monitor which of the following?
   a. Sodium levels
   b. Bone marrow function
   c. Calcium levels
   d. Potassium levels

6. When developing the plan of care for a patient with hyperaldosteronism the nurse would expect the physician to prescribe which agent?
   a. Spironolactone
   b. Furosemide
   c. Hydrochlorothiazide
   d. Acetazolamide

7. A patient with severe glaucoma who is about to undergo eye surgery would benefit from a decrease in intraocular fluid. This is often best accomplished by giving the patient
   a. a loop diuretic.
   b. a thiazide diuretic.
   c. a carbonic anhydrase inhibitor.
   d. an osmotic diuretic.

8. The nurse would instruct a patient receiving a loop diuretic to report
   a. yellow vision.
   b. weight loss of 1 pound/day.
   c. muscle cramping.
   d. increased urination.

MULTIPLE RESPONSE

Select all that apply.

1. Diuretics are currently recommended for the treatment of which of the following?
   a. Hypertension
   b. Renal disease
   c. Obesity
   d. Severe liver disease
   e. Fluid retention of pregnancy
   f. Heart failure

2. Routine nursing care of a client receiving a diuretic would include which of the following?
   a. Daily weighing
   b. Tight fluid restrictions
   c. Periodic electrolyte evaluations
   d. Monitoring of urinary output
   e. Regular IOP testing
   f. Teaching the patient to report muscle cramping

BIBLIOGRAPHY AND REFERENCES

Brunton, L., Chabner, B., & Knollman, B. (2011). *Goodman and Gilman's the pharmacological basis of therapeutics* (12th ed.). New York: McGraw-Hill.

Einhorn, P. T., Davis, B. R., Wright, J. T., et al. (2010). ALLHAT: Still providing correct answers after 7 years. *Current Opinion in Cardiology, 25*, 355–365.

Facts and Comparisons. (2015). *Drug facts and comparisons*. St. Louis, MO: Author.

Facts and Comparisons. (2015). *Professional's guide to patient drug facts*. St. Louis, MO: Author.

Fuster, V., Alexander, R. W., & Rourke, R. A. (Eds.). (2011). *Hurst's the heart* (13th ed.). New York: McGraw-Hill.

Karch, A. M. (2014). *Lippincott's nursing drug guide*. Philadelphia, PA: Lippincott Williams & Wilkins.

Peck, P. (2004). More diuretic use correlates with more end stage renal disease. *Family Practice News, 34*(16), 13.

Porth, C. M. (2013). *Pathophysiology: Concepts of altered health states* (9th ed.). Philadelphia, PA: Lippincott Williams & Wilkins.

Shafi, T., Appel, L. J., Miller, E. R., et al. (2008). Changes in serum potassium mediate thiazide-induced diabetes. *Hypertension, 52*, 1002–1029.

Stafford, R. S., Bartholomew, L. K., Cushman, W. C., et al. (2010). Impact of the ALLHAT/JNC7 dissemination project on thiazide-type diuretic use. *Archives of Internal Medicine, 170*, 851–858.

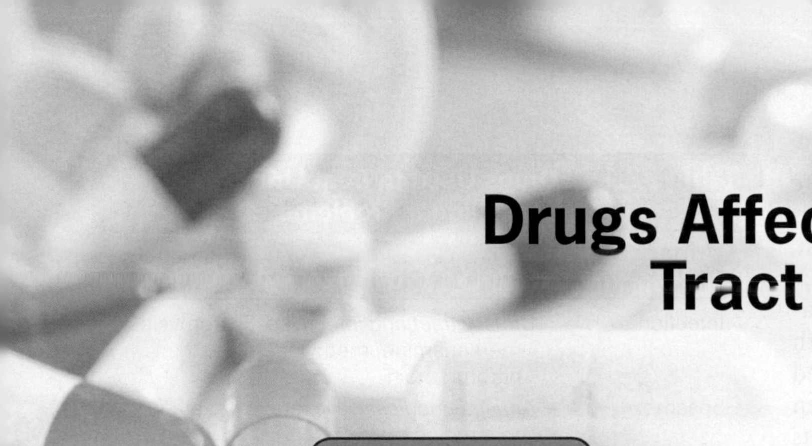

52 Drugs Affecting the Urinary Tract and the Bladder

Learning Objectives

Upon completion of this chapter, you will be able to:

1. Describe four common problems associated with the urinary tract, including the clinical manifestations of these problems.
2. Describe the therapeutic actions, indications, pharmacokinetics, contraindications and cautions, most common adverse reactions, and important drug–drug interactions associated with urinary tract anti-infectives, antispasmodics, and analgesics, bladder protectants, and drugs used to treat benign prostatic hyperplasia (BPH).
3. Discuss the use of drugs affecting the urinary tract and bladder across the lifespan.
4. Compare and contrast the prototype drugs fosfomycin, oxybutynin, and doxazosin with other agents in their class.
5. Outline the nursing considerations, including important teaching points, for patients receiving drugs affecting the urinary tract and bladder.

Glossary of Key Terms

acidification: the process of increasing the acid level; used to treat bladder infections, making the bladder an undesirable place for bacteria

antispasmodics: agents that block muscle spasm associated with irritation or neurological stimulation

benign prostatic hyperplasia (BPH): enlargement of the prostate gland, associated with age and inflammation; also called benign prostatic hypertrophy

cystitis: inflammation of the bladder, caused by infection or irritation

dysuria: painful urination

interstitial cystitis: chronic inflammation of the interstitial connective tissue of the bladder; may extend into deeper tissue

nocturia: getting up to void at night, reflecting increased renal perfusion with fluid shifts in the supine position when a person has gravity-dependent edema related to heart failure; other medical conditions, including urinary tract infection, increase the need to get up and void

pyelonephritis: inflammation of the pelves of the kidney, frequently caused by backward flow problems or by bacteria ascending the ureter

urgency: the feeling that one needs to void immediately; associated with infection and inflammation in the urinary tract

urinary frequency: the need to void often; usually seen in response to irritation of the bladder, age, and inflammation

Drug List

Urinary Tract Anti-infectives
fosfomycin
(P) methenamine
methylene blue
nitrofurantoin

Urinary Tract Antispasmodics

Anticholinergics
darifenacin
fesoterodine
flavoxate
(P) oxybutynin
solifenacin
tolterodine
trospium

Beta agonist
mirabegron

Other Drugs Used That Affect the Urinary Tract and Bladder

Urinary Tract Analgesic
(P) phenazopyridine

Bladder Protectant
(P) pentosan polysulfate sodium

Drugs for Treating Benign Prostatic Hyperplasia

Alpha-Adrenergic Blockers
alfuzosin
doxazosin
(P) silodosin
tamsulosin
terazosin

Drugs That Block Testosterone Production
dutasteride
(P) finasteride

Conditions affecting the urinary tract and bladder are common problems. These conditions include acute urinary tract infections (UTIs), bladder spasms, bladder pain, and benign prostatic hyperplasia (BPH).

Acute UTIs occur second in frequency only to respiratory tract infections in the US population. Females, with shorter urethras, are particularly vulnerable to repeated urinary tract, bladder, and even kidney infections. Children also may have frequent urinary tract problems. Patients with indwelling catheters or intermittent catheterizations often develop bladder infections or **cystitis**, which can result from bacteria introduced into the bladder by these devices. Blockage anywhere in the urinary tract can lead to backflow problems and the spread of bladder infections into the kidney (**pyelonephritis**).

The signs and symptoms of a UTI are uncomfortable and include **urinary frequency**, **urgency**, burning on urination (associated with cystitis), chills, fever, flank pain, and tenderness (associated with acute pyelonephritis), though in older adults the only presentation may be confusion, disorientation and other central nervous system (CNS) effects. To treat these infections, clinicians use specific urinary tract anti-infectives, which include antibiotics, as well as specific agents that reach antibacterial levels only in the kidney and bladder and are thought to sterilize the urinary tract.

Table 52.1 Drugs Used to Treat Urinary Tract and Bladder Problems

Urinary Tract Problem	Drugs of Choice
Infection	*Urinary tract anti-infectives:* Fosfomycin, methenamine, methylene blue, nitrofurantoin
Spasm	*Antispasmodics:* Flavoxate, oxybutynin, tolterodine
Pain	*Urinary tract analgesic:* Phenazopyridine *Bladder protectant for interstitial cystitis:* Pentosan
BPH	*Alpha-adrenergic blockers:* Doxazosin, tamsulosin, terazosin, alfuzosin *Testosterone inhibitors:* Finasteride, dutasteride

BPH, benign prostatic hyperplasia.

Drugs also are available to block spasms of the urinary tract muscles, decrease urinary tract pain, protect the cells of the bladder from irritation, and treat enlargement of the prostate gland in men. Table 52.1 summarizes urinary tract problems and the drugs of choice to treat them. Box 52.1 highlights important considerations related to urinary tract drugs based on the patient's age.

BOX 52.1 FOCUS ON Drug Therapy Across the Lifespan

Urinary Tract Agents

CHILDREN

Children may develop UTIs, including cystitis, and need to be treated with a urinary tract anti-infective. Some children, because of congenital problems or indwelling catheters, require other urinary tract agents such as urinary tract analgesics or antispasmodics. The older anti-infectives—nitrofurantoin and methenamine—have established pediatric guidelines. A child with repeated UTIs should be evaluated for potential sexual abuse.

Children need to be instructed in proper hygiene and should not be given bubble baths if UTIs occur. They should be encouraged to avoid the alkaline ash juices such as orange or grapefruit juice and urged to drink lots of water.

If an antispasmodic is needed, oxybutynin is indicated for children older than 5 years of age, and flavoxate can be used in children older than 12 years of age. Phenazopyridine is indicated as a urinary tract analgesic for children 6 to 12 years of age. The child should be cautioned about the change in urine color that might occur with phenazopyridine because it might be frightening if the child is not expecting it.

ADULTS

Adults need to be cautioned about the various measures that can be used to decrease the likelihood of UTIs. They should be encouraged to drink plenty of fluids to maintain bladder health.

If they are taking an anticholinergic to block spasm, adult patients need to be advised of other precautions to take when the parasympathetic system is blocked.

Adult men being treated for BPH need to be aware of the possibility of decreased sexual function, as well as fatigue, lethargy, and the potential for dizziness, which could interfere with working or activities of daily living.

The use of urinary tract agents during pregnancy should be approached with caution. If an antibiotic is needed the one-dose fosfomycin might be the drug of choice because of the limited exposure to the drug. Women who are nursing should use these agents with caution because of the potential for adverse effects on the baby, or they should find another method of feeding the baby.

OLDER ADULTS

Older adults often have conditions that are treated with the urinary tract agents. They are also more likely to have renal or hepatic impairment, which requires caution in the use of these drugs. Older adults should be started on the lowest possible dose of the drug, and it should be titrated slowly based on patient response. Special precautions to monitor cardiac function, intraocular pressure, blood pressure, and bladder emptying need to be taken when using alpha-adrenergic blockers with these patients. Older patients may have a difficult time maintaining fluid intake and might benefit from extra encouragement to drink fluids, including cranberry juice, and to avoid alkaline ash drinks.

Urinary Tract Anti-Infectives

Urinary tract anti-infectives (Table 52.2) are of two types. One type comprises the antibiotics, which are particularly effective against the gram-negative bacteria that cause most UTIs. The antibiotics used specifically to treat UTIs include fosfomycin (*Monurol*), and nitrofurantoin (*Furadantin*). Ciprofloxacin (*Cipro*) and cotrimoxazole (*Bactrim, Septra*) are also used frequently to treat UTIs but are not specific to UTIs and are also used for treating other infections (see Chapter 9). The other type of urinary tract anti-infective works to acidify the urine, killing bacteria that might be in the bladder. This group includes methenamine (*Hiprex*) and methylene blue (*Urolene Blue*).

Therapeutic Actions and Indications

Urinary tract anti-infectives act specifically within the urinary tract to destroy bacteria, either through a direct antibiotic effect or through **acidification** of the urine. They do not generally have an antibiotic effect systemically, being activated or effective only in the urinary tract (Figure 52.1). Those drugs with an antibiotic effect interfere with reproduction of the gram-negative bacteria and cause bacterial cell death. Those that cause acidification of the urine produce an environment that is not conducive to bacterial survival, leading to bacterial cell death. They are used to treat chronic UTIs, as adjunctive therapy in acute cystitis and pyelonephritis, and as prophylaxis with urinary tract anatomical abnormalities and residual urine disorders. See the Critical Thinking Scenario for additional information regarding teaching the patient about treatment with methenamine for cystitis.

Table 52.2 discusses Usual Indications for each of the urinary tract anti-infectives.

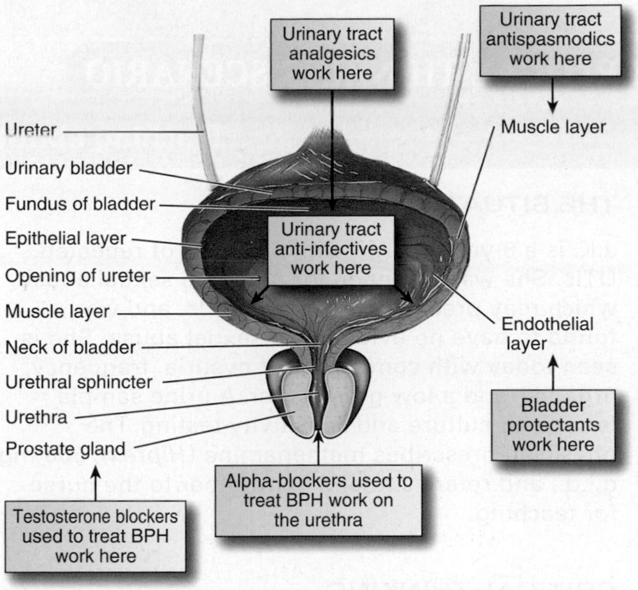

FIGURE 52.1 Sites of action of drugs acting on the urinary tract.

Pharmacokinetics

Fosfomycin, taken orally, has the convenience of only a one-time dose. It is not recommended for children younger than 18 years of age. It is rapidly absorbed, undergoes slow hepatic metabolism, and is excreted in the urine and feces. Unpleasant GI effects limit its usefulness in some patients. The dose does not need to be changed in cases of renal impairment.

Nitrofurantoin is another older drug with a very short half-life (20–60 min). It is not effective against as many gram-negative bacteria as the newer drugs, but it has been successfully used for suppression therapy in adults and children with chronic UTIs. It is well absorbed

Table 52.2 ***Drugs in Focus:* Urinary Tract Anti-Infectives**

Drug Name	Usual Dosage	Usual Indications
fosfomycin (*Monurol*)	One packet (3 g) dissolved in water PO	Treatment of UTIs caused by susceptible bacteria (one-dose drug) in patients >18 y
methenamine (*Hiprex*)	1 g b.i.d. to q.i.d. PO *Pediatric (6–12 y):* 0.5–1 g PO b.i.d. to q.i.d. *Pediatric (<6 y):* 0.25–0.5 mg/kg/d PO in divided doses	Suppression or elimination of bacteriuria associated with UTIs and anatomical abnormalities
methylene blue (*Urolene Blue*)	65–130 mg PO t.i.d.	Suppression or elimination of bacteriuria associated with UTIs and anatomical abnormalities
nitrofurantoin (*Furadantin*)	50–100 mg PO q.i.d. for 10–14 d; 50–100 mg PO at bedtime for chronic suppressive therapy Pediatric: 5–7 mg/kg/d in four divided doses; 1 mg/kg/d PO at bedtime for chronic suppressive therapy	Treatment of UTIs caused by susceptible bacteria

UTI, urinary tract infection.

CRITICAL THINKING SCENARIO

Teaching about Cystitis Treatment

THE SITUATION

J.K. is a 6-year-old girl with a history of repeated UTIs. She was screened for potential sexual abuse, which may present as repeated UTIs, and was found to have no evidence of sexual abuse. She is seen today with complaints of dysuria, frequency, urgency, and a low-grade fever. A urine sample is sent for culture and sensitivity testing. The physician prescribes methenamine (*Hiprex*), 500 mg q.i.d., and refers J.K. and her mother to the nurse for teaching.

CRITICAL THINKING

What is the best approach for this patient?

What key teaching points (at least five) should be emphasized to assist the pharmacological therapy in treating this infection? *Think about the following points: What the drug is doing, how it works, and how it works best.*

DISCUSSION

Cystitis is very difficult to treat in young girls and can become a chronic problem. Patient and parent education is very important for blocking the growth of bacteria and curing the infection. Teaching points should emphasize activities that will decrease the number of bacteria introduced into the bladder, acidify the urine to make the bladder an inhospitable environment for bacterial growth, and flush the bladder to prevent stagnant urine from encouraging bacterial growth.

To decrease the number of bacteria introduced into the bladder, patient education should cover the following hygiene measures: Always wipe from front to back and never from back to front to avoid the introduction of intestinal bacteria into the urethra; avoid baths, particularly bubble baths, which facilitate the entry of bacteria into the urethra on the bubbles; and wear dry, cotton underwear to discourage bacterial growth.

Patient education also should stress the importance of avoiding alkaline ash foods (e.g., citrus fruits, certain vegetables) and antacids and encouraging foods that acidify the urine. Cranberry juice is often recommended as a choice for fruit juice because it helps to prevent the bacteria from adhering to the bladder wall, helping to prevent infection. Fluid intake, especially water, should be encouraged as much as possible to keep the bladder flushed. Finally, the patient should be encouraged to complete the full course of medication prescribed and not to stop taking the drug when symptoms disappear. See Box 52.2, Focus on the Evidence? Cranberry for UTIs?

PATIENT TEACHING FOR J.K.: URINARY TRACT ANTI-INFECTIVE METHENAMINE

Assessment: History and Examination

Assess J.K.'s health history, particularly any allergies to antibacterial medications, and liver or renal dysfunction. (If J.K. were of childbearing age, you would assess pregnancy and breastfeeding status.)

Focus the physical examination on the following areas:

CNS: Orientation, reflexes, strength
Skin: Color, texture, edema
Gastrointestinal (GI): Liver evaluation
Genitourinary (GU): Urinary output
Laboratory tests: Liver function tests, urinalysis, urine culture, and sensitivity testing

Nursing Diagnoses

Acute pain related to GI, CNS, and skin effects of the drug
Disturbed sensory perception related to CNS effects
Deficient knowledge regarding drug therapy

Planning

The patient will receive the best therapeutic effect from the drug therapy.
The patient will have limited adverse effects to the drug therapy.
The patient will have an understanding of the drug therapy, adverse effects to anticipate, and measures to relieve discomfort and improve safety.

Implementation

Obtain urine sample for culture and sensitivity test.
Provide comfort and safety measures: Safety precautions, skin care, nutrition.
Encourage eating acidifying foods and drinking lots of fluids.
Teach hygiene measures.
Administer medication with food if GI upset is a problem.
Provide support and reassurance to deal with drug effects and lifestyle changes.

Teaching about Cystitis Treatment (continued)

Provide patient teaching to J.K. and her parents or caregivers regarding drug name, dosage, adverse effects, precautions, warnings to report, hygiene measures, and dietary changes as needed.

Evaluation

Evaluate drug effects: Relief of symptoms, resolution of infection.

Monitor for adverse effects: GI upset, headache, dizziness, confusion, dysuria, pruritus, urticaria.

Monitor for drug–drug interactions as indicated, especially use of antacids.

Evaluate the effectiveness of patient-teaching program and comfort and safety measures.

PATIENT TEACHING FOR J.K.

- A urinary tract anti-infective such as methenamine treats UTIs by destroying bacteria and by helping to produce an environment that is not conducive to bacterial growth.
- If this drug causes stomach upset, it can be taken with food. It is important to avoid foods that alkalinize the urine, such as citrus fruits and milk, because they decrease the effectiveness of the drug. Cranberry juice is one juice that can be used. As much fluid as possible (eight to ten 8-oz glasses of water a day) should be taken to help flush out the bacteria and treat the infection.
- Avoid using any over-the-counter (OTC) medication that might contain sodium bicarbonate (e.g., antacids, baking soda) because these drugs alkalinize the urine and interfere with the ability of methenamine to treat the infection. If you question the use of any OTC drug, check with your health care provider.
- Take the full course of your prescription. Do not use this drug to self-treat any other infection.
- Common adverse effects of this drug may include the following:
  - Stomach upset, nausea: *Taking the drug with food or eating small, frequent meals may help.*
  - Painful urination: If this occurs, report it to your health care provider. A dose adjustment may be needed.
- Report any of the following to your health care provider: Skin rash or itching, severe GI upset, GI upset that prevents adequate fluid intake, very painful urination (and pregnancy in older female patients).
- The following can help to decrease UTIs:
  - *Avoid bubble baths.*
  - Void whenever you feel the urge; try not to wait.
  - Always wipe from front to back, never from back to front.
  - Limit alkaline ash foods, such as citrus juices, and avoid the use of antacids.
  - Tell any doctor, nurse, or other health care provider involved in your care that you are taking this drug.

BOX 52.2 FOCUS ON The Evidence: Cranberry for UTIs?

Cranberry juice and cranberries have long been accepted as a good choice for treating and preventing UTIs. In the past, it was thought that the compounds in the cranberry caused an acidic urine, and that was what made them effective. Evidence-based research did not support that claim, finding that patients could not consume the amount of juice that would need to be consumed to make the urine acidic enough to kill bacteria. Studies did show, however, that the compounds in cranberries, A-type proanthocyanidins, inhibited the *Escherichia coli* bacteria from adhering to the bladder wall and prevented the infections from occurring. Research studies showed no efficacy in the use of cranberry to treat UTIs. Research studies vary widely, however, on supporting or not supporting the use of cranberry in preventing UTIs. In 2011, a study showed no difference between placebo and cranberry products in UTI prevention (Barbosa-Cesnik et al., 2011). A systemic review published in 2012 showed cranberry products did have a protective role in preventing UTIs, though pointed out problems with some of the trials that were evaluated (Wang et al., 2012). The bottom line is that patients with UTIs should drink fluids, six to eight glasses a day. Alkaline fluids should be avoided, so adding a juice that is not alkaline ash may be a good idea, and that may help the situation. Nurses need to be aware that there is a lot of sugar in regular cranberry juice, so patients who need to limit sugar intake need to be cautious. Many cranberry products are also relatively expensive, a problem that could be an issue for patients on fixed incomes or with other financial issues. An elderly diabetic on a fixed income may not be a candidate and making sure the patient drinks enough water every day may or may not be just as effective. Research continues.

when taken orally, metabolized in the liver, and excreted in the urine. No dose adjustment is needed with renal impairment.

Methenamine, taken orally, is well absorbed, undergoes metabolism in the liver, and is excreted in the urine. Methenamine has established dose guidelines for children and comes in a suspension form.

Methylene blue is well absorbed orally, widely distributed, metabolized in the tissues, and excreted in the urine, bile, and feces.

Nitrofurantoin and methenamine cross the placenta and enter breast milk. Fosfomycin might be the drug of choice for cystitis during pregnancy or lactation because of the short exposure to the drug.

Contraindications and Cautions

These drugs are contraindicated in the presence of any known allergy to any of these drugs *to prevent hypersensitivity reactions*. They should be used with caution in the presence of renal dysfunction, *which could interfere with the excretion and action of these drugs*, and with pregnancy and lactation *because of the potential for adverse effects on the fetus or neonate.*

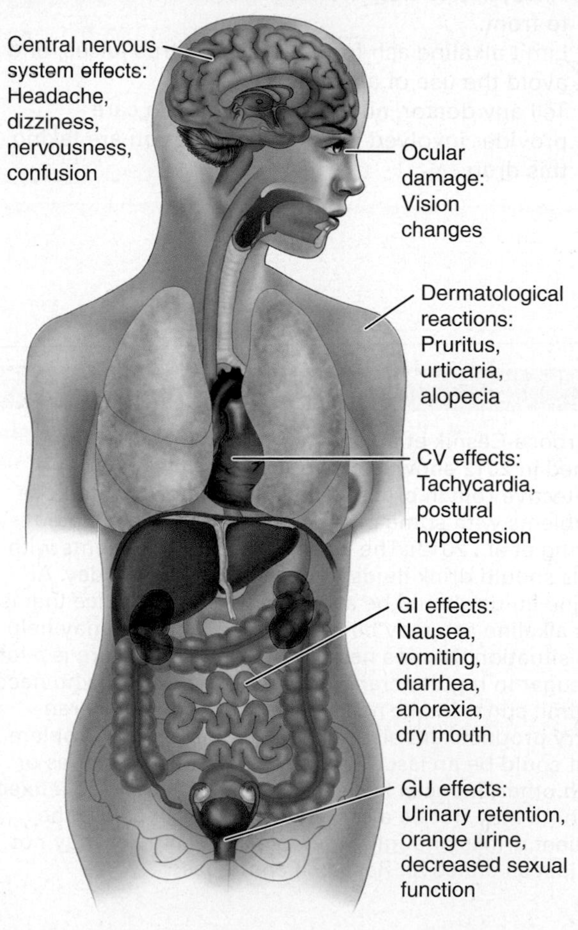

FIGURE 52.2 Variety of adverse effects and toxicities associated with drugs affecting the urinary tract and bladder.

Adverse Effects

Adverse effects associated with these drugs include nausea, vomiting, diarrhea, anorexia, bladder irritation, and dysuria (Figure 52.2). Infrequent symptoms include pruritus, urticaria, headache, dizziness, nervousness, and confusion. These effects may result from GI irritation caused by the agent, which may be somewhat alleviated if the drug is taken with food, or from a systemic reaction to urinary tract irritation. Fosfomycin is associated with unpleasant GI effects, which limit its usefulness in some patients. Methylene blue can stain the skin if it comes in contact with it.

Clinically Important Drug–Drug Interactions

Because these drugs are from several different chemical classes the drug–drug interactions that can occur are very specific to the drug being used. Consult a nursing drug guide for specific interactions.

Prototype Summary: Fosfomycin

Indications: Treatment of women with uncomplicated UTIs caused by susceptible strains of bacteria.

Actions: Interferes with cell wall formation of gram-negative bacteria, leading to cell death.

Pharmacokinetics:

Route	Onset	Peak	Duration
Oral	Varies	2 h	12 h

$T_{1/2}$: 5.7–9.5 hours; excreted unchanged in the urine.

Adverse Effects: Headache, dizziness, nausea, diarrhea, vaginitis.

Nursing Considerations for Patients Receiving Urinary Tract Anti-Infectives

Assessment: History and Examination

- Assess for *contraindications or cautions*: Any history of allergy to antibiotics or anti-infectives *to avoid hypersensitivity reactions*; liver or renal dysfunction *that might interfere with the drug's metabolism and excretion*; and current status of pregnancy and lactation, *which require cautious use of the drug.*
- Perform a physical assessment before therapy *to establish baseline data* and during therapy *to determine the effectiveness of the drug and the occurrence of any adverse effects associated with drug therapy.*
- Inspect the skin *to evaluate for the development of rash or hypersensitivity reactions.*

- Assess level of consciousness and monitor orientation and reflexes *to evaluate any CNS effects of the drug.*
- Assess urinary elimination patterns, including amount and episode frequency, and for complaints of frequency, urgency, pain, or difficulty voiding *to determine the effectiveness of therapy.*
- Monitor laboratory test results, including urinalysis and urine culture and sensitivity, *to evaluate effectiveness and appropriateness of drug choice* and renal and hepatic function tests *to determine the need for possible dose adjustment and to identify possible toxicity.*

Nursing Diagnoses

Nursing diagnoses related to drug therapy might include the following:

- Acute pain related to GI, CNS, or skin effects of drug
- Disturbed sensory perception (kinesthetic, tactile, visual) related to CNS effects
- Impaired urinary elimination related to the underlying problem necessitating drug therapy
- Risk for injury related to possible CNS effects
- Deficient knowledge regarding drug therapy

Planning

- The patient will receive the best therapeutic effect from the drug therapy.
- The patient will have limited adverse effects to the drug therapy.
- The patient will have an understanding of the drug therapy, adverse effects to anticipate, and measures to relieve discomfort and improve safety.

Implementation with Rationale

- Ensure that culture and sensitivity tests are performed before therapy begins and are repeated if the response is not as expected *to ensure appropriate treatment of the infection.*
- Administer the drugs with food *to decrease GI adverse effects if they occur.*
- Institute safety precautions if the patient experiences CNS effects *to prevent patient injury.*
- Advise patients to continue the full course of the drug ordered and not to stop taking it as soon as the uncomfortable signs and symptoms pass *to ensure eradication of the infection and prevent the emergence of resistant strains of bacteria.*
- Encourage the patient to drink lots of fluids (unless contraindicated by other conditions) *to promote flushing of the bladder and prevent urinary stasis* and to avoid citrus juices and antacids, *which promote an alkaline urine and provide opportunity for bacteria growth.*
- Provide or assist with perineal hygiene as indicated *to reduce the risk of reinfection or prevent transmission of infection.*
- Explain to patients with chronic UTIs about additional activities that can facilitate an acidic urine *to increase the effectiveness of urinary tract anti-infectives.*
- Provide thorough patient teaching, including drug name, dosage, intended effect and schedule for administration; measures to prevent or alleviate adverse effects; the need to avoid foods that cause alkaline ash and produce an alkaline urine (e.g., citrus juices, antacids); the need to take the drug with food or meals to reduce GI effects; the importance of increasing fluid intake, including the use of cranberry juice; measures to prevent the recurrence of UTIs; and the need for periodic monitoring and laboratory testing, such as urinalysis and urine culture and sensitivity, *to enhance patient knowledge about drug therapy and to promote compliance.*

Evaluation

- Monitor patient response to the drug (resolution of UTI and relief of signs and symptoms); repeat culture and sensitivity tests as recommended for evaluation of the effectiveness of all of these drugs.
- Monitor for adverse effects (skin evaluation, orientation and reflexes, GI effects).
- Evaluate the effectiveness of the teaching plan (patient can name drug, dosage, adverse effects to watch for, specific measures to avoid them, and measures to take to increase the effectiveness of the drug).
- Monitor the effectiveness of comfort and safety measures and compliance with the therapeutic regimen.

KEY POINTS

- Urinary tract anti-infectives destroy bacteria in the urinary tract that could be causing infections.
- Urinary tract specific antibiotics prevent bacterial reproduction and cause bacterial cell death.
- Some urinary tract anti-infectives kill urinary tract bacteria by acidifying the urine, making the tract a poor host for bacterial growth, or by killing the bacteria outright.
- Hygiene measures, proper diet, and extra hydration are activities that help to decrease harmful bacteria in the urinary tract, which promotes the effect of urinary tract anti-infective agents.

Urinary Tract Antispasmodics

Urinary tract **antispasmodics** (Table 52.3) block the spasms of urinary tract muscles caused by various conditions. The antispasmodics that are available include the anticholinergics flavoxate (generic), oxybutynin (*Ditropan XL*), tolterodine (*Detrol*), fesoterodine (*Toviaz*), darifenacin (*Enablex*), solifenacin (*VESIcare*), and trospium (*Sanctura*) and the beta-agonist mirabegron (*Myrbetriq*).

Therapeutic Actions and Indications

Inflammation in the urinary tract, such as cystitis, prostatitis, urethritis, and urethrocystitis/urethrotrigonitis, causes smooth muscle spasms along the urinary tract. Irritation of the urinary tract leading to muscle spasm also occurs in patients with neurogenic bladder. These spasms lead to the uncomfortable effects of **dysuria** (pain or discomfort with urination), urgency, incontinence, **nocturia** (recurrent nighttime urination), and suprapubic pain. The urinary tract antispasmodics relieve these spasms by blocking parasympathetic activity, thus suppressing overactivity, which leads to relaxation of the detrusor and other urinary tract muscles (see Figure 52.1). Because the parasympathetic system uses acetylcholine to cause its effects, these drugs are called anticholinergic drugs.

Trospium is a newer drug in this group. It also specifically blocks muscarinic receptors and reduces the muscle tone of the bladder. It is specifically indicated for the treatment of overactive bladder with symptoms of urinary incontinence, urgency, and urinary frequency.

Mirabegron (*Myrbetriq*) is the newest drug for treating an overactive bladder. It is a beta-agonist and stimulates the sympathetic nerves in the bladder which leads to detrusor muscle relaxation. This effect allows for more urine to accumulate in the bladder helping to increase muscle pressure and urine flow rate. It does not have the anticholinergic effects seen with the other drugs but does have stimulatory sympathetic effects that may cause an increase in blood pressure, heart rate, etc. See Table 52.3 for Usual Indications of other urinary tract antispasmodics.

Pharmacokinetics

All of these agents are administered orally with the exception of oxybutynin, which is given not only orally but is also available as a dermal patch and a topical gel. These drugs are rapidly absorbed, have a slow onset of action, and have a duration of action of 6 to 12 hours. Oxybutynin, when given by the transdermal system, has a duration of action of 96 hours. The system has to be replaced every 4 days. These drugs are metabolized in the liver and excreted in the urine. They cross the placenta and are found in breast milk. Mirabegron is absorbed from the GI tract with peak levels in 3.5 hours. After hepatic metabolism, it is excreted in the urine with a half-life of approximately 50 hours.

Contraindications and Cautions

These drugs are contraindicated in the presence of known allergy to the drugs *to avoid hypersensitivity reactions*; with pyloric or duodenal obstruction or recent surgery *because*

Table 52.3 ***Drugs in Focus:*** **Urinary Tract Antispasmodics**

Drug Name	Usual Dosage	Usual Indications
Anticholinergics		
darifenacin (*Enablex*)	7.5 mg/d PO; may be increased to 15 mg/d	Treatment of overactive bladder in patients with urinary urgency, incontinence, or frequency
fesoterodine (*Toviaz*)	Initial dose 4 mg/d PO, may be increased to 8 mg/d if needed	Treatment of overactive bladder with symptoms of urgency, incontinence, and frequency
flavoxate (generic)	100–200 mg PO t.i.d. to q.i.d.; reduce dose when patient improves	Symptomatic relief of urinary bladder spasm in patients >12 y
oxybutynin (*Ditropan XL, Oxytrol, Gelnique*)	*ER tablets:* 5 mg/d PO up to a maximum 30 mg/d *Transdermal patch:* Apply to dry, intact skin q3–4 d *Gel:* Apply 1 mL to thigh, abdomen, or upper arm once every 24 h *Pediatric (>5 y):* 5 mg PO b.i.d., up to a maximum 5 mg PO t.i.d.	Symptomatic relief of urinary bladder spasm; treatment of overactive bladder
solifenacin (*VESIcare*)	5–10 mg/d PO	Treatment of overactive bladder in patients with urinary urgency, incontinence, or frequency
tolterodine (*Detrol, Detrol LA*)	1–2 mg PO b.i.d.; ER capsules—4 mg/d; reduce dose in patients with hepatic impairment to 1 mg PO b.i.d.	Treatment of overactive bladder in patients with urinary urgency, frequency, or incontinence
trospium (*Sanctura*)	20 mg PO b.i.d. at least 1 h before meals; reduce dose in patients with renal or hepatic impairment	Symptomatic relief of overactive bladder with symptoms of urinary incontinence, urgency, and urinary frequency
Beta-Agonist		
mirbegron (*Myrbetriq*)	25–50 mg/d PO	Treatment of overactive bladder with symptoms of urinary incontinence, frequency, urgency

ER, extended release.

the anticholinergic effects can cause serious complications; with obstructive urinary tract problems, *which could be further aggravated by the blocking of muscle activity or relaxation of the bladder*; and with glaucoma, myasthenia gravis, or acute hemorrhage, *which could all be exacerbated by the anticholinergic effects of these drugs*. Caution should be used in patients with renal or hepatic dysfunction, *which could alter the metabolism and excretion of the drugs*, and in pregnant and lactating patients *because of potential adverse effects on the fetus or neonate secondary to the anticholinergic effects of the drugs*. Mirabegron should be used with caution in the presence of hypertension *because this could be aggravated by the drug effects*.

Adverse Effects

Adverse effects of the anticholinergic urinary tract antispasmodics are related to the blocking of the parasympathetic system and include nausea, vomiting, dry mouth, nervousness, tachycardia, and vision changes.

Flavoxate is associated with CNS effects (blurred vision, dizziness, confusion) that make it less desirable to use in certain patients, such as the elderly or patients with neurological problems.

Oxybutynin has numerous anticholinergic effects, making it undesirable in certain conditions or situations that might be aggravated by decreased sweating, urinary retention, tachycardia, and changes in GI activity.

Mirabegron stimulates the sympathetic system and may cause hypertension and urinary retention.

Clinically Important Drug–Drug Interactions

Decreased effectiveness of phenothiazines and haloperidol has been associated with the combination of these drugs with oxybutynin. If any such combinations must be used the patient should be monitored closely and appropriate dose adjustments made. If darifenacin or fesoterodine are combined with antifungals or antiviral agents, there is a risk of toxic effects. The dose of darifenacin or fesoterodine must be reduced. There is a risk of increased QT interval and serious cardiac arrhythmias if solifenacin is combined with other drugs that prolong the QT interval (antihistamines, antipsychotics); the patient must be monitored closely if this combination is used. There is also a risk of increased serum levels and toxic effects if solifenacin is combined with ketoconazole or other cytochrome P-450 (CYP) 3A4 inhibitors; the dose of solifenacin must be reduced and the patient followed closely. Tolterodine levels and toxicity can increase if it is taken with CYP2D6 inhibitors (fluoxetine); the dose of tolterodine must be reduced if this combination is used. Trospium can interfere with the excretion of drugs by tubular secretion, leading to increased serum levels of those drugs, such as digoxin, morphine, metformin, and tenofovir. The patient needs close monitoring and appropriate dose adjustments if necessary. Mirabegron should not be combined with drugs that are metabolized by the CYP2D6 system as it inhibits that system. Digoxin should be started at a lower dose in patients taking mirabegron and the patient should be monitored closely.

Ⓟ Prototype Summary: Oxybutynin

Indications: Relief of symptoms of bladder instability associated with uninhibited neurogenic and reflex neurogenic bladder; treatment of signs and symptoms of overactive bladder.

Actions: Acts directly to relax smooth muscle in the bladder; inhibits the effects of acetylcholine at muscarinic receptors.

Pharmacokinetics:

Route	Onset	Peak	Duration
Oral	30–60 min	3–6 h	6–10 h
Transdermal system	Varies	6–8 h	96 h

$T_{1/2}$: Unknown; metabolized in the liver and excreted in the urine.

Adverse Effects: Drowsiness, dizziness, blurred vision, tachycardia, dry mouth, nausea, urinary hesitancy, decreased sweating.

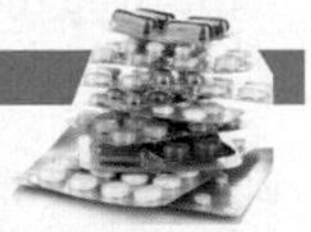

Nursing Considerations for Patients Receiving Urinary Tract Antispasmodics

Assessment: History and Examination

- Assess for *contraindications or cautions*: Any history of allergy to these drugs *to prevent hypersensitivity reactions*; pyloric or duodenal obstruction or other GI lesions or obstructions of the lower urinary tract, *which could be dangerously exacerbated by these drugs*; glaucoma, *which could increase intraocular pressure due to blockage of the parasympathetic nervous system*; and current status of pregnancy or lactation, *which would require cautious use*.
- Perform a physical assessment before therapy *to establish baseline data* and during therapy *to determine the effectiveness of the drug and the occurrence of any adverse effects associated with drug therapy*.
- Inspect the skin *to evaluate for the development of rash or hypersensitivity reactions*.
- Assess level of consciousness, orientation, and reflexes *to evaluate for any CNS effects of the drug*.
- Assess urinary elimination pattern, including amount and frequency of episodes, and for any complaints of frequency, urgency, pain, or difficulty voiding *to*

(continues on page 908)

monitor for excessive parasympathetic blockade or development of underlying UTI.
- Arrange for ophthalmological examination, including intraocular pressure, *to assess for any developing glaucoma.*
- Assess vital signs, including pulse, *to establish a baseline for evaluating the extent of parasympathetic blockade.*
- Monitor the results of laboratory tests, such as urinalysis and urine culture and sensitivity, *to evaluate the effectiveness if UTI is the problem,* and renal and hepatic function tests *to determine the need for possible dose adjustment and to evaluate for possible toxicity.*

Nursing Diagnoses

Nursing diagnoses related to drug therapy might include the following:
- Acute pain related to GI, CNS, or ophthalmological effects of drug
- Disturbed sensory perception (visual) related to CNS or ophthalmological effects
- Deficient knowledge regarding drug therapy
- Risk of impaired urinary elimination related to parasympathetic blocking

Planning

- The patient will receive the best therapeutic effect from the drug therapy.
- The patient will have limited adverse effects to the drug therapy.
- The patient will have an understanding of the drug therapy, adverse effects to anticipate, and measures to relieve discomfort and improve safety.

Implementation with Rationale

- Arrange for the appropriate treatment of any underlying UTI, *which may be causing the spasm.*
- Arrange for an ophthalmological examination at the beginning of therapy and periodically during long-term treatment *to evaluate drug effects on intraocular pressure so that the drug can be stopped if intraocular pressure increases.*
- Administer the drug with food if GI upset occurs *to alleviate GI discomfort.*
- Encourage fluid intake *to maintain urinary flow, flush the bladder, and prevent urinary stasis.*
- Offer frequent sips of water or use of sugarless hard candy *to alleviate dry mouth.*
- Monitor urinary output *to ensure adequate renal function and bladder emptying.*
- Institute safety precautions if the patient experiences CNS effects *to prevent patient injury.*
- Encourage the patient to continue treatment for the underlying cause of the spasm *to treat the cause and prevent the return of the signs and symptoms.*
- Offer support and encouragement *to help the patient deal with the discomfort of the drug therapy.*
- Provide thorough patient teaching, including drug name, dosage, rationale for use, and schedule for administration; signs and symptoms of adverse effects; measures to alleviate or prevent adverse effects; use of fluids and sugarless hard candy *to combat dry mouth;* danger signs and symptoms to report immediately; appropriate perineal hygiene measures *to reduce the risk of infection if that is the underlying cause;* and the importance of periodic monitoring, including laboratory testing and evaluation, *to enhance patient knowledge about drug therapy and to promote compliance.*

Evaluation

- Monitor patient response to the drug (resolution of urinary tract spasms and relief of signs and symptoms); repeat culture and sensitivity tests as recommended for evaluation of the effectiveness of all of these drugs.
- Monitor for adverse effects (skin evaluation, orientation and reflexes, intraocular pressure, hypertension with mirabegron).
- Monitor the effectiveness of comfort and safety measures and compliance with the regimen.
- Evaluate the effectiveness of the teaching plan (patient can name drug, dosage, adverse effects to watch for, and specific measures to avoid them).

KEY POINTS

- Smooth muscle spasms affecting the urinary tract may be caused by inflammation and irritation; effects of the spasms include dysuria, urinary urgency, incontinence, nocturia, and suprapubic pain.
- Antispasmodics block parasympathetic activity, thereby relaxing detrusor and other urinary tract muscles. The newest drug for this disorder, mirabegron, is a beta-agonist and causes the detrusor muscle to relax, allowing increased urine storage and improved muscle pressure and urine outflow.

Other Drugs Affecting the Urinary Tract and Bladder

Two other types of drugs are frequently used to alleviate problems in the urinary tract and bladder. Urinary tract analgesics are used to decrease pain, and the bladder protectant pentosan is used to prevent irritation to the bladder wall. See Table 52.4 for a complete list of these agents.

Table 52.4 *Drugs in Focus:* Other Drugs Affecting the Urinary Tract and Bladder

Drug Name	Usual Dosage	Usual Indications
Urinary Tract Analgesic		
phenazopyridine (*Azo-Standard, Baridium, Pyridium*)	200 mg PO t.i.d. for up to 2 days *Pediatric (6–12 y):* 12 mg/kg/d *or* 350 mg/m²/d PO, divided into three doses; do not exceed 2 d	Symptomatic relief of the discomforts associated with urinary tract trauma or infection
Bladder Protectant		
pentosan polysulfate sodium (*Elmiron*)	100 mg PO t.i.d.	Relief of bladder pain or discomfort associated with interstitial cystitis

Urinary Tract Analgesics

Pain involving the urinary tract can be very uncomfortable and lead to urinary retention and increased risk of infection. The agent phenazopyridine (*Azo-Standard, Baridium,* and others) is a dye that is used to relieve urinary tract pain (Table 52.4).

Therapeutic Actions and Indications

Phenazopyridine exerts a direct, topical analgesic effect on the urinary tract mucosa (see Figure 52.1). It is used to relieve symptoms (burning, urgency, frequency, pain, discomfort) related to urinary tract irritation from infection, trauma, or surgery.

Pharmacokinetics

Phenazopyridine is available for oral use and has a very rapid onset of action. It is widely distributed, crossing the placenta and entering breast milk. It is metabolized in the liver and excreted in the urine.

Contraindications and Cautions

Phenazopyridine is contraindicated in the presence of known allergy to the drug *to prevent hypersensitivity reactions* and with serious renal dysfunction, *which would interfere with the excretion and effectiveness of the drug.* These drugs should be avoided during pregnancy and lactation, but, if it is decided that they are needed, caution should be used *because of the potential for adverse effects on the fetus or neonate.*

Adverse Effects

Adverse effects associated with this drug include GI upset, headache, rash, and a reddish-orange coloring of the urine, all of which are related to the drug's chemical actions in the system. There also is a potential for renal or hepatic toxicity. Use of this drug for longer than 2 days increases the risk of toxic effects.

Clinically Important Drug–Drug Interactions

The risk of toxic effects of this drug increases if it is combined with antibacterial agents used for treating UTIs. If this combination is used the phenazopyridine should not be used for longer than 2 days.

Prototype Summary: Phenazopyridine

Indications: Symptomatic relief of pain, urgency, burning, frequency, and discomfort related to lower urinary tract irritation caused by infection, trauma, surgery, or various procedures.

Actions: Has a direct, topical analgesic effect on the urinary tract mucosa; mechanism of action is not known.

Pharmacokinetics:

Route	Onset	Peak
Oral	Rapid	Unknown

$T_{1/2}$: Unknown; metabolized in the liver and excreted in the urine.

Adverse Effects: Headache; rash; yellowish tinge to skin, sclera, urine; and GI disturbances.

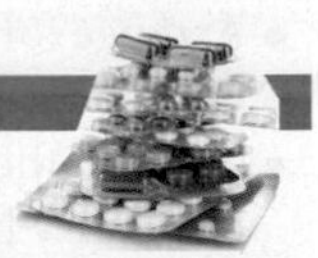

Nursing Considerations for Patients Receiving a Urinary Tract Analgesic

Assessment: History and Examination

- Assess for *contraindications or cautions*: History of allergy to these drugs *to prevent hypersensitivity reactions* or renal insufficiency, *which could interfere with the excretion and effectiveness of the drug*; and current status of pregnancy or lactation *because of the potential for adverse effects on the fetus or baby.*

(continues on page 910)

- Perform a physical assessment before therapy *to establish baseline data* and during therapy *to determine the effectiveness of the drug and the occurrence of any adverse effects associated with drug therapy.*
- Inspect the skin *to evaluate for the development of rash or hypersensitivity reactions*; check sclera *for evidence of possible jaundice.*
- Assess GI and hepatic function, including auscultating bowel sounds, *to establish baseline data to assess adverse effects of the drug.*
- Assess urinary elimination patterns, including color, amount, and complaints of frequency, dysuria, or difficulty voiding, *to identify possible underlying infection and evaluate the effectiveness of the drug.*
- Monitor the results of laboratory tests, including urinalysis and urine culture and sensitivity, *to identify possible underlying conditions such as infection or renal dysfunction,* and renal and hepatic function tests, *to determine the need for possible dose adjustment or to determine the possible risk for toxic effects.*

Nursing Diagnoses

Nursing diagnoses related to drug therapy might include the following:

- Acute pain related to GI effects of drug and headache
- Impaired urinary elimination related to the underlying condition necessitating drug therapy
- Deficient knowledge regarding drug therapy

Planning

- The patient will receive the best therapeutic effect from the drug therapy.
- The patient will have limited adverse effects to the drug therapy.
- The patient will have an understanding of the drug therapy, adverse effects to anticipate, and measures to relieve discomfort and improve safety.

Implementation with Rationale

- Arrange for appropriate treatment of any underlying UTI *that may be causing the pain.*
- Caution the patient that this drug is a dye and that urine may be reddish-brown and may stain fabrics *to prevent undue anxiety when this adverse effect occurs.*
- Administer the drug with food *to alleviate GI irritation if GI upset is a problem.*
- Urge the patient to discontinue use of the drug and contact his or her health care provider if sclera or skin become yellowish—*a sign of drug accumulation in the body and a possible sign of hepatic toxicity.*
- Provide thorough patient teaching, including drug name, dosage, rationale for use, and schedule for administration; signs and symptoms of adverse effects; measures to alleviate or prevent adverse effects; possible discoloration of urine (reddish-brown); measures to prevent or reduce the risk of recurring underlying problems such as UTI; and importance of periodic monitoring, including laboratory testing and evaluation, *to enhance patient knowledge about drug therapy and to promote compliance.*

Evaluation

- Monitor patient response to the drug (resolution of urinary tract pain).
- Monitor for adverse effects (skin evaluation, GI upset and complaints, headache).
- Evaluate the effectiveness of the teaching plan (patient can name drug, dosage, adverse effects to watch for, and specific measures to avoid them).
- Monitor the effectiveness of comfort measures and compliance with the regimen.

Bladder Protectant

The bladder protectant pentosan polysulfate sodium (*Elmiron*) is used to coat or adhere to the bladder mucosal wall and protect it from irritation related to solutes in urine.

Therapeutic Actions and Indications

Pentosan polysulfate sodium, available for oral administration, is a heparin-like compound that has anticoagulant and fibrinolytic effects. This drug adheres to the bladder wall mucosal membrane and acts as a buffer to control cell permeability, preventing irritating solutes in the urine from reaching the bladder wall cells (see Figure 52.1). It is used specifically to decrease the pain and discomfort associated with **interstitial cystitis**, a chronic inflammation of the interstitial connective tissue of the bladder that may extend into deeper tissue. See Table 52.4.

Pharmacokinetics

After oral administration, very little of this drug is absorbed (3%). It is distributed to the GI tract, liver, spleen, skin, bone marrow, and periosteum. It undergoes metabolism in the liver and spleen and is excreted in the urine. It has a half-life of 4.8 hours. It is not known whether the drug crosses the placenta or enters breast milk due to the lack of adequate studies of the effects of the drug during pregnancy or lactation; caution should be used if the drug is needed during pregnancy or lactation.

Contraindications and Cautions

Pentosan should not be used with any condition that involves an increased risk of bleeding (surgery, pregnancy, anticoagulation, hemophilia) *because of its heparin-like effects*. It is also contraindicated in the presence of a history of heparin-induced thrombocytopenia, *which could recur with use of this drug*.

Caution should be used in patients with hepatic or splenic dysfunction, *which could be affected by the heparin like actions of the drug*, and in pregnant or lactating women *because of the potential for adverse effects on the fetus or neonate*.

Adverse Effects

Adverse effects associated with pentosan use include bleeding that may progress to hemorrhage (related to the drug's heparin effects), headache, alopecia (seen with heparin-type drugs), and GI disturbances related to local irritation of the GI tract with administration.

Clinically Important Drug–Drug Interactions

There is a potential for increased bleeding risks if this drug is combined with anticoagulants, aspirin, or nonsteroidal anti-inflammatory drugs (NSAIDs). If such a combination is used the patient should be monitored very closely for any signs of bleeding, and appropriate dose adjustments should be made to the anticoagulants, aspirin, or NSAID.

Prototype Summary: Pentosan Polysulfate Sodium

Indications: Relief of bladder pain associated with interstitial cystitis.

Actions: Adheres to the bladder wall mucosal membrane and acts as a buffer to control cell permeability, preventing irritating solutes in the urine from reaching the bladder wall cells.

Pharmacokinetics:

Route	Onset
Oral	Varies

$T_{1/2}$: 4.8 hours; metabolized in the liver and spleen and excreted in the urine.

Adverse Effects: Bleeding, headache, alopecia, and GI disturbances.

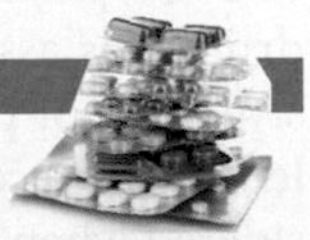

Nursing Considerations for Patients Receiving a Bladder Protectant

Assessment: History and Examination

- Assess for *contraindications or cautions*: History of allergy to these drugs *to prevent hypersensitivity reactions* or renal insufficiency, *which could interfere with excretion of the drug*; history of bleeding abnormalities, splenic disorders, or hepatic dysfunction, *which could be exacerbated by the heparin-like effects*; and current status of pregnancy and lactation, *which require cautious use of this drug*.
- Perform a physical assessment before therapy *to establish baseline data* and during therapy *to determine the effectiveness of the drug and the occurrence of any adverse effects associated with drug therapy*.
- Inspect the skin for color and note any evidence of petechiae or bruising *that may suggest coagulation problems and possible hypersensitivity reactions*.
- Assess vital signs for changes *to provide early evidence of bleeding*.
- Assess the urinary elimination pattern *to evaluate the effects of the underlying condition and the effectiveness of therapy*.
- Monitor laboratory test results, including liver function tests and coagulation studies, *to establish a baseline for monitoring safe use of the drug and the occurrence of adverse effects*.

Nursing Diagnoses

Nursing diagnoses related to drug therapy may include the following:

- Ineffective tissue perfusion related to bleeding secondary to heparin-like effects of the drug
- Acute pain related to headache and GI effects of the drug
- Alteration in body image related to alopecia
- Risk for injury related to bleeding
- Deficient knowledge regarding drug therapy

Planning

- The patient will receive the best therapeutic effect from the drug therapy.
- The patient will have limited adverse effects to the drug therapy.
- The patient will have an understanding of the drug therapy, adverse effects to anticipate, and measures to relieve discomfort and improve safety.

Implementation with Rationale

- Assist with establishing the presence of interstitial cystitis by biopsy or cystoscopy before beginning therapy *to ensure that appropriate therapy is being used*.
- Administer the drug on an empty stomach, 1 hour before or 2 hours after meals, *to relieve GI discomfort and improve absorption*.
- Obtain specimens for coagulation studies as ordered to *assess for excessive heparin-like effect*.
- Monitor urinary elimination for amount and characteristics and patient's complaints of pain or difficulty voiding *to evaluate the effectiveness of therapy*.

(continues on page 912)

- Arrange for a wig or appropriate head covering *if alopecia develops as a result of drug therapy.*
- Inspect the skin frequently for evidence of petechiae, bruising, or oozing from insertion sites *to identify increased risk for bleeding.*
- Institute safety precautions such as minimizing invasive procedures and protection from injury *to minimize the patient's risk for injury.*
- Provide thorough patient teaching, including drug name, dosage, rationale for use, and schedule for administration; signs and symptoms of adverse effects; measures to alleviate or prevent adverse effects; danger signs and symptoms to report immediately; comfort measures, such as taking the drug on an empty stomach, use of a wig if alopecia occurs, and analgesics for headache; measures to prevent or reduce the risk of recurrent interstitial cystitis; and the importance of periodic monitoring, including laboratory testing and evaluation, *to enhance patient knowledge about drug therapy and to promote compliance.*

Evaluation

- Monitor patient response to the drug (relief of bladder pain and discomfort).
- Monitor for adverse effects (skin evaluation, GI upset and complaints, headache, coagulation studies).
- Evaluate the effectiveness of the teaching plan (patient can name drug, dosage, adverse effects to watch for, and specific measures to avoid them).
- Monitor the effectiveness of comfort measures and compliance with the regimen.

KEY POINTS

- Phenazopyridine is a urinary tract analgesic that is used to decrease bladder pain that could result in changes in bladder function and emptying. This drug is a dye, and patients need to be warned about changes in the color of urine and potential for staining skin and clothing.
- Pentosan is a bladder protectant. It is a heparin-like drug that protects the inner lining of the bladder from irritation by solutes in the urine. Because it is a heparin-like drug the risk of bleeding must be considered.

Drugs for Treating Benign Prostatic Hyperplasia

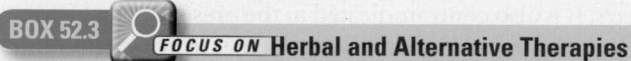

Benign prostatic hyperplasia (BPH), also called benign prostatic hypertrophy or enlarged prostate, is a common problem in men, and it increases in incidence with age. The prostate completely encircles the urethra. The enlargement of the gland surrounding the urethra leads to discomfort, difficulty in initiating a stream of urine, feelings of bloating, and an increased incidence of cystitis.

Two types of drugs are used to relieve the symptoms of BPH. These drugs include the alpha-adrenergic blockers doxazosin (*Cardura*), tamsulosin (*Flomax*), alfuzosin (*Uroxatral*), silodosin (*Rapaflo*), and terazosin (generic) and drugs that block testosterone production—finasteride (*Proscar*) and dutasteride (*Avodart*). Box 52.3 discusses an alternative therapy used to treat BPH.

BOX 52.3 FOCUS ON Herbal and Alternative Therapies

Saw palmetto is an herbal therapy that has been used very successfully for the relief of symptoms associated with BPH. Patients with BPH should be cautioned not to combine saw palmetto with finasteride because serious toxicity can occur. Patients should also be cautioned that random studies of various saw palmetto products have shown a huge variation in contents and activity of the tablets. If patients choose to use this alternative therapy, they should be cautioned to check products carefully and to avoid switching products once they have success with one.

Therapeutic Actions and Indications

Before any of these drugs are used, it is important to make sure that the prostate enlargement is benign and not caused by cancer, infection, stricture, or hypotonic bladder, which would require a different treatment. Patients receiving long-term therapy need to be reassessed periodically to make sure that they have not developed a serious underlying problem like prostate cancer. Alpha-adrenergic blockers block postsynaptic $alpha_1$-adrenergic receptors, which results in a dilation of arterioles and veins and a relaxation of sympathetic effects on the bladder and urinary tract. In addition to treating BPH, most of these drugs are also indicated for treating hypertension (see Chapter 43).

Drugs that block testosterone production—dutasteride and finasteride—inhibit the intracellular enzyme that converts testosterone to the potent androgen dihydrotestosterone (DHT), which the prostate gland depends on for its development and maintenance (see Figure 52.1). In 2011, postmarketing studies found that the use of these drugs was associated with the development of an aggressive form of prostate cancer. The incidence was small, but led to the recommendation that this information be considered when selecting an appropriate drug to treat BPH.

See Table 52.5 for Usual Indications for alpha-adrenergic blockers and drugs that block testosterone production.

See the Critical Thinking Scenario for additional information about treating a patient with BPH.

Table 52.5 *Drugs in Focus:* Drugs for Treating Benign Prostatic Hyperplasia

Drug Name	Usual Dosage	Usual Indications
Alpha-Adrenergic Blockers		
alfuzosin (*Uroxatral*)	10 mg/d PO, take after the same meal each day	Relief of symptoms of BPH
doxazosin (*Cardura*)	1 mg PO daily with titration up to 8 mg/d if needed; not for use in children	Relief of symptoms of BPH; hypertension
silodosin (*Rapaflo*)	8 mg/d PO with a meal	Relief of symptoms of BPH
tamsulosin (*Flomax*)	0.4–0.8 mg/d PO, 30 min after the same meal each day	Treatment of BPH
terazosin (generic)	1–20 mg/d PO based on patient response	Relief of symptoms of BPH; hypertension
Drugs That Block Testosterone Production		
dutasteride (*Avodart*)	0.5 mg/d PO	Long-term treatment of symptomatic BPH to shrink the prostate and relieve symptoms of hyperplasia
finasteride (*Proscar, Propecia*)	5 mg/d PO for BPH, 1 mg/d PO for male-pattern baldness (*Propecia*)	Long-term treatment of symptomatic BPH to shrink the prostate and relieve symptoms of hyperplasia; prevention of male-pattern baldness in patients with strong family history

BPH, benign prostatic hyperplasia.

CRITICAL THINKING SCENARIO

Dealing with Benign Prostatic Hyperplasia

THE SITUATION

P.F. is a 72-year-old man who has been having difficulty urinating. It has become so uncomfortable to start a stream that he has come into the clinic to be evaluated. He has a history of angina and uses sublingual nitroglycerin as needed. He also has a history of erectile dysfunction. He tells you that he does use sildenafil (*Viagra*) when he needs to but never combines it with his nitroglycerin, per physician orders. He is diagnosed with BPH and wants to learn various treatment options.

CRITICAL THINKING

What is the best approach for this patient?

What important drug interactions need to be considered when talking about drug treatment? *Think about the following points: What the drug is doing, how it works, and how it works best.*

What nondrug actions can the patient take to help with the problem and to make drug therapy more effective?

DISCUSSION

BPH is a very common problem caused by enlargement of the prostate gland. The gland responds to testosterone and slowly grows over time. Since the gland encircles the urethra, much like an inner tube, as it grows it compresses the urethra and eventually it becomes difficulty to start urine moving into the urethra (just like blowing up an inner tube makes the opening in the middle smaller and smaller). Since the growth of the prostate is a normal process that occurs over time, most men are not aware of it until they become older and the gland is compressing the urethra enough to cause urinary symptoms. This is not a cancer. However, the possibility of prostate cancer will need to be discussed and the prostate evaluated.

Two classes of drugs are available for treating BPH. Alpha-adrenergic blockers cause a relaxation of the muscles in the urethra and the vessels in the area; this may be enough to allow easier urine flow. This class of drugs must be used with caution with any other drugs that lower blood pressure, as the relaxation of muscle in the blood vessels occurs throughout the body. Since P.F. uses nitroglycerin on occasion and erectile dysfunction drugs, both of which cause vasodilation and drop in blood pressure, this class of drugs may not be the best for him. The other class of drugs block testosterone so the prostate loses the hormone influence to grow and be maintained; over time this could cause a shrinking of the gland to allow urine flow. The patient needs to know that he should not father a child and should not donate blood during and for 6 months following the use of the drug and that a woman of childbearing age should not touch the tablet. P.F felt this class of drugs could fit better with his life situation. He needs to be cautioned to avoid saw palmetto while on this drug.

(continues on page 914)

Dealing with Benign Prostatic Hyperplasia (continued)

P.F. can be encouraged to make some lifestyle changes that have been shown to help with BPH symptoms. Limiting fluid intake to about 2 quarts per day, limiting use of or avoiding alcohol and caffeine, limiting drinking fluids after dinner and before bed, trying to urinate every 3 hours, and staying active and warm have all been shown to help.

In severe cases, the prostate may be removed surgically or with ablation. There are many nerves in the area; therefore, this surgery always comes with some risk of loss of sexual function or bladder control.

NURSING CARE GUIDE FOR P.F.: BENIGN PROSTATIC HYPERPLASIA DRUG ANDROGEN HORMONE INHIBITOR

Assessment: History and Examination

Assess P.F.'s health history, particularly any allergies to finasteride or any components of the tablet, and liver dysfunction.

Focus the physical examination on the following areas:

GI: Abdominal exam, liver evaluation

GU: Prostate exam, urinary output

Laboratory tests: Renal function tests, prostate-specific antigen (PSA) level

Nursing Diagnoses

Disturbed self-image related to gynecomastia, loss of libido

Depression related to age-related changes, sexual dysfunction

Deficient knowledge regarding drug therapy

Planning

The patient will receive the best therapeutic effect from the drug therapy.

The patient will have limited adverse effects to the drug therapy.

The patient will have an understanding of the drug therapy, adverse effects to anticipate, and measures to relieve discomfort and improve safety.

Implementation

Ensure that diagnosis of BPH is accurate (rule out prostate cancer, infections, hypotonic bladder).

Administer without regard to meals.

Monitor urine flow and symptoms.

Encourage lifestyle changes to improve BPH symptoms; avoidance of alcohol, caffeine, frequent bladder emptying, limiting fluid intake and timing of fluid intake.

Provide support and reassurance to deal with drug effects and lifestyle changes.

Provide patient teaching regarding drug name, dosage, adverse effects, precautions, warnings to report, avoiding blood donation and fathering a child for 6 months, warning women of childbearing age to avoid touching the tablet; avoiding the use of saw palmetto.

Evaluation

Evaluate drug effects: Relief of symptoms, improvement in urine flow.

Monitor for adverse effects: Abdominal upset, gynecomastia, loss of libido.

Monitor for drug–drug interactions with saw palmetto.

Evaluate the effectiveness of patient-teaching program and comfort and safety measures.

PATIENT TEACHING FOR J.K.

- This drug is an androgen blocker that will stop the stimulation of prostrate growth and may shrink the prostate, which will help with urine flow.
- Take this tablet once a day without regard to food. It may take some time to see the improvement in symptoms.
- Avoid using saw palmetto while you are on this drug. This herb is often advertised to treat BPH. Combining it with this drug can lead to adverse effects.
- Take the full course of your prescription. Do not use this drug to self-treat any other infection.
- Be aware that you will not be able to donate blood and should not father a child during and for 6 months after stopping this drug because of the adverse effects it could have on a fetus. Women of childbearing age should not touch the tablets because the drug can be absorbed through the skin.
- Common adverse effects of this drug may include the following:
  - Loss of libido, impotence, decreased volume of ejaculate: *This effect usually resolves over time and will stop when the drug is stopped.*
  - Breast enlargement or tenderness: This effect is related to the hormonal effects of the drug, consult with your health care provider if this becomes too uncomfortable.
  - Report any of the following to your health care provider: Inability to pass urine, groin pain, fever, weakness.
- The following can help to decrease the symptoms of BPH:
  - Limit fluid intake to about 2 quarts a day.
  - Avoid or limit alcohol and caffeine.
  - Empty your bladder at least every 3 hours.
  - Limit fluids in the evening before bed; works best if you avoid fluid after the evening meal
  - Stay active and warm. Cold and inactivity tend to make the problem worse.
  - Tell any doctor, nurse, or other health care provider involved in your care that you are taking this drug.

Pharmacokinetics

The $alpha_1$ selective adrenergic blocking agents are well absorbed after oral administration, reaching peak levels in 2 to 8 hours, and undergo extensive hepatic metabolism. They are excreted in the urine. Finasteride and dutasteride are rapidly absorbed from the GI tract after oral administration, undergo hepatic metabolism, and are excreted in the feces and urine.

Contraindications and Cautions

Both groups of drugs are contraindicated in patients who are allergic to the drugs *to prevent hypersensitivity reactions.* Caution should be used in patients with hepatic or renal dysfunction, *which could alter the metabolism and excretion of the drugs.* The adrenergic blockers should be used with caution in patients with heart failure or known coronary disease, *which could be aggravated by the drop in blood pressure or tachycardia.* Finasteride and dutasteride have no indications for women and are rated pregnancy category X *because of androgen effects.* Women must be cautioned not to touch finasteride or dutasteride tablets *because of the risk of absorption through the skin.*

Adverse Effects

Adverse effects of alpha-adrenergic blockers include headache, fatigue, dizziness, postural dizziness, lethargy, tachycardia, hypotension, GI upset, and sexual dysfunction, all of which are effects seen with blockade of the alpha-receptors. Tamsulosin is not associated with as many adverse adrenergic-blocking effects as the other agents. Finasteride and dutasteride are associated with decreased libido, impotence, and sexual dysfunction, all of which are related to decreased levels of DHT. Patients using either finasteride or dutasteride cannot donate blood for 6 months after the last dose to protect potential blood recipients from exposure to the testosterone-blocking effects. These men should not father a child during and for 6 months following treatment and will not be able to donate blood during that same time period because of the risk of exposure to the drug.

Clinically Important Drug–Drug Interactions

There is a possibility of increased antihypertensive effects if the alpha-adrenergic blockers are combined with any other antihypertensives, nitrates, or erectile dysfunction drugs, all of which can cause lower blood pressure. The patient should be monitored and appropriate dose adjustments made to the antihypertensive agent if this combination is used; patients should be advised not to use with nitrates or erectile dysfunction drugs. The testosterone blockers should not be used with saw palmetto, an herb often used to treat BPH, as toxic adverse effects can occur.

Ⓟ Prototype Summary: Doxazosin

Indications: Treatment of BPH.

Actions: Blocks postsynaptic $alpha_1$-adrenergic receptors, which results in a dilation of arterioles and veins and a relaxation of sympathetic effects on the bladder and urinary tract.

Pharmacokinetics:

Route	Onset	Peak
Oral	Varies	2–3 h

$T_{1/2}$: 22 hours; metabolized in the liver and excreted in the urine, bile, and feces.

Adverse effects: Headache, fatigue, dizziness, postural dizziness, lethargy, vertigo, tachycardia, palpitations, nausea, dyspepsia, diarrhea, sexual dysfunction, rash.

Ⓟ Prototype Summary: Finasteride

Indications: Treatment of BPH.

Actions: Inhibits the intracellular enzyme that converts testosterone to a potent androgen that the prostate depends on for its development and maintenance.

Pharmacokinetics:

Route	Onset	Peak
Oral	Rapid	8 h

$T_{1/2}$: 6 hours; metabolized in the liver and excreted in the urine, bile, and feces.

Adverse effects: Impotence, decreased libido, abdominal upset, gynecomastia.

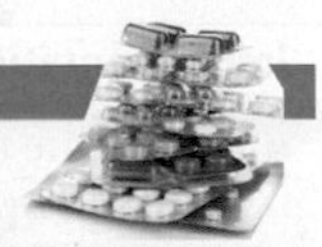

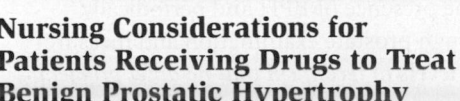

Nursing Considerations for Patients Receiving Drugs to Treat Benign Prostatic Hypertrophy

Assessment: History and Examination

- Assess for *contraindications or cautions*: History of allergy to the drug *to prevent hypersensitivity reaction;* renal or hepatic failure, *which could alter the metabolism and excretion of the drug;* or history of heart failure or coronary heart disease (with alpha-adrenergic blockers), which could *be exacerbated by the effects of the alpha-adrenergic blockers.*
- Perform a physical assessment before therapy *to establish baseline data* and during therapy *to determine the effectiveness of the drug and the occurrence of any adverse effects associated with drug therapy.*

(continues on page 916)

- Inspect the skin *to evaluate for the development of rash or hypersensitivity reactions.*
- Assess cardiopulmonary status, including vital signs especially blood pressure and pulse rate, and auscultate heart sounds and assess tissue perfusion, *to determine possible cardiovascular effects of alpha-adrenergic blockade.*
- Assess urinary elimination pattern and renal function *to assure adequate kidney function and evaluate for potential changes in drug excretion.*
- Assist with prostate examination and palpation *to establish hyperplasia and rule out other potential medical problems.*
- Monitor laboratory test results, including urinalysis, *to evaluate for possible changes*; renal and hepatic function tests *to determine the need for dose adjustment*; and PSA levels *to eliminate the diagnosis of prostate cancer.*

Nursing Diagnoses

Nursing diagnoses related to drug therapy might include the following:

- Sexual dysfunction related to drug effects
- Acute pain related to headache, CNS effects, and GI effects of the drug
- Risk for injury related to blockage of alpha-receptors
- Deficient knowledge regarding drug therapy

Planning

- The patient will receive the best therapeutic effect from the drug therapy.
- The patient will have limited adverse effects to the drug therapy.
- The patient will have an understanding of the drug therapy, adverse effects to anticipate, and measures to relieve discomfort and improve safety.

Implementation with Rationale

- Determine the presence of BPH and periodically evaluate through prostate examination and measurement of PSA levels *to reconfirm that no other problem is occurring.*
- Administer the drug without regard to meals, but give with meals *if GI upset is a problem.*
- Arrange for analgesics, *if needed, for headache.*
- Encourage the patient to change positions slowly and to sit at the edge of the bed or chair for a few minutes before rising *if low blood pressure becomes a problem.*
- Offer support and encouragement and refer for counseling if appropriate *to help the patient cope with potential decreases in sexual functioning.*
- Provide thorough patient teaching, including drug name, dosage, rationale for use, and schedule for administration; signs and symptoms of adverse effects; measures to alleviate or prevent adverse effects, such as changing positions slowly and taking drug with food if GI upset occurs; and the importance of periodic monitoring, including laboratory testing and evaluation, *to enhance patient knowledge about drug therapy and to promote compliance.*

Evaluation

- Monitor patient response to the drug (relief of signs and symptoms of BPH, improved urine flow, decrease in discomfort).
- Monitor for adverse effects (skin evaluation, GI upset and complaints, headache, cardiovascular effects).
- Monitor the effectiveness of comfort measures and compliance with the regimen.
- Evaluate the effectiveness of the teaching plan (patient can name drug, dosage, adverse effects to watch for, and specific measures to avoid them).

KEY POINTS

- BPH is a common enlargement of the prostate gland in older men.
- Drugs frequently used to relieve the signs and symptoms of prostate enlargement include alpha-adrenergic blockers, which relax the sympathetic effects on the bladder and sphincters, and finasteride and dutasteride, which block the body's production of a powerful androgen. The prostate is dependent on testosterone for its maintenance and development; blocking the androgen leads to shrinkage of the gland and relief of symptoms.

SUMMARY

- Urinary tract anti-infectives include two groups of drugs: Antibiotics that are particularly effective against gram-negative bacteria, and drugs that work to acidify the urine, ultimately killing the bacteria that might be in the bladder.
- Many activities are necessary to help decrease the bacteria in the urinary tract (e.g., hygiene measures, proper diet, forcing fluids) to facilitate the treatment of UTIs and help the urinary tract anti-infectives be more effective.
- Inflammation and irritation of the urinary tract can cause smooth muscle spasms along the urinary tract. These spasms lead to the uncomfortable effects of dysuria, urgency, incontinence, nocturia, and suprapubic pain.
- The urinary tract antispasmodics act to relieve spasms of the urinary tract muscles by blocking parasympathetic activity and relaxing the detrusor and other urinary tract muscles.

- The urinary tract analgesic phenazopyridine is used to provide relief of symptoms (burning, urgency, frequency, pain, discomfort) related to urinary tract irritation resulting from infection, trauma, or surgery.
- Pentosan polysulfate sodium is a heparin-like compound that has anticoagulant and fibrinolytic effects and adheres to the bladder wall mucosal membrane to act as a buffer to control cell permeability. This action prevents irritating solutes in the urine from reaching the cells of the bladder wall. It is used specifically to decrease the pain and discomfort associated with interstitial cystitis.
- BPH is a common enlargement of the prostate gland in older men.
- Drugs frequently used to relieve the signs and symptoms of prostate enlargement include alpha-adrenergic blockers, which relax the sympathetic effects on the bladder and sphincters, and finasteride and dutasteride, which block the body's production of a powerful androgen. The prostate is dependent on testosterone for its maintenance and development; blocking the androgen leads to shrinkage of the gland and relief of symptoms.

CHECK YOUR UNDERSTANDING

Answers to the questions in this chapter can be found in Answers to Check Your Understanding Questions on thePoint®.

MULTIPLE CHOICE

Select the best answer to the following.

1. When describing methylene blue to a patient the nurse should explain that it is a urinary tract anti-infective that acts by
- **a.** interfering with bacterial cell wall formation.
- **b.** interfering with bacterial cell division.
- **c.** alkalinizing the urine, which kills bacteria.
- **d.** acidifying the urine, which kills bacteria.

2. The antibiotic of choice for a patient with cystitis who has great difficulty following medical regimens is
- **a.** penicillin.
- **b.** fosfomycin.
- **c.** ciprofloxacin.
- **d.** nitrofurantoin.

3. Urinary tract antispasmodics block the pain and discomfort associated with spasm in the smooth muscle of the urinary tract. The numerous adverse effects associated with these drugs are related to
- **a.** their blockade of sympathetic beta-receptors.
- **b.** their stimulation of cholinergic receptors.
- **c.** their stimulation of sympathetic receptors.
- **d.** their blockade of cholinergic receptors.

4. When planning the care for an older male patient diagnosed with BPH, which two types of drugs would the nurse most likely expect the physician to prescribe?
- **a.** Alpha-adrenergic blockers and anticholinergic drugs
- **b.** Alpha-adrenergic blockers and testosterone production blockers
- **c.** Anticholinergic drugs and alpha-adrenergic stimulators
- **d.** Testosterone production stimulators and adrenal androgens

5. The drug of choice for treatment of BPH in a man with known hypertension might be
- **a.** doxazosin.
- **b.** terazosin.
- **c.** tamsulosin.
- **d.** propranolol.

6. Before administering a drug for the treatment of BPH the nurse should ensure that
- **a.** the patient has had a prostate examination, including measurement of the PSA level.
- **b.** the patient has not had a vasectomy.
- **c.** the patient is still sexually active.
- **d.** the patient is hypertensive.

7. A male who is very concerned about his hair loss and who is being treated for BPH might prefer treatment with
- **a.** doxazosin.
- **b.** finasteride.
- **c.** tamsulosin.
- **d.** terazosin.

8. After bladder surgery, many patients experience burning, urgency, frequency, and pain related to urinary tract irritation. Such patients would benefit from treatment with
- **a.** methylene blue.
- **b.** fosfomycin.
- **c.** phenazopyridine.
- **d.** flavoxate.

(continues on page 918)

MULTIPLE RESPONSE

Select all that apply.

1. In evaluating a client for the presence of a bladder infection, one would expect to find reports of which of the following?
a. Frequency of urination
b. Painful urination
c. Edema of the fingers and hands
d. Urgency of urination
e. Feelings of abdominal bloating
f. Itching, scaly skin

2. Important educational points for clients with cystitis include which of the following?
a. Avoidance of bubble baths
b. Voiding immediately after sexual intercourse
c. Always wiping from back to front
d. Avoidance of foods high in alkaline ash
e. Tight fluid restriction
f. Always wiping from front to back

BIBLIOGRAPHY AND REFERENCES

Barbosa-Cesnik C., Brown, M. B., Buxton, M., et al. (2011). Cranberry juice fails to prevent recurrent urinary tract infection: Results from a randomized placebo-controlled trial. *Clinical Infectious Diseases, 52*(1), 23–30.

Brunton, L., Chabner, B., & Knollman, B. (2011). *Goodman and Gilman's the pharmacological basis of therapeutics* (12th ed.). New York: McGraw-Hill.

Facts and Comparisons. (2015). *Drug facts and comparisons*. St. Louis, MO: Author.

Facts and Comparisons. (2015). *Professional's guide to patient drug facts*. St. Louis, MO: Author.

Gilchrist, K. (2004). Benign prostatic hyperplasia: Is it a precursor to prostate cancer? *Nurse Practitioner, 29*(6), 30–37.

Karch, A. M. (2014). *Lippincott's nursing drug guide*. Philadelphia, PA: Lippincott Williams & Wilkins.

Knezevich, E., Knezevich, J., & Spangler, M. (2011). Benign prostatic hyperplasia and the medication management of associated lower urinary tract symptoms. *US Pharmacist, 36*(6), 20–24.

McMurdo, M. E., Bissett, L. Y., Price, R. J., et al. (2005). Does ingestion of cranberry juice reduce symptomatic urinary tract infections in older people in the hospital? A double-blind, placebo-controlled trial. *Age and Ageing, 34*(3), 256–261.

Medical Letter. (2012). *The medical letter on drugs and therapeutics*. New Rochelle, NY: Author.

Mehnert-Kay, S. A. (2005). Diagnosis and management of uncomplicated urinary tract infections. *American Family Physician, 72*, 451–456.

Porth, C. (2013). *Pathophysiology: Concepts of altered health states* (9th ed.). Philadelphia, PA: Lippincott Williams & Wilkins.

Wang, C., Fang, C., Chen, N., et al. (2012). Cranberry-containing products for prevention of urinary tract infections in susceptible populations: A systematic review and meta-analysis of randomized controlled trials. *Archives of Internal Medicine, 172*(13), 988–996.

PART 10

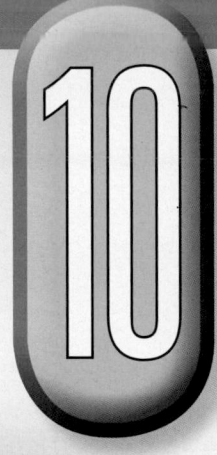

DRUGS ACTING ON THE RESPIRATORY SYSTEM

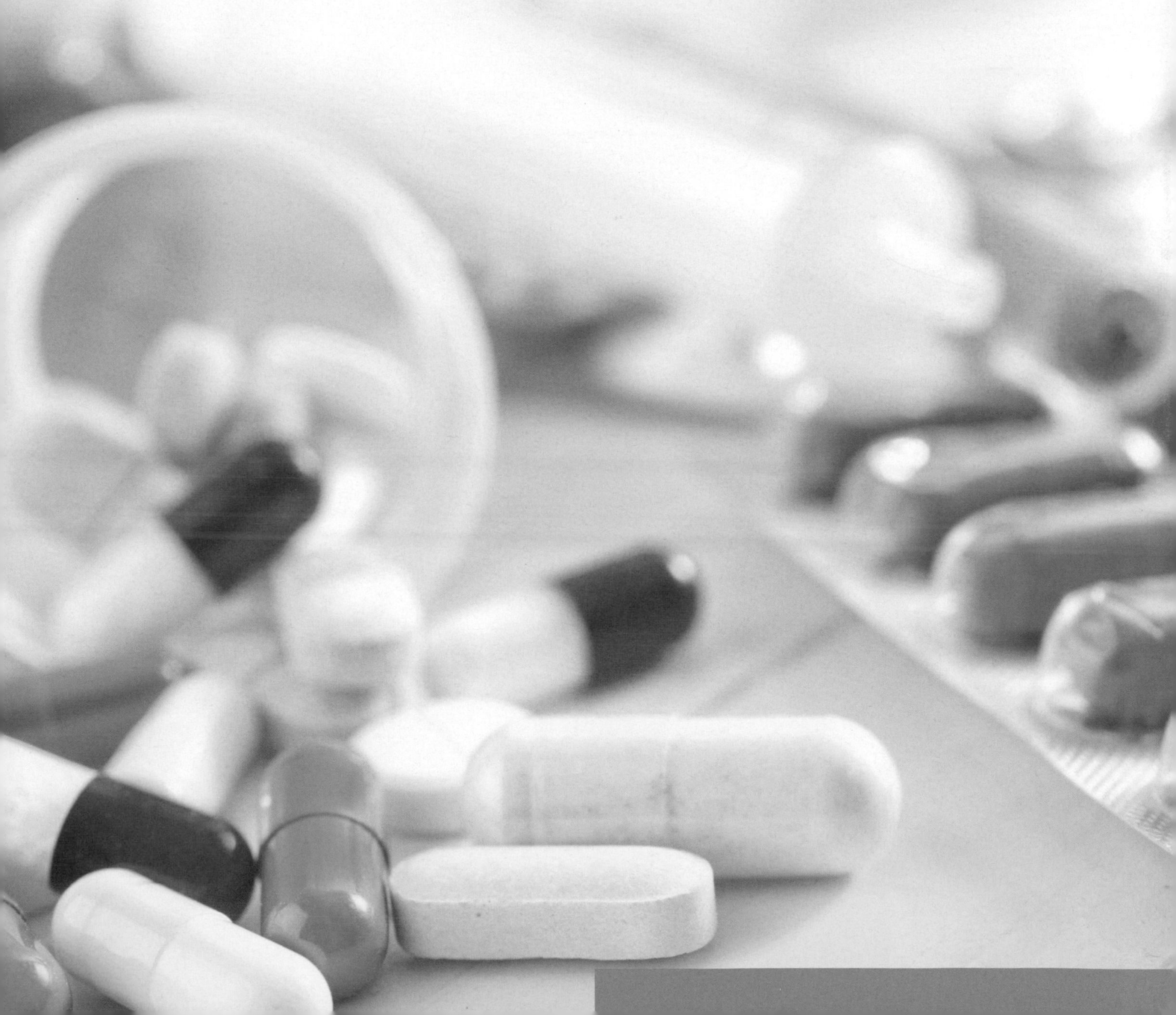

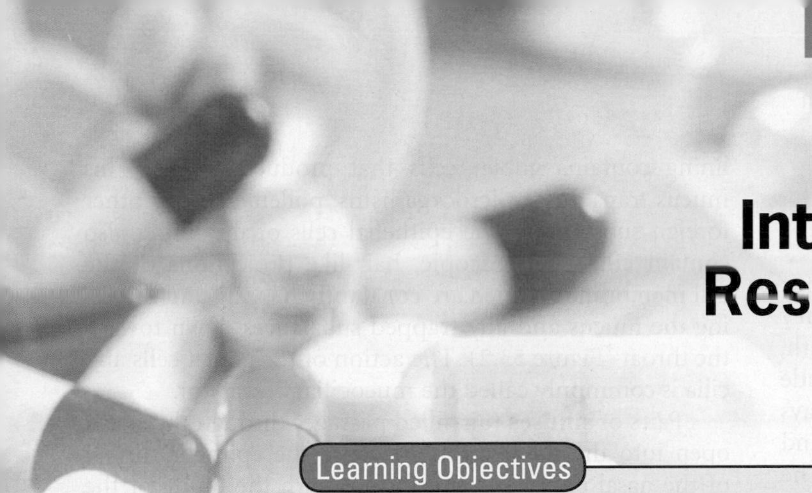

53 Introduction to the Respiratory System

Learning Objectives

Upon completion of this chapter, you will be able to:

1. Describe the major structures of the respiratory system, including the role of each in respiration.
2. Describe the process of respiration, with clinical examples of problems that can arise with alterations in the respiratory membrane.
3. Differentiate between the common conditions that affect the upper respiratory system.
4. Identify three conditions involving the lower respiratory tract, including the clinical presentations of these conditions.
5. Discuss the process involved in obstructive respiratory diseases, correlating this to the signs and symptoms of these diseases.

Glossary of Key Terms

alveoli: the respiratory sac, the smallest unit of the lungs, where gas exchange occurs

asthma: disorder characterized by recurrent episodes of bronchospasm (i.e., bronchial muscle spasm leading to narrowed or obstructed airways)

atelectasis: collapse of once-expanded alveoli

bronchial tree: the conducting airways leading into the alveoli; they branch smaller and smaller, appearing much like a tree

chronic obstructive pulmonary disease (COPD): chronic condition that occurs over time; often the result of chronic bronchitis or repeated and severe asthma attacks; leads to destruction of the respiratory defense mechanisms and physical structure

cilia: microscopic, hair-like projections of the epithelial cell membrane lining the upper respiratory tract, which are constantly moving and directing the mucus and any trapped substance toward the throat

common cold: viral infection of the upper respiratory tract that initiates the release of histamine and prostaglandins and causes an inflammatory response

cough: reflex response to irritation in the conducting airways, results in expelling of forced air through the mouth

cystic fibrosis: a hereditary disease that results in the accumulation of copious amounts of very thick secretions in the lungs, which will eventually lead to obstruction of the airways and destruction of the lung tissue

larynx: the vocal chords and the epiglottis, which close during swallowing to protect the lower respiratory tract from any foreign particles

lower respiratory tract: the bronchi and the alveoli that make up the lungs; the area where gas exchange takes place

pneumonia: inflammation of the lungs that can be caused by bacterial or viral invasion of the tissue or by aspiration of foreign substances

pneumothorax: air in the pleural space exerting high pressure against the alveoli

respiration: the act of breathing to allow the exchange of gases, a basic process for living things

respiratory distress syndrome (RDS): disorder found in premature neonates whose lungs have not had time to mature and who are lacking sufficient surfactant to maintain open airways to allow for respiration

respiratory membrane: area through which gas exchange must be made; made up of the capillary endothelium, the capillary basement membrane, the interstitial space, the alveolar basement membrane, the alveolar endothelium, and the surfactant layer

seasonal rhinitis: inflammation of the nasal cavity, commonly called hay fever; caused by reaction to a specific antigen

sinuses: air-filled passages through the skull that open into the nasal passage

sinusitis: inflammation of the epithelial lining of the sinus cavities

sneeze: reflex response to irritation to receptors in the nares, results in expelling of forced air through the nose

surfactant: lipoprotein that reduces surface tension in the alveoli, allowing them to stay open to allow gas exchange

trachea: the main conducting airway leading into the lungs

upper respiratory tract: the nose, mouth, pharynx, larynx, and trachea—the conducting airways where no gas exchange occurs

ventilation: the movement of gases in and out of the lungs.

The respiratory system is essential for survival. It brings oxygen into the body, allows for the exchange of gases, and leads to the expulsion of carbon dioxide and other waste products. The normal functioning of the respiratory system depends on an intricate balance of the nervous, cardiovascular, and musculoskeletal systems. Numerous conditions can affect the respiratory tract and interfere with the body's ability to ensure adequate oxygenation and gas exchange.

Structure and Function of the Respiratory System

The respiratory system consists of two major components: The **upper respiratory tract** and the **lower respiratory tract**. The upper portion is composed of the nose, mouth, pharynx, larynx, and trachea. The lower portion is made up of the **bronchial tree** (Figure 53.1). Conducting airways are tubes that bring air into the lungs for gas exchange and include the upper airways, bronchi, and bronchioles. The smallest bronchi and the **alveoli** (respiratory sacs), which make up the lungs, where gas exchange takes place, are called the respiratory airways.

The Upper Respiratory Tract

The upper respiratory tract is primarily involved in the movement of air in and out of the body, called **ventilation**. Air usually moves into the body through the nose and into the nasal cavity. The nasal hairs catch and filter foreign substances that may be present in the inhaled air. The air is warmed and humidified as it passes by blood vessels close to the surface of the epithelial lining in the nasal cavity. Oxygen moves more efficiently when in warm and humid air, making respiration easier. The epithelial lining contains goblet cells that produce mucus. This mucus traps dust, microorganisms, pollen, and any other foreign substances. The epithelial cells of the lining also contain **cilia**—microscopic, hair-like projections of the cell membrane—which are constantly moving and directing the mucus and any trapped substances down toward the throat (Figure 53.2). The action of the goblet cells and cilia is commonly called the mucociliary escalator.

Pairs of **sinuses** (air-filled passages through the skull) open into the nasal cavity. Because the epithelial lining of the nasal passage is continuous with the lining of the sinuses the mucus produced in the sinuses drains into the nasal cavity. From there the mucus drains into the throat and is swallowed into the gastrointestinal tract, where stomach acid destroys foreign materials.

Air moves from the nasal cavity into the pharynx and larynx. The **larynx** contains the vocal chords and the epiglottis, which closes during swallowing to protect the lower respiratory tract from any foreign particles. From the larynx, air proceeds to the **trachea**, the main conducting airway into the lungs. The trachea bifurcates, or divides, into two main bronchi, which further divide into smaller and smaller branches. All of these tubes contain mucus-producing goblet cells and cilia to entrap any particles that may have escaped the upper protective mechanisms. The

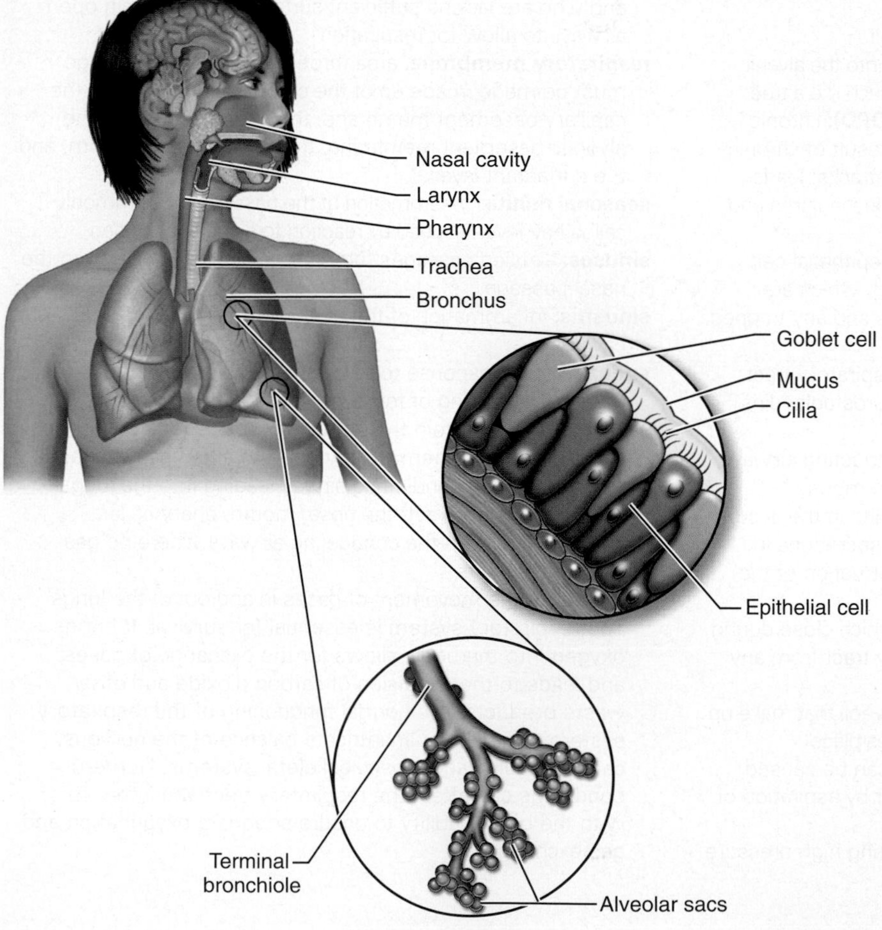

FIGURE 53.1 The respiratory tract.

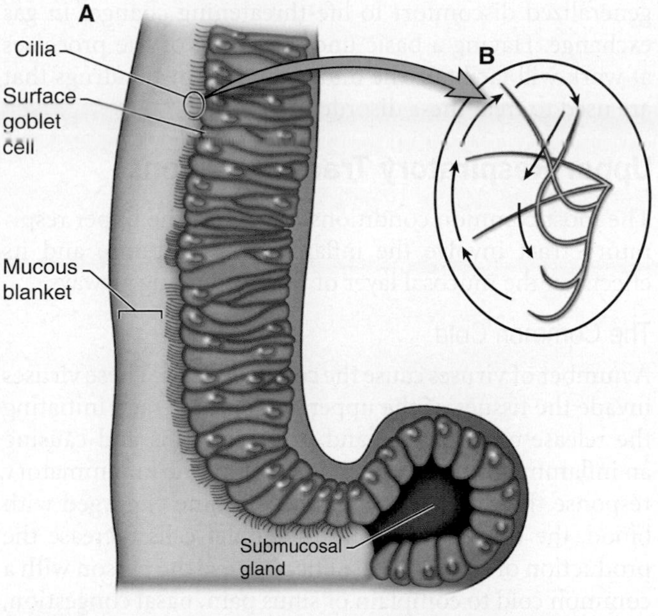

FIGURE 53.2 **A:** The mucociliary escalator. **B:** Conceptual scheme of ciliary movement, which allows forward motion to move the viscous gel layer and backward motion to occur entirely within the less viscous layer of the mucous blanket.

cilia in these tubes move the mucus up the trachea and into the throat, where again it is swallowed.

The walls of the trachea and conducting bronchi are highly sensitive to irritation. When receptors in the walls are stimulated a central nervous system reflex is initiated and a cough results. The **cough** causes air to be pushed through the bronchial tree under tremendous pressure, cleaning out any foreign irritant. This reflex, along with the similar **sneeze** reflex (which is initiated by receptors in the nasal cavity), forces foreign materials directly out of the system, opening it for more efficient flow of gas.

Throughout the airways, many macrophage scavengers freely move about the epithelium and destroy invaders. Mast cells are present in abundance and release histamine, serotonin, adenosine triphosphate, and other chemicals to ensure a rapid and intense inflammatory reaction to any cell injury. The end result of these various defense mechanisms is that the lower respiratory tract is virtually sterile—an important protection against respiratory infection that could interfere with essential gas exchange.

The Lower Respiratory Tract

The lower respiratory tract (i.e., the respiratory airways) is composed of the bronchial tree, the smallest bronchioles, and the alveoli (see Figure 53.1). The bronchial tubes are composed of three layers: Cartilage, muscle, and epithelial cells. The cartilage keeps the tube open, but it becomes progressively less abundant as the bronchi divide and get smaller. The muscles also keep the bronchi open; the muscles in the bronchi become smaller and less abundant, with only a few muscle fibers remaining in the terminal bronchi and alveoli. The epithelial cells are very similar in structure and function to the epithelial cells in the nasal passage. The alveoli at the end of the bronchioles form the respiratory membrane. These structures are the functional units of the lungs where gas exchange occurs.

The lungs are two spongy organs that fill the chest cavity. They are separated by the mediastinum, which contains the heart, esophagus, thymus gland, and various blood vessels and nerves. The lungs are made up of the bronchial tree, the alveoli, the blood supply to the lungs, the blood coming from the right ventricle to the alveoli for gas exchange, and elastic tissue, which is important in allowing the expansion and recoil of the lungs to allow ventilation. The left lung is composed of two lobes or sections, and the right lung is composed of three lobes. The lung tissue receives its blood supply from the bronchial artery, which branches directly off the aorta. The alveoli receive unoxygenated blood from the right ventricle via the pulmonary artery. The delivery of this blood to the alveoli is referred to as pulmonary perfusion.

Gas Exchange

Gas exchange occurs in the alveoli. In this process, carbon dioxide is lost from the blood and oxygen is transferred to the blood. The exchange of gases at the alveolar level is called **respiration**. The alveolar sac holds the gas, allowing needed oxygen to diffuse across the **respiratory membrane** into the capillary while carbon dioxide, which is more abundant in the capillary blood, diffuses across the membrane and enters the alveolar sac to be expired.

The respiratory membrane is made up of the capillary endothelium, the capillary basement membrane, the interstitial space, the alveolar basement membrane, the alveolar epithelium, and the surfactant layer (Figure 53.3). The sac is able to stay open because the surface tension of the cells is decreased by the lipoprotein **surfactant**. Absence of

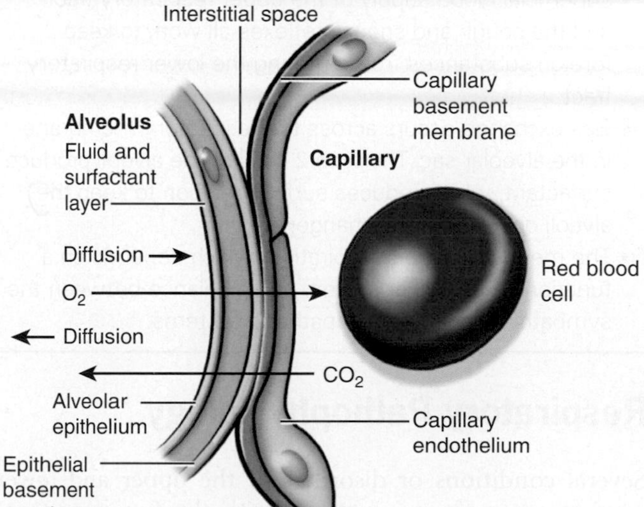

FIGURE 53.3 The respiratory membrane.

surfactant leads to alveolar collapse. Surfactant is produced by the type II cells in the alveoli. These cells have other metabolic functions, including the conversion of angiotensin I to angiotensin II by angiotensin-converting enzyme, the degradation of serotonin, and possibly the metabolism of various hormones.

The oxygenated blood is returned to the left atrium via the pulmonary veins; from there it is pumped throughout the body to deliver oxygen to the cells and to pick up waste products.

Respiration

Respiration, or the act of breathing to allow gas exchange, is controlled by the central nervous system. The inspiratory muscles—diaphragm, external intercostals, and abdominal muscles—are stimulated to contract by the respiratory center in the medulla. The medulla receives input from chemoreceptors (neuroreceptors sensitive to carbon dioxide and acid levels) to increase the rate and/or depth of respiration to maintain homeostasis in the body.

The vagus nerve, a predominantly parasympathetic nerve, plays a key role in stimulating diaphragm contraction and inspiration. Vagal stimulation also leads to a bronchoconstriction or tightening. The sympathetic system also innervates the respiratory system. Stimulation of the sympathetic system leads to increased rate and depth of respiration and dilation of the bronchi to allow freer flow of air through the system.

KEY POINTS

- The respiratory system has two parts: The upper respiratory tract, which includes the nose, pharynx, larynx, and trachea, and the lower respiratory tract, which includes the bronchial tree and alveoli. Gas exchanges occur in the alveoli.
- Nasal hairs, mucus-producing goblet cells, cilia, the superficial blood supply of the upper respiratory tract, and the cough and sneeze reflexes all work to keep foreign substances from entering the lower respiratory tract.
- Gas exchange occurs across the respiratory membrane in the alveolar sac. The type 2 cells of the alveoli produce surfactant, which reduces surface tension to keep the alveoli open for gas exchange.
- The medulla controls respiration, which depends on a functioning muscular system and a balance between the sympathetic and parasympathetic systems.

Respiratory Pathophysiology

Several conditions or disorders of the upper and lower respiratory tracts can interfere with the functioning of the respiratory system. These problems can range from generalized discomfort to life-threatening changes in gas exchange. Having a basic understanding of the processes at work will facilitate the understanding of the drugs that are used to treat these disorders.

Upper Respiratory Tract Conditions

The most common conditions that affect the upper respiratory tract involve the inflammatory response and its effects on the mucosal layer of the conducting airways.

The Common Cold

A number of viruses cause the **common cold.** These viruses invade the tissues of the upper respiratory tract, initiating the release of histamine and prostaglandins and causing an inflammatory response. As a result of the inflammatory response the mucous membranes become engorged with blood, the tissues swell, and the goblet cells increase the production of mucus. These effects cause the person with a common cold to complain of sinus pain, nasal congestion, runny nose, sneezing, watery eyes, scratchy throat, and headache. In susceptible people, this swelling can block the outlet of the eustachian tube, which drains the inner ear and equalizes pressure across the tympanic membrane. If this outlet becomes blocked, feelings of ear stuffiness and pain can occur, and the individual is more likely to develop an ear infection (otitis media).

Seasonal Rhinitis

A similar condition that afflicts many people is allergic or **seasonal rhinitis** (an inflammation of the nasal cavity), commonly called hay fever. This condition occurs when the upper airways respond to a specific antigen (e.g., pollen, mold, dust) with a vigorous inflammatory response, resulting again in nasal congestion, sneezing, stuffiness, and watery eyes.

Sinusitis

Other areas of the upper respiratory tract can become irritated or infected, with a resultant inflammation of that particular area. **Sinusitis** occurs when the epithelial lining of the sinus cavities becomes inflamed. The resultant swelling often causes severe pain due to pressure against the bone, which cannot stretch, leading to blockage of the sinus passage. The danger of a sinus infection is that, if it is left untreated, microorganisms can travel up the sinus passages and into brain tissue.

Pharyngitis and Laryngitis

Pharyngitis and laryngitis are infections of the pharynx and larynx, respectively. These infections are frequently caused by common bacteria or viruses. Pharyngitis and laryngitis are frequently seen with influenza, which is caused by a variety of different viruses and produces uncomfortable respiratory symptoms or other inflammations along with fever, muscle aches and pains, and malaise.

Lower Respiratory Tract Conditions

A number of disorders affect the lower respiratory tract, including atelectasis, pneumonia (bacterial, viral, or aspiration), bronchitis or inflammation of the bronchi (acute and chronic), bronchiectasis, and the obstructive disorders—asthma, chronic obstructive pulmonary disease (COPD), cystic fibrosis (CF), and respiratory distress syndrome (RDS). Tuberculosis, discussed in Chapter 9, is a bacterial infection. Once known as consumption, this disease has been responsible for many respiratory deaths throughout the centuries. All of these disorders involve, to some degree, an alteration in the ability to move gases in and out of the lungs.

Atelectasis

Atelectasis, the collapse of once-expanded alveoli, can occur as a result of outside pressure against the alveoli—for example, from a pulmonary tumor, a **pneumothorax** (air in the pleural space exerting high pressure against the alveoli), or a pleural effusion. Atelectasis most commonly occurs as a result of airway blockage, which prevents air from entering the alveoli, keeping the lung expanded. This occurs when a mucous plug, edema of the bronchioles, or a collection of pus or secretions occludes the airway and prevents the movement of air. Patients may experience atelectasis after surgery, when the effects of anesthesia, pain, and decreased coughing reflexes can lead to a decreased tidal volume and accumulation of secretions in the lower airways. Patients may present with crackles, dyspnea, fever, cough, hypoxia, and changes in chest wall movement. Treatment may involve clearing the airways, delivering oxygen, and assisting ventilation. In the case of a pneumothorax, treatment also involves the insertion of a chest tube to restore the negative pressure to the space between the pleura.

Pneumonia

Pneumonia is an inflammation of the lungs caused either by bacterial or viral invasion of the tissue or by aspiration of foreign substances into the lower respiratory tract. The rapid inflammatory response to any foreign presence in the lower respiratory tract leads to localized swelling, engorgement, and exudation of protective sera. The respiratory membrane is affected, resulting in decreased gas exchange. Patients complain of difficulty breathing and fatigue, and they may present with fever, noisy breath sounds, and poor oxygenation.

Bronchitis

Acute bronchitis occurs when bacteria, viruses, or foreign materials infect the inner layer of the bronchi. There is an immediate inflammatory reaction at the site of the infection, resulting in swelling, increased blood flow in that area, and changes in capillary permeability, leading to leakage of proteins into the area. The person with bronchitis may have a narrowed airway during the inflammation; this condition can be very serious in a person with obstructed or narrowed airflow. Chronic bronchitis is an inflammation of the bronchi that does not clear.

Bronchiectasis

Bronchiectasis is a chronic disease that involves the bronchi and bronchioles. It is characterized by dilation of the bronchial tree and chronic infection and inflammation of the bronchial passages. With chronic inflammation the bronchial epithelial cells are replaced by a fibrous scar tissue. The loss of the protective mucus and ciliary movement of the epithelial cell membranes, combined with the dilation of the bronchial tree, leads to chronic infections in the now-unprotected lower areas of the lung tissue. Patients with bronchiectasis often have an underlying medical condition that makes them more susceptible to infections (e.g., immune suppression, AIDS, chronic inflammatory conditions). Patients present with the signs and symptoms of acute infection, including fever, malaise, myalgia, arthralgia, and a purulent, productive cough.

Obstructive Pulmonary Diseases

As noted previously, the obstructive pulmonary diseases include asthma, CF, COPD, and RDS.

Asthma

Asthma is characterized by reversible bronchospasm, inflammation, and hyperactive airways (Figure 53.4). The hyperactivity is triggered by allergens or nonallergic inhaled irritants or by factors such as exercise and emotions. The trigger causes an immediate release of histamine, which results in bronchospasm in about 10 minutes. The later response (3–5 hours) is cytokine-mediated inflammation, mucus production, and edema contributing to obstruction. Appropriate treatment depends on understanding the early and late responses. The extreme case of

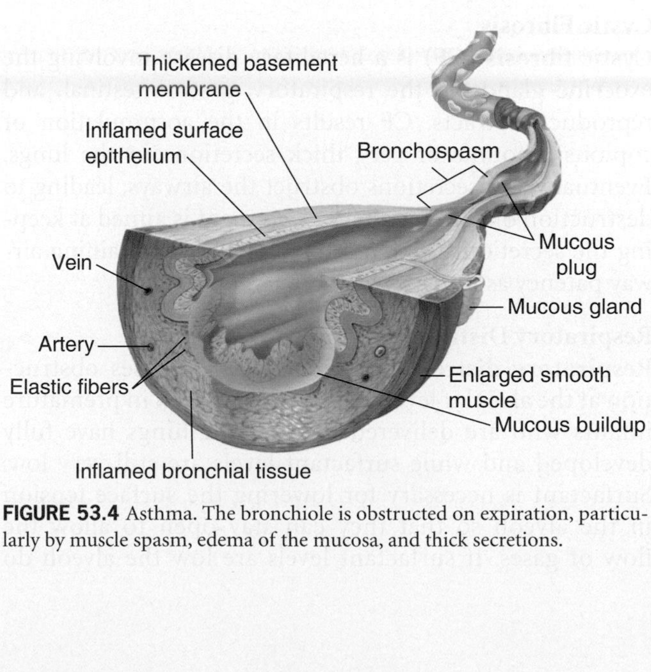

FIGURE 53.4 Asthma. The bronchiole is obstructed on expiration, particularly by muscle spasm, edema of the mucosa, and thick secretions.

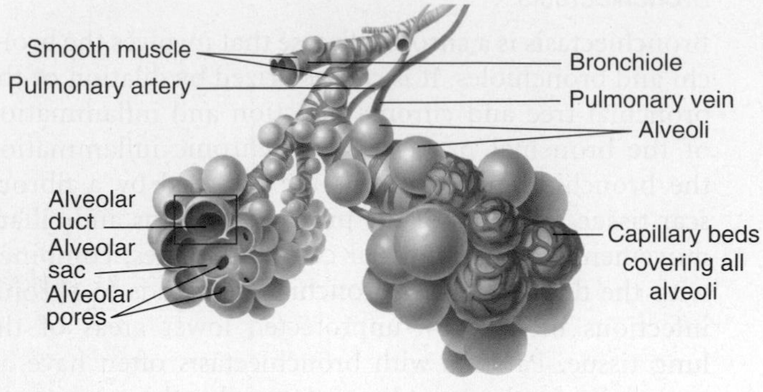

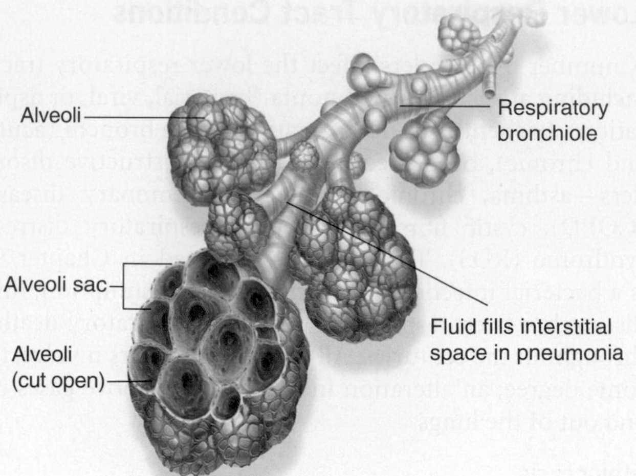

FIGURE 53.5 Normal alveoli versus distended and destroyed alveoli.

asthma is called status asthmaticus; this is a life-threatening bronchospasm that does not respond to usual treatment and occludes airflow into the lungs.

Chronic Obstructive Pulmonary Disease

Chronic obstructive pulmonary disease (COPD) is a permanent, chronic obstruction of airways, often related to cigarette smoking. It is caused by two related disorders—emphysema and chronic bronchitis—both of which result in airflow obstruction on expiration, as well as overinflation of the lungs and poor gas exchange. Emphysema is characterized by loss of the elastic tissue of the lungs, destruction of alveolar walls, and a resultant alveolar hyperinflation with a tendency to collapse with expiration. Chronic bronchitis is a permanent inflammation of the airways with mucus secretion, edema, and poor inflammatory defenses. The characteristics of both disorders often are present in a person with COPD (Figure 53.5).

Cystic Fibrosis

Cystic fibrosis (CF) is a hereditary disease involving the exocrine glands of the respiratory, gastrointestinal, and reproductive tracts. CF results in the accumulation of copious amounts of very thick secretions in the lungs. Eventually, the secretions obstruct the airways, leading to destruction of the lung tissue. Treatment is aimed at keeping the secretions fluid and moving and maintaining airway patency as much as possible.

Respiratory Distress Syndrome

Respiratory distress syndrome (RDS) causes obstruction at the alveolar level. It is frequently seen in premature infants who are delivered before their lungs have fully developed and while surfactant levels are still very low. Surfactant is necessary for lowering the surface tension in the alveoli so that they can stay open to allow the flow of gases. If surfactant levels are low the alveoli do not expand and cannot receive air, leading to decreased gas exchange, low oxygen levels, and generalized distress throughout the body as cells do not receive the oxygen that they need to survive. Treatment is aimed at instilling surfactant to prevent atelectasis and to allow the lungs to expand.

Acute respiratory distress syndrome (ARDS) is characterized by progressive loss of lung compliance and increasing hypoxia. This syndrome typically results from a severe insult to the body, such as cardiovascular collapse, major burns, severe trauma, or rapid depressurization. Treatment of ARDS involves reversal of the underlying cause of the problem combined with ventilatory support.

KEY POINTS

- Inflammation of the lower respiratory tract can result in serious disorders that interfere with gas exchange, including bronchitis and pneumonia.
- Obstructive disorders interfere with the ability to deliver gases to the alveoli because of obstructions in the conducting airways and eventually in the respiratory airways. These disorders include asthma, COPD, CF, and RDS.

SUMMARY

- The respiratory system is composed of the upper respiratory tract, which includes the nose, pharynx, larynx, and trachea, and the lower respiratory tract, which includes the bronchial tree and the alveoli.
- The respiratory system is essential for survival; it brings oxygen into the body, allows for the exchange of gases, and expels carbon dioxide and other waste products.

- The upper airways have many features to protect the fragile alveoli: Hairs filter the air; goblet cells produce mucus to trap foreign material; cilia move the trapped material toward the throat for swallowing; the blood supply close to the surface warms the air and adds humidity to improve gas movement and gas exchange; and the cough and sneeze reflexes clear the airways.
- The alveolar sac is where gas exchange occurs across the respiratory membrane. The alveoli produce surfactant to decrease surface tension within the sac and facilitate diffusion.
- Respiration is controlled through the medulla in the central nervous system and depends on a balance between the sympathetic and parasympathetic systems and a functioning muscular system.
- Inflammation of the upper respiratory tract is seen in many disorders, including the common cold, seasonal rhinitis, sinusitis, pharyngitis, and laryngitis.
- Inflammation of the lower respiratory tract can result in serious disorders that interfere with gas exchange, including bronchitis and pneumonia.
- Obstructive disorders interfere with the ability to deliver gases to the alveoli because of obstructions in the conducting airways and eventually in the respiratory airways. These disorders include asthma, COPD, CF, and RDS.

CHECK YOUR UNDERSTANDING

Answers to the questions in this chapter can be found in Answers to Check Your Understanding Questions on thePoint®.

MULTIPLE CHOICE

Select the best answer to the following.

1. The nurse emphasizes the need to take sinusitis very seriously because
   a. it can cause a loss of sleep and exhaustion.
   b. it can lead to a painful otitis media.
   c. if it is left untreated, microorganisms can travel to brain tissue.
   d. drainage from infected sinus membranes often leads to pneumonia.

2. Diffusion of CO_2 from the tissues into the capillary blood
   a. occurs if the tissue concentration of CO_2 is greater than that in the blood.
   b. decreases as blood acidity increases.
   c. increases in the absence of carbonic anhydrase.
   d. is accompanied by a decrease in plasma bicarbonate.

3. The type II cells of the walls of the alveoli function to
   a. replace mucus in the alveoli.
   b. produce serotonin.
   c. secrete surfactant.
   d. protect lungs from bacterial invasion.

4. A patient who coughs is experiencing a reflex caused by
   a. inflammation irritating the sinuses in the skull.
   b. irritants affecting receptor sites in the nasal cavity.
   c. pressure against the eustachian tube.
   d. irritation to receptors in the trachea and conducting airways

5. Which of the following is most critical for respiration to occur?
   a. Low levels of oxygen
   b. Low levels of CO_2
   c. Functioning inspiratory muscles
   d. An actively functioning autonomic system

6. After teaching a community group about the common cold the instructor determines that the teaching was successful when the group states which of the following as the cause?
   a. Bacteria that grow best in the cold
   b. Allergens in the environment
   c. Irritation of the delicate mucous membrane
   d. A number of different viruses

7. A patient with COPD would be expected to have
   a. an acute viral infection of the respiratory tract.
   b. loss of protective respiratory mechanisms due to prolonged irritation or damage.
   c. localized swelling and inflammation within the lungs.
   d. inflammation or swelling of the sinus membranes over a prolonged period.

(continues on page 928)

MULTIPLE RESPONSE

Select all that apply.

1. Which of the following would a nurse expect to assess if a patient has inflammation of the upper respiratory tract?
   a. A runny nose
   b. Laryngitis
   c. Sneezing
   d. Hypoxia
   e. Rales
   f. Wheezing

2. For gas exchange to occur in the lungs, oxygen must pass through which of the following?
   a. The conducting airways
   b. The alveolar epithelium
   c. The pleural fluid
   d. The interstitial alveolar wall
   e. The capillary basement membrane
   f. The interstitial space

3. The nose performs which of the following functions in the respiratory system?
   a. Serves as a passageway for air movement
   b. Warms and humidifies the air
   c. Cleanses the air using hair fibers
   d. Stimulates surfactant release from the alveoli
   e. Initiates the cough reflex
   f. Initiates the sneeze reflex

BIBLIOGRAPHY AND REFERENCES

Barrett, K., Barman, S., Boitano, S., et al. (2015). *Ganong's review of medical physiology* (25th ed.). New York: McGraw-Hill.

Brunton, L., Chabner, B., & Knollman, B. (2011). *Goodman and Gilman's the pharmacological basis of therapeutics* (12th ed.). New York: McGraw-Hill.

George, R. B., Light, R. W., Matthay, M. A., et al. (Eds.). (2006). *Chest medicine: Essentials of pulmonary and critical care medicine.* Philadelphia, PA: Lippincott Williams & Wilkins.

Hall, J. (2015). *Guyton and Hall's textbook of medical physiology* (13th ed.). Philadelphia, PA: W. B. Saunders

Levitzky, M. G. (2013). *Pulmonary pathophysiology* (8th ed.). New York: McGraw-Hill.

Porth, C. M. (2013). *Pathophysiology: Concepts of altered health states* (9th ed.). Philadelphia, PA: Lippincott Williams & Wilkins.

Simon, S. (2007). *Lungs: Your respiratory system.* New York: Collins.

Spiro, S. (2012). *Respiratory medicine* (4th ed.). London, UK: Manson Publishing Ltd.

West, J. B. (2012). *Pulmonary physiology and pathophysiology* (8th ed.). Philadelphia, PA: Lippincott Williams & Wilkins.

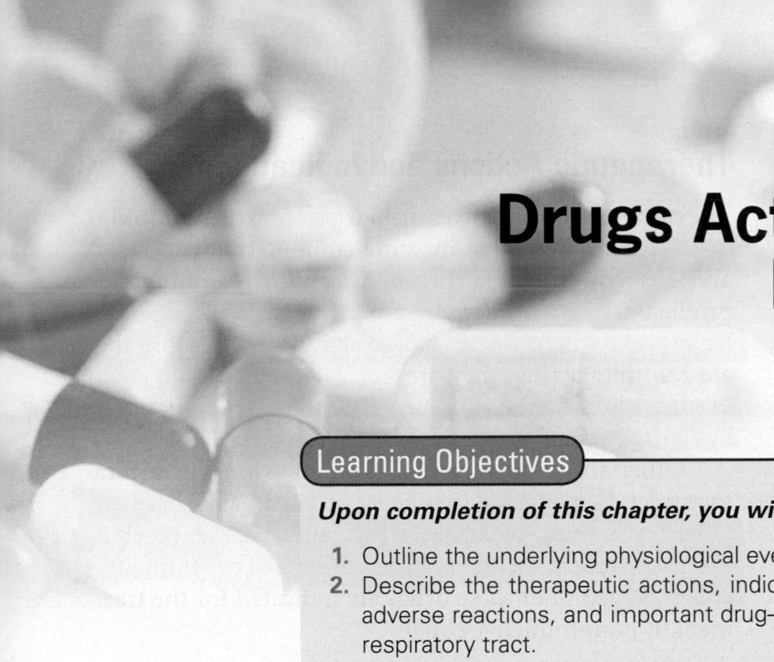

54 Drugs Acting on the Upper Respiratory Tract

Learning Objectives

Upon completion of this chapter, you will be able to:

1. Outline the underlying physiological events that occur with upper respiratory disorders.
2. Describe the therapeutic actions, indications, pharmacokinetics, contraindications, most common adverse reactions, and important drug–drug interactions associated with drugs acting on the upper respiratory tract.
3. Discuss the use of drugs that act on the upper respiratory tract across the lifespan.
4. Compare and contrast the prototype drugs with other agents in their class and with other classes of drugs that act on the upper respiratory tract.
5. Outline the nursing considerations, including important teaching points, for patients receiving drugs acting on the upper respiratory tract.

Glossary of Key Terms

antihistamines: drugs that block the release or action of histamine, a chemical released during inflammation that increases secretions and narrows airways

antitussives: drugs that block the cough reflex

decongestants: drugs that decrease the blood flow to the upper respiratory tract and decrease the overproduction of secretions

expectorants: drugs that increase productive cough to clear the airways

mucolytics: drugs that increase or liquefy respiratory secretions to aid the clearing of the airways

rebound congestion: a process that occurs when the nasal passages become congested as the effect of a decongestant drug wears off; patients tend to use more drug to decrease the congestion, and a vicious circle of congestion, drug, and congestion develops, leading to abuse of the decongestant; also called rhinitis medicamentosa

rhinitis medicamentosa: reflex reaction to vasoconstriction caused by decongestants; a rebound vasodilation that often leads to prolonged overuse of decongestants; also called rebound congestion

Drug List

Antitussives
benzonatate
codeine
(P) dextromethorphan
hydrocodone

Decongestants

Topical Nasal Decongestants
oxymetazoline
phenylephrine
(P) tetrahydrozoline
xylometazoline

Oral Decongestants
(P) pseudoephedrine

Topical Nasal Decongestants
beclomethasone
budesonide
(P) flunisolide
fluticasone
triamcinolone

Antihistamines

First Generation
brompheniramine
carbinoxamine
chlorpheniramine
clemastine
cyproheptadine
dexchlorpheniramine
dimenhydrinate
diphenhydramine
(P) hydroxyzine
meclizine
promethazine
triprolidine

Second Generation (nonsedating)
azelastine
cetirizine
desloratadine
fexofenadine
levocetirizine
loratadine

Expectorant
(P) guaifenesin

Mucolytics
acetylcysteine
(P) dornase alfa

Drugs that affect the respiratory system work to keep the airways open and gases moving efficiently. The classes discussed in this chapter mainly act on the upper respiratory tract. Figure 54.1 shows the structures of the upper respiratory tract. Figure 54.2 displays the sites of action of these drugs.

Antitussives

Antitussives are drugs that suppress the cough reflex (Table 54.1). Many disorders of the respiratory tract, including the common cold, sinusitis, pharyngitis, and pneumonia, are accompanied by an uncomfortable, unproductive cough. Persistent coughing can be exhausting and can cause muscle strain and further irritation of the respiratory tract. A cough that occurs without the presence of any active disease process or persists after treatment may be a symptom of another disease process and should be investigated before any medication is given to alleviate it. Box 54.1 discusses the use of antitussives and other drugs acting on the upper respiratory tract in various age groups.

Therapeutic Actions and Indications

The traditional antitussives include codeine (generic only), hydrocodone (available in some combination products), and dextromethorphan (generic and in combination products), which act directly on the medullary cough center of the brain to depress the cough reflex. Because they are centrally acting, they are not the drugs of choice for anyone who has a head injury or who could be impaired by central nervous system (CNS) depression.

Other antitussives have a direct effect on the respiratory tract. Benzonatate (*Tessalon*) acts as a local anesthetic on the respiratory passages, lungs, and pleurae, blocking the effectiveness of the stretch receptors that stimulate a cough reflex. All of these drugs are indicated for the treatment of nonproductive cough.

Pharmacokinetics

Codeine, hydrocodone, and dextromethorphan are rapidly absorbed, metabolized in the liver, and excreted in the urine. They cross the placenta and enter breast milk. Benzonatate is metabolized in the liver and excreted

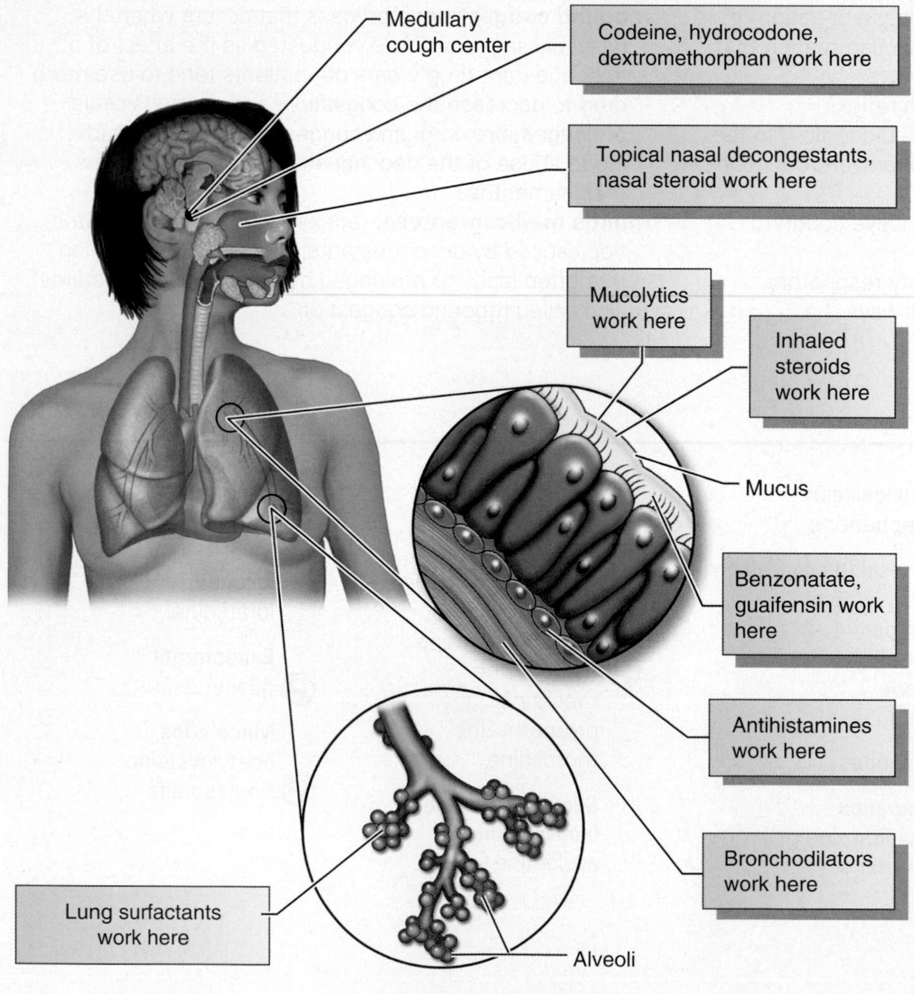

FIGURE 54.1 Sites of action of drugs acting on the upper respiratory tract.

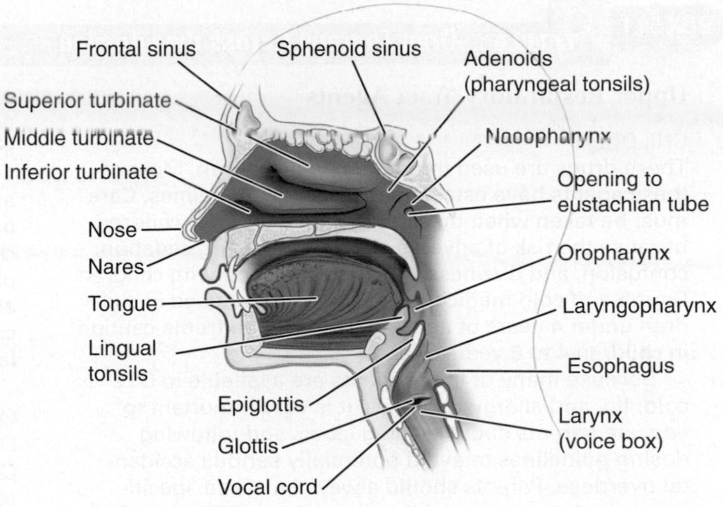

FIGURE 54.2 Structures of the upper respiratory tract.

in the urine. These drugs should not be used in pregnancy and lactation (see Contraindications and Cautions).

Contraindications and Cautions

Antitussives are contraindicated in patients who need to cough to maintain the airways (e.g., postoperative patients and those who have undergone abdominal or thoracic surgery) *to avoid respiratory distress*. Careful use is recommended for patients with asthma and emphysema *because cough suppression in these patients could lead to an accumulation of secretions and a loss of respiratory reserve.* Caution should also be used in patients who are hypersensitive to or have a history of addiction to narcotics (codeine, hydrocodone). *Codeine is a narcotic and has addiction potential.* Patients who need to drive or to be alert should use codeine, hydrocodone, and dextromethorphan with extreme caution *because these drugs can cause sedation and drowsiness.* These drugs should not be used during pregnancy and lactation *because of the potential for adverse effects on the fetus or baby, including sedation and CNS depression.* In 2010, several babies experienced serious adverse effects when their mothers nursed them after taking codeine products for cough suppression. Since then, a genetic test of codeine metabolism has become available for nursing mothers who feel the need to use a codeine product for cough suppression to determine the potential risk to the baby.

Adverse Effects

Traditional antitussives have a drying effect on the mucous membranes and can increase the viscosity of respiratory tract secretions. Because they affect centers in the brain, these antitussives are associated with CNS adverse effects, including drowsiness and sedation. Their drying effect can lead to nausea, constipation, and complaints of dry mouth (Figure 54.3). The locally acting antitussives are associated with gastrointestinal (GI) upset, headache, feelings of congestion, and sometimes dizziness.

Clinically Important Drug–Drug Interactions

Dextromethorphan should not be used with monoamine oxidase (MAO) inhibitors; hypotension, fever, nausea, myoclonic jerks, and coma could occur.

Table 54.1 ***Drugs in Focus:* Antitussives**

Drug Name	Usual Dosage	Usual Indications
benzonatate (*Tessalon*)	*Adult and pediatric (>10 y):* 100–200 mg PO t.i.d.	Treatment of nonproductive cough
codeine (generic)	*Adult:* 10–20 mg PO q4–6 h *Pediatric (6–12 y):* 5–10 mg PO q4–6 h *Pediatric (2–6 y):* 2.5–5 mg PO q4–6 h	Treatment of nonproductive cough
dextromethorphan (generic)	*Adult:* 10–30 mg PO q4–8 h; 60 mg PO b.i.d. for sustained action *Pediatric (6–12 y):* 5–10 mg PO q4 h; 30 mg PO b.i.d. for sustained action *Pediatric (2–6 y):* 2.5–7.5 mg PO q4–8 h; 15 mg PO b.i.d. for sustained action	Treatment of nonproductive cough
hydrocodone (generic)	*Adult:* 5–10 mg PO q4–6 h *Pediatric (2–12 y):* 1.25–5 mg PO q4–6 h	Treatment of nonproductive cough

BOX 54.1 FOCUS ON **Drug Therapy Across the Lifespan**

Upper Respiratory Tract Agents

CHILDREN

These drugs are used frequently with children. Most of these agents have established pediatric guidelines. Care must be taken when these drugs are used with children because the risk of adverse effects—including sedation, confusion, and dizziness—is more common with children. Cough and cold medications should not be used in children under 4 years of age and used with extreme caution in children 4 to 6 years of age.

Because many of these agents are available in OTC cold, flu, and allergy remedies, it is very important to educate parents about reading labels and following dosing guidelines to avoid potentially serious accidental overdose. Parents should always be asked specifically whether they are giving the child an OTC or herbal remedy.

Parents should also be encouraged to implement nondrug measures to help the child cope with the upper respiratory problem—drink plenty of fluids, use a humidifier, avoid smoke-filled areas, avoid contact with known allergens or irritants, and wash hands frequently during the cold and flu season.

ADULTS

Adults may inadvertently overdose on these agents when taking multiple OTC preparations to help them get through the misery of a cold or flu. They need to be questioned specifically about the use of OTC or herbal remedies before any of these drugs are advised or administered. Adults can also be encouraged to use nondrug measures to help them cope with the signs and symptoms.

The safety for the use of these drugs during pregnancy and lactation has not been established. There is a potential for adverse effects on the fetus related to blood flow changes and direct drug effects when the drugs cross the placenta. The drugs may enter breast milk and also may alter fluid balance and milk production. It is advised that caution be used if one of these drugs is prescribed during lactation.

OLDER ADULTS

Older adults frequently are prescribed one of these drugs. Older adults are more likely to develop adverse effects associated with the use of these drugs, including sedation, confusion, and dizziness. Safety measures may be needed if these effects occur and interfere with the patient's mobility and balance.

Older adults also are more likely to have renal and/or hepatic impairment related to underlying medical conditions, which could interfere with the metabolism and excretion of these drugs. The dose for older adults should be started at a lower level than recommended for younger adults. The patient should be monitored very closely, and dose adjustment should be based on the patient's response.

These patients also need to be alerted to the potential for toxic effects when using OTC preparations and should be advised to check with their health care provider before beginning any OTC drug regimen.

Prototype Summary: Dextromethorphan

Indications: Control of nonproductive cough.

Actions: Depresses the cough center in the medulla to control cough spasms.

Pharmacokinetics:

Route	Onset	Peak	Duration
Oral	25–30 min	2 h	3–6 h

$T_{1/2}$: 2 to 4 hours; metabolized in the liver and excreted in the urine.

Adverse Effects: Dizziness, respiratory depression, dry mouth.

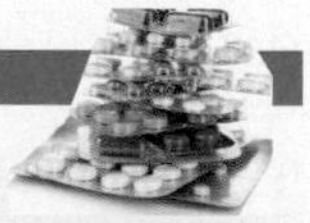

Nursing Considerations for Patients Receiving Antitussives

Assessment: History and Examination

- Assess for *possible contraindications or cautions*: Any history of allergy to any component of the drug or drug vehicle *to avoid allergic reactions*; cough that persists longer than 1 week or is accompanied by other signs and symptoms, *which could indicate a serious underlying medical condition that should be addressed before suppressing symptoms*; and pregnancy or lactation *because of the potential for adverse effects on the fetus or baby.*
- Perform a physical examination *to establish baseline data for assessing the effectiveness of the drug and the occurrence of any adverse effects associated with drug therapy.*
- Monitor temperature *to evaluate for possible underlying infection.*
- Assess respirations and adventitious sounds *to assess drug effectiveness and to monitor for accumulation of secretions.*
- Evaluate orientation and affect *to monitor for CNS effects of the drug.*

Nursing Diagnoses

Nursing diagnoses related to drug therapy might include the following:

- Ineffective airway clearance related to excessive drug effects
- Disturbed sensory perception related to CNS effects
- Deficient knowledge regarding drug therapy

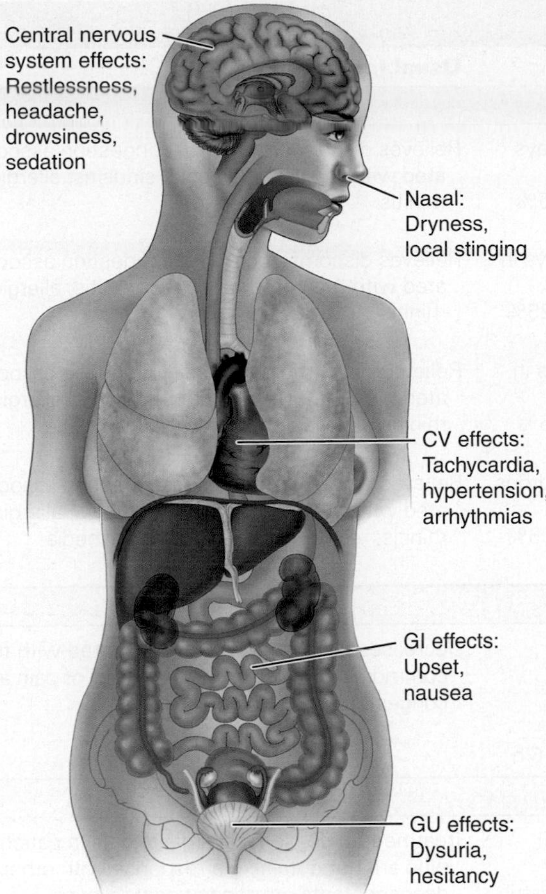

FIGURE 54.3 Variety of adverse effects and toxicities associated with drugs affecting the upper respiratory tract.

Planning

- The patient will receive the best therapeutic effect from the drug therapy.
- The patient will have limited adverse effects to the drug therapy.
- The patient will have an understanding of the drug therapy, adverse effects to anticipate, and measures to relieve discomfort and improve safety.

Implementation with Rationale

- Ensure that the drug is not taken any longer than recommended *to prevent serious adverse effects and increased respiratory tract problems.*
- Arrange for further medical evaluation for coughs that persist or are accompanied by high fever, rash, or excessive secretions *to detect the underlying cause of the cough and to arrange for appropriate treatment of the underlying problem.*
- Provide other measures *to help relieve cough* (e.g., humidity, cool temperatures, fluids, use of topical lozenges) as appropriate.
- Provide thorough patient teaching, including the drug name and prescribed dosage, measures to help avoid adverse effects, warning signs that may indicate problems, and the need for periodic monitoring and evaluation, *to enhance patient knowledge about drug therapy and to promote compliance.*
- Offer support and encouragement *to help the patient cope with the disease and the drug regimen.*

Evaluation

- Monitor patient response to the drug (control of nonproductive cough).
- Monitor for adverse effects (respiratory depression, dizziness, sedation).
- Evaluate the effectiveness of the teaching plan (patient can name drug, dosage, adverse effects to watch for, specific measures to avoid them, and measures to take to increase the effectiveness of the drug).
- Monitor the effectiveness of other measures to relieve cough.

KEY POINTS

- Antitussive drugs suppress the cough reflex by acting centrally to suppress the medullary cough center or locally as an anesthetic or to increase secretion and buffer irritation.
- Antitussive drugs can cause CNS depression, including drowsiness and sedation.
- Antitussive drugs should be used with caution in any situation in which coughing could be important for clearing the airways.

Decongestants

Decongestants decrease the overproduction of secretions by causing local vasoconstriction to the upper respiratory tract (Table 54.2). This vasoconstriction leads to a shrinking of swollen mucous membranes and tends to open clogged nasal passages, providing relief from the discomfort of a blocked nose and promoting drainage of secretions and improved airflow. An adverse effect that accompanies frequent or prolonged use of these drugs is a **rebound congestion**, technically called **rhinitis medicamentosa**. The reflex reaction to vasoconstriction is a rebound vasodilation, which often leads to prolonged overuse of decongestants.

Decongestants are usually adrenergics or sympathomimetics (see Chapter 30). Topical steroids are also used as decongestants, although they take several weeks to be really effective and are more often used in cases of chronic rhinitis.

Table 54.2 *Drugs in Focus:* Decongestants

Drug Name	Usual Dosage	Usual Indications
Topical Nasal Decongestants		
oxymetazoline (*Afrin*)	*Adult and pediatric (>6 y):* Two to three sprays or drops in each nostril b.i.d. *Pediatric (2–5 y):* Two to three drops of 0.05% solution in each nostril b.i.d.	Relieves discomfort of nasal congestion associated with the common cold, sinusitis, allergic rhinitis
phenylephrine (*Coricidin*)	*Adult and pediatric (>6 y):* One to two sprays in each nostril q3–4 h *Pediatric (2–6 y):* Two to three drops of 0.125% solution in each nostril q4 h as needed	Relieves discomfort of nasal congestion associated with the common cold, sinusitis, allergic rhinitis
tetrahydrozoline (*Tyzine*)	*Adult and pediatric (>6 y):* Two to four drops in each nostril t.i.d. to q.i.d. *Pediatric (2–6 y):* Two to three drops of 0.05% solution in each nostril q4–6 h	Relieves discomfort of nasal congestion associated with the common cold, sinusitis, allergic rhinitis; relieves pressure of otitis media
xylometazoline (*Otrivin*)	*Adult:* Two to three sprays *or* two to three drops in each nostril q8–10 h (0.17% solution) *Pediatric (2–12 y):* Two to three drops of 0.05% solution q8–12 h	Relieves discomfort of nasal congestion associated with the common cold, sinusitis, allergic rhinitis; relieves pressure of otitis media
Oral Decongestant		
pseudoephedrine (*Sudafed, Decofed*)	*Adult:* 60 mg PO q4–6 h *Pediatric (6–12 y):* 30 mg PO q4–6 h *Pediatric (2–5 y):* 15 mg PO q4–6 h *Pediatric (1–2 y):* 0.02 mL/kg PO q4–6 h *Pediatric (3–12 mo):* Three drops/kg PO q4–6 h	Decreases nasal congestion associated with the common cold, allergic rhinitis; relief of pain and congestion of otitis media
Topical Steroid Nasal Decongestants		
beclomethasone (*Beconase*)	*Adult:* One to two inhalations in each nostril b.i.d. *Pediatric (6–11 y):* One inhalation in each nostril b.i.d.	Treatment of seasonal allergic rhinitis in patients who are not obtaining a response with other decongestants or preparations; relieves inflammation following removal of nasal polyps
budesonide (*Pulmicort Respules*)	*Adult and pediatric (>6 y):* Two sprays in each nostril morning and evening *or* four sprays in each nostril in the morning	Treatment of seasonal allergic rhinitis in patients who are not obtaining a response with other decongestants or preparations; relieves inflammation following removal of nasal polyps
flunisolide (generic)	*Adult:* Two sprays in each nostril b.i.d. *Pediatric (6–14 y):* One spray in each nostril t.i.d. to two sprays in each nostril b.i.d.	Treatment of seasonal allergic rhinitis in patients who are not obtaining a response with other decongestants or preparations; relieves inflammation following removal of nasal polyps
fluticasone (generic)	*Adult and pediatric (4–11 y):* Two sprays in each nostril daily	Treatment of seasonal allergic rhinitis in patients who are not obtaining a response with other decongestants or preparations; relieves inflammation following removal of nasal polyps
triamcinolone (generic)	*Adult:* Two sprays in each nostril every day	Treatment of seasonal allergic rhinitis in patients who are not obtaining a response with other decongestants or preparations; relieves inflammation following removal of nasal polyps

Topical Nasal Decongestants

The topical nasal decongestants include oxymetazoline (*Afrin*, and others), phenylephrine (*Coricidin*, and many others), tetrahydrozoline (*Tyzine*), and xylometazoline (*Otrivin*). Many of these are available as over-the-counter (OTC) preparations. The choice of a topical nasal decongestant varies with the individual. Some patients may have no response to one and respond very well to another.

Therapeutic Actions and Indications

Topical decongestants are sympathomimetics, meaning that they imitate the effects of the sympathetic nervous system to cause vasoconstriction, leading to decreased edema and inflammation of the nasal membranes. They are available as nasal sprays that are used to relieve the discomfort of nasal congestion that accompanies the common cold, sinusitis, and allergic rhinitis. These drugs can also be used when dilation of the nares is desired to facilitate medical

BOX 54.2 FOCUS ON **Patient and Family Teaching**

Administering Nasal Medications

Proper administration technique is very important for assuring that drugs given nasally have the desired therapeutic effect. It is important to periodically check the nares for any signs of erosion or lesions, which could allow systemic absorption of the drug. Most patients prefer to self-administer nasal drugs, so patient teaching is very important. Explain the technique, and then observe the patient using the technique.

NASAL SPRAY
Teach the patient to sit upright and press a finger over one naris to close it. Hold the spray bottle upright and place the tip of the bottle about 1/2 inch into the open naris. Firmly squeeze the bottle to deliver the drug. Caution the patient not to squeeze too forcefully, which could send the drug up into the sinuses, causing more problems. Repeat with the other naris.

NASAL AEROSOL
Teach the patient to place the medication cartridge into the plastic nasal adapter and shake it well. Remove the plastic cap from the applicator and place the tip inside the nostril. Have the patient sit upright and tilt the head back. The patient should firmly press on the canister once to deliver the drug; inhale; hold his or her breath for a few seconds; and then exhale. The patient should be encouraged to keep the head tilted back for a few minutes and reminded not to blow his or her nose for at least 2 minutes.

examination or to relieve the pain and congestion of otitis media. Opening the nasal passage allows better drainage of the eustachian tube, relieving pressure in the middle ear. See Table 54.2 for Usual Indications for each of these agents.

Pharmacokinetics

Because these drugs are applied topically the onset of action is almost immediate and there is less chance of systemic effects. Although they are not generally absorbed systemically, any portion of these topical decongestants that is absorbed is metabolized in the liver and excreted in the urine. See Box 54.2 for tips on how to teach the patient to use these medications.

Contraindications and Cautions

Caution should be used when there is any lesion or erosion in the mucous membranes *that could lead to systemic absorption.* Caution should also be used in patients with any condition that might be exacerbated by sympathetic activity, such as glaucoma, hypertension, diabetes, thyroid disease, coronary disease, or prostate problems, *because these agents have adrenergic properties. Because there are no studies regarding the effects of these topical drugs in pregnancy or lactation*, if used during pregnancy or lactation, caution is advised.

Adverse Effects

Adverse effects associated with topical decongestants include local stinging and burning, which may occur the first few times the drug is used. If the sensation does not pass the drug should be discontinued because it may indicate lesions or erosion of the mucous membranes. Use for longer than 3 to 5 days can lead to a rebound congestion. (Rebound congestion occurs when the nasal passages become congested as the drug effect wears off. As a result, patients tend to use more drug to decrease the congestion, thus initiating a vicious cycle of congestion–drug–congestion, which leads to abuse of the decongestant.) Sympathomimetic effects (e.g., increased pulse and blood pressure; urinary retention) should be monitored because some systemic absorption may occur, although these effects are less likely with topical administration than with other routes.

Clinically Important Drug–Drug Interactions

The use of topical nasal decongestants is contraindicated with concurrent use of cyclopropane or halothane anesthesia because serious cardiovascular (CV) effects could occur. Combined use with any other sympathomimetic drug or sympathetic-blocking drug could result in toxic or noneffective responses. Monitor the use of these combinations carefully.

Prototype Summary: Tetrahydrozoline

Indications: Symptomatic relief of nasal and nasopharyngeal mucosal congestion due to the common cold, hay fever, or other respiratory allergies.

Actions: Sympathomimetic effects, partly due to release of norepinephrine from nerve terminals; vasoconstriction leads to decreased edema and inflammation of the nasal membranes.

Pharmacokinetics:

Route	Peak	Duration
Topical (nasal spray)	5–10 min	6–10 h

$T_{1/2}$: Unknown; metabolized in the liver and excreted in the urine; little is usually absorbed for systemic metabolism.

Adverse Effects: Disorientation, confusion, lightheadedness, nausea, vomiting, fever, dyspnea, rebound congestion.

Nursing Considerations for Patients Receiving Topical Nasal Decongestants

Assessment: History and Examination

- Assess for *possible contraindications or cautions*: Any history of allergy to the drug or a component of the drug vehicle; glaucoma, hypertension, diabetes, thyroid disease, coronary disease, and prostate problems, *all of which could be exacerbated by the sympathomimetic effects*; and pregnancy or lactation, *which require cautious use of the drug.*
- Perform a physical examination *to establish baseline data for assessing the effectiveness of the drug and the occurrence of any adverse effects associated with drug therapy.*
- Assess skin color and temperature *to assess sympathetic response.*
- Evaluate orientation and reflexes *to evaluate CNS effects of the drug.*
- Monitor pulse, blood pressure, and cardiac auscultation *to assess CV and sympathomimetic effects.*
- Evaluate respirations and adventitious breath sounds *to assess the effectiveness of the drug and potential excess effect.*
- Perform bladder percussion *to monitor for urinary retention related to sympathomimetic effects.*
- Evaluate nasal mucous membrane *to monitor for lesions that could lead to systemic absorption and to evaluate decongestant effect.*

Nursing Diagnoses

Nursing diagnoses related to drug therapy might include the following:

- Acute pain related to GI, CNS, or local effects of drug.
- Disturbed sensory perception (kinesthetic) related to CNS effects (less likely with this route of administration).
- Deficient knowledge regarding drug therapy.

Planning

- The patient will receive the best therapeutic effect from the drug therapy.
- The patient will have limited adverse effects to the drug therapy.
- The patient will have an understanding of the drug therapy, adverse effects to anticipate, and measures to relieve discomfort and improve safety.

Implementation with Rationale

- Teach patient the proper administration of the drug *to ensure therapeutic effect* (see Box 54.2). The patient should be instructed to clear the nasal passages before use, to tilt the head back when applying the drops or spray, and to keep it tilted back for a few seconds after administration. This technique *helps to ensure contact with the affected mucous membranes and decreases the chances of letting the drops trickle down the back of throat, which may lead to more systemic effects.*
- Caution the patient not to use the drug for longer than 5 days and to seek medical care if signs and symptoms persist after that time *to facilitate detection of underlying medical conditions that may require treatment.*
- Caution the patient that these drugs are found in many OTC preparations and that care should be taken not to inadvertently combine drugs with the same ingredients, *which could lead to overdose.*
- Provide safety measures if dizziness or sedation occurs as a result of drug therapy *to prevent patient injury.*
- Institute other measures *to help relieve the discomfort of congestion* (e.g., use of a humidifier, increased fluid intake, cool environment, avoidance of smoke-filled areas) as appropriate.
- Provide thorough patient teaching, including the drug name and prescribed dosage, measures to help avoid adverse effects, warning signs that may indicate problems, and the need for periodic monitoring and evaluation, *to enhance patient knowledge about drug therapy and to promote compliance.*
- Offer support and encouragement *to help the patient cope with the disease and the drug regimen.*

Evaluation

- Monitor patient response to the drug (relief of nasal congestion).
- Monitor for adverse effects (local burning and stinging; adrenergic effects such as increased pulse, blood pressure, urinary retention, cool and clammy skin).
- Evaluate the effectiveness of the teaching plan (patient can name drug, dosage, adverse effects to watch for, specific measures to avoid them, measures to take to increase the effectiveness of the drug, proper administration technique).
- Monitor the effectiveness of comfort and safety measures and compliance with the regimen.

Oral Decongestants

The only oral decongestant currently available for use is pseudoephedrine (*Triaminic Allergy Congestion*, and many combination products) (Table 54.2).

Therapeutic Actions and Indications

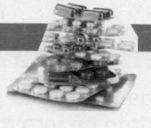

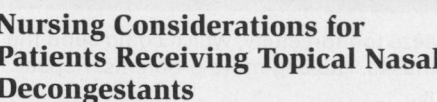

Oral decongestants are drugs that are taken orally to decrease nasal congestion related to the common cold, sinusitis, and allergic rhinitis. They are also used to relieve the pain and congestion of otitis media. Opening of the nasal passage allows better drainage of the eustachian tube, relieving pressure in the middle ear.

Oral decongestants shrink the nasal mucous membrane by stimulating the alpha-adrenergic receptors in the nasal mucous membranes. This shrinkage results in a decrease in membrane size, promoting drainage of the sinuses and improving airflow.

Pharmacokinetics

Pseudoephedrine is generally well absorbed and reaches peak levels quickly—in 20 to 45 minutes. It is widely distributed in the body, metabolized in the liver, and primarily excreted in the urine.

Contraindications and Cautions

Because pseudoephedrine has adrenergic properties, caution should be used in patients with any condition *that might be exacerbated by sympathetic activity*, such as glaucoma, hypertension, diabetes, thyroid disease, coronary disease, and prostate problems. *Because there are no adequate studies about its use during pregnancy and lactation,* such use should be reserved for situations in which the benefit to the mother outweighs any potential risk to the fetus or neonate.

Adverse Effects

Adverse effects associated with pseudoephedrine include rebound congestion. Because this drug is taken systemically, adverse effects related to the sympathomimetic effects are more likely to occur, including feelings of anxiety, tenseness, restlessness, tremors, hypertension, arrhythmias, sweating, and pallor. This drug is found in many OTC cold and flu preparations, and care must be taken to avoid inadvertent overdose when more than one such drug is used.

FOCUS ON Safe Medication Administration

In late 2000 the U.S. Food and Drug Administration (FDA) removed the oral decongestant phenylpropanolamine (PPA) from the market. This drug, which had been the center of controversy for many years, was found to be associated with an increased number of strokes in young women who took it. The drug had been an ingredient in many OTC cold, allergy, and flu remedies. After a short absence, most of these products reappeared on the market with the drug pseudoephedrine taking the place of PPA. This drug, a sympathomimetic, is also known to cause sympathetic effects, including increased blood pressure and increased heart rate. Close follow-up of the effects of this drug will be done to monitor for any increased risk associated with its use.

Clinically Important Drug–Drug Interactions

Many OTC products, including cold remedies, allergy medications, and flu remedies, may contain pseudoephedrine. Taking many of these products concurrently can cause serious adverse effects. Teach patients to read the OTC labels to avoid inadvertent overdose.

Ⓟ Prototype Summary: Pseudoephedrine

Indications: Temporary relief of nasal congestions caused by the common cold, hay fever, sinusitis; promotion of nasal and sinus drainage; relief of eustachian tube congestion.

Actions: Sympathomimetic effects, causes vasoconstriction in mucous membranes of nasal passages resulting in their shrinkage, which promotes drainage and improvement in ventilation.

Pharmacokinetics:

Route	Onset	Duration
Oral	30 min	4–6 h

$T_{1/2}$: 7 hours; metabolized in the liver and excreted in the urine.

Adverse Effects: Anxiety, restlessness, headache, dizziness, drowsiness, vision changes, seizures, hypertension, arrhythmias, pallor, nausea, vomiting, urinary retention, respiratory difficulty.

Nursing Considerations for Patients Receiving an Oral Decongestant

Assessment: History and Examination

- Assess for *possible contraindications or cautions*: Any history of allergy to the drug and pregnancy or lactation, *which are contraindications to drug use*; hypertension or coronary artery disease, *which require cautious use*; and hyperthyroidism, diabetes mellitus, or prostate enlargement, *all of which could be exacerbated by these drugs.*
- Perform a physical examination *to establish baseline data for assessing the effectiveness of the drug and the occurrence of any adverse effects associated with drug therapy.*
- Assess skin color and lesions *to monitor for adverse reactions.*
- Evaluate orientation, reflexes, and affect *to monitor CNS effects of the drug.*
- Monitor blood pressure, pulse, and auscultation *to assess CV stimulations.*

(continues on page 938)

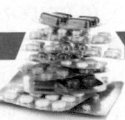

- Evaluate respiration and adventitious sounds *to monitor drug effectiveness.*
- Monitor urinary output *to evaluate for urinary retention.*

Nursing Diagnoses

Nursing diagnoses related to drug therapy might include the following:

- Acute pain related to GI, CNS, or skin effects of the drug
- Increased cardiac output related to sympathomimetic actions of the drug
- Disturbed sensory perception (kinesthetic) related to CNS effects
- Deficient knowledge regarding drug therapy

Planning

- The patient will receive the best therapeutic effect from the drug therapy.
- The patient will have limited adverse effects to the drug therapy.
- The patient will have an understanding of the drug therapy, adverse effects to anticipate, and measures to relieve discomfort and improve safety.

Implementation with Rationale

- Note that this drug is found in many OTC products, especially combination cold and allergy preparations; *care should be taken to prevent inadvertent overdose or excessive adverse effects.*
- Provide safety measures as needed if CNS effects occur *to prevent patient injury.*
- Monitor pulse, blood pressure, and cardiac response to the drug, especially in patients who are at risk for cardiac stimulation, *to detect adverse effects early and arrange to reduce dose or discontinue the drug.*
- Encourage the patient not to use this drug for longer than 1 week, and to seek medical evaluation if symptoms persist after that time, *to encourage the detection of underlying medical conditions that could be causing these symptoms and to arrange for appropriate treatment.*
- Provide thorough patient teaching, including the drug name and prescribed dosage, measures to help avoid adverse effects, warning signs that may indicate problems, and the need for periodic monitoring and evaluation, *to enhance patient knowledge about drug therapy and to promote compliance.*
- Offer support and encouragement *to help the patient cope with the disease and the drug regimen.*

Evaluation

- Monitor patient response to the drug (improvement in nasal congestion).
- Monitor for adverse effects (sympathomimetic reactions, including increased pulse, blood pressure, pallor, sweating, arrhythmias, feelings of anxiety, tension, dry skin).
- Evaluate the effectiveness of the teaching plan (patient can name drug, dosage, adverse effects to watch for, specific measures to avoid them, and measures to take to increase the effectiveness of the drug).
- Monitor the effectiveness of comfort and safety measures and compliance with the regimen.

Topical Nasal Steroid Decongestants

The topical nasal steroid decongestants (Table 54.2) include beclomethasone (*Beconase*, and others), budesonide (*Pulmicort Respules*), flunisolide (generic), fluticasone (generic), and triamcinolone (generic).

Therapeutic Actions and Indications

Topical nasal steroid decongestants are very popular for the treatment of allergic rhinitis and to relieve inflammation after the removal of nasal polyps. They have been found to be effective in patients who are no longer getting a response with other decongestants. The exact mechanism of action of topical steroids is not known. Their anti-inflammatory action results from their ability to produce a direct local effect that blocks many of the complex reactions responsible for the inflammatory response.

Pharmacokinetics

The onset of action is not immediate, and these drugs may actually require up to 1 week to cause any changes. If no effects are seen after 3 weeks the drug should be discontinued. Because these drugs are not generally absorbed systemically, their pharmacokinetics is not reported. If they were to be absorbed systemically, they would have the same pharmacokinetics as other steroids (see Chapter 36).

Contraindications and Cautions

Because nasal steroids block the inflammatory response, their use is contraindicated in the presence of acute infections. Increased incidence of *Candida albicans* infection has been reported with their use, related to the anti-inflammatory and anti-immune activities associated with steroids. Caution should be used in any patient who has an active infection, including tuberculosis, *because systemic absorption would interfere with the inflammatory and immune responses.* Patients using nasal steroids should avoid exposure to any airborne infection, such as chickenpox or measles. As with all drugs, caution should always be used when taking these drugs during pregnancy or lactation. Because the systemic absorption of these drugs is minimal, they are often used during pregnancy and lactation.

Adverse Effects

Because they are applied topically, there is less of a chance of systemic absorption and associated adverse effects. The most common adverse effects are local burning, irritation, stinging, dryness of the mucosa, and headache. Because healing is suppressed by steroids, patients who have recently experienced nasal surgery or trauma should be monitored closely until healing has occurred.

Ⓟ Prototype Summary: Flunisolide

Indications: Treatment of seasonal allergic rhinitis for patients who are not getting any response from other decongestant preparations; relief of inflammation after the removal of nasal polyps.

Actions: Anti-inflammatory action, which results from the ability to produce a direct local effect that blocks many of the complex reactions responsible for the inflammatory response.

Pharmacokinetics:

Route	Onset	Peak	Duration
Topical (nasal spray)	Immediate	10–30 min	4–6 h

$T_{1/2}$: Not generally absorbed systemically.

Adverse Effects: Local burning, irritation, stinging, dryness of the mucosa, headache, increased risk of infection.

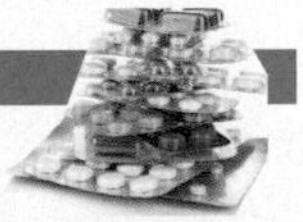

Nursing Considerations for Patients Receiving Topical Steroid Nasal Decongestants

Assessment: History and Examination

- Assess for *possible contraindications or cautions*: Any history of allergy to steroid drugs or any components of the drug vehicle, *which would be a contraindication*, and acute infection, *which would require cautious use.*
- Perform a physical examination *to establish baseline data for assessing the effectiveness of the drug and the occurrence of any adverse effects associated with drug therapy.*
- Perform an intranasal examination *to determine the presence of any lesions that would increase the risk of systemic absorption of the drug.*
- Assess respiration and adventitious sounds *to evaluate drug effectiveness.*
- Monitor temperature *to monitor for the possibility of acute infection.*

Nursing Diagnoses

Nursing diagnoses related to drug therapy might include the following:

- Acute pain related to local effects of the drug
- Risk for injury related to suppression of inflammatory reaction
- Deficient knowledge regarding drug therapy

Planning

- The patient will receive the best therapeutic effect from the drug therapy.
- The patient will have limited adverse effects to the drug therapy.
- The patient will have an understanding of the drug therapy, adverse effects to anticipate, and measures to relieve discomfort and improve safety.

Implementation with Rationale

- Teach the patient how to administer these drugs properly, *which is very important to ensure effectiveness and prevent systemic effects.* A variety of preparations are available (e.g., sprays, aerosols, powder disks). Advise the patient about the proper administration technique for whichever preparation is recommended.
- Have the patient clear the nasal passages before using the drug *to improve its effectiveness.*
- Encourage the patient to continue using the drug regularly, even if results are not seen immediately, *because benefits may take 2 to 3 weeks to appear.*
- Monitor the patient for the development of acute infection that would require medical intervention. Encourage the patient to avoid areas where airborne infections could be a problem *because steroid use decreases the effectiveness of the immune and inflammatory responses.*
- Provide thorough patient teaching, including the drug name and prescribed dosage, measures to help avoid adverse effects, warning signs that may indicate problems, and the need for periodic monitoring and evaluation, *to enhance patient knowledge about drug therapy and to promote compliance.*
- Offer support and encouragement *to help the patient cope with the disease and the drug regimen.*

Evaluation

- Monitor patient response to the drug (relief of nasal congestion).
- Monitor for adverse effects (local burning and stinging).
- Evaluate the effectiveness of the teaching plan (patient can name drug, dosage, adverse effects to watch for, specific measures to avoid them, and measures to take to increase the effectiveness of the drug).
- Monitor the effectiveness of comfort and safety measures and compliance with the regimen.

KEY POINTS

- Decongestants cause local vasoconstriction, thereby reducing blood flow to the mucous membranes of the nasal passages and sinus cavities.
- Rebound vasodilation (rhinitis medicamentosa) is an adverse effect of excessive or long-term decongestant use.
- Topical nasal decongestants are preferred for patients who need to avoid the systemic adrenergic effects associated with oral decongestants.
- Topical nasal steroid decongestants block the inflammatory response and are preferred for patients with allergic rhinitis for whom systemic steroid therapy is undesirable.

Antihistamines

Antihistamines (Table 54.3) block the release or action of histamine, a chemical released during inflammation that increases secretions and narrows airways. Antihistamines are found in multiple OTC preparations that are designed to relieve respiratory symptoms and to treat allergies. When choosing an antihistamine the individual patient's reaction to the drug is usually the governing factor. Because first-generation antihistamines have greater anticholinergic effects with resultant drowsiness a person who needs to be alert should be given one of the second-generation, less-sedating antihistamines. In some people the second-generation antihistamines are also sedating, so care must be taken until the patient knows what response will occur.

Table 54.3 ***Drugs in Focus:* Antihistamines**

Drug Name	Usual Dosage	Usual Indications
First Generation		
brompheniramine (*J-Tan*)	*Adult and pediatric (>12 y):* 6–12 mg PO q12 h *Pediatric (6–12 y):* 6 mg/d PO	Relief of symptoms of seasonal and perennial allergic rhinitis
carbinoxamine (*Histex, Palgic*)	*Adults:* 4–8 mg PO t.i.d. to q.i.d. *Pediatric (1–3 y):* 2 mg PO t.i.d. to q.i.d. *Pediatric (3–6 y):* 2–4 mg PO t.i.d. to q.i.d. *Pediatric (≥6 y):* 4–6 mg PO t.i.d. to q.i.d.	Relief of nasal and nonnasal symptoms of seasonal and perennial rhinitis
chlorpheniramine (*Aller-Chlor*, others)	*Adult and pediatric (>12 y):* 4 mg PO q4–6 h; 8–12 mg at bedtime for sustained release; use caution in elderly patients *Pediatric (6–12 y):* 2 mg PO q4–6 h *Pediatric (2–5 y):* 1 mg PO q4–6 h (sustained release) *Pediatric (6–12 y):* 8 mg PO at bedtime *Pediatric (<6 y):* Not recommended	Relief of symptoms of seasonal and perennial allergic rhinitis, allergic conjunctivitis, uncomplicated urticaria, and angioedema; amelioration of allergic reactions; relief of discomfort associated with dermographism; used as adjunctive therapy in anaphylactic reactions
clemastine (*Tavist Allery*)	*Adult and pediatric (>12 y):* 1.34 mg PO b.i.d.; use caution with elderly patients *Pediatric (6–12 y):* 0.67 mg PO b.i.d. *Pediatric (<6 y):* Not recommended	Relief of symptoms of seasonal and perennial allergic rhinitis, allergic conjunctivitis, uncomplicated urticaria, and angioedema; amelioration of allergic reactions; relief of discomfort associated with dermographism; used as adjunctive therapy in anaphylactic reactions
cyproheptadine (generic)	*Adult:* 4–20 mg/d PO in divided doses *Pediatric (7–14 y):* 4 mg PO b.i.d. to t.i.d. *Pediatric (2–6 y):* 2 mg PO b.i.d. to t.i.d.	Relief of symptoms of seasonal and perennial allergic rhinitis, allergic conjunctivitis, uncomplicated urticaria, and angioedema; amelioration of allergic reactions; relief of discomfort associated with dermographism; used as adjunctive therapy in anaphylactic reactions
dexchlorpheniramine (generic)	*Adult and pediatric (>12 y):* 4–6 mg PO at bedtime or q8–10 h during the day *Pediatric (6–12 y):* 4 mg/d PO at bedtime	Relief of symptoms of seasonal and perennial allergic rhinitis, allergic conjunctivitis, uncomplicated urticaria, and angioedema; amelioration of allergic reactions; relief of discomfort associated with dermographism; used as adjunctive therapy in anaphylactic reactions

Drug Name	Usual Dosage	Usual Indications
dimenhydrinate (*Dimentabs*, others)	*Adult and pediatric (>12 y):* 50–100 mg PO q4–6 h *or* 50 mg IM as needed *Pediatric (<2 y):* 1.25 mg/kg IM q.i.d. *Pediatric (2–6 y):* 25 mg PO q6–8 h *Pediatric (6–12 y):* 25–50 mg PO q6–8 h	Relief of nausea and vomiting associated with motion sickness
diphenhydramine (*Benadryl*, others)	*Adult:* 25–50 mg PO q4–6 h *or* 10–50 mg IM or IV *Pediatric:* 12.5–25 mg PO t.i.d. to q.i.d. *or* 5 mg/kg/d IM or IV *Geriatric:* Use caution	Relief of symptoms of seasonal and perennial allergic rhinitis, allergic conjunctivitis, uncomplicated urticaria, and angioedema; amelioration of allergic reactions; relief of discomfort associated with dermographism; also used as adjunctive therapy in anaphylactic reactions, as a sleeping aid, and for parkinsonism
hydroxyzine (*Vistaril*, others)	*Adult:* 25–100 mg PO t.i.d. to q.i.d. *or* 25–100 mg IM q4–6 h *Pediatric (>6 y):* 50–100 mg/d PO in divided doses *Pediatric (<6 y):* 50 mg/d PO in divided doses *or* 1.1 mg/kg per dose IM	Relief of symptoms of seasonal and perennial allergic rhinitis, allergic conjunctivitis, uncomplicated urticaria, and angioedema; amelioration of allergic reactions; relief of discomfort associated with dermographism; used as adjunctive therapy in anaphylactic reactions; also used for sedation
meclizine (*Antivert*)	*Adult and pediatric (>12 y):* 25–100 mg/d PO; use caution with elderly patients	Relief of nausea and vomiting associated with motion sickness
promethazine (*Phenergan*)	*Adult:* 25 mg PO, PR, IM, or IV *Pediatric:* 6.25–25 mg PO or PR	Relief of symptoms of seasonal and perennial allergic rhinitis, allergic conjunctivitis, uncomplicated urticaria, and angioedema; ameliorates allergic reactions; relief of discomfort associated with dermographism; used as adjunctive therapy in anaphylactic reactions; also used for sedation
triprolidine (generic)	*Adults and pediatric (≥12 y):* 10 mL PO q4–6 h *Pediatric (6–12 y):* 5 mL PO q4–6 h *Pediatric (4–6 y):* 3.75 mL PO q4–6 h *Pediatric (2–4 y):* 2.5 mL PO q4–6 h *Pediatric (4 mo–2 y):* 1.25 mL PO q4–6 h	Relief of signs and symptoms of seasonal and perennial allergic rhinitis
Second Generation (Nonsedating)		
azelastine (*Astelin*)	Two sprays per nostril b.i.d.	Relief of symptoms of seasonal and perennial allergic rhinitis
cetirizine (*Zyrtec*)	*Adult and pediatric (>12 y):* 5–10 mg/d PO; use 5 mg/d with hepatic or renal impairment *Pediatric (6–11 y):* 5 or 10 mg/d PO *Pediatric (6 mo–5 y):* 2.5 mg PO q12 h *or* 5 mg/d PO	Relief of symptoms of seasonal and perennial allergic rhinitis; management of chronic urticaria
desloratadine (*Clarinex*)	*Adult and pediatric (>12 y):* 5 mg/d PO *Pediatric (6–11 y):* 1 tsp, 2.5 mg/5 mL/d PO *Pediatric (12 mo–5 y):* 1/2 tsp, 1.25 mg/2.5 mL/d PO *Pediatric (6–11 mo):* 1 mg/d PO *Hepatic or renal impairment:* 5 mg PO every other day	Relief of symptoms of seasonal allergic rhinitis, chronic idiopathic urticaria
fexofenadine (*Allegra*)	*Adult and pediatric (>12 y):* 60 mg PO b.i.d. *Pediatric (6–11 y):* 30 mg PO b.i.d. *Geriatric or renal-impaired patient:* 60 mg PO every day	Relief of symptoms of seasonal and perennial allergic rhinitis
levocetirizine (*Xyzal*)	*Adults and pediatric (≥12 y):* 5 mg PO, once daily in the evening *Pediatric (6–11 y):* 2.5 mg PO once daily in the evening	Relief of signs and symptoms of seasonal and perennial allergic rhinitis; chronic idiopathic urticaria
loratadine (*Claritin*)	*Adult and pediatric (>6 y):* 10 mg/d PO *Pediatric (2–5 y):* 5 mg/d PO (syrup) *Geriatric or hepatic-impaired patient:* 10 mg PO every other day	Relief of symptoms of seasonal and perennial allergic rhinitis, allergic conjunctivitis, uncomplicated urticaria, and angioedema; amelioration of allergic reactions; relief of discomfort associated with dermographism; and as an adjunctive therapy in anaphylactic reactions

BOX 54.3 FOCUS ON Patient and Family Teaching

Following reports of serious and even fatal adverse effects when OTC cough and cold medicines were used in children under the age of 2 years, the FDA held meetings to evaluate the safety and efficacy of the use of these products in young children. In early 2008, it completed its review and came out with recommendations that these products should not be used in children 4 years of age and younger. In 2009 the FDA suggested that these products not be used in children 6 and younger. While continued research looks at the efficacy and safety of these products for children 6 to 11 years of age the FDA suggests that parents be instructed in the safe use of OTC cough and cold products. Parents should be taught the following:

- Do not give OTC cough and cold products to children younger than 4 years of age unless specifically instructed to do so by a health care provider. Use extreme caution in using these products in children 4 to 6 years of age. Check with a health care provider before deciding to use these products in this age group.
- Do not give your child OTC cough and cold medicines made for adults; look for the Children's, Infant's, or Pediatric use on the label.
- Always check the "Active Ingredients" on the drug label.
- Be very careful if you are giving your child more than one cough and cold medicine; many contain the same active ingredients, and overdose can occur.
- Carefully follow the directions in the "Drug Facts" section of the label and follow the directions for how often you can give the drug.
- Use the measuring spoons or cups that come with the medicine; do not use household spoons, which can vary widely in the amount of medicine they hold.
- Use OTC cough and cold medicines with child-proof caps and keep them out of the reach of children to avoid possible overdose.
- Consult with your health care provider; these drugs only treat signs and symptoms and do not cure any disease; contact your health care provider if the symptoms get worse.
- Do not use these products to make your child sleepy.
- Tell any health care provider taking care of your child the names of any OTC products that you are giving your child.
- Nondrug approaches to handling the symptoms of a cold include: using a humidifier, making sure the child drinks plenty of fluids, use of a bulb syringe aspirator in younger children, use of saline nasal spray or drops to help with congestion, appropriate use of analgesics to help with any pain or discomfort, positioning to promote drainage of fluids. If your child does not improve or continues to have a fever, consult with your health care provider.

Because of their OTC availability, these drugs are often misused to treat colds and influenza (see Box 54.3).

First-generation antihistamines include brompheniramine (*J-Tan*), carbinoxamine (*Histex, Palgic*), chlorpheniramine (*Aller-Chlor*, and others), clemastine (*Tavist Allergy*), cyproheptadine (generic), dexchlorpheniramine (generic), dimenhydrinate (*Dimentabs*, and others), diphenhydramine (*Benadryl*, and others), hydroxyzine (*Vistaril*, and others), meclizine (*Antivert*), promethazine (*Phenergan*), and triprolidine (generic).

Second-generation antihistamines include azelastine (*Astelin*), cetirizine (*Zyrtec*), desloratadine (*Clarinex*), fexofenadine (*Allegra*), levocetirizine (*Xyzal*), and loratadine (*Claritin*).

Therapeutic Actions and Indications

The antihistamines selectively block the effects of histamine at the histamine-1 receptor sites, decreasing the allergic response. They also have anticholinergic (atropine-like) and antipruritic effects. Antihistamines are used for the relief of symptoms associated with seasonal and perennial allergic rhinitis, allergic conjunctivitis, uncomplicated urticaria, and angioedema. They are also used for the amelioration of allergic reactions to blood or blood products, for relief of discomfort associated with dermographism, and as adjunctive therapy in anaphylactic reactions. See Table 54.3 for Usual Indications for each of these agents. Other uses that are being explored include relief of exercise and hyperventilation-induced asthma and histamine-induced bronchoconstriction in asthmatics. They are most effective if used before the onset of symptoms.

Pharmacokinetics

The antihistamines are well absorbed orally, with an onset of action ranging from 1 to 3 hours. They are generally metabolized in the liver, with excretion in the feces and urine. These drugs cross the placenta and enter breast milk (see Contraindications and Cautions).

Contraindications and Cautions

Antihistamines are contraindicated during pregnancy or lactation *unless the benefit to the mother clearly outweighs the potential risk to the fetus or baby*. They should be used with caution in renal or hepatic impairment, *which could alter the metabolism and excretion of the drug*. Special care should be taken when these drugs are used by any patient with a history of arrhythmias or prolonged QT intervals *because fatal cardiac arrhythmias have been associated with the use of certain antihistamines and drugs that increase QT intervals, including erythromycin*. Box 54.3 presents topics for parent education in the use of these OTC products.

Adverse Effects

The adverse effects most often seen with antihistamine use are drowsiness and sedation (see Critical Thinking Scenario for additional information), although second-generation antihistamines are less sedating in many people.

CRITICAL THINKING SCENARIO

Dangers of Self-Medicating for Seasonal Rhinitis

THE SITUATION

K.E. is a 46-year-old businessman who has been self-treating for seasonal rhinitis and a cold. His wife calls the physician's office; she is concerned that her husband is dizzy, has lost his balance several times, and is very drowsy. He is unable to drive to work or to stay awake. She wants to take him to the emergency department of the local hospital.

CRITICAL THINKING

What is the best approach for this patient?

What crucial patient history questions should you ask before proceeding any further?

If you do not know this patient, given his presenting story, what medical conditions would need to be ruled out before proceeding further?

If K.E. is self-medicating for the signs and symptoms of seasonal rhinitis, what could be causing his drowsiness and dizziness?

What teaching points should be emphasized with this patient and his wife?

DISCUSSION

The first impression of K.E.'s condition is that it is a neurological disorder. K.E. should be evaluated by a health care provider to rule out significant neurological problems. However, after a careful patient history and physical examination, K.E.'s condition seemed to be related to high levels of OTC medications.

There are a multitude of OTC cold and allergy remedies, most of which contain the same ingredients in varying proportions. A patient may be taking one to stop his nasal drip, another to help his cough, another to relieve his congestion, and so on. By combining OTC medications like this a patient is at great risk for inadvertently overdosing or at least allowing the medication to reach toxic levels.

In this situation, the first thing to determine is exactly what medication is being taken and how often. K.E. seems to have received toxic levels of antihistamines, decongestants, or other upper respiratory tract agents. The nurse should encourage K.E.—and all patients—to check the labels of any OTC medications being taken and to check with the health care provider if there are any questions. K.E. and his wife should receive written information about the drugs that K.E. is taking. They also should be shown how to read OTC bottles or boxes for information on the contents of various preparations. In addition, they should be encouraged to use alternative methods to relieve the discomfort of seasonal rhinitis (e.g., using a humidifier, drinking lots of liquids, and avoiding smoky areas) to allay the belief that many OTC drugs are needed. Finally, K.E. and his wife should be advised to check with their health care provider if they have any questions about OTC or prescription drugs or if they have continued problems coping with seasonal allergic reactions. Other prescription medication may prove more effective.

NURSING CARE GUIDE FOR K.E.: ANTIHISTAMINES

Assessment: History and Examination

Assess K.E.'s health history for allergies and GI stenosis or obstruction, bladder obstruction, narrow-angle glaucoma, benign prostatic hypertrophy, and concurrent use of MAO inhibitors and OTC allergy or cold products.

Focus the physical examination on the following areas:
CNS: Orientation, reflexes, affect, coordination
Skin: Lesions
CV: Blood pressure, pulse, peripheral perfusion
GI: Bowel sounds, abdominal exam
Hematological: Complete blood count
Respiratory: Respiratory rate and character, nares, adventitious sounds
Genitourinary (GU): Urinary output

Nursing Diagnoses

Acute pain related to GI effects or dry mouth
Decreased cardiac output
Impaired sensory perception (kinesthetic)
Impaired urinary elimination related to thickening mucus
Deficient knowledge regarding drug therapy

Planning

The patient will receive the best therapeutic effect from the drug therapy.

The patient will have limited adverse effects to the drug therapy.

The patient will have an understanding of the drug therapy, adverse effects to anticipate, and measures to relieve discomfort and improve safety.

Implementation

Provide comfort and safety measures (e.g., give drug with meals); teach about mouth care; increase humidity; institute safety measures if dizziness occurs.

Provide support and reassurance to deal with drug effects and allergy.

Provide patient teaching regarding drug name, dosage, adverse effects, precautions, and warning signs to report.

(continues on page 944)

Dangers of Self-Medicating for Seasonal Rhinitis (continued)

Evaluation

Evaluate drug effects (i.e., relief of respiratory symptoms).

Monitor for adverse effects: CNS effects, thickening of secretions, urinary retention, glaucoma.

Monitor for drug–drug interactions as indicated.

Evaluate the effectiveness of support and encouragement strategies, patient-teaching program, and comfort and safety measures.

PATIENT TEACHING FOR K.E.

- Antihistamines are commonly used to treat the signs and symptoms of various allergic reactions. Because these drugs work throughout the body, many systemic effects can occur with their use (e.g., dry mouth, dizziness, drowsiness).
- Take this drug only as prescribed. Do not increase the dose if symptoms are not relieved. Instead, consult your health care provider.
- Common effects of this drug include:
  - *Drowsiness, dizziness:* Do not drive or operate dangerous machinery if this occurs. Use caution to prevent injury.
  - *GI upset, nausea, vomiting, heartburn:* Taking the drug with food may help this problem.
  - *Dry mouth:* Frequent mouth care and sucking sugarless lozenges may help.
  - *Thickening of the mucus, difficulty coughing, tightening of the chest:* Use a humidifier or, if you do not have one, place pans of water throughout the house to increase the humidity of the room air; avoid smoke-filled areas; drink plenty of fluids.
  - Report any of the following to your health care provider: *Difficulty breathing, rash, hives, difficulty in voiding, abdominal pain, visual changes, disorientation or confusion.*
- Avoid the use of alcoholic beverages while you are taking this drug. Serious drowsiness or sedation can occur if these are combined.
- Avoid the use of any OTC medication without first checking with your health care provider. Several of these medications contain drugs that can interfere with the effectiveness of this drug or they can contain very similar drugs and you could experience toxic effects.
- Tell any doctor, nurse, or other health care provider involved in your care that you are taking this drug.
- Take this drug only as prescribed. Do not give this drug to anyone else, and do not take similar preparations that have been prescribed for someone else. Keep this drug, and all medications, out of the reach of children.

The anticholinergic effects that can be anticipated include drying of the respiratory and GI mucous membranes, GI upset and nausea, arrhythmias, dysuria, urinary hesitancy, and skin eruption and itching associated with dryness.

Clinically Important Drug–Drug Interactions

Drug–drug interactions vary among the antihistamines; for example, anticholinergic effects may be prolonged if diphenhydramine is taken with an MAO inhibitor, and the interaction of fexofenadine with ketoconazole or erythromycin may raise fexofenadine concentrations to toxic levels. For more information, consult a nursing drug handbook or package insert for individual details.

Prototype Summary: Diphenhydramine

Indications: Symptomatic relief of perennial and seasonal rhinitis, vasomotor rhinitis, allergic conjunctivitis, urticaria, and angioedema; also used for treating motion sickness and parkinsonism and as a nighttime sleep aid and to suppress coughs.

Actions: Competitively blocks the effects of histamine at histamine-1 receptor sites; has atropine-like antipruritic and sedative effects.

Pharmacokinetics:

Route	Onset	Peak	Duration
Oral	15–30 min	1–4 h	4–7 h
IM	20–30 min	1–4 h	4–8 h
IV	Rapid	30–60 min	4–8 h

$T_{1/2}$: 2.5 to 7 hours; metabolized in the liver and excreted in the urine.

Adverse Effects: Drowsiness, sedation, dizziness, epigastric distress, thickening of bronchial secretions, urinary frequency, rash, bradycardia.

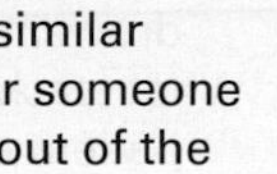

Nursing Considerations for Patients Receiving Antihistamines

Assessment: History and Examination

- Assess for *possible contraindications or cautions*: Any history of allergy to antihistamines; pregnancy or lactation; and prolonged QT interval, *which are contraindications to the use of the drug*; and renal or hepatic impairment, *which requires cautious use of the drug.*

- Perform a physical examination *to establish baseline data for assessing the effectiveness of the drug and the occurrence of any adverse effects associated with drug therapy.*
- Assess the skin color, texture, and lesions *to monitor for anticholinergic effects or allergy.*
- Evaluate orientation, affect, and reflexes *to monitor for changes due to CNS effects.*
- Assess respirations and adventitious sounds *to monitor for drug effects.*
- Evaluate liver and renal function tests *to monitor for factors that could affect the metabolism or excretion of the drug.*

Nursing Diagnoses

Nursing diagnoses related to drug therapy might include the following:

- Acute pain related to GI, CNS, or skin effects of the drug
- Disturbed sensory perception (kinesthetic) related to CNS effects
- Deficient knowledge regarding drug therapy

Planning

- The patient will receive the best therapeutic effect from the drug therapy.
- The patient will have limited adverse effects to the drug therapy.
- The patient will have an understanding of the drug therapy, adverse effects to anticipate, and measures to relieve discomfort and improve safety

Implementation with Rationale

- Administer drug on an empty stomach, 1 hour before or 2 hours after meals, *to increase the absorption of the drug*; the drug may be given with meals if GI upset is a problem.
- Note that the patient may have poor response to one of these agents but a very effective response to another; the prescriber may need to try several different agents *to find the one that is most effective.*
- Because of the drying nature of antihistamines, patients often experience dry mouth, which may lead to nausea and anorexia; suggest sugarless candies or lozenges *to relieve some of this discomfort.*
- Provide safety measures as appropriate if CNS effects occur *to prevent patient injury.*
- Increase humidity and push fluids *to decrease the problem of thickened secretions and dry nasal mucosa.*
- Have patient void before each dose *to decrease urinary retention if this is a problem.*
- Provide skin care as needed if skin dryness and lesions become a problem *to prevent skin breakdown.*
- Caution the patient to avoid excessive dose and to check OTC drugs for the presence of antihistamines, *which are found in many OTC preparations and could cause toxicity.*
- Caution the patient to avoid alcohol while taking these drugs *because serious sedation can occur.*
- Provide thorough patient teaching, including the drug name and prescribed dosage, measures to help avoid adverse effects, warning signs that may indicate problems, and the need for periodic monitoring and evaluation, *to enhance patient knowledge about drug therapy and to promote compliance.*
- Offer support and encouragement *to help the patient cope with the disease and the drug regimen.*

Evaluation

- Monitor patient response to the drug (relief of the symptoms of allergic rhinitis).
- Monitor for adverse effects (skin dryness, GI upset, sedation and drowsiness, urinary retention, thickened secretions, glaucoma).
- Evaluate the effectiveness of the teaching plan (patient can name drug, dosage, adverse effects to watch for, specific measures to avoid them, and measures to take to increase the effectiveness of the drug).
- Monitor the effectiveness of comfort and safety measures and compliance with the regimen.

KEY POINTS

- The antihistamines selectively block the effects of histamine at the histamine-1 receptor sites, decreasing the allergic response. Antihistamines are used for the relief of symptoms associated with seasonal and perennial allergic rhinitis, allergic conjunctivitis, uncomplicated urticaria, and angioedema.
- Patients taking antihistamines may react to dryness of the skin and mucous membranes. The nurse should encourage them to drink plenty of fluids, use a humidifier if possible, avoid smoke-filled rooms, and use good skin care and moisturizers.
- Antihistamines should be avoided with any patient who has a prolonged QT interval because serious cardiac complications and even death have occurred.

Expectorants

Expectorants (Table 54.4) increase productive cough to clear the airways. They liquefy lower respiratory tract secretions, reducing the viscosity of these secretions and making it easier for the patient to cough them up. Expectorants are available in many OTC preparations, making them widely available to the patient without advice from a health care provider. Currently, the only available expectorant is guaifenesin (*Mucinex*, and others).

Table 54.4 ***Drugs in Focus:* Expectorant**

Drug Name	Usual Dosage	Usual Indications
guaifenesin (*Mucinex*, others)	*Adult and pediatric (>12 y)*: 200–400 mg PO q4 h *Pediatric (6–12 y)*: 100–200 mg PO q4 h *Pediatric (2–6 y)*: 50–100 mg PO q4 h	Symptomatic relief of respiratory conditions characterized by a dry, nonproductive cough, including the common cold, acute bronchitis, and influenza

Therapeutic Actions and Indications

Guaifenesin enhances the output of respiratory tract fluids by reducing the adhesiveness and surface tension of these fluids, allowing easier movement of the less viscous secretions. The result of this thinning of secretions is a more productive cough and thus decreased frequency of coughing. See Table 54.4 for Usual Indications.

Pharmacokinetics

Guaifenesin is rapidly absorbed, with an onset of 30 minutes and a duration of 4 to 6 hours. Sites of metabolism and excretion have not been reported.

Contraindications and Cautions

This drug should not be used in patients with a known allergy to the drug *to prevent hypersensitivity reactions*, and it should be used with caution in pregnancy and lactation *because of the potential for adverse effects on the fetus or baby* and with persistent coughs, *which could be indicative of underlying medical problems.*

Adverse Effects

The most common adverse effects associated with expectorants are GI symptoms (e.g., nausea, vomiting, anorexia). Some patients experience headache, dizziness, or both; occasionally, a mild rash develops. The most important consideration in the use of these drugs is discovering the cause of the underlying cough. Prolonged use of OTC preparations could result in the masking of important symptoms of a serious underlying disorder. These drugs should not be used for more than 1 week; if the cough persists, encourage the patient to seek health care.

Ⓟ Prototype Summary: Guaifenesin

Indications: Symptomatic relief of respiratory conditions characterized by dry, nonproductive cough and in the presence of mucus in the respiratory tract.

Actions: Enhances the output of respiratory tract fluid by reducing the adhesiveness and surface tension of the fluid, facilitating the removal of viscous mucus.

Pharmacokinetics:

Route	Onset	Peak	Duration
Oral	30 min	Unknown	4–6 h

$T_{1/2}$: Unknown; metabolism and excretion are also unknown.

Adverse Effects: Nausea, vomiting, headache, dizziness, rash.

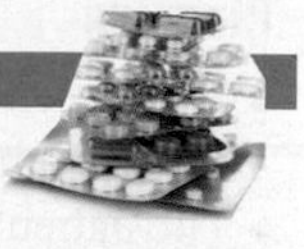

Nursing Considerations for Patients Receiving Expectorants

Assessment: History and Examination

- Assess for *possible contraindications or cautions*: Any history of allergy to the drug; persistent cough due to smoking, asthma, or emphysema, *which would be cautions to the use of the drug*; and very productive cough, *which would indicate an underlying problem that should be evaluated.*
- Perform a physical examination *to establish baseline data for assessing the effectiveness of the drug and the occurrence of any adverse effects associated with drug therapy.*
- Assess the skin *for the presence of lesions and color to monitor for any adverse reactions.*
- Monitor temperature *to assess for an underlying infection.*
- Assess respirations and adventitious sounds *to evaluate the respiratory response to the drug effects.*
- Monitor orientation and affect *to monitor CNS effects of the drug.*

Nursing Diagnoses

Nursing diagnoses related to drug therapy might include the following:

- Acute pain related to GI, CNS, or skin effects of the drug
- Disturbed sensory perception (kinesthetic) related to CNS effects
- Deficient knowledge regarding drug therapy

Planning

- The patient will receive the best therapeutic effect from the drug therapy.
- The patient will have limited adverse effects to the drug therapy.
- The patient will have an understanding of the drug therapy, adverse effects to anticipate, and measures to relieve discomfort and improve safety.

Implementation with Rationale

- Caution the patient not to use these drugs for longer than 1 week and to seek medical attention if the cough persists after that time *to evaluate for any underlying medical condition and to arrange for appropriate treatment.*
- Advise the patient to take small, frequent meals *to alleviate some of the GI discomfort associated with these drugs.*
- Advise the patient to avoid driving or performing dangerous tasks if dizziness and drowsiness occur *to prevent patient injury.*
- Alert the patient that these drugs may be found in OTC preparations and that care should be taken *to avoid excessive doses.*
- Provide thorough patient teaching, including the drug name and prescribed dosage, measures to help avoid adverse effects, warning signs that may indicate problems, and the need for periodic monitoring and evaluation, *to enhance patient knowledge about drug therapy and to promote compliance.*
- Offer support and encouragement *to help the patient cope with the disease and the drug regimen.*

Evaluation

- Monitor patient response to the drug (improved effectiveness of cough).
- Monitor for adverse effects (skin rash, GI upset, CNS effects).
- Evaluate the effectiveness of the teaching plan (patient can name drug, dosage, adverse effects to watch for, specific measures to avoid them, and measures to take to increase the effectiveness of the drug).
- Monitor the effectiveness of comfort and safety measures and compliance with the regimen.

KEY POINTS

- Expectorants are drugs that liquefy the lower respiratory tract secretions. They are used for the symptomatic relief of respiratory conditions characterized by a dry, nonproductive cough.
- Guaifenesin is the only expectorant currently available. Care should be taken to avoid inadvertent overdose when using OTC products that might contain this drug.

Mucolytics

Mucolytics (Table 54.5) increase or liquefy respiratory secretions to aid the clearing of the airways in high-risk respiratory patients who are coughing up thick, tenacious secretions. Patients may be suffering from conditions such as chronic obstructive pulmonary disease (COPD), cystic fibrosis, pneumonia, or tuberculosis. Mucolytics include acetylcysteine (generic) and dornase alfa (*Pulmozyme*).

Therapeutic Actions and Indications

Acetylcysteine is used orally to protect liver cells from being damaged during episodes of acetaminophen toxicity because it normalizes hepatic glutathione levels and binds with a reactive hepatotoxic metabolite of acetaminophen. Acetylcysteine affects the mucoproteins in the respiratory secretions by splitting apart disulfide bonds that are responsible for holding the mucus material together. The result is a decrease in the tenacity and viscosity of the secretions. See Table 54.5 for Usual Indications.

Dornase alfa is a mucolytic prepared by recombinant DNA techniques that selectively break down respiratory tract mucus by separating extracellular DNA from proteins. It is used in cystic fibrosis, which is characterized by thick, tenacious mucous production. See Table 54.5 for Usual Indications. See Box 54.4 for information about targeted treatment of cystic fibrosis.

Pharmacokinetics

The medication may be administered by nebulization or by direct instillation into the trachea via an endotracheal tube or tracheostomy.

Acetylcysteine is metabolized in the liver and excreted somewhat in the urine. It is not known whether it crosses the placenta or enters breast milk. Dornase alfa has a long duration of action, and its fate in the body is not known.

Contraindications and Cautions

Caution should be used in cases of acute bronchospasm, peptic ulcer, and esophageal varices *because the increased secretions could aggravate the problem.* There are no data on the effects of the drugs in pregnancy or lactation.

Adverse Effects

Adverse effects most commonly associated with mucolytic drugs include GI upset, stomatitis, rhinorrhea, bronchospasm, and occasionally a rash.

Table 54.5 *Drugs in Focus:* Mucolytics

Drug Name	Usual Dosage	Usual Indications
acetylcysteine (generic)	By nebulization, 2–20 mL of 10% solution q2–6 h; by direct instillation, 1–2 mL of 10–20% solution q1–4 h; 140 mg/kg PO loading dose, then 17 doses of 70 mg/kg PO q4 h as an antidote	Liquefaction of secretions in high-risk respiratory patients who have difficulty moving secretions, including postoperative patients (e.g., patients with tracheostomies to facilitate airway clearance and suctioning); clearing of secretions for diagnostic tests (e.g., diagnostic bronchoscopy); used orally to protect the liver from acetaminophen toxicity; treatment of atelectasis from thick mucus secretions
dornase alfa (*Pulmozyme*)	2.5 mg inhaled through nebulizer, may increase to 2.5 mg b.i.d. if needed	To relieve the buildup of secretions in high-risk respiratory patients who have difficulty moving secretions, including postoperative patients (e.g., patients with tracheostomies to facilitate airway clearance and suctioning); clearing of secretions for diagnostic tests (e.g., diagnostic bronchoscopy); treatment of atelectasis from thick mucus secretions as in cystic fibrosis

Ⓟ Prototype Summary: Acetylcysteine

Indications: Mucolytic adjunctive therapy for abnormal, viscid, or inspissated mucous secretions in acute and chronic bronchopulmonary disorders; to lessen hepatic injury in cases of acetaminophen toxicity.

Actions: Splits links in the mucoproteins contained in the respiratory mucus secretions, decreasing the viscosity of the secretions; protects liver cells from acetaminophen effects.

Pharmacokinetics:

Route	Onset	Peak	Duration
Instillation, inhalation	1 min	5–10 min	2–3 h
Oral	30–60 min	1–2 h	Unknown

$T_{1/2}$: 6.25 hours; metabolized in the liver and excreted in the urine.

Adverse Effects: Nausea, stomatitis, urticaria, bronchospasm, rhinorrhea.

BOX 54.4

Targeted Treatment of Cystic Fibrosis

In 2013, ivacaftor (*Kalydeco*) became available for the treatment of cystic fibrosis. It is a cystic fibrosis transmembrane conductance regulator (CFTR) that facilitates increased chloride transport at the surface of epithelial cells in multiple organs. In these cystic fibrosis patients the end result was improved lung function. It is approved for patients 6 years and older who have specific CFTR gene mutations: G551D, G1244E, G1349D, G178R, Grr1S, S1251N, S1255P, S549N, S549R, or R117H. The FDA has approved a cystic fibrosis mutation test that can be used to determine the appropriateness of this drug. It is an oral agent and needs to be used with caution in patients with liver impairment or those also using CYP3A inhibitors. The most common adverse effects include abdominal pain, rash, nausea, dizziness, headache, and sore throat.

Nursing Considerations for Patients Receiving Mucolytics

Assessment: History and Examination

- Assess for *possible contraindications or cautions:* Any history of allergy to the drugs and the presence of acute bronchospasm, *which are contraindications to the use of these drugs;* and peptic ulcer and esophageal varices, *which would require careful monitoring and cautious use.*
- Perform a physical examination *to establish baseline data for assessing the effectiveness of the drug and the occurrence of any adverse effects associated with drug therapy.*
- Assess skin color and lesions *to monitor for adverse reactions.*
- Monitor blood pressure and pulse *to evaluate cardiac response to drug treatment.*
- Evaluate respirations and adventitious sounds *to monitor drug effectiveness.*

Nursing Diagnoses

Nursing diagnoses related to drug therapy might include the following:

- Acute pain related to GI, CNS, or skin effects of the drug
- Disturbed sensory perception (kinesthetic) related to CNS effects
- Ineffective airway clearance related to bronchospasm
- Deficient knowledge regarding drug therapy

Planning

- The patient will receive the best therapeutic effect from the drug therapy.
- The patient will have limited adverse effects to the drug therapy.
- The patient will have an understanding of the drug therapy, adverse effects to anticipate, and measures to relieve discomfort and improve safety.

Implementation with Rationale

- Avoid combining with other drugs in the nebulizer *to avoid the formation of precipitates and potential loss of effectiveness of either drug.*
- Dilute concentrate with sterile water for injection *if buildup becomes a problem that could impede drug delivery.*
- Note that patients receiving acetylcysteine by face mask should have the residue wiped off the facemask and off their face with plain water *to prevent skin breakdown.*
- Review use of the nebulizer with patients receiving dornase alfa at home *to ensure the most effective use of the drug.* Patients should be cautioned to store the drug in the refrigerator, protected from light.
- Caution cystic fibrosis patients receiving dornase alfa about the need to continue all therapies for their cystic fibrosis *because dornase alfa is only a palliative therapy that improves respiratory symptoms, and other therapies are still needed.*
- Provide thorough patient teaching, including the drug name and prescribed dosage, measures to help avoid adverse effects, warning signs that may indicate problems, and the need for periodic monitoring and evaluation, *to enhance patient knowledge about drug therapy and to promote compliance.*
- Offer support and encouragement *to help the patient cope with the disease and the drug regimen.*

Evaluation

- Monitor patient response to the drug (improvement of respiratory symptoms and loosening of secretions).
- Monitor for adverse effects (CNS effects, skin rash, bronchospasm, and GI upset).
- Evaluate the effectiveness of the teaching plan (patient can name drug, dosage, adverse effects to watch for, specific measures to avoid them, and measures to take to increase the effectiveness of the drug).
- Monitor the effectiveness of comfort and safety measures and compliance with the regimen.

KEY POINTS

- Mucolytics work to break down mucus to aid high-risk respiratory patients in coughing up thick, tenacious secretions.
- Dornase alfa is specific for the treatment of patients with cystic fibrosis, which is characterized by a thick, tenacious mucus production that can block airways.

SUMMARY

- The classes of drugs that affect the upper respiratory system work to keep the airways open and gases moving efficiently.
- Antitussives are drugs that suppress the cough reflex. They can act centrally to suppress the medullary cough center or locally to increase secretion and buffer irritation or to act as local anesthetics. These drugs should not be used longer than 1 week; patients with persistent cough after that time should seek medical evaluation.
- Decongestants are drugs that cause local vasoconstriction and therefore decrease the blood flow to the irritated and dilated capillaries of the mucous membranes lining the nasal passages and sinus cavities.
- An adverse effect that accompanies frequent or prolonged use of decongestants is rebound vasodilation, called rhinitis medicamentosa. The reflex reaction to vasoconstriction is a rebound vasodilation, which often leads to prolonged overuse of decongestants.
- Topical nasal decongestants are preferable in patients who need to avoid systemic adrenergic effects. Oral decongestants are associated with systemic adrenergic effects and require caution in patients with CV disease, hyperthyroidism, or diabetes mellitus.
- Topical nasal steroid decongestants block the inflammatory response from occurring. These drugs, which take several days to weeks to reach complete effectiveness, are preferred for patients with allergic rhinitis who need to avoid the complications of systemic steroid therapy.
- The antihistamines selectively block the effects of histamine at the histamine-1 receptor sites, decreasing the allergic response. Antihistamines are used for the relief of symptoms associated with seasonal and perennial allergic rhinitis, allergic conjunctivitis, uncomplicated urticaria, or angioedema.
- Patients taking antihistamines may react to dryness of the skin and mucous membranes. The nurse should encourage them to drink plenty of fluids, use a humidifier if possible, avoid smoke-filled rooms, and use good skin care and moisturizers.
- Antihistamines should be avoided with any patient who has a prolonged QT interval because serious cardiac complications and even death have occurred.
- Expectorants are drugs that liquefy lower respiratory tract secretions. They are used for the symptomatic relief of respiratory conditions characterized by a dry, nonproductive cough.
- Mucolytics work to break down mucus to aid high-risk respiratory patients in coughing up thick, tenacious secretions.
- Many of the drugs that act on the upper respiratory tract are found in various OTC cough and allergy preparations. Patients need to be advised to always read the labels carefully to avoid inadvertent overdose and toxicity.

CHECK YOUR UNDERSTANDING

Answers to the questions in this chapter can be found in Answers to Check Your Understanding Questions on thePoint®.

MULTIPLE CHOICE

Select the best answer to the following.

1. A patient with sinus pressure and pain related to seasonal rhinitis would benefit from taking
   a. an antitussive.
   b. an expectorant.
   c. a mucolytic.
   d. a decongestant.

2. Antitussives are useful in blocking the cough reflex and preserving the energy associated with prolonged, nonproductive coughing. Antitussives are best used with
   a. postoperative patients.
   b. asthma patients.
   c. patients with a dry, irritating cough.
   d. COPD patients who tire easily.

3. Patients with seasonal rhinitis experience irritation and inflammation of the nasal passages and passages of the upper airways. Treatment for these patients might include
   a. systemic corticosteroids.
   b. mucolytic agents.
   c. an expectorant.
   d. topical nasal steroids.

4. A patient taking an OTC cold medication and an OTC allergy medicine is found to be taking double doses of pseudoephedrine. As a result, the patient might exhibit
   a. ear pain and eye redness.
   b. restlessness and palpitations.
   c. sinus pressure and ear pain.
   d. an irritating cough and nasal drainage.

5. Antihistamines should be used very cautiously in patients with
   a. a history of arrhythmias or prolonged QT intervals.
   b. COPD or bronchitis.
   c. asthma or seasonal rhinitis.
   d. angioedema or low blood pressure.

6. A patient is not getting a response to the antihistamine that was prescribed. Appropriate action might include
   a. switching to a decongestant.
   b. stopping the drug and increasing fluids.
   c. trying a different antihistamine.
   d. switching to a corticosteroid.

7. Dornase alfa (*Pulmozyme*), because of its mechanism of action, is reserved for use in
   a. clearing secretions before diagnostic tests.
   b. facilitating the removal of secretions postoperatively.
   c. protecting the liver from acetaminophen toxicity.
   d. relieving the buildup of secretions in cystic fibrosis.

MULTIPLE RESPONSE

Select all that apply.

1. Common adverse effects associated with the use of topical nasal steroids would include which of the following?
   a. Local burning and stinging
   b. Dryness of the mucosa
   c. Headache
   d. Constipation and urinary retention
   e. Fungal infections
   f. Osteonecrosis

2. An antihistamine would be the drug of choice for treating which of the following?
   a. Itchy eyes
   b. Irritating cough
   c. Nasal congestion
   d. Runny nose
   e. Idiopathic urticaria
   f. Thick, tenacious secretions

3. Additional nursing interventions for clients receiving antihistamines probably would include which of the following?
   a. Using a humidifier
   b. Advising the client to suck sugarless lozenges to help relieve the dry mouth
   c. Limiting fluid intake to decrease swelling
   d. Providing safety measures to prevent falls or injury
   e. Encouraging pushing fluids, if allowed
   f. Leaving bowls of water around the house to increase humidity

BIBLIOGRAPHY AND REFERENCES

Adkinson, F., Holgate, S., Busse., W., et al. (2009). *Middleton's allergy: Principles and practice* (7th ed.). St. Louis, MO: Mosby.

Brunton, L., Chabner, B., & Knollman, B. (2011). *Goodman and Gilman's the pharmacological basis of therapeutics* (12th ed.). New York: McGraw-Hill.

Dykewicz, M. (2011). Management of rhinitis: Guidelines, evidence basis and systematic clinical approach. *Immunology and Allergy Clinics, 31*(3), 619–634.

Facts and Comparisons. (2015). *Drug facts and comparisons*. St. Louis, MO: Author.

Facts and Comparisons. (2015). *Professional's guide to patient drug facts*. St. Louis, MO: Author.

Irwin, R. S., Baumann, M. H., Bolser, D. C., et al. (2006). Diagnosis and management of cough executive summary: ACCP evidence-based clinical practice guidelines. *Chest, 129*(1 Suppl.), 1S–23S.

Karch, A. M. (2014). *Lippincott's nursing drug guide*. Philadelphia, PA: Lippincott Williams & Wilkins.

Nguyen, P., Vickery, J., & Blaiss, M. (2011). Management of rhinitis: Allergic and non-allergic. *Allergy Asthma and Immunology Research, 3*(3), 148–156.

Tharpe, C., & Kemp, S. (2014). Pediatric allergic rhinitis. *Immunology and Allergy Clinics, 35*(1), 185–198.

The Medical Letter. (2012). *The medical letter on drugs and therapeutics*. New Rochelle, NY: Author.

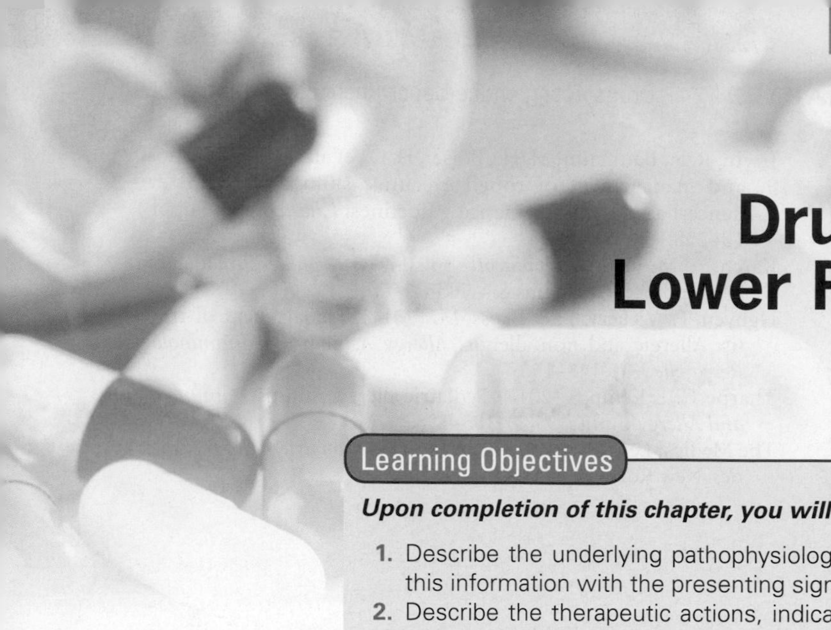

55 Drugs Acting on the Lower Respiratory Tract

Learning Objectives

Upon completion of this chapter, you will be able to:

1. Describe the underlying pathophysiology involved in obstructive pulmonary disease and correlate this information with the presenting signs and symptoms.
2. Describe the therapeutic actions, indications, pharmacokinetics, contraindications, most common adverse reactions, and important drug–drug interactions associated with drugs used to treat lower respiratory tract disorders.
3. Discuss the use of drugs used to treat obstructive pulmonary disorders across the lifespan.
4. Compare and contrast the prototype drugs used to treat obstructive pulmonary disorders with other agents in their class and with other classes of drugs used to treat obstructive pulmonary disorders.
5. Outline the nursing considerations, including important teaching points, for patients receiving drugs used to treat obstructive pulmonary disorders.

Glossary of Key Terms

bronchodilator: medication used to facilitate respirations by dilating the airways; helpful in symptomatic relief or prevention of bronchial asthma and bronchospasm associated with chronic obstructive pulmonary disease

Cheyne-Stokes respiration: abnormal pattern of breathing characterized by apneic periods followed by periods of tachypnea; may reflect delayed blood flow through the brain

leukotriene receptor antagonists: drugs that selectively and competitively block or antagonize receptors for the production of leukotrienes D_4 and E_4, components of slow-reacting substance of anaphylaxis (SRSA)

mast cell stabilizer: drug that works at the cellular level to inhibit the release of histamine (released from mast cells in response to inflammation or irritation) and the release of slow-reacting substance of anaphylaxis (SRSA)

sympathomimetics: drugs that mimic the effects of the sympathetic nervous system

xanthenes: naturally occurring substances, including caffeine and theophylline, that have a direct effect on the smooth muscle of the respiratory tract, both in the bronchi and in the blood vessels

Drug List

Bronchodilators/ Antiasthmatics

Xanthines
(P) aminophylline
caffeine
dyphylline
theophylline

Sympathomimetics
albuterol
arformoterol
ephedrine
(P) epinephrine
formoterol
indacaterol
isoproterenol
levalbuterol
metaproterenol
olodaterol
salmeterol
terbutaline

Anticholinergics
(P) ipratropium
tiotropium
umeclidinium

Drugs Affecting Inflammation

Inhaled Steroids
beclomethasone
(P) budesonide
ciclesonide
fluticasone
triamcinolone

Leukotriene Receptor Antagonists
montelukast
(P) zafirlukast
zileuton

Lung Surfactants
(P) beractant
calfactant
poractan

Drugs for Pulmonary Fibrosis
intedanib
perfenisone

The lower respiratory tract includes the bronchial tree and the alveoli, where gas exchange occurs (see Figure 55.1). Disorders of the lower respiratory tract can have a direct impact on gas exchange and oxygenation and can include infections such as bronchiectasis, bronchitis, and pneumonia and obstructive disorders that directly interfere with airflow to the alveoli.

Pulmonary obstructive diseases include asthma and chronic obstructive pulmonary disease (COPD), which includes emphysema and chronic bronchitis. (See Chapter 53 for detailed pathophysiology.) These diseases cause obstruction of the major airways and may lead to complications such as infections, pneumonia, and movement of inhaled substances deep into the respiratory system. The obstruction of asthma and COPD can be related to inflammation that results in narrowing of the interior of the airway and to muscular constriction that results in narrowing of the conducting tube (Figure 55.2). Asthma is associated with the development of immunoglobulin E (IgE) antibodies to specific antigens that, when activated, cause the immediate release of inflammatory chemicals from mast cells. The reaction to the chemicals causes rapid swelling of the inner lining of the airways and a narrowing of the conducting tubes. COPD is most often caused by chronic exposure to irritants that cause a chronic inflammation and swelling in the airway. Cigarette smoking is the leading cause of COPD. With chronic inflammation, muscular and cilial action is lost, and complications related to the loss of these protective processes can occur, such as infections, pneumonia, and movement of inhaled substances deep into the respiratory system. In severe COPD, air is trapped in the lower respiratory tract, the alveoli degenerate and fuse together, and the exchange of gases is greatly impaired. See Box 55.1 for reducing COPD exacerbations.

The first step for treatment includes reducing environmental exposure to irritants such as stopping smoking, filtering allergens from the air, and avoiding exposure to known irritants and allergens. If these efforts are not sufficient to prevent problems, treatment is aimed at either opening the conducting airways through muscular bronchodilation or decreasing the effects of inflammation on the lining of the airway. See Table 55.1 for guidelines for maintenance treatment of asthma.

Additional obstructive pulmonary diseases are respiratory distress syndrome (RDS), which causes obstruction at the alveolar level and is seen in neonates, and adult respiratory distress syndrome (ARDS), which is characterized by progressive loss of lung compliance and increasing hypoxia. This syndrome occurs as a result of a severe insult to the body, such as cardiovascular (CV) collapse, major burns, severe trauma, and rapid depressurization. The obstruction of RDS in the neonate is related to a lack of the lipoprotein surfactant, which leads to an inability to maintain an open alveolus. Surfactant is essential in decreasing the surface tension in the tiny alveolus, allowing it to expand

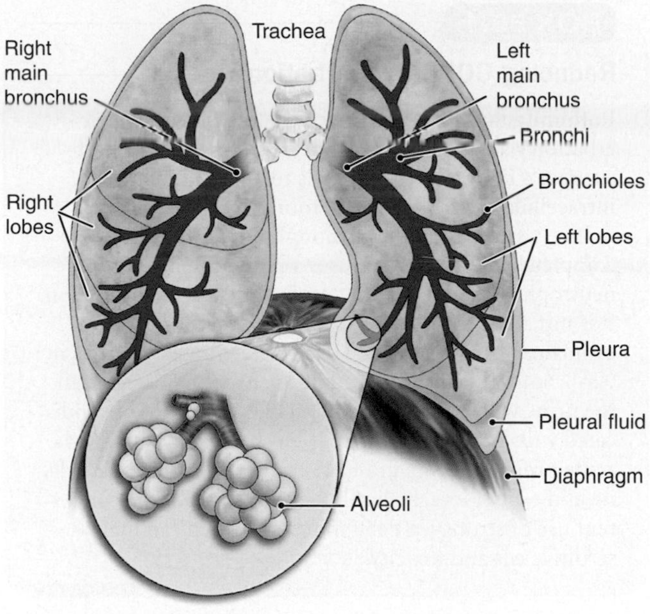

FIGURE 55.1 The lower respiratory tract.

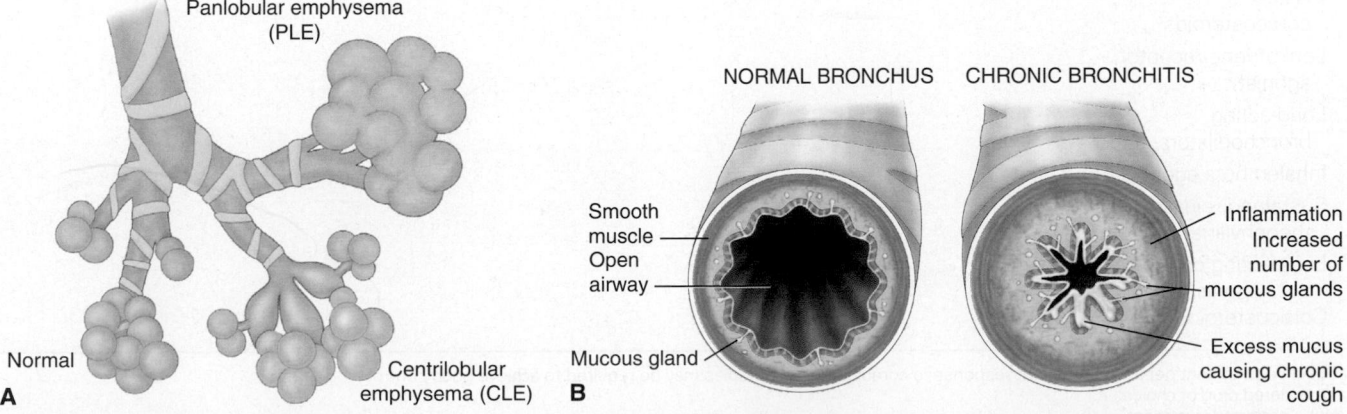

FIGURE 55.2 Changes in the airways with chronic obstructive pulmonary disease. A. Example of alveolar changes in COPD. B. Airway changes in bronchitis.

BOX 55.1

Reducing COPD Exacerbation

Roflumilast (*Daliresp*) is now available to reduce exacerbation risk in patients with COPD. It is a phosphodiesterase 4 inhibitor, which leads to an accumulation of intracellular cyclic adenosine monophosphate (AMP) in lung tissues. This effect, though the action is not completely understood, causes a reduction in sputum neutrophils and eosinophils and improved lung function. It is not a bronchodilator and cannot be used for acute bronchospasm. It is an oral agent, reaching peak levels in 0.5–1 hour. It is metabolized in the liver and excreted in the urine with a half-life of 17–30 hours. It is contraindicated with liver impairment. It has been associated with acute bronchospasm and CNS changes including suicidality and weight loss. It should be avoided with the concurrent use of strong CYP450 inducers, which can increase serum levels and toxicity.

and remain open. If surfactant is lacking the alveoli collapse and gas exchange cannot occur. Pharmacological therapy for RDS involves instilling surfactant into the alveoli. The treatment of ARDS involves reversal of the underlying cause of the problem combined with ventilatory support. See Box 55.2 for the use of lower respiratory tract agents with different age groups.

Bronchodilators/Antiasthmatics

Bronchodilators (Table 55.2), or antiasthmatics, are medications used to facilitate respiration by dilating the airways. They are helpful in symptomatic relief or prevention of bronchial asthma and for bronchospasm associated with COPD. Several of the bronchodilators are administered orally and absorbed systemically, giving them the potential for many systemic adverse effects. Other medications are administered directly into the airways by nebulizers. These medications have the advantage of fewer systemic adverse reactions. Bronchodilators include xanthines, sympathomimetics, and anticholinergics. A new type of drug used to treat alpha$_1$-protease deficiency, *Zemaira*, is discussed in Box 55.3.

Xanthines

The **xanthines**, including caffeine and theophylline, come from a variety of naturally occurring sources. These drugs were once the main treatment choices for asthma and bronchospasm. However, because they have a relatively narrow margin of safety and interact with many other drugs, they are no longer considered the first-choice bronchodilators. Xanthines used to treat respiratory disease include aminophylline (generic), caffeine (*Caffedrine*, and others), dyphylline (generic), and theophylline (generic).

Table 55.1 Guidelines for Maintenance Treatment of Asthma[a]

	Intermittent Asthma (Symptoms Less Than Once a Week, No Symptoms Between Attacks)		Mild Persistent Asthma (Symptoms at Least Once a Week But Less Than Once a Day)		Moderate Persistent Asthma (Daily Symptoms and Treatment, Attacks Affect Activities)		Severe Asthma (Continuous Symptoms, Limited Physical Activity, Frequent Exacerbations)	
Treatment	**Prevention**	**Acute**	**Prevention**	**Acute**	**Prevention**	**Acute**	**Prevention**	**Acute**
Short-acting inhaled beta-agonist[b]		×		×		×		×
Inhaled corticosteroids[b]			×		×		×	
Leukotriene receptor agonist			×					
Long-acting bronchodilators					×		×	
Inhaled beta-agonists[b]								
Sustained release theophylline			×[c]					
Long-acting oral beta-agonist								
Corticosteroids							×[d]	

[a]Effective treatment depends on patient response; a combination of therapies may be required to achieve good control.
[b]Considered drug of choice.
[c]Not a preferred treatment.
[d]Wean to inhaled preparation as soon as possible.

BOX 55.2 FOCUS ON Drug Therapy Across the Lifespan

Lower Respiratory Tract Agents

CHILDREN

Antiasthmatics are frequently used in children. The incidence of asthma in children has been rapidly increasing in the 21st century. The leukotriene receptor antagonists have been found to be especially effective for long-term prophylaxis in children. Acute episodes are best treated with a short-acting beta-agonist and then a long-acting inhaled steroid.

Parents need to be encouraged to take measures to prevent acute attacks, including avoidance of known allergens, smoke-filled rooms, and crowded or dusty areas. Parents should be cautioned about the proper way to measure liquid preparations to avoid inadvertent toxic doses or lack of therapeutic effects.

Theophylline has been used in children, but because of its many adverse effects and the better control afforded by newer agents its use is reserved for cases that do not respond to other therapies.

As the child grows and matures the disease will need to be reevaluated and dose adjustments made to meet the needs of the growing child. Puberty brings the impact of many new hormones on the body, and this frequently will change the presentation of asthma and needs to readjust treatment. Teenagers need to learn the proper administration and use of inhaled steroids for prevention of exercise-induced asthma.

As with other classes of medications, children may be more susceptible to the adverse effects associated with these drugs and need to be carefully monitored and evaluated. OTC drugs and herbal remedies should be avoided if possible; if they are used, they should be reported to the health care provider so that appropriate dose adjustments can be made where needed.

The parents of premature babies undergoing surfactant therapy will require consistent support and education to help them to cope with the stress of this event.

ADULTS

Adults may be able to manage their asthma quite well with the use of inhalers and avoidance of aggravating situations. Periodic review of the proper use of the various inhalers should be part of routine evaluation of these patients. Periodic spirometry readings should be done to evaluate the effectiveness of the therapy, and review of triggers and ways to avoid triggers should be included in each visit.

The safety of these drugs during pregnancy and lactation has not been established. There is a potential for adverse effects on the fetus related to blood flow changes and direct drug effects when the drugs cross the placenta. Use should be reserved for those situations in which the benefit to the mother outweighs the potential risk to the fetus. The drugs may enter breast milk and also may alter fluid balance and milk production. It is advised that caution be used if one of these drugs is prescribed during lactation.

OLDER ADULTS

Older adults frequently are prescribed one or more of these drugs. Older adults are more likely to develop adverse effects associated with the use of these drugs, such as sedation, confusion, dizziness, urinary retention, and CV effects. Safety measures may be needed if these effects occur and interfere with the patient's mobility and balance.

Older adults are also more likely to have renal and/or hepatic impairment related to underlying medical conditions, which could interfere with the metabolism and excretion of these drugs. The dose for older adults should be started at a lower level than that recommended for young adults. Patients should be monitored very closely and dose adjustment made based on patient response.

These patients also need to be alerted to the potential for toxic effects when using OTC preparations and should be advised to check with their health care provider before beginning any OTC drug regimen. Older adults with progressive COPD may be taking many combined drugs to help them maintain effective respirations. These patients should have an overall treatment plan involving complex pulmonary toilet, positioning, fluids, nutrition, humidified air, rest, and activity plans, as well as a complicated drug regimen to deal with the impact of this disease.

Therapeutic Actions and Indications

The xanthines have a direct effect on the smooth muscles of the respiratory tract, both in the bronchi and in the blood vessels (Figure 55.3). Although the exact mechanism of action is not known, one theory suggests that xanthines work by directly affecting the mobilization of calcium within the cell. They do this by stimulating two prostaglandins, resulting in smooth muscle relaxation, which increases the vital capacity that has been impaired by bronchospasm or air trapping. Xanthines also inhibit the release of slow-reacting substance of anaphylaxis (SRSA) and histamine, decreasing the bronchial swelling and narrowing that occurs as a result of these two chemicals. See Table 55.2 for Usual Indications for these drugs. Unlabeled uses include stimulation of respirations in **Cheyne-Stokes respiration**, an abnormal pattern of breathing characterized by apneic periods followed by periods of tachypnea that may reflect delayed blood flow through the brain, and the treatment of apnea and bradycardia in premature infants. Because the xanthines are associated with many adverse effects and management can be difficult, they are not the drug of choice when starting to treat patients with obstructive pulmonary disease. There are still some prescribers, however, that use them. They are still used in the intensive care unit (ICU) when acute asthma attacks have progressed to a critical situation.

Pharmacokinetics

The xanthines are rapidly absorbed from the gastrointestinal (GI) tract when given orally, reaching peak levels within 2 hours. They are also given IV, reaching peak effects within minutes. They are widely distributed

Table 55.2 ***Drugs in Focus:* Bronchodilators/Antiasthmatics**

Drug Name	Usual Dosage	Usual Indications
Xanthines		
aminophylline (generic)	*Adult:* 6 mg/kg PO loading dose, then 3.8 mg/kg q4 h × three doses; maintenance: 3 mg/kg q6 h *Range:* 600–1,600 mg/d PO in three to four divided doses *Rectal:* 500 mg q6–8 h *IV emergency use:* 1 mg/kg/h for the first 12 h after a loading dose of 0.6–3.2 mg/kg based on theophylline levels; 0.8 mg/kg/h should be used after 12 h of therapy *Geriatric, renal or hepatic impaired patient:* Reduce dose and monitor closely *Pediatric:* 6 mg/kg PO loading dose, then 4 mg/kg (6 mo–9 y) or 3 mg/kg (9–16 y) q4 h for three doses, then maintain at same dose q6 h *Range:* 12 mg/kg/d PO *IV emergency use:* After a loading dose, administer 1.2 mg/kg/h for children 6 mo–9 y *or* 1 mg/kg/h for children 9–16 y; if continued after 12 h, reduce dose to 1 mg/kg/h (6 mo–9 y) *or* 0.8 mg/kg/h (9–16 y) Base all doses on patient response and serum levels	Relief of symptoms or prevention of bronchial asthma and reversal of bronchospasm associated with COPD. Use usually reserved for acute bronchospasm emergency
caffeine (*Caffedrine*)	*Adult:* 500–1,000 mg IM, do not exceed 2.5 g/d *Pediatric:* 10 mg/kg IV followed by 2.5 mg/kg/d for neonatal apnea	Relief of symptoms or prevention of bronchial asthma and reversal of bronchospasm associated with COPD
dyphylline (generic)	*Adult:* Up to 15 mg/kg PO q.i.d. *or* 250–500 mg injected slowly IM *Geriatric or impaired adult:* Use caution	Relief of symptoms or prevention of bronchial asthma and reversal of bronchospasm associated with COPD
theophylline (generic)	Dosage varies widely, based on preparation and patient response *Adult:* 6 mg/kg PO loading dose followed by 3 mg/kg PO q4 h × three doses, then 3 mg/kg PO q6 h *Chronic therapy:* 400 mg/d PO in divided doses *Rectal:* 500 mg q6–8 h *IV emergency use:* 4.7 mg/kg IV loading dose followed by oral therapy *Pediatric:* 6 mg/kg PO loading dose, then 4 mg/kg (6 mo–9 y) *or* 3 mg/kg (9–16 y) PO q4 h × three doses, then the same dose q6 h *Chronic therapy:* 400 mg/d PO in divided doses	Relief of symptoms or prevention of bronchial asthma and reversal of bronchospasm associated with COPD
Sympathomimetics		
albuterol (*Proventil HFA*)	*Adult:* 2–4 mg PO t.i.d. to q.i.d. *or* two inhalations q4–6 h *or* two inhalations 15 min before exercise *Pediatric (>12 y):* adult dose *Pediatric (6–12 y):* 2 mg t.i.d. to q.i.d. oral tablets *Pediatric (6–14 y):* 2 mg t.i.d. to q.i.d. PO oral syrup *Pediatric (2–6 y):* 0.1 mg/kg PO t.i.d. oral syrup *Pediatric (2–12 y (inhalation)):* 1.25–2.5 mg; for prevention of exercise-induced bronchospasm, 200-mcg capsule inhaled 15 min before exercise	Long-acting treatment and prophylaxis of bronchospasm and prevention of exercise-induced bronchospasm in patients 2 y and older
arformoterol (*Brovana*)	*Adult:* 15 mcg b.i.d. by nebulization	Long-term maintenance treatment of bronchoconstriction in COPD
ephedrine (generic)	*Adult:* 25–50 mg IM, subcutaneous, or IV *Pediatric:* 25–100 mg/m² IM or subcutaneous divided into four to six doses	Treatment of acute bronchospasm in adults and children, although epinephrine is the drug of choice

Drug Name	Usual Dosage	Usual Indications
Sympathomimetics (Continued)		
epinephrine *(EpiPen)*	*Adult:* 0.1–0.3 mL subcutaneous q20 min for 4 h as needed; may also be given by aerosol inhalation or nebulization *Pediatric:* 0.01–0.3 mL/m^2 subcutaneous q20 min for 4 h as needed	Drug of choice for treatment of acute bronchospasm
formoterol (*Foradil*)	*Adult and pediatric (□5 y for asthma maintenance):* 12-mcg capsule q12 h, inhaled using the *Aerolizer inhaler* *Adult and pediatric (□12 y):* 12-mcg capsule inhaled using the *Aerolizer inhaler*, at least 15 min before exercising; do not use additional doses for 12 h	Maintenance treatment of asthma and prevention of bronchospasm in patients □5 y of age with reversible obstructive airway disease, prevention of exercise-induced bronchospasm in patients □12 y of age *Special considerations:* Patients taking the drug for asthma maintenance should not use additional doses of the drug for exercise-induced asthma.
indacaterol (*Arcapta*)	75 mcg inhaled using *Neohaler* only once a day	Long-term maintenance of bronchodilation in adults with COPD
isoproterenol (*Isuprel*)	*Adult:* 0.01–0.02 mg IV during anesthesia; 1:200 solution with 5–15 deep inhalations for acute bronchial asthma *or* 5–15 inhalations using nebulizer for COPD-related bronchospasm *Pediatric:* 0.25 mL *or* the 1:200 solution for each 10–15 min of nebulization	Treatment of bronchospasm during anesthesia; prophylaxis of bronchospasm (when used as inhalant) in adults and children
levalbuterol (*Xopenex HFA*)	*Adult and pediatric (>12 y):* 0.63 mg q6–8 h by nebulization *Pediatric (6–11 y):* 0.31 mg t.i.d. by nebulizer	Treatment and prevention of bronchospasm in patients >6 y of age who have reversible obstructive pulmonary disease
metaproterenol (generic)	*Adult:* 20 mg PO t.i.d. to q.i.d.; two to three inhalations q3–4 h; use caution if patient is >60 y *Pediatric (>12 y):* Inhalation and oral doses, same as adult *Pediatric (6–12 y):* Nebulizer, 0.1–0.2 mL in saline *Pediatric (6–9 y):* 10 mg PO t.i.d. to q.i.d.	Treatment and prophylaxis of bronchospasm and acute asthma attacks in children ≤6 y of age
olodaterol (*Striverdi Respimat*)	*Adult:* Two inhalations (5 mcg/d) once a day at the same time each day	LABA for treatment of airflow obstruction in patients with COPD
salmeterol (*Serevent*)	*Adult and pediatric (□12 y):* Two puffs q12 h *or* two puffs 30–60 min before exercise *Pediatric (4–12 y):* One inhalation b.i.d. at least 12 h apart; one inhalation □30 min before exercising	Prevention of exercise-induced asthma; prophylaxis of bronchospasm in selected patients >4 y of age
terbutaline (generic)	*Adult and pediatric (>15 y):* 5 mg PO q6 h while awake; 0.25 mg subcutaneous, repeat in 15 min as needed; two inhalations separated by 60 s q4–6 h *Pediatric (12–15 y):* 2.5 mg PO t.i.d.; two inhalations separated by 60 s q4–6 h as needed	Treatment and prophylaxis of bronchospasm in patients >12 y of age
Anticholinergics		
aclidinium (*Tudorza Pressair*)	400 mcg b.i.d. by oral inhalation using provided device	Long-term maintenance and treatment of bronchospasm for adults with COPD
ipratropium (*Atrovent*)	36 mcg (two inhalations) four times per day, up to 12 inhalations if needed; spacer not used *Nasal spray:* two sprays per nostril t.i.d. to q.i.d.	Maintenance and treatment of bronchospasm for adults with COPD; nasal spray for rhinorrhea associated with seasonal and perennial rhinitis or the common cold
tiotropium (*Spiriva*)	18 mcg/d (one capsule) using the *HandiHaler* inhalation device	Long-term, once-daily maintenance and treatment of bronchospasm associated with COPD in adults
umeclidinium (*Incruse Ellipta*)	62.5 mcg/d for oral inhalation using device provided	Long-term, once-daily maintenance and treatment of airflow obstruction associated with COPD in adults

COPD, chronic obstructive pulmonary disease; LABA, long-acting beta-agonist.

BOX 55.3

Enzyme Therapy: Alpha$_1$-Protease Inhibitor (Human)

An alpha$_1$-protease inhibitor, *Zemaira*, was approved in 2003 for the treatment of alpha$_1$-protease deficiency, a chronic, hereditary, autosomal dominant disorder that presents as progressive, severe emphysema, usually during a person's thirties or forties. Alpha$_1$-protease inhibitor is normally present in the lungs and acts to neutralize neutrophil elastase, which is increased by smoking or lung infection. Patients who do not produce enough alpha$_1$-protease inhibitor are at risk for progressive lung tissue destruction with smoking or lung infection. This type of emphysema and COPD does not respond well to the drug therapy usually associated with COPD. *Zemaira* is infused during a period of 15 minutes once each week at a dose of 60 mg/kg and provides protection from tissue destruction.

and metabolized in the liver and excreted in the urine. Xanthines cross the placenta and enter breast milk (see Contraindications and Cautions).

Contraindications and Cautions

Caution should be taken with any patient with GI problems, coronary disease, respiratory dysfunction, renal or hepatic disease, alcoholism, or hyperthyroidism *because these conditions can be exacerbated by the systemic effects of xanthines.* Xanthines are available for oral and parenteral use; the parenteral drug should be switched to the oral form as soon as possible *because the systemic effects of the oral form are less acute and more manageable.*

Although no studies are available of xanthine effects on human pregnancy, *they have been associated with fetal abnormalities and breathing difficulties at birth in animal studies,* so use should be limited to situations in which the benefit to the mother clearly outweighs the potential risk to

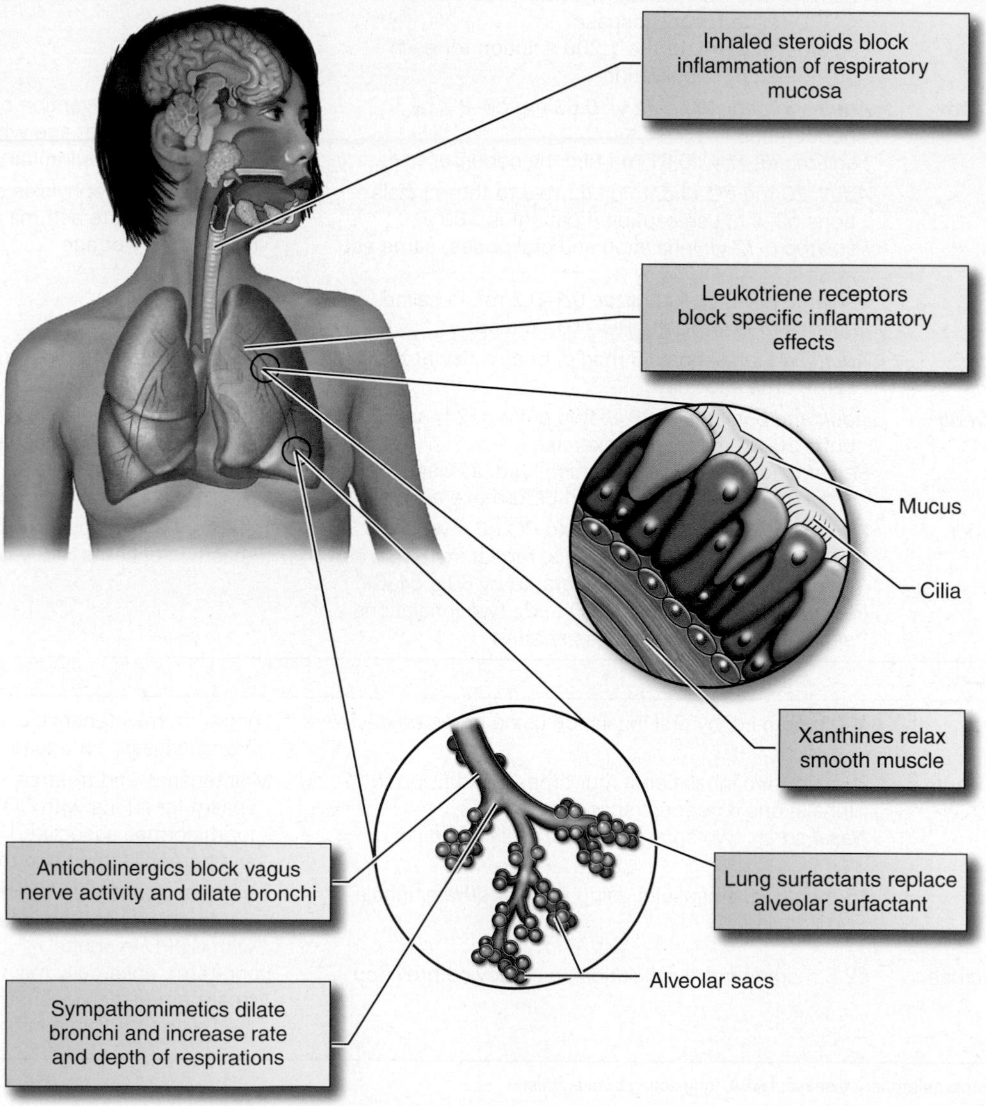
Inhaled steroids block inflammation of respiratory mucosa
Leukotriene receptors block specific inflammatory effects
Mucus
Cilia
Xanthines relax smooth muscle
Anticholinergics block vagus nerve activity and dilate bronchi
Lung surfactants replace alveolar surfactant
Alveolar sacs
Sympathomimetics dilate bronchi and increase rate and depth of respirations

FIGURE 55.3 Sites of action of drugs used to treat obstructive pulmonary disorders.

the fetus. *Because the xanthines enter breast milk and could affect the baby*, another method of feeding the baby should be selected if these drugs are needed during lactation.

Adverse Effects

Adverse effects associated with xanthines are related to theophylline levels in the blood (see the Critical Thinking Scenario for additional information on toxic reaction to theophylline). Therapeutic theophylline levels are from 10 to 20 mcg/mL. With increasing levels, predictable adverse effects are seen, ranging from GI upset, nausea, irritability, and tachycardia to seizures, brain damage, and even death (see Table 55.3).

Table 55.3 Adverse Effects Associated with Various Serum Levels of Theophylline

Serum Level (mcg/mL)	Adverse Effects
≤20	Uncommon
≤20–25	Nausea, vomiting, diarrhea, insomnia, headache, irritability
>30–35	Hyperglycemia, hypotension, cardiac arrhythmias, tachycardia, seizures, brain damage, death

CRITICAL THINKING SCENARIO

Toxic Reaction to Theophylline

THE SITUATION

R.P. has a medical diagnosis of chronic bronchitis and has been stabilized on theophylline for the past 3 years. She has been labeled as noncompliant with medical therapy because she continues to smoke cigarettes (more than three packs per day), knowing that she has a progressive pulmonary disease. R.P. was referred to a student nurse for teaching. After several sessions in which the student presented posters and pictures and gave R.P. a great deal of personal attention and encouragement, it was determined that R.P. had a good understanding of her problem and would stop or at least cut down on her smoking. Three days later, R.P. presented to the emergency department with complaints of dizziness, nausea, vomiting, confusion, grouchiness, and palpitations. Her admission heart rate was 96 beats/min with occasional to frequent premature ventricular contractions.

CRITICAL THINKING

What probably happened to R.P.?

What information should the student have known before conducting the teaching program?

How could that information have been included in the patient-teaching program?

What would the best approach be to this patient now?

DISCUSSION

R.P. probably did cut down on her smoking. However, she was not aware that cigarette smoking increases the metabolism of theophylline and that she had been stabilized on a dose that took that information into account. When she cut down on smoking, theophylline was not metabolized as quickly and began to accumulate, leading to the toxic reaction that brought R.P. into the emergency department. This is a real nursing challenge. By following the teaching program and doing what she was asked to do, R.P. became sicker and felt awful. A careful teaching approach will be necessary to encourage R.P. to continue cutting down on cigarette smoking.

Staff should be educated on the numerous variables that affect drug therapy and encouraged to check drug interactions frequently when making any changes in a patient's regimen. Regular follow-up and support will be important to help R.P. regain trust in her medical care providers and continue her progress in cutting down smoking. Frequent checks of theophylline levels should be done while R.P. is cutting back, and dose adjustments should be made by her prescriber to maintain therapeutic levels of theophylline and avoid toxic levels.

NURSING CARE GUIDE FOR R.P.: XANTHINES

Assessment: History and Examination

Assessment parameters include a health history focused particularly on allergies, peptic ulcer, gastritis, renal or hepatic dysfunction, coronary disease, cigarette use, pregnancy, and lactation, as well as concurrent use of cimetidine, erythromycin, troleandomycin, ciprofloxacin, hormonal contraceptives, ticlopidine, ranitidine, rifampin, barbiturates, phenytoin, benzodiazepines, and beta-blockers.

Focus the physical examination on the following areas:

Central nervous system (CNS): Orientation, reflexes, affect, coordination

Respiratory: Respiratory rate and character, adventitious sounds

Skin: Color, lesions

CV: Blood pressure, pulse, peripheral perfusion, baseline electrocardiogram

GI: Bowel sounds, abdominal exam

Laboratory tests: Serum theophylline levels, renal and hepatic function tests

(continues on page 960)

Toxic Reaction to Theophylline (continued)

Nursing Diagnoses

Acute pain related to GI effects or dry mouth
Decreased cardiac output
Impaired sensory perception (kinesthetic, visual)
Activity intolerance
Deficient knowledge regarding drug therapy

Planning

The patient will receive the best therapeutic effect from the drug therapy.
The patient will have limited adverse effects to the drug therapy.
The patient will have an understanding of the drug therapy, adverse effects to anticipate, and measures to relieve discomfort and improve safety.

Implementation

Provide supportive care with comfort and safety measures.
Give drug with meals.
Allow for rest periods.
Provide a quiet environment.
Ensure dietary control of caffeine.
Provide headache therapy as needed.
Provide reassurance to deal with drug effects and lifestyle changes.
Provide patient teaching regarding drug name, dosage, adverse effects, precautions, warnings to report, dietary cautions, and need for follow-up.

Evaluation

Evaluate drug effects: Relief of respiratory difficulty, improvement of air movement.
Monitor for adverse effects: GI upset, CNS effects, cardiac arrhythmias.
Monitor for drug–drug interactions as appropriate.
Evaluate the effectiveness of the patient-teaching program and comfort and safety measures.

PATIENT TEACHING FOR R.P.

- The drug that has been prescribed for you, theophylline, is called a bronchodilator. Bronchodilators work by relaxing the airways, helping to make breathing easier and to decrease wheezes and shortness of breath. To be effective, this drug must be taken exactly as prescribed.
- This drug should be taken on an empty stomach with a full 8-ounce glass of water. If GI upset is severe, you can take the drug with food. Do not chew the enteric-coated or time release capsules or tablets—they must be swallowed whole to be effective.
- Common effects of this drug include the following:
  - *GI upset, nausea, vomiting, heartburn*: Taking the drug with food may help with these problems.
  - *Restlessness, nervousness, difficulty in sleeping*: The body often adjusts to these effects over time. Avoiding other stimulants, such as caffeine, may help to decrease some of these symptoms.
  - *Headache*: This often goes away with time. If headaches persist or become worse, notify your health care provider.
  - Report any of the following to your health care provider: *Vomiting, severe abdominal pain, pounding or fast heartbeat, confusion, unusual tiredness, muscle twitching, skin rash, or hives.*
  - Many foods can change the way that your drug works; if you decide to change your diet, consult with your health care provider.
  - Adverse effects of the drug can be avoided by avoiding foods that contain caffeine or other xanthine derivatives (coffee, cola, chocolate, tea) or by using them in moderate amounts. This is especially important if you experience nervousness, restlessness, or sleeplessness.
  - Cigarette smoking affects the way your body uses this drug. If you decide to change your smoking habits, such as increasing or decreasing the number of cigarettes you smoke each day, consult with your health care provider regarding the possible need to adjust your dose.
  - Avoid the use of any over-the-counter (OTC) medication without first checking with your health care provider. Several of these medications can interfere with the effectiveness of this drug.
  - Tell any doctor, nurse, or other health care provider involved in your care that you are taking this drug.
  - Keep this drug and all medications out of the reach of children.

Clinically Important Drug–Drug Interactions

Because of the mechanism of xanthine metabolism in the liver, many drugs interact with xanthines. The list of interacting drugs should be checked any time a drug is added to or removed from a drug regimen.

Nicotine increases the metabolism of xanthines in the liver; xanthine dose must be increased in patients who continue to smoke while using xanthines. In addition, extreme caution must be used if the patient decides to decrease or discontinue smoking, because severe xanthine toxicity can occur.

Ⓟ Prototype Summary: Aminophylline

Indications: Symptomatic relief or prevention of bronchial asthma and reversible bronchospasm associated with chronic bronchitis and emphysema.

Actions: Directly relaxes bronchial smooth muscle, causing bronchodilation and increasing vital capacity; also inhibits the release of slow-reacting substance of anaphylaxis and histamine.

Pharmacokinetics:

Route	Onset	Peak	Duration
Oral	1–6 h	4–6 h	6–8 h
IV	Immediate	30 min	4–8 h

$T_{1/2}$: 3 to 15 hours (nonsmoker), 4 to 5 hours (smoker); metabolized in the liver and excreted in the urine.

Adverse Effects: Irritability, restlessness, dizziness, palpitations, life-threatening arrhythmias, loss of appetite, proteinuria, respiratory arrest, fever, flushing.

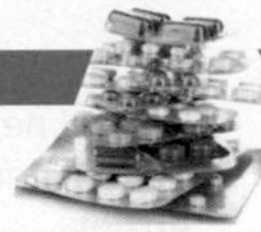

Nursing Considerations for Patients Receiving Xanthines

Assessment: History and Examination

- Assess for *possible contraindications or cautions*: Any known allergies *to prevent hypersensitivity reactions*; cigarette use, *which affects the metabolism of the drug*; peptic ulcer, gastritis, renal or hepatic dysfunction, and coronary disease, *all of which could be exacerbated and require cautious use*; and pregnancy and lactation, *which are contraindications because of the potential for adverse effects on the fetus or nursing baby.*
- Perform a physical examination *to establish baseline data for assessing the effectiveness of the drug and the occurrence of any adverse effects associated with drug therapy.*
- Perform a skin examination, including color and the presence of lesions, *to provide a baseline as a reference for drug effectiveness.*
- Monitor blood pressure, pulse, cardiac auscultation, peripheral perfusion, and baseline electrocardiogram *to provide a baseline for effects on the CV system.*
- Assess bowel sounds, do a liver evaluation, and monitor liver and renal function tests *to provide a baseline for renal and hepatic function tests.*
- Evaluate serum theophylline levels *to provide a baseline reference and identify conditions that may require caution in the use of xanthines.*

Nursing Diagnoses

Nursing diagnoses related to drug therapy might include the following:

- Acute pain related to headache and GI upset
- Disturbed sensory perception (kinesthetic, visual) related to CNS effects
- Deficient knowledge regarding drug therapy

Planning

- The patient will receive the best therapeutic effect from the drug therapy.
- The patient will have limited adverse effects to the drug therapy.
- The patient will have an understanding of the drug therapy, adverse effects to anticipate, and measures to relieve discomfort and improve safety.

Implementation with Rationale

- Administer oral drug with food or milk *to relieve GI irritation if GI upset is a problem.*
- Monitor patient response to the drug (e.g., relief of respiratory difficulty, improved airflow) *to determine the effectiveness of the drug dose and to adjust dose as needed.*
- Provide comfort measures, including rest periods, quiet environment, dietary control of caffeine, and headache therapy as needed, *to help the patient cope with the effects of drug therapy.*
- Provide periodic follow-up, including blood tests, *to monitor serum theophylline levels.*
- Provide thorough patient teaching, including the drug name and prescribed dosage, measures to help avoid adverse effects, warning signs that may indicate problems, and the need for periodic monitoring and evaluation, *to enhance patient knowledge about drug therapy and to promote compliance.*

Evaluation

- Monitor patient response to the drug (improved airflow, ease of respirations).
- Monitor for adverse effects (CNS effects, cardiac arrhythmias, GI upset, local irritation).
- Monitor for potential drug–drug interactions; consult with the prescriber to adjust doses as appropriate.
- Evaluate the effectiveness of the teaching plan (patient can name drug, dosage, adverse effects to watch for, and specific measures to avoid adverse effects).
- Monitor the effectiveness of comfort measures and compliance with the regimen.

Sympathomimetics

Sympathomimetics are drugs that mimic the effects of the sympathetic nervous system. One of the actions of the sympathetic nervous system is dilation of the bronchi with increased rate and depth of respiration. This is the desired effect when selecting a sympathomimetic as a bronchodilator. Sympathomimetics that are used as bronchodilators include albuterol (*Proventil HFA*, and others), arformoterol (*Brovana*), ephedrine (generic), epinephrine (*EpiPen*), formoterol (*Foradil*), indacaterol (*Arcapta*), isoproterenol (*Isuprel*, and others), levalbuterol (*Xopenex HFA*), metaproterenol (generic), olodaterol (*Striverdi*), salmeterol (*Serevent*), and terbutaline (generic).

Therapeutic Actions and Indications

Most of the sympathomimetics used as bronchodilators are $beta_2$-selective adrenergic agonists. That means that at therapeutic levels their actions are specific to the $beta_2$-receptors found in the bronchi (see Chapter 30). This specificity is lost at higher levels. Other systemic effects of sympathomimetics include increased blood pressure, increased heart rate, vasoconstriction, and decreased renal and GI blood flow—all actions of the sympathetic nervous system. These overall effects limit the systemic usefulness of these drugs in certain patients.

Epinephrine, the prototype drug, is the drug of choice in adults and children for the treatment of acute bronchospasm, including that caused by anaphylaxis; it is also available for inhalation. Because epinephrine is associated with systemic sympathomimetic effects, it is not the drug of choice for patients with cardiac conditions. See Table 55.2 for Usual Indications for each of these agents.

Pharmacokinetics

Sympathomimetics available only as an inhalant include arformoterol, formoterol, indacaterol, levalbuterol, olodaterol and salmeterol. They vary in their duration of action; long-acting beta adrenergics have half-lives between 45 and 126 hours.

Other sympathomimetics are available in various forms. Albuterol and metaproterenol are available in inhaled and oral forms. Terbutaline can be used as an inhalant and as an oral and parenteral agent. Isoproterenol is available for IV use. Ephedrine is used orally and in parenteral form (for IV, IM, and subcutaneous use). Its use has declined over the past few years with the availability of safer drugs.

These drugs are rapidly distributed after injection; they are transformed in the liver to metabolites that are excreted in the urine. The half-life of these drugs is relatively short—less than 1 hour. They are known to cross the placenta and to enter breast milk (see Contraindications and Cautions). The inhaled drugs are rapidly absorbed into the lung tissue. Although very little of the drug is absorbed systemically, any absorbed drug will still be metabolized in the liver and excreted in the urine.

Contraindications and Cautions

These drugs are contraindicated or should be used with caution, depending on the severity of the underlying condition, *in conditions that would be aggravated by the sympathetic stimulation*, including cardiac disease, vascular disease, arrhythmias, diabetes, and hyperthyroidism. These drugs should be used during pregnancy and lactation *only if the benefits to the mother clearly outweigh potential risks to the fetus or neonate.*

Adverse Effects

Adverse effects of these drugs, which can be attributed to sympathomimetic stimulation, include CNS stimulation, GI upset, cardiac arrhythmias, hypertension, bronchospasm, sweating, pallor, and flushing (Figure 55.4). Isoproterenol is associated with more cardiac side effects than some other drugs. The long-acting beta-agonists

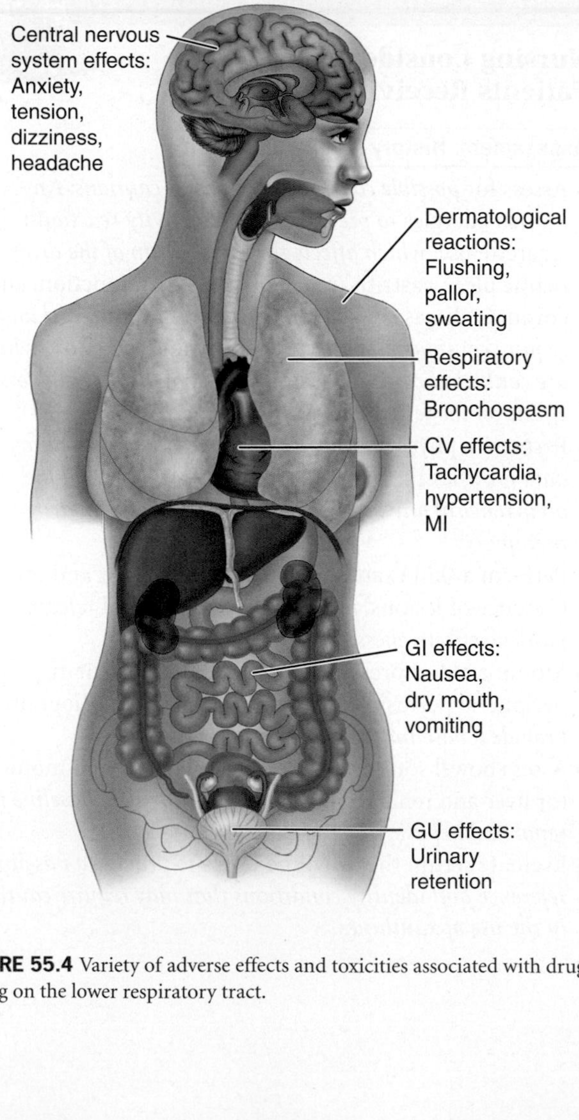

FIGURE 55.4 Variety of adverse effects and toxicities associated with drugs acting on the lower respiratory tract.

BOX 55.4 FOCUS ON Cultural Considerations

As a result of postmarketing studies the boxed warning label on the asthma drug salmeterol (*Serevent*) was changed to warn of a small but significant increase in the risk of life-threatening asthma episodes in patients using salmeterol. In the study, which involved 13,000 patients each in a salmeterol treatment group and a control group, there were 13 asthma-related deaths in a 28-week period in the salmeterol group compared with 4 asthma-related deaths in the control group. The study showed that African American patients had a greater risk of asthma-related deaths than did other groups. The U.S. Food and Drug Administration agreed that the benefit of using salmeterol for the treatment of asthma was greater than the risk that the drug poses, but cautioned health care professionals to be cautious when prescribing these drugs. Since then, black box warnings have been added to all of the LABAs to alert health care providers to the risk of asthma-related deaths with these drugs.

(LABAs) have a black box warning about the increased risk of asthma-related deaths when patients use these drugs. It is recommended that an inhaled corticosteroid also be used to decrease that risk. The LABAs alone are not recommended for treating asthma.

If the patient is taking formoterol for asthma maintenance, additional doses of drug should not be used for exercise-induced asthma because the cumulative sympathomimetic effects can cause serious CV problems. Salmeterol and the other LABAs have a greater risk of asthma-related deaths especially in older patients and African American patients (see Box 55.4). This risk is lowered when the LABAs are combined with an inhaled corticosteroid. Current recommendations are that, if using a LABA, the patient must also be prescribed an inhaled corticosteroid. The LABAs are not recommended for use in asthma.

Clinically Important Drug–Drug Interactions

Special precautions should be taken to avoid the combination of sympathomimetic bronchodilators with the general anesthetics cyclopropane and halogenated hydrocarbons. Because these drugs sensitize the myocardium to catecholamines, serious cardiac complications could occur.

Prototype Summary: Epinephrine

Indications: Treatment of anaphylactic reactions, acute asthmatic attacks; relief from respiratory distress of chronic obstructive pulmonary disease and bronchial asthma.

Actions: Reacts at alpha- and beta-receptor sites in the sympathetic nervous system to cause bronchodilation, increased heart rate, increased respiratory rate, and increased blood pressure.

Pharmacokinetics:

Route	Onset	Peak	Duration
SC	5–10 min	20 min	20–30 min
IM	5–10 min	20 min	20–30 min
IV	Instant	20 min	20–30 min
Inhalation	3–5 min	20 min	1–3 h

$T_{1/2}$: Unknown; metabolized by normal neural pathways.

Adverse Effects: Fear, anxiety, restlessness, headache, nausea, decreased renal formation, pallor, palpitation, tachycardia, local burning and stinging, rebound congestion with nasal inhalation.

Nursing Considerations for Patients Receiving Sympathomimetics

Assessment: History and Examination

- Assess for *possible contraindications or cautions*: Any known allergies to any sympathomimetic or drug vehicle *to prevent hypersensitivity reactions*; cigarette use, *which affects the metabolism of the drug*; pregnancy or lactation, *which require cautious use of the drug*; cardiac disease, vascular disease, arrhythmias, diabetes, and hyperthyroidism, *which may be exacerbated by sympathomimetic effects*; and use of the general anesthetics cyclopropane and halogenated hydrocarbons, *which sensitize the myocardium to catecholamines and could cause serious cardiac complications if used with these drugs.*
- Perform a physical examination *to establish baseline data for assessing the effectiveness of the drug and the occurrence of any adverse effects associated with drug therapy.*
- Assess reflexes and orientation *to evaluate CNS effects of the drug.*
- Monitor respirations and adventitious sounds *to establish a baseline for drug effectiveness and possible adverse effects.*
- Evaluate pulse, blood pressure, and, in certain cases, a baseline electrocardiogram *to monitor the CV effects of sympathetic stimulation.*
- Evaluate liver function tests *to assess for changes that could interfere with metabolism of the drug and require dose adjustment.*

Nursing Diagnoses

Nursing diagnoses related to drug therapy might include the following:

- Increased cardiac output related to sympathomimetic effects
- Acute pain related to CNS, GI, or cardiac effects of the drug
- Disturbed thought processes related to CNS effects
- Deficient knowledge related to drug therapy

(continues on page 964)

Planning

- The patient will receive the best therapeutic effect from the drug therapy.
- The patient will have limited adverse effects to the drug therapy.
- The patient will have an understanding of the drug therapy, adverse effects to anticipate, and measures to relieve discomfort and improve safety.

Implementation with Rationale

- Reassure patient that the drug of choice will vary with each individual. *These sympathomimetics are slightly different chemicals and are prepared in a variety of delivery systems.* A patient may have to try several different sympathomimetics before the most effective one is found.
- Advise the patient to use the minimal amount needed for the shortest period necessary *to prevent adverse effects and accumulation of drug levels.*
- Teach patients who use one of these drugs for exercise-induced asthma to use it 30 to 60 minutes before exercising *to ensure peak therapeutic effects when they are needed.*
- Alert patient that long-acting adrenergic blockers are not for use during acute attacks *because they are slower acting and will not provide the necessary rescue in a state of acute bronchospasm.*
- Provide safety measures as needed if CNS effects become a problem *to prevent patient injury.*
- Provide small, frequent meals and nutritional consultation if GI effects interfere with eating *to ensure proper nutrition.*
- Provide thorough patient teaching, including the drug name and prescribed dosage, measures to help avoid adverse effects, warning signs that may indicate problems, and the need for periodic monitoring and evaluation, *to enhance patient knowledge about drug therapy and to promote compliance.* Carefully teach the patient about proper use of the prescribed delivery system. Review that procedure periodically *because improper use may result in ineffective therapy* (Box 55.5).
- Offer support and encouragement *to help the patient cope with the disease and the drug regimen.*

Evaluation

- Monitor patient response to the drug (improved breathing).
- Monitor for adverse effects (CNS effects, increased pulse and blood pressure, GI upset).
- Evaluate the effectiveness of the teaching plan (patient can name drug, dosage, adverse effects to watch for, specific measures to avoid them, and measures to take to increase the effectiveness of the drug).
- Monitor the effectiveness of other measures to ease breathing.

Anticholinergics

Patients who cannot tolerate the sympathetic effects of the sympathomimetics might respond to the anticholinergic drugs ipratropium (*Atrovent*), tiotropium (*Spiriva*), aclidinium (*Tudorza Pressair*), and umeclidinium (*Incruse Ellipta*). These drugs are not as effective as the sympathomimetics but can provide some relief to those patients who cannot tolerate the other drugs. Tiotropium was the first drug approved for once-daily maintenance treatment of, bronchospasm associated with COPD; umeclidinium is now also available for once-a-day treatment.

Therapeutic Actions and Indications

Anticholinergics are used as bronchodilators because of their effect on the vagus nerve, which is to block or antagonize the action of the neurotransmitter acetylcholine at vagal-mediated receptor sites (see Figure 55.2). Normally, vagal stimulation results in a stimulating effect on smooth muscle, causing contraction. By blocking the vagal effect, relaxation of smooth muscle in the bronchi occurs, leading to bronchodilation. See Table 55.2 for Usual Indications for these drugs.

Pharmacokinetics

These drugs are available for inhalation, using an inhaler device. Ipratropium is also available as a nasal spray for seasonal rhinitis. Ipratropium has an onset of action of 15 minutes when inhaled. Its peak effects occur in 1 to 2 hours, and it has a duration of effect of 3 to 4 hours. Little is known about its fate in the body. It is generally not absorbed systemically.

Tiotropium has a rapid onset of action and a long duration, with a half-life of 5 to 6 days. It is excreted unchanged in the urine.

Aclidinium has an onset of 10 minutes and a half-life of 5 to 8 hours, being excreted unchanged in the urine.

Umeclidinium (*Incruse Ellipta*) has an onset of 5 to 15 minutes and a half-life of 11 hours. It is also excreted unchanged in the urine.

Contraindications and Cautions

Caution should be used in any condition *that would be aggravated by the anticholinergic or atropine-like effects of the drug*, such as narrow-angle glaucoma (*drainage of the vitreous humor can be blocked by smooth muscle relaxation*), bladder neck obstruction or prostatic hypertrophy (*relaxed muscle causes decreased bladder tone*), and conditions aggravated by dry mouth and throat. The use of ipratropium or tiotropium is contraindicated in the presence of known allergy to the drug or to soy products or peanuts (the vehicle used to make ipratropium an aerosol contains a protein associated with peanut allergies); umeclidinium is contraindicated in patients with milk protein allergies *to prevent hypersensitivity reactions.* These drugs are not

BOX 55.5 FOCUS ON **Patient and Family Teaching**

Teaching Patients to Self-Administer Medication

It is important to deliver inhaled drugs into the lungs to achieve a rapid reaction and decrease the occurrence of systemic adverse effects. Patients who are self-administering inhaled drugs may be using an inhaler or a nebulizer.

Inhalers

An inhaler is a device that allows a canister containing the drug to be inserted into a metered dose device that will deliver a specific amount of the drug when the patient compresses the canister. The inhaler has a mouthpiece and may also have a spacer, which is used to hold the dose of the drug while the patient inhales. This is advantageous if the patient has difficulty compressing the canister and inhaling at the same time or if inhaling is difficult. If a powder for inhalation is being administered a spacer is not used.

Have the patient shake the canister, exhale, and then place the spacer in his or her mouth. (If a spacer is not being used, he or she should hold the device about 1 inch from the open mouth.) The patient should then compress the canister while inhaling, hold his or her breath as long as possible, and then exhale through pursed lips. The patient should then rinse his or her mouth and wash the spacer (if used). Some drugs come with a very specific inhaling device designed just for that drug. If the patient is using one of those drugs the manufacturer's instructions should be consulted.

Nebulizers

A nebulizer uses compressed air to change a liquid drug into a fine mist for inhalation. If a patient is using a hand-held device or a mask, he or she should sit upright or in a semi-Fowler's position and place the correct amount of liquid (drug dose) in the nebulizer chamber, which is attached to a compressed gas system. The patient should breathe slowly and deeply during the treatment. After the liquid is gone the patient should rinse his or her mouth and clean the mask or device.

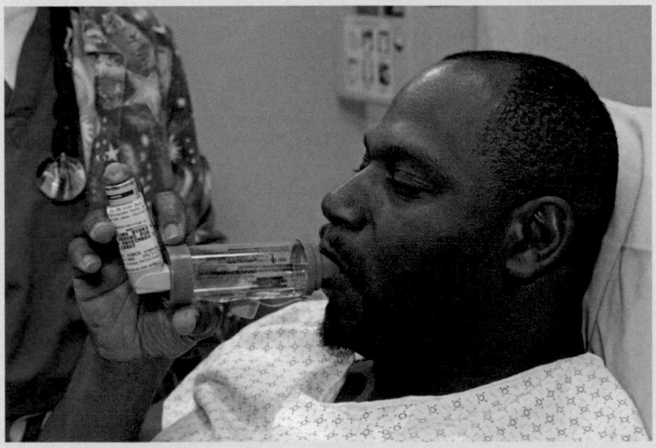

Patients may use these devices for several years. It is important to check their administration techniques periodically to ensure that the patient is getting a therapeutic dose of the drug.

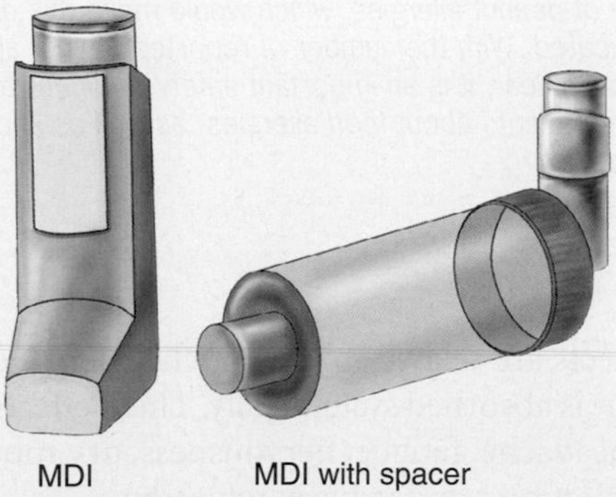

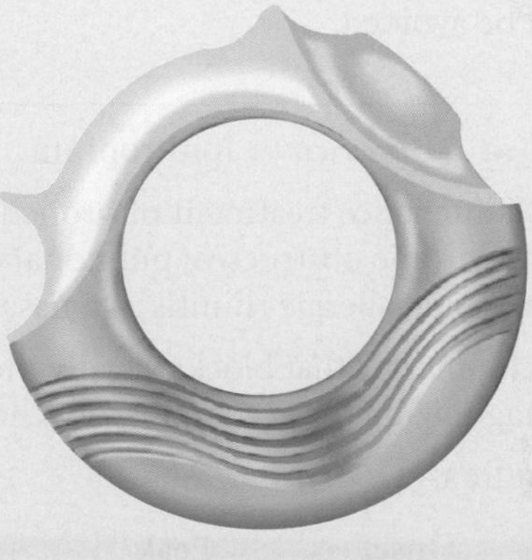

Dry-powder inhaler

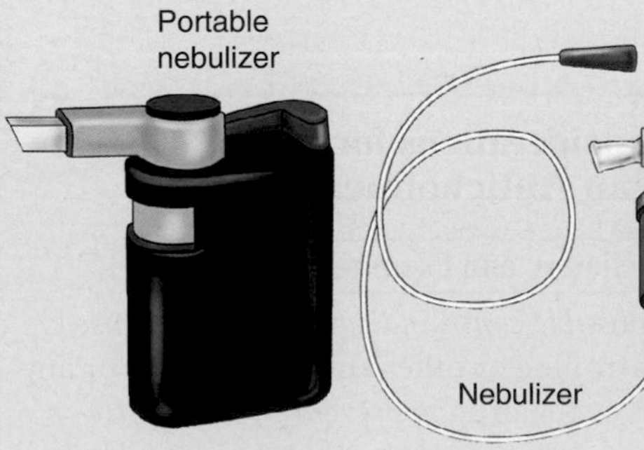

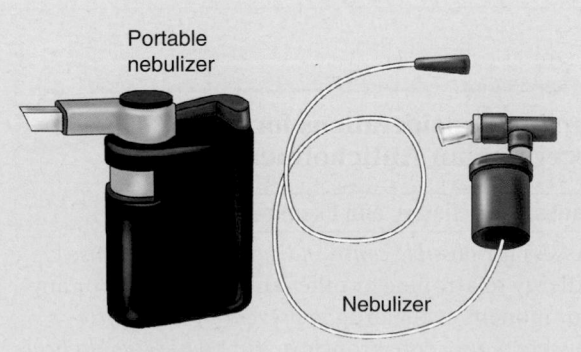

usually absorbed systemically, but as with all drugs caution should be used in pregnancy and lactation *because of the potential for adverse effects on the fetus or nursing baby.*

FOCUS ON Safe Medication Administration

*The propellant used to make ipratropium an inhaled drug has a cross-sensitivity to the antigen that causes peanut allergies. Patients who are started on inhaled ipratropium, or the combination drug **Combivent** should be questioned about the possibility of peanut allergies, which would make this drug contraindicated. With the number of reported peanut allergies growing each year, it is an important safety reminder to check with patients about food allergies, as well as known drug allergies.*

Adverse Effects

Adverse effects are related to the anticholinergic effects of the drug if it is absorbed systemically. These effects include dizziness, headache, fatigue, nervousness, dry mouth, sore throat, palpitations, and urinary retention.

Clinically Important Drug–Drug Interactions

There is an increased risk of adverse effects if these drugs are combined with any other anticholinergics; this combination should be avoided.

Prototype Summary: Ipratropium

Indications: Maintenance treatment of bronchospasm associated with chronic obstructive pulmonary disease; treatment of seasonal allergic rhinitis as a nasal spray.

Actions: Anticholinergic that blocks vagally mediated reflexes by antagonizing the action of acetylcholine.

Pharmacokinetics:

Route	Onset	Peak	Duration
Inhalation	15 min	1–2 h	3–4 h

$T_{1/2}$: Unknown; metabolized by neural pathways.

Adverse Effects: Nervousness, dizziness, headache, nausea, GI distress, cough, palpitations.

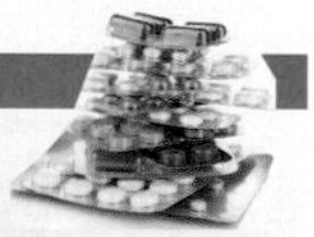

Nursing Considerations for Patients Receiving an Anticholinergic

Assessment: History and Examination

- Assess for *possible contraindications or cautions*: Allergy to atropine or other anticholinergics or any component of the drug *to prevent hypersensitivity reactions*; acute bronchospasm, *which would be a contraindication*; narrow-angle glaucoma (*drainage of the vitreous humor can be blocked by smooth muscle relaxation*), bladder neck obstruction or prostatic hypertrophy (*relaxed muscle causes decreased bladder tone*), and conditions aggravated by dry mouth and throat, *all of which could be exacerbated by the use of this drug*; and pregnancy and lactation, *which would require cautious use.*
- Perform a physical examination *to establish baseline data for assessing the effectiveness of the drug and the occurrence of any adverse effects associated with drug therapy.*
- Assess the skin color and lesions *for dryness or allergic reaction and to evaluate oxygenation.*
- Evaluate orientation, affect, and reflexes *to evaluate CNS effects.*
- Assess pulse and blood pressure *to monitor CV effects of the drug.*
- Evaluate respirations and adventitious sounds *to monitor drug effectiveness and possible adverse effects.*
- Evaluate urinary output and prostate palpation as appropriate *to monitor anticholinergic effects.*

Nursing Diagnoses

Nursing diagnoses related to drug therapy might include the following:

- Acute pain related to CNS, GI, or respiratory effects of the drug
- Imbalanced nutrition: Less than body requirements related to dry mouth and GI upset
- Deficient knowledge regarding drug therapy

Planning

- The patient will receive the best therapeutic effect from the drug therapy.
- The patient will have limited adverse effects to the drug therapy.
- The patient will have an understanding of the drug therapy, adverse effects to anticipate, and measures to relieve discomfort and improve safety.

Implementation with Rationale

- Ensure adequate hydration and provide environmental controls, such as the use of a humidifier, *to make the patient more comfortable.*
- Encourage the patient to void before each dose of medication *to prevent urinary retention related to drug effects.*
- Provide safety measures if CNS effects occur *to prevent patient injury.*
- Provide small, frequent meals and sugarless lozenges *to relieve dry mouth and GI upset.*
- Advise the patient not to drive or use hazardous machinery if nervousness, dizziness, and drowsiness occur with this drug *to prevent injury.*

- Provide thorough patient teaching, including the drug name and prescribed dosage, measures to help avoid adverse effects, warning signs that may indicate problems, and the need for periodic monitoring and evaluation, *to enhance patient knowledge about drug therapy and to promote compliance.*
- Review the use of the inhalator with the patient; caution the patient not to exceed 12 inhalations in 24 hours *to prevent serious adverse effects.*
- Offer support and encouragement *to help the patient cope with the disease and the drug regimen.*

Evaluation

- Monitor patient response to the drug (improved breathing).
- Monitor for adverse effects (CNS effects, increased pulse or blood pressure, GI upset, dry skin, and mucous membranes).
- Evaluate the effectiveness of the teaching plan (patient can name drug, dosage, adverse effects to watch for, specific measures to avoid them, and measures to take to increase the effectiveness of the drug).
- Monitor the effectiveness of other measures to ease breathing.

KEY POINTS

- Asthma; COPD, which includes emphysema and chronic bronchitis; and RDS are pulmonary obstructive diseases. All but RDS involve obstruction of the major airways; RDS obstructs the alveoli.
- Drug treatment of asthma and COPD aims to relieve inflammation and promote bronchial dilation.
- Xanthine-derived drugs affect the smooth muscles of the respiratory tract—both in the bronchi and in the blood vessels. The effects of the xanthines are directly related to blood levels of theophylline. Excessive or toxic levels can lead to coma and death. These drugs are not used as often as in the past since the approval of safer drugs.
- Sympathomimetics replicate the effects of the sympathetic nervous system; they dilate the bronchi and increase the rate and depth of respiration.
- Anticholinergics affect the vagus nerve to relax bronchial smooth muscle and thereby promote bronchodilation.

Drugs Affecting Inflammation

Bronchodilation is important in opening up the airway to allow air to flow into the alveoli. The second component of treating obstructive pulmonary disorders is to alter the inflammatory process that leads to swelling and further airway narrowing. Effective treatment of asthma and COPD targets both components. The drugs used to affect inflammation are the inhaled steroids, the leukotriene receptors, and a mast cell stabilizer (now only one OTC product is available), which can affect both bronchodilation and inflammation (Table 55.4).

Inhaled Steroids

Inhaled steroids have been found to be a very effective treatment for bronchospasm. Agents approved for this use include beclomethasone (*Beconase AQ*), budesonide (*Pulmicort Respules, Pulmicort Flexhaler*), ciclesonide (*Alvesco*), fluticasone (*FloventDiscus, Flovent HFA*), and triamcinolone (generic). The drug of choice depends on the individual patient's response; a patient may have little response to one agent and do very well on another. It is usually useful to try another preparation if one is not effective within 2 to 3 weeks.

Fixed combination drugs are also available using some of these drugs (Box 55.6).

Therapeutic Actions and Indications

Inhaled steroids are used to decrease the inflammatory response in the airway. In an airway that is swollen and narrowed by inflammation and swelling, this action will increase airflow and facilitate respiration. Inhaling the steroid tends to decrease the numerous systemic effects that are associated with steroid use. When administered into the lungs by inhalation, steroids decrease the effectiveness of the inflammatory cells. This has two effects: Decreased swelling associated with inflammation and promotion of beta-adrenergic receptor activity, which may promote smooth muscle relaxation and inhibit bronchoconstriction (see Figure 55.2). See Table 55.4 for Usual Indications.

Pharmacokinetics

These drugs are rapidly absorbed from the respiratory tract, but they take from 2 to 3 weeks to reach effective levels, and so patients must be encouraged to take them to reach and then maintain the effective levels. They are metabolized by natural systems, mostly within the liver, and are excreted in the urine. The glucocorticoids are known to cross the placenta and to enter breast milk (see Contraindications and Cautions).

Contraindications and Cautions

- Inhaled steroids are not for emergency use and not for use during an acute asthma attack or status asthmaticus. They should not be used during pregnancy or lactation *unless the benefit to the mother clearly outweighs any potential risk to the fetus or nursing baby*. These preparations should be used with caution in any patient who has an active infection of the respiratory system *because depression of the inflammatory response could result in serious illness.*

Table 55.4 *Drugs in Focus:* Drugs Affecting Inflammation

Drug Name	Usual Dosage	Usual Indications
Inhaled Steroids		
beclomethasone (*Beconase*)	*Adult:* 84–168 mcg t.i.d. to q.i.d. (two inhalations) *Pediatric (6–12 y):* One to two inhalations t.i.d. to q.i.d.; do not exceed 10 inhalations per day	Prevention and treatment of asthma; treatment of chronic steroid-dependent bronchial asthma; used as adjunctive therapy for asthma patients who do not respond to traditional bronchodilators
budesonide (*Pulmicort Respules, Pulmocort Flexhaler*)	*Adult and pediatric (>6 y):* 200–400 mcg b.i.d. (two inhalations); maximum dose 800 mcg b.i.d. *Pediatric (>6 y):* 200 mcg b.i.d.	Prevention and treatment of asthma; treatment of chronic steroid-dependent bronchial asthma; used as adjunctive therapy for asthma patients who do not respond to traditional bronchodilators
ciclesonide (*Alvesco*)	*Adult and pediatric (□12 y):* 80–320 mcg b.i.d. by inhalation	Prevention and treatment of asthma; treatment of chronic steroid-dependent bronchial asthma; used as adjunctive therapy for asthma patients who do not respond to traditional bronchodilators
fluticasone (*Flovent Discus, Flovent HFA*)	*Adult:* 88–440 mcg b.i.d. by inhalation *Pediatric (4–11 y):* 50–100 mcg b.i.d. by inhalation	Prevention and treatment of asthma; treatment of chronic steroid-dependent bronchial asthma; used as adjunctive therapy for asthma patients who do not respond to traditional bronchodilators
triamcinolone (generic)	*Adult:* Two inhalations (200 mcg) t.i.d. to q.i.d. *Pediatric (6–12 y):* one to two inhalations t.i.d. to q.i.d.	Prevention and treatment of asthma; treatment of chronic steroid-dependent bronchial asthma; used as adjunctive therapy for asthma patients who do not respond to traditional bronchodilators
Leukotriene Receptor Antagonists		
montelukast (*Singulair*)	*Adult and pediatric (>15 y):* 10 mg PO daily in the evening *Pediatric (6–23 mo):* 4-mg granules PO in the evening *Pediatric (2–5 y):* 4-mg chewable tablet PO in the evening *Pediatric (6–14 y):* 5-mg chewable tablet PO in the evening	Prophylaxis and treatment of chronic bronchial asthma in adults and children 6 mo and older
zafirlukast (*Accolate*)	*Adult and pediatric (>12 y):* 20 mg PO b.i.d. *Pediatric (5–11 y):* 10 mg PO b.i.d.	Prophylaxis and treatment of chronic bronchial asthma in adults and in children 5 y and older
zileuton (*Zyflo*)	*Adult and pediatric (□12 y):* 600 mg PO q.i.d. for a total of 2,400 mg/d	Prophylaxis and treatment of chronic bronchial asthma in patients □12 y of age

BOX 55.6

Fixed Combination Respiratory Drugs

The benefit of combining different classes of drugs for the treatment of asthma and COPD has resulted in the development of fixed combination drugs.

- *Advair Diskus* and *Advair HFA* are combinations of fluticasone (a steroid) and salmeterol (a sympathetic agent). They are approved for managing asthma in patients 4 years of age and older.
- *Combivent* is a combination of ipratropium (an anticholinergic agent) and albuterol (a sympathetic agent).
- *Symbicort* is a combination of budesonide (a corticosteroid) and formoterol (a sympathetic agent). Patients should be stabilized on each drug separately before switching to the fixed combination drug. Once the switch has been made the dosing is cut in half, and most patients find it easier to be compliant with drug therapy.
- *Anoro Ellipta* combines umeclidinium (an anticholinergic) and vilanterol (a LABA). One inhalation a day for the maintenance treatment of COPD. Not indicated with a severe sensitivity to milk proteins.
- *Breo Ellipta* combines fluticasone (a corticosteroid) with the LABA vilanterol. Once-daily inhalation for the treatment of COPD and for the treatment of asthma patients 18 years and older. Not for the relief of acute bronchospasm.

Adverse Effects

Adverse effects are limited because of the route of administration. Sore throat, hoarseness, coughing, dry mouth, and pharyngeal and laryngeal fungal infections are the most common side effects encountered. If a patient does not administer the drug appropriately or develops lesions that allow absorption of the drug the systemic side effects associated with steroids may occur.

Prototype Summary: Budesonide

Indications: Prevention and treatment of asthma; to treat chronic steroid-dependent bronchial asthma; as adjunct therapy for patients whose asthma is not controlled by traditional bronchodilators.

Actions: Decreases the inflammatory response in the airway; this action will increase airflow and facilitate respiration in an airway narrowed by inflammation.

Pharmacokinetics:

Route	Onset	Peak	Duration
Inhalation	Slow	Rapid	8–12 h

$T_{1/2}$: 2 to 3 hours; metabolized in the liver and excreted in the urine.

Adverse Effects: Irritability, headache, rebound congestion, epistaxis, local infection.

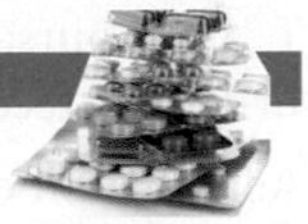

Nursing Considerations for Patients Receiving Inhaled Steroids

Assessment: History and Examination

- Assess for *possible contraindications or cautions*: Acute asthmatic attacks and allergy to the drugs, *which are contraindications*, and systemic infections, pregnancy, or lactation, *which require cautious use*.
- Perform a physical examination *to establish baseline data for assessing the effectiveness of the drug and the occurrence of any adverse effects associated with drug therapy*.
- Assess temperature *to monitor for possible infections*.
- Monitor blood pressure, pulse, and auscultation *to evaluate CV response*.
- Assess respirations and adventitious sounds *to monitor drug effectiveness*.
- Examine the nares *to evaluate for any lesions that might lead to systemic absorption of the drug*.

Nursing Diagnoses

Nursing diagnoses related to drug therapy might include the following:

- Risk for injury related to immunosuppression
- Acute pain related to local effects of the drug
- Deficient knowledge regarding drug therapy

Planning

- The patient will receive the best therapeutic effect from the drug therapy.
- The patient will have limited adverse effects to the drug therapy.
- The patient will have an understanding of the drug therapy, adverse effects to anticipate, and measures to relieve discomfort and improve safety.

Implementation with Rationale

- Do not administer the drug to treat an acute asthma attack or status asthmaticus *because these drugs are not intended for treatment of acute attack and will not provide the immediate relief that is needed*.
- Taper systemic steroids carefully during the transfer to inhaled steroids; *deaths have occurred from adrenal insufficiency with sudden withdrawal*.
- Have the patient use decongestant drops before using the inhaled steroid *to facilitate penetration of the drug if nasal congestion is a problem*.
- Have the patient rinse the mouth after using the inhaler *because this will help to decrease systemic absorption and to help reduce the risk of oral thrush and decrease GI upset and nausea*.
- Monitor the patient for any sign of respiratory infection; *continued use of steroids during an acute infection can lead to serious complications related to the depression of the inflammatory and immune responses*.
- Provide thorough patient teaching, including the drug name and prescribed dosage, measures to help avoid adverse effects, warning signs that may indicate problems, and the need for periodic monitoring and evaluation, *to enhance patient knowledge about drug therapy and to promote compliance*.
- Instruct the patient to continue to take the drug *to reach and then maintain effective levels* (drug takes 2 to 3 weeks to reach effective levels).
- Offer support and encouragement *to help the patient cope with the disease and the drug regimen*.

Evaluation

- Monitor patient response to the drug (improved breathing).
- Monitor for adverse effects (nasal irritation, fever, GI upset).
- Evaluate the effectiveness of the teaching plan (patient can name drug, dosage, adverse effects to watch for, specific measures to avoid them, and measures to take to increase the effectiveness of the drug).
- Monitor the effectiveness of other measures to ease breathing.

Leukotriene Receptor Antagonists

A newer class of drugs, the **leukotriene receptor antagonists**, was developed to act more specifically at the site of the problem associated with asthma. Zafirlukast (*Accolate*) was the first drug of this class to be developed. Montelukast (*Singulair*) and zileuton (*Zyflo*) are the other drugs currently available in this class. Because this class is relatively new, long-term effects and the benefits of one drug over another have not yet been determined.

Therapeutic Actions and Indications

Leukotriene receptor antagonists selectively and competitively block (zafirlukast, montelukast) or antagonize (zileuton) receptors for the production of leukotrienes D_4 and E_4, components of SRSA. As a result, these drugs block many of the signs and symptoms of asthma, such as neutrophil and eosinophil migration, neutrophil and monocyte aggregation, leukocyte adhesion, increased capillary permeability, and smooth muscle contraction. These factors contribute to the inflammation, edema, mucus secretion, and bronchoconstriction seen in patients with asthma. See Table 55.4 for Usual Indications of these drugs. They do not have immediate effects on the airways and are not indicated for treating acute asthma attacks.

Pharmacokinetics

These drugs are given orally. They are rapidly absorbed from the GI tract. Zafirlukast and montelukast are extensively metabolized in the liver by the cytochrome P-450 system and are primarily excreted in the feces. Zileuton is metabolized and cleared through the liver. These drugs cross the placenta and enter breast milk (see Contraindications and Cautions).

Contraindications and Cautions

These drugs should be used cautiously in patients with hepatic or renal impairment *because these conditions can affect the drug's metabolism and excretion. Fetal toxicity has been reported in animal studies*, so these drugs should be used during pregnancy only if the benefit to the mother clearly outweighs the potential risks to the fetus. No adequate studies have been done on the effects on the baby if these drugs are used during lactation; caution should be used.

These drugs are not indicated for the treatment of acute asthmatic attacks *because they do not provide any immediate effects on the airways*. Patients need to be cautioned that they should not rely on these drugs for relief from an acute asthmatic attack.

Adverse Effects

Adverse effects associated with leukotriene receptor antagonists include headache, dizziness, nausea, diarrhea, abdominal pain, elevated liver enzyme concentrations, vomiting, generalized pain, fever, and myalgia. Because these drugs are relatively new, there is little information about their long-term effects. Patients should be advised to monitor their use of these drugs and to report any increase of acute episodes or lack of response to the drug, which could indicate a worsening problem or decreased responsiveness to drug therapy.

Clinically Important Drug–Drug Interactions

Use caution if propranolol, theophylline, terfenadine, or warfarin is taken with these drugs because increased toxicity can occur. Toxicity may also occur if these drugs are combined with calcium-channel blockers, cyclosporine, or aspirin; decreased dose of either drug may be necessary.

Ⓟ Prototype Summary: Zafirlukast

Indications: Prevention and long-term treatment of asthma in adults and children 5 years of age or older.

Actions: Specifically blocks receptors for leukotrienes, which are components of slow-reacting substance of anaphylaxis, blocking airway edema and processes of inflammation in the airway.

Pharmacokinetics:

Route	Onset	Peak	Duration
Oral	Rapid	3 h	Unknown

$T_{1/2}$: 10 hours; metabolized in the liver and excreted in the urine and feces.

Adverse Effects: Headache, dizziness, nausea, generalized pain and fever, infection.

Nursing Considerations for Patients Receiving Leukotriene Receptor Antagonists

Assessment: History and Examination

- Assess for *possible contraindications or cautions*: Allergy to the drug and acute bronchospasm or asthmatic attack, *all of which would be contraindications to the use of the drug*; impaired renal or hepatic function, *which could alter the metabolism and excretion of the drug and might require a dose adjustment*; and pregnancy or lactation, *which require cautious use*.
- Perform a physical examination *to establish baseline data for assessing the effectiveness of the drug and the occurrence of any adverse effects associated with drug therapy*.
- Evaluate temperature *to monitor for underlying infection*.
- Assess orientation and affect *to monitor for CNS effects of the drug*.

- Evaluate respirations and adventitious breath sounds *to monitor the effectiveness of the drug.*
- Evaluate liver and renal function tests *to assess for impairments that could interfere with metabolism or excretion of the drugs.*
- Perform an abdominal evaluation *to monitor GI effects of the drug.*

Nursing Diagnoses

Nursing diagnoses related to drug therapy might include the following:

- Acute pain related to headache, GI upset, or myalgia
- Risk for injury related to CNS effects
- Deficient knowledge regarding drug therapy

Planning

- The patient will receive the best therapeutic effect from the drug therapy.
- The patient will have limited adverse effects to the drug therapy.
- The patient will have an understanding of the drug therapy, adverse effects to anticipate, and measures to relieve discomfort and improve safety.

Implementation with Rationale

- Administer drug on an empty stomach, 1 hour before or 2 hours after meals; *the bioavailability of these drugs is decreased markedly by the presence of food.*
- Caution the patient that these drugs are not to be used during an acute asthmatic attack or bronchospasm; *instead, regular emergency measures will be needed.*
- Caution the patient to take the drug continuously and not to stop the medication during symptom-free periods *to ensure that therapeutic levels are maintained.*
- Provide appropriate safety measures if dizziness occurs *to prevent patient injury.*
- Urge the patient to avoid OTC preparations containing aspirin, *which might interfere with the effectiveness of these drugs.*
- Provide thorough patient teaching, including the drug name and prescribed dosage, measures to help avoid adverse effects, warning signs that may indicate problems, and the need for periodic monitoring and evaluation, *to enhance patient knowledge about drug therapy and to promote compliance.*
- Offer support and encouragement *to help the patient cope with the disease and the drug regimen.*

Evaluation

- Monitor patient response to the drug (improved breathing).
- Monitor for adverse effects (drowsiness, headache, abdominal pain, myalgia).
- Evaluate the effectiveness of the teaching plan (patient can name drug, dosage, adverse effects to watch for, specific measures to avoid them, and measures to take to increase the effectiveness of the drug).
- Monitor the effectiveness of other measures to ease breathing.

Mast Cell Stabilizer

A **mast cell stabilizer** prevents the release of inflammatory and bronchoconstricting substances when the mast cells are stimulated to release these substances because of irritation or the presence of an antigen. Cromolyn (*NasalCrom*) is the only drug still available in this class, only available in an OTC form, and it is no longer considered part of the treatment standards because of the availability of more specific and safer drugs.

KEY POINTS

- Corticosteroids decrease the inflammatory response. The inhalable form is associated with many fewer systemic effects than are the other corticosteroid formulations.
- To block various signs and symptoms of asthma the leukotriene receptor antagonists block or antagonize receptors for the production of leukotrienes D_4 and E_4.

Lung Surfactants

Lung surfactants (Table 55.5) are naturally occurring compounds or lipoproteins containing lipids and apoproteins that reduce the surface tension within the alveoli, allowing expansion of the alveoli for gas exchange. Four lung surfactants available for use are beractant (*Survanta*), calfactant (*Infasurf*), the newest drug of the class, lucinactant (*Surfaxin*), and poractant (*Curosurf*).

Therapeutic Actions and Indications

These drugs are used to replace the surfactant that is missing in the lungs of neonates with RDS (see Figure 55.2). See Table 55.5 for Usual Indications.

Pharmacokinetics

These drugs are instilled directly into the trachea and begin to act immediately on instillation. They are metabolized in the lungs by the normal surfactant metabolic pathways.

Contraindications and Cautions

Because lung surfactants are used as emergency drugs in the newborn, there are no contraindications.

Table 55.5 *Drugs in Focus:* Lung Surfactants

Drug Name	Usual Dosage	Usual Indications
beractant (*Survanta*)	4 mL/kg birth weight, instilled intratracheally; may repeat up to four times in 48 h	Rescue treatment of infants who have RDS; prophylactic treatment of infants at high risk for development of RDS (birth weight of <1,350 g; birth weight >1,350 g who have evidence of respiratory immaturity)
calfactant (*Infasurf*)	3 mg/kg birth weight, as soon as possible for prophylaxis; 3 mg/kg birth weight, divided into two doses, repeat up to a total of three doses 12 h apart, for rescue; instilled into trachea	Rescue treatment of infants who have RDS; prophylactic treatment of infants at high risk for RDS (see prior entry for risks)
poractant (*Curosurf*)	2.5 mL/kg birth weight, intratracheally, half in each bronchus, may repeat with up to two 1.25-mL/kg doses at 12-h intervals	Rescue treatment of infants who have RDS; this drug is being tried in the treatment of adult RDS and with adults after near-drowning

RDS, respiratory distress syndrome.

Adverse Effects

Adverse effects that are associated with the use of lung surfactants include patent ductus arteriosus, bradycardia, hypotension, intraventricular hemorrhage, pneumothorax, pulmonary air leak, hyperbilirubinemia, and sepsis. These effects may be related to the immaturity of the patient, the invasive procedures used, or reactions to the lipoprotein.

Ⓟ Prototype Summary: Beractant

Indications: Prophylactic treatment of infants at high risk for developing RDS; rescue treatment of infants who have developed RDS.

Actions: Natural bovine compound of lipoproteins that reduce the surface tension and allow expansion of the alveoli; replaces the surfactant that is missing in infants with RDS.

Pharmacokinetics:

Route	Onset	Peak
Intratracheal	Immediate	Hours

$T_{1/2}$: Unknown; metabolized by surfactant pathways.

Adverse Effects: Patent ductus arteriosus, intraventricular hemorrhage, hypotension, bradycardia, pneumothorax, pulmonary air leak, pulmonary hemorrhage, apnea, sepsis, infection.

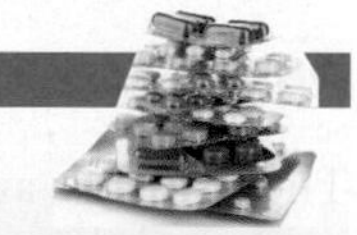

Nursing Considerations for Patients Receiving Lung Surfactants

Assessment: History and Examination

- Assess for *possible contraindications or cautions*: Screen for time of birth and exact weight *to determine appropriate doses*. Because this drug is used as an emergency treatment, there are no contraindications to screen for.
- Perform a physical examination *to establish baseline data for assessing the effectiveness of the drug and the occurrence of any adverse effects associated with drug therapy.*
- Assess the skin temperature and color *to evaluate perfusion.*
- Monitor respirations, adventitious sounds, endotracheal tube placement and patency, and chest movements *to evaluate the effectiveness of the drug and drug delivery.*
- Evaluate blood pressure, pulse, and arterial pressure *to monitor the status of the infant.*
- Evaluate blood gases and oxygen saturation *to monitor drug effectiveness.*
- Assess temperature and complete blood count *to monitor for sepsis.*

Nursing Diagnoses

Nursing diagnoses related to drug therapy might include the following:

- Decreased cardiac output related to CV and respiratory effects of the drug
- Risk for Injury related to prematurity and risk of infection
- Ineffective airway clearance related to the possibility of mucus plugs
- Deficient knowledge regarding drug therapy (for parents)

Planning

- The patient will receive the best therapeutic effect from the drug therapy.
- The patient will have limited adverse effects to the drug therapy.
- The patient will have an understanding of the drug therapy, adverse effects to anticipate, and measures to relieve discomfort and improve safety.

Implementation with Rationale

- Monitor the patient continuously during administration and until stable *to provide life support measures as needed.*
- Ensure proper placement of the endotracheal tube with bilateral chest movement and lung sounds *to provide adequate delivery of the drug.*

- Have staff view the manufacturer's teaching video before regular use *to review the specific technical aspects of administration.*
- Suction the infant immediately before administration, but do not suction for 2 hours after administration unless clinically necessary, *to allow the drug time to work.*
- Provide support and encouragement to parents of the patient, explaining the use of the drug in the teaching program, *to help them cope with the diagnosis and treatment of their infant.*
- Continue other supportive measures related to the immaturity of the infant *because this is only one aspect of medical care needed for premature infants.*

Evaluation

- Monitor patient response to the drug (improved breathing, alveolar expansion).
- Monitor for adverse effects (pneumothorax, patent ductus arteriosus, bradycardia, sepsis).
- Evaluate the effectiveness of the teaching plan and support parents as appropriate.
- Monitor the effectiveness of other measures to support breathing and stabilize the patient.
- Evaluate the effectiveness of other supportive measures related to the immaturity of the infant.

KEY POINTS

- Lung surfactants are naturally occurring compounds that reduce the surface tension in the alveoli, allowing them to expand. They are injected directly into the trachea of infants who have RDS.
- Administration of lung surfactants requires proper placement of the endotracheal tube, suctioning of the infant before administration (but not for 2 hours after administration unless necessary), and careful monitoring and support of the infant to ensure lung expansion and proper oxygenation.

Other Drugs Used to Treat Lower Respiratory Tract Disorders

The other major pathophysiology that can affect the lower respiratory tract is infection. Infection can manifest as bronchitis or pneumonia. These infections occur when pathogens are able to enter the normally well-protected airways and surrounding tissue. Stress, age, and concurrent respiratory dysfunction all increase the opportunities for these pathogens to invade the respiratory tract and cause problems. These infections can be viral, bacterial, fungal, or protozoal in origin. They are treated using the appropriate agents to affect the specific pathogen that is involved. See Chapter 9 for drugs used to treat bacterial infections, Chapter 10 for drugs used to treat viral infections, Chapter 11 for drugs used to treat fungal infection, and Chapter 12 for drugs used to treat protozoal infections. Patients with infections of the respiratory tract may have difficulty breathing, decreased oxygenation leading to fatigue, and changes in abilities to carry on the activities of daily living, including eating. These patients require support, assistance to maintain function, help with nutrition, and support to deal with the uncomfortable feeling of not being able to breathe.

See Box 55.7 for information about two drugs approved for treatment of idiopathic pulmonary fibrosis.

BOX 55.7

Drugs for Idiopathic Pulmonary Fibrosis

In 2014 the first drugs for the treatment of idiopathic pulmonary fibrosis (IPF) were approved. IPF is a disease of progressive lung scarring and decline in lung function with no known cause or treatment. These two new drugs offer treatment options to these patients. Pirfenidone (*Esbriet*), a pyridine, and nintedanib (*Ofev*), a kinase inhibitor, are both approved for the treatment of IPF. Nintedanib is a very small molecule that inhibits numerous kinase receptors including ones associated with proliferation, migration, and formation of fibroblasts that are implicated in the development of IPF. It should be used with caution with hepatic impairment and can cause embryo/fetal toxicity. Nintedanib can cause severe GI problems leading to dehydration as well as thromboembolic events including myocardial infarction (MI). Bleeding in patients with known bleeding risks and GI perforation when used after GI surgery have been reported. Pirfenidone has been shown to improve lung function in patients with IPF, but the mechanism of action is not known. It is an oral agent taken three times a day. The drug needs to be tapered to reach the desired therapeutic dosing. It has also been associated with liver toxicity and GI issues. Rash and photosensitivity have also been reported. It should be used with caution with renal impairment, liver impairment, and use of CYP1A2 inhibitors.

SUMMARY

- Pulmonary obstructive diseases include asthma and COPD, which includes emphysema and chronic bronchitis—these disorders cause obstruction of the major airways—and RDS, which causes obstruction at the alveolar level.
- Drugs used to treat asthma and COPD include drugs to block inflammation and drugs to dilate bronchi.
- The xanthine derivatives have a direct effect on the smooth muscle of the respiratory tract, both in the bronchi and in the blood vessels.

- The adverse effects of the xanthines are directly related to the theophylline concentration in the blood and can progress to coma and death.
- Sympathomimetics are drugs that mimic the effects of the sympathetic nervous system; they are used for dilation of the bronchi and to increase the rate and depth of respiration.
- Anticholinergics can be used as bronchodilators because of their effect on the vagus nerve, resulting in relaxation of smooth muscle in the bronchi, which leads to bronchodilation.
- Steroids are used to decrease the inflammatory response in the airway. Inhaling the steroid tends to decrease the numerous systemic effects that are associated with steroid use.
- Leukotriene receptor antagonists block or antagonize receptors for the production of leukotrienes D_4 and E_4, thus blocking many of the signs and symptoms of asthma.
- Lung surfactants are instilled into the respiratory system of premature infants who do not have enough surfactant to ensure alveolar expansion.

CHECK YOUR UNDERSTANDING

Answers to the questions in this chapter can be found in Answers to Check Your Understanding Questions on thePoint®.

MULTIPLE CHOICE

Select the best answer to the following.

1. Treatment of obstructive pulmonary disorders is aimed at
a. opening the conducting airways or decreasing the effects of inflammation.
b. blocking the autonomic reflexes that alter respirations.
c. blocking the effects of the immune and inflammatory systems.
d. altering the respiratory membrane to increase the flow of oxygen and carbon dioxide.

2. The xanthines
a. block the sympathetic nervous system.
b. stimulate the sympathetic nervous system.
c. directly affect the smooth muscles of the respiratory tract.
d. act in the CNS to cause bronchodilation.

3. Your patient has been maintained on theophylline for many years and has recently taken up smoking. The theophylline levels in this patient would be expected to
a. rise because nicotine prevents the breakdown of theophylline.
b. stay the same because smoking has no effect on theophylline.
c. fall because nicotine stimulates liver metabolism of theophylline.
d. rapidly reach toxic levels.

4. A person with hypertension and known heart disease has frequent bronchospasms and asthma attacks that are most responsive to sympathomimetic drugs. This patient might be best treated with
a. an inhaled sympathomimetic to decrease systemic effects.
b. a xanthine.
c. no sympathomimetics because they would be contraindicated. correct
d. an anticholinergic.

5. A patient with many adverse reactions to drugs is tried on an inhaled steroid for treatment of bronchospasm. For the first 3 days the patient does not notice any improvement. You should
a. switch the patient to a xanthine.
b. encourage the patient to continue the drug for 2 to 3 weeks.
c. switch the patient to a sympathomimetic.
d. try the patient on surfactant.

6. Leukotriene receptor antagonists act to block production of a component of slow-reacting substance of anaphylaxis. They are most beneficial in treating
a. seasonal rhinitis.
b. pneumonia.
c. COPD.
d. asthma.

7. Respiratory distress syndrome occurs in
a. babies with frequent colds.
b. babies with genetic allergies.
c. premature and low-birth-weight babies.
d. babies stressed during the pregnancy.

8. Lung surfactants used therapeutically are
  a. injected into a developed muscle.
  b. instilled via a nasogastric tube.
  c. injected into the umbilical artery.
  d. instilled into an endotracheal tube properly placed in the baby's lungs.

MULTIPLE RESPONSE

Select all that apply.

1. Clients who are using inhalers require careful teaching about which of the following?
  a. Avoiding food 1 hour before and 2 hours after dosing
  b. Storage of the drug
  c. Administration techniques to promote therapeutic effects and avoid adverse effects
  d. Lying flat for as long as 2 hours after dosing
  e. Timing of administration
  f. The difference between rescue treatment and prophylaxis

2. A child with repeated asthma attacks may be treated with which of the following drugs?
  a. A leukotriene receptor antagonist
  b. A beta-blocker
  c. An inhaled corticosteroid
  d. An inhaled beta-agonist
  e. A surfactant
  f. A mast cell stabilizer

BIBLIOGRAPHY AND REFERENCES

Bauldoff, G. (2012). When breathing is a burden: How to help patients with COPD. *American Nurse, 7*(8).

Berger, W. (2009). *Asthma*. New York: Oxford University Press.

Brunton, L., Chabner, B., & Knollman, B. (2011). *Goodman and Gilman's the pharmacological basis of therapeutics* (12th ed.). New York: McGraw-Hill.

Cobridge, S., & Cobridge, T. (2010). Asthma in adolescents and adults. *American Journal of Nursing, 110*(5), 28–38.

Donner, C., & Carone, M. (Eds.). (2007). *Clinical challenges in COPD*. New York: Clinical Publishing.

Facts and Comparisons. (2015). *Drug facts and comparisons*. St. Louis, MO: Author.

Facts and Comparisons. (2015). *Professional's guide to patient drug facts*. St. Louis, MO: Author.

Gershon, A., Campbell, M., Croxford, R., et al. (2014). Combination LABAs and inhaled corticosteroids compared with LABAs alone in older adults with COPD. *Journal of the American Medical Association, 312*(11), 1114–1121.

Karch, A. M. (2014). *Lippincott's nursing drug guide*. Philadelphia, PA: Lippincott Williams & Wilkins.

Kuehn, B. (2007). New asthma guidelines released. *Journal of the American Medical Association, 298*(13), 1503–1504.

Porth, C. M. (2013). *Pathophysiology: Concepts of altered health states* (9th ed.). Philadelphia, PA: Lippincott Williams & Wilkins.

Robinson, T., & Scullion, J. (2009). *Oxford handbook of respiratory nursing*. New York: Oxford University Press.

PART 11

DRUGS ACTING ON THE GASTROINTESTINAL SYSTEM

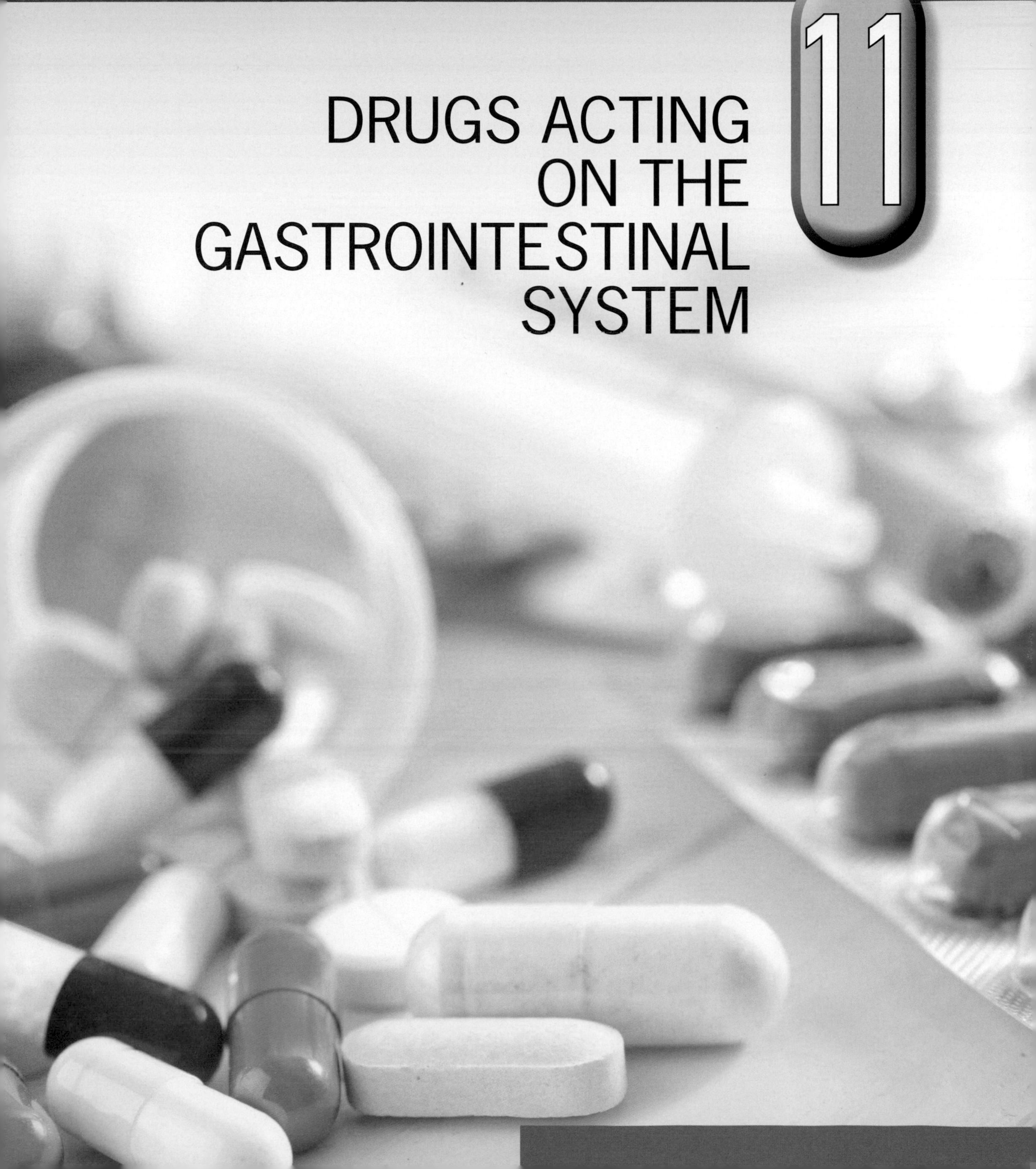

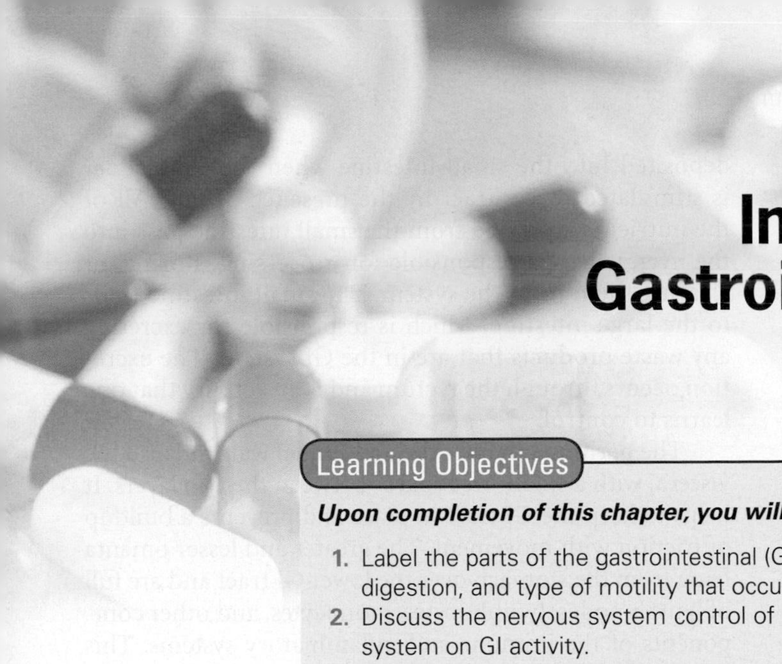

56 Introduction to the Gastrointestinal System

Learning Objectives

Upon completion of this chapter, you will be able to:

1. Label the parts of the gastrointestinal (GI) tract on a diagram, describing the secretions, absorption, digestion, and type of motility that occurs in each part.
2. Discuss the nervous system control of the GI tract, including influences of the autonomic nervous system on GI activity.
3. List three of the local GI reflexes and describe the clinical application of each.
4. Describe the steps involved in swallowing, including two factors that can influence this reflex.
5. Discuss the vomiting reflex, addressing three factors that can stimulate the reflex.

Glossary of Key Terms

bile: fluid produced in the liver and stored in the gallbladder that contains cholesterol and bile salts; essential for the proper breakdown and absorption of fats

chyme: contents of the stomach containing ingested food and secreted enzymes, water, and mucus

gallstones: hard crystals formed in the gallbladder when the bile containing many crystalline substances is concentrated

gastrin: substance secreted by the stomach in response to many stimuli; stimulates the release of hydrochloric acid from the parietal cells and pepsin from the chief cells; causes histamine release at histamine-2 receptors to effect the release of acid

histamine-2 (H_2) receptors: sites near the parietal cells of the stomach that, when stimulated, cause the release of hydrochloric acid into the lumen of the stomach; also found near cardiac cells

hydrochloric acid: acid released by the parietal cells of the stomach in response to gastrin release or parasympathetic stimulation; makes the stomach contents more acidic to aid digestion and breakdown of food products

local gastrointestinal reflex: reflex response to various stimuli that allows the GI tract local control of its secretions and movements based on the contents or activity of the whole GI system

nerve plexus: network of nerve fibers running through the wall of the GI tract that allows local reflexes and control

pancreatic enzymes: digestive enzymes secreted by the exocrine pancreas, including pancreatin and pancrelipase, which are needed for the proper digestion of fats, proteins, and carbohydrates

peristalsis: type of GI movement that moves a food bolus forward; characterized by a progressive wave of muscle contraction

saliva: fluid produced by the salivary glands in the mouth in response to tactile stimuli and cerebral stimulation; contains enzymes to begin digestion, as well as water and mucus to make the food bolus slippery and easier to swallow

segmentation: GI movement characterized by contraction of one segment of the small intestine while the next segment is relaxed; the contracted segment then relaxes, and the relaxed segment contracts; exposes the chyme to a vast surface area to increase absorption

swallowing: complex reflex response to a bolus in the back of the throat; allows passage of the bolus into the esophagus and movement of ingested contents into the GI tract

vomiting: complex reflex mediated through the medulla after stimulation of the chemoreceptor trigger zone; protective reflex to remove possibly toxic substances from the stomach

The gastrointestinal (GI) system is the only system in the body that is open to the external environment. It begins at the mouth and ends at the anus. The GI system is responsible for only a very small part of waste excretion. The kidneys and lungs are responsible for excreting most of the waste products of normal metabolism.

Structure and Function of the Gastrointestinal System

The GI system is composed of one continuous tube that begins at the mouth; progresses through the esophagus, stomach, and small and large intestines; and ends at the anus. The pancreas, liver, and gallbladder are accessory organs that support the functions of the GI system (Figure 56.1).

Structures

The tube that comprises the GI tract is continuous with the external environment, opening at the mouth and again at the anus. Because of this the GI tract contains many foreign agents and bacteria that are not found in the rest of the body. These bacteria, the normal flora of the GI tract, have a role in digestion and in protecting the body from other bacteria that might be ingested. The tube begins in the mouth, which has salivary glands that secrete digestive enzymes and lubricants to facilitate swallowing. The mouth leads to the esophagus, which produces mucus to help facilitate movement, which connects to the stomach. The stomach is responsible for mechanical and chemical breakdown of foods into usable nutrients. The stomach empties into the small intestine, where absorption of nutrients occurs. The pancreas deposits digestive enzymes and sodium bicarbonate into the beginning of the small intestine to neutralize the acid from the stomach and to further facilitate digestion. The liver produces bile, which is stored in the gallbladder. The bile is very important in the digestion of fats and is deposited into the small intestine when the gallbladder is stimulated to contract by the presence of fats. All of the nutrients absorbed from the small intestine pass into the liver, which is responsible for processing, storing, or clearing them from the system. The small intestine leads to the large intestine, which is responsible for excreting any waste products that are in the GI system. The excretion occurs through the rectum and is an activity that one learns to control.

The peritoneum lines the abdominal wall and also the viscera, with a small "free space" between the two layers. It helps to keep the GI tract in place and prevents a buildup of friction with movement. The greater and lesser omenta hang from the stomach over the lower GI tract and are full of lymph nodes, lymphocytes, monocytes, and other components of the immune and inflammatory systems. This barrier provides rapid protection for the rest of the body if any of the bacteria or other foreign agents in the GI tract should be absorbed into the body.

Layers of the GI tract

The GI tube is composed of four layers: The mucosa, the muscularis mucosa, the **nerve plexus** (a network of nerve fibers running through the wall of the GI tract that allows local reflexes and control), and the adventitia.

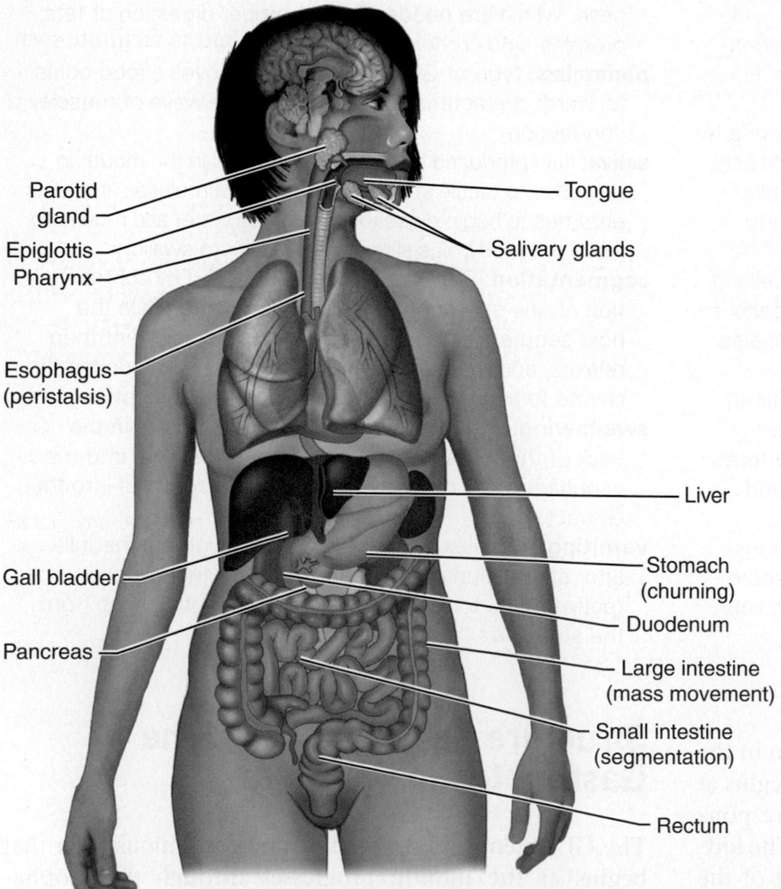

FIGURE 56.1 The gastrointestinal tract.

Mucosal Layer

The mucosal layer provides the inner lining of the GI tract. It can be seen in the mouth and is fairly consistent throughout the tube. It is important to remember when assessing a patient that, if the mouth is very dry or full of lesions, that is a reflection of the state of the entire GI tract and may indicate that the patient has difficulty digesting or absorbing nutrients. This layer has an epithelial component and a connective tissue component.

Muscularis Mucosa Layer

The muscularis mucosa layer is made up of muscles. Most of the GI tract has two muscle layers. One layer runs circularly around the tube, helping keep the tube open and squeezing the tube to aid digestion and motility. The other layer runs horizontally, which helps propel the GI contents down the tract. The stomach has a third layer of muscle, which runs obliquely and gives the stomach the ability to move contents in a churning motion.

Nerve Plexus Layer

The nerve plexus has two layers of nerves—one submucosal layer and one myenteric layer. These nerves allow the GI tract local control over movement, secretions, and digestion. The nerves respond to local stimuli and act on the contents of the GI tract accordingly. The GI tract is also innervated by the sympathetic and parasympathetic nervous systems. These systems can slow down or speed up the activity in the GI tract but cannot initiate local activity. The sympathetic system is stimulated during times of stress ("fight-or-flight" response) when digestion is not a priority. To slow the GI tract the sympathetic system decreases muscle tone, secretions, and contractions and increases sphincter tone. By shutting down GI activity the body saves energy for other activities. In contrast, the parasympathetic system ("rest-and-digest" response) stimulates the GI tract, increasing muscle tone, secretions, and contractions and decreases sphincter tone, allowing easy movement.

Adventitia Layer

The adventitia is the outer layer of the GI tract. It serves as a supportive layer and helps the tube maintain its shape and position (Figure 56.2).

Gastrointestinal Activities

The GI system has four major activities:

- *Secretion* of enzymes, acid, bicarbonate, and mucus
- *Absorption* of water and almost all of the essential nutrients needed by the body
- *Digestion* of food into usable and absorbable components
- *Motility* (movement) of food and secretions through the system (what is not used is excreted in the form of feces)

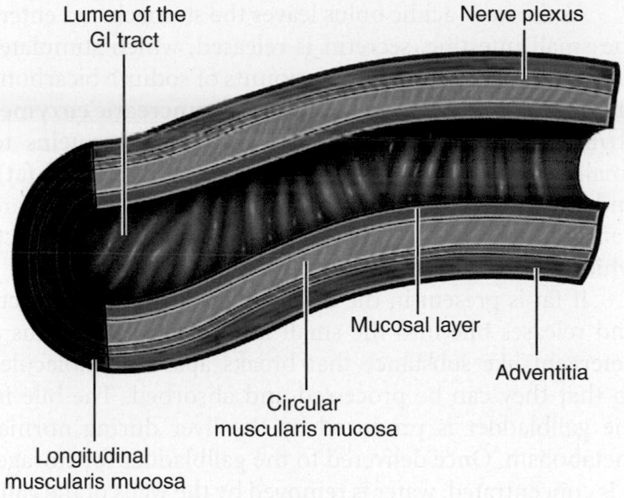

FIGURE 56.2 Layers of the gastrointestinal tract.

These functions are discussed in detail in the following sections.

Secretion

The GI tract secretes various compounds to aid the movement of the food bolus through the GI tube, to protect the inner layer of the GI tract from injury, and to facilitate the digestion and absorption of nutrients (see Figure 56.1). Secretions begin in the mouth. **Saliva**, which contains water and digestive enzymes, is secreted from the salivary glands to begin the digestive process and to facilitate swallowing by making the bolus slippery.

Mucus is also produced in the mouth to protect the epithelial lining and to aid in swallowing. The esophagus produces mucus to protect the inner lining of the GI tract and to further facilitate the movement of the bolus down the tube.

The stomach produces acid and digestive enzymes. In addition, it generates a large amount of mucus to protect the stomach lining from the acid and the enzymes. In the stomach, secretion begins with what is called the cephalic phase of digestion. The sight, smell, or taste of food stimulates the stomach to begin secreting before any food reaches the stomach. Once the bolus of food arrives at the stomach, gastrin is secreted. **Gastrin** stimulates the stomach muscles to contract, the parietal cells to release **hydrochloric acid**, and the chief cells to release pepsin. Parasympathetic stimulation also leads to acid release. Gastrin and the parasympathetic system stimulate **histamine-2 (H_2) receptors** near the parietal cells, causing the cells to release hydrochloric acid into the lumen of the stomach. Proteins, calcium, alcohol, and caffeine in the stomach increase gastrin secretion. High levels of acid decrease the secretion of gastrin. Other digestive enzymes are released appropriately, in response to proteins and carbohydrates, to begin digestion. Peptic ulcers can develop when there is a decrease in the protective mucosal layer or an increase in acid production.

As the now-acidic bolus leaves the stomach and enters the small intestine, secretin is released, which stimulates the pancreas to secrete large amounts of sodium bicarbonate (to neutralize the acid bolus), the **pancreatic enzymes** chymotrypsin and trypsin (to break down proteins to smaller amino acids), other lipases (to break down fat), and amylases (to break down sugars). These enzymes are delivered to the GI tract through the common bile duct, which is shared with the gallbladder.

If fat is present in the bolus the gallbladder contracts and releases bile into the small intestine. **Bile** contains a detergent-like substance that breaks apart fat molecules so that they can be processed and absorbed. The bile in the gallbladder is produced by the liver during normal metabolism. Once delivered to the gallbladder for storage, it is concentrated; water is removed by the walls of the gallbladder. Some people are prone to developing **gallstones** in the gallbladder when the concentrated bile crystallizes. These stones can move down the duct and cause severe pain or even blockage of the bile duct.

In response to the presence of food the small and large intestines may secrete various endocrine hormones, including growth hormone, aldosterone, and glucagon. They also secrete large amounts of mucus to facilitate the movement of the bolus through the rest of the GI tract.

Digestion

Digestion is the process of breaking food into usable, absorbable nutrients. Digestion begins in the mouth, with the enzymes in the saliva starting the process of breaking down sugars and proteins. The stomach continues the digestion process with muscular churning, breaking down some foodstuffs while mixing them thoroughly with hydrochloric acid and enzymes. The acid and enzymes further break down sugars and proteins into building blocks and separate vitamins, electrolytes, minerals, and other nutrients from ingested food for absorption. The beginning of the small intestine introduces bile to the food bolus, which is now called **chyme**. Bile breaks down fat molecules for processing and absorption into the bloodstream and the pancreatic enzymes continue the digestion of sugars, proteins, and fats. Digestion is finished at this point, and absorption of the nutrients begins.

Absorption

Absorption is the active process of removing water, nutrients, and other elements from the GI tract and delivering them to the bloodstream for use by the body. The portal system drains all of the lower GI tract, where absorption occurs, and delivers what is absorbed into the venous system directly to the liver. The liver filters, clears, and further processes most of what is absorbed before it is delivered to the body (see Figure 56.1). Some absorption occurs in the lower end of the stomach, most commonly absorption of water and alcohol. Most absorption occurs in the small intestine. It is about 8,500 mL/d, including nutrients, drugs, and anything that is taken into the GI tract, as well as any secretions. The small intestine mucosal layer is specially designed to facilitate this absorption, with long villi on the epithelial layer providing a vast surface area for absorption. The large intestine absorbs approximately 350 mL/d, mostly sodium and water.

Motility

The GI tract depends on an inherent motility to keep things moving through the system. The nerve plexus maintains a basic electrical rhythm (BER), much like the pacemaker rhythm in the heart. The cells within the plexus are somewhat unstable and leak electrolytes, leading to the regular firing of an action potential. This rhythm maintains the tone of the GI tract muscles and protects the lining of the GI tract from digestive enzymes and other toxins and is affected by local or autonomic stimuli to increase or decrease the rate of firing.

The basic movement seen in the esophagus is **peristalsis**, a constant wave of contraction that moves from the top to the bottom of the esophagus. The act of **swallowing**, a response to a food bolus in the back of the throat, stimulates the peristaltic movement that directs the food bolus into the stomach. The stomach uses its three muscle layers to produce a churning action. This action mixes the digestive enzymes and acid with the food to increase digestion. A contraction of the lower end of the stomach sends the chyme into the small intestine.

The small intestine uses a process of segmentation with an occasional peristaltic wave to clear the segment. **Segmentation** involves contraction of one segment of small intestine while the next segment is relaxed. The contracted segment then relaxes, and the relaxed segment contracts. This action exposes the chyme to a vast surface area to increase absorption. The small intestine maintains a BER of 11 contractions per minute. This regular movement is assessed when listening for bowel sounds.

The large intestine uses a process of mass movement with an occasional peristaltic wave. When the beginning segment of the large intestine is stimulated, it contracts and sends a massive peristaltic movement throughout the entire large intestine. The end result of the mass movement is usually excretion of waste products.

Rectal distention after mass movement stimulates a defecation reflex that causes relaxation of the external and internal sphincters. Control of the external sphincter is a learned behavior. The receptors in the external sphincter adapt relatively quickly and will stretch and require more and more distention to stimulate the reflex if the reflex is ignored.

KEY POINTS

- The GI system begins at the mouth and ends at the anus; a long tube extends between them and comprises the esophagus, the stomach, the small intestine, and the large intestine. Essential functions are digestion and absorption of nutrients.

- The GI tract is composed of four layers: The mucosa, the muscularis mucosa, the nerve plexus, and the adventitia.
- The GI tract has four major functions: Secretion, absorption, digestion, and motility.
- The GI system secretes enzymes, acid, bicarbonate, and mucus to facilitate the digestion and absorption of nutrients.
- The small intestine is the section of the GI tract where most absorption occurs. The veins of the small intestine carry the absorbed products to the liver for filtering, cleaning, and metabolism, or the breaking down of absorbed products into usable substances.
- The nerve plexus controls the GI system by maintaining electrical rhythm and responding to local stimuli (increasing or decreasing activity). The autonomic nervous system influences GI activity, with the sympathetic system slowing and the parasympathetic system increasing activity.

Gastrointestinal Reflexes

To function effectively, several local and central reflexes occur. Local reflexes involve stimulation of the nerves in the GI tract and cause movement and secretion. Central reflexes, which include swallowing and vomiting, are controlled by the medulla.

Local Reflexes

Stimulation of local nerves within the GI tract causes increased or decreased movement within the system, maintaining homeostasis. Loss of reflexes or stimulation can result in constipation and the lack of movement of the bolus along the GI tract or diarrhea with increased motility and excretion. The longer a fecal bolus remains in the large intestine the more sodium and water are absorbed from it and the harder and less mobile it can become. There are many **local gastrointestinal reflexes**. Some knowledge of how these reflexes operate makes it easier to understand what happens when the reflexes are blocked or overstimulated and how therapeutic measures are often used to cause reflex activity.

- *Gastroenteric reflex*: Stimulation of the stomach by stretching, the presence of food, or cephalic stimulation (the body's response to smelling, seeing, tasting, or thinking about food) causes an increase in activity in the small intestine. It is thought that this prepares the small intestine for the coming chyme.
- *Gastrocolic reflex*: Stimulation of the stomach also causes increased activity in the colon, again preparing it to empty any contents to provide space for the new chyme.
- *Duodenal–colic reflex*: The presence of food or stretching in the duodenum stimulates colon activity and mass movement, again to empty the colon for the new chyme.

It is important to remember the gastroenteric, gastrocolic, and duodenal reflexes when helping patients to maintain GI movement. Taking advantage of stomach stimulation (e.g., having the patient drink prune juice or hot water or eat bran) and providing the opportunity of time and privacy for a bowel movement after eating in the morning encourage normal reflexes to keep things in control.

Other local GI reflexes include the following:

- *Ileogastric reflex*: The introduction of chyme or stretch to the large intestine slows stomach activity, as does the introduction of chyme into the small and large intestine, allowing time for absorption. In part, this reflex explains why patients who are constipated often have no appetite: The continued stretch on the ileum that comes with constipation continues to slow stomach activity and makes the introduction of new food into the stomach undesirable.
- *Intestinal–intestinal reflex*: Excessive irritation to one section of the small intestine causes a cessation of activity above that section to prevent further irritation and an increase in activity below that section, which leads to a flushing of the irritant. This reflex is active in "Montezuma's revenge" (traveler's diarrhea): Local irritation of the intestine causes increased secretions and movement below that section, resulting in watery diarrhea and a cessation of movement above that section. Loss of appetite or even nausea may occur. An extreme reaction to this reflex can be seen after abdominal surgery, when the handling of the intestines causes intense irritation and the reflex can cause the entire intestinal system to cease activity, leading to a paralytic ileus.
- *Peritoneointestinal reflex*: Irritation of the peritoneum as a result of inflammation or injury leads to a cessation of GI activity, preventing continued movement of the GI tract and thus further irritation of the peritoneum.
- *Renointestinal reflex*: Irritation or swelling of the renal capsule causes a cessation of movement in the GI tract, again preventing further irritation to the capsule.
- *Vesicointestinal reflex*: Irritation or overstretching of the bladder can cause a reflex cessation of movement in the GI tract, again preventing further irritation to the bladder from GI movement. Many patients with cystitis or overstretched bladders from occupational constraints or neurological problems complain of constipation, which can be attributable to this reflex.
- *Somatointestinal reflex*: Taut stretching of the skin and muscles over the abdomen irritates the nerve plexus and causes a slowing or cessation of GI activity preventing further irritation. During the era when tight girdles were commonly worn, this reflex was often seen among women, and constipation was a serious problem for many women who wore such constraining garments. Tight-fitting clothing (e.g., jeans) can have the same effect. Patients who complain of chronic constipation may be suffering from overactivity of the somatointestinal reflex.

Central Reflexes

Two centrally mediated reflexes—swallowing and vomiting—are very important to the functioning of the GI tract.

Swallowing

The swallowing reflex is stimulated whenever a food bolus stimulates pressure receptors in the back of the throat and pharynx. These receptors send impulses to the medulla, which stimulates a series of nerves that cause the following actions: The soft palate elevates and seals off the nasal cavity, respirations cease in order to protect the lungs, the larynx rises and the glottis closes to seal off the airway, and the pharyngeal constrictor muscles contract and force the food bolus into the top of the esophagus, where pairs of muscles contract in turn to move the bolus down the esophagus into the stomach. This reflex is complex, involving more than 25 pairs of muscles.

This reflex can be facilitated in a number of ways if swallowing (food or medication) is a problem. Icing the tongue by sucking on a *Popsicle* or an ice cube blocks external nerve impulses and allows this more basic reflex to respond. Icing the sternal notch or the back of the neck, although not as appealing, has also proved effective in stimulating the swallowing reflex. In addition, keeping the head straight (not turned to one side) allows the muscle pairs to work together and helps the process. Providing stimulation of the receptors in the mouth through temperature variations and textured foods helps to initiate the reflex. Patients who do not produce their own saliva can be given artificial saliva to increase digestion and to lubricate the food bolus, which also helps the swallowing reflex.

Vomiting

The **vomiting** reflex is another basic reflex that is centrally mediated and important in protecting the system from unwanted irritants. The vomiting reflex is stimulated by two centers in the medulla. The more primitive center is called the emetic zone. When stimulated, it initiates projectile vomiting. This type of intense reaction is seen in young children and whenever increased pressure in the brain or brain damage allows the more primitive center to override the more mature chemoreceptor trigger zone (CTZ). The CTZ is stimulated in several ways:

- Tactile stimulation of the back of the throat, a reflex to get rid of something that is too big or too irritating to be swallowed
- Excessive stomach distention
- Increasing intracranial pressure by direct stimulation
- Stimulation of the vestibular receptors in the inner ear (a reaction often seen with dizziness after "wild" rides in amusement parks)
- Stimulation of stretch receptors in the uterus and bladder (a possible explanation for vomiting in early pregnancy and before delivery)
- Intense pain fiber stimulation
- Direct stimulation by various chemicals, including fumes, certain drugs, and debris from cellular death (a reason for vomiting after chemotherapy or radiation therapy that results in cell death)

Once the CTZ is stimulated a series of reflexes occurs. Salivation increases, and there is a large increase in the production of mucus in the upper GI tract, which is accompanied by a decrease in gastric acid production. This action protects the lining of the GI tract from potential damage by the acidic stomach contents. (Nauseated patients who start swallowing repeatedly or complain about secretions in their throat are in the process of preparing for vomiting.) The sympathetic system is stimulated, with a resultant increase in sweating, increased heart rate, deeper respirations, and nausea. This prepares the body for fight or flight and the insult of vomiting. The esophagus then relaxes and becomes distended, and the gastric sphincter relaxes. The patient takes one deep respiration; the glottis closes, and the palate rises, trapping the air in the lungs and sealing off entry to the lungs. The abdominal and thoracic muscles contract, increasing intraabdominal pressure. The stomach then relaxes, and the lower section of the stomach contracts in waves, approximately six times per minute. With nothing in the stomach, this movement is known as retching, and it can be quite tiring and uncomfortable. This action causes a backward peristalsis and movement of stomach contents up the esophagus and out the mouth. The body thus rids itself of offending irritants.

The vomiting reflex is complex and protective, but it can be undesirable in certain clinical situations, when the stimulant is not something that can be vomited or when the various components of the vomiting reflex could be detrimental to a patient's health status.

KEY POINTS

- Swallowing, a centrally mediated reflex important in delivering food to the GI tract for processing, is controlled by the medulla. It involves a complex series of timed reflexes.
- Vomiting is controlled by the CTZ in the medulla or by the emetic zone in immature or injured brains. The CTZ is stimulated by several different processes and initiates a complex series of responses that first prepare the system for vomiting and then cause a strong backward peristalsis to rid the stomach of its contents.

SUMMARY

- The GI system is composed of one long tube that starts at the mouth, includes the esophagus, the stomach, the small intestine, and the large intestine, and ends at the anus. The GI system is responsible for digestion and absorption of nutrients.
- Secretion of digestive enzymes, acid, bicarbonate, and mucus facilitates the digestion and absorption of nutrients.

- The GI system is controlled by a nerve plexus, which maintains a BER and responds to local stimuli to increase or decrease activity. The sympathetic nervous system, if stimulated, slows GI activity; stimulation of the parasympathetic nervous system increases activity. Initiation of activity depends on local reflexes.
- A series of local reflexes within the GI tract helps to maintain homeostasis within the system. Overstimulation of any of these reflexes can result in constipation (underactivity) or diarrhea (overactivity).
- Swallowing, a centrally mediated reflex important in delivering food to the GI tract for processing, is controlled by the medulla. It involves a complex series of timed reflexes.
- Vomiting is controlled by the CTZ in the medulla or by the emetic zone in immature or injured brains. The CTZ is stimulated by several different processes and initiates a complex series of responses that first prepare the system for vomiting and then cause a strong backward peristalsis to rid the stomach of its contents.

CHECK YOUR UNDERSTANDING

Answers to the questions in this chapter can be found in Answers to Check Your Understanding Questions on thePoint®.

MULTIPLE CHOICE

Select the best answer to the following.

1. After teaching a group of students about GI activity and constipation the instructor determines that the teaching was successful when the students state which of the following about constipation?
- **a.** It results from increased peristaltic activity in the intestinal tract.
- **b.** It occurs primarily when one does not have a daily bowel movement.
- **c.** It leads to decreased salt and water absorption from the large intestine.
- **d.** It can be artificially induced by increasing the volume of the large intestine.

2. In explaining the importance of the pancreas to a student nurse the instructor would explain that the pancreas
- **a.** is primarily an endocrine gland.
- **b.** secretes enzymes in response to an increased plasma glucose concentration.
- **c.** neutralizes the hydrochloric acid secreted by the stomach.
- **d.** produces bile.

3. Gastrin
- **a.** stimulates acid secretion in the stomach.
- **b.** secretion is blocked by the products of protein digestion in the stomach.
- **c.** secretion is stimulated by acid in the duodenum.
- **d.** is responsible for the chemical or gastric phase of intestinal secretion.

4. When explaining the control of the activities of the GI tract—movement and secretion—the nurse would be most accurate to state that the GI is basically controlled by
- **a.** the sympathetic nervous system.
- **b.** the parasympathetic nervous system.
- **c.** local nerve reflexes of the GI nerve plexus.
- **d.** the medulla in the brain stem.

5. The presence of fat in the duodenum causes
- **a.** acid indigestion.
- **b.** decreased acid production.
- **c.** increased gastrin release.
- **d.** contraction of the gallbladder.

6. The basic type of movement that occurs in the small intestine is
- **a.** peristalsis.
- **b.** mass movement.
- **c.** churning.
- **d.** segmentation.

7. Most of the nutrients absorbed from the GI tract pass immediately into the portal venous system and are processed by the liver. This is possible because almost all absorption occurs through
- **a.** the lower section of the stomach.
- **b.** the top section of the large intestine.
- **c.** the small intestine.
- **d.** the ileum.

(continues on page 986)

MULTIPLE RESPONSE

Select all that apply.

1. The CTZ in the brain is activated by which of the following?
a. Stretch of the uterus
b. Stretch of the bladder
c. Decreased GI activity
d. Radiation
e. Cell death
f. Extreme pain

2. Acid production in the stomach is stimulated by which of the following?
a. Protein in the stomach
b. Calcium products in the stomach
c. High levels of acid in the stomach
d. Alcohol in the stomach
e. Low levels of acid in the stomach
f. H_2 stimulation

3. When describing the action of pancreatic digestive enzymes in breaking down substances, which substances would the instructor include?
a. Gastric acid
b. Fats
c. Proteins
d. Sugars
e. Bile
f. Lipids

BIBLIOGRAPHY AND REFERENCES

Barrett, K., Barman, S., Boitano, S., et al. (2015). *Ganong's review of medical physiology* (25th ed.). New York: McGraw-Hill.

Brunton, L., Chabner, B., & Knollman, B. (2011). *Goodman and Gilman's the pharmacological basis of therapeutics* (12th ed.). New York: McGraw-Hill.

Hall, J. (2015). *Guyton and Hall's textbook of medical physiology* (13th ed.). Philadelphia, PA: W. B. Saunders.

Johnson, L. R., & Ghishan, F. K. (2012). *Physiology of the gastrointestinal tract* (5th ed.). New York: Academic Press.

Parkman, H., & Fisher, R. S. (2006). *The clinician's guide to acid/peptic disorders and motility disorders of the GI tract.* Thorofare, NJ: Slack.

Porth, C. M. (2013). *Pathophysiology: Concepts of altered health states* (9th ed.). Philadelphia, PA: Lippincott Williams & Wilkins.

Rhoades, R. A., & Bell, D. R. (2012). *Medical physiology: Principles of clinical medicine.* Philadelphia, PA: Lippincott Williams & Wilkins.

Seidel, E. (2006). *Crash course: GI system.* St. Louis, MO: Mosby.

Seifter, J., Rafnon, A., & Sloane, D. (2005). *Concepts in medical physiology.* Philadelphia, PA: Lippincott Williams & Wilkins.

57 Drugs Affecting Gastrointestinal Secretions

Learning Objectives

Upon completion of this chapter, you will be able to:

1. Describe the current theories on the pathophysiological process responsible for the signs and symptoms of peptic ulcer disease.
2. Describe the therapeutic actions, indications, pharmacokinetics, contraindications and cautions, most common adverse reactions, and important drug–drug interactions associated with drugs used to affect gastrointestinal (GI) secretions.
3. Discuss the drugs used to affect GI secretions across the lifespan.
4. Compare and contrast the prototype drugs used to affect GI secretions with other agents in their class and with other classes of drugs used to affect GI secretions.
5. Outline the nursing considerations, including important teaching points, for patients receiving drugs used to affect GI secretions.

Glossary of Key Terms

acid rebound: reflex response of the stomach to lower-than-normal acid levels; when acid levels are lowered through the use of antacids, gastrin production and secretion are increased to return the stomach to its normal acidity

antacids: group of inorganic chemicals that neutralize stomach acid

digestive enzymes: enzymes produced in the gastrointestinal tract to break down foods into usable nutrients

gastrointestinal protectant: drug that coats any injured area in the stomach to prevent further injury from acid or pepsin

histamine-2 (H_2) antagonist: drug that blocks the H_2 receptor sites; used to decrease acid production in the stomach (H_2 sites are stimulated to cause the release of acid in response to gastrin or parasympathetic stimulation)

peptic ulcer: erosion of the lining of stomach or duodenum; results from imbalance between acid produced and the mucous protection of the gastrointestinal lining or possibly from infection by *Helicobacter pylori* bacteria

prostaglandin: any one of numerous tissue hormones that have local effects on various systems and organs of the body, including vasoconstriction, vasodilation, increased or decreased GI activity, and increased or decreased pancreatic enzyme release

proton pump inhibitor: drug that blocks the H^+, K^+–ATPase enzyme system on the secretory surface of the gastric parietal cells, thus interfering with the final step of acid production and lowering acid levels in the stomach

Drug List

Drugs Used to Treat Gastroesophageal Reflux Disease and Ulcer Disease

Histamine-2 Antagonists
- (P) cimetidine
- famotidine
- nizatidine
- ranitidine

Antacids
- aluminum salts
- calcium salts
- magnesium salts
- (P) sodium bicarbonate

Proton Pump Inhibitors
- dexlansoprazole
- esomeprazole
- lansoprazole
- (P) omeprazole
- pantoprazole
- rabeprazole

Gastrointestinal Protectant
- (P) sucralfate

Prostaglandin
- (P) misoprostol

Drugs Used to Treat Digestive Enzyme Dysfunction
- (P) pancrelipase
- saliva substitute

Gastrointestinal (GI) disorders are among the most common complaints seen in clinical practice. Many products are available for the self-treatment of upset stomach, heartburn, and sour stomach. (See Box 57.1 for a list of these over-the-counter [OTC] drugs.) The underlying causes of these disorders can range from dietary excess, stress, hiatal hernia, esophageal reflux, and adverse drug effects to the more serious **peptic ulcer** disease. This chapter addresses the major conditions often requiring drug therapy: Peptic ulcer disease and disorders involving increased acid levels and digestive enzyme dysfunction (Box 57.2).

Drugs Used to Treat Gastroesophageal Reflux Disease and Ulcer Disease

Drugs typically used to affect GI secretions in treating peptic ulcer disease and disorders involving increased GI acid work to decrease GI secretory activity, block the action of GI secretions, or form protective coverings on the GI lining to prevent erosion from GI secretions. Recent research studies have begun questioning the effects that lowering acid levels might have on the homeostasis of the GI system and on total body homeostasis, including calcium and magnesium levels and the effects on normal flora bacteria (Box 57.3).

The drugs used to treat gastroesophageal reflux disease (GERD) and ulcer disease include histamine-2 (H_2) antagonists, which block the release of hydrochloric acid in response to gastrin; antacids, which interact with acids at the chemical level to neutralize them; proton pump inhibitors, which suppress the secretion of hydrochloric acid into the lumen of the stomach; GI protectants, which coat any injured area in the stomach to prevent further injury from acid; and prostaglandins, which inhibit the secretion

BOX 57.1

Over-the-Counter Drugs Affecting Gastrointestinal Secretions

aluminum hydroxide (*Amphogel*)
aluminum–magnesium combinations (*Maalox, Mylanta*, and others)
calcium carbonate (*Tums*, and others)
cimetidine (*Tagamet HB*)
esomeprazole (*Nexium24HR*)
famotidine (*Pepcid AC*)
magnesium salts (*Phillips' Milk of Magnesia*, and others)
nizatidine (*Axid*)
omeprazole (*Prilosec OTC*)
omeprazole with sodium bicarbonate (*Zegrid OTC*)
ranitidine (*Zantac*)
sodium bicarbonate (baking soda, *Bell-ans*)

BOX 57.2

Conditions That Affect Gastrointestinal Secretions

Ulcer Disease

Erosions in the lining of the stomach and adjacent areas of the GI tract are called peptic ulcers. Ulcer patients present with a predictable description of gnawing, burning pain often occurring a few hours after meals. Many of the drugs that are used to affect GI secretions are designed to prevent, treat, or aid in the healing of these ulcers. The cause of chronic peptic ulcers is not completely understood. For many years, it was believed that ulcers were caused by excessive acid production, and treatment was aimed at neutralizing acid or blocking the parasympathetic system to decrease normal GI activity and secretions. Further research led many to believe that, because acid production was often normal in ulcer patients, ulcers were caused by a defect in the mucous lining that coats the inner lumen of the stomach to protect it from digestive enzymes. The leading cause of peptic ulcers in the United States is the use of NSAIDs. NSAIDS inhibit cyclooxygenase receptors, and one of the functions of these sites is the production of the mucous lining in the stomach. A thinner protective coat is more susceptible to the erosive action of acid. Treatment is now aimed at improving the balance between the acid produced and the mucous layer that protects the stomach lining. Currently, it is believed that chronic ulcers may be the result of impaired mucous lining and infection by *Helicobacter pylori* bacteria. Combination antibiotics have been found to be quite effective in treating some patients with chronic ulcers.

Acute ulcers, or "stress ulcers," are often seen in situations that involve acute physiological stress, such as trauma, burns, or prolonged illness. The activity of the sympathetic nervous system during stress decreases blood flow to the GI tract, leading to less blood flow to the inner layer of the GI tract and weakening of the mucosal layer of the stomach and erosion by acid in the stomach. Many of the drugs available for treating various peptic ulcers act to alter the acid-producing activities of the stomach to decrease the erosive action.

Digestive Enzyme Dysfunction

Some patients require a supplement to the production of digestive enzymes. Patients with strokes, salivary gland disorders, or extreme surgery of the head and neck may not be able to produce saliva. Saliva is important in beginning the digestion of sugars and proteins and is essential in initiating the swallowing reflex. Artificial saliva may be necessary for these patients. Patients with common bile duct problems, pancreatic disease, or cystic fibrosis may not be able to produce or secrete pancreatic enzymes. These enzymes may need to be administered to allow normal digestion and absorption of nutrients.

BOX 57.3 FOCUS ON The Evidence

Drugs That Decrease Acid May Affect More Than Acid Levels

In December 2005 the *Journal of the American Medical Association* published a study that followed patients taking proton pump inhibitors (*Nexium, Prevacid, Protonix,* and others) over a period of 10 years. This report was verified with follow-up studies published in 2009 and 2010. The report showed that patients using these drugs had *Clostridium difficile* infections leading to diarrhea at three times the rate of patients not using these drugs. There was also a reported two-time increase in these infections in patients using H_2 antagonists (*Tagamet, Pepcid, Axid,* and others). *C. difficile* is a significant cause of diarrhea in the community. Other studies have reported similar findings. Drugs that lower acid levels change the normal environment of the GI tract, perhaps allowing bacteria to thrive that would normally be destroyed by the acid. Most of these acid-lowering drugs are available in OTC preparations and may be used in excessive doses for prolonged periods of time without the health care provider's knowledge. This information should alert health care providers and patients to the need for caution in using these drugs. If a patient is complaining about diarrhea the health care provider should specifically ask about the use of acid-lowering products (sometimes patients do not even think of these products as drugs because they can buy them without a prescription). During health care teaching sessions, it is important to remind people to read the labels of OTC drugs carefully and to follow instructions. If a patient feels the need to take one of these products for a prolonged period of time, he or she should be advised to obtain a medical evaluation because the symptoms being treated with these drugs could have an underlying medical cause that should be evaluated.

When evaluating the data from these studies, the researchers also noted a similar increase in these GI infections in patients using NSAIDs (ibuprofen, ketoprofen, and others) for a prolonged period of time. The researchers suggested that further study be done on that group of patients to verify the finding.

It is important to keep current with long-term studies on drugs and to remember that changing a normal function or environment in the body will change the balance of homeostasis in the body and could potentially cause other problems. In 2007 and again in 2013, studies reported an increase in osteoporosis and bone fractures in patients on long-term proton pump inhibitor use. Changing the acidity of the GI tract seems to affect calcium absorption. Other studies have linked the use of proton pump inhibitors to lower serum magnesium levels, which can cause hypertension, also linked to inability to be absorbed in a low-acid environment; loss of vitamin B_{12} absorption (this vitamin requires intrinsic factor in the lining of the stomach to facilitate absorption), linking that absorption to acidity levels; and an increase in pneumonia (loss of normal flora that require a certain acidity to survive might lead to the overgrowth of other bacteria in the GI tract that can go back up the esophagus and enter the airways). Many studies have linked altered GI acidity to a change in oral drug absorption. Oral drugs are tested in subjects or patients with normal stomach acidity and when that is not present the drugs may not be broken down as expected. Other studies of long-term antacid use highlight the change to a more alkaline urine because the alkaline byproducts of antacids filtered into the kidney can cause an alteration in drug excretion. The result of all of these studies is that we have developed over the years a new appreciation of the GI tract and the precarious balance that is needed to keep it functioning normally. Teaching patients to limit use, only use these products for a short term and then encourage follow-up to evaluate the cause of signs and symptoms, can have an important impact on patient safety and the therapeutic effectiveness of these products.

of gastrin and increase the secretion of the mucous lining of the stomach, providing a buffer.

Figure 57.1 depicts the sites of actions of these drugs used to treat GERD and ulcer disease. Box 57.4 highlights important considerations related to use of these drugs across the lifespan.

Histamine-2 Antagonists

Histamine-2 (H_2) antagonists (Table 57.1) block the release of hydrochloric acid in response to gastrin. These drugs include cimetidine (*Tagamet HB*), ranitidine (*Zantac*), famotidine (*Pepcid*), and nizatidine (*Axid*).

Therapeutic Actions and Indications

The H_2 antagonists selectively block H_2 receptors located on the parietal cells. Blocking these receptors prevents the release of gastrin, a hormone that causes local release of histamine (due to stimulation of histamine receptors), ultimately blocking the production of hydrochloric acid. This action also decreases pepsin production by the chief cells. H_2 receptor sites are also found in the heart, and high levels of these drugs can produce cardiac arrhythmias (see Adverse Effects).

These drugs are used in the following conditions:

- Short-term treatment of active duodenal ulcer or benign gastric ulcer (reduction in the overall acid level can promote healing and decrease discomfort).
- Treatment of pathological hypersecretory conditions such as Zollinger-Ellison syndrome (blocking the overproduction of hydrochloric acid that is associated with these conditions).
- Prophylaxis of stress-induced ulcers and acute upper GI bleeding in critical patients (blocking the production of

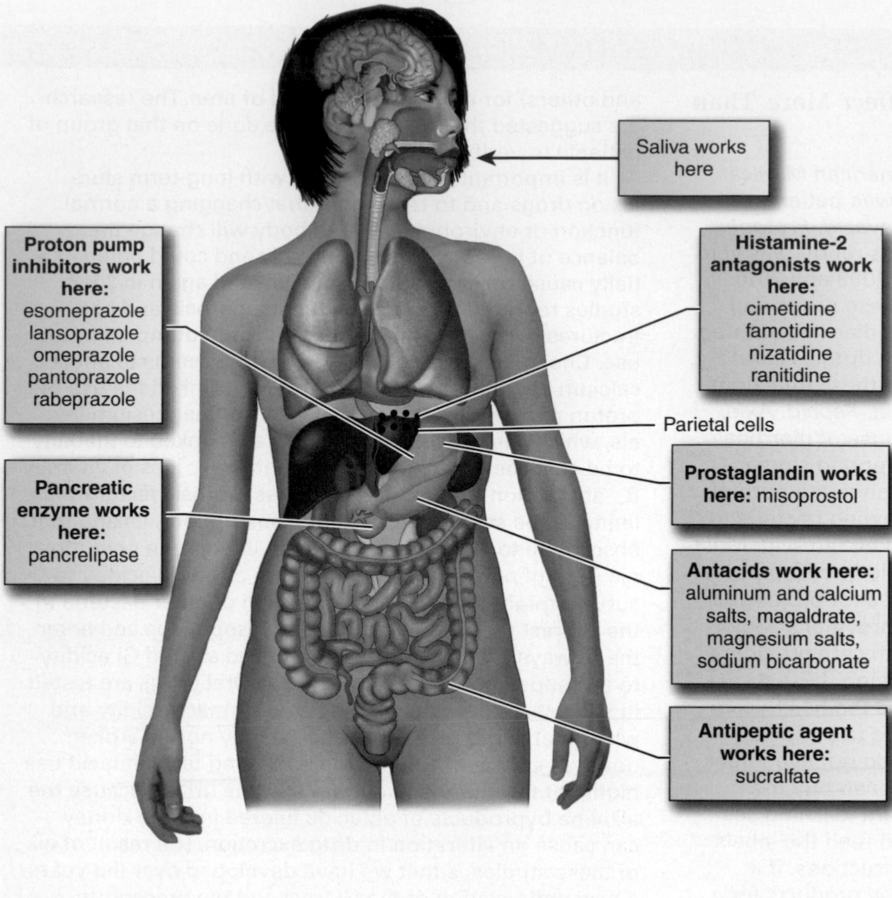

FIGURE 57.1 Sites of action of drugs affecting gastrointestinal secretions.

BOX 57.4 FOCUS ON **Drug Therapy Across the Lifespan**

Agents that Affect Gastrointestinal Secretions

CHILDREN

Famotidine is the only H_2 antagonist approved for use in children. The proton pump inhibitors, although not specifically indicated for use in children, have been very successfully used to decrease ulcer formation related to stress or drug therapy. Dose should be determined by the age and weight of the child. Lansoprazole has established pediatric doses if a proton pump inhibitor is most appropriate.

Antacids may be used in children who complain of upset stomach or who are receiving therapy known to increase acid production; 5 to 15 mL every 1 to 3 hours is usually an effective dose.

Special caution should be used with any of these agents to prevent electrolyte disturbances or any interference with nutrition, which could be especially detrimental to children.

ADULTS

Adults should be cautioned not to overuse any of these agents and to check with their health care provider if GI discomfort continues after repeated use of any of these drugs. Patients should be monitored for any electrolyte disturbances or interference with the absorption or action of other drugs. If antacids are used, they should be spaced 1 to 2 hours before or after the use of other drugs. In 2005 and again in 2007 and 2012, some studies were published that linked prolonged use of these agents with an increased incidence of colitis and other GI infections, electrolyte imbalance, bone loss, hypertension, and other systemic issues. Patients should be cautioned to limit the use of these drugs and to seek medical help for persistent symptoms.

The safety of these drugs during pregnancy and lactation has not been established, so they should be used with caution during pregnancy or lactation.

Misoprostol is an abortifacient and should never be used during pregnancy. Women of childbearing age who use misoprostol should be advised to use barrier-type contraceptives. Use of the other agents should be reserved for those situations in which the benefit to the mother outweighs the potential risk to the fetus. The drugs may enter breast milk and also may alter electrolyte levels or gastric secretions in the neonate. It is advised that caution be used if one of these drugs is prescribed during lactation.

OLDER ADULTS

Older adults frequently are prescribed one or more of these drugs. Older adults are more likely to develop adverse effects associated with the use of these drugs, including sedation, confusion, dizziness, urinary retention, and CV effects. Safety measures may be needed if these effects occur and interfere with the patient's mobility and balance. Because of changes that occur within the

BOX 57.4 FOCUS ON Drug Therapy Across the Lifespan *(continued)*

GI tract with age, absorption of nutrients can be affected when any of these drugs is used. The use of proton pump inhibitors and H_2 blockers in older adults has been associated with decreased absorption of vitamin B_{12} and the development of pernicious anemia.

Older adults are also more likely to have renal and/or hepatic impairment related to underlying medical conditions, which could interfere with the metabolism and excretion of these drugs. The dose for older adults should be started at a lower level than recommended for younger adults. Patients should be monitored very closely, and dose adjustment should be made based on patient response.

These patients also need to be alerted to the potential for toxic effects when using OTC preparations that may contain the same ingredients as many of these agents. They should be advised to check with their health care provider before beginning any OTC drug regimen.

Proton pump inhibitors may be the best choice for treating GERD in older patients because of fewer adverse effects and better therapeutic response with these drugs.

Table 57.1 *Drugs in Focus:* Drugs Used to Treat Gastroesophageal Reflux Disease and Ulcer Disease

Drug Name	Usual Dosage	Usual Indications
Histamine-2 Antagonists		
cimetidine (*Tagamet HB*)	300 mg PO q.i.d. at meals and at bedtime *or* 800 mg PO at bedtime; 300 mg IV or IM q6–8 h *or* 200 mg PO for heartburn; reduce dose with geriatric patients or patients with renal impairment *Pediatric (1–16 y):* 0.5–1 mg/kg/d PO *or* 0.25 mg/kg IV q12 h	Treatment of duodenal ulcer, benign gastric ulcer, pathological hypersecretory syndrome, GERD; prophylaxis of stress ulcers; relief of symptoms of heartburn, acid indigestion, sour stomach *Special considerations:* Not for children <16 y old
famotidine (*Pepcid, Pepcid AC*)	20–40 mg PO or IV at bedtime *or* 20 mg PO b.i.d., 10 mg PO for prevention or relief of heartburn; reduce dose in renal-impaired or geriatric patients	Treatment of duodenal ulcer, benign gastric ulcer, pathological hypersecretory syndrome, GERD; relief of symptoms of heartburn, acid indigestion, sour stomach
nizatidine (*Axid*)	150–300 mg PO at bedtime *or* 150 mg PO b.i.d., 75 mg PO 30 min before food to prevent heartburn; reduce dose in renal-impaired or geriatric patients	Treatment of duodenal ulcer, benign gastric ulcer, pathological hypersecretory syndrome, GERD; relief of symptoms of heartburn, acid indigestion, sour stomach in adults *Special considerations:* Not recommended for use in children
ranitidine (*Zantac*)	150 mg daily to b.i.d. PO IM or IV; 75 mg PO as needed for heartburn; reduce dose in renal-impaired or geriatric patients	Treatment of duodenal ulcer, benign gastric ulcer, pathological hypersecretory syndrome, GERD; relief of symptoms of heartburn, acid indigestion, sour stomach in adults *Special considerations:* Not recommended for use in children
Antacids		
aluminum salts (*AlternaGEL*)	*Adult:* 500–1,500 mg three to six times per day between meals and at bedtime *Pediatric:* 50–150 mg/kg PO q24 h in divided doses q4–6 h	Symptomatic relief of GI hyperacidity, treatment of hyperphosphatemia, prevention of formation of phosphate urinary stones
calcium salts (*Oystercal, Tums*)	0.5–2 g PO as needed as an antacid	Symptomatic relief of GI hyperacidity, treatment of calcium deficiency, prevention of hypocalcemia
magnesium salts (*Milk of Magnesia*, others)	280–1,500 mg PO q.i.d., dose based on salt used *Pediatric:* One half of the adult dose	Symptomatic relief of GI hyperacidity, prophylaxis of stress ulcers, relief of constipation
sodium bicarbonate (*Bell-ans*)	*Adult:* 300–2,000 mg PO daily to q.i.d.	Symptomatic relief of GI hyperacidity, minimization of uric acid crystalluria, adjunctive treatment in severe diarrhea

(table continues on page 992)

Table 57.1 *Drugs in Focus:* Drugs Used to Treat Gastroesophageal Reflux Disease and Ulcer Disease (continued)

Drug Name	Usual Dosage	Usual Indications
Proton Pump Inhibitors		
dexlansoprazole (*Kapidex*)	30–60 mg/d PO for 4–8 wk	Treatment and maintenance of erosive esophagitis, treatment of heartburn associated with GERD
esomeprazole (*Nexium*)	*Acute:* 20–40 mg/d PO for 4–8 wk; 20–40 mg/d PO for maintenance	Treatment of GERD, severe erosive esophagitis, duodenal ulcers, and pathological hypersecretory conditions
lansoprazole (*Prevacid*)	15–30 mg/d PO based on condition and response, 30 mg IV over 30 min for up to 7 d *Pediatric (1–11 y) (≤30 kg):* 15 mg/kg/d PO *Pediatric (1–11 y) (>30 kg):* 30 mg/kg/d PO *Pediatric (12–17 y):* 15–30 mg/d PO	Treatment of gastric ulcer, GERD, pathological hypersecretory syndromes; maintenance therapy for healing duodenal ulcers and esophagitis; in combination therapy for the eradication of *Helicobacter pylori* infection; approved for use in children for treatment of GERD, peptic ulcer, and Zollinger-Ellison syndrome
omeprazole (*Prilosec*)	20–40 mg/d PO for 4–8 wk based on condition and response	Treatment of gastric ulcers, GERD, pathological hypersecretory syndromes; maintenance therapy for healing duodenal ulcers and esophagitis; in combination therapy for the eradication of *H. pylori* infection; available OTC for relief of heartburn symptoms
pantoprazole (*Protonix*)	40 mg PO daily to b.i.d. *or* 40 mg/d IV for 7–10 d	Treatment of GERD in adults, healing of erosive esophagitis, treatment of hypersecretory syndromes
rabeprazole (*Aciphex*)	20–60 mg/d PO based on condition and response	Treatment and maintenance of GERD; treatment of duodenal ulcers, pathological hypersecretory conditions; used as combination therapy for the eradication of *H. pylori* infection
GI Protectant		
sucralfate (*Carafate*)	1 g PO b.i.d. to q.i.d.	Short-term treatment of duodenal ulcers; maintenance of duodenal ulcers (at reduced dose) after healing in adults; treatment of oral and esophageal ulcers due to radiation, chemotherapy, or sclerotherapy; currently under investigation for treatment of gastric ulcers, gastric damage induced by NSAIDs, prevention of stress ulcers in acutely ill individuals
Prostaglandin		
misoprostol (*Cytotec*)	200 mcg PO q.i.d., reduce dose in patients with renal impairment	Prevention of NSAID-induced ulcers in adults at high risk for development of these gastric ulcers, under investigation for treatment of duodenal ulcers in patients who are not responsive to H_2 antagonists, used in combination therapy with mifepristone as an abortifacient

GERD, gastroesophageal reflux disease; GI, gastrointestinal; OTC, over the counter; NSAID, nonsteroidal anti-inflammatory drug.

acid protects the stomach lining, which is at risk because of decreased mucus production associated with extreme stress).

- Treatment of erosive gastroesophageal reflux (decreasing the acid being regurgitated into the esophagus will promote healing and decrease pain).
- Relief of symptoms of heartburn, acid indigestion, and sour stomach (OTC preparations).

See the Critical Thinking Scenario for additional information on H_2 antagonists.

Pharmacokinetics

Cimetidine, ranitidine, and famotidine are available in oral and parenteral forms. Nizatidine is available only in oral form. Cimetidine was the first drug in this class to be developed. It has been associated with antiandrogenic effects, including gynecomastia and galactorrhea. It reaches peak levels in 1 to 1.5 hours and is metabolized mainly in the liver; it can slow the metabolism of many other drugs that use the same metabolizing enzyme system. It is excreted in the urine. It has a half-life of 2 hours and is known to cross the placenta and enter breast milk.

CRITICAL THINKING SCENARIO

Histamine-2 Antagonists

THE SITUATION

W.T., a 48-year-old traveling salesman, had experienced increasing epigastric discomfort during a 7-month period. When he finally sought medical care the diagnosis was a peptic ulcer. He began taking calcium carbonate (*Tums*) for relief of his immediate discomfort, as well as ranitidine (*Zantac*), 150 mg b.i.d. W.T. was referred to the nurse for patient teaching and given an appointment for a follow-up visit in 3 weeks.

CRITICAL THINKING

Think about the physiology of duodenal ulcers and the various factors that can contribute to aggravating the problem. What patient-teaching points should be covered with this patient regarding diet, stress factors, and use of alcohol and tobacco?

What adverse effects of the drugs should this patient be aware of?

What lifestyle changes may be necessary to ensure ulcer healing, and how can W.T. be assisted in making these changes fit into the demands of his job?

DISCUSSION

Further examination indicated that W.T. is a healthy man except for the ulcer. He admits to smoking cigarettes, drinking alcohol regularly at business lunches and dinners, and eating a great deal of fast food and drinking a lot of coffee when he is on the road. He states that his job has become increasingly stressful as the economy has worsened. Because he is basically healthy and does not seek medical care unless very uncomfortable (7 months of pain), he may find it difficult to comply with his drug therapy and any suggested lifestyle changes.

W.T. needs patient education, which for purposes of building trust should preferably be with the same nurse. The instruction should include information on duodenal ulcer disease, ways to decrease acid production (such as avoiding cigarettes, acid-stimulating foods, alcohol, and caffeine), and ways to improve the protective mucous layer of the stomach by decreasing stress and anxiety-causing situations. In addition, spacing of the ranitidine and antacid doses should be stressed. Ranitidine should be taken 1 hour before or 2 hours after any antacids because they can interfere with the absorption of ranitidine and the patient may not receive a therapeutic dose. W.T. should be encouraged to avoid OTC medications and self-medication because several of these products contain ingredients that could aggravate his ulcer or interfere with the effectiveness of the drugs that have been prescribed. W.T. should be encouraged to return for regular medical evaluation of his drug therapy and his underlying condition.

Finally, W.T. should feel that he has some control over his situation. Because he does not routinely seek medical care, he may be more comfortable with a medical regimen that he has participated in planning. Allow him to suggest ways to decrease stress, ways to cut down on smoking or the use of alcohol without interfering with the demands of his job, and the best times to take the drugs in his schedule. He will learn in time which foods and situations irritate his condition. However, research has not shown that bland or restrictive diets are particularly effective in decreasing ulcer pain or spread, and they may actually increase patient anxiety. W.T. should be encouraged to jot down the situations or times of day that seem to cause him the most problems. This information can help to provide a guide for adjusting lifestyle and/or dietary patterns to aid ulcer healing and prevent further development of ulcers.

NURSING CARE GUIDE FOR W.T.: HISTAMINE-2 ANTAGONISTS

Assessment: History and Examination

Assess W.T.'s health history for allergies to any of these drugs, renal or hepatic failure, and other drugs being taken, such as antimetabolites, alkylating agents, oral anticoagulants, phenytoin, beta-blockers, alcohol, quinidine, lidocaine, theophylline, benzodiazepines, nifedipine, tricyclic antidepressants, and carbamazepine.

Focus the physical examination on the following areas:
CNS: Orientation, affect
Skin: Color, lesions
CV Cardiovascular (CV): Pulse, cardiac auscultation
GI: Liver evaluation
Laboratory tests: Complete blood count, liver, renal function tests

Nursing Diagnoses

Acute pain related to GI or CNS effects
Disturbed sensory perception (kinesthetic, auditory) related to CNS effects
Decreased cardiac output related to cardiac effects
Deficient knowledge regarding drug therapy

Planning

The patient will receive the best therapeutic effect from the drug therapy.

The patient will have limited adverse effects to the drug therapy.

(continues on page 994)

Histamine-2 Antagonists (continued)

The patient will have an understanding of the drug therapy, adverse effects to anticipate, and measures to relieve discomfort and improve safety.

Implementation

Administer with meals and at bedtime.
Provide comfort and safety measures: Analgesics, access to bathroom, safety precautions.
Arrange for decreased dose in renal/hepatic disease.
Provide support and reassurance to deal with drug effects and lifestyle changes.
Provide patient teaching regarding drug name, dosage, adverse effects, precautions, and warnings to report.

Evaluation

Evaluate drug effects: Relief of GI symptoms, ulcer healing, prevention of ulcer progression.
Monitor for adverse effects: Headache, dizziness, insomnia, gynecomastia, arrhythmias, GI alterations.
Monitor for drug–drug interactions as listed.
Evaluate the effectiveness of the patient-teaching program.
Evaluate the effectiveness of comfort and safety measures.

PATIENT TEACHING FOR W.T.

- The drug that has been prescribed for you, ranitidine, is called an H_2 antagonist. An H_2 antagonist decreases the amount of acid that is produced in the stomach. It is used to treat conditions that are aggravated by excess acid.
- Some of the following adverse effects may occur with this drug:
  - *Diarrhea:* Have ready access to bathroom facilities. This usually becomes less severe over time.
  - *Dizziness, headache:* These usually lessen as your body adjusts to the drug. Change positions slowly. If you fell drowsy, avoid driving or dangerous activities.
  - Report any of the following to your health care provider: *Sore throat, unusual bleeding or bruising, confusion, muscle or joint pain, tarry stools.*
- Avoid taking any OTC medication without first checking with your health care provider. Several of these medications can interfere with the effectiveness of this drug.
- If an antacid has been ordered for you, take it exactly as prescribed, spaced apart from your ranitidine.
- Tell any physician, nurse, or other health care provider involved in your care that you are taking this drug.
- If you are taking any other medications, do not vary the drug schedules. Consult with your primary health care provider if anything should happen to change any of these drugs or your scheduled doses.
- It is important to have regular medical follow-up while you are taking this drug to evaluate your response to the drug and any possible underlying problems.
- Keep this drug, and all other medications, out of the reach of children.

Ranitidine, which is longer acting and more potent than cimetidine, is not associated with the antiandrogenic adverse effects or the marked slowing of metabolism in the liver as cimetidine is. It reaches peak levels in 5 to 15 minutes when given parenterally and 1 to 3 hours when given orally. It has a duration of 8 to 12 hours and a half-life of 2 to 3 hours. Ranitidine is metabolized by the liver and excreted in urine. It crosses the placenta and enters breast milk.

Famotidine is similar to ranitidine, but it is much more potent than either cimetidine or ranitidine. It reaches peak effects in 1 to 3 hours and has a duration of 6 to 15 hours. Famotidine is metabolized in the liver and excreted in the urine with a half-life of 2.5 to 3.5 hours. Famotidine crosses the placenta and enters breast milk. Famotidine is approved for use in children aged 1 to 16 years old.

Nizatidine, the newest drug in this class, is similar to ranitidine in its effectiveness and adverse effects. It differs from the other three drugs in that it is eliminated by the kidneys, with no first-pass metabolism in the liver. It is the drug of choice for patients with liver dysfunction and for those who are taking other drugs whose metabolism is slowed by the hepatic activity of the other three H_2 antagonists. It reaches peak effects in 0.5 to 3 hours and has a half-life of 1 to 2 hours. Like the other three drugs, it crosses the placenta and enters the breast milk.

Contraindications and Cautions

The H_2 antagonists should not be used with known allergy to any drugs of this class *to prevent hypersensitivity reactions.* Caution should be used during pregnancy or lactation *because of the potential for adverse effects on the fetus or nursing baby* and with hepatic or renal dysfunction, *which could interfere with drug metabolism and excretion.* (Hepatic dysfunction is not as much of a problem with nizatidine.) Care should also be taken if prolonged or continual use of these drugs is necessary *because they may be masking serious underlying conditions.*

Adverse Effects

The adverse effects most commonly associated with H_2 antagonists include the following: GI effects of diarrhea or constipation; CNS effects of dizziness, headache, somnolence, confusion, or even hallucinations (thought to be related to possible H_2 receptor effects in the CNS); cardiac arrhythmias and hypotension (related to H_2 cardiac receptor blocking; more commonly seen with IV or IM administration or with prolonged use); and gynecomastia (more common with long-term use of cimetidine) and impotence.

Clinically Important Drug–Drug Interactions

Cimetidine, famotidine, and ranitidine can slow the metabolism of the following drugs, leading to increased serum levels and possible toxic reactions: Warfarin anticoagulants, phenytoin, beta-adrenergic blockers, alcohol, quinidine, lidocaine, theophylline, chloroquine, benzodiazepines, nifedipine, pentoxifylline, tricyclic antidepressants (TCAs), procainamide, and carbamazepine. There is a risk of increased salicylate levels if nizatidine is taken with aspirin.

Prototype Summary: Cimetidine

Indications: Short-term treatment of active duodenal or benign gastric ulcers; treatment of pathological hypersecretory conditions; prophylaxis of stress-induced ulcers; treatment of erosive gastroesophageal reflux; relief of symptoms of heartburn and acid indigestion.

Actions: Inhibits the actions of histamine at H_2 receptor sites of the stomach, inhibiting gastric acid secretion and reducing total pepsin output.

Pharmacokinetics:

Route	Onset	Peak	Duration
Oral	Varies	1–1.5	4–5 h
IM, IV	Rapid	1–1.5	4–5 h

$T_{1/2}$: 2 hours, metabolized in the liver and excreted in the urine.

Adverse Effects: Dizziness, confusion, headache, somnolence, cardiac arrhythmias, cardiac arrest, diarrhea, impotence, gynecomastia, rash.

Nursing Considerations for Patients Receiving Histamine-2 Antagonists

Assessment: History and Examination

- Assess for *possible contraindications or cautions*: History of allergy to any H_2 antagonists *to prevent potential allergic reactions*; impaired renal or hepatic function, *which could affect metabolism and excretion of the drug*; a detailed description of the GI problem, including length of time of the disorder and medical evaluation, *to evaluate appropriate use of the drug and possibility of underlying medical problems*; and current status of pregnancy or lactation *because of the potential for adverse effects on the fetus or newborn*.
- Perform a physical examination *to establish baseline data before beginning therapy, determine effectiveness of the therapy, and evaluate for any adverse effects associated with drug therapy*.
- Inspect the skin for evidence of lesions or rash to *monitor for adverse reactions*.
- Evaluate neurological status, including orientation and affect, *to assess CNS effects of the drug and to plan for protective measures*.
- Assess cardiopulmonary status, including pulse, blood pressure, and electrocardiogram (if IV use is needed), *to evaluate the cardiac effects of the drug*.
- Perform abdominal examination, including assessment of liver, *to establish a baseline and rule out underlying medical problems*.
- Monitor the results of laboratory tests, including liver and renal function tests, *to predict changes in metabolism or excretion of the drug that might require dose adjustment*.

Nursing Diagnoses

Nursing diagnoses related to drug therapy might include the following:

- Acute pain related to CNS and GI effects
- Disturbed sensory perception (kinesthetic, auditory) related to CNS effects
- Risk for injury related to CNS effects
- Decreased cardiac output related to cardiac arrhythmias
- Deficient knowledge regarding drug therapy

Planning

- The patient will receive the best therapeutic effect from the drug therapy.
- The patient will have limited adverse effects to the drug therapy.
- The patient will have an understanding of the drug therapy, adverse effects to anticipate, and measures to relieve discomfort and improve safety.

Implementation with Rationale

- Administer oral drug with or before meals and at bedtime (exact timing varies with product) *to ensure therapeutic levels when the drug is most needed*.
- Arrange for decreased dose in cases of hepatic or renal dysfunction *to prevent serious toxicity*.

(continues on page 996)

- Monitor the patient continually if giving IV doses *to allow early detection of potentially serious adverse effects, including cardiac arrhythmias.*
- Assess the patient carefully for any potential drug–drug interactions if given in combination with other drugs *because of the drug effects on liver enzyme systems.*
- Provide comfort, including analgesics, ready access to bathroom facilities, and assistance with ambulation, *to minimize possible adverse effects.*
- Periodically reorient the patient and institute safety measures if CNS effects occur *to ensure patient safety and improve patient tolerance of the drug and drug effects.*
- Arrange for regular follow-up *to evaluate drug effects and the underlying problem.*
- Offer support and encouragement *to help patients cope with the disease and the drug regimen.*
- Provide patient teaching regarding drug name, dosage, and schedule for administration; importance of spacing administration appropriately as ordered; need for readily available access to bathroom; signs and symptoms of adverse effects and measures to minimize or prevent them; danger signs that necessitate notifying the health care provider immediately; safety measures, such as avoiding driving and asking for assistance when ambulating, to deal with possible effects of dizziness, somnolence, or confusion; the need for compliance with therapy to achieve the intended results; and the importance of periodic monitoring and evaluation, including laboratory testing, *to determine drug effectiveness and to enhance patient knowledge about drug therapy and to promote compliance.*

Evaluation

- Monitor patient response to the drug (relief of GI symptoms, ulcer healing, prevention of progression of ulcer).
- Monitor for adverse effects (dizziness, confusion, hallucinations, GI alterations, cardiac arrhythmias, hypotension, gynecomastia).
- Evaluate the effectiveness of the teaching plan (patient can name drug, dosage, adverse effects to watch for, and specific measures to avoid them).
- Monitor the effectiveness of comfort measures and compliance with the regimen.

KEY POINTS

- Agents affecting GI secretion include H_2 antagonists, antacids, proton pump inhibitors, GI protectants, and prostaglandins. Digestive enzymes replace missing GI enzymes.
- Among the most common complaints addressed in clinical practice are GI symptoms.
- Increased acid production, decrease in the protective mucous lining of the stomach, infection with *Helicobacter pylori* bacteria, or a combination of these is the likely cause of peptic ulcers.
- H_2 antagonists block the release of acid in response to gastrin or parasympathetic release; adverse effects can include dizziness, confusion, cardiac arrhythmias, and galactorrhea.

Antacids

Antacids (Table 57.1) are a group of inorganic chemicals that neutralize stomach acid. Antacids are available OTC, and many patients use them to self-treat a variety of GI symptoms. There is no one perfect antacid (see Adverse Effects). The choice of an antacid depends on adverse effect and absorption factors. Available agents are sodium bicarbonate (*Bell-ans*), calcium carbonate (*Oystercal*, *Tums*, and others), magnesium salts (*Milk of Magnesia*, and others) and aluminum salts (*Amphojel*, and others).

Therapeutic Actions and Indications

Antacids neutralize stomach acid by direct chemical reaction (see Figure 57.1). They are recommended for the symptomatic relief of upset stomach associated with hyperacidity, as well as the hyperacidity associated with peptic ulcer, gastritis, peptic esophagitis, gastric hyperacidity, and hiatal hernia. See Table 57.1 for Usual Indications for each antacid.

Pharmacokinetics

Sodium bicarbonate, the oldest drug in this group, is readily available in many preparations, including baking soda powder, tablets, solutions, and as an injectable for treating systemic acidosis. This drug is widely distributed when absorbed orally, reaching peak levels in 1 to 3 hours, crossing the placenta, and entering breast milk. It is excreted in the urine and can cause serious electrolyte imbalance in people with renal impairment.

Calcium carbonate is actually precipitated chalk and is available in tablet and powder forms. The main drawbacks to this agent are constipation and acid rebound. It has an onset of action in about 3 to 5 minutes. It can be absorbed systemically and cause calcium imbalance. When absorbed, it is metabolized in the liver and excreted in the urine and feces, with a half-life of 1 to 3 hours. Calcium carbonate is known to cross the placenta and enter breast milk.

Magnesium salts are very effective in buffering acid in the stomach but have been known to cause diarrhea; they are sometimes used as laxatives. They are available as tablets, chewable tablets, and capsules and in liquid forms. Although these agents are not generally absorbed systemically and are excreted in the feces, absorbed magnesium can lead to nerve damage and even coma, if absorbed; it is excreted in the urine.

Aluminum salts, available as tablets, capsules, suspensions, and in a liquid form, do not cause acid rebound but are not very effective in neutralizing acid. They are bound in the feces for excretion. They have been related to severe constipation. Aluminum binds dietary phosphates and causes hypophosphatemia, which can then cause calcium imbalance throughout the system.

Many of these antacids are available in combination forms to take advantage of the acid-neutralizing effect and block adverse effects. For example, a combination of calcium and aluminum salts (*Maalox*) buffers acid and produces neither constipation nor diarrhea.

Contraindications and Cautions

The antacids are contraindicated in the presence of any known allergy to antacid products or any component of the drug *to prevent hypersensitivity reactions.* Caution should be used in the following instances: Any condition that can be exacerbated by electrolyte or acid–base imbalance *to prevent exacerbations and serious adverse effects;* any electrolyte imbalance, *which could be exacerbated by the electrolyte-changing effects of these drugs;* GI obstruction, *which could cause systemic absorption of the drugs and increased adverse effects;* renal dysfunction, *which could lead to electrolyte disturbance if any absorbed antacid is not neutralized properly;* and pregnancy and lactation *because of the potential for adverse effects on the fetus or neonate.*

Adverse Effects

The adverse effects associated with these drugs relate to their effects on acid–base and electrolyte balance. Administering an antacid frequently causes **acid rebound**, in which the stomach produces more acid in response to the alkaline environment. Neutralizing the stomach contents to an alkaline level stimulates gastrin production to cause an increase in acid production and return the stomach to its normal acidic state. In many cases, acid rebound causes an increase in symptoms, which results in an increased intake of the antacid. This leads to more acid production and an ongoing cycle. When more and more antacid is used the risk for systemic effects rises. Alkalosis with resultant metabolic changes (nausea, vomiting, neuromuscular changes, headache, irritability, muscle twitching, and even coma) may occur. The use of calcium salts may lead to hypercalcemia and milk–alkali syndrome (seen as alkalosis, renal calcium deposits, or severe electrolyte disorders). Constipation or diarrhea may result, depending on the antacid being used. Hypophosphatemia can occur with the use of aluminum salts. Finally, fluid retention and heart failure can occur with sodium bicarbonate because of its high sodium content.

Clinically Important Drug–Drug Interactions

Antacids can greatly affect the absorption of drugs from the GI tract. Most drugs are prepared for an acidic environment, and an alkaline environment can prevent them from being broken down for absorption or can actually neutralize them so that they cannot be absorbed. Patients taking antacids should be advised to separate them from any other medications by 2 hours.

If the pH of urine is affected by large doses of antacids the levels of drugs, such as quinidine, may increase and the levels of salicylates may decrease.

(P) Prototype Summary: Sodium Bicarbonate

Indications: Symptomatic relief of upset stomach from hyperacidity; prophylaxis for GI bleeding and stress ulcers; adjunctive treatment of severe diarrhea; also used for treatment of metabolic acidosis; may also be used to treat certain drug intoxications to minimize uric acid crystallization.

Actions: Neutralizes or reduces gastric acidity, resulting in an increase in gastric pH, which inhibits the proteolytic activity of pepsin.

Pharmacokinetics:

Route	Onset	Peak	Duration
Oral	Rapid	30 min	1–3 h
IV	Immediate	Rapid	Unknown

$T_{1/2}$: Unknown; excreted unchanged in the urine.

Adverse Effects: Gastric rupture, systemic alkalosis (headache, nausea, irritability, weakness, tetany, confusion), hypokalemia (secondary to intracellular shifting of potassium), gastric acid rebound.

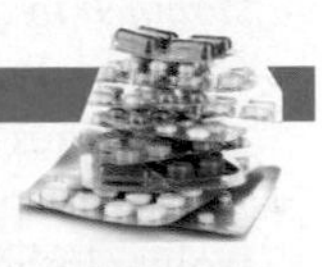

Nursing Considerations for Patients Receiving Antacids

Assessment: History and Examination

- Assess for *possible contraindications or cautions:* Any history of allergy to antacids *to prevent hypersensitivity reactions;* renal dysfunction, *which might interfere with the drug's excretion;* electrolyte disturbances, *which could be exacerbated by the effects of the drug;* and current status of pregnancy or lactation *due to possible effects on the fetus or newborn.*
- Perform a physical examination *to establish baseline data before beginning therapy, determine the effectiveness of the therapy, and evaluate for any potential adverse effects associated with drug therapy.*
- Inspect the abdomen. Auscultate bowel sounds to *ensure GI motility.*
- Assess mucous membrane status *to evaluate potential problems with absorption and hydration.*
- Monitor laboratory test results, including serum electrolyte levels and renal function tests, *to monitor*

(continues on page 998)

for adverse effects of the drug and potential alterations in excretion that may necessitate dose adjustment.

Nursing Diagnoses

Nursing diagnoses related to drug therapy might include the following:

- Diarrhea related to GI effects
- Risk for constipation related to GI effects
- Imbalanced nutrition: Less than body requirements related to GI effects
- Risk for imbalanced fluid volume related to systemic effects
- Deficient knowledge regarding drug therapy

Planning

- The patient will receive the best therapeutic effect from the drug therapy.
- The patient will have limited adverse effects to the drug therapy.
- The patient will have an understanding of the drug therapy, adverse effects to anticipate, and measures to relieve discomfort and improve safety.

Implementation with Rationale

- Administer the drug apart from any other oral medications approximately 1 hour before or 2 hours after *to ensure adequate absorption of the other medications.*
- Have the patient chew tablets thoroughly and follow with water *to ensure that therapeutic levels reach the stomach to decrease acidity.*
- Obtain specimens for periodic monitoring of serum electrolytes *to evaluate drug effects.*
- Assess the patient for any signs of acid–base or electrolyte imbalance *to ensure early detection and prompt interventions.*
- Monitor the patient for diarrhea or constipation *to institute a bowel program before severe effects occur.*
- Monitor the patient's nutritional status if diarrhea is severe or constipation leads to decreased food intake *to ensure adequate fluid and nutritional intake to promote healing and GI stability.*
- Offer support and encouragement *to help the patient cope with the disease and the drug regimen.*
- Provide thorough patient teaching, including the drug name and prescribed dosage, schedule for administration, signs and symptoms of adverse effects and measures to minimize or prevent them, warning signs that may indicate possible problems and the need to notify the health care provider immediately, the importance of maintaining fluid and nutritional intake if diarrhea or constipation occurs, possible bowel-training programs to deal with constipation or diarrhea if severe, cautions related to prolonged chronic use of drug and increased risk for acid rebound, the importance of checking with the health care provider before using any OTC medications, differences associated with the various OTC antacid formulations, and the need for periodic monitoring and evaluation *to enhance patient knowledge about drug therapy and to promote compliance.*

Evaluation

- Monitor patient response to the drug (relief of GI symptoms caused by hyperacidity).
- Monitor for adverse effects (GI effects, imbalances in serum electrolytes, and acid–base status).
- Evaluate the effectiveness of the teaching plan (patient can name the drug and dosage, as well as describe adverse effects to watch for, specific measures to avoid them, and measures to take to increase the effectiveness of the drug).
- Monitor the effectiveness of comfort measures and compliance with the regimen.

KEY POINTS

- Antacids are used to chemically react with and neutralize acid in the stomach. They can provide rapid relief from increased acid levels. They are known to cause GI alterations such as diarrhea or constipation and can alter the absorption of many drugs.
- Acid rebound occurs when the stomach produces more gastrin and more acid in response to lowered acid levels in the stomach, which commonly occurs with the use of antacids. Balancing the reduction of the stomach acid without increasing acid production is a clinical challenge.

Proton Pump Inhibitors

Proton pump inhibitors (Table 57.1) suppress the secretion of hydrochloric acid into the lumen of the stomach. Six proton pump inhibitors are available: Omeprazole (*Prilosec*), esomeprazole (*Nexium*), lansoprazole (*Prevacid*), dexlansoprazole (*Kapidex*), pantoprazole (*Protonix*), and rabeprazole (*Aciphex*).

Therapeutic Actions and Indications

The gastric acid pump or proton pump inhibitors suppress gastric acid secretion by specifically inhibiting the hydrogen–potassium adenosine triphosphatase (H^+, K^+–ATPase) enzyme system on the secretory surface of gastric parietal cells. This action blocks the final step of acid production, lowering the acid levels in the stomach (see Figure 57.1). They are recommended for the short-term treatment of active duodenal ulcers, GERD, erosive esophagitis, and benign active gastric ulcer; for the long-term treatment of pathological hypersecretory conditions; as maintenance therapy for healing of erosive esophagitis and ulcers;

and in combination with amoxicillin and clarithromycin for the treatment of *Helicobacter pylori* infection. See Table 57.1 for Usual Indications for each of these agents.

FOCUS ON Safe Medication Administration

With many patients taking nonsteroidal anti-inflammatory drugs (NSAIDs) over a long term for a variety of conditions, including arthritis and cancers, the incidence of GI ulceration and bleeding could increase. In 2011 the U.S. Food and Drug Administration (FDA) approved ***Duexis****, a combination of ibuprofen (800 mg) for relieving arthritis pain and famotidine (26.6 mg) for protecting the stomach from the adverse effects of the NSAID on the mucosal lining. Many prescribers will prescribe a proton pump inhibitor when using an NSAID long term. This combination makes it easier for the patient by combining them both in one tablet.*

Pharmacokinetics

Esomeprazole, lansoprazole, and pantoprazole are available in delayed release oral forms and as IV preparations. Rabeprazole, dexlansoprazole, and omeprazole are available only in delayed release oral forms.

These drugs are acid labile and are rapidly absorbed from the GI tract, reaching peak levels in 3 to 5 hours. They undergo extensive metabolism in the liver and are excreted in the urine. Omeprazole is faster acting and more quickly excreted than the other proton pump inhibitors. It has a half-life of 30 to 60 minutes. Esomeprazole is a longer acting drug; it has a half-life of 60 to 90 minutes and a duration of 17 hours. It is not broken down as rapidly in the liver as the parent drug omeprazole. Lansoprazole has a half-life of 2 hours and a duration of 12 hours.

Pantoprazole and rabeprazole have half-lives of 90 minutes and durations of 12 to 14 hours. Dexlansoprazole is available in a delayed capsule that offers two releases, having peak effects in 1 to 2 hours and then 4 to 5 hours, offering longer protection throughout the day. There are no adequate studies about whether these drugs cross the placenta or enter breast milk.

Contraindications and Cautions

These drugs are contraindicated in the presence of known allergy to either the drug or the drug components *to prevent hypersensitivity reactions.* Caution should be used in pregnant or lactating women *because of the potential for adverse effects on the fetus or neonate.* The safety and efficacy of these drugs have not been established for patients younger than 18 years of age, except for lansoprazole, which is the proton pump inhibitor of choice if one is needed for a child.

Adverse Effects

The adverse effects associated with these drugs are related to their effects on the H^+, K^+–ATPase pump on the parietal and other cells. CNS effects of dizziness and headache are commonly seen; asthenia (loss of strength), vertigo, insomnia, apathy, and dream abnormalities may also be observed. GI effects can include diarrhea, abdominal pain, nausea, vomiting, dry mouth, and tongue atrophy. Upper respiratory tract symptoms, including cough, stuffy nose, hoarseness, and epistaxis, are frequently seen (Figure 57.2). Other, less common adverse effects include rash, alopecia, pruritus, dry skin, back pain, and fever. In preclinical studies, long-term effects of proton pump inhibitors included the development of gastric cancer. Recent studies show an increase in bone loss and decreased calcium levels, decreased magnesium levels leading to hypertension, and increased incidence of *Clostridium difficile* diarrhea and pneumonia in patients using these drugs long term. These effects are thought to be related to changing the normal acidity in the stomach that changes the environment for absorbing calcium or magnesium and the environment of normal flora bacteria, which can lead to infection from those previously friendly bacteria.

Clinically Important Drug–Drug Interactions

There is a risk of increased serum levels and increased toxicity of benzodiazepines, phenytoin, and warfarin if

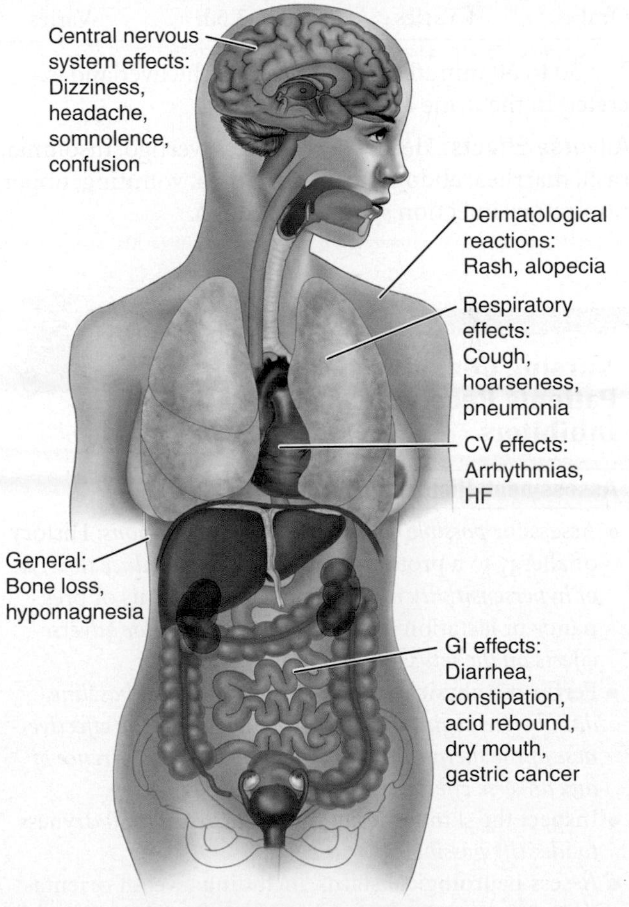

FIGURE 57.2 Variety of adverse effects and toxicities associated with drugs affecting gastrointestinal secretions.

these are combined with these drugs; patients should be monitored closely. Decreased levels of ketoconazole and theophylline have been reported when combined with these drugs, leading to loss of effectiveness. Sucralfate is not absorbed well in the presence of these drugs, and doses should be spaced at least 30 minutes apart if this combination is used. There is an increased risk of CV events if proton pump inhibitors are combined with clopidogrel; this combination should always be avoided.

Prototype Summary: Omeprazole

Indications: Short-term treatment of active duodenal ulcer or active benign gastric ulcer; treatment of heartburn or symptoms of gastroesophageal reflux; treatment of pathological hypersecretory syndromes; eradication of *Helicobacter pylori* infection as part of combination therapy.

Actions: Specifically inhibits the H^+, K^+–ATPase enzyme system on the secretory surface of gastric parietal cells, blocking the final step in acid production and decreasing gastric acid levels.

Pharmacokinetics:

Route	Onset	Peak	Duration
Oral	Varies	0.5–3.5 h	Varies

$T_{1/2}$: 30 to 60 minutes; metabolized in the liver and excreted in the urine and bile.

Adverse Effects: Headache, dizziness, vertigo, insomnia, rash, diarrhea, abdominal pain, nausea, vomiting, upper respiratory infection symptoms, cough.

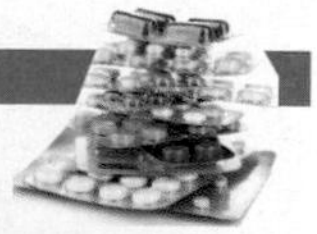

Nursing Considerations for Patients Receiving Proton Pump Inhibitors

Assessment: History and Examination

- Assess for *possible contraindications or cautions*: History of allergy to a proton pump inhibitor *to reduce the risk of hypersensitivity reaction* and current status of pregnancy or lactation *because of the potential for adverse effects on the fetus or nursing baby.*
- Perform a physical examination *to establish baseline data before beginning therapy to determine the effectiveness of the therapy and to evaluate for the occurrence of any adverse effects associated with drug therapy.*
- Inspect the skin for lesions, rash, pruritus, and dryness *to identify possible adverse effects.*
- Assess neurological status, including level of orientation, affect, and reflexes, *to evaluate for CNS effects of the drug.*
- Inspect and palpate the abdomen *to determine potential underlying medical conditions*; assess for changes in bowel elimination and GI upset *to identify possible adverse effects.*
- Assess respiratory status, including respiratory rate and rhythm; note evidence of cough, hoarseness, and epistaxis, *to monitor for potential adverse effects of the drug.*

Planning

- The patient will receive the best therapeutic effect from the drug therapy.
- The patient will have limited adverse effects to the drug therapy.
- The patient will have an understanding of the drug therapy, adverse effects to anticipate, and measures to relieve discomfort and improve safety.

Nursing Diagnoses

Nursing diagnoses related to drug therapy might include the following:

- Diarrhea related to GI effects
- Risk for constipation related to GI effects
- Imbalanced nutrition: Less than body requirements related to GI effects
- Disturbed sensory perception (kinesthetic, auditory) related to CNS effects
- Risk for injury related to CNS effects
- Deficient knowledge regarding drug therapy

Implementation with Rationale

- Administer drug before meals to ensure that the patient does not open, chew, or crush capsules; they should be swallowed whole *to ensure the therapeutic effectiveness of the drug.*
- Provide appropriate safety and comfort measures if CNS effects occur *to prevent patient injury.*
- Monitor the patient for diarrhea or constipation *to institute an appropriate bowel program as needed.*
- Monitor the patient's nutritional status; use of small frequent meals may be helpful *if GI upset is a problem.*
- Arrange for medical follow-up if symptoms are not resolved after 4 to 8 weeks of therapy *because serious underlying conditions could be causing the symptoms.*
- Offer support and encouragement *to help the patient cope with the disease and the drug regimen.*
- Provide thorough patient teaching, including the drug name and prescribed dosage; the importance of taking the drug whole without opening, chewing, or crushing it; signs and symptoms of possible adverse effects and measures to minimize or prevent them; danger signs that need to be reported to the health care provider immediately; nutritional measures, such as small, frequent meals; safety measures, such as avoiding driving and getting assistance with ambulation as needed;

methods for dealing with constipation or diarrhea; and the need for periodic monitoring and evaluation, *to enhance patient knowledge about drug therapy and to promote compliance.*

Evaluation

- Monitor patient response to the drug (relief of GI symptoms caused by hyperacidity, healing of erosive GI lesions).
- Monitor for adverse effects (GI effects, CNS changes, dermatological effects, respiratory effects).
- Monitor the effectiveness of comfort and safety measures and compliance with the regimen.
- Evaluate the effectiveness of the teaching plan (patient can name the drug and dosage and describe adverse effects to watch for, specific measures to avoid them, and measures to take to increase the effectiveness of the drug).

KEY POINTS

- The gastric acid pump or proton pump inhibitors suppress gastric acid secretion by specifically inhibiting the H^+, K^+–ATPase enzyme system on the secretory surface of the gastric parietal cells. This action blocks the final step of acid production, lowering the acid levels in the stomach.
- Proton pump inhibitors are indicated for the short-term treatment of active duodenal ulcer or active benign gastric ulcer, treatment of heartburn or symptoms of gastroesophageal reflux, treatment of pathological hypersecretory syndromes, and eradication of *Helicobacter pylori* infection as part of combination therapy.

Gastrointestinal Protectant

Gastrointestinal protectants (Table 57.1) coat any injured area in the stomach to prevent further injury from acid. Sucralfate (*Carafate*) is the only GI protectant currently available.

Therapeutic Actions and Indications

Sucralfate forms an ulcer-adherent complex at duodenal ulcer sites, protecting the sites against acid, pepsin, and bile salts. This action prevents further breakdown of the area and promotes ulcer healing. The drug also inhibits pepsin activity in gastric juices, preventing further breakdown of proteins in the stomach, including the protein wall of the stomach (see Figure 57.1). See Table 57.1 for Usual Indications.

Pharmacokinetics

Sucralfate is rapidly absorbed after oral administration, metabolized in the liver, and excreted in the feces. It crosses the placenta and may enter breast milk.

Contraindications and Cautions

Sucralfate should not be given to any person with known allergy to the drug or any of its components *to prevent hypersensitivity reactions.* It should not be given to individuals with renal failure or undergoing dialysis *because a buildup of aluminum may occur if it is used with aluminum-containing products.* Caution should be used in patients who are pregnant or lactating *because of the potential adverse effects on the fetus or neonate.*

Adverse Effects

The adverse effects associated with sucralfate are primarily related to its GI effects. Constipation is the most frequently seen adverse effect. Diarrhea, nausea, indigestion, gastric discomfort, and dry mouth may also occur. Other adverse effects that have been reported with this drug include dizziness, sleepiness, vertigo, skin rash, and back pain.

Clinically Important Drug–Drug Interactions

If aluminum salts are combined with sucralfate, there is a risk of high aluminum levels and aluminum toxicity. Extreme care should be taken if this combination is used.

In addition, if phenytoin, fluoroquinolone antibiotics (e.g., ciprofloxacin, norfloxacin), or penicillamine is combined with sucralfate, decreased serum levels and drug effectiveness may result. In such combinations the individual agents should be administered separately, with at least 2 hours between drugs.

(P) Prototype Summary: Sucralfate

Indications: Short-term treatment and maintenance treatment of active duodenal ulcer; treatment of oral and esophageal ulcers due to radiation, chemotherapy, or sclerotherapy.

Actions: Forms an ulcer-adherent complex at the duodenal ulcer site, protecting the ulcer from acid, bile salts, and pepsin, promoting healing of the ulcer; also inhibits pepsin activity in gastric juices.

Pharmacokinetics:

Route	Onset	Duration
Oral	30 min	5 h

$T_{1/2}$: 6 to 20 hours; metabolized in the liver and excreted in the feces.

Adverse Effects: Sleeplessness, dizziness, vertigo, insomnia, rash, constipation, diarrhea, nausea, indigestion, dry mouth, back pain.

Nursing Considerations for Patients Receiving a Gastrointestinal Protectant

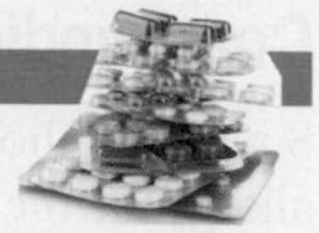

Assessment: History and Examination

- Assess for *possible contraindications or cautions*: Any history of allergy to sucralfate *to prevent hypersensitivity reactions*; renal dysfunction or dialysis, *which can lead to a buildup of aluminum*; and current status of pregnancy or lactation.
- Perform a physical examination *to establish baseline data before beginning therapy, to determine the effectiveness of therapy, and to evaluate for any adverse effects associated with drug therapy.*
- Inspect the skin for color and evidence of lesions or rash *that might indicate adverse drug effects.*
- Assess the patient's neurological status, including level of orientation, affect, and reflexes, *to monitor for CNS effects of the drug.*
- Examine the abdomen; auscultate bowel sounds *to evaluate GI motility*; evaluate bowel elimination pattern or changes *that could suggest possible adverse effects.*
- Assess mucous membrane status *to evaluate potential problems with absorption.*
- Monitor the results of laboratory tests such as renal function studies *to identify the need for possible dose adjustments and toxic effects.*

Nursing Diagnoses

Nursing diagnoses related to drug therapy might include the following:

- Diarrhea related to GI effects
- Risk for constipation related to GI effects
- Imbalanced nutrition: Less than body requirements related to GI effects
- Disturbed sensory perception (kinesthetic) related to CNS effects
- Deficient knowledge regarding drug therapy

Planning

- The patient will receive the best therapeutic effect from the drug therapy.
- The patient will have limited adverse effects to the drug therapy.
- The patient will have an understanding of the drug therapy, adverse effects to anticipate, and measures to relieve discomfort and improve safety.

Implementation with Rationale

- Administer the drug on an empty stomach, 1 hour before or 2 hours after meals and at bedtime, *to ensure the therapeutic effectiveness of the drug.*
- Monitor the patient for GI pain *and arrange to administer antacids to relieve pain if needed.*
- Administer antacids or antibiotics, if ordered, between doses of sucralfate, not within 30 minutes of a sucralfate dose, *because sucralfate can interfere with the absorption of oral agents.*
- Provide comfort and safety measures if CNS effects occur *to prevent patient injury.*
- Provide frequent mouth care, including sugarless lozenges to suck, *to alleviate dry mouth.*
- Ensure ready access to bathroom facilities *if diarrhea occurs*, institute bowel training as needed, and provide small, frequent meals *if GI effects are uncomfortable.*
- Offer support and encouragement *to help the patient cope with the disease and the drug regimen.*
- Provide thorough patient teaching, including the drug name and prescribed dosage; schedule for administration; importance of taking the drug on an empty stomach; use of antacids if ordered and the need to separate doses by at least 2 hours; signs and symptoms of possible adverse effects and measures to minimize or prevent their occurrence; danger signs that need to be reported to the health care provider immediately; safety measures, such as avoiding driving and asking for help with ambulation, *to minimize injury secondary to CNS effects*; dietary measures such as small, frequent meals *to minimize diarrhea*; increased fluid and fiber in the diet *to reduce the risk of constipation*; small, frequent meals *to help with GI upset*; comfort measures, such as mouth care and use of sugarless lozenges, *to alleviate dry mouth*; the importance of compliance with therapy *to achieve the intended effects*; measures to help avoid adverse effects; warning signs that may indicate problems; and the need for periodic monitoring and evaluation *to evaluate the effectiveness of therapy, enhance patient knowledge about therapy, and promote compliance.*

Evaluation

- Monitor the patient response to the drug (relief of GI symptoms, healing of erosive GI lesions).
- Monitor for adverse effects (GI effects, CNS changes, dermatological effects).
- Monitor the effectiveness of comfort and safety measures and compliance with the regimen.
- Evaluate the effectiveness of the teaching plan (patient can name drug and dosage and describe the adverse effects to watch for, specific measures to avoid them, and measures to take to increase the effectiveness of the drug).

KEY POINTS

- The GI protectant sucralfate forms a protective coating over the eroded stomach lining to protect it from acid and digestive enzymes to aid healing.
- Constipation is a common occurrence with this drug.

Prostaglandins

Prostaglandins are used to protect the stomach lining. The prostaglandin available for this use is the synthetic prostaglandin E_1 analogue misoprostol (*Cytotec*).

Therapeutic Actions and Indications

Prostaglandin E_1 inhibits gastric acid secretion and increases bicarbonate and mucus production in the stomach, thus protecting the stomach lining (see Figure 57.1). Misoprostol is primarily used to prevent NSAID-induced gastric ulcers in patients who are at high risk for complications from a gastric ulcer (e.g., elderly or debilitated patients, patients with a past history of ulcer). See Table 57.1 for more information and Usual Indications about this drug.

Pharmacokinetics

Misoprostol is given orally. It is rapidly absorbed from the GI tract, metabolized in the liver, and excreted in the urine. Misoprostol crosses the placenta and enters breast milk.

Contraindications and Cautions

Misoprostol is contraindicated with allergy to any part of the drug *to prevent hypersensitivity reactions*. This drug is also contraindicated during pregnancy *because it is an abortifacient*. Women of childbearing age should be advised to have a negative serum pregnancy test within 2 weeks of beginning treatment, and they should begin the drug on the second or third day of their next menstrual cycle. In addition, they should be instructed to use barrier contraceptives during therapy. Caution should be used during lactation *because of the potential for adverse effects on the newborn*. Caution also is necessary in patients with hepatic or renal impairment, *which could interfere with the effective metabolism and excretion of the drug*.

Adverse Effects

The adverse effects associated with this drug are primarily related to its GI effects—nausea, diarrhea, abdominal pain, flatulence, vomiting, dyspepsia, and constipation. Genitourinary effects, which are related to the actions of prostaglandins on the uterus, include miscarriages, excessive bleeding, spotting, cramping, hypermenorrhea, dysmenorrhea, and other menstrual disorders. Women taking this drug should be notified, both in writing and verbally, of these potential effects of this drug.

Prototype Summary: Misoprostol

Indications: Prevention of NSAID-induced or aspirin-induced gastric ulcers in patients at risk for complications of gastric ulcers; as an abortifacient with mifepristone.

Actions: Inhibits gastric acid secretion and increases bicarbonate and mucous production, protecting the lining of the stomach; increases stimulatory effects in the uterus.

Pharmacokinetics:

Route	Onset	Peak
Oral	Rapid	12–15 min

$T_{1/2}$: 20 to 40 minutes; metabolized in the liver and excreted in the urine.

Adverse Effects: Nausea, diarrhea, abdominal pain, flatulence, vomiting, excessive bleeding or spotting, hypermenorrhea, dysmenorrhea, miscarriage.

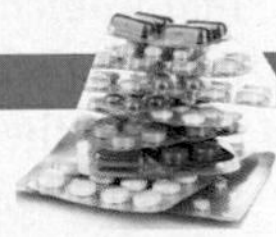

Nursing Considerations for Patients Receiving Prostaglandin

Assessment: History and Examination

- Assess for *possible contraindications or cautions*: Any history of allergy to misoprostol *to prevent hypersensitivity reactions* and current status of pregnancy or lactation *because of the potential for adverse effects on the fetus or nursing baby*.
- Perform a physical examination *to establish baseline data before beginning therapy and during therapy to determine the effectiveness of the drug and to evaluate for the occurrence of any adverse effects associated with drug therapy*.
- Examine the abdomen for possible changes to *rule out medical conditions*.
- Perform a pregnancy test and assess normal menstrual activity *to make sure that the woman is not pregnant*.
- Monitor the results of laboratory tests, including renal and hepatic function tests, *to determine the need for possible dose adjustment and identify toxic effects*.

Nursing Diagnoses

Nursing diagnoses related to drug therapy might include the following:

- Diarrhea related to GI effects
- Risk for constipation related to GI effects
- Imbalanced nutrition: Less than body requirements related to GI effects
- Ineffective sexuality pattern related to genitourinary effects
- Deficient knowledge regarding drug therapy

Planning

- The patient will receive the best therapeutic effect from the drug therapy.

(continues on page 1004)

- The patient will have limited adverse effects to the drug therapy.
- The patient will have an understanding of the drug therapy, adverse effects to anticipate, and measures to relieve discomfort and improve safety.

Implementation with Rationale

- Administer to patients at high risk for NSAID-induced ulcers during the full course of NSAID therapy *to prevent the development of gastric ulcers.* Administer four times a day, with meals and at bedtime, *to ensure maximum benefit of the drug.*
- Arrange for a serum pregnancy test within 2 weeks before beginning treatment and begin therapy on the second or third day of the menstrual period *to ensure that women of childbearing age are not pregnant and to prevent the abortifacient effects associated with this drug.*
- Provide the patient with both written and oral information regarding the associated risks of pregnancy *to ensure that the patient understands the risks involved;* advise the use of barrier contraceptives during therapy *to ensure the prevention of pregnancy.*
- Evaluate nutritional status if GI effects are severe *to arrange for appropriate measures to relieve discomfort and ensure nutrition,* such as small, frequent meals, and increased fluid intake if appropriate.
- Explain the risk of menstrual disorders and pain, miscarriage, and excessive bleeding *related to the drug effects on prostaglandin activity in the uterus.*
- Offer support and encouragement *to help the patient cope with the disease and the drug regimen.*
- Provide thorough patient teaching, including the drug name and prescribed dosage; schedule for administration; the need to take the drug with meals and at bedtime; signs and symptoms of adverse effects and measures to minimize or prevent them; the importance of avoiding pregnancy while taking drug; the use of barrier contraceptives to prevent pregnancy; dietary measures such as small, frequent meals and increased fluid intake to alleviate or minimize adverse GI effects; danger signs to report to the health care provider immediately; support to deal with changes in sexuality patterns that may occur; and the importance of periodic monitoring and evaluation *to enhance patient knowledge about drug therapy and to promote compliance.*

Evaluation

- Monitor the patient response to the drug (prevention of GI ulcers related to NSAIDs).
- Monitor for adverse effects (GI, genitourinary).
- Monitor the effectiveness of comfort and safety measures and compliance with the regimen.
- Evaluate the effectiveness of the teaching plan (patient can name drug and dosage and describe adverse effects to watch for, specific measures to avoid them, and measures to take to increase the effectiveness of the drug).

KEY POINTS

- The prostaglandin misoprostol is used to inhibit gastric acid secretion and increase bicarbonate and mucus production in the stomach; this action will protect the lining of the stomach.
- This drug increases prostaglandin effects in the uterus, causing increased contractions, excessive bleeding, and cramping. This drug is pregnancy category X and cannot be used during pregnancy.

Digestive Enzymes

Digestive enzymes (Table 57.2) are substances produced in the GI tract to break down foods into usable nutrients. Some patients—those who have suffered strokes, salivary gland disorders, or extreme surgery of the head and neck and those with cystic fibrosis or pancreatic dysfunction—may require a supplement to the production of digestive enzymes. Two digestive enzymes are available for replacement in conditions that result in lower-than-normal levels of these enzymes: Saliva substitute (*MouthKote, Salivart*) and pancrelipase (*Creon, Pancrease*).

Therapeutic Actions and Indications

Saliva substitute contains electrolytes and carboxymethylcellulose to act as a thickening agent in dry mouth conditions. This makes the food bolus easier to swallow and begins the early digestion process. Saliva substitute helps in conditions that result in dry mouth—stroke, radiation therapy, chemotherapy, and other illnesses. The pancreatic enzymes are replacement enzymes that help the digestion and absorption of fats, proteins, and carbohydrates (see Figure 57.1). See Table 57.2 for Usual Indications for each agent.

Pharmacokinetics

Saliva substitute is available as a solution, in lozenge form, and on swab sticks for oral administration. It is not generally absorbed systemically. It works when applied to the mouth. Pancrelipase, which is available in capsules, delayed release capsules, powder, and tablet form, is thought to be processed through normal metabolic systems in the body. Little is known about its pharmacokinetics.

Contraindications and Cautions

Saliva substitute is contraindicated in the presence of known allergy to parabens or any component of the drug *to prevent hypersensitivity reactions.* It should be used cautiously in patients with heart failure, hypertension, or renal failure *because there may be an abnormal absorption of electrolytes, including sodium, leading to increased CV load.* Pancreatic enzymes should not be used with known allergy to the product or to pork products *to prevent*

Table 57.2 *Drugs in Focus:* Drugs Used to Treat Digestive Enzyme Dysfunction

Drug Name	Usual Dosage	Usual Indications
Digestive Enzymes		
pancrelipase (*Creon, Pancrease*)	*Adult:* 4,000–48,000 units PO with each meal and snacks *Pediatric (6 mo–1 y):* 2,000 units PO per meal *Pediatric (1–6 y):* 4,000–8,000 units PO with meals, 4,000 units with snacks *Pediatric (7–12 y):* 4,000–12,000 units PO with each meal and snack	Aids digestion and absorption of fats, proteins, and carbohydrates in conditions that result in a lack of this enzyme; used as replacement therapy in patients with cystic fibrosis, chronic ductal obstruction, pancreatic insufficiency, steatorrhea, or malabsorption syndrome and after pancreatectomy or gastrectomy
saliva substitute (*MouthKote, Salivart*)	Spray or apply to oral mucosa	Aids in conditions resulting in dry mouth—stroke, radiation therapy, chemotherapy, and other illnesses

hypersensitivity reactions. In addition, both saliva substitute and pancreatic enzymes should be used cautiously in pregnancy and lactation *because of the risk for adverse effects on the fetus or baby.*

Adverse Effects

The adverse effects most commonly seen with saliva substitute involve complications from abnormal electrolyte absorption, such as increased levels of magnesium, sodium, or potassium. The adverse effects that most often occur with pancreatic enzymes are related to GI irritation and include nausea, abdominal cramps, and diarrhea.

Prototype Summary: Pancrelipase

Indications: Replacement therapy in patients with deficient exocrine pancreatic secretions.

Actions: Replaces pancreatic enzymes to aid in the digestion and absorption of fats, proteins, and carbohydrates.

Pharmacokinetics: Generally not absorbed systemically.

$T_{1/2}$: Generally not absorbed systemically.

Adverse Effects: Nausea, abdominal cramps, diarrhea, hyperuricosuria.

Nursing Considerations for Patients Receiving Digestive Enzymes

Assessment: History and Examination

- Assess for *possible contraindications or cautions*: Any history of allergy to any of the drugs or to pork products (pancreatic enzymes) *to prevent hypersensitivity reactions*; heart failure or hypertension (saliva substitute) *because there may be an abnormal absorption of electrolytes, including sodium, leading to increased CV load*; and current status of pregnancy or lactation *because of the potential for adverse effects on the fetus or nursing baby.*
- Perform a physical examination *to establish baseline data before beginning therapy and during therapy to evaluate the effectiveness of the drug and determine the occurrence of any adverse effects associated with drug therapy.*
- Perform an abdominal examination *to rule out underlying medical conditions and assess for adverse effects of the drug*; auscultate bowel sounds *to evaluate GI motility.*
- Monitor mucous membranes *to assess for their condition and for any indication of the need for saliva substitute.*
- Assess cardiopulmonary status, including blood pressure and cardiac rate and rhythm, *to identify changes that may indicate electrolyte imbalances.*
- Monitor the results of laboratory tests, including renal function tests, *to determine the need for possible dose adjustment and identify toxic effects* and pancreatic enzyme levels *to assure correct dose and to monitor patient response.*

Nursing Diagnoses

Nursing diagnoses related to drug therapy might include the following:

- Diarrhea related to GI effects
- Imbalanced nutrition: Less than body requirements related to GI effects
- Deficient knowledge regarding drug therapy

Planning

- The patient will receive the best therapeutic effect from the drug therapy.
- The patient will have limited adverse effects to the drug therapy.

(continues on page 1006)

- The patient will have an understanding of the drug therapy, adverse effects to anticipate, and measures to relieve discomfort and improve safety.

Implementation with Rationale

- Have the patient swish a saliva substitute around the mouth as needed for dry mouth and throat *to coat the mouth and ensure therapeutic effectiveness of the drug.*
- Monitor swallowing *because it may be impaired due to the underlying medical conditions or decrease in lubricating effects related to low saliva levels, and additional therapy may be needed.*
- Administer pancreatic enzymes with meals and snacks so that enzyme is available when it is needed. Avoid spilling powder on the skin *because it may be irritating.* Do not crush the capsule or allow the patient to chew it; it must be swallowed whole *to ensure full therapeutic effects.*
- Assess nutritional status if there are GI effects *to arrange for appropriate measures to relieve discomfort and ensure nutrition, such as frequent small meals.*
- Obtain laboratory specimens as indicated *to evaluate electrolyte levels and pancreatic enzyme levels.*
- Offer support and encouragement *to help the patient cope with the disease and the drug regimen.*
- Provide thorough patient teaching, including the drug name and prescribed dosage; schedule for administration; the technique for using saliva substitute; the importance of taking pancreatic enzymes with meals and snacks; the need to take the pancreatic enzyme whole and not to crush or chew the capsule; dietary measures to follow; signs and symptoms of adverse effects and measures to minimize or prevent them; danger signs that need to be reported to the health care provider immediately; the need for periodic monitoring, including laboratory tests to evaluate electrolyte levels (with saliva substitute) to evaluate for possible imbalances, or pancreatic enzyme levels (with pancreatic enzymes) to evaluate the effectiveness of therapy; and the importance of complying with therapy and follow-up *to enhance patient knowledge about drug therapy and to promote compliance.*

Evaluation

- Monitor the patient response to the drug (e.g., relief of dry mouth and throat; digestion of fats, proteins, and carbohydrates).
- Monitor for adverse effects (e.g., electrolyte imbalance, GI effects).
- Monitor the effectiveness of comfort and safety measures and compliance with the regimen.
- Evaluate the effectiveness of the teaching plan (patient can name the drug and dosage and describe adverse effects to watch for, specific measures to avoid them, and measures to take to increase the effectiveness of the drug).

KEY POINTS

- Digestive enzymes such as substitute saliva and pancreatic enzymes may be needed if normal enzyme levels are very low and proper digestion cannot take place.
- Patients receiving replacement enzymes will need to be monitored to ensure that the dose is correct for their particular situation to avoid adverse effects.

SUMMARY

- GI complaints are some of the most common symptoms seen in clinical practice.
- Peptic ulcers may result from increased acid production, decrease in the protective mucous lining of the stomach, infection with *Helicobacter pylori* bacteria, or a combination of these.
- Agents used to decrease the acid content of the stomach include H_2 antagonists, which block the release of acid in response to gastrin or parasympathetic release; antacids, which chemically react with the acid to neutralize it; proton pump inhibitors, which block the last step of acid production to prevent release; and prostaglandins, which block gastric acid secretion and increase bicarbonate production.
- Acid rebound occurs when the stomach produces more gastrin and more acid in response to lowered acid levels in the stomach, which commonly occurs with the use of antacids. Balancing the reduction of the stomach acid without increasing acid production is a clinical challenge.
- The GI protectant sucralfate forms a protective coating over the eroded stomach lining to protect it from acid and digestive enzymes to aid healing.
- The prostaglandin misoprostol blocks gastric acid secretion while increasing the production of bicarbonate and mucous lining in the stomach.
- Digestive enzymes such as substitute saliva and pancreatic enzymes may be needed if normal enzyme levels are very low and proper digestion cannot take place.

CHECK YOUR UNDERSTANDING

Answers to the questions in this chapter can be found in Answers to Check Your Understanding Questions on thePoint®.

MULTIPLE CHOICE

Select the best answer to the following.

1. Which of the following would a nurse include when describing the action of H_2 antagonists to a patient?
   a. They block the release of gastrin and pepsin, leading to a decrease in protein digestion.
   b. They selectively block histamine receptors, reducing swelling and inflammation at numerous sites.
   c. They selectively block specific histamine receptor sites, leading to a reduction in gastric acid secretion.
   d. They are effective primarily for long-term use because of their slow onset of action.

2. H_2 receptors are found throughout the body, including
   a. in the nasal passages, upper airways, and stomach.
   b. in the CNS and upper airways.
   c. in the respiratory tract and the heart.
   d. in the heart, CNS, and stomach.

3. Which H_2 antagonist would the nurse expect to be ordered for a patient with known liver dysfunction?
   a. Cimetidine
   b. Famotidine
   c. Nizatidine
   d. Ranitidine

4. The nurse would monitor a patient receiving IV cimetidine (generic) for an acute ulcer problem for
   a. GI upset.
   b. gynecomastia.
   c. cardiac arrhythmias.
   d. constipation.

5. Acid rebound is a condition that occurs when
   a. lowering gastric acid to an alkaline level stimulates the release of gastric acid.
   b. raising gastric acid levels causes heartburn.
   c. combining protein, calcium, and smoking greatly elevates gastric acid levels.
   d. eating citrus fruit neutralizes gastric acid.

6. A nurse taking care of a patient who is receiving a proton pump inhibitor should teach the patient to
   a. take the drug after every meal.
   b. chew or crush tablets to increase their absorption.
   c. swallow tablets or capsules whole.
   d. stop taking the drug after 3 weeks of therapy.

7. Misoprostol (*Cytotec*) is a prostaglandin that is used to
   a. prevent uterine contractions.
   b. prevent NSAID-related gastric ulcers in patients at high risk.
   c. decrease hyperacidity with meals and at bedtime.
   d. relieve the burning associated with hiatal hernia at night.

8. A nurse caring for a patient receiving pancreatic enzymes as replacement therapy should be assessing the patient for
   a. hypertension.
   b. cardiac arrhythmias.
   c. excessive weight gain.
   d. signs of GI irritation.

MULTIPLE RESPONSE

Select all that apply.

1. Patients who use antacids frequently can be expected to experience which of the following adverse effects?
   a. Systemic alkalosis
   b. Electrolyte imbalances
   c. Hypokalemia
   d. Metabolic acidosis
   e. Constipation or diarrhea
   f. Muscular weakness

2. Saliva substitute (*Moi-Stir*) may be useful in which of the following circumstances?
   a. Cancer radiation therapy
   b. Stroke
   c. Parkinson's disease
   d. Brain injury
   e. Situational anxiety
   f. Hypertension

BIBLIOGRAPHY AND REFERENCES

Broeren, M., Geerdink, E., & Vader, H., et al. (2009). Hypomagnesemia induced by several proton-pump inhibitors. *Annals of Internal Medicine, 151*, 755–756.

Brunton, L., Chabner, B., & Knollman, B. (2011). *Goodman and Gilman's the pharmacological basis of therapeutics* (12th ed.). New York: McGraw-Hill.

Chan, F. (2009). *Peptic ulcer disease, an issue of gastroenterology clinics*. Philadelphia, PA: W. B. Saunders.

Charlot, M., Ahlehoff, O., & Norgaard, M. (2010). Proton pump inhibitors are associated with cardiovascular risk independent of clopidogrel use: A nationwide cohort study. *Annals of Internal Medicine, 153*, 378–386.

Chinitis, A., & Holtzbauer, S. (2013). Epidemiology of community-associated Clostridium difficile infection. *JAMA Internal Medicine, 173*(14), 1359–1367.

Facts and Comparisons. (2015). *Drug facts and comparisons*. St. Louis, MO: Author.

Facts and Comparisons. (2015). *Professional's guide to patient drug facts*. St. Louis, MO: Author.

Karch, A. M. (2014). *Lippincott's nursing drug guide*. Philadelphia, PA: Lippincott Williams & Wilkins.

Khalli, H., Huang, E., Jacobson, B., et al. (2012). Proton pump inhibitors and risk of hip fracture in relation to dietary and life style factors: A prospective cohort study. *British Medical Journal, 344*, e372.

Lam, J., Schneider, J., Zhao, W., et al. (2013). Proton pump inhibitor and histamine 2 receptor antagonist use and vitamin B_{12} deficiency. *Journal of the American Medical Association, 310*(16), 1765–1774.

Porth, C. M. (2013). *Pathophysiology: Concepts of altered health states* (9th ed.). Philadelphia, PA: Lippincott Williams & Wilkins.

Voelker, R. (2010). Proton pump inhibitors linked to fracture risk. *Journal of the American Medical Association, 304*(1), 29.

Yu-Xiao, Y., Lewis, S. D., Epstein, S., et al. (2007). Long term proton pump inhibitor therapy and risk of hip fracture. *Journal of the American Medical Association, 296*, 2947–2953.

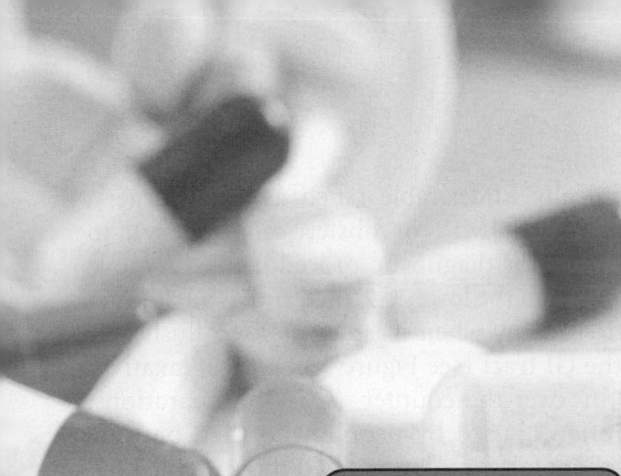

58 Drugs Affecting Gastrointestinal Motility

Learning Objectives

Upon completion of this chapter, you will be able to:

1. Describe the underlying processes in diarrhea and constipation and correlate them with the types of drugs used to treat these conditions.
2. Describe the therapeutic actions, indications, pharmacokinetics, contraindications and cautions, most common adverse reactions, and important drug–drug interactions associated with laxatives and antidiarrheal drugs.
3. Discuss the use of laxatives and antidiarrheal agents across the lifespan.
4. Compare and contrast the prototype laxatives and antidiarrheals with other agents in their class and with other classes of laxatives and antidiarrheals.
5. Outline the nursing considerations, including important teaching points, for patients receiving laxatives and antidiarrheal agents.

Glossary of Key Terms

antidiarrheal: drug that blocks the stimulation of the gastrointestinal (GI) tract, leading to decreased activity and increased time for absorption of needed nutrients and water

bulk stimulant: agent that increases in bulk, frequently by osmotic pull of fluid into the feces; the increased bulk stretches the GI wall, causing stimulation and increased GI movement

cathartic dependence: overuse of laxatives that can lead to the need for strong stimuli to initiate movement in the intestines; local reflexes become resistant to normal stimuli after prolonged use of harsher stimulants, leading to further laxative use

chemical stimulant: agent that stimulates the normal GI reflexes by chemically irritating the lining of the GI wall, leading to increased activity in the GI tract

constipation: slower-than-normal evacuation of the large intestine, which can result in increased water absorption from the feces and can lead to impaction

diarrhea: more-frequent-than-normal bowel movements, often characterized as fluid-like and watery because not enough time for absorption is allowed during the passage of food through the intestines

lubricant: agent that increases the viscosity of the feces, making it difficult to absorb water from the bolus and easing movement of the bolus through the intestines

Drug List

Laxatives

Chemical Stimulants
- bisacodyl
- (P) cascara
- castor oil
- senna

Bulk Stimulants
- lactulose
- (P) magnesium citrate
- magnesium hydroxide
- magnesium sulfate
- polycarbophil
- polyethylene glycol
- polyethylene glycol electrolyte solution
- psyllium
- sodium picosulfate with magnesium oxide

Lubricants
- docusate
- glycerin
- (P) mineral oil

Other Laxatives
- methylnaltrexone
- naloxegol

Gastrointestinal Stimulants
- dexpanthenol
- (P) metoclopramide

Antidiarrheals
- bismuth subsalicylate
- crofelemer
- (P) loperamide
- opium derivatives

Irritable Bowel Syndrome Drugs
- alosetron
- lubiprostone
- hyoscyamine

Drugs used to affect the motor activity or motility of the gastrointestinal (GI) tract can do so in several different ways. They can be used to speed up or improve the movement of intestinal contents along the GI tract when movement becomes too slow or sluggish to allow for proper absorption of nutrients and excretion of wastes, as in **constipation.** Drugs are also used to increase the tone of the GI tract and to stimulate motility throughout the system. They can also be used to decrease movement along the GI tract when rapid movement decreases the time for the absorption of nutrients, leading to a loss of water and nutrients and the discomfort of **diarrhea.** This chapter addresses three major categories of drugs: Laxatives, GI stimulants, and antidiarrheal agents. See Figure 58.1 for sites of action of these drugs on GI motility. Box 58.1 highlights important considerations related to laxatives and other drugs affecting GI motility, based on the patient's age.

Laxatives

Laxative, or cathartic, drugs (Table 58.1) are indicated for the short-term relief of constipation, to prevent straining when it is clinically undesirable (such as after surgery, myocardial infarction [MI], or obstetrical delivery), to evacuate the bowel for diagnostic procedures, to remove ingested poisons from the lower GI tract, and as an adjunct in anthelmintic therapy when it is desirable to flush helminths from the GI tract (see Figure 58.1). Most laxatives are available in over-the-counter (OTC) preparations, and they are often abused by people who then become dependent on them for stimulation of GI movement. Such individuals may develop chronic intestinal disorders as a result. Measures such as instituting proper diet and exercise, increasing fluid intake, and taking advantage of the actions of the intestinal reflexes have eliminated the need for laxatives in many situations; therefore, these agents are used less frequently than they once were in clinical practice.

Kinds of laxatives include chemical stimulants (which chemically irritate the lining of the GI tract), bulk stimulants (which cause fecal matter to increase in bulk), and lubricants (which help the intestinal contents move more slowly). Newer laxatives are available for very specific needs and alter sodium absorption or affect opioid receptors in the GI tract.

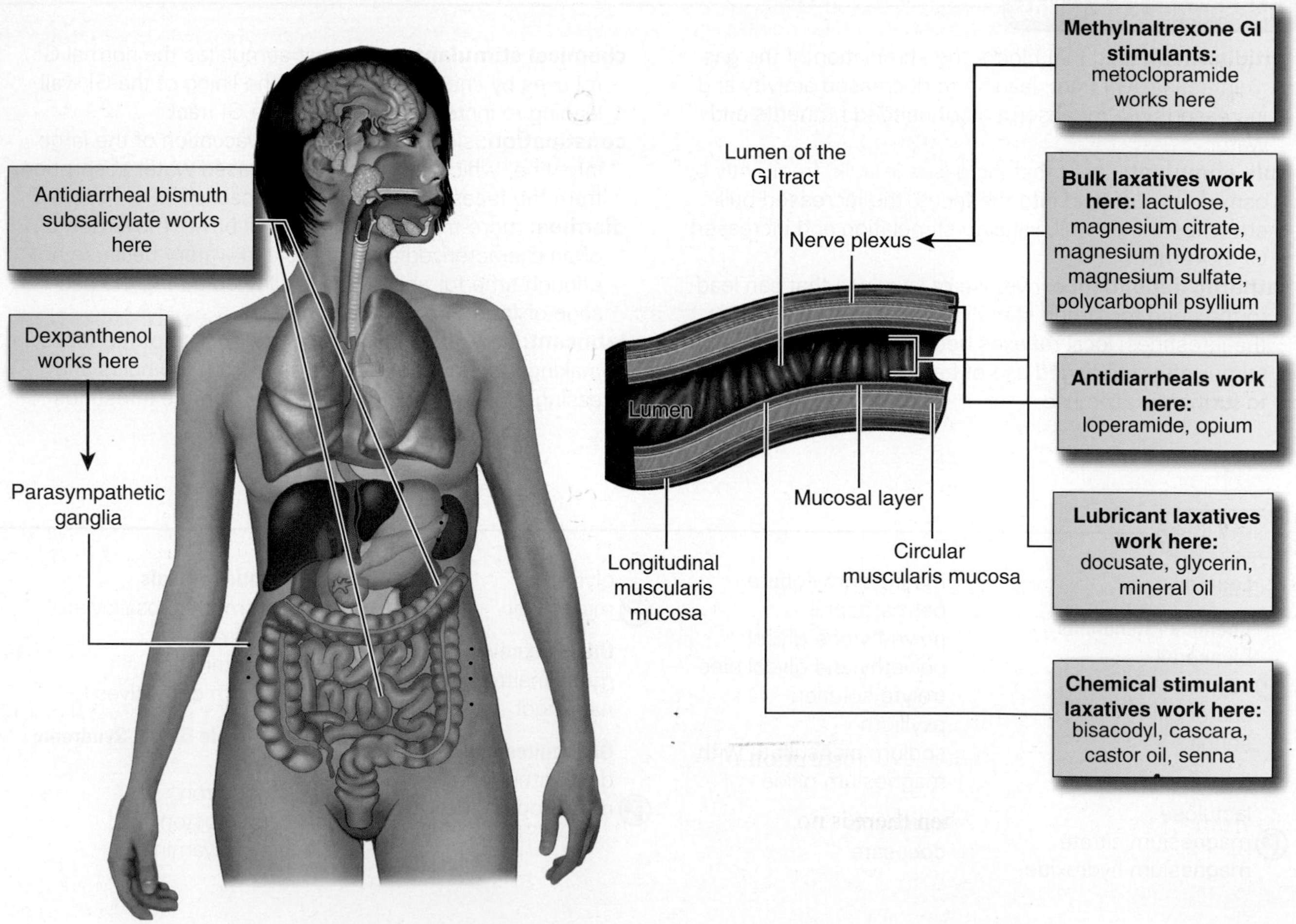

FIGURE 58.1 Sites of action of drugs affecting gastrointestinal motility.

BOX 58.1 FOCUS ON Drug Therapy Across the Lifespan

Laxatives and Antidiarrheal Agents

CHILDREN

Laxatives should not be used in children routinely. Proper diet, including roughage, plenty of fluids, and exercise, should be tried first if a child has a tendency to become constipated. If a laxative is needed, glycerin suppositories are the best choice for infants and young children. Lubricants can be used in older children; harsh stimulants should be avoided. Children with encopresis, however, are often given senna preparations or mineral oil to help them to evacuate the massive stool.

Children receiving these agents should use them for only a short period and should be evaluated for potential underlying medical or nutritional problems if they are not able to return to normal function.

Loperamide may be the antidiarrheal of choice in children older than 2 years of age if such a drug is needed. Special precautions need to be taken to monitor for electrolyte and fluid disturbances and supportive measures taken as needed.

ADULTS

Adults who use laxatives need to be cautioned not to become dependent. Proper diet, exercise, and adequate intake of fluids should keep the GI tract functioning normally. If an antidiarrheal is needed, adults should be carefully instructed in the proper dosing of the drug and monitoring of their total use to avoid excessive dose.

The safety for the use of these drugs during pregnancy and lactation has not been established. Use should be reserved for those situations in which the benefit to the mother outweighs the potential risk to the fetus. A mild stool softener is often used after delivery. The drugs may enter breast milk and also may affect GI activity in the neonate. It is advised that caution be used if one of these drugs is prescribed during lactation.

OLDER ADULTS

Older adults are more likely to develop adverse effects associated with the use of these drugs, including sedation, confusion, dizziness, electrolyte disturbances, fluid imbalance, and cardiovascular effects. Safety measures may be needed if these effects occur and interfere with the patient's mobility and balance.

Older patients also may be taking other drugs that are associated with constipation and may need help to prevent severe problems from developing.

Older adults are more likely to have renal and/or hepatic impairment related to underlying medical conditions, which could interfere with the metabolism and excretion of the antidiarrheal drugs. The dose for older adults should be started at a lower level than recommended for younger adults. The patient should be monitored very closely, and dose adjustment should be made based on patient response.

These patients also need to be alerted to the potential for toxic effects when using OTC preparations and should be advised to check with their health care provider before beginning any OTC drug regimen.

A psyllium product is the agent of choice with older adults because there is less risk of adverse reactions. The patient needs to be cautioned to drink plenty of fluid after taking one of these agents to prevent problems that can occur if the drug starts to pull in fluid while still in the esophagus.

The older adult should be encouraged to drink plenty of fluids, to exercise every day, and to get plenty of roughage in the diet. Many older adults have established routines, such as drinking warm water or prune juice at the same time each morning, that are disrupted with illness or hospitalization. These patients should be encouraged and helped to try to maintain their usual protocol as much as possible.

Chemical Stimulants

Chemical stimulants directly stimulate the nerve plexus in the intestinal wall, causing increased movement and the stimulation of local reflexes. Laxatives classified as chemical stimulants include bisacodyl (*Dulcolax*), cascara (generic), castor oil (generic), and senna (*Senokot*).

Therapeutic Actions and Indications

Castor oil, an old standby, is used when a thorough evacuation of the intestine is desirable. All of these agents begin working at the beginning of the small intestine and increase motility throughout the rest of the GI tract by irritating the nerve plexus. Because castor oil blocks absorption of fats (including fat-soluble vitamins) and may lead to constipation from GI tract exhaustion when there is no stimulus to movement, its frequent use is not desirable. Bisacodyl acts in a similar manner but is somewhat milder in effect; it can also be given in a water enema to stimulate the activity in the lower GI tract. Cascara is somewhat milder than castor oil and is often used when effects are needed overnight. Senna is available orally in tablet and syrup form and as a rectal suppository.

Pharmacokinetics

Most of these agents are only minimally absorbed and exert their therapeutic effect directly in the GI tract. Changes in absorption, water balance, and electrolytes resulting from GI changes can have adverse effects on patients with underlying medical conditions that are affected by volume and electrolyte changes (see Adverse Effects). Castor oil has an onset of action of 2 to 6 hours; the remaining chemical stimulants have an onset of action of 6 to 8 hours, making them preferable if one wants the drug to work overnight and see effects in the morning.

Contraindications and Cautions

Chemical stimulant laxatives are contraindicated with allergy to any component of the drug *to prevent hypersensitivity reactions* and in acute abdominal disorders,

Table 58.1 *Drugs in Focus:* Laxatives

Drug Name	Usual Dosage	Usual Indications
Chemical Stimulants		
bisacodyl (*Dulcolax*)	10–15 mg PO *or* 2.5 g in water via enema	Emptying of the GI tract before some surgeries or diagnostic tests (e.g., barium enema); prevention of constipation and straining after GI surgery, MI, obstetrical delivery; short-term treatment of constipation
cascara (generic)	325–650 mg PO	Short-term treatment of constipation, evacuation of the large intestine for diagnostic examination *Special considerations:* May have a slow, steady effect or may cause severe cramping and rapid evacuation of the contents of the large intestine; patient should be advised of the possibilities and the need to maintain ready access to bathroom facilities
castor oil (generic)	15–30 mL PO	Emptying of the GI tract for diagnostic testing, short-term treatment of constipation *Special considerations:* Avoid frequent use to prevent constipation from GI tract exhaustion when there is no stimulus to movement.
senna (*Senokot*)	One to eight tablets per day at bedtime *or* 10–25 mL of syrup	Short-term treatment of constipation, treatment of encopresis, found in many OTC preparations
Bulk Stimulants		
lactulose (*Constilac*)	15–30 mL PO	Short-term treatment of constipation, alternative choice for patients with cardiovascular disorders
magnesium citrate (*Citrate of Magnesia*)	One glassful, 1/2 glass for pediatric patients	Stimulates bowel evacuation before GI diagnostic tests and examinations
magnesium hydroxide (*Milk of Magnesia*)	15–30 mL PO	Short-term treatment of constipation, prevention of straining after GI surgery, obstetrical delivery, MI
magnesium sulfate (*Epsom salts*)	10–25 mg PO	Very potent laxative used for total, rapid evacuation of the GI tract (e.g., for treatment of GI poisoning)
polycarbophil (*FiberCon*)	1 g PO, one to four times per day as needed; do not exceed 6 g/d for adults or 3 g/d for children	Short-term treatment of constipation (mild laxative)
polyethylene glycol (*MiraLax*)	17 gm PO in 8 oz water daily, for up to 2 wk	Short-term treatment of constipation (mild laxative)
polyethylene glycol electrolyte solution (*GoLYTELY*, and others)	4 L of oral solution at a rate of 240 mL every 10 min	Stimulates bowel evacuation prior to GI examination (e.g., colonoscopy, sigmoidoscopy)
psyllium (*Metamucil*)	1 tsp or packet in cold water, one to three times per day; 1/2 packet for children	Mild laxative, short-term treatment of constipation
sodium picosulfate/magnesium oxide (*Prepopik*)	Reconstitute with cold water, swallow immediately, and repeat	Stimulates bowel evacuation prior to colonoscopy
Lubricants		
docusate (*Colace*)	50–240 mg PO	Prophylaxis for patients who should not strain (such as after surgery, MI, or obstetrical delivery)
glycerin (*Sani-Supp*)	4 mL of liquid suppository	Short-term treatment of constipation
mineral oil (*Agoral Liquid*)	5–45 mL PO	Short-term treatment of constipation

GI, gastrointestinal; MI, myocardial infarction; OTC, over the counter.

including appendicitis, diverticulitis, and ulcerative colitis, *when increased motility could lead to rupture or further exacerbation of the inflammation.* Laxatives should be used with caution in heart block, coronary artery disease (CAD), or debilitation, *which could be affected by the decrease in absorption and changes in electrolyte levels that can occur* and with great caution during pregnancy and lactation *because, in some cases, stimulation of the GI tract can precipitate labor and many of these agents cross the placenta and are excreted in breast milk.*

Castor oil should not be used during pregnancy *because its irritant effect has been associated with induction of premature labor*. Magnesium laxatives can cause diarrhea in the neonate if used during lactation.

Adverse Effects

The adverse effects most commonly associated with chemical stimulant laxatives are GI effects such as diarrhea, abdominal cramping, and nausea. Central nervous system (CNS) effects, including dizziness, headache, and weakness, are not uncommon and may relate to loss of fluid and electrolyte imbalances that may accompany laxative use. Sweating, palpitations, flushing, and even fainting have been reported after laxative use. These effects may be related to a sympathetic stress reaction to intense neurostimulation of the GI tract or to the loss of fluid and electrolyte imbalance.

A very common adverse effect that is seen with frequent laxative use or laxative abuse is **cathartic dependence.** This reaction occurs when patients use laxatives over a long period of time and the GI tract becomes dependent on vigorous stimulation of the laxative. Without this stimulation the GI tract does not move for a period of time (i.e., several days), which could lead to constipation and drying of the stool and ultimately to impaction.

Specifically related to chemical stimulants, cascara, although a reliable agent, may have a slow, steady effect or may cause severe cramping and rapid evacuation of the contents of the large intestine. Castor oil blocks absorption of fats (including fat-soluble vitamins) and may lead to constipation from GI tract exhaustion when there is no stimulus to movement.

Clinically Important Drug–Drug Interactions

Because laxatives increase the motility of the GI tract and some interfere with the timing or process of absorption, it is advisable not to take laxatives with other prescribed medications. The administration of laxatives and other medications should be separated by at least 30 minutes.

Prototype Summary: Castor Oil

Indications: To evacuate the bowel for diagnostic procedures; to remove ingested poisons from the lower GI tract; an adjunct in anthelmintic therapy when it is desirable to flush helminths from the GI tract.

Actions: Directly stimulates the nerve plexus in the intestinal wall, causing increased movement and the stimulation of local reflexes.

Pharmacokinetics: Not absorbed systemically.

$T_{1/2}$: Not absorbed systemically.

Adverse Effects: Diarrhea, abdominal cramps, perianal irritation, dizziness, cathartic dependence.

Bulk Stimulants

Bulk stimulants (also called mechanical stimulants) are rapid-acting, aggressive laxatives that cause the fecal matter to increase in bulk. They increase the motility of the GI tract by increasing the fluid in the intestinal contents, which enlarges bulk, stimulates local stretch receptors, and activates local activity. Available bulk stimulants include the following agents: Magnesium sulfate (*Epsom salts*), magnesium citrate (*Citrate of Magnesia*), magnesium hydroxide (*Milk of Magnesia*), lactulose (*Constilac*), polycarbophil (*FiberCon*), psyllium (*Metamucil*), polyethylene glycol (*MiraLax*), polyethylene glycol electrolyte solution (*GoLYTELY*), and sodium picosulfate with magnesium oxide (*Prepopix*)

Therapeutic Actions and Indications

Bulk stimulants increase the motility of the GI tract by increasing the fluid in the intestinal contents, which enlarges bulk, stimulates local stretch receptors, and activates local activity.

Lactulose is a saltless osmotic laxative that pulls fluid out of the venous system and into the lumen of the small intestine.

Magnesium citrate is a milder and slower-acting laxative. It works by a saline pull, bringing fluids into the lumen of the GI tract.

Magnesium hydroxide is a milder and slower-acting laxative. It also works by a saline pull, bringing fluids into the lumen of the GI tract.

Magnesium sulfate acts by exerting a hypertonic pull against the mucosal wall, drawing fluid into the intestinal contents.

Polycarbophil is a natural substance that forms a gelatin-like bulk out of the intestinal contents. This agent stimulates local activity. It is considered milder and less irritating than many other bulk stimulants. Patients must use caution and take polycarbophil with plenty of water (see Adverse Effects).

Polyethylene glycol and polyethylene glycol electrolyte solution are hypertonic fluids containing many electrolytes that pull fluid out of the intestinal wall to increase the bulk of the intestinal contents.

Psyllium, another gelatin-like bulk stimulant, is similar to polycarbophil in action and effect.

Sodium picosulfate with magnesium oxide provides a combination stimulant laxative with a bulk laxative. It is used to cleanse the colon in adults before colonoscopy procedures.

See Table 58.1 for Usual Indications for each of these agents.

Pharmacokinetics

These drugs are all taken orally. They are directly effective within the GI tract and are not generally absorbed systemically. They are rapidly acting, causing effects as they pass through the GI tract.

Contraindications and Cautions

Bulk laxatives are contraindicated with allergy to any component of the drug *to prevent hypersensitivity reactions* and in acute abdominal disorders, including appendicitis, diverticulitis, and ulcerative colitis, *when increased motility could lead to rupture or further exacerbation of the inflammation*. Laxatives should be used with caution in heart block, CAD and debilitation, *which could be affected by the decrease in absorption and changes in electrolyte levels that can occur*, and with great caution during pregnancy and lactation *because, in some cases, stimulation of the GI tract can precipitate labor and many of these agents cross the placenta and are excreted in breast milk*. Polyethylene glycol electrolyte solution should be used with caution in any patient with a history of seizures *because of the risk of electrolyte absorption causing neuronal instability and precipitating seizures*.

Adverse Effects

The adverse effects most commonly associated with bulk laxatives are GI effects such as diarrhea, abdominal cramping, and nausea (Figure 58.2). CNS effects, including dizziness, headache, and weakness, are not uncommon and may relate to loss of fluid and electrolyte imbalances that may accompany laxative use. Sweating, palpitations, flushing, and even fainting have been reported after laxative use. These effects may be related to a sympathetic stress reaction to intense neurostimulation of the GI tract or to the loss of fluid and electrolyte imbalance. Patients must use caution and take bulk laxatives with plenty of water. If only a little water is used the laxative may absorb enough fluid in the esophagus to swell into a gelatin-like mass that can obstruct the esophagus and cause severe problems.

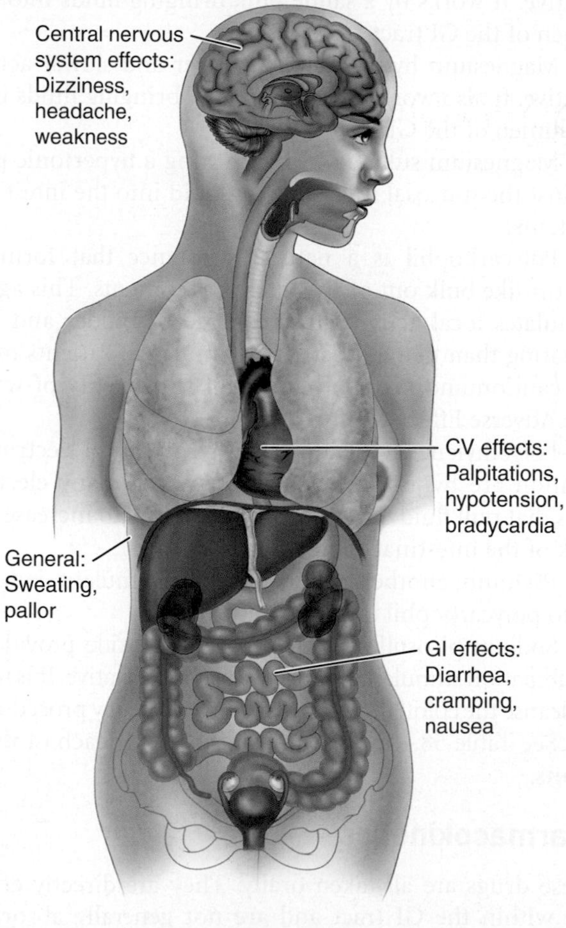

FIGURE 58.2 Variety of adverse effects and toxicities associated with drugs affecting gastric motility.

Clinically Important Drug–Drug Interactions

Bulk laxatives increase the motility of the GI tract, and some interfere with the timing or process of absorption. It is advisable not to take laxatives with other prescribed medications. The administration of laxatives and other medications should be separated by at least 30 minutes. There is an increased risk of neuromuscular blockade when using nondepolarizing neuromuscular junction blockers with magnesium salts; if this combination is used the patient must be closely monitored and appropriate life support provided.

> **Ⓟ Prototype Summary: Magnesium Citrate**
>
> **Indications:** Short-term relief of constipation; to prevent straining when it is clinically undesirable; to evacuate the bowel for diagnostic procedures; to remove ingested poisons from the lower GI tract; as an adjunct in anthelmintic therapy when it is desirable to flush helminths from the GI tract.
>
> **Actions:** Increases the motility of the GI tract by increasing the fluid in the intestinal contents, which enlarges bulk, stimulates local stretch receptors, and activates local activity.
>
> **Pharmacokinetics:** Not absorbed systemically.
>
> **$T_{1/2}$:** Not absorbed systemically.
>
> **Adverse Effects:** Diarrhea, abdominal cramps, bloating, perianal irritation, dizziness.

Lubricants

Sometimes it is desirable to make defecation easier without stimulating the movement of the GI tract. This is done using **lubricants**. Patients with hemorrhoids and those who have recently had rectal surgery may need lubrication of the stool. Some patients who could be harmed by straining might also benefit from this type of laxative. The type of laxative recommended depends on the condition of the patient, the speed of relief needed, and the possible implication of various adverse effects. Lubricating laxatives include docusate (*Colace*), glycerin (*Sani-Supp*), and mineral oil (*Agoral Liquid*).

Therapeutic Actions and Indications

Docusate has a detergent action on the surface of the intestinal bolus, increasing the admixture of fat and water and making a softer stool.

Glycerin is a hyperosmolar laxative that is used in suppository form to gently evacuate the rectum without systemic effects higher in the GI tract.

Mineral oil is the oldest of these laxatives. It is not absorbed and forms a slippery coat on the contents of the intestinal tract. When the intestinal bolus is coated with mineral oil, less water is absorbed out of the bolus, and the bolus is less likely to become hard or impacted.

Pharmacokinetics

These drugs are not absorbed systemically and are excreted in the feces. Docusate and mineral oil are given orally. Glycerin is available as a rectal suppository or as a liquid for rectal retention.

Contraindications and Cautions

These laxatives are contraindicated with allergy to any component of the drug *to prevent hypersensitivity reactions* and in acute abdominal disorders, including appendicitis, diverticulitis, and ulcerative colitis, *when increased motility could lead to rupture or further exacerbation of the inflammation.* Laxatives should be used with caution in heart block, CAD, and debilitation, *which could be affected by the decrease in absorption and changes in electrolyte levels that can occur*; caution should be used during pregnancy and *lactation because, in some cases, stimulation of the GI tract can precipitate labor and many of these agents cross the placenta and are excreted in breast milk.*

Adverse Effects

The adverse effects most commonly associated with lubricant laxatives are GI effects such as diarrhea, abdominal cramping, and nausea. In addition, leakage and staining may be a problem when mineral oil is used and the stool cannot be retained by the external sphincter. CNS effects, including dizziness, headache, and weakness, are not uncommon and may relate to loss of fluid and electrolyte imbalances that may accompany laxative use. Sweating, palpitations, flushing, and even fainting have been reported after laxative use. These effects are less likely to happen with the lubricant laxatives than with the chemical or mechanical stimulants.

Clinically Important Drug–Drug Interactions

Frequent use of mineral oil can interfere with absorption of the fat-soluble vitamins A, D, E, and K.

Ⓟ Prototype Summary: Mineral Oil flat enema

Indications: Short-term relief of constipation; to prevent straining when it is clinically undesirable; to remove ingested poisons from the lower GI tract; an adjunct in anthelmintic therapy when it is desirable to flush helminths from the GI tract.

Actions: Forms a slippery coat on the contents of the intestinal tract; less water is absorbed out of the bolus, and the bolus is less likely to become hard or impacted.

Pharmacokinetics: Not absorbed systemically.

$T_{1/2}$: Not absorbed systemically.

Adverse Effects: Diarrhea; abdominal cramps; bloating; perianal irritation; dizziness; interference with absorption of the fat-soluble vitamins A, D, E, and K; leakage of stool and staining.

Other Laxatives

The newest laxatives to be approved do not fit into the categories usually used for laxatives. These drugs are discussed in Box 58.2.

BOX 58.2

Other Laxatives

Two other drugs that do not fit into the categories usually used for laxatives have been approved for the treatment of a specific form of constipation.

- Methylnaltrexone (*Relistor*) was approved in 2008 for the treatment of opioid-induced constipation in patients with advanced disease who are receiving palliative care and are no longer responsive to traditional laxatives. Opioids bind to various receptors in the body, including the mu-receptors, which leads to decreased GI motility and constipation. Patients on long-term opioid treatment frequently have a very difficult time with constipation. Methylnaltrexone is a selective antagonist to opioid binding at the mu-receptor. It does not cross the blood–brain barrier and therefore acts specifically at peripheral opioid receptor sites, like the GI tract, but does not affect the analgesic effects of opioids in the CNS. This drug is given by daily subcutaneous injections. It reaches peak levels in 1/2 hour and is eliminated primarily unchanged in the urine. The half-life of the drug is about 8 hours. Patients may experience abdominal pain, flatulence, nausea, dizziness, and diarrhea. Severe or continued diarrhea should be reported. Use of this drug for beyond 4 months has not been studied.

(continues on page 1016)

BOX 58.2

Other Laxatives (continued)

- Naloxegel (*Movantik*) was approved in 2014. This drug is also a mu-receptor opioid agonist approved for the treatment of patients with opioid-induced chronic constipation and in adults with chronic, noncancer pain. It is rapidly absorbed after oral administration, reaches peak levels in less than 2 hours, is metabolized in the liver, and excreted primarily in the feces. Naloxegel has a half-life of 6 to 11 hours. Any maintenance laxative needs to stopped before starting naloxegel. It is taken once daily and the tablets must be swallowed whole, not cut, crushed, or chewed. There is a risk of opioid withdrawal with this drug and GI perforation has been reported. Patients should be monitored closely. The most common adverse effects relate to the effects on the GI tract, diarrhea, flatulence, nausea, vomiting, and abdominal pain. It is not approved for use for any other indication.

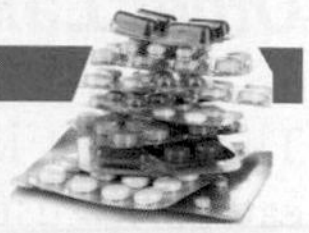

Nursing Considerations for Patients Receiving Laxatives

Assessment: History and Examination

- Assess for *possible contraindications or cautions*: History of allergy to laxatives *to prevent hypersensitivity reaction*; fecal impaction or intestinal obstruction, *which could be exacerbated by increased GI activity*; acute abdominal pain, nausea, or vomiting, *which could represent an underlying medical condition*; and current status of pregnancy or lactation, *which could be contraindications or require cautious use.*
- Perform a physical examination *to establish baseline data before beginning therapy and during therapy to determine the effectiveness of the drug and to evaluate for any adverse effects associated with drug therapy.*
- Inspect the skin for rash to *monitor for adverse reactions.*
- Assess the patient's neurological status, including level of orientation and affect, *to evaluate any CNS effects of the drug.*
- Obtain a baseline pulse rate *to assess for any cardiovascular effects of the drug.*
- Assess bowel elimination patterns, including the patient's perception of normal frequency, actual frequency, and stool characteristics, *to determine the need for therapy.*
- Investigate the patient's nutritional intake, including fluid intake and ingestion of fiber-containing foods, *to evaluate for possible contributing factors related to the need for the drug.*
- Assess the patient's level of activity *to determine possible contributing factors for decreased bowel motility.*
- Perform an abdominal examination, including inspecting abdomen for distention, palpating for masses, and auscultating for bowel sounds, *to establish adequate bowel function, rule out underlying medical conditions, and assess the effectiveness of the drug.*
- Monitor results of laboratory tests, including serum electrolyte levels, *to detect any changes related to altered absorption.*

Nursing Diagnoses

Nursing diagnoses related to drug therapy may include the following:

- Acute pain related to CNS and GI effects
- Diarrhea related to drug effects
- Deficient knowledge regarding drug therapy

Planning

- The patient will receive the best therapeutic effect from the drug therapy.
- The patient will have limited adverse effects to the drug therapy.
- The patient will have an understanding of the drug therapy, adverse effects to anticipate, and measures to relieve discomfort and improve safety.

Implementation with Rationale

- Administer a laxative only as a temporary measure *to prevent the development of cathartic dependence.*
- Arrange for appropriate dietary measures, exercise, and environmental controls *to encourage the return of normal bowel function.*
- Administer the oral form with a full glass of water and caution the patient not to chew tablets *to ensure that the laxative reaches the GI tract to allow for therapeutic effects.* Encourage fluid intake throughout the day as appropriate *to maintain fluid balance and improve GI movement.*
- Administer bulk laxatives with plenty of water. *If only a little water is used, it may absorb enough fluid in the esophagus to swell into a gelatin-like mass that can* obstruct the esophagus and cause severe problems.
- Insert rectal suppositories high into the rectum; encourage patients to retain enemas or rectal solution as long as possible *to improve effectiveness.*
- Do not administer in the presence of acute abdominal pain, nausea, or vomiting, *which might indicate a serious underlying medical problem that could be exacerbated by laxative use.*
- Monitor bowel function *to evaluate drug effectiveness.* If diarrhea or cramping occurs, discontinue the drug *to relieve discomfort and to prevent serious fluid and electrolyte imbalance.*
- Provide comfort and safety measures *to improve patient compliance and to ensure patient safety*, including ready access to bathroom facilities, assistance with ambulation, and periodic orientation if CNS effects occur.

- Offer support and encouragement *to help the patient deal with the discomfort of the condition and drug therapy.*
- Offer support and encouragement *to help the patient deal with the diagnosis and the drug regimen.*
- Provide thorough patient teaching, including the drug name, dosage, and schedule for administration; method of administration, such as taking the oral form with a full glass of water, thoroughly mixing the powdered or granular form with water or juice to ensure complete dissolution, inserting the suppository form, or using and retaining an enema; approximate time for achievement of results and importance of having bathroom facilities readily available; safety measures, such as changing positions slowly and using assistance with ambulation if dizziness or weakness occurs; signs and symptoms of possible adverse effects and measures to minimize or prevent them; possible leakage and staining when mineral oil is used and the stool cannot be retained by the external sphincter; danger signs and symptoms to be reported to a health care provider immediately; the importance of daily activity *to promote bowel function*; the need for the ingestion of high-fiber foods and adequate fluids *to stimulate GI motility*; the importance of avoiding the overuse of laxatives *to prevent chronic or long-term problems with elimination*; a bowel-training program if indicated *to prevent dependence on laxatives*; and importance of periodic monitoring and evaluation *to evaluate the effectiveness of therapy, enhance patient knowledge about drug therapy, and promote compliance.*

Evaluation

- Monitor patient response to the drug (relief of GI symptoms, absence of straining, evacuation of GI tract).
- Monitor for adverse effects (dizziness, confusion, GI alterations, sweating, electrolyte imbalance, cathartic dependence).
- Monitor the effectiveness of comfort measures and compliance with the regimen.
- Evaluate the effectiveness of the teaching plan (patient can name the drug and dosage, describe adverse effects to watch for, and specific measures to use to avoid them).

KEY POINTS

- Laxative drugs stimulate GI motility and assist in bowel elimination.
- Laxatives can be chemical or bulk stimulants or lubricants.
- In many cases, implementing diet and exercise strategies and promoting natural intestinal reflexes have decreased the need to use laxatives.
- Chronic use of laxatives can lead to dependence on them and on external stimuli for normal GI function.

Gastrointestinal Stimulants

Some drugs are available for more generalized GI stimulation that results in an overall increase in GI activity and secretions (Table 58.2). These drugs stimulate parasympathetic activity or make the GI tissues more sensitive to parasympathetic activity. Such stimulants include dexpanthenol (*Ilopan*) and metoclopramide (*Reglan*).

Therapeutic Actions and Indications

By stimulating parasympathetic activity within the GI tract, these drugs increase GI secretions and motility on a general level throughout the tract (see Figure 58.1). They do not have the local effects of laxatives to increase activity only in the intestines. These drugs are indicated when more rapid movement of GI contents is desirable. Dexpanthenol works by increasing acetylcholine levels and stimulating the parasympathetic system. Metoclopramide works by blocking dopamine receptors and making the GI cells more sensitive to acetylcholine, which leads to increased GI activity and rapid movement of food through the upper GI tract. See Table 58.2 for Usual Indications for each of these agents. Metoclopramide is also being studied for improvement of lactation in doses of 30 to 45 mg/d. Its effectiveness in improving lactation may be linked to its dopamine-blocking effect, which is often associated with increased prolactin levels.

Pharmacokinetics

Dexpanthenol is given by IM injection and reaches peak levels within 4 hours. Metoclopramide is given orally or

Table 58.2 *Drugs in Focus:* Gastrointestinal Stimulants

Drug Name	Usual Dosage	Usual Indications
dexpanthenol (*Ilopan*)	250–500 mg IM or IV, repeat in 2 h and then q6 h as needed	Prevention of intestinal atony or loss of intestinal muscle tone in postoperative situations in adults
metoclopramide (*Reglan*)	10–20 mg IM, IV, or PO *Pediatric (6–14 y):* 2.5–5 mg IV over 1–2 min *Pediatric (<6 y):* 0.1 mg/kg IV over 1–2 min	Relief of symptoms of gastroesophageal reflux disease, prevention of nausea and vomiting after emetogenic chemotherapy or postoperatively, relief of symptoms of diabetic gastroparesis, promotion of GI movement during small-bowel intubation or promotion of rapid movement of barium, currently under investigation for improvement of lactation in doses of 30–45 mg/d

GI, gastrointestinal.

by IM injection or IV infusion and has a peak effect by all routes in 60 to 90 minutes. They are metabolized in the liver and excreted in the feces and urine. Metoclopramide crosses the placenta and enters breast milk; dexpanthenol may cross the placenta and enter breast milk.

Contraindications and Cautions

GI stimulants should not be used in patients with a history of allergy to any of these drugs *to prevent hypersensitivity reactions* or with any GI obstruction or perforation, *which could be exacerbated by the GI stimulation.* They should be used with caution during pregnancy or lactation and only if the *benefit to the mother clearly outweighs the potential risk to the fetus or neonate.*

Adverse Effects

The most common adverse effects seen with GI stimulants include nausea, vomiting, diarrhea, intestinal spasm, and cramping. Other adverse effects, such as declining blood pressure and heart rate, weakness, and fatigue, may be related to parasympathetic stimulation, extrapyramidal effects, and Parkinson-like syndrome.

Clinically Important Drug–Drug Interactions

Metoclopramide has been associated with decreased absorption of digoxin from the GI tract; patients taking this combination should be monitored carefully.

Decreased immunosuppressive effects and increased toxicity of cyclosporine have occurred when combined with metoclopramide. This combination should be avoided.

Increased sedation can occur if either of these drugs is combined with alcohol or other CNS sedative drugs.

Ⓟ Prototype Summary: Metoclopramide

Indications: Relief of acute and chronic diabetic gastroparesis; short-term treatment of gastroesophageal reflux disorder in adults who cannot tolerate standard therapy; prevention of postoperative or chemotherapy-induced nausea and vomiting; facilitation of small-bowel intubation; stimulation of gastric emptying; promotion of intestinal transit of barium.

Actions: Stimulates movement of the upper GI tract without stimulating gastric, pancreatic, or biliary secretions; appears to sensitize tissues to the effects of acetylcholine.

Pharmacokinetics:

Route	Onset	Peak	Duration
Oral	30–60 min	60–90 min	1–2 h
IM	10–15 min	60–90 min	1–2 h
IV	1–5 min	60–90 min	1–2 h

$T_{1/2}$: 5 to 6 hours; metabolized in the liver and excreted in the urine.

Adverse Effects: Restlessness, drowsiness, fatigue, extrapyramidal effects, Parkinson-like reactions, nausea, diarrhea.

Nursing Considerations for Patients Receiving Gastrointestinal Stimulants

Assessment: History and Examination

- Assess for *possible contraindications or cautions:* Any history of allergy to these drugs *to prevent hypersensitivity reactions;* intestinal obstruction, bleeding, or perforation, *which could be exacerbated by stimulating the GI tract;* and current status of pregnancy or lactation, *which require cautious use.*
- Perform a physical examination *to establish baseline data before beginning therapy and during therapy to determine the effectiveness of the drug and to evaluate for the occurrence of any adverse effects associated with drug therapy.*
- Perform an abdominal examination, including inspecting for distention, palpating for masses, and checking bowel sounds, *to ensure adequate GI function and motility.*
- Assess cardiopulmonary status, including pulse and blood pressure, *to monitor for possible cardiovascular adverse effects.*
- Inspect skin for color and evidence of lesions or rash *to assess for hypersensitivity reactions.*

Nursing Diagnoses

Nursing diagnoses related to drug therapy may include the following:

- Diarrhea related to drug effects
- Acute pain related to GI effects
- Deficient knowledge regarding drug therapy

Planning

- The patient will receive the best therapeutic effect from the drug therapy.
- The patient will have limited adverse effects to the drug therapy.
- The patient will have an understanding of the drug therapy, adverse effects to anticipate, and measures to relieve discomfort and improve safety.

Implementation with Rationale

- Administer at least 15 minutes before each meal and at bedtime *to ensure therapeutic effectiveness.*
- Monitor blood pressure carefully if giving the drug IV *to detect changes in blood pressure indicating the need to consult with the prescriber.*
- Monitor diabetic patients, who will have increased speed of transit through the GI tract, which could alter absorption and glucose levels, *to arrange for alteration in insulin dose or timing as appropriate.*
- Offer support and encouragement *to help the patient deal with the diagnosis and the drug regimen, including the discomfort of cramping and pain.*

- Provide thorough patient teaching, including the drug name and prescribed dosage, measures to help avoid adverse effects, warning signs that may indicate problems, and the need for periodic monitoring and evaluation, *to enhance patient knowledge about drug therapy and to promote compliance.*
- Provide thorough patient teaching, including the drug name, prescribed dosage, and schedule for administration; method for oral administration (15 minutes before meals and at bedtime); signs and symptoms of adverse effects and measures to minimize or prevent them; danger signs that need to be reported to the health care provider immediately; importance of avoiding alcohol or other CNS depressants; safety measures, such as avoiding driving and obtaining assistance with ambulation as needed; and the importance of periodic monitoring and evaluation *to enhance patient knowledge about drug therapy and to promote compliance.*

Evaluation

- Monitor patient response to the drug (increased tone and movement of GI tract).
- Monitor for adverse effects (GI effects, parasympathetic activity).
- Monitor the effectiveness of comfort measures and compliance with the regimen.
- Evaluate the effectiveness of the teaching plan (patient can name the drug and dosage, as well as describe adverse effects to watch for and specific measures to take to avoid them and to increase the effectiveness of the drug).

KEY POINTS

- GI stimulants act to increase parasympathetic stimulation in the GI tract and to increase tone and general movement throughout the GI system.
- Patients receiving GI stimulants should be monitored for generalized increases in parasympathetic activity.

Antidiarrheals

Antidiarrheals block stimulation of the GI tract for symptomatic relief from diarrhea. Available agents include bismuth subsalicylate (*Pepto-Bismol*), crofelemer (*Fulyzag*), loperamide (*Imodium*), and opium derivatives (*Paregoric*). Several antidiarrheal products are available in combination (Box 58.3). There is also a drug approved strictly for use in treating traveler's diarrhea (Box 58.4).

Therapeutic Actions and Indications

Antidiarrheal agents slow the motility of the GI tract through direct action on the lining of the GI tract to inhibit local reflexes (bismuth subsalicylate), through direct action on the muscles of the GI tract to slow activity (loperamide), or through action on CNS centers that cause GI spasm and slowing (opium derivatives; see Figure 58.1). These drugs are indicated for the relief of

BOX 58.3

Combination Antidiarrheal Products

Two very popular antidiarrheal agents combine atropine with a meperidine-like compound. Meperidine (*Demerol*) has a local effect on the GI wall, causing a slowing of intestinal motility. Difenoxin and diphenoxylate are chemically related to meperidine and are used at doses that decrease GI activity without having analgesic or respiratory effects. These drugs, which are controlled substances—difenoxin is category C-IV and diphenoxylate is category C-V—are combined with atropine to discourage deliberate use of excessive doses to get the euphoric effects associated with meperidine.

difenoxin with atropine (*Motofen*)	*Adult:* Two tablets PO, then one tablet after each loose stool; do not exceed eight tablets in 24 h *Pediatric:* Not for use in children <12 y
diphenoxylate with atropine (*Lomotil*)	*Adult:* 5 mg PO q.i.d. *Pediatric 2–12 y:* Use liquid form only, start with 0.3–0.4 mg/kg/d PO in four divided doses

BOX 58.4

Treating Traveler's Diarrhea

Rifaximin (*Xifaxan*) was the first antibiotic approved by the U.S. Food and Drug Administration (FDA) specifically for treating traveler's diarrhea. A new antibiotic, rifaximin, acts locally in the GI tract against noninvasive strains of *Escherichia coli*, the most common cause of traveler's diarrhea. About 80 to 90% of the drug is delivered to the intestines without being absorbed through the GI tract.

Rifaximin acts locally in the GI tract to destroy the *E. coli* that causes the signs and symptoms associated with traveler's diarrhea. The drug is taken in 200-mg tablets, three times a day for 3 days once the signs and symptoms of the disorder occur. It should not be used if the patient has bloody diarrhea or if diarrhea persists more than 48 hours or worsens during treatment with the drug. Destroying the causative agent will relieve the GI symptoms of diarrhea, nausea, and anorexia. Prevention remains the best intervention for traveler's diarrhea.

Because of its local effect in the GI tract and impact on GI bacteria that produce ammonia, rifaximin has been found to be effective in reducing the risk of overt hepatic encephalopathy recurrence in patients 18 and older with hepatic cirrhosis. Hepatic encephalopathy is associated with high ammonia levels. For this use the drug is given orally twice a day.

Table 58.3 *Drugs in Focus:* Antidiarrheals

Drug Name	Usual Dosage	Usual Indications
bismuth subsalicylate (*Pepto-Bismol*)	*Adult:* 524 mg PO q30–60 min as needed, up to eight doses per day *Pediatric (<3 y):* Not recommended *Pediatric (3–6 y):* 1/3 tablet *or* 5 mL PO *Pediatric (6–9 y):* 2/3 tablet *or* 10 mL PO *Pediatric (9–12 y):* One tablet *or* 15 mL PO	Treatment of traveler's diarrhea, prevention of cramping and distention associated with dietary excess and some viral infections
crofelemer (*Fulyzag*)	*Adult:* One 125 mg DR tablet PO b.i.d.	Symptomatic relief of noninfectious diarrhea in adults on HIV/AIDS antiretroviral medication
loperamide (*Imodium*)	*Adult:* 4 mg PO, then 2 mg PO after each loose stool *Pediatric (2–12 y):* 1–2 mg PO t.i.d. *Pediatric (<2 y):* Not recommended	Short-term treatment of diarrhea associated with dietary problems, viral infections
opium derivatives (*Paregoric*)	*Adult:* 5–10 mL PO once to four times daily *Pediatric:* 0.25–0.5 mL/kg PO once to four times daily as needed	Short-term treatment of cramping and diarrhea

DR, delayed release.

symptoms of acute and chronic diarrhea, reduction of volume of discharge from ileostomies, and prevention and treatment of traveler's diarrhea (Table 58.3; Box 58.4). Bismuth subsalicylate has been found to be very helpful in treating traveler's diarrhea (see the Critical Thinking Scenario for additional information) and in preventing cramping and distention associated with dietary excess and some viral infections. Crofelemer works in the inner lining of the GI tract to block specific chloride channels leading to less water loss as diarrhea and return to more balance between water and chloride and sodium in the cells. This drug is specifically for symptomatic relief of noninfectious diarrhea in adult patients on HIV/AIDS antiretroviral therapy.

Pharmacokinetics

Bismuth subsalicylate is absorbed from the GI tract after oral administration, metabolized in the liver, and excreted in the urine. It crosses the placenta, but it is not known whether it enters breast milk. Loperamide is slowly absorbed after oral administration, metabolized in the liver, and excreted in the urine and feces. It may cross the placenta and enter breast milk. Opium derivative (*Paregoric*), a category C-III controlled substance, is readily absorbed after oral administration, metabolized in the liver, and excreted in the urine. It crosses the placenta and enters breast milk. Crofelemer is minimally absorbed and its half-life, metabolism, and excretion are unknown.

CRITICAL THINKING SCENARIO

Traveler's Diarrhea

THE SITUATION

P.F. received an all-expenses-paid trip to Mexico to celebrate his graduation from college. He was very excited about getting away for a week of sun and fun, and arranged to stay in the same hotel as two college friends who were also celebrating. The three men had a wonderful time visiting the beaches, bars, and nightclubs in the area. On the third day of the trip, P.F. began experiencing nausea, some vomiting, and a low-grade fever. Several hours later, he began experiencing intense cramping and diarrhea. For the next 2 days, P.F. felt so ill he was unable to leave his hotel room. The next morning, he arranged for an emergency trip home.

CRITICAL THINKING

What is probably happening to P.F.? *Think about the GI reflexes and explain the underlying cause for his signs and symptoms.*

What treatment should be started now?

What could have been done to prevent this problem from occurring?

What possible drug therapy might have been helpful for P.F.?

Traveler's Diarrhea (continued)

DISCUSSION

P.F. is probably experiencing the common disorder called traveler's diarrhea. This disorder occurs when pathogens found in the food and water of a foreign environment are ingested. (Because these pathogens are commonly found in the environment, they do not normally cause problems for the people who live in the area.) When the pathogen, usually a strain of *Escherichia coli*, enters a host that is not accustomed to the bacteria, it releases enterotoxins and sets off an intestinal–intestinal reaction in the host.

The intestinal–intestinal reaction results in a reduction of activity above the point of irritation (which causes nausea and in some cases vomiting) and an increase in activity below the point of irritation. The body is trying to flush the invader from the body. A low-grade fever may occur as a reaction to the toxins released by the bacteria. Muscle aches and pains, malaise, and fatigue are often common symptoms. It is important at this stage of the disease to maintain fluid intake to prevent dehydration from occurring.

P.F. may want to return home, but with intense cramping and diarrhea it might not be a good idea. Bismuth subsalicylate (*Pepto-Bismol*), taken four times a day, has been effective in preventing traveler's diarrhea and associated problems. It is available OTC and readily accessible for travelers. Taken during a course of traveler's diarrhea, it may relieve the stomach upset and nausea and some of the discomfort of the diarrhea. Some patients respond to the prophylactic antibiotics *Bactrim* and *Septra*, combinations of trimethoprim and sulfamethoxazole that are often prescribed as prophylactic measures for patients who are traveling to areas known to be associated with traveler's diarrhea and for those who are known to be very susceptible to the disorder. However, it is not recommended that people use antibiotic prophylaxis unless they are very high risk, because of the increasing development of resistant strains of bacteria. Once traveler's diarrhea is diagnosed, rifaximin (*Xifaxan*) can be taken. The 200-mg tablets are taken three times a day. It should not be used if the patient has bloody diarrhea or diarrhea that worsens or persists for more than 48 hours. In the past, antidiarrheals, like loperamide, have been used to help patients with traveler's diarrhea. It is now thought that these slow the GI tract enough to allow longer exposure to the offending bacteria, which could make the situation worse. The Centers for Disease Control and Prevention (CDC) now advises the use of antidiarrheals only if needed to allow travel out of the area.

The best course of action, however, is prevention. Several measures can be taken to avoid ingestion of the local bacteria: Drinking only bottled or mineral water; avoiding fresh fruits and vegetables that may have been washed in the local water, unless they are peeled; avoiding ice cubes in drinks because the ice cubes are made from the local water; avoiding any food that might be undercooked or rare, including shellfish; and even being cautious about using water to brush the teeth or gargle. People who have suffered a bout of traveler's diarrhea are very cautious about exposure to local bacteria when they travel again, often combining prophylactic drug therapy with careful avoidance of local pathogens. P.F. can be reassured that in a few days the diarrhea and associated signs and symptoms should pass and he will regain his strength and energy.

NURSING CARE GUIDE FOR P.F.: ANTIDIARRHEALS

Assessment: History and Examination

Assess the patient's health history for allergies to any of these drugs, acute abdominal pain, concurrent use of aspirin products, methotrexate, valproic acid, corticosteroids, oral tetracyclines, oral antidiabetic agents, or sulfinpyrazone.

Focus the physical examination on the following:
CNS: Orientation, reflexes
GI: Abdominal evaluation, bowel sounds
Respiratory: Respiratory rate and depth
Laboratory tests: Serum electrolyte levels
Other: Temperature

Nursing Diagnoses

Acute pain related to GI and CNS effects
Diarrhea related to GI effects
Deficient knowledge regarding drug therapy

Planning

The patient will receive the best therapeutic effect from the drug therapy.
The patient will have limited adverse effects to the drug therapy.
The patient will have an understanding of the drug therapy, adverse effects to anticipate, and measures to relieve discomfort and improve safety.

Implementation

Administer an antidiarrheal agent only as a temporary measure.
Provide comfort and safety measures, including assistance, access to bathroom, and safety precautions if necessary.
Monitor bowel function.
Provide support and reassurance for coping with drug effects and discomfort.
Provide patient teaching regarding drug name and dosage, adverse effects and precautions, and warning signs of serious adverse effects to report.

(continues on page 1022)

Traveler's Diarrhea (continued)

Evaluation

Evaluate drug effects: Relief of GI symptoms.
Monitor for adverse effects: GI alterations, dizziness, confusion, salicylate toxicity.
Monitor for drug–drug interactions as indicated.
Evaluate the effectiveness of patient-teaching program and comfort and safety measures.

PATIENT TEACHING FOR P.F.

- The drug you are taking is called bismuth subsalicylate (*Pepto-Bismol*). This drug is called an antidiarrheal agent. It forms a protective coating over the inner lining of the intestine and soothes the irritated areas.
- Take this drug exactly as indicated. Shake the bottle well before using the liquid preparation. If you are using tablets, make sure that you chew them thoroughly; do not swallow them whole.
- Common effects of this drug include:
  - *Darkening of the stools:* Do not become concerned; this is a normal effect that will go away when you stop taking the drug.
  - *Ringing in the ears, rapid respirations:* This is more likely to occur if you are taking other products that contain aspirin, which is also a salicylate.
- Report any of the following conditions to your health care provider: *Diarrhea that does not stop within 2 days, ringing in the ears, rapid respirations, fever, and/or intense abdominal pain.*
- Stay away from any food or beverage that may be contaminated with bacteria. Use bottled water for drinking, as well as for brushing your teeth. Do not wash fruit or vegetables with water from the local supply.
- Do not use any other medication that contains aspirin; inadvertent overdose may occur.
- Tell any doctor, nurse, or other health care provider involved in your care that you are taking this drug.
- Keep this drug and all medications out of the reach of children.

Contraindications and Cautions

Antidiarrheal drugs should not be given to anyone with known allergy to the drug or any of its components *to prevent hypersensitivity reactions*. Caution should be used in pregnancy and lactation *because of the potential adverse effects to the fetus or baby*. Care should also be taken in individuals with any history of GI obstruction; acute abdominal conditions, *which could be exacerbated by the effects of the drugs*, or diarrhea due to poisonings, *which could be worsened by slowing of the GI tract, allowing increased time for absorption of the poison*; or with hepatic impairment, *which could alter the metabolism of the drugs*.

Adverse Effects

The adverse effects associated with antidiarrheal drugs, such as constipation, distention, abdominal discomfort, nausea, vomiting, dry mouth, and even toxic megacolon, are related to their effects on the GI tract. Other adverse effects that have been reported include fatigue, weakness, dizziness, and skin rash. Opium derivatives are also associated with light-headedness, sedation, euphoria, hallucinations, and respiratory depression related to effect on the opioid receptors.

Clinically Important Drug–Drug Interactions

Drug interactions vary depending on the antidiarrheal agent. Consult the drug package insert for specific interactions.

Ⓟ Prototype Summary: Loperamide

Indications: Control and symptomatic relief of acute, nonspecific diarrhea and chronic diarrhea associated with irritable bowel syndrome; reduction of volume of discharge from ileostomies

Actions: Inhibits intestinal peristalsis through direct effects on the longitudinal and circular muscles of the intestinal wall, slowing motility and movement of water and electrolytes

Pharmacokinetics:

Route	Onset	Peak
Oral (capsule)	Varies	5 h

$T_{1/2}$: 10.8 hours; metabolized in the liver and excreted in the urine and feces

Adverse Effects: Abdominal pain, distention, or discomfort; dry mouth; nausea; constipation; dizziness; tiredness; drowsiness

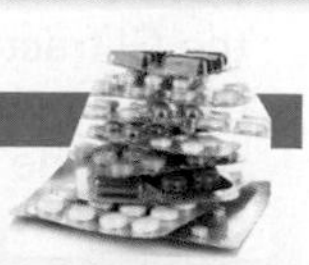

Nursing Considerations for Patients Receiving Antidiarrheals

Assessment: History and Examination

- Assess for *possible contraindications or cautions*: Any history of allergy to these drugs *to prevent hypersensitivity reactions*; acute abdominal conditions, *which could be exacerbated by these drugs*; poisoning, *which is a contraindication to slowing GI activity*; hepatic impairment, *which could alter the metabolism of the drug*; and current status of pregnancy or lactation, *which require cautious use.*

- Perform a physical examination *to establish baseline data before beginning therapy and during therapy to determine the effectiveness of the drug and to evaluate for the occurrence of any adverse effects associated with drug therapy.*
- Inspect the skin for color and evidence of lesions or rash *to monitor for potential hypersensitivity reactions.*
- Perform an abdominal examination, including inspecting for distention, palpating for masses, and auscultating bowel sounds, to evaluate GI function and *to rule out potential underlying medical conditions.*
- Assess bowel elimination pattern, including frequency and characteristics of stool, *to assist in determining appropriateness for drug therapy.*
- Assess the patient's neurological status, including level of orientation and affect, *to monitor for CNS effects of the drug.*

Nursing Diagnoses

Nursing diagnoses related to drug therapy may include the following:

- Constipation related to GI slowing caused by antidiarrheal agent
- Acute pain related to GI effects
- Disturbed sensory perception (kinesthetic, gustatory) related to CNS effects
- Deficient knowledge regarding drug therapy

Planning

- The patient will receive the best therapeutic effect from the drug therapy.
- The patient will have limited adverse effects to the drug therapy.
- The patient will have an understanding of the drug therapy, adverse effects to anticipate, and measures to relieve discomfort and improve safety.

Implementation with Rationale

- Administer the drug after each unformed stool *to ensure therapeutic effectiveness.* Keep track of the exact amount given *to ensure that the dose does not exceed the recommended daily maximum dose.* If using crofelemer the drug is taken twice a day *to maintain effectiveness against anti-HIV drug actions, which can cause diarrhea.*
- Monitor the response carefully; note the frequency and characteristics of the stool. If no response is seen within 48 hours *the diarrhea could be related to an underlying medical condition.* Arrange to discontinue the drug and arrange for medical evaluation *to allow for the diagnosis of underlying medical conditions.*
- Provide appropriate safety and comfort measures if CNS effects occur *to prevent patient injury.*
- Offer support and encouragement *to help the patient deal with the diagnosis and the drug regimen.*
- Provide thorough patient teaching, including the drug name and prescribed dosage; schedule for administration; use of drug after each loose stool; recommended daily maximum dose and the need not to exceed it; signs and symptoms of adverse effects, including measures to minimize or prevent them; safety measures, such as avoiding driving and obtaining assistance with ambulation as needed *to reduce the risk of injury due to weakness or dizziness*; danger signs and symptoms that need to be reported immediately; the importance of notifying the health care provider if diarrhea is not controlled within 48 hours; and the need for follow-up *to enhance patient knowledge about drug therapy and to promote compliance.*

Evaluation

- Monitor the patient response to the drug (relief of diarrhea).
- Monitor for adverse effects (GI effects, CNS changes, dermatological effects).
- Monitor the effectiveness of comfort and safety measures and compliance with the regimen.
- Evaluate the effectiveness of the teaching plan (patient can name the drug and dosage, as well as describe adverse effects to watch for, specific measures to use to avoid them, and measures to take to increase the effectiveness of the drug).

KEY POINTS

- Antidiarrheal drugs are used to soothe irritation to the intestinal wall, block GI muscle activity to decrease movement, or affect CNS activity to cause GI spasm and stop movement.
- Antidiarrheal drugs can cause GI discomfort and constipation.

Irritable Bowel Syndrome Drugs

Irritable bowel syndrome (IBS) is a very common disorder. It strikes three times as many women as men and reportedly accounts for half of all referrals to GI specialists. The disorder is characterized by abdominal distress, bouts of diarrhea or constipation, bloating, nausea, flatulence, headache, fatigue, depression, and anxiety. No anatomical cause has been found for this disorder. Underlying causes might be stress related. Patients with this disorder have often suffered for years, not enjoying meals or activities because of their GI pain and discomfort. Lubiprostone is the most recent drug used to treat this condition. Lubiprostone and other drugs used to treat IBS are discussed in Box 58.5.

BOX 58.5

Treating Irritable Bowel Syndrome

Alosetron Returns

Alosetron (*Lotronex*) was the first drug to provide relief to this patient population. This drug, a serotonin 5-HT antagonist, blocks specific serotonin receptors in the enteric nervous system of the GI tract, which leads to decreased perception of abdominal pain and discomfort, decreased GI motility, and increased colon transit time. In late 2000, alosetron was pulled from the market after less than 1 year of availability. Reports of ischemic colitis, mesenteric colitis, and even death in patients who were using the drug led to this decision. In July 2002, after hearing lots of testimony and reading many petitions from patients, the FDA agreed to approve the release of the drug for marketing. This is the first time in the history of the FDA that a drug pulled from the market because of safety concerns has been rereleased. The prescribing information now includes a black box warning alerting users to the proper use and a patient medication guide. Restrictions have been applied to the use of the drug, and patients who use it must read and sign a Patient–Physician Agreement. The use of *Lotronex* should be discontinued immediately if the patient develops constipation or symptoms of ischemic colitis. It is approved for women with IBS with diarrhea being the predominant complaint.

Lubiprostone

Lubiprostone (*Amitiza*) is a locally acting chloride-channel activator that increases the secretion of a chloride-rich intestinal fluid without changing sodium or potassium levels. Increasing the intestinal fluid leads to increased motility. Lubiprostone is approved for the treatment of chronic, idiopathic constipation and for the treatment of IBS with constipation in adult women. This drug has very little systemic absorption. It is taken orally with plenty of water and food at a dose of 8 mcg twice a day for IBS or 24 mcg twice a day for chronic constipation. Lubiprostone frequently causes nausea; taking the drug with food helps to decrease this effect. Patients may also experience diarrhea and increased bowel sounds. Patients should report continued or severe diarrhea.

Hyoscyamine

Hyoscyamine (*Anaspaz*), an anticholinergic agent that was found to decrease GI spasm, was approved in 2001 as an adjunctive therapy for the treatment of IBS.

Support and symptomatic relief remain the mainstays of treating this disorder. Stress management and a consistent relationship with a health care provider may help to relieve some of the problems associated with this common, although not entirely understood, disorder.

SUMMARY

- Laxatives are drugs used to stimulate movement along the GI tract and to aid bowel evacuation. They may be used to prevent or treat constipation.
- Laxatives can be chemical stimulants, which directly irritate the local nerve plexus; bulk stimulants, which increase the size of the food bolus and stimulate stretch receptors in the wall of the intestine; or lubricants, which facilitate movement of the bolus through the intestines.
- Using proper diet and exercise, as well as taking advantage of the actions of the intestinal reflexes, has eliminated the need for laxatives in many situations.
- Cathartic dependence can occur with the chronic use of laxatives, leading to a need for external stimuli for normal functioning of the GI tract.
- GI stimulants act to increase parasympathetic stimulation in the GI tract and to increase tone and general movement throughout the GI system.
- Antidiarrheal drugs are used to soothe irritation to the intestinal wall, block GI muscle activity to decrease movement, or affect CNS activity to cause GI spasm and stop movement.
- Drugs used to treat IBS are specific for the main underlying complaint, either diarrhea or constipation, and patient selection must be carefully matched to the effect of the drug.

CHECK YOUR UNDERSTANDING

Answers to the questions in this chapter can be found in Answers to Check Your Understanding Questions on thePoint®.

MULTIPLE CHOICE

Select the best response to the following.

1. Laxatives are drugs that are used to
   a. increase the quantity of wastes excreted.
   b. speed the passage of the intestinal contents through the GI tract.
   c. increase digestion of intestinal contents.
   d. increase the water content of the intestinal contents.

2. The laxative of choice when mild stimulation is needed to prevent straining is
   a. senna.
   b. castor oil.
   c. bisacodyl.
   d. magnesium citrate.

3. Cathartic dependence can occur when
   a. patients do not use laxatives routinely and experience severe bouts of constipation.
   b. chronic laxative use leads to a reliance on the intense stimulation of laxatives.
   c. patients maintain a nutritious high-fiber diet.
   d. patients start an exercise program to promote bowel elimination.

4. Drugs that stimulate parasympathetic activity are used to increase GI activity and secretions. For which of the following would this group be most likely used?
   a. Duodenal ulcers
   b. Gastric ulcers
   c. Gastroesophageal reflux disease
   d. Poisoning, to induce nausea and vomiting

5. The drug of choice for treating/preventing traveler's diarrhea is
   a. loperamide.
   b. opium.
   c. rifaximin.
   d. bisacodyl.

MULTIPLE RESPONSE

Select all that apply.

1. A nurse is preparing a teaching plan for a client who has been prescribed a laxative. The teaching plan should include which of the following?
   a. The importance of proper diet and fluid intake
   b. The need to take the drug for several weeks to get the full effect
   c. The importance of exercise
   d. The need to take advantage of natural reflexes by providing privacy and time to allow them to work
   e. The need to limit fluids
   f. The importance of limiting the duration of laxative use

2. A nurse might expect an order for mineral oil for which patient?
   a. A debilitated patient low on nutrients
   b. A patient with hemorrhoids
   c. A patient with recent rectal surgery
   d. A child with encopresis
   e. A postpartum woman
   f. A patient with Crohn's disease

3. When explaining the actions of laxatives to a client the nurse would state that they can work by
   a. acting as chemical stimulants.
   b. acting as lubricants of the intestinal bolus.
   c. acting to increase bulk of the intestinal bolus and stimulate movement.
   d. stimulating CNS centers in the medulla to cause GI movement.
   e. blocking the parasympathetic nervous system.
   f. causing CNS depression.

BIBLIOGRAPHY AND REFERENCES

Baker, D. E. (2007). Lubiprostone: A new drug for the treatment of idiopathic chronic constipation. *Reviews in Gastroenterological Disorders, 7*(4), 214–222.

Bisanz, A. (2007). Chronic constipation. *American Journal of Nursing, 107*(4), 72B–72H.

Brunton, L., Chabner, B., & Knollman, B. (2011). *Goodman and Gilman's the pharmacological basis of therapeutics* (12th ed.). New York: McGraw-Hill.

Facts and Comparisons. (2015). *Drug facts and comparisons*. St. Louis, MO: Author.

Karch, A. M. (2014). *Lippincott's nursing drug guide*. Philadelphia, PA: Lippincott Williams & Wilkins.

Leung, L., Riutta, T., Kotecha, J., et al. (2011). Chronic constipation: An evidence-based review. *Journal of the American Board of Family Medicine, 24*(4), 436–451.

Porth, C. M. (2013). *Pathophysiology: Concepts of altered health states* (9th ed.). Philadelphia, PA: Lippincott Williams & Wilkins.

Shah, S. B., & Hanauer, S. B. (2007). Treatment of diarrhea in patients with inflammatory bowel disease: Concepts and cautions. *Reviews in Gastroenterological Disorders, 7*(Suppl. 3), S3–S10.

Steffen, R., Hill, D., & DuPont, H. (2015). Travelers diarrhea: A clinical review. *Journal of the American Medical Association, 313*(1), 71–80.

The Medical Letter. (2015). *The medical letter on drugs and therapeutics*. New Rochelle, NY: Author.

Thomas, J., Karver, S., Cooney, G. A., et al. (2008). Methlynatrexone for opioid-induced constipation in advanced illness. *New England Journal of Medicine, 358*, 2332–2343.

Tobias, N., Mason, D., Lutkenhoff, M., et al. (2008). Management and principles of organic causes of childhood constipation. *Journal of Pediatric Health Care, 22*(1), 12–23.

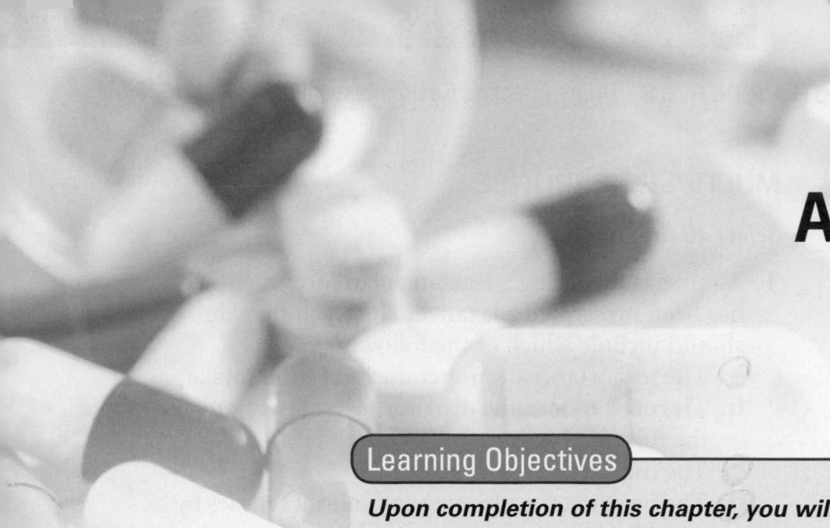

59 Antiemetic Agents

Learning Objectives

Upon completion of this chapter, you will be able to:

1. Outline the vomiting reflex, including factors that stimulate it and mechanisms for measures used to block it.
2. Describe the therapeutic actions, indications, pharmacokinetics, contraindications and cautions, most common adverse reactions, and important drug–drug interactions associated with each of the classes of antiemetic agents.
3. Discuss the use of antiemetics across the lifespan.
4. Compare and contrast the prototype antiemetics with other agents in their class and with other classes of antiemetics.
5. Outline the nursing considerations, including important teaching points, for patients receiving antiemetics

Glossary of Key Terms

antiemetic: agent that blocks the hyperactive response of the chemoreceptor trigger zone (CTZ) to various stimuli, the response that produces nonbeneficial nausea and vomiting

emetic: agent used to induce vomiting to rid the stomach of toxins or drugs

intractable hiccough: repetitive stimulation of the diaphragm that leads to hiccough, a diaphragmatic spasm that persists over time

phenothiazine: antianxiety drug that blocks the responsiveness of the CTZ to stimuli, leading to a decrease in nausea and vomiting

photosensitivity: hypersensitive reaction to the sun or ultraviolet light, seen as an adverse reaction to various drugs; can lead to severe skin rash and lesions, as well as damage to the eye

Drug List

Antiemetic Agents

Phenothiazines
chlorpromazine
perphenazine
(P) prochlorperazine

Nonphenothiazine
(P) metoclopramide

5-HT$_3$ Receptor Blockers
dolasetron
granisetron
(P) ondansetron
palonosetron

Substance P/Neurokinin 1 Receptor Antagonist
(P) aprepitant
rolapitant

Miscellaneous Agents
dronabinol
hydroxyzine
nabilone
trimethobenzamide

One of the most common and most uncomfortable complaints encountered in clinical practice is that of nausea and vomiting. Vomiting is a complex reflex reaction to various stimuli (see Chapter 56). In some cases of overdose or poisoning, it may be desirable to induce vomiting to rapidly rid the body of a toxin. This can be accomplished by physical stimuli, often to the back of the throat. In some cases, gastric lavage is used to clear the contents of the stomach. **Emetics**, or drugs that cause vomiting, are no longer recommended for at-home poison control (Box 59.1).

In many clinical conditions the reflex reaction of vomiting is not beneficial in ridding the body of any toxins but is uncomfortable and even clinically hazardous to the patient's condition. In such cases an **antiemetic** is used to decrease or prevent nausea and vomiting. Antiemetic agents can be centrally acting or locally acting, and they have varying degrees of effectiveness. See Figure 59.1 for sites of action of antiemetics. Box 59.2 highlights important considerations related to the use of antiemetics across the lifespan.

Antiemetic Agents

Drugs used in managing nausea and vomiting are called antiemetics (Table 59.1). All of them work by reducing the hyperactivity of the vomiting reflex in one of two ways: Locally, to decrease the local response to stimuli that are being sent to the medulla to induce vomiting, or centrally, to block the chemoreceptor trigger zone (CTZ) or suppress the vomiting center directly. Locally acting antiemetics may be antacids, local anesthetics, adsorbents, protective drugs that coat the gastrointestinal (GI) mucosa, or drugs that prevent distention and stretch stimulation of the GI tract. These agents are often reserved for use in mild nausea. Many of these drugs are discussed in Chapter 57. See Box 59.3 for information about combination drugs used to treat nausea and vomiting.

BOX 59.1 FOCUS ON The Evidence

Ipecac Syrup No Longer Recommended

In the summer of 2003 the U.S. Food and Drug Administration released the results of efficacy and toxicity studies done with the emetic drug syrup of ipecac and ruled that the drug was not effective for its intended use.

In November 2003 the American Academy of Pediatrics (AAP) revised its long-standing recommendation that parents be advised to keep and use ipecac for ingestion of toxic substances. Study findings showed that ipecac did not fully empty the stomach, that inducing vomiting in many cases was more toxic than what was ingested, and that the poison that was ingested needed to be carefully evaluated before the proper treatment was recommended.

History

Until November 2003, syrup of ipecac was the standard emetic agent in use in the United States. It was purchased in prepackaged 1-ounce containers without a prescription to have on hand in case of emergency. Parents were encouraged to keep one of these prepackaged doses at home, just in case it was needed. Ipecac syrup was thought to irritate the GI mucosa locally, which stimulated the CTZ in the brain to induce vomiting within 20 minutes. Parents were cautioned not to use ipecac syrup in the following situations: When caustic alkali or corrosive mineral acids were ingested because the potential for serious damage to the upper GI tract and airways overrode any benefit; when a volatile petroleum distillate such as kerosene was swallowed because the risk of aspiration into the lungs, with a resultant fulminant and untreatable pneumonia, was serious; when a patient was comatose or semicomatose or showed signs of convulsing, again because the risk of aspiration was too great; or when a rapid-acting and specific antidote to the poison was available and that treatment would be the most appropriate.

New Guidelines

The new guidelines set forth by the AAP for anticipatory counseling for prenatal and well-infant visits include:

- Keep potential poisons out of sight and out of reach.
- Always return any childproof caps to the locked position after they are used.
- Never transfer a substance to a different container; it is important to have the information on the original container in case of emergency.
- Safely dispose of all unused or no-longer-needed medication.
- Never refer to medications as candy or a treat.
- Post the telephone number of the poison control center near the phone. If a local poison control center is not available, post 1-800-222-1222.

The AAP recommends that parents be advised to dispose of any ipecac that they may have at home. The organization stresses the importance of prevention and calling an authority if accidental ingestion occurs. Additional information on the AAP policy and position, ipecac study and results, and teaching guidelines and brochures are available online at: http://aappolicy.org.

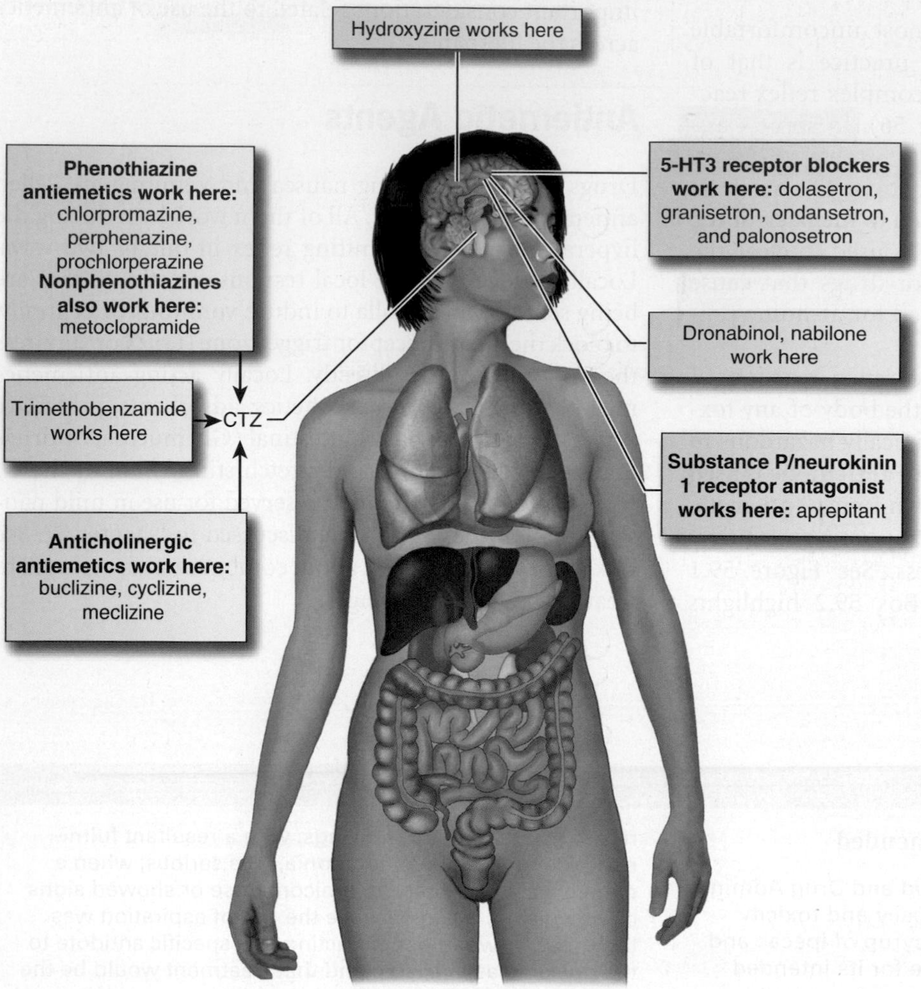

FIGURE 59.1 Sites of action of emetics/antiemetics. CTZ, chemoreceptor trigger zone.

BOX 59.2 FOCUS ON **Drug Therapy across the Lifespan**

Antiemetic Agents

CHILDREN

Parents should be taught to call their health care provider or a local poison control center if their children ingest potentially toxic substances. The professionals will advise them of the best treatment in each individual case.

Antiemetics should be used with caution in children who are at higher risk for adverse effects, including CNS effects, as well as fluid and electrolyte disturbances.

Prochlorphenazine is often the drug of choice with children, and it has established oral, rectal, and parenteral doses. The serotonin 5-HT$_3$ agents have been used very successfully in children younger than 2 years of age. Palonosetron is approved for use in children 1 month and older. Care should be used when determining dose and timing of dose. Dronabinol does not have established guidelines for children, but if it is used the child should be constantly supervised and dose should be calculated very carefully based on age and weight.

ADULTS

Antiemetics are often used after surgery or chemotherapy, and precautions should be used to ensure that CNS effects do not interfere with mobility or other activities.

The safety of these drugs during pregnancy and lactation has not been established. Use should be reserved for those situations in which the benefit to the mother outweighs the potential risk to the fetus. The drugs may enter breast milk and also may cause fluid imbalance that could interfere with milk production. It is advised that caution be used if one of these drugs is prescribed during lactation.

OLDER ADULTS

Older adults are more likely to develop adverse effects associated with the use of these drugs, including sedation, confusion, dizziness, fluid imbalance, and CV effects. Safety measures may be needed if these effects occur and interfere with the patient's mobility and balance.

Older adults are also more likely to have renal and/or hepatic impairment related to underlying medical conditions, which could interfere with the metabolism and excretion of these drugs. The dose for older adults should be started at a lower level than that recommended for young adults. The patient should be monitored very closely, and dose adjustment should be made based on patient response.

If dronabinol is used with older patients, special safety precautions should be in place because the older patient is more likely to experience CNS effects and related problems when using this drug.

Table 59.1 *Drugs in Focus:* Antiemetic Agents

Drug Name	Usual Dosage	Usual Indications
Phenothiazines		
chlorpromazine (generic)	*Adult:* 10–25 mg PO q4–6 h *or* 50–100 mg PR *or* 25 mg IM *Pediatric:* 0.5 mg/kg PO q4–6 h, 1.1 mg/kg PR q6–8 h *or* 0.5 mg/kg IM q6–8 h	Treatment of nausea and vomiting, including that specifically associated with anesthesia; severe vomiting; intractable hiccoughs
perphenazine (generic)	8–16 mg/d PO in divided doses; 5–10 mg IM for rapid control; 5 mg IV in divided doses, slowly	Treatment of severe nausea and vomiting, intractable hiccoughs in patients >12 y
prochlorperazine (generic)	*Adult:* 5–10 mg PO t.i.d. to q.i.d.; 25 mg PR b.i.d.; 5–10 mg IM q3–4 h, up to 40 mg/d; 5–10 mg IM 1–2 h before, during, or after anesthesia, may repeat in 30 min *Pediatric (9.1–13.2 kg):* 2.5 mg PO or PR daily to b.i.d., do not exceed 7.5 mg/d *Pediatric (13.6–17.7 kg):* 2.5 mg PO or PR b.i.d. to t.i.d., do not exceed 10 mg/d *Pediatric (18.2–38.6 kg):* 2.5 mg PO or PR t.i.d. to 5 mg b.i.d., do not exceed 15 mg/d *or* 0.132 mg/kg IM as a single dose	Treatment of severe nausea and vomiting, including that specifically associated with anesthesia
Nonphenothiazine		
metoclopramide (*Reglan*)	10–20 mg IM at the end of surgery; 2 mg/kg IV over not <15 min given 30 min before chemotherapy, then q2 h for two doses, then q3 h for three doses	Treatment of nausea and vomiting, especially related to chemical stimulation of the CTZ in adults
5-HT_3 Receptor Blockers		
dolasetron (*Anzemet*)	*Adult:* 100 mg PO within 1 h of procedure, 12.5 mg IV for postoperative vomiting, 1.8 mg/kg IV *or* 100 mg IV injection before chemotherapy *Pediatric (2–16 y):* 1.8 mg/kg PO 1 h before chemotherapy, diluted in apple or apple–grape juice; 1.8 mg/kg IV 30 min before chemotherapy; 1.2 mg/kg IV for postoperative vomiting	Treatment of nausea and vomiting associated with emetogenic chemotherapy, prevention of postoperative nausea and vomiting
granisetron (generic)	*Adult and pediatric (>2 y):* 10 mcg/kg IV over 5 min starting within 30 min of chemotherapy *or* 1 mg PO b.i.d. beginning up to 1 h before chemotherapy and giving the second dose 12 h after, use only on days of chemotherapy	Treatment of nausea and vomiting associated with emetogenic chemotherapy
ondansetron (*Zofran*)	*Adult:* 8 mg PO t.i.d. *or* 24 mg PO 30 min before chemotherapy; three 0.15-mg/kg doses IV over 15 min beginning before chemotherapy *or* one 32-mg dose infused over 30 min, given 30 min before chemotherapy; 4 mg IV or IM *or* 16 mg PO 1 h before surgery to prevent postoperative vomiting *Pediatric (4–12 y):* 4 mg PO t.i.d., use same IV dose as adults	Treatment of severe nausea and vomiting associated with emetogenic chemotherapy, radiation therapy, postoperative situations
palonosetron (*Aloxi*)	*Adult:* 0.25 mg IV as a single dose over 30 s given 30 min before the start of chemotherapy, do not repeat dose for 7 d *Pediatric (1 mo to <17 y):* 20 mcg/kg IV over 15 min given 30 min before the start of chemotherapy	Treatment of acute and delayed vomiting associated with highly emetogenic chemotherapy
Substance P/Neurokinin 1 Receptor Antagonist		
aprepitant (*Emend*)	125 mg PO 1 h before chemotherapy (day 1); then 80 mg PO in the morning, on days 2 and 3, with dexamethasone 12 mg PO on day 1 and 8 mg PO on days 2–4, and 32 mg ondansetron IV on day 1 only	Prevention of acute and delayed nausea and vomiting associated with highly emetogenic cancer chemotherapy
rolapitant (*Varubi*)	180 mg PO, 1–2 h before start of chemotherapy with dexamethasone and any 5-HT3 receptor inhibitor	Prevention of delayed nausea and vomiting associated with emetogenic cancer chemotherapy

(table continues on page 1030)

Table 59.1 *Drugs in Focus:* Antiemetic Agents (continued)

Drug Name	Usual Dosage	Usual Indications
Miscellaneous Agents		
dronabinol (*Marinol*)	5 mg/m^2 PO 1–3 h before chemotherapy, repeat q2–4 h as needed for a total of four to six doses per day	Management of nausea and vomiting associated with cancer chemotherapy in adults
hydroxyzine (*Vistaril*)	*Adult:* 25–100 mg IM *Pediatric:* 1.1 mg/kg IM	Treatment of prepartum, postpartum, and postoperative nausea and vomiting
nabilone (*Cesamet*)	1–2 mg PO b.i.d.; initial dose given 1–3 h before chemotherapy begins, continue through chemotherapy and for 48 h after last dose	Treatment of nausea and vomiting associated with cancer chemotherapy in adults
trimethobenzamide (*Tigan*)	*Adult:* 250 mg PO t.i.d. to q.i.d., 200 mg PR t.i.d. to q.i.d., 200 mg IM t.i.d. to q.i.d. *Pediatric (≥30 lb):* 100–200 mg PO or PR t.i.d. to q.i.d. *Pediatric (<30 lb):* 100 mg PR t.i.d. to q.i.d.	Treatment of nausea and vomiting (not sedating)

CTZ, chemoreceptor trigger zone; 5-HT_3, serotonin.

BOX 59.3

Combination Drugs for Nausea/Vomiting

Diclegis is a combination of doxylamine succinate (an antihistamine) and pyridoxine (vitamin B6 analog). It is approved for the treatment of nausea and vomiting of pregnancy in women who do not respond to nondrug management. This is the only drug approved for this use. Two tablets are taken at bedtime; if the nausea persists, one additional tablet can be taken in the morning and another in the afternoon (a total of four a day).

Akynzeo is a combination of netupitant, a substance P/NK1 antagonist, and palonosetron. It is approved for prevention of acute and delayed nausea and vomiting associated with initial and repeat courses of cancer chemotherapy. The palonosetron prevents the nausea and vomiting during the acute phase while netupitant prevents the nausea and vomiting during the acute and delayed phase. This is an oral agent taken an hour before the start of chemotherapy.

Centrally acting antiemetics can be classified into several groups: Phenothiazines, nonphenothiazines, serotonin (5-HT_3) receptor blockers, substance P/neurokinin 1 (NK1) receptor antagonist, and a miscellaneous group.

Phenothiazines

The **phenothiazine** most commonly used as an antiemetic is prochlorperazine (generic), which has rapid onset and limited adverse effects. Other drugs in this group include chlorpromazine (generic) and perphenazine (generic). Chapter 22 discusses the phenothiazines in greater detail. (See the Critical Thinking Scenario for additional information about nursing care of a patient taking prochlorperazine.)

CRITICAL THINKING SCENARIO

Handling Postoperative Nausea and Vomiting

THE SITUATION

A.J. is a 16-year-old boy who has undergone reconstructive knee surgery after a football injury. After the surgery, A.J. complains of nausea and vomits three times in 2 hours. A.J. becomes increasingly agitated. Rectal prochlorperazine (*generic*) is ordered to relieve the nausea, to be followed by an oral order when tolerated. The prochlorperazine is somewhat helpful in relieving the nausea, but A.J. expresses a desire to try cannabis, which he has read is good for the relief of nausea.

CRITICAL THINKING

What are the important nursing implications in this case? What other measures could be taken to relieve A.J.'s nausea?

Handling Postoperative Nausea and Vomiting (continued)

What explanation could be given to the request for cannabis?

DISCUSSION

It is often impossible to pinpoint an exact cause of a patient's nausea and vomiting in a hospital setting. For example, the underlying cause may be related to the pain, a reaction to the pain medication being given, or a response to what A.J. described as the "awful hospital smell." A combination of factors should be considered when dealing with nausea and vomiting. A.J., as a teenager, may become increasingly agitated by the discomfort and possible embarrassment of vomiting. The administration of rectal prochlorperazine may "take the edge off" the nausea. A.J. will have to be reminded that the drug he is being given may make him dizzy, weak, or drowsy and that he should ask for assistance if he needs to move.

Once the nausea and vomiting diminish somewhat, it will be possible to try other interventions to help stop the vomiting reflex. One such intervention is removing the offending odor that A.J. described, if possible, because doing so may relieve a chemical stimulus to the CTZ. Administration of pain medication, as prescribed, may relieve the CTZ stimulus that comes with intense pain. Other interventions include providing a serene, quiet environment and encouraging A.J. to take slow, deep breaths, which stimulate the parasympathetic system (vagus nerve) and partially override the sympathetic activity stimulated by the CTZ to activate vomiting. For many patients, mouth care, ice chips, or small sips of water may also help to relieve the discomfort and ease the sensation of nausea.

After A.J. has relaxed a bit and his nausea has abated the use of cannabis for treating nausea can be discussed. This may be a good opportunity to explain the many effects of cannabis to A.J. The drug does relieve nausea and vomiting, especially in patients undergoing chemotherapy. It also decreases activity in the respiratory tract, affects the development of sperm in males, and alters thinking patterns and brain chemistry. The U.S. Food and Drug Administration has approved the use of the active ingredient in cannabis, delta-9-tetrahydrocannabinol, in an oral form—dronabinol (*Marinol*) and nabilone (*Cesamet*) —for the relief of nausea and vomiting in cancer patients who have not responded to other therapies and for the treatment of anorexia associated with AIDS. It is not approved for use in the postoperative setting.

NURSING CARE GUIDE FOR A.J.: ANTIEMETICS

Assessment: History and Examination

Assess A.J.'s health history for allergies to any antiemetic, coma, central nervous system (CNS) depression, severe hypotension, liver dysfunction, bone marrow depression, epilepsy, and concurrent use of alcohol, anticholinergic drugs, barbiturate anesthetics, and guanethidine. Determine the type and amount of anesthesia used.

Focus the physical examination on the following areas:

CNS: Orientation, affect

Skin: Color, lesions

CV: Pulse, blood pressure, orthostatic blood pressure

GI: Abdominal and liver evaluation

Laboratory tests: Hematological, complete blood count, liver function tests

Nursing Diagnoses

Acute pain related to GI, skin, and CNS effects

Risk for injury related to CNS and CV effects

Deficient knowledge regarding drug therapy

Planning

The patient will receive the best therapeutic effect from the drug therapy.

The patient will have limited adverse effects to the drug therapy.

The patient will have an understanding of the drug therapy, adverse effects to anticipate, and measures to relieve discomfort and improve safety.

Implementation

Administer antiemetics only as a temporary measure.

Provide comfort and safety measures, including assistance with mobility, access to bathroom, safety precautions, mouth care, and ice chips.

Monitor A.J. for dehydration and provide remedial measures as needed.

Provide support and reassurance for coping with drug effects and discomfort.

Provide patient teaching regarding drug name, dosage, adverse effects, precautions, and warning to report.

Evaluation

Evaluate drug effects (e.g., relief of nausea and vomiting).

Monitor for adverse effects, including GI alterations, orthostatic hypotension, dizziness, confusion, sensitivity to sunlight, and dehydration.

Monitor for drug–drug interactions as appropriate.

Evaluate the effectiveness of the patient-teaching program and comfort and safety measures.

PATIENT TEACHING FOR A.J.

- The drug that has been prescribed for you is called prochlorperazine. It belongs to a class of drugs called antiemetics. An antiemetic helps to prevent nausea and vomiting and the discomfort they cause.

(continues on page 1032)

Handling Postoperative Nausea and Vomiting (continued)

- Common effects of this drug include:
  - *Dizziness, weakness*: Change positions slowly. If you feel drowsy, avoid driving or dangerous activities for at least 24 hours after the last dose of this drug (such as the use of heavy machinery or tasks requiring coordination).
  - *Sensitivity to the sun*: Avoid exposure to the sun and ultraviolet light because serious reactions may occur. If exposure cannot be prevented, use sunscreen and protective clothing to cover the skin.
  - *Dehydration*: Avoid excessive heat exposure, and try to drink fluids as much as possible, because you will have an increased risk for heat stroke.
- Report any of the following conditions to your health care provider: *Fever, rash, yellowing of the eyes or skin, dark urine, pale stools, easy bruising, rash, and vision changes.*
- Avoid over-the-counter (OTC) medications. If you feel that you need one, check with your health care provider first.
- Tell any doctor, nurse, or other health care provider that you are taking this drug.
- Keep this drug and all medications out of the reach of children.

Therapeutic Actions and Indications

Phenothiazines are centrally acting antiemetics that change the responsiveness or stimulation of the CTZ in the medulla (Figure 59.1). The phenothiazines are recommended for the treatment of nausea and vomiting, including that specifically associated with anesthesia, severe vomiting, and **intractable hiccoughs**, which occur with repetitive stimulation of the diaphragm and lead to persistent diaphragm spasm. See Table 59.1 for Usual Indications for each of these agents.

Pharmacokinetics

These drugs are available as tablets or as syrup for oral administration, as rectal suppositories, and as solution for IM or IV use. The route of choice is determined by the condition of the patient. They have a rapid onset of action of 5 to 20 minutes and a duration of action of 3 to 12 hours, depending on the route of administration. They are metabolized in the liver and excreted in the urine. They are known to cross the placenta and enter breast milk.

Contraindications and Cautions

In general, antiemetics should not be used in patients with coma or severe CNS depression or in those who have experienced brain damage or injury *because of the risk of further CNS depression.* Other contraindications include severe hypotension or hypertension and severe liver dysfunction, *which might interfere with the metabolism of the drug.* Caution should be used in individuals with renal dysfunction, moderate liver impairment, active peptic ulcer, or during pregnancy and lactation *because of the potential for adverse effects on the fetus or baby.* See Chapter 22 for details about the phenothiazines.

Adverse Effects

Adverse effects associated with antiemetics are linked to their interference with normal CNS stimulation or response. Drowsiness, dizziness, weakness, tremor, and headache are common adverse effects. Other, not uncommon adverse effects include hypotension, hypertension, and cardiac arrhythmias. Autonomic effects such as dry mouth, nasal congestion, anorexia, pallor, sweating, and urinary retention often occur with phenothiazines (Figure 59.2). Patients should be cautioned that their urine may be tinged pink

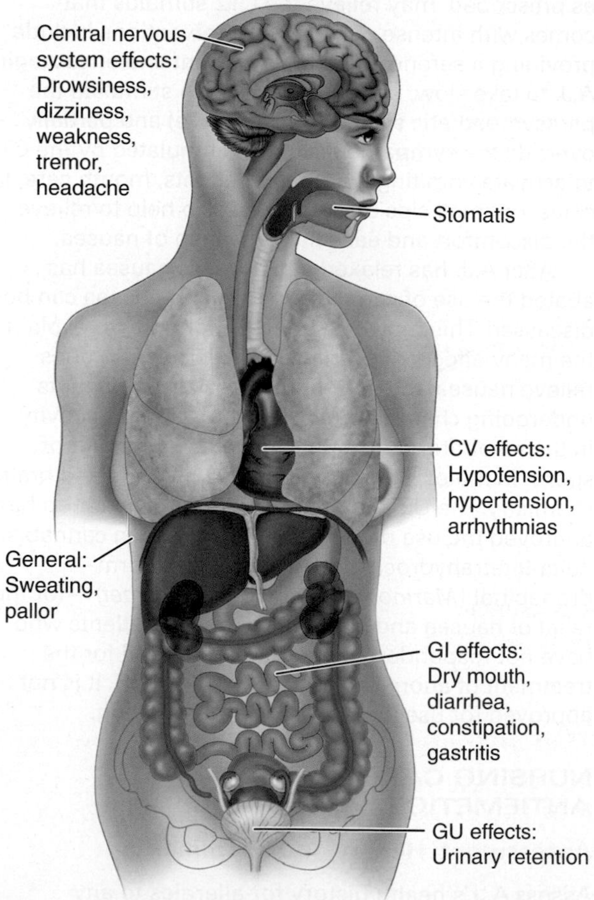

FIGURE 59.2 Variety of adverse effects and toxicities associated with antiemetic agents.

to red–brown. This is a drug effect but can cause concern if the patient is not expecting it. Endocrine effects such as menstrual disorders, galactorrhea, and gynecomastia have been reported with phenothiazine use. **Photosensitivity** (increased sensitivity to the sun and ultraviolet light) is a common adverse reaction with these antiemetics. Patients should be advised to use sunscreens and protective garments if exposure cannot be avoided.

Clinically Important Drug–Drug Interactions

Additive CNS depression can be seen with any of the antiemetics if they are combined with other CNS depressants, including alcohol. Patients should be advised to avoid this combination and any OTC preparation unless they check with their health care provider. Other drug–drug interactions are specific to each drug (refer to a nursing drug guide).

Prototype Summary: Prochlorperazine

Indications: Control of severe nausea and vomiting.

Actions: Mechanism of action not understood; depresses various areas of the CNS, including the CTZ in the medulla.

Pharmacokinetics:

Route	Onset	Peak	Duration
Oral	30–40 min	Unknown	3–4 h
Rectal	60–90 min	Unknown	3–4 h
IM	10–20 min	10–30 min	3–4 h
IV	Immediate	10–30 min	3–4 h

$T_{1/2}$: Unknown; metabolized in the liver and excreted in the urine.

Adverse Effects: Drowsiness, dystonia, photophobia, blurred vision, urine discolored pink to red–brown.

Nonphenothiazine

The only nonphenothiazine currently available for use as an antiemetic is metoclopramide (*Reglan*), which acts to reduce the responsiveness of the nerve cells in the CTZ to circulating chemicals that induce vomiting. Chapter 58 discusses metoclopramide, which is also commonly used to treat gastroparesis, in greater detail.

Prototype Summary: Metoclopramide

Indications: Prevention of nausea and vomiting associated with emetogenic cancer chemotherapy, prevention of postoperative nausea and vomiting.

Actions: Slows GI activity, sedating.

Pharmacokinetics:

Route	Onset	Peak	Duration
Oral	30–60 min	60–90 min	1–2 h
IM	10–15 min	60–90 min	1–2 h
IV	1–3 min	60–90 min	1–2 h

$T_{1/2}$: 5 to 6 hours; metabolized in the liver and excreted in the urine.

Adverse Effects: Drowsiness, fatigue, restlessness, extrapyramidal symptoms, diarrhea.

5-HT$_3$ Receptor Blockers

The 5-HT$_3$ receptor blockers block those receptors associated with nausea and vomiting in the CTZ and locally. These drugs include dolasetron (*Anzemet*), granisetron (generic), ondansetron (*Zofran*), and palonosetron (*Aloxi*).

Therapeutic Actions and Indications

The 5-HT$_3$ receptor blockers have proven especially helpful in treating the nausea and vomiting associated with antineoplastic chemotherapy and radiation therapy and postoperative nausea and vomiting. They are specific for the treatment of nausea and vomiting associated with emetogenic chemotherapy. These are relatively new drugs, and the drug of choice depends on personal preference and experience. Palonosetron is approved for use in children 1 month of age and older.

Pharmacokinetics

The 5-HT$_3$ receptor blockers are rapidly absorbed, reaching peak levels within 1 hour. They are metabolized in the liver and excreted in the urine. Ondansetron, dolasetron, and granisetron are available in oral and IV forms; palonosetron is only available in an IV form.

Contraindications and Cautions

These drugs are contraindicated with known allergy to any component of the drug *to prevent hypersensitivity reactions*. Caution should be used during pregnancy and lactation *because of the potential for adverse effects on the fetus or nursing baby*.

Adverse Effects

The adverse effects most frequently seen with these drugs are headache, dizziness, and myalgia related to their CNS effects. Pain at the injection site, rash, constipation, hypotension, and urinary retention have also been reported.

Prototype Summary: Ondansetron

Indications: Control of severe nausea and vomiting associated with emetogenic cancer chemotherapy, radiation therapy; treatment of postoperative nausea and vomiting. morning sickness for pregnant

Actions: Blocks specific receptor sites associated with nausea and vomiting, peripherally and in the CTZ.

Pharmacokinetics:

Route	Onset	Peak	Duration
Oral	30–60 min	60–90 min	1.7–2.2 h
IV	Immediate	60–90 min	Duration of infusion

$T_{1/2}$: 3.5 to 6 hours; metabolized in the liver and excreted in the urine.

Adverse Effects: Headache, dizziness, drowsiness, myalgia, urinary retention, constipation, pain at injection site.

Substance P/Neurokinin 1 Receptor Antagonist

The first drug in the newest class of drugs for treating nausea and vomiting is the substance P/NK1 receptor antagonist aprepitant (*Emend*). Rolapitant (*Varubi*) was approved as the second drug in this class in 2015.

Therapeutic Actions and Indications

These drugs act directly in the CNS to block receptors associated with nausea and vomiting with little to no effect on serotonin, dopamine, or corticosteroid receptors. Aprepitant is approved for use in treating the nausea and vomiting associated with highly emetogenic antineoplastic chemotherapy, including cisplatin therapy. It is given orally, in combination with dexamethasone. Rolapitant is used in combination with other antiemetics for prevention of delayed nausea and vomiting associated with emetogenic antineoplastic chemotherapy.

Pharmacokinetics

Both drugs are metabolized in the liver and excreted in the urine and feces. These drugs are known to cross the placenta and to enter breast milk.

Contraindications and Cautions

Neither drug should be used during pregnancy and lactation *because of the potential for adverse effects on the fetus or nursing baby* or with known allergy to any component of the drug *to prevent hypersensitivity reactions.* Rolapitant cannot be combined with thioridazine or pimozide.

Adverse Effects

The adverse effects associated with both drugs include GI effects of diarrhea, constipation, and gastritis; nausea; anorexia; headache; and fatigue.

Clinically Important Drug–Drug Interactions

There is a risk of serious increase in serum levels of pimozide if these drugs are used together; this combination should be avoided. There is a decrease in effectiveness of warfarin if it is combined with aprepitant, and the patient must be monitored very closely and adjustments made in the warfarin dose if this combination must be used. There is a decrease in the effectiveness of hormonal contraceptives if they are taken concurrently with aprepitant; use of a barrier contraceptive should be suggested.

Prototype Summary: Aprepitant

Indications: In combination with other agents for the prevention of acute and delayed nausea and vomiting associated with severely emetogenic cancer chemotherapy.

Actions: Selectively blocks human substance P/NK1 receptors in the CNS, blocking the nausea and vomiting caused by highly emetogenic chemotherapeutic agents.

Pharmacokinetics:

Route	Onset	Peak
Oral	Rapid	4 h

$T_{1/2}$: 9 to 13 hours; metabolized in the liver and excreted in the urine and feces.

Adverse Effects: Anorexia, fatigue, constipation, diarrhea, liver enzyme elevations, dehydration.

Miscellaneous Agents

Miscellaneous agents used as antiemetics include dronabinol (*Marinol*) and nabilone (*Cesamet*), which contain the active ingredient of cannabis (marijuana); hydroxyzine (*Vistaril*), which may suppress cortical areas of the CNS; and trimethobenzamide (*Tigan*), which is similar to the antihistamines but is not as sedating.

Trimethobenzamide, available in oral, parenteral, and suppository form, is often the drug of choice in this group because it is not associated with as much sedation and CNS suppression as other agents. It is rapidly absorbed, metabolized in the liver, and excreted in the urine. It crosses the placenta and enters breast milk, and use should be reserved for situations in which the benefit to the mother outweighs any potential risk to the fetus or neonate.

Hydroxyzine is used for nausea and vomiting before or after obstetrical delivery or surgery. It is rapidly absorbed, metabolized in the liver, and excreted in the urine. It has not been associated with fetal problems during pregnancy and is not thought to enter breast milk; however, as with all drugs, caution should be used during pregnancy and lactation.

Dronabinol and nabilone are only approved for use in managing the nausea and vomiting associated with cancer chemotherapy in cases that have not responded to other treatment. The exact mechanisms of action of dronabinol and nabilone are not understood. They are readily absorbed and metabolized in the liver, with excretion through the bile and in the urine. They are controlled substances; dronabinol is a category C-III controlled substance, and nabilone is a category C-II substance. They must be used under close supervision because of the possibility of altered mental status.

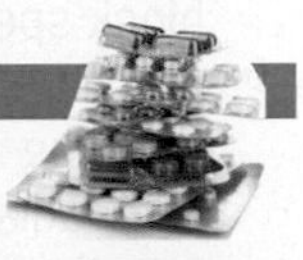

Nursing Considerations for Patients Receiving an Antiemetic Agent

Assessment: History and Examination

- Assess for possible contraindications or cautions: History of allergy to antiemetic *to avoid potential hypersensitivity reactions*; impaired renal or hepatic function, *which could interfere with the metabolism or excretion of the drug*; coma or semiconscious state, CNS depression, or CNS injury, *which could be exacerbated by the CNS-depressing effects of the drug*; hypotension or hypertension, *which could be affected by the CNS effects of the drug*; active peptic ulcer, *which could be exacerbated by the GI effects of the drug*; and current status of pregnancy and lactation *because of the potential for adverse effects on the fetus or nursing baby.*
- Perform a physical examination to establish baseline data before beginning therapy and during therapy *to determine the effectiveness of the drug and evaluate for the occurrence of any adverse effects associated with drug therapy.*
- Assess the patient's neurological status, including level of orientation, affect, and reflexes, *to monitor for CNS effects and to rule out underlying CNS problems that could be a contraindication.*
- Assess cardiopulmonary status, including baseline pulse and blood pressure, *to evaluate effects on the CV system.*
- Inspect the skin for color and evidence of lesion or rash *to evaluate for photosensitivity and adverse effects of the drug.*
- Examine the abdomen, including the liver, and auscultate bowel sounds *to evaluate GI function and motility, rule out underlying medical problems, and identify possible adverse drug effects.*
- Assess complaints of nausea and evaluate emesis; note color, amount, and frequency of vomiting episodes *to determine the need for therapy.*
- Monitor laboratory test results, including liver and renal function tests, *to monitor for potential problems with metabolism or excretion.*

Nursing Diagnoses

Nursing diagnoses related to drug therapy might include the following:

- Acute pain related to CNS, skin, and GI effects
- Risk for injury related to CNS effects
- Decreased cardiac output related to cardiac effects
- Deficient knowledge regarding drug therapy

Planning

- The patient will receive the best therapeutic effect from the drug therapy.
- The patient will have limited adverse effects to the drug therapy.
- The patient will have an understanding of the drug therapy, adverse effects to anticipate, and measures to relieve discomfort and improve safety.

Implementation with Rationale

- Assure that the route of administration is appropriate for each patient *to ensure therapeutic effects and decrease adverse effects*: If used to prevent motion sickness, should be given 30 minutes before activity that involves motion; some oral tablets can be placed in the mouth and allowed to dissolve slowly; rectal suppositories should be inserted high into the rectum; IV infusions should be run slowly, monitoring the patient for CNS depression.
- Assess the patient carefully for any potential drug–drug interactions if giving antiemetics in combination with other drugs *to avert potentially serious drug–drug interactions.*
- Provide comfort and safety measures, including mouth care, ready access to bathroom facilities, assistance with ambulation and periodic orientation, ice chips to suck, protection from sun exposure, and remedial measures to treat dehydration if it occurs, *to protect the patient from injury and to increase patient comfort.*
- Provide support and encouragement, as well as other measures (quiet environment, carbonated drinks, deep breathing), *to help the patient cope with the discomfort of nausea and vomiting and drug effects.*
- Provide thorough patient teaching, including the drug name and prescribed dosage; the schedule and method for administration; the need to avoid alcohol and other CNS depressants (if the patient is not hospitalized); signs and symptoms of adverse effects and measures to minimize or prevent them; the use of sunscreen and protective clothing when outside; comfort measures

(continues on page 1036)

to reduce feelings of nausea, such as adequate ventilation, deep breathing, and a quiet environment; the importance of fluid intake and signs and symptoms of dehydration that should be reported to the health care provider; safety measures, such as assistance with ambulation and gradual position changes; the need to notify the health care provider before using any OTC medications; and the importance of periodic monitoring and evaluation *to enhance patient knowledge about drug therapy and to promote compliance.*

Evaluation

- Monitor the patient response to the drug (relief of nausea and vomiting).
- Monitor for adverse effects (dizziness, confusion, GI alterations, cardiac arrhythmias, hypotension, gynecomastia, pink- to brown-tinged urine, photosensitivity).
- Monitor the effectiveness of comfort measures and compliance with the regimen.
- Evaluate the effectiveness of the teaching plan (patient can name the drug and dosage as well as describe adverse effects to watch for and specific measures to avoid them).

KEY POINTS

- Antiemetics are used to manage nausea and vomiting in situations in which these actions are not beneficial and could cause harm to the patient.
- Antiemetics act by depressing the hyperactive vomiting reflex, either locally or through alteration of CNS actions.
- The choice of an antiemetic depends on the cause of the nausea and vomiting and the expected actions of the drug.
- Antiemetics include the phenothiazines and centrally acting nonphenothiazine metoclopramide, anticholinergic/antihistamines, the 5-HT_3 receptor blockers, and the newest class of antiemetic, the substance P/NK1 antagonist.
- Other drugs used as antiemetics include cannabinoids, hydroxyzine, and trimethobenzamide.

SUMMARY

- Phenothiazines and the nonphenothiazine metoclopramide are used as antiemetics to depress the CNS, including the CTZ. Patients must be monitored for CNS depression. Photosensitivity and pink to red–brown color of the urine are common adverse effects of these drugs.
- The 5-HT_3 blockers are newer antiemetics that directly block specific receptors in the CTZ to prevent nausea and vomiting. They are used in cases of nausea and vomiting associated with antineoplastic chemotherapy and radiation therapy and postoperative nausea and vomiting.
- Most antiemetics cause some CNS depression, with resultant dizziness, drowsiness, and weakness. Care must be taken to protect the patient and advise him or her to avoid dangerous situations.
- Photosensitivity is another common adverse effect with antiemetics. Patients should be protected from exposure to the sun and ultraviolet light. Sunscreens and protective clothing are essential if exposure cannot be prevented.

CHECK YOUR UNDERSTANDING

Answers to the questions in this chapter can be found in Answers to Check Your Understanding Questions on thePoint®.

MULTIPLE CHOICE

Select the best answer to the following.

1. The nurse anticipates that prochlorperazine (*Compazine*) would be the antiemetic of choice for which of the following?
   a. Nausea and vomiting after anesthesia
   b. Nausea and vomiting due to cancer chemotherapy
   c. Motion sickness
   d. Intractable hiccoughs
2. Most antiemetics work with the CNS to decrease the activity of
   a. the medulla.
   b. the chemoreceptor trigger zone.
   c. the respiratory center.
   d. the sympathetic nervous system.

3. Which of the following instructions would be most appropriate to give to a patient to reduce the risk of photosensitivity related to the use of antiemetic agents?
   a. Avoid having their picture taken.
   b. Cover the head at extremes of temperature.
   c. Take extra precautions to avoid heat stroke.
   d. Wear protective clothing when in the sun.

4. The 5-HT3 receptor blockers, including ondansetron (*Zofran*) and granisetron (*Kytril*), are particularly effective in decreasing the nausea and vomiting associated with
   a. vestibular problems.
   b. cancer chemotherapy.
   c. pregnancy.
   d. severe pain.

5. A parent calls with concerns that a 2-year-old child ate a bottle full of baby aspirin. The nurse would advise the parent to
   a. administer ipecac immediately.
   b. induce vomiting by inserting a finger against the back of the child's throat.
   c. force fluids as the parent brings the child in for evaluation.
   d. feed the child charcoal.

MULTIPLE RESPONSE

Select all that apply.

1. Nursing interventions for the client receiving an antiemetic drug would include which of the following?
   a. Frequent mouth care
   b. Bowel program to deal with constipation
   c. Protection from falls or injury
   d. Fluids to guard against dehydration
   e. Protection from sun exposure
   f. Quiet environment and temperature control

2. Palonosetron (*Aloxi*) would be the drug of choice for a client with which of the following problems?
   a. Nausea and vomiting associated with cancer chemotherapy
   b. A prolonged QT interval
   c. Delayed nausea and vomiting associated with antineoplastic chemotherapy
   d. Difficulty swallowing
   e. Hypokalemia
   f. Hypomagnesemia

BIBLIOGRAPHY AND REFERENCES

American Association of Pediatrics Committee on Injury, Violence, and Poison Prevention. (2003). Poison treatment in the home. *Pediatrics, 112*, 1182–1185.

Brunton, L., Chabner, B., & Knollman, B. (2011). *Goodman and Gilman's the pharmacological basis of therapeutics* (12th ed.). New York: McGraw-Hill.

Facts and Comparisons. (2015). *Drug facts and comparisons*. St. Louis, MO: Author.

Forbes, D., & Fairbrother, S. (2008). Cyclic nausea and vomiting in childhood. *Australian Family Physician, 27*(1/2), 33–36.

Gutierrez-Williams, G., & Goldman, M. (2008). Cost effective management of postoperative vomiting. *Connecticut Medicine, 72*(1), 21–24.

Karch, A. M. (2014). *Lippincott's nursing drug guide*. Philadelphia, PA: Lippincott Williams & Wilkins.

Kerr, C. L. (2008). What goes in must come out. *Journal of Pediatric Health Care, 22*(1), 44–48.

Pectasides, D., Dafni, U., Arvantinos, G., et al. (2007). A randomized trial to compare the efficacy and safety of antiemetic treatment with ondansetron and ondansetron zydis in patients with breast cancer treated with high-dose epirubicin. *Anticancer Research, 27*(6C), 4411–4417.

Porth, C. M. (2013). *Pathophysiology: Concepts of altered health states* (9th ed.). Philadelphia, PA: Lippincott Williams & Wilkins.

The Medical Letter. (2015). *The medical letter on drugs and therapeutics*. New Rochelle, NY: Author.

Ware, M., Daeninck, P., & Maida, V. (2008). A review of nabilone in the treatment of chemotherapy-induced nausea and vomiting. *Therapeutics and Clinical Risk Management, 4*(1), 99–107.

Parenteral Agents A

Parenteral preparations are fluids that are given either IV or through a central line.

Therapeutic Actions and Indications

Parenteral agents are used for the following purposes: To provide replacement fluids, sugars, electrolytes, and nutrients to patients who are unable to take them in orally; to provide ready access for administration of drugs in an emergency situation; to provide rehydration; and to restore electrolyte balance. The composition of the IV fluids needed for a patient depends on the patient's fluid and electrolyte status.

Parenteral nutrition (PN) is the administration of essential proteins, amino acids, carbohydrates, vitamins, minerals, trace elements, lipids, and fluids. PN is used to improve or stabilize the nutritional status of cachectic or debilitated patients who cannot take in or absorb oral nutrition to the extent required to maintain their nutritional status. The exact composition of the PN solution is determined after a nutritional assessment and must take into account the patient's current health status, age, and metabolic needs.

Contraindications and Cautions

PN is contraindicated in anyone with known allergies to any component of the solution. Multiple combination products are available, so a suitable solution may be found *to avoid adverse reactions.* PN should be used with caution in patients with unstable cardiovascular status *because of the change in fluid volume that might occur and the resultant increased workload on the heart.* These preparations also should be used with caution in patients with unstable fluid and electrolyte status, *who could react adversely to sudden changes in fluids and electrolytes.*

Adverse Effects

Adverse effects associated with the use of PN include IV irritation, extravasation of the fluid into the tissues, infection of the insertion site, fluid volume overload, vascular problems related to fluid shifts, and potential electrolyte imbalance related to dilution of the blood. PN also is associated with mechanical problems related to insertion of the line, such as pneumothorax, infections, or air emboli; emboli related to protein or lipid aggregation; infections related to nutrient-rich solution and invasive administration; metabolic imbalances related to the composition of the solution; gallstone development (especially in children); and nausea (especially related to the administration of lipids).

Clinically Important Drug–Drug Interactions

Some IV drugs can be diluted only with particular IV solutions to avoid precipitation or inactivation of the drug. A drug guide should be checked before diluting any IV drug in solution.

Nursing Considerations

Assessment: History and Examination

- Obtain a nutritional assessment. Screen for any medical conditions and drugs being taken.
- Evaluate the insertion site; skin hydration; orientation and affect; height and weight; pulse, blood pressure, and respirations; and blood chemistries, complete blood count with differential, and glucose levels.

Nursing Diagnoses

The patient receiving a parenteral agent might have the following nursing diagnoses related to drug therapy:

- Acute pain related to administration of the fluid
- Risk for infection related to invasive delivery system
- Risk for imbalanced nutrition related to fluid composition
- Risk for fluid Imbalance related to fluid compositions
- Deficient knowledge regarding drug therapy

Planning

- The patient will receive the best therapeutic effect from the parenteral therapy.
- The patient will have limited adverse effects to the parenteral therapy.
- The patient will have an understanding of the parenteral therapy, adverse effects to anticipate, and measures to relieve discomfort and improve safety.

Implementation

- Assess the patient's general physical condition before beginning infusion *to decrease the potential for adverse effects.*

- Monitor the IV insertion site or central line and regularly consult with the prescriber *to discontinue the site of infusion and treat any infection or extravasation as soon as it occurs.*
- Follow these administration guidelines *to provide the most therapeutic use of PN with the fewest adverse effects*:
  - Refrigerate PN solutions until ready to use.
  - Check contents before hanging to ensure that no precipitates are present.
  - Do not hang bag for longer than 24 hours.
  - Suggest the use of on-line filters to decrease bacterial invasion and infusion of aggregate.
- Discontinue PN only after an alternative source of nutrition has been established *to ensure continued nutrition for the patient*; taper slowly *to avoid severe reactions.*
- Provide comfort measures *to help the patient tolerate drug effects* (e.g., provide proper skin care as needed, analgesics, hot soaks to extravasation sites).
- Include information about the solution being used (e.g., what to expect, adverse effects that may occur, follow-up tests that may be needed) *to enhance patient knowledge about parenteral therapy and promote compliance with the treatment.*

Evaluation

- Monitor patient response to the parenteral therapy (stabilization of nutritional state, fluid and electrolyte balance, laboratory values).
- Monitor for adverse effects (local irritation, infection, fluid and electrolyte imbalance).
- Evaluate the effectiveness of the teaching plan (patient can name adverse effects to watch for and specific measures to avoid them; patient understands the importance of follow-up that will be needed).
- Monitor the effectiveness of comfort measures and compliance with the regimen.

Table A Parenterals

Solution	Caloric Content (cal/L)	Osmolarity (mOsm/L)	Usual Indications
In Solutions			
Dextrose Solutions			
2.5% (25 g/L)	85	126	Provides calories and fluid
5% (50 g/L)	170	253	Provides calories and fluid, keeps vein open for administration of IV drugs; frequent choice for dilution of IV drugs
10% (100 g/L)	340	505	Hypertonic solution used after admixture with other fluids; provides calories and fluid
20% (200 g/L)	680	1,010	Hypertonic solution used after admixture with other fluids; provides calories and fluid
25% (250 g/L)	850	1,330	Hypertonic solution used after admixture with other fluids; provides calories and fluid; treatment of acute hypoglycemic episodes in infants to restore glucose levels and suppress symptoms; sclerosing agent for varicose veins
30% (300 g/L)	1,020	1,515	Hypertonic solution used after admixture with other fluids; provides calories and fluid
40% (400 g/L)	1,360	2,020	Hypertonic solution used after admixture with other fluids; provides calories and fluid
50% (500 g/L)	1,700	2,525	Hypertonic solution used after admixture with other fluids; provide calories and fluid; treatment of hyperinsulinemia; sclerosing agent for varicose veins
60% (600 g/L)	2,040	3,030	Hypertonic solution used after admixture with other fluids; provides calories and fluid
70% (700 g/L)	2,380	3,535	Hypertonic solution used after admixture with other fluids; provides calories and fluid

Solution	Sodium Content (mEq/L)	Chloride Content (mEq/L)	Osmolarity (mOsm/L)	Usual Indications
Saline Solutions				
0.45% (1/2 normal saline)	77	77	155	Hydrating solution; may be used to evaluate kidney function; treatment of hyperosmolar diabetes
0.9% (normal saline)	154	154	310	Replacement of fluid, sodium, and chloride; flushing lines and catheters; dilution of IV medications; priming of dialysis machines; neonate blood transfusions

(table continues on page 1040)

Table A Parenterals (continued)

Solution	Caloric Content (cal/L)	Osmolarity (mOsm/L)	Usual Indications	
Saline Solutions				
3%	513	513	1,030	Hypertonic solution to treat sodium and chloride depletion; emergency treatment of water intoxication or severe salt depletion
5%	855	855	1,710	Hypertonic solution to treat sodium and chloride depletion; emergency treatment of water intoxication or severe salt depletion

Commonly Used Combination Fluids[a]

Solution	Na Content (mEq/L)	K Content (mEq/L)	Cl Content (mEq/L)	Ca Content (mEq/L)	Mg Content (mEq/L)	Lactate (mEq/L)	Acetate (mEq/L)	Osmolarity (mOsm/L)
Plasma-Lyte-56	40	13	40	–	3	–	18	111
Ringer's Injection	147	4	156	4	–	–	–	310
Lactated Ringer's	130	4	109	3	–	28	–	273
Normosol-R	140	5	96	–	3	–	27	295

Typical Central Parenteral Nutrition Solution[a,b]—1 Liter

Component	Purpose	Dose	Special Considerations
10% Amino acids	Provides 50-g protein for growth and healing	500 mL	Monitor blood pressure, cardiac output, blood chemistries, and urine to determine the effect of intravascular protein pull
50% Dextrose	Provides 850 cal for energy	500 mL	Monitor blood sugar; evaluate injection site for any sign of infection, irritation
20% Fat emulsion	Provides 500 fat calories, ready energy	250 mL	Monitor for any sign of emboli (e.g., shortness of breath, chest pain, deep leg pain, neurological changes); carefully monitor patients for any sign of increased vascular workload, especially very young and geriatric patients
Sodium chloride	Provides sodium and chloride needed for various chemical reactions within the body	40 mEq	Monitor cardiac rhythm, serum electrolytes
Calcium gluconate	Provides essential calcium for muscle contraction, blood clotting, numerous chemical reactions	4.8 mEq	Monitor cardiac rhythm, muscle strength, serum electrolytes
Magnesium sulfate	Provides magnesium for various chemical reactions within the body	8 mEq	Monitor blood pressure, deep tendon reflexes, and serum electrolytes.
Potassium phosphate	Provides needed potassium for nerve functioning, muscle contractions, etc.	9 mM	Monitor pulse, including rhythm, muscle function, and serum electrolytes
Multivitamins	Provide a combination of essential vitamins to maintain cell integrity, promote healing	10 mL	Monitor for signs of vitamin deficiency or toxicity
Trace elements	Provide small amounts of elements essential for numerous chemical reactions in the body and maintenance of cell integrity and healing		Periodically monitor blood chemistries to determine adequacy of replacement
Zinc		3 mg	
Copper		1.2 mg	
Manganese		0.3 mg	
Chromium		12 mcg	
Selenium		20 mcg	

Total nonprotein calories: 1,350
Total volume of solution: 1,250 mL
Dextrose concentration: 25%
Amino acid concentration: 5%
Osmolarity: 1,900 mOsm/L

Component	Purpose	Dose	Special Considerations
Typical Peripheral Parenteral Nutrition Solution[a,b,c]—1 Liter			
8.5% Amino acids	Provides 41-g protein for growth and healing	500 mL	Monitor blood pressure, cardiac output, blood chemistries, urine to determine effect of intravascular protein pull
20% Dextrose	Provides 340 cal for energy	500 mL	Monitor blood sugar; evaluate injection site for any sign of infection or irritation
20% Fat emulsion	Provides 500 fat calories, ready energy	250 mL	Monitor for any sign of emboli (e.g., shortness of breath, chest pain, deep leg pain, neurological changes); carefully monitor patients for any sign of increased vascular workload, especially very young and geriatric patients
Sodium chloride	Provides sodium and chloride needed for various chemical reactions within the body	40 mEq	Monitor cardiac rhythm, serum electrolytes
Calcium gluconate	Provides essential calcium for muscle contraction, blood clotting, numerous chemical reactions	4.8 mEq	Monitor cardiac rhythm, muscle strength, serum electrolytes
Magnesium sulfate	Provides magnesium for various chemical reactions within the body	8 mEq	Monitor blood pressure, deep tendon reflexes, and serum electrolytes
Potassium phosphate	Provides needed potassium for nerve functioning, muscle contractions, etc.	9 mM	Monitor pulse, including rhythm, muscle function, and serum electrolytes
Multivitamins	Provide a combination of essential vitamins to maintain cell integrity, promote healing, etc.	10 mL	Monitor for signs of vitamin deficiency or toxicity
Trace elements	Provide small amounts of elements essential for numerous chemical reactions in the body and maintenance of cell integrity and healing		Periodically monitor blood chemistries to determine adequacy of replacement
Zinc		3 mg	
Copper		1.2 mg	
Manganese		0.3 mg	
Chromium		12 mcg	
Selenium		20 mcg	

Total nonprotein calories: 840
Total volume of solution: 1,250 mL
Dextrose concentration: 10%
Amino acid concentration: 4.25%
Osmolarity: 900 mOsm/L

[a]Multiple combination preparations are available commercially. Each preparation varies in the concentration of one or more components and should be checked carefully before hanging.
[b]Actual concentration of solution and components of any particular solution will be determined by assessment of the patient's current status and nutritional needs.
[c]Solutions used for peripheral therapy are usually less concentrated and less irritating to the vessel.

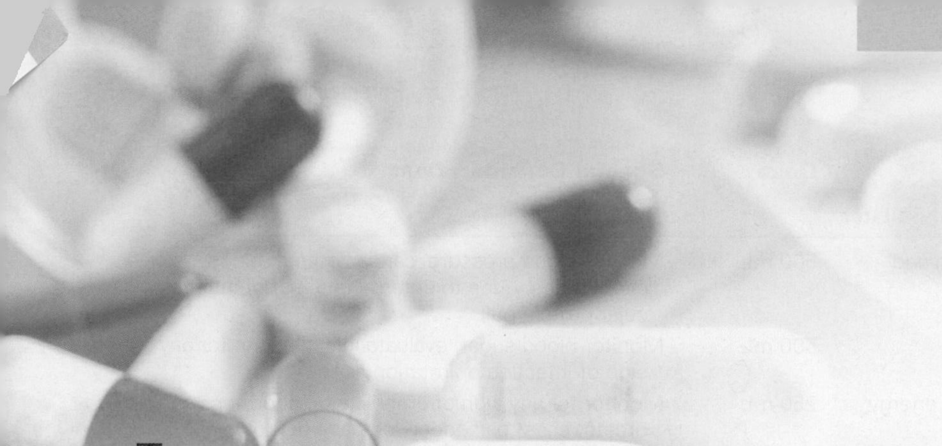

Topical Agents B

Topical agents are intended for surface use only and are not meant for ingestion or injection. They may be toxic if absorbed into the system, but they have several useful purposes when applied to the surface of the skin or mucous membranes. Some forms of drugs are prepared to be absorbed through the skin for systemic effects. These drugs may be prepared as transdermal patches (e.g., nitroglycerin, estrogens, nicotine), which are designed to provide a slow release of the drug from the vehicle. Drugs prepared for this type of administration are discussed with the specific drug in the text and are not addressed in this appendix.

Therapeutic Actions and Indications

Topical agents are used to treat a variety of disorders in a localized area. Table B describes the usual uses for the many different types of topical agents. Because these drugs are designed for topical application, they are minimally absorbed systemically and, if used properly, should have minimal systemic effects.

Contraindications and Cautions

The use of topical agents is contraindicated *in cases of allergy to the drugs* and in the presence of open wounds or abrasions, *which could lead to the systemic absorption of the drugs*. Caution should be used during pregnancy *if there is any possibility that the agent might be absorbed*. Caution should also be used *in the presence of any known allergy to the vehicles of preparation* (creams, lotions).

Adverse Effects

Because these drugs are not intended to be absorbed systemically the adverse effects usually associated with topical agents are local effects, including local irritation, stinging, burning, or dermatitis. Toxic effects are associated with inadvertent systemic absorption.

Nursing Considerations

Assessment: History and Examination

- Screen for the presence of *any known allergy to the drug*, which would be a contraindication to its use.
- Include *screening for baseline status before beginning therapy and for any potential adverse effects*. Assess the following: Condition of area to be treated.

Nursing Diagnoses

The patient receiving a topical agent might have the following nursing diagnoses related to drug therapy:

- Risk for injury related to toxic effects associated with absorption
- Acute pain related to local effects of the drug
- Deficient knowledge regarding drug therapy

Planning

- The patient will receive the best therapeutic effect from the drug therapy.
- The patient will have limited adverse effects to the drug therapy.
- The patient will have an understanding of the drug therapy, adverse effects to anticipate, and measures to relieve discomfort and improve safety.

Implementation

- Ensure proper administration of the drug *to provide best therapeutic effect and least adverse effects as follows*:
  - Apply sparingly. Some preparations come with applicators, some should be applied while wearing protective gloves, and others are dropped onto the site with no direct contact. Consult information regarding the individual drug being used for specific procedures.

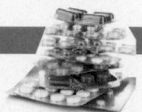

- Do not use with open wounds or broken skin, *which could lead to systemic absorption and toxic effects.*
- Avoid contact with the eyes, *which could be injured by the drug.*
- Do not use with occlusive dressings, *which could increase the risk of systemic absorption.*
- Monitor the area being treated *to evaluate drug effects on the condition being treated.*
- Provide comfort measures *to help the patient tolerate drug effects* (e.g., analgesia as needed for local pain, itching).
- Provide patient teaching *to enhance patient knowledge about drug therapy and promote compliance with the drug regimen*:
  - Teach the patient the proper administration technique for the topical agent ordered.
  - Caution the patient that transient stinging or burning may occur.
  - Instruct the patient to report severe irritation, allergic reaction, or worsening of the condition being treated.

Evaluation

- Monitor patient response to the drug (improvement in condition being treated).
- Monitor for adverse effects (local stinging or inflammation).
- Evaluate the effectiveness of the teaching plan (patient can name drug, dosage, adverse effects to watch for, and specific measures to avoid them; patient understands the importance of continued follow-up).
- Monitor the effectiveness of comfort measures and compliance with the regimen.

Table B Topical Agents

Drug	Brand Name	Dosage	Usual Indications/Special Considerations
Emollients			
dexpanthenol	*Panthoderm*	Apply once or twice daily as needed	Relieves itching and aids in healing for mild skin irritations
urea	*Aquacare, Carmol, Gordon's Urea, Nutraplus, Ureacin*	Apply b.i.d. to q.i.d. to area affected	Rub in completely; used to restore nails—cover with plastic wrap; keep dry and remove in 3, 7, or 14 d
vitamins A and D	generic	Apply locally with gentle massage b.i.d. to q.i.d.	Relieves minor burns, chafing, skin irritations; consult health care provider if not improved within 7 d
zinc oxide	*Borofax Skin Protectant*	Apply as needed	Relieves burns, abrasion, diaper rash
Growth Factor			
becaplermin	*Regranex*	Apply to diabetic foot ulcers b.i.d. to q.i.d.	Increases the incidence of healing of diabetic foot ulcers as adjunctive therapy; must have an adequate blood supply
Lotions and Solutions			
Burow's solution aluminum acetate	*Domeboro Powder*	Dissolve one packet in a pint of water; apply q15–30 min for 4–8 h	Astringent wet dressing for relief of inflammatory conditions, insect bites, athlete's foot, bruises, sores; do not use occlusive dressing
calamine lotion	generic	Apply to affected area t.i.d. to q.i.d.	Relieves itching, pain of poison ivy, poison sumac, and poison oak, insect bites, and minor skin irritations
hamamelis water	*Witch Hazel, A.E.R.*	Apply locally up to six times per day	Relieves itching and irritation of vaginal infection, hemorrhoids, postepisiotomy discomfort, posthemorrhoidectomy care
Antiseptics			
benzalkonium chloride	*Benza, Mycocide NS, Zephiran*	Mix in solution as needed; spray for preoperative use	Thoroughly rinse detergents and soaps from skin before use; add antirust tablets for instruments stored in solution; dilute solution as indicated for use
chlorhexidinegluconate	*BactoShield, Dyna-Hex, Exidine, Hibistat, Hibiclens*	Scrub or rinse; leave on for 15 s; for surgical scrub—3 min	Use for surgical scrub, preoperative skin preparation, wound cleansing; preoperative bathing and showering

(table continues on page 1044)

Table B Topical Agents (continued)

Drug	Brand Name	Dosage	Usual Indications/Special Considerations
Antiseptics			
hexachlorophene	*pHisoHex*	Apply as wash	Surgical wash, scrub; do not use with burns or on mucous membranes; rinse thoroughly
iodine	generic	Wash affected area	Highly toxic; avoid occlusive dressings; stains skin and clothing; iodine allergy is common
povidone–iodine	*ACU-dyne, Betadine, Betagen, Exodine, Iodex, Minidyne, Operand, Polydine*	Apply as needed	Treated areas may be bandaged; HIV is inactivated in this solution; causes less irritation than iodine; less toxic
sodium hypochlorite	*Dakin's*	Apply as antiseptic	Caution—chemical burns can occur
Antibiotics			
ciprofloxacin/ dexamethasone	*Ciprodex*	Apply drops to ears or outer ear canal	Treatment of acute otitis media with tympanostomy tubes; acute otitis externa
ciprofloxacin/ hydrocortisone	*Cipro-HC Otic drops*	Apply drops to ears or outer ear canal	Treatment of acute otitis media with tympanostomy tubes; acute otitis externa
mupirocin	*Bactroban, Centany*	Apply small amount to affected area t.i.d.	Used to treat impetigo caused by *Staphylococcus aureus, Streptococcus* pathogens; may be covered with a gauze pad; monitor for signs of superinfection, reevaluate if no clinical response in 3–5 d
mupirocin calcium	*Bactroban Nasal*	Apply one-half of the single-use ointment tube between nostrils b.i.d. for 5 d	Eradication of nasal colonization or methicillin-resistant *Staphylococcus aureus*
retapamulin	*Altabax*	Apply thin layer of ointment to affected area b.i.d. for 5 d for patients □9 mo	Treatment of impetigo
Antivirals			
acyclovir	*Zovirax*	Apply 0.5-in. ribbon to affected area six times per day for 7 d	Treatment of herpes simplex cold sores and fever blisters (cream); initial herpes simplex virus genital infections (ointment)
acyclovir/ hydrocortisone	*Xerese*	Apply five times a day for 5 d; begin as soon as cold sore becomes apparent	Treatment of herpes simplex cold sores in patients aged 6 y and older
docosanal	*Abreva*	Apply daily to b.i.d.	Used for treatment of oral and facial herpes simplex cold sores and fever blisters; caution patient not to overuse
imiquimod	*Aldara*	Apply thin layer to warts and rub in three times per week at bedtime for 16 wk	For treatment of genital warts and perianal warts; remove with soap and water after 6–10 h
imiquimod	*Zyclara*	Apply daily at bedtime for 2 wk, may repeat after a 2-wk break	Treatment of genital, perianal warts in patients 12 and older
kunecatechins (sinecatechins)	*Veregen*	Apply thin layer to each wart t.i.d. for up to 16 wk	Treatment of external and perianal warts in immune competent patients older than 18 y
penciclovir	*Denavir*	Apply thin layer to affected area q2 h while awake for 4 d	Treatment of cold sores in healthy patients; begin use at first sign of cold sore; reserve use for herpes labialis on lips and face; avoid mucous membranes
Antipsoriatics			
anthralin	*Balnetar, Dithro-Scalp, Fototar, Zithranol*	Apply daily only to psoriatic lesions	May stain fabrics, skin, hair, fingernails; use protective dressing
calcipotriene	*Dovonex*	Apply thin layer twice a day	Monitor serum calcium levels with extended use; use only for disorder prescribed; may cause local irritation; is a synthetic vitamin D_3
calcipotriene/ betamethasone	*Taclonex, Taclonex Scalp*	Apply once daily for up to 4 wk	Monitor serum calcium levels and check for endocrine imbalance

Drug	Brand Name	Dosage	Usual Indications/Special Considerations
Antiseborrheics			
selenium sulfide	*Selsun Blue*	Massage 5–10 mL into scalp; rest 2–3 min, rinse	May damage jewelry, remove before use; discontinue if local irritation occurs
Antifungals			
butenafine HCl	*Mentax*	Apply to affected area once a day for 4 wk	Treatment of athlete's foot (intradigitalpedia), tineacorporis, ringworm, tineacruris
ciclopirox	*Loprox, Penlac, Penlac Nail Lacquer*	Apply directly to affected fingernails or toenails	Treatment of onychomycosis of the fingernails and toenails in immunocompromised patients
clotrimazole	*Cruex, Desenex, Lotrimin, Mycelex*	Gently massage into affected area b.i.d.	Cleanse area before applying; use for up to 4 wk; discontinue if irritation or worsening of condition occurs
econozole nitrate	generic	Apply locally daily to b.i.d.	Treatment of athlete's foot (intradigitalpedia), tineacorporis, ringworm, tineacruris; cleanse area before applying; treat for 2–4 wk; for athlete's foot, change socks and shoes at least once a day
efinaconazole	*Jublia*	Apply daily for 48 wk using flow brush applicator	Topical treatment of onychomycosis of the toenails
gentian violet	generic	Apply locally b.i.d.	May stain skin and clothing; do not apply to active lesions
ketoconazole	*Extina, Nizora, Xolegel*	Shampoo daily	Reduction of scaling due to dandruff; burning may occur
luliconazole	*Luzu*	Apply locally once a day for 1 wk, 2 wk for tinea pedis	Treatment of athlete's foot (intradigitalpedia), tinea corporis
naftifine HCl	*Naftin*	Gently massage into affected area b.i.d.	Avoid occlusive dressings; wash hands thoroughly after application; do not use longer than 4 wk
oxiconazole	*Oxistat*	Apply daily to b.i.d.	May be needed for up to 1 mo
sertaconazole nitrate	*Ertaczo*	Apply to affected areas and surrounding tissue b.i.d. for 4 wk	Treatment of tinea pedis
terbinafine	*Lamisil*	Apply to area b.i.d. until clinical signs are improved; 1–4 wk	Do not use occlusive dressings; report local irritation; discontinue if local irritation occurs
tolnaftate	*AbsorbineAftate, Genaspor, Quinsana Plus, Tinactin, Ting*	Apply small amount b.i.d. for 2–3 wk; 4–6 wk may be needed if skin is very thick	Cleanse skin with soap and water before applying drug, dry thoroughly; wear loose, well-fitting shoes; change socks at least q.i.d.
Pediculocides/Scabicides			
benzyl alcohol	generic	Apply to scalp or hair near scalp	Single application is usually sufficient, for treatment of head lice in patients 6 mo and older
crotamiton	*Eurax*	Thoroughly massage into skin over entire body, repeat in 24 h; patient should take a cleansing bath or shower 48 h after last application	Change all bed linens and clothing the next day; contaminated clothing can be dry-cleaned or washed in hot water; shake well before using
ivermectin	*Sklice*	Apply once to head for 10 min, no need for nit picking	Treatment of head lice in patients 6 mo and older
lindane	generic	Apply thin layer to entire body; leave on 8–12 h; wash thoroughly; shampoo 1–2 oz into dry hair and leave in place for 4 min	Single application is usually sufficient; reapply after 7 d at signs of live lice; teach hygiene and prevention; treat all contacts; advise parents that this is a readily communicable disease

(table continues on page 1046)

Table B Topical Agents (continued)

Drug	Brand Name	Dosage	Usual Indications/Special Considerations
Pediculocides/Scabicides			
malathion	*Ovide Lotion*	Apply to dry hair and leave on for 8–12 h; repeat in 7–9 d	Avoid use with open lesions; change bed linens and clothing daily; treat all contacts
permethrin	*Acticin, Elimite, Nix*	Thoroughly massage into all skin areas; wash off after 8–14 h; shampoo into freshly washed, rinsed, and towel-dried hair, leave on for 10 min, rinse	Single application is usually curative; notify health care provider if rash, itch becomes worse; approved for prophylactic use during head lice epidemics
spinosad	*Natroba*	Apply to dry scalp and hair, leave on for 10 min, rinse; may be repeated every 7 d as needed	Treatment of head lice in patients 4 y and older
Keratolytics			
podophyllum resin	*Podocon-25, Podofin*	Applied only by physician	Do not use if wart is inflamed or irritated; very toxic; use minimum amount possible to avoid absorption
podofilox	*Condylox*	Apply q12 h for 3 consecutive days	Allow to dry before using area; dispose of used applicator; may cause burning and discomfort
Topical Hemostatics			
absorbable gelatin	*Gelfoam*	Smear or press to cut surface; when bleeding stops, remove excess; apply sponge and allow to remain in place; will be absorbed	Prepare paste by adding 3–4 mL of sterile saline to contents of jar; apply sponge dry or saturated with saline; assess for signs of infection; do not use in presence of infection
absorbable fibrin sealant	*TachoSil*	Apply yellow side of patches directly to bleeding area	For cardiovascular surgery when usual techniques to control bleeding are ineffective
human fibrin sealant	*Evicel, Artiss*	Spray or drop onto tissue in short bursts to produce a thin layer	Adjunct used to reduce bleeding in vascular and liver surgery; used to adhere autologous skin grafts
microfibrillar collagen	*Hemopad, Hemostat, Hemotene*	Use dry; apply directly to source of bleeding, apply pressure for 3–5 min; discard leftover product	Monitor for infection; remove any excess material once bleeding has stopped
thrombin	*Thrombinar, Thrombostat*	Prepare in sterile distilled water; mix freely with blood on the surface of the injury	Contraindicated in the presence of any bovine allergies; watch for severe allergic reactions in sensitive individuals
thrombin, recombinant	*Recothrom*	Apply solution directly to bleeding site with absorbable gelatin sponge	Control of minor bleeding and oozing; do not use with allergy to hamster or snake proteins
Pain Relief			
capsaicin	*Axsain, Capsin, Pain Doctor, Pain-X, Zostrix*	Do not apply more than three to four times per day	Provides temporary relief from the pain of osteoarthritis, rheumatoid arthritis, neuralgias; do not bandage tightly; stop use and seek medical help if condition worsens or persists after 14–28 d
Burn Preparations			
mafenide	*Sulfamylon*	Apply to a clean, debrided wound, one to two times per day; cover burns at all times with drug; reapply as needed	Bathe patient in a whirlpool daily to debride wound; continue debridement with a gloved hand; cover; continue until healing occurs Monitor for infection and toxicity, especially acidosis; may cause severe discomfort requiring premedication before application
silver sulfadiazine	*Silvadene, SSD Cream, Thermazene*	Apply daily to b.i.d. to a clean, debrided wound; use 1/16-in. thickness	Bathe patient in a whirlpool to aid debridement; dressings are not necessary but may be used; reapply when necessary; monitor for fungal infections

Drug	Brand Name	Dosage	Usual Indications/Special Considerations
Estrogens			
estradiol hemihydrate	*Vagifem*	Insert one tablet intravaginally daily for 2 wk, then one tablet intravaginally two times per week	Treatment of atrophic vaginitis; attempt to taper every 3–6 mo
Acne, Rosacea, and Melasma Products			
adapalene	*Differin*	Apply a thin film to affected area after washing	Do not use near cuts or open wounds; avoid sun-burned areas; do not combine with other products; limit exposure to the sun; less drying than most acne products
alitretinoin	*Panretin*	1% gel; apply as needed to cover lesion b.i.d.	Treatment of lesions of Kaposi sarcoma; inflammation, peeling, redness may occur
azelaic acid	*Azelex, Finevin (20%)*	Wash and dry skin; massage thin layer into skin b.i.d.	Wash hands thoroughly after application; improvement usually seen within 4 wk; initial irritation usually passes with time
brimonidine	*Mirvaso*	Apply pea size to forehead, chin, cheeks daily	Risk of vascular insufficiency; for treatment of persistent facial erythema of rosacea in adults
clindamycin	*Clindesse, Evoclin*	Wash and dry area; massage into area morning and evening	Do not use occlusive dressings; may cause transient burning
clindamycin with benzoyl peroxide	*Acanya, BenzaClin*	Apply to affected area b.i.d.	Wash and pat dry area before application
clindamycin with tretinoin	*Ziana, Veltin*	Rub pea-sized amount over entire face once daily at bedtime	Do not use in patients with colitis
dapsone	*Aczone Gel*	Apply thin layer to affected areas b.i.d.	Follow hemoglobin and reticulocyte counts; do not use with patients with glucose-6-phosphate dehydrogenase deficiencies
fluocinolone, hydroquinone, tretinoin	*Triluma*	Apply to depigmented area of melasma once each evening at least 30 min before bed	Treatment of melasma; not for use in pregnancy; skin peeling can occur; wear protective clothing when outside
ingenolmebutate	*Picato*	Apply gel once a day to face/scalp for 5 d; to trunk for 2 d	Treatment of acne
ivermectin	*Soolantra*	Apply to affected areas daily	Treatment of rosacea
metronidazole	*MetroGel, MetroLotion, Noritate*	Apply cream to affected area	Treatment of rosacea
sodium sulfacetamide	*Klaron*	Apply a thin film b.i.d.	Wash affected area with mild soap and water, pat dry; avoid use in denuded or abraded areas
tazarotene	*Tazorac*	Apply thin film daily in the evening	Avoid use in pregnancy; drying, causes photosensitivity; do not use with products containing alcohol
tretinoin, 0.025% cream	*Avita*	Apply thin layer daily	Discomfort, peeling, redness, and worsening of acne may occur for first 2–4 wk
tretinoin, 0.05% cream	*Renova*	Apply thin coat in evening	Use for the removal of fine wrinkles
tretinoin, gel	*Retin-A-Micro*	Apply to cover daily, after cleansing	Exacerbation of inflammation may occur at first; therapeutic effects usually seen in first 2 wk
Antihistamine			
azelastine HCl	*Astelin*	Two sprays per nostril b.i.d.	Avoid use of alcohol and OTC antihistamines; dizziness and sedation may occur.
Hair Removal			
eflornithine	*Vaniqa*	Apply to unwanted facial hair b.i.d. for up to 24 wk	Approved for use in women only

(table continues on page 1048)

Table B Topical Agents (continued)

Drug	Brand Name	Dosage	Usual Indications/Special Considerations
Immune Modulator			
pimecrolimus	*Elidel*	Apply locally b.i.d.	Treatment of mild to moderate atopic dermatitis in nonimmunosuppressed patients over 2 y old
Antidiaper Rash Drug			
miconazole/zinc oxide, petrolatum	*Vusion*	Apply gently for 7 d	Culture for *Candida* before treatment. Treatment of diaper rash
Local Anesthetics			
lidocaine/tetracaine	*Synera*	Apply one patch to intact skin 20–30 min before procedure	Dermal analgesia for superficial venous access, dermatological procedures
Topical Corticosteroids			
These drugs enter cells and bind to cytoplasmic receptors, initiating complex reactions that are responsible for the anti-inflammatory, antipruritic, and antiproliferative effects of these drugs. They are used to relieve the inflammation and pruritic manifestations of corticosteroid-sensitive dermatoses and for temporary relief of minor skin irritations and rashes. These agents should always be applied sparingly because of the risk of systemic corticosteroid effects if absorbed systemically. Occlusive dressings and tight coverings should be avoided. Prolonged use should also be avoided because of the risk of systemic effects and local irritation and breakdown. These agents are applied topically two to three times daily.			
alclometasone dipropionate	generic	Ointment, cream: 0.05% concentration	Occlusive dressings may be used for the management of refractory lesions of psoriasis and deep-seated dermatoses
beclomethasone	*Beconase AQ, Qnasl*	Nasal spray	Treatment of rhinitis
betamethasone dipropionate	generic	Ointment, cream, lotion, aerosol: 0.05% concentration	
betamethasone dipropionate, augmented	*Diprolene*	Ointment, cream, lotion: 0.05% concentration	
betamethasone valerate	*Beta-Val, Luxiq, Valisone*	Ointment, cream, lotion: 0.01% concentration	
ciclesonide	*Alvesco, Omnaris, Zetonna*	Inhalation: 80 mcg, 160 mcg per actuation	
clobetasol propionate	*Cormax, Temovate, Olux*	Ointment, cream: 0.05% concentration	
	Clobex	Spray 0.05%	
clocortolone pivalate	*Cloderm*	Cream: 0.1% concentration	
desonide	*DesOwen, Verdeso*	Ointment, cream: 0.05% concentration	
desoximetasone	*Topicort*	Ointment, cream: 0.25% concentration	
		Gel: 0.05% concentration	
dexamethasone	*Aeroseb-Dex*	Gel: 0.1% concentration	
		Aerosol: 0.01%, 0.04% concentration	
diflorasone diacetate	generic	Ointment, cream: 0.05% concentration	
		Cream: 0.5% concentration	
fluocinolone acetonide	*Synalar*	Ointment: 0.025% concentration	
		Cream: 0.01% concentration	
fluocinonide	*Lidex*	Ointment: 0.05% concentration	
	Fluonex, Lidex	Cream: 0.05% concentration	
	Lidex, Vanos	Solution, gel: 0.05% concentration	
		Cream: 0.1%	
fluticasone fumarate	*Veramyst*	35 mcg/spray, nasal spray	

Drug	Brand Name	Dosage	Usual Indications/Special Considerations
Topical Corticosteroids			
fluticasone propionate	*Cutivate*	Cream: 0.05% concentration	
	Flonase, FloventDiskus, Flovent HFA	Ointment: 0.005% concentration Nasal spray; 88–220 mcg b.i.d. using nasal inhalation	
halcinonide	*Halog*	Ointment, cream, solution: 0.1% concentration	
halobetasol propionate	*Ultravate*	Ointment, cream: 0.05% concentration	
hydrocortisone	*Bactine, Hydrocortisone, Cort-Dome, Dermolate, Dermtex HC, Cortizone 10, Hycort, Tegrin-HC*	Lotion: 0.25% concentration Cream, lotion, ointment, aerosol: 0.5%, 1% concentration	
	Hytone	Cream, lotion, ointment, solution: 1% concentration	
hydrocortisone acetate	*Cortaid, Lanacort-5*	Ointment: 0.5% concentration (OTC preparations)	
	Gynecort, Lanacort 5	Cream: 0.5% concentration (OTC preparations)	
	Anusol-HC	Cream: 1% concentration	
	Cortaid with Aloe	Cream: 0.5%, 1% concentration (OTC preparations)	
hydrocortisone buteprate	generic	Cream: 0.1% concentration	
hydrocortisone butyrate	*Locoid*	Ointment, cream: 0.1% concentration	
hydrocortisone valerate	*Westcort*	Ointment, cream: 0.2% concentration	
mometasone furoate	*Elocon*	Ointment, cream, lotion: 0.1% concentration	
	Nasonex	Nasal spray: 0.2% concentration	
	AsmanexTwisthaler	Solution for inhalation: 220 mcg/actuation	
prednicarbate	*Dermatop*	Cream: 0.1% concentration(preservative free)	
triamcinolone acetonide			
	Triacet, Triderm	Cream: 0.025%, 0.5% concentration Cream: 0.1% concentration Lotion: 0.025%, 0.1% concentration	

OTC, over the counter.

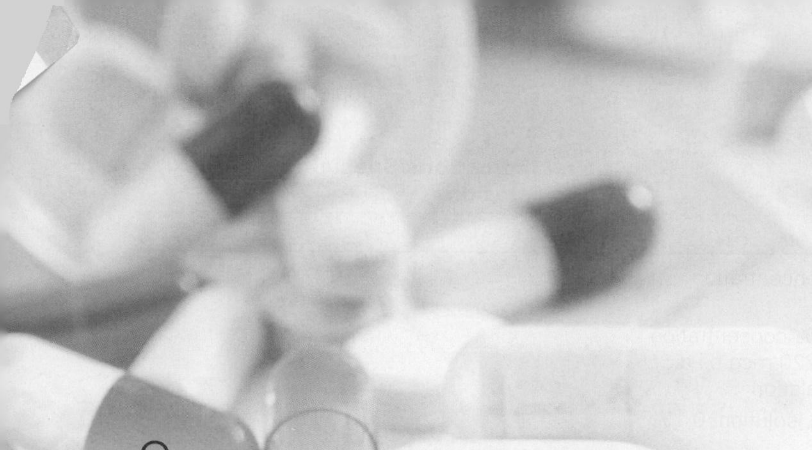

Ophthalmic Agents C

Ophthalmic agents are drugs that are intended for direct administration into the conjunctiva of the eye. These drugs are used to treat glaucoma (miotics constrict the pupil and decrease the resistance to aqueous flow), to aid in the diagnosis of eye problems (mydriatics dilate the pupil for examination of the retina; cycloplegics paralyze the muscles that control the lens to aid refraction); to treat local ophthalmic infections or inflammation; and to provide relief from the signs and symptoms of allergic reactions.

These drugs are not generally absorbed systemically because of their method of administration. They are classified in pregnancy category C, and caution should always be used when giving drugs during pregnancy or lactation.

Contraindications and Cautions

These drugs are contraindicated in the presence of allergy to the specific drug or to any component of the product being used. Although they are seldom absorbed systemically, caution should be used in any patient who would have problems with the systemic effects of the drugs if they were absorbed systemically.

Adverse Effects

Adverse effects of these drugs include local irritation, stinging, burning, blurring of vision (prolonged when using ointments), tearing, and headache.

Clinically Important Drug–Drug Interactions

Because of their actions on the eye or because of the components of the drug, many of these drugs cannot be given at the same time but should be spaced 1 to 2 hours apart. Check the specific drug being used for details.

Dosage

The usual dosage for any of these drugs is one to two drops in each eye or in the affected eye two to four times daily, or 0.25 to 0.5 inches of ointment in the affected eye or eyes.

Nursing Considerations

Assessment

- Screen for the following: Allergy to the specific drug or components of the preparation; underlying medical conditions *that would be affected if the drug were absorbed systemically.*
- Evaluate eye, conjunctival color; note any lesions. A vision examination may be appropriate.

Nursing Diagnoses

The patient receiving an ophthalmic agent may have the following nursing diagnoses related to drug therapy:

- Acute pain related to administration of the drug
- Risk for injury related to changes in vision
- Deficient knowledge regarding drug therapy

Planning

- The patient will receive the best therapeutic effect from the drug therapy.
- The patient will have limited adverse effects to the drug therapy.
- The patient will have an understanding of the drug therapy, adverse effects to anticipate, and measures to relieve discomfort and improve safety.

Implementation

- Assess the patient's general physical condition before beginning the test *to decrease the potential for adverse effects.*
- Follow these administration guidelines *to provide the most therapeutic use of the drug with the fewest adverse effects:*
  - *Solution or drops:* Wash hands thoroughly before administering; do not touch the dropper to the patient's eye or to any other surface. Have the patient tilt the head backward or lie down, and have the patient stare upward. Gently grasp the lower eyelid and pull the eyelid away from the eyeball;

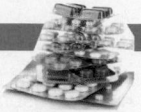

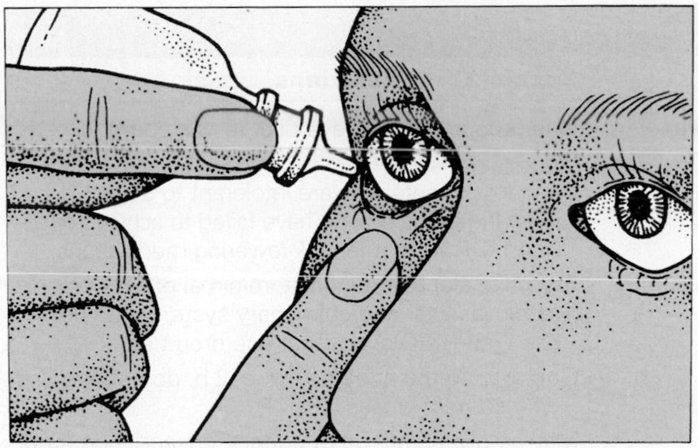

FIGURE C.1 Administration of ophthalmic drops.

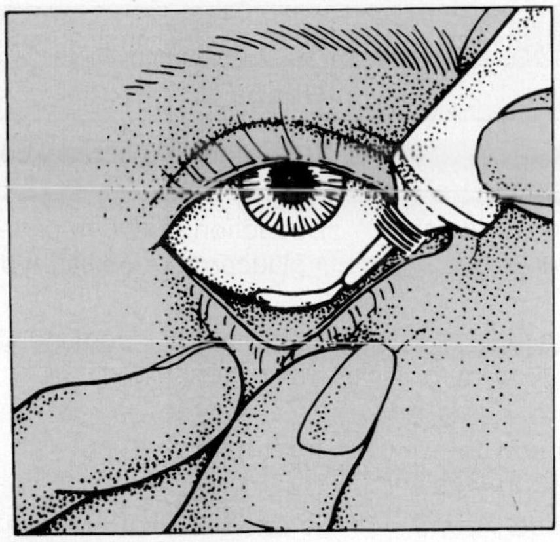

FIGURE C.2 Administration of ophthalmic ointment.

instill drops into the pouch formed by the eyelid. Release the lid slowly; have the patient close the eye and look downward. Apply gentle pressure to the inside corner of the eye for 3 to 5 minutes to retard drainage. Do not rub the eyes; do not rinse the eyedropper. Do not use eye drops that have changed color; if more than one type of eye drop is used, wait at least 5 minutes between administrations. See Figure C.1.

- *Ointment:* Wash hands thoroughly before administering; hold the tube between the hands for several minutes to warm the ointment; discard the first centimeter of ointment when opening the tube for the first time. Tilt the patient's head backward or have the patient lie down and stare upward. Gently pull out the lower lid to form a pouch; place 0.25 to 0.5 inches of ointment inside the lower lid. Have the patient close the eye for 1 to 2 minutes and roll the eyeball in all directions; remove any excess ointment from around the eye. If using more than one kind of ointment, wait at least 10 minutes between administrations. See Figure C.2.

- *Provide comfort measures to help the patient tolerate drug effects* (e.g., control light, administer analgesics as needed).
- Include the following information—in addition to the proper administration technique for the drug—in the teaching program for the patient *to improve compliance and provide safety and comfort measures as necessary:* Safety measures may need to be taken if blurring of vision should occur; burning and stinging may occur on administration but should pass quickly; the pupils will dilate with mydriatic agents and the eyes may become very sensitive to light (the use of sunglasses is recommended); any severe eye discomfort, palpitations, nausea, or headache should be reported to the health care provider.

Evaluation

- Monitor patient response to the drug (changes in pupil size, relief of pressure of glaucoma, relief of itching and tearing related to allergic reaction).
- Monitor for adverse effects (local irritation, blurring of vision, headache).
- Evaluate the effectiveness of the teaching plan (patient can name adverse effects to watch for and specific measures to avoid them; the patient understands the importance of the follow-up that will be needed).
- Monitor the effectiveness of comfort measures and compliance with the regimen.

Table C Ophthalmic Agents

Drug	Usage	Special Considerations
alcaftadine (*Lastacaft*)	Prevention of itching associated with allergic conjunctivitis	One drop in each eye daily; remove contacts; not for treatment of contact lens irritation.
apraclonidine (*Iopidine*)	To control or prevent postsurgical elevations of IOP after argon laser eye surgery	Monitor for the possibility of vasovagal attack; do not give to patients with allergy to clonidine
azelastine HCl (*Optivar*)	Treatment of ocular itching associated with allergic conjunctivitis	Antihistamine, mast cell stabilizer; dosage (≥3 y): one drop b.i.d.; rapid onset, 8-h duration
azithromycin (*Azasite*)	Treatment of bacterial conjunctivitis	Treatment of bacterial conjunctivitis, one drop b.i.d. 8–12 h apart for 2 d, then once a day for 5 d
bepotastine HCl (*Bepreve*)	Treatment of ocular itching associated with allergic rhinitis	Apply twice daily for patients 2 y and older

(table continues on page 1052)

Table C Ophthalmic Agents (continued)

Drug	Usage	Special Considerations
besifloxacin (*Besivance*)	Treatment of bacterial conjunctivitis (pink eye)	One drop in affected eye t.i.d. (6–8 h apart) for 7 d
bimatoprost (*Latisse, Lumigan*)	Reduction of IOP in patients with open-angle glaucoma or ocular hypertension	Used for patients who are intolerant to other IOP-lowering drugs or who have failed to achieve optimum IOP with other IOP-lowering medications
brimonidine tartrate (*Alphagan P*)	Treatment of open-angle glaucoma and ocular hypertension	Selective $alpha_2$-antagonist; minimal effects on cardiovascular and pulmonary systems; do not use with MAOIs; dosage: one drop t.i.d.
brimonidine with timolol (*Combigan*)	Treatment of IOP	One drop to the affected eye q12 h; do not use with contact lenses
brinzolamide (*Azopt*)	To decrease IOP in open-angle glaucoma	May be given with other agents; dosage: one drop t.i.d.; give 10 min apart from any other agents
bromfenac (*Xibrom*)	Treatment of postoperative inflammation following cataract surgery	One drop in affected eye b.i.d. starting 24 h after surgery for 2 wk
carbachol (*Miostat*)	Direct-acting miotic; for treatment of glaucoma; miosis during surgery	Surgical dose: a one-use-only portion; for glaucoma: 1–2 drops up to t.i.d. as needed
carteolol (generic)	Reduction of IOP in chronic open-angle glaucoma	One drop in affected eye(s) b.i.d.
cyclopentolate (*Cyclogyl, Pentolair*)	Mydriasis/cycloplegia in diagnostic procedures	Individuals with dark-pigmented irises may require higher doses; compress lacrimal sac for 1–2 min after administration to decrease any systemic absorption.
cyclosporine emulsion (*Restasis*)	Increases tear production in patients with decreased tear production related to inflammation or keratoconjunctivitis sicca	One drop in each eye b.i.d., approx. 12 h apart; remove contact lenses during use
dexamethasone intravitreal (*Ozurdex*)	Treatment of macular edema following branch retinal artery occlusion or central retinal artery occlusion	Monitor for infection and retinal detachment following injection; use caution with a history of ocular herpes simplex
diclofenac sodium (*Voltaren Ophthalmic*)	Photophobia: for use in patients undergoing incisional refractive surgery	Apply 1 drop q.i.d. beginning 24 h after cataract surgery; continue through the first 2 wk after surgery
difluprednate (*Durezol*)	Treatment of photophobia in patients undergoing incisional refractory surgery	Administer 1 drop into the affected eye q.i.d., beginning 2 wk before surgery and continuing for 2 wk after surgery
dorzolamide (*Trusopt*)	Treatment of elevated IOP in open-angle glaucoma or ocular hypertension	A sulfonamide; monitor patients taking parenteral sulfonamides for possible adverse effects
dorzolamide 2% and timolol 0.5% (*Cosopt*)	To decrease IOP in open-angle glaucoma or ocular hypertension in patients who do not respond to beta-blockers alone	Administer 1 drop in affected eye b.i.d.; monitor for cardiac failure; if absorbed, may mask symptoms of hypoglycemia or thyrotoxicosis
echothiophate (generic)	Treatment of glaucoma; irreversible cholinesterase inhibitor; long acting; accommodative esotropia	Given only once a day because of long duration of action; tolerance may develop with prolonged use but efficacy usually returns after a rest period
emedastine (*Emadine*)	Temporary relief of signs and symptoms of allergic conjunctivitis	One drop in affected eye up to q.i.d.; patient should not wear contact lenses if eyes are red; may cause headache, blurred vision
epinastine (*Elestat*)	Prevention of itching caused by allergic conjunctivitis	One drop in each eye b.i.d. for entire time of exposure; remove contact lenses before use
fluocinolone (*Retisert*)	Treatment of noninfectious uveitis in posterior segment of eye	One implant every 3 mo
fluorometholone (*Flarex, FML*)	Topical corticosteroid used for treatment of inflammatory conditions of the eye	Improvement should occur within several days; discontinue if no improvement is seen; discontinue if swelling of the eye occurs
ganciclovir (*Zirgan*)	Treatment of acute herpetic keratitis	Apply gel in lower conjunctival sac daily
gatifloxacin (*Zymar, Zymaxid*)	Treatment of bacterial conjunctivitis caused by susceptible strains	Contacts should not be worn; can cause blurred vision
homatropine (*Isopto Homatropine, Homatropine HBr*)	Long-acting mydriatic and cycloplegic used for refraction and treatment of inflammatory conditions of the uveal tract	Individuals with dark-pigmented irises may require larger doses; 5–10 min is usually required for refraction
ketorolac (*Acuvail*)	Treatment of pain and inflammation following cataract surgery	Apply to affected eye twice daily

Drug	Usage	Special Considerations
ketotifen (*Aliway, Zaditor*)	Temporary relief of itching due to allergic conjunctivitis	Remove contact lenses before use—may be replaced 10 min after administration; an antihistamine/mast cell stabilizer
latanoprost (*Xalatan*)	Treatment of open-angle glaucoma or ocular hypertension in patients intolerant or unresponsive to other agents	Remove contact lenses before use and for 15 min after use; allow at least 5 min between this and the use of any other agents; expect blurring of vision
levobunolol (*AK Beta, Betagan Liquifilm*)	Lowering of IOP with chronic open-angle glaucoma, ocular hypertension	One to two drops b.i.d.; do not combine with beta-blockers
levofloxacin (*Quixin*)	Treatment of bacterial conjunctivitis caused by susceptible bacteria	One to two drops per day in affected eye
lodoxamide (*Alomide*)	Treatment of vernal conjunctivitis and keratitis	Patients should not wear contact lenses while using this drug; discontinue if stinging or burning persists after instillation One to two drops q.i.d.
loteprednoletabonate (*Lotemax* [0.5%]), (*Alrex* [0.2%])	Treatment of steroid-resistant ocular disease Treatment of postoperative inflammation after ocular surgery	One to two drops q.i.d. beginning 24 h after surgery and continuing for 2 wk Shake vigorously before use; discard after 14 d; prolonged use may cause nerve or eye damage
loteprednol with tobramycin (*Zylet*)	Treatment of inflammatory ocular conditions with risk of bacterial ocular infection	Apply one to two drops every 4–6 h
metipranolol (*OptiPranolol*)	Beta-blocker; used in treating chronic open-angle glaucoma and ocular hypertension	Concomitant therapy may be needed; caution patient about possible vision changes
mitomycin-C (*Mitosol*)	Control of scarring following trabeculotomy	Applied topically intraoperatively
moxifloxacin (*Moxeza, Vigamox*)	Treatment of bacterial conjunctivitis caused by susceptible strains	Contact lenses should not be worn; can cause blurred vision
natamycin (*Natacyn*)	Antibiotic used to treat fungal blepharitis, conjunctivitis, and keratitis; drug of choice for *Fusarium solani* keratitis	Shake well before each use; store at room temperature; failure to improve in 7–10 d suggests a nonsusceptible organism; reevaluate
nedocromil (*Alocril*)	Treatment of itching of allergic conjunctivitis	One to two drops in each eye b.i.d. for entire allergy season
olopatadine hydrochloride (*Pataday, Patanol, Pazeo*)	Mast cell stabilizer and antihistamine; provides fast onset of relief of itching due to conjunctivitis and has prolonged action	Not for use with contact lenses; headache is a common side effect
phenylephrine/ketorolac (*Omidra*)	Prevention of intraoperative midrosis; pain relief with cataract surgery	4 mL in 500 mL ophthalmic irrigating solution used when needed during surgery
pilocarpine (*Adsorbocarpine, Piloptic, Pilostat*)	Chronic and acute glaucoma; treatment of mydriasis caused by drugs; direct-acting mitotic	Can be stored at room temperature for up to 8 wk, then discard; may use one to two drops up to six times per day, based on patient response
rimexolone (*Vexol*)	Corticosteroid; postoperative ocular surgery for the treatment of anterior uveitis	Monitor for signs of steroid absorption.
sulfacetamide (*Bleph-10*)	Treatment of ocular infections	One to two drops every 2–3 h; gradually taper over 7–10 d
tafluprost (*Zioptan*)	Reduction of IOP in patients with open-angle glaucoma or ocular hypertension	One drop in affected eye(s) once daily in the evening
timolol (*Timoptic-XE*)	Treatment of elevated IOP in ocular hypertension or open-angle glaucoma	One drop in affected eye(s) each day in the morning
travoprost (*Travatan Z*)	Reduction of IOP in patients with open-angle glaucoma or ocular hypertension	Reserve for patients who are intolerant of other IOP-lowering medications or who have failed to achieve optimum IOP with other IOP-lowering medications
trifluridine (*Viroptic*)	Antiviral; used to treat primary keratoconjunctivitis and recurrent epithelial keratitis due to herpes simplex virus types 1 and 2	Transient burning or stinging may occur; reconsider drug choice if improvement is not seen within 7 d; do not administer longer than 21 d at a time
tropicamide (*Mydriacyl, Tropicacyl*)	Mydriatic and cyclopegic for refraction	One to two drops, repeat in 5 min; may repeat in 30 min for prolonged effects

IOP, intraocular pressure; MAOI, monoamine oxidase inhibitor.

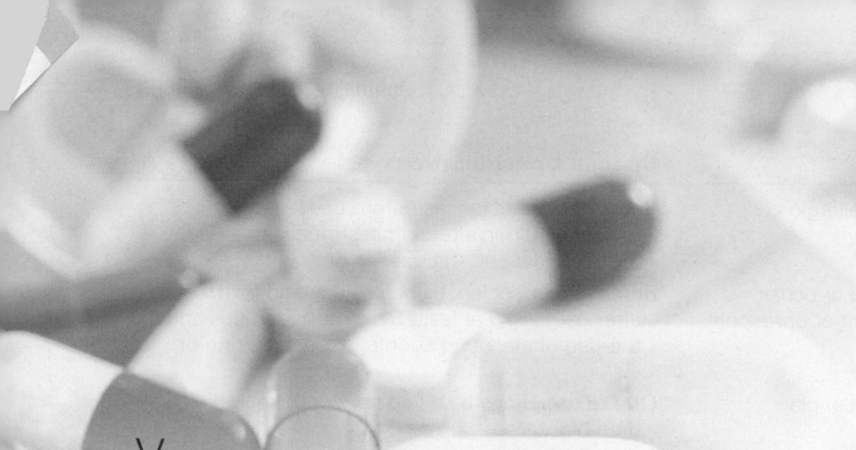

Vitamins D

Vitamins are substances that the body requires for carrying out essential metabolic reactions. The body cannot synthesize enough of these components to meet all of its needs; therefore, they must be obtained from animal and vegetable tissues taken in as food. Vitamins are needed only in small amounts because they function as coenzymes that activate the protein portions of enzymes, which catalyze a great deal of biochemical activity. Many recent studies have found that too high a level of certain vitamins can be toxic and cause health problems. Since 2014, national guidelines caution patients and providers about the use of supplemental vitamins. Studies do not support the use of vitamins in situations without a documented vitamin deficiency noting that the risk of too much of a vitamin and the adverse effects associated with that do not outweigh any benefit. Vitamins are either water soluble and excreted in the urine, or they are fat soluble and capable of being stored in adipose tissue in the body.

Therapeutic Actions and Indications

Vitamins act as coenzymes to activate a variety of proteins on enzymes that catalyze biochemical activity. They are indicated for the treatment of vitamin deficiencies, as dietary supplements when needed, and as specific therapy related to the activity of the vitamin.

Contraindications and Cautions

These drugs are contraindicated in the presence of any known allergy to the drug or the colorants, additives, or preservatives used in the drug. They are categorized as pregnancy category C and are used to maintain adequate vitamin levels during pregnancy and lactation.

Adverse Effects

The adverse effects primarily associated with these drugs are related to gastrointestinal upset and irritation, which is caused by direct gastrointestinal contact with the drugs.

Clinically Important Drug–Drug Interactions

Pyridoxine—vitamin B_6—interferes with the effectiveness of levodopa. Fat-soluble vitamins may not be absorbed if given concurrently with mineral oil, cholestyramine, or colestipol.

Nursing Considerations

Assessment

- Obtain a nutritional assessment. Ensure that the patient has an actual vitamin deficiency. Screen for any medical conditions and drugs being taken and for any known allergies.
- Evaluate skin and mucous membranes, as well as pulse, respirations, and blood pressure. Complete blood count (CBC) and clotting times may need to be evaluated with specific vitamins.

Nursing Diagnoses

The patient receiving vitamins might have the following nursing diagnoses related to drug therapy:

- Acute pain related to GI discomfort
- Risk for imbalanced nutrition related to replacement therapy
- Deficient knowledge regarding drug therapy

Planning

- The patient will receive the best therapeutic effect from the drug therapy.
- The patient will have limited adverse effects to the drug therapy.
- The patient will have an understanding of the drug therapy, adverse effects to anticipate, and measures to relieve discomfort and improve safety.

Implementation

- Assess the patient's general physical condition before beginning test to *decrease the potential for adverse effects and ensure need for the drug.*
- Advise the patient to avoid the use of over-the-counter preparations that contain the same vitamins *to prevent inadvertent overdose of the vitamin.*
- Provide comfort measures *to help the patient tolerate drug effects* (e.g., take drug with meals to alleviate gastrointestinal distress).
- Include information about the solution being used in a test (e.g., what to expect, adverse effects that may occur, follow-up tests that may be needed) *to enhance patient*

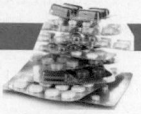

knowledge about drug therapy and promote compliance with drug regimen.

Evaluation

- Monitor patient response to the drug (adequate vitamin intake).
- Monitor for adverse effects (GI upset).
- Evaluate the effectiveness of the teaching plan (patient can name adverse effects to watch for and specific measures to avoid them; patient understands the importance of follow-up that will be needed).
- Monitor the effectiveness of comfort measures and compliance with the regimen.

Table D Vitamins

Vitamin	Solubility Type	Recommended Dietary Allowance	Therapeutic Uses/Special Considerations
A (*Aquasol A*)	Fat	1,000 mcg (male) 800 mcg (female) 1,300 mcg (lactation) 500 mcg (pediatric)	Severe deficiency: 500,000 IU/d for 3 d, then 50,000 IU/d for 2 wk given IM or PO; Protect IM vial from light; hypervitaminosis A can occur, including cirrhotic-like liver syndrome with CNS effects; GI drying, rash, and liver changes; treat by discontinuing the vitamin and give saline, prednisone, and calcitonin IV; liver damage may be permanent
ascorbic acid (*Dull C, Vita-C, N'Ice*)	Water	45–60 mg (male) 45–60 mg (female) 70–90 mg (lactation) 70 mg (pregnancy) 40–45 mg (pediatric)	May be given PO, IM, slow IV, or SC; treatment of scurvy: 300–1,000 mg/d; enhanced wound healing: 300–500 mg/d for 7–10 d; burns: 1–2 g/d; also being studied for treatment of common cold, asthma, CAD, cancer, and schizophrenia; may be very toxic at high doses
calcifediol (D_3) (*Calderol*)	Fat		Management of metabolic bone disease or hypocalcemia in patients receiving chronic renal dialysis: 300–350 mcg/wk daily or on alternate days; discontinue if hypercalcemia occurs
cholecalciferol (D_3) (*Delta-D*)	Fat	400 IU (male) 400–800 IU (female) 400 IU (lactation) 400 IU (pregnancy) 400 IU (pediatric 1–12 mo) 600 IU (pediatric 1–18 yr)	Vitamin D deficiency: 400–1,000 IU/d; may be useful for the treatment of hypocalcemictetany and hypoparathyroidism
cyanocobalamin (B_{12}) (*Big Shot B_{12}, Twelve Resin-K*)	Water	2 mcg (male) 2 mcg (female) 2.6 mcg (lactation) 2.2 mcg (pregnancy) 0.9–1.2 mcg (pediatric)	Deficiency: 25–250 mcg/d (note: oral route is not for the treatment of pernicious anemia); pernicious anemia: 100 mcg IM each month for life; given with folic acid; nasal route is preferable.
D	Fat	400 IU (male) 400–800 IU (female) 400 IU (lactation) 400 IU (pregnancy) 400 IU (pediatric)	Vitamin D deficiency: 400–1,000 IU/d; may be useful for the treatment of hypocalcemictetany and hypoparathyroidism; encourage balanced diet and exposure to sunlight; do not use with mineral oil
E (*Aquavit-E, Vita-Plus E Softgels*)	Fat	15 IU (male) 12 IU (female) 16–18 IU (lactation) 15 IU (pregnancy) 4–10 IU (pediatric)	Used in certain premature infants to reduce the toxic effects of oxygen on the lung and retina; do not give IV; report fatigue, weakness, nausea, or headache.
ergocalciferol (D_2) (*Calciferol, Drisdol Drops*)	Fat	200–400 IU (male) 200–400 IU (female) 400 IU (lactation) 400 IU (pregnancy) 300–400 IU (pediatric)	Give IM in GI, biliary, or liver disease; refractory rickets: 12,000–500,000 IU/d; hypoparathyroidism: 50,000–2,000,000 IU/d; familial hypophosphatemia: 10,000–80,000 IU/d plus 1–2 g phosphorus

(table continues on page 1056)

Table D Vitamins (continued)

Vitamin	Solubility Type	Recommended Dietary Allowance	Therapeutic Uses/Special Considerations
niacin (B_3) (*Niacor, Nicotinic Acid, Nicotinex, Slo-Niacin, Niaspan*)	Water	15–20 mg (male) 13–15 mg (female) 20 mg (lactation) 17 mg (pregnancy) 5–13 mg (pediatric)	Prevention and treatment of pellagra: up to 500 mg/d; niacin deficiency: up to 100 mg/d; also used for the treatment of hyperlipidemia if no response to diet and exercise: 1–2 g t.i.d.; do not exceed 6 g/d; feelings of warmth or flushing may occur with administration but usually pass within 2 h
nicotinamide (B_3) (*Niacinamide*)	Water	15–20 mg (male) 13–15 mg (female) 20 mg (lactation) 17 mg (pregnancy) 5–13 mg (pediatric)	Prevention and treatment of pellagra: up to 50 mg, 3 to 10 times per day
P (bioflavonoids) (*Amino-Opti-C, Bio-Acerola C, Flavons 500, Pan C 500, Peridin-C, Quercetin, Span C*)	Water	Unknown	Used to treat bleeding, abortion, poliomyelitis, diabetes, and other conditions; there is little evidence that these uses have any clinical efficacy
phytonadione (K) (*Mephyton*)	Fat	45–80 mcg (male) 45–65 mcg (female) 65 mcg (lactation) 65 mcg (pregnancy) 5–30 mcg (pediatric)	Hypoprothrombinemia due to anticoagulant use: 2.5–10 mg PO, IM; hemorrhagic disease of the newborn: 0.5–1 mg IM within 1 h of birth; 1–5 mg IM may be given to the mother before delivery; hypoprothrombinemia in adult: 2.5–25 mg PO or IM
pyridoxine HCl (B_6) (*Aminoxin*)	Water	1.7–2 mg (male) 1.4–1.6 mg (female) 2.1 mg (lactation) 2.2 mg (pregnancy) 0.3–1.4 mg (pediatric)	Deficiency: 10–20 mg/d PO or IM for 3 wk; vitamin B_6 deficiency syndrome: up to 600 mg/d for life; isoniazid poisoning (give an equal amount of pyridoxine): 4 g IV followed by 1 g IM q30 min; reduces the effectiveness of levodopa and leads to serious toxic effects—avoid this combination
riboflavin	Water	1.4–1.8 mg (male) 1.2–1.3 mg (female) 1.7–1.8 mg (lactation) 1.6 mg (pregnancy) 0.4–1.2 mg (pediatric)	Treatment of deficiency: 5–15 mg/d; may cause a yellow or orange discoloration to the urine
Thiamine HCl (B_1) (*Thiamilate*)	Water	1.2–1.5 mg (male) 1–1.1 mg (female) 1.6 mg (lactation) 1.5 mg (pregnancy) 0.3–1 mg (pediatric)	Treatment of wet beriberi: 10–30 mg IV t.i.d.; treatment of beriberi: 10–20 mg IM t.i.d. for 2 wk with multivitamin containing 5–10 mg/d for 1 mo; do not mix in alkaline solutions; used orally as a mosquito repellant, alters body sweat composition; feeling of warmth and flushing may occur with administration but usually passes within 2 h

CNS, central nervous system; GI, gastrointestinal; CAD, coronary artery disease.

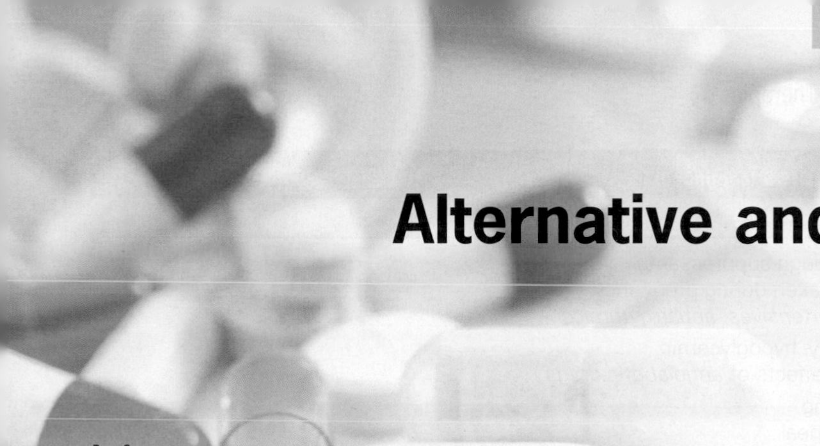

Alternative and Complementary Therapies E

Many dietary supplements and "natural" remedies are used by the public for self-treatment. These substances, many derived from the folklore of various cultures, commonly contain ingredients that have been identified and that have known therapeutic activities. Some of these substances have unknown mechanisms of action but over the years have been reliably used to relieve specific symptoms. There is an element of the placebo effect in using some of these substances. The power of believing that something will work and that there is some control over the problem is often beneficial in achieving relief from pain or suffering. Some of these substances may contain yet-unidentified ingredients that eventually may prove useful in the modern field of pharmacology. Because these products are not regulated or monitored, there is always a possibility of toxic effects. Some of these products may contain ingredients that interact with prescription drugs. A history of the use of these alternative therapies may explain unexpected reactions to some drugs.

Table E Alternative and Complementary Therapies

Substance	Reported Uses and Possible Risks
acidophilus (probiotics)	*Oral:* Prevention or treatment of uncomplicated diarrhea Decreased effectiveness of *warfarin*
alfalfa	*Topical:* Healing ointment, relief of arthritis pain *Oral:* Treatment of arthritis, hot flashes; strength giving; reduction of cholesterol level Increased risk of bleeding with *warfarin*; increased photosensitivity with *chlorpromazine*; increased risk of hypoglycemia with *antidiabetic drugs*; loss of effectiveness with *hormonal contraceptives* or *hormone replacement*
allspice	*Topical:* Anesthetic for teeth and gums; soothes sore joints and muscles *Oral:* Treatment of indigestion, flatulence, diarrhea, fatigue Risk of seizures with excessive use; decreased *iron* absorption
aloe leaves	*Topical:* Treatment of burns, healing of wounds *Oral:* Treatment of chronic constipation *Caution:* Oral use may cause serious hypokalemia; risk of spontaneous abortion if used in third trimester
androstenedione	*Oral, spray:* Anabolic steroid to increase muscle mass and strength *Caution:* May increase risk of cardiovascular disease and certain cancers
angelica	*Oral:* "Cure all" for gynecological problems, headaches, backaches, loss of appetite, and gastrointestinal spasms; increases circulation in the periphery Risk of bleeding if combined with *anticoagulants*
anise	*Oral:* Relief of dry cough, treatment of flatulence May increase *iron* absorption and cause toxicity
apple	*Oral:* Control of blood glucose, constipation May interfere with *antidiabetic drugs*, *fexofenadine*
arnica	*Topical:* Relief of pain from muscle or soft-tissue injury *Oral:* Immune system stimulant May decrease effects of *antihypertensives* and increase effects of *anticoagulants* and *platelet drugs*; very toxic to children
ashwagandha	*Oral:* To improve mental and physical functioning; general tonic; to protect cells during cancer chemotherapy and radiation therapy May increase bleeding with *anticoagulants*; may interfere with *thyroid replacement* therapy; discourage use during pregnancy and lactation
astragalus	*Oral:* To increase stamina, energy; to improve immune function, resistance to disease; to treat upper respiratory tract infection, common cold May increase effects of *antihypertensives*; caution against use during fever or acute infection

(table continues on page 1058)

Table E Alternative and Complementary Therapies (continued)

Substance	Reported Uses and Possible Risks
barberry	*Oral:* Antidiarrheal, antipyretic, cough suppressant Risk of spontaneous abortion if taken during pregnancy May increase effects of *antihypertensives, antiarrhythmics*
basil	*Oral:* Analgesic, anti-inflammatory, hypoglycemic Risk of increased hypoglycemic effects of *antidiabetic drugs*
bayberry	*Topical:* To promote wound healing *Oral:* Stimulant, emetic, antidiarrheal May block effects of *antihypertensives*
bee pollen	*Oral:* To treat allergies, asthma, impotence, prostatitis; suggested use to decrease cholesterol levels Risk of hyperglycemia; discourage use by diabetic patients or with *antidiabetic drugs*; may cause allergic reaction in patients allergic to bees
betel palm	*Oral:* Mild stimulant, digestive aid Increased risk of hypertensive crisis with *monoamine oxidase inhibitors (MAOIs)*; blocks heart-rate reduction of *beta-blockers, digoxin*; alters effects of *antiglaucoma drugs*
bilberry	*Oral:* Treatment of diabetes; cardiovascular problems; lowers cholesterol and triglycerides; treatment of diabetic retinopathy; treatment of cataracts, night blindness Increased risk of bleeding with *anticoagulants*; disulfiram-like reaction with *alcohol*
birch bark	*Topical:* Treatment of infected wounds, cuts *Oral:* As tea for relief of stomach ache Topical form very toxic to children
blackberry	*Oral:* As tea for generalized healing; treatment of diabetes Risk of interaction with *antidiabetic drugs*
black cohosh root	*Oral:* Treatment of premenstrual syndrome (PMS), menopausal disorders, rheumatoid arthritis Contains estrogen-like components; caution against use with *hormone replacement therapy* or *hormonal contraceptives*; discourage use during pregnancy and lactation; may lower blood pressure with *sedatives, antihypertensives, anesthetics*; increased risk of fungal infection with *immunosuppressants*
bromelain	*Oral:* Treatment of inflammation, sports injuries, upper respiratory tract infection, PMS, and adjunctive therapy in cancer treatment May cause nausea, vomiting, diarrhea, menstrual disorders
burdock	*Oral:* Treatment of diabetes; atropine-like adverse effects, uterine stimulant May increase hypoglycemic effects of *antidiabetic drugs*
capsicum	*Topical:* External analgesic *Oral:* Treatment of bowel disorders, chronic laryngitis, peripheral vascular disease May increase bleeding with *warfarin, aspirin*; increases cough with *angiotensin-converting enzyme inhibitors (ACEIs)*; increases toxicity with *MAOIs*; increases sedation with *sedatives*
catnip leaves	*Oral:* Treatment of bronchitis, diarrhea
cat's claw	*Oral:* Treatment of allergies, arthritis; adjunct in the treatment of cancers and AIDS Discourage use during pregnancy and lactation and use by transplant recipients; increased risk of bleeding episodes if taken with oral *anticoagulants*; increased hypotension with *antihypertensives*
cayenne pepper	*Topical:* Treatment of burns, wounds, relief of toothache
celery	*Oral:* Lowers blood glucose, acts as a diuretic; may cause potassium depletion Advise caution when taken with *antidiabetic drugs*
chamomile	*Topical:* Treatment of wounds, ulcer, conjunctivitis *Oral:* Treatment of migraines, gastric cramps, relief of anxiety Contains coumarin—closely monitor patients taking *anticoagulants*; may cause depression; monitor patients on *antidepressants*; cross-reaction with ragweed allergies may occur; discourage use during pregnancy and lactation
chaste-tree berry	*Oral:* Progesterone-like effects; used to treat PMS and menopausal problems and to stimulate lactation Advise caution when taken with *hormone replacement therapy* and *hormonal contraceptives*
chicken soup	*Oral:* Breaks up respiratory secretions, bronchodilator, relieves anxiety
chicory	*Oral:* Treatment of digestive tract problems, gout; stimulates bile secretions
Chinese angelica (dong quai)	*Oral:* General tonic; treatment of anemias, PMS, menopause; antihypertensive, laxative Use caution with the flu, hemorrhagic diseases; monitor patients on *antihypertensives, vasodilators*, or *anticoagulants* for toxic effects; advise caution when taken with *hormone replacement therapy*
chondroitin	*Oral:* Treatment of osteoarthritis and related disorders (usually combined with glucosamine) Risk of increased bleeding if combined with *anticoagulants*
chong cao fungi	*Oral:* Antioxidant; promotes stamina, sexual function Discourage use by children

Substance	Reported Uses and Possible Risks
Coleus forskohlii	*Oral:* Treatment of asthma, hypertension, eczema Urge caution when taken with *antihypertensives* or *antihistamines*; severe additive effects can occur; discourage use if patient has hypotension or peptic ulcer
comfrey	*Topical:* Treatment of wounds, cuts, ulcers *Oral:* Gargle for tonsillitis Warn against using with *eucalyptus*; monitor liver function
coriander	*Oral:* Weight loss, lowers blood glucose Advise caution when taken with *antidiabetic drugs*
creatine monohydrate	*Oral:* Enhancement of athletic performance Warn against using with *insulin*; do not use with *caffeine*
dandelion root	*Oral:* Treatment of liver and kidney problems; decreases lactation (after delivery or with weaning); lowers blood glucose Advise caution when taken with *antidiabetic drugs, antihypertensives*, and *quinolone antibiotics*
DHEA (dehydroepiandrosterone)	*Oral:* Slows aging, improves vigor ("Fountain of Youth"); androgenic side effects Risk of interactions with *alprazolam, calcium-channel blockers*, and *antidiabetic drugs*; screen patients older than 40 y for hormonally sensitive cancers before use
dihuang	*Oral:* Treatment of diabetes mellitus Risk of hypoglycemia with *antidiabetic drugs*
dried root bark of *Lycium chinense* Miller	*Oral:* Lowers cholesterol, lowers blood glucose; advise caution with *antidiabetic drugs*
echinacea (cone flower)	*Oral:* Treatment of colds, flu; stimulates the immune system, attacks viruses; causes immunosuppression if used long term May be liver toxic; discourage use longer than 12 wk; caution against taking with *liver-toxic drugs* or *immunosuppressants* Discourage use with *antifungals*; serious liver injury could occur; advise against use by patients with systemic lupus erythematosus, tuberculosis, AIDS
elder bark and flowers	*Topical:* Gargle for tonsillitis, pharyngitis *Oral:* Treatment of fever, chills
ephedra	*Oral:* Increases energy, relieves fatigue May cause serious complications, including death; increased risk of hypertension, stroke, myocardial infarction; interacts with many drugs; *banned by the U.S. Food and Drug Administration*
ergot	*Oral:* Treatment of migraine headaches, treatment of menstrual problems, hemorrhage Monitor patients who take ergot with *antihypertensives*
eucalyptus	*Topical:* Treatment of wounds *Oral:* Decreases respiratory secretions; suppresses cough Warn against using with *comfrey*; very toxic in children
evening primrose	*Oral:* Treatment of PMS, menopause, rheumatoid arthritis, diabetic neuropathy Discourage use with *phenothiazines, antidepressants, including selective serotonin reuptake inhibitors (SSRIs)*—increases risk of seizures; discourage use by those with epilepsy, schizophrenia
false unicorn root	*Oral:* Treatment of menstrual and uterine problems Advise against use during pregnancy and lactation
fennel	*Oral:* Treatment of colic, gout, flatulence; enhances lactation Significantly decreases levels of *ciprofloxacin*
fenugreek	*Oral:* Lowers cholesterol level; reduces blood glucose; aids in healing Advise caution when taken with *antidiabetic drugs, anticoagulants*
feverfew	*Oral:* Treatment of arthritis, fever, migraine Advise caution when taken with *anticoagulants*; may increase bleeding; discourage use before or immediately after surgery because of bleeding risk
fish oil	*Oral:* Treatment of coronary diseases, arthritis, colitis, depression, aggression, attention-deficit disorder
gamboge	*Oral:* Appetite suppressant, lowers cholesterol, promotes weight loss Oral use may be unsafe; discourage use
garlic	*Oral:* Treatment of colds; diuretic; prevention of coronary artery disease; intestinal antiseptic; lowers blood glucose; anticoagulant effects; decreases blood pressure Advise caution if patient has diabetes or takes *oral anticoagulants, antidiabetic agents* Known to affect blood clotting; anemia reported with long-term use
ginger	*Oral:* treatment of nausea, motion sickness, postoperative nausea (may increase risk of miscarriage) Affects blood clotting; warn against use with *anticoagulants*

(table continues on page 1060)

Table E Alternative and Complementary Therapies (continued)

Substance	Reported Uses and Possible Risks
ginkgo	*Oral:* Vascular dilation; increases blood flow to the brain, improving cognitive function; used in treating Alzheimer disease; antioxidant Can inhibit blood clotting; seizures reported with high doses; warn against use with *anticoagulants, aspirin*, or *nonsteroidal anti-inflammatory drugs (NSAIDs)*; can interact with *phenytoin, carbamazepine, phenobarbital, tricyclic antidepressants, MAOIs*, and *antidiabetic drugs*; advise caution
ginseng	*Oral:* Aphrodisiac, mood elevator, tonic; antihypertensive; decreases cholesterol levels; lowers blood glucose; adjunct in cancer chemotherapy and radiation therapy May cause irritability if combined with *caffeine*; inhibits clotting; warn against use with *anticoagulants, aspirin, NSAIDs*; warn against use for longer than 3 mo; may cause headaches, manic episodes if used with *phenelzine, MAOIs*; additive effects of *estrogens* and *corticosteroids*; may also interfere with cardiac effects of *digoxin*; monitor patient closely if he or she takes these drugs or an *antidiabetic drug*
glucosamine	*Oral:* Treatment of osteoarthritis and joint diseases, usually combined with chondroitin Monitor glucose levels in diabetic patients
goldenrod leaves	*Oral:* Treatment of renal disease, rheumatism, sore throat, eczema May decrease effects of *diuretics* by increasing sodium retention; advise caution if patient has a history of allergies
goldenseal	*Oral:* Lowers blood glucose, aids healing; treatment of bronchitis, colds, flu-like symptoms, cystitis May cause false-negative test results in those who use such drugs as marijuana and cocaine; large amounts may cause paralysis; affects blood clotting; warn against use with *anticoagulants*; may interfere with *antihypertensives, acid blockers, barbiturates*; may increase effects of *sedatives*; death can result from overdose
gotu kola	*Topical:* Chronic venous insufficiency Warn against using with *antidiabetic drugs, cholesterol-lowering drugs, sedatives*
grape seed extract	*Oral:* Treatment of allergies, asthma; improves circulation; decreases platelet aggregation Advise caution with *oral anticoagulants*; may increase bleeding
green tea leaf	*Oral:* Antioxidant, to prevent cancer and cardiovascular disease, to increase cognitive function (caffeine effects) Advise caution with *oral anticoagulants*; may increase bleeding; may increase blood pressure; caution against using with *milk*
guarana	*Oral:* Decreases appetite, promotes weight loss Advise caution; increases blood pressure, risk of cardiovascular events
guayusa	*Oral:* Lowers blood glucose; promotes weight loss Advise caution with *antihypertensives*; decreases absorption of *iron* May decrease clearance of *lithium*
hawthorn	*Oral:* Treatment of angina, arrhythmias, blood pressure problems; decreases cholesterol Advise caution with *digoxin, ACEIs, central nervous system (CNS) depressants*; may potentiate effects
hop	*Oral:* Sedative; aids healing; alters blood glucose Discourage use with *CNS depressants, antipsychotics*
horehound	*Oral:* Expectorant; treatment of respiratory problems, gastrointestinal disorders Use caution with *antidiabetic drugs, antihypertensives*
horse chestnut seed	*Oral:* Treatment of varicose veins, hemorrhoids Advise caution with oral *anticoagulants*; may increase bleeding
hyssop	*Topical:* Treatment of cold sores, genital herpes, burns, wounds *Oral:* Treatment of coughs, colds, indigestion, and flatulence Warn against use by pregnant patients and those with seizures; toxic in children and pets
jambul	*Oral:* Treatment of diarrhea, dysentery; lowers blood glucose Use caution with *CNS depressants, Java plum*
java plum	*Oral:* Treatment of diabetes mellitus Advise caution with *antidiabetic drugs*
jojoba	*Topical:* Promotion of hair growth, relief of skin problems Toxic if ingested
juniper berries	*Oral:* Increases appetite, aids digestion; diuretic; urinary tract disinfectant; lowers blood glucose level Advise caution when taken with *antidiabetic drugs*; not for use in pregnancy
kava	*Oral:* Treatment of nervous anxiety, stress, restlessness; tranquilizer Warn against use with *alprazolam*; may cause coma; advise against use with Parkinson disease or history of stroke; discourage use with *St. John's wort, anxiolytics, alcohol*; risk of serious liver toxicity
kudzu	*Oral:* Reduces cravings for *alcohol*; being researched for use with alcoholics Interacts with *anticoagulants, aspirin, antidiabetic drugs, cardiovascular drugs*

Substance	Reported Uses and Possible Risks
lavender	*Topical:* Astringent for minor cuts, burns *Oral:* Treatment of insomnia, restlessness Advise caution with *CNS depressants*; oil is potentially poisonous
Ledum tincture	*Topical:* Treatment of insect bites, puncture wounds; dissolves some blood clots and bruises
licorice	*Oral:* Prevents thirst, soothes coughs; treats "incurable" chronic fatigue syndrome; treatment of duodenal ulcer Acts like aldosterone; blocks *spironolactone* effects; can lead to *digoxin* toxicity because of effects of lowering aldosterone; advise extreme caution; contraindicated with renal or liver disease, hypertension, coronary artery disease, pregnancy, lactation; warn against taking with *thyroid drugs, antihypertensives, hormonal contraceptives*
ma huang	*Oral:* Treatment of colds, nasal congestion, asthma Contains ephedrine; warn against use with *antihypertensives, antidiabetic drugs, MAOIs, digoxin*; serious adverse effects could occur
mandrake root	*Oral:* Treatment of fertility problems
marigold leaves and flowers	*Oral:* Relief of muscle tension, increases wound healing; advise against use during pregnancy and breastfeeding
melatonin	*Oral:* Relief of jet lag; treatment of insomnia, jet lag Advise caution with *antihypertensives, benzodiazepines, beta-blockers, methamphetamine*
milk thistle	*Oral:* Treatment of hepatitis, cirrhosis, fatty liver caused by alcohol or drug use May affect metabolism and increase toxicity of *drugs using cytochrome P450 (CYP450), CYP3A4*, and *CYP2C9* systems
milk vetch	*Oral:* Improves resistance to disease; adjunct therapy in cancer chemotherapy and radiation therapy
mistletoe leaves	*Oral:* Promotes weight loss; relief of signs and symptoms of diabetes Advise caution with *antihypertensives, CNS depressants, immunosuppressants*
Momordica charantia (karela)	*Oral:* Blocks intestinal absorption of glucose; lowers blood glucose; weight loss Advise caution when taken with *antidiabetic drugs*
nettle	*Topical:* Stimulation of hair growth, treatment of bleeding *Oral:* Treatment of rheumatism, allergic rhinitis; antispasmodic; expectorant Advise against use during pregnancy and breastfeeding; increases effects of *diuretics*
nightshade leaves and roots	*Oral:* Stimulates circulatory system; treatment of eye disorders
octacosanol	*Oral:* Treatment of parkinsonism, enhancement of athletic performance Advise against use during pregnancy and lactation; avoid use with *carbidopa–levodopa*
parsley seeds and leaves	*Oral:* Treatment of jaundice, asthma, menstrual difficulties, urinary infections, conjunctivitis Risk of serotonin syndrome with *SSRIs, lithium, opioids*; increased hypotension with *antihypertensives*
passionflower vine	*Oral:* Sedative and hypnotic May increase sedation with other *CNS depressants, MAOIs*; advise against drinking *alcohol* while taking this herb; advise patient not to use with *anticoagulants*
peppermint leaves	*Oral:* Treatment of nervousness, insomnia, dizziness, cramps, coughs *Topical:* Rubbed on forehead to relieve tension headaches
psyllium	*Oral:* Treatment of constipation; lowers cholesterol Can cause severe gas and stomach pain; may interfere with nutrient absorption; avoid use with *warfarin, digoxin, lithium*—absorption of *oral drugs* may be blocked; do not combine with *laxatives*
raspberry	*Oral:* Healing of minor wounds; control and treatment of diabetes, gastrointestinal disorders, upper respiratory disorders Advise caution with *antidiabetic drugs*; disulfiram-like reaction with *alcohol*
red clover	*Oral:* Estrogen replacement in menopause, suppresses whooping cough, asthma Risk of bleeding with *anticoagulants, antiplatelets*; discourage use in pregnancy
red yeast rice	*Oral:* Cholesterol-lowering agent Increased risk of rhabdomyolysis with *cyclosporine, fibric acid, niacin, lovastatin, grapefruit juice*
rose hips	*Oral:* Laxative, to boost the immune system and prevent illness Advise caution with *estrogens, iron, warfarin*
rosemary	*Topical:* Relief of rheumatism, sprains, wounds, bruises, eczema *Oral:* Gastric stimulation, relief of flatulence, stimulation of bile release, relief of colic Disulfiram-like reaction with *alcohol*
rue extract	*Topical:* Relief of pain associated with sprains, groin pulls, whiplash Advise caution with *antihypertensive drugs, digoxin, warfarin*
saffron	*Oral:* Treatment of menstrual problems, abortifacient

(table continues on page 1062)

Table E Alternative and Complementary Therapies (continued)

Substance	Reported Uses and Possible Risks
sage	*Oral:* Lowers blood pressure; lowers blood glucose Advise caution with *antidiabetic drugs, anticonvulsants, alcohol*
SAM-e (*AdoMet*)	*Oral:* Promotion of general well-being and health May cause frequent gastrointestinal complaints and headache Risk of serotonin syndrome with *antidepressants*
sarsaparilla	*Oral:* Treatment of skin disorders, rheumatism Advise caution with *anticonvulsants*
sassafras	*Topical:* Treatment of local pain, skin eruptions *Oral:* Enhancement of athletic performance, "cure" for syphilis Oil may be toxic to fetus, children, and adults when ingested; *interacts with many drugs*
saw palmetto	*Oral:* Treatment of benign prostatic hyperplasia Warn against use with estrogen replacement or hormonal contraceptives—may greatly increase adverse effects; may decrease iron absorption; advise against use with *finasteride*; toxicity could occur
schisandra	*Oral:* Health tonic, liver protectant; adjunct in cancer chemotherapy and radiation therapy Warn against use during pregnancy; causes uterine stimulation; advise caution with all *drugs metabolized in the liver*
squaw vine	*Oral:* Diuretic, tonic, aid in labor and childbirth, treatment of menstrual problems May cause liver toxicity; increased toxicity of *digoxin*; disulfiram-like reaction with *alcohol*
St. John's wort	*Oral:* Treatment of depression, PMS symptoms; antiviral *Topical:* To treat puncture wounds, insect bites, crushed fingers or toes Discourage tyramine-containing foods; hypertensive crisis is possible Thrombocytopenia has been reported; can increase sensitivity to light; advise against taking with drugs that cause photosensitivity; severe photosensitivity can occur in light-skinned people; serious interactions have been reported with *SSRIs, MAOIs, kava, digoxin, theophylline, AIDS antiviral drugs, sympathomimetics, antineoplastics, hormonal contraceptives*; advise against these combinations
sweet violet flowers	*Oral:* Treatment of respiratory disorders; emetic Increases effects of *laxatives*
tarragon	*Oral:* Weight loss; prevents cancer; lowers blood glucose Advise caution with *antidiabetic drugs*
tea tree oil	*Topical:* Antifungal, antibacterial; used to treat burns, insect bites, irritated skin, acne; used as a mouthwash
thyme	*Topical:* As liniment, gargle; to treat wounds *Oral:* Antidiarrheal, relief of bronchitis, laryngitis May increase sensitivity to light; warn against combining with *photosensitivity-causing drugs*; also warn against combining with *MAOIs* or *SSRIs*; may cause serious adverse effects
turmeric	*Oral:* Antioxidant, anti-inflammatory; used to treat arthritis May cause gastrointestinal distress; warn against use with known biliary obstruction; may cause increased bleeding with oral *anticoagulants, NSAIDs*; advise caution with *immunosuppressants*
valerian	*Oral:* Sedative and hypnotic; reduces anxiety, relaxes muscles Can cause severe liver damage; warn against use with *barbiturates, alcohol, CNS depressants*, or *antihistamines*; can cause serious sedation
went rice	*Oral:* Cholesterol- and triglyceride-lowering effects Warn against use in pregnancy, liver disease, alcoholism, or acute infection
white willow bark	*Oral:* Treatment of fevers Advise caution with *anticoagulants, NSAIDs, diuretics*
xuan shen	*Oral:* Lowers blood glucose; slows heart rate; treatment of heart failure Advise caution when taken with *antidiabetic drugs* *Oral:* Treatment of erectile dysfunction Can affect blood pressure; CNS stimulant; has cardiac effects; manic episodes have been reported in psychiatric patients; warn against use with *SSRIs*, tyramine-containing foods; advise caution with *tricyclic antidepressants*

From Karch, A. M. (2015). *2016 Lippincott pocket drug guide for nurses.* Philadelphia, PA: Lippincott Williams & Wilkins.

Diagnostic Agents F

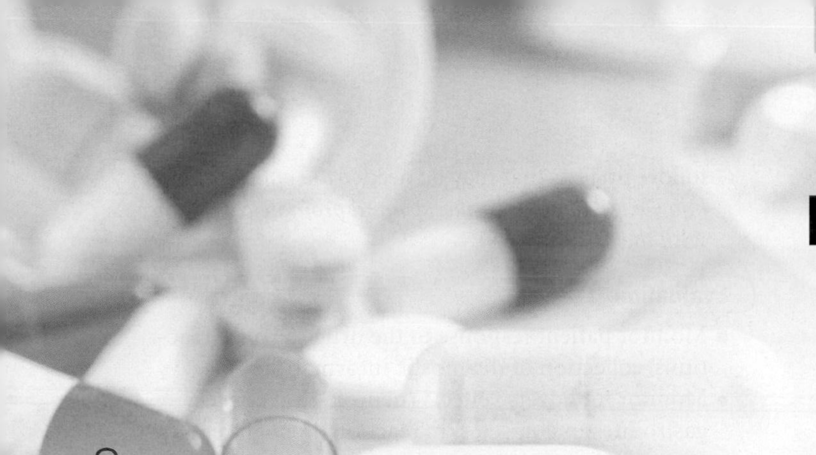

Some pharmacological agents are used solely to diagnose particular conditions. Diagnostic tests that use these agents include the following:

- In vitro tests, which are done outside the body to measure the presence of particular elements (e.g., proteins, blood glucose, bacteria).
- In vivo tests, which introduce drugs into the body to evaluate specific physiological functions (e.g., cardiac output, intestinal absorption, gastric acid secretion).

Therapeutic Actions and Indications

In vitro tests are often performed as part of the nursing evaluation of a patient, or they may be done at home by the patient as part of a medical regimen. These drugs can include reagents that react with specific enzymes or chemicals, such as glucose, blood, or human chorionic gonadotropin (HCG). Drugs used for in vivo tests may stimulate or suppress normal body reactions, such as a glucose challenge to evaluate insulin release or thyroid suppression tests to evaluate thyroid response. Specific tests of blood, urine, or other bodily fluids are often needed to evaluate the body's response to these drugs and to make a diagnosis. Drugs given as part of in vivo tests are administered under the supervision of medical personnel who are either conducting the test or making the diagnosis. They are usually given only once or used over a short period of time. Their use is part of an overall diagnostic plan to determine the underlying source of a particular problem.

Contraindications and Cautions

The use of any of the in vivo drugs is contraindicated *in cases of allergy to the drugs themselves or to the colorants or preservatives used in them*. Specific agents may be contraindicated *in conditions that could be exacerbated by the stimulation of particular body responses*. These drugs should be used cautiously during pregnancy or lactation.

Adverse Effects

The adverse effects seen with diagnostic agents are usually associated with the suppression or stimulation of the response they are being used to test. Because these drugs are given as only part of a test, the adverse effects usually last for a short period and can be tolerated by the patient.

Clinically Important Drug–Drug Interactions

Drug interactions vary with the particular agent that is being used. Consult a drug guide for specific information before giving any diagnostic agent.

Clinically Important Drug–Food Interactions

Because these tests are designed to elicit very specific responses, there is often the possibility that food will interfere with the actions or sensitivity of the test. Consult a drug guide for specific information about drug–food interactions before giving any diagnostic agent.

Nursing Considerations

Assessment: History and Examination

- Screen for the following conditions, which could be contraindications to use of the agent: Presence of known allergy to any of these drugs or to the colorants or preservatives used in these drugs.
- Include screening for baseline status before beginning therapy and for any potential adverse effects. Assess the following: Skin and mucous membrane condition; orientation, affect, and reflexes; pulse, blood pressure, and respirations; abdominal examination; bowel sounds; and blood and urine tests required for the particular test being performed.

Nursing Diagnoses

The patient receiving a diagnostic agent might have the following nursing diagnoses related to drug therapy:

- Acute pain related to effects of the drugs
- Fear related to the test being done and possible test results
- Disturbed body Image related to testing procedure and related tests that must be done
- Deficient knowledge regarding drug therapy

Planning

- The patient will receive the best therapeutic effect from the drug therapy.

(continues on page 1064)

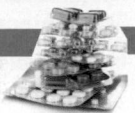

- The patient will have limited adverse effects to the drug therapy.
- The patient will have an understanding of the drug therapy, adverse effects to anticipate, and measures to relieve discomfort and improve safety.

Implementation

- Assess the patient's general physical condition before beginning the test *to decrease the potential for adverse effects.*
- Provide comfort measures *to help patient tolerate drug effects* (e.g., give the drug with food to decrease gastrointestinal upset, provide proper skin care as needed, administer analgesics for headache as appropriate, provide privacy for the collection and storage of urine samples).
- Include information about the drug being used in a test (e.g., what to expect, adverse effects that may occur, follow-up tests that may be needed) *to enhance patient knowledge about drug therapy and promote compliance with the drug regimen.*

Evaluation

- Monitor patient response to the drug (adverse reactions, collection of diagnostic information).
- Monitor for adverse effects (neurological effects, gastrointestinal upset, skin reaction, hypoglycemia, constipation).
- Evaluate the effectiveness of teaching plan (patient can name adverse effects to watch for and specific measures to avoid them; patient understands importance of follow-up that will be needed).
- Monitor the effectiveness of comfort measures and compliance with the regimen.

Table F Diagnostic Agents

Test Object	Brand Names	Usual Indications	Special Considerations
In Vitro Tests			
Acetone	*Acetest*	Test for ketones in urine, blood, serum, or plasma	Most frequently used to test urine; *Acetest* is the only product that is also used for blood products
Albumin	*Albustix, Chemstrip Micral*	At-home urine test for the presence of proteins	Advise patient to follow product storage instructions
Urine bacteria	*Azo Test Strips, Microstix-3, Uricult, Isocult for Bacteriuria*	Test for urine nitrates, uropathogens, gram-negative bacteria	Most accurate if used with a clean catch urine sample
Bilirubin	*Ictotest*	Test for urine bilirubin levels	Most accurate if used with a clean catch urine sample
Blood urea nitrogen (BUN)	*Azostix*	Estimate of BUN	Used as a reagent strip with whole blood
Candida tests	*Isocult for Candida*	Culture paddles or reagent slides for testing vaginal smears	Rapid test for the presence of *Candida* with vaginal examination
Chlamydia trachomatis	*Amplicor, Chlamydiazyme, MicroTrak for Chlamydia, Surecell Chlamydia, Clearview Chlamydia*	Kits and slides for testing urogenital, rectal, conjunctival, and nasopharyngeal specimens for the presence of *Chlamydia*	Kits are specific for testing specimens
Cholesterol	*Advanced Care Cholesterol Test, Cholestrak Total Home Testing Kit*	At-home cholesterol test	Kit includes audio cassette with instructions; patient should be cautioned to seek medical care and advice
Glucose, blood	*Glucostix Glucometer Elite, Accu-Chek, Advantage,* and others	At-home testing of blood glucose levels	Patient should be taught how to calibrate the machine, proper blood-drawing technique, and importance of seeking follow-up medical care
Glucose, urine	*Diastix, Keto-Diastix*	At home testing of urine glucose, ketones	Used as reagent strip for urine; discard after 6 mo
Gonorrhea	*Biocult-GC, Isocult for Neisseria gonorrhoeae*	Kits and culture paddles for the detection of *N. gonorrhoeae* on endocervical, rectal, urethral, and oropharyngeal specimens	Test kits containing reagents, preservatives as needed for detection of *N. gonorrhoeae* during physical examination

Test Object	Brand Names	Usual Indications	Special Considerations
In Vitro Tests			
Mononucleosis	*Mono-Plus*, *Mono-Diff*, *Mono-Spot*, and others	Kits, reagents, and slides for the testing of serum and blood for mononucleosis	Rapid tests for suspected cases of mononucleosis; all necessary reagents and preservatives are included in the kit
Occult blood	*CEZ Detect*, *Hemoccult II*, and others	Kits and slides for the testing of fecal swabs for the presence of occult blood	Card forms can be used by patient at home in routine screening programs
Ovulation	*Answer*, *OvuQuick Self-Test*, *First Response Ovulation Predictor*, and others	Kits to determine the levels of luteinizing hormone in the urine as a predictor of ovulation	Used at home by patient as part of fertility program; patient may need instruction
Pregnancy	*Advance*, *First Response Pregnosis*, and others	Kits or urine strips to detect the presence of HCG as a predictor of pregnancy	May be used at home; patient may need instruction and should be advised to seek follow-up medical care
Rheumatoid factor	*Rheumatoid Factor Test*, *Rheumaton*	Slide tests for the presence of rheumatoid factor in blood, serum, or synovial fluid	An aid in the diagnosis of autoimmune diseases
Sickle cell	*Sickledex*	Kit for the testing of blood for the presence of hemoglobin S	Diagnostic for sickle cell anemia
Streptococci	*Sure Cell Streptococci*, *Culturette 10 Minute Group A Strep ID*, *Bactigen B Streptococcus*, and others	Kits, slides, and culture paddles for the identification of streptococcal infection in blood, serum, urine, throat, and cerebrospinal fluid	Early detection of streptococcal infection to facilitate beginning of treatment before culture and sensitivity results are known
In Vivo Tests			
Arginine	*R-Gene 10*	Diagnostic aid to assess pituitary reserve of growth hormone	IV infusion, followed by blood tests to monitor response
Benzylpenicilloyl polylysine	*Pre-Pen*	Skin test to evaluate sensitivity to penicillin and safety of administering penicillin in potentially sensitive individuals	Intradermal or scratch test is used; positive reaction is usually seen within 10–15 min
Indocyanine green	Generic	Determining cardiac output, hepatic function, and liver blood flow; also used for ophthalmic angiography	Use caution in patient with known allergy to dyes
Methacholine chloride	*Provocholine*	Diagnosis of bronchial airway hypersensitivity in patients without documented asthma	Inhaled with pulmonary function test immediately; may cause hypotension, chest pain, or gastrointestinal upset
Secretin	*SecroFlo*	Diagnosis of pancreatic exocrine disease; diagnosis of gastrinoma	Requires a 12-h to 15-h fast; passing of a radiopaque tube for pancreatic function or repeated blood samples for gastrinoma diagnosis
Sincalide	*Kinevac*	Stimulation of gallbladder contractions, pancreatic secretion to evaluate for stones, enzyme activity	*Gallbladder:* Given IV over 30–60 s *Pancreatic function:* Given IV over 60 min
Sodium iodide	*Sodium Iodide I-123*	Diagnosis of thyroid function or morphology	Handle with care; oral capsules are radioactive, dispose of properly; thyroid can be evaluated for radiation content within 6 h of dose
Thyrotropin alpha	*Thyrogen*	Differentiation of thyroid function to estimate thyroid reserve	Given IM every 24 h for two doses; follow with radioactive iodine and thyroid scan

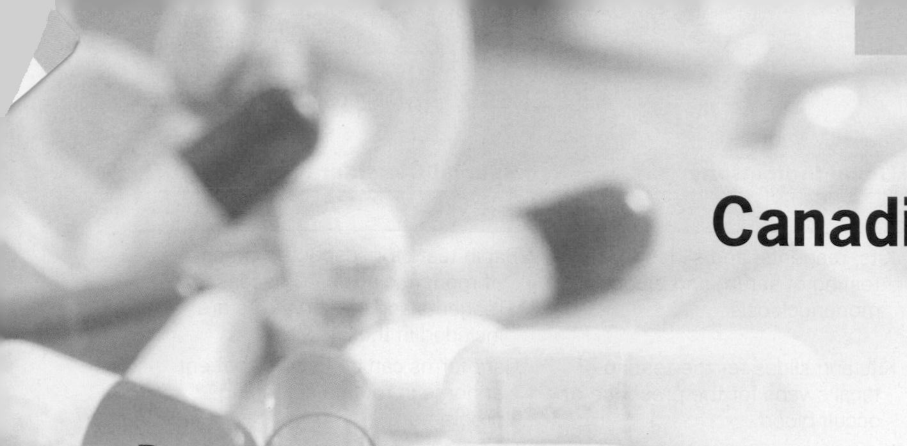

Canadian Drug Names G

Presented here is a list of Canadian brand names for frequently used drugs. The brand name appears in italics with the corresponding generic name listed in parentheses.

A

Abenol (acetaminophen)
Acet (acetaminophen)
Acid Control (cimetidine)
Acid Reducer (cimetidine)
Aclasta (zoledronic acid)
Activasert-PA (alteplase)
Adalat XL (nifedipine)
Airomir (albuterol)
Akcarpine (pilocarpine)
AK-Con (naphazoline)
AK-Dex (dexamethasone)
AK-Dilate (phenylephrine)
AK Mycin (gentamicin)
AK Pentolate (cyclopentolate)
AK Trol (dexamethasone)
Alcomicin (gentamicin)
Alertec (modafinil)
Aller-Aid (diphenhydramine)
Allerdryl (diphenhydramine)
Allergy Formula (diphenhydramine)
Allerject (epinephrine)
Allernix (diphenhydramine)
Aller Relief (cetirizine)
Alloprin (allopurinol)
Alugel (aluminum hydroxide)
Anapen (epinephrine)
Ancalixir (phenobarbital)
Androcur (cyproterone)
Anexate (flumazenil)
Apo-Cal (calcium carbonate)
Apo-Cloxi (cloxacillin)
Apo-Diclo (diclofenac)
Apo-Erythro (erythromycin)
Apo-Folic (folic acid)
Apo-Indomethacin (indomethacin)
Apo-Keto (ketoprofen)
Apo-Keto-E (ketoprofen)
Apo-Salvent (albuterol)
Apo-Triazo (triazolam)
Apprilon (tetracycline)
Aristocort C (triamcinolone)
Aristocort R (triamcinolone)
Arthrinol (aspirin)
Arthrisin (aspirin)
Artria S.R. (aspirin)
Artritol (acetaminophen)
Asaphen (aspirin)
Astrin (aspirin)
Atacand Plus (candesartan/hydrochlorothiazide)
Atasol (acetaminophen)
Atridox (tetracycline)
Anamys (fluticasone)
Aventyl (nortriptyline)

B

Balminil DM (dextromethorphan)
Balminil Expectorant (guaifenesin)
Barriere-HC (hydrocortisone)
Bentylol (dicyclomine)
Benylin (diphenhydramine)
Betaderm (betamethasone)
Betaject (betamethasone)
Betaloc IV (metoprolol)
Betaxin (thiamine)
Bronchophan Expectorant (guaifenesin)
Bronchophan Forte DM (dextromethorphan)
Buckley's DM (dextromethorphan)
Burinex (bumetanide)
Bustab (buspirone)

C

Caelyx (doxorubicin)
Calcite (calcium carbonate)
Calglycine (calcium)
Calmex (diphenhydramine)
Calsan (calcitonin)
Caltine (calcitonin, salmon)
Canesoral (fluconazole)
Canesten Topical (clotrimazole)
Canesten Vaginal (clotrimazole)
Carbolith (lithium)
Carter's Little Pills (bisacodyl)
Ceclor (cephalosporin)
Celestoderm (betamethasone)
Celesentri (maraviroc)
C.E.S. (estrogen)
Champix (varenicline)
Citamycin (gentamicin)
Cipralex (escitalopram)
Citro-Mag (magnesium)
Clarus (isotretinoin)
Clavulin (amoxicillin/clavulanate)
ClearLax (polyethylene glycol)
Clinda-T (clindamycin)
Clonopam (clonazepam)
Clotrimaderm (clotrimazole)
Codulax (bisacodyl)
Congest (estrogen)
Cortate (hydrocortisone)
Cortoderm (hydrocortisone)
Coryphen (aspirin)
Coversyl (perindopril)
Crystapen (penicillin G)
Cyclocort (amcinonide)
Cytosar (cytarabine)

D

Dalacin C (clindamycin)
Dalacin T (clindamycin)
Dermovate (clobetasol)
Desocort (desonide)
Desoxi (desoximetasone)
Dexasone (dexamethasone)
Dexiron (iron dextran)
Diazemuls (diazepam)

Diodex (dexamethasone)
Diogent (gentamicin)
Diomycin (erythromycin)
Dionephrin (nephazoline)
Diopentolate (cyclopentolate)
Diopred (prednisolone)
Diopticon (nephazalone)
Diosulf (sulfacetamide)
Diotrope (tropicamide)
Dioval Plus (magnesium hydroxide/ aluminum hydroxide)
Diprosone (betamethasone)
Dixarit (clonidine)
Doloral (morphine)
Dormex (diphenhydramate)
Dormiphen (diphenhydramate)
Dosolax (docusate)
Doxycin (doxycycline)
Doxytab (doxycycline)
Drymira (ciclesonide)
Durela (tramadol)

E

Ebixa (memantine)
Elavil (amitriptyline)
Elocom (mometasone)
Eltroxin (levothyroxine)
Emocort (hydrocortisone)
Entrophen (aspirin)
Epimorph (morphine)
Epival (valproic acid)
Eprex (epoetin)
Erybid (erythromycin)
Erysol (erythromycin)
Erythro EC (erythromycin)
Erythro ES (erythromycin)
Erythro-S (erythromycin)
Estradot (estradiol)
Etibi (ethambutol)
Euglucon (glyburide)
Euthyrox (levothyroxine)
Ezetrol (ezetimibe)

F

Fampyra (dalfampridine)
Fasturtec (rasburicase)
Fenomax (fenofibrate)
Fluanxol (flupentixol)
Fluoderm (fluocinolone)
Formulex (dicyclomine)
Fortolin (acetaminophen)
Fungizone (amphotericin B)
Furantoin (nitrofurantoin)

G

Gen-Triazolam (triazolam)
Gluconorm (repaglinide)
Glycon (metformin)

H

Hepalean (heparin)
Heptovir (lamivudine)
Hexit (lindane)
Histanil (promethazine)
Hycodan (hydrocodone)
Hycort (hydrocortisone)
Hyderm (hydrocortisone)
Hydromorph Contin (hydromorphone)
Hydroval (hydrocortisone)

I

Imovane (zopiclone)
Impril (imipramine)
Indameth (indomethacin)
Indocid P.D.A. (indomethacin)
Infacol (simethicone)
Infufer (iron dextran)
Insomnal (diphenhydramine)
Insulin Toronto (insulin)
Isotamine (isoniazid)

J

Jurnista (hydromorphone)

K

Karacil (psyllium)
K-Exit (sodium polystyrene sulfonate)
Klean Prep (polyethylene glycol/ electrolytes)
Koffex DM (dextromethorphan)

L

Lax-A-Day (polyethylene glycol)
Levate (amitriptyline)
Levocarb CR (carbidopa/levodopa)
Lidemol (fluocinonide)
Lipidil (fenofibrate)
Lithane (lithium)
Lithmax (lithium)
Lodalis (colesevelam)
Lopresor (metoprolol)
Lopresor SR (metoprolol)
Losec (omeprazole)
Lotriderm (clotrimazole)
Lyderm (flucinonide)

M

Mazepine (carbamazepine)
Medroxy (medroxyprogesterone)
Megace OS (megestrol)
M-Eslon (morphine)
Mestinon SR (pyridostigmine)
Metadol (methadone)
Metonia (metoclopramide)
Micozole (miconazole)
Midamor (amiloride)
Mobicox (meloxicam)
Monicure (fluconazole)
Morphine HP Injection (morphine)
MOS (morphine)
MOS SR (morphine)
Mucomyst (acetylcysteine)
Multipax (hydroxyzine)
Mydifrin (phenylephrine)
Myocet (doxorubicin)

N

Nadostine (nystatin)
Nadril (diphenhydramine)
Naphcon A (naphazoline)
Naprosyn (naproxen)
Natulan (procarbazine)
Neocitran Thin Strips Cough (dextromethorphan)
Nimotop (nimodipine)
Nitrogard SR (nitroglycerin)
Nolvadex-D (tamoxifen)
Norventyl (nortriptyline)
Novamoxin (amoxicillin)
Novasen (aspirin)
Novofolacid (folic acid)
Novolin ge NPH (insulin)
Novo-Methacin (indomethacin)
Novonidazol (metronidiazole)
Novorapid (insulin)
Novo-Trialom (triazolam)
Novoxapam (oxazepam)
Nu-Cal (calcium carbonate)
Nu-Indo (indomethacin)
Nu-Triazo (triazolam)
Nyaderm (nystatin)

O

Oesclim (estradiol)
Oleptro (trazodone)
Onbrez Breezhaler (indacaterol)
Ondissolve ODF (ondansetron)
Opcon A (naphazoline)
Opticrom (cromolyn)
Orudis-E (ketoprofen)
Orudis-SR (ketoprofen)
Ovol (simethicone)
Oxy-IR (oxycodone)
Oxyneo (oxycodone)

P

Pancrease V (pancrelipase)
Panto IV (pantoprazole)
Pantoloc (pantoprazole)
Pariet (rabeprazole)
Parvolex (acetylcysteine)
Pediacol (simethicone)
Pediaphen (acetaminophen)
Pediatrix (acetaminophen)
Pediazole (erythromycin)
Pegalax (polyethylene glycol)
Peptic Guard (famotidine)
Pharmorubicin PFS (epirubicin)
Phenazo (phenazopyridine)
Pitrex (tolnaftate)
PMS Egozinc (zinc)
PMS Isoniazid (isoniazid)
PMS Lindane (lindane)
PMS Nystatin (nystatin)
PMS Pyrazinamide (pyrazinamide)
Polylax (polyethylene glycol/ electrolytes)
Posanol (posaconazole)
Prefrin (phenylephrine)
Presyn (vasopressin)
Prevex (betamethasone)
Prevex HC (betamethasone)
Prochlorazine (prochlorperazine)
Procytox (cyclophosphamide)
Prodiem (psyllium)
Propyl-Thyracil (propylthiouracil)
Protrin DF (trimethoprim/ sulfamethoxazole)
Protylol (dicyclomine)

R

Ralivia (tramadol)
Rasilez (alikiren)
Reactine (cetirizine)
Relaxa (polyethylene glycol)
Reminyl ER (galantamine)
Renedil (felodipine)
RestoraLax (polyethylene glycol)
Revimine (dopamine)
Rhinalar (flunisolide)
Rhodis (ketoprofen)
Rivanase AQ (beclomethasone)
Rivasa (aspirin)
Rivasone (betamethasone)
Rivotril (clonazepam)
Robaxacet (methocarbamol/ acetaminophen)
Robitussin AC Liquid (dextromethorphan)
Rofact (rifampin)
Rogitine (phentolamine)
Rolene (betamethasone)
Rosone (betamethasone)
Rylosol (sotalol)

S

Salazopyrin EN-Tabs (sulfasalazine)
Salbutamol (salbuterol)
Sarna HC (hydrocortisone)
Sedatuss (dextromethorphan)
Selax (docusate)
Sinequan (doxepin)
Soflax (docusate)
Soflax Ex (bisacodyl)
Statex (morphine)
Stieprox (ciclopirox)
Sulcrate (sucralfate)
Syn-Nadolol (nadolol)

T

Taminol (acetaminophen)
Tamofen (tamoxifen)
Tamone (tamoxifen)
Tamoplex (tamoxifen)
Tazocin (pipercillin/tazoactam)
Tebrazid (pyrazinamide)
Tecnal (butalbital, aspirin, caffeine)
Tecta (pantoprazole)
Tegretol CR (carbamazepine)
Telzir (fosamprenavir)
Tempra (acetaminophen)
Tiamol (fluocinonide)
Toloxin (digoxin)
Topactin (fluocinonide)
Topiderm (hydrocortisone)
Toradol (ketorolac)
Trajenta (linagliptin)
Trandate (labetalol)
Transderm-V (scopolamine)
Trazorel (trazodone)
Tremytoine (phenytoin)
Triaderm (triamcinolone)
Triaminic DM (dextromethorphan)
Triaminic Long-Acing Children's Cough (dextromethorphan)
Tridesilon (desonide)
Tridural (tramadol)
Trikacide (metronidazole)
Trisulfa (trimethoprim/ sulfamethoxazole)
Trisulfa S (trimethoprim/ sulfamethoxazole)
Trosec (trospium)

U

Ulcidine (famotidine)
Uremol HC (hydrocortisone)
Uromitexan (mesna)
Urozide (hydrochlorothiazide)

V

Velbe (vinblastine)
Ventolin Diskus (albuterol)
Ventolin Nebules (albuterol)
Vibra-Tabs (tetracycline)

W

Winpred (prednisone)

X

Xatral (alfuzosin)
Xerese (acyclovir)
Xylocard (lidocaine)

Z

Zeldox (ziprasidone)
Zytram Xl (tramadol)
Zyvoxam (linezolid)

Tables of Normal Values H

Note: Values and units of measurement listed in these tables are derived from several resources. Substantial variation exists in the ranges quoted as "normal" and may vary depending on the assay used by different laboratories. Therefore, these tables should be considered as directional only. Some values (e.g., hormones) vary by gender, age, time of day, and condition (e.g., pregnancy) so a text on endocrinology should be consulted for complete data. Where possible, Canadian sources are used; globalrph.com was used to provide non-SI unit conversions.

Abbreviations: CCS, Canadian Cardiovascular Society; CHEP, Canadian Hypertension Education Program; HDL, high-density lipoprotein; LDL, low-density lipoprotein; MCC, Medical Council of Canada; PSA, prostate-specific antigen; TIBC, total iron-binding capacity.

Table H.1 Vital Signs and Body Mass Index

Parameter	Normal Values
Blood Pressure (Systolic/Diastolic) ***CHEP 2012***	
At physician's office (average five measurements)	<140/90 mm Hg
Ambulatory BP monitor	<135/85 mm Hg
With diabetes	<130/80 mm Hg
Heart Rate (HR) or Pulse	
Bradycardia	<60 beats/min
Normal	60–80 beats/min
Tachycardia	>100 beats/min
Respiration Rate (RR)	
Bradypnea	<12 breaths/min
Normal (eupnea)	12–18 breaths/min
Tachypnea	>18 breaths/min
Body Temperature	
Fever	>37.5°C
Normal	36.5–37.5°C (approximate)
Hypothermia	<35.0°C
Body Mass Index (BMI)	
Underweight	<18.5 kg/m^2
Normal (Health Canada 2012)	18.5–24.9 kg/m^2 (Caucasian)
Overweight	25.0–29.9 kg/m^2
Obesity class I	30.0–34.9 kg/m^2
Obesity class II	35.0–39.9 kg/m^2
Obesity class III (extreme, morbid)	≥40.0 kg/m^2

Table H.2 Common Blood Chemistries

Parameter	SI Units (Canada)	Traditional Units (USA)
Albumin (MCC 2012)	35–50 g/L	3.5–5.0 g/dL
Alanine aminotransferase (ALT) (MCC 2012)	3–36 U/L	3–36 U/L
Alkaline phosphatase(ALP serum) (MCC 2012)	35–100 U/L	35–100 U/L
Ammonia (NH_3)	12–41 µmol/L	20–70 mcg/dL
Amylase (serum) (MCC 2012)	<160 U/L	<160 U/L
Aspartate aminotransferase (AST) (MCC 2012)	0–35 U/L	0–35 U/L
Bicarbonate (HCO_3)(serum) (MCC 2012)	24–30 mmol/L	24–30 mEq/L
Bilirubin serum (MCC 2012), total	<26 µmol/L	<1.5 mg/dL
Bilirubin, conjugated (direct)	<7 µmol/L	<0.4 mg/dL
Blood urea nitrogen (BUN) (MCC 2012)	2.5–8.0 mmol/L	7–22 mg/dL
Calcium serum (MCC 2012)		
— Total	2.18–2.58 mmol/L	8.7–10.3 mg/dL
— Ionized	1.05–1.3 mmol/L	4.2–5.2 mg/dL
Carbon dioxide pressure, arterial ($PaCO_2$)	35–45 mm Hg	35–45 mm Hg
Chloride serum (MCC 2012)	98–106 mmol/L	98–106 mEq/L
Cholesterol, Total		
— Desirable	<5.2 mmol/L	<200 mg/dL
— Borderline high	5.2–6.2 mmol/L	201–240 mg/dL
— High	>6.2 mmol/L	>241 mg/dL
Cholesterol, LDL (CCS 2012)		
— High-risk patients (Framingham risk score)	<2.0 mmol/L or >50% reduction	<77.3 mg/dL or >50% reduction
— Intermediate-risk patient if LDL >3.5	<2.0 mmol/L or 50% reduction	<77.3 mg/dL or 50% reduction
— Low-risk patient if LDL >5.0	>50% reduction from baseline	>50% reduction from baseline
Cholesterol, HDL low	<1.00 mmol/L	<40 mg/dL
Creatine kinase serum (CK also CPK) (MCC 2012)	5–130 U/L	5–130 U/L
Copper	11.0–25.0 µmol/L	70–155 mcg/dL
Creatinine, serum		
— Male	70–120 µmol/L	0.8–1.4 mg/dL
— Female	50–90 µmol/L	0.56–1.0 mg/dL
Creatinine clearance (adult)	75–125 mL/min	75–125 mL/min
Ferritin	22–561 pmol/L	10–250 ng/mL
Folic acid (folate) (MCC 2012)	7–36 nmol/L	3–16ng/mL
Gamma glutamyl transferase (GGT)		
— Female	5–36 U/L	5–36 U/L
— Male	8–61 U/L	8–61 U/L
Glucose, fasting		
— Normal	3.3–5.8 mmol/L	59–105 mg/dL
Glucose, postprandial		
— Normal	<6.5 mmol/L	<120 mg/dL
Glycosylated hemoglobin—HbA1C normal (MCC 2012)	4%–6%	4%–6%
beta-Hydroxybutyrate	<270 µmol/L	<2.8 mg/dL
Iron (MCC 2012)	11–32 µmol/L	60–178 pg/dL
Iron-binding capacity, total—TIBC	45–82 µmol/L	251–460 pg/dL
Lactic acid (lactate plasma venous)	0.9–1.8 mmol/L	9–16 mg/dL
Lactate dehydrogenase serum (LDH) (MCC 2012)	95–195 U/L	95–195 IU/L
Magnesium serum	0.75–0.95 mmol/L	1.82–2.31 mg/dL
Osmolality serum (MCC 2012)	280–300 mmol/kg	280–300 mOsm/kg
Oxygen partial pressure, arterial—PaO_2 (MCC 2012)	85–105 mm Hg	85–105 mm Hg
pH—arterial	7.35–7.45 pH	7.35–7.45 pH
Phosphorus, inorganic (MCC 2012)	0.80–1.50 mmol/L	2.5–4.5 mg/dL
Potassium	3.5–5.0 mmol/L	3.5–5.0 mEq/L

Parameter	SI Units (Canada)	Traditional Units (USA)
Protein, total		
— Plasma	60–80 g/L	6.0–8.0 g/dL
— Urine	<0.15 g/d	<150 mg/24 h
PSA serum (MCC 2012)		
— 40 years or older	0–4 mcg/L	0–4 mcg/L
Pyruvate (pyruvic acid)	31–102 μmol/L	0.30–0.90 mg/dL
Sodium serum	135–145 mmol/L	135–145 mEq/L
Transferrin serum	1.88–3.41 g/L	188–341 mg/dL
Transferrin saturation	0.2–0.5	20%–50%
Triglyceride (MCC 2012)	<2.20 mmol/L	<195 mg/dL
Troponin T	<0.01 mcg/L	<0.01 mcg/L
Uric acid (MCC 2012)	180–420 μmol/L	3.0–7.0 mg/dL
— Blood urea nitrogen (BUN)	2.5–8.0 mmol/L	7–22.4 mg/dL
Vitamin B_{12} (*Cyanocobalamin*)	74–516 pmol/L	100–700 pg/mL
Zinc	9.2–19.9 μmol/L	60–130 mcg/dL

Table H.3 Hematological Parameters

Parameter	SI Units (Canada)	Traditional Units (USA)
Red Blood Cells		
Erythrocytes (RBC) (MCC 2012)		
— Female	4.0–5.2 $\times 10^{12}$/L	4.0–5.2 $\times 10^{6}$/mm^3
— Male	4.4–5.7 $\times 10^{12}$/L	4.4–5.7 $\times 10^{6}$/mm^3
Reticulocyte count (MCC 2012)	20–84 $\times 10^{9}$/L	0.5%–2.5%
Hematocrit (MCC 2012)		
— Female	0.370–0.460 g/L	37%–46%
— Male	0.420–0.520 g/L	42%–52%
Hemoglobin		
— Female	123–157 g/L	12.3–15.7 g/dL
— Male	140–174 g/L	14.0–17.4 g/dL
Erythrocyte sedimentation rate (ESR Westergren) (MCC 2012)		
— Female	<10 mm/h	<10 mm/h
— Male	<6 mm/h	<6 mm/h
White Blood Cells (WBC)		
White blood cell count	4.0–10.0 $\times 10^{9}$/L	4.0–10.0 $\times 10^{3}$/mm^3
WBC differential (MCC 2012)		
Segmented neutrophils	2–7 $\times 10^{9}$/L	45%–75%
Lymphocytes	1.5–3.4 $\times 10^{9}$/L	16%–46%
Monocytes	0.14–0.86 $\times 10^{9}$/L	4%–11%
Band neutrophils	<0.7 $\times 10^{9}$/L	0%–5%
Eosinophils	<0.45 $\times 10^{9}$/L	0%–8%
Basophils	<0.10 $\times 10^{9}$/L	0%–3%
Coagulation		
Bleeding time (Ivy) (MCC 2012)	<9 min	<9 min
Clotting time	5–15 min	5–15 min
Fibrinogen	5.1–11.8 μmol/L	175–400 mg/dL
International normalized ratio (INR) (MCC 2012)	0.9–1.2	0.9–1.2
Plasminogen	75%–140%	75%–140%
Platelet count (thrombocytes) (MCC 2012)	130–400 $\times 10^{9}$ /L	130–400 $\times 10^{3}$/mm^3
Prothrombin time (PT) (MCC 2012)	10–13 s	10–13 s
Partial thromboplastin time (PTT) (MCC 2012)	28–38 s	28–38 s
Thrombin time	14–16 s	14–16 s

Table H.4 Hormones

Parameter	SI Units (Canada)	Traditional Units (USA)
Adrenocorticotropin (ACTH)	1.3–16.7 pmol/L	6.0–76.0 pg/mL
Aldosterone (normal sodium diet adult)	0.52–0.94 nmol/L	19–34 ng/dL
Calcitonin		
— Female	<6.4 ng/L	<6.4 pg/mL
— Male	<13.8 ng/L	<13.8 pg/mL
Cortisol serum		
—Time: AM	110–607 nmol/L	5–25 mcg/dL
—Time: PM	83–469 nmol/L	3.1–16.7 mcg/dL
Estrogens (such as estradiol)		
— Female (premenopausal)	185–1,625 pmol/L	50–450 pg/mL
— Male	<200	<55
Follicle-stimulating hormone (FSH)		
— Female (premenopausal)	2–12 IU/L	2–12 IU/L
— Male	1–12	1–12
Glucagon	50–200 ng/L	50–200 pg/mL
Growth hormone	<8 mcg/L	<8 ng/mL
Insulin	36–179 pmol/L	5–25 μU/L
Luteinizing hormone (LH)		
— Female (premenopausal)	0.0–76 IU/L	0.0–76 IU/L
— Male	1.5–9.3 IU/L	1.5–9.3 IU/L
Parathyroid hormone (PTH)	1.2–5.8 pmol/L	11–54 pg/mL
Progesterone		
— Female (mid-luteal phase)	14.3–64 nmol/L	4.5–25.2 ng/mL
— Male	0.95–3.18 nmol/L	0.3–1.0 ng/mL
Prolactin	<1.29 nmol/L	<30 ng/mL
Renin activity		
— Normal sodium diet	0.5–4.0 ng/mL/h	0.5–4.0 ng/mL/h
—Thyroxine (T4 free serum)	8.5–15.2 pmol/L	0.66–1.18 ng/dL
—Triiodothyronine (T3 free serum) (MCC 2012 for SI units)	3.5–6.5 pmol/L	227–422 ng/dL
Testosterone		
— Female	<2.1 nmol/L	<62 ng/dL
— Male	6.7–28.9 nmol/L	300–1000 ng/dL
Thyroid-stimulating hormone (TSH) (MCC 2012)	0.4–5.0 μU/mL	0.4–5.0 μU/mL
Vitamin D3	60–105 nmol/L	24–40 ng/mL
— Cholecalciferol		
— 25-Hydroxy-cholecalciferol	25–137 nmol/L	10–55 ng/mL
— 1,25-Dihydroxy-cholecalciferol	58–156 pmol/L	24–65 pg/mL

I

Canadian Recommended Immunization Schedules

This is based on an update of the National Advisory Committee on Immunization (NACI) Recommended Routine Immunization Schedule for Infants and Children published in the *Canadian Immunization Guide*, 2012–2014 updates. Publicly funded immunization programs may vary by province and territory. For more information on specific vaccines and on the NACI recommended immunization schedules for children who did not commence their immunization in early infancy, consult the *Canadian Immunization Guide*, 2013 (http://www.phac-aspc.gc.ca/publicat/cig-gci/index.html) and the vaccine manufacturer's package insert. Yearly recommendations are available online at http://www.phac-aspc.gc.ca/im/is-cv/index-eng.php#a.

General Recommendations

Administration of vaccines in accordance with the immunization schedules summarized in the following tables will provide optimal protection from vaccine-preventable diseases for most individuals. However, modifications of the recommended schedule may be necessary due to missed appointments or illness. **In general, interruption of an immunization series does not require restarting the vaccine series, regardless of the interval between doses. Individuals with interrupted immunization schedules should be vaccinated to complete the appropriate schedule for their *current* age.** See Timing of Vaccine Administration in Part 1 and vaccine-specific chapters in Part 4 of *Canadian Immunization Guide* for additional information.

Similar, but not identical, vaccines may be available from different manufacturers; therefore, it is useful to review the relevant chapters in the *Canadian Immunization Guide* as well as the manufacturer's product leaflet or product monograph before administering a vaccine. See Principles of Vaccine Interchangeability in Part 1 for information about the interchangeability of similar vaccines from different manufacturers. Product monographs are continually updated; it is best practice to consult the product monographs for vaccines which can be found in Health Canada's Drug Product Database (http://www.hc-sc.gc.ca/dhp-mps/prodpharma/databasdon/index-eng.php).

Table I.1 Routine Childhood Immunization Schedule: Infants and Children (birth to 17 years of age)

- For children at risk due to underlying medical conditions, see Table I.4 for additional recommendations for immunization.
- [·] = dose(s) may not be required depending upon age of child and/or vaccine used (see the relevant vaccine-specific chapter in Part 4 and provincial/territorial schedule).
- See Table I.8 for abbreviations and brand names for vaccines. See Timing of Vaccine Administration and Vaccine Administration Practices in Part 1 regarding administration of multiple injections. See vaccine-specific chapters in Part 4 for additional information.

	Age															
Vaccine	Birth	2 mo	4 mo	6 mo	12 mo	15 mo	18 mo	23 mo	2 y	4 y	5 y	6 y	9 y	12 y	14–16 y	17 y

Table 1—Footnote A

Diphtheria toxoid–tetanus toxoid–acellular pertussis–inactivated polio–*Haemophilus influenzae* type b (DTaP-IPV-Hib): For infants and children beginning primary immunization at 7 months of age and older, the number of doses of Hib vaccine required varies by age.

Table 1—Footnote B

Diphtheria toxoid–tetanus toxoid–acellular pertussis–hepatitis B–inactivated polio–*Haemophilus influenzae* type b (DTaP-HB-IPV-Hib): An alternative schedule may be used at 2, 4 and 12 to 23 months of age with DTaP-IPV-Hib vaccine at 6 months of age.

Table 1—Footnote C

Diphtheria toxoid–tetanus toxoid–acellular pertussis–inactivated polio (DTaP-IPV) *or* **tetanus toxoid–reduced diphtheria toxoid–reduced acellular pertussis–inactivated polio** (Tdap-IPV).

Table 1—Footnote D

Tetanus toxoid–reduced diphtheria toxoid–reduced acellular pertussis (Tdap): 10 years after last dose.

Table 1—Footnote E

Rotavirus: Rot-5 vaccine—3 doses, at least 4 weeks apart; Rot-1 vaccine—2 doses, at least 4 weeks apart. Give first dose between 6 weeks and 14 weeks and 6 days of age. Do not initiate series in infants aged 15 weeks or older. Administer all doses by age 8 months plus 0 days.

Table 1—Footnote F

Pneumococcal conjugate 13-valent: Healthy infants, consider a 3-dose schedule—2, 4, and 12 months of age. Infants beginning primary immunization at 7–11 months of age—2 doses, at least 8 weeks apart followed by a third dose after 12 months of age, at least 8 weeks after the second dose. Children who have received age-appropriate pneumococcal vaccination with a conjugate pneumococcal vaccine but not Pneu-C-13: 12–35 months of age—1 dose; 36–59 months of age and of aboriginal origin or attend group child care—1 dose; other healthy children 36–59 months of age—consider 1 dose.

Table 1—Footnote G

Meningococcal conjugate monovalent: Healthy children, 1 dose at 12 months of age. Meningococcal immunization may begin in infancy depending on provincial/territorial schedule; schedule for infants depends on age at first dose and vaccine used. If Men-C-C first received at less than 12 months of age, give a booster dose at 12–23 months of age. If Men-C-C first received at 12 months of age or older, only 1 dose required until adolescence. See Table I.4 for alternate recommended meningococcal immunization for children considered at risk.

Table 1—Footnote H

Meningococcal conjugate monovalent or quadrivalent: Early adolescence (around 12 years of age)—1 dose, even if meningococcal conjugate vaccine received at a younger age. Vaccine chosen depends on local epidemiology and programmatic considerations.

Table 1—Footnote I

Measles–mumps–rubella: First dose at 12–15 months of age; second dose at 18 months of age or anytime thereafter, typically before school entry.

Table 1—Footnote J

Varicella: First dose at 12–15 months of age; second dose at 18 months of age or anytime thereafter, typically before school entry.

Table 1—Footnote K

Measles–mumps–rubella–varicella: First dose at 12–15 months of age; second dose at 18 months of age or anytime thereafter, typically before school entry.

Table 1—Footnote L

Hepatitis B: Preferred schedule—months 0, 1, and 6 (first dose = month 0) with at least 4 weeks between the first and second dose, 2 months between the second and third dose, and 4 months between the first and third dose. Alternatively, HB may be routinely administered in infancy as DTaP-HB-IPV-Hib vaccine, with first dose at 2 months of age. See Table I.4 for recommended HB immunization for newborns considered at risk.

Table 1—Footnote M

Hepatitis B: 9–17 years of age—preferred 3-dose schedule, months 0, 1, and 6 (first dose = month 0) with at least 4 weeks between the first and second dose, at least 2 months between the second and third dose, and at least 4 months between the first and third dose; 11–15 years of age—2-dose schedule (months 0 and 4–6, depending on product used).

Table 1—Footnote N

Human papillomavirus: Girls—HPV2 vaccine—months 0, 1, and 6 (first dose = month 0) *or* HPV4 vaccine—months 0, 2, and 6 (first dose = month 0). Boys—HPV4 vaccine—months 0, 2, and 6 (first dose = month 0).

Table 1—Footnote O

Influenza: Recommended annually for children 6–59 months of age (fifth birthday) and encouraged for older children. Children (6 months–8 years of age, previously immunized with Inf) and children (9 years of age and older) —1 dose. Children (6 months–less than 9 years of age, receiving Inf for the first time)—2 doses, at least 4 weeks apart.

DTaP-IPV-Hib		Footnote A	Footnote A	Footnote A	Footnote A Generally at 18 months				
					OR				
DTaP-HB-IPV-Hib *followed by* **DTaP-IPV-Hib**		Footnote B	Footnote B	Footnote B	Footnote A Generally at 18 months				
DTaP-IPV *or* **Tdap-IPV**							Footnote C		
Tdap									Footnote D
Rot		Footnote E	Footnote E	Footnote [E] Complete series by 8 months + 0 days					
Pneu-C-13		Footnote F	Footnote F	Footnote [F]	Footnote F	Footnote F			
Men-C-C		Footnote [G]	Footnote [G]	Footnote [G]	Footnote G Generally at 12 months				
Men-C-C								Footnote H	
					OR				
Men-C-ACYW-135								Footnote H	
MMR					Footnote I	Footnote I Generally at 4–6 years			
Var					Footnote J	Footnote J Generally at 4–6 years			
					OR				
MMRV					Footnote K	Footnote K Generally at 4–6 years			
HB	Footnote L 3-dose schedule Generally at months 0, 1, and 6 (first dose = month 0)								
					OR				
HB								Footnote M 2- or 3-dose schedule	
HPV								Footnote N 3-dose schedule	
Inf				Footnote O Recommended annually 1- or 2-dose schedule			Footnote O Encouraged annually	1 dose	

Table I.2 Recommended Immunization Schedule: Children (less than 7 years of age) NOT Previously Immunized as Infants

- For children at risk due to underlying medical conditions, see Table I.4 for additional recommendations for immunization.
- [ ] = dose(s) may not be required depending upon age of child and/or vaccine used (see the relevant vaccine-specific chapter in Part 4 and provincial/territorial schedule).
- See Table I.8 for abbreviations and brand names for vaccines. See Timing of Vaccine Administration and Vaccine Administration Practices in Part 1 regarding administration of multiple injections. See vaccine-specific chapters in Part 4 for additional information.

Table 2—Footnote A

Diphtheria toxoid–tetanus toxoid–acellular pertussis–inactivated polio–*Haemophilus influenzae* type b (DTaP-IPV-Hib) *or* **diphtheria toxoid–tetanus toxoid–acellular pertussis–inactivated polio combination vaccine** (DTaP-IPV): The number of doses of Hib-containing vaccine required varies by age at first dose. If first visit at 12–14 months of age: 1 dose of Hib-containing vaccine at first visit and booster dose at least 2 months after the previous dose. If first visit at 15 months to less than 5 years of age: 1 dose of Hib-containing vaccine. If first visit at 60 months of age (5 years of age) or older, Hib-containing vaccine is not required.

Table 2—Footnote B

Diphtheria toxoid–tetanus toxoid–acellular pertussis–inactivated polio (DTaP-IPV) *or* **tetanus toxoid–reduced diphtheria toxoid–reduced acellular pertussis–inactivated polio** (Tdap-IPV): Omit the dose at 4–6 years of age if the fourth dose of DTaP-IPV vaccine was given after the fourth birthday.

Table 2—Footnote C

Pneumococcal conjugate 13-valent: 12–23 months of age at first visit—2 doses, at least 8 weeks apart. 24–59 months of age (fifth birthday) at first visit—1 dose.

Table 2—Footnote D

Meningococcal conjugate monovalent: 12 months to less than 5 years of age—1 dose; 5–11 years of age—consider 1 dose. See Table I.4 for alternate recommended meningococcal immunization for children considered at risk.

Table 2—Footnote E

Measles–mumps–rubella: 2 doses, at least 4 weeks apart.

Table 2—Footnote F

Varicella: 2 doses, at least 3 months apart. A minimum interval of 6 weeks between doses may be used if rapid, complete protection is required.

Table 2—Footnote G

Measles–mumps–rubella–varicella: 2 doses, at least 3 months apart. A minimum interval of 6 weeks between doses may be used if rapid, complete protection is required.

Table 2—Footnote H

Hepatitis B: Preferred 3-dose schedule—months 0, 1, and 6 (first dose = month 0) with at least 4 weeks between the first and second dose, 2 months between the second and third dose, and 4 months between the first and third dose.

Table 2—Footnote I

Influenza: Recommended annually for children 6–59 months of age (fifth birthday) and encouraged for older children. Children (6 months to less than 9 years of age receiving Inf for the first time)—2 doses, at least 4 weeks apart.

		Time After First Visit						
Vaccine	**First Visit**	**4 wk**	**8 wk**	**3 mo**	**4 mo**	**6 mo**	**6–12 Months After Last Dose**	**4–6 Years of Age**
DTaP-IPV-Hib *or* **DTaP-IPV**	Footnote A		Footnote A		Footnote A		Footnote A	
DTaP-IPV *or* **Tdap-IPV**								Footnote [B]
Pneu-C-13	Footnote [C]		Footnote [C]					
Men-C-C	Footnote D							
MMR	Footnote E	Footnote E Generally at 4–6 years						
Var	Footnote F			Footnote F **OR**				
MMRV	Footnote G			Footnote G Generally at 4–6 years				
[HB]	Footnote [H]	Footnote [H]				Footnote [H]		
Inf	Footnote I	Footnote I						

Table I.3 Recommended Immunization Schedule: Children (7 to 17 years of age) NOT Previously Immunized

- For children at risk due to underlying medical conditions, see Table I.4 for additional recommendations for immunization.
- [·] = dose(s) may not be required depending upon age of child and/or vaccine used (see the relevant vaccine-specific chapter in Part 4 and provincial/territorial schedule). See Table I.8 for abbreviations and brand names for vaccines. See Timing of Vaccine Administration and Vaccine Administration Practices in Part 1 regarding administration of multiple injections. See the vaccine-specific chapters in Part 4 for additional information.

Vaccine	First Visit	Time After First Visit					6–12 Months After Last Dose	10 Years After Last Dose	9–11 Years of Age	12 Years of Age	13–17 Years of Age
		4 wk	6 wk	8 wk	3 mo	6 mo					

Table 3—Footnote A

Tetanus toxoid–reduced diphtheria toxoid–reduced acellular pertussis–inactivated polio: 2 doses, 8 weeks apart; third dose 6–12 months after second dose.

Table 3—Footnote B

Tetanus toxoid–reduced diphtheria toxoid–reduced acellular pertussis: 10 years after last dose.

Table 3—Footnote C

Meningococcal conjugate monovalent: 5–11 years of age—consider 1 dose.

Table 3—Footnote D

Meningococcal conjugate monovalent or quadrivalent: Early adolescence (around 12 years of age)—1 dose, even if meningococcal conjugate vaccine received at a younger age. Vaccine chosen depends on local epidemiology and programmatic considerations. See Table I.4 for alternate recommended meningococcal immunization for children considered at risk.

Table 3—Footnote E

Measles–mumps–rubella: 2 doses, at least 4 weeks apart.

Table 3—Footnote F

Varicella: 7–12 years of age—2 doses, at least 3 months apart. A minimum interval of 6 weeks between doses may be used if rapid, complete protection is required. 13 years of age and older—2 doses, at least 6 weeks apart; immunity should be evaluated prior to vaccination.

Table 3—Footnote G

Measles–mumps–rubella–varicella: 7–12 years of age—2 doses, at least 3 months apart. A minimum interval of 6 weeks between doses may be used if rapid, complete protection is required.

Table 3—Footnote H

Hepatitis B: Preferred 3-dose schedule—months 0, 1, and 6 (first dose = month 0) with at least 4 weeks between the first and second dose, 2 months between the second and third dose, and 4 months between the first and third dose. 11–15 years of age—2-dose schedule (months 0 and 4–6, depending on the product used).

Table 3—Footnote I

Human papillomavirus: Girls, 9 years of age and older—HPV2 vaccine—months 0, 1, and 6 (first dose = month 0) or HPV4 vaccine—months 0, 2, and 6 (first dose = month 0). Boys, 9 years of age and older—HPV4 vaccine—months 0, 2, and 6 (first dose = month 0).

Table 3—Footnote J

Influenza: Encouraged annually for all children. Children (6 months–8 years of age, previously immunized with Inf) and children (9 years of age and older)—1 dose. Children (6 months–less than 9 years of age, receiving Inf for the first time)—2 doses, at least 4 weeks apart.

(table continues on page 1078)

Table I.3 Recommended Immunization Schedule: Children (7 to 17 years of age) NOT Previously Immunized (continued)

		Time After First Visit									
Vaccine	**First Visit**	**4 wk**	**6 wk**	**8 wk**	**3 mo**	**6 mo**	**6–12 Months After Last Dose**	**10 Years After Last Dose**	**9–11 Years of Age**	**12 Years of Age**	**13–17 Years of Age**
Tdap								Footnote B			
Men-C-C	Footnote [C]										
Men-C-C										Footnote D	
						OR					
Men-C-ACYW-135										Footnote D	
MMR	Footnote E	Footnote E									
Var	Footnote F		Footnote F								
						OR					
MMR	Footnote G				Footnote G						
HB	Footnote H	Footnote [H]				Footnote H					
HPV									Footnote I 3-dose schedule		
Inf	Footnote J Encouraged annually 1- or 2-dose schedule										

Table I.4 Additional Recommended Immunizations: Children (birth to 17 years of age) Considered at Risk Due to Underlying Medical Conditions

- [·] = dose(s) may not be required depending upon age of child and/or vaccine used (see vaccine-specific chapter in Part 4 and provincial/territorial schedule). See Immunization of Travellers and Immunization of Workers in Part 3 for additional information about vaccines recommended for travellers and workers. See Immunization of Immunocompromised Persons and Immunization of Persons with Chronic Diseases in Part 3 for additional condition-specific recommendations. See Table I.8 for abbreviations and brand names for vaccines. See Timing of Vaccine Administration and Vaccine Administration Practices in Part 1 regarding administration of multiple injections. See to the vaccine-specific chapters in Part 4 for additional information

Table 4—Footnote A
***Haemophilus influenzae* type b**: 5 years of age and older with increased risk of invasive Hib disease—1 dose regardless of prior history of Hib vaccination and at least 1 year after any previous dose.

Table 4—Footnote B
Pneumococcal polysaccharide 23-valent: 2 years of age or older, at high risk of invasive pneumococcal disease—1 dose. If Pneu-C-13 is also required, give Pneu-C-13 first followed by Pneu-P-23, at least 8 weeks later. Reimmunize children at highest risk of invasive pneumococcal disease—give 1 booster dose after 3 years if first vaccinated with Pneu-P-23 at 10 years of age or younger, give 1 booster dose after 5 years if first vaccinated with Pneu-P-23 at 11 years of age and older.

Table 4—Footnote C
Pneumococcal conjugate 13-valent: Infants at high risk of invasive pneumococcal disease—in addition to the routine doses at 2, 4, and 12 months of age, give an extra dose at 6 months to make a 4-dose primary series. Children aged 3 and older at high risk of invasive pneumococcal disease who have not previously received Pneu-C-13—1 dose.

Table 4—Footnote D
Meningococcal conjugate quadrivalent: Children at high risk of invasive meningococcal disease: 2–11 months of age—2 or 3 doses of Menveo™, 8 weeks apart with another dose between 12–23 months of age and at least 8 weeks after the previous dose; 12–23 months of age–2 doses of Menveo™, 8 weeks apart; 24 months of age and older—2 doses of either Men-C-ACYW-135 vaccine, 8 weeks apart. Give a booster dose every 3 to 5 years if vaccinated at less than 7 years of age and every 5 years if vaccinated at 7 years of age and older.

Table 4—Footnote E
Hepatitis A: 12 months of age and older in high-risk groups—2 doses, given 6–36 months apart (depending on product used).

Table 4—Footnote F
Hepatitis B: Higher dose of monovalent HB vaccine recommended for those with certain immunocompromising conditions, chronic renal failure, and dialysis (3 or 4 doses). Premature infants weighing less than 2,000 grams at birth vaccinated because born to HB-infected mothers—4 doses. 2-dose schedule an option (months 0 and 4–6, depending on product used).

Table 4—Footnote G
Hepatitis A–hepatitis B: Combined vaccine preferred for children 12 months of age and older if both HA and standard dosage HB vaccines are recommended—2- or 3-dose schedule.

Table 4—Footnote H
Influenza: Recommended annually for children at risk of influenza-related complications. Children (6 months–8 years of age, previously immunized with Inf) and children (9 years of age and older)—1 dose. Children (6 months–less than 9 years of age, receiving Inf for the first time)—2 doses, at least 4 weeks apart.

	Age									
Vaccine	**Birth**	**2 mo**	**6 mo**	**12 mo**	**15 mo**	**18 mo**	**23 mo**	**2 y**	**3 y**	**5–17 y**
HiB										Footnote A 1 dose
Pneu-P-23								Footnote B 1 dose + 1 booster dose if at highest risk		
Pneu-C-13			Footnote C							Footnote [C]
Men-C-ACYW-135		Footnote D 2-, 3-, or 4 dose schedule + booster doses								
HA				Footnote E 2-dose schedule						
HB	Footnote F 2-, 3-, or 4-dose schedule									
				OR						
HAHB				Footnote G 2- or 3-dose schedule						
Inf			Footnote H 1- or 2-dose schedule							

Table I.5 Recommended Immunization Schedule: Adults (18 years of age and older) NOT Previously Immunized

- For adults considered at risk, see Table I.7 for additional recommendations for immunization.
- [·] = dose(s) may not be required depending upon age of vaccinee and/or vaccine used (see vaccine-specific chapter in Part 4 and provincial/territorial schedule). See Immunization of Travellers and Immunization of Workers in Part 3 for additional information about vaccines recommended for travellers and workers. See Table I.8 for abbreviations and brand names for vaccines. Refer to Timing of Vaccine Administration and Vaccine Administration Practices in Part 1 regarding administration of multiple injections. See vaccine-specific chapters in Part 4 for further information.

Table 5—Footnote A

Tetanus toxoid–reduced diphtheria toxoid–reduced acellular pertussis–inactivated polio (Tdap-IPV): 1 dose for pertussis protection.

Table 5—Footnote B

Tetanus toxoid–reduced diphtheria toxoid–inactivated polio (Td-IPV): First dose, 8 weeks after the dose of Tdap-IPV; second dose, 6–12 months after the previous dose.

Table 5—Footnote C

Tetanus toxoid–reduced diphtheria toxoid (Td): 10 years after last dose.

Table 5—Footnote D

Measles–mumps–rubella: Adults born in 1970 or later—1 dose, except—travellers to destinations outside of North America, health care workers, students in post-secondary educational settings, and military personnel—2 doses, at least 4 weeks apart. Adults born before 1970 can be assumed to have acquired natural immunity to measles and mumps and do not need MMR vaccination except—nonimmune military personnel or health care workers (2 doses, at least 4 weeks apart), nonimmune travellers (1 dose), nonimmune students in post-secondary educational settings (consider 1 dose). Rubella-susceptible adults, regardless of age—1 dose.

Table 5—Footnote E

Varicella: Adults 18–49 years of age—2 doses, at least 6 weeks apart; immunity should be evaluated prior to vaccination. Adults 50 years of age and older are generally presumed to be immune.

Table 5—Footnote F

Herpes zoster: Adults 50–59 years of age—may receive 1 dose; adults 60 years of age and older—1 dose.

Table 5—Footnote G

Pneumococcal polysaccharide 23-valent: Adults 65 years of age and older—1 dose

Table 5—Footnote H

Meningococcal conjugate monovalent or quadrivalent: Adults less than 25 years of age—1 dose (vaccine chosen depends on local epidemiology). See Table I.7 for alternate recommended meningococcal immunization for adults considered at risk.

Table 5—Footnote I

Human papillomavirus: Recommended for women to 26 years of age, may be given to women 27 years of age and older at ongoing risk of exposure—HPV2 vaccine—months 0, 1, and 6 (first dose = month 0) or HPV4 vaccine—months 0, 2, and 6 (first dose = month 0). Recommended for men to 26 years of age, may be given to men 27 years of age and older at ongoing risk of exposure—HPV4 vaccine—months 0, 2, and 6 (first dose = month 0).

Table 5—Footnote J

Influenza: Adults at high risk of influenza-related complications (including pregnant women, adults 65 years of age and older); adults capable of transmitting influenza to individuals at high risk; adults who provide essential community services—1 dose annually. Encouraged for all adults.

		Time After First Visit					
Vaccine	**First Visit**	**4 wk**	**6 wk**	**8 wk**	**6 mo**	**6–12 Months After Last Dose**	**10 Years After Last Dose**
Tdap-IPV *followed by* **Td-IPV**	Footnote A			Footnote B		Footnote B	
Td							Footnote C
MMR	Footnote [D]						
Var	Footnote [E]		Footnote [E]				
				OR			
Zos	Footnote [F]						
Pneu-P-23	Footnote [G]						
Men-C-C	Footnote [H]						
				OR			
Men-C-ACYW-135	Footnote [H]						
HPV	Footnote I 3-dose schedule						
Inf	Footnote J Annually						

Table I.6 Recommended Immunizations: Adults (18 years of age and older) Previously Immunized

- For adults considered at-risk, see Table I.7 for additional recommendations for immunization.
- [·] = dose may not be required.
- See Immunization of Travellers and Immunization of Workers in Part 3 for additional information about vaccines recommended for travellers and workers. See Table I.8 for abbreviations and brand names for vaccines. See Timing of Vaccine Administration and Vaccine Administration Practices in Part 1 regarding administration of multiple injections. See vaccine-specific chapters in Part 4 for additional information.

Table 6—Footnote A
Tetanus toxoid–reduced diphtheria toxoid (Td): 1 booster dose every 10 years.

Table 6—Footnote B
Tetanus toxoid–reduced diphtheria toxoid–reduced acellular pertussis (Tdap): 1 dose in adulthood for pertussis protection regardless of interval from last dose of Td.

Table 6—Footnote C
Pneumococcal polysaccharide 23-valent: Adults 65 years of age and older—1 dose.

Table 6—Footnote D
Herpes zoster: 50–59 years of age—may receive 1 dose; 60 years of age and older—1 dose. If dose given before 60 years of age, additional dose at 60 years of age or older is not currently recommended.

Table 6—Footnote E
Influenza: Adults at high risk of influenza-related complications (including pregnant women, adults 65 years of age and older); adults capable of transmitting influenza to individuals at high risk; adults who provide essential community services—1 dose annually. Encouraged for all adults.

	Age				
Vaccine	**18–26 y**	**27–49 y**	**50–59 y**	**60 y**	**65 y and older**
Td	Footnote A 1 dose every 10 years				
Tdap	Footnote B 1 dose				
Pneu-P-23					Footnote C 1 dose
Zos			Footnote [D] 1 dose	Footnote [D] 1 dose	
Inf	Footnote E Annually				Footnote E Annually

Table I.7 Additional Recommended Immunizations: Adults (18 years of age and older) Considered at Risk

- See Immunization of Travellers and Immunization of Workers in Part 3 for information about vaccines recommended for travellers and workers. See Immunization of Immunocompromised Persons and Immunization of Persons with Chronic Diseases in Part 3 for additional condition-specific immunization recommendations. See Table I.8 for abbreviations and brand names for vaccines. See Timing of Vaccine Administration and Vaccine Administration Practices in Part 1 regarding administration of multiple injections. See vaccine-specific chapters in Part 4 for additional information.

	Age
Vaccine	**18 y of age and older**

Table 7—Footnote A
***Haemophilus influenzae* type b**: Adults with increased risk of invasive Hib disease—1 dose regardless of prior history of Hib vaccination and at least 1 year after any previous dose.

Table 7—Footnote B
Inactivated polio: 1 booster dose for adults at increased risk of exposure to polio.

Table 7—Footnote C
Measles–mumps–rubella: Adults born in 1970 or later—1 dose, except—travellers to destinations outside of North America, health care workers, students in post-secondary educational settings, and military personnel—2 doses, at least 4 weeks apart. Adults born before 1970 can be assumed to have acquired natural immunity to measles and mumps and do not need MMR vaccination except—nonimmune military personnel or health care workers (2 doses, at least 4 weeks apart), nonimmune travellers (1 dose), nonimmune students in post-secondary educational settings (consider 1 dose). Rubella-susceptible adults, regardless of age—1 dose.

Table 7—Footnote D
Pneumococcal polysaccharide 23-valent: Adults at high risk of invasive pneumococcal disease—1 dose. Adults at highest risk of invasive pneumococcal disease if at least 5 years from first vaccination with Pneu-P-23—1 booster dose.

(table continues on page 1082)

Table I.7 Additional Recommended Immunizations: Adults (18 years of age and older) Considered at Risk (continued)

Vaccine	Age 18 y of age and older
Table 7—Footnote E **Pneumococcal conjugate 13-valent**: Adults with HIV or immunocompromising conditions (except hematopoietic stem cell transplant recipients)—1 dose of Pneu-C-13 followed 8 weeks later by 1 dose of Pneu-P-23. Administer Pneu-C-13 dose at least 1 year after any previous dose of Pneu-P-23.	
Table 7—Footnote F **Meningococcal conjugate quadrivalent**: Adults at high risk of invasive meningococcal disease—2 doses, 8 weeks apart. Reimmunize every 5 years.	
Table 7—Footnote G **Hepatitis A**: Adults in high-risk groups—2 doses, 6–36 months apart (depending on product used).	
Table 7—Footnote H **Hepatitis B**: Adults in high-risk groups—3- or 4-dose schedule (depending on product used). Higher dose of monovalent HB vaccine recommended for those with certain immunocompromising conditions, chronic renal failure, and dialysis.	
Table 7—Footnote I **Hepatitis A–hepatitis B**: Combined vaccine preferred if both HA and standard dosage HB vaccines are recommended—3- or 4-dose schedule.	
Table 7—Footnote J **Influenza**: Adults at high risk of influenza-related complications—1 dose annually.	
Table 7—Footnote K **Typhoid**: Adults with ongoing or intimate exposure to a chronic carrier of *Salmonella typhi*—1 dose injectable typhoid vaccine or 4 doses oral typhoid vaccine; reimmunization recommended if at continuing risk.	
Table 7—Footnote L **Bacillus Calmette–Guérin**: 1 dose may be considered in exceptional circumstances for adults at high risk of repeated exposure to tuberculosis.	
Table 7—Footnote M **Rabies**: Adults at high risk of close contact with rabid animals—3 doses for preexposure immunization. Periodic serology testing and booster doses (if required) for those at continuing high risk.	
HiB	Footnote A 1 dose
IPV	Footnote B 1 booster dose
MMR	Footnote C Second dose
Pneu-P-23	Footnote D 1 dose + 1 booster dose if at highest risk
Pneu-C-13	Footnote E 1 dose
Men-C-ACYW-135	Footnote F 2-dose schedule + booster doses
HA	Footnote G 2-dose schedule
HB	Footnote H 3- or 4-dose schedule **OR**
HAHB	Footnote I 3- or 4-dose schedule
Inf	Footnote J Annually
Typh-I	Footnote K 1 dose + booster doses if at ongoing risk **OR**
Typh-O	Footnote K 1 dose + booster doses if at ongoing risk
BCG	Footnote L 1 dose
Rab	Footnote M 3-dose schedule + booster doses if required

Table I.8 Abbreviations and Brand Names of Vaccines Used in Immunization Schedules

Abbreviation	Vaccine	Brand Names*
Table 1—Footnote * See vaccine-specific chapters in Part 4 for brand-specific recommendations.		
BCG	Bacillus Calmette-Guérin	BCG Vaccine
DTaP-HB-IPV-Hib	Diphtheria, tetanus, acellular pertussis, hepatitis B, inactivated polio, *Haemophilus influenzae* type b (pediatric)	INFANRIX hexa™
DTaP-IPV	Diphtheria, tetanus, acellular pertussis, inactivated polio (pediatric)	QUADRACEL®
DTaP-IPV-Hib	Diphtheria, tetanus, acellular pertussis, inactivated polio, *Haemophilus influenzae* type b (pediatric)	PEDIACEL®
HA	Hepatitis A	AVAXIM® AVAXIM®–Pediatric HAVRIX® 1440 HAVRIX® 720 Junior VAQTA®
HAHB	Hepatitis A, hepatitis B	TWINRIX® TWINRIX® Junior
HB	Hepatitis B	ENGERIX®-B RECOMBIVAX HB®
Hib	*Haemophilus influenzae* type b	Act-HIB®
HPV2	Human papillomavirus	CERVARIX™
HPV4	Human papillomavirus	GARDASIL®
Inf	Influenza	AGRIFLU® FLUAD® FLUMIST® FLUVIRAL® INFLUVAC® INTANZA® VAXIGRIP®
IPV	Polio (inactivated)	IMOVAX® Polio
Men-C-ACYW-135	Meningococcal conjugate quadrivalent	Menactra® Menveo™
Men-C-C	Meningococcal conjugate monovalent	Meningitec® Menjugate® NeisVac-C®
MMR	Measles, mumps, rubella	M-M-R® II PRIORIX®
MMRV	Measles, mumps, rubella, varicella	PRIORIX-TETRA®
Pneu-C-13	Pneumococcal conjugate 13-valent	Prevnar® 13
Pneu-P-23	Pneumococcal polysaccharide 23-valent	PNEUMOVAX® 23 PNEUMO 23®
Rab	Rabies	IMOVAX® Rabies RabAvert®
Rot-1	Rotavirus monovalent	ROTARIX™
Rot-5	Rotavirus pentavalent	RotaTeq®
Td	Tetanus, diphtheria (reduced)	Td ADSORBED
Tdap	Tetanus, diphtheria (reduced), acellular pertussis (reduced)	ADACEL® BOOSTRIX®
Tdap-IPV	Tetanus, diphtheria (reduced), acellular pertussis (reduced), inactivated polio	ADACEL®-POLIO BOOSTRIX®-POLIO
Td-IPV	Tetanus, diphtheria (reduced), inactivated polio	Td POLIO ADSORBED
Typh-I	Typhoid (injection)	TYPHIM Vi® TYPHERIX
Typh-O	Typhoid (oral)	Vivotif®
Var	Varicella (chickenpox)	VARILRIX® VARIVAX® III
Zos	Herpes zoster (shingles)	ZOSTAVAX®

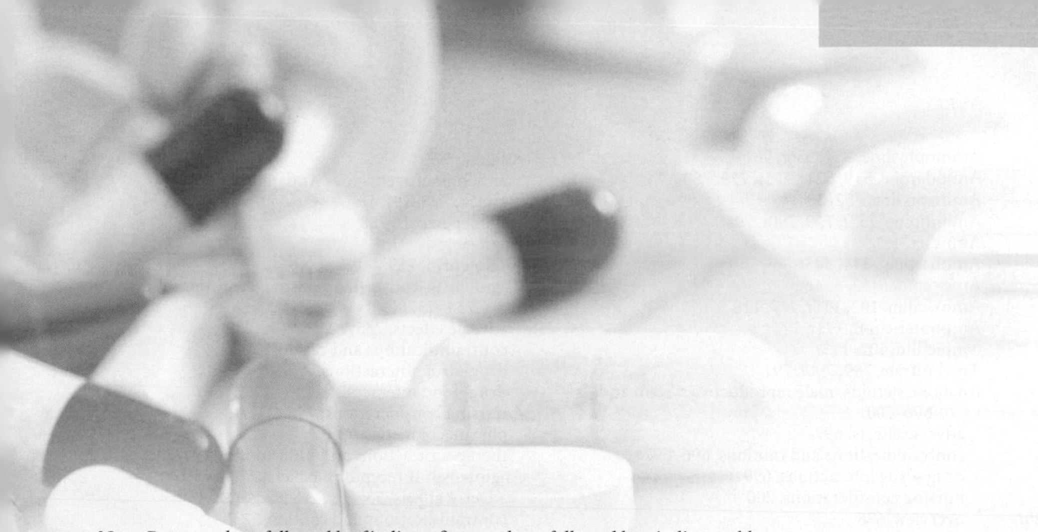

Index

Note: Page numbers followed by *f* indicate figures; those followed by *t* indicate tables.

H

J

K

L

Q

R

S

T